Textbook of Neurointensive Care

A. Joseph Layon • Andrea Gabrielli
William A. Friedman

Editors

Textbook of Neurointensive Care

Second Edition

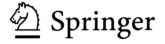 Springer

Editors
A. Joseph Layon, MD, FACP
Critical Care Medicine
Pulmonary and Critical Care Medicine
The Geisinger Health System
Danville
PA
USA

Temple University School of Medicine
Philadelphia
PA
USA

Andrea Gabrielli, MD, FCCM
Departments of Anesthesiology and Surgery
University of Florida College of Medicine
Gainesville
FL
USA

William A. Friedman, MD
Department of Neurological Surgery
University of Florida College of Medicine
Gainesville
FL
USA

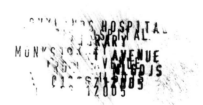

ISBN 978-1-4471-5225-5   ISBN 978-1-4471-5226-2   (eBook)
DOI 10.1007/978-1-4471-5226-2
Springer London Heidelberg New York Dordrecht

Library of Congress Control Number: 2013945859

*To my family—Susana Picado, Maria Layon-Taylor, Nicolas Layon,
Daniel Layon—all in the service of our people and country. All of whom have
sacrificed.*
To those who are in search of a home, family, country: may you find them.
To those who struggle to become: may you be.

—A. Joseph Layon

*To my father Pietro and my mother Giuliana, now walking the family dog
between the clouds, for being my role models and the inspiration behind all
my efforts.*
To my brother and friend Marco, the real smart guy of the family.
To my students, friends, and colleagues worldwide.
*To our patients, our inspiration for compassionate care, our reason to try
harder.*

—Andrea Gabrielli

*To my many colleagues, friends, and patients who have taught me so much
about neurosurgery.*

—William A. Friedman

Foreword to the Second Edition

During the 9 years since the publication of the first edition of this *Textbook of Neurointensive Care*, considerable developments have evolved in the critical care of the neurologically injured patient. This second edition captures such advances presented by more than 100 leading authorities, offering a clear and comprehensive update. It represents a collective accomplishment of clinician scientists dedicated to providing such enormous material and thereby extensive knowledge in the care of the brain injured from the emergency department to the ICU, to the operating room, and through the postoperative period. This edition is the only textbook providing such a comprehensive offering throughout the continuum of care.

Such a continuum of critical care is exemplified throughout this second edition in its extensive chapters. A presentation of key concepts of brain physiology essential to the understanding of intracranial hypertension is offered in the chapter on elevated intracranial hypertension. Despite recent advances in the treatment, diagnosis, and management of aneurysms and cerebral vasospasm, morbidity and mortality remain high and are addressed in the chapter on treatment of aneurysmal subarachnoid hemorrhage. The chapter on intracranial hemorrhage is an essential presentation. Such hemorrhage remains formidable as patient outcome is still poor, despite recent advances that have led to extensive research establishing evidence-based management. This chapter notes the disparate incidence of stroke in African-Americans and discusses possible risk factors in this population. Neuroradiologic imaging is discussed in a substantial chapter, providing an understanding of how such images are created utilizing MRI and CT modalities though technical presentation. The chapter on pharmacotherapy in the neurosurgical ICU is a further example of the comprehensive approach to such care extended by this second edition. Knowledge of pharmacokinetics and pharmacodynamics of neuroactive drugs is provided for the optimal management of neuroinjured patients. In addition to these chapters, all the contributions provide evidenced-based data and algorithms for decision making and illustrate key points; multiple supporting references are provided for documentation and reviews.

This second edition is improved in its sectioning with the provision of an Introduction (Part I) which presents fundamentals of neurocritical care issues of organization, quality improvement, and the emerging ICU subspecialty of Neurointensive Care Medicine. Part II addresses Neuroanatomy and Neurophysiology; Part III covers Neuromonitoring; Part IV addresses in detail the Neuroinjured Patient; Part V details Special Situations such as traumatic brain injury in the adult and as well as in the pediatric population, the treatment of spinal cord injury, and the treatment of seizures; Part VI provides Situations of Special Interest such as intraoperative neuroanesthesia, neurorehabilitation, and brain death and the management of potential organ donation. This section also reviews the ongoing concerns of ethical issues in the neurointensive care unit.

In 2003, the year prior to the publication of the first edition of the *Textbook of Neurocritical Care*, the Joint Commission (JC, formerly JCAHO) launched the Primary Stroke Center Certification Program. During the 9 years since the First Edition, more than 925 certified primary stroke centers have been established in 48 states, with comprehensive stroke centers now being certified by JC in several states. The *Get With The Guidelines-Stroke National Quality Improvement and Registry Program* of the American Heart/American Stroke Association has grown rapidly over these 9 years. Over 1,400 hospitals are participating in this program. The first edition of this textbook and its editors and authors have contributed immensely to the quality and outcomes of stroke care of these programs. Interim and current developments so comprehensively provided now in this second edition will further enhance such care. It is a pleasure and privilege to continue to work with such accomplished investigators. This second edition is a tribute and an essential contribution to the care of the neurologically injured.

Danville, PA, USA   Edgar J. Kenton III, MD, FAAN, FAHA

Preface to the Second Edition

We claimed, in the Preface to the First Edition of *Textbook of Neurointensive Care*, that in the near future our hospitals would be composed of EDs, ICUs, and operating rooms. Studies of hospitals seem to have borne this out. And while we still are not sure of the precise dimensions and shape it will take, health care (maybe better put, health *insurance*) reform will impact our work and work environment significantly. Even those of us who hoped for a reformed health system when the First Edition went to press had no idea, even in our heart of hearts, that in 2013 we would see the beginnings—just that—of the reform of our health-care system.

In this context, we have attempted to change and improve our *Textbook of Neurointensive Care*. In this second edition, there is more emphasis on evidence-based medicine—our jump-off point, not our end point—and best practice. We have improved chapters on the organization of neurocritical care (Chap. 1) and quality improvement (Chap. 2); enhanced chapters on neuromonitoring (Chaps. 7 and 8) and on the prehospital care of the neurologically injured patient (Chap. 9); and added chapters on neuroendocrine function (Chap. 15), on hematological/thrombotic issues (Chaps. 16 and 17), and on acute kidney injury and the neurologically injured patient (Chap. 19). Additionally, there is an entire chapter (Chap. 36) on temperature regulation. Finally, we have added a chapter on brain death and the management of the potential organ donor (Chap. 44).

The reader will note that we eliminated the section on "The Future of NeuroCritical Care." We are good, but not that good! We cannot see into the future any better than anyone else can!

We thank our contributors for their hard work. We are in debt to them in a manner that will never be paid. And the same goes for our editor and publisher, Elizabeth Corra and Grant Weston: they have the patience of saints.

Let us know what you think of this second edition. As always, the errors in this book belong to the three editors.

Gainesville, FL, USA
Gainesville, FL, USA
Gainesville, FL, USA

A. Joseph Layon, MD, FACP
Andrea Gabrielli, MD, FCCM
William A. Friedman, MD

Preface to the First Edition

Whether apocryphal or not, it is said that in the near future, hospitals will be composed of three areas: the emergency department, the operating rooms, and the intensive care unit (ICU). The rationale for such a statement is that managed care is driving medicine in the United States toward outpatient care except in cases of very ill patients, who are admitted into the ICU. Our experience is that the severity of illness of the patients we care for is greater every year. This is as true in the general ICU population as it is in those individuals with neurologic disease. Partly because of this increased severity of illness in patients with neurologic injury, we conceived the project that led to this book.

The book before you is unusual in several respects. It is a textbook, rather than a monograph, of neurointensive care. We initiate the book with a solid review of neurophysiology and neuroanatomy, including anatomy as seen through the "eyes" of our radiology colleagues. We remind the reader of the problems that our neurosurgical colleagues *expect to see*, even in a well-performed procedure. The body of the book then follows, first with general topics and then with specific disease states. Difficult ethical issues, including topics such as access to health care, alterations of a do-not-resuscitate order in patients going to the operating room, withdrawal and withholding of therapy, physician-assisted suicide, and brain death, are embraced and discussed. We finish the book with clinically relevant research issues that are present on the horizon, beckoning us forward with the unfulfilled promises that make up their potential. The use of evidence-based medicine when such data exist, provision of protocols and algorithms, and honesty when our best approximations and biases are the only data available have served as our credo.

As any authors should, we undertook this book with some hesitation. To write a book—any book—means laying open, for the world to see, one's biases, flaws, and inadequacies. This is especially true when dealing with an area as broad and complex as treatment of the critically ill patient with neurologic injuries. While others might have written a different book, we undertook this project and offer it, with humility, to our colleagues.

Although we live in a society that lionizes—at least rhetorically—the individual and individual exploits, work of any quality is of necessity the culmination of a collective effort. This is true in the case of our textbook. Our coauthors are dedicated clinicians and scientists with whom we are honored to be associated. They have worked diligently in the process of creation of this work. The publishers and printers are remarkable people and true professionals who put up with our foibles and ideas of cover art (we lost on that one). To Allan Ross, Executive Editor, Natasha Andjelkovic, Senior Editor, and Peter McEllhenney, Assistant Editor, at Elsevier; Jesamyn Angelica; and Nancy Lombardi at PM Gordon Associates, we offer our heartfelt thanks and appreciation. To Poppy Meehan, the hand that guided the entire project, we can only say thank you.

While this is a work of many, we are responsible for any errors or other flaws. We hope you find this text useful. Let us know what you think. There should, after all, be a second edition.

Danville, PA, USA	A. Joseph Layon, MD, FACP
Gainesville, FL, USA	Andrea Gabrielli, MD, FCCM
Gainesville, FL, USA	William A. Friedman, MD

Contents

Contributors

Muhammad M. Abd-El-Barr, MD, PhD Department of Neurosurgery, Brigham and Women's Hospital, Harvard Medical School, Boston, MA, USA

William Allen, JD, MD Program for Bioethics, Law, and Medical Professionalism, University of Florida College of Medicine, Gainesville, FL, USA

Mourad M. Alsabbagh, MD Division of Nephrology, Hypertension, and Transplantation, University of Florida College of Medicine, Gainesville, FL, USA

Lennox K. Archibald, MD, PhD, FRCP Department of Medicine, College of Medicine, University of Florida College of Medicine and the Malcom Randall VA Medical Center, Gainesville, FL, USA

Abdo Asmar, MD Department of Clinical Science, University of Central Florida, Orlando, FL, USA

Eva Azicnuda, PsyD IRCCS Sanata Lucia Foundation, Rome, Italy

Jeffrey A. Bennett, MD Department of Radiology, University of Florida College of Medicine, Gainesville, FL, USA

Azra Bihorac, MD, PhD Division of Critical Care Medicine, Department of Anesthesiology, University of Florida College of Medicine, Gainesville, FL, USA

Umberto Bivona, PhD IRCCS Sanata Lucia Foundation, Rome, Italy

Thomas P. Bleck, MD, FCCM Department of Neurological Sciences, Neurosurgery, Medicine, and Anesthesiology, Rush Medical College, Chicago, IL, USA

Novella Bonaffini, MD Department of Neurology and Stroke Unit, Ospedale S. Eugenio-ASL RMC, Rome, Italy

M. Ross Bullock, MD, PhD Department of Neurosurgery, University of Miami/Jackson Memorial Hospital, Miami, FL, USA

Jennifer R. Bushwitz, PharmD Department of Pharmacy Services, Shands at the University of Florida, Gainesville, FL, USA

Clifton W. Callaway, MD, PhD Department of Emergency Medicine, University of Pittsburgh, Pittsburgh, PA, USA

Lawrence J. Caruso, MD Department of Anesthesiology, University of Florida College of Medicine, Gainesville, FL, USA

Sheila Catani, MD IRCCS Sanata Lucia Foundation, Rome, Italy

Cherylee W. J. Chang, MD, FACP, FCCM Department of Medicine and Surgery, Neuroscience Institute/Neurocritical Care, The Queen's Medical Center, University of Hawaii, John A. Burns School of Medicine, Honolulu, HI, USA

Jean E. Cibula, MD Department of Neurology, University of Florida College of Medicine, Gainesville, FL, USA

Giuseppe Citerio, MD Neuro-Anesthesia and Neuro-Intensive Care Unit, Department of Anesthesia and Critical Care, Ospedale San Gerardo, Monza, Italy

Maria Paola Ciurli, PsyD IRCCS Sanata Lucia Foundation, Rome, Italy

Janice M. Cohen, MD Department of Neuroscience/Physical Medicine and Rehabilitation, Memorial Regional Hospital South/Memorial Healthcare System, Hollywood, FL, USA

Douglas B. Coursin, MD Department of Medicine, University of Wisconsin School of Medicine and Public Health, Madison, WI, USA

Erin M. Dunbar, MD Department of Neurosurgery, University of Florida College of Medicine, Gainesville, FL, USA

Stephan Eisenschenk, MD Department of Neurology, University of Florida College of Medicine, Gainesville, FL, USA

A. Ahsan Ejaz, MD, FASN Division of Nephrology, Hypertension, and Transplantation, University of Florida College of Medicine, Gainesville, FL, USA

F. Kayser Enneking, MD Department of Anesthesiology, University of Florida College of Medicine, Shands Quality Committee, Shands at the University of Florida, Gainesville, FL, USA

Kyle M. Fargen, MD, MPH Department of Neurological Surgery, University of Florida College of Medicine, Gainesville, FL, USA

Andres Fernandez, MD Division of Neurocritical Care, Department of Neurology, Columbia University, New York, NY, USA

Rita Formisano, MD, PhD IRCCS Sanata Lucia Foundation, Rome, Italy

William A. Friedman, MD Department of Neurological Surgery, University of Florida College of Medicine, Gainesville, FL, USA

Andrea Gabrielli, MD, FCCM Department of Anesthesiology Surgery, University of Florida College of Medicine, Gainesville, FL, USA

David Garcia, MD Department of Hematology, University of New Mexico, Albuquerque, NM, USA

Achille Gaspardone, MPhil, MD, FESC, FACC, EAPCI Division of Cardiology, Department of Medicine, Ospedale S. Eugenio-ASL RMC, Rome, Italy

Romergryko G. Geocadin, MD ACCM-Neurology, Johns Hopkins University and Hospital, Baltimore, MD, USA

Robin L. Gilmore, MD Department of Neurology, Maury Regional Medical Center, Columbia, TN, USA

Dietrich Gravenstein, MD Department of Anesthesiology, University of Florida College of Medicine, Gainesville, FL, USA

Nikolaus Gravenstein, MD Departments of Anesthesiology and Neurological Surgery, University of Florida College of Medicine, Gainesville, FL, USA
Department of Periodontology, University of Florida College of Dentistry, Gainesville, FL, USA

Steven B. Greenberg, MD Department of Anesthesiology, NorthShore University HealthSystem, University of Chicago, Evanston, IL, USA

Ahmed N. Hassan, MD Department of Neurology/Neurocritical Care, Washington University School of Medicine, St. Louis, MI, USA

Kevin W. Hatton, MD Division of Critical Care Medicine, Department of Anesthesiology, University of Kentucky, Lexington, KY, USA

Vishnumurthy Shushrutha Hedna, MD Department of Neurology, University of Florida College of Medicine, Gainesville, FL, USA

Mary A. Herman, MD, PhD Department of Anesthesiology, University of Florida College of Medicine, Gainesville, FL, USA

Brian L. Hoh, MD, FACS, FAHA, FAANS Department of Neurological Surgery, University of Florida College of Medicine, Gainesville, FL, USA

Daniel J. Hoh, MD Department of Neurological Surgery, University of Florida College of Medicine, Gainesville, FL, USA

Cesare Iani, MD Department of Neurology and Stroke Unit, Ospedale S. Eugenio-ASL RMC, Rome, Italy

R. Patrick Jacob, MD Department of Neurological Surgery, University of Florida College of Medicine, Gainesville, FL, USA

Sayona John, MD Department of Neurology, Rush University Medical Center, Chicago, IL, USA

Jeffrey P. Keck Jr., MD Virginia Commonwealth University, Richmond, VA, USA

Departments of Anesthesia and Critical Care, Pikeville Medical Center, Pikeville, KY, USA

Matthew M. Kimball, MD Department of Neurological Surgery, University of Florida College of Medicine, Gainesville, FL, USA

Nathan Kohler, MD, PhD Department of Radiology, Florida Hospital, Orlando, FL, USA

Aaron N. LacKamp, MD Department of Anesthesiology and Critical Care Medicine, Johns Hopkins University School of Medicine, Baltimore, MD, USA

Matthew F. Lawson, MD Tallahassee Neurological Clinic, Tallahassee, FL, USA

A. Joseph Layon, MD, FACP Critical Care Medicine, Pulmonary and Critical Care Medicine, The Geisinger Health System, Danville, PA, USA

Temple University School of Medicine, Philadelphia, PA, USA

Aimée C. LeClaire, PharmD, BCPS Clinical Pharmacy Services, Critical Care Clinical Pharmacy Services, Department of Pharmacy Services, Shands at the University of Florida, Gainesville, FL, USA

Peter Le Roux, MD Department of Neurosurgery, University of Pennsylvania, Philadelphia, PA, USA

Chamisa MacIndoe, DO Department of Neurosurgery, University of New Mexico, Albuquerque, NM, USA

Elizabeth Brady Mahanna, MD Division of Critical Care Medicine, Department of Anesthesiology, University of Florida College of Medicine, Gainesville, FL, USA

Michael E. Mahla, MD Division of Neuroanesthesia, Department of Anesthesiology, University of Florida College of Medicine, Gainesville, FL, USA

Stephan A. Mayer, MD, FCCM Neurocritical Care Division, Columbia University Medical Center, New York, NY, USA

Leah Meisterling, DO, MBA Surgical Intensive Care Unit, Hartford Hospital, Hartford, CT, USA

Department of Anesthesiology, University of Connecticut School of Medicine, Farmington, CT, USA

David Meurer, MD Department of Emergency Medicine, University of Florida College of Medicine, Gainesville, FL, USA

J.D. Mocco, MD, MS, FAANS, FAHA Department of Neurosurgery, Vanderbilt University Medical Center, Nashville, TN, USA

Ennio Montinaro, MD Department of Neurology and Stroke Unit, Ospedale S. Eugenio-ASL RMC, Rome, Italy

Jan S. Moreb, MD Division of Hematology and Oncology, Department of Medicine, University of Florida College of Medicine, Gainesville, FL, USA

Thomas C. Mort, MD Department of Anesthesiology and Critical Care Medicine, Hartford Hospital, University of Connecticut, Glastonbury, CT, USA

Alan K. Novick, MD Department of Neuroscience/Physical Medicine and Rehabilitation, Memorial Regional Hospital South/Memorial Healthcare System, Hollywood, FL, USA

Michael S. Okun, MD Department of Neurology, University of Florida College of Medicine, Gainesville, FL, USA

Seth F. Oliveria, MD, PhD Department of Neurological Surgery, University of Florida College of Medicine, Gainesville, FL, USA

Kristine H. O'Phelan, MD Neurocritical Care Division, Department of Neurology, University of Miami Miller School of Medicine, Miami, FL, USA

Sandip Patel, MD Department of Radiology, University of Florida College of Medicine, Gainesville, FL, USA

David W. Pincus, MD, PhD Department of Neurological Surgery, University of Florida College of Medicine, Gainesville, FL, USA

Ronald G. Quisling, MD Department of Radiology, Neuroradiology Section, University of Florida College of Medicine, Gainesville, FL, USA

Maryam Rahman, MD, MS Department of Neurological Surgery, University of Florida College of Medicine, Gainesville, FL, USA

Albert L. Rhoton Jr., MD Department of Neurological Surgery, University of Florida College of Medicine, Gainesville, FL, USA

Bryan D. Riggeal, MD Rockdale Neurology Associates, Conyers, GA, USA

Fred Rincon, MD, MSc, MBE, FACP, FCCP, FCCM Department of Neurosurgery, Thomas Jefferson University, Philadelphia, PA, USA

Steven A. Robicsek, MD, PhD Department of Anesthesiology, University of Florida College of Medicine, Gainesville, FL, USA

Steven N. Roper, MD Department of Neurological Surgery, University of Florida College of Medicine, Gainesville, FL, USA

Jack C. Rose, MD Department of Neurosciences, California Pacific Medical Center, San Francisco, CA, USA

Arash Salardini, BSc, MBBS Department of Radiology, University of Florida College of Medicine, Gainesville, FL, USA

Adam Schiavi, PhD, MD Division of Neuroanesthesia and Neurosciences Critical Care, Anesthesiology and Critical Care Medicine, Johns Hopkins University and Hospital, Baltimore, MD, USA
ACCM-Neurology, Johns Hopkins University and Hospital, Baltimore, MD, USA

Christoph N. Seubert, MD, PhD Division of Neuroanesthesia, Department of Anesthesiology, University of Florida College of Medicine, Gainesville, FL, USA
Intraoperative Neurophysiologic Monitoring Laboratory, Shands Hospital, Gainesville, FL, USA

Michiko Shimada, MD, PhD Division of Cardiology, Respiratory Medicine, and Nephrology, Hirosaki University Graduate School of Medicine, Hirosaki City, Japan

Robert D. Stevens, MD Department of Anesthesiology, Critical Care Medicine, Neurology, and Neurosurgery, Johns Hopkins University School of Medicine, Baltimore, MD, USA

Alexander Taghva, MD Department of Neurological Surgery, Ohio State University, Columbus, OH, USA

Robert C. Tasker, MA, MBBS, MD Division of Critical Care Medicine, Department of Anesthesiology, Perioperative and Pain Medicine, Boston Children's Hospital, Boston, MA, USA
Department of Neurology, Boston Children's Hospital, Boston, MA, USA

Shelly D. Timmons, MD, PhD, FACS, FAANS Department of Neurological Surgery, Geisinger Health System, Danville, PA, USA

Arthur J. Tokarczyk, MD Department of Anesthesiology, NorthShore University HealthSystem, University of Chicago Pritzker School of Medicine, Evanston, IL, USA

William J. Triggs, MD Department of Neurology, University of Florida College of Medicine, Gainesville, FL, USA

Joseph A. Tyndall, MD, MPH Department of Emergency Medicine, University of Florida College of Medicine, Gainesville, FL, USA

Christine Van Dillen, MD Department of Emergency Medicine, University of Florida College of Medicine, Gainesville, FL, USA

Gregory J. Velat, MD Department of Neurosurgery, Lee Memorial Hospital, Fort Myers, FL, USA

Federico A. Villa, MD Neuro-Anesthesia and Neuro-Intensive Care Unit, Department of Anesthesia and Critical Care, Ospedale San Gerardo, Monza, Italy

Candice S. Waked, DO Department of Neurology, Emory University, Atlanta, GA, USA

Chad W. Washington, MS, MPHS, MD Department of Neurological Surgery, Washington University in St. Louis, St. Louis, MO, USA

Michael F. Waters, MD, PhD Department of Neurology, McKnight Brain Institute, University of Florida College of Medicine, Gainesville, FL, USA

Hung Tzu Wen, MD Department of Neurosurgery, Hospital das Clinicas, College of Medicine, University of São Paulo, São Paulo, Brazil

Peggy White, MD Department of Anesthesiology, University of Florida College of Medicine, Gainesville, FL, USA

Larissa D. Whitney, PA-C, BS, MS Department of Critical Care Medicine, Geisinger Medical Center, Danville, PA, USA

Kenneth E. Wood, DO Department of Critical Care Medicine, The Geisinger Medical Center, Danville, PA, USA

Anthony T. Yachnis, MD Department of Pathology and Laboratory Medicine, University of Florida College of Medicine, Gainesville, FL, USA

Cameron Zahed, MD, MS Department of Anesthesiology, Internal Medicine, and Critical Care, University of Wisconsin Hospital and Clinics, Madison, WI, USA

Gregory J. Zipfel, MD Department of Neurosurgery, Barnes-Jewish Hospital, St. Louis, MO, USA

Neurocritical Care Organization

1

Sayona John and Thomas P. Bleck

Contents

Abstract

Neurocritical Care Organization gives a brief introduction into the history, need, and development of Neuro ICUs. This chapter describes the different models of ICUs that currently exist and the pros and cons of these models. It also describes staffing models for physicians and physician extenders. A special note has been made of workflows in an ICU and quality metrics of importance.

Keywords

ICU • Neurocritical care • ICU staffing • ICU quality metrics • Unit organization • Physician extenders

History and Evolution of Intensive Care Medicine

Intensive care medicine is the science and the art of detecting and managing critically ill patients while preventing further deterioration, in order to achieve the best possible outcomes. Intensive care medicine emerged as a specialty in the 1950s with its beginnings in Copenhagen during the poliomyelitis epidemic, where patients with respiratory failure were artificially ventilated [1].

The ICU is commonly located in proximity to other acute areas in the hospital such as the emergency room and the operating rooms as most situations in the ICU are critically time dependent. This also permits optimization of the timing of admissions to the ICU and safe, effective discharge of patients to a less intensive area of the hospital for the continued monitoring of resolving organ dysfunction [2].

The concept of levels of care was defined by a National Institute of Health (NIH) consensus conference of critical care medicine at the Bethesda Conference in 1983 [3]. Based on differences in staffing, available technology, and professional organizational structure of ICUs, the Bethesda Conference proposed the division of intensive care facilities into four groups: intensive care, high care, medium care, and

S. John, MD (✉)
Department of Neurology, Rush University Medical Center,
1725 West Harrison, Chicago, IL 60521, USA
e-mail: sayona_john@rush.edu

T.P. Bleck, MD, FCCM
Department of Neurological Sciences, Neurosurgery,
Medicine, and Anesthesiology, Rush Medical College,
600 S Paulina Street, 544AF, Chicago, IL 60612, USA
e-mail: tbleck@gmail.com

A.J. Layon et al. (eds.), *Textbook of Neurointensive Care*,
DOI 10.1007/978-1-4471-5226-2_1, © Springer-Verlag London 2013

3

low care. The two main criteria used in this classification were the availability of technological resources (type and intensity of use of specific monitoring and therapeutic interventions) and the availability of human resources (training and coverage by medical leadership and nurse-to-patient ratio).

The limiting factor in the practice of intensive care at ICU level is the amount of work that can be performed and not the complexity. This implies that a given number of nurses in an ICU can take care of patients with varying complexity if other variables such as occupancy rate and length of stay are taken into account. The care of critically ill patients by intensivists and critical care nurses can improve patient-related outcomes as well as achieve a more efficient use of available resources. Improved outcomes include reduction in rates of infections, decreased complications, reduced length of stay, and decreased mortality.

The concept of life support now extends to include other acute, potentially reversible disorders. Care now includes prevention of secondary complications of critical illness such as pressure ulcers, deep vein thrombosis, and stress ulcers. In the USA, a separate subspecialty of intensive care medicine has been created with specific training requirements and accreditation as an extension of internal medicine, anesthesiology, general surgery, pediatrics, and neurology training. In many other countries, critical care is either a subspecialty of anesthesiology or, increasingly, an independent specialty.

Neurocritical Care as a Subspecialty

In the 1970s, stroke units began to appear which were dedicated to the care of stroke patients and are some of the direct precursors to modern neurocritical care units. Advances in anesthesiology for neurosurgery also generated a need for specialized postoperative care units. In the 1980s, research in neurology and neurosurgery began to take root, leading to improved diagnosis and therapy, and prompting the inception of the first specialized neurocritical care units. This led to the need for physicians with expertise not only in the neurologic and neurosurgical aspects of these patients but also in the principles of hemodynamic monitoring, mechanical ventilation, and management of multiple organ dysfunctions.

In spite of the existence of specialized neurointensive care units, presence of specialists in the area was not obligatory. In the last decade steps have been taken toward the recognition of this expertise. Neurocritical care as a subspecialty was accepted in the USA by the United Council of Neurological Subspecialties (UCNS) in 2006 [4]. Medical training standards were established, and a period of 2 years was determined as the period needed in training of which 1 year must compromise continuous clinical work in an ICU [5].

The Neurocritical Care Society was founded in the USA in 2002 with the mission of promoting better quality of care of critically ill neurological and neurosurgical patients. The mission is to promote better quality of care of these patients, professional collaboration, research, training, and education.

Need for Specialized Units

Several studies have now shown that it is important that patients in the ICU are cared for by physicians specialized in critical care medicine. Units with intensivists present lower mortality, better resource allocation with lower costs, and also shorter length of stay than the units without permanent doctors or specialists [6].

A recent meta-analysis of 12 studies encompassing 24,520 patients presented original data comparing models of care for critically ill neurologic patients and revealed clear reduction in mortality and improved neurologic outcomes for patients cared for in a specialized critical care unit [7].

Intensive Care Unit Organization

There are three common models of ICU organization:

Open Unit: Any physician with privileges to admit patients to the hospital can admit and care for patients in the ICU. Medical decisions are made by the admitting physician, often with the input of consultants which may include intensivists. The perceived benefit of this model is continuity of care.

Closed Unit: All patients entering the ICU are admitted to the care of an intensivist for the duration of the ICU stay. The admitting physician may or may not remain closely involved in the care of the patient while in the ICU. This model is gaining acceptance in the United States based on research findings and response to Leapfrog standard [8] and has shown lower mortality, fewer complications, and shorter ICU and hospital length of stay.

Semiclosed Unit: In this model, the intensivist may participate in some or all of the patients care while in the ICU, in conjunction with the patients attending physician. The intensivist's role may be limited to triage functions and emergency response but more often includes hemodynamic, respiratory, fluid, and nutritional management. This model is common in surgical practices where the attending surgeon addresses the operative aspects of a patient's care, with the rest of the management being delegated to the intensivist [9].

Pronovost and colleagues [6] conducted a systematic review examining physician staffing patterns and clinical outcomes. The model of care in each of 17 studies was classified as low intensity (no intensivist or elective consultation) or high intensity (mandatory critical care consultation or closed ICU). The high-intensity model was associated with lower ICU and hospital mortality. There is also evidence that hospital investment in the physician intensivist services is recouped with better patient flow and lower utilization of pharmacy, laboratory, and radiology services. Having an intensivist round on postoperative patients shortens length of stay, reduces complications, and lowers total hospital cost.

ICU Physician Staffing

The Leapfrog Organization ICU physician staffing (IPS) standards [8] were established after reviewing published literature and have since been reviewed and revised incorporating current data and input from hospital and physician communities. Hospitals fulfilling the IPS standard operate ICUs that are managed or comanaged by:

1. Intensivists who are present during daytime hours and provide clinical care exclusively in the ICU.
2. Intensivists who, when not present on site or via telemedicine, return pages at least 95 % of the time within 5 min and arrange for a physician, physician assistant, nurse practitioner, or an FCCS-certified nurse to reach ICU patients within 5 min [8] (FCCS is the course on Fundamental Critical Care Support of the Society of Critical Care Medicine.)

The number of physicians needed to adequately staff an ICU depends on the number of beds, the severity of illness, the number of hours spent in-house and on-call, the intensity of services provided, the availability of consultants, nursing, and patient and family expectations. A clinical full-time equivalent (FTE) represents the amount of work done by one individual working only on patient-care tasks in the intensive unit with in-house coverage for the ICU 24 h of the day, 7 days a week for 365 days; 4.2 FTEs would be needed to cover the work load. This workload might be met by five FTE physicians [9].

Physician Extenders

The term physician extender refers to mid-level health providers such as nurse practitioners (NPs) and physician assistants (PAs). PAs have to complete an accredited training program, usually 2 years in duration, and pass a national examination to obtain a license. PAs have to practice medicine under a physician's supervision. NPs generally complete a 2-year masters degree after a 4-year registered nursing degree and are licensed in the state where practicing. NPs have the ability to practice independently [9].

The need for physician extenders in the recent years has been driven primarily by cutbacks in federal funding for residency training, by the Accreditation Council on Graduate Medical Education standards placing limits on the duty hours for medical trainees, and by increasing patient-care needs [9].

A few studies have shown that introduction of collaborative care by NPs and an intensivist is beneficial to patient outcomes, financial outcomes, length of stay, and patient satisfaction. In one study, patients managed by acute care nurse practitioners had significantly shorter overall length of stay, shorter mean length of stay in the ICU, lower rates of urinary tract infection and skin breakdown, and shorter time to discontinuation of the Foley catheter and mobilization with a total cost savings [10].

Workflow in an ICU

Optimal patient care in an ICU involves complex interplay between multiple medical services utilizing a wide range of medicines, treatments, and procedures. Communication and information transfer within the team and between teams are key. Workflow describes a sequence of specific tasks performed by a single person or a team and is generally based on a set of procedural rules and aims at realization of an objective. Process is a specific notion that has a well-defined input, output, and purpose. Analyzing the workflow may help to redesign work allocation strategies and improve productivity. Various scoring systems have been used to analyze nursing activities and workload. In contrast, few studies have been done evaluating physicians activities and work load [11].

Quality Metrics in an ICU

Quality of health care and intensive care unit care in particular has become a national and international policy issues. Practice patterns and quality of medical care vary widely and health-care providers are interested in having objective information about their performance. Publicly reported measures of quality of care are readily available for patients to review about the quality of care available to them.

Health-care quality is defined as "the degree to which health services for individuals and populations increase the likelihood of desired health outcomes and are consistent with current professional knowledge." The Institute of Medicine (IOM) definition suggests a broad approach to measuring health-care quality, desired outcomes, and related processes of care. Outcomes are relative improvement in health and in experience/satisfaction that are achieved by the use of processes of care that are supported by scientific evidence and consumer preference [12].

Global quality measures include readmission to the ICU, ICU length of stay greater than 7 days, and ICU mortality rates. Complication measures include ventilator-associated pneumonia, infections related to central venous catheter and indwelling urinary catheter, gastrointestinal bleeding, prolonged mechanical ventilation, transfusion-related complications, postoperative myocardial infarctions or cardiac death, deep vein thrombosis and pulmonary embolism, decubitus ulcers, and medication errors per ICU days. Economic measures include patient and family satisfaction.

To improve quality of care, performance must be measured. By improving ICU quality measures, it is possible to reduce mortality, morbidity, and ICU length of stay. Controversy exists regarding whether quality measures should be interventions (process or structural) or outcome measures. Process measures are easier to measure than outcome measures and can be used to provide immediate feedback to providers regarding their performance and provide validity of performance. Outcome measures are ultimately what patients care about. It is more important to select measures in which evidence regarding the association between the intervention and outcome is strong. Quality of care cannot improve in the absence of an intervention that can improve patient outcomes [13].

Pronovost and coworkers [14] focused on developing and implementing measures of ICU quality of care aimed at improving quality, noticing that many patients were not receiving the right therapy which resulted in significant and preventable morbidity, mortality, and increased costs (Table 1.1). Their results included suggestions on how to design and implement measures of quality using primary data collection. Suggested mechanisms to reduce errors included implementation of protocols, checklists, and scheduled multiple physicians' rounds. Protocols have been promoted as enhancing the efficiency, safety, and efficacy of care, as enabling more rigorous clinical research, and as facilitating education. Although protocols are easily applied to simple processes, their usefulness is debatable when more complex issues are involved [15]. An alternative to the protocol is the checklist. Vincent [16] created the "Fast Hug" checklist which highlights seven key aspects in the general care of all critically ill patients listing feeding, analgesia, sedation, thromboembolic prevention, head of the bed elevation, stress ulcer prophylaxis, and glucose control. Checklists such as this may help improve quality of care in ICUs.

Table 1.1 Quality measures, definitions, and design specifications

Quality measure	Definition	Specifications
Outcome measures		
ICU mortality rate	% of ICU discharges who die in the ICU (no risk adjustment; to be used for comparison over time within an ICU)	Numerator: Total no. of ICU deaths
		Denominator: Total no. of ICU discharges (including deaths and transfers)
% of ICU patients, with ICU LOS >7 days	% of ICU discharges with ICU LOS >7 days	Numerator: All ICU patients with ICU LOS >7 days
		Denominator: Total no. of ICU discharges (including deaths and transfers)
Average ICU LOS	Average ICU LOS	Numerator: Sum of ICU length of stay for all discharges
		Denominator: Total no. of ICU discharges (including deaths and transfers)
Average days on mechanical ventilation	Average days on mechanical ventilation	Numerator: Total no. ventilator days
		Denominator: Total number of intubated/trached patients, who where mechanically ventilated
Suboptimal management of pain	% of 4-hintervals with a pain score >3	Numerator: No. of 4-h intervals in which the pain score was >3
		Denominator: Total no. of 4-h intervals
Patient/family satisfaction	To be developed	To be developed
Access measures		
Rate of delayed admissions	Rate of delay admissions to the ICU	Numerator: Number of admissions that are delayed for ≥4 h to ICU (exclude transfers from outside hospitals)
		Denominator: Total number of ICU admissions (exclude transfers from outside hospitals)
Rate of delayed discharges	Rate of delay discharges from the ICU	Numerator: Number of discharges that are delayed for ≥4 from ICU
		Denominator: Total number of ICU discharges
Cancelled OR cases	Number of canceled OR cases due to lack of ICU bed	Numerator: Number of canceled OR cases owing to lack of ICU bed
		Denominator: None (if total number of OR cases are available, than these data can be presented as a rate)
Emergency department by-pass hours	Emergency department by-pass hours per month owing to lack of ICU bed	Numerator: Total by-pass hours per month that are caused by a lack of ICU bed
		Denominator: None

Table 1.1 (continued)

Quality measure	Definition	Specifications
Complication measures		
Rate of unplanned ICU readmissions	Rate of unplanned ICU readmission	Numerator: No of patients who had an unplanned ICU readmission within 48 h ICU discharge
		Denominator: Total no. of ICU discharges
Rate of catheter-related bloodstream infections	Rate of catheter-related bloodstream infections per 1,000 catheter days	Numerator: No of patients with catheter-related blood stream Infections as defined by CDC
		Denominator: Total no. of catheter days in the ICU
Rate of resistant infections	Rate of new-onset resistant infections per ICU patient day	Numerator: No of patients who developed resistant infections in the ICU (defined as MRSA or VRE infections)
		Denominator: Total ICU patient days
Process measures		
Appropriate sedation	The percent of ventilator days on which: (1) sedation was held for at least 12 h or until patient could follow commands or (2) if patient followed commands without the need to hold sedation	Numerator: No of ventilator days on which (1) sedation was held for $\geq$12 h or until patient followed commands or (2) patient followed commands without sedation held
		Denominator: Total ventilator days
Prevention of ventilator-associated pneumonia	The percent of ventilator days on which the head of bed is elevated $\geq$30°	Numerator: No of ventilator days on which the head of the bed was elevated $\geq$30°
		Denominator: Total no. of ventilator days
Appropriate PUD prophylaxis	The percent of ventilator days on which patient received PUD prophylaxis	Numerator: No of ventilator days on which patients received PUD prophylaxis
		Denominator: Total ventilator days
Appropriate DVT prophylaxis	The percent of ventilator days on which patient received DVT prophylaxis	Numerator: No of ventilator days on which patients received DVT prophylaxis
		Denominator: Total ventilator days
Appropriate use of blood transfusions	The percent of packed red blood cell transfusions for which the hemoglobin level before transfusion was less than 8 g/dL	Numerator: No of packed red blood cell transfusions for which the hemoglobin level immediately before transfusion was less than 8 g/dL (include transfusions during episodes of massive bleeding ($\geq$4 U-h) and assume that these transfusions all had hemoglobin levels <8)
		Denominator: Total no. of transfusions
Effective assessment of pain	% of 4-h intervals for which each patient had a pain score documented with the visual analogue scale	Numerator: No of 4-h intervals for which patients had a pain score measured with the visual analogue scale
		Denominator: Total number of 4-h intervals

Reprinted with permission of Elsevier from Pronovost et al. [14]

Abbreviations: *LDS* length of stay, *OR*, operating room, *MRSA* methacillin resistant staph aureus, *VRE* vancomycin resistant enterococcus

References

1. Lassen HCA. A preliminary report on the 1952 epidemic of poliomyelitis in Copenhagen with special reference to the treatment of acute respiratory insufficiency. Lancet. 1953;1:37–41.
2. Moreno R, Miranda DR, Matos R, Fevereiro T. Mortality after discharge from intensive care: the impact of organ system failure and nursing workload use at discharge. Intensive Care Med. 2001;27:999–1004.
3. Lockward HJ, Giddings L, Thomas EJ. Progressive patient care: a preliminary report. JAMA. 1960;172:132–7.
4. Mayer SA, Coplin WM, Chang C, et al. Core Curriculum and competencies for advanced training in neurological intensive care: United Council for Neurologic Subspecialties guidelines. Neurocrit Care. 2006;5:166–71.
5. Mayer SA, Coplin WM, Chang C, et al. Core Curriculum and competencies for advanced training in neurological intensive care: United Council for Neurologic Subspecialties guidelines. Neurocrit Care. 2006;5:159–65.
6. Pronovost PJ, Angus DC, Dorman T, et al. Physician staffing patterns and clinical outcomes in critically ill patients: a systematic review. JAMA. 2002;288:2151–62.
7. Kramer AH, Zygun DA. Do Neurocritical Care units save lives? Measuring the impact of specialized ICU's. Neurocrit Care. 2011;14:329–33.
8. The Leapfrog Group. Available at http://www.leapfroggroup.org
9. Irwine RS, Rippe JM, editors. Irwine and Rippe's intensive care medicine. 6th ed. Philadelphia: Lippincott Williams & Wilkins; 2007.
10. Russell D, VorderBruegge M, Burns SM. Effect of an outcomes-managed approach to care of neuroscience patients by acute care nurse practitioners. Am J Crit Care. 2002;11:353–62.
11. Flaatten H, Moreno RP, Putensen C, Rhodes A, editors. Organisation and management of intensive care. Berlin: Medical Scientific Publishing GmbH; 2010.
12. Palmer RH. Process based measures of quality: the need for detailed clinical data in large health care databases. Ann Intern Med. 1997;127:733–8.

13. Berenholtz S, Dorman T, Ngo K, Pronovost P. Qualitative review of intensive care unit quality indicators. J Crit Care. 2002;17(1): 1–15.
14. Pronovost PJ, Berenholtz SM, Ngo K, et al. Developing and pilot testing quality indicators in the intensive care unit. J Crit Care. 2003;18(3):145–55.
15. Brattebo G, Hofoss D, Flaatten H, et al. Effect of a scoring system and protocol for sedation on duration of patients' need for ventilator support in a surgical intensive care unit. BMJ. 2002;324: 1386–9.
16. Vincent J-L. Give your patient a fast hug (at least) once a day. Crit Care Med. 2005;33(6):1225–9.

Quality Improvement and Neurocritical Care

2

Matthew F. Lawson, F. Kayser Enneking, and J.D. Mocco

Contents

M.F. Lawson, MD
Tallahassee Neurological Clinic, 1401 Centerville Road,
Suite 300, Tallahassee, FL 52308, USA
e-mail: mlawsonmd@yahoo.com

F.K. Enneking, MD
Department of Anesthesiology,
University of Florida College of Medicine,
Shands Quality Committee,
Shands at the University of Florida,
1600 SW Archer Road,
100254, Gainesville, FL 32610, USA
e-mail: enneking@ufl.edu

J.D. Mocco, MD, MS, FAANS, FAHA (✉)
Department of Neurosurgery,
Vanderbilt University Medical Center,
1161 21st Ave S, RM T4224 MCN, Nashville, TN 37232, USA
e-mail: j.mocco@vanderbilt.edu

Abstract

In 1998 the Institute of Medicine established the Committee on the Quality of Healthcare in America in response to growing concern over the quality, safety, efficacy, and efficiency of healthcare in the USA. The primary motivation behind this committee was the belief that despite technological and scientific advances, very small gains had been made in quality of care and patient outcome. Quality improvement is the process by which we critically evaluate care provided by a practitioner in the context of the health system in which they work and enact changes in processes that moves us toward the goal of providing care that is patient and family centered, reproducible, safe, and evidence based; where there are no or inadequate data upon which to base care decisions, quality improvement encourages discovery to generate such information. Additionally, the emphasis on quality in medicine is intimately related to cost-effectiveness and cost reduction. There are a number of ICU-specific quality measures being reported to the UHC, CMS, and other reporting agencies. These measures include development of practices to prevent hospital-acquired conditions and have an emphasis on patient safety. In addition to these specific measures, other factors impact quality of care in a modern ICU, including team communication skills and effective information handoff. Communication is a critically important skill in the NeuroICU, linking physicians, advanced practitioners, nurses, respiratory therapists, physical and occupational therapists, clerks, pharmacists, dietitians, and most importantly, the patient and their family. We expect the role of quality improvement to grow over the next decade, and it will make a significant impact on how we practice medicine in the future.

Keywords

Quality • Safety • PSI • AHRQ • Indicator • IOM

Spotlight on Quality and Safety

In 1998, the Institute of Medicine established the Committee on the Quality of Healthcare in America in response to growing concern over the quality, safety, efficacy, and efficiency of healthcare in the USA. This group's mission was to enact changes that would substantially improve the quality of care within 10 years. The primary motivation behind this committee was the belief that, despite technological and scientific advances, very small gains had been made in quality of care and patient outcome.

The committee wasted no time in identifying several quality issues in healthcare, and the first major publication, *To Err Is Human: Building a Safer Health System* [1], was published in 1999. This landmark monograph put a spotlight on healthcare in America, with an eye toward quality, safety, and the prevention of medical errors. The IOM report contended that "more people die in a given year from medical errors that from motor vehicle accidents (43,458), breast cancer (42,297), or AIDS (16,516)" and estimated the total number of deaths due to medical errors to be 44,000–98,000 deaths per year. These graphic descriptions of medical errors and dramatic statements comparing medical errors to conditions like breast cancer and AIDS, conditions familiar to most Americans, catapulted quality and safety into the national healthcare debate.

As dramatic as the IOM report sounded, the goal was not to incite fear in the public or anger in the healthcare community – although, to some extent these occurred – but to identify problems with healthcare delivery in the USA in a manner that would result in action. The focus on safety served two major purposes: first, improving patient safety is an admirable goal and in line with the mission of the healthcare system; second, it resonates with the public and is recognized by them as critically important to their own care. The first step toward quality improvement, according to the IOM, was to "break the cycle of inaction" and develop a "comprehensive approach to improving patient safety" [1].

The IOM hoped to improve quality and safety by implementing systems that would enable healthcare professionals and institution to learn from mistakes. Instead of focusing on assignment of blame, they advocated using every error, regardless of whether or not there was patient injury or harm, as a tool to learn *why* the error occurred. In this manner, institutions and professionals could focus action on developing processes of care that would reduce medical errors and increase the reliable delivery of safe care. Ultimately, *To Err Is Human* included four recommendations for improving quality and safety:

- Establishing a national focus to create leadership, research, tools, and protocols to enhance the knowledge base about safety.

- Identifying and learning from errors through immediate and strong mandatory reporting efforts, as well as the encouragement of voluntary efforts, both with the aim of making sure the system continues to be made safer for patients.
- Raising standards and expectations for improvements in safety through the actions of oversight organizations, group purchasers, and professional groups.
- Creating safety systems inside healthcare organizations through the implementation of safe practices at the delivery level, which is the ultimate target of all the recommendations [1].

This approach was successful in advancing discussion and scholarly activity in the areas of quality and safety. Stelfox and colleagues, in 2006, reviewed the number of medical publications, including guidelines, editorials, original research, and news items related to quality and safety both before and after the publication of *To Err Is Human* [2]. They concluded that the IOM report was associated with a significant increase in publications relating to patient safety, but there was little evidence that safety had actually improved.

Patient safety and error prevention can be thought of as a "systems" issue. Complex medical information must flow efficiently between physician, nurse, technologist, clerk, pharmacist, patient, and a variety of other professionals. Breakdowns, failures, and inconsistencies in this flow of information can lead to preventable medical errors. The focus on patient safety after the IOM report led many institutions to perform a top to bottom review of patient care systems and protocols with the aim of anticipating errors, refining systems to avoid these, and improving communication and data handoffs. Tools common to many institutions include patient safety committees, hiring patient safety or chief quality officers, performing root cause analyses when errors occur, and patient safety rounds. The purpose is to create an environment where care processes can be continuously reviewed and refined.

Unfortunately, putting quality and safety initiatives in place and making meaningful improvements in patient safety is both difficult and not amenable to simple "top-down" leadership. Longo and colleagues, in 2005, published "The Long Road to Patient Safety," studying all acute care hospitals in Utah and Missouri between 2002 and 2004 to identify changes in hospital patient safety systems [3]. The authors surveyed these institutions at two points in time with a 91 question survey to assess how the institution's patient safety systems had changed over time. Overall response rates were high, 76.8 % for the 2002 survey and 78.0 % for the 2004 survey. One hundred seven hospitals responded in both 2002 and 2004.

The results were surprising. Nine percent of hospitals in the study still had no written patient safety plans in 2004, and only 74 % of responding institutions reported having a fully implemented safety plan. Fewer than 39 % of responding institutions had budgeted funds dedicated for patient safety initiatives. Despite these shortcomings, their study illustrated several bright spots in safety initiatives including relatively high rates of adoption of patient safety strategies in surgical units and in medication prescription and dispensing mechanisms. Examples include mandatory operative "time-out" before starting a procedure, mandatory preoperative anesthesia evaluations, surgical checklists, and pharmacy procedures for look-alike and soundalike drug names. Ultimately, Longo concluded that as of 2004, patient safety systems were not sufficient to meet IOM recommendations.

Just 2 years after publishing *To Err Is Human*, the IOM committee on Healthcare in America published its second book, *Crossing the Quality Chasm: A New Health System for the 21st Century* [4]. The book's purpose was to aid in the development of dialogue and focus for an agenda for quality improvement going forward. *To Err Is Human* brought national attention to quality issues and patient safety and developed a public appetite for change. *Crossing the Quality Chasm* identified areas for change and proposed a national agenda for improvement.

Major Players in Quality

The roots of the IOM date back to 1863, when President Lincoln established the National Academy of Sciences. In 1970, the IOM was created as the health science arm of the National Academy of Sciences, which has evolved into the National Academies. Presently, the IOM's mission is to "serve as advisor to the nation to improve health" [5].

Another major player in the national quality in healthcare movement is the Agency for Healthcare Research and Quality (AHRQ). This government agency is the health service arm of the US Department of Health and Human Services. Its mission is "to improve the quality, safety, efficiency, and effectiveness of health care for all Americans" [6]. Perhaps the most important facet of the AHRQ is the quality indicators (QIs) this agency develops; they are the benchmark for measuring quality at many institutions. To facilitate their use, the QIs utilize administrative (coding and billing) data, since it is uniform and readily available across health institutions.

One of the major classes of Quality Indicators developed by the AHRQ are the Patient Safety Indicators (PSIs), which "reflect quality of care inside hospitals, as well as geographic areas, to focus on potentially avoidable complications and iatrogenic events" [6]. The focus of the PSIs is to identify inpatient complications as well as complications and adverse events that occur as a result of a procedure, surgery, or childbirth. These were developed by the AHRQ in conjunction with researchers at the University of California, San Francisco (UCSF), UC Davis, and Stanford University after a thorough review of the literature and study of ICD-9 coding data [7]. A list of PSIs can be found in Table 2.1. The PSIs have been an invaluable tool for monitoring ICU quality and safety and identifying areas in need of improvement.

Table 2.1 Patient safety indicators

The PSIs include the following provider-level indicators:	
Patient safety indicators – provider	PSI number
Complications of anesthesia	1
Death in low-mortality DRGs	2
Decubitus ulcer	3
Failure to rescue	4
Foreign body left during procedure	5
Iatrogenic pneumothorax	6
Selected infections due to medical care	7
Postoperative hip fracture	8
Postoperative hemorrhage or hematoma	9
Postoperative physiologic and metabolic derangements	10
Postoperative respiratory failure	11
Postoperative pulmonary embolism or deep vein thrombosis	12
Postoperative sepsis	13
Postoperative wound dehiscence	14
Accidental puncture or laceration	15
Transfusion reaction	16
Birth trauma – injury to neonate	17
Obstetric trauma – vaginal with instrument	18
Obstetric trauma – vaginal without instrument	19

Reprinted with permission from AHRQ [23]

The healthcare quality movement has literally hundreds of interested parties, including patient rights groups, medical societies and physician organizations, hospital systems, health insurance companies, device and pharmaceutical corporations, and federal and state governments. Undoubtedly, these diverse stakeholders have different ideas about the definition of quality, as well as how to measure and improve upon it. The National Quality Forum (NQF) was founded in 1999 as a federally mandated body to bring together the diverse stakeholders. This not-for-profit organization, funded by both private and public sources, strives to improve healthcare by bringing stakeholders to the table, building consensus, and endorsing national consensus standards for measuring quality and for public reporting quality metrics. The NQF has more than 350 member organizations, of which there are over 30 medical specialty societies, including the American Association of Neurological Surgeons (AANS), Society of Critical Care Medicine, American Society of Anesthesiologists, and Anesthesia Quality Institute [8].

Another major institutional player in the national quality movement is the University HealthSystem Consortium (UHC). This body is an alliance of 113 academic medical centers and 254 affiliated institutions, accounting for over 90 % of the nation's academic healthcare systems. The unique aspect of the UHC is that it collects quality data from member organizations, performs analyses, and then provides members the data by which they may compare and rank themselves to similar institutions. In this way, the UHC "provides the lens through which the (member) organization assesses all that it does" [9]. The goal is to promote excellence in quality, safety, and cost-effectiveness by allowing members to see their relative strengths and weaknesses in several areas. Institutions can download a composite score and quality report from the UHC. Not surprisingly, safety represents 30 % of the composite score and is based largely on the AHRQ Patient Safety Indicators (PSIs).

Evaluating Quality Improvement

What is quality improvement? Other than a popular buzz word used by hospital administrators, insurance executives, department chairs, and textbook authors, quality improvement is difficult to define. The AHRQ defined quality as "doing the right thing, at the right time, in the right way, for the right person with the best possible results" [10]. In our eyes, quality improvement is the process by which we critically evaluate care provided by a practitioner in the context of the health system in which they work and enact changes in processes that move us toward the goal of providing care that is patient and family centered, reproducible, safe, and evidence based; where there are no or inadequate data upon which to base care decisions, quality improvement encourages discovery to generate such information.

While both the AHRQ definition and our variation on that theme resonate with patients and providers, how is one to measure and improve quality? There are two major analytic processes by which quality can be evaluated: process and outcome. Broadly speaking, *process* of care evaluation focuses on whether hospitals and physicians provide care that is known to be efficacious, such as using DVT prophylaxis in high-risk ICU patients. *Outcome* evaluation focuses on the concrete outcomes related to care, such as ICU mortality due to PE or DVT. Both of these strategies have merits and drawbacks [11].

Process-based evaluation is useful because many of these measures are based on strong scientific evidence for use, such as the DVT prophylaxis example above. It is also relatively easy to evaluate a wide cross section of facilities and providers to see if they are adhering to the process; it is easy to determine if the provider wrote for subcutaneous heparin, if the pharmacy dispensed it and if the nurse gave it. However, there are a number of serious drawbacks. The most glaring is that many facets of medicine cannot be broken down to a standard regimen and definitive best practices may not be applicable to entire populations. Process of care evaluation cannot account for "physician judgment," where a physician decides between two acceptable treatment strategies. Finally, meeting process measures does not necessarily ensure that a high level of quality is being met [11].

Outcome measures are appealing, as they align the interests of the patients and providers more closely. Therefore, measuring outcome after traumatic brain injury would be in the interest of the patients and care providers and may be a better indicator of overall quality than process measures. However, there can be significant confounding factors, such as patient demographics, comorbidities, and locations that do not allow for fair comparison of these outcome measures between different physicians or institutions [11].

Both process and outcome measures are important in evaluating quality in the current quality improvement movement. Process measures have become critical in evaluating hospital- and unit-based adherence to evidence-based guidelines and standards, while outcome measures help physicians and hospitals keep their eye on the ball. The debate between process and outcome measures was summarized by Dr. Jha:

> Although the US health care system is now committed to quality measurement and the public reporting of such data, debates will continue about what to measure, who collects the data, and what to report publicly. More information is needed on processes and outcomes across a large number of conditions for hospitals, physician practices, and other health care settings and practitioners. Much of these data are on their way, led by major payers such as Medicare and coalitions of employers who want greater accountability for the care they purchase and to stimulate improvements in quality of care. In the most expensive health care system in the world, patients and physicians should expect nothing less [11].

Mortality and Length of Stay

Ahead of their time, the Healthcare Financing Administration (HCFA) published inpatient mortality rates for Medicare patients in the 1980s. These data were hospital specific and gave citizens their first glimpse at in-hospital mortality. However, physician groups and hospital associations felt the data were misleading and inaccurately reflected of the quality of care provided at a given institution [12].

It is generally accepted that patients with different medical comorbidities, age, demographics, and family risk factors may have different outcomes for a similar medical condition. Thus, the overall mortality rates for myocardial infarction could be quite different between a rural Midwest community hospital and a large, inner city tertiary care facility. The tertiary care facility may be caring for older individuals, sicker individuals, who may be from very different socioeconomic backgrounds than the patients in the community hospital. The tertiary facility may provide outstanding care, but if the overall mortality of its arguably sicker patient exceeds that of the community facility, the tertiary facility may appear to be a low quality institution. Many argued that the HCFA overall mortality data was limited because it did not account for these factors.

In the late 1980s, with the rise of electronic billing databases, the solution to this problem was developed. If patients' risk of mortality could be stratified in some way, based on their age, medical comorbidities, and other factors, one could estimate the expected risk of mortality for a given hospital population. The Commission on Professional and Hospital Activities (CPHA) developed computer models to estimate risk of death based on the existing billing data from inpatient admissions. This computer model was then used to calculate *expected mortality rates* at particular hospitals for a given diagnosis that would reflect the relative sickness of the patients at that facility. The expected mortality rates were based on patients' comorbid conditions, age, and the complexity of the procedure being performed. The results of this computer model were expressed as a ratio of observed mortality to expected mortality. This ratio, the observed-to-expected mortality ratio is known as the *mortality index,* and its use was validated in a study involving 300 hospitals and thousands of admissions [12].

The goal for any facility, practice, or intensive care unit is to have a low mortality index, much less than one. If the mortality index for a given institution is above one, this represents mortality rates in excess of those expected, or calculated, based the patients' comorbidities. A mortality index of one represents a mortality rate equal to the expected mortality rate, and an index less than one represents an observed mortality rate that is lower than expected. One might think that any mortality index value below one would be an acceptable number. However, due to the trailing method of data collection and continuous improvement strategies, for academic centers the average value for mortality index in neurosurgical populations is closer to 0.6.

In a similar manner, length of stay for a given type of admission or procedure can be followed with the *length of stay index.* This vale is the observed length of stay compared to the expected length of stay, calculated from the coding data. As with mortality index, length of stay index values below one represent a length of stay in the hospital that is shorter than expected. Both mortality index and length of stay index are important quality markers that are reported to facilities as a part of the UHC data.

While mortality and length of stay indices are important markers for quality, it is important to recognize their limitations. The main limitation, which is also a major strength, is the fact that these values are based on billing codes. The data calculated for mortality and length of stay index are therefore only as accurate as the medical coding at the hospital of interest. Coding variation can artificially worsen or improve both of these indexes.

Klugman and colleagues published a report in 2010 in which they reported the use of palliative care ICD-9 codes made a dramatic difference in their hospital's mortality index [13]. They became concerned in 2008 due to a rather high mortality index at their institution. Their own internal review revealed that many of the patients that expired had active palliative care orders, but the palliative care codes were infrequently applied to the admission by the hospital coding staff. Once they had corrected this coding error, they had a dramatic reduction in mortality index. They concluded that there are limitations to using coding data and that providers, hospitals, and the public should be aware of these limitations when reviewing publicly reported quality data.

Financial Implications of Quality in Medicine

The emphasis on quality in medicine is intimately related to cost-effectiveness and cost reduction. Perhaps due to the recent worldwide economic slowdown, combined with – in the USA – the historical and ongoing increased cost of medical services, cost-effectiveness in the context of quality has become a major topic in medicine and at all levels of government. Indeed, to paraphrase one of the leaders of the quality movement: expensive care may well be poor-quality care (Steele G, personal communication with AJ Layon, 2011). There have been many attempts by private payers and government payers to modify payment structures to include elements that reward providers for providing high-quality and cost-effective care, while penalizing those that cannot.

Another trend in quality in medicine is the public reporting of hospital and physician quality data. While this is not a direct financial incentive, the implication is that an empowered consumer base will choose providers and institutions

Table 2.2 PQRI/PQRS quality measures for neurosurgery, neurology, and neurocritical care

Only a fraction of the 153 quality measures apply
Perioperative care (similar to SCIP measures)
Timing of antibiotic prophylaxis
Appropriate antibiotic choice (1st/2nd cephalosporin)
Discontinuation of prophylactic antibiotics
Venous thromboembolism prophylaxis
Stroke
Venous thromboembolism prophylaxis
Anticoagulant for AFIB prescribed at discharge
Dysphagia screening
Consideration/evaluation for rehab services
Thrombolytic therapy for ischemic stroke

Reprinted with permission from AHRQ [23]

that demonstrate high-quality care. In fact, in 2009 at least 22 states had legislation in some form that mandated reporting of some quality metrics [14]. An important question is whether individuals needing healthcare services can function as "consumers," at least for urgent care issues.

In 2006, the Tax Relief and Healthcare Act (TRHCA) required that CMS establish a voluntary system of quality reporting for physicians. In this system, called the Medicare Physician Quality Reporting Initiative (PQRI), participating physicians who submitted quality data about their patients would receive incentive payments and be publically recognized on the CMS website. This completely voluntary system began data collection in 2007. It grew rapidly, and by 2009 it had 153 self-reportable quality measures. Only a fraction of the reportable quality measures are applicable to neurosurgery, neurology, or neurocritical care, and an example of these can be seen in Table 2.2. In 2010 the system continued to evolve and is now called the Physician Quality Reporting System (PQRS) [15].

Quality reporting systems are also in place at the hospital level. Hospitals have had the opportunity to voluntarily contribute quality data to CMS since 2004. Up until 2008, most of these programs were designed as "pay for reporting" type systems, where hospitals and physicians received incentive payments to participate and report quality data. In 2008, pay for reporting morphed into "pay for performance," as CMS began the practice of reduced reimbursement for hospital-acquired conditions.

Pay for performance is not only part of the CMS landscape, as private payers have had quality-based payment schedules in place for several years. In fact, a 2005 study found that nearly 50 % of HMOs had pay for performance quality-based incentives worked into contracts with providers and hospitals [16]. This move toward pay for performance is seen as a way for payers to influence and improve quality care by mandating provider adherence to treatment algorithms and evidence-based guidelines.

This move has had serious consequences, particularly in surgical and medical ICUs, as these units are at high risk for hospital-acquired conditions. Examples of such conditions include catheter-associated UTI (CA-UTI), respiratory failure, ventilator-associated pneumonia, central-line-associated infection, deep venous thrombosis, and surgical site infection. Overall, ICUs are relative high-cost providers of medical care. As the focus on cost reduction intensifies, it is expected that there will be more emphasis on pay for performance systems in ICU settings. A review of the topic in 2009 concluded that participation in these new pay for performance systems, while unpopular with many physicians, had the potential benefit of dramatically improving care for ICU patients [17].

Quality Improvement in the NeuroICU

There are a number of ICU-specific quality measures being reported to the UHC, CMS, and other reporting agencies. The focus on quality in a neurocritical care unit can be broken down into several key areas: (1) development and adherence to standardized evidence-based practices for preventing hospital-acquired conditions and emphasis on patient safety; (2) regular review of quality metrics, particularly our AHRQ PSI data, to identify areas in need of improvement; and (3) development of quality projects and initiatives to correct deficiencies. This process is possible by participating in the UHC, or similar quality registries, where one can view their quality data and compliance rates and compare the data with similar institutions. Using this tool, one can identify strengths and weaknesses and focus resources to areas of critical need and improve patient outcome.

In 2009, Krimsky described a single institution experience implementing a patient safety program in an intensive care setting. The motivation behind the project was a hospital wide quality analysis that identified several deaths due to PE in patients who were not receiving routine DVT prophylaxis. These preventable deaths prompted a patient safety project for the ICU. The project tracked implementation of the safety program as well as three specific interventions for improving patient safety: routine DVT prophylaxis in non-ambulatory patients, ventilator-associated pneumonia prophylaxis for intubated patients, and stress-ulcer prophylaxis. The program included nursing and physician education, team building exercises, enhancing communication and handoffs, and mandatory documentation of implementation of these measures on progress notes [18].

The authors found the implementation of their patient safety initiatives to be very successful. Objectively, they tracked the compliance rates with the evidence-based prophylactic measures and found a significant increase in compliance. They nearly achieved the goal of 100 % compliance for these measures and developed processes for implementing safety measures that could be repeated in the future as other initiatives were started.

The focus on preventing hospital-acquired complications is a major focus of quality improvement movements in intensive care settings nationwide. There are two major motivations for this: first, preventing line infections, DVTs, and UTIs is a relatively straightforward mission, with easily identifiable patient end points that markedly impact patient care in a positive manner; second, CMS reimbursement to hospitals is reduced for hospital-acquired conditions, so there is considerable financial incentive for institutions to reduce these events. The hospital-acquired central venous catheter infection event has been well studied and has documented success in a variety of ICU settings.

National Quality Initiatives in ICUs

In 2011, Pronovost and coworkers published "Preventing Bloodstream Infections: A Measurable National Success Story in Quality Improvement." They describe a program called "On the CUSP: Stop BSI," where CUSP stands for Comprehensive Unit-Based Safety Program. This effort started as a collaboration with the Johns Hopkins University Quality and Safety Research Group, the American Hospital Association, and the Michigan Health and Hospital Association. It was partially funded by the AHRQ and now has operations in 45 states. The goal of this program was to eradicate central venous catheter-related bloodstream infections using a multifaceted intervention system that involved convincing physicians and staff of the need for change, providing tools to enact change, and using external "levers" to help enact change. This program was one of many that helped reduce the national central-line infection rate by 63 % between 2001 and 2009 [14].

An important aspect of the Pronovost paper is the authors' analysis of *why* the central-line infection reduction program was successful. They attribute this to a number of factors, including the ability to convince providers that minimizing these infections was an important and attainable goal. There was a mature scientific basis for monitoring and diagnosing central-line infections. Several large studies demonstrated that elimination of central-line infection in a variety of settings was possible, thus forcing providers to acknowledge that it was achievable in their own patients. Finally, they cite the ability to leverage several external factors, including social pressure to enact change, economic pressure from the CMS, and regulatory pressure from the Joint Commission. Together, the educational program, clinical tools, and external "levers" helped dramatically reduce central-line infections in participating institutions. Several of the early adopters have up to 3 years

of follow-up data that demonstrate a *durable* reduction in central-line infection rates [14].

Single Institution Quality Projects

Equally important to the national movements and quality improvement initiatives in neurocritical care are single institution quality projects focused on correcting a local quality issue. A review of our own quality data revealed an unacceptably high rate of Foley catheter-associated urinary tract infections (CA-UTI). We found that the Foley catheter utilization rate in our neurointensive care unit was nearly 100 % and that catheters were being used for a diverse set of indications. Many of these indications were outdated, such as decreased bedside nursing time devoted to toileting patients. Furthermore, catheters were placed in a variety of settings, including other facilities, the operating room, other ICU settings, and the floor, and a variety of different products were used.

Armed with this data, a group of physicians and nurses worked together on a quality task force to reduce our CA-UTI rate. They reviewed the literature and developed an evidence-based UTI prevention bundle. The focus of this bundle was to reduce Foley catheter use, avoid insertion of a catheter without a clear medical indication, maintain sterility of the system, and encourage early removal. After this bundle was developed, we instituted a study period to track the results over a 30 month period (20,394 catheter days) [19].

The results were dramatic. We reduced our overall Foley catheter utilization rate from 100 to 73.3 %, and there was a substantial reduction in the CA-UTI rate, from 13.3 to 4.0 per 1,000 catheter days. Both of these reductions were highly significant, with p values less than 0.001. Importantly, there was no concomitant increase in sacral decubitus ulcer, potentially an unforeseen consequence of decreasing urinary catheter use due to potential incontinence. We concluded that an evidence-based UTI prevention bundle and continuous quality improvement strategy can have a significant impact on quality in the NeuroICU.

Communication and Handoffs

Communication is a critically important skill in the NeuroICU, linking physicians, advanced practitioners, nurses, respiratory therapists, physical and occupational therapists, clerks, pharmacists, dietitians, and, most importantly, the patient and their family. Without effective communication, the delivery of healthcare breaks down and quality care is impossible. Recent changes in resident work hours have impacted the physician-staffing abilities at academic centers across the USA, which has led to "shift work" setups in many critical care units. In this setting, effective communication and patient care handoffs is critical in the provision of high-quality care.

In any hospital unit, communication with patient families is a very important aspect of care. It is in this setting that the diagnosis and prognosis can be discussed with the family, and medical providers can learn about the patients' wishes regarding aggressive and end-of-life care. In the NeuroICU – indeed any ICU – many patients cannot communicate with their medical providers, making effective communication with family more important. A recent review by Scheunemann and colleagues looked at different communication strategies in the ICU setting. They reviewed over 2,800 papers published since 1995 on communication with families in the ICU. Ultimately, they concluded that printed materials for family education, daily communication by the ICU team, as well as selective ethics consultation and palliative care consultation resulted in improved emotional outcomes for families, reduced LOS, and appropriate treatment intensity [20].

More important is the role of communication between physician teams providing care in the NeuroICU setting. With multiple teams of neurologists, neurosurgeons, and intensivists caring for patients, effective communication between the teams is critical. Most organizations promoting quality in medicine have advocated for standardizing and improving this important form of medical communication. Methodologies to improve communication between teams may take several directions. One of perhaps the most obvious is a structured handoff between teams. Unfortunately, the available literature on the appropriate structure, setting, format, and content of an effective handoff is lacking. A recent review of all published literature on physician handoffs concluded that there is no scientific basis for a standard format for this type of communication [21].

In one study of handoffs in the NeuroICU, Lyons and colleagues concluded that specific physician education on handoffs, minimization of interruptions, a standard location, and adequate time were crucial for an effective transmission of information and communication [22]. There is considerable need for further study of effective handoff techniques and procedures, with review of NeuroICU outcomes when using those techniques. A second method by which communication is "forced" is by closing the unit to order writing; in this manner, the teams must discuss the plan together as only one of the groups – usually the intensivist team – is allowed to write orders.

Summary and Future Directions

Quality improvement is here to stay, and the social motivation behind this movement is growing. No physician would ever board an aircraft if they knew the airline did not have a safety policy or continuous improvement program. Why would our patients expect less from us? It is not only our duty as physicians to provide the best care possible but also our duty to provide "the right thing, at the right time, in the right way, for the right person with the best possible results" [10].

There is a perfect storm of social demand for improvement in quality and safety as well as economic and regulatory pressures, partially due to our recent recession and soaring healthcare expenditures that will evoke significant change in our health system in the coming decade. Some physicians view this with fear and apprehension, while others see it as an opportunity of unparalleled importance and opportunity. The decade after the IOM report *To Err Is Human* was met with only limited success in improving patient quality. The current environment is a direct result of the work of the IOM, and the health system is just starting to make significant gains in quality and safety. The potential exists for the coming decade to be known as the era of quality in medicine.

References

1. Kohn LT, Corrigan J, Donaldson MS. To err is human: building a safer health system. Washington, D.C.: National Academy Press; 2000.
2. Stelfox HT, Palmisani S, Scurlock C, Orav EJ, Bates DW. The "To Err is Human" report and the patient safety literature. Qual Saf Health Care. 2006;15:174–8.
3. Longo DR, Hewett JE, Ge B, Schubert S. The long road to patient safety. JAMA. 2005;294:2858–65.
4. Institute of Medicine (U.S.). Committee on Quality of Health Care in America. Crossing the quality chasm: a new health system for the 21st century. Washington, D.C.: National Academy Press; 2001.
5. Institute of Medicine. About the IOM; 2011. http://www.iom.edu/About-IOM.aspx. Accessed 16 July 2013.
6. AHRQ. Agency for Healthcare Research and Quality. Mission and Budget; 2011. http://www.ahrq.gov/about/mission/index.html. Accessed 25 June 2013.
7. AHRQ. Agency for Healthcare Research and Quality. AHRQ quality indicators: patient safety indicators; 2010. http://www.ahrq.gov/health-care-information/topics/topic-patient-safety-indicators.html. Accessed 25 June 2013.
8. NQF. National Quality Forum; 2011. http://www.qualityforum.org/Home.aspx. Accessed 25 June 2013.
9. UHC. University HealthSystem Consortium; 2011. https://www.uhc.edu. Accessed 25 June 2013.
10. AHRQ. Agency for Healthcare Research and Quality. Your guide to choosing quality healthcare; 2010. http://www.ahrq.gov/index.html. Accessed 25 June 2013.
11. Jha AK. Measuring hospital quality: what physicians do? How patients fare? Or both? JAMA. 2006;296:95–7.
12. DesHarnais SI, Chesney JD, Wroblewski RT, Fleming ST, McMahon Jr LF. The risk-adjusted mortality index: a new measure of hospital performance. Med Care. 1988;26:1129–48.
13. Klugman R, Allen L, Benjamin EM, Fitzgerald J, Ettinger W. Mortality rates as a measure of quality and safety, "caveat emptor". Am J Med Qual. 2010;25:197–201.
14. Pronovost PJ, Marsteller JA, Goeschel CA. Preventing bloodstream infections: a measurable national success story in quality improvement. Health Aff. 2011;30:628–34.

15. CMS. Centers for Medicare and Medicaid services. Physician Quality Reporting System; 2011. http://www.cms.gov/Medicare/Quality-Initiatives-Patient-Assessment-Instruments/PQRS/index.html?redirect=/PQRS/. Accessed 25 June 2013.

16. Rosenthal MB, Landon BE, Normand SL, Frank RG, Epstein AM. Pay for performance in commercial HMOs. N Engl J Med. 2006;355:1895–902.

17. Khanduja K, Scales DC, Adhikari NK. Pay for performance in the intensive care unit – opportunity or threat? Crit Care Med. 2009; 37:852–8.

18. Krimsky WS, Mroz IB, McIlwaine JK, Surgenor SD, Christian D, Corwin HL, Houston D, Robison C, Malayaman N. A model for increasing patient safety in the intensive care unit: Increasing the implementation rates of proven safety measures. Qual Saf Health Care. 2009;18:74–80.

19. Titsworth W, Hester J, Correia T, Reed R, Williams M, Guin P, Layon A, Archibald L, Mocco J. Reduction of catheter associated urinary tract infections among neurosurgical intensive care unit patients: a single institution's success. J Neurosurg. 2012;116(4): 911–20.

20. Scheunemann LP, McDevitt M, Carson SS, Hanson LC. Randomized, controlled trials of interventions to improve communication in intensive care. Chest. 2011;139:543–54.

21. Cohen MD, Hilligoss PB. The published literature on handoffs in hospitals: deficiencies identified in an extensive review. Qual Saf Health Care. 2010;19:493–7.

22. Lyons MN, Standley TDA, Gupta AK. Quality improvement of doctors' shift-change handover in neuro-critical care. Qual Saf Health Care. 2010;19:1–7.

23. AHRQ. Agency for Healthcare Research and Quality. AHRQ quality indicators: guide to patient safety indicators; 2007. http://qualityindicators.ahrq.gov/Downloads/Modules/PSI/V43/Composite_User_Technical_Specification_PSI_4.3.pdf. Accessed 25 June 2013.

Neurointensive Care Medicine as an Emerging ICU Subspecialty

3

Cherylee W.J. Chang

Contents

C.W.J. Chang, MD, FACP, FCCM
Department of Medicine and Surgery,
Neuroscience Institute/Neurocritical Care,
The Queen's Medical Center,
University of Hawaii,
John A. Burns School of Medicine,
1301 Punchbowl Street, QET 5,
Honolulu, HI 96813, USA
e-mail: chang@queens.org

Abstract

Critical care developed as a specialty in the 1800s. Its evolution has been facilitated by a recognition of the need for more intensive observation and nursing of sicker patients and by advances in technology starting with the ability to mechanically ventilate patients. Critical care specialty training began primarily in the postoperative setting with anesthesiologists and surgeons. Internal medicine and pulmonary medicine managed the medical patients with respiratory failure. Neurologists although initially involved with patients during the polio epidemic have traditionally had little to no training in managing critically ill patients and have been relegated to a primarily consultative and diagnostician role in the ICU. In the last few decades, however, acute stroke therapies and new research that increases the understanding of the pathophysiology of primary and secondary brain injury and the interplay of the neurological system and its disorders and other organ systems put neurologists into an active role in patient care in the ICU. Neurocritical care or intensive care neurology is a growing field with a growing body of knowledge that has shown to improve patient care. This chapter reviews the history of critical care as a subspecialty and the means for critical care certification both in the USA and internationally. It reviews the evolution of neurocritical care and the accreditation of training programs and certification of individuals, which currently is only available to North American candidates. With people living longer, the world has an aging population and faces a critical care workforce shortage. Neurocritical care is attracting a multiprofessional group of practitioners into this workforce. These individuals play an important role not only in the delivery of care to neurological critically ill patients but are key to the advocacy, education, prevention, and research to help improve outcomes.

Keywords

Evolution • History • Intensive care neurology • Neurocritical care • Neurointensive care

A.J. Layon et al. (eds.), *Textbook of Neurointensive Care*,
DOI 10.1007/978-1-4471-5226-2_3, © Springer-Verlag London 2013

History of Neurology and Critical Care

Critical care in the modern age is a multiprofessional specialty that acknowledges the need for many individuals with different skill sets that contribute to the care and survival of a patient with unstable vital signs and life-threatening medical conditions. This typically occurs in a localized area where patients can be grouped and managed by a specialized team. The beginnings of critical care, i.e., the delivery of care to sicker patients who require intensive nursing, are universally credited to the work of Florence Nightingale in the mid-1800s [1]. During the Crimean War (1853–1856), there were reports of unsanitary and poor conditions for the sick and wounded in the British camps. The British War Minister requested Nightingale, then the superintendent of the Hospital for Invalid Gentlewomen in London, to use a team of nurses to improve the conditions in the barrack hospitals in Turkey [2, 3]. In 1854, Nightingale and her colleagues improved the sanitation and hygiene and also created an area near the nursing station where the sickest and most injured soldiers were observed and managed closely. These were the beginnings of intensive care medicine.

The next reference to the critical care concept emerged in the 1920s when Walter Dandy, a neurosurgeon, established two adjacent two-bed rooms that served as a neurosurgical ICU and the first intensive care unit (ICU) at the Johns Hopkins Hospital in Baltimore, Maryland. These beds were staffed at all times with one specially trained nurse for craniotomy patients during their first 24 h after surgery [4, 5]. This postoperative model evolved to the surgical intensive care unit where these patients were managed by surgeons or anesthesiologists.

The universal adoption of mechanical ventilation solidified the need for areas of a hospital where patients needed closer monitoring and skilled nursing care. The polio epidemic hastened the use of the negative pressure, Drinker ventilator, or "iron lung" in the 1920s [6]. The invention of an improved and less expensive iron lung by Emerson in 1931 allowed its widespread use to create large polio wards in the 1940s and 1950s [7]. During this time, intensive care was required to keep the patient's airway clear of secretions, and there was a recognized need for proper airway humidification and fluid resuscitation to prevent hypotension and awareness of the dangers of hypoventilation and hyperventilation. Since these patients suffered from a neuromuscular disease, neurologists were often the primary caregivers [8]. However, anesthesiologists soon assumed an important role in the care of these patients.

In Sweden, despite tracheostomy and the use of negative pressure cuirass ventilators, the mortality of in polio patients with respiratory failure remained at 85 % due to swallowing difficulties and aspiration. The use of the Engström positive pressure ventilator dropped the mortality rate of respiratory failure-complicated poliomyelitis to 27 % [9]. A red rubber endotracheal tube was first developed by Irish anesthetist Sir Ivan Magill in the 1920s, and the plastic disposable endotracheal tube was introduced by David Sheridan in 1959 [10]. With endotracheal intubation, prolonged mechanical ventilation became popularized with the use of positive pressure ventilators in the 1950s. These units were typically directed by anesthesiologists [11]. Peter Safar, an Austrian anesthesiologist, best known for his work in cardiopulmonary cerebral resuscitation, created the first general intensive care unit in the USA in 1961 at the Baltimore City Hospital [12].

Critical Care as a Subspecialty

As the physical premise of an intensive care unit developed, the practitioners working within them began to coalesce as a team. The critical care-trained nurse, respiratory therapist, physician, dietitian, and pharmacist become integral to a patient's holistic care.

With the advent of the Salk vaccine for polio in the 1950s, neurologists were no longer primary caregivers for critically ill patients [13]. And as the initial intensive care units typically focused on postoperative care, patients were primarily managed by anesthesiologists. Trauma units, however, were run predominantly by surgeons. ICUs with patients with primary cardiac or pulmonary issues were more commonly managed by internists. In the USA, the training of physicians in critical care mirrored the specialty units. Peter Safar offered the first critical care medicine (CCM) training for anesthesiology. General surgery and internal medicine followed suit.

In the 1970s, three physicians with common goals of advancement of critical care—Max Harry Weil, an internist and cardiologist based in Los Angeles; Peter Safar, an anesthesiologist and pioneer of the general ICU at Pittsburgh; and William Shoemaker, a trauma surgeon—gathered a group of 28 individuals to found the Society of Critical Care Medicine (SCCM) [14]. Ake Grenvik, a Swedish-trained intensivist with a background in general surgery, thoracic and cardiovascular surgery, and anesthesiology, joined Safar in Pittsburgh. Through the efforts of Grenvik and the support of the SCCM, a recommendation was made in the late 1970s to establish a common board certification process in CCM through the American Board of Medical Specialties (ABMS) [15, 16]. A national committee was formed to address this issue; however, representatives from the specialty boards of anesthesiology, internal medicine, pediatrics, and surgery could not agree to the details of required training. Each of these specialties applied for separate ABMS certification examinations with separate training programs. Surgical critical care currently offers fellowship training to candidates who have completed at least 3 clinical years at an accredited graduate education program not only in general surgery but also in neurosurgery, urology, and obstetrics and gynecology (OB/GYN) [17]. Of these latter three, only OB/GYN offers subspecialty certificates in critical care. In 1999, the American Board of Internal Medicine and American Board of Emergency Medicine worked together to offer a 6-year combined training in internal medicine, emergency medicine, and critical care medicine. As of 2011, the ABMS offers subspecialty certificates in critical care through anesthesiology, emergency medicine, internal medicine, obstetrics and gynecology, and pediatrics.

In Canada, trainees who have completed 3 years in their primary specialty—including anesthesia, cardiac surgery, emergency medicine, general surgery, internal medicine, and pediatrics—are allowed admission to subspecialty training in critical care. Entrance from other specialties are allowed after completion of the primary specialty, as long as prior training includes 3 months in a general care medicine or surgical ICU (SICU) and 15 months of clinical rotations in internal medicine and/or surgery [18]. In 2011, Canada had 13 adult critical care training programs and seven pediatric critical care medicine programs accredited by the Royal College of Physicians and Surgeons of Canada [19, 20]. There, unlike the USA, agreement exists as to the core curriculum and requirement of 2 years of adult critical care training. Experience in internal medicine, anesthesiology, cardiology, transfusion medicine, trauma, and radiology provides the core foundation. The pediatric CCM examination is different, but the adult CCM certification examination is uniform across the specialties. Certification in the primary specialty is also required.

In an effort to harmonize the training in intensive care medicine globally, an international Competency-Based Training Program in Intensive Care Medicine for Europe (CoBaTrICE) and other world regions has been established [21]. This is a collaborative effort supported by the European Critical Care Research network and is spearheaded by Professor Julian Bion. The program involves 102 core competencies in 12 domains with syllabi, assessment tools, and educational resources [22]. In 2011, 28 countries are participating in CoBaTrICE. Countries with national coordinators include Austria, Belgium, Bulgaria, Croatia, Cyprus, Czech Republic, Denmark, Estonia, Finland, France, Germany, Greece, Hungary, Ireland, Israel, Italy, Latvia, the Netherlands, Norway, Poland, Portugal, Slovakia, Slovenia, Spain, Sweden, Switzerland, Turkey, and the UK. Other countries and regions that have expressed interest include Argentina, Australia, New Zealand, Brazil, Canada, Chile, China, Columbia, Costa Rica, East Africa, Egypt, Hong Kong, India, Indonesia, Japan, Malaysia, Philippines, South America, USA, and West Africa.

While establishing its program, in 2004, the CoBaTrICE Collaboration published an international survey taken of national intensive care medicine representatives, with responses from 41 countries. Twenty-nine were from the European region [23]. Countries that shared common training programs were grouped together, i.e., Denmark, Norway, and Sweden (Scandinavia) and Australia and New Zealand (ANZ). Twenty programs (53 %) allowed multiple specialty access to a common critical care training program. Critical care was only available through anesthesia in nine (24 %). The minimal duration of critical care training varied from 3 to 72 months with a mode of 24 months. The core curriculum was nationally standardized in 75 % of the respondents. A certification examination was required in 29 (76 %).

The European Union of Medical Specialists (UEMS) is a non-statutory body that represents medical specialties across the European Union. With the information from Barrett study that showed the diverse routes from different primary specialties to intensive care medicine training, the UEMS established a Multidisciplinary Joint Committee for Intensive Care Medicine (MJCICM) that would represent the diversity of national specialty structures. From members of the MJCICM and the ESICM, the UEMS also created a specialty Board for ICM to facilitate the harmonization of ICM training in Europe. The Board could accommodate the various models of training that includes ICM as a (1) supraspecialty (following primary specialty base training), (2) primary specialty, and (3) subspecialty. The MJCICM acts as the executive committee for this Board [24]. At a meeting of the MJCICM in April 2008, the nine medical disciplines involved in ICM (i.e., anesthesiology, cardiac surgery, cardiology, internal medicine, neurology, neurosurgery, pediatrics, respiratory medicine, and surgery) voted against the idea that ICM become an independent primary specialty. The rationale is that critical care medicine is too complex to be a single specialty and a multidisciplinary approach with different expertise promotes a higher level of care [25]. In 2011, only Spain and Switzerland have made ICM an independent specialty.

To promote quality standards in education and the practice of intensive care medicine (ICM) in Europe, the European Society of Intensive Care Medicine (ESICM) awards a European Diploma in Intensive Medicine (EDIC) to candidates who pass a 100 questions multiple choice written examination followed by an oral/clinical exam [26].

Another evaluation of the training environment by CoBaTrICE in 2009 showed that half of the EU countries modified their training programs, with seven adopting the CoBaTrICE program [27]. Fifty-seven percent of the countries have multidisciplinary access to critical care after base specialty training. Fifty percent required 24 months of critical care training with a range of 10–60 months. National examinations were given in 26 countries (93 %). Ten utilized the EDIC as a mandatory exit exam. This makes the EDIC the first international certifying examination for CCM.

To date, there is no international neurocritical care certification.

Critical Care Training Saves Lives

In 2008, the US Centers for Disease Control and Prevention reported that, of 124 million emergency department visits, over 2.1 million patients were admitted to a critical care area [28]. It is estimated that 1 % of the US gross domestic product is utilized in the cost of care of these critically ill patients [29]. These patients have acutely life-threatening illnesses, and evidence supports the positive impact of critical care-trained specialists to decrease mortality. In an early study by Brown and Sullivan in Canada in 1986, management by critical care-trained physicians was added to the care team of an attending physician or surgeon. This change reduced ICU mortality rate by 52 % (27.8–13.4 %, $p<0.01$) [30]. Other studies support the concept of improved outcome with full-time intensivist staffing [31–33]. In 2002, Pronovost reviewed 26 studies and 7 published abstracts of intensive care unit physician staffing [34]. A high-intensity model was compared to a low intensity staffing model. The high-intensity staffing required all critical care to be directed by an intensivist by either a closed unit model or mandatory intensivist consultation. Low intensity was defined as no intensivist or an elective intensivist consultation. The high-intensity model showed a 40 % reduction in ICU mortality and a 30 % reduction in hospital mortality and in ICU length of stay (LOS). Since that time, other studies continue to support that continuous 24-h, on-site presence of a critical care specialist improves quality and decreased LOS [35]. In one study, a full-time intensivist increased adherence to evidence-based care processes from 76 to 84 % ($p=0.002$) and decreased ICU complications from 11 to 7 % ($p=0.023$) and hospital LOS by 1.4 days (95 % CI, −0.3 to −2.5 days, $p=0.17$) [36].

Quality Issues in the ICU

Although full-time staffing by an intensivist positively impacts quality of care and mortality, the majority of hospitals have not adopted this model. In 1999, the Institute of Medicine estimated that up to 98,000 Americans die annually from preventable medical errors and noted that large employers could provide more market reinforcement for the quality and safety of healthcare [37]. As a result, in November 2000, the Business Roundtable, the United States's association of Fortune 500 chief executive officers, and the Robert Wood Johnson Foundation, which is focused on improving health and healthcare in the USA, helped support and launch the Leapfrog Group, a consortium of major purchasers of healthcare. This consortium represents 130 employers and 65 Fortune 500 companies that purchase healthcare for its employees. Its members only utilize and reward hospitals that implement significant improvements in quality and safety. Approximately 1,300 hospitals (58 % of all hospital beds) in the USA participate in the Leapfrog survey which provides a report card of performance measures that allows for a comparative rating among hospitals [38]. The Leapfrog Group proposed three initial safety leaps that are also endorsed by the National Quality Forum. These include computer physician order entry, evidence-based hospital referral, and critical care-certified physician staffing in the intensive care unit (IPS). A fourth leap includes the Leapfrog Safe Practices Score based on 31 other National Quality Forum-Endorsed Safe Practices.

It is estimated that if non-rural hospitals in the USA were to adopt the full-time intensivist physician staffing, 54,000 lives and $5.3 billion dollars might be saved [39–41]. Despite this, in 2004, 79 % (1,473,085) of admissions to adult ICUs and 51 % (73,500) of pediatric critically ill patients were being managed by non-intensivists [40].

In a telephone survey by Kahn and colleagues in 2007 of 72 hospitals, 47 responded and only 45 % of these could identify an ICU director in charge of physician staffing in the ICU [42]. Only 25 % of hospitals cited full compliance of the Leapfrog initiative. The major barriers were perceived as a potential lack of control of the primary physician in providing care to the critically ill patient and loss of income to the primary physician. The cost to a hospital for salaries of intensivists, nurse practitioners, and physician assistants was also a factor. This cost could be offset by reductions in inappropriate ICU admissions and shortened ICU and hospital length of stay [43]. Adherence to evidence-based practice would have cost savings as well as improved quality [44]. Another barrier to the Leapfrog Group IPS implementation also includes a workforce shortage of intensivists.

Critical Care Workforce Shortage

In 1976, the Graduate Medical Education National Advisory committee predicted a 22 % physician surplus by 2000 [45]. By 1995, fellowship training directors and the leadership of the American College of Chest Physicians, the Society of Critical Care Medicine, and the American Thoracic Society met in 1995 to address this issue. Representatives from these groups formed the Committee on Manpower of Pulmonary and Critical Care Societies (COMPACCS) [46]. In 2000, COMPACCS concluded that, as of 1997, intensivists provided care to 36.8 % of all ICU patients and the ratio of supply and demand of intensivists would remain in balance until 2007 but that thereafter, due to an aging population, demand of critical care work hours would outstrip an unchanging supply by 22 % in 2020 and by 35 % in 2030 [47]. Since this report was published in 2000 and the Leapfrog Group was being established at that time, they would not have accounted for the demand increased by the Leapfrog mandate for full intensivist coverage in non-rural hospitals. Thus, they likely greatly underestimated predicted shortfalls. Based on concerns that arose from the COMPACCS findings, in 2003, Congress requested the Health Resources and Services Administration to prepare a report to study the supply and demand for critical care physicians [48]. The results, published in 2006, estimated the increase in the more optimal level of patients whose care was directed by an intensivist from one-third to two-thirds. HRSA estimated an increase in supply from 1,900 to 2,800 between 2000 and 2020 and a need of 3,100 FTE intensivists in 2000 and 4,300 by 2020. This projects a shortage of 1,200 intensivists in 2000 and 1,500 in 2020. This 35 % shortfall of critical care manpower in 2020 is attributed to lifestyle issues and poor reimbursement which makes CCM a less attractive specialty for newly trained physicians [49].

More specialists in the field of critical care are needed. Before certification in neurocritical care was available in 2007, only internal medicine, anesthesiology, pediatrics, and surgery offered critical care certification. There is a small but increasing number of emergency medicine physicians who have completed critical care fellowships. In a recent survey, 12 emergency physicians had completed a CCM fellowship between 1974 and 1989, 15 between 1990 and 1999, and 43 between 2000 and 2007 [50]. However, until 2011 when the American Board of Internal Medicine and the American Board of Emergency Physicians reached an accord, these physicians were not able to obtain CCM certification.

Neurocritical Care and Emergency Neurology as an Emerging Subspecialty

Neurologists played an important role for their patients with neuromuscular disease and subsequent bulbar dysfunction and respiratory failure during the polio epidemics. In the subsequent decades, however, the neurologist's role became that of a diagnostician rather than an active participant in critical care management. Postoperative neurosurgical care for elective surgeries and aneurysmal subarachnoid hemorrhage clipping was provided by the anesthesiologists and neurosurgeons. In the traumatically brain-injured patients, trauma surgeons also assisted in the critical care. For the other critically ill neurologic patients such as those with neuromuscular diseases (Guillain-Barré and myasthenia gravis, status epilepticus, ischemic or hemorrhagic stroke, or postcardiac arrest hypoxic-ischemic patients), the medical intensivists or pulmonologists managed the ventilator and neurologists had a consultative role.

Active interventions in the form of intravenous thrombolysis for acute ischemic stroke changed the field of neurology [51]. Early recognition of an ischemic event and rapid evaluation for treatment gave neurologists an active role in acute care and made neurology a more dynamic specialty [52]. In the 1980s, burgeoning research in the understanding of secondary brain injury that includes hypoperfusion from hypotension, persistent intracranial hypertension, or vasospasm; hypoxia; reperfusion injury; inflammation; and prolonged seizures made active intervention and attention to details of medical management for an acutely neurologically ill patient a new priority. Neurointerventional techniques for managing subarachnoid hemorrhage also created a need for neurointensive care for patients with endovascular rather than surgical procedures. This helped drive the need for an intensive care with a nursing and physician team focused on the neurological exam and nuances of care that helped prevent further brain injury.

The backbone of the neurointensive care unit is the nursing staff. Nurses in these units not only master the general skills needed in intensive care medicine, but they are proficient in a detailed neurological examination typically administered hourly or bihourly, and their ability to detect early signs of neurological deterioration can make a difference in further brain injury and survival. From the physician standpoint, the diagnosis and management of life-threatening neurological diseases and recognitions of the interplay with other medical conditions and organ systems are essential. Traditionally, most care teams for a neurological critically injured patient would include a neuroscience-trained physician (i.e., a neurologist or neurosurgery) as a consultant with an intensivist trained in pulmonary or internal medicine, surgery, or anesthesiology. In the 1980 and 1990s, a new model, neurocritical care, emerged as a subspecialty where the neuroscience expert was also the intensivist. This required a new training program for physicians that focused on a core curriculum of both general critical care and neurological disease states. In addition, a means to certify individual expertise in this new subspecialty was needed.

With more advanced diagnostic capabilities, potential treatment, and research, neurology has seen the development of many subspecialties within its own specialty. In 2000, a survey of graduating neurology residents showed that 75 % sought fellowship training to develop subspecialty expertise [53]. Yet, under the ABMS requirements, small, developing subspecialties have no means to objectively mandate program curriculum or certify individual competence until they are more established and can apply for ABMS recognition. Under the direction of Stephen Sergay and the American Academy of Neurology Commission on Subspecialty Certification, the leaders of the American Academy of Neurology, American Neurological Association, Association of University Professors of Neurology, Child Neurology

Society, and the Professors of Child Neurology addressed this issue, and in 2003, they became the parent organizations of a new entity: the United Council for Neurologic Subspecialties (UCNS). With input from the American Board of Psychiatry and Neurology, the UCNS has created standards for accreditation of subspecialty training programs and certification of individuals with the mission to improve the safety and quality of care to patients. The UCNS Board of Directors includes representatives from the American Board of Psychiatry and Neurology and the Accreditation Council for Graduate Medical Education [54]. As of 2011, the UCNS has nine subspecialty members in autonomic disorders, behavioral neurology and neuropsychiatry, clinical neuromuscular pathology, geriatric neurology, headache medicine, neural repair and rehabilitation, neuroimaging, neuro-oncology, and neurocritical care.

In 2005, neurocritical care became the sixth subspecialty member of the UCNS under the sponsorship of the American Academy of Neurology Critical Care and Emergency Neurology (AAN CCEN), the Neurocritical Care Society (NCS), and the Society for Neuroscience in Anesthesiology and Critical Care (SNACC). The core curriculum of fellowship training as well as the examination covers the cognitive skill sets of the pathology, pathophysiology, and therapy of neurological disease states, such as stroke, neurotrauma, seizures, neuromuscular disease, central nervous system infections, inflammatory and demyelinating diseases, toxic-metabolic disorders, neuroendocrine, neuro-oncology, encephalopathies, and clinical syndromes (e.g., coma, herniation syndromes, death by neurologic criteria). The general critical care curriculum includes not only the body of knowledge needed to manage any patient found in ICU setting but also the particular entities that confound neurological disease states, such as neurogenic pulmonary edema and autonomic dysfunction associated with traumatic brain injury (TBI) [55]. The skill sets also include administrative and ICU management skills and the ethical and legal aspects of critical care medicine (Table 3.1). Diplomates are expected to not only understand the technology and devices used in general medical or surgical critical care but also master the management and interpretation of intracranial pressure monitoring devices, transcranial Doppler, continuous electroencephalography, jugular bulb and brain tissue oxygenation monitoring, and interpretation of computerized tomography, magnetic resonance imaging, and contrast cerebral angiography. The UCNS neurocritical care exam content is evenly split between general critical care and neurological disease states [56].

It is well recognized that intensivists trained in many disciplines could obtain the cognitive and procedural skill sets necessary to be a neurointensivist. For this reason, UCNS eligible candidates for neurocritical care fellowship and examination include physicians who hold primary specialty

ABMS certification in neurology, neurosurgery, internal medicine, anesthesiology, surgery, emergency medicine, and pediatrics. In the initial 5 years of UCNS certification, similar to a new ABMS specialty, a practice track has been offered to be eligible to sit for the examination. Since its first examination in 2007, 389 diplomates have been certified in neurocritical care by the UCNS. As of 2011, 37 UCNS-accredited fellowships are offered.

Does Neurocritical Care Expertise Make a Difference?

A neurointensive care unit is a multiprofessional team of nurses, physicians, and pharmacists specially trained for neuroscience critical care. The development of a subspecialty that requires additional training by physicians and nurses and that demonstrates its value to patients and hospitals supports and validates the need to adopt and foster this subspecialty. The recent implementation of neurocritical care teams in ICUs without previous subspecialty expertise provides an opportunity to evaluate changes in ICU and hospital length of stay and outcomes such as mortality and discharge disposition and other impact on patient care. Discharge disposition is often utilized as a surrogate outcome measures since patients who are able to perform their own activities of daily living (ADLs) or those who need minimal assistance will be more likely to be discharged home. Those that have good potential for recovery will be discharged to a rehabilitation facility, while those with worse outcomes who need full assistance will be discharged to a skilled nursing facility. Both single and multicenter studies have looked at this issue in patient populations such as intracerebral hemorrhage (ICH), head trauma, and subarachnoid hemorrhage (SAH) and a mixed population including patients with cerebral neoplasm, stroke, SAH, SDH, and status epilepticus (Table 3.2).

Between 1995 and 1997, Mirski compared ICH patients admitted to a newly developed 8-bed neuroscience ICU to ICH patients admitted the previous year to the surgical ICU and medical ICU which were also staffed by intensivists, but these intensivists did not have neuroscience training [57]. There was no difference in patient age, admission Glasgow Coma Scale (GCS), comorbidities, and location and size of the hemorrhage, but mortality dropped from 36 to 19 % ($p<0.05$). The number of patients who returned home or were discharged to a rehabilitation facility increased from 48 to 69 % ($p<0.05$). In addition, the neurocritical care model appeared to improve efficiency of care as the number of consultants decreased to 0.4 ± 0.5 per patient from 3.4 ± 0.7 for those being cared in the SICU and from 2.8 ± 1.1 per patient for those cared for in the medical ICU (MICU) $p<0.05$. The authors compared the study hospital to 80 institutions of

Table 3.1 Knowledge-based and United Council for Neurologic Subspecialties core curriculum for neurocritical care

Neurological disease states: pathology, pathophysiology, and therapy	General critical care: pathology, pathophysiology, and therapy
Cerebrovascular diseases	Cardiovascular, e.g., shock, myocardial infarction, neurogenic cardiac changes, arrhythmias
Neurotrauma	Pulmonary, e.g., acute respiratory failure, neuromuscular respiratory failure, mechanical ventilation, neurogenic breathing patterns, COPD, asthma.
Seizures and epilepsy	Renal, e.g., acute and chronic renal failure, acid-base disorder, derangement in electrolytes, osmolality, neurogenic disorders of sodium regulation
Neuromuscular diseases	Metabolic and endocrine
Cerebral infections	Infectious disease
Toxic-metabolic disorders	Hematologic disorders
Inflammatory and demyelinating diseases	Gastrointestinal and genitourinary
Neuroendocrine disorders	Immunology and transplantation
Neuro-oncology	General trauma and burns
Encephalopathies	Postoperative care
Clinical syndromes, e.g., coma, intracranial hypertension, death by neurologic criteria	
Postoperative neurosurgical care	
Management: barbiturate coma, induced hypothermia, cerebral thrombolysis	
Monitoring and imaging	
Prognosis and severity scores	ECG
ICP monitoring: fluid-coupled, fiber-optic, strain gauge	Invasive and noninvasive hemodynamic monitoring
Continuous EEG	Respiratory and metabolic monitoring
Transcranial Doppler	General imaging, e.g., chest and abdomen films
Brain tissue oxygenation	
Cerebral blood flow	
CT scan, MRI, cerebral angiogram, cerebral perfusion	
Administrative	
Organization and staffing of a unit	
Triage and bed allocation	
Collaborative practice including multidisciplinary rounds	
Performance improvement and quality assurance	
Ethical, legal, and end-of-life care	

Data from American Academy of Neurology and Association of University Professors of Neurology, Graduating Neurology Residency Survey [53] and from United Council of Neurologic Specialities [54]

similar size and level of care in HBSI, a national hospital database. The neurointensive care unit in the study hospital was the only patient care area in the medical center that surpassed national HBSI benchmark expectations for ICU LOS. For postoperative craniotomy patients with and without hemorrhage (A-DRGs 001 and 002) and patients with skull fracture with and without coma (A-DRGs 027 and 028), ICU LOS were 25–45 % below benchmark. This represented a 28 % cost savings to the hospital (not hospital charge) for A-DRGs 001 and 002. For A-DRGs 027 and 028, the cost differential was 35 %. For instance, in A-DRG 001, LOS was decreased by an average of 1.5 days per case, with cost saving exceeding $5,900 per case.

Diringer and Edwards evaluated 266 ICH patients admitted to two dedicated neuroscience ICUs compared to 772 patients admitted to general ICUs over a period of 3 years [58]. They primarily utilized information from Project Impact, the national critical care data system of the Society of Critical Care Medicine launched in 1996. Independent predictors for higher mortality included not being admitted to a neuroscience ICU (OR 3.43, 95 % CI, 1.65–7.6, $p=0.002$), lower admission GCS, older age, and being admitted to hospitals with smaller ICUs or hospitals that admitted fewer ICH patients. The mortality rates in the two neuroscience units were 28 and 39 %. The units were similar, had 16 and 18 beds, and admitted 91 and 175 patients per year.

In one study of ischemic and hemorrhagic stroke, and subarachnoid hemorrhage, Varelas utilized historical controls with 174 patients admitted to a general ICU before the

Table 3.2 Outcomes after the establishment of a neurocritical care team

	Decreased mortality	Decreased ICU LOS	Decreased hospital LOS	Better discharge disposition	Decreased total cost of care	Adherence to protocols
ICH						
Mirski et al. [57]	X		X	X	X	
Diringer and Edwards [58]	X					
Knopf et al. [59]		X	X			
SAH						
Samuels et al. [60]				X		
Knopf et al. [59]	X			X		
Ischemic stroke						
Bershad et al. [61]		X	X	X		
Knopf et al. [59]				X[a]		
Combined stroke						
Varelas et al. [62]		X	X	X		
Head trauma						
Varelas et al. [63]	X		X	X		X
Mixed neuro population						
Suarez et al. [64]	X	X	X			

[a]Indicates 3-month outcome

institution of a 10-bed neuroscience ICU compared to 259 patients thereafter [62]. Although mortality did not differ, more patients were discharged home, 75 % vs. 54 % ($p=0.003$), and after adjusting for covariates, both ICU LOS and hospital LOS were significantly shortened by 1.9 days (95 % CI, 1.5–2.43, $p<0.0001$) and 1.7 days (95 % CI, 1.28–2.25, $p=0.0002$), respectively.

In a mixed population of neurosurgical and neurology ICU patients primarily with intracranial or spinal cord neoplasm, ischemic and hemorrhagic stroke, subdural hematoma, and subarachnoid hemorrhage, Suarez and colleagues reviewed 1,201 patients in 20 months before the implementation of a neurocritical care team and 1,180 patients 19 months afterward [64]. They showed a significant decrease to in-hospital mortality (OR 0.7, 95 % CI, 0.5–1.0, $p=0.044$) and decreased ICU and hospital LOS without worsening in readmission.

Bershad and colleagues studied 400 acute ischemic stroke patients before and after the institution of a full-time neurocritical care team and demonstrated decreased ICU and hospital LOS with an increased proportion of home discharges [61]. Samuels and coworkers performed a retrospective review of 703 aneurysmal subarachnoid hemorrhage patients treated before and after the development of a neurocritical care team that showed no difference in the severity on admission as measured by the Hunt and Hess scale but demonstrated a significant increase in those discharged home (25.2–36.5 %) $p<0.001$ [60]. Knopf evaluated a total of 2,096 ischemic, hemorrhagic stroke, and SAH patients in an 18-bed ICU before the recruitment of a neurointensivist, during his tenure and after his departure without a replacement [59]. After adjustment for age, severity of stroke, and receipt of thrombolysis in the ischemic stroke patients, the presence

of a neurointensivist predicted good outcome at a 3-month follow-up. After adjusting for age, ICH score on admission, and presence of IVH, ICH patients had a shorter ICU and hospital LOS (OR 0.625, 95 % CI, 0.427–0.915, $p=0.016$ and OR 0.649, 95 % CI, 0.444–0.947, $p=0.025$), although there was no impact on short- or long-term outcomes. For patients with SAH, the presence of a neurointensivist improved discharge disposition and decreased in-hospital mortality in a multivariate analysis adjusted for age, Hunt and Hess scale, and presence of IVH.

The appointment of a neurointensivist has also shown advantages in the head trauma patients. Varelas and colleagues evaluated 328 patients before and 264 patients after a neurointensivist began primary management in a 10-bed neuroscience ICU at a level 1 trauma center in Wisconsin [63]. In this 38-month period, there was a 51 % reduction in mortality ($p=0.01$), a 12 % decrease in hospital LOS ($p=0.026$), and a 57 % increased likelihood of being discharged to home or to rehabilitation. The presence of a neurointensivist also showed an improvement in adherence to protocols, with improved documentation of GCS from 60.5 to 82 % ($p=0.02$). The same author showed that the presence of a neurointensivist team improved compliance with medical documentation of severity of injury from 32.5 to 57.5 % (OR 2.8, 95% CI, 1.9–4.2). Documentation included the GCS in TBI patients, clot volume in ICH patients, and Hunt and Hess scale, GCS, and Fisher grade of CT scan findings within 48 h of admission [65].

The benefit of the neurointensivist does not lie solely in the direct patient care but also in the neuroscience education that occurs with the nursing staff, respiratory therapists, pharmacists, and house staff focusing on a team approach to the implementation and adherence to guidelines for improved patient care and outcomes. Authors nearly uniformly describe that establishing a dedicated neurocritical unit included not only the bedside attention of a neurointensivist but the neurointensivist's implementation of neuroscience education for the nursing, implementation, and adherence to guidelines and to advanced neuromonitoring protocols [57, 58, 60–62]. In 2002, Patel and colleagues showed that establishment of protocol-driven therapy in TBI patients in a neurocritical care unit trended toward improved favorable outcomes at 6 months from 56 to 66.4 % but reached significance in patients with severe TBI (GCS 3–8) with an improvement from 40.4 to 59.6 % ($p=0.43$) [66]. Fewer patients were left severely disabled or in a persistent vegetative state. Lerch and coworkers described that structured treatment protocols for elevated intracranial pressure and detection and treatment of cerebral vasospasm in patients with aneurysmal subarachnoid hemorrhage improved outcomes in the patients with a higher severity grade [67].

Kramer and Zygun evaluated 12 studies comparing 24,520 brain-injured patients and showed that mortality was lower in specialized neurologic ICUs (OR 0.78, 95 % CI, 0.64–0.95, $p=0.01$). Neurologic outcomes were also improved (OR 1.29, 95 % CI, 1.11–1.51, $p=0.001$) [68]. There was a large heterogeneity to the studies which was expected due to the wide variability in the methodology of these studies. Despite limitations and bias of the studies, these studies strongly suggest that a specialized neurocritical care team of nurses, respiratory therapists, pharmacists, social workers, and rehabilitation staff, led by the neurointensivist, improves patient outcomes and decreases mortality.

An online survey in 2007 of physicians practicing neurology or critical care medicine had 980 of 7,524 respondents that included 41.4 % neurologists, 18.8 % internists, 11.9 % pediatric intensivists, 9.4 % anesthesiologist, and 18.5 % from other specialties. Over 70 % of respondents agreed that neurocritical care units staffed by neurointensivists would improve the quality of care of neurology and neurosurgical patients with critical illness [69]. The subspecialty is becoming widely recognized as being of value to patients. In 2008, the Leapfrog Group formally recognized UCNS-certified neurointensivists as meeting the ICU Physician Staffing (IPS) requirement. Prior to this, Leapfrog recognized intensivists as ABMS board-certified physicians, with (1) additional subspecialty critical care certification, (2) emergency medicine critical care fellowship training, or (3) training before critical care certification with at least 6 weeks of full-time ICU care annually since 1987 [70].

Pediatric neurocritical care is yet another aspect of subspecialty expertise that combines the area of pediatric neurology with pediatric neurocritical care. Various models of training and delivery of care are being proposed for this emerging new subspecialty [71, 72].

The Neurocritical Care Society

Neurocritical care involves the dedication of multiple specialties and multiprofessional healthcare providers to patients with the unique needs that can be found in neurological critical illness. In 2003, the Neurocritical Care Society (NCS) was established as a nonprofit multiprofessional, international society whose mission statement focuses on quality of patient care, professional collaboration, research, training and education, and advocacy to improve outcomes. In 2003, with Thomas Bleck as its first president, the NCS had 70 members. In 2011, the NCS has over 1,100 members from 49 countries. The membership includes trainees and physicians from a multitude of specialties, nurses, nurse practitioners, physician assistants, pharmacists, respiratory therapists, and other healthcare providers. This organization provides a strong platform for collaboration and from which to promote advocacy in brain injury prevention, research, and education to improve the outcomes for patients.

Summary

There is a critical care manpower crisis facing the USA as advances in technology and treatment increase life-span and create an aging population. The specialized critical training of clinicians clearly impacts the quality of care by improving mortality and decreasing length of stay both in the ICU and the hospital. Intensivists have proposed solutions to address this shortage which include (1) adopting common standards including guidelines for clinical care, level of care, regionalization and triage, and end-of-life issues to improve efficiency and quality in manpower and resources; (2) using information technology to facilitate these standards to improve efficiency and improve safety; (3) government support for incentives of graduate medical education in critical care and for adequate reimbursement for critical care professional services; and (4) support from the government for research into the optimal role of intensivists, matching need to location, technology (e.g., telemedicine and ICUs), and training expertise [73].

As to this last solution, neurocritical care has evidence to support that further subspecialty neuroscience expertise in critical care can benefit a subset of patients. The immediate and future crisis, however, is whether the supply of critical care practitioners in general can meet the demand of the population. Some argue that further subspecialization of critical care fellowships will worsen the shortage [74]. Yet, the intent of neurocritical care fellowships is to increase the number of clinicians trained in leadership and research, and well educated in the delivery of general critical care, in addition to bringing the benefit of subspecialty critical care neurologic training to their patients. Neurointensivists can help increase the much needed number of clinicians in intensive care medicine. Kaplan and Shaw pointed out in a recent commentary that "The challenge now exists for certifying organizations to adopt a single critical care medicine examination. Critical care medicine is no longer the purview of only a few specialty-trained individuals just as intensive care is no longer a rarity" [75].

Perhaps the need to create the separate track of UCNS accreditation of programs and certification of individuals could have been avoided had the initiative in the 1970s to create a common board certification in critical care been adopted. However, the difference in and advantage of the UCNS is that it not only allows certification in critical care but also embraces the multidisciplinary nature of practitioners who master the body of knowledge needed to manage a neurologically critically ill patient. It is a certification that is similar to the European model of critical care by embracing trainees and diplomats from different primary specialties. In Europe, the CoBaTrICE Collaborative is working to standardize training, and the European Diploma in Intensive Care Medicine provides a universal certification; however, it does not yet address the subspecialty of neurocritical care expertise.

Neurointensive care medicine has emerged as a promising area that has established itself as an accepted and valid subspecialty that can improve care for the neurological critically ill patient. Studies show that it can improve mortality and outcomes and decrease ICU and hospital length of stay and total cost of care. Its challenges remain in advancing research and using this information to create guidelines to optimize care. Also, the standards of training programs and certification of practitioners must remain rigorous so that trainees in neurocritical care can also contribute to the expanding need for intensivists. A more universal and even an international means of critical care certification, and neurocritical care certification, represent a worthy, though lofty, challenge.

References

1. Florence Nightingale. BBC history (1820–1910), http://www.bbc.co.uk/hitory/historic_figures/nightingale_florence.shtml. Accessed 3 Oct 2011.
2. Bloy M. Florence Nightingale. 1820–1910. The Victorian Web http://www.victorianweb.org/history/crimea/florrie.html. Accessed 3 Oct 2011.
3. Nightingale F. Notes on hospitals. 3rd ed. London: Longman, Roberts-Green; 1863.
4. Rizzoli HV. Dandy's brain team. Clin Neurosurg. 1985;32:23–37.
5. Sherman IJ, Ketzer RM, Tamrgo RJ. Personal recollections of Walter E. Dandy and his Brain Team. J Neurosurg. 2006;105:487–93.
6. Drinker P, Shaw L. An apparatus for the prolonged administration of artificial respiration: a design for adults and children. J Clin Invest. 1929;7:229–47.
7. Geddes LA. The history of artificial respiration. IEEE Eng Med Biol Mag. 2007;26:38–41.
8. Bleck TP. Historical aspects of critical care medicine and the nervous system. Crit Care Clin. 2009;25:153–64.
9. Engström CG. Treatment of severe cases of respiratory paralysis by the Engström universal respirator. Br Med J. 1954;2:666–9.
10. Heinz WC. Inventor: the Dave Sheridan story. Albany: The Albany Medical Center; 1988.
11. Holmdahl MH. Respiratory care unit. Anesthesiology. 1962;23:559–68.
12. Safar P, DeKornfeld TJ, Pearson JW, Redding JS. The intensive care unit. A three-year experience at Baltimore City Hospitals. Anaesthesia. 1961;16:275–84.
13. Salk JE. Studies in human subjects on active immunization against poliomyelitis: a preliminary report of experiments in progress. JAMA. 1953;151:1081–9.
14. Grenvik A, Pinsky MR. Evolution of the intensive care unit as a clinical center and critical care medicine as a discipline. Crit Care Clin. 2009;25:239–50.
15. Grenvik A. Certification of specialty competence in critical care medicine as a new subspecialty: a status report. Crit Care Med. 1978;6:335–59.
16. Grenvik A, Leonard JJ, Arens JF, Carey LC, Disney FA. Critical care medicine. Certification as a multidisciplinary subspecialty. Crit Care Med. 1981;9:117–25.
17. Program Requirements for Residency Education in Surgical Critical Care. www.acgme.org. Accessed 5 Oct 2011.
18. Royal College of Physicians and Surgeons of Canada Critical Care Program Directors. http://rcpsc.medical.org/residency/accreditation/arps/critical-care_e.php. Accessed 5 Oct 2011.
19. Galvin I, Steel A. In Critical Care in Canada: an overview of critical care medicine training and the clinical and research fellowship opportunities for international medical graduates. 2nd ed. Toronto: Interdepartmental Division of Critical Care Medicine, Toronto General Hospital, University of Toronto; 2010.
20. The Royal College of Physicians and Surgeons of Canada. Subspecialty training requirements in adult critical care medicine. 2007.http://rcpsc.med.org/residency/certification/training/criticare-ad_e.pdf. Accessed 6 Oct 2011.
21. CoBaTrICE: An International Competency Based Training programme in Intensive Care Medicine. http://www.cobatrice.org/en/index.asp. Accessed 6 Oct 2011.
22. The CoBaTrICE Collaboration, Bion JF, Barrett H. Development of core competencies for an international training programme in intensive care medicine. Intensive Care Med. 2006;32:1371–83.
23. Barrett H, Bion JF. An international survey of training in adult intensive care medicine. Intensive Care Med. 2005;31:553–61.
24. EBICM: European Board of Intensive Care Medicine. http://ebicm.esicm.org/training/. Accessed 7 Oct 2011.
25. Van Aken H, Melin-Olsen J, Pelosi P. Intensive care medicine: a multidisciplinary approach! Eur J Anaesthesiol. 2011;28:313–5.
26. European Society of Intensive Care Medicine. European Diploma in Intensive Care Medicine (EDIC). http://www.esicm.org/Data/ModuleGestionDeConenu/PagesGenerees/03-education/0A-european-diploma/11.asp. Accessed 6 Oct 2011.
27. The CoBaTrICE Collaboration. The educational environment for training in intensive care medicine: structures, processes, outcomes and challenges in the European region. Intensive Care Med. 2009;35:1575–83.
28. Center for Disease Control. National Hospital Ambulatory Medical Care Survey: 2008 Emergency Department Summary Tables. http://www.cdc.gov/nchs/ahcd.htm. Accessed 6 Oct 2011.
29. Halpern NA, Bettes L, Greenstein R. Federal and nationwide intensive care units and healthcare costs: 1986-1992. Crit Care Med. 1994;22:2001–7.
30. Brown JJ, Sullivan G. Effect on ICU mortality of a full-time critical care specialist. Chest. 1989;95:127–9.

31. Manthous CA, Amoateng-Adjepong Y. al-Kharrat T et al. Effects of a medical intensivist on patient care in a community teaching hospital. Mayo Clin Proc. 1997;72:391–9.

32. Zimmerman JE, Wagner DP, Draper EA, Wright L, Alzola C, Knaus WA. Evaluation of acute physiology and chronic health evaluation III predictions of hospital mortality in an independent database. Crit Care Med. 1998;26:1317–26.

33. Ghorra S, Reinert SE, Cioffi W, Buczko G, Simms HH. Analysis of the effect of conversion from open to closed surgical intensive care unit. Ann Surg. 1999;229:163–71.

34. Pronovost PJ, Angus DC, Dorman T, Robinson KA, Dremsizov TT, Young TL. Physician staffing patterns and clinical outcomes in critically ill patients. JAMA. 2002;288:2151–62.

35. Young MP, Birkmeyer JD. Potential reduction in mortality rates using an intensivist model to manage intensive care units. Eff Clin Pract. 2000;3:284–9.

36. Gajic O, Afessa B, Hanson AC, et al. Effect of 24-hour mandatory versus on-demand critical care specialist presence on quality of care and family and provider satisfaction in the intensive care unit of a teaching hospital. Crit Care Med. 2008;36:36–44.

37. Kohn LT, Corrigan J, Donaldson MS, Institute of Medicine (US), Committee on Quality of Health Care in America. To Err is human: building a safer healthcare system. Washington, DC: Institute of Medicine, National Academy Press; 1999.

38. The Leapfrog Group. http://www.leapfroggroup.org. Accessed 3 Dec 2011.

39. Birkmeyer JD, Birkmeyer CM, Skinner JS. Economic implications of the Leapfrog Safety Standards. Washington, DC: The Leapfrog; 2001.

40. Pronovost PJ, Needham DM, Water H, et al. Intensive care unit physician staffing: financial modeling of the Leapfrog standard. Crit Care Med. 2004;32:1247–53.

41. Birkmeyer JD, Dimick JB. The Leapfrog Group's patient safety practices 2003: The potential benefits of universal adoption, http://leapfroggroup.org/media/file/Leapfrog-Birkmeyer.pdf. Accessed 4 Dec 2011.

42. Kahn JM, Matthews FA, Angus DC, Barnato AE, Rubenfeld GD. Barriers to implementing the Leapfrog Group recommendations for intensivist physician staffing: a survey of intensive care unit directors. J Crit Care. 2007;22:97–103.

43. Logani S, Green A. Gasperino J. Crit Care Res Pract: Benefits of high-intensity intensive care unit physician staffing under the Affordable Care Act; 2011. doi:10.1155/2011/170814.

44. Gasperino J. The Leapfrog initiative for intensive care unit physician staffing and its impact on intensive care unit performance: a narrative review. Health Policy. 2011;102:223–8.

45. Graduate Medical Education Advisory Committee. Report of the Graduate Medical Education National Advisory Committee: summary report. Washington, DC: US Department of Health and Human Services (HAS); 1981. p. 81–651.

46. Pingleton SK. Committee on Manpower of Pulmonary and Critical Care Societies: a report to membership. Chest. 2001;120:327–8.

47. Angus DC, Kelley MA, Schmitz RJ, White A, Popovich J, Committee on Manpower for Pulmonary and Critical Care Societies. Current and projected workforce requirements for care of the critically ill and patients with pulmonary disease: can we meet the requirements of an aging population. JAMA. 2000; 284:2762–70.

48. Ewart GW, Marcus L, Gaba MM, Bradner JD, Medina JL, Chandler EB. The critical care medicine crisis: a call for federal action – a white paper from the critical care professional societies. Chest. 2004;125:1518–21.

49. Health Resources and Services Administration. Report to Congress: The Critical Care Workforce: a study of the supply and demand for critical care physicians. Senate Report 108–81. Washington, DC: Health Resources and Services Administration; 2006.

50. Mayglothling JA, Gunnerson KJ, Huang DT. Current practice, demographics, and trends of critical care trained emergency physicians in the United States. Acad Emerg Med. 2010;17:325–9.

51. The National Institute of Neurological Disorders and Stroke rt-PA Stroke Study Group. Tissue plasminogen activator for acute ischemic stroke. N Engl J Med. 1995;333:1581–7.

52. Adams HP, del Zoppo G, Alberts MJ, et al. Guidelines for the early management of adults with ischemic stroke. A guideline from the American Heart Association/American Stroke Association Stroke Council, Clinical Cardiology Council, Cardiovascular Radiology and Intervention Council, and the Atherosclerotic Peripheral Vascular Disease and Quality of Care Outcomes in Research Interdisciplinary Working Groups. Stroke. 2007;38:1655–711.

53. American Academy of Neurology and Association of University Professors of Neurology, Graduating Neurology Residency Survey. 2000. www.ucns.org/go/about/background. Accessed 6 Dec 2011.

54. United Council of Neurologic Specialities. http://www.ucns.org/go/about/background. Accessed 6 Dec 2011.

55. Neurocritical Care Core Curriculum. http://www.ucns.org/globals/axon/assets/3656.pdf. Accessed 6 Dec 2011.

56. Neurocritical Care Written Examination Content Outline. http://www.ucns.org/globals/axon/assets/3657.pdf. Accessed 6 Dec 2011.

57. Mirski MA, Chang CWJ, Cowan R. Impact of a neuroscience intensive care unit on neurosurgical patient outcomes and cost of care: evidence-based support for an intensivist-directed specialty ICU model of care. J Neurosurg Anesthesiol. 2001;13:83–92.

58. Diringer MN, Edwards DF. Admission to a neurologic/neurosurgical intensive care unit is associated with reduced mortality rate after intracerebral hemorrhage. Crit Care Med. 2001;29: 635–40.

59. Knopf L, Staff I, Gomes J, McCullough L. Impact of a neurointensivist on outcomes in critically ill stroke patients. Neurocrit Care. 2012;16(1):63–71.

60. Samuels O, Webb A, Culler S, Martin K, Barrow D. Impact of a dedicated neurocritical care team in treating patients with aneurysmal subarachnoid hemorrhage. Neurocrit Care. 2011;14: 334–40.

61. Bershad EM, Feen ES, Hernandez OH, Fareed M, Suri K, Suarez JI. Impact of a specialized neurointensive care team on outcomes of critically ill acute ischemic stroke patients. Neurocrit Care. 2008;9:287–92.

62. Varelas PN, Schultz L, Conti M, Spanaki M, Genarrelli T, Hacein-Bey L. The impact of a neuro-intensivist on patients with stroke admitted to a neurosciences intensive care unit. Neurocrit Care. 2008;9:293–9.

63. Varelas PN, Eastwood D, Yun HJ, et al. Impact of a neurointensivist on outcomes in patients with head trauma treated in a neurosciences intensive care unit. J Neurosurg. 2006;104:713–9.

64. Suarez JI, Zaidat OO, Suri MF, et al. Length of stay and mortality in neurocritically ill patients: impact of a specialized neurocritical care team. Crit Care Med. 2004;32:2311–7.

65. Varelas PN, Spanaki MV, Hacein-Bey L. Documentation in medical records improves after a neurointensivist's appointment. Neurocrit Care. 2005;3:234–6.

66. Patel HC, Menon DK, Tebbs S, Hawker R, Hutchinson PJ, Kirkpatrick PJ. Specialist neurocritical care and outcome from head injury. Intensive Care Med. 2002;28:547–53.

67. Lerch C, Yonekawa Y, Muroi C, Bjeljac M, Keller E. Specialized neurocritical care, severity grade, and outcome of patients with aneurysmal subarachnoid hemorrhage. Neurocrit Care. 2006;5: 85–92.

68. Kramer AH, Zygun DA. Do neurocritical care units save lives? Measuring the impact of specialized ICUs. Neurocrit Care. 2011;14:329–33.

69. Markandaya M, Thomas KP, Jahromi B, et al. The role of neuro-critical care: a brief report on the survey results of neurosciences and critical care specialists. Neurocrit Care. 2012;16(1):72–81.

70. The Leapfrog Group. Factsheet: ICU Physician Staffing (IPS). 2008. http://www.leapfroggroup.org/media/file/Leapfrog-ICU_Physician_Staffing_Fact_Sheet.pdf. Accessed 4 Dec 2011.

71. Tasker RC. Pediatric neurocritical care: is it time to come of age? Curr Opin Pediatr. 2009;21:724–30.

72. Scher M. Proposed cross-disciplinary training in pediatric neurointensive care. Pediatr Neurol. 2008;39:1–5.

73. Kelley MA, Angus D, Chalfin DB, et al. The critical care crisis in the United States: a report from the profession. Chest. 2004;125:1514–7.

74. Krell K. Critical care workforce. Crit Care Med. 2008;36:1350–3.

75. Kaplan LJ, Shaw AD. Standards for education and credentialing in critical care medicine. JAMA. 2011;305:296–7.

Part II

Neuroanatomy and Pathophysiology

Basic Neuroanatomy for the Neurointensivist

4

Hung Tzu Wen and Albert L. Rhoton Jr.

Contents

H.T. Wen, MD
Department of Neurosurgery,
Hospital das Clinicas, College of Medicine,
University of São Paulo, Rua Conselheiro Brotero,
1505, cj. 52, Higienopolis, São Paulo, São Paulo 01232-010, Brazil
e-mail: wenht@uol.com.br

A.L. Rhoton Jr., MD (✉)
Department of Neurological Surgery,
University of Florida College of Medicine,
100265, Gainesville, FL 32611, USA
e-mail: rhoton@neurosurgery.ufl.edu

Abstract

The goal of this chapter is to provide information not only about the anatomy of the brain that comprises neural, arterial, and venous structures but also to establish their functional and, at some extent, radiological correlations, to enable the neurointensive care unit staff to (1) perform a concise but precise neurologic examination and be able to establish the anatomic diagnosis; (2) understand the major vascular (arterial and venous) territories of the brain and correlate them with the neurological and radiological findings (computed tomography (CT), angiography, or magnetic resonance imaging (MRI)); (3) understand the anatomical localization, the risks, and the potential neurologic complications of the most commonly used intracranial neurosurgical procedures; and (4) establish the prevention or early detection and treatment of those complications.

The topics covered in this chapter are the sulci and gyri of the lateral, basal, and medial surfaces of the cerebrum; sylvian fissure, insula, lateral ventricles, foramen of Monro, internal capsule, corpus callosum, basal ganglia, thalamus, hippocampus, amygdala, choroidal fissure, anterior perforated substance, and third ventricle; the middle, posterior, and anterior cerebral arteries and their supply territories; major veins of the superficial and deep venous system of the cerebrum; the contents of the posterior fossa (midbrain, pons, medulla oblongata, fourth ventricle, cerebellum, and the spinal cord); the basilar and the vertebral arteries; the superior, anterior inferior, and posterior inferior cerebellar arteries and their supply territories; the galenic, petrosal, and tentorial venous draining systems and major clinical brainstem syndromes; and the cranial nerves and the major sensory and motor pathways.

A.J. Layon et al. (eds.), *Textbook of Neurointensive Care*,
DOI 10.1007/978-1-4471-5226-2_4, © Springer-Verlag London 2013

Keywords

Neuroanatomy • Cerebrum • Brainstem • Brain anatomy
Cerebral arteries • Cerebrovascular disease • Cerebral
vein • Posterior fossa anatomy • Cerebellar arteries
Spinal cord

Introduction

The goal of this chapter is to provide the necessary information of the neuroanatomy that enables the neurointensive care unit staff to (1) perform a concise but precise
neurologic examination and be able to establish the anatomic diagnosis; (2) understand the major vascular (arterial and venous) territories of the brain and correlate them
with the findings of the neurological examination and the
radiological findings (computed tomography [CT], angiography, or magnetic resonance imaging [MRI]); (3)
understand the anatomical localization, the risks, and the
potential neurologic complications of the most commonly
used intracranial neurosurgical procedures; and (4) establish the prevention or early detection and treatment of
those complications.

The adult central nervous system can be divided into eight
major components: (1) cerebral hemisphere, (2) basal ganglia, (3) diencephalon, (4) midbrain, (5) pons, (6) medulla
oblongata, (7) cerebellum, and (8) spinal cord. The cerebral
hemisphere plus basal ganglia and the thalamus are collectively called forebrain.

In describing the anatomy of the brain, some confusion
can arise when terms such as rostral, caudal, or both are used
instead of anterior or superior and inferior or posterior. The
term "rostral" means nose, mouth, or face region and "caudal" means tail. As for spinal cord and the brainstem, ventral
means anterior, dorsal means posterior, rostral means superior, and caudal means inferior. However, because of the
110° flexure that the human brain undergoes during development, for the cerebrum and diencephalon, rostral means
anterior, caudal means posterior, ventral means inferior, and
dorsal means superior (Fig. 4.1).

The Cerebrum

Lateral Surface

The cerebrum is arbitrarily divided into five lobes: frontal, temporal, parietal, occipital, and the hidden insula [1].
On the lateral surface, the central sulcus and the posterior
ramus of the sylvian fissure separate the frontal lobe from
the parietal and temporal lobes. Posteriorly, the lateral

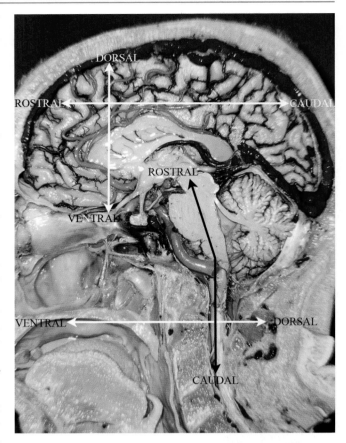

Fig. 4.1 Midsagittal section displaying the differences between the
spatial orientation of the cerebrum and the brainstem

parietotemporal line, which runs from the impression of the
parieto-occipital sulcus on the lateral surface to the preoccipital notch, separates the occipital lobe from the parietal
and temporal lobes. The parietal and the temporal lobes are
separated by the posterior ramus of the sylvian fissure and
by the temporo-occipital line, which runs from the posterior end of the posterior ramus of the sylvian fissure to the
midpoint of the lateral parietotemporal line (Fig. 4.2a). The
central sulcus starts from the medial surface of the hemisphere and extends on the lateral surface of the hemisphere
from medial to lateral, superior to inferior, and from posterior to anterior. Usually it does not intercept the posterior
ramus of the sylvian fissure and leaves a "bridge" connecting the precentral to the postcentral gyrus, known as "Pli
de passage frontoparietal inferior or opercule rolandique"
or subcentral gyrus [2]. As a characteristic of its trajectory,
the central sulcus presents a sinuous silhouette, forming a
well-defined superior knee with its convexity directed posteriorly "Ɔ" and a nonconstant inferior knee with its convexity directed anteriorly "C." Together they resemble the
shape of an inverted letter "S" that is best identified near the
midline [1] (Fig. 4.2a).

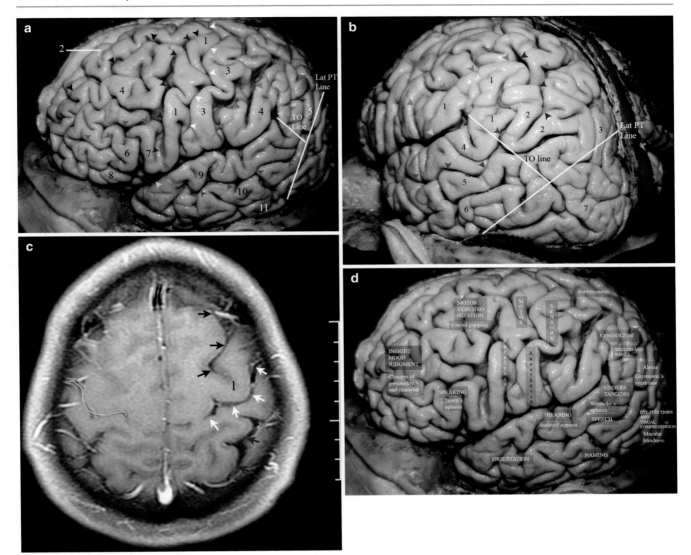

Fig. 4.2 (**a**) Lateral surface of the left cerebral hemisphere. The *white arrowheads* indicate the central sulcus; the *black arrowheads* indicate the superior frontal sulcus; the *blue arrowheads* indicate the precentral sulcus; the *red arrowheads* indicate the inferior frontal sulcus; the *green arrowheads* indicate the postcentral sulcus; the *yellow arrowheads* indicate the posterior ramus of the sylvian fissure; the *purple arrowheads* indicate the superior temporal sulcus. *1* Precentral gyrus, *2* superior frontal gyrus, *3* postcentral gyrus, *4* supramarginal gyrus, *5* angular gyrus, *6* pars triangularis, *7* pars opercularis, *8* pars orbitalis, *9* superior temporal gyrus, *10* middle temporal gyrus, *11* inferior temporal gyrus, *TO Line* temporo-occipital line, *Lat PT Line* lateral parietotemporal line. (**b**) Posterolateral view of the left cerebral hemisphere. The *green arrowheads* indicate the postcentral sulcus; the *blue arrowheads* indicate the intraparietal sulcus; the *yellow arrowheads* indicate the posterior ramus of the sylvian fissure; the *purple arrowheads* indicate the superior temporal sulcus; *1* supramarginal gyrus, *2* angular gyrus, *3* superior parietal lobule, *4* superior temporal gyrus, *5* middle temporal gyrus, *6* inferior temporal gyrus, *7* occipital lobe, *TO Line* temporo-occipital line, *Lat PT Line* lateral parietotemporal line. (**c**) MRI axial cut. The *black arrows* indicate the superior frontal sulcus; the *white arrows* indicate the central sulcus that limits posteriorly the "omega sign"; the *green arrows* indicate the postcentral sulcus; the *blue arrows indicate* the intraparietal sulcus; the *yellow line* on the opposite hemisphere displays the "omega sign"; *1* hand area of the precentral gyrus. (**d**) The functional mapping of the lateral surface of the left hemisphere (in *light blue*) and the expected symptoms which result from injury to those areas (in *light red*)

Frontal Lobe

The frontal lobe presents two main sulci: the superior and the inferior frontal sulci, which are anteroposteriorly oriented and extend from the precentral sulcus to the frontal pole. At their posterior end, these two sulci are intercepted perpendicularly by the precentral sulcus, which has a very similar direction to that of the central sulcus. The precentral sulcus forms the anterior limit of the precentral gyrus. These two frontal sulci divide the lateral surface of the frontal lobe into three gyri: the superior, the middle, and the inferior frontal gyri. The anterior horizontal, the anterior ascending, and the posterior rami of the sylvian fissure divide the inferior frontal gyrus into three parts: pars orbitalis, triangularis, and opercularis. The apex of the pars triangularis is usually retracted superiorly leaving a space in the sylvian fissure that is usually the largest space in the superficial compartment of the sylvian fissure. The apex of the pars triangularis is directed inferiorly toward the junction of three rami of the sylvian fissure; this junctional point coincides with the anterior limiting sulcus of the insula in the depth of the sylvian fissure. It marks the anterior limit of the basal ganglia and the location of the anterior horn of the lateral ventricle (Fig. 4.2a). At the intercepting point between the superior frontal and the precentral sulci, the precentral gyrus often presents the morphology of the Greek letter "Ω" (omega) with its convexity pointing posteriorly. This is the most easily identifiable landmark of the motor strip and corresponds to the hand area (Fig. 4.2c).

Parietal Lobe

The parietal lobe is limited anteriorly by the central sulcus, medially by the interhemispheric fissure, inferolaterally by the sylvian fissure and the temporo-occipital line, and posteriorly by the lateral parietotemporal line. Its two main sulci are the postcentral and the intraparietal sulci. The postcentral sulcus is very similar to the central sulcus, except for its variable continuity. The postcentral sulcus is the posterior limit of the postcentral gyrus, and sometimes it can be double. The intraparietal sulcus starts at the postcentral sulcus and is directed posteriorly and inferiorly toward the occipital pole; its direction is often parallel and is 2–3 cm lateral to the midline. The bottom of the intraparietal sulcus is related to both the roof of the atrium and the occipital horn. The intraparietal sulcus divides the lateral surface of the parietal lobe into two parts: the superior and the inferior parietal lobules. The superior parietal lobule, the superomedial and smaller part, continues as precuneus in the medial surface of the parietal lobe. The inferior parietal lobule is constituted by the supramarginal and the angular gyri. The supramarginal gyrus is the posterior continuation of the superior temporal gyrus and turns around the posterior ascending ramus of the sylvian fissure. The angular gyrus is the posterior continuation of the middle temporal gyrus and turns superiorly and medially behind the posterior ramus of the sylvian fissure up to the intraparietal sulcus; it is sometimes limited between the two posterior terminations of the superior temporal sulcus, the angular and the anterior occipital rami (Fig. 4.2a, b).

The postcentral and the intraparietal sulci and the superior parietal lobule are a "mirror image" of the precentral and the superior frontal sulci, and the superior frontal gyrus, having the central sulcus as the mirror.

Temporal Lobe

It is limited superiorly by the posterior ramus of the sylvian fissure and posteriorly by the temporo-occipital and the lateral parietotemporal lines. It presents two main sulci: the superior and the inferior temporal sulci that divide the lateral surface of the temporal lobe into three gyri, the superior, the middle, and the inferior temporal gyri. The inferior temporal gyrus occupies the lateral and the basal surfaces of the cerebrum. The superior and the inferior temporal gyri converge anteriorly to form the temporal pole (Fig. 4.2a, b).

Occipital Lobe

It is located behind the lateral parietotemporal line and is composed of a number of irregular convolutions that are divided by a short horizontal sulcus and the lateral occipital sulcus into the superior and the inferior occipital gyri (Fig. 4.2b).

The functional map of the lateral surface of the hemisphere is shown in Fig. 4.2d, and the functional mapping of the precentral gyrus (homunculus of the primary motor strip) is shown in Fig. 4.3a.

Sylvian Fissure

The sylvian fissure is not merely a complex fissure that carries the middle cerebral artery and its branches, and separates the frontal and the parietal lobes from the temporal lobe. From the neurosurgical viewpoint, the sylvian fissure is the gateway connecting the surface of the anterior part of the brain to its depth with all the neural and vascular components along the way. The extensive spectrum of the neural and the vascular structures within the reach of the transylvian approach includes insula, basal ganglia, lateral ventricle, middle cerebral artery, temporal operculum, frontal and parietal opercula, uncus, orbit, anterior cranial fossa, optic nerve, internal carotid artery and branches, anterior portion of the third ventricle, and interpeduncular fossa. The sylvian fissure is the space between the frontal, parietal, temporal opercula, and the insula and extends from the basal to the lateral surface of the brain. It is constituted by a superficial and a deep part (cisternal part). The superficial part presents a stem and three rami; the stem extends medially from the uncus to the lateral end of the sphenoid ridge, where the stem divides into the anterior horizontal, the anterior ascending, and the posterior rami (Fig. 4.2a). The deep part is divided into a "sphenoidal compartment" and an "operculoinsular compartment." The sphenoidal compartment arises in the region of the limen insulae, lateral to the anterior perforated substance, and extends posteriorly to the sphenoid ridge between the basal frontal and the temporal lobes. The operculoinsular compartment is formed by two narrow clefts, the opercular cleft between the opposing lips of the frontoparietal and the temporal opercula, and the insular cleft, which has a superior limb located between the insula and the frontoparietal operculum, and an inferior limb between the insula and the temporal operculum [3] (Fig. 4.3b). The gyri that constitute the frontal and parietal opercula of the sylvian fissure are from

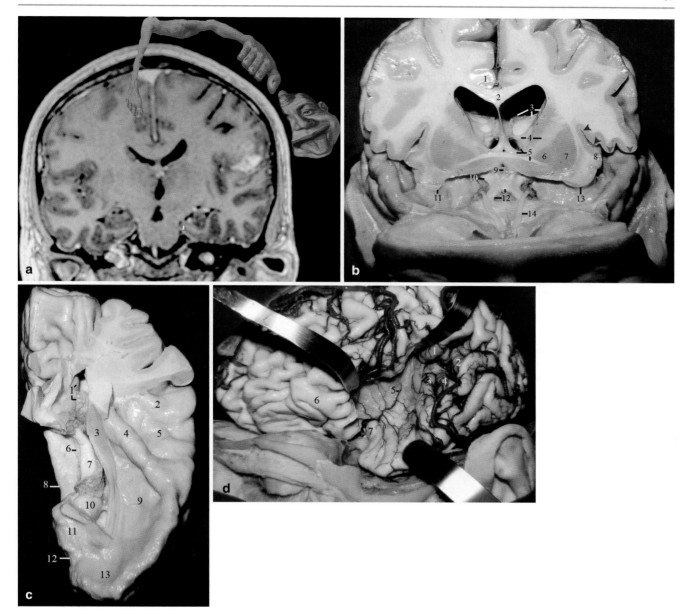

Fig. 4.3 (**a**) Coronal section through the primary motor strip to show the motor homunculus. (**b**) Coronal section of a specimen just anterior to the level of the foramen of Monro. *1* Cingulated gyrus, *2* body of the corpus callosum, *3* choroid plexus of the lateral ventricle, thalamus and the body of the caudate nucleus, *4* thalamostriate vein (not filled with dye) and the anterior limb of the internal capsule, *5* foramen of Monro, column of the fornix, and anterior commissure, *6* globus pallidus, *7* putamen, *8* insula, *9* lamina terminalis, *10* optic tract, *11* limen insulae, *12* optic nerve and chiasm, *13* insular pole, *14* olfactory tract. The *red arrowheads* indicate the opercular compartment of the sylvian fissure; the *blue* and *green arrowheads* indicate the insular compartment of the sylvian fissure. (**c**) Anterosuperior view of the left temporal lobe. *1* Calcar avis and the

choroid plexus of the atrium, *2* posterior transverse temporal gyrus, *3* temporal stem, *4* Heschl's gyrus (anterior transverse temporal gyrus), *5* middle transverse temporal gyrus, *6* dentate gyrus, *7* body of the hippocampus, *8* parahippocampal gyrus, *9* planum polare, *10* head of the hippocampus, *11* anterior segment of the uncus, *12* rhinal incisura, *13* temporal pole. (**d**) Anterolateral view of the left cerebral hemisphere. The sylvian fissure has been wide opened to display the insula and the insular veins (in this specimen the insula is rather atrophic); two retractors have been placed to retract superiorly the frontal and the parietal opercula; the planum polare has been retracted inferiorly. *1* Postcentral gyrus, *2* posterior transverse temporal gyrus, *3* Heschl's gyrus, *4* middle transverse temporal gyrus, *5* insular veins, *6* frontal lobe, *7* anterior segment of the uncus

posterior to anterior: the supramarginal, the postcentral, and the precentral gyri; pars opercularis; triangularis; and orbitalis (Fig. 4.2a); the gyri that constitute the temporal operculum of the sylvian fissure are from posterior to anterior:

planum temporale, Heschl's gyrus, and planum polare [4] (Fig. 4.3c). Each gyrus of the frontoparietal opercula is related to its counterpart on the temporal side: the supramarginal gyrus is in contact with the planum temporale; the postcentral gyrus with Heschl's gyrus, and the precentral gyrus, pars opercularis, triangularis, and orbitalis are related to the planum polare [5]. The medial wall of the sylvian fissure is the insula or island of Reil, which can only be seen when the lips of the sylvian fissure are widely separated (Fig. 4.3d). The insula has the shape of a pyramid with its apex directed inferiorly and presents an anterior and a lateral surface. The anterior surface presents triangular shape and is

constituted by the transverse and the accessory gyri, and the insular pole. The medial portion of the insular pole is marked by an arched ridge of variable prominence, the limen insulae, which is composed of fibers of uncinate fasciculus covered by a thin layer of gray matter that connects the frontal basal area to the temporal lobe. "Limen" means threshold, and the limen insulae is the threshold between the carotid cistern medially and the sylvian fissure laterally (Fig. 4.3b). The

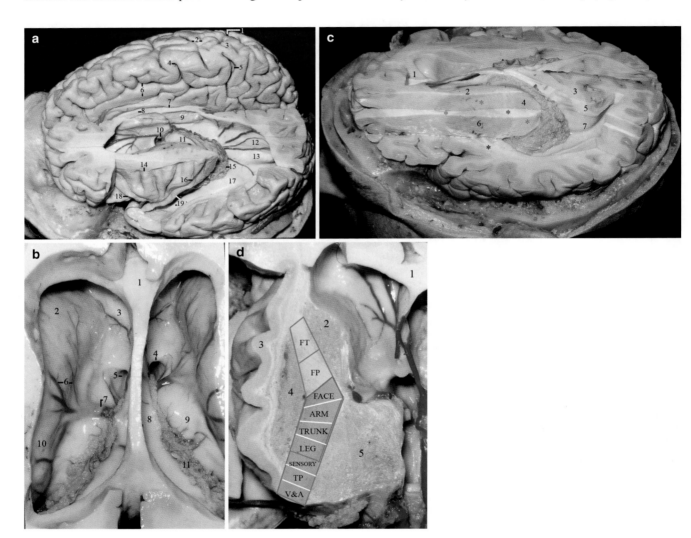

Fig. 4.4 (**a**) Superolateral view of the left cerebral hemisphere to display the lateral ventricle. *1* Central sulcus, *2* precentral sulcus and gyrus, *3* postcentral gyrus, *4* paracentral ramus of the cingulate sulcus, *5* marginal ramus of the cingulate sulcus, *6* cingulate sulcus and gyrus, *7* callosal sulcus, *8* corpus callosum, *9* septum pellucidum, *10* foramen of Monro, *11* thalamus, *12* bulb of the callosum, *13* calcar avis, *14* superior limiting sulcus of the insula, *15* choroid plexus of the atrium, *16* central sulcus of the insula, *17* collateral trigone, *18* anterior limiting sulcus of the insula, *19* inferior limiting sulcus of the insula and the temporal horn. (**b**) Superior view of the frontal horn and the body of the lateral ventricle. *1* Corpus callosum, *2* head of the caudate nucleus, *3* rostrum of the corpus callosum, *4* column of the fornix, *5* foramen of Monro, *6* caudate veins, *7* thalamostriate vein, *8* body of the fornix, *9* thalamus, *10* body of the caudate nucleus, *11* choroid plexus. (**c**) Superolateral view of the left

hemisphere. *1* Forceps minor, *2* caudate nucleus, *3* forceps major, *4* thalamus, *5* bulb of the callosum, *6* lentiform nucleus, *7* calcar avis; the *purple star* indicates the anterior limb of the internal capsule (IC); the *green star* indicates the genu of the IC; the *blue star* indicates the posterior limb of the IC; the *red star* indicates the retrolentiform part of the IC; the *black star* indicates the sublentiform part of the IC. (**d**) An axial section has been made through the left central core to display the distribution of the fibers in the internal capsule; the fibers from the corticospinal tract occupy approximately the anterior half of the posterior limb of the internal capsule. In *yellow*, the anterior limb; in *red*, the corticospinal tract; in *green*, the posterior half of the posterior limb. *1* Corpus callosum, *2* head of the caudate nucleus, *3* insula, *4* lentiform nucleus, *5* thalamus; *FT* frontothalamic fibers, *FP* frontopontine fibers, *TP* temporopontine fibers, *V&A* visual and auditory fibers

insula is encircled and separated from the opercula by a deep furrow called the circular or limiting sulcus of the insula, which presents three parts, the superior, anterior, and inferior parts (Fig. 4.4a). From the limen insulae the sulci and gyri of the insula are directed superiorly in a radial manner. The deepest sulcus, the central sulcus of insula, is a constant sulcus that extends upward and backward across the insula. It divides the lateral surface of the insula into a large anterior zone that is divided by several shallow sulci into three to five short gyri and a posterior zone that is formed by anterior and posterior long gyri [6] (Fig. 4.4a). From microsurgical and radiological viewpoints, the insula represents the external covering of the central core, constituted by the extreme, external and internal capsules, claustrum, basal ganglia, and thalamus (Fig. 4.4d). The anterior, inferior, and posterior limits of the insula on the lateral projection correspond to anterior, inferior, and posterior limits of the central core. The superior limit of the central core (caudate nucleus) is higher than the upper limit of the insula (Fig. 4.3b).

Lateral Ventricles

The lateral ventricles are two C-shaped cavities that wrap around the central core of the hemisphere (Fig. 4.4a). Each ventricle has five components: frontal horn, body, atrium, occipital, and temporal horns [7]. The frontal horn is located in front of the foramen of Monro and presents roof, floor, anterior, lateral, medial, and posterior walls. The genu of the corpus callosum forms the anterior wall, the transition between the genu and the body of the corpus callosum forms the roof, the rostrum of the corpus callosum forms the narrow floor, the septum pellucidum forms the medial wall, and the thalamus forms the posterior wall. The head of the caudate nucleus forms the majority of the lateral wall, but the most anterior part is constituted by the most anterior part of the anterior limb of the internal capsule, and it is in close relation to the anterior limiting sulcus of the insula. The body of the lateral ventricle is located behind the foramen of Monro and extends to the point where the septum pellucidum, the corpus callosum, and the fornix meet. It presents the roof, floor, lateral, and medial walls. The body of the corpus callosum forms the roof, the septum pellucidum above and the body of the fornix below form the medial wall, the body of the caudate nucleus forms the lateral wall, and the thalamus forms the floor (Fig. 4.5d). The caudate nucleus and the thalamus are separated by the striothalamic sulcus, the groove in which the stria terminalis and the thalamostriate vein course (Fig. 4.4b). The atrium has roof, floor, anterior, medial, and lateral walls. The roof is formed by the body, the splenium, and the tapetum of the corpus callosum; the floor is formed by the collateral trigone, a triangular area that bulges upward over the posterior end of the collateral sulcus; the medial wall is formed by two roughly horizontal prominences; the upper prominence, the bulb of the callosum, is formed by the large

bundle of fibers called forceps major that connects the two occipital lobes; the lower prominence, calcar avis, overlies the deepest part of the calcarine sulcus; the lateral wall has an anterior part, formed by the caudate nucleus as it wraps the lateral margin of the pulvinar, and a posterior part, formed by the fibers of the tapetum as they sweep anteroinferiorly along the lateral margin of the ventricle and separate the ventricular cavity from the optic radiation; and the anterior wall has a medial part composed of the crus of the fornix as it wraps the posterior part of the pulvinar and a lateral part formed by the pulvinar of the thalamus. The occipital horn extends posteriorly into the occipital lobe from the atrium. It varies in size from being absent to extending far posteriorly in the occipital lobe. The bulb of the callosum and the calcar avis form its medial wall, the tapetum forms the roof and the lateral wall, and the collateral trigone forms the floor (Figs. 4.4a and 4.5a) [7]. The temporal horn extends forward and inferiorly from the atrium into the medial part of the temporal lobe and presents roof, floor, and anterior, lateral, and medial walls. The tapetum, the tail of the caudate nucleus, the part of the retrolentiform and sublentiform components of the internal capsule, and the amygdaloid nucleus form the roof. The retrolentiform component is the posterior thalamic radiation that includes the optic radiation (Fig. 4.4c); the sublentiform component is formed mainly by the acoustic radiation. The amygdaloid nucleus constitutes the most anterior part of the roof of the temporal horn, and is located above and in front of the head of the hippocampus (Fig. 4.5c), anterior to the inferior choroidal point, which is the most anterior site of attachment of the choroid plexus in the temporal horn [8]. There is no clear separation between the roof of the temporal horn and the thalamus, since all fibers of the optic radiation come from the lateral geniculate body. Therefore it is reasonable to consider the roof of the temporal horn as a lateral extension of the thalamus [8]. The attachment site of the choroids plexus can be a surgical landmark to separate the thalamus from the roof of the temporal horn (Fig. 4.5b). The tapetum and the optic radiation form the lateral wall, the amygdaloid body forms the anterior wall, the head of the hippocampus forms the anterior third of the medial wall, and the choroidal fissure forms the posterior 2/3 [8]. The floor is formed medially by the hippocampus and laterally by the collateral eminence (Fig. 4.5a). The temporal horn is projected on to the middle temporal gyrus on the lateral view.

The structures related to the lateral ventricle are foramen of Monro, internal capsule, corpus callosum, fornix, thalamus, caudate nucleus, hippocampus, temporal amygdala, and choroidal fissure.

Foramen of Monro

The foramen of Monro communicates the lateral ventricle to the third ventricle. It is bounded anteriorly and superiorly by the fornix and posteriorly by the thalamus; the elements that

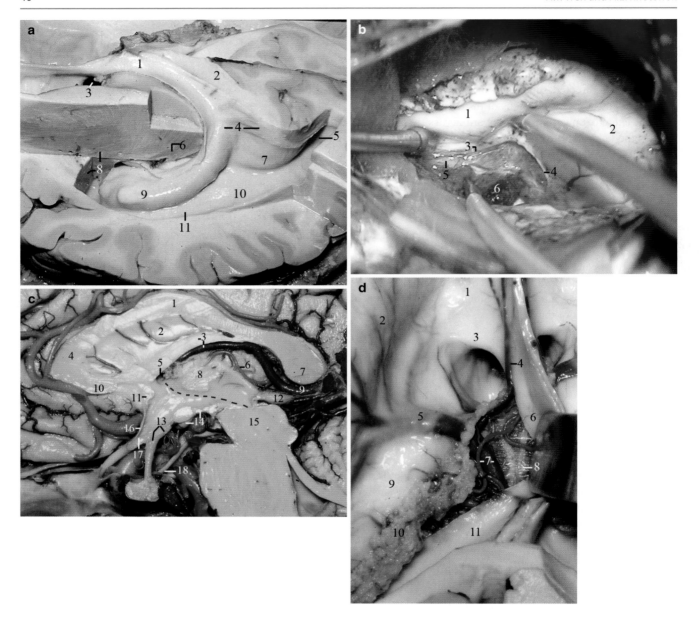

Fig. 4.5 (**a**) Lateral view of the left hippocampus. *1* Fornix, *2* forceps major (corpus callosum), *3* foramen of Monro, *4* tail of the hippocampus and the bulb of the callosum, *5* occipital horn, *6* lateral geniculate body, *7* calcar avis, *8* globus pallidus (*above*) and amygdala (*below*), *9* head of the hippocampus, *10* collateral trigone, *11* collateral eminence. (**b**) Intraoperative photograph of the left hippocampus. The choroidal fissure has been split by detaching the choroid plexus from the fimbria of the fornix. The choroid plexus is now attached to the thalamus. *1* Body of the hippocampus, *2* head of the hippocampus, *3* fimbria of the fornix, *4* fimbria of the fornix, *5* thalamus (under the arachnoid membrane), *6* choroid plexus attached to the thalamus. (**c**) Midsagittal section. *1* Body of the corpus callosum, *2* septum pellucidum, *3* body of the fornix and the internal cerebral vein, *4* genu of the corpus callosum, *5* foramen of Monro, *6* medial posterior choroidal artery, *7* splenium of the corpus callosum, *8* massa intermedia, *9* vein of Galen, *10* rostrum of the corpus callosum, *11*

anterior commissure, *12* pineal gland, *13* infundibular recess (anterior) and the tuber cinereum (posterior), *14* mamillary body (anterior) and the posterior perforated substance (posterior), *15* midbrain, *16* lamina terminalis, *17* optic recess, *18* oculomotor nerve. The *blue dotted line* indicates the hypothalamic sulcus. (**d**) Superior view of the frontal horn and the body of the lateral ventricle. The choroidal fissure has been split through the taenia fornicis to display the layers of the roof of the third ventricle: the superior membrane of the tela choroidea has been opened to display the velum interpositum and the vessels, the inferior membrane of the tela choroidea, and two strands of the choroid plexus. *1* Rostrum of the corpus callosum, *2* head of the caudate nucleus, *3* column of the fornix, *4* anterior septal vein, *5* thalamostriate vein, *6* body of the fornix, *7* internal cerebral vein and the medial posterior choroidal artery, *8* inferior membrane of the tela choroidea and the choroid plexus, *9* thalamus, *10* choroid plexus of the lateral ventricle, *11* body of the fornix

run close to the foramen of Monro are the anterior septal vein superior and medially, choroidal plexus posterior and medially,

and the thalamostriate vein lateral and posteriorly (Figs. 4.3b, 4.4a, b, and 4.5d).

Internal Capsule

The internal capsule has five parts [9, 10]: anterior and posterior limbs, genu, retrolentiform, and sublentiform parts. The anterior limb is located between the head of the caudate nucleus and the lentiform nucleus, and it contains frontopontine fibers; the posterior limb is located between the thalamus and the lentiform nucleus and contains corticospinal tract, frontopontine, corticorubral fibers, and fibers of the superior thalamic radiation (somesthetic radiation). The genu comes directly to the ventricular surface and touches the wall of the lateral ventricle immediately lateral to the foramen of Monro, and contains corticonuclear fibers and anterior fibers of the superior thalamic radiation (Fig. 4.4d). The retrolentiform part is located posteriorly to the lentiform nucleus and contains mainly parietopontine, occipitopontine, occipitocollicular, and occipitotectal fibers and the posterior thalamic radiation that includes the optic radiation. The sublentiform part is located below the lentiform nucleus and contains temporopontine, parietopontine fibers, and acoustic radiation from the medial geniculate body to the superior temporal and transverse temporal gyri (Fig. 4.4c).

Corpus Callosum

The corpus callosum is the largest transverse commissure connecting the two cerebral hemispheres. It contributes to the wall of each of the five parts of the lateral ventricle. The corpus callosum has two anterior parts, the rostrum and genu; a central part, the body; and a posterior part, the splenium (Fig. 4.5c). The rostrum is located below and forms the floor of the frontal horn (Figs. 4.4b and 4.5d). The genu forms the anterior wall of the frontal horn as it sweeps obliquely forward and laterally to connect the frontal lobes. The genu gives rise to a large fiber tract, the forceps minor, which forms the anterior wall of the frontal horn; the genu and the body of the corpus callosum form the roof of both the frontal horn and the body of the lateral ventricle. The splenium gives rise to a large tract, the forceps major, which forms a prominence called bulb in the upper part of the medial wall of the atrium and occipital horn as it sweeps posteriorly to connect the occipital lobes (Fig. 4.4c). Another fiber tract, the tapetum, which arises in the posterior part of the body and splenium, sweeps laterally and inferiorly to form the roof and lateral wall of the atrium and the temporal and occipital horn.

Basal Ganglia

Although macroscopically fused and gathered into a "central core," the basal ganglia and the thalamus are embryologically and functionally distinct structures. The basal ganglia are telencephalic structures and the thalamus is a diencephalic structure. The basal ganglia consist of four nuclei: (1) striatum (caudate nucleus, putamen, and nucleus accumbens), (2) globus pallidus, (3) substantia nigra, and (4) subthalamic nucleus. The basal ganglia play a major role in voluntary motor movements; however, they do not have direct input or output with the spinal cord. They receive their primary input from the cerebral cortex and send their output to the brainstem, and, via the thalamus, back to the prefrontal, premotor, and motor cortices. The motor activity of the basal ganglia is therefore mostly mediated by motor areas of the frontal lobe. The disturbance of the basal ganglia is usually characterized by (1) tremor and other involuntary movements, (2) changes in posture and muscle tone, and (3) poverty and slowness of movement without paralysis.

The caudate nucleus is another C-shaped structure that wraps around the thalamus; it has head, body, and tail. The head and body are lateral walls of the frontal horn and the body of the lateral ventricle. The tail extends from the atrium into the roof of the temporal horn and is continuous with the amygdaloid nucleus (Figs. 4.3b and 4.4b–d).

Thalamus

The thalamus is located in the center of the lateral ventricle. Each lateral ventricle wraps around the superior, inferior, and posterior surfaces of the thalamus. The anterior tubercle of the thalamus is the posterior limit of the foramen of Monro (Figs. 4.3b, 4.4a–d, and 4.5d).

The thalamus is not a relay station where information is simply passed on to the neocortex—the thalamus acts as a gatekeeper for information to the cerebral cortex, preventing or enhancing the passage of specific information depending on the behavioral state of the person. The thalamus is composed of more than 50 nuclei, which can be divided into specific or relay or nonspecific or diffusely projecting nuclei. The relay nuclei have a specific relationship with particular region of the neocortex and are classically divided into four groups, depending on their position in relation to the internal medullary lamina: the anterior group receives input from the mamillary bodies and from the subiculum of the hippocampal formation; the medial group receives input from the basal ganglia, amygdala, and midbrain and has been implicated in memory, with its major output to the frontal cortex; and the nuclei from ventral group are named according to their position within the thalamus. The ventral anterior and ventral lateral nuclei are important for motor control and carry information from the basal ganglia and cerebellum to the motor cortex. The ventral posterior lateral conveys somatosensory information to the neocortex. The posterior group includes the medial and lateral geniculate nuclei, lateral posterior nucleus, and pulvinar. The medial geniculate nucleus is a component of the auditory system; the lateral geniculate nucleus receives information from the retina and conveys it to the primary visual cortex; the pulvinar seems to be interconnected with parietal, temporal, and occipital lobes.

The nonspecific or diffusely projecting nuclei are either located in the midline (midline nuclei) or within the internal medullar lamina (intralaminar nuclei). The largest intralaminar nucleus is the centromedian nucleus, and it projects to the amygdala, hippocampus, and basal ganglia. These nuclei are also thought to mediate cortical arousal.

Hippocampus

The hippocampus occupies the medial part of the floor of the temporal horn and is divided into three parts: head, body, and tail (Fig. 4.5a). The head of the hippocampus, the anterior and the largest part, is directed anterior and inferiorly, and then medially. At the medial end of the tip of the temporal horn, it turns up vertically and bends over laterally forming the medial wall of the tip of the temporal horn, ahead of the choroidal fissure; the head of the hippocampus is free of the choroid plexus, and it is characterized by three or four hippocampal digitations; its overall shape resembles a feline paw and is directed toward the posterior segment of the uncus [11]. Its posterior limit is characterized by the initial segment of the fimbria and the choroidal fissure. Superiorly, the head of the hippocampus is related to the posteroinferior portion of the amygdala. The emergence of the choroid plexus, the fimbria, and the choroidal fissure marks the beginning of the body of the hippocampus. The body of the hippocampus has an anteroposterior and inferosuperior direction and narrows as it approaches the atrium of the lateral ventricle. Posterior to the head of the hippocampus, the medial wall of the temporal horn is the choroidal fissure. At the atrium of the lateral ventricle, the body of the hippocampus changes its direction and has its longitudinal axis oriented transversely to become the tail of the hippocampus. The tail of the hippocampus is slender and constitutes the medial part of the floor of the atrium; medially the tail of the hippocampus fuses with the calcar avis. Histologically the terminal segment of the hippocampal tail continues as the subsplenial gyrus, which covers the inferior splenial surface (Fig. 4.5a).

Amygdala

The amygdala and the hippocampus constitute the core of the limbic system [12]. The temporal amygdala is composed by a series of gray matter nuclei classified into three main groups: basolateral, corticomedial, and central groups. From the neurosurgical viewpoint, the temporal amygdala can be considered as being entirely located within the boundaries of the uncus: superiorly, the amygdala blends into the globus pallidus; inferiorly, the temporal amygdala bulges inferiorly into the most anterior portion of the roof of the temporal horn above the hippocampal head and the uncal recess; medially, it is related to the anterior and the posterior segments of the uncus; it also constitutes the anterior wall of the temporal horn [8] (Fig. 4.5a).

Choroidal Fissure

The choroidal fissure is one of the most important intraventricular surgical landmarks for neurosurgeons. The choroidal fissure is a cleft located between the thalamus and the fornix. It is the site of attachment of the choroid plexus in the lateral ventricle. It is a C-shaped arc that extends from the foramen of Monro through the body, to the atrium, to the temporal horn [13, 14]. The body part of the choroidal fissure is between the body of the fornix and the thalamus; the atrial part is between the crus of the fornix and the pulvinar of the thalamus (Figs. 4.4b and 4.5d); the temporal part is between the fimbria of the fornix and the stria terminalis of the thalamus. The choroid plexus is attached to the fornix and to the thalamus via ependymal covering called taenia fornicis and taenia choroidea, respectively; in the temporal part, the taenia fimbriae attaches the choroidal plexus to the fimbria. The choroidal fissure is one of the most important landmarks in microneurosurgeries involving the temporal lobe: it separates temporal structures that can be removed from thalamic structures that should be preserved (Fig. 4.5b).

Third Ventricle

The third ventricle is a narrow, funnel-shaped, unilocular, midline cavity. It communicates at its anterosuperior margin with each lateral ventricle through the foramen of Monro and posteriorly with the fourth ventricle through the aqueduct of Sylvius (Fig. 4.5c). It has a roof, a floor, an anterior, a posterior, and two lateral walls [15, 16]. The roof extends from the foramen of Monro anteriorly to the suprapineal recess posteriorly and is constituted by five layers [14] (Fig. 4.5d): from superior to inferior, they are (1) the fornix, (2) the superior membrane of the tela choroidea, (3) the velum interpositum which is the vascular layer located in a space between the superior and the inferior membranes of the tela choroidea and contains internal cerebral veins and branches of the medial posterior choroidal arteries, (4) the inferior membrane of the tela choroidea, which forms the floor of the velum interpositum, and (5) the choroid plexus of the third ventricle, usually represented by two parallel strands of choroid plexus projecting backward on each side of the midline. The floor extends from the optic chiasm anteriorly to the orifice of the aqueduct of Sylvius posteriorly, and it is constituted from anterior to posterior by the optic and infundibular recesses, tuber cinereum, mamillary bodies, posterior perforated substance, midbrain, and aqueduct (Fig. 4.5c). The anterior wall is constituted by the lamina terminalis, and the posterior wall is represented from inferior to superior by the posterior commissure, pineal recess, habenular commissure, pineal gland, and suprapineal recess. At the inner angle formed by the roof and the anterior wall is the anterior commissure. Frequently there is another commissure in the cavity of the third ventricle located posteriorly to the foramen of Monro called massa intermedia, which connects both thalami. The lateral wall of the third ventricle is constituted by thalamus above and by hypothalamus below, both separated by hypothalamic sulcus, a shallow groove extending from the foramen of Monro to the aqueduct. The hypothalamic sulcus is the rostral continuation of the sulcus limitans of the brainstem and the central canal in the spinal cord. During the development of the central nervous system, the neural tube is divided by the sulcus limitans into two plates: dorsal to the sulcus limitans is the alar plate, and ventral to the sulcus limitans is the basal plate. In the spinal cord and the brainstem, the structures evolved from the alar plate bear sensory and coordination functions; the structures evolved from the basal plate bear motor function. However, only the alar plate is evolved in the development of the telencephalon and diencephalon; in the diencephalon, the alar plate is further divided by the hypothalamic sulcus into a ventral and a dorsal part: the dorsal part becomes the thalamus (sensory and coordination) and the ventral part becomes hypothalamus (motor).

Even though the neural control of emotion involves several regions, including the amygdala and the limbic association areas of the cerebral cortex, they all work through the hypothalamus to control the autonomic nervous system. The hypothalamus coordinates behavioral response to ensure bodily homeostasis, the constancy of the internal environment, by working through three major systems: the autonomic nervous system, the endocrine system, and an ill-defined neural system concerned with motivation (Fig. 4.5b).

The third ventricle can be approached from the front, through the lamina terminalis via interhemispheric or pterional approaches; from behind, through the velum interpositum via supracerebellar infratentorial approach; or from above, through its roof as in transcallosal interforniceal [17] and transcallosal transchoroidal approaches (Fig. 4.5d) [14].

Lateral Surface: Venous Relationships

The superficial venous system drains the superficial one-fifth of the thickness of the cerebrum, while the deep venous system drains the rest four-fifths of the depth of the cerebrum [18]. On the lateral surface of the cerebrum, the superficial venous drainage system is accomplished to venous channels adjacent to the lobes. In the frontal and parietal lobes, the venous drainage can direct superiorly toward the superior sagittal sinus or inferiorly toward the superficial sylvian vein; in the temporal lobe, the veins can drain superiorly toward the superficial sylvian vein or inferiorly toward the dural sinuses below the temporal lobe [19]. There are three main anastomotic veins on the lateral surface of the cerebrum: (1) The superficial sylvian vein that begins at the posterior part of the posterior ramus of the sylvian fissure and runs inferiorly and anteriorly along the fissure and commonly anastomoses with veins of Trolard and Labbé. It may arise as two trunks or present several variations. In the region of the pterion, it enters the dura and runs along the lesser wing of the sphenoid, in the sphenoparietal sinus, or sinus of the lesser wing of the sphenoid [20] to enter the anterior end of the cavernous sinus via medial end of the superior orbital fissure, then drains into the

basilar sinus and the inferior petrosal sinus. (2) The vein of Trolard or superior anastomotic vein is the largest anastomotic vein crossing the lateral surface of the brain between the superior sagittal sinus and the sylvian fissure. It is more frequently located at the parietal lobe. (3) The vein of Labbé or inferior anastomotic vein is the largest anastomotic vein that crosses the temporal lobe between the sylvian fissure and the transverse sinus. It usually arises from the middle portion of the sylvian fissure and is directed posterior and inferiorly toward the anterior part of the transverse sinus, at the level of the preoccipital notch (Fig. 4.6a).

The deep part of the sylvian fissure is related to the deep sylvian or middle cerebral vein and its tributaries. The tributaries of the deep sylvian vein come mainly from the sulci of the insula. The deep middle cerebral vein begins as a vein in the central sulcus of insula, and runs anterior and inferiorly toward the limen insulae where it joins other insular veins to form a common trunk [6] (Fig. 4.3d).

The deep venous system is divided in ventricular and cisternal groups; the cisternal group will be discussed under the basal surface. The most important ventricular veins are the thalamostriate and the internal cerebral vein. The thalamostriate vein courses in the striothalamic sulcus (between the caudate nucleus and the thalamus) in the body of the lateral ventricle; the internal cerebral vein receives the venous drainage from the anterior septal, thalamostriate, and veins from the superior surface of the thalamus, then courses posteriorly in the velum interpositum to drain into the vein of Galen [21] (Figs. 4.4b and 4.5d).

Lateral Surface: Arterial Relationships

Most of the lateral surface of the cerebral hemisphere is supplied by the middle cerebral artery. The middle cerebral artery (MCA) [3] is divided into four segments (Fig. 4.6b):

1. The M1 or sphenoidal segment extends from the bifurcation of the internal carotid artery to the limen insulae. The M1 presents two types of branches: the lateral lenticulostriate arteries that arise mostly from the superior or posterosuperior aspect of the M1 and penetrate the anterior perforated substance to supply the basal ganglia and early branches that course toward the temporal lobe to supply the temporal pole.

2. The M2 or insular segment extends from the limen insulae to the superior and inferior circular (limiting) sulci of insula; it runs in the insular compartment of the sylvian fissure, and it is constituted by the superior and the inferior trunks and their branches. After reaching the superior or inferior circular (limiting) sulcus of insula, the M2 branches enter the opercular compartment and are called M3 segment.

3. The M3 or opercular segment runs in the opercular compartment and is related to the frontal and parietal opercula

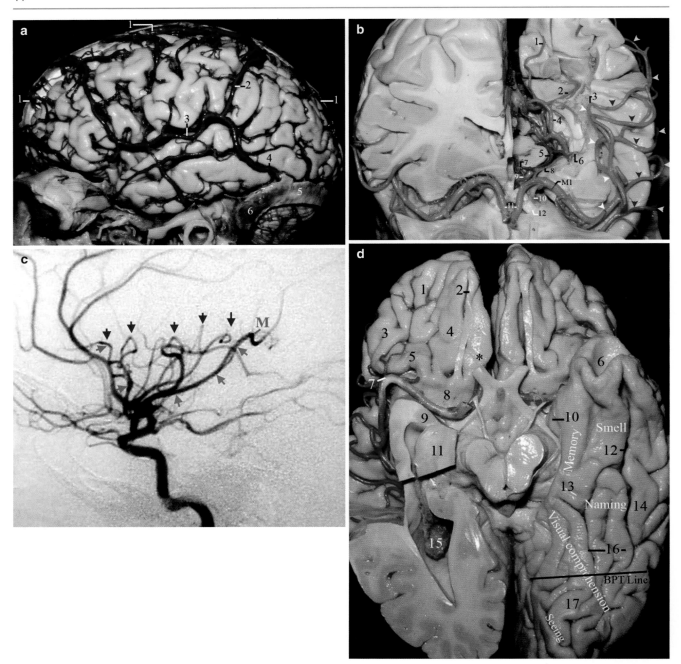

Fig. 4.6 (**a**) Lateral view of the left cerebral hemisphere. *1* Superior sagittal sinus, *2* vein of Trolard, *3* superficial sylvian vein, *4* vein of Labbé, *5* transverse sinus, *6* sigmoid sinus. (**b**) Frontal view. *1* Parieto-occipital artery, *2* calcarine artery, *3* sylvian point, *4* posterior cerebral artery (PCA), *5* basal vein, *6* inferior choroidal point, *7* P1 segment of the PCA, *8* anterior choroidal artery, *9* posterior communicating artery, *10* supraclinoid carotid artery, *11* anterior cerebral artery (A1 segment), *12* optic nerve; the *white arrowheads* indicate the M2 segment of the MCA; the *blue arrowheads* indicate the M3; the *yellow arrowheads* indicate the M4. (**c**) Lateral projection of a carotid angiography. The *green arrows* indicate the M2 segment of the MCA and the location of the inferior limiting sulcus of the

insula; the *blue arrows* indicate the transition between the M2 and M3 segment, and the location of the superior limiting sulcus of the insula; the *red arrows* indicate the M2 segment and the anterior limiting sulcus of the insula. *M* sylvian point. (**d**) Basal view of the cerebrum with its functional mapping. *1* Anterior orbital gyrus, *2* olfactory tract, *3* lateral orbital gyrus, *4* medial orbital gyrus, *5* posterior orbital gyrus, *6* temporal pole, *7* genu of the middle cerebral artery, *8* anterior perforated substance, *9* amygdala, *10* uncus, *11* head of the hippocampus, *12* occipitotemporal sulcus, *13* parahippocampal gyrus, *14* inferior temporal gyrus, *15* choroid plexus of the atrium, *16* collateral sulcus and fusiform gyrus, *17* lingual gyrus; *BPT Line* basal parietotemporal line; * rectus gyrus

superiorly and to the temporal operculum inferiorly. The loop of the most posterior M3 segment branch that exits

from the sylvian fissure is called "M point" or "sylvian point" [22]. Anatomically the sylvian point is located behind the insula, above the medial end of the Heschl's gyrus. The angiographic sylvian point or "M point" displays the location of the medial end of the Heschl's gyrus, the posterior end of the insula, and the central core, atrium, and pulvinar of the thalamus. On lateral projection, the M2 and M3 segments form the "sylvian triangle" that depicts the shape of the insula and the anterior, inferior, and posterior limits of the central core (Fig. 4.6c). The caudate nucleus is projected above the superior level of the sylvian triangle on lateral projection.

4. The fourth segment is the M4 or cortical segment; it extends from the sylvian fissure to the lateral surface of the cerebrum.

Basal Surface: Neural Relationships

The basal surface comprises of frontal, temporal, and occipital lobes. The olfactory tract and sulcus divide the basal surface of the frontal lobe in two uneven parts, a smaller and medial part is the rectus gyrus, and a larger and lateral part, the orbital surface, which is located above the orbit and is composed by orbital gyri. The orbital surface is divided by the orbital sulcus, a complex sulcus that presents a rough configuration of the letter "H," into four quadrants: anterior, medial, posterior, and lateral orbital gyri. The temporal lobe is separated posteriorly from the occipital lobe by the basal parietotemporal line (from the preoccipital notch to the junction between the parieto-occipital and calcarine fissures) and presents from lateral to medial, the inferior temporal gyrus, occipitotemporal sulcus, fusiform gyrus, collateral sulcus, and parahippocampal gyrus (Fig. 4.6d). The collateral sulcus is an inferior-to-superior, medial-to-laterally oriented sulcus that bulges into the lateral part of the floor of the temporal horn (collateral eminence) and the atrium (collateral trigone). These gyri are kept separated anteriorly by the rhinal sulcus that separates the uncus medially from the temporal pole laterally. The rhinal sulcus can be considered an anterior continuation of the collateral sulcus, and it continues superiorly on the surface of the planum polare to separate this from the uncus medially (Fig. 4.6d).

Anterior Perforated Substance (APS)

The APS is the entry site for the perforating arteries from the internal carotid, the anterior choroidal, and the anterior and the middle cerebral arteries to the basal ganglia, the anterior portion of the thalamus, the genu, and the anterior and the posterior limbs of the internal capsule. It is also the exit site for the inferior striate veins. APS is a convex cavity extending upward at the posterior end of the basal surface of the frontal lobe. The APS can be considered as the "floor" of the anterior half of the basal ganglia (Fig. 4.6d).

Basal Surface: Venous Relationships

The most important deep venous channel on the basal surface is the basal vein of Rosenthal. The basal vein originates below the APS and is divided into three segments (Fig. 4.7a): the first, or anterior or striate segment, originates from the junction of the anterior cerebral, inferior striate, olfactory, frontoorbital, and deep middle cerebral veins under the APS and runs posteriorly under the optic tract, medially to the anterior portion of the crus cerebri. The second, or middle or peduncular segment, starts from the most medial point in the course of the basal vein, usually correspondent to the site where the peduncular vein joins the basal vein. It runs laterally between the upper part of the posteromedial surface of the uncus and the upper part of the crus cerebri, and under the optic tract to reach the most lateral part of the crus cerebri, which corresponds to the most lateral point of the vein as it turns around the crus cerebri, usually where the inferior ventricular vein joins the basal vein; this is called the anterior peduncular segment by Huang and Wolf [23]; it then turns medially, superiorly, and posteriorly to the plane of the lateral mesencephalic sulcus behind the crus cerebri to constitute the posterior peduncular segment. The main tributaries of the second segment are the peduncular or interpeduncular vein, the inferior ventricular, the inferior choroidal, the hippocampal, and the anterior hippocampal veins. The third or posterior mesencephalic segment runs medially, superiorly, and posteriorly from the lateral mesencephalic sulcus, and under the pulvinar of the thalamus to penetrate the quadrigeminal cistern and generally drain into the vein of Galen. The main tributaries of the third segment are the lateral mesencephalic vein, the posterior thalamic, the posterior longitudinal hippocampal, the medial temporal, and the medial occipital veins (Fig. 4.7a).

Basal Surface: Arterial Relationships

The internal carotid artery and its branches, and the posterior cerebral artery are better visualized from this surface. The internal carotid artery (ICA) is divided into five parts: cervical, petrous, cavernous, clinoid, and the supraclinoid portions. The supraclinoid portion has been divided into three segments based on the origin of its major branches [24] (Fig. 4.7b): the ophthalmic segment extends from the origin of the ophthalmic artery to the origin of the posterior communicating artery (PCom); the communicating segment extends from the origin of the PCom to the origin of the anterior choroidal artery (AChA); and the choroidal segment extends from the origin of the AChA to the bifurcation of the ICA. Each segment gives off a series of perforating branches with a relatively constant site of termination.

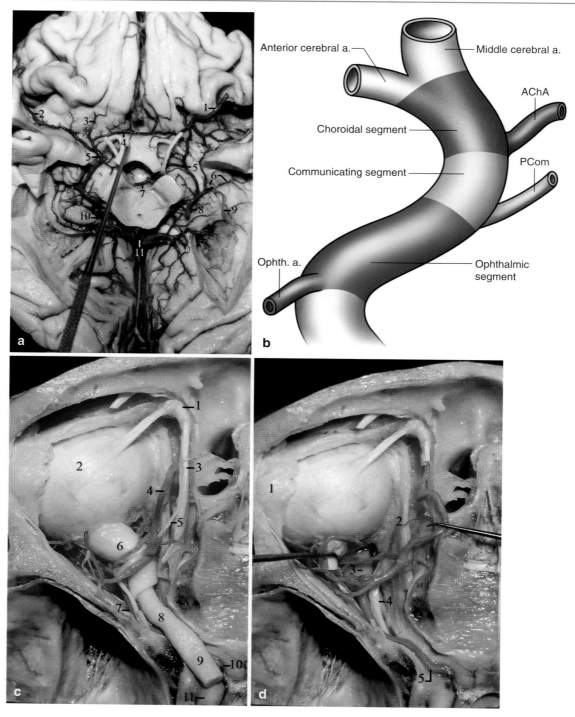

Fig. 4.7 (**a**) Basal view. *1* Frontoorbital vein, *2* deep middle cerebral vein, *3* olfactory vein, *4* anterior cerebral vein, *5* transition between the first and the second segment of the basal vein, *6* inferior ventricular vein and the inferior choroidal point, *7* peduncular vein, *8* transition between the second and the third segment of the basal vein, *9* anterior choroidal artery, *10* posterior mesencephalic segment, *11* vein of Galen. (**b**) Lateral view of the left supraclinoid internal carotid artery and its main branches. *AChA* anterior choroidal artery, *PCom* posterior communicating artery; *Ophth A* ophthalmic artery. (**c**) Superior view of the left orbit; the roof has been removed. *1* Trochlea of the superior oblique

muscle, *2* tendon of the superior oblique muscle and the eye globe, *3* superior oblique muscle, *4* anterior ethmoidal artery, *5* trochlear nerve to the superior oblique muscle, *6* optic nerve inside the orbit, *7* ophthalmic artery, *8* optic nerve inside the optic canal, *9* optic nerve inside the intracranial cavity, *10* ophthalmic artery, *11* supraclinoid carotid artery. (**d**) Same specimen of the (**c**); the superior oblique muscle and the optic nerve have been cut. *1* Lacrimal gland, *2* medial rectus muscle, *3* inferior rectus muscle, *4* inferior division of the oculomotor nerve to the medial rectus muscle, *5* ophthalmic artery

The ophthalmic artery arises under the optic nerve, usually from the medial one-third of the superior surface of the ICA, then it passes anteriorly and laterally to become superolateral to the ICA to enter the optic canal and the orbit. The anterior and the posterior ethmoidal arteries, both branches from the ophthalmic artery directed to the nose, are the main communicating channel between the internal and the external carotid arteries (Fig. 4.7c, d). The perforating arteries from this segment are distributed to the stalk of the pituitary gland, the optic chiasm, and less commonly to the optic nerve, premamillary portion of the floor of the third ventricle, and the optic tract. The superior hypophyseal arteries, which can range from 1 to 5 in number, pass medially to supply the pituitary stalk and the anterior lobe of the pituitary gland. The inferior hypophyseal artery from the meningohypophyseal trunk of the cavernous ICA supplies the posterior lobe. The infundibular arteries are another group of arteries that arise from the PCom and supply the same area as the superior hypophyseal artery. The posterior communicating artery (PCom) arises from the posteromedial or the posterior or the posterolateral aspect of the ICA and passes posteromedially to join the posterior cerebral artery (PCA) (Fig. 4.8a). In the embryo, the PCom continues as PCA, but in the adult the PCA becomes part of the basilar system. If PCom remains the major origin of the PCA, the configuration of the PCom is termed "fetal." The largest branch from the PCom is the premamillary artery or "anterior thalamoperforating artery." The anterior choroidal artery (AChA) arises either from the posterolateral or the posterior aspect of the ICA, and courses posteriorly below the optic tract toward the temporal horn by passing through the choroidal fissure (Fig. 4.8a). The AChA sends off branches to the optic tract, crus cerebri, lateral geniculate body, and uncus and supplies the optic radiation, globus pallidus, midbrain, thalamus, and the retrolenticular and posterior portion of the posterior limb of the internal capsule [25].

The choroidal segment of the ICA is the most frequent site of perforating arteries (range 1–9), arising from the posterior aspect of the ICA. They terminate in the posterior half of the central region of the APS, optic tract, and uncus.

The anterior perforating arteries are those arising from the ICA, MCA, AChA, and anterior cerebral arteries; they enter the brain through the APS.

Embryologically the posterior cerebral artery (PCA) arises as a branch of the ICA, but up to birth its most often origin is the basilar artery. The PCA is classified in four segments [26] (Fig. 4.8a): the P1 extends from the basilar bifurcation to the site where the PCom joins the PCA. The P2 extends from the PCom to the posterior aspect of the midbrain. The P2 is further divided into P2A (anterior) and P2P (posterior) segments. P2A begins at the PCom and courses around the crus cerebri; inferiorly to the optic tract, AChA,

and basal vein; and medially to the posteromedial surface of the uncus, up to the posterior margin of the crus cerebri. The P2P begins at the posterior margin of the crus cerebri and runs laterally to the tegmentum of the midbrain within the ambient cistern, parallel and inferiorly to the basal vein, inferolaterally to the geniculate bodies and pulvinar, and medially to the parahippocampal gyrus to enter the quadrigeminal cistern. The P3 begins under the posterior part of the pulvinar in the lateral aspect of the quadrigeminal cistern and ends at the anterior limit of the anterior calcarine sulcus. The P3 is often divided into its major terminal branches: the calcarine and the parieto-occipital arteries before reaching the anterior limit of the anterior calcarine sulcus. The P4 segment is the cortical branches of the PCA.

The main branches arising from the PCA are the posterior thalamoperforating, the direct perforating, the short and long circumflex, the thalamogeniculate, the medial and the lateral posterior choroidal, the inferior temporal, the parieto-occipital, the calcarine, and the posterior pericallosal arteries. The posterior thalamoperforating arteries, which arise from P1 and enter the brain through the posterior perforated substance, interpeduncular fossa, and medial crus cerebri, supply the anterior and part of the posterior thalamus, hypothalamus, subthalamus, substantia nigra, red nucleus, oculomotor and trochlear nuclei, oculomotor nerve, mesencephalic reticular formation, pretectum, rostromedial floor of the third ventricle, and the posterior portion of the internal capsule. The direct perforating arteries to the crus cerebri arise mainly from the P2A segment and supply the crus cerebri. The short and long circumflex arteries to the brainstem arise mainly from the P1 and less frequently from the P2A; the short circumflex artery courses around the midbrain and terminates at the geniculate bodies; the long circumflex artery courses around the midbrain and reaches the colliculi. The thalamogeniculate arteries arise equally from the P2A or the P2P segments, perforate the inferior surface of the geniculate bodies, and supply the posterior half of the lateral thalamus, posterior limb of the internal capsule, and optic tract. The medial posterior choroidal arteries (MPChA) arise mainly from the P2A and less frequently from the P2P and P1 segments, and course around the midbrain, medial to the main trunk of the PCA, turn around the pulvinar of the thalamus to proceed superiorly at the lateral side of colliculi and pineal gland, to enter the roof of the third ventricle through the velum interpositum, and finally course through the foramen of Monro to enter the choroid plexus in the lateral ventricle (Figs. 4.5c, d and 4.8b). The MPChA supplies the crus cerebri, tegmentum, geniculate bodies (mainly the medial), colliculi, pulvinar, pineal gland, and medial thalamus. Angiographically on lateral projection, the MPChA describes the shape of the number "3." The inferior curve of the "3" is when it turns around the pulvinar and the superior curve is

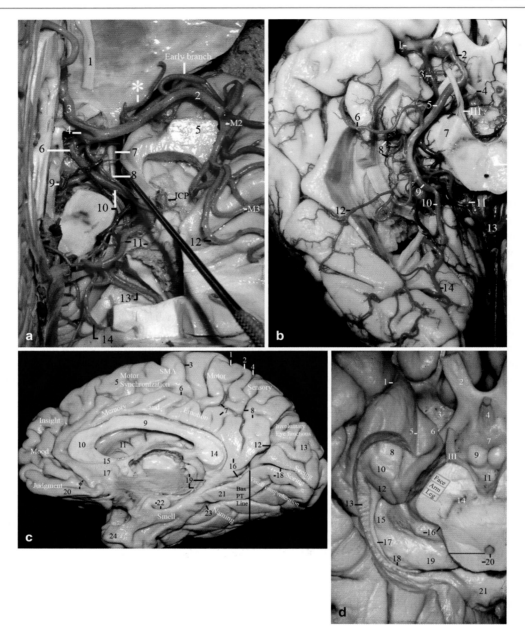

Fig. 4.8 (**a**) Superior view. *1* Olfactory tract, *2* genu of the middle cerebral artery (MCA), *3* anterior cerebral artery, *4* supraclinoid ICA, *5* insular pole, *6* PCom, *7* tentorial edge, *8* AChA, *9* P1 segment of the posterior cerebral artery (PCA), *10* P2A segment of the PCA, *11* P2P segment of the PCA and lateral posterior choroidal artery (LPChA), *12* sylvian point, *13* calcarine artery, *14* parieto-occipital artery, * lesser wing of the sphenoid; early branch, early branch of the MCA, *M2* insular segment of the MCA, *M3* opercular segment of the MCA, *ICP* inferior choroidal point. (**b**) Basal view of the right temporal lobe. *1* M1 segment of the MCA, *2* PCom, *3* AChA, *4* P1, *5* P2A, *6* anterior group of the inferior temporal arteries, *7* crus cerebri, *8* hippocampal arteries, *9* P2P, *10* P3, *11* MPChA, *12* middle group of the inferior temporal arteries, *13* vein of Galen, *14* posterior group of the inferior temporal arteries. (**c**) Medial surface of the right cerebral hemisphere and its functional mapping. *1* Central sulcus, *2* postcentral gyrus, *3* paracentral ramus, *4* postcentral sulcus, *5* medial frontal gyrus, *6* cingulate sulcus, *7* marginal ramus and the cingulate gyrus, *8* subparietal sulcus and precuneus, *9* body of the corpus callosum, *10* genu of the corpus callosum, *11* head of the caudate nucleus, *12* parieto-occipital sulcus, *13* cuneus,

14 splenium of the corpus callosum, *15* rostrum of the corpus callosum, *16* isthmus of the cingulate gyrus and the anterior calcarine sulcus, *17* paraterminal gyrus, *18* posterior calcarine sulcus and the lingual gyrus, *19* dentate gyrus, fornix and the thalamus, *20* rectus gyrus, *21* parahippocampal gyrus, *22* uncus and uncal notch, *23* collateral sulcus, *24* temporal pole, *Bas PT Line* basal parieto-occipital line, * superior and inferior rostral sulci, *SMA* supplementary motor area. (**d**) Basal view. Part of the parahippocampal gyrus has been removed from the uncal notch. The location of the corticospinal tract in the crus cerebri also is shown. *1* Rhinal sulcus, *2* optic nerve, *3* anterior perforated substance, *4* pituitary stalk, *5* impression of the tentorium, *6* anterior segment of the uncus, *7* tuber cinereum, *8* uncinate gyrus, *9* mamillary body, *10* band of Giacomini, *11* posterior perforated substance, *12* intralimbic gyrus, *13* dentate gyrus, *14* substantia nigra, *15* lateral geniculate body, *16* medial geniculate body and the lateral mesencephalic sulcus, *17* fimbria of the fornix, *18* choroidal fissure, *19* pulvinar of the thalamus, *20* aqueduct and the tectum of the midbrain, *21* splenium of the corpus callosum. The *blue line* indicates the plane at the level of the aqueduct; the tegmentum is anterior and the tectum is posterior to that plane when it contours the colliculi before entering the roof of the third ventricle. Lateral posterior choroidal arteries (LPChA) arise mainly from the P2P, and less frequently from the P2A segment, and pass laterally to enter the ventricular cavity directly through the choroidal fissure, to supply the choroid plexus in the atrium and the temporal horn. It anastomoses with the AChA (Fig. 4.8a). Inferior temporal arteries are distributed to the basal surface of the temporal and occipital lobes. They include hippocampal artery and three groups of temporal arteries, namely, anterior, middle, and posterior temporal arteries (Fig. 4.8b). The anterior temporal artery arises mainly from the P2A, while the middle and posterior temporal arteries arise mainly from the P2P segment. Parieto-occipital and calcarine arteries are usually terminal branches of the PCA; they arise predominantly from P3, however sometimes may also arise from the P2P segment and course respectively in parieto-occipital fissure and the calcarine fissure. As the calcarine fissure reaches laterally to bulge into the medial wall of the atrium and the occipital horn, the calcarine artery also follows laterally into the depth of the calcarine fissure (Figs. 4.6b and 4.8a). Splenial or posterior pericallosal artery supplies the splenium of the corpus callosum and arises from the parieto-occipital artery in 62 % of the cases, but it also can arise from calcarine, MPChA, posterior temporal, P2P, P3, and LPChA.

Medial Surface: Neural Relationships

The medial surface of the cerebrum comprises the sulci and gyri of the frontal, parietal, occipital, and temporal lobes (Fig. 4.8c). The general organization of the gyri of the frontal, parietal, and occipital lobes on this surface can be compared to that of a three-layer roll; the inner layer is represented by the corpus callosum, the intermediate layer by the cingulate gyrus, and the outer layer by the medial frontal gyrus, paracentral lobule, precuneus, cuneus, and lingual gyrus. The cingulate gyrus is separated inferiorly from the corpus callosum by the callosal sulcus and superiorly from the outer layer by cingulate sulcus. Several secondary rami ascend from the cingulate sulcus in a radiate pattern and divide the outer layer into several sections; there are two secondary rami of particular importance: the paracentral ramus, which ascends from the cingulate sulcus at the level of the midpoint of the corpus callosum and separates the medial frontal gyrus anteriorly from the paracentral lobule posteriorly, and the marginal ramus, which ascends from the cingulate sulcus at the level of the splenium of the corpus callosum and separates the paracentral lobule anteriorly from the precuneus posteriorly. The marginal ramus intercepts the postcentral gyrus in almost 100 % of the cases, and it is an important landmark to determine the location of the sensory or motor areas in the lateral convexity through a midsagittal MRI (Fig. 4.9a). The parieto-occipital sulcus separates the precuneus superiorly from the cuneus inferiorly, and the calcarine sulcus separates the cuneus superiorly from the lingual gyrus inferiorly. The paracentral ramus along with the marginal ramus determines the paracentral lobule, which is concerned with movements of the contralateral lower limb and perineal region, and is involved in voluntary control over defecation and micturition. The paracentral lobule comprises the anterior part of the postcentral, precentral gyri, and the posterior portion of the superior frontal gyrus. The precuneus along with the part of the paracentral lobule behind the central sulcus forms the medial part of the parietal lobe; the precuneus corresponds to the superior parietal lobule on the lateral surface. The precuneus presents the subparietal sulcus, a vaguely H-shaped sulcus where the vertical arm of the H tends to align with the marginal ramus, and the parieto-occipital sulcus, which separates the precuneus above from the cingulated gyrus below (Fig. 4.8c). The parieto-occipital and the calcarine sulci determine the cuneus; the cuneus along with the medial part of the lingual gyrus is the medial portion of the occipital lobe. The calcarine sulcus starts at the occipital pole and directs anteriorly, presenting a slightly curved course with its characteristic upward convexity. The calcarine sulcus joins the parieto-occipital sulcus (only superficially) at an acute angle behind the isthmus of the cingulate gyrus and continues anteriorly to intercept the isthmus of the cingulate gyrus. The portion of the calcarine sulcus anterior to the junction is called anterior calcarine sulcus, and it is crossed by a buried anterior cuneo-lingual gyrus and bulges into the medial wall of the atrium of the lateral ventricle as calcar avis. It presents the visual cortex only on its lower lip. The part of the calcarine sulcus posterior to the union is called posterior calcarine sulcus and presents the striate (visual) cortex on its upper and lower lips (Fig. 4.8c). Anteriorly, the cingulate and the medial frontal gyri wrap around the genu and the rostrum of the corpus callosum. At the inferior end of these two gyri, under the rostrum of the corpus callosum, and in front of the lamina terminalis is a narrow triangle of gray matter, the paraterminal gyrus, separated from the rest of the cortex by a shallow posterior paraolfactory sulcus. Slightly anterior to this sulcus, a short vertical sulcus may occur, the anterior paraolfactory sulcus; the cortex between the posterior and anterior paraolfactory sulci is the subcallosal area or paraolfactory gyrus. Frequently two anteroposteriorly directed sulci, the superior and inferior rostral sulci, which are parallel to the floor of the anterior fossa, divide the inferior portion of the medial frontal gyrus into three parts. Posteriorly the cingulate gyrus continues inferiorly with the parahippocampal gyrus through the isthmus of the cingulate gyrus. The mesial portion of the temporal lobe presents intra- and extraventricular elements. The intraventricular elements are hippocampus, fimbria, amygdala, and choroidal fissure; the extraventricular elements are parahippocampal gyrus, uncus, and dentate gyrus (Figs. 4.6d

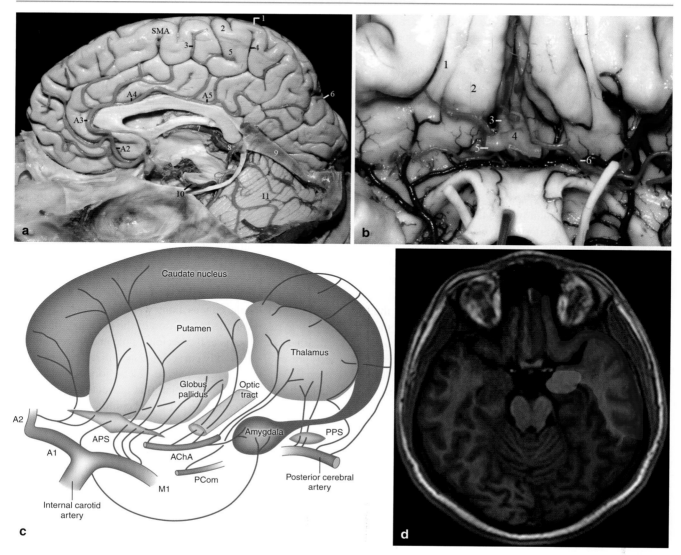

Fig. 4.9 (**a**) Midsagittal view. *1* Postcentral gyrus, *2* precentral gyrus, *3* paracentral ramus, *4* marginal ramus, *5* paracentral lobule, *6* parieto-occipital sulcus, *7* internal cerebral vein, *8* vein of Galen, *9* straight sinus, *10* basal vein, *11* tentorial surface of the cerebellum, *A2, A3, A4,* and *A5* are segments of the anterior cerebral artery, *SMA* the supplementary motor area. (**b**) Basal view. *1* Olfactory tract, *2* rectus gyrus, *3* A2, *4* ACom, *5* A1 (cut), *6* recurrent artery. (**c**) Vascularization of the basal ganglia and the thalamus. The caudate nucleus: the lower portion of the head is supplied by the medial lenticulostriate arteries (including the recurrent artery); the upper portion of the head and the body are supplied by the medial and the lateral lenticulostriate arteries; the tail and part of the body are supplied by the lateral posterior choroidal arteries. Putamen: most of the putamen is supplied by the lateral lenticulostriate arteries; its anterior portion is supplied by the medial lenticulostriate arteries, and its posterior portion is supplied by the anterior choroidal artery (*AChA*). Globus pallidus: its vascular pattern is similar to that of putamen. Amygdala: it receives branches from the supraclinoid internal carotid

artery and from the anterior choroidal artery. Thalamus: most of the thalamus is supplied by the branches (thalamoperforating, thalamogeniculate) from the posterior cerebral artery; its anterior and inferior portions are supplied by branches from PCom and AChA; its anterior and superior portion can be supplied by lateral posterior choroidal artery, and its superior and posterior portion are supplied by the medial posterior choroidal artery. Internal capsule: the anterior limb is predominately supplied by medial lenticulostriate arteries; the genu is supplied predominantly by perforators from the choroidal segment of the internal carotid artery, and the posterior limb is predominately supplied by the anterior choroidal artery. (**d**) The approximate vascular territory of the main cerebral arteries. In *green*, anterior cerebral artery and its perforators (in *gray*, perforators from the anterior communicating artery); in *red*, middle cerebral artery (its perforators are in *pink*); in *blue*, posterior cerebral artery (in *violet*, thalamoperforating arteries; in *light blue*, posterior choroidal arteries; in *light violet*, thalamogeniculate arteries); in *brown*, perforators from PCom; in *orange*, perforators from the ICA; in *yellow*, AChA

and 4.8c, d). The parahippocampal gyrus extends from anterior to posteriorly, and at its anterior extremity, it deviates medially and bends posteriorly to constitute the uncus. Posteriorly, just below the splenium of the corpus callosum,

the parahippocampal gyrus is often intersected by the anterior calcarine sulcus, which divides the posterior portion of the parahippocampal gyrus into the isthmus of the cingulate gyrus superiorly, and the parahippocampal gyrus inferiorly, which continues posteriorly as the lingual gyrus. Superiorly the parahippocampal gyrus is separated from the dentate gyrus by the hippocampal sulcus. Laterally, parahippocampal gyrus is limited by the collateral sulcus posteriorly and the rhinal sulcus anteriorly. The rhinal sulcus marks the lateral limit of the entorhinal area of the parahippocampal gyrus; the parahippocampal gyrus is separated from the inferior surface of the posterior segment of the uncus by the uncal notch. Medially the parahippocampal gyrus is related to the tentorium edge and to the contents of the ambient cistern. The various components of the parahippocampal gyrus are the subiculum, presubiculum, parasubiculum, and entorhinal area, being the subiculum its medial round edge. The name uncus means "hook." It is formed by the anterior portion of the parahippocampal gyrus, which has deviated medially and folded posteriorly. Inferiorly, the uncus is separated from the parahippocampal gyrus by the uncal notch. Anteriorly, the uncus continues with the anterior portion of the parahippocampal gyrus without a sharp limit; superiorly, the uncus is continuous with the globus pallidus. At the basal surface, the uncus is separated laterally from the temporal pole by the rhinal sulcus, and its medial part is normally herniated medially to the tentorial edge. When viewed from its basal surface, the uncus presents the shape of an arrowhead with its apex pointing medially, featuring an apex, an anterior segment, and a posterior segment (Figs. 4.6d and 4.8c, d). The anterior segment or anteromedial surface belongs to the parahippocampal gyrus and presents the semilunar and the ambient gyri. The anteromedial surface is related to the proximal sylvian fissure and carotid cistern, and is the posterolateral limit of the APS. The posterior segment is related to the hippocampus and has two surfaces: a posteromedial and an inferior surface (Figs. 4.6d and 4.8c, d). The posterior segment is occupied by three small gyri; from anterior to posterior, they are the uncinate gyrus, the band of Giacomini, and the intralimbic gyrus. Posteriorly and superiorly to the uncus is the inferior choroidal point, where the choroid plexus of the temporal horn begins. The inferior choroidal point corresponds to the site where the AChA enters and the inferior ventricular vein leaves the temporal horn through the choroidal fissure (Figs. 4.6b, 4.7a, and 4.8a). The dentate gyrus bears this name because of its characteristic toothlike elevations; the margo denticulatus is prominent mainly in its anterior and middle portions. The dentate gyrus continues anteriorly with the band of Giacomini, also called the tail of the dentate gyrus, and continues posteriorly with the fasciolar gyrus, a smooth grayish band that is located posteriorly to the splenium of the corpus callosum; the fasciolar gyrus continues above the corpus callosum as the indusium griseum to finally end as the paraterminal gyrus. The fimbrodentate and hippocampal sulci separate the dentate gyrus, respectively, from the fimbria superiorly and the parahippocampal gyrus inferiorly (Fig. 4.8d).

The extraventricular and the intraventricular structures of the mesial temporal lobe are intimately related. The anterior segment of the uncus is related to M1, ICA, and amygdala. The apex of the uncus passes above the oculomotor nerve and is related to the uncal recess and the amygdala laterally; the posterior segment is related to the head of the hippocampus and the amygdala laterally, to the P2A inferomedially, and to the AChA superomedially.

Medial Surface: Venous Relationships

The medial frontal veins drain the medial surface of the frontal lobe. They can either empty superiorly into the superior sagittal sinus, or inferiorly into the inferior sagittal sinus or into the veins that pass around the corpus callosum to drain into the anterior end of the basal vein. The medial parietal veins drain the medial surface of the parietal lobe; they can empty superiorly into the superior sagittal sinus or course around the splenium of the corpus callosum and drain inferiorly into the vein of Galen or its tributaries. The posterior pericallosal veins, one on each side, arise from tributaries that drain the posterior part of the cingulate gyrus and the precuneus, and course side by side around the splenium of the corpus callosum to terminate in either the vein of Galen or the internal cerebral vein. The anterior and the posterior calcarine veins drain the occipital lobe. The anterior calcarine or internal occipital vein arises from tributaries that drain the anterior portion of the cuneus and lingual gyrus and passes forward to join the posterior pericallosal vein near the splenium before terminating in either the internal cerebral or in the vein of Galen. The posterior calcarine vein arises from tributaries that drain the area bordering the posterior part of the calcarine fissure and then curves sharply upward on the cuneus to reach the superior sagittal sinus.

The deep venous system of the mesial temporal region drains into the basal vein of Rosenthal.

Medial Surface: Arterial Relationships

The anterior cerebral artery (ACA) is classified in five segments [27]: A1 segment extends from the bifurcation of the ICA to the anterior communicating artery (ACom). A2 segment extends from the ACom to the junction between the rostrum and the genu of the corpus callosum. A3 segment extends from the genu of the corpus callosum to the point where the artery turns sharply and posteriorly above the genu of the corpus callosum. The A2 and A3 segments together are also called ascending segment. A4 and A5 segments extend above the corpus callosum, from the genu to the splenium. These two segments together are also called horizontal segment, and the point bisected in the lateral view close behind the coronal suture separates them. The segment of the ACA distal to the ACom (A2–A5) has also been called pericallosal artery (Fig. 4.9a). The junction of the ACom with the A1 segment occurs above the chiasm in 70 % and above the nerve in 30 %. The shorter A1 segments are usually stretched tightly over the chiasm; the longer ones pass anteriorly over the optic nerve and can be elongated and tortuous and reach either the tuberculum sellae or the planum sphenoidale (Fig. 4.6b). The medial lenticulostriate perforators, ranging from 1 to 11 branches (average of 6.4), arise from the superior, the posterior, or the posterior-superior aspect of the proximal half of A1 segment and pursue a direct posterior and superior course to enter the medial half of APS. Embryologically the ACom develops from a multichanneled vascular network that coalesces to a variable degree by the time of birth. Only in 20 % of the cases, the ACom communicates 2 A1 segments of equal size. The ACom complex probably exists as a single channel in about 75 % of the cases [28]. The perforators from ACom, ranging from 0 to 4 (average 1.6), usually arise from its posteroinferior aspect to supply the infundibulum, the APS, the optic chiasm, the subcallosal area, and the preoptic areas of the hypothalamus. The recurrent artery of Heubner of the ACA arises in 78 % of the cases from the proximal A2, and it doubles back on its parent vessel and courses anteriorly to the A1 segment in 60 % of the cases; it is the largest and longest branch directed to the APS. After its origin, it passes above the carotid bifurcation and accompanies the M1 into the medial part of the sylvian fissure before entering the anterior and middle portions of the full mediolateral extent of the APS [29] (Fig. 4.9b). The A2 segment is also the source of the central or the basal perforating arteries, which pass posteriorly to enter the optic chiasm, the lamina terminalis, and the anterior forebrain, below the corpus callosum. The two first cortical branches of the ACA supplying the medial surface, the orbitofrontal and the frontopolar arteries, usually arise from the A2 segment. The segments A3–A5 give rise to other cortical branches to supply the medial surface of the hemisphere. All the cortical branches arise more frequently from the pericallosal than from the callosomarginal artery (Fig. 4.9a).

The anterior cerebral artery syndromes include (1) paracentral lobule syndrome, (2) supplementary motor area (SMA) syndrome, (3) anterior cingulated syndrome, (4) callosal syndrome, (5) basal forebrain syndrome, and (6) total ACA territory infarction [30].

The paracentral syndrome is characterized by weakness of the contralateral lower limb, most intense in the foot and ankle, with or without sensory loss. The transient or permanent incontinence of urine can also be present. The SMA occupies the medial surface of the superior frontal gyrus immediately anterior to the paracentral lobule (Figs. 4.8c and

4.9a); the SMA syndrome can be characterized by dysphasia (when the dominant hemisphere is affected), akinesia in the contralateral limb, contralateral hand grasping or groping, contralateral alien hand signs (when the dominant hemisphere is affected, the right hand consistently interrupts manual tasks performed by the left hand), and dyspraxia. The anterior cingulate syndrome is more evident when the cingulated cortex is bilaterally and extensively affected; this might cause akinetic mutism, complex behavioral changes, loss of sphincter control, and autonomic dysfunctions (temperature, cardiac, and respiratory irregularities). The callosal syndrome can be characterized by "split brain" sign and symptoms: left hand apraxia (inability to perform actions with left hand on verbal command), alien hand syndrome (left hand behaving like a foreigner or an alien, and acts uncooperatively), and left hand agraphia. The basal forebrain syndrome occurs when the territories of the orbitofrontal and frontopolar arteries and the septal region are affected, and the signs and symptoms include amnesia, emotional disinhibition, inappropriate social conduct, and autonomic disturbances. The total ACA infarction syndrome is a combination of the previously mentioned syndromes.

Vascularization of the Basal Ganglia and the Thalamus

The complex vascularization pattern of the central core of the cerebrum (the basal ganglia, the internal capsule, and the thalamus) can be summarized in Fig. 4.9c [31, 32].

The vascular territories of the cerebrum can be seen in Figs. 4.9d and 4.10a–c [33].

The Posterior Fossa

The posterior fossa is the largest and deepest of the three cranial fossae. It comprises one-eighth of the intracranial space and contains the pathways regulating consciousness, vital autonomic functions, and motor activities, in addition to the center for controlling balance and gait. Only 2 of the 12 pairs of the cranial nerves are located entirely outside the posterior fossa. The posterior fossa extends from the tentorial incisura, through which it communicates with the supratentorial space, to the foramen magnum, through which it communicates with the spinal cord. The posterior fossa is separated from the supratentorial space by the tentorium cerebella.

The intracranial surface of the posterior fossa presents jugular foramen, internal acoustic meatus, hypoglossal canal, vestibular and cochlear aqueducts, and several venous emissary foramina. The posterior fossa also presents neural (the cerebellum, the brainstem, and the cranial nerves) and vascular elements (arteries and veins), which can be characterized

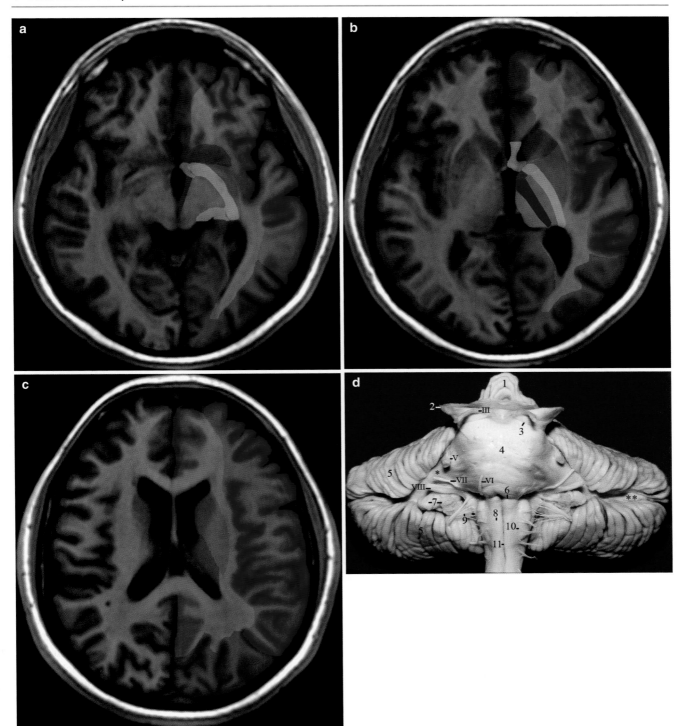

Fig. 4.10 (**a–c**) The approximate vascular territory of the main cerebral arteries. In *green*, anterior cerebral artery and its perforators (in *gray*, perforators from the anterior communicating artery); in *red*, middle cerebral artery (its perforators are in *pink*); in *blue*, posterior cerebral artery (in *violet*, thalamoperforating arteries; in *light blue*, posterior choroidal arteries; in *light violet*, thalamogeniculate arteries); in *brown*, perforators from PCom; in *orange*, perforators from the ICA; in *yellow*,

AChA. (**d**) Frontal view. *1* Culmen, *2* crus cerebri, *3* pontomesencephalic sulcus, *4* basilar sulcus, *5* petrosal surface of the cerebellum, *6* pontomedullary sulcus, *7* flocculus and the choroid plexus (foramen of Luschka), *8* pyramid, *9* IX, X, and XI nerves, *10* preolivary sulcus, *11* anterior median fissure. *V* trigeminal nerve, *VI* abducent nerve, *VII* facial nerve, *VIII* vestibulocochlear nerve, * middle cerebellar peduncle, ** petrosal fissure

by the "rule of three," where the brainstem presents three parts (midbrain, pons, and medulla) and the cerebellum presents three surfaces (petrosal, tentorial, and suboccipital), three cerebellar peduncles (superior, middle, and inferior), three fissures (cerebellomesencephalic, cerebellopontine, and cerebellomedullary), three main arteries (SCA, AICA, and PICA), and three main venous drainage groups (petrosal, galenic, and tentorial) [34].

Brainstem

The brainstem cannot be considered simply a connecting structure between the diencephalon and the spinal cord. Through the long projection systems of its reticular formation, the brainstem modulates sensory and motor pathways, and modulates arousal and conscious states (ascending projections to the diencephalon and the cerebrum); the brainstem presents the nuclei of ten cranial nerves that supply the sensory and motor functions of the face and head and the autonomic functions of the body; the brainstem also coordinates reflexes and simple behavior mediated by the cranial nerves. As a general rule, the descending motor system occupies the anterior portion of the brainstem, while the long ascending and descending sensory tracts (the medial lemniscus, spinothalamic tract, and auditory, vestibular, and visceral sensory pathways) run within the reticular formation, which is located at the core (tegmentum) of the brainstem.

The brainstem is divided into three parts: midbrain, pons, and medulla.

The midbrain is separated superiorly from the diencephalon by the optic tract, lateral geniculate body, and the pulvinar of the thalamus; inferiorly the midbrain is separated from the pons by the pontomesencephalic sulcus and by the emergence of the trochlear nerve, which is a mesencephalic structure. The midbrain is divided by a midline sagittal plane into two cerebral peduncles; each peduncle is further divided into three parts (an anterior part, crus cerebri, or basis pedunculi); an intermediate part, the tegmentum; and a posterior part located behind the aqueduct, the tectum; the substantia nigra and the lateral mesencephalic sulcus separate the crus cerebri from the tegmentum (Fig. 4.8d). The oculomotor nerves emerge from the medial side of the crura cerebri in the interpeduncular fossa (Figs. 4.5c, 4.6d, 4.8d, and 4.10d). The pontomesencephalic sulcus, which separates the midbrain from the pons, originates in the depth of the interpeduncular fossa and runs around the inferior margin of the crus cerebri to join the lateral mesencephalic sulcus behind the crus cerebri. The posterior aspect of the midbrain presents superior and inferior colliculi (quadrigeminal plate). The superior colliculi are connected to the lateral geniculate bodies via brachium of the superior colliculus, and the inferior colliculi are connected to the medial geniculate bodies via brachium

of the inferior colliculus. The trochlear nerve exits the brainstem below the inferior colliculus (Figs. 4.11c, 4.12b, 4.13b, and 4.14a, d).

The pons or protuberance presents a prominent anterior surface that is considerably convex from side to side, and it consists of transverse fibers that cross the median plane and converge on each side to form the middle cerebellar peduncles. The basilar sulcus is a shallow median groove on the anterior surface of the pons and usually lodges the basilar artery; this sulcus is bounded on each side by an eminence caused by the descent of the corticospinal fibers through the substance of the pons. The middle cerebellar peduncle is separated from the belly of the pons by a vertical shallow groove, the lateral pontine sulcus. Just lateral to the lateral pontine sulcus is the emergence of the trigeminal nerve, with its smaller superomedial motor root and a larger inferolateral sensory root (Fig. 4.10d). Posteriorly the pons constitutes the upper portion of the floor of the fourth ventricle (Figs. 4.12b and 4.13b).

The medulla presents at its anterior aspect three longitudinal fissures, being one median and two paramedian: the median one is the anterior median fissure, which continues inferiorly as the anterior median fissure of the spinal cord. The paramedian sulci of the anterior aspect of the medulla are the anterolateral sulci. At the medulla, the anterolateral sulcus is located medially to the olive; because of that it is also called preolivary sulcus. The preolivary sulcus is the upper continuation of the anterolateral sulcus of the spinal cord. The rootlets of the hypoglossal nerve that exit from the preolivary sulcus are analogous to the ventral motor rootlets that exit from the anterolateral sulcus of the spinal cord. The pyramid characterizes the anterior region, located between the anterior median fissure and the preolivary sulcus (Fig. 4.10d).

The rootlets of the accessory, the vagus, and the glossopharyngeal nerves exit from the postolivary sulcus, the continuation of the posterolateral sulcus of the spinal cord in the medulla; therefore these cranial nerve rootlets are analogous to the dorsal spinal rootlets. These rootlets emerge from the brainstem and extend almost straight laterally to the jugular foramen. The pontomedullary sulcus separates the pons from the medulla, and its junction with the preolivary sulcus marks the apparent origin of the abducent nerve (Fig. 4.10d).

Among all structures located in the brainstem, the reticular formation deserves special consideration. The reticular formation of the brainstem is located in the tegmentum (core) of the brainstem, and it modulates sensation, movement, consciousness, reflexive behavior, and the activities of ten cranial nerves. By convention, the reticular formation is defined only for the brainstem, and it contains specific groups of cells extending from the upper pons to the hypothalamus that are responsible for "activating" the cerebral

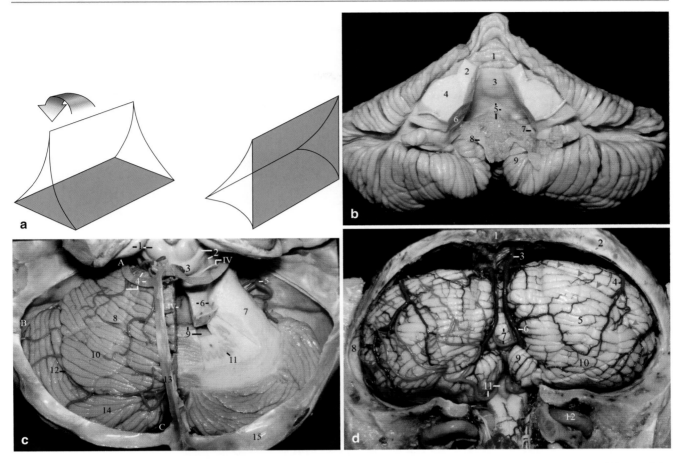

Fig. 4.11 (**a**) A normal tent is shown on the *left*. The fourth ventricle resembles a turned over tent with its floor (in *green*) facing forward (*right*). (**b**) Frontal view. The brainstem has been removed to display the roof of the fourth ventricle. *1* Central lobule, *2* superior cerebellar peduncle, *3* lingula (covered by superior medullary velum), *4* middle cerebellar peduncle, *5* fastigium, nodule, and the choroid plexus of the fourth ventricle, *6* inferior cerebellar peduncle, *7* inferior medullary velum, *8* tela choroidea, *9* tonsil. (**c**) Superior view. The cortex of the right cerebellar hemisphere has been removed up to the postclival fissure. *1* Thalamus and the superior colliculus, *2* brachium of the inferior colliculus and the lateral mesencephalic sulcus, *3* inferior colliculus, *4* wing of the central lobule, tentorial edge, and the branches of the superior cerebellar artery, *5* internal acoustic meatus and the anterior inferior cerebellar artery, *6* superior cerebellar peduncle and the interpeduncular sulcus, *7* middle

cerebellar peduncle, *8* quadrangular lobule, *9* nodule (midline) and the superior pole of the tonsil (lateral), *10* simple lobule, *11* dentate nucleus, *12* postclival fissure, *13* straight sinus, *14* superior semilunar lobule, *15* transverse sinus. *A–B* anterolateral margin, *B–C* posterolateral margin. *C* posterior cerebellar incisura. The *small red dots* on the superior cerebellar peduncle and on the dentate nucleus are the precentral arteries. (**d**) Posterior view of the suboccipital surface of the cerebellum. *1* Torcula, *2* transverse sinus, *3* inferior vermian vein draining into the torcula, *4* inferior hemispheric vein, *5* inferior semilunar lobule, *6* inferior vermian vein coursing on the secondary fissure, *7* pyramid and the vermian branch of the posterior inferior cerebellar artery (PICA), *8* sigmoid sinus, *9* tonsil, *10* biventral lobule, *11* hemispheric branch of PICA and the floor of the fourth ventricle, *12* vertebral artery; the *green arrowheads* indicate the great horizontal fissure or suboccipital fissure

cortex and thalamus, increasing wakefulness, vigilance, and the responsiveness of cortical and thalamic neurons to sensory stimuli, a state known as arousal; those cell groups constitute the ascending reticular activating system (ARAS). The ARAS reaches the cerebral cortex through two major branches at the junction of the midbrain and diencephalon. One is through the thalamus, where it activates and modulates thalamic relay nuclei as well as intralaminar and related nuclei with extensive diffuse cortical projections. The second branch is through the lateral hypothalamic area and is joined by the ascending output from the hypothalamic and basal forebrain cell groups that diffusely innervate the

cerebral cortex. Damage to either branch of the ARAS and/or its projections to the cerebral cortex or bilateral damage of the cerebral cortex can impair consciousness.

Cerebellum

The cerebellum (from the Latin for little brains) is made up primarily of white matter covered with a thin layer of gray matter (cerebellar cortex) and three pairs of deep nuclei: the fastigial, the interposed (composed by two nuclei, the globose and emboliform), and the dentate.

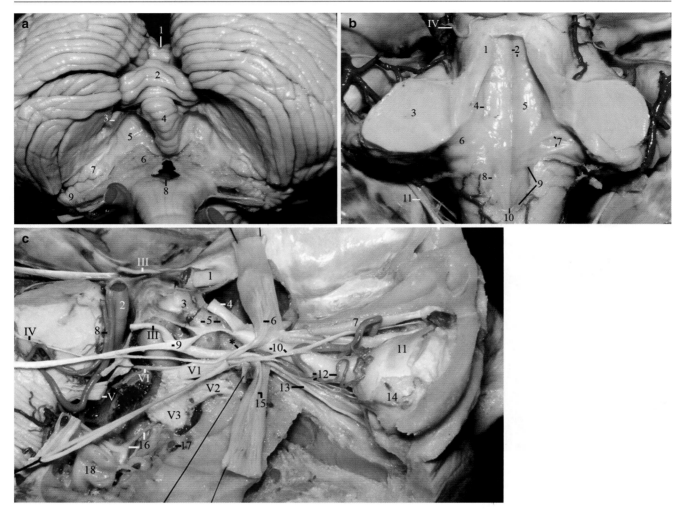

Fig. 4.12 (**a**) Posterior view of the suboccipital surface of the cerebellum; the tonsils and the biventral lobule have been removed. *1* Tuber, *2* pyramid, *3* peduncle of the tonsil, *4* uvula, *5* inferior medullary velum, *6* tela choroidea of the fourth ventricle, *7* peduncle of the flocculus, *8* foramen of Magendie, *9* flocculus. (**b**) Posterior view of the floor of the fourth ventricle. *1* Superior cerebellar peduncle, *2* median sulcus and median eminence, *3* middle cerebellar peduncle, *4* superior fovea, *5* facial colliculus, *6* inferior cerebellar peduncle, *7* stria medullary, *8* inferior fovea, *9* calamus scriptorius, *10* obex, *11* spinal accessory nerve. (**c**) Superolateral view of the right cavernous sinus and the orbit. *1* Left optic nerve, *2* basilar artery, *3* pituitary gland, *4* right optic nerve (intracranial portion), *5* supraclinoid internal carotid artery and the ophthalmic artery, *6* superior division of the oculomotor nerve to the superior rectus muscle, *7* superior oblique muscle, *8* superior cerebellar artery (double), *9* tentorial edge, *10* nasociliary nerve, *11* insertion of the superior oblique muscle on the eye globe, *12* ophthalmic artery, ciliary ganglion and nerves, and ciliary arteries, *13* inferior division of the oculomotor nerve to the inferior oblique muscle, *14* lacrimal gland, *15* abducent nerve to the lateral rectus muscle, *16* geniculate ganglion and the greater superficial petrosal nerve, *17* foramen spinosum and the middle meningeal artery, *18* semicircular canals, *III* oculomotor nerve, *IV* trochlear nerve, *V* trigeminal nerve (cut), *VI* abducent nerve, *V1* ophthalmic division of the trigeminal nerve, *V2* maxillary division of the trigeminal nerve, *V3* mandibular division of the trigeminal nerve, *** the trochlear nerve courses above the annulus of Zinn

The cerebellum plays an important role in motor function by evaluating disparities between the intended movement and the actual action, and by adjusting the operation of motor centers in the cortex and brainstem while a movement is in progress, as well as during repetition of the same movement. The cerebellum is provided with extensive information about the goals, commands, and feedback signals associated with the programming the execution of movement. There are therefore 40 times more axons projecting into the cerebellum than exiting from it [35].

From a morphologic viewpoint, the cerebellum is composed of three parts: a small, median portion called the vermis and two large, lateral cerebellar hemispheres. Both the vermis and the hemispheres are divided, by fissures and sulci, into lobules. The cerebellum is connected to the brainstem through the three cerebellar peduncles, and through the brainstem, the cerebellum establishes its connections with the cerebrum and the spinal cord. However, at its central portion, the cerebellum is separated from the brainstem by the fourth ventricle.

From a functional viewpoint, the cerebellum presents three distinct regions: one is the vermis, and other two regions are located in the intermediate and in the lateral parts of the cerebellar hemisphere. These regions and the flocculonodular lobe receive different afferent inputs, project to different parts of the motor systems, and represent distinct functional subdivisions. The flocculonodular lobule or vestibulocerebellum is related to controlling eye movements

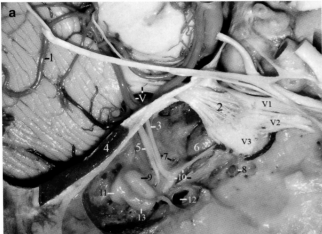

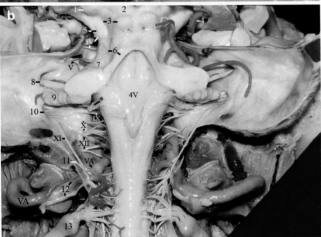

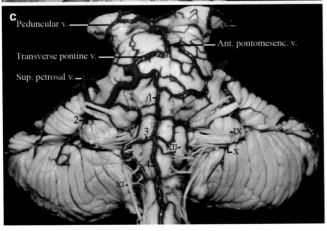

and balance via the cranial nerve VIII to the lateral vestibular nuclei. The vermis and the intermediate part of the cerebellar hemisphere constitute the spinocerebellum; the vermis is related to controlling proximal muscles of the body and limbs via fastigial nucleus; the intermediate part of the hemisphere is related to controlling the more distal muscles of the limbs via the interposed nucleus. The lateral part of the cerebellar hemisphere is called the cerebrocerebellum, and it is involved in planning and mental rehearsal of complex motor actions and in the conscious assessment of movement errors, via the dentate nucleus.

All the cerebellar output comes from the deep nuclei and from the flocculonodular lobule. The superior cerebellar peduncle contains most of the cerebellar efferent projections.

The cerebellum presents three surfaces: petrosal, tentorial, and suboccipital surfaces. The petrosal surface is related anteriorly to the petrous part of the temporal bone; the tentorial surface is related superiorly to the tentorium cerebelli and inferiorly to the upper part of the roof of the fourth ventricle; the suboccipital surface is related inferiorly to the squamosal part of the occipital bone and anteriorly to the inferior part of the roof of the fourth ventricle. Since the fourth ventricle and the cerebellum are closely related, their anatomy will be considered together.

The fourth ventricle is often described as a tent-shaped midline structure surrounded mainly by the vermian components of the cerebellum. A regular tent has a roof that is divided into two halves, a floor and two lateral walls; the fourth ventricle resembles a turned over tent with its base facing forward and two open lateral walls: the floor is represented by the pons and medulla; the superior cerebellar peduncles, the superior medullary velum, and the adjacent

Fig. 4.13 (**a**) Superior view of the right middle fossa. *1* Hemispheric branch of the superior cerebellar artery, *2* Gasserian ganglion, *3* beginning of the meatal segment of the facial nerve, *4* superior petrosal sinus, *5* superior vestibular nerve, *6* petrosal carotid artery, *7* beginning of the labyrinthine segment of the facial nerve and the cochlea, *8* middle meningeal artery, *9* superior semicircular canal, *10* greater superficial petrosal nerve, tensor tympani muscle, and geniculate ganglion, *11* posterior semicircular canal, *12* tympanic cavity, *13* lateral semicircular canal, *V* trigeminal nerve, *V1* ophthalmic division of the trigeminal nerve, *V2* maxillary division of the trigeminal nerve, *V3* mandibular division of the trigeminal nerve. (**b**) Posterior view. *1* Medial geniculate body, *2* superior colliculus, *3* inferior colliculus and lateral mesencephalic sulcus, *4* posterior cerebral artery, *5* crus cerebri, *6* superior cerebellar peduncle and interpeduncular sulcus, *7* middle cerebellar peduncle, *8* internal acoustic meatus, facial nerve, and vestibulocochlear nerve, *9* flocculus, *10* jugular foramen, glossopharyngeal, vagus, and accessory nerves, *11* triangular process of the dentate ligament, *12* posterior inferior cerebellar artery (extradural origin) and C1 nerve, *13* dorsal ganglion of C2, * choroid plexus of the foramen of Luschka, *4V* floor of the fourth ventricle, *IX* glossopharyngeal nerve, *X* vagus nerve, *XI* accessory nerve, *XII* hypoglossal nerve, *VA* vertebral artery. (**c**) Frontal view. *1* Anterior pontomesencephalic vein, *2* vein of the great horizontal fissure, *3* transverse medullary vein, *4* anterior medullary vein

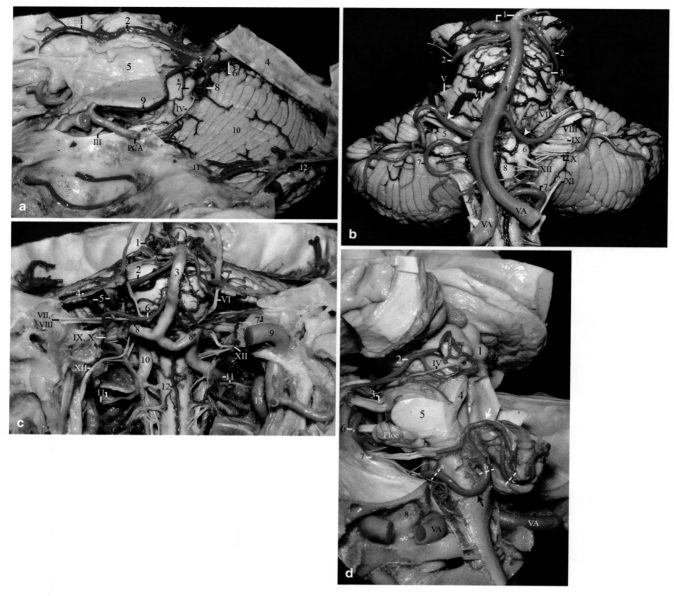

Fig. 4.14 (**a**) Lateral view. *1* Anterior septal vein, *2* internal cerebral vein, *3* vein of Galen, *4* straight sinus, *5* thalamus, *6* superior vermian vein, *7* superior and inferior colliculi, *8* precentral cerebellar vein, *9* basal vein, *10* tentorial surface of the cerebellum, *11* superior petrosal sinus, *12* transverse sinus, *III* oculomotor nerve, *PCA* posterior cerebral artery, *IV* trochlear nerve. (**b**) Anterior view of the brainstem and the cerebellum. *1* PCA, *2* SCA, *3* transverse pontine artery, *4* basilar artery, *5* flocculus, *6* olive, *7* PICA, *8* pyramid, *V* trigeminal nerve, *VI* abducent nerve, *VII* facial nerve, *VIII* vestibulocochlear nerve, *IX* glossopharyngeal nerve, *X* vagus nerve, *XI* spinal accessory nerve, *XII* hypoglossal nerve, *VA* vertebral artery. The *white arrowhead* indicates AICA. Please note the direct branches from the posterior wall of the basilar artery to the brainstem. (**c**) Frontal view. The lateral mass of the C1 has been removed. *1* Cerebellomesencephalic segment of the superior cerebellar artery (SCA), *2* pontomesencephalic segment of the SCA, *3* basilar artery, *4* superior

petrosal sinus, *5* trigeminal nerve and the superior petrosal vein, *6* anterior inferior cerebellar artery (AICA), *7* meatal loop of the AICA, *8* origin of the posterior inferior cerebellar artery (PICA), *9* petrous carotid artery, *10* intradural vertebral artery, *11* extradural vertebral artery and the C1 nerve (the lateral mass of the C1 has been removed), *12* anterior spinal artery, *13* vertebral artery (from C2 to C1), *VI* abducent nerve, *VII* facial nerve, *VIII* vestibulocochlear nerve, *IX* glossopharyngeal nerve, *X* vagus nerve, *XI* accessory nerve, *XII* hypoglossal nerve. (**d**) Left posterolateral view. *1* Inferior colliculus, *2* SCA, *3* trigeminal nerve, *4* superior cerebellar peduncle, *5* middle cerebellar peduncle, *6* internal acoustic meatus and AICA, *7* jugular foramen, *8* lateral mass of C1, *VA* vertebral artery. Proximal to "a," lateral medullary segment of PICA; from "a" to "b," tonsillomedullary segment of PICA; from "b" to "c," telovelotonsillar segment of PICA. The *white arrow* indicates the cranial loop of PICA; the *black arrow* indicates the caudal loop of PICA. *Floc* flocculus

lingula constitute the superior part of the roof; the inferior part of the roof is composed of the inferior medullary velum, tela choroidea, choroid plexus, uvula, and nodule; the two

open lateral walls are represented by the lateral recesses that communicate the fourth ventricle with the cerebellopontine angle through the foramen of Luschka (Fig. 4.11a).

Petrosal Surface of the Cerebellum and Fourth Ventricle

Each half of the petrosal surface is intersected by the great horizontal fissure, or petrosal fissure, that circumscribes the cerebellum. The choroid plexus and the rhomboid lip of the foramen of Luschka are located anteriorly and inferiorly to the flocculus. The glossopharyngeal nerve is the most superior rootlet; single, it is located immediately in front of the choroid plexus. The flocculus is located below the lateral extension of the pontomedullary sulcus, and it is the hemispheric correspondent of the nodule (Fig. 4.10d).

The upper half of the roof of the fourth ventricle is constituted by neural elements: the superior cerebellar peduncles, the superior medullary velum, and the lingual [36].

The lower half of the roof is composed by nonneural elements and presents a horizontal portion: the inferior medullary velum, which covers the nodule and the superior pole of the tonsils, and a vertical portion, the tela choroidea and the choroid plexus, covering the anterior aspect of the nodule, uvula, and partly the tonsils. At the midline, the upper and the lower halves of the roof converge at the fastigium (Fig. 4.11b).

The lateral recess is the lateral extension of the fourth ventricle and connects the fourth ventricle to the cerebellopontine angle. The lateral recess presents an anterior, a superior, and a posterior wall and a floor. The anterior and superior walls are constituted by the inferior cerebellar peduncle as it runs upward and then turns backward toward the cerebellum. The floor of the lateral recess is constituted by the tela choroidea anteriorly, the choroid plexus in the middle, and the inferior medullary velum posteriorly; at the foramen of Luschka, the inferior medullary velum becomes thicker and is called the peduncle of the flocculus and constitutes the posterior wall of the foramen of Luschka. The tonsils are two reniform structures that are hemispheric components of the uvula and are attached to the cerebellum through the peduncles of the tonsil, located at the superolateral aspect of each tonsil (Fig. 4.11b).

Tentorial Surface of the Cerebellum and Fourth Ventricle

The tentorial surface faces the tentorium and presents two cerebellar incisurae and three margins. The cerebellar incisurae are the anterior and posterior cerebellar incisurae; the brainstem fits into the anterior cerebellar incisura and the falx cerebelli fits into the posterior cerebellar incisura. The margins are the anterosuperior margin, the posterior wall of the cerebellomesencephalic fissure; the anterolateral margin, which separates the tentorial from the petrosal surfaces; and the posterolateral margin, which separates the tentorial from the suboccipital surfaces. The vermis and the hemispheric counterpart of the tentorial surface are from anterior to posteriorly: lingula (without hemispheric correspondent), central lobule (wing of the central lobule), culmen (quadrangular lobule), declive (simple lobule), and folium (part of the superior semilunar lobule), being the primary fissure between the quadrangular and simple lobule, and the most prominent fissure, the postclival fissure located between the simple and the superior semilunar lobules. The tentorial surface presents the cerebellomesencephalic or precentral cerebellar fissure, which is located between the cerebellum and the midbrain. The interpeduncular or interbrachial sulcus, which separates the superior from the middle cerebellar peduncles, ascends from the bottom of the cerebellomesencephalic fissure toward the lateral aspect of the pons, where it is joined by the pontomesencephalic sulcus to proceed superiorly as the lateral mesencephalic sulcus to the medial geniculate body; the lateral mesencephalic sulcus separates the crus cerebri or from the tegmentum (Fig. 4.11c).

Among the cerebellar nuclei (fastigial, globose, emboliform, and dentate), the dentate nucleus is the most laterally located and the largest one. As the majority of the fibers that constitutes the superior cerebellar peduncle arise from the dentate nucleus, this nucleus is located at the posterior projection of the superior cerebellar peduncle (Fig. 4.11c).

Suboccipital Surface of the Cerebellum and Fourth Ventricle

It is located below the transverse and the sigmoid sinuses, and its surface faces inferiorly, almost parallel to the ground; therefore, for a better visualization of this surface either in surgery or for anatomical studies, the head or the cerebellum has to be bended forward.

The suboccipital surface presents the posterior cerebellar incisura, and the vermohemispheric or paravermian fissure, which separates the inferior vermis from the cerebellar hemisphere. The components of the inferior vermis and its hemispheric correspondents are folium (superior semilunar lobule), tuber (inferior semilunar lobule), pyramid (biventral lobule), uvula (tonsil), and nodule (flocculus). In the anatomical position, the most inferior part of the inferior vermis is the pyramid. The most prominent fissure on the suboccipital surface is the great horizontal fissure or suboccipital fissure, which is a circumferential fissure that begins in the posterior cerebellar notch between the folium and the tuber and runs forward and slightly downward on the suboccipital surface, between the superior and the inferior semilunar lobules, and then onto the petrosal surface as the petrosal fissure. The secondary fissure is located between the tonsils and the biventral lobule (Fig. 4.11d).

After the removal of the tonsils, the inferior portion of the roof of the fourth ventricle comes to the view (Fig. 4.12a). After the removal of the inferior portion of the roof of the fourth ventricle, the floor of the fourth ventricle is exposed.

The floor of the fourth ventricle has a rhomboid shape and presents a strip between the lower margin of the cerebellar peduncles and the site of attachment of the tela choroidea; this strip called junctional part is characterized by the striae medullary that extends into the lateral recesses. The junctional part divides the floor of the fourth ventricle into two unequal triangles, the superior and larger one, with its apex directed to the aqueduct, is the pontine part, and the inferior and smaller one with its apex directed toward the obex, is the medullary part of the floor. These three parts of the floor are also divided longitudinally into two symmetrical halves by the median sulcus. The sulcus limitans, another longitudinal sulcus, divides each half of the floor into a raised median strip called the median eminence and a lateral strip called area vestibular. The motor nuclei of the cranial nerves are located medially to the sulcus limitans, and the sensory nuclei are located laterally to it. The pontine part is characterized by two rounded prominences, facial colliculi, located on the median eminence, one on each side of the median sulcus. The facial colliculi is limited laterally by the superior fovea, a dimple formed by the sulcus limitans. The medullary part presents the configuration of a feather, or pen nib, called calamus scriptorius, with three triangular areas overlying the hypoglossal and vagus nuclei (hypoglossal and vagal trigones), and the area postrema; just lateral to the hypoglossal trigone, the sulcus limitans presents another dimple called inferior fovea. At the junctional part the sulcus limitans is discontinuous (Figs. 4.12b and 4.13b).

Veins of the Posterior Fossa

The posterior fossa venous system can be divided into three groups: (1) anterior or petrosal group that drains into the superior and inferior petrosal sinuses, (2) superior or galenic group that drains into the vein of Galen, and (3) posterior or tentorial group that drains into the sinuses near the torcula [37, 38].

There is a tendency for the veins to empty into the nearest draining system. The veins running on the petrosal surface of the cerebellum and the anterior surface of the brainstem tend to drain into the petrosal sinuses via superior petrosal veins (Fig. 4.14c), except those veins running on the surface of the midbrain that drain to the vein of Galen (Fig. 4.13d).

The tentorial surface of the cerebellum and the posterior aspect of the brainstem are enclosed within the three draining systems: the anterior portion of the tentorial surface tends to drain into the galenic system; the lateral portion of the tentorial surface of the cerebellum tends to drain into the superior petrosal sinus; the posterior portion of the tentorial surface of the cerebellum tends to drain into the tentorial sinus located in the tentorium cerebella (Fig. 4.14a).

The veins draining the suboccipital surface of the cerebellum tend to empty into the torcula or into the transverse sinus or into the sinuses located in the tentorium cerebelli (Fig. 4.11d).

Arteries of the Posterior Fossa

The arteries supplying the posterior fossa are vertebral artery, posterior inferior cerebellar artery (PICA), basilar artery, anterior inferior cerebellar artery (AICA), and superior cerebellar artery (SCA).

The Vertebral Artery (VA)

The vertebral artery arises on each side from the subclavian artery, then enters the transverse foramen of the C6 and ascends through the transverse foramina of the upper cervical vertebrae up to the C2. After exiting from the transverse foramen of the C2, the VA deviates laterally to enter the transverse foramen of C1. The VA then turns behind the lateral mass of C1, above the posterior arch of the C1 to course medially and superiorly to pierce the dura at the foramen magnum (Figs. 4.11d, 4.13b, and 4.14d). At this point, the VA usually gives off the posterior meningeal and posterior spinal arteries. The intradural segment of VA is divided into lateral segment and anterior medullary segments before joining its contralateral mate to form the basilar artery (Fig. 4.14b–d).

The lateral medullary segment extends from its entrance into the posterior fossa to the preolivary sulcus, and it is related to the rootlets of the IX, X, and XI nerves.

The anterior medullary segment begins at the preolivary sulcus, and it is related to the rootlets of the hypoglossal nerve and crosses the pyramid to join with the other VA at or near the pontomedullary sulcus to form the basilar artery (Fig. 4.14b, c).

The main branches of the VA are the posterior spinal, anterior spinal, PICA, and anterior and posterior meningeal arteries. The VA also sends off branches to supply the lateral and anterior parts of the medulla along its way around the medulla.

The Posterior Inferior Cerebellar Artery (PICA)

The PICA supplies the medulla, the inferior vermis, the inferior portion of the fourth ventricle, the tonsils, and the inferior aspect of the cerebellum. It is the most important branch of the VA (Fig. 4.14c), and its area of supply is the most variable of the cerebellar arteries. The PICA gives off perforating, choroidal, and cortical arteries.

The "normal" PICA has the most complex and variable course of the cerebellar arteries and is divided into five segments [39] (Fig. 4.14d): (1) anterior medullary segment which extends from its origin to the inferior olive; (2) lateral medullary segment, which extends from the inferior olive to the origin of the IX, X, and XI nerves; (3) tonsillomedullary or posterior medullary segment, which begins at the level of the lower cranial nerves and loops below the inferior pole of the cerebellar tonsil and upward along the medial surface of the tonsil; (4) telovelotonsillar or supratonsillar segment, which courses in the cleft between the tela choroidea of the fourth ventricle and the medial surface of the tonsil, loops over the superior pole of the tonsil (cranial loop), and divides into vermian and hemispheric branches; and (5) cortical segment, which begins a short distance distal to the cranial loop, where it usually divides into two major branches (tonsillohemispheric (to the cerebellar hemisphere) and inferior vermian (to the inferior vermis) branches) (Fig. 4.11d).

The Basilar Artery

The basilar artery is formed by the junction of the two vertebral arteries. As a single vascular trunk, it usually courses superiorly in a shallow median groove on the anterior surface of the pons. It extends from the pontomedullary sulcus, which demarcates the rostral medulla and caudal pons, to the level of the emerging oculomotor nerves from the caudal midbrain. The basilar artery is often tortuous and may be slightly curved in its rostral course along the brainstem. The basilar artery may deviate a short distance off the midline, but a few will deviate laterally as far as the origin of the abducent nerve or the facial and vestibulocochlear nerves. Its length varies from 2.5 to 4.0 cm, and after passing between the two oculomotor nerves, the artery terminates by dividing into the two posterior cerebral arteries (Fig. 4.14b, c).

In its course the basilar artery gives off the following branches on both sides: pontine, labyrinthine, anterior inferior cerebellar, superior cerebellar, and posterior cerebral arteries. The pontine branches of the basilar artery consist of a number of small vessels that supply the pons and midbrain. Median vessels arise at right angles from the posterior aspect of the basilar and enter the pons along its anterior median groove (Fig. 4.14b, c). The transverse branches arise from the posterolateral and lateral aspects of the basilar artery, and in their circumferential course around the brainstem, they send penetrating vessels into the pons.

Anterior Inferior Cerebellar Artery (AICA)

The AICA and PICA are defined according to their origin rather than by the portion of the cerebellum that they supply. The AICA by definition is originated from the basilar artery (usually at it lower third) and the PICA from the vertebral artery. The AICA usually supplies the base and the tegmentum of the pons, and the most anterior undersurface of the cerebellum. The AICA originates from the basilar artery, usually as a single trunk, and encircles the pons near the abducent, facial, and vestibulocochlear nerve. After coursing near and sending branches to the nerves entering the internal acoustic meatus and to the choroid plexus protruding from the foramen of Luschka, it passes around the flocculus on the middle cerebellar peduncle to supply the lips of the cerebellopontine fissure and the petrosal surface of the cerebellum.

The AICA presents the following segments: anterior pontine, lateral pontine, flocculonodular, and cortical segments [40]:

The anterior pontine segment begins at the origin from the basilar artery and ends at the level of a line drawn through the long axis of the inferior olive and extending upward on the pons, and is located between the clivus and the belly of the pons; the AICA usually lies in contact with the rootlets of the abducent nerve.

The lateral pontine segment begins at the anterolateral margin of the pons and passes through the cerebellopontine angle, above, below, or between the facial and vestibulocochlear nerves and is intimately related to the internal auditory meatus, to the lateral recess, and to the choroid plexus protruding from the foramen of Luschka. This segment gives rise to the nerve-related branches that course near or within the internal acoustic meatus in close relationship to the facial and vestibulocochlear nerves: the labyrinthine arteries that are the one or more branches of the AICA that enter the internal auditory canal and send branches to the bone and dura lining the internal auditory canal, to the nerve within the canal, and terminate by giving rise to the vestibular, cochlear, and vestibulocochlear arteries that supply the organs of the inner ear (Fig. 4.14b, c). The recurrent perforating arteries arise from the nerve-related vessels and often travel from their origin toward the meatus, occasionally looping into the meatus before taking a recurrent course along the facial and vestibulocochlear nerves to reach the brainstem. They send branches to these nerves and to the brainstem surrounding the entry zone of those nerves. The subarcuate artery usually originates medial to the porus, penetrates the dura covering the subarcuate fossa, and enters the subarcuate canal. This artery supplies the petrous bone in the region of the semicircular canals. The subarcuate canal is recognized as a potential route of extension of infections from the mastoid region to the meninges and to the superior petrosal sinus.

The flocculonodular segment begins where the artery passes rostral or caudal to the flocculus to reach the middle cerebellar peduncle and the cerebellopontine fissure. The trunks that course along the peduncle may be hidden beneath the flocculus or in the lips of the cerebellopontine fissure (Fig. 4.14b, d).

The cortical segment is composed of the cortical branches to the petrosal surface of the cerebellum.

The AICA is divided into the rostral and caudal trunks near the facial-vestibulocochlear nerve complex. After crossing the nerves, the rostral trunk usually courses laterally above the flocculus to reach the surface of the middle cerebellar peduncle and the petrosal fissure to be distributed to the superior lip of the cerebellopontine fissure and to the adjoining part of the petrosal surface. The caudal trunk supplies the inferior part of the petrosal surface, including a part of the flocculus and the choroid plexus and is frequently related to the lateral portion of the fourth ventricle. If the bifurcation is proximal to the facial and vestibulocochlear nerve, the caudal trunk courses caudal to the flocculus to supply the inferior part of the petrosal surface, including a part of the flocculus and the choroid plexus. If the bifurcation is distal to the nerves, the caudal trunk courses posteriorly in the inferior limb of the cerebellopontine fissure near the foramen of Luschka. The distal branches of the caudal trunk often anastomose with the PICA, and those from the rostral trunk anastomose with the SCA. The most common pattern is for the AICA to supply the majority of the petrosal surface of the cerebellum, but the cortical area of the supply is quite variable. It can vary from a small area on the flocculus and adjacent part of the petrosal surface to include the whole petrosal surface and adjacent part of the tentorial and suboccipital surfaces of the cerebellum.

The Superior Cerebellar Artery (SCA)

The SCA is the most rostral of the infratentorial vessels, and it arises near the apex of the basilar artery and encircles the pons and the lower midbrain. It supplies the tentorial surface of the cerebellum, the midbrain tegmentum, the deep cerebellar nuclei, and the inferior colliculus [41]. The SCA presents the following segments (Figs. 4.12c, 4.13a, and 4.14b–d):

The anterior pontomesencephalic segment extends from its origin to the anterolateral margin of the brainstem. It courses laterally on the anterior aspect of the upper pons, usually in an arcuate curve convex inferiorly; at the anterolateral margin of the brainstem, it lies inferior to the oculomotor nerve (Figs. 4.12c, 4.13a, and 4.14c).

The lateral pontomesencephalic segment begins at the anterolateral margin of the brainstem and follows caudally onto the lateral side of the upper pons in the infratentorial portion of the ambient cistern to terminate into the cerebellomesencephalic fissure. The bifurcation of the SCA into its rostral and caudal trunks often occurs in this segment; while the rostral trunk supplies the vermis, and a variable portion of the adjacent tentorial surface, the caudal trunk supplies the tentorial surface lateral to the area supplied by the rostral trunk.

The cerebellomesencephalic segment courses in the cerebellomesencephalic fissure through a series of hairpin-like curves; it then passes upward to reach the anterosuperior margin of the cerebellum. Inside the cerebellomesencephalic fissure, the cortical branches from the rostral and caudal trunks send off small arterial twig branches called precentral arteries. Those precentral arteries arising from the rostral trunk supply the inferior colliculus, and those arising from the inferior trunk supply the deep cerebellar nuclei (Fig. 4.11c). The cortical segment supplies the tentorial surface of the cerebellum and is divided into hemispheric and vermian groups. The cortical surface of each half of the vermis is divided into median and paramedian segments, and each hemisphere lateral to the vermis is divided into medial, intermediate, and lateral segments (Fig. 4.11c).

Acknowledgment We want to acknowledge that Dr. Antônio CM Mussi was a coauthor on the previous edition of this chapter. This first edition chapter served as inspiration for this second edition chapter.

References

1. Ono M, Kubik S, Abernathey CD. Atlas of the cerebral sulci. Stuttgart: Georg Thieme Verlag; 1990.
2. Naidich T, Valavanis A, Kubik S. Anatomic relationships along the low-middle convexity. I. Normal specimens and magnetic resonance imaging. Neurosurgery. 1995;36:517–32.
3. Gibo H, Caarver CC, Rhoton Jr AL. Microsurgical anatomy of the middle cerebral artery. J Neurosurg. 1981;54:151–69.
4. Szikla G, Bourvier T, Hori T, et al. Angiography of the human brain cortex. Berlin: Springer; 1977.
5. Wen HT, Mussi ACM, Rhoton Jr AL. Surgical anatomy of the brain. In: Winn HR, editor. Youmans neurological surgery. 5th ed. Philadelphia: Saunders; 2003. p. 5–44.
6. Wolf BS, Huang YP. The insula and deep middle cerebral venous drainage system: normal anatomy and angiography. Am J Roentgenol Radium Ther Nucl Med. 1963;90:472–89.
7. Timurkaynak E, Rhoton Jr AL, Barry M. Microsurgical anatomy and operative approaches to the lateral ventricles. Neurosurgery. 1986;19:685–723.
8. Wen HT, Rhoton Jr AL, de Oliveira E, et al. Microsurgical anatomy of the temporal lobe: Part 1 Mesial temporal lobe and its vascular relationship as applied to amygdalohippocampectomy. Neurosurgery. 1999;45:549–92.
9. Warwick R, Williams PL. Gray's anatomy. 35th ed. Philadelphia: WB Saunders; 1973.
10. Williams PL. Gray's anatomy. 38th ed. London: Churchill Livingstone; 1995.
11. Duvernoy HM. The human hippocampus: an atlas of applied anatomy. Munich: JF Bergmann Verlag; 1988.
12. Gloor P. The temporal lobe and limbic system. New York: Oxford University Press; 1997.
13. Nagata S, Rhoton Jr AL, Barry M. Microsurgical anatomy of the choroidal fissure. Surg Neurol. 1988;30:3–59.
14. Wen HT, Rhoton Jr AL, de Oliveira E. Transchoroidal approach to the third ventricle: an anatomic study of the choroidal fissure and its clinical application. Neurosurgery. 1998;42:1205–19.

15. Yamamoto I, Rhoton Jr AL, Peace D. Microsurgery of the third ventricle: Part 1. Microsurgical anatomy. Neurosurgery. 1981;8:334–56.

16. Rhoton Jr AL. Microsurgical anatomy of the third ventricular region. In: Apuzzo MLJ, editor. Surgery of the third ventricle region. Baltimore: Williams & Wilkins; 1987. p. 570–90.

17. Apuzzo MLJ, Giannotta SL. Transcallosal interforniceal approach. In: Apuzzo MLJ, editor. Surgery of the third ventricle region. Baltimore: Williams & Wilkins; 1987. p. 354–80.

18. Yasargil MG. Microneurosurgery: AVM of the brain, vol. IIIB. Stuttgart: Georg Thieme Verlag; 1988.

19. Oka K, Rhoton Jr AL, Barry M, et al. Microsurgical anatomy of the superficial veins of the cerebrum. Neurosurgery. 1985; 17:711–48.

20. Wolf BS, Huang YP, Newman CM. The superficial sylvian venous drainage system. Am J Roentgenol Radium Ther Nucl Med. 1963;89:398–410.

21. Ono M, Rhoton Jr AL, Peace D, et al. Microsurgical anatomy of the deep venous system of the brain. Neurosurgery. 1984;15:621–57.

22. Taveras JM, Wood EH. Diagnostic neuroradiology. Baltimore: Williams & Wilkins; 1964.

23. Huang YP, Wolf BS. The basal cerebral vein and its tributaries. In: Newton TH, Potts DG, editors. Radiology of the skull and brain, vol. 2, book 3. St. Louis: C.V. Mosby; 1974. p. 2111–54.

24. Gibo H, Lenkey C, Rhoton Jr AL. Microsurgical anatomy of the supraclinoid portion of the internal carotid artery. J Neurosurg. 1981;55:560–74.

25. Rhoton Jr AL, Fujii K, Fradd B. Microsurgical anatomy of the anterior choroidal artery. Surg Neurol. 1979;12:171–87.

26. Zeal AA, Rhoton Jr AL. Microsurgical anatomy of the posterior cerebral artery. J Neurosurg. 1978;48:534–59.

27. Lin JP, Kricheff II. The anterior cerebral artery complex: 1. Normal anterior cerebral artery complex. In: Newton TH, Potts DG, editors. Radiology of the skull and brain, vol. 2, book 2. St. Louis: C.V. Mosby; 1974. p. 1391–410.

28. Yasargil MG. Microneurosurgery: microsurgical anatomy of the basal cisterns and vessels of the brain, vol. 1. Stuttgart: Georg Thieme Verlag; 1984.

29. Perlmutter D, Rhoton Jr AL. Microsurgical anatomy of the anterior cerebral-anterior communicating-recurrent artery complex. J Neurosurg. 1976;45:259–72.

30. Hung TP, Ryu SJ. Anterior cerebral artery syndromes. In: Vinken PJ, Bruyn GW, Klawans HL, editors. Handbook of clinical neurology, vol. 53, part 1. Amsterdam: Elsevier Science; 1988. p. 339–52.

31. Salamon G, Lazorthes G. Tumors of the basal ganglia: an angiographic study. Neuroradiology. 1971;2:80–9.

32. Westberg G. Arteries of the basal ganglia. Acta Radiol Diagn. 1966;5:581–96.

33. Salamon G, Huang YP. Radiologic anatomy of the brain. Berlin: Springer; 1976. p. 332–44.

34. Rhoton Jr AL. The posterior cranial fossa: microsurgical anatomy and surgical approaches. Neurosurgery. 2000;47:S7–27.

35. Ghez C, Thach WT. The cerebellum. In: Kandel ER, Schwartz JH, Jessel TM, editors. Principles of neuroscience. 4th ed. New York: Mc Graw Hill; 2000. p. 832–52.

36. Matsushima T, Rhoton Jr AL, Lenkey C. Microsurgery of the fourth ventricle: part 1. Microsurgical anatomy. Neurosurgery. 1982; 11:631–67.

37. Matsushima T, Rhoton Jr AL, de Oliveira E. Microsurgical anatomy of the veins of the posterior fossa. J Neurosurg. 1983;59:63–105.

38. Huang YP, Wolf BS. The veins of the posterior fossa-superior or galenic draining group. Am J Roentgenol. 1965;95:808–21.

39. Lister JR, Rhoton Jr AL, Matsushima T, et al. Microsurgical anatomy of the posterior inferior cerebellar artery. Neurosurgery. 1982;10:170–99.

40. Martin RG, Grant JL, Peace D, et al. Microsurgical relationships of the anterior inferior cerebellar artery and the facial vestibulocochlear nerve complex. Neurosurgery. 1980;6:483–507.

41. Hardy DG, Peace D, Rhoton Jr AL. Microsurgical anatomy of the superior cerebellar artery. Neurosurgery. 1980;6:10–28.

The Functional Organization of the Nervous System

William A. Friedman

5

Contents

Abstract

The nervous system is organized in such a way that a careful history and physical will almost always allow the clinician to localize the site of disease. This requires a basic knowledge of the neurological exam and the anatomy that underlies that exam. In this chapter we will review the examination of mental status, cranial nerves, motor, reflex, and sensory systems. We will then illustrate the application of those exams in multiple example cases.

Keywords

Neurological examination • Cranial nerves • Reflexes
Mental status • Motor function

Introduction

Central and peripheral nervous system diseases are different from most other medical problems in one fascinating and important way: The precise site of the neurological disorder can almost always be determined from a careful history and neurological examination. Once the site of disease is elucidated, a differential diagnosis, drawing from the basic categories of neurological illness, can be constructed. The history is particularly valuable in ordering the differential diagnosis from most to least probable. When this intellectual process is finished, appropriate diagnostic tests can be ordered. And, it is hoped, the precise diagnosis will then be established.

The Neurological Examination

The neurological examination is generally divided into the following parts: mental status, cranial nerves, motor examination (including cerebellar function), reflexes, and sensory examination. As in other parts of the physical exam, adhering to a strict order helps the physician avoid errors of omission.

W.A. Friedman, MD
Department of Neurological Surgery,
University of Florida College of Medicine,
Gainesville, FL 32010, USA
e-mail: friedman@neurosurgery.ufl.edu

A.J. Layon et al. (eds.), *Textbook of Neurointensive Care*,
DOI 10.1007/978-1-4471-5226-2_5, © Springer-Verlag London 2013

Mental Status

Examination of mental status focuses on level of consciousness, orientation, memory, emotional state, and higher cortical functions (including language). Orientation is typically tested to person, place, and time. Patients are frequently described as "oriented times three." Typically, recent memory is tested by asking the patient to remember three objects and then testing them 2 and 5 min later for recall. Long-term memory may be tested by asking for their address, phone number, the names of presidents, capitals, etc.

Altered states of consciousness are described by a variety of terms including, in order of severity, clouded, lethargic, obtunded, stuporous, and comatose. Clouding of consciousness refers to a mildly depressed level of awareness and slowing of mentation. A "lethargic" patient will lie quietly or sleep in the absence of stimulation but can interact fairly well when prompted. An "obtunded" patient will sleep in the absence of stimulation, can be aroused with some difficulty, and has generally depressed intellectual function. A "stuporous" patient requires vigorous stimulation to provoke any arousal and is incapable of meaningful verbal exchange. A "comatose" patient fits the following precise definition: "incapable of following commands, does not speak, and does not open eyes to pain." Dementia, unlike the previous descriptors, refers only to a loss of intellectual function and does not imply any alteration of consciousness.

Unfortunately, the terms described previously are rather imprecise. In order to eliminate interobserver variability in describing decreased levels of consciousness, the Glasgow Coma Scale was developed. It relies upon three simple tests: best eye opening response, best verbal response, and best motor response (Fig. 5.1). The worst score is 3 and the best score is 15. The definition of coma cited earlier corresponds to a GCS score of 8 or less.

The differential diagnosis of coma is broad. It includes toxic/metabolic disorders like electrolyte imbalance, endocrine dysfunction, toxin ingestion, infection, nutritional deficiency, organ failure, and epilepsy. A wide variety of structural disorders can also cause coma, including hemorrhage, ischemic stroke, brain abscess, brain tumor, and trauma.

A variety of disorders of "higher cortical function" can occur without alteration of consciousness. The most important are those which disturb language function. Disorders affecting the ability to use speech are called aphasias. Broca's aphasia refers to a disorder affecting the posterior inferior left frontal lobe (Brodmann's area 45). It produces difficulty with speech output but has little effect of speech understanding. Wernicke's aphasia involves the posterior superior left temporal lobe (Brodmann's area 22). It causes loss of ability to understand spoken or written language, but speech output remains fluent (although nonsensical). A rarer disorder, called conduction aphasia, refers to a condition where understanding a spontaneous speech is relatively preserved,

Fig. 5.1 The Glasgow Coma Scale (Modified with permission of Elsevier from Teasdale and Jennett [1])

Eye opening

Spontaneous	⟹	4
To speech	⟹	3
To pain	⟹	2
None	⟹	1

Best verbal response

Oriented	⟹	5
Confused speech	⟹	4
Inappropriate	⟹	3
Incomprehensible	⟹	2
None	⟹	1

Best motor response

Obeys commands	⟹	6
Localizes pain	⟹	5
Withdraws	⟹	4
Abnormal flexion	⟹	3
Extension	⟹	2
None	⟹	1

with loss of the ability to repeat. This results from lesion in the pathways which connect Broca's and Wernicke's areas (Figs. 5.2 and 5.3). In general, perisylvian lesions are associated with loss of the ability to repeat, while deeper lesions produce the so-called "transcortical aphasias" which are associated with preserved repetition.

Gerstmann's syndrome refers to a constellation of four neurological findings: finger agnosia, alexia, acalculia, and agraphia. It is usually found with lesions of the left inferior parietal lobe. Alexia without agraphia can be seen with lesions of the dominant occipital lobe, when they extend into the splenium of the corpus callosum.

A detailed discussion of the fascinating varieties of higher cortical dysfunction and their localization is beyond the scope of this chapter.

Cranial Nerves (Fig. 5.4)

The Olfactory Nerve

The olfactory nerve mediates the sense of smell. This can be tested by asking the patient to identify vials containing common substances (coffee, orange extract, etc.) by smell alone while alternately occluding each nostril. The olfactory

Fig. 5.2 Brodmann's cytoarchitectonic map. Most cerebral cortex consists of six layers. The anatomy of each layer may vary depending on whether that area is more sensory, motor, or associative in function. Brodmann sliced the brain horizontally, starting from the *top*, and assigned *numbers* to each new area of cortex. These "Brodmann's numbers" are still used to refer to different anatomical areas of the brain (With permission of David Peace, Illustrator. Reproduced with permission from Friedman et al. [2])

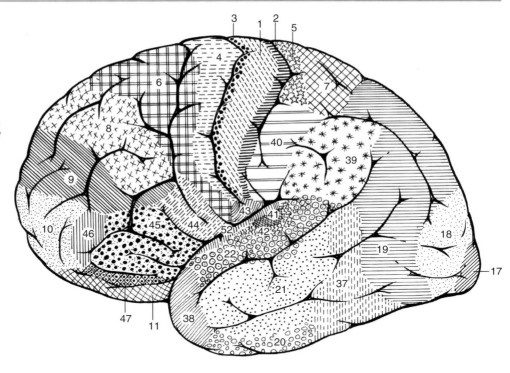

Fig. 5.3 A "functional" map of the brain shows the expected deficit from focal lesions. Lesions in Wernicke's area (Brodmann 22) tend to produce an aphasia where comprehension is lost but speech is fluent. Lesions in Broca's area (Brodmann 45) produce an aphasia with relatively preserved comprehension but lack of speech output (With permission of David Peace, Illustrator. Reproduced with permission from Friedman et al. [2])

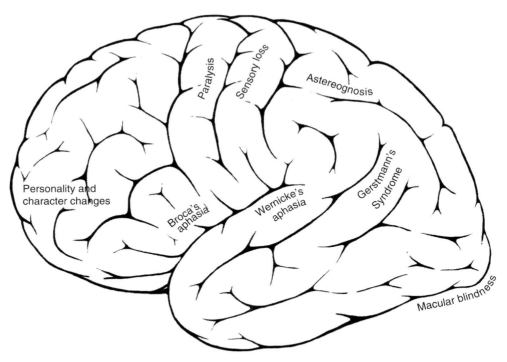

nerve is the most frequently injured by head trauma. It can also be affected by neoplasms growing near the olfactory groove area intracranially, including meningiomas and esthesioneuroblastomas.

The Optic Nerve

The optic nerve connects the retina to the optic chiasm and, hence, to the posterior visual pathways (Fig. 5.5). Unlike other cranial nerves, it can be directly viewed via the fundoscopic examination. Increased intracranial pressure will often be manifest as papilledema of the optic nerve head. Longstanding pressure or inflammation of the optic nerve will produce fundoscopically visible optic pallor (optic atrophy). The most valuable localizing test of visual pathway function involves "visual fields." Visual fields are tested in the clinic by having the patient occlude one eye. The examiner then directs the patient to look straight ahead and tests his ability to count fingers in the

Fig. 5.4 Anterior inferior view of the brain shows the 12 paired cranial nerves (With permission of David Peace, Illustrator. Reproduced with permission from Friedman et al. [2])

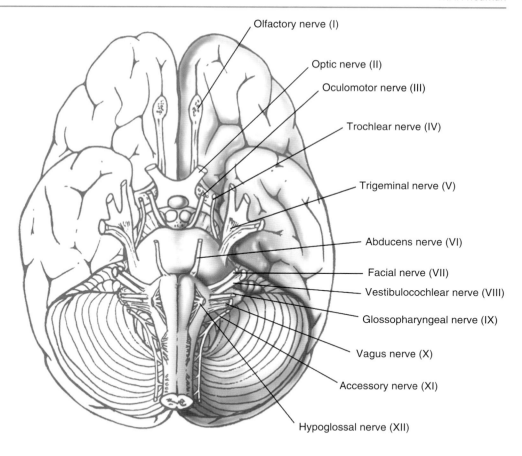

Olfactory nerve (I)

Optic nerve (II)

Oculomotor nerve (III)

Trochlear nerve (IV)

Trigeminal nerve (V)

Abducens nerve (VI)

Facial nerve (VII)

Vestibulocochlear nerve (VIII)

Glossopharyngeal nerve (IX)

Vagus nerve (X)

Accessory nerve (XI)

Hypoglossal nerve (XII)

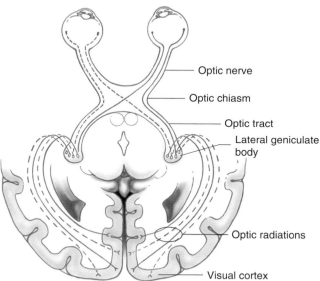

Optic nerve

Optic chiasm

Optic tract

Lateral geniculate body

Optic radiations

Visual cortex

Fig. 5.5 The optic nerves meet at the optic chiasm. The optic tracts run from the chiasm to the lateral geniculate nuclei of the thalamus. The optic radiations run from these nuclei to the primary visual cortex in the occipital lobe. The nasal retinal fibers cross in the chiasm, so a lesion there tends to produce the characteristic "bitemporal visual field cut." Lesions of the tract, radiations, or occipital lobe tend to produce complete loss of vision on the opposite side (a homonymous hemianopia) (With permission of David Peace, Illustrator. Reproduced with permission from Friedman et al. [2])

four quadrants of that eye's visual field. Formal visual fields can be performed by an ophthalmologist if this is abnormal. A variety of visual field abnormalities are described, which very accurately localize the site of the lesion within the nervous system (Fig. 5.6): unilateral visual loss, junctional scotoma, bitemporal hemianopia, and homonymous hemianopia.

The Oculomotor Nerve

The oculomotor nerve innervates the levator palpebrae, the medial rectus, the superior rectus, the inferior oblique, the inferior rectus, the pupilloconstrictor muscle, and the muscle which controls accommodation of the lens within the eye (Fig. 5.7). Lesions of the third nerve result in movement of the globe into a "down and out" position, ptosis, and pupillary dilatation. Temporal lobe herniation can produce a unilateral third nerve injury with, usually, contralateral hemiplegia. Direct compression of the third nerve by an aneurysm or tumor can produce these findings, as can diabetes or stroke.

The Trochlear Nerve

The trochlear nerve innervates the superior oblique muscle (Fig. 5.8). Lesions of this nerve result in vertical diplopia, with the affected eye elevated and externally rotated. The patient will attempt to correct the condition by tilting their head away from the affected side (to internally rotate the eye). The trochlear nerve is rarely affected in isolation, but frequently affected in combination with the III nerve and VI nerve by lesions of the cavernous sinus area.

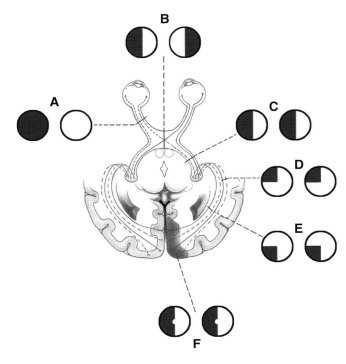

Fig. 5.6 Lesions in various parts of the visual pathways lead to very characteristic and localizing visual field defects: *A* optic nerve, *B* optic chiasm, *C* optic tract, *D* temporal optic radiations, *E* parietal optic radiations, *F* primary visual cortex (With permission of David Peace, Illustrator. Reproduced with permission from Friedman et al. [2])

The Trigeminal Nerve

The trigeminal nerve provides sensation to the face (Fig. 5.9). It has three divisions: The ophthalmic division innervates the forehead and eye; the maxillary division innervates the upper jaw and side of nose; and the mandibular division innervates the lower jaw, teeth, and tongue. The trigeminal nerve also innervates the muscles of mastication. Injuries to this nerve will result in ipsilateral loss of facial sensation and atrophy and weakness of the masseter muscle. This most frequently results from tumors (acoustic schwannoma, trigeminal schwannoma, nasopharyngeal carcinoma, etc.). The trigeminal nerve is also involved in a severe, lancinating pain disorder, called trigeminal neuralgia, which is frequently treated with surgery.

The Abducens Nerve

The abducens nerve innervates the lateral rectus muscle which moves the globe laterally (Fig. 5.10). Lesions of the nerve will produce inward deviation of the eye. Because of its long subarachnoid course, this nerve is commonly affected by increased intracranial pressure which can produce unilateral or bilateral sixth nerve palsy (a so-called false localizing sign).

The Facial Nerve

The facial nerve innervates the muscles of facial expression (Fig. 5.11). It is also responsible for salivary gland activity, lacrimation, and taste over the anterior two thirds of the tongue. Peripheral lesions of the nerve (such as trauma or Bell's palsy) cause weakness of the upper and lower face. Lesions of the upper motor neuron pathways from the motor cortex innervating the facial nerve nucleus in the brainstem cause weakness of the contralateral lower face only. The upper face receives bilateral cortical innervation and remains normal. This type of facial paralysis is called a "central seventh."

Fig. 5.7 The oculomotor nerve exits the brainstem between the mesencephalon and pons and travels to the cavernous sinus and on to the orbit. The motor nucleus innervates multiple extraocular muscles. The Edinger–Westphal nucleus provides parasympathetic innervation to the pupil and the lens of the eye (With permission of David Peace, Illustrator. Reproduced with permission from Friedman et al. [2])

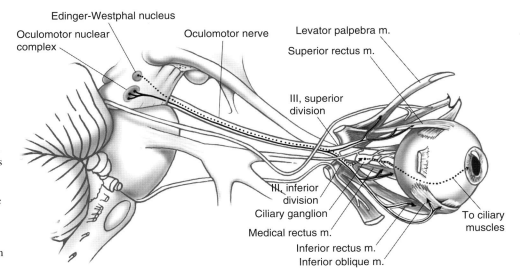

Edinger-Westphal nucleus

Oculomotor nuclear complex

Oculomotor nerve

Levator palpebra m.

Superior rectus m.

III, superior division

III, inferior division

Ciliary ganglion

Medical rectus m.

Inferior rectus m.

Inferior oblique m.

To ciliary muscles

The Vestibulocochlear Nerve

The vestibulocochlear nerve innervates the cochlea (the organ of hearing) and the vestibular complex (the organ of balance). Lesions of this nerve are seen after basilar skull fractures and with tumors of the cerebellopontine angle (usually acoustic schwannomas). Hearing is usually tested in clinic by determining whether a patient can hear fingers rubbing together outside the external ear canal. Formal audiometry is performed if this is abnormal.

The Glossopharyngeal Nerve

The glossopharyngeal nerve innervates the stylopharyngeus muscle, which is involved in swallowing (Fig. 5.12). This nerve supplies taste sensation to the posterior tongue. Lesions of the ninth nerve rarely occur in isolation, and section of the nerve usually does not result in any significant deficit.

The Vagus Nerve

The vagus nerve innervates most of the muscles responsible for swallowing and supplies sensory input to the pharynx as well (Fig. 5.13). Lesions of the nerve result in asymmetry of palatal movement. Of course, the vagus also supplies parasympathetic input to the heart and GI tract. The ninth, tenth, and eleventh nerves exit through the jugular foramen, where they can be jointly affected by tumors (especially jugular foramen schwannomas and meningiomas).

The Spinal Accessory Nerve

The spinal accessory nerve innervates the trapezius and sternocleidomastoid muscles (Fig. 5.14). These muscles are tested by shoulder shrug and head turning. Trauma is the most frequent cause of an isolated XI nerve injury; not infrequently, it is iatrogenic during surgery in the posterior cervical triangle.

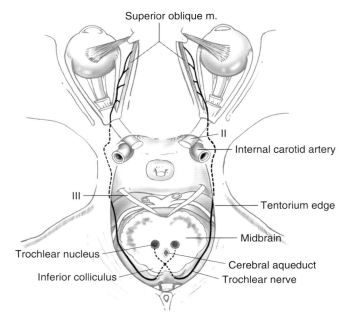

Fig. 5.8 The fourth cranial nerve is the only one which decussates (crosses midline). It exits just below the collicular plate and travels along the tentorium to the cavernous sinus. It enters the orbit and innervates one extraocular muscle – the superior oblique (With permission of David Peace, Illustrator. Reproduced with permission from Friedman et al. [2])

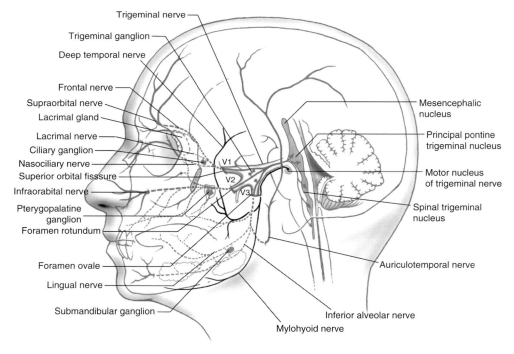

Fig. 5.9 The trigeminal nerve exits the brainstem at the pontine level. The trigeminal (Gasserian) ganglion is just lateral to the cavernous sinus. Three branches enter the cavernous sinus and innervate the face: the ophthalmic branch (V1), the maxillary branch (V2), and the mandibular branch (V3). The trigeminal nerve also mediates motor function (the muscles of mastication and the tensor tympani) (With permission of David Peace, Illustrator. Reproduced with permission from Friedman et al. [2])

Fig. 5.10 The sixth nerve nucleus is in the floor of the fourth ventricle. The nerve exits the *midline* at the junction of the pons and medullar. It travels along the clivus and through Dorello's canal to reach the cavernous sinus. This nerve innervates one extraocular muscle – the lateral rectus (With permission of David Peace, Illustrator. Reproduced with permission from Friedman et al. [2])

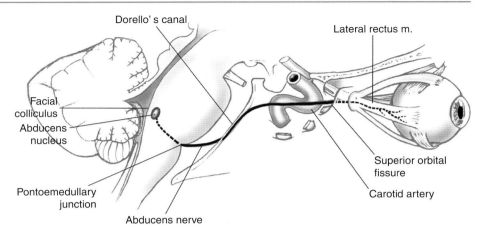

Fig. 5.11 The seventh nerve exits lateral to six, in the pontomedullary groove. It innervates the muscles of facial expression through multiple branches after exiting the stylomastoid foramen. This nerve also provides parasympathetic innervation to the geniculate and sphenopalatine ganglia and, hence, to the lacrimal and salivary glands. The chorda tympani branch provides taste sensation to the anterior two-thirds of the tongue (With permission of David Peace, Illustrator. Reproduced with permission from Friedman et al. [2])

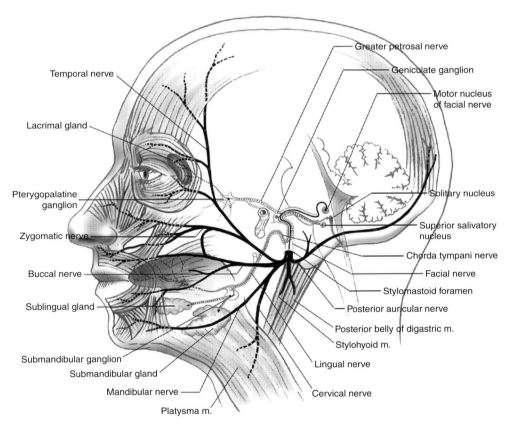

The Hypoglossal Nerve

The hypoglossal nerve innervates the muscles of the tongue. Dysfunction leads to protrusion of the tongue toward the affected side and atrophy of the affected side. This nerve may be affected by tumor, trauma, or stroke.

Motor Function

Motor function involves motor cortex of the brain, the corticospinal (and other descending) tracts, the motor pathways within the spinal cord, the motor neurons within the brainstem and spinal cord, the nerve roots, peripheral nerves, neuromuscular junction, and muscles. In addition, normal motor function is heavily dependent on complex circuitry within the basal ganglia and the cerebellum. Disease at any of these sites will lead to alterations in the motor examination and, in many cases, will clearly localize to a specific part of the nervous system (Fig. 5.15).

Diseases of the motor cortex and descending motor pathways are called "upper motor neuron" disorders and are characterized by weakness of the opposite side of the body,

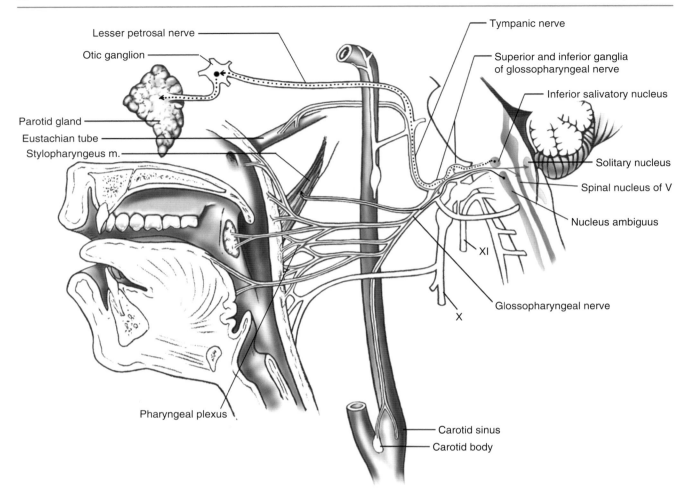

Fig. 5.12 The glossopharyngeal nerve provides motor innervation to the stylopharyngeus muscle and parasympathetic innervation to the parotid gland and carotid body (With permission of David Peace, Illustrator. Reproduced with permission from Friedman et al. [2])

lack of atrophy, spasticity, and increased reflexes (Fig. 5.16). Diseases of the motor neurons in the brainstem and spinal cord, as well as the peripheral and cranial nerves, are called "lower motor neuron" disorders (Fig. 5.17). They are characterized by weakness, atrophy, decreased tone, and decreased reflexes. Diseases of the neuromuscular junction (such as myasthenia gravis) result in fluctuating weakness affecting cranial and limb muscles, normal tone and reflexes, and no atrophy. Diseases affecting the muscle (like polymyositis) result in atrophy, weakness, and decreased reflexes and tone. Diseases affecting the basal ganglia and its related pathways (like Parkinson's disease) are called "extrapyramidal" disorders. They are frequently associated with normal strength, increased tone, unchanged reflexes, and tremor. Diseases of the cerebellar pathways can result in decreased tone and reflexes, normal strength, limb incoordination, and gait ataxia.

Examination of the motor systems should include evaluation for atrophy, changes in tone, strength, and coordination.

Strength is usually tabulated on a 0–5 scale: 0 is total paralysis; 1 is a visible flicker of movement only; 2 is movement weaker than antigravity; 3 is full movement against gravity; 4 is full movement overcome by resistance; and 5 is normal strength.

Coordination is tested by having the patient touch finger tip to nose and by observing gait. Lateral cerebellar lesions tend to affect extremity coordination. Vermian lesions tend to produce ataxic gait. In Parkinson's disease and other extrapyramidal disorders, gait tends to be stooped and shuffling. A hemiparesis will typically cause a spastic gait. Waddling gait is associated with muscular dystrophy affecting the hips.

Reflexes

The reflex examination centers on determination of the deep tendon reflex responses at the elbows, knees, and ankles.

Fig. 5.13 The vagus nerve provides motor innervation to the pharyngeal muscles and parasympathetic innervation to the heart and gut (With permission of David Peace, Illustrator. Reproduced with permission from Friedman et al. [2])

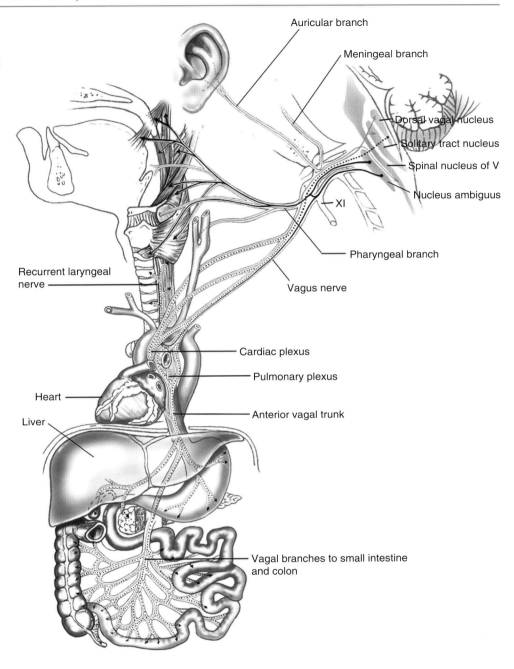

This reflex arc requires integrity of sensory neurons, motor neurons, and muscle. The rating is 0–4, with 0 signifying absence, 2+ being normal, and 4+ being very hyperactive. Hyperactive reflexes may be seen with upper motor neuron disease. Hypoactive reflexes may be seen with diseases of the peripheral nerve (i.e., polyneuritis), sensory root (i.e., tabes dorsalis), anterior horn cell (i.e., polio), proximal nerve root (i.e., lumbar disc herniation), peripheral motor nerve (i.e., trauma), and muscle (i.e., myopathy).

Various superficial (cutaneous) reflexes are "released" in upper motor neuron disease. The most commonly tested are the Babinski (Fig. 5.18), a dorsiflexion of the toes to plantar stimulation, and the Hoffman, twitching of the distal thumb in response to "flicking" the distal fingers (Fig. 5.19a, b).

Sensation

Pain and temperature sensation are mediated via the spinothalamic tracts, which cross in the spinal cord and ascend to the opposite side of the brainstem and cortex (Figs. 5.20 and 5.21). Touch and proprioception are mediated by the dorsal

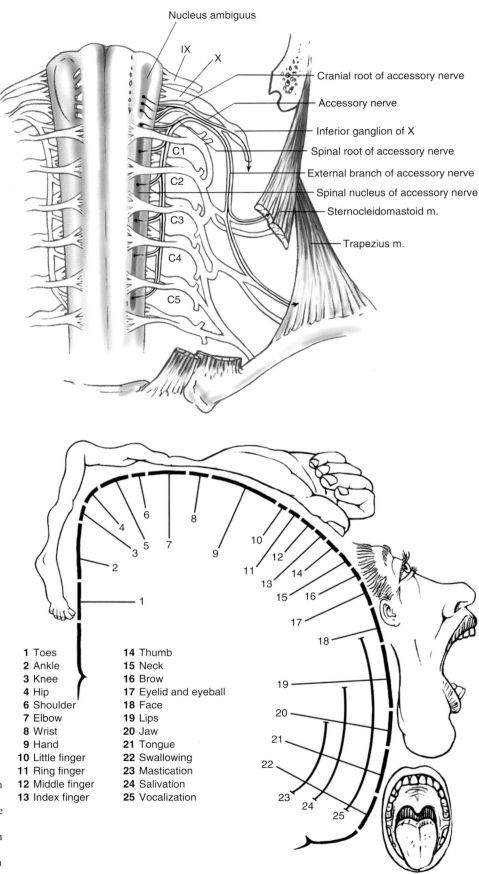

Fig. 5.14 The spinal accessory nerve has branches from the brainstem (nucleus ambiguous) and the upper cervical spinal cord. It provides motor innervation to the trapezius and sternocleidomastoid muscles (With permission of David Peace, Illustrator. Reproduced with permission from Friedman et al. [2])

Fig. 5.15 This coronal section through the primary motor strip of the brain illustrates the "motor homunculus." The parts of the body which are innervated by different motor strip areas are shown (With permission of David Peace, Illustrator. Reproduced with permission from Friedman et al. [2])

1 Toes	**14** Thumb
2 Ankle	**15** Neck
3 Knee	**16** Brow
4 Hip	**17** Eyelid and eyeball
6 Shoulder	**18** Face
7 Elbow	**19** Lips
8 Wrist	**20** Jaw
9 Hand	**21** Tongue
10 Little finger	**22** Swallowing
11 Ring finger	**23** Mastication
12 Middle finger	**24** Salivation
13 Index finger	**25** Vocalization

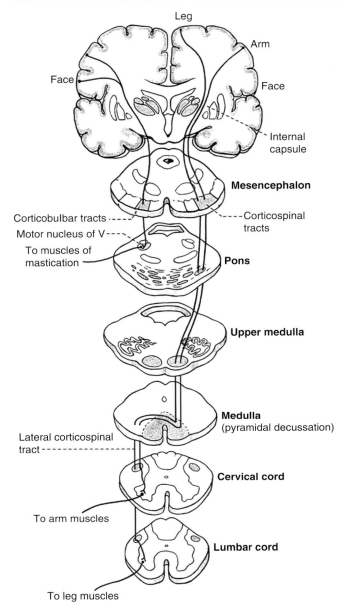

Fig. 5.16 The upper motor neuron fibers descend through the internal capsule into the ventral mesencephalon to the pyramids of the medulla. There the pathways decussate and form the corticospinal tracts in the posterolateral spinal cord (With permission of David Peace, Illustrator. Reproduced with permission from Friedman et al. [2])

columns of the spinal cord. These pathways remain ipsilateral until they reach the sensory decussation in the lower brainstem. Consequently, lesions of the hemispinal cord will result in loss of pain and temperature on the opposite side of the body and loss of touch and proprioception on the ipsilateral side of the body.

The sensory exam should include tests of pain fibers (pin), light touch (fingers), proprioception (checking that the patient can tell whether toes or fingers are being moved up or down), and vibration (tuning fork). Various patterns of sensory loss can localize to specific areas of the nervous system and/or to certain well-known disease processes (Figs. 5.22 and 5.23). For example: Loss of all sensory modalities in the distribution of one peripheral or cranial nerve clearly localizes to that nerve. Loss of all modalities below a given spinal level localizes to the spinal cord. Loss of sensation on one side of the face and the opposite side of the body localizes to the brainstem. Loss of sensation of one side of the body and face localizes to the opposite cerebrum. Loss of dorsal column modalities only usually indicates a metabolic disease such as B_{12} deficiency.

Clinical Anatomical Correlation in Neurological Disease

In this section of the chapter, we will briefly review the neurologic functions that commonly localize to the major anatomic divisions of the nervous system.

Brain

Frontal Lobe

The frontal lobes of the brain subserve many important neurologic functions. First, the frontal association areas are responsible for personality and level of energy. Frontal lobe lesions can result in apathy, inactivity, depression, changes in personality, inappropriate actions, etc. Severe bilateral frontal lobe injury leads to a condition called akinetic mutism. Alternatively, some frontal lesions lead to a sense of euphoria accompanied by inappropriate jocularity (witzelsucht).

The frontal eye fields (Brodmann's area 8) direct both eyes to the opposite side of the body. Damage to this area of the brain will frequently result in head and eye turning toward the side of injury. This is seen after trauma and stroke.

The posterior portion of the frontal lobes contains the primary motor cortex (Brodmann's area 4). This strip is organized in a somatotopic pattern, with face most inferior, then hand, then arm. Hip and shoulder are near the top of the strip. Leg function is localized to the mesial hemisphere. Injury to this area will result in paralysis of an "upper motor neuron" variety.

The inferior posterior surface of the dominant (usually left) frontal lobe is called Broca's area (Brodmann's area 45). This area of the brain mediates speech output. Injury to this area results in "Broca's aphasia," which is characterized by loss of spontaneous speech, inability to write, inability to repeat, but relatively preserved speech comprehension and reading ability.

Fig. 5.17 The corticospinal (and other) axons synapse with the motor neurons of the ventral spinal gray matter. The lower motor neuron axons exit through the ventral root and travel through the spinal roots and peripheral nerves to reach the neuromuscular junction. This diagram also illustrates the basic spinal reflex arc whereby stretch of the muscle spindle leads to synaptic connections with the motor neurons leading to the muscle involved in the reflex (With permission of David Peace, Illustrator. Reproduced with permission from Friedman et al. [2])

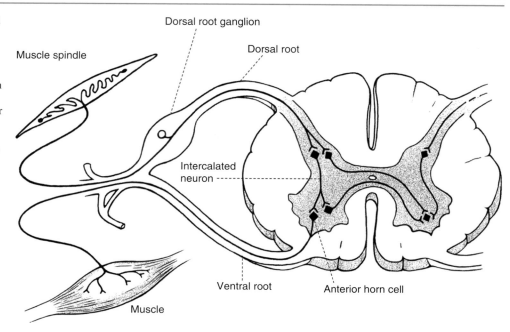

Fig. 5.18 The Babinski sign (With permission of David Peace, Illustrator. Reproduced with permission from Friedman et al. [2])

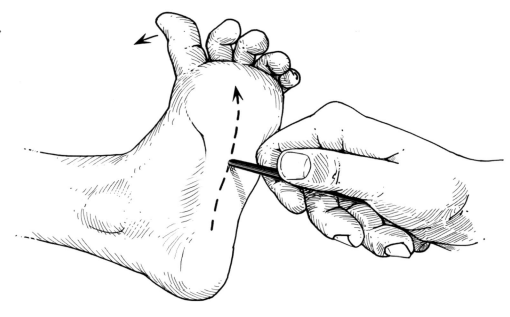

Temporal Lobe

The temporal lobes, especially the mesial limbic structures (including the hippocampus), are an important part of the neurologic circuits involved in memory. Disease of the temporal lobes, especially when bilateral, can lead to profound recent memory loss.

The dominant temporal lobe (usually left) is involved in language function. The posterior superior temporal gyrus is called Wernicke's area (Brodmann's area 22). Lesions of this area cause Wernicke's aphasia which is characterized by inability to understand spoken or written speech. Speech output is fluent but is nonsensical.

Lesions of both temporal tips can produce a condition called the Kluver–Bucy syndrome, which is characterized by oral automatisms and hypersexuality. This condition is rare and is most commonly seen with head trauma.

Parietal Lobe

The anterior parietal lobes contain the primary somatosensory cortex (Brodmann's areas 3,1,2). Like the motor strip, this area is organized somatotopically. Lesions of the primary sensory cortex cause loss of all sensory modalities in the corresponding opposite body parts. Posterior to the

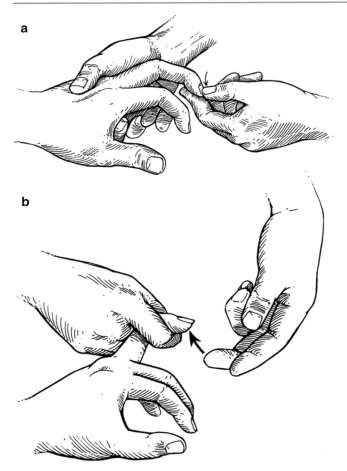

Fig. 5.19 The Hoffman (**a**) and Tromner (**b**) reflexes produce flexion of the distal thumb if upper motor neuron disease is present (With permission of David Peace, Illustrator. Reproduced with permission from Friedman et al. [2])

primary sensory cortex, in the superior parietal lobules, are the sensory association areas. Lesions of this area produce "agnosias" wherein objects cannot be recognized by sensory input even though the primary sensory modalities are intact. Parietal lesions can produce "neglect" of the opposite hemibody, wherein the patient tends to ignore stimuli to that side. Severe neglect can lead to autotopagnosia, or inability to recognize one's own body. Anosognosia refers to ignorance of the existence of disease and has been specifically applied to denial of hemiplegia. A more subtle test for parietal lobe dysfunction involves simultaneous stimulation of bilateral body parts. With parietal lesions, the sensation over the opposite body will frequently not be perceived.

The left inferior parietal lobe integrates many sensory modalities. Lesions in this area can produce Gerstmann's syndrome, which is characterized by finger agnosia, acalculia, left–right confusion (allochiria), and agraphia. Lesions in the angular gyrus area of the inferior parietal lobe are particularly likely to cause anomia, the inability to remember the names of objects.

The right parietal lobe is implicated in higher sensory processing as well. Lesions in this area can produce "dressing apraxia," wherein a patient cannot figure out how to properly put on clothing because of inability to integrate sensory information.

Occipital Lobe

The occipital lobes contain primary visual cortex. Lesions of the occipital lobe tend to produce loss of vision in the opposite visual fields of both eyes (homonymous hemianopia). The macular (central) fields may be spared.

Fig. 5.20 All sensory neurons reside in the dorsal root or brainstem ganglia. Sensory fibers enter the spinal cord through the dorsal root. Those mediating proprioception, vibration, and fine touch enter the dorsal columns and ascend ipsilaterally. Those mediating pain and temperature sensation cross the midline and ascend in the spinothalamic tracts (With permission of David Peace, Illustrator. Reproduced with permission from Friedman et al. [2])

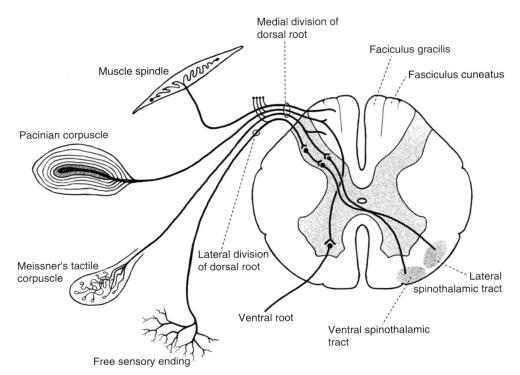

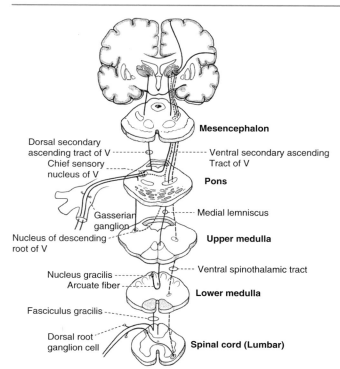

Fig. 5.21 The spinothalamic tracts ascend to the sensory thalamic nuclei and on to the sensory cortex. The dorsal column fibers synapse in the dorsal column nuclei of the medulla, decussate, and ascend to the thalamus and then to the cortex (With permission of David Peace, Illustrator. Reproduced with permission from Friedman et al. [2])

More anterior occipital areas contain visual association cortex. Lesions here will produce a variety of "visual agnosias." Inability to recognize faces is called "prosopagnosia."

Brainstem

The brainstem is usually divided into three parts: mesencephalon, pons, and medulla. The brainstem connects the cerebral hemispheres and deep structures to the spinal cord, so it contains the long motor and sensory tracts which connect these structures as well as all of the cranial nerve nuclei. Because so many important structures are crowded into such a small area, even small injuries to the brainstem produce highly localizable deficits. Large brainstem insults frequently produce coma or death.

Ventral mesencephalic lesions tend to produce an ipsilateral third nerve palsy and contralateral hemiplegia. This symptom complex, called Weber's syndrome, can be seen with stroke and tumors. Dorsal mesencephalic lesions often are associated with Parinaud's syndrome. Parinaud's syndrome is characterized by decreased papillary light reflex, preserved pupillary constriction to accommodation, paralysis of upgaze,

retraction–convergence nystagmus, and other anomalies. Parinaud's is most often seen with pineal region tumors but can also be seen with severe hydrocephalus.

Ventral pontine lesions produce an ipsilateral sixth nerve palsy and contralateral weakness (Millard–Gubler syndrome). This is most often seen with stroke. More dorsolateral lesions are associated with hearing loss, vertigo, facial weakness, and ataxia.

Ventral medullary lesions produced an ipsilateral twelfth nerve palsy and contralateral hemiplegia (Hughlings Jackson syndrome). Dorsal lateral lesions produce Wallenberg's syndrome. Wallenberg's syndrome is usually associated with vertebral artery occlusion and is characterized by dysphonia, Horner's syndrome, dysphagia, ataxia, ipsilateral facial numbness, and contralateral body numbness.

Many other brainstem syndromes have been described; a comprehensive review is beyond the scope of this chapter.

Spinal Cord

The spinal cord may be injured by trauma, tumor, degenerative disease, vascular lesions, infection, and metabolic disorders. A complete spinal cord injury results in loss of all motor and sensory function below the level of the lesion. If the thoracic cord is involved, this results in paraplegia. If the cervical cord is involved, quadriplegia is seen. In the acute phase of an injury, all reflexes are lost; this is termed "spinal shock." Because sympathetic outflow to the body is interrupted, hypotension associated with bradycardia is often seen. Gradually, reflexes return and, because of the upper motor neuron nature of the injury, become hyperactive.

A variety of partial spinal cord injury syndromes are commonly described. Brown-Sequard syndrome refers to a "hemispinal cord" injury, which can be produced by trauma or by neoplasm. This is characterized by loss of ipsilateral motor function, as well as proprioception and vibratory sensation below the lesion. Contralateral pain and temperature sensation are lost.

The anterior spinal artery syndrome is usually associated with trauma but can be caused by vascular disease of the aorta. It can be seen after prolonged clamp times during aortic aneurysm or coarctation repair. It is characterized by bilateral paralysis and loss of pain and temperature sensation, with preservation of dorsal column function (touch and proprioception).

The dorsal column syndrome refers to isolated injury of the dorsal columns, most commonly associated with metabolic disease. This results in loss of touch and proprioception below the lesion, with preservation of other function.

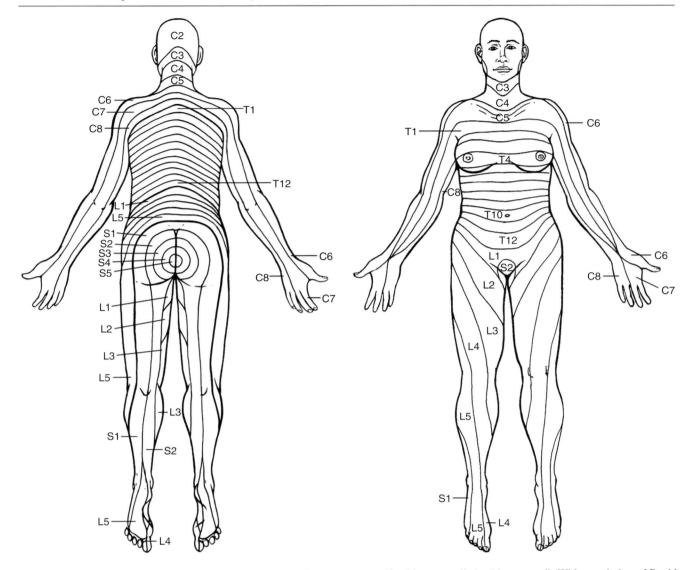

Fig. 5.22 Each spinal sensory root, from C2 to coccygeal 5, innervates a specific skin area, called a "dermatome" (With permission of David Peace, Illustrator. Reproduced with permission from Friedman et al. [2])

The motor neurons of the spinal cord can be selectively injured in certain diseases, including poliomyelitis, and some forms of amyotrophic lateral sclerosis. This results in weakness and atrophy of the associated muscles, without sensory loss.

Peripheral Nerve

The peripheral nerves contain motor and sensory axons. The cell bodies of origin of the sensory axons are found in the dorsal root ganglia. The cell bodies of origin of the motor axons are found in the ventral horn of the spinal cord. The

sensory axons subserve the many peripheral sensory organs, which convey pain, temperature, touch, special sensory function, etc. The motor axons conduct impulses from the lower motor neurons to the muscles.

Hundreds of disorders can affect the peripheral nerves. Peripheral nerve disease typically leads to weakness and atrophy of the involved muscles. Disease of a specific nerve will lead to sensory loss in the known distribution of that nerve. Generalized peripheral neuropathy tends to cause loss of sensation in a "stocking-glove" distribution, although there are many exceptions.

The reader is referred to several excellent texts for a detailed discussion of peripheral neuropathy [3–8].

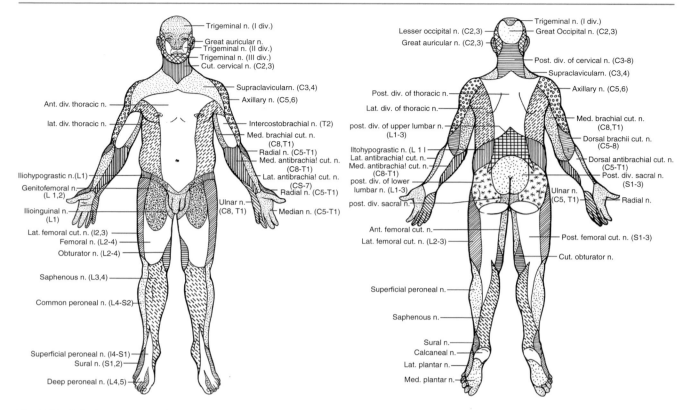

Fig. 5.23 Spinal nerves combine to form a multiple of peripheral nerves. Each peripheral nerve also has a known sensory skin representation. Careful attention to the sensory exam can localize the nervous system lesion to a peripheral nerve, a spinal nerve, the spinal cord, the brainstem, or the cerebrum (With permission of David Peace, Illustrator. Reproduced with permission from Friedman et al. [2])

Neuromuscular Junction

The synapse between the motor axon and the muscle is called the neuromuscular junction. It is probably the best studied and understood synapse in the body. Diseases of the neuromuscular junction (like myasthenia gravis) tend to produce fluctuating weakness, no signs of atrophy, and involvement of cranial and peripheral muscles and respond to anticholinesterase inhibitors.

Muscle

Diseases of muscle are called "myopathies." Myopathy can be congenital, metabolic, inflammatory, infectious, or can present as a remote effect of carcinoma. Myopathies are characterized by weakness, most frequently affecting the proximal more than the distal musculature. Often, atrophy is present, and reflexes are reduced. Muscle pain may be present, and muscle enzymes may be elevated.

Putting It All Together: Patient Examples

Case 1

An 80-year-old white male presents to the emergency room. His family says that he took a fall 1 month ago. His past medical history is significant for atrial fibrillation, for which he is anticoagulated with Coumadin. He and they have noticed progressive headache and, more recently, weakness of the right arm. Your neurological exam reveals 4/5 weakness of all muscles in the right arm and a right central seventh nerve paralysis.

Analysis

Where is the lesion? A right central seventh nerve paralysis means the lesion must affect the descending corticobulbar fibers to the seventh nerve nucleus, from the left brain. Likewise, the right arm weakness points to a left brain lesion affecting the motor pathways.

What is the lesion? The history tells us that he is anticoagulated and he took a fall. This strongly suggests traumatic hemorrhage. The fact that it has evolved is much more typical of subdural blood than epidural or intracerebral blood.

Management: You order a CT scan (Fig. 5.24). It confirms the presence of a large chronic and subacute subdural hematoma. The patient is taken to surgery for burr hole drainage and makes a complete recovery.

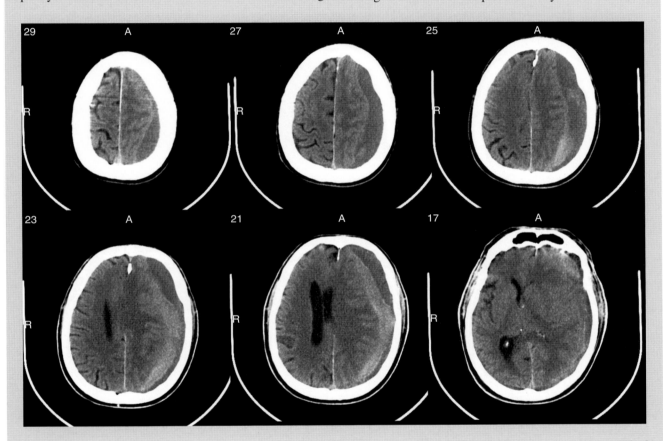

Fig. 5.24 Noncontrast computed tomography shows a chronic and subacute panhemispheric left subdural hematoma, producing shift of the ventricles from left to right

Case 2

A 53-year-old male presents to the emergency room with the history of sudden onset of severe headache, followed by nausea, vomiting, rapid onset of right-sided weakness, and decreased level of consciousness. His past medical history is significant for poorly controlled hypertension. Your neurological examination reveals coma (GCS < 7), with anisocoria (left pupil bigger than right) and right-sided decerebration.

Analysis

Where is the lesion? The sudden onset of symptoms is suggestive of a vascular event (stroke). The neurological exam shows a herniation syndrome, with dilated left pupil and right-sided decerebration. This localized to the left brain, above the level of the third nerve nucleus.

What is the lesion? The history of hypertension suggests the possibility of hypertensive intracerebral hemorrhage. Aneurysmal subarachnoid hemorrhage with an intracerebral component and/or hydrocephalus is another possibility. Less likely would be a tumor that bled or a vascular malformation.

Management: You order a CT scan (Fig. 5.25). It reveals intracerebral hemorrhage involving the left thalamus, basal ganglia, and midbrain, with spread to the left lateral ventricle. This patient, after detailed discussion with the family, underwent withdrawal of care and rapidly succumbed.

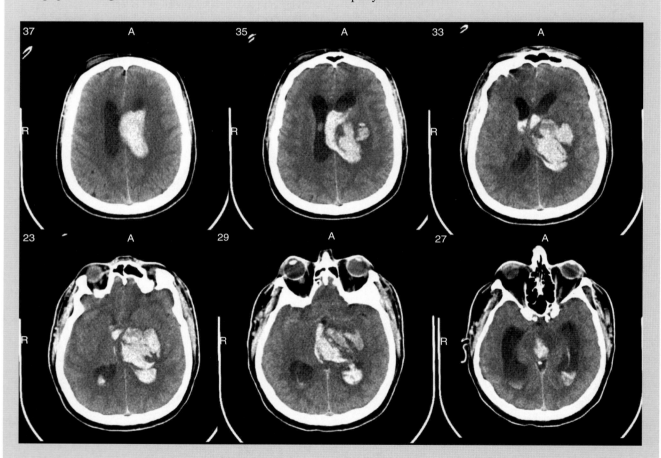

Fig. 5.25 Noncontrast computed tomography shows a large acute intracerebral hematoma involving the left lateral ventricle, thalamus, basal ganglia, and midbrain. The ventricles are dilated bilaterally due to hydrocephalus

Case 3

An 8-year-old boy presents to the emergency room. His parents noted poor vision about 2 months earlier. That day, an ophthalmologist found severe papilledema on fundoscopic exam and sent him to the ER. Your neurological exam reveals a bilateral bitemporal field cut and is otherwise normal.

Analysis

Where is the lesion? The bilateral field cut localizes the lesion to the inferior optic chiasm.

What is the lesion? Lesions known to occur in this area (suprasellar) in this age group include craniopharyngioma, germinoma, optic nerve/hypothalamic glioma, pituitary tumor, and teratoma.

Management: You obtain an MRI scan (Fig. 5.26). It shows a ring-enhancing, internally cystic suprasellar lesion, with a normal sized sella. This is most consistent with craniopharyngioma. You perform a craniotomy and aggressive subtotal resection of tumor. In the NICU, he has diabetes insipidus, which is easily managed with DDAVP.

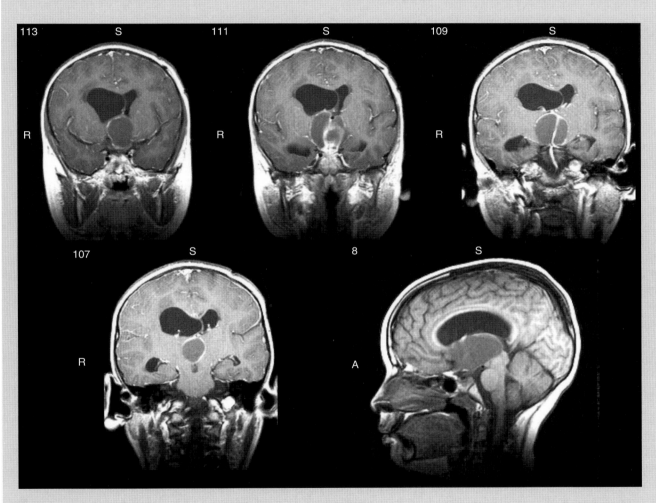

Fig. 5.26 Enhanced magnetic resonance imaging shows a ring-enhancing, cystic-appearing mass in the suprasellar space, extending into and filling the third ventricle. This causes hydrocephalus

Case 4

A 15-year-old boy presents with gradually increasing headache and double vision over the past 3 months. Your neurological examination is remarkable for dilated pupils, poorly reactive to light, but briskly reactive to accommodation (Fig. 5.27). He is unable to look up.

Analysis

Where is the lesion? This combination of ocular findings is called Parinaud's syndrome. It localized to the dorsal midbrain/pineal region.

What is the lesion? Lesions most likely to occur in this area, at this age, are pineal region tumors: germinoma, non-germinomatous germ cell tumors, pineocytoma, and pineoblastoma.

Management: You obtain an MRI. It reveals a contrast-enhancing lesion near the pineal gland. CSF markers are negative. A stereotactic biopsy confirms a germinoma. The patient is cured with a combination of craniospinal RT and chemotherapy.

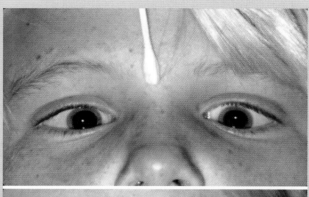
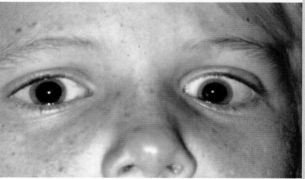
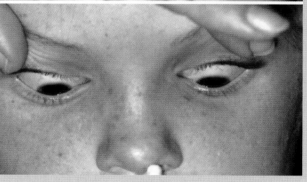

Fig. 5.27 The patient is able to converge (*top panel*). When looking straight ahead, one can see that the pupils are large and poorly reactive to light (*middle panel*). The patient is able to look down (*bottom panel*), but not up. These findings are part of "Parinaud's syndrome"

Case 5

A 22-year-old male falls at work, striking his forehead and hyperextending his neck. In the emergency room, he complains of weakness in his arms and severe burning pain in the arms and hands. Your examination reveals complete paralysis of biceps, triceps, and hand muscles but normal strength in the legs. He has no upper extremity reflexes and 3+ lower extremity reflexes. Light touch produces a hyperpathic (exaggerated painful) response in the arms and chest.

Analysis

Where is the lesion? This is one of the partial spinal cord injury syndromes, called the "central cord syndrome." It localizes to the central cord, at the C5–6 level (since deltoid is intact but biceps is paralyzed).

What is the lesion? This injury is due to hyperextension with narrowing of the spinal canal. Other lesions, like intramedullary tumors or hydromyelia, can present with similar findings, but are not, obviously, associated with trauma.

Management: The patient undergoes plain x-rays, CT, and MRI of the cervical spine. The MRI (Fig. 5.28) shows T2 hyperintensity behind C3–4 and C4–5, associated with a very narrow spinal canal and bulging/herniated cervical discs. The patient is treated medically for several days and improves. He then undergoes C3–4, C4–5 anterior cervical discectomy and fusion, to prevent future spinal cord injury.

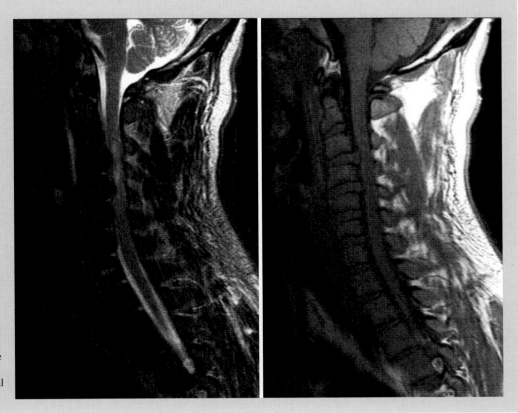

Fig. 5.28 Sagittal T2 (*left*) and T1 (*right*) MRI images show hyperintensity in the cord behind C3–4 and C4–5 bulging/herniated discs. The overall diameter of the spinal canal is small. This is compatible with a central cervical spinal cord injury

Case 6

A 72-year-old female presents to your office with a 3-year history of increasingly severe stabbing right facial pain. It is primarily in the V2 and V3 distributions. It is brought on by talking, teeth brushing, and eating. Tegretol was initially helpful but now is not preventing severe breakthrough episodes. Your neurological examination is normal, and the patient brings a normal MRI with her.

Analysis

Where is the lesion? The lesion involves the right trigeminal nerve.

What is the lesion? This set of historical findings – lancinating facial pain, with trigger points, and relief with Tegretol – is diagnostic of trigeminal neuralgia. Most cases of trigeminal neuralgia are idiopathic and are usually caused by arterial compression of the trigeminal nerve at the point where it enters the pons. Other causes include multiple sclerosis and tumors, but these are ruled out by the normal MRI.

Management: Management options include microvascular decompression, radiofrequency nerve lesioning, and radiosurgery. MVD produces most durable results and usually does not cause facial numbness. Note that this disease is diagnosed from history alone, with confirmation coming from the normal exam and MRI.

Case 7

A 75-year-old woman complains of a 3-month history of visual blurring in the right eye. She also notes intermittent intense electrical feelings over her entire body, with constant tingling in both hands. Your neurological examinations disclose impaired recent memory, diminished light touch over the arms, and greatly diminished proprioception and vibration in the arms and legs.

Analysis

Where is the lesion? The patient's symptoms and signs are consistent with lesions in several areas of the CNS. The greatly diminished proprioception and vibration in the arms and legs localize to the dorsal cervical spinal cord (the posterior columns). Diminished memory localizes to the brain, and decreased visual acuity in one eye only localizes to the optic nerve.

What is the lesion? Diseases that affect the dorsal spinal cord are usually metabolic or infectious. They include vitamin B_{12} deficiency, Wilson's disease, and neurosyphilis. The neurological manifestations of B_{12} deficiency are also known to cause memory and visual problems (combined systems disease).

Management: A vitamin B_{12} level was very low. The patient responded well to monthly B_{12} injections. MRI imaging (Fig. 5.29) of the cervical spine confirmed the presence of localized dorsal column disease.

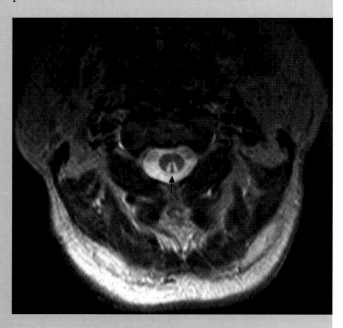

Fig. 5.29 Axial MRI imaging shows hyperintensity in the dorsal columns of the spinal cord (*arrow*). This is compatible with B_{12} deficiency

Case 8

A 45-year-old male complains of increasingly severe tingling and numbness in the right little and ring finger. Your examination reveals mild weakness of the interossei of the right hand, with mild atrophy of the first dorsal interosseus muscle. Sensation is mildly decreased in the ulnar nerve distribution. There is a positive Tinel's sign at the right cubital tunnel.

Analysis

Where is the lesion? The sensory and motor findings are in the distribution of one nerve, the ulnar nerve. The positive Tinel's sign at the elbow suggests cubital tunnel entrapment.

What is the lesion? Most cubital tunnel syndromes (like carpal tunnel syndromes) are due to repetitive motion. Prior arm fracture, diabetes, or hypothyroidism can be contributing factors.

Management: You order a nerve conduction velocity test, which confirms slowing across the cubital tunnel syndrome. You perform a neurolysis of the ulnar nerve, with excellent relief of symptoms.

Acknowledgment We wish to acknowledge that Dr. Kelly D. Foote and Mr. David Peace were coauthors on this chapter with Dr. Friedman in the first edition of this title; this new chapter, totally revised and updated, was inspired by the original chapter.

References

1. Teasdale G, Jennett B. Assessment of coma and impaired consciousness. A practical scale. Lancet. 1974;2:81–4.
2. Friedman WA, Foote KD, Peace D. Neurologic disease: an overview. In: Layon AJ, Gabrielli AG, Friedman WA, editors. Textbook of neurointensive care. Philadelphia: W.B. Saunders; 2004.
3. Aronson AE, et al. Clinical examination in neurology. 4th ed. Philadelphia: W.B. Saunders; 1977. p. 1–235.
4. Heilman KM, Watson RT, Greer M. Differential diagnosis of neurologic signs and symptoms. London: Appleton; 1977. p. 1–231.
5. Newman NJ. Practical neuro-ophthalmology. In: Tindall GT, Cooper PR, Barrow DL, editors. The practice of neurosurgery. Baltimore: Williams and Wilkins; 1996. p. 159–85.
6. Rengachary SS. Cranial nerve examination. In: Wilkins RH, Rengachary SS, editors. Neurosurgery. New York: McGraw-Hill; 1985. p. 50–70.
7. Ropper AH, Samuels M. Adams and Victor's principles of neurology. 9th ed. New York: McGraw-Hill; 2001. p. 1–1572.
8. Winn HR. Youman's neurological surgery, vol. I. Philadelphia: W.B. Saunders; 2011.

Introduction to Basic Neuropathology

6

Anthony T. Yachnis

Contents

Abstract

A basic understanding of nervous system pathology is integral to providing high-quality, safe, evidence-based care to patients with neurological diseases. This is particularly important in the field of critical care medicine. Although the manner in which disorders may affect the brain and spinal cord is quite varied (as are clinical and radiologic manifestations of disease), special structural features of the central nervous system give rise to unique patterns of vulnerability that produce reproducible morphologic patterns of neuropathology. Some types of pathological changes are unique to the nervous system such as demyelination and neurodegeneration, while others, such as trauma, neoplasms, and vascular diseases that occur elsewhere in the body, will have characteristic structural and functional effects on the brain and spinal cord. This chapter will cover basic reactions of the central nervous system to injury and then review some typical anatomic patterns of CNS disease.

Keywords

Hypoxia/ischemia • Edema • Herniation • Contusion • Glioblastoma • Demyelination • Abscess

Basic Central Nervous System Reactions

Unique structural features of nervous system organization include both microscopic and macroscopic anatomic specializations. These include special characteristics of neurons and their "selective" vulnerabilities, the unique but nonspecific reactions of astrocytes, and the blood-brain barrier. Gross anatomic features of critical importance in routine care of an ICU patient include encasement of the brain within a rigid compartment (i.e., "brain in a box") and the production, circulation, and resorption of the cerebrospinal fluid (CSF).

The neuron is the fundamental functional unit of the nervous system. Physiologically related groups of neurons are

A.T. Yachnis, MD
Department of Pathology and Laboratory Medicine,
University of Florida College of Medicine,
100265, Gainesville, FL 32610, USA
e-mail: yachnis@pathology.ufl.edu

A.J. Layon et al. (eds.), *Textbook of Neurointensive Care*,
DOI 10.1007/978-1-4471-5226-2_6, © Springer-Verlag London 2013

arranged in anatomic and functional units or groups, and pathology may affect not only a single set of neurons but an entire functional pathway. Cortical neurons have a characteristic pyramidal shape and contain cytoplasmic Nissl substance (corresponding to rough endoplasmic reticulum), variable amounts of lipofuscin, and vesicular nuclei with prominent nucleoli (Fig. 6.1a). The highly polarized morphology of diverse groups of CNS neurons with dendrites and axons emanating from the cell body or soma is supported by a variety of cytoskeletal elements including microtubules, microfilaments, and the three subtypes of intermediate filaments (low, medium, and high molecular weight neurofilament proteins) [1]. Immunohistochemical detection of the latter is often used in neuropathology to detect cells with mature neuronal phenotype (Fig. 6.1b). Synaptophysin is a synaptic vesicle protein that is widely expressed in gray matter neuropil and is another commonly used antigen used to demonstrate neuronal or neuroendocrine lineage [2]. The neuronal nuclear antigen is expressed in the nuclei and cell bodies of a wide variety of neurons

with a few notable exceptions (Purkinje cells and cerebellar dentate neurons) [3].

One of the most common neuronal changes occurs in the setting of focal or diffuse hypoxia or ischemia [4]. Thus, the acute ischemic cell change occurs when the insult is severe enough to cause irreversible cell death and becomes evident 18–24 h after severe hypoxia, ischemia, or hypotension. The neurons undergo shrinkage with a change from cytoplasmic basophilia to eosinophilia and nuclear shrinkage with hyperchromasia (pyknosis) (Fig. 6.1c). Other classic neuronal cytoplasmic alterations include the accumulation (or storage) of a metabolic product resulting from loss or dysfunction of a catabolic enzyme due to a specific gene defect. Here, cytoplasmic swelling will occur followed in many cases by neuronal death. Neuronal cytoplasmic accumulations are characteristic of the neurodegenerative diseases: hyperphosphorylated forms of tau are major constituents of neurofibrillary tangles in Alzheimer's disease and the frontotemporal dementias, while discrete Lewy bodies are typical of idiopathic Parkinson's disease (Fig. 6.1d). In contrast to

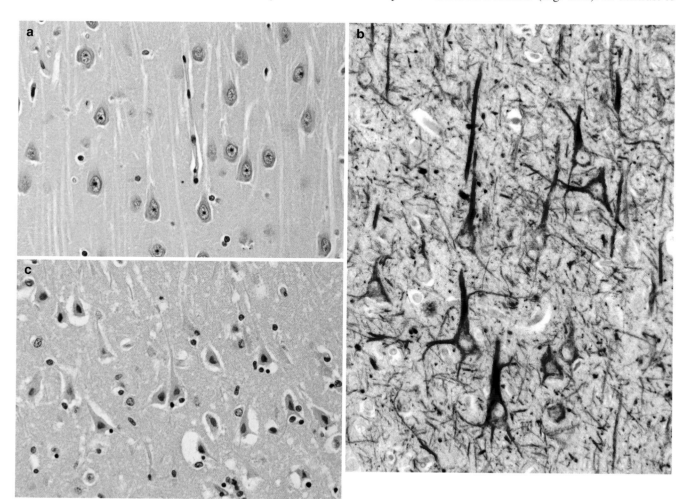

Fig. 6.1 Basic reactions. (**a**) Normal pyramidal neurons of the hippocampus. (**b**) Cortical neurons: immunohistochemical study for neurofilament protein. (**c**) Neurons of hippocampal region CA1 (Sommer's sector) showing acute ischemic cell change ("red-dead" neurons). (**d**) Lewy body (*arrow*) within a substantia nigra neuron in a case of idiopathic Parkinson's disease. (**e**) Fibrous astrocytes immunohistochemically stained for GFAP. (**f**) Piloid gliosis with abundant hypereosinophilic Rosenthal fibers

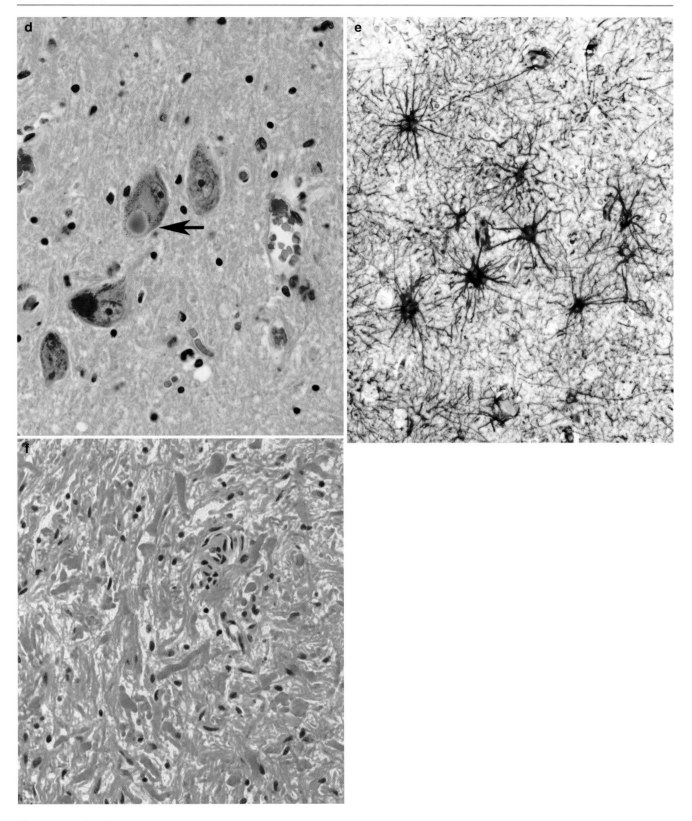

Fig. 6.1 (continued)

the pathological cytoplasmic accumulations mentioned previously, neurons may accumulate the age-related lipochrome pigment (lipofuscin), which, except for the various forms

neuronal lipofuscinosis, accumulates normally with age [5]. While many neuronal types accumulate lipofuscin, large neurons of the cerebellar dentate nucleus, globus pallidus, inferior olivary nuclei, and anterior horn neurons of the spinal cord and brain stem are most prominently affected.

Neurons respond to axonal transection by the cytoplasmic accumulation of axoplasmic constituents ("central chromatolysis"), while the distal axon segment undergoes degeneration and phagocytosis (Wallerian degeneration). Axoplasmic material including neurofilaments, microtubules, and mitochondria may also accumulate at sites of axonal shearing or transection. Amyloid precursor protein (APP) may be detected in axons by immunohistochemistry as early as 3–4 h after traumatic axonal injury [6]. In the central nervous system, the capacity for axonal regeneration remains limited, while peripheral nerves retain regenerative capacity if the basal lamina of Schwann cells remains intact.

Astrocytes are the major supportive cells of the central nervous system and provide diverse functions including glial-guided neuronal migration during development, interstitial fluid and electrolyte homeostasis, and trophic effects on the cerebral microvasculature [4]. Fibrous astrocytes, which reside primarily in the white matter, express glial fibrillary acidic protein (GFAP) in the perinuclear cytoplasm and in markedly attenuated cell processes (Fig. 6.1e). The latter extend to the endothelial basal laminae of capillaries and other small cerebral blood vessels. Of note, the water channel protein aquaporin 4 is localized to astrocytic foot processes that are intimately associated with brain microvessels and is believed to function in fluid and electrolyte homeostasis [7]. Antibodies to aquaporin 4 have been identified in association with the neuromyelitis optica (Devic's disease) spectrum of demyelinating disorders [8].

Reaction to brain injury, in general, results in reactive changes of astrocytes. "Fibrous" astrocytosis is the most common type of reactive gliosis and may be encountered in early organizing phases of injuries such as cerebral infarctions, infections, or demyelinating conditions. Astrocytes may develop a hypertrophic (or gemistocytic) appearance in early and pronounced tissue reactions. Later stages of fibrous astrocytosis are dominated by an abundance of highly elongated cell processes, which form the glial "scar." Some astrocytic reactions ("piloid gliosis") contain an abundance of Rosenthal fibers (Fig. 6.1f), which are elongated hypereosinophilic proteinaceous deposits composed of GFAP and αB-crystallin [9]. Rosenthal fibers are characteristically seen in cystic areas of pilocytic astrocytomas but may also be seen in gliotic brain tissue comprising walls of cysts associated with non-glial tumors such as craniopharyngiomas and hemangioblastomas or in syringomyelic cysts and pineal cysts. Alexander's disease is a genetic disorder caused by specific mutations in the GFAP gene in which there is extensive leukoencephalopathy with widespread deposition of Rosenthal fibers [10]. Systemic metabolic disturbances (i.e., liver failure) can affect the CNS causing a characteristic reaction of protoplasmic astrocytes that are located in the gray matter. Under conditions of systemic hyperammonemia, the nuclei of protoplasmic astrocytes undergo chromatin clearing often with enlarged nucleoli. This "protoplasmic astrocytosis" is called "Alzheimer type II cell change."

Oligodendrocytes generate and maintain myelin ensheathment of the larger axons, which mediates rapid neurotransmission. Their degeneration results in local interruption in formation and maintenance of myelin (demyelination), resulting in impaired or blocked impulse conduction along axons. Specific oligodendrocyte injury due to a papovavirus occurs in progressive multifocal leukoencephalopathy (PML).

Microglia are resident histiocytes of the central nervous system that interface with the immune system. A specialized type of perivascular microglial cell functions as the antigen-presenting cell of the brain [11]. Activation results in morphologic transformation to so-called pleomorphic microglia (or "rod-cell" microglia), which respond to low-grade, incomplete necrosis, or chronic infections, and have already become capable of ingesting destroyed nerve cell fragments ("neuronophagia") or myelin. Activation to fully developed macrophages occurs with acute, severe tissue destruction and with active demyelination. Reactive macrophages in brain, however, arise not only from tissue microglia but also from circulating monocytes.

Ependyma and choroid plexus in the ventricle lining play a role in CSF production/homeostasis, respectively. Ependymal cells undergo necrosis and are not replaced, leaving a subependymal glial nodule (scar).

Central nervous system cells display a striking differential or *selective vulnerability* to injurious insults [4]. For example, acute, severe local perfusion failure leads to ischemic infarction in which regions of complete anoxia undergo necrosis of virtually all cellular elements including neurons, glia, and myelin. However, at the edges of an ischemic lesion or with only partial ischemia, there may be subtotal or incomplete destruction, with neurons (the most sensitive cells) being affected first followed by oligodendroglia, astrocytes, microglia, and finally blood vessels. Individual subtypes of neurons also display differential vulnerability, with hippocampal pyramidal cells of Sommer's sector (CA1) and cerebellar Purkinje cells being most sensitive to hypoxic-ischemic injury followed by large neurons of cortical layers 3, 5, and 6, with smaller interneurons being less sensitive.

Blood-Brain Barrier

Proper function of central nervous system neurons in chemical and electrical transmission is highly regulated by the local ionic microenvironment of synapses and axons [12, 13]. Maintaining the delicate homeostatic balance of neuronal microenvironments requires a blood-brain barrier, which represents a unique anatomic and physiologic separation of the brain interstitial (extracellular) and cerebrospinal fluid compartments from the blood (intravascular compartment). The major anatomic substrates of this barrier are capillary endothelial tight junctions extending in a collar-like fashion around each cell, forming a complete "seal," without fenestrations found in endothelium elsewhere in the body. Basal lamina of endothelial cells forms a distinct extracellular matrix around brain capillaries. Astrocytes form an intricate network surrounding brain capillaries and promote the induction and maintenance of barrier properties. As previously noted, aquaporin 4, which is localized to astrocyte end feet, may also play a role in fluid homeostasis [7].

A second interface between the blood and CSF occurs within choroid plexus epithelial cells that functionally create an ultrafiltrate of the plasma: the cerebrospinal fluid (CSF). The arachnoid epithelium of the leptomeninges forms a third barrier between brain extracellular fluid and that of the remainder of the body.

Brain Swelling, Hydrocephalus, and Herniation

In adults and children after closure of the cranial sutures, the brain is encased within a rigid bony skull with a fixed intracranial space that is further subdivided by tough sheetlike dura mater. Normally, the skull, dura, and CSF provide physical protection and buffer the enclosed brain. However, with diffuse or focal expanding intracranial lesions such as edema, hemorrhage, tumor, abscess, or severe trauma, the brain will swell against the non-expansile skull or herniate around prominent edges of the dura (falx cerebri, tentorium cerebelli) or bone (foramen magnum) [4]. The rate of expansion is critical and correlates with clinical signs and symptoms. For example, slowly growing masses such as meningiomas allow for compensatory changes, and there may be little neurological until the mass is large. In contrast, a rapidly growing process such as an acute hypertensive hemorrhage may be rapidly lethal.

Cerebral edema, a major cause of brain swelling and herniation, is the accumulation of fluid within extracellular or intracellular CNS elements and may occur by three fundamental mechanisms [14]. BBB breakdown leads to *vasogenic edema* with leakage of protein, fluid, and electrolytes into the cerebral extracellular (interstitial) space and is encountered in trauma, tumors, infections, hemorrhage, and in the later stages of infarction. This type of edema tends to be more prominent in the white matter, although gray matter is also affected. In contrast, *cytotoxic edema* results from intracellular fluid accumulation within the cellular elements themselves. This occurs most classically in the early stages of focal or diffuse hypoxic/anoxic/ischemic injury where

loss of cellular ATP production disrupts the energy-dependent Na+/K+ membrane pump. Neurons are most sensitive to hypoxia/ischemia, and swelling of individual cells with the influx of Na+ and water leads to focal or diffuse brain swelling that primarily affects the gray matter. *Interstitial edema* results most often from passive diffusion of periventricular CSF from the ventricles under conditions of hydrocephalus.

Hydrocephalus most often occurs because of obstruction of CSF flow but can rarely occur due to increased production by a choroid plexus papilloma [4, 15, 16]. Obstruction can occur anywhere along the pathway of flow from the lateral ventricles through the foramina of Monro, in the third ventricle, cerebral aqueduct, fourth ventricle, and its outflow foramina of Luschka and Magendie. The normal CSF volume is approximately 140 ml of which only 20–25 ml is located within the ventricular system. The remainder fills the subarachnoid space including the major cisterns, fissures, and around the cerebral surfaces. Absorption occurs mostly through the arachnoid villi of the dural sinuses (mostly the superior sagittal sinus). Hemorrhage, tumor, or infectious/inflammatory processes involving the meninges and subarachnoid space can cause hydrocephalus after the CSF exits the ventricular system ("communicating hydrocephalus"). The latter form of hydrocephalus may also result from superior sagittal sinus thrombosis which impairs CSF absorption by arachnoid villi. With *noncommunicating hydrocephalus*, obstruction occurs within the ventricular system. One of the most common sites of obstruction is due to atresia, stenosis, or obstruction of the aqueduct of Sylvius (Fig. 6.2).

Cerebral *herniation* occurs as a consequence of mass increase within the protective but non-expansile skull and dura [4]. Mass lesions (e.g., abscesses, tumors, hemorrhages, and hydrocephalus) compress adjacent structures, displacing them (after CSF and blood volumes are first adjusted). The volume of the mass itself and any added volume of associated edema are additive. Brain tissue, if compressed sufficiently, will become edematous, largely vasogenic in type. Space-occupying lesions produce pressure differentials between adjacent intracranial or between intracranial and extracranial compartments. The relatively elastic brain tissue herniates from high- to low-pressure compartments along resultant pressure gradients.

The types of herniations are defined by whether the pathological process is focal or diffuse and by the anatomic site that has herniated [4]. Thus, *transtentorial herniation* refers to downward shifting as a result of an expanding space-occupying lesion in one or both supratentorial compartments. As the herniation progresses, the compressive force is transmitted downward through the brain stem producing progressively deepening coma and functional deterioration. *Uncal herniation* occurs with a unilateral space-occupying lesion in which structures shift downward from one side resulting in the anteromedial portion of the temporal lobe

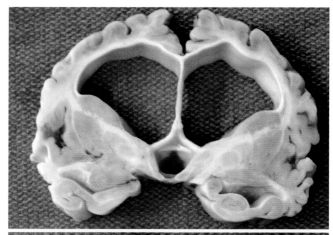

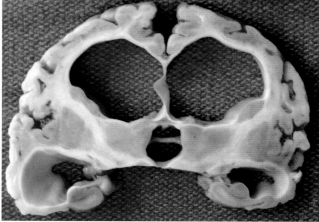

Fig. 6.2 Hydrocephalus

moving downward over the adjacent ipsilateral free edge (incisura) of the tentorium cerebelli. As it evolves, uncal herniation may lead to a variety of neurological changes. Ipsilateral compression of third cranial nerve, especially the superficial parasympathetic fibers, leads to a dilated, fixed, or "blown" pupil on the side of the lesion. Compression of reticular formation in midbrain leads to decerebrate rigidity and coma. Decerebrate posture involves rigid extension of the arms and legs, downward pointing of the toes, and backward arching of the head. Stretching or tearing of small branches of the posterior cerebral or basilar arteries supplying the midbrain and upper pons results in *Duret hemorrhages* in these areas. Ipsilateral compression of the posterior cerebral artery will cause ipsilateral medial occipital lobe infarction. Hemorrhage or softening of the contralateral cerebral peduncle (Kernohan's notch) may occur as it is compressed against the contralateral incisura causing a hemiparesis ipsilateral (paradoxically) to the lesion.

Central herniation refers to a symmetrical downward displacement, most importantly of hypothalamic and thalamic structures, due to generalized and/or symmetrical swelling of both hemispheres (e.g., massive bilateral cerebral swelling in

severe anoxia). Compression of the diencephalon causes stupor. *Cingulate herniation*, also called subfalcine herniation, refers to mesial shift of cingulate gyrus across the midline under the free edge of the falx cerebri as a result of a unilateral space-occupying lesion. *Cerebellar tonsillar herniation* occurs with diffuse swelling or mass lesions of the cerebellum and posterior fossa or may be due to progressive expansion of a large supratentorial lesion. Downward displacement of the inferior vermis and mesial cerebellar tonsils through the foramen magnum typically is seen. Medullary compression may result eventually in respiratory arrest. Less commonly, a posterior fossa mass will also force the superior cerebellar vermis and rostral pons upward through the incisura of the tentorium compressing the midbrain and obstructing the cerebral aqueduct. Outward displacement of swollen brain through a traumatic skull defect is called *transcalvarial herniation*.

Traumatic Brain Injury (TBI)

Two fundamental forms of damage can be identified in the development of brain injury following head trauma: (1) *primary damage* occurs at the moment of injury and (2) *secondary damage* results from subsequent associated phenomena such as cerebral edema and herniation. With severe brain trauma, both forms of injury may be present. Furthermore, the rate of accumulation and volume of intracranial hemorrhage that accompanies the injury will have profound effects on clinical course. Elevated intracranial pressure, hypoxia, and brain swelling represent common complications in significant head trauma with secondary infection being more likely in penetrating head injury than in non-penetrating closed head injury.

Closed head injury is a general form of brain trauma that can result from direct contact at a site of impact or indirectly from related acceleration/deceleration forces acting on the head and brain in which penetration of the skull does not occur [17]. Thus, despite the considerable protection provided by the skull and meninges, non-penetrating trauma to the skull can be associated with significant indirect brain injury. *Concussion* is a clinical syndrome defined as a transient alteration of consciousness secondary to head injury, usually caused by change in momentum or rotational acceleration of the head [18]. The patient may experience loss of consciousness, temporary respiratory arrest, or loss of reflexes. Experimental neuropathological studies of concussion have shown minimal and nonspecific neuronal changes [19, 20]. When unconsciousness lasts for 24 h or longer, more significant diffuse anatomic brain injury is more likely to have occurred.

More recent studies suggest that some degree of axonal injury (discussion follows) may occur with relatively mild forms of brain trauma, and such injury is likely to be irreversible and cumulative even with repeated minor trauma. Furthermore, autopsy studies of former professional football players and boxers who have sustained significant head trauma, much of the time associated with periods of unconsciousness, appear to be at risk for the subsequent development of *chronic traumatic encephalopathy* [21, 22]. This neurodegenerative disease occurs later in the lives of some individuals with a history of repeated head trauma. The exact relationship between recurring mild TBI, with or without concussion, and CTE is not completely understood at present. Published neuropathological features of CTE include extensive tau-immunoreactive inclusions scattered throughout the cerebral cortex in a patchy, superficial distribution, with focal epicenters at the depths of sulci and around the cerebral vasculature and widespread TDP-43-immunoreactive inclusions that may occasionally be associated with symptoms of motor neuron disease [21, 22].

Contusion/laceration injury of the brain results from direct contact at the site of impact or from relative movement of the brain inside the skull, related to acceleration/deceleration of the head [17]. Contusion is essentially a "bruise" of the brain that by definition should have an intact superficial pia mater, while laceration results from more severe tissue injury that results in tearing of the pia. Laceration often accompanies contusion and is associated with more significant bleeding than contusion alone. The most superficial or exposed portions of the brain (most commonly gyral crests in adults) suffering the injury undergo necrosis, often with eventual overlying meningeal fibrocollagenous scarring and underlying parenchymal gliosis.

Coup contusions are located directly beneath or adjacent to the site of traumatic contact of the head with an impacting object. By contrast, *contrecoup contusions*, in the literal sense, are located opposite to the site of traumatic contact of the head with an object. However, contrecoup contusions most commonly occur characteristically at along the inferior-lateral surfaces of frontal and temporal lobes and along the orbital frontal gyri (Fig. 6.3a, b). They result from shearing forces related to rotational acceleration of the brain "over" the rough underlying bony surfaces of anterior and middle fossae.

Diffuse axonal injury (*DAI*) results from shearing or tensile forces acting on axons within the transiently distorted brain during head trauma. These transient distortions of the brain occur as it moves within the skull as a result of traumatic acceleration/deceleration forces, usually in the lateral plane. The distribution of the characteristic axonal breaks and swellings ("spheroids") varies somewhat according to the specific circumstances, but the changes are most commonly found in parasagittal white matter, corpus callosum, internal capsule, and in brain stem (including the reticular

formation). Diffuse axonal injury results in the abnormal accumulation of many axoplasmic constituents [23]. Among the more important is *amyloid precursor protein* (*APP*), which can be detected by immunohistochemistry [24–26]. When this form of primary injury is substantial, the patient will typically be comatose immediately after the traumatic event and may remain in a persistent vegetative state until death [27].

Traumatic intracranial hemorrhage may involve the CNS tissue (parenchymal hemorrhage) or any of the actual or potential spaces within or around the brain or spinal cord [17]. Hemorrhage accumulates immediately following the traumatic event, and its effects depend not only on volume but also the rate of accumulation and location. *Epidural hemorrhage* usually results from skull fracture involving temporal or parietal bones in which the fracture crosses an arterial groove (usually that of the middle meningeal artery), tearing the vessel and resulting in brisk bleeding. Blood dissects between the inner surface of the skull and the outer surface of the dura. Such bleeding is often associated with a so-called lucid interval during which the patient appears to have recovered while epidural blood continues to accumulate. However, significant brain compression and herniation can occur with continued epidural blood accumulation.

Subdural hemorrhage occurs when blood accumulates in the potential space between the inner surface of the dura and outer surface of the arachnoid membrane and results from tearing of bridging veins, which pass from the cerebral surface through the subdural space to drain into the superior sagittal sinus. Hemorrhage occurs as a consequence of traumatic anterior/posterior movements of the brain with respect to the relatively fixed dura. Large tears in bridging veins or dural venous sinuses result in *acute subdural hemorrhage* with rapid accumulation of blood and a rapidly developing "mass effect," which puts the patient at a significant risk of herniation. *Chronic subdural hematoma* involves more gradual accumulation of blood. Recurrent bleeding over a period of days, weeks, or even months may occur, often with a history of apparently trivial trauma. When subdural hematomas organize, they do so by fibrovascular invasion of the hematoma from the dural surface. The resulting fibrovascular neomembrane eventually covers both outer and inner surfaces of the blood clot. The sequence of events in the organization of a chronic subdural hematoma includes lysis of the recent blood clot during the first week of trauma followed by growth of fibroblasts from the inner dural surface into the hematoma by 2–3 weeks. Early formation of vascularized connective tissue occurs by about 1–3 months post-trauma. Rebleeding of the fibrovascular neomembrane may result in significant mass effect with compression and/or herniation.

Traumatic *subarachnoid hemorrhage* resulting from head injury is a common phenomenon and is usually associated

Fig. 6.3 Contrecoup contusions. (**a**) Acute contrecoup contusions
of the inferior frontal and temporal regions. (**b**) Acute contrecoup
contusions showing hemorrhagic necrosis of the inferior frontal lobes

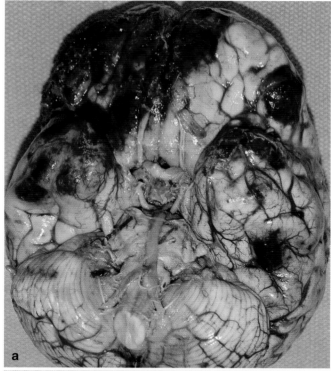

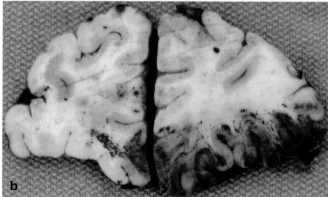

with contusion/laceration of the brain and/or subdural hemorrhage. Bleeding within brain parenchyma is due to contu-
sion/laceration or penetrating brain injury.

Not all skull fractures (perhaps the minority) are associated with true penetration of the skull. In a significant number of instances, the skull has been, at least transiently,
deformed during impact. Vascular or meningeal tearing with
cortical contusion/laceration may accompany significant
skull fracture, but not invariably, since considerable energy is
absorbed during the process of breaking the skull bone.
Conversely, as alluded to above, fatal brain injury can occur
in the absence of skull fracture. With *penetrating head
injury*, external forces exerted on the head are applied in such
a way as to cause penetration of the skin/mucous membranes
and skull. For example, with open/compound skull fracture
or missile injuries, the direct injury to the brain tissue can be

further complicated by the effects of the ensuing opening to
the environment, especially entry of microorganisms.

Traumatic spinal cord injury may result from both closed
and penetrating injuries. Fractures and subluxations, unique
to the bony spinal column, can markedly distort or disrupt
the underlying spinal cord and nerve roots. Both concussion
and contusion/laceration of spinal cord are encountered,
sometimes complicated by significant parenchymal hemorrhage. In addition, epidural, subdural, and subarachnoid
hemorrhages can also occur, with effects dependent on the
rate, volume, and location of blood accumulation, as within
the cranium. At the level of an acute spinal injury, there may
be hemorrhage, necrosis, and axonal swelling. The lesion
tapers above and below the level of injury. Over time, the
lesion undergoes liquefaction and cavitation with axonal
degeneration above and below the lesion.

Cerebrovascular Disease

Cerebrovascular disease ranks third behind heart disease and cancer as a cause of death in the United States and Europe [28]. The causes of CNS ischemia typically may be categorized as regional or global. *Regional ischemic injury* may result from occlusive diseases of arteries and arterioles, e.g., atherosclerosis, thromboembolism, vasospasm, malformation, vasculitis, dissection, and hypertension, or as a complication of diseases that do not primarily damage vessels, e.g., blood dyscrasias and hypercoagulability. The terms "stroke," "brain attack," or "cerebrovascular accident" (CVA) refer to an acute, non-epileptic, persistent alteration in neurological status that lasts more than 24 h and correlates with a sudden disruption of blood flow to a focal area of the brain. This can occur in two basic ways, both related to blood vessel pathology: Obstructed or stenotic blood vessels deprive the brain of oxygen and nutrients, while hemorrhage of diseased vessels may cause tissue destruction and oxygen deprivation. *Global hypoxia/ischemia* of the brain occur with hypotension, most often due to cardiac or pulmonary disease or in conditions of reduced oxygen-carrying capacity of the blood (as in carbon monoxide poisoning). In global hypoxia/ischemia, watershed zones between two vascular territories are preferentially susceptible in addition to the aforementioned vulnerable neuronal populations such as Sommer's sector (hippocampal region CA1), cerebellar Purkinje cells, and cortical layers 3 and 5 [29].

Ischemic "strokes" due to atherothrombotic or embolic disease account for about 70 % of all CVAs [28]. Risk factors are the same as for coronary heart disease: hypertension, diabetes, smoking, and hyperlipidemia. *Ischemic infarcts* occur within the distributions of the major cerebral arteries [30– 32]. Classic changes of a 1- to 2-day-old infarct include congestion, swelling, and dusky discoloration of the gray matter with slight softening in a well-defined vascular territory. Large acute infarcts may be associated with a significant mass effect and herniation (Fig. 6.4). If reperfusion occurs, as is the case for most embolic infarcts, the area of ischemia will appear hemorrhagic. With organization of the lesion, macrophages enter the tissue to remove necrotic material (liquefaction). Such removal results in softening and disruption of the tissues and a circumscribed pattern of laminar necrosis in which the cortex appears detached from the underlying white matter.

While ischemic cerebrovascular diseases most often arise from arterial thromboembolism, *venous thrombosis* is an important cause of cerebral ischemia. Superior sagittal sinus thrombosis occurs with some infections and various hypercoagulation states, including systemic malignancies. Here, venous outflow from superficial veins of the superior median aspect of the cerebral hemispheres is obstructed, resulting in marked congestion and hemorrhagic infarction in this region.

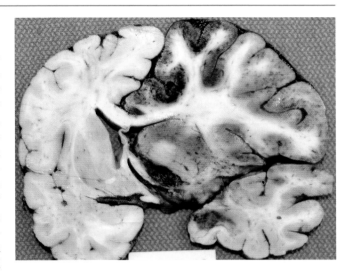

Fig. 6.4 Acute cerebral infarct. Massive acute cerebral infarct in distributions of anterior and middle cerebral arteries with significant mass effect and right cingulate gyrus herniation

In addition to being a risk factor for atherosclerosis, *systemic hypertension* is associated with cerebrovascular changes such as lipohyalinosis and lacunar lesions and may contribute to dementia [33]. Hypertension is the most important underlying etiology of acute nontraumatic intracerebral hemorrhage (ICH) and accounts for 10–20 % of all strokes [28]. Such hemorrhages occur most commonly in the deep nuclei, cerebellum, or pons and are associated with high mortality. Lacunar infarcts are located in the deep nuclei, particularly the putamen, and can involve the posterior limb of the internal capsule resulting in motor deficits of varying severity [30, 32] (Fig. 6.4). Accumulation of lacunar infarctions can lead to a stepwise decline in cognition often referred to as *multi-infarct dementia*. Chronic hypertension affects deep penetrating arteries and arterioles and is associated with lacunar lesions by promoting microvascular fibrinoid necrosis [33]. Healing of such a lesion includes the transient appearance of foamy or lipid-laden macrophages (lipohyalinosis) and eventually progresses to fibrosis and hyalinization. With acute hypertension, "onion-skinning" of the vessel wall occurs. The idea that massive deep nuclear hemorrhages were caused by rupture of Charcot-Bouchard aneurysms (rarely if ever observed in clinical practice) remains controversial [28]. Hypertensive CNS bleeds most likely have a multifactorial etiology with vascular hyalinization and fibrinoid changes causing decreased wall compliance and increased fragility. The *posterior reversible encephalopathy syndrome (PRES)* [34, 35] usually occurs in the setting of extreme hypertension and another risk factor, such as exposure to certain medications (e.g., FK506), pregnancy (as part of eclampsia), or drug abuse (e.g., cocaine).

Cerebral amyloid angiopathy (CAA) accounts for 12–15 % of all cerebral hemorrhages in the elderly and is due to the accumulation of amyloid in the walls of leptomeningeal and superficial cortical blood vessels [36–39]. Thus, in contrast to the deep cerebral hemorrhages of chronic hypertension, hemorrhages associated with amyloid angiopathy are more peripheral and involve the cerebral cortex and adjacent structures. Clinical symptoms reflect the anatomic extent and location of the hemorrhage. Lobar hemorrhage can occur acutely as a massive acute stroke, most often involving the frontal or frontoparietal regions, or as recurrent hemorrhagic infarctions that take place over a period of years. Large hemorrhages of the right parietal lobe may result in a classic contralateral neglect syndrome in which patients fail to recognize the left side of their body as their own. The most common form of amyloid associated with sporadic and some familial forms of CAA is the Aβ-amyloid peptide (Aβ), which is a cleavage product of the amyloid precursor protein encoded on chromosome 21 and is the same type of amyloid found in neuritic (senile) plaques of Alzheimer's disease. Rarely, CAA may occur together with CNS vasculitis.

Cerebral autosomal dominant arteriopathy with subcortical infarcts and leukoencephalopathy (CADASIL) is an inherited vasculopathy that has the cardinal symptoms of migraine headaches with aura, ischemic attacks (transient or strokes), depression, and eventual progression of the disease to dementia [40]. MRI typically reveals hyperintense lesions of the subcortical and deep white matter, and lacunar infarcts of the basal ganglia may also be present. Affected parenchymal and leptomeningeal contain granular, PAS-positive material, which replaces smooth muscle cells of the media and corresponds to pathognomonic accumulation of granular osmiophilic material (GOM) by electron microscopy. Involvement of systemic arteries has allowed for definitive diagnosis of CADASIL by skin biopsy with characteristic GOM in dermal arterioles. CADASIL is caused by mutations in the *Notch 3* gene on chromosome 19p13, and NOTCH 3 protein may be detected in affected blood vessels [41].

Aneurysms and Vascular Malformations

An *aneurysm* is defined as an abnormally dilated segment of a blood vessel. Included in this group of CNS vascular diseases are saccular (congenital), fusiform (atherosclerotic), infectious (mycotic), and traumatic types [28, 42, 43]. Most often, the first sign of an intracranial aneurysm is subarachnoid hemorrhage, with an annual incidence of about 10–15 per 100,000 [43] and a peak incidence in the sixth decade. Risk factors for the development of saccular (berry) aneurysms, which are the most common type, include chronic hypertension, cigarette smoking, female sex, and African American race. There are well-known associations of berry aneurysms with autosomal dominant polycystic kidney disease, Ehlers-Danlos syndrome type IV, neurofibromatosis type I, and Marfan's syndrome. About 6–9 % of arteriovenous malformations (AVMs) may occur together with one or more saccular aneurysms.

Typically occurring at branch points in large arteries of the circle of Willis, turbulent flow may contribute to aneurysmal dilatation. The most common locations include branch points between the anterior cerebral and anterior communicating arteries (40 %), the M1 and M2 divisions of the middle cerebral artery within the Sylvian fissure (34 %), and the internal carotid and posterior communicating arteries (20 %). The most sensitive and specific method of identifying a saccular aneurysm is cerebral angiography.

Variable amounts of basal subarachnoid hemorrhage are found in patients dying acutely. A berry aneurysm consists of a thin-walled saclike structure that is attached to an arterial branch point via a narrow neck. The sac may be spherical, oval, or lobulated, and multiple aneurysms may be present. The rupture site is usually apparent at the apex of the sac, and there may be evidence of previous surgical clipping. If the bleeding point of the ruptured aneurysm is oriented toward the cerebral surface, hemorrhage under arterial pressure dissects into the brain parenchyma and may extend into the ventricular system. Most saccular aneurysms are between 0.1 and 2.5 cm in diameter. Those measuring more than 2.5 cm are called giant aneurysms.

Fusiform aneurysms exceed 4.5 mm in diameter and may cause significant brain compression and mass effect. They do not usually produce subarachnoid hemorrhage and most often involve the vertebrobasilar system. Symptoms relate to brain stem and cranial nerve compression and ischemia as a result of atherothrombotic occlusion and/or mass effect of the lesion. Despite surgical intervention, the mortality rate is high.

Vascular invasion by infectious organisms and the associated inflammatory reaction can lead to focal dilatations of cerebral blood vessels and symptomatic hemorrhage [44]. Referred to as *infective or mycotic aneurysms*, such lesions may be caused by bacteria as well as fungi. They account for 3–5 % of all intracranial aneurysms and may rupture and result in subarachnoid hemorrhage or multiple hemorrhagic infarcts with disseminated disease. Vasoinvasive fungi such as *Aspergillus* species directly invade the vessel wall and cause thrombosis and hemorrhage. The clinical course can be rapidly progressive with high mortality.

Vascular malformations are traditionally classified into four groups: AVMs, cavernous angiomas, capillary telangiectasia, and venous angiomas. The basis for classification takes into account the caliber and configuration of the component blood vessels, the relationship of abnormal vessels to brain parenchyma, and the presence or absence of arteriovenous shunting.

Arteriovenous malformations (AVMs) account for 1.5–4 % of all brain masses, with a peak incidence in adults between ages 20 and 40 years [45–47]. Most AVMs are supratentorial and occur within the distributions of the major cerebral arteries (middle cerebral artery > anterior > posterior). Less common sites may include the corpus callosum, choroid plexus, or the optic nerve (the latter associated with Wyburn-Mason syndrome) [28]. AVMs consist of a tangled mass of blood vessels of varying diameter and wall thickness. Superficial AVMs tend to have a broad base near the cortical surface where they drain into surface veins, whereas deeper lesions drain into the deep venous system. Microscopically, abnormal arterial and venous channels are variable in size and configuration, and gliotic CNS tissue is typically between the abnormal blood vessels. Arterial elements may have variable amounts of smooth muscle proliferation, collagen deposition, and reduplication of the internal elastic lamina, whereas large arterialized veins are thick walled and collagenized. Thrombosis with varying stages of recanalization and sometimes calcification may be present. If embolization was performed before surgery, there will be evidence of endovascular material, which may incite a foreign body giant cell reaction. Two-thirds of patients with AVMs suffer clinically significant hemorrhage, and the risk is higher in younger individuals (<45 years of age). Treatment options include surgical resection, endovascular embolization, or radiosurgery.

Cavernous angiomas (also called cavernous malformations, cavernous hemangiomas, and cavernomas) arise most commonly in young adults, with a slight male preponderance. A third of patients present with focal epilepsy, and surgery is performed to control symptoms. Cavernous angiomas may occur anywhere in the nervous system and leptomeninges, but most typically cause seizures when the cerebral cortex is involved. Although the cause is not known, some familial forms of cavernous angioma are associated with mutations of the *CCM1* gene on chromosome 7q11-21. This gene encodes KRIT1, which interacts with proteins of the RAS family of guanine triphosphatases (GTPases). Other possible genetic disease-related loci have been identified on chromosomes 7p15-p13 (*CCM2*) and 3q25.2-27 (*CCM3*) [48]. MRI is pathognomonic and typically reveals a compact focus of increased vascularity with variable density that is surrounded by a ring of hypodensity. The latter corresponds to hemosiderin deposition in the adjacent brain tissue (ferruginous penumbra). In contrast to AVMs, cavernous angiomas have no direct arterial contribution. They consist of a compact mass of dilated, thin-walled, variably hyalinized vascular channels with little intervening brain tissue. There is no muscular hypertrophy or elastic lamina, but vessels may be calcified or thrombosed. The surrounding brain tissue is gliotic and shows evidence of remote hemorrhage with scattered hemosiderin-laden macrophages. The prognosis is usually excellent after surgical resection. Cavernous malformations are not typically embolized, and the role of radiosurgery for such lesions is uncertain.

Capillary telangiectases are typically incidental findings of little clinical significance and only rarely become symptomatic. *Venous angiomas* are dilated veins of the superficial or subcortical cerebral vasculature, which are similar to varicose veins elsewhere in the body but may be associated with other vascular malformations in the same patient. Venous angiomas are functional blood vessels, and their removal would result in extensive hemorrhagic infarction of the underlying brain.

Brain Tumors

Tumors of the nervous system may arise from brain tissue, its coverings, or adjacent structures or may metastasize from distant systemic sites. CNS tumors may exert local effects by infiltration, invasion, and destruction of neural tissue or by compressive effects on the brain, spinal cord, and local blood vessels. Associated cerebral edema occurs with many brain tumors. As expanding intracranial masses, CNS tumors result in raised intracranial pressure and/or compressive effects, which may lead to herniation. Acute hemorrhage in a brain tumor may result in altered or acute symptoms. Only a few of the more common tumors of adults (gliomas, meningiomas, schwannomas, metastases) and children (medulloblastoma) will be considered here.

Gliomas are the most common type of primary intra-axial brain tumors of adults [49]. All gliomas extensively infiltrate brain tissue such that complete surgical removal is generally not possible. Tumors of the astrocytoma group are classified as astrocytoma (WHO Grade II), anaplastic astrocytoma (WHO Grade III), and glioblastoma multiforme (WHO Grade IV) on the basis of pleomorphism, mitotic activity, and the presence or absence of microvascular proliferation and necrosis [50].

Diffuse astrocytomas (*WHO Grade II*) consist of highly infiltrative, pleomorphic cells with fibrillary processes that are most common in the cerebral hemispheres. Mitotic activity is low or absent, and there is no microvascular proliferation or necrosis [51]. While such tumors generally display slow growth with survival being measured in years, they may progress to higher-grade gliomas through successive stages of anaplastic transformation [52]. In contrast, the *glioblastoma (GBM, WHO Grade IV)* is the most highly malignant glioma and also the most common primary tumor of adults (Fig. 6.5a, b) [49, 50]. Of the 22,070 new cases of GBM reported by the National Cancer Institute in 2009, an estimated 12,920 individuals died of the disease. GBM is a mitotically active tumor with microvascular proliferation and necrosis, often of the pseudopalisading type (Fig. 6.4). In addition, tumor cells may extensively infiltrate the brain, especially along white matter tracts, far beyond the apparent site of origin. Such tumors often cross the corpus callosum producing the so-called butterfly glioma appearance. Areas of active tumor growth and microvascular proliferation produce the characteristic rim or ring enhancement on the T1 post-contrast MRI. Associated edema adds to the mass effect produced by such tumors.

One molecular subtype of GBM occurs spontaneously (arises de novo) in older individuals (fifth to sixth decades), has a short duration of symptoms, and is associated with epidermal growth factor receptor (EGFR) gene amplification and overexpression [52, 53]. Another subtype of GBM is believed to arise as a result of progressive anaplastic transformation from less malignant forms of astrocytoma. This subtype has frequent *IDH-1* (isocitrate dehydrogenase-1) and *p53* mutations as an early tumorigenic event [54, 55]. Further molecular subtypes of GBM with prognostic significance have been identified by large-scale gene profiling [56, 57].

Oligodendrogliomas (*WHO Grades II and III*) account for about 5–15 % of all gliomas and arise in the cerebral hemispheres, most often in the frontal lobes. Such tumors often extensively infiltrate the cerebral cortex in a gyriform growth pattern and may be associated with seizures. Oligodendrogliomas (WHO Grade II) present a monomorphous histology with round hyperchromatic nuclei, perinuclear haloes, and background chicken-wire-like vasculature [58]. Microcalcifications are common. *Anaplastic oligodendrogliomas* (*WHO Grade III*) show increased cellularity, mitotic activity, microvascular proliferation, and sometimes necrosis. Co-deletions of chromosomes 1p and 19q due to an unbalanced translocation are correlated with longer survival and better prognosis than the other infiltrating gliomas [59–61].

A subset of glioblastomas have a mutation of the NADP+-dependant isocitrate dehydrogenase-1 (IDH1) gene, which mostly affects a single codon (IDHR132H). This mutation has been identified in 50–80 % of secondary glioblastomas but in only 3–12 % of primary glioblastomas and occurs in around 70 % of diffuse WHO Grade II gliomas (astrocytomas, oligodendrogliomas, and mixed gliomas) [62]. Antibodies have recently been raised against mutated variants of IDH1 (R132H) that have proven useful in distinguishing infiltrating glioma cells from native of reactive CNS elements [63] (Fig. 6.5a, b). In addition, early reports indicating that the presence of IDH-1 mutations correlates with a better outcome in patients with WHO Grade II–IV gliomas suggest that testing for such mutations may be important prognostically [64].

Meningiomas are believed to arise from arachnoidal cells of the leptomeninges and are typically dural based. As such, they typically compress the adjacent brain and have an arachnoid plane, allowing for complete surgical removal in most cases. Compression of adjacent vascular structures in some case may give the radiologic appearance of perilesional edema, thus suggesting a higher-grade tumor. However, more than 90 % of meningiomas are histologically benign

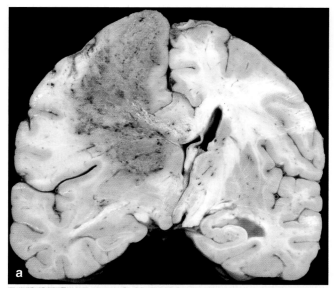

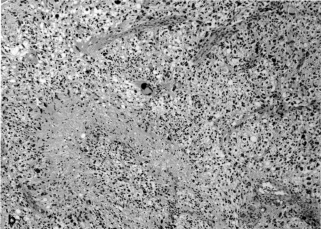

Fig. 6.5 Glioblastoma multiforme. (**a**) Large glioblastoma of left cerebral hemisphere with mass effect and right cingulate gyrus herniation. (**b**) Histological section (H&E stain) of glioblastoma (WHO Grade IV) with pseudopalisading necrosis (*lower left*) and microvascular proliferation (*upper right*)

(WHO Grade I), and, although several distinct histological subtypes have been described, clinical effects are largely based on location and the specific brain regions that are compressed [65]. While small meningiomas may be found in 1–2 % of patients as incidental findings at autopsy, slow growth in neurologically silent areas may allow some tumors to attain a large size before significant symptoms develop. *Atypical meningiomas* (*WHO Grade II*) display an increased risk of recurrence and are defined by increased mitotic activity (four or more mitoses per ten high-power fields) and three or more of the following: architectural sheeting, hypercellularity, small cell collections, macronucleoli, and spontaneous geographic necrosis [65, 66]. Brain invasion is also a current criterion for atypical meningioma. The clear cell and chordoid subtypes of meningioma are also classified as WHO Grade II. *Anaplastic (malignant) meningiomas (WHO Grade III)* account for less than 2 % of meningiomas and may invade the brain, having a high risk of recurrence but also carry an added risk of late metastasis [67]. High mitotic rates (20 or more mitoses per 10 high-power fields) or malignant sarcomatous or carcinomatous histology defines these tumors. The papillary and rhabdoid variants of meningiomas are currently classified as WHO Grade III.

Schwannomas (WHO Grade I) account for about 8 % of all intracranial tumors and about 30 % of primary intraspinal tumors [68]. Intracranial schwannomas most often arise in the cerebellopontine angle from the vestibular branch of the eighth cranial nerve. Symptoms include unilateral hearing loss and tinnitus, and, while such tumors are histologically benign and well demarcated from surrounding structures, large tumors may cause significant compression of the adjacent brain stem.

Metastatic tumors represent the most common form of brain neoplasia in adults with an annual incidence of about 4–10 per 100,000, and the incidence increases with age [50]. About 30 % of patients with disseminated disease will have brain metastases as a result of hematogenous spread to the brain parenchyma, dura, or meninges. While intra-axial spinal cord metastases are relatively rare, pathological fractures from osseous spinal metastases may result in significant neurological compromise. Bronchogenic carcinomas remain the most common primary neoplasms that metastasize to the brain followed by ductal breast carcinoma, melanoma, and primary cancers of the gastrointestinal and genitourinary tract (especially clear cell renal cell carcinoma) [50]. Brain metastases are most often found at the junction between gray and white matter and are often well demarcated from the adjacent brain. There may be extensive central necrosis, and perilesional edema, which can be extensive, adds to the overall mass effect of the tumor. The classic hemorrhagic metastases include melanoma, renal cell carcinoma, and choriocarcinoma. Rarely, diffuse invasion of the meninges (carcinomatosis) occurs, with multiple cranial nerve and spinal root signs, without a focal lesion.

The most common malignant brain tumor in children is the *medulloblastoma (WHO Grade IV)*, an embryonal tumor of the cerebellum [69]. The classic variant occurs in the fourth ventricle, typically arising from the cerebellar vermis as a solid, contrast-enhancing mass with restricted diffusion. In this site, symptoms of nausea, vomiting, and headache are related to obstruction and hydrocephalus. Histologically, medulloblastomas are highly cellular mitotically active tumors with little associated cytoplasm, nuclear molding, and occasional Homer-Wright rosettes. Patient outcome is related to the tendency of such tumors to disseminate along CSF pathways. The desmoplastic medulloblastoma tends to occur in older children and more commonly arises in a lateral cerebellar hemisphere. This variant displays a histologically nodular growth pattern, contains stromal reticulin, is associated with *PTCH1* gene mutations (9q22 loss), and carries a better prognosis than the classic variant. A large/cell anaplastic medulloblastoma with poor prognosis has a high frequency of *c-myc* amplification and features increased nuclear size and molding with significant pleomorphism and atypical mitotic figures [70]. The *atypical teratoid/rhabdoid tumor (AT/RT)* is another embryonal brain tumor that occurs in young children, typically less than 2 years of age. Such tumors are characterized by loss of the *INI1* gene on chromosome 22, which encodes a chromatin remodeling nuclear protein. Lack of detection of INI1 protein by immunohistochemistry is useful to distinguish the AT/RT from other CNS embryonal tumors which express this antigen [71].

Demyelinating Conditions

In addition to classic *multiple sclerosis (MS)* with its chronic relapsing remitting clinical course with involvement of multiple level of the neuraxis, some instances of acute inflammatory demyelination present as focal tumorlike mass lesions (tumefactive MS). Rare monophasic forms of inflammatory demyelination (*acute disseminated encephalomyelitis*) may follow viral infections or vaccinations, and fulminant forms of demyelination such as *acute hemorrhagic leukoencephalopathy* also fall within this category of disease [72–74]. Inflammatory demyelinating diseases all share the common pathological feature that a presumably autoimmune reaction is primarily directed against central nervous system myelin with, at least initially, relative sparing of axons. More recent studies have suggested that axonal loss also occurs as the disease progresses, and this certainly correlates with progression of neurological deficits [75, 76].

The lesions of multiple sclerosis (MS) are classically multiple, asymmetric, and randomly distributed plaques that are found in white matter of brain stem, spinal cord, optic nerves, cerebrum, and cerebellum [72–74]. Periventricular demyelination is particularly striking in some cases. In early lesions, there is a rapid breakdown of myelin with relative preservation of axons. Perivascular cuffing by lymphocytes and plasma cells is usually found along local small veins and postcapillary venules. Later, especially after repeated attacks, myelin has virtually been eliminated, but axons will also be lost. It is presumed that partial recovery from early attacks depends upon initial sparing of axons. Gliosis can become more dense over time, moderate numbers of macrophages can still be present, and perivenous mononuclear infiltration may still be prominent. Areas of demyelination can vary from microscopic in size to several centimeters in diameter. They are characteristically sharply circumscribed with abrupt margins representing a boundary where fibers become abruptly devoid of myelin. Smaller foci of demyelination are often clearly perivenular.

One notable subtype of demyelinating disease is *neuromyelitis optica* (NMO; Devic's disease), in which the lesions are most prominent in spinal cord and optic nerves, and a rapid clinical course is typical. 70–75 % of patients have serum antibodies to *aquaporin 4* water channel [77, 78]. This molecule is located on astrocyte foot processes of the blood-brain barrier (BBB). NMO may represent an autoimmune channelopathy that adversely affects the BBB. Acute or subacute necrotizing myelopathy is a severe, often necrotizing, demyelinating disorder that predominantly affects the spinal cord. Some of these acute forms may represent cases of acute necrotizing hemorrhagic encephalomyelopathy or acute disseminated encephalomyelitis.

Progressive multifocal leukoencephalopathy (PML) is an opportunistic infection by a papovavirus (JC virus) in which demyelination results from lytic infection of oligodendrocytes [79]. Coalescence of multiple foci of demyelination may result in a tumorlike mass lesion. Infection of astrocytes often results in a bizarre or transformed appearance of such cells that may further suggest a neoplasm. PML lesions typically do not produce much lymphocytic inflammation, which is characteristic other viral encephalitides. However, in patients with the *immune reconstitution syndrome*, treatment of an immunocompromised AIDS patient with evolving PML may result in a striking inflammatory reaction that presumably represents a host response to the JC virus infection [80]. PML has occurred as a rare complication of natalizumab therapy for multiple sclerosis [81].

Central Nervous System Infections

Although the brain and spinal cord are well protected from infection, pathogens may gain access to the CNS in several ways [82]. Blood borne spread from septic foci outside the nervous system may result in both meningeal (meningitis) and parenchymal infections (cerebritis, abscess). Infectious agents may be introduced by penetrating trauma or open fractures or extend from adjacent infected sinuses as in otitis media, mastoiditis, or paranasal sinuses. Developmental defects such as meningomyelocele may also provide a pathway for infection. Some viruses (herpes, rabies) may travel to the CNS in a retrograde fashion within axons of infected nerve cells. Infectious agents may be introduced via ventriculoperitoneal shunts, indwelling catheters, or by neurosurgical procedures.

Patterns of CNS involvement by specific infections depend in large part on specific pathogenic features of the infecting organism and the immune status of the host. Only a few specific illustrative patterns of infection will be discussed here.

Acute purulent (bacterial) meningitis may occur after trauma, during septicemia or bacteremia from systemic sources of infection, or as direct extension from sinus or skin (facial cellulitis) infections. While the availability of effective vaccines has reduced the incidence of acute bacterial meningitis over the past 10–15 years, the disease remains an important clinical problem and often results in death, with an overall fatality rate remaining at about 15 % [83, 84]. Causative agents differ with patient age, with *S. pneumoniae* being a major offender in adults and children, while Group B streptococci, *L. monocytogenes*, and coliforms continue to be important causes in neonates [82]. Acute meningitis due to *N. meningitides* occurs in localized outbreaks in children and young adults in day-care centers, dorms, or military barracks. Initial stages of hyperemia and moderate edema are typically followed by a fibrinopurulent exudate that accumulates in the subarachnoid space, around blood vessels, and in the Virchow-Robin spaces. Congestion and edema may be marked in meningococcal meningitis, and very little leptomeningeal exudate is typically seen in patients dying of disseminated disease (Waterhouse-Friderichsen syndrome). Complications include vascular thrombosis with ischemia, cranial nerve deficits, ventriculitis, and hydrocephalus.

Brain abscesses may present insidiously with signs and symptoms of an expanding intracranial mass, thus mimicking a brain tumor [85]. Hematogenous spread is most common as with suppurative bronchopulmonary, cardiac (infectious endocarditis), or periodontal sources of infection. Blood borne spread to the brain often results in abscesses located within the distribution of the middle cerebral artery at the gray-white matter junction. In contrast, extension of infection from adjacent sinuses or from retrograde thrombophlebitis results in lesions near such sites of origin. For example, abscesses complicating mastoiditis in patients with otitis media are often located in the temporal lobe or cerebellum.

Organisms associated with brain abscess include anaerobic or microaerophilic streptococci, staphylococci, bacteroides, and various gram-negative bacilli [85]. *Nocardia* and *Actinomycetes* species are also occasionally found in brain abscesses. Opportunistic organisms may cause abscesses in chronically debilitated or immunosuppressed patients. Abscesses arise as small necrotic foci that contain bacteria and polymorphonuclear leukocytes (focal cerebritis). The organizing abscess wall consists of granulation tissue that will progress to a fibrous capsule and associated capillary proliferation that can lead to significant perilesional edema. This can result in increased intracranial pressure, herniation, and death. Rupture of an abscess into a ventricle may result in ventriculitis and meningitis.

A wide range of fungi may infect the central nervous system, mostly in the immunocompromised host [82]. CNS cryptococcal infections, however, are exceptions, as they can affect immunocompetent as well as immunocompromised individuals. In the former, meningeal infection by cryptococcus causes a chronic granulomatous reaction, while in the latter, fungi spread along Virchow-Robin spaces to form characteristic gelatinous cysts in the basal ganglia. Isolated cryptococcosis may also occur. CNS infection by vasoinvasive fungi such as rhinocerebral mucormycosis or *Aspergillus* and related species may result in hemorrhagic cerebral infarctions (Fig. 6.6a, b)

The most common cause of focal cerebral mass lesions in AIDS patients results from infection by *Toxoplasma gondii* [86]. CNS involvement results in vasculitis, which leads to a focal necrotizing process in which free tachyzoites and encysted bradyzoites may be found at the periphery of the lesion (Fig. 6.5). Imaging studies reveal an enhancing destructive-appearing process that tends to localize to the deep cerebral nuclei. Similar changes may be observed in primary CNS lymphoma, which should be considered in patients not responding to empiric therapy for CNS toxoplasmosis.

Viruses may cause a variety of characteristic CNS pathologies ranging from self-limiting lymphocytic meningitis to widespread encephalitis affecting particular regions of the brain depending on specific neurotropisms [87]. Common tissue reactions to viral infection include lymphocytic meningitis, perivascular cuffing by lymphocytes, and variable amounts of neuronal loss, gliosis, and microglial nodules. The most common sporadic encephalitis in the USA is caused by *Herpes simplex*, which in adults causes a severe acute necrotizing encephalitis that typically involves the cerebral cortex of the temporal lobes and adjacent frontal cortex in an asymmetrical pattern. Opportunistic cytomegalovirus infections of immunocompromised patients typically affect the ventricular surfaces (ventriculitis) or the spinal cord (myelitis). Rabies virus attacks large neurons such as Purkinje cells and hippocampal pyramidal cells. Arbovirus encephalitides may affect more widespread areas of the brain. HIV1 infection may affect the nervous system directly (giant cell encephalitis, leukoencephalitis, vacuolar myelopathy) or secondarily via a number of opportunistic CNS infections [88].

Prion diseases result from pathogenic conformational changes of a normally expressed prion protein (cellular PrP) that results in misfolding into a toxic form that destroys neurons and is resistant to conventional thermal or chemical destruction [89]. While most cases are sporadic, about 10–15 % of prion disease is inherited, and less than 1 % of cases has been transmitted by neurosurgical procedures, dural or corneal grafts, and cadaveric pituitary extracts. Creutzfeldt-Jakob disease (CJD) occurs sporadically with an incidence of one per million population and is characterized by a rapidly progressive dementia, myoclonus, and characteristic EEG finding (spike-wave phenomenon). At autopsy, there are widespread spongiform change, neuronal loss, and

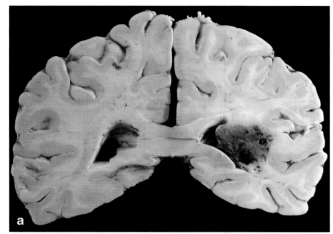

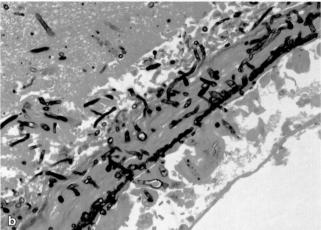

Fig. 6.6 CNS aspergillosis. (**a**) Hemorrhagic lesion next to right atrium of the lateral ventricle. (**b**) Histological section (GMS stain) showing large septate fungal hyphae consistent with *Aspergillus* species

reactive astrocytosis with minimal lymphocytic inflammation. Other rare inherited human prion diseases include Gerstmann-Straussler-Scheinker disease (autosomal dominant inheritance with cerebellar ataxia) and fatal familial insomnia (autosomal dominant with progressive insomnia). A new variant CJD (vCJD) was reported in the United Kingdom in 1996 that is now believed to have been transmitted by consumption of beef during the bovine spongiform encephalopathy outbreak in the UK during the 1980s.

Toxic Metabolic Diseases

Acute or chronic alcoholism is associated with a number of CNS changes [90, 91]. Blood levels of 150–200 mg/dl are associated with problems of equilibrium and coordination, while levels between 250 and 400 mg/dl may cause coma or death. In addition to changes associated with repeated head trauma (subdural hematomas, contusions, etc.), chronic alcohol abuse may result in atrophy of the anterior superior cerebellar vermis, which may be a direct toxic effect of alcohol or may be due to associated thiamine (vitamin B1) deficiency. The *Wernicke-Korsakoff syndrome* is also due to thiamine deficiency, is most common in alcoholics, but may also occur with malnutrition of other causes [91]. This disorder consists of two disorders that often coexist, especially in patients coming to autopsy. Wernicke's encephalopathy is a clinical syndrome of disordered consciousness, psychosis, ataxia, and cranial nerve palsies, including ophthalmoplegia. The condition is potentially reversible by thiamine administration but fatal if not treated. At autopsy, hemorrhagic lesions in periventricular regions of the third ventricle and aqueduct are typical, with the mammillary bodies being characteristically involved. Patients with Korsakoff syndrome, which usually occurs in untreated or chronic cases, develop profound irreversible memory disturbances with confabulation usually related to a lesion of the medial dorsal thalamus. *Central pontine myelinolysis* is an acquired syndrome of electrolyte-induced demyelination that may occur with alcoholism but is due to rapid overcorrection of hyponatremia. Careful attention to current guidelines for the treatment of hyponatremia will help prevent this devastating disorder [92]. Alzheimer type II reactive astrocytosis is a general effect that is associated with chronic liver disease and hyperammonemia.

Vitamin B$_{12}$ deficiency may cause *subacute combined degeneration of the spinal cord*. In addition to anemia, B$_{12}$ deficiency may produce severe and irreversible effects on long tracts of the spinal cord. Symptoms develop over a few weeks' time and are due to degeneration of lateral (motor) and posterior columns (sensory) of spinal cord (especially mid-thoracic in early stages). Acute *methanol (methyl alcohol)* toxicity causes a metabolic acidosis that may result in blindness, due to degeneration of retinal ganglion cells. A major metabolite of methanol is formic acid, which is believed to play a role in retinal toxicity. Selective putaminal necrosis and focal white matter changes may also be seen with severe exposure. *Carbon monoxide (CO)* is toxic because of its strong affinity for hemoglobin (binds 100–200 times more avidly than oxygen). Carboxyhemoglobin decreases the oxygen-carrying capacity of the blood, resulting in anemic hypoxia and a bright red appearance of the brain in patients dying acutely of CO poisoning. In more chronic cases, there is characteristic bilateral necrosis of the globus pallidus, with neuronal necrosis in many cortical areas, and white matter destruction can be prominent in some cases.

Neurodegenerative Disease

Neurodegenerative diseases are a diverse group of disorders with slowly progressive clinical deficits and variable clinico-pathological features [93]. These disorders are becoming increasingly prevalent as life expectancy increases and tend to include features suggesting exaggerated deficits of the type associated with aging, e.g., dementia (Alzheimer's disease) or slowness and loss of dexterity (idiopathic Parkinson's disease) [94, 95]. Particular groups of neurons are affected in a relatively selective fashion and are characterized pathologically by the accumulation of abnormal peptides or proteins within neurons or the neuropil. This has led to the current concept of neurodegenerative diseases representing forms of proteinopathies due at least in part to fundamental disorders of protein synthesis, processing, and elimination [93]. Numerous regressive anatomic changes in neurons—such as reduction in dendritic extent, degeneration of axons, disordered neurotransmitter function (including excitotoxicity), free radical toxicity, environmental toxicity, and disordered trophic factors—have all been implicated in the context of neurodegenerative disorders. The severity of dementia is also related to the severity and extent of concurrent cerebrovascular disease, especially microscopic infarcts [33, 96].

On postmortem study, brains from patients with neurodegenerative disease will show variable degrees of atrophy, which may be striking in particular regions such as frontotemporal atrophy in Alzheimer's disease and the frontotemporal lobar dementias (FTLDs). Histological examination typically reveals the abnormal accumulation of protein inclusions. Thus, Alzheimer's disease is an amyloid proteinopathy in which the Aβ-amyloid peptide accumulates in neuritic plaques within frontal and temporal association areas [97] and hyperphosphorylated tau accumulates in neuronal cytoplasmic neurofibrillary tangles (especially in the temporal lobe) [98]. The most consistent risk factor for late-onset AD is the apolipoprotein E genotype, especially the ε4 allele [94]. Abnormal tau aggregates are also prominent in some FTLDs (Pick disease, FTDP 17), progressive supranuclear palsy (PSP), and corticobasal degeneration, to name a few. In contrast, the Lewy body disorder spectra—including idiopathic Parkinson's disease, dementia with Lewy bodies (DLB), and the multiple system atrophies—all feature abnormal α-synuclein deposition [99]. As mentioned previously, some FTLDs and motor neuron degenerations like amyotrophic lateral sclerosis (ALS) feature prominent aggregates of TDP-43. Individual cases may show multiple types of the proteinaceous aggregates described earlier, and rare cases of clinical dementia will show little or no apparent neuropathology. Finally, abnormal protein aggregates may be associated with genetic neurodegenerations associated with trinucleotide repeats (Huntington disease, spinocerebellar degenerations).

References

1. Stiess M, Bradke F. Neuronal polarization: the cytoskeleton leads the way. Dev Neurobiol. 2011;71:430–44.
2. Perry A, Brat D. Neuropathology patterns and introduction. In: Perry A, Brat D, editors. Practical surgical neuropathology. Philadelphia: Elsevier; 2010. p. 1–14.

3. Sarnat HB, Nochlin D, Born DE. Neuronal nuclear antigen (NeuN): a marker of neuronal maturation in early human fetal nervous system. Brain Dev. 1998;20:88–94.

4. Vinters HV, Kleinschmidt-DeMasters BK. General pathology of the central nervous system. In: Love S, Louis DN, Ellison DW, editors. Greenfield's neuropathology. 8th ed. London: Hodder Arnold; 2008. p. 1–62.

5. Gray DA, Woulfe J. Lipofuscin and aging: a matter of toxic waste. http://sageke.sciencemag.org/cgi/content/full/2005/5/re1. Published 2 Feb 2005.

6. Reichard RR, Smith C, Graham DI. The significance of beta-APP immunoreactivity in forensic practice. Neuropathol Appl Neurobiol. 2005;31:304–13.

7. Benfenati V, Ferroni S. Water transport between CNS compartments: functional and molecular interactions between aquaporins and ion channels. Neuroscience. 2010;168:926–40.

8. Graber DJ, Levy M, Kerr D, Wade WF. Neuromyelitis optica pathogenesis and aquaporin 4. J Neuroinflammation. 2008;5:1–22.

9. Wisniewski T, Goldman JE. Alpha B-crystallin is associated with intermediate filaments in astrocytoma cells. Neurochem Res. 1998;23:385–92.

10. Quinlan RA, Brenner M, Goldman JE, Messing A. GFAP and its role in Alexander disease. Exp Cell Res. 2007;313:2077–87.

11. Hickey WF, Kimura H. Perivascular microglial cells of the CNS are bone-marrow-derived and present antigen in vivo. Science. 1988;230:290–2.

12. Abbott NJ, Ronnback L, Hansson E. Astrocyte-endothelial interactions at the blood-brain barrier. Nat Rev Neurosci. 2006;7:41–53.

13. Abbott NJ, Patabendige AAK, Dolman DEM, et al. Structure and function of the blood-brain barrier. Neurobiol Dis. 2010;37:13–25.

14. Nag S, Manias JL, Stewart DJ. Pathology and new players in the pathogenesis of brain edema. Acta Neuropathol. 2009;118:197–217.

15. Del Bigio MR. Neuropathological changes caused by hydrocephalus. Acta Neuropathol. 1993;85:573–85.

16. Del Bigio MR. Cellular damage and prevention in childhood hydrocephalus. Brain Pathol. 2004;14:317–24.

17. Blumbergs P, Reilly P, Vink R. Trauma. In: Love S, Louis DN, Ellison DW, editors. Greenfield's neuropathology. 8th ed. London: Hodder Arnold; 2008. p. 733–832.

18. Bruns JJ, Jagoda AS. Mild traumatic brain injury. Mt Sinai J Med. 2009;76:129–37.

19. Povlishock JT, Katz DI. Update of neuropathology and neurological recovery after traumatic brain injury. J Head Trauma Rehabil. 2005;2:76–94.

20. Povlishock JT, Becker DP, Cheng CL, Vaughan GW. Axonal change in minor head injury. J Neuropathol Exp Neurol. 1983; 42:225–42.

21. Gavett BE, Stern RA, McKee AC. Chronic traumatic encephalopathy: a potential late effect of sport-related concussive and subconcussive head trauma. Clin Sports Med. 2011;30:179–88.

22. McKee AC, Gavett BE, Stern RA, et al. TDP-43 proteinopathy and motor neuron disease in chronic traumatic encephalopathy. J Neuropathol Exp Neurol. 2010;69:918–29.

23. Uryu K, Chen XH, Martinez D, et al. Multiple proteins implicated in neurodegenerative diseases accumulate in axons after brain trauma in humans. Exp Neurol. 2007;208:185–92.

24. Gorrie C, Oakes S, Duflou J, et al. Axonal injury in children after motor vehicle crashes: extent, distribution, and size of axonal swellings using beta-APP immunohistochemistry. J Neurotrauma. 2002; 19:1171–82.

25. Sherriff FE, Bridges LR, Sivaloganathan S. Early detection of axonal injury after human head trauma using immunocytochemistry for beta-amyloid precursor protein. Acta Neuropathol. 1994;87:55–62.

26. Smith DH, Chen XH, Iwata A, et al. Amyloid beta accumulation in axons after traumatic brain injury in humans. J Neurosurg. 2003; 98:1072–7.

27. Gennarelli TA. Animate models of human head injury. J Neurotrauma. 1994;11:357–68.

28. Decker DA, Perry A, Yachnis AT. Vascular and ischemic brain disorders. In: Perry A, Brat D, editors. Practical surgical neuropathology. Philadelphia: Elsevier; 2010. p. 527–50.

29. Auer RN, Dunn JF, Sutherland GR. Hypoxia and related conditions. In: Love S, Louis DN, Ellison DW, editors. Greenfield's neuropathology. 8th ed. London: Hodder Arnold; 2008. p. 63–119.

30. Hazrati LN, Bergeron C, Butany J. Neuropathology of cerebrovascular diseases. Semin Diagn Pathol. 2009;26:103–15.

31. Vinters HV. Cerebrovascular disease—practical issues in surgical and autopsy pathology. Curr Top Pathol. 2001;95:51–99.

32. DeGirolami U, Seilhean D, Hauw JJ. Neuropathology of central nervous system arterial syndromes. Part I: the supratentorial circulation. J Neuropathol Exp Neurol. 2009;68:113–24.

33. Lammie GA. Hypertensive cerebral small vessel disease and stroke. Brain Pathol. 2002;12:358–70.

34. Schiff D, Lopes MB. Neuropathological correlates of reversible posterior leukoencephalopathy. Neurocrit Care. 2005;2:303–5.

35. Feske SK. Posterior reversible encephalopathy syndrome: a review. Semin Neurol. 2011;31:202–15.

36. Thal DR, Griffin WS, de Vos RA, Ghebremedhin E. Cerebral amyloid angiopathy and its relationship to Alzheimer's disease. Acta Neuropathol. 2008;115:599–609.

37. Love S, Miners S, Palmer J, et al. Insights into the pathogenesis and pathogenicity of cerebral amyloid angiopathy. Front Biosci. 2009;1:4778–92.

38. Revesz T, Holton JL, Lashley T, et al. Genetics and molecular pathogenesis of sporadic and hereditary cerebral amyloid angiopathies. Acta Neuropathol. 2009;118:115–30.

39. Weller RO, Boche D, Nicoll JA. Microvasculature changes and cerebral amyloid angiopathy in Alzheimer's disease and their potential impact on therapy. Acta Neuropathol. 2009;118: 87–102.

40. Chabarit H, Joutel A, Dichgans M, et al. CADASIL. Lancet Neurol. 2009;8:643–53.

41. Joutel A, Dodick DD, Parisi JE, et al. De novo mutation in the Notch 3 gene causing CADASIL. Ann Neurol. 2000;47:388–91.

42. Rhoton Jr AL. Aneurysms. Neurosurgery. 2002;51(4 Suppl): S121–58.

43. Seibert B, Tummala RP, Chow R, et al. Intracranial aneurysms: review of current options and outcomes. Front Neurol. 2011;2:1–11.

44. Ducruet AF, Hickman ZL, Zacharia BE, et al. Intracranial infectious aneurysms: a comprehensive review. Neurosurg Rev. 2010; 33:37–46.

45. Al-Shahi R, Bhattacharya JJ, Currie DG, et al. Prospective, population-based detection of intracranial vascular malformations in adults: the Scottish Intracranial Vascular Malformation Study (SIVMS). Stroke. 2003;34:1163–9.

46. Fleetwood IG, Steinberg GK. Arteriovenous malformations. Lancet. 2002;359:863–73.

47. Friedlander RM. Clinical practice. Arteriovenous malformations of the brain. N Engl J Med. 2007;356:2704–12.

48. Labauge P, Denier C, Bergametti F, Tounier-Lasserve E. Genetics of cavernous angiomas. Lancet Neurol. 2007;6:237–44.

49. Brat DJ, Perry A. Astrocytic and oligodendroglial tumors. In: Perry A, Brat D, editors. Practical surgical neuropathology—a diagnostic approach. Philadelphia: Churchill Livingstone/Elsevier; 2010. p. 63–102.

50. Louis DN, Ohgaki H, Wiestler OD, Cavenee WK. WHO classification of tumours of the central nervous system. Lyon: International Agency for Research; 2007.

51. Brat DJ, Prayson RA, Ryken TC, Olsen JJ. Diagnosis of glioma: role of neuropathology. J Neurooncol. 2008;89:287–311.

52. Ohgaki H, Kleihues P. Genetic pathways to primary and secondary glioblastoma. Am J Pathol. 2007;170:1445–53.

53. Purow B, Schiff D. Advances in genetics of glioblastoma: are we reaching a critical mass? Nat Rev Neurol. 2009;5:419–26.

54. Nikiforova MN, Hamilton RL. Molecular diagnostics of gliomas. Arch Pathol Lab Med. 2011;135:558–68.

55. Riemenschneider MJ, Jeuken JW, Wesseling P, et al. Molecular diagnostics of gliomas: state of the art. Acta Neuropathol. 2010; 120:567–84.

56. Phillips HS, Kharbanda S, Chen R, et al. Molecular subclasses of high-grade glioma predict prognosis, delineate a pattern of disease progression, and resemble stages in neurogenesis. Cancer Cell. 2006;9:157–73.

57. Colman H, Zhang L, Sulman EP, et al. A multigene predictor of outcome in glioblastoma. Neuro Oncol. 2010;12:49–57.

58. Dunbar E, Yachnis AT. Glioma diagnosis: immunohistochemistry and beyond. Adv Anat Pathol. 2010;17:187–201.

59. Aldape K, Burger PC, Perry A. Clinicopathologic aspects of 1p/19q loss and the diagnosis of oligodendroglioma. Arch Pathol Lab Med. 2007;131:242–51.

60. Gianinni C, Burger PC, Berkey BA, et al. Anaplastic oligodendroglial tumors: refining the correlation among histopathology, 1p 19q deletion and clinical outcome in Intergroup Radiation Therapy Oncology Group Trial 9402. Brain Pathol. 2008;18:360–9.

61. Jenkins RB, Blair H, Ballman KV, et al. A t(1;19)(q10;p10)mediates the combined deletions of 1p and 19q and predicts a better prognosis of patients with oligodendroglioma. Cancer Res. 2006;66:9852–61.

62. Yan H, Parsons DW, Jin G, et al. IDH1 and IDH2 mutations in gliomas. N Engl J Med. 2009;360:765–73.

63. Houillier C, Wang X, Kaloshi G, et al. IDH1 or IDH2 mutations predict longer survival and response to temozolomide in low-grade gliomas. Neurology. 2010;75:1560–6.

64. Capper D, Weibert S, Balss J, et al. Characterization of R132H mutation-specific IDH1 antibody binding in brain tumors. Brain Pathol. 2010;20:245–54.

65. Perry A. Meningiomas. In: Perry A, Brat DJ, editors. Practical surgical neuropathology—a diagnostic approach. Philadelphia: Churchill Livingstone/Elsevier; 2010. p. 185–217.

66. Lohmann CM, Brat DJ. A conceptual shift in the grading of meningiomas. Adv Anat Pathol. 2007;7:153–7.

67. Perry A, Scheithauer BW, Stafford SL, et al. "Malignancy" in meningiomas: a clinicopathological study of 116 patients with grading implications. Cancer. 1999;85:2046–56.

68. Scheithauer BW, Woodruff JM, Spinner RJ. Peripheral nerve sheath tumors. In: Perry A, Brat DJ, editors. Practical surgical neuropathology—a diagnostic approach. Philadelphia: Churchill Livingstone/Elsevier; 2010. p. 235–85.

69. Yachnis AT, Perry A. Embryonal (primitive) tumors of the central nervous system. In: Perry A, Brat D, editors. Practical surgical neuropathology. Philadelphia: Elsevier; 2010. p. 165–84.

70. Parsons DW, Li M, Zhang X, et al. The genetic landscape of the childhood cancer medulloblastoma. Science. 2011;331:435–9.

71. Dunham C. Pediatric brain tumors: a histologic and genetic update on commonly encountered entities. Semin Diagn Pathol. 2010; 27:147–59.

72. Frohman EM, Racke MK, Raine CS. Multiple sclerosis—the plaque and its pathogenesis. N Engl J Med. 2006;354:942–55.

73. Love S. Demyelinating diseases. J Clin Pathol. 2006;59:1151–9.

74. Schmidt RE. White matter and myelin disorders. In: Perry A, Brat DJ, editors. Practical surgical neuropathology—a diagnostic approach. Philadelphia: Churchill Livingstone/Elsevier; 2010. p. 485–513.

75. Trapp BD, Peterson J, Ransahoff RM, et al. Axonal transaction in the lesions of multiple sclerosis. N Engl J Med. 1998;338:278–85.

76. Moore GR. Current concepts in the neuropathology and pathogenesis of multiple sclerosis. Can J Neurol Sci. 2010;37:S5–15.

77. Jarius S, Wildemann B. AQP4 antibodies in neuromyelitis optica: diagnostic and pathogenetic relevance. Nat Rev Neurol. 2010;6:383–92.

78. Marignier R, Giraudon P, Vukusic S, et al. Anti-aquaporin-4 antibodies in Devic's neuromyelitis optica: therapeutic implications. Ther Adv Neurol Disord. 2010;3:311–21.

79. White MK, Khalili K. Pathogenesis of progressive multifocal leukoencephalopathy—revisited. J Infect Dis. 2011;203:578–86.

80. Johnson T, Nath A. Immune reconstitution inflammatory syndrome and the central nervous system. Curr Opin Neurol. 2011;24:284–90.

81. Hellwig K, Gold R. Progressive multifocal leukoencephalopathy and natalizumab. J Neurol. 2011;258(11):1920–8.

82. Kleinschmidt-DeMasters BK, Tyler KL. Infections and inflammatory disorders. In: Perry A, Brat DJ, editors. Practical surgical neuropathology—a diagnostic approach. Philadelphia: Churchill Livingstone/Elsevier; 2010. p. 455–84.

83. Thigpen MC, Whitney CG, Messonnier NE, et al. Bacterial meningitis in the United States, 1998–2007. N Engl J Med. 2011;21: 2016–25.

84. Edberg M, Furebring M, Sjölin J, Enblad P. Neurointensive care of patients with severe community-acquired meningitis. Acta Anaesthesiol Scand. 2011;55:732–9.

85. Honda H, Warren DK. Central nervous system infections: meningitis and brain abscess. Infect Dis Clin North Am. 2009;23:609–23.

86. Walker M, Zunt JR. Parasitic central nervous system infections in the immunocompromised host. Clin Infect Dis. 2005;40:1005–15.

87. Love S, Wiley CA. Viral infections. In: Graham DI, Lantos PL, editors. Greenfield's neuropathology. 8th ed. London: Hodder Arnold; 2008. p. 1105–15.

88. Del Valle L, Pina-Oviedo S. HIV disorders of the brain: pathology and pathogenesis. Front Biosci. 2006;11:718–32.

89. Norrby E. Prions and protein folding diseases. J Intern Med. 2011;270:1–14.

90. Harris J, Chimelli L, Kril J, Ray D. Nutritional deficiencies, metabolic disorders, and toxins affecting the nervous system. In: Graham DI, Lantos PL, editors. Greenfield's neuropathology. 8th ed. London: Hodder Arnold; 2008. p. 675–731.

91. Harper C. The neuropathology of alcohol-related brain damage. Alcohol Alcohol. 2009;44:136–40.

92. Rahman M, Friedman WA. Hyponatremia in neurosurgical patients: clinical guidelines development. Neurosurgery. 2009;65:925–35.

93. Lowe J, Mirra SS, Hyman BT, Dickson DW. Ageing and dementia. In: Graham DI, Lantos PL, editors. Greenfield's neuropathology. 8th ed. London: Hodder Arnold; 2008. p. 1105–15.

94. Berg L, McKeel DW, Miller P, et al. Clinicopathologic studies in cognitively healthy aging and Alzheimer disease. Relation of histologic markers to severity, age, sex, and apolipoprotein E genotype. Arch Neurol. 1998;55:326–35.

95. Sonnen JA, Larson EB, Crane PK, et al. Pathological correlates of dementia in a longitudinal, population-based sample of aging. Ann Neurol. 2007;62:406–13.

96. Jellinger KA, Attems J. Prevalence and impact of cerebrovascular pathology in Alzheimer disease and parkinsonism. Acta Neurol Scand. 2006;114:38–46.

97. Mirra SS. The CERAD neuropathology protocol and consensus recommendations for the postmortem diagnosis of Alzheimer disease: a commentary. Neurobiol Aging. 1997;18:S91–4.

98. Braak H, Braak E. Neuropathological staging of Alzheimer-related changes. Acta Neuropathol. 1991;82:239–59.

99. Leverenz J, McKeith I. Dementia with Lewy bodies. Med Clin North Am. 2002;86:519–35.

Part III

Neuromonitoring

Noninvasive Monitoring in the Neurointensive Care Unit: EEG, Oximetry, TCD

7

Christoph N. Seubert, Jean E. Cibula, and Michael E. Mahla

Contents

Abstract

Noninvasive monitoring modalities in the neurointensive care unit fall into two broad categories. The first aims to assess function of the nervous system. Examples of such monitoring modalities are the clinical exam, the electroencephalogram, and the recording of evoked potentials. Since neurological function is disrupted before cellular integrity is lost, monitors of function provide early warning of inadequate oxygen supply and provide opportunity to correct this problem before irreversible damage occurs. The second category aims to determine the adequacy of cerebral perfusion. Examples are transcranial Doppler ultrasonography, near-infrared spectroscopy, tissue pO_2, and brain or jugular venous oximetry. No single monitoring technique is without its limitations or addresses all questions raised by a given patient.

Keywords

Electroencephalography • EEG • Transcranial Doppler • TCD • Jugular bulb oximetry • Brain tissue oxygen • Brain death • Coma • Prognosis

C.N. Seubert, MD, PhD (✉)
Division of Neuroanesthesia, Department of Anesthesiology,
University of Florida College of Medicine,
1600 SW Archer Rd, Rm M509, 100254,
Gainesville, FL 32610-0254, USA

Intraoperative Neurophysiologic Monitoring Laboratory,
Shands Hospital, Gainesville, FL, USA
e-mail: cseubert@anest.ufl.edu

J.E. Cibula, MD
Department of Neurology,
University of Florida College of Medicine,
Gainesville, FL 32611, USA
e-mail: jean.cibula@neurology.ufl.edu

M.E. Mahla, MD
Division of Neuroanesthesia, Department of Anesthesiology,
University of Florida College of Medicine,
1600 SW Archer Rd, Rm M509, 100254,
Gainesville, FL 32610-0254, USA
e-mail: mahla@ufl.edu

Introduction

Monitoring the brain is a natural extension of medical care in neurointensive care units (NICU). Careful, repeated, and reliable assessment of the patient's neurological status underlies therapeutic decisions and thus underpins ultimate outcome. Improvements in the disease process present opportunities to decrease the level of physiologic support and to initiate interventions aimed towards rehabilitation. Conversely, progression of the disease processes may necessitate increased levels of physiologic support and additional medical or neurosurgical interventions in order to mitigate secondary injury to the central nervous system (CNS).

A.J. Layon et al. (eds.), *Textbook of Neurointensive Care*,
DOI 10.1007/978-1-4471-5226-2_7, © Springer-Verlag London 2013

Neurophysiologic monitoring is done on the premise that normal function and the ability to compensate for pathophysiologic processes cease *before* irreversible structural damage ensues. Removal of the secondary insult should allow continued structural integrity and eventual recovery of function. In the CNS, this therapeutic window may extend from a few minutes to a few hours depending on the pathophysiologic reason why function failed and on the monitoring modality used to assess the change.

Monitoring modalities fall into two broad categories. The first aims to assess function of the nervous system. Examples of such monitoring modalities are the clinical exam, the electroencephalogram, and the recording of evoked potentials. The second category aims to determine the adequacy of cerebral perfusion. Examples are transcranial Doppler ultrasonography, near-infrared spectroscopy, tissue pO_2, and brain or jugular venous oximetry. No single monitoring technique is without its limitations or addresses all questions raised by a given patient. As clinicians decide what monitoring is used to help with patient management, neurological monitoring should not be held to a higher standard than other monitors. In fact, no monitor in either operating room or ICU has been shown to change outcome. Multimodal approaches that combine assessment of cerebral blood flow, cerebral function, and intracranial pressure with appropriate imaging and respiratory and cardiac monitoring show the greatest promise of prospectively aiding therapeutic decision making. Ultimately, any contribution made by monitoring will be tied to implementation of appropriate therapies.

Monitoring of Neurological Function

When O_2 delivery to the brain falls below a level sufficient to meet the cerebral metabolic requirement for oxygen ($CMRO_2$), function fails. Since function is disrupted *before* cellular integrity is lost, monitors of function provide early warning of inadequate O_2 supply and provide opportunity to correct this problem before irreversible damage occurs. Such monitors can be used to guide therapy when the CNS may be compromised by the natural progression of a disease process, e.g., worsening cerebral edema after cardiac arrest or head trauma, or by a complication of a disease, e.g., vasospasm in the wake of a subarachnoid hemorrhage.

Alternatively, brain function may be abnormal despite adequate O_2 supply due to factors intrinsic or extrinsic to the brain. Examples of the former include convulsive or nonconvulsive seizures and postictal states; examples of the latter include metabolic abnormalities such as hepatic encephalopathy or intoxications. In a given patient, such depressant factors may coexist with inadequate O_2 supply. For example, seizure activity, which frequently occurs after delayed resuscitation from cardiac arrest, may coexist with and compound post-hypoxic cerebral edema.

The Neurological Examination

Overview
Of all neurophysiologic monitoring modalities, the neurological examination of an awake and cooperative patient allows for the most comprehensive assessment of CNS function. It requires no special equipment or technologists to operate the equipment and can be applied continually, as needed. It should include a repeated focused assessment of CNS structures at risk in a given patient and a general overview such as the documentation of the level of consciousness, e.g., by the Glasgow Coma Scale, motor responses to verbal and/or painful stimuli, and evaluation of brainstem reflexes.

In practice, however, the neurological examination has important limitations. First, patients in neurointensive care frequently present in an altered state or with diseases that severely limit the information obtainable by a neurological exam. Second, neurological evaluations are usually done discontinuously and by examiners of varying skill or may be variably documented. Therefore, they may miss evolving changes and/or give variable results. Third, the results of neurological exams are confounded and constrained by therapeutic interventions that are frequently used in the ICU such as endotracheal intubation, sedatives/hypnotics, analgesics, or neuromuscular blocking agents. For example, the decrease and eventual absence of a pupillary light response in the syndrome of a transtentorial herniation will be preceded by extensive changes in the level of consciousness and higher cortical functions, which will be missed in an intubated patient treated with neuromuscular blocking agents.

Level of Consciousness
The first step in the neurological examination is the assessment of the level of consciousness. The standard tool is the *Glasgow Coma Scale (GCS)*, which grades the patient's best efforts in the categories of *eye opening* (4–1 points), *motor response* (6–1 point), and *verbal response* (5–1 points), with higher scores indicating better CNS function. One obvious limitation in the use of the GCS for repeated assessments is the requirement of a verbal response, which will be unobtainable in intubated patients. Clinicians have devised various ways to overcome this limitation, such as a combined eye opening/motor response score marked with a "T" subscript to indicate endotracheal intubation or a best clinical guess at the response that a patient would give, if he/she were extubated. Regardless of the method used to adapt the GCS to intubated patients, it retains most of its diagnostic and prognostic utility [1].

Because of the limitations of the GCS for repeated assessment, a host of other scales have been developed to grade disorders of consciousness, with a particular emphasis on the potential for rehabilitation. Their utility has been systematically reviewed recently [2], but their detailed discussion exceeds the scope of this chapter.

Brain Death

One area, which has brought both the merits as well as the limitations of the neurological exam into clear focus, is determination of brain death for purposes of organ donation or withdrawal of support, which is discussed in detail in Chap. 44. Because the clinical determination of brain death requires a comprehensive and methodical clinical assessment of the patient [3], it may also serve as a guide to the neurological exam of a comatose patient in the NICU. Its steps, with the exception of the apnea test, will be briefly summarized here.

In the case of brain death, the GCS by definition assumes the lowest possible value, because brain death is characterized by coma and unresponsiveness [4–6]. Motor responses *elicited by the exam* need to be differentiated from spontaneous movements *during the exam*. The latter are typically brief, slow movements, which originate from the spinal cord, and do not become integrated into decerebrate or decorticate responses. Only rarely are they reproducible upon repeat testing. Reproducible partial eye opening that failed to reveal the iris has been described in response to a peripheral painful stimulus in a patient who fulfilled clinical criteria of brain death [4, 6]. Conditions that may confound the clinical diagnosis of coma are listed in Table 7.1 [5]. In addition to considering such confounding conditions, the diagnosis of coma should be consistent with imaging studies and/or the overall clinical picture.

The next step in the neurological examination is the assessment of brainstem function. As in the assessment of the level of consciousness, direct trauma to either afferent or efferent structures needs to be considered before any of the tests of brainstem function are interpreted as consistent with brain death. Typical tests, their afferent and efferent pathways, and potentially interfering clinical conditions other than direct trauma to the tested pathways are summarized in Table 7.2.

Monitoring Spontaneous Electrical Activity: Electroencephalography

Theory

Electroencephalography (EEG) is a graphical representation of voltage differences over certain areas of the cortex over time. The electrical signal is a summation of the excitatory postsynaptic potentials and the inhibitory postsynaptic potentials under each electrode and may be recorded anywhere from the scalp over the cerebral cortex. Each EEG channel has two input electrodes, the second of which is subtracted from the first by inverting the signal polarity of the second input, which is known as differential amplification. If the voltage difference is negative, the tracing goes upward, and if the difference is positive, the tracing is deflected downward by convention. In modern digital recordings, all of the electrodes are recorded with respect to a particular referential electrode and are subsequently digitally processed into montages, or combinations, of electrodes, some of which is referential (where the second input is a common electrode that minimizes local input such as one placed on the ipsilateral

Table 7.1 Neurological states resembling brain death

Disease state	Diagnostic aids	Comments
Hypothermia	Core temperature <32 °C	May cause central nervous system depression up to clinical brain death
	Osborne waves on ECG	
Acute poisoning	Drug screening	In differentiating from brain death, consider antidote and/or document subtherapeutic drug concentration and/or wait for four elimination half-lives
	Serum concentration Measurements	Direct central nervous system depressants may confound confirmatory testing of brain death because of CMRO$_2$/CBF coupling
Metabolic encephalopathy	Laboratory testing	Imaging studies should document structural central nervous system changes
Akinetic mutism	Intact lower brainstem function	Imaging study shows frontal or mesencephalic brain lesion
	Intact sleep-wake cycle	
Locked-in syndrome	Clinical course and imaging studies	Central locked-in syndrome: corticobulbar and corticospinal tracts are interrupted at the level of the base of the pons; vertical eye movements are intact
		Peripheral locked-in syndrome: Guillain-Barré syndrome, advanced amyotrophic lateral sclerosis, neuromuscular blocking agents, organophosphate poisoning

Data from Wijdicks [5]. Reproduced with permission from Seubert and Mahla [92]

Abbreviations: *CMRO$_2$* cerebral metabolic requirement for oxygen, *CBF* cerebral blood flow, *ECG* electrocardiogram

Table 7.2 Neurological exam of brainstem function

Brainstem reflex	Afferent path	Efferent path	Caveats
Pupillary light reaction	II	III	Not confounded by systemic drugs, absence may be caused by prolonged administration of neuromuscular blocking agents [6]
Ocular movements (oculocephalic reflex or caloric nystagmus)	VIII	III, VI	Confounded by damage from ototoxic drugs, cervical spine trauma may preclude testing of the oculocephalic reflex; voluntary ocular movements are sometimes the only finding that differentiates a "locked-in" syndrome from brain death
Corneal reflex/pressure on supraorbital nerve	V	VII	
Gag	IX	IX, X	May be difficult to assess in orotracheally intubated patient
Cough	X	X, cervical roots	Best tested by assessing the response to tracheal suctioning

Reproduced with permission from Seubert and Mahla [92]

ear or in the sagittal midline) or differential (where there may be a chain or sequence of electrodes comparing EEG signals point to point). In the former, the amplitude differences provide localizing information, and in the latter, localization is by phase reversals where polarity changes. The interpreting physician may change from one montage to another while reading the study in order to assess artifact or polarity, an ability not found in the old analog/paper EEG machines. The EEG technologist is an essential part of the team, monitoring signals, monitoring electrode integrity, and ensuring that impedances are balanced between electrodes. Failure to maintain good impedances can result in significant contamination by artifact, which may obscure important findings or lead to a false interpretation of the EEG. Differential amplification (see previous discussion) allows for common mode rejection: the elimination of identical signals from the output if they are present in both inputs. Common mode rejection assists with the elimination of 60 Hz artifact from an electrical device at the bedside that is poorly shielded. Mismatch of impedances impairs the ability of common mode rejection to eliminate some artifacts. Proper grounding also aids in reducing electrical interference. Grounding also reduces the risk of direct electrical shock to the patients and caregivers. The ICU electrical environment is particularly challenging, with multiple monitors, IV pumps, ventilators, specialty beds, and cardiac equipment all providing potential artifact sources. Since intracranial electrodes tend to be less subject to environmental artifact and record from a much more localized area, some centers use invasive electrodes and monitors routinely for patients in the ICU [7].

It is generally impractical for the ICU staff to be expected to interpret the raw EEG signal except for a few select cases, such as the monitoring of burst suppression (Fig. 7.1) and when titration of sedation such as in pentobarbital coma is required. Reviewing the entire EEG takes a significant amount of time for the skilled technologist or physician, and, typically, the technologist will review the data and sample them for the physician's review. A two-channel EEG may not record over an area of interest, and artifact identification

may be problematic. When more electrodes are used, there is greater sensitivity for detecting abnormalities and spatial localization of abnormalities, but the review and interpretation of such a record require more time and expertise. Changes that occur over hours may be subtle and missed on a raw EEG. Reviews may only be performed once or twice a day, and, thus, feedback may be delayed. In large centers, technologists may be able to watch live streaming EEG remotely, but since they may be watching multiple patients, some events may be missed even in this setting [8].

Drug Effects

It is crucial for the physician interpreting the EEG to know the medications the patient is receiving, as they may have a profound effect on the EEG patterns observed. Medications such as carbapenems or fluoroquinolones may lower the seizure threshold. Levetiracetam may cause EEG changes resembling subclinical seizures. Prominent, so-called drug spindles, for example, are seen with benzodiazepines, propofol, and other sedating medications. Withdrawal from pentobarbital coma can result in a transiently sharply contoured background which can be of concern for seizures in the unwary. Sedation with anesthetics such as pentobarbital and propofol can cause burst-suppression patterns, which carry a grave prognosis if seen in unmedicated patients following cardiopulmonary arrest [9].

Clinical Applications
Monitoring

Nevertheless, if the patient has persistently altered mental status or develops clinical seizures, EEG monitoring is an important component of patient care and should be considered early in the patient's ICU stay [10]. A routine EEG (less than 1 h) may be sufficient if the patient is neurologically stable. In the patient with an unstable or deteriorating neurological examination, a prolonged EEG study, even lasting overnight or days (long-term EEG), may be needed to determine whether or not subclinical seizures or nonconvulsive status epilepticus may be the culprit. Please see Chap. 39

Fig. 7.1 Electroencephalogram recorded from a patient in a pharmacologic coma. All channels show a pattern of burst suppression, i.e., periods of EEG activity followed by periods of EEG silence

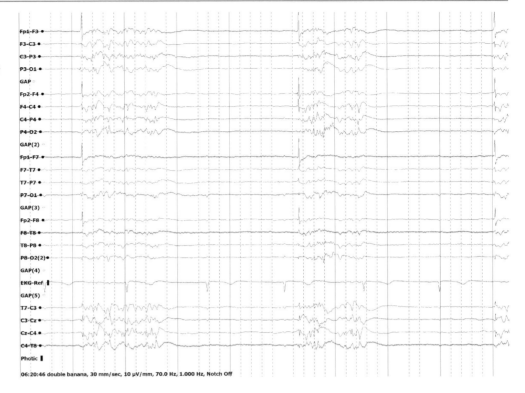

on Seizures for further discussion of seizures and status epilepticus, which is considered a neurological emergency requiring immediate intervention. Other clinical events that are reflected in the EEG are sedative drugs, physiological states such as sleep and arousal, as well as pathological states such as sleep deprivation or cerebral ischemia [11]. Of note, both ischemia and increasing concentrations of anesthetics cause a slowing of EEG activity and ultimately burst suppression (Fig. 7.2). Conversely, EEG reactivity to environmental stimuli and persistence or reappearance of sleep architecture portend a better neurological prognosis. When in doubt, discuss the testing with the monitoring neurologist to determine what type of EEG study best fits the patient's needs. Some tertiary centers routinely use long-term EEG monitoring on alert patients for 24 h and stuporous or comatose patients for 48 h on admission to the neuro-ICU, particularly those with hemorrhages in order to detect subclinical seizures or status epilepticus. A normal EEG does not exclude the possibility of a seizure, but a longer study (and larger sample size) may help ensure that a subclinical presentation is not missed.

In order to improve bedside utility of ICU EEG recording, trending software has been developed using quantitative EEG techniques to provide an overview of the EEG which may be interpretable at the bedside with relatively minimal training. Most currently available digital EEG machines can have such software added if it is not available as an initial option. Hirsch and Brenner's *Atlas of EEG in Critical Care*

provides an excellent overview and detailed introduction to this topic and methods [12]. The displayed options can be customized for the patient, so that a continuous overview of the EEG data is readily seen. These techniques do not replace the expert review of the raw EEG data because the software is not able to completely address artifact or detect more subtle abnormalities. Quantitative bedside EEG analysis may, however, help improve timeliness of feedback to the patient care team and responsiveness to changes in the patient's condition. Commonly used quantitative techniques include:

- *Fourier transform* changes the EEG displayed from amplitude over time to frequency over time and displays the resulting data as a *power spectrum* where the frequencies making up a particular segment of EEG are displayed. *Compressed spectral arrays* may represent these data as a stack of successive tracings and can also use colored bands to represent the EEG power at different frequencies as a *color density spectral array*. Individual EEG channels are typically displayed, but topographical maps may also be used.
- *Envelope trending* uses the median peak-to-peak amplitude in a particular block of time to create a graph over time for a specific electrode pair. Selection of the area of interest is crucial to detecting changes.
- *The spectral edge frequency* is the frequency below which a predetermined percentage of the study's EEG power lies.

Fig. 7.2 EEG ischemia. This is part of the long-term EEG performed on a 68-year-old patient with severe neurovascular disease. The patient was admitted to the neuro ICU because of a thrombosis of the mid-basilar artery resulting in midbrain and bilateral thalamic infarcts. The patient had a prior history of a left internal carotid artery occlusion and an old left cortical stroke in the territory of the posterior middle cerebral artery The EEG shows a poorly organized background with some degree of generalized slowing, likely due to the new thalamic strokes. EEG slowing is maximal in the area of old infarction on the left

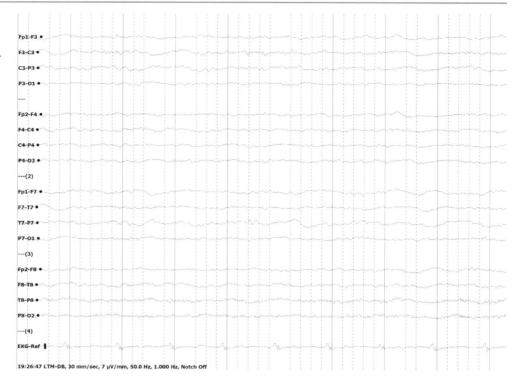

- *Asymmetry indices* may be used in a patient at high risk for vasospasm, for example, and compares the EEG frequency of homologous pairs of electrodes averaged over the entire hemisphere. A shift from one side to another could indicate vasospasm or ischemia from another cause [13, 14].
- The *brain symmetry index* (*BSI*) is a numerical value between 0 (perfect symmetry) and 1 (maximal asymmetry) over all frequencies at a homologous electrode pair which has been shown to correlate with stroke scales and has been used to follow progress after tPA administration [15, 16].
- *Automated spike and seizure detection* is available on digital EEG systems, but since these largely rely on frequency and amplitude algorithms, artifact may have a significant impact and the study must still be reviewed by an expert. Seizures without an EEG correlate are not detected by such software, and many will falsely detect a seizure if the patient is moving or being moved [17].

Brain Death

Because EEG monitors only the cerebral cortex, other types of neurodiagnostic tools must be used to evaluate subcortical structures. In general, the best tool is the neurological examination itself, performed by an experienced clinician. For cerebral death evaluations, evidence has not shown that electrophysiologic tools are necessary for the diagnosis and, thus, they are considered confirmatory or ancillary only [3]. While both somatosensory evoked potentials (SSEPs) and

bispectral index (BIS) will typically show specific patterns associated with brain death, there is insufficient evidence to show that these modalities will accurately document cessation of the function of *the entire* brain. The ancillary tests most commonly used in this clinical setting include EEG, cerebral angiography, nuclear perfusion scanning, transcranial Doppler (TCD), CT angiography (CTA), and magnetic resonance imaging and angiography (MRI/MRA). Ancillary tests do not replace the core examination but may help shorten the observation period and are often used if there is uncertainty regarding the neurological examination.

Sedation

Sedation of patients in the ICU is done to relieve patient's anxiety and discomfort and facilitate supportive care. Recent work highlighting the morbidity and cost of excessive sedation has led to the adoption of sedation protocols that incorporate interruption of sedation, efforts towards weaning from mechanical ventilation, and mobilization [18, 19]. Such an approach needs to be adapted to patients in the NICU, because the pharmacologic target of the sedatives – the brain – is frequently affected by the disease process that brought the patient to intensive care in the first place [20]. For example, sedation of NICU patients interferes on the one hand with their neurological exam, while on the other hand, sedation is a therapeutic intervention in the setting of elevated intracranial pressure.

Assessment of the adequacy of sedation is typically done clinically by applying sedation scales such as the Richmond Agitation-Sedation Scale, which assesses the spectrum from sedation to agitation over a range from unarousable (a value of −5) to alert/calm (a value of 0) to combative (a value of +5) [21]. Processed frontal EEG in the form of the "depth-of-anesthesia" monitors such as the bispectral index (BIS) or EEG-entropy has also been studied as a tool to facilitate appropriate titration of sedation. While these monitors may accurately reflect anesthetic drug effect [22] – a BIS value <30, for example, predominately reflects the degree of EEG suppression [23] – level of sedation includes parameters other than measurable drug effects on the frontal cortex. For example, analgesia, a very important component of sedation, is not well monitored by either BIS or EEG-entropy [24]. The main utility of EEG-based monitors of sedation may therefore lie in guiding administration of sedatives, if patients require deep sedation or administration of neuromuscular blocking agents. In both these settings, artifacts that typically confound EEG recording are reduced, and standard sedation scales are of limited utility.

Evoked Electrical Activity

Theory

Evoked potentials can be used to evaluate the sensory and motor systems. Motor evoked potentials are recorded at the level of the muscles and do not have to be extracted from background EEG activity. Sensory evoked potentials, in contrast, are recorded from scalp surface electrodes placed in standard EEG positions. They represent the response to a series of repeated sensory stimuli and are signal averaged over time to extract the evoked response from the EEG background. Signal averaging is necessary because evoked potentials are typically one to two orders of magnitude smaller than EEG. Thus, the signal-to-noise ratio precludes recording of responses evoked by individual stimuli. Characteristic waves are produced, and then latencies are measured which can be compared to normative data in order to provide localizing information for neurological deficits. Naming conventions vary, but generally they are based on latency of the response and designated positive or negative polarity (Fig. 7.3). Sensory evoked responses are generally much less vulnerable to medication/sedation effects (but are reduced or absent in hypothermia) and are most frequently used for specific diagnostic questions.

VEPs

For example, visual evoked potentials (VEPs) are commonly used to evaluate the visual pathways in patients with demyelinating disorders. The patient focuses on the center of a screen showing an alternating checkerboard pattern. The latency of the responses produced can help to demonstrate the presence of a lesion in the optic pathway, even in the absence of a deficit in visual acuity. VEPs are not commonly used in the ICU setting.

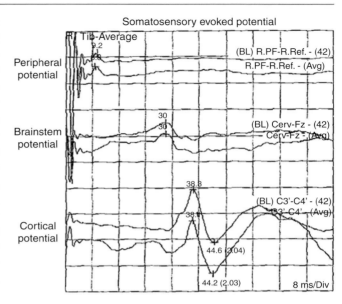

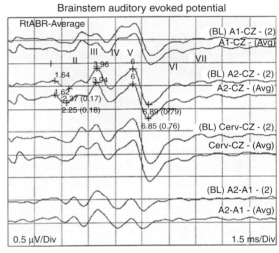

Fig. 7.3 Sensory evoked potentials in response to somatosensory and auditory stimulation. The *top panel* shows three pairs of traces in response to posterior tibial nerve stimulation. Potentials are recorded along the somatosensory pathway peripherally in the popliteal fossa, at the level of the brainstem, and over the contralateral somatosensory cortex. The *bottom panel* shows brainstem auditory evoked potentials along the neural pathway of the brainstem recorded from different electrodes. Wave I represents neural activity in the inner ear. Waves III–V represent rostral conduction of the auditory impulse in the brainstem

AEPs

Brainstem auditory evoked potentials (BAEPs) are used routinely to test hearing in infants but can also be used intraoperatively for brainstem and cranial nerve VIII surgeries and in comatose patients as a prognostication tool (see section "Clinical Application"). The sensory stimulus for BAEPs is a brief "click" applied via headphones at a volume that exceeds the hearing threshold. If hearing is intact, changes may be seen after brainstem compression or infarction [25].

SSEPs

Somatosensory evoked potentials (SSEPs) are evoked by electrical stimulation of median and posterior tibial nerves and recorded along the conducting pathway as well as over the contralateral somatosensory cortex (Fig. 7.3). SSEPs have been studied in the setting of anoxic-ischemic encephalopathy, and the absence of the bilateral N20 with median nerve stimulation 1–3 days after CPR was predictive of a poor outcome [26]; however, the hypothermia protocol may confound the predictive value of this, as can other metabolic derangements. Conversely, the bilateral persistence of a cortical response to SSEPs from median nerve stimulation has so far consistently predicted eventual awakening (albeit with varying degrees of function) from hypoxic coma [27].

MEPs

Motor evoked potentials (MEPs) may be used in spinal cord or aortic surgeries where the anterior spinal artery may be threatened. Traditional SSEP monitoring serves as a surrogate for monitoring the motor pathways but may not always detect motor deficits, so MEPs have been used in parallel [28]. Transcranial stimulation is the preferred method, which produces D waves by direct pyramidal cell activation and I waves by indirect activation through interneurons as well as polyphasic compound muscle action potentials [29]. MEP recording can be performed outside the operating room setting using a magnetic coil but is impossible in patients requiring complete neuromuscular blockade and may be more difficult in children. There is ongoing interest in magnetic stimulation in the field of neurorehabilitation research, but use in the ICU is investigational.

Clinical Application

As the use of evoked potentials spread from the diagnostic setting to the operating room, there was also enthusiasm for evaluating their role in the neuro-ICU. Because continuous high-quality recordings require the presence of trained technologists and because evoked potentials can only be recorded from selected pathways of the CNS, their adoption as monitors of subcortical function to complement EEG was not realized. Their current clinical application is restricted to specific diagnostic questions and to prognostication in coma.

Somatosensory evoked potentials in combination with brainstem auditory evoked potentials are helpful in the management of comatose patients [30–38]. In general, if both brainstem auditory evoked potentials and cortical somatosensory evoked potentials are intact at presentation and remain intact, ultimate outcome is good. A relatively good outcome may occur in this case even if all clinical signs indicate a very poor prognosis [31]. If the cortical somatosensory evoked potentials at presentation are absent and the brainstem auditory evoked potentials are present, the best outcome expected is a chronic vegetative state. If both cortical somatosensory evoked potentials and all brainstem auditory evoked potential waves beyond wave I are absent, brain death is very likely. It is important to note that drug overdose will not eliminate either the brainstem auditory evoked potential or the early and intermediate latency components of the somatosensory evoked potential. While the electroencephalogram may be entirely absent in the case of drug overdose or therapy such as in barbiturate coma, the brainstem auditory evoked potential and somatosensory evoked potential should be present if the patient has brain function.

Slight differences in sensitivity, specificity, and predictive value of evoked potentials exist that depend on the etiology of the comatose state. In anoxic-ischemic coma, absence of cortical SEPs 24 h after the precipitating event was found to be the best method to predict poor outcome [27]. Similarly, bilateral loss or absence of cortical SEPs is always associated with a poor outcome in comatose patients, whose EEG reveals alpha, theta, or alpha-theta coma [38]. Conversely, presence of cortical SEPs is associated with a favorable outcome. Auditory evoked potentials are less useful in anoxic-ischemic coma. Brainstem responses may initially be absent, due to cochlear ischemia, but are otherwise only affected very late in the course of anoxia/ischemia. Presence of mid-latency or late auditory potentials is predictive of a good outcome but is subject to the same modulating influences as the EEG. In coma due to head trauma, both the cerebral hemispheres and the brainstem may be involved in a pattern of lesions that reflects more the mechanism of injury and less the intrinsic tolerance to hypoxia/ischemia of a given brain structure. Presence of cortical EPs such as the N20 of the median SSEP or mid-latency AEPs is still associated with favorable outcomes even if the latency of the peaks is increased [39]. Conversely, absence of cortical peaks and progressive rostro-caudal deterioration of BAEPs, as occurs with transtentorial herniation, leads to brain death [40]. The decreased predictive power of absent cortical responses in posttraumatic coma is demonstrated by the fact that all cases of good clinical outcomes despite absent cortical SSEPs stem from such trauma patients [41, 42].

Monitors of Cerebral Blood Flow

Cerebral ischemia is one of the most common pathophysiologic mechanisms of secondary injury in NICU patients with a variety of CNS diseases. Therefore, maintenance of adequate cerebral blood flow is a critical therapeutic objective. The most frequent modality used is the invasive measurement of arterial blood pressure either by itself or augmented by simultaneous measurement of intracranial pressure, as discussed in Chaps. 8 and 35. Patient management

Table 7.3 Techniques for measuring cerebral blood flow

Category	Technique	Resolution		Invasiveness	Cost
		Temporal	Spatial		
Indirect	Neurological exam	>3 min	Eloquent areas	No	+
	Electroencephalogram/evoked potentials	1–3 min	Cortex/sensory pathway	No	++
	Cerebral perfusion pressure	<1 min	Global	Subdural, intraventricular, or intraparenchymal probe	+
Bedside	Kety-Schmidt	15 min	Hemispheric	Jugular catheter	+
	^{133}Xenon washout	3–15 min	3–4 cm	Jugular catheter, radiation	+
	AVDO$_2$, jugular venous oxygen saturation (S$_{Jv}$O$_2$)	<1 min	Global	Jugular catheter	+
	Double indicator dilution	3 min	Global	Jugular catheter, descending thoracic aortic catheter	+
	Near-infrared spectroscopy	<1 min	Local, bifrontal	No	+
	Thermal clearance probe	<1 min	Local, 1–2 cm	Exposed cortex	+
	Laser Doppler flow probe	<1 min	Local, 1–2 cm	Exposed cortex	+
Tomographic	Positron emission tomography (PET)	4–6 min/section	<1 cm	Radiation from positron emitter	+++++
	Stable xenon computed tomogram (CT)	4–6 min/section	<1 cm	Radiation from CT scan	+++
	Single-photon emission tomography (SPECT)	4–6 min/section	<1 cm	Radiation from gamma emitter	+++
	Magnetic resonance imaging (MRI)	4–6 min/section	<1 cm	No	+++

Data from Martin and Doberstein [43], Madsen and Secher [44], Cottrell [45], and Keller et al. [46]. Reproduced with permission from Seubert and Mahla [92]

according to the principle of maintaining cerebral perfusion pressure is, however, limited to a global approach that accounts neither for the specific needs of an individual patient nor for regional variation within a given patient's brain. Regional variation in perfusion can be assessed through the imaging of the transit of a bolus of contrast medium during CT or MRI imaging. While the great benefit of imaging is its good spatial resolution, a significant downside of imaging is the increase in the risk of complications associated with the need to move critically ill patients to the scanners. Conversely, the prominent role of imaging is confirmed by the trend to make CT scanners sufficiently portable to allow deployment at the bedside and to move MRI scanners close to neuro-ICUs. Details on neuroradiological techniques are provided in Chap. 40.

Indicator Dilution Methods

Bedside techniques of determining cerebral blood flow rely on a variety of techniques and provide either crude estimates of global cerebral blood flow or highly localized information. They measure cerebral blood flow by determining either the wash-in or washout of a relatively inert indicator substance such as a dye, isotope, or a pulse of heat, in a variation of an idea that dates back to the early studies of Kety and Schmidt. Available techniques are summarized in Table 7.3 [43–46]. Some modalities that are in more widespread use will be discussed next in some detail.

Transcranial Doppler

A unique bedside approach to the study of cerebral perfusion is the determination of cerebral blood flow velocities in major intracranial arteries using transcranial Doppler ultrasound. Older instrumentation was restricted to measurements of flow velocity at a particular depth and required the operator to assemble a mental image of the intracranial circulation as successive arterial segments were interrogated. Newer machines combine pulsed-wave Doppler measurements of flow velocity with ultrasound imaging capacities, which greatly facilitates anatomic orientation, correct attribution of flow velocities to particular vessels, and correction of flow velocities for the angle of insonation [47]. Transcranial Doppler studies are typically done once daily during vulnerable periods in the course of a CNS disease but can also be used continuously, for example, to detect embolic events.

Theory

Transcranial Doppler (TCD) uses ultrasound waves to measure the velocity of blood flow in the basal arteries of the brain and the extracranial internal carotid artery. Ultrasound is transmitted through the relatively thin temporal bone and at reduced intensity through the orbit or the foramen magnum [48]. In approximately 10 % of patients, particularly elderly females, technically satisfactory recordings cannot be obtained because of a limited temporal bone window [48].

When the ultrasound waves contact moving red blood cells, they are reflected back towards the transducer at a changed frequency. The change in frequency is an example of the Doppler effect and is related to velocity and direction of flow. Velocity increases during systole and decreases during diastole. Blood cells in the center of the lumen move faster than blood cells near the vessel wall, producing a spectrum of flow velocities. This flow spectrum resembles the shape of the waveform produced by an intra-arterial pressure transducer (Fig. 7.4). The TCD probe emits ultrasound waves as short pulses and thus represents an application of pulsed-wave Doppler. Because ultrasound travels through tissue at a constant velocity, assessment of flow at different distances from the transducer becomes possible by varying the time window during which the reflected ultrasound waves are received. Thus, each segment of the arteries at the base of the brain has a distinct signature in terms of depth of insonation, direction of flow, and shape of the waveform (Fig. 7.4).

Although TCD allows interrogation of all arteries that supply the brain, TCD cannot provide a simple assessment of global or hemispheric blood flow. In the setting of acute stroke or traumatic arterial dissection, the mere patency of a vessel is an important question that has diagnostic, therapeutic, and prognostic implications [48, 49]. Beyond the question of vessel patency, the link between TCD measurements and cerebral blood flow is indirect. From a technical point of view, the angle of insonation needs to be kept constant between assessments. Furthermore, two assumptions have to be met for TCD-measured blood flow velocity to correspond to CBF: First, the diameter of the artery must remain constant. Only then is flow proportional to flow velocity. Second, the blood flow in the basal arteries of the brain must be directly related to cortical CBF. These assumptions likely represent an oversimplification and have not been supported adequately by evidence. Specifically, radioactive xenon-measured CBF does not correlate well with TCD-derived MCA velocity during carotid endarterectomy or cardiopulmonary bypass [50–52]. Likewise, normal variations in blood flow velocities are large [53]. Despite this limitation, TCD has found many applications in the NICU, particularly in combination with other monitoring modalities that assess CBF.

Clinical Applications
Vasospasm
TCD has been very helpful in identifying vasospasm following aneurysmal subarachnoid hemorrhage. As the diameter of the arterial lumen decreases with vasospasm, the velocity of blood flowing through the narrowed vessel must increase if flow is to be maintained (Fig. 7.5). Importantly, such increases

in flow velocity precede neurological deficits and thus provide a window of opportunity for intervention. Using absolute flow velocity alone, detection and documentation of the severity and duration of vasospasm is possible with a specificity that approaches 100 % but with limited sensitivity [53–55]. Sensitivity may be improved by normalizing the flow velocity to a patient-specific baseline measured prior to the time of vasospasm [53]. A way of accounting for changes in global cerebral blood flow, e.g., during induced hypertension, the intracranial flow velocity of the middle cerebral artery can be divided by the flow velocity of the ipsilateral extracranial internal carotid artery (Lindegaard ratio) [56]. A Lindegaard ratio greater than 3 is consistent with the presence of vasospasm. One important setting, wherein absolute TCD flow velocity may underestimate the severity of vasospasm, is that of increased ICP [57]. Increases in ICP, however, lead to characteristic changes in the TCD waveform and increase the pulsatility index, which relates the difference between peak systolic and end-diastolic velocity either to the mean or to the systolic velocity. Interpreting TCD flow velocities also needs to take localized therapeutic interventions into account. Specifically, TCD flow velocities may remain elevated despite successful dilation as a result of impaired autoregulation in the poststenotic vascular bed [58].

TBI
TCD in combination with determinations of CBF has identified phases of hyperemia and cerebral arterial vasospasm in traumatic brain injury as important mechanisms that underlie increased ICP and secondary injury, respectively [59–62]. Similar to vasospasm after aneurysmal subarachnoid hemorrhage, the severity of posttraumatic vasospasm correlates with the radiological severity of tissue damage, although the onset of posttraumatic vasospasm may be earlier than that after subarachnoid hemorrhage [63]. TCD has also been used in traumatic brain injury to assess the degree to which cerebral blood flow regulation is disrupted. Whereas normal CO_2-reactivity, pressure autoregulation, and flow/metabolism coupling are associated with a good outcome, disrupted CBF regulation carries a bad prognosis [64, 65].

Brain Death
The TCD-generated waveform exhibits sequential characteristic changes as intracranial pressure increases (Fig. 7.4) [66]. As ICP increases, the systolic waveform becomes more peaked. As ICP nears diastolic blood pressure, diastolic flow diminishes and subsequently ceases. Once ICP exceeds diastolic blood pressure, TCD shows a pattern of to-and-fro movement of blood that indicates imminent intracranial circulatory arrest (Fig. 7.6). This change in waveforms can be used to calculate a pulsatility index by relating the difference between peak systolic and end-diastolic velocity either to the mean or to the systolic velocity. Such waveform analyses

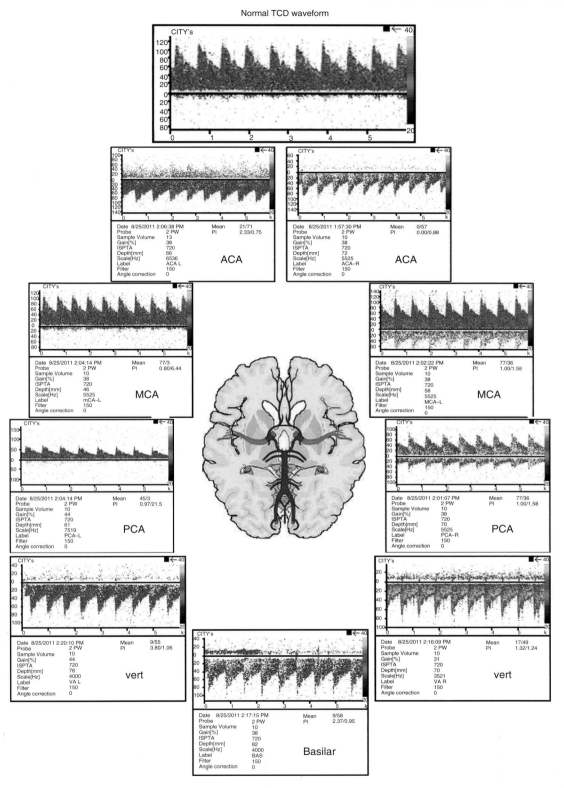

Fig. 7.4 Normal transcranial Doppler (TCD) exam. The *top panel* shows a normal flow pattern in a middle cerebral artery (MCA) with a spectrum of flow velocities. The *bottom panel* shows a complete exam of anterior (ACA), middle (MCA), and posterior (PCA) cerebral arteries insonated through a temporal bone window. From the temporal window flow in posterior and middle cerebral arteries is towards the transducer (depicted as positive values), and flow in the anterior cerebral arteries is away from the transducer (depicted as negative values). Vertebral arteries (vert) and basilar artery are insonated from the back of the flexed neck through the foramen magnum. All flow is away from the transducer, depicted as negative values (Courtesy of Michael Waters, MD)

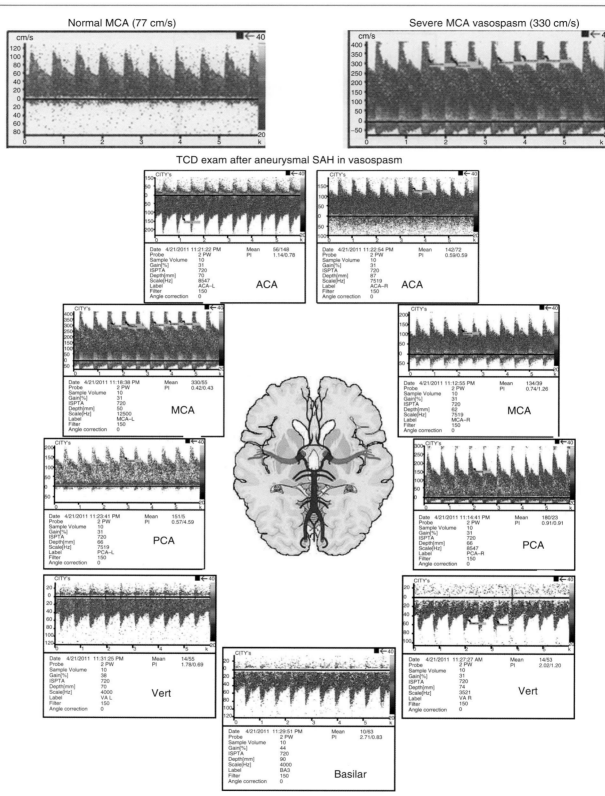

Fig. 7.5 Transcranial Doppler (TCD) exam in severe vasospasm. The *top panel* compares flow velocities in normal and severely narrowed middle cerebral arteries. Note the different velocity scales. The *bottom panel* shows the complete exam with vasospasm in the left posterior, middle, and anterior cerebral arteries as well as the right posterior and middle cerebral arteries. The exam also illustrates the operator dependence of the exam, because the right anterior cerebral artery is not captured (Courtesy of Michael Waters, MD)

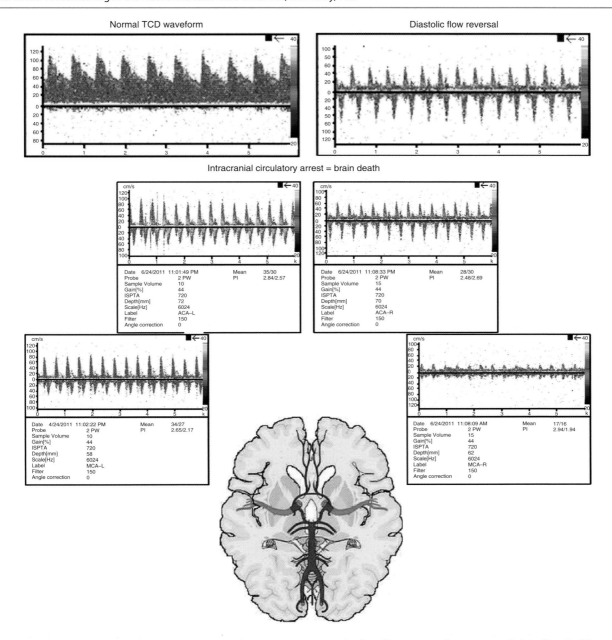

Fig. 7.6 Transcranial Doppler (TCD) exam in brain death. As intracranial pressure rises, diastolic flow becomes compromised first, resulting in a more peaked appearance of the TCD waveform. Once intracranial exceeds diastolic pressure, flow reverses during diastole (Courtesy of Michael Waters, MD)

correlate well with the intracranial pressure [57, 67, 68], especially if they take the arterial blood pressure curve into account [69]. However, serial TCD cannot replace ICP monitoring because, in a given patient, factors such as autoregulation, vasospasm, or proximal arterial stenosis may alter the TCD signal independent of the ICP [48].

Clinical brain death demonstrates a characteristic blood flow velocity pattern (Fig. 7.6). There is a short systolic inflow of blood followed by an exit of blood (flow direction reverses) from the cranium during diastole. TCD is a validated confirmatory test in the diagnosis of brain death, with a sensitivity that exceeds 90 % and a specificity of near 100 % [70]. While TCD can ascertain the diagnosis in most patients at the bedside, a large craniotomy or an inadequate bone window may preclude the complete examination necessary to confirm brain death.

Thermal Diffusion Flowmetry

Thermal diffusion flowmetry measures local cerebral blood flow through a probe inserted into the white matter. The probe consists of two thermistor elements. One thermistor measures brain temperature. The other is held at a slightly higher temperature than the first thermistor. The energy required to maintain the temperature differential between the two thermistors is proportionate to the heat-conducting properties of white matter, which stays constant as long as the probe is properly placed and does not move, and to the convective cooling of cerebral blood flow, which is reported in the conventional units of ml/100 g/min. Local CBF measured by thermal diffusion agrees well with CBF measured by stable xenon CT [71]. An example of a clinical application of thermal diffusion flowmetry is the determination of presence or absence of cerebral autoregulation in traumatic brain injury [72], which may impact the management strategy and ultimately outcome in these patients [73]. One limitation of thermal diffusion flowmetry is that the measurement will cease if the patient becomes febrile beyond a temperature of 39.5 °C. This reflects a built-in safety feature that prevents tissue heating beyond 41 °C.

Laser Doppler Flowmetry

The second technique that is transitioning from bench to bedside is the measurement of local CBF by using a fiberoptic laser Doppler flow probe. Because it measures local blood flow velocity based on the Doppler principle discussed previously, it only presents relative cerebral blood flow and thus gives just trending information.

Monitors of Oxygen Supply/Demand Balance

The average oxyhemoglobin saturation can be used, in a manner analogous to mixed venous oxygen saturation, to determine whether oxygen supply and demand are in balance. As long as changes in $CMRO_2$ are matched by concomitant changes in cerebral blood flow, oxygen extraction will stay the same as will oxyhemoglobin saturation. If demand outstrips supply, oxygen extraction will increase, thereby decreasing oxyhemoglobin saturation. Jugular bulb oximetry and cerebral oximetry are two approaches that aim to measure oxygen saturation. Both technologies use reflectance oximetry to determine saturation values. Reflectance oximetry relies on the fact that near-infrared light penetrates tissue for several centimeters and that hemoglobin, in its oxygenated and deoxygenated form, is the major tissue compound absorbing near-infrared light [44]. Near-infrared light of at least two different wavelengths is emitted, and the reflected light of each wavelength is quantified to determine an oxygen saturation value. While the technologies of jugular bulb oximetry and cerebral oximetry are similar in concept,

different assumptions underlie the validity of jugular bulb oximetry and cerebral oximetry as monitors of global and regional oxygen supply/demand balance, respectively.

Direct measurements of oxygen partial pressure in brain tissue (PbO_2) can be derived from a modified Clark electrode implanted into the brain. The technology is relatively robust and provides information about actual tissue oxygenation, albeit only from a highly localized area of metabolically heterogeneous brain. If the probe is situated in normal brain, PbO_2 correlates with jugular bulb saturation [74]. Severe or prolonged tissue hypoxia is associated with worse functional outcomes [75]. As familiarity with this technique improves, it may supplant jugular bulb oximetry, which has greater rates of failure and complications.

Jugular Venous Oximetry ($S_{JV}O_2$)

The measurement of jugular bulb oxygen saturation requires placement of a catheter into the jugular vein. That catheter is advanced from a puncture site in the neck retrograde under fluoroscopic guidance until its tip lies in the jugular bulb. Oxygen saturation can be determined continuously by using a fiberoptic catheter or intermittently by blood gas analysis. Due to its invasive nature and potential interference with cerebral venous drainage, cannulation is usually only done on one side.

There are several theoretical problems with this technique. The measurement technique evaluates the *global* balance between cerebral O_2 supply and demand. The amount of brain that must be affected for $S_{JV}O_2$ to change is thought to be on the order of 10–15 %. Inadequate CBF to a small area of cortex may be masked by blood, which has a higher SvO_2 from areas of adequately perfused brain in either hemisphere. Thus, a high saturation can be falsely reassuring. Similarly, admixture of extracerebral venous blood e.g., through catheter malposition, may falsely increase $S_{JV}O_2$. Although virtually all blood from the brain drains via the jugular veins, mixing of venous blood is incomplete and results in differences between right- and left-sided measurements [76–78]. Specifically, the dominant jugular vein, i.e., the right jugular vein in the majority of patients, drains predominantly cortical venous blood, whereas the contralateral jugular vein drains mostly blood from subcortical structures [78, 79]. To account for this asymmetry, many clinicians cannulate the jugular bulb on the side where jugular vein compression causes the largest increase in intracranial pressure [78, 79]. Placement of a catheter in the jugular vein may diminish jugular outflow or cause thrombosis after prolonged use and thus raise ICP in patients with decreased intracranial elastance. However, in clinical practice, such complications are rare [80, 81] and should be weighed against the benefit of the information obtained. Despite these limitations, $S_{JV}O_2$ monitoring is an integral part of multimodality monitoring in many NICUs.

Although $S_{JV}O_2$ monitoring has been used after cardiac surgery and subarachnoid hemorrhage, most reports involve management of severely head-injured patients. In head-injured patients, $S_{JV}O_2$ values of <50 or >75 % are associated with worse outcomes. Episodes of jugular venous oxygen desaturation, thought to reflect episodes of relative ischemia, were associated with worse neurological deficits even after adjusting for confounding factors such as age, Glasgow Coma Scale, or type of injury [82, 83]. Similarly, $S_{JV}O_2$ values of >75 %, which may reflect the decreased demand of traumatized tissue rather than true hyperemia, were associated with worse patient outcomes [84, 85]. $S_{JV}O_2$ monitoring appears to be helpful in detecting cerebral ischemia associated with excessive hyperventilation. Although hyperventilation may lower ICP, the accompanying decrease in CBF can cause O_2 delivery to fall below demand. Falling $S_{JV}O_2$ suggests that another technique to control ICP, e.g., drug-induced reduction of $CMRO_2$ or CSF drainage, might be safer. The prompt feedback and straightforward conceptual framework for interpretation provided by $S_{JV}O_2$ monitoring has played an important role in limiting hyperventilation and shifting the focus away from controlling ICP towards maintaining CPP.

Cerebral Oximetry

The cerebral oximeter was developed as a noninvasive assessment of the adequacy of cerebral oxygenation [85]. In addition to the brain tissue underlying the oximetry probe, the light also passes through the scalp and skull. The exact light path is not known. Therefore, the relative contribution of extracranial and intracranial blood to the measured saturation may vary according to sensor design and placement. The sensor is usually placed on the skin overlying the frontopolar portion of the cerebral cortex (forehead). Arterial, capillary, and venous hemoglobin within the light path contributes to the measured saturation value. Because two-thirds to four-fifths of the cerebral blood volume is on the venous side, cerebral oximetry determines predominantly local S_vO_2 [44].

Cerebral oximetry is most widely used in the care of cardiac surgery patients, particularly during complex surgical procedures such as those requiring circulatory arrest. The perceived utility in this setting may derive from the fact that the majority of changes seen in cardiac surgery affect all of the cerebral inflow and hence overcome some of the conceptual limitations of the device. More germane to the situation in the NICU may be the experience with cerebral oximetry during carotid endarterectomy. Cerebral oximetry has been compared to transcranial Doppler and $S_{JV}O_2$ as a means to assess global cerebral perfusion [86, 87]. While neither of these monitors is currently considered a gold standard for measuring the adequacy of CBF during carotid endarterectomy, the relationships demonstrated were interesting.

Decreases in cerebral oxygen saturation were accompanied by significant decreases in middle cerebral artery flow velocity (MCAv). The converse was not always true, however. Significant falls in MCAv could occur without any change in oxygen saturation at all, suggesting the presence of collateral circulation. There was also a strong correlation between JvO_2 and cerebral oxygen saturation. The degree of change in the two monitors was not necessarily similar, however. Placement of the probe over the parietal cortex produced a more similar degree of change in the two monitors than the standard frontal placement. Compared to accepted tests of adequate cerebral blood flow during carotid artery occlusion such as the neurological exam of the awake patient, the EEG, or SSEPs, cerebral oximetry showed good sensitivity but relatively poor specificity. The poor specificity makes it difficult to define a relative or absolute threshold below which cerebral oxygen saturation indicates ischemia [88].

Perhaps the greatest limitation of this monitor is the lack of multichannel capability. There is no reason to expect that oxygen saturation in one portion of the brain would reflect oxygen saturation in other areas of the brain. Indeed, EEG changes during ischemia are sometimes limited to a few channels. Likewise, many patients in the NICU are at risk for secondary focal or multifocal rather than generalized damage to CNS structures. Studies of cerebral oximetry in patients with traumatic brain injury failed to document consistent utility of the monitor. Thus, although $S_{JV}O_2$ and cerebral oximetry provide complementary information on the cerebral oxygen supply/demand balance, further study and technical development will be required before cerebral oximetry can claim a place in the multimodal assessment of NICU patients.

Tissue Probes

In contrast to most other techniques for evaluating brain oxygenation, tissue monitoring and microdialysis offer both the advantage and disadvantage of monitoring a very discrete region of tissue. Most centers place such probes into uninjured white matter on the side of the brain with more severe pathology [89]. Continuous brain tissue oxygen monitoring measures the balance of oxygen delivery and cerebral metabolism by reporting the partial pressure of oxygen at the probe site [89]. The value thus differs from both arterial and mixed venous oxygen partial pressures. Normal values are between 20 and 50 mmHg. Values less than 20 mmHg identify cerebral hypoxia and ischemia in patients with brain injury, aneurysmal subarachnoid hemorrhage, malignant stroke, or other patients at risk for secondary brain injury. Intraparenchymal direct oxygen partial pressure measurements ($PbrO_2$) have been shown to be of value in the management of cerebral perfusion and management of patients with traumatic brain injury [90].

Many studies over the past decade support that subthreshold levels of PbrO$_2$ are associated with increased morbidity and mortality in patients with severe brain injury. In 2007, Guidelines for the Management of Severe Head Injury [91] (intervention based on a brain tissue oxygenation threshold of less than 15 mmHg) were adopted as a level III recommendation. While the exact significance of local partial pressure of brain tissue oxygen continues to be debated, evidence for inclusion in multimodal monitoring is increasing.

Brain microdialysis can also be performed through an implanted tissue probe. Energy metabolites such as the lactate to pyruvate ratio, neurotransmitters involved in excitotoxicity, or molecules indicative of cell damage can be measured over time. This monitor provides the unique opportunity to interrogate the pathophysiologic process that underlies changed neurological function. It is currently used mostly in the context of research protocols.

References

1. Kornbluth J, Bhardwaj A. Evaluation of coma: a critical appraisal of popular scoring systems. Neurocrit Care. 2011;14:134–43.
2. Seel RT, Sherer M, Whyte J, Katz DI, Giacino JT, Rosenbaum AM, Hammond FM, Kalmar K, Bender-Pape TL, Zafonte R, Biester RC, Kaelin D, Kean J, Zasler N. Assessment scales for disorders of consciousness: evidence-based recommendations for clinical practice and research. Arch Phys Med Rehabil. 2010;91: 1795–813.
3. Wijdicks EF, Varelas PN, Gronseth GS, Greer DM. Evidence–based guideline update: determining brain death in adults: report of the Quality Standards Subcommittee of the American Academy of Neurology. Neurology. 2010;74:1911–8.
4. Santamaria J, Orteu N, Iranzo A, Tolosa E. Eye opening in brain death. J Neurol. 1999;246:720–2.
5. Wijdicks EF. Brain death. Philadelphia: Lippincott Williams & Wilkins; 2001.
6. Schmidt JE, Tamburro RF, Hoffman GM. Dilated nonreactive pupils secondary to neuromuscular blockade. Anesthesiology. 2000;92:1476–80.
7. Fisch BJ. Digital and analog EEG instruments: parts and functions, chapter 3. In: Fisch BJ, editor. Fisch and Spehlmann's EEG primer. Amsterdam: Elsevier; 1999.
8. Pauri F, Pierelli F, et al. Long-term EEG-video-audio monitoring: computer detection of focal EEG patterns. Electroencephalogr Clin Neurophysiol. 1992;82:1–9.
9. Wijdicks EF, Hijdra A, Young GB, Bassetti CL, Wiebe S. Practice parameter: prediction of outcome in comatose survivors after cardiopulmonary resuscitation (an evidence-based review): report of the Quality Standards Subcommittee of the American Academy of Neurology. Neurology. 2006;67:203–10.
10. Hirsch LJ. Continuous EEG, monitoring in the ICU. J Clin Neurophysiol. 2004;21:332–40.
11. Friedman D, Claasen J, Hirsch LJ. Continuous electroencephalogram monitoring in the intensive care unit. Anesth Analg. 2009;109: 506–23.
12. Hirsch L, Brenner RP. Atlas of EEG in critical care. Hoboken: Wiley-Blackwell; 2010.
13. Claasen J, Mayer SA, Hirsch LJ. Continuous EEG monitoring in patients with subarachnoid hemorrhage. J Clin Neurophysiol. 2005;22:92–8.
14. Vespa P, Nuwer MR, et al. Early detection of vasospasm after acute subarachnoid hemorrhage using continuous EEG ICU monitoring. Electroencephalogr Clin Neurophysiol. 1997;103:607–15.
15. van Putten MJ. The revised brain symmetry index. Clin Neurophysiol. 2007;118:2362–7.
16. de Vos CC, van Maarseveen SM, Brouwers PJ, van Putten MJ. Continuous EEG monitoring during thrombolysis in acute hemispheric stroke patients using the brain symmetry index. J Clin Neurophysiol. 2008;25:77–82.
17. Scheuer ML, Wilson SB. Data analysis for continuous EEG monitoring in the ICU: seeing the forest and the trees. J Clin Neurophysiol. 2004;21:353–78.
18. Morandi A, Brummel NE, Ely EW. Sedation, delirium and mechanical ventilation: the "ABCDE" approach. Curr Opin Crit Care. 2011;17:43–9.
19. Jackson DL, Proudfoot CW, Cann KF, Walsh T. A systematic review of the impact of sedation practice in the ICU on resource use, costs and patient safety. Crit Care. 2010;14:R59. 1–12.
20. Beretta L, DeVitis A, Grandi E. Sedation in neurocritical patients: is it useful? Minerva Anestesiol. 2011;77:828–34.
21. Ely EW, Truman B, Shintani A, Thomason JWW, Wheeler AP, Gordon S, et al. Monitoring sedation status over time in ICU patients: the reliability and validity of the Richmond Agitation Sedation Scale (RASS). JAMA. 2003;289:2983–91.
22. Cottenceau V, Petit L, Masson F, Guehl D, Asselineau J, Cochard JF, Pinaquy C, Leger A, Sztark F. The use of bispectral index to monitor barbiturate coma in severely brain injured patients with refractory intracranial hypertension. Anesth Analg. 2008;107:1676–82.
23. Bruhn J, Bullion TW, Shafer SL. Bispectral Index (BIS) and burst suppression: revealing a part of the BIS algorithm. J Clin Monit Comput. 2000;16:593–6.
24. Sackey PV. Frontal EEG, for intensive care unit sedation: treating numbers or patients? Crit Care. 2008;12:186.
25. Legatt AD, Arezzo JC, Vaughn Jr HG. The anatomic and physiologic basis of brainstem auditory evoked potentials. Neurol Clin. 1988;6:681–704.
26. Young GB. Clinical practice. Neurologic prognosis after cardiac arrest. N Engl J Med. 2009;361:605–11.
27. Zandbergen EG, de Haan RJ, Stoutenbeek CP, Koelman JH, Hijdra A. Systematic review of early prediction of poor outcome in anoxic-ischaemic coma. Lancet. 1998;352:1808–12.
28. Legatt A, Ellen R. Grass lecture: motor evoked potential monitoring. Am J Electroneurodiagnostic Technol. 2004;44:223–43.
29. Hallett M. Transcranial magnetic stimulation: a primer. Neuron. 2007;55:187–99.
30. Goodwin SR, Toney KA, Mahla ME. Sensory evoked potentials accurately predict recovery from prolonged coma caused by strangulation. Crit Care Med. 1993;21:631–3.
31. Goodwin SR, Friedman WA, Bellefleur M. Is it time to use evoked potentials to predict outcome in comatose children and adults? Crit Care Med. 1991;19:518–24.
32. Greenberg RP, Newlon PG, Hyatt MS, Narayan RK, Becker DP. Prognostic implications of early multimodality evoked potentials in severely head-injured patients. A prospective study. J Neurosurg. 1981;55:227–36.
33. Greenberg RP, Becker DP, Miller JD, Mayer DJ. Evaluation of brain function in severe human head trauma with multimodality evoked potentials. Part 2: localization of brain dysfunction and correlation with posttraumatic neurological conditions. J Neurosurg. 1977;47:163–77.
34. Greenberg RP, Mayer DJ, Becker DP, Miller JD. Evaluation of brain function in severe human head trauma with multimodality evoked potentials. Part 1: evoked brain-injury potentials, methods, and analysis. J Neurosurg. 1977;47:150–62.
35. Greenberg RP, Newlon PG, Becker DP. The somatosensory evoked potential in patients with severe head injury: outcome prediction and monitoring of brain function. Ann N Y Acad Sci. 1982;388:683–8.

36. Machado C. Multimodality evoked potentials and electroretinography in a test battery for an early diagnosis of brain death. J Neurosurg Sci. 1993;37:125–31.

37. Machado C, Valdes P, Garcia-Tigera J, Virues T, Biscay R, Miranda J, Coutin P, Roman J, Garcia O. Brain-stem auditory evoked potentials and brain death. Electroencephalogr Clin Neurophysiol. 1991;80:392–8.

38. Guerit JM, Fischer C, Facco E, Tinuper P, Murri L, Ronne-Engstrom E, Nuwer M. Standards of clinical practice of EEG and EPs in comatose and other unresponsive states. The International Federation of Clinical Neurophysiology. Electroencephalogr Clin Neurophysiol Suppl. 1999;52:117–31.

39. Guerit JM, de Tourtchaninoff M, Soveges L, Mahieu P. The prognostic value of three-modality evoked potentials (TMEPs) in anoxic and traumatic comas. Neurophysiol Clin. 1993;23:209–26.

40. Sleigh JW, Havill JH, Frith R, Kersel D, Marsh N, Ulyatt D. Somatosensory evoked potentials in severe traumatic brain injury: a blinded study. J Neurosurg. 1999;91:577–80.

41. Schwarz S, Schwab S, Aschoff A, Hacke W. Favorable recovery from bilateral loss of somatosensory evoked potentials. Crit Care Med. 1999;27:182–7.

42. Lindsay K, Pasaoglu A, Hirst D, Allardyce G, Kennedy I, Teasdale G. Somatosensory and auditory brain stem conduction after head injury: a comparison with clinical features in prediction of outcome. Neurosurgery. 1990;26:278–85.

43. Martin NA, Doberstein C. Cerebral blood flow measurement in neurosurgical intensive care. Neurosurg Clin N Am. 1994;5: 607–18.

44. Madsen PL, Secher NH. Near-infrared oximetry of the brain. Prog Neurobiol. 1999;58:541–60.

45. Cottrell JE. Cerebral blood flow. In: Cottrell JE, editor. Anesthesia and neurosurgery. New York: Mosby Year Book, Inc; 2001. p. 800–25.

46. Keller E, Wietasch G, Ringleb P, Scholz M, Schwarz S, Stingele R, Schwab S, Hanley D, Hacke W. Bedside monitoring of cerebral blood flow in patients with acute hemispheric stroke. Crit Care Med. 2000;28:511–6.

47. Nedelmann M, Stolz E, Gerriets T, Baumgartner RW, Malferrari G, Seidel G, Kaps M. Consensus recommendations for transcranial color-coded duplex sonography for the assessment of intracranial arteries in clinical trials on acute stroke. Stroke. 2009;40:3238–44.

48. Manno EM. Transcranial Doppler ultrasonography in the neurocritical care unit. Crit Care Clin. 1997;13:79–104.

49. Ringelstein EB, Biniek R, Weiller C, Ammeling B, Nolte PN, Thron A. Type and extent of hemispheric brain infarctions and clinical outcome in early and delayed middle cerebral artery recanalization. Neurology. 1992;42:289–98.

50. Halsey JH, McDowell HA, Gelmon S, Morawetz RB. Blood velocity in the middle cerebral artery and regional cerebral blood flow during carotid endarterectomy. Stroke. 1989;20:53–8.

51. Nuttall GA, Cook DJ, Fulgham JR, Oliver Jr WC, Proper JA. The relationship between cerebral blood flow and transcranial Doppler blood flow velocity during hypothermic cardiopulmonary bypass in adults. Anesth Analg. 1996;82:1146–51.

52. Weyland A, Stephan H, Kazmaier S, Weyland W, Schorn B, Grune F, Sonntag H. Flow velocity measurements as an index of cerebral blood flow. Validity of transcranial Doppler sonographic monitoring during cardiac surgery. Anesthesiology. 1994;81:1401–10.

53. Sloan MA, Haley Jr EC, Kassell NF, Henry ML, Stewart SR, Beskin RR, Sevilla EA, Torner JC. Sensitivity and specificity of transcranial Doppler ultrasonography in the diagnosis of vasospasm following subarachnoid hemorrhage. Neurology. 1989;39:1514–8.

54. Wozniak MA, Sloan MA, Rothman MI, Burch CM, Rigamonti D, Permutt T, Numaguchi Y. Detection of vasospasm by transcranial Doppler sonography. The challenges of the anterior and posterior cerebral arteries. J Neuroimaging. 1996;6:87–93.

55. Sloan MA, Burch CM, Wozniak MA, Rothman MI, Rigamonti D, Permutt T, Numaguchi Y. Transcranial Doppler detection of vertebrobasilar vasospasm following subarachnoid hemorrhage. Stroke. 1994;25:2187–97.

56. Lindegaard KF, Nornes H, Bakke SJ, Sorteberg W, Nakstad P. Cerebral vasospasm after subarachnoid haemorrhage investigated by means of transcranial Doppler ultrasound. Acta Neurochir Suppl (Wien). 1988;42:81–4.

57. Klingelhofer J, Dander D, Holzgraefe M, Bischoff C, Conrad B. Cerebral vasospasm evaluated by transcranial Doppler ultrasonography at different intracranial pressures. J Neurosurg. 1991;75:752–8.

58. Giller CA, Purdy P, Giller A, Batjer HH, Kopitnik T. Elevated transcranial Doppler ultrasound velocities following therapeutic arterial dilation. Stroke. 1995;26:123–7.

59. Kelly DF, Kordestani RK, Martin NA, Nguyen T, Hovda DA, Bergsneider M, McArthur DL, Becker DP. Hyperemia following traumatic brain injury: relationship to intracranial hypertension and outcome. J Neurosurg. 1996;85:762–71.

60. Kordestani RK, Counelis GJ, McBride DQ, Martin NA. Cerebral arterial spasm after penetrating craniocerebral gunshot wounds: transcranial Doppler and cerebral blood flow findings. Neurosurgery. 1997;41:351–9.

61. Lee JH, Martin NA, Alsina G, McArthur DL, Zaucha K, Hovda DA, Becker DP. Hemodynamically significant cerebral vasospasm and outcome after head injury: a prospective study. J Neurosurg. 1997;87:221–33.

62. Martin NA, Patwardhan RV, Alexander MJ, Africk CZ, Lee JH, Shalmon E, Hovda DA, Becker DP. Characterization of cerebral hemodynamic phases following severe head trauma: hypoperfusion, hyperemia, and vasospasm. J Neurosurg. 1997;87:9–19.

63. Sander D, Klingelhofer J. Cerebral vasospasm following posttraumatic subarachnoid hemorrhage evaluated by transcranial Doppler ultrasonography. J Neurol Sci. 1993;119:1–7.

64. Lee JH, Kelly DF, Oertel M, McArthur DL, Glenn TC, Vespa P, Boscardin WJ, Martin NA. Carbon dioxide reactivity, pressure autoregulation, and metabolic suppression reactivity after head injury: a transcranial Doppler study. J Neurosurg. 2001;95:222–32.

65. Klingelhofer J, Sander D. Doppler CO2 test as an indicator of cerebral vasoreactivity and prognosis in severe intracranial hemorrhages. Stroke. 1992;23:962–6.

66. Hassler W, Steinmetz H, Gawlowski J. Transcranial Doppler ultrasonography in raised intracranial pressure and in intracranial circulatory arrest. J Neurosurg. 1988;68:745–51.

67. Goraj B, Rifkinson-Mann S, Leslie DR, Lansen TA, Kasoff SS, Tenner MS. Correlation of intracranial pressure and transcranial Doppler resistive index after head trauma. AJNR Am J Neuroradiol. 1994;15:1333–9.

68. Klingelhofer J, Conrad B, Benecke R, Sander D, Markakis E. Evaluation of intracranial pressure from transcranial Doppler studies in cerebral disease. J Neurol. 1988;235:159–62.

69. Schmidt B, Klingelhofer J, Schwarze JJ, Sander D, Wittich I. Noninvasive prediction of intracranial pressure curves using transcranial Doppler ultrasonography and blood pressure curves. Stroke. 1997;28:2465–72.

70. Monteiro LM, Bollen CW, van Huffelen AC, Ackerstaff RG, Jansen NJ, van Vught AJ. Transcranial Doppler ultrasonography to confirm brain death: a meta-analysis. Intensive Care Med. 2006; 32:1937–44.

71. Vajkoczy P, Roth H, Horn P, Luecke T, Thomé C, Huebner U, Martin GT, Zappletal C, Klar E, Schilling L, Schmiedek P. Continuous monitoring of regional cerebral blood flow—experimental and clinical validation of a novel thermal diffusion microprobe. J Neurosurg. 2000;93:265–74.

72. Rosenthal G, Sanchez-Mejia RO, Phan N, Hemphill 3rd JC, Martin C, Manley GT. Incorporating a parenchymal thermal diffusion cerebral blood flow probe in bedside assessment of cerebral

autoregulation and vasoreactivity in patients with severe traumatic brain injury. J Neurosurg. 2011;114:62–70.

73. Howells T, Elf K, Jones PA, Ronne-Engström E, Piper I, Nilsson P, Andrews P, Enblad P. Pressure reactivity as a guide in the treatment of cerebral perfusion pressure in patients with brain trauma. J Neurosurg. 2005;102:311–7.

74. Gupta AK, Hutchinson PJ, Al Rawi P, Gupta S, Swart M, Kirkpatrick PJ, Menon DK, Datta AK. Measuring brain tissue oxygenation compared with jugular venous oxygen saturation for monitoring cerebral oxygenation after traumatic brain injury. Anesth Analg. 1999;88:549–53.

75. Valadka AB, Gopinath SP, Contant CF, Uzura M, Robertson CS. Relationship of brain tissue PO2 to outcome after severe head injury. Crit Care Med. 1998;26:1576–81.

76. Latronico N, Beindorf AE, Rasulo FA, Febbrari P, Stefini R, Cornali C, Candiani A. Limits of intermittent jugular bulb oxygen saturation monitoring in the management of severe head trauma patients. Neurosurgery. 2000;46:1131–8.

77. Lam JM, Chan MS, Poon WS. Cerebral venous oxygen saturation monitoring: is dominant jugular bulb cannulation good enough? Br J Neurosurg. 1996;10:357–64.

78. Macmillan CS, Andrews PJ. Cerebrovenous oxygen saturation monitoring: practical considerations and clinical relevance. Intensive Care Med. 2000;26:1028–36.

79. Goetting MG, Preston G. Jugular bulb catheterization does not increase intracranial pressure. Intensive Care Med. 1991;17:195–8.

80. Coplin WM, O'Keefe GE, Grady MS, Grant GA, March KS, Winn HR, Lam AM. Thrombotic, infectious, and procedural complications of the jugular bulb catheter in the intensive care unit. Neurosurgery. 1997;41:101–7.

81. Gopinath SP, Robertson CS, Contant CF, Hayes C, Feldman Z, Narayan RK, Grossman RG. Jugular venous desaturation and outcome after head injury. J Neurol Neurosurg Psychiatry. 1994;57:717–23.

82. Fandino J, Stocker R, Prokop S, Trentz O, Imhof HG. Cerebral oxygenation and systemic trauma related factors determining neurological outcome after brain injury. J Clin Neurosci. 2000;7:226–33.

83. Cormio M, Valadka AB, Robertson CS. Elevated jugular venous oxygen saturation after severe head injury. J Neurosurg. 1999;90:9–15.

84. Macmillan CS, Andrews PJ, Easton VJ. Increased jugular bulb saturation is associated with poor outcome in traumatic brain injury. J Neurol Neurosurg Psychiatry. 2001;70:101–4.

85. Highton D, Elwell C, Smith M. Noninvasive cerebral oximetry: is there light at the end of the tunnel? Curr Opin Anaesthesiol. 2010;23:576–81.

86. Cho H, Nemoto EM, Yonas H, Balzer J, Sclabassi RJ. Cerebral monitoring by means of oximetry and somatosensory evoked potentials during carotid endarterectomy. J Neurosurg. 1998;89:533–8.

87. Duffy CM, Manninen PH, Chan A, Kearns CF. Comparison of cerebral oximeter and evoked potential monitoring in carotid endarterectomy. Can J Anaesth. 1997;44:1077–81.

88. Pennekamp CW, Bots ML, Kappelle LJ, Moll FL, de Borst GJ. The value of near-infrared spectroscopy measured cerebral oximetry during carotid endarterectomy in perioperative stroke prevention. A review. Eur J Vasc Endovasc Surg. 2009;38:539–45.

89. Maloney-Wilensky E, Le Roux P. The physiology behind direct brain oxygen monitors and practical aspects of their use. Childs Nerv Syst. 2010;26:419–30.

90. Maloney-Wilensky E, Gracias V, Itkin A, Hoffman K, Bloom S, Yang W, Christian S, LeRoux PD. Brain tissue oxygen and outcome after severe traumatic brain injury: a systematic review. Crit Care Med. 2009;37:2057–63.

91. Brain Trauma Foundation; American Association of Neurological Surgeons; Congress of Neurological Surgeons; Joint Section on Neurotrauma and Critical Care, AANS/CNS, Bratton SL, Chestnut RM, Ghajar J, McConnell Hammond FF, Harris OA, Hartl R, Manley GT, Nemecek A, Newell DW, Rosenthal G, Schouten J, Shutter L, Timmons SD, Ullman JS, Videtta W, Wilberger JE, Wright DW. Guidelines for the management of severe traumatic brain injury. X. Brain oxygen monitoring and thresholds. J Neurotrauma. 2007;24 Suppl 1:S65–70.

92. Seubert CN, Mahla ME. Neurologic monitoring in the neurointensive care unit. In: Layon AG, Gabrielli A, Friedman WA, editors. Textbook of neurointensive care. Philadelphia: WB Saunders; 2004.

Invasive Neurological and Multimodality Monitoring in the NeuroICU

8

Peter Le Roux

Contents

Abstract

Patients admitted to the neurocritical care unit (NCCU) are at risk for secondary brain injury that frequently can exacerbate outcome. Consequently, current NCCU management strategies focus on the identification, prevention, and management of secondary brain injury, since there are few pharmacological agents that demonstrate efficacy in these patients. In the last decade, techniques to monitor brain function have evolved and, in the modern NCCU, play an important role in patient care and in particular in a patient-specific targeted approach. Monitors include radiologic techniques that provide information about a specific point in time or bedside monitors that provide continuous or noncontinuous physiologic information. In turn, these bedside techniques may be subdivided into invasive or noninvasive monitors. In this review we will discuss invasive intracranial monitors including (1) intracranial pressure; (2) monitors of cerebral oxygenation (direct measurement of brain oxygen [PbtO₂] and jugular venous catheters); (3) metabolic monitors, i.e., cerebral microdialysis; and (4) cerebral blood flow monitors such as thermal diffusion flowmetry and laser Doppler flowmetry.

Keywords

Brain injury • Brain oxygen • Brain metabolism • Cerebral microdialysis • Cerebral blood flow • Intracranial pressure Monitoring • Intensive care

Introduction

A fundamental goal of neurocritical care is the identification, prevention, and management of secondary brain injury (SBI), i.e., pathological events that occur after the primary insult. Secondary brain injury includes intracranial events such as increased intracranial pressure (ICP); altered cerebral blood flow (CBF) that leads to ischemia; brain hypoxia;

P. Le Roux, MD
Department of Neurosurgery, University of Pennsylvania,
235 S. 8th Street, Philadelphia, PA 19106, USA
e-mail: lerouxp@uphs.upenn.edu

metabolic dysfunction, e.g., excitotoxicity or mitochondrial dysfunction; and seizures including nonconvulsive seizures among others. Each of these is known to adversely affect outcome in a variety of acute neurologic disorders, e.g., traumatic brain injury (TBI), stroke, or subarachnoid hemorrhage (SAH). In addition, systemic insults such as hypotension, hypoxia, anemia, fever, hyperglycemia, and hypoglycemia all exacerbate the underlying neurologic disorder and outcome. Clinical studies suggest that up to 90 % of patients with acute brain injury who require admission to the neurocritical care unit (NCCU) develop SBI [1].

There are few pharmacological neuroprotective agents that have shown efficacy in the clinical environment despite success in animal studies [2]. Current NCCU management therefore is directed towards providing an optimal physiological environment to reduce the burden of secondary insults. The foundation of this strategy is monitoring, the goal of which is to detect harmful pathophysiological events before they cause irreversible damage to the brain. In turn, this permits early treatment and real-time feedback about the treatment effect.

In the past decade, multimodality monitoring that attempts to integrate cerebral physiological data derived from a variety of sources has become increasingly popular in the NCCU. Multimodality monitoring can be defined as the simultaneous collection of data from multiple diverse (and complimentary) sources associated with a single patient when no one single method can provide complete information. Ideally, this information needs to be viewed and interpreted in a time-synchronized and integrated manner. This concept is very important when monitoring the brain since it is a complex system with interrelated hemodynamic, metabolic, and electrical subsystems, i.e., one monitor (or imaging study) is unlikely to tell the entire physiological story. A variety of monitors are available, and these can be considered in two broad categories: (1) radiologic techniques that provide a snapshot in time and (2) bedside monitors that in turn may be subdivided into (a) invasive or noninvasive or (b) continuous or noncontinuous monitors. Monitors may be further divided into those that provide quantitative data or qualitative or trend data on cerebral pressure, flow, metabolism, and function. This classification can be used when considering how to use the various monitors described later in this chapter. However, there presently is no Level I evidence how use of any one or combination of monitors influences patient care; most information is derived from clinical observational studies or based on physiological principles.

It is important to recognize that monitoring should be interpreted with the clinical examination and monitoring itself does alter outcome. Instead, it is what is done with the information that contributes to patient well-being. In particular, data from monitoring help guide individualized management of SBI, targeted to patient-specific pathophysiology. In this chapter, we will review invasive intracranial monitors including (1) intracranial pressure (ICP); (2) monitors of cerebral oxygenation including direct measurement of brain oxygen ($PbtO_2$) and jugular venous catheters; (3) metabolic monitors, i.e., cerebral microdialysis (CMD); and (4) cerebral blood flow monitors such as thermal diffusion flowmetry and laser Doppler flowmetry.

Intracranial Pressure

ICP monitoring is considered the "basic" intracranial monitor for comatose patients admitted to the NCCU after an acute brain injury, either traumatic or vascular, and has the longest history of use [3–5]. Multiple clinical studies have demonstrated a clear relationship between mortality and increased ICP (>20 mmHg) [6–10], and treatment of elevated ICP makes sound physiological sense [11]. How ICP influences outcome, however, depends in large part on how effective treatment for increased ICP is and the potential adverse effect of the treatment proposed. Indeed, even brief episodes of elevated ICP can adversely affect outcome [10]. For example, Treggiari and colleagues [12] in a systematic literature observed that, compared to normal ICP, the response of elevated ICP to treatment predicted outcome better than absolute ICP values: (1) increased ICP is associated with a 3.5–6.9-fold increase of death; (2) increased ICP that responds to treatment is associated with a three to fourfold increase in death or poor neurological outcome; whereas (3) increased ICP that does not respond to treatment has a relative risk odds ratio >100 of death. Similar observations have been made in SAH, particularly when ICP is >50 [13]. Recently Stein and coworkers [14] reviewed the literature over a 40-year period and using meta-analytic techniques compared outcome in more than 120,000 patients with and without ICP monitoring and intensive therapy. ICP monitoring and treatment was associated with better outcome that remained independent of time. Using a decision-analytical model, Whitmore and colleagues [15] also demonstrated that aggressive TBI treatment that includes invasive intracranial monitoring and decompressive craniectomy is cost-effective and associated with better outcome at all ages than "routine care," in which Brain Trauma Foundation guidelines are not followed, or comfort care. There are, however, some studies that question how an ICP monitor influences outcome [16–18].

Pathophysiology

Two fundamental aspects of brain physiology—(1) the Monro-Kellie doctrine and (2) cerebral autoregulation [19]—provide a framework for management of abnormal ICP.

The Monro-Kellie Doctrine and Compliance

The Monro-Kellie doctrine states that the total volume of the intracranial contents, i.e., brain, blood, and CSF, is constant provided the cranial vault is intact. The combined volumes of these compartments determine the ICP, i.e., ICP=brain+blood+CSF. When there is an increase in volume in one of the compartments or a mass lesion develops, the blood and CSF can shift some of their volume outside of the skull through natural means, i.e., there can be some degree of compensation. ICP therefore will remain normal if there are reductions in volume of the other compartments when a mass lesion, e.g., an acute hematoma or cerebral edema, develops. In this compensated state, the volume increase is offset by shifting venous blood out of the intracranial space and CSF into the spinal subarachnoid space. However, ICP will increase rapidly once compensation is exhausted, and, when ICP is >20 mmHg, brain tissue begins to herniate from areas of high pressure to areas of low pressure.

Allied to the Monro-Kellie doctrine is compliance that describes how the intracranial contents are able to compensate for volume changes. Cerebral compliance represents the ICP response (ΔP) to a change in volume (ΔV) described by the pressure-volume index. When compliance becomes compromised (i.e., there is a rightward shift of the pressure-volume index), the pressure response for a given volume increases. Once compliance is exhausted, a small change in volume can result in a rapid increase in ICP or cause acute herniation. Hence, when compliance is reduced, even minor events, e.g., nasotracheal suctioning, a change in head position, patient turning, pain, a seizure (including a nonconvulsive seizure), and hypoventilation or altered ventilation that increases $PaCO_2$ (increased cerebral blood volume), can increase ICP. Rapid volume challenges are less buffered and can influence ICP more than slow changes since compensation for a volume change is time dependent.

Autoregulation and Cerebral Perfusion Pressure

Cerebral perfusion pressure (CPP) that is necessary to maintain cerebral blood flow (CBF) is defined as mean arterial pressure (MAP) minus intracranial pressure (CPP=MAP−ICP). Therefore, changes in ICP or blood pressure can influence CPP. The optimal CPP is not precisely defined and may be patient and disease specific but is considered to be 50–70 mmHg. There are regional differences in CBF, but, in general, normal CBF is about 50 ml/100 g brain/min. When CBF is <20 ml/100 g brain/min, cerebral ischemia results and cell death occurs when CBF is <5 ml/100 g brain/min. The healthy brain is able to maintain a constant CBF through cerebral autoregulation (CAR). There are two forms of CAR: (1) metabolic that is influenced by cellular requirements and (2) pressure. In pressure CAR, vasoconstriction or dilation of the cerebral vasculature helps maintain a constant CBF across a broad range of blood pressures (about 50–150 mmHg) in the normal individual. However, in a variety of acute neurologic disorders, CAR is impaired or absent. CBF then may simply parallel changes in CPP and lead to inadequate tissue oxygen and glucose delivery. Vascular autoparalysis occurs when ICP equals CPP and CBF can no longer be maintained. Cerebral autoregulation and CO_2 vasoreactivity can be assessed using a CBF probe to calculate changes in local cerebrovascular resistance (CPP/local CBF) in response to blood pressure and hyperventilation challenges [20]. This can help determine the patient's optimal CPP. Alternatively, the moving correlation index between ICP and MAP (PRx) can be used to evaluate cerebral vasomotor reactivity. A PRx greater than 0.3 suggests impaired reactivity [21].

The Rationale for an ICP Monitor

Much of the poor outcome after acute neurologic disorders including TBI and SAH is associated with secondary brain injury that evolves over time. This includes increased ICP that develops in about 50 % of severe TBI patients [7] and SAH patients, including those in good grade [13]. In particular, an ICP >20 mmHg is significantly associated with increased mortality [22]. It is difficult to diagnose elevated ICP by clinical means alone. In addition, findings on an admission CT suggest who is at risk for increased ICP, but the relationship between these CT findings and the subsequent ICP course during ICU care is not reliable [23]. Late ICP increases, particularly in a sedated patient, can only be detected by pupil dilation or changes in blood pressure and pulse, i.e., often after herniation occurs. This means early treatment is impossible without an ICP monitor, i.e., an ICP monitor is essential to permit timely diagnosis and targeted ICP treatment. In addition, continuous ICP monitoring will trigger prompt imaging that prevents surgical delays for mass lesions and also prevents blind prophylactic ICP treatment or unnecessary empiric therapies. This is important since each ICP therapy (and also treatment of reduced CPP) has potential deleterious effects [24, 25]. In general, an ICP monitor should be considered in a patient with a Glasgow Coma Scale ≤8 [3]; the specific indications for an ICP monitor that are best defined in TBI are listed in Table 8.1.

Table 8.1 Indications for an ICP monitor

GCS 3–8 and abnormal CT scan
GCS 3–8 with normal CT and two or more of the following:
Age >40 years
Motor posturing
SBP <90 mmHg
GCS 9–15 and CT scan:
Mass lesion (Extra-axial >1 cm thick, temporal contusion, ICH >3 cm)
Effaced cisterns
Shift >5 mm
Following a craniotomy
Neurological examination cannot be followed, e.g., requires another surgical procedure, sedation

Adapted with permission from Bratton et al. [22]. Copyright © Mary Ann Liebert, Inc., Publishers

GCS Glasgow Coma Scale

Types of ICP Monitors

The use of ICP monitors in best described in adults after TBI, and there are several published guidelines on ICP technology and use, e.g., the European Neurointensive Care and Emergency Medicine consensus on neurological monitoring [26] and the Brain Trauma Foundation (BTF) Guidelines [3], among others [27, 28]. There is less specific information available on ICP monitor use in pediatrics [29]. A variety of noninvasive ICP monitors are available, but at present these devices are not reliable and generally are used as a screening tool for elevated ICP in select patients, e.g., those with coagulopathy or liver failure. In the NCCU, ICP is best monitored invasively. These devices usually are placed by neurosurgeons, but, in some institutions, neurointensivists may insert ICP monitors with neurosurgical backup [30].

There are no clinical outcome studies that demonstrate that one monitoring technology is superior to others. Three technologies—(1) a ventricular catheter connected to an external strain gauge, (2) catheter-tip strain gauge devices, and (3) catheter-tip fiber-optic technology—are considered accurate and interchangeable in use. Each of these technologies can be placed into the ventricle. Strain gauges or fiber optics also can be inserted into the brain parenchyma. The most commonly used ICP monitors include the Camino® or the Ventrix® (Integra Neurosciences, Plainsboro, NJ, USA; integralife.com), Codman® Microsensor® (Codman, Raynham, MA, USA; www.depuy.com), the Spiegelberg ICP sensor and compliance device (Spiegelberg KG, Hamburg, Germany; www.spiegelberg.de), and the Raumedic ICP sensor and multiparameter probe (Raumedic AG, Germany; www.raumedic.de). The Spiegelberg device also allows in vivo calibration and compliance monitoring. Fluid-coupled or pneumatic devices placed in the subarachnoid, subdural, or epidural space are less accurate [3] and infrequently used.

The most frequently used ICP monitors (and most accurate) are a ventricular catheter or an intraparenchymal monitor [3, 5]. Both can be inserted at the patient's bedside in the NCCU, and significant complications are rare. Hemorrhage is the most common procedural complication and occurs in 1 % of parenchymal monitors and 5 % of ventricular catheter. Most of these are of little or no clinical importance and usually identified only on imaging. A platelet count of >100,000 and an INR ≤1.6 are necessary to place an ICP monitor although there is little specific literature on this topic [31, 32].

Ventricular Catheter

A ventriculostomy or external ventricular drain (EVD) often is referred to as the "gold standard" ICP monitor. However, this designation may stem from it being the first monitoring system that was available. An EVD also allows therapeutic CSF drainage [33]. However, an EVD can miss episodes of increased ICP when it is draining [34], and, when using a traditional "ventricular catheter with an external transducer," only intermittent ICP measurements when the drain is closed are feasible. There are other potential disadvantages when using EVDs. First, ventricular catheters can be difficult to insert after acute brain injury because of small ventricular size or shift. Second, catheter blockage or displacement can occur, and, when it does, ICP is underestimated during simultaneous ICP monitoring and ventricular CSF drainage [35]. Third, infection can be identified in 5–20 % of patients [36, 37]. This risk is associated with catheter manipulation, e.g., flushing with normal saline to restore catheter patency or CSF sampling.

Intraparenchymal ICP Monitors

Intraparenchymal devices are easier to place than EVDs. A specifically designed cranial access device or "bolt" inserted through a burr hole in the skull is used to secure these monitors. Many of these bolts also allow insertion of other monitors, e.g., brain oxygen, brain temperature, microdialysis, and CBF probes. Parenchymal ICP monitors usually are placed into normal-appearing white matter on the admission CT in the nondominant frontal lobe in diffuse injuries or on the side of maximal pathology when there is focal abnormality. ICP values should be interpreted with the clinical examination and imaging studies since the values may depend on device location and its proximity to a focal abnormality. Continuous ICP recording over several days is feasible, and drift over time is very rare in fiber-optic catheters [31]. The risk associated with an intraparenchymal ICP monitor is significantly less than that associated with

Table 8.2 Physiological parameters to maintain in the NCCU as part of goal-directed therapy after acute brain injury

Pulse oximetry ≥90 %

$PaO_2 \geq 100$ mmHg

$PaCO_2$ 35–45 mmHg

$SBP \geq 100$ mmHg

pH 7.35–7.45

ICP < 20 mmHg

$PbtO_2 \geq 15$ mmHg

CPP ≥ 60 mmHg

Temp 36.0–38.3 °C

Glucose 80–180 mg/dl

Na + 135–145—if using HTS 145–160

INR ≤ 1.4

Platelets ≥ 75 × 10^3/mm^3

Hgb ≥ 8 g/dl

Table 8.3 A suggested approach to the management of elevated ICP (ICP > 20 mmHg × > 2 min)

1. Elevate HOB 30° (as tolerated by MAP, ICP, $PbtO_2$)

2. Loosen the cervical collar or any device about the neck

3. Medication: continuous short-acting agents are preferable
   Analgesia, e.g., fentanyl or morphine
   Sedation, e.g., propofol × 24–48 h, then lorazepam
   Paralytics only *if shivering or bucking ventilator*

4. Control body temperature; avoid fever

5. Osmotherapy (in sequence):
   Mannitol bolus (0.25–1.0 g/kg)
   Repeat mannitol bolus
   If no effect on ICP within 20 min and BP normal—5 % HTS bolus
   3 % NaCl infusion titrated according to Na level
   (HTS may be given first if ICP increased in hypotensive patient)

6. Drain CSF through an external ventricular drain (if available)
   Open drainage until:
      ICP is < 20 mmHg, or
      5 ml CSF drains, or
      Drainage stops
      Repeat as needed; do not actively withdraw CSF

7. Hyperventilate[a] to reduce $PaCO_2$ as tolerated by $PbtO_2$ or $SjvO_2$

8. If ICP remains elevated despite these measures, consider one of the following:
   Additional propofol to burst suppression
   Induced normothermia
   Decompressive craniectomy
   Pentobarbital bolus then continuous infusion: requires cEEG and monitor of cardiac function

[a]Hyperventilation should not be used prophylactically. In the absence of a monitor that allows assessment of how the vasoconstriction associated with hyperventilation affects cerebral blood flow or metabolism, it should only be used transiently in patients with signs of herniation (rapidly decreasing consciousness, particularly with changes in pupil reactivity) to target a $PaCO_2$ of 28–35 mmHg

a ventricular catheter; hemorrhage is reported in about 1 % of parenchymal monitors and infections less frequently. Technical complications, e.g., catheter breakage or dislodgement, may occur in about 4 % of cases. These often occur during transport, nursing maneuvers, or patient activities but usually are of little clinical consequence.

Treatment of Increased ICP

In the NCCU intracranial pressure is best treated with an ICP monitor in place. *The current consensus is to treat ICP that is greater than 20 mmHg* [3]. This recommendation is based on very sound clinical observations and physiological data mainly in TBI patients, but, to date, there is no level I evidence for this management [6–9, 11]. Similar observations have been made in other conditions, e.g., SAH [13]. The Monro-Kellie doctrine and an understanding of autoregulation provide the framework for management. For example, if a large mass lesion is present, then surgery is required, whereas in cerebral edema, osmotherapy is indicated to manage ICP. CPP (i.e., ICP and MAP) also is an important physiological parameter to follow in the NCCU. *Consensus recommendations suggest CPP should be maintained between 50 and 70 mmHg* [3], although, when using multimodality monitoring, patient- and disease-specific targets can be established. To facilitate ICP and CPP management, careful attention to a variety of physiological parameters is required as part of goal-directed care (Table 8.2). A suggested approach to management of elevated ICP is provided in Table 8.3.

Duration of ICP Monitoring

TBI patients who develop intracranial hypertension usually do so in the first week [38]. Many ICP increases occur within the first 2–3 days, but a first ICP elevation is observed after 72 h in about 20 % of patients [39]. The course of ICP in other disorders is less well-defined. An ICP monitor usually can be removed once the patient follows commands. In the comatose patient, monitor removal may be considered if ICP is normal during the first 72 h, i.e., no ICP spikes are observed. If ICP is elevated, the monitor should only be removed once the ICP is normal for at least 24 h without any specific treatment other than sedation for mechanical ventilation. A follow-up CT scan to confirm reduced mass effect is a useful guide for this decision.

ICP Is More than a Number

Brain multimodality monitoring is increasingly used in neurocritical care. These studies indicate that normal ICP < 20 mmHg can still be associated with inadequate CPP, secondary brain injury, brain hypoxia, or other evidence for

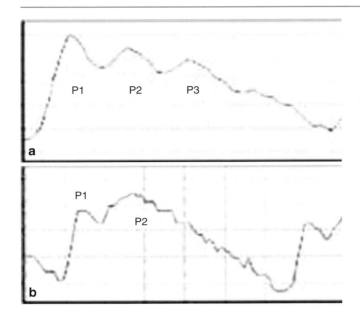

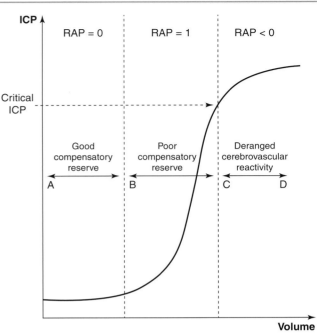

Fig. 8.1 (**a**) Normal ICP waveform: P1 > P2 > P3. (**b**) Reduced compliance: P2 and P3 amplitude increases. The normal ICP waveform has three components: (1) percussion wave (P1), (2) tidal wave (P2), and (3) dicrotic wave (P3). In a normal waveform (*left*) P1 is >P2 and >P3. When compliance is reduced (*right*) the P2 and P3 amplitude increase and P2 is >P1

Fig. 8.2 Intracranial pressure (*ICP*) volume curve (Modified with permission from www.neurosurg.cam.ac.uk/pages/brainphys: Brain Physics in 30 short lectures (not only for engineers) by Dr. Marek Czosnyka (University of Cambridge Reader in Brain Physics). Copyright © 2011 Neurosurgery Unit, Department of Clinical Neurosciences, University of Cambridge)

cellular dysfunction [40–45], i.e., ICP treatment can be more than a single threshold. Other parameters to consider include (1) the ICP trend over time, (2) ICP waveform analysis, (3) compliance, and (4) whether the ICP value is associated with other detrimental effects, e.g., an alteration in CBF, brain metabolism, or brain oxygen delivery.

A reproducible volume challenge and measurement of the ICP change is needed to quantify cerebral compliance, e.g., injection of a small (1 cc) volume of fluid through an EVD. The immediate ICP response provides the volume-pressure response (VPR = ICP change/volume injected). Logarithmic conversion of the VPR or the pressure-volume index (PVI) then defines the volume change that would produce a tenfold ICP increase. This assessment is very rarely performed in clinical practice since it requires manipulation of an EVD that may adversely alter intracranial hemodynamics or increase the infection risk. Instead, compliance usually is examined by qualitative assessment including waveform analysis, derived indices, or calculation of the therapeutic intensity level (TIL).

In the ICP waveform, the three most prominent wavelets are labeled P1, P2, and P3. Under normal conditions, i.e., good compliance, P1 is the highest component (Fig. 8.1a, b). As compliance decreases, the P2 amplitude may increase, and this often precedes an ICP increase. Eventually, the P2 wavelet may equal or exceed P1, and the ICP waveform resembles the arterial pulse waveform, i.e., compromised or absent compliance. The brain's compensatory reserve also

may be estimated from the therapeutic intensity level (TIL) that is a quantitative measure of treatment needed to control ICP [46]. A greater TIL implies worse compliance and a "sicker" patient since multiple or more complex therapies are needed for ICP control. In addition, a patient with an abnormal ICP waveform but normal ICP may require greater vigilance or different treatment than a patient with normal ICP and a normal waveform.

Compliance assessment can be supplemented with other monitors, e.g., TCD or near-infrared spectroscopy (NIRS), and continuous automated digital computations can be used to describe the interdependence between ICP regulatory processes. In particular, the derived indices of cerebrovascular reactivity (PRx) and cerebrospinal compensatory reserve (RAP) help describe the intracranial compensatory reserve and cerebrovascular autoregulatory reserve [47–53]. When the RAP index is near 0, there is a good compensatory reserve. A negative PRx (−1 to 0) suggests preserved autoregulation, but an increased RAP index (+1) or PRx (>0.3) suggests there is little intracranial compensatory reserve, i.e., small volume changes may cause a rapid ICP increase (Fig. 8.2). Rap and Prx also can be used to choose optimal CPP thresholds for each patient and in outcome prediction.

Continuous multimodality monitoring, e.g., brain oxygen, cEEG, microdialysis, or CBF, can complement the information from an ICP monitor. This allows various therapies, including those for ICP, to be used in a targeted fashion in individual patients and, in some patients, allows for permissive intracranial hypertension in which mild elevations in ICP do not always require treatment, provided other physiological parameters are normal. These monitors also allow detection of deleterious effects associated with ICP therapy, e.g., reduced CBF from hyperventilation. Anecdotal evidence suggests that a combination of monitors and management based on all the information may help predict when ICP increases may occur, improve outcome or better predict outcome than use of an ICP monitor alone [44, 54–57].

Oxygenation in Brain

Monitoring of cerebral oxygenation after brain injury can help detect and so prevent secondary brain injury. There are four methods to measure brain oxygenation: jugular venous bulb oximetry, direct brain tissue oxygen tension measurement, near-infrared spectroscopy (NIRS), and oxygen-15 positron emission tomography (PET). NIRS and PET are beyond the scope of this chapter.

Jugular Venous Oximetry

Placement of a catheter in the jugular bulb permits assessment of global brain oxygenation. The jugular bulb is the final common pathway for venous blood that drains the cerebral hemispheres, cerebellum, and brain stem. The contribution by the extracranial circulation is between 0 and 6.6 % but can be greater when blood is contaminated with blood from the facial vein that joins the internal jugular vein just below the jugular bulb (i.e., inadequate catheter placement). Therefore, jugular bulb oxygen saturation ($SjvO_2$) reflects the balance between supply and oxygen consumption by the brain.

$SjvO_2$ can be measured by intermittent sampling or continuously (jugular venous oximetry) through a fiber-optic oximetric catheter. Two fiber-optic catheters, the Oximetrix® (Abbott Laboratories, North Chicago, IL, USA) and the Edslab II (Baxter Healthcare Corporation, Irvine, CA, USA) are commercially available. Intermittent sampling through a retrograde jugular catheter is cheaper and permits calculation of the arteriovenous difference in oxygen ($AVDO_2$), glucose, or lactate based upon the Fick principle [58]. When the cerebral metabolism is stable, $AVDO_2$ changes represent CBF changes and so can reflect global CBF adequacy [59]. However, jugular bulb catheters cannot be used for quantitative or regional CBF measurements and may not detect regional ischemia or hypoxia in the brain [60].

The cerebral metabolic rate for oxygen ($CMRO_2$) is calculated from the CBF and the $AVDO_2$ according to the equation

$$CMRO_2 = CBF \times (\text{arterial oxygen content} - \text{jugular venous bulb oxygen content})$$

$$\text{Arterial oxygen content} = [(Hb \times 1.34 \times SaO_2) + (PaO_2 \times 0.0031)]$$

$$\text{Jugular venous oxygen content} = \begin{bmatrix} (Hb \times 1.34 \times SjvO_2) \\ + (PjvO_2 \times 0.0031) \end{bmatrix}$$

where Hb = hemoglobin in g/dl, SaO_2 = arterial saturation, $SjvO_2$ = jugular venous bulb saturation, PaO_2 = oxygen partial pressure in arterial blood in mmHg, and $PjvO_2$ = oxygen partial pressure in jugular venous blood in mmHg.

Since Hb concentration should be the same in arterial and venous blood, and the amount of dissolved oxygen is minimal, CMRO also can be estimated from CBF and the difference in arterial and jugular oxygen saturation.

$$CMRO_2 = CBF \times k(SaO_2 - SjvO_2)$$

Therefore, the $AVDO_2$ (or $SjvO_2$) may be used to relate changes in metabolism to changes in CBF. Hypoperfusion and ischemia are associated with increased $AVDO_2$ and hyperemia with a reduced $AVDO_2$ (Table 8.4). The same principle can be applied to other metabolites such as glucose and lactate. Normal jugular venous oximetry ($SjvO_2$) ranges between 55 and 75 %. An $SjvO_2$ <50 % for at least 10 min is considered the threshold for ischemia [61]. Low $SjvO_2$ indicates reduced oxygen delivery (e.g., vasospasm, excessive hyperventilation, inadequate CPP) or increased oxygen demand (e.g., fever or seizures). Increased $SjvO_2$ (>70 %) suggests that CBF is greater than brain needs (hyperemia) or there is decreased metabolic demand.

$SjvO_2$ provides insight about global cerebral oxygenation but only when the catheter tip is placed in the dominant jugular bulb. Flow often is greater in the right jugular venous bulb [62, 63], but two methods can help distinguish which jugular bulb is dominant. First, the jugular foramen on CT is larger

Table 8.4 Values of $AVDO_2$ and $SjvO_2$

$SjvO_2$
Normal: 60 (55)–75 (80) %
Ischemia: <50–55 %
Hyperemic: >75 %
Arteriovenous difference of oxygen ($AVDO_2$)
Normal: 5–7.5 vol. % (5.1–8.3 vol. %)
Ischemia: $AVDO_2$ >7.5 vol. % (CBF<$CMRO_2$)
Hyperemia: $AVDO_2$ <5 vol. % = (CBF>$CMRO_2$)

Table 8.5 Potential limitations of retrograde jugular catheters

Changes in $SvjO_2$ associated with increased ICP may only occur after herniation

Artifacts associated with catheter movement are common

Incorrect placement can result in extracerebral contamination

Single jugular bulb assessed

Anemia may narrow $AVDO_2$

Accuracy: 45–50 % sensitivity, 98–100 % specificity

Recalibration is required at least every 24 h

May miss regional hypoxia

Risk of infection and thrombosis

on the dominant jugular bulb side. Second, when an ICP monitor is present, each internal jugular vein can be compressed in turn. Compression of the dominant jugular vein causes a greater ICP increase. This can be important because up to a 15 % difference between right and left SjO_2 has been observed in TBI patients [64].

To ensure accurate use, the catheter must be placed in the jugular bulb to avoid facial vein contamination; ultrasound (US) guidance may help [65]. A lateral skull or cervical spine X-ray or an anteroposterior chest X-ray that includes the neck must be obtained to confirm catheter position [66]. The catheter tip should lie at the level of and just medial to the mastoid bone above the lower edge of C1. To maintain patency and decrease the chance of wall artifacts, the catheter is connected to a slow continuous infusion of 0.9 % saline and flush system [67]. For continuous monitoring, a fiber-optic catheter is passed through a 4-F introducer into the jugular bulb. Recalibration is needed after insertion and every 8–12 h [68, 69].

Like all monitors, data from jugular bulb catheters are best interpreted with data from other monitors, the clinical exam, and radiologic findings. Jugular bulb catheters provide bedside information about CBF changes over time and CBF adequacy relative to the cerebral metabolism. Episodes of $SjvO_2$ desaturation (relative CBF decrease) are common in comatose TBI or SAH patients and may occur despite careful hemodynamic and ICP management [70, 71]. These $SjvO_2$ desaturations (particularly $SjvO_2$ <50 % for >15 min) are associated with poor neurological outcome in TBI [71]. Jugular bulb catheters can be used to guide patient care, e.g., titrate hyperventilation for increased ICP [71], and during surgical procedures, e.g., cerebral aneurysm surgery, carotid endarterectomy, or cardiac surgery, to detect intraoperative ischemia [59, 72, 73].

Jugular bulb catheters have several potential limitations (Table 8.5). First, sensitivity is low, and a relatively large brain volume (approximately 13 %) must be affected before $SjvO_2$ levels decrease <50 % [74]. Second, heterogeneity in CBF or metabolism may give misleading information, e.g., when hyperemic areas overshadow focally ischemic areas. Third, $SjvO_2$ reliability can be compromised by changes in arterial oxygen content, hemodilution, catheter position, the need for frequent calibrations, or an ICP increase. Fourth, complications such as arterial puncture, venous air embolism, and venous thrombosis may occur at catheter insertion [68]. The commonest complications are carotid artery puncture and hematoma formation, which occur in about 1–4 % of insertions. Pneumothorax and damage to adjacent structures, such as vagus and phrenic nerves or the thoracic duct, are infrequent complications. There is an increased risk of local and systemic infection with long-term placement.

Brain Tissue Oxygen (PbtO₂) Monitoring

Brain tissue oxygen is defined as the partial pressure of oxygen in the brain interstitial space and reflects the availability of oxygen for oxidative energy production. Several abbreviations have been used to describe brain oxygen. However, at the 13th International Symposium on Intracranial Pressure and Brain Monitoring held in July 2007 in San Francisco, it was recommended that $PbtO_2$ be used as the standard abbreviation.

Today, direct $PbtO_2$ monitors are the most frequently used technique in the NCCU to assess cerebral oxygenation. In this technique, a fine catheter (approximately 0.5 mm in diameter) is placed into the brain parenchyma, specifically the white matter. Usually the monitors are secured in a multiple lumen bolt with other monitors, e.g., ICP and brain temperature that is inserted into a burr hole. This procedure can be performed at bedside in the NCCU, and, in general, $PbtO_2$ monitors are placed when the Glasgow Coma Scale (GCS) is ≤8, i.e., consistent with ICP monitor indications. There remains much debate on where in the brain a $PbtO_2$ monitor should be placed since it is a regional monitor. This is true also of parenchymal ICP monitors. In TBI patients, $PbtO_2$ catheters usually are placed into the right frontal lobe white matter in diffuse brain injury or on the side of maximal pathology when there is focal injury. In SAH, the $PbtO_2$ monitor may be placed in the vascular distribution of where maximal vasospasm is expected. Probe location should be confirmed with a CT scan since $PbtO_2$ values often are less when the monitor is adjacent to a contusion or other pathology [75, 76]. However, when the probe is in "normal-appearing" frontal subcortical white matter, there is evidence that this local measurement provides insight into global oxygenation [77–79]. Once the monitor is inserted, about 30–60 min of stabilization is required, and then probe function can be confirmed with an oxygen challenge test, particularly if the initial $PbtO_2$ reading is abnormal. In an oxygen challenge, the FIO_2 is increased from baseline to 1.0 for approximately 5 min; a $PbtO_2$ increase should occur with a functioning probe. The response is less robust when the probe is in an underperfused (CBF is < 20 ml/100 g/min) region [80]. Complications associated with use are very rare; overall the incidence of device-associated contusion is less than 2 %, and most of these are of no clinical consequence [45, 81]. Infection is even less frequent even with long-term monitoring. Technical complications, e.g., device displacement or malfunction, may complicate up to 10 % of device insertions, but there is little if any drift with time [82].

There are two primary technologies used for $PbtO_2$ measurement: one is based on the Clark principle that uses the electrochemical properties of noble metals; the other is an optical technique. Several systems have been commercially available: Licox® (Integra Neuroscience, Plainsboro, NJ) and Neurotrend™ (Diametrics Medical, St Paul, MN) have been most frequently used. There is a greater body of literature that describes the Licox system, and the Neurotrend device is no longer commercially available in most countries. Less frequently used $PbtO_2$ monitors include the Neurovent-P Temp® (Raumedic AG, Munchberg, Germany), which uses the same polarographic technique as the Licox, and the OxyLab pO_2® (Oxford Optronix Ltd., Oxford, UK) that measures $PbtO_2$ using optical fluorescence technology. These devices and $PbtO_2$ have been validated against fiber-optic jugular oxygen saturation monitoring, xenon-enhanced CT scanning, PET, and SPECT.

The Licox monitor is the most frequently used $PbtO_2$ monitor in critical care. It is a modified Clark electrode that uses the electrochemical properties of noble metals to measure the oxygen content of tissue. The Neurovent uses the same technique, but there are important differences, and so the values obtained by these devices cannot be used interchangeably [83, 84]. Similarly, there are several differences between the Neurotrend and Licox devices that limit direct comparison. In particular, the thresholds for hypoxia are different. The Neurotrend also changed design in 1998, making it difficult to compare studies before and after this date that describe this technology [79]. $PbtO_2$ measurement using the Clark principle is an oxygen-consuming process and temperature dependent and so requires constant calibration of the system to patient temperature. The Licox monitor has a separate temperature probe that is inserted through a triple lumen bolt alongside the $PbtO_2$ probe. If brain temperature is not measured (e.g., a microdialysis catheter is inserted rather than the temperature probe), the $PbtO_2$ monitor must be calibrated manually preferable every 30 min by using core body temperature.

Oxygen content usually is expressed in units of concentration (ml O_2/100 cc), and oxygen delivery and $CMRO_2$ are expressed in ml O_2/100 g brain/min. The Licox monitor, however, provides a measure of $PbtO_2$ in units of tension (mmHg); to compare this to standard oxygen concentration measurements, the following conversion factor is used: 1 mmHg = 0.003 ml O_2/100 g brain. There are many factors that influence $PbtO_2$ [79]. $PbtO_2$ values vary not only with CBF (and factors that regulate it, e.g., CO_2 and MAP) but also with changes in arterial oxygen tension (PaO_2) [85–88]. Hence, a $PbtO_2$ monitor is not an "ischemia" monitor. Rather, it likely is a marker of the balance between regional oxygen supply and cellular oxygen consumption and may be best described by the equation $PbtO_2 = CBF \times AVTO_2$, i.e., the interaction between plasma oxygen tension and CBF [86]. Some studies suggest $PbtO_2$ may reflect oxygen diffusion or be a measure of the oxygen that accumulates in brain tissue [42, 87, 89, 90], while PET studies suggest $PbtO_2$ may correlate inversely with oxygen extraction fraction (OEF) [90]. Together, these various observations suggest, importantly, that $PbtO_2$ is not the same as $SjvO_2$, i.e., a $PbtO_2$ monitor is different from a jugular bulb catheter.

Brain oxygen monitors have been used in the clinical environment in Europe since 1993. The Licox was FDA approved in 2001, and $PbtO_2$ was first included in the treatment guidelines for severe TBI in 2007. Normal values have been established in animal studies and in humans undergoing awake, functional neurosurgical procedures (e.g., deep brain stimulation); a $PbtO_2$ between 25 and 30 mmHg may be considered normal [91, 92]. Normal mitochondria require an oxygen level of about 1.5 mmHg to function; this corresponds to a $PbtO_2$ between 15 and 20 mmHg in normal white matter [89]. Threshold values for hypoxia vary slightly depending on what type of $PbtO_2$ monitor is used. In addition trends over time may be more important than a threshold. A $PbtO_2 < 20$ mmHg (on the Licox) is considered compromised $PbtO_2$ and a threshold at which to consider or initiate therapy. The 2007 Guidelines for Severe TBI recommend that $PbtO_2$ values <15 mmHg be considered as the critical threshold for "ischemia" [93]. Decreases in $PbtO_2$ are not benign, and microdialysis studies show that these decreases are associated with independent chemical markers of brain ischemia [94]. In SPECT studies, $PbtO_2$ averages 10 ± 5 mmHg during episodes of cerebral ischemia and 37 ± 12 mmHg in normal brain [95]. Values of 0 mmHg that persist longer than 30 min and show no response to an oxygen challenge are consistent with brain death [96, 97]. The number, duration, and intensity of brain hypoxic episodes ($PbtO_2 < 15$ mmHg) and any $PbtO_2$ values ≤5 mmHg are associated with poor outcome after TBI [77, 79, 82, 95, 98–103]. Indeed pooled analysis of observational data indicates that a $PbtO_2 < 10$ mmHg after TBI is associated with a significant increase in both mortality and unfavorable outcome [45]. This relationship is independent of intracranial hypertension, i.e., brain hypoxia is not simply a marker of disease severity [44]. The exact relationship with outcome, however, may vary with where the probe is placed: in normal white matter, the penumbra, or in a contusion [75, 76, 89]. The outcome relationship appears more robust when the device is located adjacent to pathology. Treatment paradigms, however, are based on the probe being in white matter that appears normal on head CT.

Brain oxygen monitoring is useful in a variety of clinical situations where secondary brain injury is likely [90, 104], and it is best used in an integrated fashion with other monitors including clinical evaluation and imaging studies. Several lines of evidence suggest that $PbtO_2$ monitors may be an ideal complement to ICP monitors. First episodes of brain hypoxia are common and may occur even when ICP and CPP are normal [41, 44, 105, 106]. Second, there is a strong relationship between $PbtO_2$ and several drivers of brain perfusion, e.g., MAP, CPP, temperature, Hgb, and end-tidal carbon dioxide (CO_2) [103, 107, 108]. This can help clinicians understand individual pathophysiology and autoregulation in each patient and determine optimal physiologic targets, e.g., CPP or Hgb [21, 109, 110]. Third, $PbtO_2$ data can help identify the need for or effects (including side effects) of various therapies, e.g., hyperventilation, hyperoxia, induced hypothermia or hypertension, transfusion, hypertonic saline, and decompressive craniectomy among others [78, 90, 107, 108, 111–124]. Finally, $PbtO_2$-based care has evolved as a potential management strategy in severe acute brain injury. Some but not all observational series suggest that the addition of $PbtO_2$-based care to ICP and CPP-based care is associated with improved outcome after severe TBI [56, 125–127]; this question is now being evaluated in a multicenter Phase II trial.

Metabolic Monitoring: Cerebral Microdialysis

Cerebral microdialysis (CMD) is an in vivo technique to sample and collect small-molecular-weight substances from the interstitial space (i.e., brain extracellular fluid). It is a well-established laboratory tool that was introduced into the clinical neurosciences in the 1990s and approved for use in Europe in 1995 and the United States in 2002. The subsequent introduction of the CMA 600 bedside analyzer (CMA Microdialysis, Solna, Sweden) significantly enhanced CMD's clinical application. The newest analyzer, the ISCUS^flex (Dipylon Medical, Solna, Sweden), was introduced in late 2008 and uses enzymatic reagents and colorimetric measurements to monitor glucose, lactate, pyruvate, glycerol, glutamate, and urea levels in microdialysis samples at the bedside. (Dipylon now is the clinical arm of CMA.) This third-generation analyzer is much smaller than the CMA 600, has batch processing capability (if needed up to 30 measurements may be made each hour), and permits simultaneous data monitoring on up to eight patients. The results are shown as trend curves on the analyzer; with appropriate software (e.g., ICUpilot), they can be integrated with other monitors [128].

The use of clinical microdialysis is now well established in several institutions worldwide where it can be used as a bedside monitor in the NCCU to examine brain tissue biochemistry. A consensus statement about CMD use in the ICU was published in 2004 [129], and, while it has largely been a research tool, CMD now is being incorporated into "point of care" testing in some institutions [130–132]. It has been used most frequently in TBI and SAH patients, and, when used with other monitors (e.g., PET, electrophysiology, and brain oxygen), CMD has improved understanding and insight into the complex biochemical and pathophysiological processes that occur in the injured brain [43, 57, 133, 134]. Since CMD measures change at the cellular level, changes in microdialysis analytes associated with compromised brain function often may precede changes in other physiological variables, e.g., ICP [55, 135]. Hence, monitoring with CMD may widen the therapeutic window. Consistent with this CMD evidence for cerebral compromise may be observed even when ICP and CPP are normal [136, 137].

The principle behind microdialysis is to imitate the function of a blood capillary. In the NCCU, this requires a sterile microdialysis catheter, a microdialysis pump, and a bedside biochemical analyzer; this equipment is all commercially available. The microdialysis catheter with the dialysis membrane at its tip is 0.6 mm in diameter. This catheter usually is placed through a triple lumen bolt, often with two other parenchymal monitors, fixed to the cranium, or it may be tunneled under the scalp and inserted into the brain tissue through a burr hole. A microdialysis pump perfuses artificial cerebrospinal fluid through the catheter, which equilibrates with the interstitial tissue around the catheter. The dialysis tubing permits diffusion of water and solutes that depend on the concentration gradient between the surrounding interstitial fluid and perfusate. The pore size of the dialysis membrane limits the size of the sampled molecules that may pass through (the cutoff) [138]. Two commercial catheters are available: (1) the CMA 70 Brain MD catheter has a relatively low cutoff of 20 kDa; (2) the CMA 71 high cutoff catheter has a cutoff of 100 kDa. The perfusion flow is kept constant, and a rate of 0.3 μl/min leads to dialysate concentrations of lactate, pyruvate, glucose, and glutamate that are approximately 70 % of those in the interstitial fluid [139].

In clinical use, MD is focused primarily on markers of cerebral energy metabolism (glucose, lactate, and pyruvate), neurotransmitters (glutamate), and cell damage (glycerol). In particular, measurements of glucose, pyruvate, and lactate provide information about the relative contributions of aerobic and anaerobic metabolism to bioenergetics and are a useful complement to $PbtO_2$ monitors, since the adult brain depends primarily on glucose and oxygen for its metabolic function and neuronal integrity. The concentration of these analytes in the dialysate fluid depends upon the equilibration between the perfusate and interstitial fluid and is called the "relative recovery," defined as dialysate/interstitial concentration ratio. Several factors, including area of the

Table 8.6 Threshold values for cerebral microdialysis

Dialysate concentration	Reinstrup et al. [141]	Schulz et al. [142]	Clinical use
Glucose (mmol/l)	1.7 (± 0.9)	2.1 (± 0.2)	<2.0
LPR	23 (± 4)	19 (± 2)	>25
Glycerol (μmol/l)	82 (± 44)	82 (± 12)	>100
Glutamate (μmol/l)	16 (± 16)	14 (± 3.3)	>15

semipermeable membrane, flow rate, and diffusion in the surrounding interstitial fluid, may affect recovery in vivo. In addition, unless it is calibrated in vivo, CMD does not provide the absolute concentration of the studied analytes. These factors generally do not affect the lactate to pyruvate ratio (LPR) that reflects the cytoplasmatic redox state and so gives information about tissue oxygenation and energetics. An LPR >25 is considered abnormal and an LPR >40 is considered to represent cell energy dysfunction. This elevated LPR may result from many causes that may be hypoxic, ischemic, or non-hypoxic/ischemic [43, 57, 140], i.e., CMD can provide insight into and "classify" both ischemic and nonischemic causes of cerebral distress.

The microdialysis catheter ideally should be placed in "at-risk" tissue since it can only measure the local metabolic product in the catheter area. While threshold values for various CMD markers are described (Table 8.6) [141, 142], trend interpretation is more useful than absolute measures since there can be considerable patient variation. The most commonly assayed CMD substances are associated with the aerobic and anaerobic glucose metabolism. CMD glucose levels are reduced in patients with severe TBI, and consistently low concentrations (<0.66 mmol l^{-1}) are associated with poor outcome [143]. Similarly, reduced CMD glucose, including that associated with intensive insulin therapy, is associated with mortality in SAH [144]. Very low brain glucose may be observed during severe hypoxia or ischemia after TBI and SAH [145, 146]. However, the determinants of CMD glucose concentration are complex, and in some patients a reduced CMD glucose may result from hyperglycolysis rather than reduced supply of glucose and oxygen [147].

The measurement of lactate and pyruvate concentrations provides further information about bioenergetics (i.e., the state of aerobic or anaerobic glycolysis). A CMD lactate concentration >4 mmol/l indicates cellular distress, but absolute brain lactate values alone do not always indicate the degree of anaerobic metabolism [57, 138]. During brain hypoxia or ischemia, there is a decrease in pyruvate concentration. A low pyruvate concentration is defined as <119 μmol/l. By contrast, normal or high extracellular pyruvate levels indicate activated aerobic glycolysis (*cerebral hyperglycolysis*) that is nonischemic in origin. Consequently, elevated CMD lactate can be classified as *hyperglycolytic* or *non-hyperglycolytic* and further classified as hypoxic or not depending on $PbtO_2$ levels. This may be important since

several lines of evidence suggest that extracellular lactate may be a preferential fuel and even a protectant for the brain under certain conditions [148–150]. Indeed, recent clinical studies demonstrate that a hyperglycolytic rather than hypoxic elevation in cerebral lactate was associated with good recovery after SAH [133]. The state of aerobic or anaerobic metabolism can be further examined with the lactate to pyruvate and lactate to glucose [142, 145] ratios. In humans, an LPR increase is associated with increased ICP, ischemia, vasospasm, or DIND after SAH, reduced $PbtO_2$, increased OEF on PET, a variety of nonischemic causes, and poor outcome after TBI and SAH [54, 57, 135, 140, 151, 152]. In this manner, CMD can be used to identify optimal physiologic targets including CPP, Hgb, or temperature and the effects of various therapies including glycemic control, hyperventilation, induced normothermia, and surgery [116, 118, 124, 144, 153].

Glycerol and glutamate are less commonly assayed CMD substances. Glycerol levels increase with membrane breakdown, and consequently it is a useful marker of cell damage [154]. Increased CMD glycerol levels are observed in severe or complete ischemia and are associated with unfavorable TBI outcome [141, 155]. However, increased glycerol can be observed when the blood–brain barrier is compromised, and so caution is needed when interpreting an elevated brain glycerol unless there is control CMD catheter, e.g., in the abdominal subcutaneous adipose tissue for a comparison [154]. Increased MD-glutamate concentrations have been associated with hypoxia, ischemia, and reduced $PbtO_2$ or CPP. In addition, increased MD glutamate is observed in TBI and SAH patients with poor outcome [57, 94, 156–158]. In recent years, the role of glutamate in outcome has been challenged, and so its measurement is less frequently performed [159]. A variety of other biomarkers, e.g., interleukins, *N*-acetylaspartate (NAA), nitric oxide, and neurofilaments, also can be examined using CMD; these markers usually are assayed in research protocols [135, 160–162].

Cerebral Blood Flow

While much of neurocritical care is focused on maintaining adequate CBF, it is important to recognize that a CBF measurement alone may not always fully describe brain physiology since flow and metabolism are coupled, i.e., a measurement about the adequacy (or not) of CBF is incomplete without some measure of metabolism. In the normal brain, when there is an increase in metabolism ($CMRO_2$), whether globally or regionally, it is matched by a CBF increase. If supply (CBF) is limited, i.e., metabolism is unmatched, there is a compensatory increase in oxygen extraction. This compensatory mechanism often is impaired in acute brain injury. On the other hand, when $CMRO_2$ is decreased, CBF, when matched, also is decreased and, while the value is low, may be adequate for metabolism.

CBF monitors can be classified as (1) those that provide a point-in-time value that may not always be repeated (radiographic or tomographic techniques), (2) noncontinuous (usually noninvasive) bedside devices that can be used daily (e.g., TCD examination), and (3) continuous (usually invasive) bedside monitors, e.g., laser Doppler and thermal diffusion techniques. Radiographic or tomographic methods provide a snapshot view of CBF in time that can be used to complement bedside monitors. These imaging techniques may be quantitative, e.g., PET, Xe-CT, and qMRA, or qualitative, e.g., SPECT, CT-P, and MRI perfusion. A variety of monitors, e.g., jugular oximetry, direct brain oxygen, microdialysis, NIRS, and EEG, provide indirect or surrogate information but are better used with a CBF monitor to help decide about flow-metabolism coupling. Finally, use of an ICP monitor and continuous blood pressure (i.e., cerebral perfusion pressure) provides useful information since CPP is an important driving force behind CBF and a factor in the autoregulatory response of the cerebral vasculature. In this section, we will discuss CPP and invasive CBF monitors, i.e., laser Doppler and thermal diffusion.

Cerebral Perfusion

The principal determinants of CPP that can be measured in the ICU are MAP and ICP, i.e., patients require an ICP monitor (see previous discussion), and an arterial pressure catheter or continuous cuff monitoring. The optimal position of the arterial pressure transducer, e.g., at the level of the foramen of Monroe or the heart, is unclear but may depend on what type of ICP monitor is used. Under normal physiologic conditions, a MAP of 80–100 mmHg and an ICP of 5–10 mmHg generate a CPP of 70–85 mmHg. However, true CPP may vary by up to 30 mmHg from measurements with MAP [48, 163, 164]. In addition, the "optimal CPP" is debated. A CPP of 60 mmHg is generally considered a minimum threshold. However, optimal CPP may vary in each patient and over time in an individual. Continuous multimodality monitoring allows optimal CPP to be determined and hence targeted to each individual [165].

When autoregulation fails, adequate brain perfusion depends even more on CPP. However, once the CPP reaches the lower threshold of the autoregulatory breakthrough zone, hyperemia and secondary ICP increase may result [166]. On the other hand, evidence for brain hypoxia can be observed despite an adequate CPP or normal ICP in TBI patients [40, 41]. Consequently, to best understand the adequacy of CPP, ICP and CPP monitoring can be supplemented with other monitors such as an SjO_2 monitor, microdialysis (e.g., lactate/pyruvate ratio), or $PbtO_2$.

Laser Doppler Flowmetry

Laser Doppler flowmetry (LDF) was introduced in 1977 to measure cutaneous blood flow. The main manufacturers of laser Doppler instruments used in clinical practice today are Perimed AB (Stockholm, Sweden), Moor Instruments Ltd. (Axminster, UK), Vasamedics Inc. (St. Paul, MN), Transonic Systems Inc. (Ithaca, NY, USA), Oxford Optronix Ltd (Oxford, UK), and LEA Medizintechnik (Giessen, Germany). LDF can be used intraoperatively or in the ICU as a bedside monitoring device that provides continuous, qualitative measurements of microvascular perfusion. It provides only regional information [167] but has excellent temporal and dynamic resolution with very short time-response changes into regional CBF.

In LDF, a small (diameter 0.5–1 mm) fiber-optic laser probe, in or on the brain, uses monochromatic laser light of wavelengths between 670 and 810 nm to illuminate a tissue volume about 1 mm^3. When light strikes the tissue that includes moving red blood cells and stationary tissue, i.e., the brain, photons are scattered and Doppler shifted in a random fashion. Photoreceptors detect a fraction of these scattered photons that generates an electric signal proportional to the volume and velocity of red blood cells. Commercially available LDF devices use Bonner and Nossal's algorithm to analyze the signal and to produce a flow output that is expressed in arbitrary units (AU), since LDF measures erythrocyte flux rather than actual CBF [168–170]. However, there is a good correlation between LDF measurements and other techniques that measure CBF, e.g., xenon clearance method, radioactive microspheres, hydrogen clearance technique, iodoantipyrine method, and thermal diffusion [171, 172].

The LDF probe is best placed in a relatively normal brain region without large vessels to limit disturbances of the flow values. In the ICU, this is usually achieved through a bolt secured in the skull. When working well, LDF provides continuous information about rCBF and can be used to assess autoregulation, CO_2 reactivity, detect ischemic insults, evaluate the response to various therapies, or help predict outcome [173, 174]. For example, in TBI, LDF determined autoregulation or the transient hyperemic response is associated with patient outcome [175, 176].

LDF has several limitations. First, LDF only measures CBF in a semiquantitative manner and in a small brain volume. Second, LDF probes require frequent calibrations to obtain reproducible and comparable LDF data. Third, errors may result from external factors, e.g., room temperature, strong external light, and sound, or internal factors, e.g., microvascular heterogeneity, hematocrit changes, or tissue or probe motion. Finally, LDF does not provide absolute CBF values. Therefore, LDF is best used as a trend monitor since it is difficult to define a threshold LDF value that indicates cerebral ischemia.

Thermal Diffusion Flowmetry

Thermal diffusion (TD) was introduced to clinical practice in 1973 and is based on thermal conductivity of brain tissue: the temperature difference between the neutral plate and the heated element indicates local CBF [177]. Validation studies show that TD-obtained rCBF values agree with rCBF values obtained in Xe-CT studies and hydrogen clearance method [178, 179]. TD probes can be placed on the brain surface, e.g., the Flowtronics probe (Flowtronics, AZ, USA) that has two gold discs on the cortex to measure superficial rCBF. Alternatively, the probe may be secured with a metal bolt through a burr hole and positioned in the parenchyma (e.g., Hemedex Inc, Cambridge, MA). The Hemedex probe is placed in normal brain tissue about 25 mm below the dura and provides a quantitative measure in the spherical volume of tissue surrounding the sensor that is at the probe tip. Compared to other continuous monitors, up to a third of CBF measurements may be lost because automatic recalibration occurs approximately every 30 min, and CBF measurements are prevented for safety reasons when temperature is >39 °C [110]. Fever also may affect measurement reliability [20, 177]. In addition, loss of tissue contact or when the probe is positioned near large vessels can compromise TD accuracy.

Superficial (cortical) TD rCBF values between 40 and 70 ml/100 g/min are considered normal, whereas values <20 ml/100 g/min or >70 ml/100 g/min represent ischemia and hyperemia, respectively [180]. Hemedex measures perfusion in subcortical white matter where a mean TD value of 18–25 ml/100 g/min is considered normal [110, 181]. Although the TD values represent local measures, serial changes can be used to detect early neurological deterioration, assess responses to therapy, guide adequate perfusion, or help predict outcome. For example, patients with an increase in rCBF from baseline tend to have a good outcome after brain injury, whereas patients with very low initial values or no increase in baseline have a poor outcome [180, 182]. In SAH, TD can be used to detect vasospasm [181], provided the probe is in the distribution of the narrowed vessel. Then, a CBF threshold of 15 ml/100 g/min and a cerebrovascular resistance of 10 have a sensitivity of 90 % and specificity of 75 % for symptomatic vasospasm.

Bioinformatics and Making Sense of the Numbers in the Future

Prevention, detection, and management of secondary brain injury are the primary purpose of neurocritical care. This is accomplished through frequent neurological examination and assessment of consciousness; imaging studies, e.g., head CT or chest X-ray; assessment of systemic and laboratory variables; and monitoring of neurophysiological parameters.

The NCCU, therefore, is a very data-intense environment. In addition, while much of current-day management is threshold oriented and based on a single parameter (i.e., treat when ICP is >20 mmHg or CPP <60 mmHg), these variables are more than a number and much can be learned from trend analysis, waveform analysis, or integration of several variables [133]. For example, valuable information about compliance, CBF autoregulation, and CSF absorption capacity may be obtained from ICP waveform analysis or evaluation of derived indices of cerebrovascular reactivity (PRx) or cerebrospinal compensatory reserve (RAP) [47, 48, 164, 183]. Recent advances in data processing and computerized bedside monitoring now make it possible to perform online, real-time analysis of indices such as PRx and RAP. This provides insight into a patient's compensatory reserve even when the numerical value of ICP is normal.

The art of neurocritical care is to use the various data derived from the clinical examination, imaging, and various monitoring parameters for patient care decision-making in real time (multimodal monitoring). However, this is complicated in part because the ability to record physiological data exceeds our ability to fully integrate it into patient care. In addition, the interaction of multiple parameters may be more relevant than any individual factor. However, the human brain has difficulty judging the interaction between more than two variables, but significantly more potential interactions are present each time a physician evaluates a patient.

Many efforts today are centered on bioinformatics in neurocritical care to bring order to the potential information overload and through integration of variables gain greater insight into disease pathophysiology and treatment [184, 185]. There are several basic requirements for this. First, continuous monitoring is required so as not to miss clinically significant events. However, the frequency of monitoring needs to be greater than the duration of the events to be detected. This raises important questions: what parameters should be monitored and how often are measurements required? Second, monitoring should be comprehensive. By its nature, multimodality monitoring comes from diverse sources, and the data varies (e.g., numeric, imaging, text, continuous, ordinal). Ideally, the necessary data for an individual patient need to be collected simultaneously, time synchronized, and displayed in an integrated fashion. There are major challenges in neurocritical care bioinformatics:

- Is every piece of information valuable or can some be discarded and, if so, which and when [85]?
- Many commercial devices are stand-alone and there are challenges in ensuring device interoperability, e.g., standardization of terminology, or do the device clocks run together?
- How are artifacts detected and how are data cleaned?
- How are missing data, e.g., during device disconnection, dealt with?

Finally, monitoring needs to be communicative and be able to plot time-synchronized trends on a single display and integrate waveforms, images, and other formats, e.g., the clinical examination or laboratory data. Several devices that begin to do this already exist, e.g., ICM+, ICUpilot, Bedmaster XA, Axon Systems Eclipse Neurological Workstation, and the CNS Monitor. The next step and the challenge for the coming years, once the data are recorded, are to create a bedside knowledge environment to couple decision support to patient care. This may come about through exploring statistical relationships between variables, discriminate function analysis, neural networks, decision tree analysis, complex systems analysis, or model-based systems, e.g., dynamic Bayesian networks have evolved from engineering and mathematics [186, 187]. With more sophisticated analysis, monitoring then will allow identification of patient transitions towards favorable or unfavorable physiological states rather than having to wait for a particular "threshold" to be reached for treatment (i.e., prediction) while taking into consideration the variability among patients [188–190]. In so doing, monitoring in the NCCU in the future can help provide individualized, targeted care and proactive restoration of normal physiology rather than reactive treatment of abnormal pathology.

References

1. Jones PA, Andrews PJ, Midgley S, et al. Measuring the burden of secondary insults in head-injured patients during intensive care. J Neurosurg Anesthesiol. 1994;6:4–14.
2. Maas AI, Menon DK, Lingsma HF, Pineda JA, Sandel ME, Manley GT. Re-orientation of clinical research in traumatic brain injury: report of an international workshop on comparative effectiveness research. J Neurotrauma. 2012;29(1):32–46.
3. Bratton SL, Chestnut RM, Ghajar J, McConnell Hammond FF, Harris OA, Hartl R, Manley GT, Nemecek A, Newell DW, Rosenthal G, Schouten J, Shutter L, Timmons SD, Ullman JS, Videtta W, Wilberger JE, Wright DW, Brain Trauma Foundation; American Association of Neurological Surgeons; Congress of Neurological Surgeons; Joint Section on Neurotrauma and Critical Care, AANS/CNS. Guidelines for the management of severe traumatic brain injury. VII. Intracranial pressure monitoring technology. J Neurotrauma. 2007;24 Suppl 1:S45–54.
4. Citerio G, Andrews PJ. Intracranial pressure. Part two: clinical applications and technology. Intensive Care Med. 2004;30:1882–5.
5. Smith M. Monitoring intracranial pressure in traumatic brain injury. Anesth Analg. 2008;106:240–8.
6. Marshall LF, Smith RW, Shapiro HM. The outcome with aggressive treatment in severe head injuries. Part I: the significance of intracranial pressure monitoring. J Neurosurg. 1979;50(1):20–5.
7. Narayan RK, Kishore PR, Becker DP, et al. Intracranial pressure: to monitor or not to monitor? A review of our experience with severe head injury. J Neurosurg. 1982;56:650–9.
8. Marmarou A, Anderson RL, Ward JD, et al. Impact of ICP instability and hypotension on outcome in patients with severe head trauma. J Neurosurg. 1991;75(Suppl):S159–66.
9. Vik A, Nag T, Fredriksli OA, Skandsen T, Moen KG, Schirmer-Mikalsen K, Manley GT. Relationship of "dose" of intracranial hypertension to outcome in severe traumatic brain injury. J Neurosurg. 2008;109(4):678–84.
10. Stein DM, Hu PF, Brenner M, Sheth KN, Liu KH, Xiong W, Aarabi B, Scalea TM. Brief episodes of intracranial hypertension and cerebral hypoperfusion are associated with poor functional outcome after severe traumatic brain injury. J Trauma. 2011;71(2):364–74.
11. Marmarou A. A review of progress in understanding the pathophysiology and treatment of brain edema. Neurosurg Focus. 2007;22(5):E1.
12. Treggiari MM, Schutz N, Yanez ND, Romand JA. Role of intracranial pressure values and patterns in predicting outcome in traumatic brain injury: a systematic review. Neurocrit Care. 2007;6:104–12.
13. Heuer G, Smith MJ, Elliott JP, Winn HR, Le Roux P. The relationship between intracranial pressure and other clinical variables in patients with aneurysmal subarachnoid hemorrhage. J Neurosurg. 2004;101:408–16.
14. Stein SC, Georgoff P, Meghan S, Mirza KL, El Falaky OM. Relationship of aggressive monitoring and treatment to improved outcomes in severe traumatic brain injury. J Neurosurg. 2010;112(5):1105–12.
15. Whitmore RG, Thawani JP, Grady MS, Levine JM, Sanborn MR, Stein SC. Is aggressive treatment of traumatic brain injury cost-effective? J Neurosurg. 2012;116(5):1106–13.
16. Cremer OL, van Dijk GW, van Wensen E, Brekelmans GJ, Moons KG, Leenen LP, Kalkman CJ. Effect of intracranial pressure monitoring and targeted intensive care on functional outcome after severe head injury. Crit Care Med. 2005;33(10):2207–13.
17. Shafi S, Diaz-Arrastia R, Madden C, Gentilello L. Intracranial pressure monitoring in brain-injured patients is associated with worsening of survival. J Trauma. 2008;64(2):335–40.
18. Forsyth RJ, Wolny S, Rodrigues B. Routine intracranial pressure monitoring in acute coma. Cochrane Database Syst Rev. 2010;(2):CD002043.
19. Oddo M, Le Roux P. What is the etiology, pathogenesis and pathophysiology of elevated intracranial pressure? In: Neligan P, Deutschman CS, editors. The evidenced based practice of critical care. Philadelphia: Elsevier Science; 2009. p. 399–405.
20. Rosenthal G, Sanchez-Mejia RO, Phan N, et al. Incorporating a parenchymal thermal diffusion cerebral blood flow probe in bedside assessment of cerebral autoregulation and vasoreactivity in patients with severe traumatic brain injury. J Neurosurg. 2011;114:62–70.
21. Lang EW, Lagopoulos J, Griffith J, Yip K, Yam A, Mudaliar Y, Mehdorn HM, Dorsch NW. Cerebral vasomotor reactivity testing in head injury: the link between pressure and flow. J Neurol Neurosurg Psychiatry. 2003;74(8):1053–9.
22. Bratton SL, Chestnut RM, Ghajar J, McConnell Hammond FF, Harris OA, Hartl R, Manley GT, Nemecek A, Newell DW, Rosenthal G, Schouten J, Shutter L, Timmons SD, Ullman JS, Videtta W, Wilberger JE, Wright DW, Brain Trauma Foundation; American Association of Neurological Surgeons; Congress of Neurological Surgeons; Joint Section on Neurotrauma and Critical Care, AANS/CNS. Guidelines for the management of severe traumatic brain injury. VI. Indications for intracranial pressure monitoring. J Neurotrauma. 2007;24 Suppl 1:S37–44.
23. Katsnelson M, Mackenzie L, Frangos S, Oddo M, Levine JM, Pukenas B, Faerber J, Dong C, Kofke WA, Leroux PD. Are initial radiographic and clinical scales associated with subsequent intracranial pressure and brain oxygen levels after severe traumatic brain injury? Neurosurgery. 2012;70(5):1095–105.
24. Muizelaar JP, Marmarou A, Ward JD, et al. Adverse effects of prolonged hyperventilation in patients with severe head injury: a randomized clinical trial. J Neurosurg. 1991;75(5):731–9.

25. Robertson CS, Valadka AB, Hannay HJ, et al. Prevention of secondary ischemic insults after severe head injury. Crit Care Med. 1999;27(10):2086–95.

26. Andrews PJ, Citerio G, Longhi L, Polderman K, Sahuquillo J, Vajkoczy P, Neuro-Intensive Care and Emergency Medicine (NICEM) Section of the European Society of Intensive Care Medicine. NICEM consensus on neurological monitoring in acute neurological disease. Intensive Care Med. 2008;34(8):1362–70.

27. Maas AI, Dearden M, Teasdale GM, Braakman R, Cohadon F, Iannotti F, Karimi A, Lapierre F, Murray G, Ohman J, Persson L, Servadei F, Stocchetti N, Unterberg A. EBIC-guidelines for management of severe head injury in adults. European Brain Injury Consortium. Acta Neurochir (Wien). 1997;139(4):286–94.

28. Procaccio F, Stocchetti N, Citerio G, Berardino M, Beretta L, Della Corte F, D'Avella D, Brambilla GL, Delfini R, Servadei F, Tomei G. Guidelines for the treatment of adults with severe head trauma (part I). Initial assessment; evaluation and pre-hospital treatment; current criteria for hospital admission; systemic and cerebral monitoring. J Neurosurg Sci. 2000;44(1):1–10.

29. Padayachy LC, Figaji AA, Bullock MR. Intracranial pressure monitoring for traumatic brain injury in the modern era. Childs Nerv Syst. 2010;26(4):441–52. Review.

30. Ehtisham A, Taylor S, Bayless L, et al. Placement of external ventricular drains and intracranial pressure monitors by neurointensivists. Neurocrit Care. 2009;10:241–7.

31. Martinez-Manas RM, Santamarta D, de Campos JM, Ferrer E. Camino intracranial pressure monitor: prospective study of accuracy and complications. J Neurol Neurosurg Psychiatry. 2000;69: 82–6.

32. Bauer DF, McGwin Jr G, Melton SM, George RL, Markert JM. The relationship between INR and development of hemorrhage with placement of ventriculostomy. J Trauma. 2011;70(5): 1112–7.

33. Timofeev I, Dahyot-Fizelier C, Keong N, Nortje J, Al-Rawi PG, Czosnyka M, Menon DK, Kirkpatrick PJ, Gupta AK, Hutchinson PJ. Ventriculostomy for control of raised ICP in acute traumatic brain injury. Acta Neurochir Suppl. 2008;102:99–104.

34. Exo J, Kochanek PM, Adelson PD, Greene S, Clark RS, Bayir H, Wisniewski SR, Bell MJ. Intracranial pressure-monitoring systems in children with traumatic brain injury: combining therapeutic and diagnostic tools. Pediatr Crit Care Med. 2011;12(5): 560–5.

35. Birch AA, Eynon CA, Schley D. Erroneous intracranial pressure measurements from simultaneous pressure monitoring and ventricular drainage catheters. Neurocrit Care. 2006;5:51–4.

36. Lozier AP, Sciacca RR, Romagnoli MF, Connolly Jr ES. Ventriculostomy-related infections: a critical review of the literature. Neurosurgery. 2002;51(1):170–81; discussion 181–2.

37. Beer R, Lackner P, Pfausler B, Schmutzhard E. Nosocomial ventriculitis and meningitis in neurocritical care patients. J Neurol. 2008;255:1617–24.

38. Bremmer R, de Jong BM, Wagemakers M, et al. The course of intracranial pressure in traumatic brain injury: relation with outcome and CT-characteristics. Neurocrit Care. 2010;12:362–8.

39. O'Phelan KH, Park D, Efird JT, Johnson K, Albano M, Beniga J, Green DM, Chang CW. Patterns of increased intracranial pressure after severe traumatic brain injury. Neurocrit Care. 2009;10(3): 280–6.

40. Le Roux P, Lam AM, Newell DW, Grady MS, Winn HR. Cerebral arteriovenous difference of oxygen: a predictor of cerebral infarction and outcome in severe head injury. J Neurosurg. 1997;87: 1–8.

41. Stiefel MF, Udoetek J, Spiotta A, Gracias VH, Goldberg AH, Maloney-Wilensky E, Bloom S, Le Roux P. Conventional neurocritical care and cerebral oxygenation after traumatic brain injury. J Neurosurgery. 2006;105:568–75.

42. Menon DK, Coles JP, Gupta AK, Fryer TD, Smielewski P, Chatfield DA, Aigbirhio F, Skepper JN, Minhas PS, Hutchinson PJ, Carpenter TA, Clark JC, Pickard JD. Diffusion limited oxygen delivery following head injury. Crit Care Med. 2004;32:1384–90.

43. Vespa PM, O'Phelan K, McArthur D, Miller C, Eliseo M, Hirt D, Glenn T, Hovda DA. Pericontusional brain tissue exhibits persistent elevation of lactate/pyruvate ratio independent of cerebral perfusion pressure. Crit Care Med. 2007;35(4):1153–60.

44. Oddo M, Levine JM, Mackenzie L, Frangos S, Feihl F, Kasner SE, Katsnelson M, Pukenas B, Macmurtrie E, Maloney-Wilensky E, Kofke WA, LeRoux PD. Brain hypoxia is associated with short-term outcome after severe traumatic brain injury independently of intracranial hypertension and low cerebral perfusion pressure. Neurosurgery. 2011;69(5):1037–45; discussion 1045.

45. Maloney-Wilensky E, Gracias V, Itkin A, Hoffman K, Bloom S, Yang W, Christian S, Le Roux P. Brain tissue oxygen and outcome after severe traumatic brain injury: a systematic review. Crit Care Med. 2009;37(6):2057–63.

46. Maset AL, Marmarou A, Ward JD, et al. Pressure-volume index in head injury. J Neurosurg. 1987;67:832–40.

47. Steiner LA, Czosnyka M, Piechnik SK, et al. Continuous monitoring of cerebrovascular pressure reactivity allows determination of optimal cerebral perfusion pressure in patients with traumatic brain injury. Crit Care Med. 2002;30:733–8.

48. Czosnyka M, Guazzo E, Whitehouse M, et al. Significance of intracranial pressure waveform analysis after head injury. Acta Neurochir. 1996;138:531–41; discussion 41–2.

49. Balestreri M, Czosnyka M, Steiner LA, et al. Association between outcome, cerebral pressure reactivity and slow ICP waves following head injury. Acta Neurochir Suppl. 2005;95:25–8.

50. Zweifel C, Lavinio A, Steiner LA, Radolovich D, Smielewski P, Timofeev I, Hiler M, Balestreri M, Kirkpatrick PJ, Pickard JD, Hutchinson P, Czosnyka M. Continuous monitoring of cerebrovascular pressure reactivity in patients with head injury. Neurosurg Focus. 2008;25(4):E2.

51. Kim DJ, Czosnyka Z, Kasprowicz M, Smieleweski P, Baledent O, Guerguerian AM, Pickard JD, Czosnyka M. Continuous monitoring of the Monro-Kellie doctrine: is it possible? J Neurotrauma. 2012;29(7):1354–63.

52. Aries MJ, Czosnyka M, Budohoski KP, Kolias AG, Radolovich DK, Lavinio A, Pickard JD, Smielewski P. Continuous monitoring of cerebrovascular reactivity using pulse waveform of intracranial pressure. Neurocrit Care. 2012;17(1):67–76.

53. Sorrentino E, Diedler J, Kasprowicz M, Budohoski KP, Haubrich C, Smielewski P, Outtrim JG, Manktelow A, Hutchinson PJ, Pickard JD, Menon DK, Czosnyka M. Critical thresholds for cerebrovascular reactivity after traumatic brain injury. Neurocrit Care. 2012;16(2):258–66.

54. Belli A, Sen J, Petzold A, Russo S, Kitchen N, Smith M. Metabolic failure precedes intracranial pressure rises in traumatic brain injury: a microdialysis study. Acta Neurochir (Wien). 2008;150: 461–9.

55. Adamides AA, Rosenfeldt FL, Winter CD, Pratt NM, Tippett NJ, Lewis PM, Bailey MJ, Cooper DJ, Rosenfeld JV. Brain tissue lactate elevations predict episodes of intracranial hypertension in patients with traumatic brain injury. J Am Coll Surg. 2009; 209(4):531–9.

56. Nangunoori R, Maloney-Wilensky E, Stiefel MDM, Park S, Kofke WA, Levine J, Yang W, Le Roux P. Brain tissue oxygen based therapy and outcome after severe traumatic brain injury: a systematic literature review. Neurocrit Care. 2012;17(1):131–8.

57. Timofeev I, Carpenter KL, Nortje J, Al-Rawi PG, O'Connell MT, Czosnyka M, Smielewski P, Pickard JD, Menon DK, Kirkpatrick PJ, Gupta AK, Hutchinson PJ. Cerebral extracellular chemistry and outcome following traumatic brain injury: a microdialysis study of 223 patients. Brain. 2011;134(Pt 2):484–94.

58. Ketty SS, Schmidt CF. The nitrous oxide method for the quantitative determination of cerebral blood flow in man: theory, procedure and normal values. J Clin Invest. 1948;27:476–83.

59. Matta BF, Lam AM, Mayberg TS, Shapira Y, Winn HR. A critique of the intraoperative use of jugular venous bulb catheters during neurosurgical procedures. Anesth Analg. 1994;79:745–50.

60. Feldman Z, Robertson CS. Monitoring of cerebral hemodynamics with jugular bulb catheters. Crit Care Clin. 1997;13(1):51–77.

61. Robertson CS, Gopinath SP, Goodman JC, et al. SjvO2 monitoring in head injured patients. J Neurotrauma. 1995;12:891–6.

62. Gibbs EL, Gibbs FA. The cross sectional areas of the vessels that form the torcular and the manner in which blood is distributed to the right and to the left lateral sinus. Anat Rec. 1934;54:419.

63. Gibbs FA. A thermoelectric blood flow recorder in the form of a needle. In: Proceedings of the Society for Experimental Biology and Medicine, San Francisco, 1933, p. 141–6.

64. Stocchetti N, Paparella A, Brindelli F, Bacchi M, Piazza P, Zuccoli P. Cerebral venous oxygen saturation studied with bilateral samples in the internal jugular veins. Neurosurgery. 1994;34:38–44.

65. National Institute for Clinical Excellence. NICE technology appraisal guidance No 49: guidance on the use of ultrasound locating devices for placing central venous catheters. 2002. London NICE. Available from www.nice.org.uk/pdf/ultrasound_49_GUIDANCE.pdf.

66. Bankier AA, Fleischmann D, Windiscch A, et al. Position of jugular oxygen saturation catheter in patients with head trauma: assessment by use of plain films. Am J Radiol. 1995;164:437–41.

67. Gunn HC, Matta BF, Lam AM, Mayberg TS. Accuracy of continuous jugular bulb venous oximetry during intracranial surgery. J Neurosurg Anesthesiol. 1995;7:174–7.

68. Goetting MG, Preston G. Jugular bulb catheterization: experience with 123 patients. Crit Care Med. 1990;18(11):1220–3.

69. Sheinberg GM, Kanter MJ, Robertson CS, et al. Continuous monitoring of jugular venous oxygen saturation in head-injured patients. J Neurosurg. 1992;76:212–7.

70. Gopinath SP, Rogertson CS, Constant CF, et al. Jugular venous desaturation and outcome after head injury. J Neurol Neurosurg Psychiatry. 1994;57:717–23.

71. Thiagarajan A, Goverdhan P, Chari P, Somasunderam K. The effect of hyperventilation and hyperoxia on cerebral venous oxygen saturation in patients with traumatic brain injury. Anesth Analg. 1998;87:850–3.

72. Crossman J, Banister K, Bythell V, Bullock R, Chambers I, Mendelow AD. Predicting clinical ischaemia during awake carotid endarterectomy: use of the SJVO2 probe as a guide to selective shunting. Physiol Meas. 2003;24:347–54.

73. Croughwell ND, Newman MF, Blumenthal JA, White WD, Lewis JB, Frasco PE, Smith LR, Thyrum EA, Hurwitz BJ, Leone BJ, Schell RM, Reves JG. Jugular bulb saturation and cognitive dysfunction after cardiopulmonary bypass. Ann Thorac Surg. 1994;58:1702–8.

74. Artru F, Dailler F, Burel E, et al. Assessment of jugular blood oxygen and lactate indices for detection of cerebral ischemia and prognosis. J Neurosurg Anesthesiol. 2004;16:226–31.

75. Longhi L, Pagan F, Valeriani V, et al. Monitoring brain tissue oxygen tension in brain-injured patients reveals hypoxic episodes in normal-appearing and in perifocal tissue. Intensive Care Med. 2007;33:2136–42.

76. Ponce LL, Pillai S, Cruz J, Li X, Hannay HJ, Gopinath S, Robertson CS. Position of probe determines prognostic information of brain tissue pO2 in severe traumatic brain injury. Neurosurgery. 2012;70(6):1492–502; discussion 1502–3.

77. Kiening KL, Unterberg AW, Bardt TF, Schneider GH, Lanksch WR. Monitoring of cerebral oxygenation in patients with severe head injuries: brain tissue PO2 versus jugular vein oxygen saturation. J Neurosurg. 1996;85:751–7.

78. Gupta AK, Hutchinson PJ, Al-Rawi P, et al. Measuring brain tissue oxygenation compared with jugular venous oxygen saturation for monitoring cerebral oxygenation after traumatic brain injury. Anesth Analg. 1999;88:549–53.

79. Maloney-Wilensky E, Le Roux P. The physiology behind direct brain oxygen monitors and practical aspects of their use. Childs Nerv Syst. 2010;26(4):419–30.

80. Hlatky R, Valadka AB, Gopinath SP, Robertson CS. Brain tissue oxygen tension response to induced hyperoxia reduced in hypoperfused brain. J Neurosurg. 2008;108(1):53–8.

81. Bailey RL, Quattrone F, Curtain C, Frangos S, Maloney-Wilensky E, Park S, Le Roux P. The safety of multimodal monitoring in severe brain injury. Neurocritical Care Society meeting, Montreal, 2011.

82. Dings J, Meixensberger J, Jager A, et al. Clinical experience with 118 brain tissue oxygen partial pressure catheter probes. Neurosurgery. 1998;43:1082–95.

83. Orakcioglu B, Sakowitz OW, Neumann JO, Kentar MM, Unterberg A, Kiening KL. Evaluation of a novel brain tissue oxygenation probe in an experimental swine model. Neurosurgery. 2010;67(6):1716–22; discussion 1722–3.

84. Dengler J, Frenzel C, Vajkoczy P, et al. Cerebral tissue oxygenation measured by two different probes: challenges and interpretation. Intensive Care Med. 2011;37:1809–15.

85. Hemphill 3rd JC, Knudson MM, Derugin N, Morabito D, Manley GT. Carbon dioxide reactivity and pressure autoregulation of brain tissue oxygen. Neurosurgery. 2001;48:377–83.

86. Rosenthal G, Hemphill III JC, Sorani M, et al. Brain tissue oxygen tension is more indicative of oxygen diffusion than oxygen delivery and metabolism in patients with traumatic brain injury. Crit Care Med. 2008;36:1917–24.

87. Scheufler KM, Rohrborn HJ, Zentner J. Does tissue oxygen-tension reliably reflect cerebral oxygen delivery and consumption? Anesth Analg. 2002;95:1042–8.

88. Scheufler K-M, Lehnert A, Rohrborn H-J, et al. Individual values of brain tissue oxygen pressure, microvascular oxygen saturation, cytochrome redox level and energy metabolites in detecting critically reduced cerebral energy state during acute changes in global cerebral perfusion. J Neurosurg Anesthesiol. 2004;16:210–9.

89. Longhi L, Valeriani V, Rossi S, De Marchi M, Egidi M, Stocchetti N. Effects of hyperoxia on brain tissue oxygen tension in cerebral focal lesions. Acta Neurochir Suppl. 2002;81:315–7.

90. Johnston AJ, Steiner LA, Coles JP, et al. Effect of cerebral perfusion pressure augmentation on regional oxygenation and metabolism after head injury. Crit Care Med. 2005;33:189–95; discussion 255–7.

91. Pennings FA, Schuurman PR, van den Munckhof P, Bouma GJ. Brain tissue oxygen pressure monitoring in awake patients during functional neurosurgery: the assessment of normal values. J Neurotrauma. 2008;25:1173–7.

92. Zauner A, Bullock R, Di X, Young HF. Brain oxygen, CO2, pH, and temperature monitoring: evaluation in the feline brain. Neurosurgery. 1995;37:1168–76; discussion 76–7.

93. Bratton SL, Chestnut RM, Ghajar J, et al. Guidelines for the management of severe traumatic brain injury. X. Brain oxygen monitoring and thresholds. J Neurotrauma. 2007;24 Suppl 1: S65–70.

94. Hlatky R, Valadka AB, Goodman JC, Contant CF, Robertson CS. Patterns of energy substrates during ischemia measured in the brain by microdialysis. J Neurotrauma. 2004;21(7):894–906.

95. Hoffman WE, Charbel FT, Edelman G. Brain tissue oxygen, carbon dioxide, and pH in neurosurgical patients at risk for ischemia. Anesth Analg. 1996;82(3):582–6.

96. Smith ML, Counelis GJ, Maloney-Wilensky E, Stiefel MF, Donley K, LeRoux PD. Brain tissue oxygen tension in clinical brain death: a case series. Neurol Res. 2007;29:755–9.

97. Figaji AA, Kent SJ. Brain tissue oxygenation in children diagnosed with brain death. Neurocrit Care. 2010;12(1):56–61.

98. van Santbrink H, Maas AIR, Avezaat CJJ. Continuous monitoring of partial pressure of brain tissue oxygen in patients with severe head injury. Neurosurgery. 1996;38:21–31.

99. van den Brink WA, van Santbrink H, Steyerberg EW, et al. Brain oxygen tension in severe head injury. Neurosurgery. 2000;46:868–78.

100. Bardt TF, Unterberg AW, Hartl R, et al. Monitoring of brain tissue PO2 in traumatic brain injury: effect of cerebral hypoxia on outcome. Acta Neurochir Suppl. 1998;71:153–6.

101. Doppenberg EM, Zauner A, Watson JC, et al. Determination of the ischemic threshold for brain oxygen tension. Acta Neurochir Suppl. 1998;71:166–9.

102. Chang JJ, Youn TS, Benson D, Mattick H, Andrade N, Harper CR, Moore CB, Madden CJ, Diaz-Arrastia RR. Physiologic and functional outcome correlates of brain tissue hypoxia in traumatic brain injury. Crit Care Med. 2009;37(1):283–90.

103. Gopinath SP, Valadka AB, Uzura M, Robertson CS. Comparison of jugular venous oxygen saturation and brain tissue PO2 as monitors of cerebral ischemia after head injury. Crit Care Med. 1999; 27:2337–45.

104. Nortje J, Gupta AK. The role of tissue oxygen monitoring in patients with acute brain injury. Br J Anaesth. 2006;97:95–106.

105. Gracias VH, Guillamondegui OD, Stiefel MF, Wilensky EM, Bloom S, Pryor JP, Reilly PM, Le Roux P, Schwab CW. Cerebral cortical oxygenation: a pilot study. J Trauma. 2004;56:469–74.

106. Rohlwink UK, Zwane E, Graham Fieggen A, Argent AC, le Roux PD, Figaji AA. The relationship between intracranial pressure and brain oxygenation in children with severe traumatic brain injury. Neurosurgery. 2012;70(5):1220–31.

107. Tolias CM, Reinert M, Seiler R, et al. Normobaric hyperoxia–induced improvement in cerebral metabolism and reduction in intracranial pressure in patients with severe head injury: a prospective historical cohort-matched study. J Neurosurg. 2004; 101(3):435–44.

108. Gupta AK, Hutchinson PJ, Fryer T, et al. Measurement of brain tissue oxygenation performed using positron emission tomography scanning to validate a novel monitoring method. J Neurosurg. 2002;96(2):263–8.

109. Jaeger M, Schuhmann MU, Soehle M, Meixensberger J. Continuous assessment of cerebrovascular autoregulation after traumatic brain injury using brain tissue oxygen pressure reactivity. Crit Care Med. 2006;34:1783–8.

110. Jaeger M, Soehle M, Schuhmann MU, et al. Correlation of continuously monitored regional cerebral blood flow and brain tissue oxygen. Acta Neurochir. 2005;147:51–6.

111. Menzel M, Doppenberg EM, Zauner A, Soukup J, Reinert MM, Bullock R. Increased inspired oxygen concentration as a factor in improved brain tissue oxygenation and tissue lactate levels after severe human head injury. J Neurosurg. 1999;91:1–10.

112. al-Rawi PG, Hutchinson PJ, Gupta AK, et al. Multiparameter brain tissue monitoring correlation between parameters and identification of CPP thresholds. Zentralbl Neurochir. 2000;61(2): 74–9.

113. Coles JP, Minhas PS, Fryer TD, et al. Effect of hyperventilation on cerebral blood flow in traumatic head injury: clinical relevance and monitoring correlates. Crit Care Med. 2002;30:1950–9.

114. Dohmen C, Bosche B, Graf R, et al. Identification and clinical impact of impaired cerebrovascular autoregulation in patients with malignant middle cerebral artery infarction. Stroke. 2007;38(1): 56–61.

115. Sakowitz OW, Stover JF, Sarrafzadeh AS, Unterberg AW, Kiening KL. Effects of mannitol bolus administration on intracranial pressure, cerebral extracellular metabolites, and tissue oxygenation in severely head-injured patients. J Trauma. 2007;62:292–8.

116. Oddo M, Milby A, Chen I, Frangos S, MacMutrie E, Maloney-Wilensky E, Stiefel MF, Kofke A, Levine JM, Le Roux P. Hemoglobin concentration and cerebral metabolism in patients with aneurysmal subarachnoid hemorrhage: a microdialysis study. Stroke. 2009;40(4):1275–81.

117. Oddo M, Levine JM, Frangos S, et al. Effect of mannitol and hypertonic saline on cerebral oxygenation in patients with severe traumatic brain injury and refractory intracranial hypertension. J Neurol Neurosurg Psychiatry. 2009;80(8):916–20.

118. Oddo M, Frangos S, Milby A, Chen I, Maloney-Wilensky E, Murtrie EM, Stiefel M, Kofke WA, Le Roux P, Levine JM. Induced normothermia attenuates cerebral metabolic distress in patients with aneurysmal subarachnoid hemorrhage and refractory fever. Stroke. 2009;40(5):1913–6.

119. Oddo M, Frangos S, Maloney-Wilensky E, Andrew Kofke W, Le Roux P, Levine JM. Effect of shivering on brain tissue oxygenation during induced normothermia in patients with severe brain injury. Neurocrit Care. 2010;12(1):10–6.

120. Weiner GM, Lacey MR, Mackenzie L, Shah DP, Frangos SG, Grady MS, Kofke WA, Levine J, Schuster J, Le Roux P. Decompressive craniectomy for elevated intracranial pressure and its effect on the cumulative ischemic burden and therapeutic intensity levels after sever traumatic brain injury. Neurosurgery. 2010; 66:1111–9.

121. Figaji AA, Zwane E, Fieggen AG, Argent AC, Le Roux P, Siesjo P, Peter JC. Pressure autoregulation, intracranial pressure and brain tissue oxygenation in children with severe traumatic brain injury. J Neurosurg Pediatr. 2009;4(5):420–8.

122. Smith MJ, Maggee S, Stiefel M, Bloom S, Gracias V, Le Roux P. Packed red blood cell transfusion increases local cerebral oxygenation. Crit Care Med. 2005;33:1104–8.

123. Muench E, Horn P, Bauhuf C, Roth H, Philipps M, Hermann P, Quintel M, Schmiedek P, Vajkoczy P. Effects of hypervolemia and hypertension on regional cerebral blood flow, intracranial pressure, and brain tissue oxygenation after subarachnoid hemorrhage. Crit Care Med. 2007;35:1844–51.

124. Nortje J, Coles JP, Timofeev I, et al. Effect of hyperoxia on regional oxygenation and metabolism after severe traumatic brain injury: preliminary findings. Crit Care Med. 2008;36:273–81.

125. Spiotta AM, Stiefel MF, Gracias VH, et al. Brain tissue oxygen-directed management and outcome in patients with severe traumatic brain injury. J Neurosurg. 2010;113:571–80.

126. Narotam PK, Morrison JF, Nathoo N. Brain tissue oxygen monitoring in traumatic brain injury and major trauma: outcome analysis of a brain tissue oxygen-directed therapy. J Neurosurg. 2009; 111:672–82.

127. Martini RP, Deem S, Yanez ND, et al. Management guided by brain tissue oxygen monitoring and outcome following severe traumatic brain injury. J Neurosurg. 2009;111(4):644–9.

128. Nordström CH. Cerebral energy metabolism and microdialysis in neurocritical care. Childs Nerv Syst. 2010;26:465–72.

129. Bellander BM, Cantais E, Enblad P, et al. Consensus meeting on microdialysis in neurointensive care. Intensive Care Med. 2004;30:2166–9.

130. Tisdall MM, Smith M. Cerebral microdialysis: research technique or clinical tool. Br J Anaesth. 2006;97:18–25.

131. Goodman JC, Robertson CS. Microdialysis: is it ready for prime time? Curr Opin Crit Care. 2009;15:110–7.

132. Cecil S, Chen PM, Callaway SE, Rowland SM, Adler DE, Chen JW. Traumatic brain injury: advanced multimodal neuromonitoring from theory to clinical practice. Crit Care Nurse. 2011;31(2): 25–36, quiz 37.

133. Oddo M, Levine J, Frangos S, Maloney-Wilensky E, Carrera E, Daniel R, Magistretti PJ, Le Roux P. Brain lactate metabolism in humans with subarachnoid haemorrhage. Stroke. 2012;43(5): 1418–21.

134. Marcoux J, McArthur DA, Miller C, Glenn TC, Villablanca P, Martin NA, Hovda DA, Alger JR, Vespa PM. Persistent metabolic crisis as measured by elevated cerebral microdialysis lactate-pyruvate ratio predicts chronic frontal lobe brain atrophy after traumatic brain injury. Crit Care Med. 2008;36(10):2871–7.

135. Belli A, Sen J, Petzold A, Russo S, Kitchen N, Smith M, Tavazzi B, Vagnozzi R, Signoretti S, Amorini AM, Bellia F, Lazzarino G. Extracellular N-acetylaspartate depletion in traumatic brain injury. J Neurochem. 2006;96(3):861–9.

136. Chen HI, Stiefel MF, Oddo M, Milby AH, Maloney-Wilensky E, Frangos S, Levine JM, Kofke WA, Le Roux P. Detection of cerebral compromise with multimodality monitoring in patients with subarachnoid hemorrhage. Neurosurgery. 2011;69:53–63.

137. Stein NR, McArthur DL, Etchepare M, Vespa PM. Early cerebral metabolic crisis after TBI influences outcome despite adequate hemodynamic resuscitation. Neurocrit Care. 2012;17(1):49–57.

138. Hillered L, Vespa PM, Hovda DA. Translational neurochemical research in acute human brain injury: the current status and potential future for cerebral microdialysis. J Neurotrauma. 2005;22:3–41.

139. Hutchinson PJ, O'Connell MT, Al-Rawi PG, et al. Clinical cerebral microdialysis: a methodological study. J Neurosurg. 2000;93:37–43.

140. Larach DB, Kofke WA, Le Roux P. Potential non-hypoxic/ischemic causes of increased cerebral interstitial fluid lactate/pyruvate ratio: a review of available literature. Neurocrit Care. 2011;15(3):609–22.

141. Reinstrup P, Stahl N, Mellergard P, et al. Intracerebral microdialysis in clinical practice: baseline values for chemical markers during wakefulness, anesthesia, and neurosurgery. Neurosurgery. 2000;47(3):701–9.

142. Schulz MK, Wang LP, Tange M, et al. Cerebral microdialysis monitoring: determination of normal and ischemic cerebral metabolisms in patients with aneurysmal subarachnoid hemorrhage. J Neurosurg. 2000;93(5):808–14.

143. Vespa PM, McArthur D, O'Phelan K, et al. Persistently low extracellular glucose correlates with poor outcome 6 months after human traumatic brain injury despite a lack of increased lactate: a microdialysis study. J Cereb Blood Flow Metab. 2003;23(7):865–77.

144. Oddo M, Schmidt JM, Carrera C, Badjatia N, Connolly ES, Presciutti M, Ostapkovich ND, Levine JM, Le Roux P, Mayer SA. Impact of tight glycemic control on cerebral glucose metabolism after severe brain injury: a microdialysis study. Crit Care Med. 2008;36:3233–8.

145. Goodman JC, Valadka AB, Gopinath SP, et al. Extracellular lactate and glucose alterations in the brain after head injury measured by microdialysis. Crit Care Med. 1999;27(9):1965–73.

146. Unterberg AW, Sakowitz OW, Sarrafzadeh AS, et al. Role of bedside microdialysis in the diagnosis of cerebral vasospasm following aneurysmal subarachnoid hemorrhage. J Neurosurg. 2001;94(5):740–9.

147. Vespa P, Bergsneider M, Hattori N, et al. Metabolic crisis without brain ischemia is common after traumatic brain injury: a combined microdialysis and positron emission tomography study. J Cereb Blood Flow Metab. 2005;25(6):763–74.

148. Berthet C, Lei H, Thevenet J, Gruetter R, Magistretti PJ, Hirt L. Neuroprotective role of lactate after cerebral ischemia. J Cereb Blood Flow Metab. 2009;29(11):1780–9.

149. Wyss MT, Jolivet R, Buck A, Magistretti PJ, Weber B. In vivo evidence for lactate as a neuronal energy source. J Neurosci. 2011;31(20):7477–85.

150. Suzuki A, Stern SA, Bozdagi O, Huntley GW, Walker RH, Magistretti PJ, Alberini CM. Astrocyte-neuron lactate transport is required for long-term memory formation. Cell. 2011;144(5):810–23.

151. Skjoth-Rasmussen J, Schulz M, Kristensen SR, et al. Delayed neurological deficits detected by an ischemic pattern in the extracellular cerebral metabolites in patients with aneurysmal subarachnoid hemorrhage. J Neurosurg. 2004;100(1):8–15.

152. Kett-White R, Hutchinson PJ, Al-Rawi PG, et al. Adverse cerebral events detected after subarachnoid hemorrhage using brain oxygen and microdialysis probes. Neurosurgery. 2002;50(6):1213–21.

153. Nordstrom CH, Reinstrup P, Xu W, et al. Assessment of the lower limit for cerebral perfusion pressure in severe head injuries by bedside monitoring of regional energy metabolism. Anesthesiology. 2003;98(4):809–14.

154. Hillered L, Valtysson J, Enblad P, et al. Interstitial glycerol as a marker for membrane phospholipid degradation in the acutely injured human brain. J Neurol Neurosurg Psychiatry. 1998;64(4):486–91.

155. Peerdeman SM, Girbes AR, Polderman KH, et al. Changes in cerebral interstitial glycerol concentration in head-injured patients; correlation with secondary events. Intensive Care Med. 2003;29(10):1825–8.

156. Vespa P, Prins M, Ronne-Engstrom E, et al. Increase in extracellular glutamate caused by reduced cerebral perfusion pressure and seizures after human traumatic brain injury: a microdialysis study. J Neurosurg. 1998;89(6):971–82.

157. Staub F, Graf R, Gabel P, et al. Multiple interstitial substances measured by microdialysis in patients with subarachnoid hemorrhage. Neurosurgery. 2000;47(5):1106–15.

158. Gopinath SP, Valadka AB, Goodman JC, Robertson CS. Extracellular glutamate and aspartate in head injured patients. Acta Neurochir Suppl. 2000;76:437–8.

159. Obrenovitch TP, Urenjak J. Is high extracellular glutamate the key to excitotoxicity in traumatic brain injury? J Neurotrauma. 1997;14(10):677–98.

160. Folkersma H, Brevé JJ, Tilders FJ, Cherian L, Robertson CS, Vandertop WP. Cerebral microdialysis of interleukin (IL)-1beta and IL-6: extraction efficiency and production in the acute phase after severe traumatic brain injury in rats. Acta Neurochir (Wien). 2008;150(12):1277–84; discussion 1284.

161. Tisdall MM, Rejdak K, Kitchen ND, Smith M, Petzold A. The prognostic value of brain extracellular fluid nitric oxide metabolites after traumatic brain injury. Neurocrit Care. 2011 [Epub ahead of print].

162. Petzold A, Tisdall MM, Girbes AR, Martinian L, Thom M, Kitchen N, Smith M. In vivo monitoring of neuronal loss in traumatic brain injury: a microdialysis study. Brain. 2011;134(Pt 2):464–83.

163. Czosnyka M, Matta BF, Smielewski P, et al. Cerebral perfusion pressure in head-injured patients: a noninvasive assessment using transcranial Doppler ultrasonography. J Neurosurg. 1998;88(5):802–8.

164. Czosnyka M, Smielewski P, Kirkpatrick P, et al. Continuous monitoring of cerebrovascular pressure-reactivity in head injury. Acta Neurochir Suppl. 1998;71:74–7.

165. Robertson CS. Management of cerebral perfusion pressure after traumatic brain injury. Anesthesiology. 2001;95(6):1513–7.

166. Vespa P. What is the optimal threshold for cerebral perfusion pressure following traumatic brain injury? Neurosurg Focus. 2003;15(6):E4.

167. Frerichs KU, Feuerstein GZ. Laser-Doppler flowmetry. A review of its application for measuring cerebral and spinal cord blood flow. Mol Chem Neuropathol. 1990;12:55–70.

168. Bonner RF, Nossal R. Principles of laser-Doppler flowmetry. In: Shepherd AP, Oberg PA, editors. Laser Doppler flowmetry. Boston: Kluwer Academic; 1990. p. 17–45.

169. Bolognese P, Miller JI, Heger IM, et al. Laser Doppler flowmetry in neurosurgery. J Neurosurg Anesthesiol. 1993;5:151–8.

170. Klaessens JHGM, Kolkman RGM, Hopman JCW, et al. Monitoring cerebral perfusion using near-infrared spectroscopy and laser Doppler flowmetry. Physiol Meas. 2003;24:N35–40.

171. Eyre JA, Essex TJH, Flecknell PA, et al. A comparison of measurements of cerebral blood flow in the rabbit using laser Doppler spectroscopy and radionuclide labelled microspheres. Clin Phys Physiol Meas. 1988;9:65–74.

172. Fakuda O, Endo S, Kuwayama N, et al. The characteristics of laser-Doppler flowmetry for the measurement of regional cerebral blood flow. Neurosurgery. 1995;36:358–64.

173. Kirkpatrick PJ, Smielweski P, Czosnyka M, et al. Continuous monitoring of cortical perfusion by laser Doppler flowmetry in ventilated patients with head injury. J Neurol Neurosurg Psychiatry. 1994;57:1382–8.

174. Kirkpatrick PJ, Smielweski P, Piechnik S, et al. Early effects of mannitol in patients with head injuries assessed using bedside multimodality monitoring. Neurosurgery. 1996;39:714–20.

175. Lam JMK, Hsiang JNK, Poon WS. Monitoring of autoregulation using laser Doppler flowmetry in patients with head injury. J Neurosurg. 1997;86:438–45.

176. Smielewski P, Czosnyka M, Kirkpatrick P, et al. Evaluation of the transient hyperemic response test in head injured patients. J Neurosurg. 1997;86:773–8.

177. Lee SC, Chen JF, Lee ST. Continuous regional cerebral blood flow monitoring in the neurosurgical intensive care unit. J Clin Neurosci. 2005;12:520–3.

178. Gaines C, Carter LP, Crowell RM. Comparison of local cerebral blood flow determined by thermal and hydrogen clearance. Stroke. 1983;14:66–9.

179. Vajkoczy P, Roth H, Horn P, et al. Continuous monitoring of regional cerebral blood flow: experimental and clinical validation of a novel thermal diffusion microprobe. J Neurosurg. 2000;93:265–74.

180. Sioutos PJ, Orozco JA, Carter LP, Weinand ME, Hamilton AJ, Williams FC. Continuous regional cerebral cortical blood flow monitoring in head-injured patients. Neurosurgery. 1995;36(5): 943–9.

181. Vajkoczy P, Horn P, Thome C, et al. Regional cerebral blood flow monitoring in the diagnosis of delayed ischemia following aneurysmal subarachnoid hemorrhage. J Neurosurg. 2003;98: 1227–34.

182. Miller JI, Chou MW, Capocelli A, et al. Continuous intracranial multimodality monitoring comparing local cerebral blood flow, cerebral perfusion pressure, and microvascular resistance. Acta Neurochir Suppl. 1998;71:82–4.

183. Lang EW, Czosnyka M, Mehdorn HM. Tissue oxygen reactivity and cerebral autoregulation after severe traumatic brain injury. Crit Care Med. 2003;31:267–71.

184. Chambers IR, et al. BrainIT: a trans-national head injury monitoring research network. Acta Neurochir Suppl. 2006;96:7–10.

185. Sorani MD, Hemphill 3rd JC, Morabito D, Rosenthal G, Manley GT. New approaches to physiological informatics in neurocritical care. Neurocrit Care. 2007;7:45–52.

186. Peelen L, et al. Using hierarchical dynamic Bayesian networks to investigate dynamics of organ failure in patients in the Intensive Care Unit. J Biomed Inform. 2010;43:273–86.

187. Hemphill JC, Andrews P, De Georgia M, Medscape. Multimodal monitoring and neurocritical care bioinformatics. Nat Rev Neurol. 2011;7(8):451–60.

188. Buchman TG. Novel representation of physiologic states during critical illness and recovery. Crit Care. 2010;14:127.

189. Jacono FF, DeGeorgia MA, Wilson CG, Dick TE, Loparo KA. Data acquisition and complex systems analysis in critical care: developing the intensive care unit of the future. J Healthc Eng. 2010;1:337–56.

190. AVERT-IT project. Avert-IT [online]. 2011. http://www.avert-it.org/

Prehospital Care of the Neurologically Injured Patient

Christine Van Dillen, David Meurer,
and Joseph A. Tyndall

Contents

C. Van Dillen, MD • D. Meurer, MD
J.A. Tyndall, MD, MPH (✉)
Department of Emergency Medicine,
University of Florida College of Medicine, 1329 SW 16th Street,
100186, Gainesville, FL 32608, USA
e-mail: c.vandillen@ufl.edu; meurer@ufl.edu; tyndall@ufl.edu

Abstract

The neurologically injured patient presents several unique challenges to the clinician. Of importance is a full understanding of the role of early intervention and the impact of every stage of clinical care – from the prehospital environment to the intensive care unit. As Emergency Medical Systems grow in sophistication, so does the ability to intervene with time sensitive measures that will improve outcomes. This chapter provides an overview of prehospital care systems development and early interventions (both in the prehospital and emergency department environments) that impact the outcomes of neurologically injured patient.

Keywords

Prehospital • EMS • Resuscitation • Therapeutic Hypothermia • ACLS • Stroke • Traumatic pediatric Injury • Spinal cord • Cerebral • Brain

Introduction

Essential to the care of the neurologically injured patient is an early recognition and a complete understanding of the time sensitive nature for intervention. One of the primary determinants of optimal outcomes depends on the initiation of timely and effective care. In many cases, care may start with a bystander or first responder who could intervene, especially if cardiovascular collapse is a presenting feature. In the case of cardiac arrest, early, rapid, and effective intervention is necessary to maximize preservation of neurological functioning assuming survival. Therefore, many principles applicable to prehospital care in general can be used in the approach to the neurologically injured patient, regardless of whether the neurological injury is a primary insult or a complication of an initial traumatic injury or an acute medical condition.

Since 2010, the American Heart Association (AHA) has republished policy statements and guidelines that emphasize regionalized systems of care that are viewed as critical to maximizing out-of-hospital cardiac arrests.

The Role of Prehospital Care in the Emergency Medical Services System

In the USA, the National Highway Traffic Safety Act of 1966 and the Emergency Medical Services Systems act of 1973 were two landmark legislative efforts that gave rise to the modern era of prehospital care and the Emergency Medical Services System. During the period of 1967 through 1968, special commissions set up through the Lyndon B. Johnson administration and several other congressional initiatives propelled the development of the 911 dispatch system, which is the means by which a significant number of patients first initiate contact with Emergency Medical Services. In the USA, activation of the Emergency Medical Services System initiates a cascade of events that results in the response of specifically trained prehospital care personnel. Prehospital care personnel present a variety of skills in clinical recognition and intervention. Early EMS activation may result in the initial arrival of a first responder who would be trained in basic life support, the fundamentals of airway and ventilation, and controlling external bleeding. Over the last decade, the skill level of prehospital care providers has continued to evolve so that, today, advanced practice paramedics come prepared with a sophisticated array of tools that have been proven to be useful and lifesaving in the out-of-hospital environment [1].

The prehospital care environment has also substantially evolved to where networks of aeromedical transportation as well as ground transportation are deployed to ensure that patients needing emergent care can be transported to the closest, most appropriate facility.

Much of the decision making that determines the final destination for patients through the EMS system are governed by protocols that help to guide on-scene prehospital care providers with appropriate triage decisions based upon their assessments. This initial first link in the care of the acutely ill or injured patient is crucial to patient survival.

As neurological emergencies require extremely specialized care, the primary determinant for an optimal outcome depends on the quality of initial management. This initial management is influenced by the first clinician in these patient encounters, which in most cases are paramedics from the local Emergency Medical Services (EMS) department. These paramedics have 1–2 years of training and make split-second decisions based on a limited history and physical exam. These decisions are based on a standard set of protocols set forth by their local medical director. Many patients who have suffered severe neurological injury also experience cardiac arrest. These patients must be resuscitated quickly and flawlessly to ensure the best possible neurological survival.

The American Heart Association (AHA) assembled a panel of 356 experts to review thousands of resuscitation articles to produce a new set of guidelines in 2010 [2]. These guidelines determine the necessary points of focus when resuscitating victims of cardiac arrest. Particularly important is that the EMS system must include:

- A dispatch call center with the ability to instruct a caller in the performance of CPR.
- A prompt first responder arrival.
- Paramedics who are able to recognize early signs of respiratory, neurological, or cardiovascular distress, that are also well trained in high quality ACLS focusing on non-stop compressions, early defibrillation, and provide safe transport [3–7].
- A community that is well educated on the prevention of coronary artery disease, identification of early symptoms of myocardial infarction, the performance of CPR, and the use of an AED when available.

Since 2010, the American Heart Association (AHA) has republished policy statements and guidelines that emphasize regionalized systems of care that are viewed as critical to maximizing out-of-hospital cardiac arrests.

Transportation of neurotrauma patients to the emergency department (ED) is usually provided with destination priority given to a certified trauma center. However, distance, geographical, logistic, and patient condition factors may determine the choice of transport and site of transport destination. For example, it may be in the patient's interest to have hemodynamic stabilization initiated in a smaller hospital if transportation to a major center is not readily available [3]. Even if the destination hospital is not a designated trauma center, outcome is enhanced with the use of the acute CNS injury clinical pathway, in which an emergency physician, neuroradiologist, neurosurgeon, and intensivist are promptly available as the victim reaches the ED [4, 5].

There is, however, evidence demonstrating that it may be vital for trauma patients who have potential neurological injury be transported to a trauma center with neurotrauma capabilities. In a study by Hart and colleagues, patients who had suffered severe traumatic brain injury (TBI) who were transported directly to a trauma center rather than initially to a non-trauma center for stabilization before a delayed transfer had decreased mortality rates [8, 9]. This decrease in mortality is thought to be associated with advanced neurosurgical capabilities, including computed tomography scanners, prompt surgical care, and the ability to monitor intracranial pressure. The only indication to stop at a hospital or emergency department (ED) without trauma or neurotrauma capability would be for hemodynamic stabilization of a patient who has progressed into cardiac arrest.

Generally, ambulances are used for transport within a 50-mile radius. Depending upon available resources, rotary-wing aircraft will often be used for distances between 51 to about 150 miles. More remote locations and longer transportation times present specific challenges, and, in many circumstances, fixed wing aircraft would be used when available to cover even longer distances in order to reduce transportation times [10]. The organization of EMS systems varies considerably throughout the world. Many European-based EMS systems utilize physicians in the prehospital care environment who can be dispatched to the scene at the time of the initial event. Improved resuscitation and survival to discharge when cardiac arrest is present have been reported when physicians accompany ambulances. In a Danish study of cardiac arrest patients, the presence of a physician in the ambulance increased the hospital discharge rate after cardiac arrest from 1 to 13 % [11]. The presence of a physician in the field seems of less importance for major trauma, regardless of the presence of CNS injury [12]. A 2001 European study of patients with major trauma (injury severity score [ISS] > 16) and severe head injury attempted to resolve the controversy between the advantage of prolonged ACLS in the field managed by physicians versus a short BLS resuscitation with immediate transport to a hospital via helicopter with EMS personnel on board. No differences in outcome could be demonstrated in this study [13]. This is likely attributed to earlier operative management. Controversial evidence was found in a systematic review of all controlled studies published in 2009. This study noticed increased survival for trauma and cardiac arrest patients where physician treatment in the field was available [14]. However, in this systematic review, the quality and strength of the literature varied and revealed many areas that would require further study. In summary, the majority of studies suggest that the advantage of a physician in the field is limited to patients who had suffered from a cardiac arrest and that health resources for trauma patients should be focused on providing rapid transport to the ED. Due to high cost, lack of availability, and insufficient data, the USA continues to rely on EMT and paramedic first responders.

Cerebral Resuscitation and the 2010 AHA CPR Guidelines

The 2010 AHA Guidelines were developed after careful review of thousands of resuscitation articles by many international experts. These guidelines are a combination of reaffirmed old guidelines as well as new recommendations [2]. The guidelines emphasize the importance of all aspects of cardiac care beginning with prevention of disease, educating the community, ensuring quality prehospital and hospital care, as well as post-arrest rehabilitation. The overall goal is to improve neurological outcome. More emphasis has been placed on first aid, CPR, and defibrillation in the workplace, so that bystanders will more likely intervene and start resuscitation. ACLS assessment and management for both lay rescuer and prehospital personnel have been simplified to ensure adherence. A better outcome was noted in cardiac arrest patients when compressions were started early, continued without interruption, were of adequate rate and depth, allowed for complete chest recoil, and where excessive ventilation was prevented [7]. This evidence led to a change in BLS sequence of steps from "ABC" (airway-breathing-chest compressions) to "CAB" (chest compressions, airway, breathing) in all patients suffering from cardiac arrest with the exclusion of newborn infants. This change in sequence is thought to be ideal for patients in cardiac arrest due to cardiac arrhythmias and ischemia (the majority of cardiac arrest cases). In patients who have sustained severe trauma, ATLS evaluation sequence should be used. This consists of primary survey (airway (open), breathing (two breaths), circulation (chest compressions), and defibrillation (use automatic external defibrillation (AED))) and secondary survey (airway (advanced airway techniques), breathing (placement confirmation, check effectiveness), circulation (access the circulation; administer drugs as indicated), and differential diagnosis). It is important to remember that if a patient suffers from a cardiac arrest, focus should be to restart perfusion to the brain no matter what the cause of this arrest.

Ethical Concerns in Resuscitation

The family's presence during resuscitation is encouraged and valuable. In the prehospital setting when a "Do Not Attempt Resuscitation" (DNAR) is noted and family is in agreement with this decision, a prehospital provider will not attempt resuscitation.

Basic Life Support: Adult and Pediatric

When a layperson recognizes a victim of sudden adult cardiac arrest, the emergency response system should be activated, an AED/defibrillator obtained, if available, and chest compressions started; early defibrillation is still emphasized. The evidence supporting whether compressions should precede defibrillation or vice versa remains controversial. Some studies have shown improved survival when 1.5–3 min of compressions was performed prior to defibrillation if the cardiac arrest occurred more than 4–5 min prior to EMS arrival. Others did not show any improvement in overall outcome whether compressions or defibrillation occurred first [15–18]; clearly, if an AED is not close, the rescuer should start compressions immediately.

Several studies have recognized the difficulty for both laypersons and trained providers to identify a pulse [19–28]. For the lay bystander, a pulse check is no longer recommended, and it should be assumed that a victim who loses conscious-ness without any evidence of effective respirations is in arrest, and chest compressions should be initiated immedi-ately without the need to deliver rescue breaths. The trained rescuer or healthcare provider should take no more than 10 s to check for a pulse before initiating compressions. For all layperson bystanders, "hands only" compressions (CPR per-formed without mouth-to-mouth ventilation) has been reviewed and is preferred, because of the overwhelming con-cerns of communicable disease transmission during mouth-to-mouth contact, and thus the elimination of this requirement in bystander CPR may increase the likelihood of bystander intervention. The opening of an airway to oxygenate and ventilate can be challenging and may also lead to a delays in the initiation of compressions. When two or more BLS trained providers are present, ventilation with bag valve mask (BVM) is appropriate. These providers are expected to have mastered proper BVM ventilation to increase resuscitation efficacy and reduce complications. When supplementary oxygen is available, the skilled rescuer should provide approximately 500–600 mL, giving one breath every 6–8 s. In victims with an asphyxial cause for arrest (e.g., infant, child, or drowning victim), ventilations should be provided as soon as possible. When a full complement of resources is available, many of these actions are simultaneously performed.

Once compressions have been initiated, checking for a pulse leads to unnecessary interruptions and is deempha-sized in current BLS algorithms. Instead, the trained pro-vider should look for other "signs of spontaneous return of circulation" which may include a change in patient color, breathing, coughing, or movement. Effective chest compres-sions are also central to the resuscitative effort. It is, again, essential that continual compressions be performed at a rapid rate of (100/min) with a technique that allows for adequate recoil of the chest to allow for filling of the heart chambers. In adults, a compression-ventilation ratio of 30:2 is recom-mended with a trained provider initiating rescue breaths with sufficient tidal volume over 1 s (after the initiation of chest compressions). Despite conceptual similarities, there are notable technical differences between adult and pediatric BLS. For example, in infants, the two-thumb-encircling-hands chest compression technique is recommended. Automatic external defibrillators (AEDs) can be used for patients older than 8 years of age, or heavier than 25 kg (55 lb). Evidence to support the use of AEDs in pediatric cardiac arrest victims is limited. The AHA currently recom-mends the use of a manual defibrillator in infants when a treatable dysrhythmia is noted by a healthcare provider. If a manual defibrillator is not available, an AED equipped with a pediatric attenuator is preferred for infants and for children less than 8 years of age. If neither is available, an AED without a dose attenuator may be used.

Managing the Airway

As previously noted, continuous effective chest compres-sions must be the primary focus in the initiation of cardiopul-monary resuscitation. After 5 min of compressions, if multiple rescuers are present, one team member can continue compressions while another manages the airway. It is an acceptable alternative to continue the use of bag-valve-mask ventilation until arrival at an emergency department. Due to increasing numbers of paramedics with advanced practice skills in the prehospital environment, individual experience in the performance of procedures such as endotracheal intu-bations has declined [29]. As a result, alternative airway devices that require less technical skill to achieve success at managing the airway have been developed and deployed as a routine alternative to endotracheal intubation under direct laryngoscopy. These alternatives include laryngeal mask air-way LMA™ (LMA, North America, San Diego, CA), Combitube™ (The Kendall Company, Mansfield, USA), King LT® (King Systems, Noblesville, IN), and the SALT™ device (MDI Microtek Medical, St. Paul, MN).

Any EMS system that extends privileges to advanced pre-hospital care practitioners to perform endotracheal intubations must ensure proper initial training, monitoring of skill reten-tion through ongoing professional practice evaluations, and must perform quality assurance to confirm appropriate use of this intervention. Providers should confirm placement of an endotracheal tube by physical examination techniques, quanti-tative and continuous CO_2 measurement (capnometry and cap-nography), or by use of devices that specifically detect tubes located in the esophagus. Capnography should also help to ensure recognition of tube displacement. Due to the frequent movement of patients in this setting, use of commercially manufactured tube holders and continuous is recommended.

Advanced Cardiac Life Support

As mentioned previously, one of the most important recent changes to the out-of-hospital resuscitation algorithm is the initiation of compressions before assessing airway and breath-ing (C-A-B) as opposed to the traditional focus on airway, breathing, then circulation (A-B-C). Again, the focus of care is on quality uninterrupted compressions followed by an eval-uation with an AED, if available without delay, and then air-way and breathing done simultaneously with compressions. In ventricular fibrillation and pulseless ventricular tachycar-dia, electrical defibrillation with a single dose of 120-200 J (depending on manufacturer's recommendations) should be administered. CPR should be resumed immediately after each shock delivery for 2 min before the next rhythm check. The optimal timing for the administration of vasopressor is also not yet established. Once compressions have begun, electrical therapy has been administered, IV/IO (intraosseous) access has been established, and there are multiple available providers present, then intravascular epinephrine 1 mg or vasopressin 40 U should be administered for refractory ventricular fibrillation (VF) or pulseless ventricular tachycardia (VT). The adult dose of epinephrine is 1 mg every 3–5 min, higher doses of epinephrine are no longer recommended [30, 31]. Vasopressin has a longer half-life, therefore only one dose is recommended. At this time, no placebo-controlled trials have shown that any vasopressor agent at any stage in cardiac arrest management increases neurologically intact survival to discharge. The evidence does show an increase in short-term return of spontaneous circulation (ROSC) [32–36]. The use of amiodarone as an antidysrhythmic is recommended for use in shock-refractory VF/pulseless VT. Recent studies noted better results with amiodarone as compared to lidocaine [37–41]. Lidocaine remains acceptable for the treatment of shock-refractory VF when amiodarone is not available.

The algorithm for pulseless electrical activity and asystole includes the administration of a vasopressor as soon as possible. Available evidence suggests that the routine use of atropine during PEA or asystole is unlikely to have a therapeutic benefit, and therefore atropine has been removed from this algorithm [42–45]. Also of note, giving all cardiac arrest victims magnesium sulfate, sodium bicarbonate, and calcium chloride is no longer recommended unless there are known underlying conditions that would improve with their administration. PEA can also be caused by reversible conditions. During each 2-min period of CPR, the provider needs to consider specific underlying factors that may have caused the arrest. These include the familiar mnemonics of the Hs (hypovolemia, hypoxia, hydrogen ion-acidosis, hyper/hypokalemia, and hypothermia) and the Ts (toxins, tamponade, tension pneumothorax, thrombosis). Due to the association of PEA with hypoxemia, an advanced airway is theoretically more important than during VF/pulseless VT.

Pediatric Advanced Life Support

The algorithm change to C-A-B from A-B-C must also be addressed in children and infants. Compressions are the focus in adult VF/VT arrest due to improved outcome with earlier emphasis of early initiation of high-quality continuous chest compressions. Asphyxial arrest is more common in infants and children; therefore, adequate ventilation is extremely important in these types of resuscitations. Beginning CPR with 30 compressions rather than two ventilations leads to a shorter delay to first compression. Evidence is insufficient to show whether a sequence beginning with ventilations (ABC) or with chest compressions (CAB) leads to a better outcome in children. Starting CPR with 30 compressions followed by two ventilations should theoretically delay ventilations by

about 18 s for the lone rescuer and even less when two rescuers are present [46, 47]. At this time, the C-A-B sequence for infants and children is recommended in order to simplify training. In trained prehospital providers, compressions and ventilations occur simultaneously.

The intraosseous (IO) route has been recommended when no intravenous (IV) access is promptly available in cardiac arrest. Two prospective trials in children and adults suggest that IO access can be established efficiently, safely, and effectively for resuscitation in all age groups [48–50]. PALS suggests vascular access to be obtained within 90 s. The recommended initial resuscitation dose of epinephrine for pediatric cardiac arrest is 0.01 mg/kg, given by the intravenous or intraosseous route or 0.1 mg/kg by the endotracheal route. Repeated doses are recommended every 3–5 min for ongoing arrest. The same dose of epinephrine is recommended for second and subsequent doses for unresponsive patients in asystole or PEA arrest. Pediatric institutions should have AED programs with a high specificity to recognize pediatric rhythms that require defibrillation or cardioversion, and a pediatric attenuating system that can be used for infants and children up to approximately 25 kg [51–55].

Treatment of supraventricular tachycardia (SVT) can start with vagal maneuvers in an attempt to convert this rhythm as long as this does not delay cardioversion in an unstable child. The administration of 0.1 mg/kg adenosine IV/ IO is recommended for the pharmacological conversion of SVT with a narrow complex in children which are hemodynamically stable. In dealing with Wolff-Parkinson-White (WPW) syndrome, the use of adenosine in children is contraindicated, and procainamide 15 mg/kg is recommended. If a patient is unstable, synchronized cardioversion at 0.5–1 J/kg should be administered then, if unsuccessful, repeated at 1–2 J/kg; this should be attempted for both SVT and wide complex tachycardia. If these interventions have proven unsuccessful, the administration of amiodarone 5 mg/kg IV/IO or procainamide 15 mg/kg along with expert consultation is recommended.

Neonatal Resuscitation

Neonates usually require resuscitation due to respiratory distress rather than cardiac issues. Therefore, ventilation is extremely important in the newly born infant with heart rate less than 100 beats/min. Chest compressions should be initiated anytime the heart rate is absent or less than 60 beats/min after 30 s of adequate assisted ventilation. Chest compressions should be coordinated with ventilation at a ratio of 3:1, at a rate of 120 events/min (90 compressions and 30 ventilations). Compression should be performed with two thumbs and encircling fingers with hands placed at the lower third of the sternum. The LMA™ is now available and acceptable for newborns who weigh more than 2,000 g or are more than

34 weeks gestation. Secondary confirmation of appropriate placement of the endotracheal tube must be done, and there are specific approaches to prevent tube dislodgment, such as the use of commercially manufactured tube holders. This is particularly true in the prehospital setting where there is greater risk of dislodgment. Continuous capnography is recommended for ETT placement confirmation with a negative result suggesting esophageal intubation. At any point that there is concern that the endotracheal tube was placed in the esophagus, the tube should be removed immediately. In this population, due to absent pulmonary flow or low cardiac output, you can see false-negative results. The fluid of choice for volume expansion in the prehospital phase for patients of all ages is an isotonic crystalloid solution such as 0.9 % saline or Ringer's lactate solutions.

Special Issues in Neonatal CPR

There are circumstances in which noninitiation or discontinuation of resuscitation in the delivery room may be appropriate. Specific situations are suggested in the AHA guidelines and include infants with confirmed gestation less than 23 weeks or birth weight less than 400 g, anencephaly, or confirmed trisomy 13 or 18. Therapeutic hypothermia during neonatal resuscitation cannot be recommended until more evidence is available.

Other Circulatory Adjuncts Approved for Clinical Use During CPR

There is continuous innovation in the design and manufacturing of new devices to attempt to improve outcome of resuscitation. These devices include the CPR plunger (active compression-decompression CPR), interposed abdominal compression device, vest CPR, mechanical piston, and impedance threshold valve. There is no evidence to date that any of these or other adjunctive devices contribute to improved neurological outcome over standard chest compressions.

Therapeutic Hypothermia in Cardiac Arrest and Neurological Survival

Hypothermia is widely accepted as the gold standard method for brain protection [56–63]. Therapeutic cooling is also called targeted temperature management or TTM. Even though there is mounting evidence to widen the application of this modality of treatment, implementation for effective patient care is not uncomplicated and carries risk. This technique is currently the most powerful method to date to prevent secondary brain injury. The neuroprotective mechanisms of targeted temperature control have been studied for several decades.

The mechanisms of action of targeted temperature control are multiple and synergistic. It is known that brain metabolism is slowed during hypothermia, and for every 1° reduction in brain temperature, there is a concomitant 6 % reduction in cerebral metabolic rate [64]. This limitation of metabolism is significant in that it limits the consumption of glucose in the brain which in turn reduces the risk of energy failure, preventing the failure of sodium-potassium pumps and calcium influx that could lead to cell death. There is a broad range of additional synergistic effects of hypothermia that have been identified that include modulation of gene expression and microRNA processes. There is also a reduction in the release of excitotoxic neurotransmitters and a reduction in free radical formation which helps to protect the brain. This along with a reduction in sustained electrical depolarizations is thought to help preserve the blood brain barrier and decrease edema thereby reducing injury from increased intracranial pressure. Translating these mechanisms to knowledge and understanding of how hypothermia exerts neuroprotection in the clinical setting require careful monitoring and advance imaging. There is, however, robust clinical evidence to show that a temperature below 35.5 °C provides the greatest clinical benefit in terms of neuroprotection. Two randomized clinical trials in 2002 showed that targeted temperature management improved neurological outcomes in patients who had suffered cardiac arrest [62, 63]. There is also consistent preclinical data that shows that the therapeutic effect of TTM may be conferred to patients with acute ischemic stroke and traumatic brain injury. There is good evidence to show that mild to moderate hypothermia reduces ICP in patients where other standard methods may be refractory, but most clinical trials to date have provided mixed results. In one study, hypothermia when compared to normal methods (hyperventilation, barbiturates, and mannitol) was more effective than all three combined in reducing intracranial pressure.

Implementing hypothermia consists of three distinct phases – induction, maintenance, and rewarming – each of which can have separate and sometimes significant complications.

Induction

Induction refers to the technique of rapid cooling. There are two categories for cooling. Surface methods use conductive loss of heat and can range from a low-technology application of ice packs in strategic areas to lower body core temperature. More sophisticated equipment would use surface cooling pads containing circulatory forced cold air or fluid applied to the patient's skin. Intravascular methods involve the use of heat exchange central line catheters. One of the complications of the induction process is shivering which will be discussed later. Some investigators are of the opinion that induction using endovascular methods may blunt the body's thermoregulatory response, but there has been so far no head-to-head comparison between surface methods and endovascular techniques with regard to this commonly encountered complication. Regardless of the method of induction, it should be applied as rapidly as possible to minimize or halt ongoing ischemic neurological injury. Application of ice packs and infusion of cold intravenous fluids (Ringer's lactate or normal saline at 4 °C) at rate of 30–40 mL/kg over 1 h is the simplest and least expensive method [65–67]. On a cautionary note, large volumes of cold fluid should not be administered to patients with congestive heart failure because of the significant risk of worsening pulmonary edema.

Maintenance

Maintenance of hypothermia is one of the more critical areas of the application of this therapeutic method. Advance cooling technology can be used to maintain core body temperature with insignificant fluctuations. Hypothermia does blunt the detection of fever in patients with potential underlying infections, so changes in temperature of circulating fluid in the more advanced monitoring technologies can be used as a proxy for temperature and can provide clues to development or progression of underlying infections.

Rewarming

Rewarming is probably the most dangerous phase of the hypothermia intervention. Too rapid an increase in core body temperature can cause systemic vasodilation and hypotension. These changes can trigger cerebral vasodilation and increased intracranial pressure. Although beyond the immediate scope of this chapter, it should be noted that rewarming would typically occur after 24 h of the initiation of induction and should occur at a rate of 0.25°/h with slower rates of rewarming should there be concerns for ICP [68]. Temperature overshoot during rewarming is also a complication that must be avoided.

The Complications of Hypothermia

Mild hypothermia can cause a profound reaction by the body in an attempt to maintain the set point body temperature established by the hypothalamus. Peripheral vasoconstriction is triggered at 36.5 °C in the physiologically normal human being. Absence of the shivering response can be a clue to the possibility of neurological injury because of the loss of the thermoregulatory response. Control of shivering is paramount in the induction process, and without adequate control the targeted temperature attainment may prove difficult. In addition, the thermoregulatory response increases systemic metabolic demand and energy consumption which can lead to further brain injury. The best known and most reliable validated method of assessing shivering is the bedside shivering assessment scale. This is a validated four-point scale that can be easily used to assess the degree of shivering and can be used as a guide in the initiation of therapy [69] (Table 9.1).

Therapy for shivering should focus on suppression rather than decoupling of the response as in paralysis. Uncoupling of the shivering response through paralysis does not change the increased neurological metabolic demands and thus can prove to be detrimental to the care of the patient. A strategy for countering these deleterious effects during induction is published in the literature as the Columbia Anti-Shivering Protocol [70] (Table 9.2).

There are number of methods that can be used to blunt the shivering response. The simplest approach is non-pharmacological and involves forcing warm air at about 40 °C over the body's surface. This increases the surface temperature without increasing the core temperature reducing or blunting the shivering response because of the sensation of warmth. First-line pharmacological therapy includes the use of acetaminophen, buspirone, and magnesium. Approximately 50 % of patients would require additional pharmacological therapy to control the shivering response. In such cases, the use of Dexmedetomidate, alpha 2 receptor agonist centrally acting, decreases the shivering threshold [71]. Propofol, fentanyl, and meperidine can also decrease the shivering thresholds. Obvious complications of using these medications at higher doses are the risk of respiratory depression. Midazolam, although less effective when compared to other

Table 9.1 The Bedside Shivering Assessment Scale (BSAS)

Score	Shivering status	Description	Action
0	None	No shivering noted (Palpation of chest wall or masseter muscle)	None
1	Mild	Shivering localized to neck and/or thorax	Monitor closely
2	Moderate	Shivering involving gross movement of upper and lower extremities as well as neck and thorax	Intervention to maintain BSAS score of ≤1
3	Severe	Shivering involves gross movements of the trunk as well as upper and lower extremities	Consider sedation and intervention to maintain BSAS score of ≤1

Reproduced with permission from Badjatia et al. [69]

Table 9.2 The Columbia Anti-Shivering Protocol

Step	Level of sedation	Pharmacological intervention for shivering	Dosages
0	None	Acetaminophen	650–1,000 mg every 4–6 h
		Buspirone	30 mg every 8 h
		Magnesium sulfate	0.5–1 mg/h IV (goal 3–4 mg/dL)
		Skin counter rewarming	Maximum temperature to 43 °C
1	Mild	Dexmedetomidate	0.2–1.5 µgm/kg/h
2	Moderate	Opioids	Fentanyl 25 µgm/h
			Meperidine 50–100 mg IM or IV
3	Deep	Propofol	50–75 µgm/kg/min
4	Neuromuscular blockade	Vecuronium	0.1 mg/kg IV

Reproduced with kind permission of Springer Science+Business Media from Choi et al. [70]

agents, can be used as pharmacological therapy to reduce the incidence of shivering [72].

Paralysis is a last resort. The use of nondepolarizing paralytic agents may become necessary in cases of severe shivering response. This form of pharmacological intervention can become necessary in cases of severe shivering responses involving the trunk as well as upper and lower extremities. Use of paralytic agents, however, uncouples the overt musculoskeletal response to shivering from the significant metabolic demands and the body's stress response. As a result, even though the physical appearance of shivering ceases, the clinician must recognize the ongoing metabolic effects and continue other simultaneous measures to reduce the metabolic effects.

Other Complications of Induction

Many other complications can arise when a state of hypothermia is first induced. The cooling effect can result in both cardiac and renal dysfunction. Bradycardia and reduced cardiac contractility as a result of lowered temperature will reduce cardiac output and blood pressure. There is also a greater risk for developing both dysrhythmias, which may manifest commonly as atrial or ventricular tachydysrhythmias or fibrillation. Renal dysfunction may also occur as cold diuresis is induced when peripheral vasoconstriction shunts blood to the kidneys; as a result, mild tubular dysfunction may also occur.

Rapid cooling causes decreases in extracellular magnesium, phosphate, and potassium. These electrolytes must be carefully monitored and supplemented. Of note, the rewarming phase can result in the release of potassium from intracellular stores, which may result in a significant hyperkalemia. Acid–base status can change significantly during induction of hypothermia. During the cooling process, carbon dioxide becomes far more soluble in the serum, reducing the partial pressure of CO_2 ($PaCO_2$), and resulting in an alkaline shift. Closely monitoring and interpreting arterial blood gases

values at hypothermic temperatures is essential. The impact of compensating for blood gas values through techniques of hypoventilation and persistent relative hypercarbia can have significant effects on cerebral blood flow and ICP.

Insulin resistance is another feature of hypothermia induction, resulting in hyperglycemia which should be actively managed. The converse is true during the rewarming stages where heightened sensitivity to insulin and a predilection for hypoglycemia occurs. Impaired immune system response, resulting from leukocyte phagocytic dysfunction can result in increased risk for pneumonia and sepsis. Mild coagulopathies and platelet dysfunction can also increase the risk of bleeding and intracranial hemorrhage.

Evidence for Application

As mentioned, there is convincing evidence data for the use and promise of hypothermia in the setting of cardiac arrest. The loss of spontaneous circulation and blood flow causes abrupt cerebral ischemia. Additionally, the return of spontaneous circulation can lead to added injury from reperfusion injury. Prior to the advent of hypothermia, the rate of survival with good neurological outcome after cardiac arrest was less than 5 %. Two-landmark studies illustrated the dramatic improvement in outcomes for patients who were treated with hypothermia at a target temperature of 33 °C [57, 58]. Other guidelines (Advanced Life Support Task Force and the International Liaison Committee on resuscitation in conjunction with the American Heart Association) recommend intervention for patients who are post-arrest due to ventricular fibrillation or tachycardia with a targeted temperature of between 32 and 34 °C.

The use of targeted temperature management in stroke has had the benefit of many decades of empiric research evidence. A large number of animal studies have shown significant neuroprotective benefits of hypothermia in models of focal cerebral ischemia. One large meta-analysis of the research work done in animal models demonstrated a mean reduction of 44 % in infarct size [73]. Most of these findings were noted in models where the ischemia was transient, with evidence of hypothermic benefit as long as 3 h after the original insult. Although there is significant basic science evidence to suggest a neuroprotective mechanism with the induction of hypothermia in ischemic brain injury, there are no large-scale clinical trials or significant enough supportive evidence to warrant hypothermia induction in stroke as standard of care. A significant recent pilot study was completed which attempted to examine this issue. The Cooling for Acute ischemic Brain Damage (COOL-AID) trial [74] was underpowered to determine efficacy of targeted temperature management in stroke but uncovered the significant challenges with the management of ischemic stroke patients. These patients are awake and not in an ICU setting under strictly controlled measures as may be the case in a post-cardiac arrest unresponsive patients. The challenges of clinical care with regard to the institution of targeted temperature management in these subsets of patients proved to be substantial and thus less amendable to adequate study.

In intracerebral hemorrhage, much of the focus in targeted temperature management is on the mass effect associated with peri-hematomal edema, as well as the control and management of increased intracranial pressure. Although a paucity of research exists on the pursuit of this particular application of targeted temperature management, recent work has shown promise. An observational study done in 2010 by Kollmar and colleagues demonstrated some impact of hypothermia on cerebral edema seen on CT imaging after 10 days of targeted temperature management, with evidence of improved outcomes compared to historical controls [75]. The time course of resolution for this category of brain injury would suggest the need for prolonged exposure to targeted temperature management, with hypothermia significantly increasing the risk for underlying infection and increased morbidity.

Subarachnoid Hemorrhage

The literature has been mixed when considering TTM in the setting of subarachnoid hemorrhage. Given that the greatest benefit of therapeutic hypothermia is conferred when hypothermia is induced prior to ischemic injury and damage, it could clearly be postulated that, in the case of subarachnoid hemorrhage and the complicating conditions of vasospasm, therapeutic hypothermia may play a role in rescue therapy. The practical concerns are, however, that when treatment for vasospasm has been initiated, as in rescue therapy, ischemia is probably well underway, limiting the potential benefits of inducing hypothermia. There have been no good studies indicating that early initiation of hypothermia in the setting of subarachnoid hemorrhage has clear beneficial effects.

Traumatic Brain Injury

In traumatic brain injury, there is no substantive data to show clinical benefit of TTM. There are many potential reasons for the apparent lack of benefit, most likely related to the underlying conditions of axonal shearing and hemorrhage that frequently occur in significant injuries. Other major concerns regarding TTM is the rewarming period which, occurring 24 h into the traumatic brain injury, just when maximal cerebral edema and increased intracranial pressure are likely to occur, creates the potential for further complications. Protocols looking at prolonging the period of hypothermia for up to 40 h are a likely next step in the investigation of the hypothermia in traumatic brain injury.

A case study, published in 2010, brought attention to the possibility of the use of targeted temperature management in treatment of spinal cord injury [76]. The evidence, however, has been scant, and there are significant limitations in the study of this area of application, given the relative paucity of patients presenting to any single institution for the high level of care needed.

Traumatic Central Nervous System Injury and Prehospital Care

Central nervous system injuries are the leading cause of morbidity and mortality in trauma. After the CNS has suffered primary injury from direct insult, it is particularly susceptible to secondary injury due to its high metabolic demand and lack of reserve. In particular, hypoxemia and hypoperfusion are the main mechanisms of secondary injury. Interventions to prevent these two mechanisms of secondary injury in the prehospital and early resuscitation phases will prevent worsening of the primary CNS insult and resulting morbidity and mortality.

Guidelines have been established and adopted regarding the prehospital management of traumatic brain injury by the Brain Trauma Foundation [77]. Furthermore, there are guidelines for management of combat-related traumatic brain injury, pediatric traumatic brain injury, and the surgical management of traumatic brain injury [78–80]. These guidelines attempt to minimize secondary brain injury by paying careful attention to specific interventions; utilization of these guidelines has been associated with decreased mortality and improved outcomes.

Severity of Head Injuries

Head injuries can be subdivided into mild, moderate, and severe categories. Mild traumatic brain injuries (TBIs), also known as concussions, involve temporary impairment of brain function which may or may not be associated with a loss of consciousness and is associated with a Glasgow Coma Score (GCS) of between 14 and 15. Moderate TBI is seen in individuals with brain trauma and swelling but who remain arousable (GCS 9–13). Severe TBIs are associated with persistent loss of consciousness (GCS 8 or less). According to the American *College of Surgeons Advanced Trauma Life Support* (8th ed), 70 % of TBI can be categorized as minor, while moderate and severe TBI represent 15 % each. The classic resuscitation paradigm of the ABCs will be utilized in the following discussion of TBI. It is noted that, in the special circumstance of exsanguinating injury, circulation may be considered before airway, as hemorrhage control via application of a tourniquet can be lifesaving and help maintain perfusion of an injured brain.

Airway

Definitive management of the airway by endotracheal intubation has long been the standard of care in advanced life-support prehospital services. It is also long been held that endotracheal intubation is mandatory for those with severe traumatic brain injury ("GCS less than 8 means intubate"). Hypoxemia and hypercapnia associated with hypoventilation are two mechanisms of secondary injury in the patient with TBI. However, prehospital intubation in patients with traumatic brain injury is controversial, based upon outcomes data. Early studies noted worse outcomes with ground EMS using rapid sequence intubation routinely in TBI patients, while outcomes were improved in a similar population transported by air EMS but without intubation [80, 81]. Because of these findings, current guidelines recommend against the routine use of rapid sequence intubation technique for ground EMS units in urban settings when the patient is spontaneously breathing and has SpO_2 greater than 90 %. It has been postulated that operator experience and attention to avoiding hypoxemia and hypercapnia by aircrews may explain this difference. However, more recent data suggest that prehospital intubation of patients with TBI is associated with improved outcomes [82].

Regardless of the technique used to secure the airway, any head-injured patient with altered mentation must be treated as if they have a concurrent spinal cord injury.

Breathing

The scope of discussion of "breathing" includes both oxygenation and maintenance of appropriate CO_2 levels. Avoidance of a hypoxic insult after TBI makes such intuitive sense that randomized controlled trials to confirm this have not been, and will not be, forthcoming. However, in one study, measurement of SpO_2 on scene of greater than 90 % was associated with mortality of approximately 15 % and severe disability of 5 %; when measured saturation was less than 60 %, it correlated with mortality of 50 % and severe disability of 50 % [83].

There is also a theoretical concern that inappropriate hyperoxia may be associated with free radical formation and secondary cellular metabolic injury. It is for this reason that some authorities recommend avoiding excess supplemental oxygenation for non-traumatic neurological injuries when saturations are greater than 94 %. Monitoring and close attention to maintaining adequate SpO_2 is recommended for all trauma patients with suspected brain injury.

Development of portable capnography and capnometry units and their utilization in the prehospital environment allows for greater attention to detail while ventilating patients. Inappropriate hyperventilation can have multiple undesirable effects. In the hypotensive patient, hyperventilation leads to increased intrathoracic pressure with subsequent decreased venous return. This leads to hypotension which, in turn, leads to inadequate perfusion of the injured brain. As will be discussed next, systemic hypotension doubles mortality in brain injured patients. Furthermore, hyperventilation causes cerebral vasoconstriction, further decreasing perfusion of the brain. Hyperventilation, with its concurrent vasoconstriction and decreased perfusion of the injured brain, is only indicated when herniation of the brain is strongly suspected, as a temporizing measure pending definitive neurosurgical intervention.

Circulation

In general, hypotension doubles the mortality in TBI patients [84]. Even one episode of prehospital hypotension is associated with a significant increase in morbidity in TBI patients. Cerebral perfusion pressure, defined as the difference between mean arterial pressure and intracranial pressure, is affected not only by poor systemic perfusion but also by increased intracranial pressure caused by diffuse edema or local mass effects from hemorrhage. Treatment with fluid resuscitation in the prehospital environment is important, requiring rapid intravenous or interosseous access and resuscitation with isotonic fluid. Despite the potential benefit, there has not been any demonstrated benefit to fluid resuscitation with hypertonic solutions over isotonic solutions in the prehospital arena [85].

Disability and Destination

Rapid assessment and recognition of those with severe TBI is vital in that it allows the appropriate therapies to be instituted. Both the American College of Surgeons and the

Brain Trauma Foundation recognize the importance of early assessment with the Glasgow Coma Score, which helps to segregate injury severity of patients. The assessment of pupillary asymmetry and reaction, along with lateralizing motor findings and signs of decreased mentation, may be the only evidence of impending herniation in the prehospital environment. Early recognition of the severely brain-injured patient not only serves to determine therapy but should also determine transport destination. Trauma centers, in particular those with immediate neurosurgical intervention capacity, improve outcomes for patients with severe TBI. In general, patients with severe TBI should be transported directly to a trauma center, even if it is not the closest medical facility. It has been demonstrated that appropriate transportation of neurologically injured pediatric patients to hospitals with pediatric critical care capabilities, such as pediatric trauma centers, improves neurological outcome [86]. Similarly, improved survival has been demonstrated in adult patients transported to trauma centers [15]. Although not specifically demonstrated in an adult neurologically injured population, transport to a facility which follows evidence-based guidelines through a continuum of care from the resuscitation suite through the ICU to the inpatient step down unit and finally to rehabilitation should improve the overall quality of focused care in this population.

With regard to mode of transport, the patient should be transported as rapidly as possible to the appropriate level of care. When ground transport to local medical resources may not be able to provide the necessary level of care, strong consideration should be given for the use of air EMS when it provides rapid transport to a specialized level of care. Transport by air EMS is associated with improved outcomes in severely injured trauma patients transported from the scene of injury [16, 17]. However, given the negative impact of hypotension on secondary brain injury, early transport to a specialty center must be balanced with hemodynamic stabilization at a local facility in the multi-trauma patient.

Other Interventions

Hyperventilation

Therapeutic hyperventilation should be considered only in patients in whom impending brain herniation is suspected [87, 88]. Typically, these patients would have a GCS consistent with severe brain injury (GCS 8 or less) and some evidence of lateralizing injury such as an asymmetric, dilated, nonreactive pupil. Although end-tidal CO_2 (PetCO$_2$) does not completely correlate with PaCO$_2$, because of the ease with which excessive ventilation has had, therapeutic hyperventilation should be monitored by capnometry in the prehospital environment. The goal is for PetCO$_2$ of 30–35 mmHg, as lower values may lead to decreased cerebral perfusion

with no outcome benefit. Mannitol, while not routinely available in the prehospital environment, may be considered by sophisticated EMS systems.

Hypoglycemia

With the advent of portable glucose monitors, empiric treatment for postulated hypoglycemia is not necessary. Hyperglycemia does not improve outcome and may be harmful [89].

Hyperbaric Oxygen

Hyperbaric oxygen, while not a prehospital therapy, may affect destination decisions. Hyperbaric oxygen has not been proven to improve outcomes when compared to conventional therapies but remains a topic of investigational interest, particularly if available closer to time of initial insult [90]. Current evidence does not support its routine use or preferential transfer to a facility with availability of emergent hyperbaric therapy.

Pediatric Considerations

Pediatric patients with severe TBI are vulnerable to secondary metabolic insult and injury due to hypotension and hypoxia. While definitive airway management by an experienced and skilled provider is important in an injured child with TBI, due to technical issues and no proven benefit to outcome, endotracheal intubation is not preferred over bag-valve-mask ventilation [78]. In the prehospital setting, care must be taken not to hyperventilate the pediatric patient. Because of age-related variability, the interpretation of blood pressure correlating with hypotension varies with age, and the prehospital provider must be aware of the appropriate norms. Appropriate resuscitation with isotonic fluids should not be delayed due to technical issues with IV access. Intraosseous access in an unfractured bone is a rapid and reasonable alternative.

Prehospital Care of Spinal Cord Injury

Spinal cord injury affects approximately 12,000 people/year in the USA, leading to a total of 250,000 Americans living with this devastating injury. The majority of these patients are previously healthy young men who are contributing members to our nation. These injuries have devastating effects on the patients, their families, and society. Many clinical trials have attempted to develop treatments to improve outcome without success. These trials evaluated the administration of steroids, gangliosides, and excitatory amino acid antagonists [91–93]. More recent studies have begun to evaluate the safety of systemic hypothermia for spinal cord injury patients in a controlled manner, but larger studies will be required to show the true safety and efficacy [94]. Further research also needs to address the therapeutic window in which hypothermia may still be effective and to decide if this therapy will need to be started in the field by EMS personnel or later in the hospital. Until phase III clinical trials have been completed, hypothermia will remain an experimental treatment for these patients [95].

Prehospital care of spinal cord injury patients follows the guidelines used for all trauma patients. Treatment starts with stabilization of the airway, breathing, and circulation while simultaneously stabilizing the cervical spine. When moving patients onto the stretcher, a long spinal board and several straps should be used to ensure immobility/stabilization of the patient's entire body. The phrenic nerve is supplied from cervical levels three through five; therefore, if the injury occurs above the level of the third cervical vertebrae, the patient may experience respiratory paralysis requiring intubation to assist oxygenation and ventilation. Spinal cord injuries below this level may also experience some respiratory distress and failure. Multiple other issues can worsen respiratory status, including failure of respiratory muscles, flail chest, hemothorax, tension pneumothorax, and open pneumothorax. In the critical care setting, a negative inspiratory force (NIF) is measured to help to assess respiratory muscle strength and, hence, need for intubation. If the NIF is greater than negative 25–30 cm H_2O – that is, the number is LESS negative – ventilatory support may be needed. SpO_2 persistently at or below about 90 % or $PetCO_2$ above 50 mmHg will most often require respiratory support, typically through endotracheal intubation. All prehospital personnel must be aware of these concerns and intubate early in order to prevent critical hypoxia leading to further injury.

In securing the airway, a gentle chin lift and forward jaw thrust should be used to open the airway with a strong focus on in-line stabilization of the cervical spine. If the patient is unconscious, then prehospital personnel must take over oxygenation and ventilation of these patients. This may be accomplished in several ways: Oral endotracheal intubation with in-line manual cervical immobilization and cricoid pressure (the Sellick maneuver) may be performed. Cricoid pressure in a patient not in arrest protects against aspiration of gastric contents; if this occurs it may massively magnify the difficulty one has with oxygenation but may also make ventilation more difficult and may impede placement of a supraglottic airway. While it is argued that routine use of cricoid pressure in cardiac arrest is not needed [96–102], many will utilize the Sellick maneuver while intubating any patient; the risk of aspiration is simply too great. Alternatively, if the prehospital provider is able to oxygenate and ventilate the patient with a bag-valve-mask device and the transport time is less than 20 min, this is an acceptable way to control the airway during transport to the ED. One may also place a King LT, LMA, or endotracheal tube through a SALT device. If these devices are used instead of an endotracheal tube, cricoid pressure should not be used as it will compromise

placement/seal. These patients must be quickly transported to a trauma center to receive specialized care, so time should not be spent on scene with multiple attempts at endotracheal intubation. In addition, multiple attempts at airway manipulation may cause deleterious increases in intracranial pressure in TBI patients, which may severely worsen prognosis.

The prehospital personnel not only provide medical care for the injured patient but also assess the security of the environment in which the patient was found. Depending on the type of accident, many times patients require extrication. Fire fighters and first responders with specific machinery receive special training in order to safely extricate these patients. If extrication is required, the patient's head must be aligned with the axis of the body, with the eyes facing forward. Patients must be secured to a rigid backboard as soon as possible. If these patients have an obvious cervical spine deformity or significant pain with movement, then other, more complex, extrication techniques may need to be applied.

If a patient is found with a helmet in place, this should remain until the patient is delivered to the ED. Some newer helmets are equipped with special pneumatic devices which allow for easy helmet removal when the devices are insufflated. If, for example, the patient has on protective football pads, the helmet should only be removed after the removal of the pads in order to prevent neck extension [13]. Helmet removal necessitates two providers, with one holding the neck and mandible in place while the other slowly removes the helmet without a twisting motion.

A problem further complicating care of spinal cord injury patients is the presence of neurogenic shock. Spinal cord injury causes a decrease, or absence, of sympathetic, along with unopposed parasympathetic, outflow. These patients may, therefore, experience bradycardia and decreased cardiac contractility leading to hypotension. Many of these patients sustain multisystem trauma, so clinicians must also consider other possible causes of instability including hypovolemic shock, cardiogenic shock from tension pneumothorax, cardiac tamponade, myocardial contusion, air embolus, and myocardial infarction. Patients with spinal cord injury should first receive IV crystalloid, Ringer's lactate or 0.9 % saline solution; 250–500 mL in repeated boluses up to 2 L for the adult, or 20 mL/kg in the child, is initially appropriate. In a critical care setting, adrenergic agonists such as neosynephrine and norepinephrine may be used if needed, while in the prehospital setting, mixed alpha and beta agonists such as dopamine or epinephrine are most often used. In the field and initially in the ED, positive signs of perfusion, such as normal mental status in awake patients or urine output of 0.5 mL/kg/h should be used to titrate vasopressor support. In an unconscious patient, a target mean arterial pressure of 65–70 mmHg can be used.

The findings on an initial neurological exam are important. This neurological evaluation should include the level of sensory impairment and muscle strength on a six-point scale, where: 0=paralysis, 1=palpable, visual contractions, 2=range of motion with gravity eliminated, 3=range of motion with gravity, 4=active range of motion with moderate resistance, and 5=active range of motion with full resistance. Transportation to the ED should be provided rapidly and safely. Any patient with whom there is concern for spinal cord injury should be transported to the nearest trauma center with advance notice to the receiving facility. Upon arrival to the ED, the prehospital personnel will give a detailed history of what was found at the scene, what interventions were performed, and a general summary of the patient's status starting from their initial contact.

Prehospital Management of Stroke

With the advent of thrombolysis and acute vascular intervention for acute ischemic stroke, rapid recognition and transport to an acute stroke center has become a key factor in the management and transport of stroke patients by Emergency Medical Services (EMS). Just as in trauma patients, rapid recognition of the disorder and transport to a stroke center, especially comprehensive stroke centers, improves outcome [103]. Similarly, as triage criteria for prioritizing patient transport to trauma centers have been developed, preferential transport of patients with acute stroke symptoms to stroke centers are being developed. For example, the State of Florida has passed legislation (Florida Statute 395.3041) requiring EMS agencies to transport patients with evidence of acute stroke to a local stroke center capable of acute intervention preferentially over the nearest medical facility. To facilitate this, a prehospital stroke checklist has been developed for EMS providers to identify patients who should be transported to such a stroke center [104]. More recently, it has been demonstrated that the transport of acute stroke patients to a comprehensive stroke center improves outcomes, not only for those who may qualify for intervention outside the thrombolytic window, but also in patients who arrive at week's end, when some institutions are "winding down," a phenomenon that does not occur in a stroke center

[103]. To aid in rapid recognition of patients exhibiting symptoms of acute stroke, several prehospital stroke assessment scores have been developed. While the National Institutes of Health (NIH) Stroke Score is comprehensive and, perhaps, the standard for neurologists, its precise complexity and comprehensiveness may lead to delay in transport of a patient for acute intervention. The Cincinnati stroke score [105], the LA prehospital stroke score [106, 107], and the MEND (Miami Emergency Neurologic Deficit) [108] scores have been developed to rapidly select patients who may benefit from early stroke intervention (Table 9.3).

Early notification of transport to the destination medical center is a key step so that rapid evaluation and imaging can be attained in patients who may be a candidate for acute intervention. The LA Motor Score has been developed to rapidly detect large arterial occlusions that may benefit from transport to a comprehensive stroke center capable of interventions in patients who may be out of the thrombolytic window (Table 9.4) [109]. The goal of these prehospital stroke scores is to identify patients who may be candidates for acute stroke interventions and transport them appropriately, not to try to exclude those who may not meet thrombolysis criteria, as further assessment and decision making will be performed at the receiving emergency department.

Once identified, the patient with symptoms suggestive of an acute stroke should be rapidly transported to a stroke center without delay for intervention – known in EMS as a "load and go" transport. Airway control and intervention in a patient with profound neurological deficit (e.g., GCS less than or equal to 8) would be the only intervention that would prioritize immediate, on-scene treatment. A thorough history, including key information such as time the patient was last seen normal, allergies, and medications – especially antiplatelet or anticoagulant therapy and diabetic medications – must be obtained. Other pertinent information to obtain includes any history of recent trauma, seizure, or myocardial infarction, as well as past medical history of prior stroke, intracerebral hemorrhage, gastrointestinal hemorrhage, or irregular heart rhythm/atrial fibrillation. All of this information obtained by prehospital care personnel will impact deci-

Table 9.3 The Cincinnati Prehospital Stroke Scale

Facial droop (have patient show teeth or smile)
Normal – both sides of face move equally
Abnormal – one side of face does not move as well as the other side
Arm drift (patient closes eyes and holds both arms straight out for 10 s)
Normal – both arms move the same or both arms do not move at all (other findings, such as pronator grip, may be helpful)
Abnormal – one arm does not move or one arm drifts down compared with the other
Abnormal speech (have the patient say "you cannot teach an old dog new tricks")
Normal – patient uses correct words with no slurring
Abnormal – patient slurs words, uses the wrong words, or is unable to speak

Reproduced with permission of Elsevier from Kothari et al. [105]

Interpretation: if any of these three signs is abnormal, the probability of a stroke is 72 %

Table 9.4 A Los Angeles Motor Score (LAMS) greater than or equal to 4 significantly increases the likelihood of large vessel involvement

Facial droop	
Absent	0
Present	1
Arm drift	
Absent	0
Drifts down	1
Falls rapidly	2
Grip strength	
Normal	0
Weak grip	1
No grip	2

Reproduced with permission from Nazeil et al. [109]

sion making as regarding thrombolysis. If possible, a family member should accompany the patient to the hospital to help with critical information that may impact therapy, particularly if the patient has speech symptoms. The presence of next of kin or healthcare proxy would also be helpful when issues of consent for treatment occur. Should a family member not be transported with the patient, attempts should be made to obtain a telephone number, preferably a cell phone, to facilitate communication between family and healthcare providers.

Treatment of the acute stroke patient should begin en route to the appropriate destination. Evaluation of the patient during transport includes obtaining blood pressure and blood glucose levels if not obtained on scene, as well as cardiac monitoring, pulse oximetry, and establishment of IV access as allowed by local EMS protocols. Hypoglycemia can be a stroke mimic and should be treated, with euglycemia preferred over hyperglycemia. Patients without hypoglycemia should not receive IV fluids containing dextrose [110]. Hypertension should not be treated in the prehospital environment as it may facilitate perfusion of an ischemic penumbra in thrombotic and embolic strokes [111]. Supplemental oxygen should only be administered to maintain SpO2 above 94 % [111] to avoid hyperoxia and potential superoxide radical formation at the cellular level.

In addition to rapid transport to an appropriate stroke center, early notification of the receiving facility has been associated with significantly decreased times from patient arrival to initial hospital assessment [112]. This early recognition and initial assessment is central to the reduction of door-to-treatment times in patients who are candidates for acute intervention. Appropriate use of air transport can reduce prehospital times, particularly for patients who may not have local access to a stroke center and may allow for transport to comprehensive stroke centers with expanded treatment time windows [111, 113]. Local transport protocols may also dictate transport to a comprehensive stroke center where other interventional modalities may be available, should the patient's symptom duration be near the cutoff for thrombolysis. Critical care interfacility transport, by ground or by air

transport, may provide access to more comprehensive care for patients who may be candidates for thrombolysis at a non-stroke center. Systems have been designed to begin treatment at non-stroke centers, often in consultation with a stroke neurologist, possibly by telemedicine, and then transport, so-called "drip and ship".

Summary

Emergency medical service systems are critical to the care of the neurologically injured patient. As part of the continuum of care, the first moments of intervention at the time of injury can be directly linked to lives saved and improved outcomes at the end of hospitalization and rehabilitation. Continued research and development in the prehospital care environment will only serve to strengthen the essential link between the first provider to encounter an ill or injured patient, the system of prehospital care response, and the provision of definitive care in an acute care setting.

References

1. Ramzy AI, Parry JM, Greenberg J. Head and spinal injury: prehospital care. In: Greenberg J, editor. Handbook of head and spine trauma. New York: Marcel Dekker; 1993. p. 29–44.
2. Field JM, Hazinski MF, Sayre MR, et al. 2010 American Heart Association guidelines for cardiopulmonary resuscitation and emergency cardiovascular care science. Circulation. 2010;122 Suppl 3:18.
3. Hollenberg J, Herlitz J, Lindqvist J, Riva G, Bohm K, Rosenqvist M, Svensson L. Improved survival after out-of-hospital cardiac arrest is associated with an increase in proportion of emergency crew–witnessed cases and bystander cardiopulmonary resuscitation. Circulation. 2008;118:389–96.
4. Lund-Kordahl I, Olasveengen TM, Lorem T, Samdal M, Wik L, Sunde K. Improving outcome after out-of-hospital cardiac arrest by strengthening weak links of the local chain of survival: quality of advanced life support and post-resuscitation care. Resuscitation. 2010;81:422–6.
5. Iwami T, Nichol G, Hiraide A, Hayashi Y, Nishiuchi T, Kajino K, Morita H, Yukioka H, Ikeuchi H, Sugimoto H, Nonogi H, Kawamura T. Continuous improvements in "chain of survival"

increased survival after out-of-hospital cardiac arrests: a large-scale population-based study. Circulation. 2009;119:728–34.

6. Rea TD, Helbock M, Perry S, Garcia M, Cloyd D, Becker L, Eisenberg M. Increasing use of cardiopulmonary resuscitation during out-of-hospital ventricular fibrillation arrest: survival implications of guideline changes. Circulation. 2006;114: 2760–5.

7. Bobrow BJ, Clark LL, Ewy GA, Chikani V, Sanders AB, Berg RA, Richman PB, Kern KB. Minimally interrupted cardiac resuscitation by emergency medical services for out-of-hospital cardiac arrest. JAMA. 2008;299:1158–65.

8. Hartl R, Gerber LM, Iacono L, et al. Direct transport within an organized state trauma system reduces mortality in patients with severe traumatic brain injury. J Trauma. 2006;60:1250–6; discussion 1256.

9. Minardi J, Crocco T, et al. Management of traumatic brain injury: first link in chain of survival. Mt Sinai J Med. 2009;76:138–44.

10. Crosby LA, Lewallen DG, editors. Emergency care and transportation of the sick and injured. 6th ed. Rosemont: American Academy of Orthopaedic Surgeons; 1995.

11. Frandsen F, Nielsen JR, Gram L, et al. Evaluation of intensified prehospital treatment in out-of-hospital cardiac arrest: survival and cerebral prognosis – the Odense ambulance study. Cardiology. 1991;79:256–64.

12. Nicholl JP, Brazier JE, Snooks HA. Effects of London helicopter emergency medical service on survival after trauma. BMJ. 1995; 311:217–22.

13. Bartolomeo SD, Sanson G, Nardi G, Scian F, et al. Effects of 2 patterns of pre-hospital care on the outcome of patients with severe head injury. Arch Surg. 2001;136:1–15.

14. Botker M, Bakke S, Christensen E, et al. A systematic review of controlled studies: do physicians increase survival with prehospital treatment? Scand J Trauma Resusc Emerg Med. 2009;17:12.

15. Nirula R, Brusel K. Do trauma centers improve functional outcomes: a national trauma databank analysis? J Trauma. 2006;61: 268–71.

16. Brown JB, Stassen NA, Bankey PE, et al. Helicopters and the civilian trauma system: national utilization patterns demonstrate improved outcomes after trauma. J Trauma. 2010;69:1030–6.

17. Brown JB, Stassen NA, Bankey PE, et al. Helicopters improve survival in seriously injured patients requiring interfacility transfer for definitive care. J Trauma. 2011;70:310–4.

18. Rivera-Laura L, Zhang J, Muehlschlegel S. Therapeutic hypothermia for acute neurological injuries. Neurotherapeutics. 2012;9:73–86.

19. Bahr J, Klingler H, Panzer W, Rode H, Kettler D. Skills of lay people in checking the carotid pulse. Resuscitation. 1997;35:23–6.

20. Brennan RT, Braslow A. Skill mastery in public CPR classes. Am J Emerg Med. 1998;16:653–7.

21. Chamberlain D, Smith A, Woollard M, Colquhoun M, Handley AJ, Leaves S, Kern KB. Trials of teaching methods in basic life support : comparison of simulated CPR performance after first training and at 6 months, with a note on the value of re-training. Resuscitation. 2002;53:179–87.

22. Eberle B, Dick WF, Schneider T, Wisser G, Doetsch S, Tzanova I. Checking the carotid pulse check: diagnostic accuracy of first responders in patients with and without a pulse. Resuscitation. 1996;33:107–16.

23. Frederick K, Bixby E, Orzel MN, Stewart-Brown S, Willett K. Will changing the emphasis from 'pulseless' to 'no signs of circulation' improve the recall scores for effective life support skills in children? Resuscitation. 2002;55:255–61.

24. Lapostolle F, Le Toumelin P, Agostinucci JM, Catineau J, Adnet F. Basic cardiac life support providers checking the carotid pulse: performance, degree of conviction, and influencing factors. Acad Emerg Med. 2004;11:878–80.

25. Moule P. Checking the carotid pulse: diagnostic accuracy in students of the healthcare professions. Resuscitation. 2000;44: 195–201.

26. Nyman J, Sihvonen M. Cardiopulmonary resuscitation skills in nurses and nursing students. Resuscitation. 2000;47:179–84.

27. Owen CJ, Wyllie JP. Determination of heart rate in the baby at birth. Resuscitation. 2004;60:213–7.

28. Sarti A, Savron F, Ronfani L, Pelizzo G, Barbi E. Comparison of three sites to check the pulse and count heart rate in hypotensive infants. Paediatr Anaesth. 2006;16:394–8.

29. Wang HE, Kupas DF, Paris PM, Bates RR, Yealy DM. Preliminary experience with a prospective, multi-centered evaluation of out-of-hospital endotracheal intubation. Resuscitation. 2003;58: 49–58.

30. Callaham M, Madsen CD, Barton CW, Saunders CE, Pointer J. A randomized clinical trial of high-dose epinephrine and norepinephrine vs. standard-dose epinephrine in prehospital cardiac arrest. JAMA. 1992;268:2667–72.

31. Gueugniaud PY, Mols P, Goldstein P, Pham E, Dubien PY, Deweerdt C, Vergnion M, Petit P, Carli P. A comparison of repeated high doses and repeated standard doses of epinephrine for cardiac arrest outside the hospital. European Epinephrine Study Group. N Engl J Med. 1998;339:1595–601.

32. Lindner KH, Prengel AW, Brinkmann A, et al. Vasopressin administration in refractory cardiac arrest. Ann Intern Med. 1996;124: 1061–4.

33. Wenzel V, Lindner KH, Krismer AC, et al. Repeated administration of vasopressin but not epinephrine maintains coronary perfusion pressure after early and late administration during prolonged cardiopulmonary resuscitation in pigs. Circulation. 1999;99: 1379–84.

34. Prengel AW, Lindner KH, Keller A. Cerebral oxygenation during cardiopulmonary resuscitation with epinephrine and vasopressin in pigs. Stroke. 1996;27:1241–8.

35. Wenzel V, Linder KH, Augenstein S, Prengel AW, Strohmenger HU. Vasopressin combined with epinephrine decreases cerebral perfusion compared with vasopressin alone during cardiopulmonary resuscitation in pigs. Stroke. 1998;29:1462–8.

36. Stiell IG, Hebert PC, Wells GA, Vandemheen KL, Tang AS, Higginson LA, Dreyer JF, Clement C, Battram E, Watpool I, Mason S, Klassen T, Weitzman BN. Vasopressin versus epinephrine for in hospital cardiac arrest: a randomized controlled trial. Lancet. 2001;358:105–9.

37. Dorian P, Cass D, Schwartz B, Cooper R, Gelaznikas R, Barr A. Amiodarone as compared with lidocaine for shock-resistant ventricular fibrillation. N Engl J Med. 2002;346:884–90.

38. Somberg JC, Bailin SJ, Haffajee CI, Paladino WP, Kerin NZ, Bridges D, Timar S, Molnar J. Intravenous lidocaine versus intravenous amiodarone (in a new aqueous formulation) for incessant ventricular tachycardia. Am J Cardiol. 2002;90:853–9.

39. Somberg JC, Timar S, Bailin SJ, Lakatos F, Haffajee CI, Tarjan J, Paladino WP, Sarosi I, Kerin NZ, Borbola J, Bridges DE, Molnar J. Lack of a hypotensive effect with rapid administration of a new aqueous formulation of intravenous amiodarone. Am J Cardiol. 2004;93:576–81.

40. Paiva EF, Perondi MB, Kern KB, Berg RA, Timerman S, Cardoso LF, Ramirez JA. Effect of amiodarone on haemodynamics during cardiopulmonary resuscitation in a canine model of resistant ventricular fibrillation. Resuscitation. 2003;58:203–8.

41. Herlitz J, Ekstrom L, Wennerblom B, Axelsson A, Bang A, Lindkvist J, Persson NG, Holmberg S. Lidocaine in out-of-hospital ventricular fibrillation. Does it improve survival? Resuscitation. 1997;33:199–205.

42. Stueven HA, Tonsfeldt DJ, Thompson BM, Whitcomb J, Kastenson E, Aprahamian C. Atropine in asystole: human studies. Ann Emerg Med. 1984;13:815–7.

43. Coon GA, Clinton JE, Ruiz E. Use of atropine for brady-asystolic prehospital cardiac arrest. Ann Emerg Med. 1981;10:462–7.

44. Tortolani AJ, Risucci DA, Powell SR, Dixon R. In-hospital cardiopulmonary resuscitation during asystole. Therapeutic factors associated with 24-hour survival. Chest. 1989;96:622–6.

45. Stiell IG, Wells GA, Hebert PC, Laupacis A, Weitzman BN. Association of drug therapy with survival in cardiac arrest: limited role of advanced cardiac life support drugs. Acad Emerg Med. 1995;2:264–73.

46. Dorph E, Wik L, Steen PA. Effectiveness of ventilation-compression ratios 1:5 and 2:15 in simulated single rescuer paediatric resuscitation. Resuscitation. 2002;54:259–64.

47. Hwang SO, Kim SH, Kim H, Jang YS, Zhao PG, Lee KH, Choi HJ, Shin TY. Comparison of 15:1, 15:2, and 30:2 compression-to-ventilation ratios for cardiopulmonary resuscitation in a canine model of a simulated, witnessed cardiac arrest. Acad Emerg Med. 2008;15:183–9.

48. Banerjee S, Singhi SC, Singh S, Singh M. The intraosseous route is a suitable alternative to intravenous route for fluid resuscitation in severely dehydrated children. Indian Pediatr. 1994;31:1511–20.

49. Brickman KR, Krupp K, Rega P, Alexander J, Guinness M. Typing and screening of blood from intraosseous access. Ann Emerg Med. 1992;21:414–7.

50. Fiser RT, Walker WM, Seibert JJ, McCarthy R, Fiser DH. Tibial length following intraosseous infusion: a prospective, radiographic analysis. Pediatr Emerg Care. 1997;13:186–8.

51. Atkinson E, Mikysa B, Conway JA, Parker M, Christian K, Deshpande J, Knilans TK, Smith J, Walker C, Stickney RE, Hampton DR, Hazinski MF. Specificity and sensitivity of automated external defibrillator rhythm analysis in infants and children. Ann Emerg Med. 2003;42:185–96.

52. Cecchin F, Jorgenson DB, Berul CI, Perry JC, Zimmerman AA, Duncan BW, Lupinetti FM, Snyder D, Lyster TD, Rosenthal GL, Cross B, Atkins DL. Is arrhythmia detection by automatic external defibrillator accurate for children? Sensitivity and specificity of an automatic external defibrillator algorithm in 696 pediatric arrhythmias. Circulation. 2001;103:2483–8.

53. Atkins DL, Scott WA, Blaufox AD, Law IH, Dick II M, Geheb F, Sobh J, Brewer JE. Sensitivity and specificity of an automated external defibrillator algorithm designed for pediatric patients. Resuscitation. 2008;76:168–74.

54. Bar-Cohen Y, Walsh EP, Love BA, Cecchin F. First appropriate use of automated external defibrillator in an infant. Resuscitation. 2005;67:135–7.

55. Konig B, Benger J, Goldsworthy L. Automatic external defibrillation in a 6 year old. Arch Dis Child. 2005;90:310–1.

56. Deasy C, Bernard S, Cameron P, et al. Design of the RINSE trial: the rapid infusion of cold normal saline by paramedics during CPR. BMC Emerg Med. 2011;13:11–7.

57. Bernard SA, Smith K, Cameron P, et al. Induction of therapeutic hypothermia by paramedics after resuscitation from out-of-hospital ventricular fibrillation cardiac arrest: a randomized controlled trial. Circulation. 2010;122:737–42.

58. Bernard S. Hypothermia after cardiac arrest: expanding the therapeutic scope. Crit Care Med. 2009;37:S227–33.

59. Holzer M, Bernard SA, Hachimi-Idrissi S, et al. Hypothermia for neuro protection after cardiac arrest: systematic review and individual patient data meta-analysis. Crit Care Med. 2005;33:414–8.

60. Scolletta S, Taccone FS, et al. Intra-arrest hypothermia during cardiac arrest: a systematic review. Crit Care. 2012;16:R41.

61. Choi HA, Badjatia N, Mayer SA. Hypothermia for acute brain injury-mechanisms and practical aspects. Nat Rev Neurol. 2012;8:214–22.

62. Bernard SA, Gray TW, Buist MD, et al. Treatment of comatose survivors of out-of-hospital cardiac arrest with induced hypothermia. N Engl J Med. 2002;346:557–63.

63. The Hypothermia after cardiac arrest Study Group. Mild therapeutic hypothermia to improve neurologic outcome after cardiac arrest. N Engl J Med. 2002;346:549–56.

64. Steen PA, Newberg LD. Hypothermia and barbituates: individual and combined effects on canine cerebral oxygen consumption. Anesthesiology. 1983;58:527–32.

65. Shreckinger M, Marion DW. Contemporary management of traumatic intracranial hypertension: is there a role for therapeutic hypothermia? Neurocrit Care. 2009;11:427–36.

66. Kliegel A, et al. Cold simple intravenous infusions preceding special endovascular cooling for faster induction of mild hypothermia after cardiac arrest – a feasibility study. Resuscitation. 2005;64:347–51.

67. Bernar S, Buist N, Monteiro O, Smith K. Induced hypothermia using large volume, ice-cold intravenous fluid in comatose survivors of out of hospital cardiac arrest- a preliminary report. Resuscitation. 2003;56:9–13.

68. Badjatia N. Fever control in the neuro – ICU: why, who and when? Curr Opin Crit Care. 2009;15:79–92.

69. Badjatia N, Strongilis E, Gordon E, et al. Metabolic impact of shivering during therapeutic temperature modulation: the bedside shivering assessment scale. Stroke. 2008;39:3242–7.

70. Choi HA, Ko SB, Presciutti M, et al. Prevention of shivering during therapeutic temperature modulation: the Columbia anti-shivering protocol. Neurocrit Care. 2011;14:389–94.

71. Doufas AG, Lin CM, Suleman MI, et al. Dexmetetomidate and meperidine additively reduce the shivering threshold in humans. Stroke. 2003;34:1218–23.

72. Kurz A, Sessler DI, Annadata R, et al. Midazolam minimally impairs thermoregulatory control. Anesth Anal. 1995;81:393–8.

73. Van der Worp HB, Sena ES, Donnan GA, Howells DW, Macleod MR. Hypothermia in animal models of acute ischemic stroke: a systematic review and meta-analysis. Brain. 2007;130:3063–74.

74. De Georgia MA, Kreiger DW, Abou-Chebl A, et al. Cooling for acute ischemic brain damage (COOL AID) a feasibility trial of endovascular cooling. Neurology. 2004;63:312–7.

75. Kollmar R, et al. Hypothermia reduces peri-hemorrhagic edema after intracerebral hemorrhage. Stroke. 2010;41:1684–9.

76. Cappuccino A, Bisson LJ, Carpenter B, et al. The use of systemic hypothermia for the treatment of an acute cervical spinal cord injury in a professional foot ball player. Spine (Philadelphia PA 1976). 2010;35:E57–62.

77. Knuth T. Guidelines for the field management of combat related head injury. Brain Trauma Foundation. 2005. Available online at https://www.braintrauma.org/coma-guidelines/. Last accessed 13 June 2012.

78. Adelson PD, Bratton SL, Carney NA, et al. Guidelines for the acute medical management of severe traumatic brain injury of infants, children, and adolescents. Pediatr Crit Care Med. 2003;4 (3 Suppl):S72–5.

79. Bullock MR, Chestnut R, Ghajar J, et al. Guidelines for the surgical management of traumatic brain injury. Neurosurgery. 2006;58(3 Suppl):S2-1–62.

80. Davis DP, Hoyt DB, Ochs M, et al. The effect of paramedic rapid sequence intubation on outcome in patients with severe traumatic brain injury. J Trauma. 2003;54:444–53.

81. Wang HE, Peitzman AB, Cassidy LD, et al. Out-of-hospital endotracheal intubation and outcome after traumatic brain injury. Ann Emerg Med. 2004;44:439–60.

82. Bernard S, Nguyen V, Cameron P. Prehospital rapid sequence intubation improves functional outcome for patients with severe traumatic brain injury. Ann Surg. 2010;252:959–65.

83. Stocchetti N, Furlan A, Volta F. Hypoxemia and arterial hypotension at the accident scene in head injury. J Trauma. 1996;40:764–7.

84. Chestnut RM, Marshall LF, Klauber MR, et al. The role of secondary brain injury in determining outcome from severe brain injury. J Trauma. 1993;34:216–22.

85. Bulger EM, May S, Kerby JD, et al. Out-of-hospital hypertonic resuscitation after traumatic hypovolemic shock: a randomized, placebo controlled trial. Ann Surg. 2011;253:431–41.

86. Farrell LS, Hannan EL, Cooper A. Severity of injury and mortality associated with pediatric blunt injuries: hospitals with pediatric intensive care units versus other hospitals. Pediatr Crit Care Med. 2004;5:5–9.

87. Muizelaar JP, Marmarou A, Ward JD, et al. Adverse effects of prolonged hyperventilation in patients with severe head injury: a randomized clinical trial. J Neurosurg. 1991;75:731–9.

88. Thomas SH, Orf J, Wedel SK, Conn AK. Hyperventilation in traumatic brain injury patients: inconsistency between consensus guidelines and clinical practice. J Trauma. 2002;52:47–53.

89. Bullock R, Chesnut RM, Clifton G, et al. Guidelines for the management of severe head injury. New York: Brain Trauma Foundation; 1995.

90. Rocksworld SB, Rockswold GL, Defillo A. Hyperbaric oxygen in traumatic brain injury. Neurol Res. 2007;29:162–72.

91. Cortez R, Levi AD. Acute spinal cord injury. Curr Treat Options Neurol. 2007;9:115–25.

92. Geisler FH, Coleman WP, Grieco G, et al. The Sygen multicenter acute spinal cord injury study. Spine. 2001;26:S87–98.

93. Kwon BK, Mann C, Sohn HM, et al. Hypothermia for spinal cord injury. Spine. 2008;8:859–74.

94. Levi AD, Casella G, Green B, et al. Spinal cord injury and modest hypothermia. J Neurotrauma. 2009;26:407–15.

95. Dietrich 3rd WD. Therapeutic hypothermia for spinal cord injury. Crit Care Med. 2009;37(Supp 7):S238–42.

96. Asai T, Goy RW, Liu E, et al. Cricoid pressure prevents placement of the laryngeal tube and laryngeal tube-suction II. Br J Anaesth. 2007;99:282–5.

97. Turgeon AF, Nicole PC, Trepanier CA, Marcoux S, Lessard MR. Cricoid pressure does not increase the rate of failed intubation by direct laryngoscopy in adults. Anesthesiology. 2005;102:315–9.

98. Allman KG. The effect of cricoid pressure application on airway patency. J Clin Anesth. 1995;7:197–9.

99. Brimacombe J, White A, Berry A. Effect of cricoid pressure on ease of insertion of the laryngeal mask airway. Br J Anaesth. 1993;71:800–2.

100. McNelis U, Syndercombe A, Harper I, Duggan J. The effect of cricoid pressure on intubation facilitated by the gum elastic bougie. Anaesthesia. 2007;62:456–9.

101. Hartsilver EL, Vanner RG. Airway obstruction with cricoid pressure. Anaesthesia. 2000;55:208–11.

102. Hocking G, Roberts FL, Thew ME. Airway obstruction with cricoid pressure and lateral tilt. Anaesthesia. 2001;56:825–8.

103. McKinney JS, Deng Y, Kasner SE, et al. Comprehensive stroke centers overcome the weekend vs. weekday gap in stroke treatment and mortality. Stroke. 2011;42:2403–9.

104. Florida Bureau of EMS Stroke Alert Checklist (Sample Document). http://www.doh.state.fl.us/demo/ems/Forms/Forms.html#formsother. Last accessed 13 June 2012.

105. Kothari RU, Pancioli A, Liu T, et al. Cincinnati prehospital stroke scale: reproducibility and validity. Ann Emerg Med. 1999;33:373–8.

106. Kidwell CS, Saver JL, Schubert GB, Eckstein M, Starkman S. Design and retrospective analysis of the Los Angeles Prehospital Stroke Screen (LAPSS). Prehosp Emerg Care. 1998;2:267–73.

107. Kidwell CS, Starkman S, Eckstein M, Weems K, Saver JL. Identifying stroke in the field: prospective validation of the Los Angeles Prehospital Stroke Screen (LAPSS). Stroke. 2000;31:71–6.

108. Advanced Stroke Life Support MEND Examination. http://www.asls.net/mend.html. Last accessed 13 June 2012.

109. Nazeil B, Starkman S, Liebeskind D, et al. A brief prehospital stroke severity scale identifies ischemic stroke patients harboring persisting large arterial occlusions. Stroke. 2008;39:2264–7.

110. Adams Jr HP, Zoppo G, Alberts MJ, et al. Guidelines for the early management of adults with ischemic stroke: a guideline from the American Heart Association/American Stroke Association Stroke Council, Clinical Cardiology Council, Cardiovascular Radiology and Intervention Council, and the Atherosclerotic Peripheral Vascular Disease and Quality of Care Outcomes in Research Interdisciplinary Working Groups. Stroke. 2007;38:1655–711.

111. Jauch EC, Cucchiara B, Adeoye O, et al. Adult stroke: 2010 American Heart Association guidelines for cardiopulmonary resuscitation and emergency cardiovascular care. Circulation. 2010;122 Suppl 3:S818–28.

112. Mosley I, Nicol M, Donnan G, et al. The impact of ambulance practice on acute stroke care. Stroke. 2007;38:2765–70.

113. Croco TJ, Grotta JC, Jauch EC, et al. EMS management of acute stroke—prehospital triage (resource document to NAEMSP position statement). Prehosp Emerg Care. 2007;11:313–7.

Airway Management in the Neurointensive Care Unit

10

Thomas C. Mort, Jeffrey P. Keck Jr., and Leah Meisterling

Contents

T.C. Mort, MD (✉)
Department of Anesthesiology and Critical Care Medicine,
Hartford Hospital, University of Connecticut,
37 Heather Glen Road, Glastonbury, CT 06033, USA
e-mail: tmort@harthosp.org

J.P. Keck Jr., MD
Virginia Commonwealth University, Richmond, VA, USA

Departments of Anesthesia and Critical Care,
Pikeville Medical Center, Pikeville, KY 41501, USA
e-mail: jeffkeck09@gmail.com

L. Meisterling, DO, MBA
Surgical Intensive Care Unit, Hartford Hospital,
Hartford, CT 06102, USA

Department of Anesthesiology,
University of Connecticut School of Medicine,
Farmington, CT, USA
e-mail: leahmeisterling@hotmail.com

A.J. Layon et al. (eds.), *Textbook of Neurointensive Care*,
DOI 10.1007/978-1-4471-5226-2_10, © Springer-Verlag London 2013

Abstract

Airway management in the critical care setting encompasses a wide, diverse range of topics, well beyond simply tracheal intubation. The delivery of oxygen and effective ventilation is affected by a multitude of clinical situations in the intensive care arena that can be lifesaving but equally could threaten the patient's outcome if not properly executed in a timely manner. From noninvasive ventilation devices extending to an accidently decannulated "fresh" bleeding tracheostomy site, it is imperative that the ICU offers the ability to deploy an experienced airway team equipped with basic and advanced airway adjuncts coupled with primary and secondary rescue strategies in the pursuit of improved patient safety.

Keywords

Airway • Extubation • Intubation • Larynx • Respiration Ventilation • Laryngeal mask airway

Table 10.1 Tolerance to hypoxia of various tissue

Tissue	Survival time
Brain	<3 min
Kidney and liver	15–20 min
Skeletal muscle	60–90 min
Vascular smooth muscle	24–72 h
Hair and nails	Several days

Reproduced with permission of the BMJ Publishing Group, LTD from Leach and Treacher [5]

Introduction

It is clear that a systematic disciplined approach to airway management will reduce the likelihood of an adverse outcome in the operating room [1–4]; this is no less true in the neurointensive care unit (NeuroICU). Conversely, each patient and their airway-related issue should be viewed as a unique event. The systemic approach provides a foundation upon which the specific needs of the patient may be met by offering the airway team guidelines that can be adaptable to the patient's unique airway challenges.

General Consequences of Hypoxia and Hypercapnia

Tissue oxygen delivery (DO_2), in mL/min, represents the bulk movement of oxygen in the blood and is proportional to cardiac output (CO) and arterial oxygen content (CaO_2). It is described by the equation

$$DO_2 = \left[(CO \times CaO_2) + 0.003(PaO_2) \right]$$

Thus, while the arterial partial pressure of oxygen (PaO_2) is an essential component of DO_2, it is clearly the least important element.

However, the presence of bulk O_2 delivered to tissue does not guarantee tissue oxygenation, as the passive movement of O_2 down a concentration gradient to the mitochondria is ultimately responsible for cellular O_2 delivery. Nevertheless, when ventilation fails, both PaO_2 and systemic O_2 delivery rapidly fall, resulting in hypoxemia. As a consequence, progressive, global hypoxia will rapidly follow. The tolerance to hypoxia of various tissues is different (Table 10.1) [5] with the central nervous system being the most sensitive organ. Irreversible damage starts about 3 min after the PaO_2 falls below 30 mmHg [5]. The neurovegetative response to hypoxia often manifests as a brief period of hypertension and concurrent tachycardia. However, if not promptly corrected, the worsening hypoxia can lead to cardiac dysrhythmias resulting in a low cardiac output state, severe bradycardia, peripheral vasodilatation, systemic hypotension, metabolic acidosis, and death.

Adequate ventilation is necessary to remove CO_2 from the tissues. The immediate consequence of hypoventilation is hypercapnia with acute respiratory acidosis and acidemia (pH < 7.35). In an apneic non-hypermetabolic patient, the increase in arterial partial pressure of CO_2 ($PaCO_2$) is predictable with time, at about 3 mmHg/min.

Respiratory acidosis, in the absence of hypoxia, may also provoke sympathetic nervous system activity, with consequent hypertension, tachycardia, cerebral vasodilatation, and increased intracranial pressure (ICP). However, in healthy individuals, altered mental status, severe acidemia, and cardiac arrest may only occur with significant hypercapnia ($PaCO_2$ greater than 80–100 mmHg). However, even small increases in $PaCO_2$ above physiologic norms may cause a significant worsening of ICP and lead to hemodynamic instability in patients with CNS injuries. Further, combined hypercarbia and hypoxia in this patient subset result in severe bradycardia and rapid deterioration of neurological status, particularly when PaO_2 falls below 60 mmHg.

Hypoxia and Secondary CNS Injury

While the CNS may be immediately damaged by the primary pathology, secondary injury from hypoxia (PaO_2 less than 60 mmHg) can be responsible for further rapid clinical deterioration. Hypoxia may originate from one of three mechanisms (or worse, a combination of the three). One has to clinically differentiate ischemic hypoxia (reduced cerebral blood flow) from anemic hypoxia (reduced O_2 delivery secondary to very low hemoglobin levels or cellular [mitochondrial] poisoning). When hypoxia is associated with neurological injury, secondary damage may result, leading to a complex cascade of inflammatory and biochemical processes involving both neurons and supportive cells. In general, CNS damage from decreased O_2 delivery has a multifactorial pathogenesis:

1. Failure of the Na^+/K^+ pump
2. Intracellular shift of Na^+, H_2O, and ionized calcium as the subsequent events [6]
3. A severe inflammatory reaction triggered by the intracellular release of O_2 free radicals, free fatty acid, and proteolytic enzymes
4. All these lead to intracellular, and then intravascular, lactic acidosis

Though restoration of blood flow and oxygen delivery is in the best interest of patient care, it has its consequences [6]. Restoration of perfusion of previously ischemic CNS cells that resulted in ionic membrane pump inefficiency may result in the following:

1. Osmotic edema (interstitial or vasogenic)
2. Disruption of the blood–brain barrier (BBB)
3. Further brain hypoperfusion leading to oxygen free radical burst
4. Activation of lipase, nucleases, and proteases
5. Potentiation of DNA injury and programmed cell death (apoptosis)

The Importance of an Organized Approach to the Airway

The importance of delivering O_2 and controlling $PaCO_2$ when dealing with the injured CNS is apparent. The first step to accomplishing ventilation and perfusion is airway management. The technique chosen for securing an airway depends on the anatomic characteristics of the airway itself and specific clinical factors associated with the injury. An organized treatment algorithm can provide immediate correction of oxygenation and ventilation while minimizing iatrogenic events. Commencing with the American Society of Anesthesiologists' publication of guidelines to manage the difficult airway, its counterparts in Canada, the UK, Germany, and Scandinavia, as well as other individual and regional societies, have published their own version of an organized approach to airway management. Though not specifically intended solely for the NeuroICU population, these guidelines provide general management tactics in regard to predicting a difficult airway, oxygenation and ventilation options, and intubation and extubation strategies with rescue alternatives [2, 3, 7].

Predicting a Difficult Airway

The awake, elective patient allows a comprehensive airway examination to assist in the recognition of factors that may result in a difficult airway (ventilation, laryngoscopy, intubation, and extubation) management [8]. A comprehensive review of airway anatomy and factors such as weight, head and neck movement, jaw movement, receding mandible, and upper incisor angulation affords improved predictability of difficulty (Table 10.2) [8]. A thorough airway examination in the NeuroICU patient, however, is rarely compatible with the elective setting. Additional airway-compromising, congenital, or acquired clinical conditions such as distortion, swelling, bleeding, and limited access to the airway further challenge the airway team (Table 10.3). These factors, combined with a hurried, abridged history and physical examination, plague the emergency encounter and clearly compromise patient safety. A rapid airway evaluation may miss more subtle pertinent findings and may only allow superficial appreciation of obvious abnormalities such as a short and stout neck, a hard cervical collar, dressings, arch bars, the dentition and the condition of the teeth, and the presence of a beard. It may be impossible to accurately check the Mallampati classification as it is not well studied in the urgent/emergent population in the supine position. The airway cared for under urgent or emergent circumstances in the NeuroICU setting is several magnitudes more complicated than the typical elective surgical patient presenting for an OR procedure (Table 10.4).

Anatomical observation of the upper airway should be integrated with knowledge of other possible airway alterations. Mallampati originally described the clinical correlation between the anatomy of the oropharyngeal structures and the degree of difficulty of laryngeal exposure. The basis of the Mallampati airway classification (three classes) is the relative size of the tongue to the size of the oropharyngeal opening. The updated version currently in use, the "modified Mallampati classification," has four classes (Fig. 10.1). For example, class IV describes a condition in which the oropharynx/posterior pharyngeal wall is completely obscured by the tongue when the mouth is wide open, strongly suggesting difficulty with laryngeal viewing with conventional laryngoscopy (Fig. 10.2). A class IV view is quite variable since the tongue may completely obliterate the mouth opening, and the class IV remains the same despite the marked increased risk of difficulty (Fig. 10.3). The ability to view the tonsillar bed and uvula (Fig. 10.4) suggests less difficulty with periglottic viewing with conventional laryngoscopy but certainly does not guarantee ease. A clear clinical correlation exists between this classification and the difficulty of direct laryngoscopy in both prospective and retrospective studies; however, it should not be the sole examining factor to base and implement an airway strategy [9]. An evaluation which utilizes multiple clinical predictors is best but may be time consuming, inexact, and impractical in an emergency. While physical examination of the airway has been the gold standard, recent research into pre-intubation fiber-optic nasopharyngoscopy, neck circumference, and ultrasound

Table 10.2 Preoperative airway examinations, acceptable endpoints, and significance of endpoints

Preop examination	Acceptable endpoints	Significance of endpoints
1. Dental		
(a) Length of upper incisors with mouth fully open	Qualitative/short incisors	Long incisors. Blade enters mouth in cephalad direction
(b) Involuntary: maxillary teeth anterior to mandibular teeth (buck teeth)	No overriding of maxillary teeth anterior to the mandibular teeth	Overriding maxillary teeth. Blade enters mouth in a more cephalad direction
(c) Voluntary: protrusion of mandibular teeth anterior to the maxillary teeth	Anterior protrusion of the mandibular teeth relative to the maxillary teeth	Test of TMJ function: means good mouth opening and jaw, will displace anteriorly with laryngoscopy
	>3 cm	2 cm phalange on blade can be easily inserted between teeth
2. Pharynx		
(a) Oropharyngeal class	≤Class II	Tongue is small in relation to size of oropharyngeal cavity
Samsoon and Young		
(b) Narrowness of palate	Should not appear very narrow and/or highly arched	A narrow palate decreases the oropharyngeal volume and room for both blade and ETT
(c) Mandibular space length (thyromental distance)	≥5 cm or ≥3 ordinary-sized finger breadths	Larynx is relatively posterior to other upper airway structures
(d) Mandibular space compliance (MS)	Qualitative palpation of normal resistance/softness	Laryngoscopy retracts tongue into the MS. Compliance of the MS determines if tongue fits into MS
3. Neck		
(a) Length of neck	Qualitative. A quantitative index is not yet available	A short neck decreases the ability to align the upper airway axes
(b) Thickness of neck	Qualitative. A quantitative index is not yet available	A thick neck decreases the ability to align the upper airway axes
(c) Range of motion of head and neck	Neck flexed and chest 35°+head extended on neck 80°=sniff position	The sniff position aligns the oral, pharyngeal, and laryngeal axes to create a favorable line of sight

Modified with permission from Practice Guidelines for Management of the Difficult Airway [3]

Table 10.3 Airway-compromising conditions

Pathologic condition	Principal pathologic/clinical features
A. Supralaryngeal	
1. Pierre Robin syndrome	Micrognathia, macroglossia, cleft soft palate
2. Treacher Collins syndrome	Auricular and ocular defects; malar and mandibular hypoplasia
3. Goldenhar's syndrome	Auricular and ocular defects; malar and mandibular hypoplasia; occipitalization of atlas
4. Down syndrome	Poorly developed or absent bridge of the nose; macroglossia
5. Klippel–Feil syndrome	Congenital fusion of a variable number of cervical vertebrae; restriction of neck movement
B. Sublaryngeal	
1. Goiter	Compression, deviation, tracheal softening
A. Infections	
1. Supraglottis	Laryngeal edema
2. Croup	Laryngeal edema
3. Abscess (intraoral, retropharyngeal)	Distortion of the airway and trismus
4. Ludwig's angina	Distortion of the airway and trismus
B. Arthritis	
1.Rheumatoid arthritis	Temporomandibular joint ankylosis, cricoarytenoid arthritis, deviation of larynx, restricted mobility of cervical spine
2. Ankylosing spondylitis	Ankylosis of cervical spine; less commonly, ankylosis of temporomandibular joints; lack of mobility of cervical spine
C. Benign tumors	
1. For example, cystic hygroma, lipoma, adenoma, goiter	Stenosis or distortion of the airway
D. Malignant tumors	
1. For example, carcinoma of tongue, larynx or thyroid	Stenosis or distortion of the airway; fixation of larynx or adjacent tissues secondary to infiltration or fibrosis from irradiation

Table 10.3 (continued)

Pathologic condition	Principal pathologic/clinical features
E. Trauma	
1. For example, facial injury, cervical spine injury and laryngeal–tracheal trauma	Edema of the airway, hematoma, ongoing nose/sinus/laryngeal bleeding, unstable fracture(s) of the maxillae, mandible, and cervical vertebrae
F. Obesity	Short, thick neck; redundant tissue in the oropharynx; sleep apnea, reduced extension due to adiposity, fat pad
G. Acromegaly	Macroglossia; prognathism
H. Acute burns	Edema of airway

Modified with permission of Elsevier from Benumof [97]

Table 10.4 Major considerations in emergent/urgent airway management

Acute cardiopulmonary/systemic pathology (MI, CHF, CVA, PE, shock, herniation, allergic reaction, cardiac arrest)

Hypoxia, hypercarbia, acidotic, electrolyte derangements

Limited airway examination at the bedside

Secretions, vomitus, bleeding, full stomach concerns, uncertain NPO status

Positioning issues, bed/mattress variety contributing to airway management difficulties

Dressings, hardware, hard cervical collar, halo vest interfere with airway access

Hemodynamic alterations; tachycardia, bradycardia, dysrhythmias, hypotension, hypertension

Airway team unfamiliar with care providers (and vice versa)

Altered mental status: agitation, belligerent, uncontrollable, anxiety, coma

Recent procedures (CVP placement → pneumothorax, NGT placement → oropharyngeal blood)

Hematologic alterations: coagulopathy, anemia, thrombocytopenia, "poisoned platelets"

Airway-related trauma (NGT, TEE probe, traumatic self-extubation, previous intubation)

Excessive volume resuscitation contributing to airway edema

Unknown or unavailable updated laboratory[a]

Conventional and advanced airway equipment shortfalls[a]

Abbreviated, incomplete gathering of medical/surgical history, review of systems[a]

No time to review or unavailable records of previous airway encounters[a]

Previous difficult airway management (unknown or unrecognized by team)[a]

[a]Designates clinical factors that may be changed by advanced planning, e.g., a well-developed and deployed difficult airway cart in the ICU setting or remote location; a system of identifying difficult airway patients by notation on the medical record, computer printouts, wristbands, and signs at the bedside; and the printing of a brief patient summary for the responding airway team that outlines medical/surgical problems, allergies, medications, recent procedures, radiographs, laboratory values, DNR status, and previous difficult airway encounters

evaluation of the airway may provide a more concrete evaluation of potential difficulties and allow improved planning [10]. However, even brief maneuvers may be impossible to implement in an emergency or crisis, e.g., cardiac arrest.

Classification of the laryngeal anatomy upon direct laryngoscopy (DL) can also be divided into four grades, 1–4 with grades 2 and 3 subdivided into "a" and "b." Originally designated by Cormack and Lehane, but updated by Cook and Yentis to more precisely describe airway views typically confronted (Fig. 10.5), this grading system can provide a standardized metric by which future interventions can be compared and practitioners can describe their observations so others will immediately understand their view [11, 12].

When the patient is comatose or uncooperative, the distance between the chin and the laryngeal cartilage prominence (thyromental distance, TMD) can be used as a rapid measurement to evaluate the airway. The TMD is a surrogate of the amount of potential free space into which the hypopharynx can be advanced when performing a DL, thereby creating a better pathway for visualization. A TMD of *greater than or equal to 3* fingerbreadths (roughly 6 cm) suggests adequate room for a successful DL and has been validated as a single-point predictor. Ostensibly, a quick review of a previous anesthesia or intubation record is also an invaluable tool to evaluate the airway in an emergency situation because many of these parameters will have been documented. However, successful previous interventions do not always guarantee positive outcomes since the upper airway anatomy is dynamic and will change with prior manipulation and comorbid conditions. In the NeuroICU setting, dynamic alterations in the airway structure may occur over minutes and hours to days; hence, a previously "EZ" airway may not be so tame the next time around due to the unpredictable dynamic alterations. One adage to remember: "Difficult in the past and likely difficult now, easy in the past does not guarantee easy now."

Electively, the overall failure to intubate the trachea with DL is reported to be uncommon, one to three cases per 10^3 attempts, though the authors feel this clearly understates the actual rate in the current milieu of obesity and other pathologic alterations of the airway [2]. Moreover, failure to bag-valve-mask (BVM) ventilate can be estimated at one to three cases per 10^4 attempts [1–5]. This is not to be interpreted that a difficult airway is rare, but should allow appreciation that, after all reasonable attempts/maneuvers by skilled practitioners, the failure rate in elective OR patients is uncommon. However, difficulty with ventilation and/or intubation is more likely in 5–10 % range, and this rate is multiplied in the urgent/emergent ICU setting. The introduction of the LMA and its variant supraglottic airway (SGA) devices has most likely altered

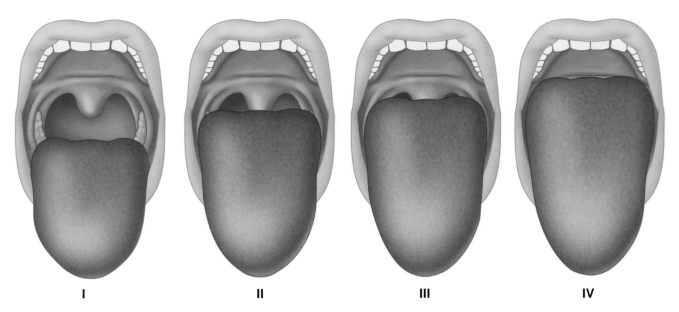

| I | II | III | IV |

Fig. 10.1 Mallampati classification I–IV (after Samsoon and Young) based on mouth opening and viewing the posterior wall of the pharynx and the relationship of the tongue, soft palate, and tonsillar bed/pillars. The classification was originally described with the patient sitting upright, non-phonating. This may be very difficult in the ICU emergent/urgent setting. Assuming difficulty is probably the most prudent course of action with the ICU airway. Note that class IV offers no view of the tonsillar bed, uvula, or soft palate. Yet, class IV can vary widely by the tongue blocking the view of the oral cavity significantly worse than what is depicted in this figure. Unfortunately, there is no class V or VI to appreciate the escalating degree of difficulty as the class worsens

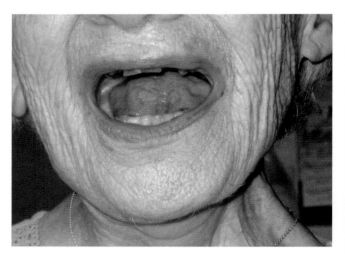

Fig. 10.2 Mallampati IV 2° radiation therapy and radical neck surgery with 1.5 fingerbreadths opening (trismus). Note that tongue obstructs view of soft and hard palate

this conservative figure based on practitioner encouragement to deploy an SGA device rapidly when BVM proves difficult or impossible. However, the incidence of intubation and BVM failure in the critically ill patient in general, and the NeuroICU patient, specifically, has not been determined.

Given the unpredictability of the airway in the urgent/emergent setting, the airway team should proceed cautiously

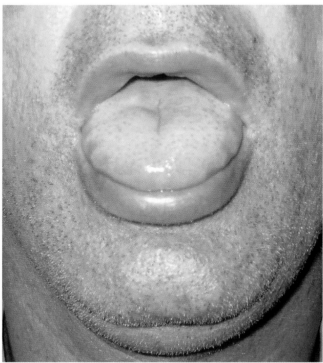

Fig. 10.3 View of Mallampati IV with tongue completely obstructing view of any oral contents. Compared to the sketched Mallampati IV, and theoretically speaking, this airway should be rated as a Mallampati class VI

armed with a primary plan with backup strategies complimented by immediate access to advance airway devices and personnel capable of performing such procedures.

Complications of Airway Management

The common consequence of most airway-related complications is hypoxemia. Various airway-related complications such as esophageal intubation (EI), regurgitation, aspiration, multiple intubation attempts, and mainstem bronchus

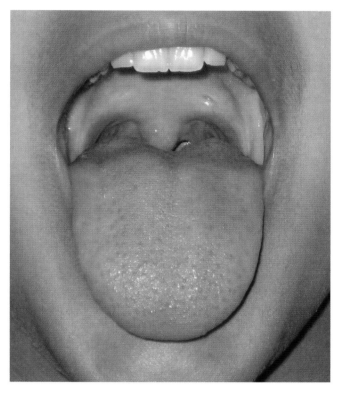

Fig. 10.4 Mallampati class II with near full view of the tonsillar bed, uvula, and soft and hard palate. This suggests a relatively easy laryngoscopy view with DL but other physical airway factors must be considered in developing a management strategy

intubation (MSBI) may each, singly or in combination, lead to various degrees of hemoglobin desaturation including significant reductions in the PaO_2 that may be catastrophic and, in the extreme circumstance, usher in a hypoxia-driven bradycardic cardiac arrest [13].

In an attempt to thwart or limit desaturation during the intubation process and provide a margin of safety for the patient in the event of airway difficulties, efforts to provide adequate oxygen reserve is considered a standard. Preoxygenation in the operating room (OR) under elective conditions incorporating either four to eight maximal forced vital capacity breaths of 100 % oxygen or 4 min of 100 % oxygen via a tight fitting facemask effectively elevates the PaO_2 to greater than 400 mmHg reliably in the healthy patient. Unfortunately, this is not the case with the critically ill patient who requires emergent intubation and who may be recalcitrant to standard noninvasive oxygen therapy; in these patients, despite optimal preoxygenation, the SpO_2 may only marginally clear the 90 % range [14, 15]. Desaturation may accompany even the easily managed airway but is magnified if multiple attempts are required, especially if esophageal intubation, regurgitation, aspiration, an unrecognized and this uncorrected mainstem bronchus intubation or loss of the airway takes place. Pre-intubation positive-pressure ventilation (BIPAP, CPAP) and positioning to optimize preoxygenation efforts (ramping in the obese, head-up position) are excellent adjuncts in the operating room, but have not been clearly defined in the urgent/emergent setting [14].

Adding to the recalcitrant efforts to optimize preoxygenation and following induction, mask ventilation may be extremely problematic with obesity, limited jaw and cervical spine mobility, a lack of dentition, a bearded face, obstructive sleep apnea, cachexia, facial bone overgrowth, facial trauma, dressing and bandages, as well as edema (external and internal) and age over 60 years [16].

Elective and urgent/emergent situations certainly differ, but an SpO_2 less than 90 % equates with a PaO_2 of between about 58 and 61 mmHg and may represent a reasonable cutoff for clinical reference. This level of hemoglobin saturation may not be life threatening in its own right, but rapid desaturation

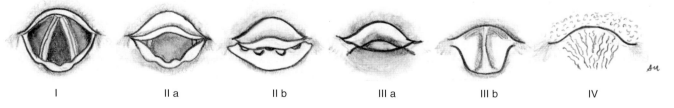

I	II a	II b	III a	III b	IV

Fig. 10.5 Laryngeal grades from conventional direct laryngoscopy based on the Cook–Yentis modification of the Lehane–Cormack categories. Grade *I* is a full view of the periglottic anatomy. Grades *II* and *III* have been subdivided into "a" and "b." Grade *IIa* shows the posterior ½ of the glottis, *IIb* reveals edge of epiglottis and arytenoids with minimal glottis, *IIIa* reveals only the leading edge of the epiglottis, *IIIb* shows a floppy and overhanging epiglottis, and grade *IV* reveals "no view" of periglottic structures or only the posterior pharyngeal wall (Courtesy of Anna Mort, AM)

beyond this point represents a very risky clinical situation for the critically ill patient with marginal cardiopulmonary reserve. Unrecognized airway management difficulties, combined with suboptimal oxygen reserves and marginal baseline PaO_2, with the added problem of a difficult mask ventilation with or without a difficult intubation, place the acutely ill patient at a much higher risk for hypoxemia and its related complications [16, 17]. Whether these are considered by the airway manager as major or minor, alone or in combination, they may lead to hypoxemia and initiate a rapid downward cascade toward patient injury. Hypoxemia, often the consequence of an airway-related event, is the one common link to altering the patient's already fragile physiologic state [13, 17].

Esophageal Intubation

Esophageal intubation (EI) is relatively common and usually without consequence in the elective setting. Its lack of recognition, however, is a primary factor in the occurrence of hypoxemia, regurgitation, and aspiration and, most notably, death and severe central neurological damage. The ASA Closed Claim Analysis and others considered the majority cases of unrecognized EI as preventable with better monitoring [1–4]. Indirect clinical signs of detecting tracheal tube location are imprecise and should be augmented by capnography or other similar technology such as a bulb syringe, esophageal detector device, or the passing of a bougie (to distinguish the tracheobronchial tree from the esophagus) [18]. Clinical signs such as auscultation of breath sounds, tube condensation, chest wall excretions, reservoir bag compliance and refilling, and tactile confirmation of the tube entering trachea each have shortcomings and difficulty with interpretation even under normal circumstances; this is reduced further in the difficult airway situation under emergent or urgent circumstances [18]. Capnography is considered "near failsafe" since it can be misinterpreted in the presence of low cardiac output, soiling of the detector, poor lighting conditions, bronchospasm, and the recent ingestion of carbonated beverages. "Failsafe" methods include viewing the tracheal tube pass between the vocal cords (impractical in 10–20 % of emergency patients) and fiber-optic verification (limitation based on blood/secretions, equipment availability, and experienced personnel). These two methods are only failsafe under perfect conditions. If esophageal intubation occurs by one intubation method, consideration should be given to an alternative intubation method or technique.

Regurgitation and Aspiration

Tracheobronchial aspiration of oral or gastric contents is always a concern with airway management, especially in the urgent/emergent setting. This higher incidence is achieved when the situation is emergent, the number of comorbidities and the severity of illness increase, the intubation occurs outside of the controlled setting of the operating room, or the person performing the intubation is less experienced. Usually, the aspirated material represents saliva or blood and has minimal clinical consequences. In the neurologically injured patient, aspiration of gastric contents may be seen secondarily due to regurgitation in a patient with incompetent laryngeal reflexes, often because of altered mental status, or the use of an anesthetic induction agent to facilitate intubation. In the operating room, the incidence of pulmonary aspiration of gastric contents ranged from 1.1 % in a series of 10,000 elective anesthetics of ASA Physical Status class I to 29 % in 10,000 emergency anesthetics in ASA Physical Status classes IV and V [19]. Although no specific data have been described in the neurologically injured patient, the incidence of gastric aspiration may be up to 30-fold more likely in emergency cases given the nature of these injuries, the higher degree of obtundation, and the lack of protective laryngeal reflexes. Hypoxemia from severe ventilation–perfusion (V/Q) mismatch is the most serious consequence of pulmonary aspiration of gastric contents. As a consequence of aspiration-induced alveolar capillary membrane damage, capillary leak can occur with an increasing loss of intravascular volume into the lung [20]. This fluid shift results in increased extravascular lung water, systemic hemoconcentration, hypotension, and tachycardia, potentially leading to hypovolemic shock further exacerbating the hypoxemia. The increase in pulmonary edema can also lead to coincident pulmonary hypertension and potential right-sided heart failure. Additionally, pulmonary hypertension may occur secondarily because of bronchospasm or the loss of functioning alveoli and subsequent increasing peak airway pressures eventually leading to left ventricular dysfunction [20]. In neurologically injured patients, pulmonary aspiration can contribute to secondary CNS injury through mechanisms of hypoxemia, hypotension, and pulmonary hypertension, leading to decreased cerebral venous return, thereby causing an acute increase in ICP.

As noted previously, aspiration of gastric contents into the tracheobronchial tree is fortunately a rare occurrence in the elective anesthesia setting. The frequency of perioperative pulmonary aspiration in adults and pediatric patients is approximately 1:2,600, with the risk 30-fold higher in the emergency setting and 5× higher in those with a higher anesthesia risk classification [21]. Though all ICU patients are at risk for this complication, for some the risk is much greater, such as those individuals receiving gastric feedings, with active vomiting and retching, upper GI bleeding, bowel obstruction, or other abdominal pathology and recent food ingestion. Though a rapid sequence intubation (RSI) is indicated in these clinical situations, certain patient presentations may supersede the rationale of rapidly obtaining the airway since difficulty may be predicted, e.g., the morbidly obese patient with a beard and a hard cervical collar (C3 burst fracture) with respiratory distress. The overall rate of regurgitation in the Hartford Hospital (1990–2011) emergency airway database was 4 %, with aspiration at 1.6 %. This substantially increases the risk of severe hypoxemia, bradycardia, and cardiac arrest. A risk reduction strategy including immediate availability of accessory airway devices and ETT verifying equipment influenced a reduction of regurgitation by 50 % and the rate of aspiration by 75 % at the authors' institution [13, 17, 21].

Mainstem Bronchus Intubation

Intubation of a mainstem bronchus (MSBI) occurs relatively frequently but is detected by initial chest auscultation and determining the appropriate depth of the ETT. If uncorrected, it may lead to hypoxemia, atelectasis, bronchospasm, coughing, and elevated peak inspiratory pressures. Fiber-optic evaluation is definitive and any of the referenced clinical signs should prompt its use. Chest radiography is quite helpful at the time the film is taken; however, an old radiograph is old news and a new radiograph is accurate at the time of development. Patient movement, e.g., following a portable radiograph, may be a significant contributing factor to ETT displacement [21].

Multiple Intubation Attempts

As the number of attempts increases, so does the incidence of airway complications: trauma, bleeding, edema, mucosal disruption, and the transformation of an airway that may be "ventilated but not intubated" to one that becomes "cannot ventilate, cannot intubate" (CVCI). Limiting the number of laryngoscopic attempts to two or three, at which point alternative airway techniques or the use of accessory airway devices is incorporated to secure the airway, is a prudent strategy [13, 17]. It has been demonstrated that the rate of complications is directly related to the number of laryngoscopic attempts during emergency airway management, specifically increasing markedly with the second attempt and beyond [13, 17, 22–24].

A high level of suspicion should be given to all critically ill patients who require emergency airway management, and each should be regarded as potentially an "unrecognized difficult airway." A limit of one or two attempts by the junior airway manager under "optimal conditions" before moving to a secondary plan, if appropriate, or allowing one or two attempts by the senior level airway manager before turning to an alternative strategy seems prudent in light of the complications associated with repetitive laryngoscopy. Indeed, one may argue that a difficult intubation is not the place for a relative novice to learn how to handle the airway; we might consider allowing them to watch, but not to be the operator.

If laryngoscopy and intubation fails on the first or second attempts, aborting conventional intubation methods and pursuing a rescue approach are warranted [13, 17, 22–24]. Further, the consequences of repetitive laryngoscopic attempts, e.g., swelling, may lower the success rate of the alternative airway rescue techniques, e.g., LMA, Combitube, and FOB, and may impinge on successful mask ventilation.

Multiple laryngoscopic attempts may eventually yield a secure airway, but the price for obtaining such an airway is the possibility of tissue edema, bleeding, worsening mask ventilation capabilities, and potentially the loss of the airway [13]. The risk of intervening hypoxia, regurgitation, esophageal intubation(s), and aspiration and the hemodynamic consequences of these airway mishaps, i.e., bradycardia, hypertension, tachycardia, hypotension, dysrhythmias, and cardiac arrest, are reasons enough to consider limiting attempts to two or three [13, 17].

The Hemodynamic Response to Airway Management

Hyperdynamic Response

A hyperdynamic response may reflect wakefulness; the magnitude, vigor, and extent of the airway procedure; underlying hypertension and cardiovascular disease; intravascular volume status; the underlying sympathetic outflow; any related renal and cerebral pathology; preoperative medication; and/or the functional reserve of the patient. Other clinical causes and the underlying pathophysiology of the patient are certainly relevant.

A brief increase in heart rate (HR) and blood pressure (BP) immediately after commencing with the manipulation of their airway, followed by a brief hyperdynamic response usually, leads to one of three hemodynamic outcomes: (1) continued hyperdynamic parameters, (2) return toward pre-intubation baseline, or (3) a sudden or gradual reduction in the BP, often to the point that volume administration and/or vasopressors are required. It is noteworthy that the young, the traumatized, and the neurological-based disease patients tend to experience an impressive hyperdynamic response (hypertension and tachycardia) to laryngoscopy and intubation [22].

Ongoing pain, anxiety, and wakefulness or general underlying pathology (e.g., CVA, renal, cardiovascular, or diabetic disease) may contribute to persistent tachycardia and/or hypertension. Careful titration of nitroglycerin, sodium nitroprusside, calcium channel blockers, or beta-blockers may be required. Reduced dosing is imperative in the presence of preexisting hypovolemia, an exaggerated response to cardiovascular depression, and in those who are experiencing only a brief upswing in blood pressure. Aggressive treatment may introduce further hemodynamic compromise when the therapy outlasts the self-limited post-intubation hypertension. The hyperdynamic response to airway instrumentation frequently accompanies head injury, intracerebral bleed, cerebral vascular accident, or an active seizure disorder.

Mindful of the preexisting comorbidities and the current clinical deterioration prompting intubation, the airway manager's judgment and experience will influence the medication choices and techniques to prepare the patient for airway instrumentation. The major challenge is to select the agents that will achieve the goal of blunting, attenuating, or blocking the laryngoscopy-related hyperdynamic response—typically for only a brief period of time—with minimal subsequent influence on post-intubation hypotension. Strategies are best tailored to the individual patient's needs, based on the experience and judgment of the airway manager, rather a standard intubation protocol (i.e., etomidate and succinylcholine) being utilized with each and every patient. Neuromuscular blocking agents (NMBAs) may have a major impact on the dosing of induction agents and the subsequent need for vasoactive support independent of any direct or indirect vasodilatory effects. In the critically ill patient who is able to maintain blood pressure by concurrent agitation, struggling, straining, and work of breathing, elimination of these efforts through the use of NMBAs may drop their BP independent of any direct or indirect vasodilatory effects of the NMB [24].

Hypotension

The incidence of post-intubation hypotension in the emergency setting is the most common of the hemodynamic alterations. The aggressive use of induction agent may potentiate the reduction in BP following airway manipulation, particularly if no additional stimulation is provided post-intubation. Positive-pressure ventilation and the application of PEEP plus any vasodilatation and myocardial depression from induction/anesthetic agents may contribute to post-intubation hypotension. This response is accentuated in incidence and magnitude in the critically ill patient who is struggling with underlying cardiopulmonary deterioration, acid–base imbalance, septic-induced hemodynamic alterations, hemorrhage, hypovolemia, and other maladies. Post-intubation hypotension may require crystalloid resuscitation or a vasoactive agent (ephedrine, phenylephrine, dopamine, norepinephrine) [24].

Post-intubation hypotension appears more frequent in the sickest of the critically ill ICU patients, especially those with sepsis and cardiovascular injury or dysfunction (MI, CHF, and cardiac tamponade). Conversely, the patient with any form of CNS injury tends to suffer less frequently from post-intubation hypotension but is hampered by the hypertensive-tachycardic response [24].

Bradycardia and Cardiac Arrest

Though tachycardia is much more common with airway manipulation, patients taking certain cardiac medications, propofol, and narcotics and with a reactive gag/cough reflex may react to airway manipulation with mild to abrupt slowing of the heart rate. Pre-intubation bradycardia may exist in hypertensive disease of the elderly, the physically fit, and those with severe hypoxemia or with the Cushing reflex. Vigorous laryngoscopy and/or intubation, inadvertent esophageal intubation, stimulation of the gag reflex, or when significant airway-related complications arise during the course of securing the emergent airway with severe or prolonged hypoxemia may lead to bradycardia and cardiac arrest [13, 17, 24]. Moreover, progressive bradycardia has been noted to precede intraoperative cardiac arrests in the majority of cases. Post-intubation bradycardia may portend catastrophic pathology, such as a tension pneumothorax or an unrecognized esophageal intubation [17].

As the number of airway-associated complications mount during difficult laryngoscopy and intubation, with concurrent hypoxemia, the incidence of bradycardia dramatically increases, often accompanying severe hypotension requiring therapy. The initial sympathetic outflow stimulated by a moderate reduction in oxygen tension is overwhelmed by the parasympathetic influence with medullary ischemia if hypoxemia is ongoing or worsening (PaO_2 less than 30 mmHg).

The aggressive teaching of airway management techniques and incorporating the standards of a designated algorithm (i.e., ASA Difficult Airway Algorithm) outside of the operating room may decrease the incidence of hypoxemic-related bradycardia and cardiac arrest. One simple strategy—prior to the introduction of video laryngoscopy—involving direct laryngoscopy supplemented by an airway catheter (bougie), the LMA, Combitube, and fiber-optic bronchoscopy as needed, reduced the incidence of bradycardic episodes and cardiac arrest by 50 % [17].

A difficult airway, complicated by severe, prolonged hypoxemia and its resultant bradycardic response, will often culminate in full cardiac arrest. The Hartford Hospital database suggests that while bradycardia occurs in 3 % of the emergency intubations, overall, 85 % of these episodes are associated with hypoxemia typically associated with multiple laryngoscopic attempts (3+), esophageal intubation, regurgitation, and aspiration. The incidence of cardiac arrest remains around 1.5 %, clearly 150-fold higher than the incidence in the more controlled operating room. Contributing factors for cardiac arrest include profound hypoxemia and the same events that result in bradycardia [13, 17, 22, 24].

Conversely, non-airway-related arrest may be incited by ETT obstruction due to secretions or displacement, tension pneumothorax, massive pulmonary thromboembolism, medication-induced cardiovascular collapse, and hemodynamic deterioration in the cardiac population.

Airway Management Strategy in the Neuro ICU

A management strategy organized in algorithmic form should facilitate a systematic approach to the airway in the NeuroICU, decrease response time, and reduce the potential for an adverse outcome. An organized plan of attack is helpful for patients with a known or recognized difficult airway prior to the first intubation attempt. Likewise, the uncooperative patient who refuses airway intervention or those who are rapidly deteriorating due to CNS pathology or hypoxia will benefit from a plan. An airway management strategy is, however, more crucial and particularly beneficial when a difficult airway is unrecognized or underappreciated by the airway team, yet becomes problematic following induction of anesthesia/unconsciousness/paralysis. An abridged algorithmic airway management strategy based on several established sources such as the 2003 iteration of the American Society of Anesthesiologist Difficult Airway Algorithm is summarized in Fig. 10.6 [2, 3, 7].

The ASA algorithm can be categorized into three separate brackets of decision making based on the patient's clinical condition, the airway status, equipment available, and the skill and judgment of the airway manager. Firstly, the airway team should consider the likelihood and impact of basic airway management problems regarding (1) difficult mask ventilation, (2) difficult intubation, (3) the patient's ability to cooperate (especially if an awake/lightly sedated approach is required), and (4) estimating any difficulty obtaining surgical airway access. It is abundantly clear that the providers should make every effort to continue oxygen delivery throughout the timeframe that airway manipulation is taking place. Following one's assessment of the previously discussed four clinical situations, one should consider the merits and relative feasibility of basic management schema, namely, three primary factors to consider that will determine one' approach to securing the airway (Table 10.5).

Following assessment of these factors, the primary and backup strategies may be developed and then executed. For example, in an obese patient with a halo vest for cervical instability and known to be difficult to manage, one might strategize that an awake approach using a noninvasive method (e.g., fiber-optic bronchoscopy [FOB]) while maintaining spontaneous ventilation would be warranted. Conversely, an acutely dyspneic patient with a fungating oral cancer invading the mandible and floor of mouth causing restricted access to the airway may best be managed awake, maintaining spontaneous ventilation coupled with an elective/urgent surgical access to secure the airway.

Following one's development of a primary and backup strategy, the ASA algorithm suggests the pursuit of management choices be essentially based on the teams' ability to provide adequate mask ventilation. If, following induction of anesthesia (assuming unconsciousness, apnea, with or without neuromuscular blockade), intubation attempts are unsuccessful, the defining moment that directs further airway care is whether or not life-sustaining mask ventilation can be maintained with SpO_2 greater than 90–93 %. If mask ventilation is adequate (facemask or LMA-SGA), then one enters the "nonemergent pathway" by virtue of the fact that one has time to obtain equipment or use a method that may consume several minutes for setup and execution, e.g., retrograde wire and FOB (Fig. 10.6). Otherwise the lack of, or suboptimal, ventilation/oxygenation places one in the "emergency pathway" since securing the airway by any means is required immediately; only those methods that can be accomplished rapidly are warranted (retrograde wire and FOB take too long to setup and execute). Thus, the inability to successfully utilize a BVM device and/or intubate (emergency pathway) may be salvaged by the LMA-SGA. If the LMA-SGA is successful, the patient then enters the nonemergency pathway. The LMA could be used solely for oxygenation and then VL or an optical stylet could be attempted (but would require LMA removal), or the LMA-SGA may provide access to the trachea via FOB or blinds attempts, if appropriate Fastrach LMA™ (LMA North America, San Diego, CA). When seconds count and one encounters a "cannot ventilate, cannot intubate" (CVCI, emergency pathway) scenario, meaning ventilation outright fails or is nonlife supporting (including use of BVM or LMA-SGA) and intubation attempts fail (DL, VL), then few options other than rapid surgical access to the airway are indicated.

Patient Preparation Before Attempting Intubation

Regardless of the intubation technique planned or the urgency for intubation, preoxygenation and denitrogenation with 100 % oxygen, to maximize the time to hemoglobin desaturation, should be always be attempted before using an induction agent. The apnea time necessary to reach a critical

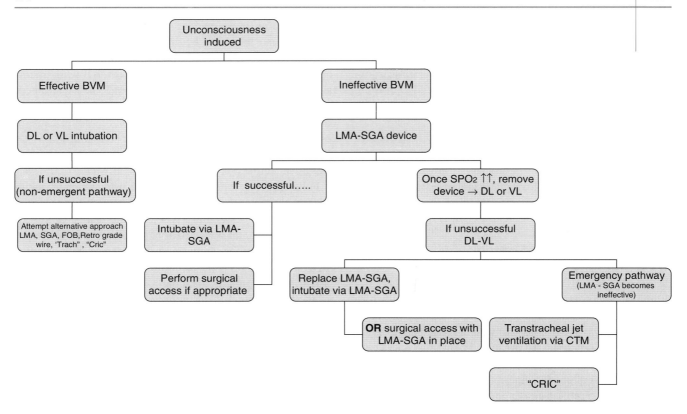

Fig. 10.6 Airway management algorithm for the NeuroICU patient population with its foundation based on the ASA Difficult Airway Algorithm but modified to reflect the role of video laryngoscopy and advanced techniques of intubating via the LMA-SGA devices. *LMA* laryngeal mask airway, *SGA* supraglottic airway, *DL* direct laryngoscopy, *VL* video laryngoscopy, *BVM* bag-valve-mask ventilation, *Cric* cricothyrotomy, *Trach* tracheostomy, *CTM* cricothyroid membrane

Table 10.5 Initial considerations of a difficult airway strategy

Awake intubation versus intubation following induction of anesthesia/sedation
Noninvasive approach to intubation (DL, VL, FOB, LMA, etc.) versus invasive (surgical access)
Preserve spontaneous ventilation versus ablate spontaneous ventilation (paralysis, heavy sedation)

SpO_2 (less than 90 %) after an induction dose of an hypnotic agent cannot always be predicted with ease, and it is expected to be decreased in the critically ill and neurologically injured patient due to a decreased functional residual capacity (FRC), pulmonary dysfunction, or increased metabolic rate. An FiO_2 of 1.0 is used to attempt rapid and full tissue denitrogenation. Commonly used techniques of 3–4 min of preoxygenation with 100 % oxygen are quite effective in the elective setting but often fail to raise the oxygen tension above the 80–120 mmHg level in the critically ill. Extension of the preoxygenation period to 6 or 8 min provides little improvement [16, 17]. This limitation of oxygenation highlights the significant risk of hypoxemia when mask ventilation or intubation proves difficult or is delayed. The likelihood of recovery of spontaneous ventilation following the ultrashort-acting succinylcholine should give the operator pause since even in patients with healthy lungs, the average time to critical desaturation (less than 90 %) is usually shorter than the mean recovery time from an intubating dose of succinylcholine.

The desired physiologic change may require several minutes to achieve (less time with controlled ventilation than with spontaneous ventilation) and is only possible with a tight mask fit on the patient to prevent entrainment of any nitrogen-rich air. Measurements of end-tidal oxygen concentration (EtO_2) are an excellent indicator of the adequacy of denitrogenation, but are typically not available in the ICU setting. Adequate preoxygenation and denitrogenation are particularly important if the use of an NMB agent, including the ultrashort-acting succinylcholine, to facilitate intubation is contemplated.

The mean duration of apnea until critical desaturation is typically between 3 and 5 min, under optimal conditions. This time to desaturation is obviously less than even the mean recovery time from an intubating dose of succinylcholine, approximately 10 min for the standard 1 mg/kg intubating dose [25]. Using smaller than standard doses of succinylcholine—remember that the ED_{95} of this agent is

0.25 mg/kg and this is the dose we recommend—may allow adequate intubating conditions and possibly hasten the return to spontaneous ventilatory efforts. However, the time may still be greater than the time to critical desaturation even in the adequately preoxygenated patient. One simply cannot trust that the return of life-sustaining spontaneous ventilation following succinylcholine will occur in a timely manner; hence, the use of an LMA or other advanced device is often needed. One will quickly move to a surgical airway if reasonable efforts at securing ventilation and oxygenation fail or remain suboptimal.

Other factors that influence rapid desaturation when intubation is attempted in the neurologically impaired patient must be factored into the equation. Critically ill patients are at higher risk of rapid desaturation because of the combination of increased oxygen consumption, V/Q mismatch, and decreased oxygen delivery [25]. Obese patients, as well as those with underlying pulmonary disease, will have a decreased FRC and some degree of concurrent V/Q mismatch. A low FRC may be further complicated by the supine position, the induction of general anesthesia, and the neuromuscular blockade. In the pediatric population and the critically ill, especially those septic or febrile, metabolic rate and oxygen consumption rates are always higher.

Aspiration Prophylaxis

Aspiration precautions should be considered in all critically ill patients from the time of admission and certainly before intubation. Many recommendations exist to minimize aspiration potential: gastric acid neutralization, elevation of the head of the bed, post-pyloric tube feedings, and subglottic suctioning are a few of the clinically proven methods in intubated and extubated patients. Chemical neutralization of gastric secretions with sodium citrate (15–30 mL by mouth) before intubation is often impossible due to a lack of adequate level of consciousness and/or protective airway reflexes; hence, the aforementioned measures are of greater importance.

The immediate use of H_2 blockers, proton pump inhibitors, or metoclopramide does not provide adequate suppression of acid production or superior gastric emptying in these patients because of the drugs' slower onset of action. Therefore, protection against acid aspiration relies mainly upon effective mechanical interventions such as cricoid pressure, whose effectiveness is questionable but has been maintained as a standard of care. Additionally, a patient's NPO status should be ascertained to further minimize the risk of aspiration. Adherence to the standards of NPO status based on offerings of the American Society of Anesthesiologists guidelines should be adhered to when possible. When clinical deterioration is taking place at a slower, yet predictable, pace and intubation is anticipated, then oral intake and enteral feedings should be suspended prior to any intubation attempt.

Achieving Effective Mask Ventilation

Ventilation by BVM is the fundamental step in managing the airway. While not protective of the airway, effective mask ventilation will prevent hypoxia and hypercapnia; patients do not die because they cannot be intubated; they die because they were not oxygenated and ventilated. A high-flow, 100 % oxygen source must be available to provide sufficient gas to compensate for facemask leaks and allow for the generation of sufficient positive pressure to overcome respiratory system resistance to gas flow. In preparation for mask ventilation and intubation, adequate positioning, including a jaw thrust maneuver and neck extension to facilitate a "sniffing position," is imperative in most patients. Aligning the oropharyngeal axis, laryngeal axis, and tracheal axis (Fig. 10.7) is typically necessary to optimize visualization with conventional laryngoscopy. Improving one's "line of sight" is imperative with DL (Fig. 10.8). Adjusting the patient's position in bed and ramping of the (obese) patient in bed with towels or pillows will also facilitate access to the airway to optimize bag ventilation (Fig. 10.9a, b). These options are not always feasible, particularly if neck injury is present or suspected, a condition which will be discussed separately. Proper seal of the facemask is paramount and should be obtained by properly seating the correct size mask on the face and adjusting the cushion tension by adding or removing air with a syringe via the valve in the mask. The mask should be sized to cover the nose at the level of the bridge of the nose and the mouth just above the chin and held tightly. While purely theoretical, circumferential mask straps should not be applied in situations involving increased ICP because of a potential risk of venous outflow obstruction from the brain, thus further increasing ICP. Similar to the use of CPAP or BiPAP masks, the accumulation of positive pressure from the application of a mask without a "pop-off" valve can further decrease venous return.

A number of alternative methods can be used to overcome lack of seal due to facial hair. Applying gauze soaked in petroleum jelly or matting the hair with a water-based lubricant can help to fill facial contours under the mask cushion. "Homemade" devices have also been used, such as plastic film over the facial hair or even a defibrillator contact pad with a small hole cut in the middle at the level of the mouth opening. While ventilating the patient, one must pay careful attention that the chest does not rise excessively, as this usually implies lung overinflation. The increased insufflation pressures created serve to increase the risk of gastric insufflation due to iatrogenic mechanical incompetence of the

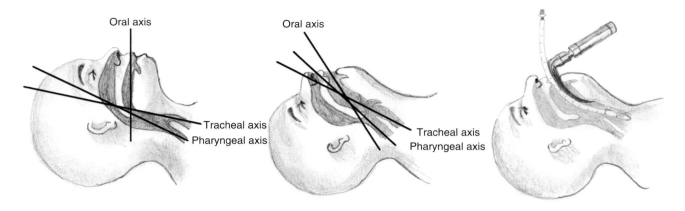

Fig. 10.7 The three airway axes that are best aligned but often are restricted due to trauma and preexisting diseases such as rheumatoid arthritis, osteoarthritis, prior surgical fixation, and obesity (Courtesy of Anna Mort, AM)

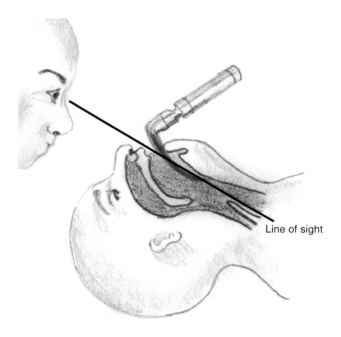

Fig. 10.8 "Line of sight" offered by conventional laryngoscopy. This may appear adequate in this view; however, the confined and narrowed view in even the "normal" airway due to reliance on the human eye's field of vision limits one's ability to visualize a full view of the glottic structures in many cases. This is particularly true with a small mouth, large teeth, large tongue, and a narrowed pharyngeal opening due to a short neck, edema, swelling, secretions, or redundant tissues seen in the obese and those with obstructive sleep apnea. VL technology widens one's "line of sight" (Courtesy of Anna Mort, AM)

lower esophageal sphincter (LES) and decreased venous return with hypotension due to rising intrathoracic pressures.

The addition of a pressure manometer to the ventilation circuit allows for real-time airway pressure monitoring in an effort to keep airway pressures less than 20 cm H_2O, thus minimizing the risk of gastric insufflation, because the LES

is assumed to be intact at pressures below this. Increasing gastric insufflation volumes will displace the diaphragm cranially, further decreasing the FRC prior to the intubation attempt. An inspiratory time of at least 1.5 s and an I:E ratio of at least 1:2.5 minimize peak airway pressures (PIP) and decrease the risk of breath stacking and auto-PEEP, thereby lowering intrathoracic pressures, as well as decreasing the risk of aspiration. Finally, even though it remains somewhat questionable as far as effectiveness in preventing regurgitation, and despite its potential contribution to difficulty with ventilation and intubation in some patients, cricoid pressure should be considered standard of care. It is perceived to be the most effective maneuver to limit gastric insufflation during ventilation of the unprotected airway.

Overcoming Airway Obstruction Due to Soft Tissue Collapse

The upper airway of the patient with altered mental status often obstructs, particularly in the obese and in those with obstructive sleep apnea (OSA). Obtundation, stupor, or unconsciousness only further complicates the anatomical issues associated with obesity, such as decreased FRC, redundant oropharyngeal tissues, increased neck circumference, and decreased range of motion in the cervical spine. Various clinical signs may be noted during airway obstruction (Table 10.6). A rocking motion of the chest wall and abdomen (paradoxical breathing), along with visual evidence of "accessory muscle" use, such as neck retraction when spontaneous ventilation is present, correlates well with airway obstruction. Except in cases of cardiopulmonary arrest, the presence of expired CO_2 (EtCO$_2$) reliably demonstrates ventilation regardless of the presence of partial obstruction.

Several methods may be used to overcome upper airway obstruction, although some are limited to the patient without

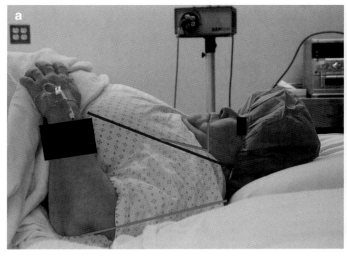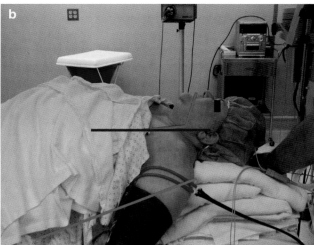

Fig. 10.9 (**a**) This super morbidly obese patent (BMI of 54, ht 5'2" 295 lb) is in standard "sniff" position with pillow under her head. *Green bar* represents angle of torso on bed. *Red bar* represents the oro-hypopharyngeal axis. *Blue bar* represents the "ear (tragus) to sternum angle." Limited access to the airway is evident in this picture. (**b**) The same patient in an optimal induction position by building an angled torso–neck–head ramp with blankets. Note the exaggerated *green bar* showing the improved torso angle. Note the marked improvement in access to the mouth, oral cavity, oropharynx, and neck structures (*red* and *blue bars*) compared to (**a**) Note the level *blue bar* representing the more optimized "ear to sternum angle"

Table 10.6 Clinical signs of airway obstruction during positive- and negative-pressure ventilation

Auditory	Gurgling in epiglottic area (esophageal ventilation)
	Crowing or stridor (laryngeal)
	Stridor (laryngeal)
	Snoring (pharyngeal)
	Wheezing (small airway)
	Absent breath sounds
Tactile	Decreased reservoir compliance
	Decreased expiratory return
	Airway vibration
	Large facemask leak
Visual	Decreased chest wall/inward abdominal excursion
	Accessory muscle recruitment
	Puffed cheeks/neck
	Abdominal rocking
	Abdominal distention
	Cyanosis
	Nasal flaring
	Suprasternal notch retraction
Objective	Increased airway pressure
	Absence of CO_2 waveform on capnograph
	Low measured expired volume
	Hypoxemia (pulse oximeter)

Reproduced with permission of Elsevier from Gravenstein and Kirby [98]

significant neck pathology or trauma. Lifting the chin pad while applying a jaw thrust can straighten the oropharyngeal axis and mobilize the anterior pharyngeal soft tissue to facilitate ventilation (Figs. 10.10a, b and 10.11). Early insertion of a plastic oral airway or nasal airway (if not contraindicated) may reduce the risk of the tongue falling backward against the soft palate. Finally, two-person (or three-person if needed) BVM ventilation may allow for a more rapid establishment of a combination of successful interventions especially in edentulous patients, the obese, OSA patients, those with facial abnormalities, and those who challenge the airway manager with difficult mask fit. Removing the pillows from behind the head may markedly improve patency.

Assuming that noninvasive maneuvers have been attempted, failed or difficult mask ventilation should yield to the early placement of a supraglottic airway device, e.g., LMA, before significant desaturation takes place. Moreover, a difficult or failed mask ventilation may be immediately remedied by attempting tracheal intubation assuming the patient is accepting of laryngoscopy [2, 3, 7, 8].

Achieving the Best Laryngoscopic View

The patient should always be placed in optimal position before any airway procedure. In most patients, the "sniffing" position (slight flexion of the cervical spine and extension of the atlantooccipital joint) is the best way to align the oropharyngeal, laryngeal, and tracheal axes (Fig. 10.7). In an obese patient, the sniffing position can be better obtained by placing an inclined pad under both the shoulders and the head, the so-called ramping (Fig. 10.9a, b). Elevation of the shoulders and scapulae, to the point where the sternum is parallel with the tragus of the ear, allows for better extension of the

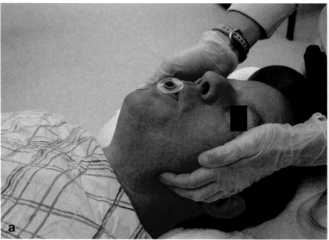
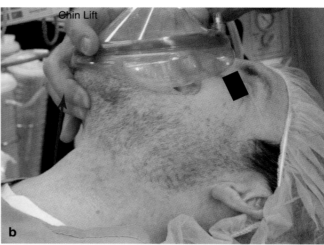

Fig. 10.10 (a) To optimize placement of the oral airway, advancement of the mandible often allows the device to "fall" in behind the tongue. (b) Following application of the facemask, a chin lift is essentially a lifting action to bring the face and mandible to the mask rather than pushing the mask onto the facial structures

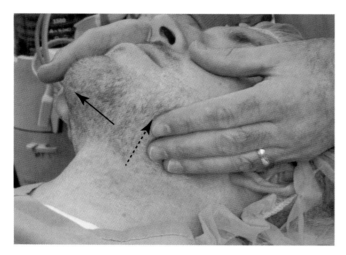

Fig. 10.11 Noninvasive maneuvers to assist with mask ventilation efforts include. *1* Neck extension at the atlantooccipital joint, *2* chin lift (*solid arrow*) with mask application, and *3* jaw thrust (*dashed arrow*) by placement of the hands at the angle of the mandible with force applied to advance the mandible forward (anteriorly)

neck in obese patients with redundant subcutaneous tissue. Current mattress choices in the ICU that help avert skin breakdown and/or improve wound healing are typically detrimental to the patient's optimal positioning, especially in the presence of obesity. In the ICU or ED, temporary removal of the bed rails or frames and the head of the bed should always be done to facilitate operator access to the airway. Additionally, with time, patients have a tendency to "change" their position in bed—that is, sliding toward the foot of the bed—placement should be adjusted to optimize operator success. Each encounter will differ due to many types of bed in use throughout critical care. It is helpful to familiarize yourself with each bed's operations before an emergency occurs.

Visualization of the larynx can be optimized through external manipulation of the trachea and thyroid cartilage, usually applied by the operator's right hand or by an assistant. Though this maneuver is distinctly different from the application of cricoid pressure, the end result may be the same. The so-called optimal external laryngeal manipulation (OELM) and the backward, upward, rightward laryngeal pressure (BURP) [26] maneuvers describe, respectively, the American and Canadian approaches to external manipulation of the larynx in order to improve vocal cord visualization during laryngoscopy; either of these can be a very useful maneuver to enhance visualization of the larynx under difficult conditions (Fig. 10.12). OELM is described as posterior and cephalic pressure over the thyroid or cricoid cartilage. The majority of the time, the best view is obtained simply by pressing the thyroid cartilage posteriorly. The BURP maneuver implies the manual displacement of the larynx posteriorly against the cervical vertebrae, then superiorly and as far as possible to the right. Both these maneuvers are indicated in direct, indirect, and video laryngoscopy grades 2 through 4, usually improving the view by at least one grade. Of note, the application of "cricoid pressure" may, indeed, deter ventilation or viewing of the periglottic anatomy. In such cases, release of the applied pressure to assist with identification of the larynx or improved ventilation is warranted.

Choosing the Laryngoscope Blade

If you ask ten anesthesiologists, you will likely receive ten differing opinions as to which laryngoscope blade is appropriate. Two simple answers exist. First, the blade with which you are most comfortable is your first choice. Secondly, the blade which the patient requires is your

ultimate blade for success. Macintosh (curved) blades are recommended when the patient has an adequate mouth opening, larger tongue, or redundant subcutaneous tissue with adequate anterior laryngeal free space. On the other hand, Miller (straight) blades—due to the blade's low profile—may be optimal for visualization of the vocal cords in patients with a small mouth opening, a smaller anterior free space, large incisors, or a large (whatever the reason), floppy epiglottis. A commonly used adjunct device for direct laryngoscopy is the gum elastic stylet or bougie. The tip of the bougie may be blindly passed under the epiglottis and through the glottis into the trachea to provide "Seldinger" access to the airway but must be performed in a gentle non-forceful manner (Fig. 10.13). Counterclockwise rotation of the ETT by 90–180° is recommended when passing over the bougie so as to avoid impingement of the ETT tip on the right vocal cord or arytenoid. Passage of the bougie with subsequent intubation of the esophagus may occur since it is typically incorporated when glottic visualization is obscured (grade 3a, 3b, Fig. 10.5). Tactile feedback from the bougie "clicking" on the tracheal rings may be helpful but is unreliable and inconsistent. An assistant applying cricoid pressure or OELM may help to bring the glottis into view. However, appreciation of the carinal (about 28–34 cm depth) or bronchial divisions (about 30–38 cm) while gently passing the bougie tip consistently differentiates trachea from esophagus. Excessive force to place the ETT should never be applied, as doing so may result in cord displacement, arytenoid dislocation, or even penetration of the pyriform fossa or tracheal rupture. The gum elastic bougie can be used to limit the extension of the neck in patients with a neck injury in the

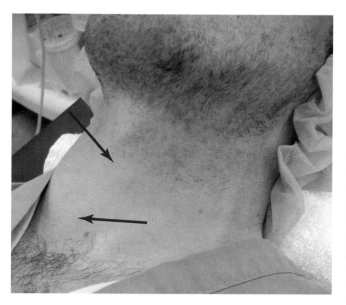

Fig. 10.12 Illustration of the location of two key landmarks on the neck. The thyroid prominence (*upper arrow*) is visible and easily palpable in most males and less so in females. The glottic opening sits behind the thyroid cartilage hence during laryngoscopy, optimal external laryngeal manipulation (of the thyroid cartilage) helps to improve laryngeal viewing. This is also true of backward, upward, and rightward external displacement of the larynx or BURP (modified). Conversely, the cricoid cartilage (*lower arrow*) is where Sellick's maneuver (cricoid pressure) is applied to potentially reduce passive regurgitation but may either improve or worsen glottic viewing and/or mask ventilation

Fig. 10.13 Airway catheter or "bougie" alongside an ETT. Note the 30° angulated "coude" tip that assists with advancement underneath the posterior surface of the epiglottis. It should only be used when anatomical landmarks exist such as the leading edge of the epiglottis. An overhanging or floppy epiglottis (grade IIIb) is less forgiving than grade IIIa since the bougie must be either used to lift the epiglottis or maneuvered past it on its way toward the glottic opening

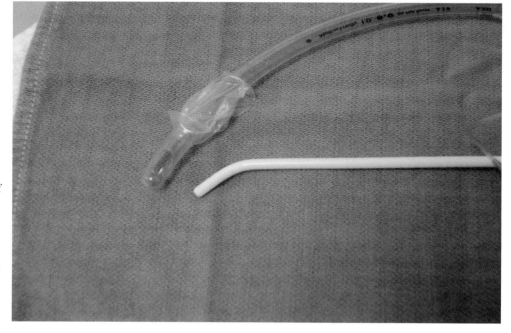

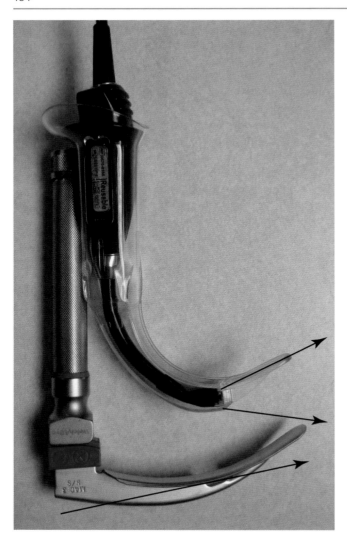

Fig. 10.14 Comparison of the "line of sight" of DL versus VL. The confined view with the curved Macintosh blade is limited in many respects to the more panoramic, expanded viewing on the video monitor (not shown) of the GlideScope® (Verathon, Bothell, WA) by virtue of the video chip technology located in the distal tip of the GlideScope baton which lies within the disposable clear plastic intubating blade. VL offers an improved ability to "see around the corner"

presence of a hard cervical collar. A number of laryngoscopic blades have recently been developed to improve access to the vocal cords when the larynx is anterior; these are often advantageous in difficult airway cases. Video laryngoscopy has evolved to offer the practitioner an improved angle of viewing when compared to the typical "line of sight" offered by conventional DL methods (Fig. 10.14). While their explosion onto the market occurred subsequent to the release of the current ASA difficult airway algorithm, they have become an integral part of many specialists' management techniques when a difficult airway is encountered. This omission will likely be rectified with the next difficult airway management algorithm update [27].

Video Laryngoscopy

A conventional laryngoscope has become the standard airway management tool despite the limitation of providing only a limited view through the mouth and being dependent on the operator's "line of sight." Secondly, this view is available only to the operator, thus limiting teaching airway management with a student. Moreover, an assistant applying OLEM or the BURP maneuver may not receive needed feedback of their attempts to improve glottic visualization. The advent of rigid fiber-optic laryngoscope (Bullard laryngoscope® (Gyrus ACMI, Southborough, MA), the UpsherScope® (Mercury Medical, Clearwater, FL), and the Wu scope® (Achi Corp., Fremont, CA, and Asahi Optical Co.-Pentax, Tokyo, Japan)) offered a great advance in glottic visualization in the difficult airway patient when compared to DL. While they are relatively easy to use, the cost may have suppressed their use. More recently, conventionally shaped blades and those with angles of 25–65° have been equipped with a camera incorporated into the blade so that the image may be displayed on a monitor (Fig. 10.15a–c). The advantages of the video display are magnification of airway anatomy, better coordination between airway team members with airway manipulation, and the ability to actually teach the student, as both parties may observe airway anatomy. Further refinements include blade shape (50–65° as compared to 25–30° with conventional blades) to improve viewing, combined with improved video and hardware components—altering size and thus portability—quality of imaging, battery source, and cost that have led to increased deployment of video laryngoscopy (VL). Further modifications include non-channeled (requiring free-handed passing of ETT as in the Storz C-MAC® (Karl Storz, Tuttlingen, Germany), GlideScope® (Verathon, Bothell, WA), and McGrath® (Aircraft Medical, Edinburgh, Scotland) models (Fig. 10.16)) versus channeled models (built-in channel on the blade to assist with passage of the ETT, e.g., Airtraq® Optical Laryngoscope (Prodol, Vizcaya, Spain), Pentax AWS (Fig. 10.17)).

A third category of advanced airway devices are those based on an optical stylet design. Essentially a "bougie with an eyepiece," these devices allow the practitioner to view airway anatomy and guide the ETT into the trachea. While designed to be advanced into the airway with only a jaw thrust and lingual (tongue) retraction using one's hand, while the stylet is piloted into the hypopharynx and trachea, redundant tissues and an enlarged tongue, which may impede placement, are easily displaced by the lifting action of conventional laryngoscopy and may improve the ease of optical stylet placement. Several manufacturers have produced relatively low-cost models, compared to the VL devices, offering everything from basic eyepiece visualization through the stylet to more advanced video screen technology (Fig. 10.18a, b).

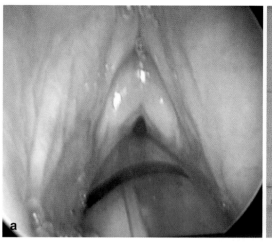
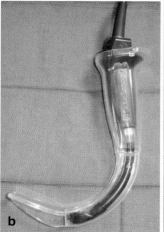
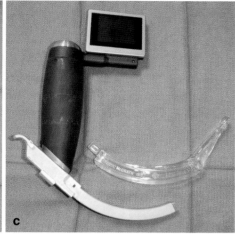

Fig. 10.15 (**a–c**) Two of the many VL models on the market. The GlideScope® (**a, b**) (Verathon, Bothell, WA) disposable blade encasing the video baton with its separate video screen. The McGrath® VL (**c**) (Aircraft Medical, Edinburgh, Scotland) is portable and easily carried, has a detachable blade, and is battery powered. Its attached video screen is much smaller but conveniently located to minimize looking away from the patient and their airway

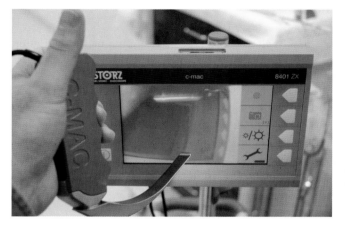

Fig. 10.16 The Storz C-MAC® (Karl Storz, Tuttlingen, Germany) video system provides a less extreme angle of its curved blade as compared to what GlideScope® (Verathon, Bothell, WA) and McGrath® (Aircraft Medical, Edinburgh, Scotland) offer. Subsequently, the other manufacturers now are offering VL blades that replicate the more conventional "curved" Macintosh blade. This combines the gold standard curved blade with video imaging

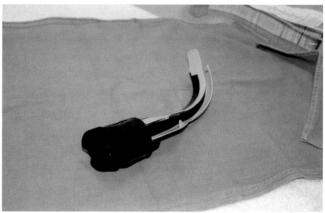

Fig. 10.17 Airtraq® Optical Laryngoscope (Prodol, Vizcaya, Spain). This single-use, transportable channeled VL device is loaded with an ETT within its channel. The operator must maneuver the ETT a much shorter distance compared to the non-channeled models. Though disposable and inexpensive, it offers a clip-on video camera for group viewing and recording

Further, the VL and optical stylets offer wide-spectrum 2D imaging when compared to the restricted view with conventional laryngoscopy methods. In addition to the extreme-angled blades (50–65°) that improve viewing in most difficult airways, VL manufacturers are offering devices with the standard angle of the DL blades. Their role in teaching airway skills will be immense, yet their use in the difficult airway remains to be determined [28–30]. An important airway caveat regarding this advanced technology is each device requires instruction, education, and practice to understand its limitations and indications and to learn how to trouble shoot. They should not be used in an urgent or emergent setting by the inexperienced operator.

VL technology allows improved viewing with less reliance on accurate aligning of the oral, pharyngeal, and laryngeal axes as we do with standard laryngoscopy. Of note, the relatively expensive up-front purchase price of most VL devices with the ongoing purchase of disposable blades can be cushioned by a disposable device that is relatively inexpensive, the Airtraq® Optical Laryngoscope (Prodol, Vizcaya, Spain) (Fig. 10.17). It is a single-use, channeled, optical laryngoscope designed to provide a view of the glottic opening without aligning the oral, pharyngeal, and laryngeal axes. Three main advantages with this device are that it is relatively cost effective, portable, and disposable.

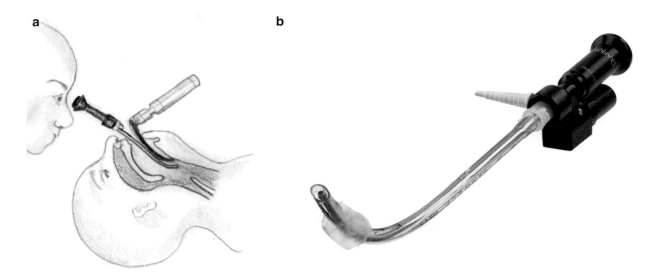

Fig. 10.18 (**a**, **b**) Clarus® Levitan optical airway scope (**b**) (Clarus Medical). Its placement into the airway (**a**) may be eased with DL assistance. The ability to "see around the corner" is a much needed advancement in management of the difficult laryngoscopy patient (**a**, Courtesy of Anna Mort, AM; **b**, Courtesy of Clarus Medical, Golden Valley, MN)

In addition to its role in intubation, VL technology has multiple uses in the ICU setting: bedside airway evaluations for potential extubation and ETT exchange, assist with passing devices into the aerodigestive tract (TEE probe, endoscope, NGT, feeding tube), assessing a cuff leak, retrieval of a foreign body, and the search for bleeding sources within the mouth–oropharynx [31]. VL technology has revolutionized airway management, especially in the difficult airway patient. However, its use must be tempered by operator understanding and the mastering of VL fundamentals. This technology should not be utilized in the known or suspected difficult airway case except by those who have reasonable experience with its use. Learning during a crisis is not warranted. Standard rescue (backup) equipment should be available in the event VL is inappropriate or proves unsuccessful in securing the airway.

When to Consider Alternatives to DL After an Unsuccessful Attempt

Numerous attempts at DL, residual edema from previous intubation attempts, or other direct trauma may degrade the quality of airway visualization due to laryngeal edema and bleeding. These physiologic and anatomic changes may also make conventional mask ventilation and SGA-LMA devices more difficult or even impossible to use. A degraded airway after numerous attempts at DL is the most common reason for the "cannot ventilate" scenario and adverse respiratory events [1, 4, 13, 17]. It is generally accepted that *three attempts* at DL are the maximum number before altering the plan or resuming mask ventilation [2, 3, 13]. It is well documented that the number of DL attempts, as well as the magnitude of the subsequent complications, such as hypoxia and bradycardia, is often proportional to the experience of the operator [13, 17]. Make your first attempt an optimal attempt and if this reveals a "failed view," quickly move to an alternative rescue device (plan B) whether it involves VL, FOB, the LMA, or other devices [7, 8, 27]. It is prudent to select the appropriate patient for the inexperienced operator since it is best, in the emergent or urgent setting, to have a more seasoned operator manage the known or suspected difficult airway (Fig. 10.19).

To limit the possibility of adverse respiratory events, we recommend that an expert laryngoscopist should be present to assure the patient's safety in any critically ill or difficult airway scenario [32–34].

Developing a Difficult Airway Algorithm in the NeuroICU

A systematic approach to the difficult airway in the NeuroICU is the key to prevent disastrous secondary injuries caused by hypoxemia. As a general rule, a provider skilled in nonsurgical and surgical airway manipulation should be immediately available in the NeuroICU. Anesthesiologists or surgical intensivists are a natural first choice to staff this role.

A difficult airway algorithm that is basically founded on the recommendation of the various published management

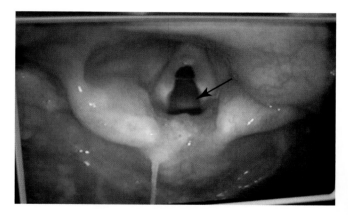

Fig. 10.19 Typically glottic view offered by video laryngoscopy (VL) on a video screen GlideScope® (Verathon, Bothell, WA). The panoramic nature VL devices allow compared to the confined view of DL is a distinct advantage for glottic viewing, diagnostic evaluation of the airway, and overcoming many of the challenges the difficult airway patient presents to the ICU practitioner. The cricoid ring is easily visualized below the vocal cord (*arrow*)

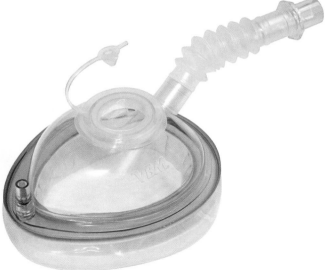

Fig. 10.20 This facemask has a silicon diaphragm (pluggable) that an FOB can be passed through while ventilation and oxygenation continue (Courtesy of VBM, Sulz, Germany)

guidelines and adapted to the patient population in the NeuroICU applies to three general categories of airway patients (Fig. 10.6):

Part 1: Predicted/recognized difficult airway

Part 2: Unpredicted difficult airway with ability to ventilate by mask

Part 3: Unpredicted difficult airway, "cannot ventilate, cannot intubate" (CVCI):

    A. Prior to pharmacologic intervention

    B. Immediately after the use of induction or paralytic agents

Part One: Strategy for the Predicted Difficult Airway

Satisfactory management of patients with a predicted difficult airway often entails endotracheal intubation by means other than conventional DL. VL, SGA devices, or utilizing an FOB, and maintaining spontaneous ventilation are all possibilities. In cases where the airway is known to be difficult, discretion tends to lead us to an awake or lightly sedated approach while maintaining spontaneous breathing. Typically, FOB is the "gold standard" with the awake intubation, but several techniques coupled with adequate airway topicalization with local anesthetics may be tried while the patient is awake (VL, DL, LMA, retrograde wire, optical stylet). FOB, due to its time constraints, is not an emergency technique, but can be applied in the urgent setting by skilled personnel. However, the time factor may dictate that supportive measures, e.g., BVM ventilation, be applied while the patient is properly and safely prepped for an awake approach, if clinically indicated (Fig. 10.20) [7, 8, 32]. As previously

stated, this technique is usually feasible only in awake or cooperative patients; it can, however, with optimal planning, equipment, personnel, and positioning, be extended to the obtunded patient with central nervous system injury. Optimal positioning for FOB typically involves sitting the patient upright, near 90° if tolerated; otherwise any head elevation is a better choice than supine, especially if the patient is obtunded and obese or has airway edema.

Every effort should be made to minimize the risk of aspiration of gastric secretions. While there is usually insufficient time to administer H_2 blockers or proton pump inhibitors and receive maximum benefit, the awake patient may be given a small amount of sodium citrate (15–30 mL) to neutralize gastric acid just prior to initiating the procedure. Additionally, a small dose (0.2 mg) of glycopyrrolate given intravenously 15–30 min before intubation may improve fiber-optic visualization of the airway due to its antisialagogue properties. The tip of the FOB is wetted with an antifogging agent and lubricated proximal to the tip with a water-based lubricant to facilitate passage of the endotracheal tube. If possible, though difficult in the urgent setting, the ETT should be preheated in warm saline for 30 s to several minutes to maximize flexibility and minimize trauma due to its thermolability. Similar to advancing an ETT over a bougie or airway catheter, there is a tendency for ETT tip to impinge on the right arytenoid/vocal cord due to the orientation of the ETT's bevel. Counterclockwise (CCW) rotation is helpful to limit tip impingement. Similarly, utilization of an ETT with a soft-tipped bird beak tip design, with its bevel oriented 90° CCW to the standard ET, offers an alternative

Fig. 10.21 (**a**, **b**) Parker FlexTip ETT™ (Parker Medical, Highland Ranch, CO). Comparing the Parker ETT design to the conventional ETT reveals the bird peak tip and a bevel that is oriented 90° CCW to the standard bevel. Note how the Parker tip design reduces ETT wobble when placed on the FOB and offers a less traumatic tip design that glides past tissues rather than impales tissue like the standard ETT tip

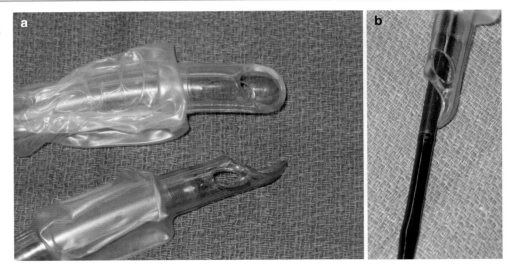

ETT choice for use in difficult airway situation when incorporating FOB or VL methods (Fig. 10.21a, b).

Our topical anesthetic of choice is viscous 4 % lidocaine (4–6 mL or up to 4 mg/kg) gargled, if applicable, or liberally applied to the oral cavity, oropharynx, and hypopharynx. Anesthesia can be achieved by placing lidocaine-soaked pledgets or tonsillar packing in the bilateral recesses of the oropharynx and having the patient clench their mandible to "squeeze" the pledget to deliver the local anesthetic. Bilateral superior laryngeal nerve and glossopharyngeal nerve blocks (2–3 mL of 1 % lidocaine) can also be performed when feasible but are rarely necessary if adequate local anesthetic administration is provided to the pharynx by the gargle method or atomizer spray to the oropharyngeal and hypopharyngeal areas. The total amount of local anesthetic should not exceed the calculated toxic dose. Local anesthesia may also be provided on a "spray as you go" basis, using aerosolized 2 or 4 % lidocaine through the operative channel while advancing the FOB. Glottic and trachea anesthesia may be achieved by several routes: (1) gargling and swallowing of local anesthetics, (2) "spray as you go" delivery via the FOB, (3) delivery of local anesthetic via an epidural catheter passed via the FOB suction port, (4) puncture and instillation of local anesthetic via the cricothyroid membrane, and (5) local application via a malleable atomizer while viewing the airway with a VL or DL device (Fig. 10.22).

The Berman, Ovassapian, and Williams specialized oral airways may be placed in the mouth prior to inserting the FOB to protect the device from being bitten but also to facilitate advancement of the ETT into the hypopharynx (the Ovassapian should be removed prior to ETT passage). Gentle external pressure on the larynx without neck extension may facilitate the exposure of the vocal chords. Since conscious sedation may not be an option for many neurosurgical

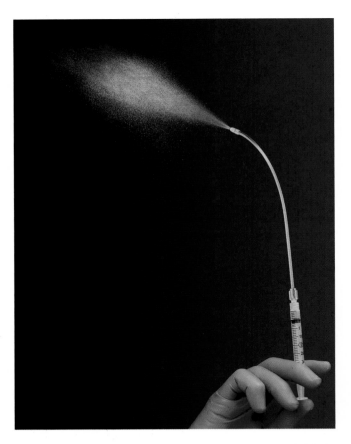

Fig. 10.22 Laryngotracheal atomizer (Wolfe Tory Medical, Salt Lake City, UT) is a malleable, directable syringe adapter capable of spraying mucosal surfaces (Courtesy of Wolfe Tory Medical, Salt lake City, UT)

patients, we cannot overemphasize the need for adequate topical anesthesia of the pharynx before attempting intubation by any of the methods discussed. As previously stated, most assume FOB is an automatic choice when an "awake" approach is contemplated, yet the LMA, DL, optical stylet, the bougie, VL, retrograde wire, and other techniques can be performed if proper preparation and operator skill are present. Potential agents for sedative use during this procedure which have little or no intrinsic effects on ICP, and may blunt iatrogenic procedural increases in ICP, include dexmedetomidine and remifentanil. Beta-adrenergic blockade can also help to minimize the increase in ICP from increased sympathetic outflow. These shorter-acting, highly titratable agents allow for optimal sedation and maintenance of spontaneous ventilation. Ketamine, while favored for its ability to maintain airway reflexes and encourage continued spontaneous ventilation, intrinsically increases ICP due its sympathomimetic effects and therefore should be avoided.

Nasotracheal intubation is an alternative to the oral route for patients without access to the mouth, a large tongue, or edema of the oropharynx and is an equally valid alternative for the spontaneously breathing, uncooperative patient or when the patient's secretions are excessive. The straighter pathway from the nasopharynx to the glottic opening may facilitate tube placement, but is not without risks. The presence of facial or posterior fossa trauma and coagulopathy is absolute contraindications to this approach. Absent these conditions, however, the mucosa of both nostrils can safely be treated with a solution of 0.1 % phenylephrine or a commercially available nasal decongestant spray, e.g., oxymetazoline (Afrin™), followed by progressive dilation, utilizing nasal trumpets lubricated with 2 % lidocaine jelly. Additional local anesthetic can be delivered via the nasal trumpet to cover the pharynx. Short-acting beta-blocker and remifentanil or dexmedetomidine should be available to blunt the sympathetic response to manipulation of the airway, which is often greater than when intubation is performed orally. Oxygen can be delivered by placing a nasal cannula between the lips or via a facemask (the facemask can be modified to accommodate FOB passage, or a commercially available device, specifically designed to perform bronchoscopy through, can be employed). When awake intubation is not feasible in the neurologically injured patient with imminent respiratory failure, part two and three of the difficult airway algorithm should be immediately executed, as discussed later in this chapter.

Part Two: Strategy for "Cannot Intubate" When Ventilation Is Possible

If DL does not result in visualization of the glottis after one to three attempts, despite use of OELM/BURP and bougie placement, the patient should be mask ventilated to improve oxygenation and denitrogenation, and a preplanned alternative route of intubation immediately carried out [7, 8, 34]. If VL or an optical stylet device is available and was not

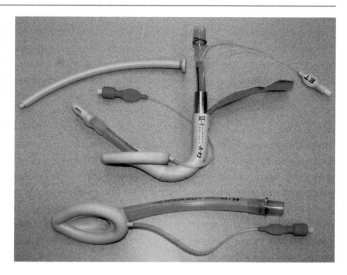

Fig. 10.23 Contrasting two of the LMA devices: LMA Fastrach™ (LMA North America, San Diego, CA) (*top*) with its distinct shorter, curved barrel to assist with blind or FOB-guided intubation compared to the LMA Classic™ (LMA, North America, San Diego, CA) model (*bottom*) which serves as an intubating conduit with FOB assistance

previously demonstrated to be ineffective on preliminary attempts, it is reasonable to make repeated attempts at laryngoscopy utilizing VL by a skilled practitioner. While this recommendation is a departure from the ASA difficult airway algorithm as it is currently written, we are confident that updated guidelines will delineate this choice. If VL is not available, a specialized LMA, the intubating LMA (ILMA) is our primary choice to facilitate placement of the endotracheal tube (Fig. 10.23). The ILMA is a supraglottic airway device that permits single-handed insertion from a neutral position, without substantial cervical manipulation or greater stimulation than direct laryngoscopy. It is designed to have an endotracheal tube advanced blindly through the device with a very high first-pass success rate. The LMA brand provides a straight, silicone wire-reinforced cuffed endotracheal tube, sized 7–8 mm internal diameter, for placement through the ILMA. The ILMA can also be used as a conduit to facilitate FOB-assisted ETT placement. Our second alternative is the classic laryngeal mask airway (LMA) placement (Fig. 10.23). If intubation is the goal, then intubation via the classic LMA should be performed with FOB assistance. Continued ventilation and oxygenation may be provided during the procedure through a bronchoscopic swivel adapter. Another option that is favored by the authors is covering the FOB with an Aintree catheter (Cook Critical Care, Bloomington, IN) followed by the delivery of the Aintree catheter to the trachea via the LMA due to the adequate exposure the LMA-SGA offers in many cases (Figs. 10.24a, b and 10.25). Once placed, the FOB and LMA are removed and a new ETT is navigated over the Aintree, which acts as a bougie [35]. To minimize air trapping and

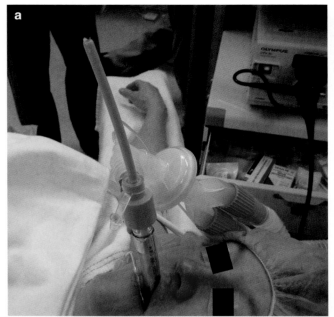

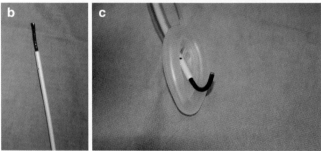

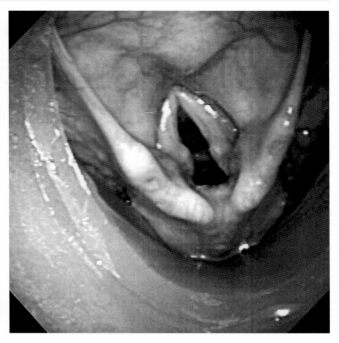

Fig. 10.25 FOB view of the glottis via the LMA Classic™ (LMA, North America, San Diego, CA). Though a full glottic view is apparent in this photo, this full view is present in less than 50 % of LMA placements. Thus, FOB is strongly recommended for ETT placement via the LMA Classic™

Fig. 10.24 (**a–c**) LMA Classic™ (LMA, North America, San Diego, CA), FO, and Aintree catheter (Cook Critical Care, Bloomington, IN). Figure (**b**) shows the Aintree catheter encasing the FOB with its placement within the distal end of the LMA Classic™ (**c**). Aintree within the LMA following FOB removal (**a**). The swivel adapter on the LMA allows continued ventilation during the procedure

barotrauma, ventilation should be provided manually rather than mechanically. However, positive-pressure-assisted ventilation via the LMA with an attached swivel adapter can be used to augment spontaneous efforts, possibly improving visualization of the laryngeal structures due to stenting of the previously collapsed soft tissue. This application is basically an exploitation of the same principles surrounding the use of CPAP or BiPAP for obstructive sleep apnea (Fig. 10.26a–c).

Part Three: Strategy for the "Cannot Ventilate, Cannot Intubate" (CVCI)

The "cannot ventilate, cannot intubate" (CVCI) scenario is the neurointensivist's worst nightmare. Hemoglobin desaturation is increasingly rapid, dependent upon the duration of the period from initial preoxygenation, the patient's oxygen consumption, intrapulmonary shunting due to increasing

hypoxia and hypercapnia, and finally decreasing FRC for reasons previously discussed. As noted earlier, the pediatric, obese, pregnant, and critically ill populations are particularly prone to rapid and profound desaturation. Undoubtedly, the first step in this scenario is to immediately request more help, including a surgical backup to immediately be present in the room. In many cases, this one step may be lifesaving. Other personnel may be delegated to perform cricoid pressure or in-line manual axial stabilization, obtain supplies, or pharmacologically control hemodynamic parameters.

The presence of large masses or severe swelling above the vocal cords (including tumor masses or facial trauma) may preclude the successful use of noninvasive alternative airway devices. This problem will be reviewed in the paragraph dedicated to the transtracheal approach to the airway.

In general, the "cannot ventilate, cannot intubate" scenario situation can be resolved only with one of the following [2, 3, 7, 8]:

1. *Placement of a Laryngeal Mask Airway* (*LMA*)
   Placing an LMA should be attempted first, as the track record of successful positioning of an LMA is excellent even in nonexpert hands. The LMA has proved to be relatively easy to use in the case of difficult intubations, including classes III and IV airways and laryngoscopy grades three or four [36]. A unique advantage of the LMA for neurosurgical patient is minimal stimulation of laryngeal reflexes associated with its insertion. While the LMA

Fig. 10.26 (**a**, **b**) Periglottic area of a swollen, edematous airway resultant from failed attempts at blind LMA Fastrach™ (LMA North America, San Diego, CA) intubation. FOB view via the LMA revealed the airway view on the left. Concern of the exact identification of the glottic opening led to the application of 8–10 cm H_2O CPAP airway pressurization to lateralize the boggy true–false cords permitting identification of the glottic opening. Passage of the FOB Aintree (Cook Critical Care, Bloomington, IN) afforded tracheal intubation

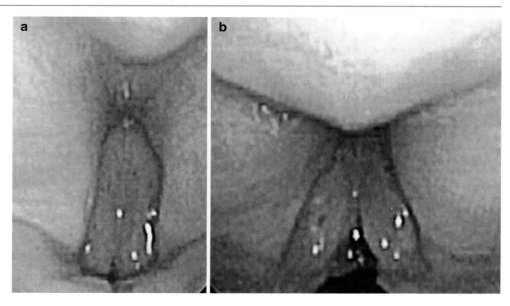

Fig. 10.27 LMA supraglottic airway devices. Several options are available for LMA-SGA devices. Pictured is the disposable LMA Classic™ (LMA, North America, San Diego, CA) (*bottom*), reusable LMA Classic™ (LMA, North America, San Diego, CA) (*middle*), and the disposable LMA Supreme™ (LMA, North America, San Diego, CA) (*top*)

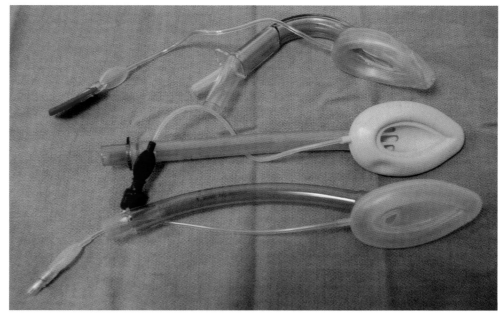

is a supraglottic device, and theoretically should not stimulate a laryngeal response, it is a large device and has been noted to be more stimulating in the oropharynx due to its higher cuff occlusion pressures. Additionally, the LMA may not protect the airway from regurgitation. The risks of aspiration may also be increased because regurgitated gastric contents cannot be expelled from the mouth. Cricoid pressure may be applied, but it may interfere with ventilation. A specialized LMA device (LMA Supreme™ or LMA ProSeal®, LMA, North America, San Diego, CA) has a gastric suctioning port, but this has yet to be proven to negate the risk of aspiration in the critically ill patient population (Fig. 10.27).

Despite these limitations, the LMA is our first backup airway device in the NeuroICU when DL and/or VL fails or is deemed inappropriate or unlikely to succeed. As we reference the "LMA," there are many variations commercially available to date that can, collectively, be referred as a group as "supraglottic airway, SGA."

2. *Placement of a Combitube®* (*Tyco Healthcare, Gosport, UK*)

The Combitube® has a lengthy track record in the prehospital environs but a more limited one within the hospital setting as an alternative device in difficult airway management. The other variants of the Combitube model (EZ tube® by Rusch, Limerick, PA; Laryngeal Tube® by King

Fig. 10.28 Combitube® (Tyco Healthcare, Gosport, UK), an esophagotracheal airway device with dual ventilating ports, allows oxygen delivery depending on its position within the esophagus (most likely) or trachea (unlikely). The dual inflatable cuffs seals the hypopharynx (*upper*) and the trachea/esophagus (*lower*)

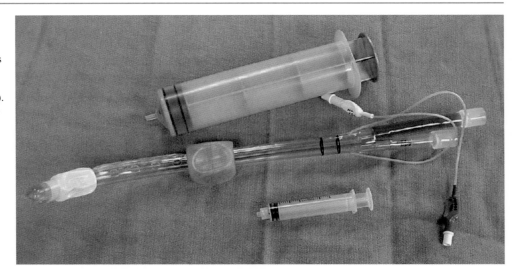

Systems, Noblesville, IN) have replaced some of the non-surgical techniques for airway control that do not rely on direct visualization of the airway and serve as a rescue device if the LMA or DL-bougie techniques fail [37].

The Combitube® is a double-lumen tube with distal and proximal cuffs (Fig. 10.28), presently available in sizes 37 French (women and smaller adults) and 41 French (adult male). Despite its bulky appearance, the Combitube® has a good safety record with only rare case reports of esophageal rupture [38]. It has been successfully used in hospitalized patients with sustained, non-traumatic cardiopulmonary arrest, as well as in patients undergoing elective surgery under general anesthesia. Another indication for the Combitube® is facial burn or massive upper airway bleeding. Admittedly, this device will be much farther down any algorithm due to its lack of availability and familiarity in most in-house facilities.

3. *Placement of Another Type of Supraglottic Device*
   The growing market for supraglottic devices is booming. It is sufficient to say that, when available, if nothing else has worked and surgical airway placement is not an option, these other devices can be attempted. The reason for discussing the LMA and Combitube® separately is due to their prevalence in the clinical settings and their documented safety and efficacy in the literature.

4. *Alternatives for the "Cannot Ventilate, Cannot Intubate" Scenario Due to Supraglottic Pathology*
   When the airway is compromised by trauma or when significant oropharyngeal or hypopharyngeal pathology is present, emergency access to the airway may only be obtained via emergency surgical airway (tracheostomy or cricothyrotomy) or a percutaneous cricothyroidotomy (Fig. 10.29):

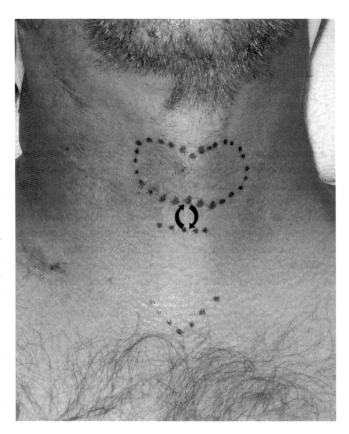

Fig. 10.29 Landmarks of the cricothyroid membrane (CTM). The lower "V" is the sternal angle; the *straight dotted line* is the upper pole of the cricoid, just below the thyroid cartilage. The CTM is marked as an *arrowed circle*

- *Emergency tracheostomy* is usually performed via a vertical incision from the cricoid cartilage down, approximately 1 cm long in the direction of the sternal notch. A #11 surgical blade should be used due to its smaller footprint and subsequent precise cut. A trained, surgically skilled operator can rapidly approach the trachea through this route. However, serious bleeding may occur via laceration of the anterior jugular and superior thyroid veins, the cricothyroid artery, or other vessels of the thyroid isthmus. If the procedure is successful and tracheal intubation is confirmed, as soon as the patient is stabilized, the next step is to immediately surgically revise the tracheostomy.

- *Emergency cricothyrotomy* is a valid alternative to the emergency tracheostomy for the neurointensivist not skilled or trained in the surgical approach to the airway. This technique requires identification of the cricothyroid membrane. The cricothyroid membrane (ligament) is directly under the skin and is composed primarily of elastic tissue. It covers the cricothyroid *space*, which averages 9 mm in height and 3 cm in width. The membrane is located in the anterior neck between the thyroid cartilage superiorly and the cricoid cartilage inferiorly. It consists of a central triangular portion (conus elasticus) and two lateral portions. It is often crossed horizontally in its upper third by the superior cricothyroid arteries.

Because the vocal cords are usually located approximately 1 cm above the cricothyroid space, they are usually not injured, even during emergency cricothyrotomy. Additionally, the anterior jugular veins run vertically in the lateral aspect of the neck and are usually spared injury during the procedure. There is, however, a considerable anatomic variation in both the arterial and venous vessel patterns of the thyroid and anterior neck. While the arteries are always located deep to the pretracheal fascia and are easily avoided during a skin incision, veins may be found in both the pretracheal fascia and above the superficial cervical fascia. To minimize the possibility of bleeding, the cricothyroid membrane should be incised at its inferior third.

To locate the cricothyroid membrane, external visible and palpable anatomic landmarks are utilized (Fig. 10.29). The laryngeal prominence and the hyoid bone above it are readily palpable. The cricothyroid membrane usually lies 1–1.5 fingerbreadths below the laryngeal prominence. The cricoid cartilage is also easily felt caudal to the cricothyroid membrane. The importance of these landmarks must be emphasized, as it can be disastrous to surgically manipulate the thyroid space instead of the cricothyroid space. There will be instances in which the normal anatomy is distorted and identification of any of the landmarks is difficult or impossible. In such cases, all attempts must be made to identify the anatomy, keeping in mind that the primary goal is salvaging the patient's life.

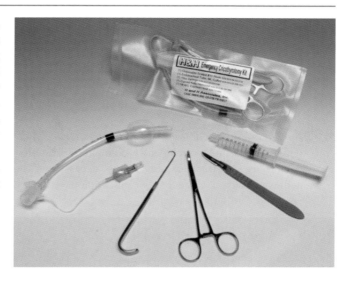

Fig. 10.30 Commercially available "cric" kit that could easily be assembled by the facility due to its simplicity. However, it must be prepared for in advance (Courtesy of H& H Associates, Ordinary, VA)

The incision is placed vertically, preferably with a #11 surgical blade, over the cricothyroid membrane. A simple kit containing basic instruments will suffice, especially in an emergency, by keeping it simple (Fig. 10.30). A small endotracheal tube, preferably armored, is placed through the membrane and aimed downward. This technique has the advantage of achieving access to the airway through a relatively avascular part of the neck. However, the cricothyroid membrane is not always easy to appreciate in obese patients or those with a short neck. In any event, the successful placement of cricothyroidotomy should be followed by an elective tracheostomy, or FOB intubation, as soon as possible, since long-term cricothyroidotomy may be associated with cricoid erosion or ulceration, tracheomalacia, subglottic stenosis, laryngeal webbing, and lesions of the vocal cords.

- *Percutaneous cricothyroidotomy* was described by Melker using the Seldinger technique (Fig. 10.31) and is our airway salvage technique of choice. The initial approach to the trachea is with a needle as opposed to a scalpel. The main advantage of this technique is the subsequent blunt dissection of the subcutaneous tissues down to the cricothyroid membrane. After locating the airway with a needle, a wire is introduced caudad in the airway and an airway catheter is then introduced over a dilator threaded over the guide wire. This technique allows the ultimate insertion of an airway considerably larger than the initial needle, often with sufficient internal diameter to allow suctioning and even spontaneous ventilation [39, 40].

While this technique is relatively atraumatic, it does require some knowledge of the anatomy of the neck and previously established proficiency in using the kit. Thus, this technique is not recommended for the physician unfamiliar with this device. When established successfully, the ultimate airway placed is a cuffed tracheostomy tube.

- *Needle cricothyroidotomy* is a rapid, *temporary* alternative to the more technically demanding cricothyroidotomy or tracheostomy. This access can be achieved with a large caliber intravenous catheter,

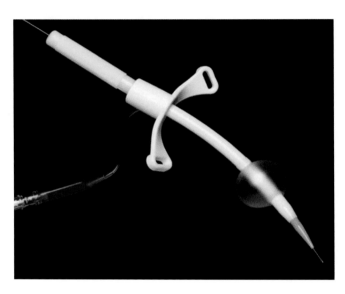

Fig. 10.31 Melker emergency cricothyrotomy catheter kit available with or without a cuffed airway (Courtesy Cook Medical, Bloomington, IN)

usually #12 or #14 gauge, or a specialized armored catheter. Needle cricothyroidotomy always requires the use of a jet device to provide ventilation (Fig. 10.32a, b). Ventilation via a high-pressure assembly must be performed by a knowledgeable practitioner who understands and adheres to the common sense practice of a low number of breaths (6–10 breaths/min) and prolonged I:E ratio of 1:4–1:6, minimizing the level of applied oxygen pressure to that which is effective to maintain life-sustaining oxygen saturations and pursue continuous efforts of maintaining airway patency so any administered high-pressure inflow is allowed the opportunity to egress out during exhalation.

Transtracheal catheter ventilation is a relatively easy method to *temporarily* oxygenate patients who cannot be mask ventilated or intubated but is highly dangerous in inexperienced hand. The use of this technique for more than short "bridging" intervals is inappropriate. It should only be used until the patient can be awakened or a definitive airway can be secured. Although oxygenation may be adequate with transtracheal catheter ventilation, passive exhalation is often insufficient to sustain ventilation. The resultant hypercapnia (causing increased cerebral blood flow) and significant air trapping (causing increased intrathoracic pressure and therefore increased cerebral venous outflow obstruction) may lead to disastrous consequences for the patient with already increased ICP or poor intracranial compliance. Other complications can occur, including those directly related to needle trauma, needle displacement in the subcutaneous

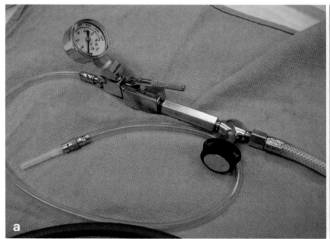

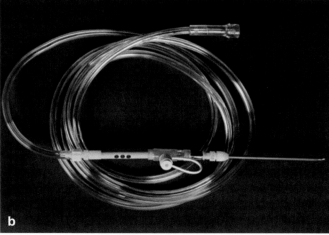

Fig. 10.32 (**a**, **b**) Two options for CTM needle puncture. Manual jet ventilator with pressure regulator (**a**) to be connected to a wall oxygen source or to an oxygen tank regulator. Figure (**b**) shows a low-pressure alternative that is the ENK Oxygen Flow Modulator™ system (Cook Medical, Bloomington, IN) that requires oxygen flow from an oxygen tank or wall source (5–15 L/min) (**b** courtesy of Cook Medical, Bloomington, IN)

tissue with resultant massive subcutaneous emphysema, catheter kinking, barotrauma with pneumothorax or tension pneumothorax, air trapping with severe hemodynamic instability due to impeded venous return, and right to left ventricular septal shift resulting in diminished cardiac output. The needle or catheter may break or bend if the patient coughs or moves, resulting in displacement. Subcutaneous air injection—sometimes massive—with loss of anatomical landmarks and tension pneumothorax appears to be the most serious and widely encountered complications.

In order to minimize barotrauma, airway patency should be maintained with head extension, jaw thrust, and chin lift by an assistant. For this reason, needle-jet ventilation is very risky in patients with a spinal cord injury, and provisions should be rapidly made to secure the airway in a more permanent fashion, such as with a surgical approach. Oral and/or nasal airway placement may also improve upper airway patency to facilitate passive exhalation. The problem in the CVCI scenario is that despite placement of a jet ventilation catheter, upper airway anatomy will not change and so only transient oxygenation can occur, because its usefulness will be limited by rising airway pressures due to lack of upper airway patency.

In summary, a systematic approach to airway management in the NeuroICU is necessary and provides a stepwise analysis of the best alternative options to avoid hypoxia and hypoventilation [2, 3, 7, 8]. A comprehensive difficult airway management program that includes education, training, scenario building, debriefing, and immediate accessibility to advanced airway devices may reduce the need for an emergency surgical airway [41].

Confirming Endotracheal Intubation

Several methods to confirm tracheal intubation have been recommended. These are described next.

Visual Inspection of the Airway After Passage of the Tube

Despite best efforts, direct observation of the ETT tip and cuff passing through the vocal cords is not always possible, especially in the patient with an anterior larynx or redundant epiglottis. Several other maneuvers can be used to assess proper placement of the endotracheal tube. When the use of these maneuvers is rapid and systematic, they do not substantially increase the time to confirm endotracheal intubation [18]. Individually, many of these methods are unreliable; in fact, collectively many of the methods used simultaneously can still prove unreliable but still better than assumption of correct placement [18]. Indirect methods such as chest rise, chest wall auscultation, gastric auscultation, bag compliance, oxygen saturation, and ETT moisture condensation may be incorrectly interpreted; hence, additional adjuncts include $ETCO_2$ detection and the esophageal detector device [18].

Esophageal Bulb Detector Device (EDD)

Recently, a suction bulb connected to the proximal end of the ETT has been utilized to confirm tracheal intubation during CPR (Fig. 10.33). If the ETT is properly placed, negative pressure will result in the bulb filling with air. If the ETT is placed into the esophagus, when negative bulb pressure is applied, the esophagus will collapse and the bulb will not re-expand. The device is disposable, small, and lightweight. The compressed self-inflating bulb is attached to the

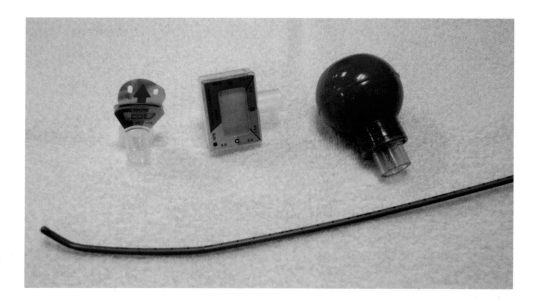

Fig. 10.33 Disposable $ETCO_2$ detection adjuncts (*left, middle*) and the esophageal detector device (EDD, *right*)

endotracheal tube through the standard 15 mm plastic fitting. The biggest advantage of this method is that it does not rely upon end-tidal CO_2 to confirm intubation of the trachea, an advantage in situations of extremely low cardiac output, cardiac arrest, or sudden increases of dead space ventilation (e.g., pulmonary embolism) [42, 43]. The same principles can be applied by using a large volume syringe to apply the negative pressure. If the endotracheal tube is properly placed, it will freely aspirate air without resistance. If the tube is esophageal, aspiration will yield resistance due to the collapse of soft tissue [43].

Detection of Exhaled CO_2

Besides direct visualization or fiber-optic confirmation of tube placement in the tracheobronchial tree, the most reliable method of ensuring tracheal intubation is the sustained presence of carbon dioxide in gas sampled from the endotracheal tube. This verification may be appreciated using a pH-sensitive indicator, the so-called colorimetry (the most common and least expensive method (Fig. 10.33)), or analytically measured via capnometry [43]. On occasion, in an esophageal placed tube, a transient presence of CO_2 in exhaled gas may be seen, possibly due to gastric insufflation during mask ventilation or the recent consumption of carbonated soft drinks. More difficult is the interpretation of correct endotracheal intubation in patients with a severe reduction of cardiac output or total circulatory arrest. As the amount of the CO_2 exhaled is directly proportional to the cardiac output, it may not be displayed at all in cases of total circulatory arrest or with resuscitative efforts insufficient to generate any sustained cardiac output [43]. The esophageal detector device methods previously discussed are a fairly reliable, rapid method or verification in these cases. On the horizon is another option to assist in the detection of ETT location, namely, tracheal rapid ultrasound exam (TRUE) for confirming endotracheal tube placement during emergency intubation [44].

Oxygen Saturation

Oxygen saturation by pulse oximeter is somewhat insensitive, as previously effective efforts oxygenation may delay the time of onset of desaturation, even in the presence of prolonged respiratory arrest. Conversely, prolonged desaturation may take a long time to recover despite endotracheal intubation and proper ventilation. Delays in response time of the oximeter may lead to false assumptions of a correctly or incorrectly placed ETT. Some consider this should be the last maneuver used to evaluate for proper ETT placement [18].

Management of the ETT After Detected Esophageal Misplacement

Once an esophageal intubation is detected, allowing the ETT to remain in place may be advantageous on several accounts; first, it provides a large caliber conduit for the directed passage of vomitus. The misplaced tube may also be used to facilitate suctioning with a larger-bore catheter. More importantly, it delineates the incorrect hole through which to place the endotracheal tube so that subsequent errors are less likely. It is possible for the presence of an esophageal tube to interfere with visualization of the larynx or manipulation of the airway in a difficult airway scenario. Thus, the physician in charge must quickly evaluate the risks versus benefits of removal prior to manipulating the tube. Airway suction with a large-bore Yankauer should be always available and used if regurgitation of gastric material follows the extubation of the esophagus.

Alternatives to Bag-Valve-Mask Ventilation and DL

The Laryngeal Mask Airway (LMA) in Management of a Difficult Airway

The LMA now has a primary role in achieving airway control, oxygenation, and ventilation in an unpredictable difficult airway when endotracheal intubation has failed.

Once placed, the LMA may be left in position to provide ventilation and oxygenation. The LMA already has a solid track record in the operating room for "saves" in the established difficult airway and in specific unpredictable situations, such as emergency Caesarian sections, airway trauma, and the newborn infant, with few reports of failure [2, 3, 7, 8, 45]. The LMA is now being adopted by practitioners in remote locations, by anesthesiologists and non-anesthesiologists alike. It has also become a recommended device for prehospital intervention and first-responder airways. In our experience, the LMA has been invaluable on many occasions when endotracheal intubation was impossible in the NeuroICU or ED. Given its ease of use and flexibility to facilitate other more definitive methods, the LMA should be considered first among the alternative airway devices to be used in the management of the difficult airway.

The presence of known pathology at the level of or above the vocal cords may be a contraindication to the use of this airway device, since it is normally inserted blindly into the pharynx. However, a random survey of 1,000 active members of the ASA showed that experienced anesthesiologists (more than 10 years in practice, age greater than 50 years) would consider use of the LMA even in these cases [45]. This predilection may be due to the familiarity of anesthesiologists with the technique and its relative simplicity to master compared to the alternatives.

The LMA should be considered a temporary airway to facilitate the introduction of an endotracheal tube with the aid of an FOB. A modified version of the LMA, the intubating LMA was developed to solve some of the disadvantages of the LMA when it is used to facilitate endotracheal intubation, with or without an FOB [46–48]. These limitations include the relatively small caliber of ETT allowed through the conventional LMA (# 6 mm internal diameter), the difficulty in passing the ETT cuff through the grill of the LMA, and the possible laryngeal injury caused by an endotracheal tube inserted blindly through an off-center LMA [46, 47].

Another modification of the LMA, the reusable LMA ProSeal® or newer disposable LMA Supreme® has been designed to limit regurgitation and pulmonary aspiration of gastric contents while the LMA is being used [49, 50]. Furthermore, it is marketed as the first device of this type that specifically allows positive-pressure ventilation in patients without spontaneous minute ventilation. The devices differ from previous versions of the LMA in that it has a rear cuff that improves the hypopharyngeal seal and a drainage tube providing a conduit to the stomach (Fig. 10.27). When they are properly placed (Fig. 10.24a–c), the orifice of the drainage port is aligned with the upper esophageal sphincter. Thus, a standard gastric tube can be inserted blindly into the esophagus to decompress the stomach and allow suctioning of liquid gastric contents [49, 50].

The increased protection from gastroesophageal reflux is not due to higher sealing pressure but rather to the innovative design of the new airway (e.g., a larger and different cuff). In fact, when the pharyngeal pressure from an LMA ProSeal® is compared with that of the classic LMA, no significant difference could be demonstrated [50]. The popularity of the Supreme reflects its ease of use, excellent sealing capabilities, and the ability to rescue the airway with Aintree-assisted FOB intubation via this LMA variation.

Main Contraindications to the Use of the LMA

The LMA offers little or no protection against pulmonary aspiration of gastric contents. The LMA is also associated with relaxation of the lower esophageal sphincter through distention of the hypopharyngeal muscles. In conditions such as glottic edema, it is possible that the laryngeal mask's low-pressure cuff may seal around the laryngeal inlet, molding to the edema. Nonetheless, and we wish to emphasize this, there are no absolute contraindications to the LMA if the alternative is loss of the airway.

Role of the LMA in Prehospital Airway Management of the Neurologically Injured Patient

In the United States, paramedics perform airway management in the field. While there is no controversy that control of the airway via an endotracheal tube is recommended in patients with Glasgow Coma Scale *less than or equal to* 8 or post-cardiac arrest, intubation of the severely traumatized patient can often be a difficult task for the paramedics. A prospective comparison between LMA and ETT management by respiratory therapists medical and paramedic students showed successful first attempt LMA placement 94 % of the time, compared with 69 % in the ETT group ($p < 0.01$) [51,

52]. We believe that the LMA should always be available for EMS providers on the street for physicians in the ED and the in the NeuroICU as first-line backup alternative to a failed intubation.

Techniques to Establish an Airway by ETT After LMA Insertion

While placement of an LMA in the NeuroICU can be a life-saving maneuver, the usual LMA peak airway pressure limitation is approximately 20 cm H_2O, coincidently that of the lower esophageal sphincter pressure as well. Neurocompromised critically ill patients often present with conditions that cause abnormal pulmonary mechanics such as chest trauma, aspiration pneumonia, and pulmonary edema, each of which may significantly decrease lung compliance. Furthermore, increased airway resistance can be associated with both cardiogenic and non-cardiogenic pulmonary edema. Together with decreased lung compliance, either type of edema can increase peak inspiratory pressures with a subsequent decrement in tidal volumes and increased risk of gastric distension in patients with LMAs [53].

Therefore, as soon as the patient is stabilized and appropriately oxygenated, the LMA should be replaced with an endotracheal tube. The blind passage of an ETT through the conventional LMA has been associated with a low rate of success, as the LMA can fail to negotiate the hypopharynx up to 65 % of the time [54]. We believe that any ETT being placed through the classic model of the LMA, or its variants, should be so placed with FOB assistance. The rate of success in placement of an endotracheal tube in this manner has been close to 100 % [54, 55].

There are two limitations to this technique: (1) cricoid pressure that may further displace the LMA and (2) the ETT size that can be used is limited due to the LMA barrel diameter. The largest ETT which can be placed inside the LMA is # 3.5 for LMA size 1, # 4.5 for size 2, # 5.0 size 2.5, # 6 cuffed for size 3 and 4, and #7.0 cuffed for size 5. In adults, we recommend using a small-caliber Rae tube, as it is approximately 3–5 cm longer than the standard endotracheal tube and is thus easier to pass, or the Mallinckrodt brand MLT 6.0 ETT. Using a bronchoscopic swivel adapter on the ETT during placement of the endotracheal tube while using the fiberoptic technique is advantageous in the critically ill patient as it—in the first instance—allows ventilation and oxygenation and is coupled with the added benefit of lateralizing edematous tissue with the goal of improving glottic visualization and hastening intubation (Fig. 10.26a, b). Another option we favor is the passing of an Aintree catheter over the FOB and its placement into the airway via an SGA device. Following removal of the SGA, with the Aintree remaining in the trachea, a larger ETT can be delivered to the trachea over the Aintree catheter (Fig. 10.24a–c).

Introduction of the intubating LMA (ILMA) has greatly facilitated endotracheal intubation in patients with difficult airways. The ILMA, either the reusable or disposable model, has a shortened, pre-curved barrel and a guiding handle (Fig. 10.23). Disposable models are now available which have similar efficacy rates and may be placed in a variety of airway situations, whether awake or asleep, primarily or as a rescue backup for other methods. It sports an excellent success rate by those skilled in its use [46–48, 56]. The ILMA is available in sizes 3, 4, and 5 corresponding, respectively, to small, normal, and large adult. The largest endotracheal tube that can be placed through ILMA is a number 8.0 ID; it can be placed either blindly or with an FOB. For safety, we recommend the use of the FOB, if the instrument is available, when an ETT is placed, though blind placement via the ILMA has an impressive track record when used by practitioners familiar with the technique.

To summarize, the ILMA is an improvement in design of the LMA, particularly adapted to management of patients with difficult airway. Experience with this device is well established in both the operating room and emergency departments, and its use is ever expanding in remote locations [46–48].

Use of the Combitube® in the Management of the Difficult Airway

The Combitube®, an evolutionary step in the design of the esophageal obturator airway, essentially seals the upper airway and therefore should be used in patients at high risk of regurgitation and aspiration of gastric contents. The main indication for the Combitube® has been in the rapid establishment of an airway during cardiopulmonary resuscitation (CPR) or difficult airway management when DL fails, typically in the prehospital setting. Its in-hospital use appears to be more limited, yet it plays an important role in the remote hospital location emergent intubation as a backup for DL, bougie, and LMA failures [37].

The Combitube® has the same limitations as the LMA and thus may not be easily inserted in patients with hypopharyngeal pathology. Although its safety record has been good, it can potentially exacerbate preexisting esophageal pathologies such as those seen with cancer, prior surgical manipulation, esophagitis, or esophageal varices in the upper portion of the esophagus.

Until recently, the Combitube® has found its widest use in prehospital cardiac arrest in which paramedics managed the airway. Direct laryngoscopy is unnecessary and there is minimal risk of aspiration. The Combitube® has also been used with success in managing difficult intubations in simulated combat situations and in obese, pregnant patients with difficult airways where risk of aspiration is high. The Combitube® is available in a standard size and "SA" (small adult) version. The most common reason for failure to ventilate with this device is advancement of the device too deeply, so that the perforated pharyngeal tube section has entirely entered the esophagus. Pulling the device back 3–4 cm usually resolves the problem. The use of the smaller version for patients less than 5 f in height is recommended by the manufacturer in order to minimize this problem. While our experience with this device is limited, that of others seems to suggest that the smaller version has a higher chance of success and a lower risk of damaging the hypopharynx and the esophagus. The Combitube® can be inserted safely in patients with cervical spine injuries, because flexion of the neck is not required. However, it should not be placed in the awake patient or even one lightly or moderately sedated as it is a strong stimulant of the gag reflex. The device has been used as a temporary means of airway control while FOB placement of an ETT through the nose is carried out. It has also been effectively used for airway maintenance during elective percutaneous dilation tracheostomy and emergent surgical airways.

While the Combitube® has been successfully used to rescue the airway in prehospital and in-hospital patients, its insertion certainly provides a great deal of sympathetic stimulation due to its bulk and the presence of a large cuff in the pharynx. This sympathetic outflow would undoubtedly increase ICP and thus would need to be treated preemptively. Stimulation of the gag reflex would manifest similar problems, including aspiration risk. While its possible role as a rescue technique of the airway in the NeuroICU has not yet been defined, the Combitube® can provide an effective way to control the airway after failed rapid sequence intubation or when a cervical collar is in place. The Combitube® or its variants are a viable next step in caring for the critically ill patient when bougie-assisted DL or LMA ventilation or intubation proves difficult or impossible [37].

Providing Ventilation After Placement of a Transtracheal Airway

Transtracheal ventilation can be a quick and inexpensive way to solve the issue of a "cannot ventilate, cannot intubate" (CVCI) difficult airway, but it contains many hidden dangers. The oxygen pressure from the wall is normally 50 pounds per square inch (psi), so a direct connection from the wall to the transtracheal catheter is not acceptable, as it may be associated with volutrauma and barotrauma. Additionally, catheter whipping and an increased incidence of catheter displacement into subcutaneous tissue may occur, with consequent massive subcutaneous emphysema. Several commercially available downregulators of wall oxygen pressure are available to titrate gas flow through a transtracheal airway [57].

In the NeuroICU, the source of high-pressure oxygen is usually a wall flow meter turned up to 15–20 L/min ("flush"); as an alternative, an oxygen tank with a dual stage regulator can be used. Low flow regulators usually necessitate a longer inspiratory to expiratory ratio. Although transtracheal ventilation may be temporarily lifesaving, adequate control of ventilation is often impossible and we recommend establishing a surgical airway as soon as possible after placement of the catheter.

When transtracheal jet ventilation (TTJV) is the only choice available, it should, if at all possible, be performed by two people, one to hold the catheter in place and the other to titrate the oxygen flow. The driving pressure of the regulator should be titrated slowly up from 5 psi to maintain a steady chest rise with each inhalation. Ventilation should be provided starting with an approximate inspiratory time (T_i) of 0.5 s, maintaining an $I{:}E$ ratio of at least 1:5 to minimize air trapping and to allow exhalation. After the procedure has been initiated, a third assistant or the placement of an oral or nasal airway may be needed to maintain patency of the upper airway. In fact, transtracheal ventilation without a patent upper airway inevitably results in progressive air trapping and barotrauma. Energetic jaw thrust, chin lift, placement of oral and nasal airways, an LMA, or an ETT placed into the hypopharynx may be tried to maintain airway patency [57].

We cannot overemphasize that in TTJV the catheter must be kept steady and aimed slightly downward to avoid kinking at the posterior wall of the trachea. Accidental dislodgment of the catheter into the subcutaneous space or perforation of the posterior wall of the trachea will result in several liters of oxygen being injected into the subcutaneous tissue and mediastinum in a fraction of a second, distorting all landmarks of the neck and leading to potential pneumothorax or pneumomediastinum as well as loss of the airway.

Aspiration of gastric or oropharyngeal secretions during TTJV has not been well studied. It is expected to be higher in unconscious, neurologically injured patients. While we have used TTJV, our preference, in an airway disaster in which an LMA or Combitube® is not appropriate or has failed, is the immediate use of a cricothyroidotomy kit or a surgical cricothyroidotomy with insertion of a number 5 or 6 endotracheal tube through the cricothyroid membrane. Although accidental perforation of the posterior tracheal wall has been described, cricothyroidotomy has a long track record of success both in trauma victims and in-house emergency use, and ready-to-use kits should always be available in the neurointensive care unit [58].

The Role of the Rigid Fiber-Optic Laryngoscope and Retrograde Intubation

These devices may be used in a "can ventilate, cannot intubate" situation because these devices are not meant for true emergencies, but rather as alternative methods for establishing endotracheal access. They may be used in a crisis if it is at the bedside and the practitioner has the skill set to execute its proper use. In general, these techniques apply to the neurologically injured patient in the more controlled operating room environment and have minimal applicability to the NeuroICU:

1. *Rigid fiber-optic laryngoscopes*: The Bullard laryngoscope® (Gyrus ACMI, Southborough, MA), the UpsherScope® (Mercury Medical, Clearwater, FL), and the Wu scope® (Achi Corp., Fremont, CA, and Asahi Optical Co., Pentax, Tokyo, Japan) remain invaluable adjuncts for difficult airway management, but they have essentially been replaced by newer video laryngoscopic technologies and deserve no further mention.

2. *Retrograde intubation*: This can be achieved with the use of a long, J-tip guide wire (usually 100–120 cm in length), a flexible epidural catheter, or a kit such as the retrograde guide wire kit (Cook Critical Care, Inc., Bloomington, IN). Known pathology above or below the vocal cords is a contraindication to this technique. In the retrograde technique, the guide wire is inserted through the cricothyroid membrane with the same technique as cricothyroid puncture described for the dilational cricothyroidotomy. However, the needle is aimed upward at an angle of approximately 45° once inserted through the cricothyroid membrane. The wire is then passed cephalad through the needle, and once it is located in the mouth (or less commonly, the nose), it is secured so that it may be used as a direct guide for the endotracheal tube or indirectly through use of an intubating stylet or airway exchange catheter. As described with other blind techniques, possible problems on insertion include failure to proceed beyond the vocal cords because the tube may impinge on the (right) vocal cord. Maneuvers recommended to overcome this problem include:

    (a) Twisting the endotracheal tube 90–180° counterclockwise.

    (b) Gentle direct laryngoscopy to displace the tongue anteriorly.

    (c) When a simple guide wire or an epidural catheter is used, threading the guide wire through the Murphy eye end of the endotracheal tube instead of the distal opening will allow an additional 1 cm of the endotracheal tube to pass beyond the vocal cords and facilitate the passage of the tip of the ETT in the trachea.

    (d) An additional step, in a graded fashion, would be to advance a smaller caliber airway exchange catheter over the wire first and then the endotracheal tube to facilitate passage.

    (e) Another modification (the authors' preference) of this technique provides for passing the J-wire, once retrieved from the oropharynx, into the suction port of an FOB and then advancing the ETT—loaded onto the FOB—via the FOB and under direct vision, into the airway. Use of the Patil-Syracuse or the VBM mask allows ventilation to be continued during the procedure (Fig. 10.20).

Specific Airway Problems in the NeuroICU

Airway Management and CNS Trauma

Management of patients with blunt/closed (CHI) or penetrating head injury requires specific skills. Elevated ICP can severely depress the level of consciousness and rapidly evolve to a herniation syndrome or be associated with decreased function of other vital organs. Some form of respiratory failure is associated in 20 % of patients with isolated head injury, regardless of the GCS score. Overall, respiratory failure is directly responsible for 25 % of all surgical deaths associated with CHI and is a contributing factor in about 50 %. Hypoxemia (PaO_2 less than 60 mmHg) is the most powerful determinant of comorbidity-related outcome from severe head injury, along with hypotension (systolic blood pressure less than 95 mmHg). In fact, approximately 90 % of adults suffering brain injury show some evidence of hypoxemic ischemia at autopsy [59].

Characteristically, autopsies of patients affected by post-traumatic severe intracranial hypertension can be associated with medial occipital necrosis from posterior cerebral artery compression against the tentorium cerebelli and boundary zone ischemia between the anterior and middle cerebral arteries. However, in many cases, secondary brain insult from hypoxemia (systemic insult) cannot be differentiated from intracranial hypertension (intracranial insult). Therefore, effective management of the airway and prevention of respiratory failure is essential in these patients. Traumatic brain injury is often associated with respiratory dysfunction, leading to hypoxia and hypercarbia.

Furthermore, CHI patients may demonstrate several abnormal patterns of breathing. *Central neurogenic hyperventilation* is the most common breathing pattern associated with head injury. However, regular cycles of hyperpnea and apnea (*Cheyne–Stokes*), ataxic or chaotic breathing, and central apnea may all be observed after head trauma. While the presence of abnormal respiratory patterns is usually only seen with a Glasgow Coma Scale score less than 8, specific patterns of breathing are unreliable at predicting the type and severity of brain damage. Absence of airway (gag and cough) reflexes, as well as intermittent obstructive apnea in stuporous or comatose patients, is common and requires immediate control and protection of the airway.

The onset of acute hypoxemia in head injury patients may also be secondary to other respiratory dysfunction. Acute respiratory failure can be secondary to direct pulmonary injury in the setting of blunt chest trauma. Pneumonia secondary to aspiration because of depressed gag and cough reflexes can be particularly severe if aspiration of particulate matter or gastric contents with a pH of less than 2.5 and volume of more than 25 mL are involved; it may lead rapidly to ARDS and severe hypoxia. Even when the airway is immediately secured, pneumonia can be common in these patients, occurring within the first week of hospitalization and contributing to increased ICU as well as hospital stay and poor long-term outcomes. In selected cases, patients with a mild alteration of mental status can be observed in the ICU without intubation if they are maintained in a 45° head-up position, are provided with aggressive control of gastric pH with H_2 blockers and/or proton pump inhibitors, undergo aggressive pulmonary toilet, are maintained in an NPO status, or are provided post-pyloric tube feedings and given proper oral hygiene and frequently have their oropharynx suctioned.

Hypoxia in patients with head injury is common in the ICU and can also be seen without aspiration. Neurogenic pulmonary edema can be observed shortly after the brain insult and is probably caused by a generalized sympathetic response. A massive catecholamine discharge secondary to traumatic stress causes transient peripheral vasoconstriction, systemic arterial hypertension, pulmonary hypertension, and altered pulmonary capillary permeability. Some cases of increased extravascular lung water in head trauma may be related to negative-pressure pulmonary edema from intermittent airway obstruction due to altered mental status. Finally, hypoxia can be due to pulmonary dysfunction from fibrin deposition, pulmonary microemboli, or a large thromboembolism.

In all of the previously discussed conditions, rapid control of the airway and correction of hypoxia are fundamental to minimize a secondary brain injury. Emergency airway management techniques in patients who have sustained severe head injury should be quick and effective, minimizing the adverse effect of intubation and permissive of rapid and decisive management of elevated ICP and associated injuries. Nevertheless, endotracheal intubation in the head-injured patient should avoid worsening a potentially injured cervical spinal cord. While effective resuscitation is taking place, preoxygenation with cricoid pressure is always recommended. Direct stimulation of the hypopharynx by DL is expected to increase the intracranial pressure through release of endogenous catecholamines and, in the case of succinylcholine use, muscular fasciculation. Lidocaine at 1.5 mg/kg has been shown to minimize the increase of intracranial pressure in response to intubation and blunt the effect of airway suctioning. Equally, short-acting beta-blocker or short-acting intravenous sedative analgesics such as remifentanil or dexmedetomidine are effective at minimizing this response [60].

The most common hypnotic agents used in airway manipulation of the head-injured patient are propofol and etomidate. Propofol is a short-acting hypnotic agent often used for induction of general anesthesia and associated with decreased cerebral blood flow, cerebral metabolic rate, and intracranial pressure. While these features are desirable upon intubation of the patient with poor intracranial compliance, the use of propofol may be associated with unacceptable hypotension in patients who are hypovolemic, septic, or affected by myocardial dysfunction, secondary to propofol's vasodilatory and myocardial depression effects. Propofol may be administered as a bolus dose between 2 and 3 mg/kg; dosage may be modified to 0.5–2 mg/kg in the elderly or when cardiac dysfunction and relative hypovolemia are conditions preexisting the intubation. The continuous infusion dosage ranges between 5 and 50 mcg/kg/min. Additional doses—or a continuous infusion—to control the post-intubation hyperdynamic response may be helpful. Etomidate is a hemodynamically better tolerated induction agent that has been extensively used in patients with increased intracranial pressure; it does have the most unfortunate effect of blocking the 11-beta hydroxylase step of steroid biosynthesis, thus putting the patient at risk for adrenocortical insufficiency. Succinylcholine remains the most rapid-onset agent to induce paralysis in order to facilitate intubation. Remarkably, the acetylcholine-like activity of succinylcholine has the potential to dangerously increase the ICP. While pretreatment with a small dose of an intravenous nondepolarizing neuromuscular blocking agent has been described to attenuate the ICP increase, by defasciculating the patient upon succinylcholine administration, we strongly discourage its use because it can be associated with unpredictable and potentially life-threatening muscle weakness and potential hypoxia if unable to intubate or ventilate. One must remember that the ED_{95} for succinylcholine is 0.25 mg/kg; the large dose—1–1.5 mg/kg—usually recommended is most often not necessary. Ketamine has been shown to be associated with hypertension, tachycardia, increased cerebral blood flow, higher oxygen consumption, and increased intracranial pressure and is therefore not recommended.

Endotracheal intubation in head trauma patients can cause a significant hemodynamic response. Maintenance of the cerebral perfusion pressure [CPP = mean arterial pressure (MAP)—intracranial pressure (ICP)] of 65–70 mmHg is always desirable and associated with a good long-term cerebral outcome. However, in the context of a disrupted blood–brain barrier, uncontrolled increases of arterial blood pressure may potentially increase cerebral edema and worsen the intracranial pressure; thus, a CPP greater than 65–70 mmHg should not be allowed in the acute stage of injury.

Drugs used to blunt hypertensive response to intubation include (1) intravenous lidocaine (see dosing discussed previously); (2) beta-blockers, such as the ultrashort-acting esmolol (0.5–2.0 mg/kg) or mixed alpha-/beta-blocker labetalol (10–20 mg iv); (3) fentanyl 3–5 mcg/kg iv); and (4) dexmedetomidine, an alpha-2 agonist also capable of providing a blunted response to the hemodynamic fluctuations of intubation, as well as providing sedation [60].

Airway Management and Spinal Cord Injury

The incidence of spinal cord injury (SCI) in patients sustaining major trauma is 1.5–4 % and up to 10 % in high-speed motor vehicle accidents, most often from concurrent fracture–dislocation [61]. Emergency management of the airway may be necessary due to diaphragmatic failure from high cervical spine injury, associated head injury, or hemodynamic instability. Although intubation is usually performed in the field, the patient may become hypoxic on arrival to the emergency department or in the NeuroICU.

Prompt, assisted ventilation should be via BVM ventilation. Cricoid pressure should be applied to prevent gastric insufflation or passive regurgitation. While anteroposterior pressure is held on the cricoid cartilage, gentle posteroanterior support should be provided with the assistant's other hand at the dorsal aspect of the cervical spine to prevent inadvertent movement of a potentially injured cervical spine. The most appropriate route of intubation is still controversial. Nasal intubation has been advocated to eliminate any movement of the neck. However, nasal intubation is not feasible and possibly dangerous if the patient is intermittently apneic, has a basilar skull fracture and profuse bleeding from multiple facial fractures, or is simply combative or uncooperative. If oral intubation is attempted, manual, in-line stabilization of the cervical spine/spinal cord is necessary. The absence of radiological evidence of cervical spine trauma should not obviate the need to stabilize the spinal cord, because significant injuries can be missed in up to 20 % of the cases of patients with negative cervical spine radiographic series. Overall, it should be appreciated that displacement of cervical segments may occur during mask ventilation, laryngoscopy oral intubation, and LMA and Combitube® placement; thus, pre-intubation maneuvers differ little from intubation techniques except with FOB.

Despite the lack of uniform approval of spinal cord immobilization protocols for suspected injury, we believe that the use of the sniffing position to improve laryngeal view during tracheal intubation can be extremely dangerous and should be avoided in any potential cervical spine injury. Neurological deterioration after endotracheal intubation is difficult to evaluate in trauma patients and is probably underreported. To our knowledge, very few cases of a neurological deterioration associated with airway management in a cervical spine injury patient have been published [61]. One case described new paraplegia that was noticed postoperatively after a *routine* approach to airway management that turned unpredictably difficult and required multiple laryngoscopes and, eventually, cricothyroidotomy [61]. The new onset of paraplegia was retrospectively attributed to an unrecognized disruption of the anterior longitudinal ligament at the C6 to C7 level.

Several alternatives have been evaluated to gain access to the airway in patients with suspected or established SCI.

While the LMA has been proven easy to use in cases of difficult intubation, including classes III and IV airways and laryngoscopy grades II through IV, its use in patients with cervical spine injury requires some caution.

In fact, it has been noted that both the LMA and ILMA, once seated into the airway, typically exert pressure against the tissue overlying the C2 to C6 vertebral bodies. A prospective study in fresh cadavers showed that the cervical pressure generated by laryngeal mask devices can produce posterior displacement of a normal cervical spine [62]. It is anticipated that such displacement would be greater in the injured cervical spine. In particular, the original ILMA, with its stiff metal arm, greatly increases vertebral pressure at the C2 to C3 level during positioning. This pressure can be almost totally relieved by forward handle elevation, but it is likely unavoidable during insertion. The same observation was reported when the standard LMA was used, but the compression pressure was less. Although the limitation of this study on fresh cadavers is clear, we believe that use of a laryngeal mask device should be recommended only when a difficult airway is anticipated or encountered in an unstable cervical spine and no other viable option is present. If ILMA placement is planned in a patient with cervical spine injury, we recommend removal of the anterior portion of the collar, forward displacement of the ILMA, and in-line manual axial stabilization. In fact, when the neck collar is in place, the strap under the chin typically lifts up and tips the larynx anteriorly, making intubation by ILMA very difficult or impossible.

The esophageal–tracheal Combitube® has been used to facilitate airway control in trauma patients with possible cervical spinal injury and has been considered an effective prehospital airway device, a backup to the ETT and a potential permanent airway [37]. We believe that elective use of the Combitube® in a patient whose neck is immobilized in a rigid cervical collar should be limited to out-of-hospital management, when routine use of the ETT is unfeasible or has failed, and there is a need to provide ventilation while protecting against aspiration. As an out-of-hospital airway device, the Combitube® can be considered an evolution of similar devices that have been used extensively in a prehospital arena for many years to ventilate the lungs, providing protection against gastric regurgitation.

In summary despite its good track record in prehospital airway care, there is little indication for the use of the Combitube® in the NeuroICU at this time except as a second-tier backup device for DL-bougie, VL, or LMA failures [37]. If encountered in a patient admitted to the NeuroICU, it should be exchanged for a definitive airway upon transfer to the ICU from the field or ED. Our preference is to use oral fiber-optic intubation after proper preparation, possibly when the patient is awake and cooperative. Otherwise, exchanges with the assistance of VL, DL-bougie, or ILMA are alternatives. No matter what the planned approach to establish the airway in these patients, manual in-line stabilization should be carefully considered for all patients.

The airway management of penetrating neck injuries needs special consideration since the incidence of tracheal–bronchial injury in patients with penetrating neck trauma is significant and death from direct airway complications is real. Ideally, endotracheal intubation should be achieved early with FOB to avoid further injury by placement of the ETT. Blind nasal intubation should be avoided at all costs, and cricothyroidotomy should be avoided in the presence of an anterior hematoma or performed only in the presence of a surgeon able to achieve immediate control of the bleeding. The use of muscle relaxants deserves early consideration because coughing, stimulation of the gag reflex, or the Valsalva maneuver may severely worsen vascular airway injury. However, their use must be balanced against the feasibility of endotracheal intubation. Finally, any air bubbling through the wound should be treated with immediate coverage with occlusive gauze in an effort to minimize entrainment of air and thereby avoid massive mediastinal and subcutaneous emphysema. While immediate surgical exploration of a penetrating neck trauma is now being challenged by a more conservative, selective approach, the presence of exsanguinating hemorrhage or expanding hematoma unresponsive to resuscitation measures should require immediate definitive airway placement and subsequent surgical exploration.

In any case, the presence of cervical spine injury adds a formidable challenge to airway management in the trauma patient. While the algorithmic approach remains somewhat debated in the literature, it is clear that the skill and personal experience of the airway operator are the most important aspects in decision making and outcome.

Elective Neurosurgical Procedures: Special Problems

Intracranial Vascular Procedure
Hemodynamic control during intubation is a fundamental goal of the intensivist, who plans to manipulate the airway in patients with intracranial vascular pathology. The threshold of blood pressure tolerance is somewhat higher in arteriovenous malformation (AVM) than in subarachnoid hemorrhage (SAH). While hypertension in an AVM is usually inconsequential, because of the presence of ectatic vessels at lower pressures, any change in stress on the vascular wall of an intracranial aneurysm which has bled or may bleed may trigger a disastrous (recurrent) hemorrhage. An arterial line should be placed before manipulation of the airway and special attention should be focused to maintain systolic blood pressure within baseline limits.

Carotid Endarterectomy (CEA)

The management of a difficult airway in this condition can be summarized in three major points. The use of succinylcholine in patients with previous stroke or major neurological injury should generally be avoided due to an increased release of potassium from upregulation of skeletal neuromuscular receptors. A consistent time period between onset of the stroke and the hyperkalemic response to succinylcholine is not well established. Because alternative nondepolarizing muscle relaxants are available, an agent like rocuronium should be considered if there is any doubt.

The frequent association between carotid arteriosclerotic disease and coronary disease, including left ventricular systolic dysfunction, should be considered. While the general recommendation is to maintain mean arterial pressure within a 20 % range of the baseline pressure, careful attention should be focused on avoiding severe blood pressure swings on intubation. Short-acting beta-blockers are likely the best choice due to their ability blunt the hyperdynamic response associated with intubation and concurrently reduce myocardial oxygen demand, thereby decreasing overall cardiac stress.

Airway manipulation may be necessary on an emergent basis in the NeuroICU, recovery room, or ward when an expanding wound hematoma compromises the patency of the airway. Surgical manipulation of large neck vessels, the intraoperative use of heparin without subsequent reversal, and the presence of a close anatomic relationship between the carotid artery and the trachea put these patients at higher risk for airway compromise due to an expanding wound hematoma. The rapid formation of a wound hematoma is often an airway and surgical emergency. Vigilance and recognition of the problem are the keys to prevent a possible airway disaster. Worsening incisional pain, voice changes, worsening dysphagia, and obvious wound swelling require immediate attention. Quick reexploration of the wound may be necessary, even in absence of the surgeon. If repeat surgical investigation is planned, as one option for preserving the airway status, an immediate direct laryngoscopy should be performed after rapid application of a topical anesthetic to the airway to evaluate the feasibility of a regular induction.

Release of the hematoma may be justified, but it must be understood that while removal of the clot mass may allow the deviated trachea to align more centrally, the airway distortion due to edema formation will remain, thus contributing to a potential airway nightmare. When the patient is already dyspneic or stridulous, rapid application of 4 % lidocaine to the airway and awake oral intubation may be the safest choice, with DL, VL, optical stylet, and FOB as options. In any case, when reexploration of the wound with evacuation of hematoma is planned, a surgeon with expertise in emergency tracheostomy or cricothyroidotomy should

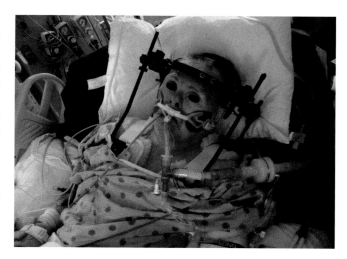

Fig. 10.34 The halo vest for cervical spine immobility

stand by as the patient is being intubated. A tracheostomy kit and a difficult airway cart should always be available at bedside or in the operating room [63].

The Acromegalic Patient

Abnormal airway anatomy is common in the acromegalic patient and hypophysectomy is a common neurosurgical procedure requiring postoperative admission to the ICU. Several acquired modifications of the bone and soft tissue can make an endotracheal intubation very challenging [64, 65]. Anatomical abnormalities interfering with endotracheal intubation include prognathism, macroglossia, and redundant soft tissue at the lips, epiglottis, and pharyngeal mucosa. Reduced mobility of the vocal cords and cricoarytenoid cartilage, as well as cervical spine fibrosis, may also inhibit DL [64, 65]. Subglottic stenosis can be suspected in patients with a history of hoarseness or stridor. When the intubation is elective, an awake approach may be prudent. A backup technique to endotracheal intubation should be readily available to control this potentially difficult airway.

Patients with a Head Frame

The presence of a head frame (halo, halo vest (Fig. 10.34)) represents a formidable obstacle to not only direct laryngoscopy but most other techniques, even FOB. Strong consideration should be given, in elective manipulations of the airway in these patients, to awake fiber-optic intubation. A well-stocked difficult airway cart *must be immediately available*, as well as an extra pair of expert hands and a neurosurgeon geared with the proper tools for quick removal of the frame, if necessary. Once again, awake intubation should always be considered first, if there is opportunity. The awake approach with adequate topicalization with local anesthetic is compatible with DL, VL, optical stylet, LMA, and retrograde techniques (2,3 7,8).

The Pediatric Neurosurgical Patient

Severe abnormality of both intracranial and extracranial structures, interfering with airway management, has been described in approximately 60 congenital syndromes associated with craniofacial defects. Airway management of these patients is especially difficult because some of these syndromes have associated increased ICP and often concurrent congenital heart disease. Management of the airway in these patients should be limited to anesthesia personnel with special expertise in pediatric neuroanesthesia and in-depth knowledge of the neurological features of the congenital disease. The new additions to the airway manager's armamentarium of rescue devices provide pediatric and neonatal sizes to accommodate the anatomical differences between the adult and the young.

Airway Management in Patients with Neuromuscular Disease

Respiratory muscle weakness, alterations of respiratory system mechanics, and impairment of the central control of ventilation can all be associated with respiratory failure requiring airway manipulation and admission into the NeuroICU. Several noninvasive alternatives are available to provide positive-pressure ventilation in a patient with neuromuscular diseases—all employing the use of special airway devices [66]. Three different devices are commonly used: (1) a mouthpiece with or without a lip seal, (2) a nasal CPAP mask, and (3) a full BiPAP facemask. Generally, the use of noninvasive positive-pressure ventilation results in effective ventilation if the patient cooperates, and it may prolong or prevent the placement of a tracheostomy. However, common contraindications exist, such as coexisting severe lung disease where secretions are a constant problem, altered mental status, lack of cooperation, poor oropharyngeal muscle strength, uncontrolled seizure disorder, history of severe esophageal regurgitation, recent upper GI surgery with intestinal anastomosis, and any orthopedic condition interfering with placement of the device. In all these cases, the patient will usually require a tracheostomy and long-term mechanical ventilation.

Extubation of the Difficult Airway

The percentage of patients requiring reintubation in the NeuroICU following tracheal decannulation is not known. However, it is reasonable to consider that altered neurological status (level of consciousness, gag and cough reflex, cognition, waxing and waning status) can increase the rate of recurrent respiratory failure post-extubation. Among other reasons, neurosurgical patients have a poor ability to handle secretions and increased work of breathing. It is known that reintubation of patients with a difficult airway carries a high

Table 10.7 Risk factors for difficult extubation

1. Known difficult anatomy confirmed on intubation
2. Any patient with an unexpected difficult airway on intubation
3. Airway edema 2° surgical manipulation or massive volume resuscitation
4. Prolonged prone position
5. Tongue, lips, or facial swelling
6. Cervical immobility or instability, trauma, surgery
7. Head frame
8. Obesity, morbid obesity (body mass index greater than 30 or 40, respectively)
9. Altered mental status, even in the presence of strong gag reflex
10. Posterior fosse surgery and brainstem surgery
11. Any condition where standard extubation criteria cannot be evaluate
12. Prolonged mechanical ventilation (more than 2 weeks)
13. Copious tracheobronchial secretions in patients without brisk cough reflex
14. Residual analgesia and/or anesthesia postsurgical procedure
15. Residual neuromuscular paralysis and respiratory weakness
16. Accidental extubation

Modified with permission from Gabrielli and Layon [99]

rate of complications [1, 4, 25]. Therefore, when tracheal extubation in a patient with a history of known or suspected difficult intubation is anticipated, a plan is necessary to minimize risk to the patient needing to be reintubated. The risk factors (Table 10.7) for difficult extubation are based on those patients who are known or suspected as having a difficult airway (mask ventilation, difficult laryngoscopy, or intubation) currently or in the past or who have risk factors that place the patient at an elevated airway management risk.

An extubation strategy should be developed which allows the airway manager to [1] replace the ETT in a timely manner and [2] ventilate and oxygenate the patient while the patient is being prepared for reintubation, as well as during the reintubation itself [2, 3, 7, 67–69]. The practitioner should assess the patient's risk on two levels: the patient's predicted ability to tolerate the extubated state and ability (or inability) to reestablish the airway if reintubation becomes necessary.

The ability to tolerate extubation assesses the systemic readiness of the patient based on extubation criteria (forced vital capacity, rapid shallow index, negative inspiratory force, cough, gag, mental status, pain management, cardiovascular stability, etc.) However, one must ask: "is the airway ready for extubation?" since the status regarding its patency (swelling, secretions, prior trauma) is a primary factor in successful extubation. Remember, any airway *may* be extubated, but *should* it be extubated? The three phase of the extubation strategy can be reviewed in Table 10.8.

To determine if the airway itself is "ready" for extubation, it can be very helpful to examine the periglottic area to determine if, at least, the airway at the level of the glottis and supraglottic suggests patency following extubation. VL plays a key role in examination of the airway since the evaluator is severely restricted in their ability when using DL (Fig. 10.35a-c). Nonetheless, the subglottic region is out of view; thus, its assessment is limited without full tracheal extubation and view with FOB [70].

The "cuff-leak" test has been used to determine upper airway patency and potential for successful extubation.

Table 10.8 Three phases of extubation strategy

Phase 1

Medical record review—assess for useful information

1. Previous airway interventions
2. Surgical/medical implications affecting the airway:
   (a) Previous surgery on the airway or neighboring structures
   (b) Medical conditions with airway implications
3. Postoperative/miscellaneous conditions
4. Current and past medical illnesses (impacting extubation tolerance)
5. Review current ventilatory requirements
6. Current vital signs and neuro/mental status, NPO status

Phase 2

1. Discussion with care providers (physicians, nursing, respiratory therapists, MLP)
2. Comprehensive airway evaluation
3. External evaluation, direct or indirect airway assessment
4. Discussion of plan with the patient (and family, if appropriate)
5. Acquisition of basic/advanced airway equipment at the bedside, as well as experienced personnel

Phase 3. Strategy for the high-risk extubation

1. Standard extubation
   Extubation/evaluation via FOB
2. Extubation followed by SGA placement for airway patency, oxygenation, ventilation, a portal to visualize anatomy and reintubation
3. Extubation over an AEC
4. Delay extubation
5. Surgical airway option

Unfortunately, qualitative and quantitative variations exist when performing the cuff leak; thus, its interpretation should be questioned rather than relied upon as a sole determining factor for extubatability. Overhydration, airway- or intubation-related trauma, positioning, generalized edema, systemic reactions, sepsis, angioedema, infections, head and neck venous drainage impingement, and too large an ETT may all account for the lack of a cuff leak. This could lead to a delay in extubation or performance of a tracheotomy. Obligating the patient to these two choices should prompt evaluation to determine if a treatable etiology of the "no cuff leak" exists. The cuff-leak test has multiple variations; thus, its performance and interpretation needs standardization [71–73]. The cuff-leak test may be performed quantitatively (measuring volume of leak) or nonquantitatively (audible air leak with ear versus stethoscope) with passive airflow (patient generated) or active airflow (ventilator/manually generated). In general, the lack of a cuff leak may suggest a higher likelihood of post-extubation stridor, reintubation, or the need for tracheotomy, though this has been refuted [71–73]. Pre-extubation steroid administration may hold promise in reducing stridor and reintubation in select patients based on specific cuff-leak criteria [74]. If no cuff leak is present, VL examination may detect reversible etiologies such as glue-like supraglottic secretions, airway swelling, excessive ETT size (too large relative to the airway), or a collapsible airway. Conversely, the presence of a cuff leak in the presence of massive facial/neck swelling would warrant VL examination to assess airway patency as well as the worthiness of placing the VL device if reintubation was required [71].

In complex airways, we most frequently use the Cook disposable airway exchange catheter (AEC), placed through the ETT as the ETT is removed [2, 3, 68, 75] to allow continuous access to the airway following extubation: a so-called "reversible extubation" (Table 10.9, Fig. 10.36). Typically, the 11 F is used in women and men of shorter stature (less

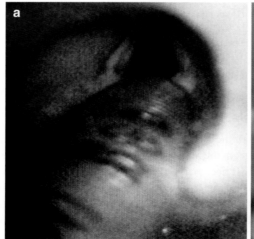
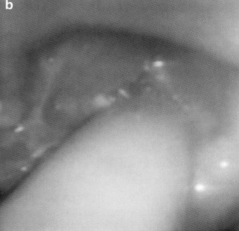

Fig. 10.35 (**a–c**) VL evaluation of the difficult airway for extubation. Figure (**a**) depicts a relatively normal appearing ICU airway as compared to (**b**) with "moderate periglottic edema" and (**c**) showing significant airway edema

Fig. 10.35 (continued)

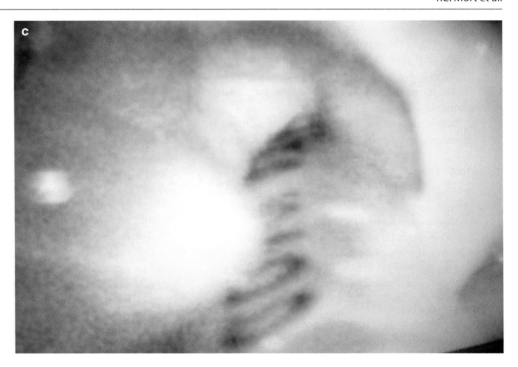

Table 10.9 Suggested method for AEC-assisted extubation

1. Upright position, discuss with patient, assemble DA cart/ equipment/personnel, monitors, NPO
2. Administer 100 % oxygen, assemble post-extubation oxygen source
3. Suction via ETT and oral cavity, oropharynx
4. Prepare securing tape, deflate cuff (expect coughing and the need for repeat suctioning)
5. Cut/loosen existing tape or ETT securing apparatus, maintain ETT position
6. Insert a lubricated AEC through the ETT to predetermined depth
7. Extubate the patient over the AEC, maintain AEC position until secured
8. Apply oxygen source
9. Wipe lubrication/secretions from AEC, secure with circumferential tape (21–26 cm depth)
10. Tape the proximal end to the patient's shoulder, assure AEC is not used for enteral feeding
11. Continued explanation/encouragement to the patient, maintain NPO status
12. Remove AEC when appropriate, continued vigilant observation in a monitored setting

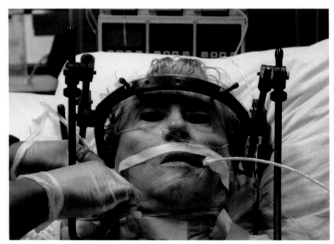

Fig. 10.36 "Reversible" extubation by placement of the airway exchange catheter (AEC) in a patient who presented with a formidable FOB challenge for intubation

than 68 in.). The medium-sized 14 F would be appropriate in their taller counterparts; the largest Cook AEC (19 F) is poorly tolerated in most patients for extubation of the airway. The catheter is taped into position the distance from the alveolar ridge of the upper incisors as was the ETT. If necessary, the one-time use of aerosolized 4 % lidocaine (3–4 mL) may increase tolerance to an airway exchange catheter, without compromising airway reflexes or increasing the risk of pulmonary aspiration. Post-extubation airway evaluation may

be performed to determine the "airway status" once the ETT has been removed from the view and may contribute valuable clinical information if stridor or respiratory distress occurs (Fig. 10.37a–c).

Post-extubation oxygen supplementation for a "reversible extubation" may be as simple as nasal cannula, a disposable facemask, nasal high flow, or even a CPAP or BiPAP mask (Fig. 10.38). It is strongly recommended not to deliver oxygen via the AEC itself since barotrauma has occurred when flow rates exceed 2 L/min (with limited egress of gas and pressure). Delivery of oxygen via the AEC (up to 2 L/min) may be

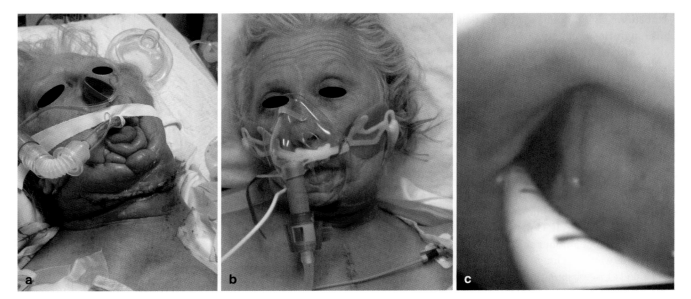

Fig. 10.37 (a–c) Known difficult airway patient for extubation (a). Extubation via AEC (b) with post-extubation endoscopy (c) showing AEC in normal appearing glottis

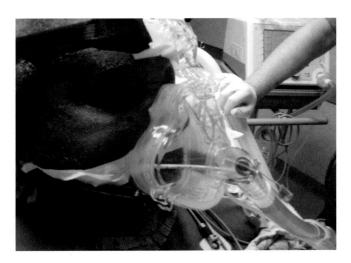

Fig. 10.38 CPAP combined with the AEC for extubation. A CPAP mask with AEC within the airway is possible by passing the AEC into the respiratory tubing

Table 10.10 Technique of reintubation via AEC

1. Optimal positioning, e.g., ramping
2. Oxygen support:
(a) Via luminal portal—must be interrupted to pass ETT
(b) Anesthesia mask with resuscitation bag (AEC to corner of mouth)
3. If stridor is present or airway swelling is suspected, choose a smaller caliber ETT (5.0–6.5 ID)
4. Determine need for induction medications—sedatives, analgesics, or topical anesthetics
5. Remove tape from AEC, maintain AEC in secure position
6. Open mouth (jaw thrust–chin lift for edentulous patient or DL to open pathway to glottis)
7. Advance smaller caliber ETT (AEC-ETT gap is best minimized) to optimize 1st-pass success
8. If unable to advance ETT into airway, back up ETT from resistance level, turn ETT CCW to realign bevel, then advance. If unsuccessful, move to a smaller caliber ETT
9. Confirm ETT using standard techniques
10. Incorporate rescue devices if AEC-assisted intubation fails

performed if readying the patient for reintubation as long as attention is paid directly to the airway. If reintubation is necessary (Table 10.10), laryngoscopy is performed to facilitate the passage of the ETT through the glottis. Impingement of the ETT tip on the right vocal cord or arytenoid (similar to passing the ETT over a bougie, bronchoscope, or tube exchanger) may be corrected by counterclockwise rotation of the ETT between 90° and 180°, plentiful lubrication, and/or laryngoscopy. Before removal of the AEC, successful tracheal position may be confirmed by VL viewing or by CO_2 detection connected to the endotracheal tube via a 15 mm adapter.

Successful reintubation over the AEC is excellent (greater than 90 %) but rescue options must be available for cases of difficulty or failure.

Duration of the Indwelling AEC?

Evidence-based studies that support a safe timeframe to keep the AEC in place are lacking. Experts suggest 30–60 min or until the likelihood of reintubation is minimized [76–78]. However, the largest series of DA extubation (nonrandomized) found that nearly one-half of those high-risk extubation who succumbed to reintubation failed within 2 h and the remaining patients failed their extubation trial generally between 2 and 10 h post-extubation [68]. Predicting when the need for reintubation is minimized can be difficult, particularly in the ICU population, who may suffer acute alterations in their cardiopulmonary, metabolic, or neurological status. The clinician's experience, judgment, and assessment of the patient should be the basis for determining the duration of AEC placement. That said, current recommendations for 30–60 min may be appropriate for the operating room extubation with no underlying cardiopulmonary issues. However, the debilitated and weakened ICU patient with a DA and recovering from bronchopneumonia and 5 days of mechanical ventilation would warrant a longer timeframe [78, 79]. Regardless, continued close observation post-extubation and immediate availability of advanced airway devices and skilled personnel is key. We recommend in high-risk patients that 1–2 h minimum is appropriate with a range to up to 24 h for those with airway concerns coupled with cardiopulmonary/neuro/systemic alterations that markedly increase the risk of extubation intolerance.

Extubation Following Cervical Spine Surgery/Trauma

Mechanical airway compromise following cervical spine injury, fracture, or surgery is a relatively uncommon, yet known, entity. Retropharyngeal hematoma, prevertebral soft tissue edema, periglottic edema, limited airway access due to a hard cervical collar or a halo vest, and vocal cord dysfunction, paresis, or paralysis lend to the challenge of these patients. Airway obstruction leading to respiratory distress and emergent need for airway management and possible surgical intervention is the ultimate catastrophe related to this clinical group. These potentially life-threatening airway difficulties warrant special emphasis due to their extreme nature and potential for a disastrous outcome. Tracheal intubation may be relatively straightforward especially under elective controlled circumstances; however, the subsequent condition of the airway may be altered significantly following an extensive resuscitation, surgical manipulation, and ICU care. The presence of risk factors (Table 10.11) suggests that immediate postoperative extubation may be best managed on a delayed basis. Meticulous postoperative fluid management with the goal of negative fluid balance (if clinically appropriate), elevation of the head of bed, diuresis, and possibly steroid administration, combined with the passage of time, continue to be the best counterbalance for induced airway deformities. In extreme cases, a surgical airway will supplant tracheal extubation.

Table 10.11 Risk factors for delayed extubation and management difficulties

Duration of surgical procedure, e.g., greater than 4 h
Intraoperative volume administration, e.g., greater than 4,000 mL
"Complicated surgical procedure"
Intraoperative blood loss, e.g., greater than 500 mL
Transfusion requirements, more than 2 units packed cells
Multilevel (3 or more) repair compared to single level repair
Anterior/posterior > anterior > posterior surgical site
Prone > supine
Trauma surgery >> elective surgical manipulation
Difficult airway management at intubation
Halo vest >> hard cervical collar >> soft collar
Obesity, OSA
Discectomy–fusion > fusion > discectomy
Obvious external airway alterations: lip/tongue/face swelling

Data from Epstein et al. [100], Manski et al. [101], Kwon et al. [102], Mazzon et al. [103], Personal Communications with Carin Hagberg MD, UT Houston, Herman Hospital and the Society for Airway Management (SAM) Forum Discussion group

Accidental Extubation in the NeuroICU

Accidental extubation in the ICU can be patient initiated (self) (uncontrolled agitation or knowingly pulling the ETT out) or inadvertent displacement of the ETT during patient positioning or transfer; proper taping of the endotracheal tube minimizes accidental extubation. Skin adhesives have merit in securing tape to the face and neck and shaving of facial hair may be necessary to facilitate the adhesiveness of the tape. Head elevation and persistent oral care, e.g., suctioning, may be helpful to reduce secretion buildup that undermines the tapes' security. Optimally, the ETT is secured with a circumferential taping around the neck with the understanding that "tight" taping might interfere with venous return leading to passive venous congestion from internal jugular compression with potential consequences in the presence of elevated ICP. New tube securing devices have been introduced to replace standard taping.

Accidental extubation is an airway emergency by definition, because many of these patients have severe underlying respiratory dysfunction or altered neurological/mental status. Inadvertent extubation more frequently requires rapid reintubation as compared to patient-initiated extubation [80–83]. Nonetheless, the armamentarium needed to successfully manipulate the airway in a "cannot intubate, cannot ventilate" situation, post "self-extubation," should be promptly available not only in the operating rooms but also in the ICU setting. Despite the presence of a well-stocked difficult airway cart available in the ICU, the intensivist without experience in advanced airway devices and emergency cricothyrotomy should immediately seek the help of surgical and anesthesia colleagues.

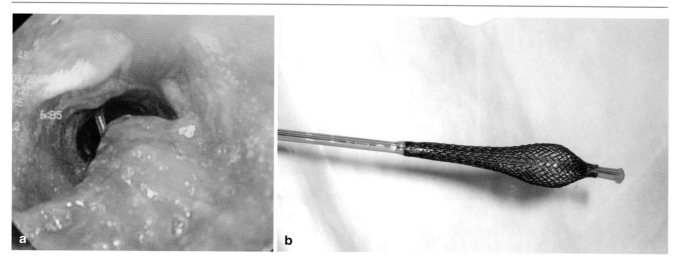

Fig. 10.39 (**a, b**) Occluding biofilm in ETT of ICU patient exhibiting acute airway obstruction (**a**) at multiple levels on lumen wall. Figure (**b**) shows an inflatable cuffed catheter with lattice covering (CAM Rescue Cath™, Omneotech, Tavernier, FL) to assist in removal of biofilm and concretions from the luminal wall

Biofilm Management in the Intubated ICU Patient

Biofilm and adherence of secretions to the ETT lumen have been implicated in the development of VAP, increased work of breathing, delays in extubation, as well as other complications. Thick copious secretions are a common problem in intubated patients that may slowly or rapidly accumulate leading to luminal narrowing or obstruction. Pulmonary secretions, blood, and aspiration soilage promote the development of a luminal biofilm at a single site or multiple levels. It may remain unappreciated by the care providers until acute partial or complete obstruction takes place. Standard suctioning techniques may fail to remove such accumulations since the suction catheter simply slides past the narrowing and is unable to remove the residual "concretions" [84, 85] (Fig. 10.39a, b).

Diagnosing the presence of biofilm may require bronchoscopy. Saline lavage and direct bronchoscopic suctioning of the accumulated concretions is possible but is time consuming and labor intensive and may obstruct the ETT lumen during attempted biofilm removal. If bronchoscopic attempts fail, the ETT may need to be exchanged. Exchange has its own intrinsic risks especially in the known or suspected difficult airway patient. Recently introduced luminal hygiene products such as the CAM Rescue Cath™ (Omneotech, Tavernier, FL) may prove effective in biofilm removal and avert high-risk ETT exchange. As a balloon-tipped catheter that is advanced to the distal end of the ETT, the mesh-covered balloon is inflated and then the catheter is withdrawn from the ETT while removing the accumulated debris (Fig. 10.39a, b).

Another common problem encountered is damage to the ETT or tracheostomy cuff or the pilot balloon-tubing assembly. If the cuff has been damaged, the ETT will have to be exchanged. However, an intact cuff may deflate due to an incompetent pilot balloon valve or a failure of the pilot balloon-tubing assembly due to perforation or breakage. An incompetent valve may be remedied by (1) ETT exchange, (2) pilot balloon inflation followed by clamping of the balloon-valve tubing, (3) placing a three-way stopcock on the end of the pilot balloon valve to resecure the incompetent valve, and (4) cutting the pilot balloon–valve tubing and replacing it with a manufactured replacement pilot balloon-tubing assembly (Fig. 10.40a–c).

Criteria for and Timing of Elective Tracheostomy in the NeuroICU

If the patient does not fulfill the criteria for safe extubation, a tracheostomy should be planned. Indication and timing of tracheostomy in the NeuroICU patient may differ from those in other ICUs [86–89]. Catastrophic neurological problems requiring NeuroICU admission are often associated with severe respiratory failure. Pulmonary infection as a result of aspiration or nosocomial infection is common, and concurrent factors include severely altered mental status, the inability to clear secretions, poor cough reflex, or continuous trachea trauma secondary to severe agitation while on mechanical ventilation. Timing of extubation in the NeuroICU can be difficult to evaluate and recurrent respiratory failure postextubation is common due to fluctuating mental status and compromised airway reflexes. Furthermore, central hyperventilation and Cheyne–Stoke breathing are common in these patients and may be misinterpreted as a clinical index of increased work of breathing, delaying extubation. While

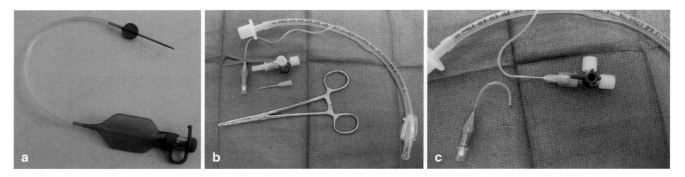

Fig. 10.40 (**a–c**) Pilot balloon repair. Replacement pilot balloon–line assembly (**a**), homemade repair kit (**b**), and final result (**c**)

the early application of elective tracheostomy may raise concerns of unnecessary surgical procedures in subjects with the potential for rapid neurological recovery, many extubated patients require reintubation and an increased ICU and hospital length of stay. Many patients who undergo early creation of a surgical airway are weaned from mechanical ventilation within 48 h of tracheostomy [89]. Another possible advantage of early tracheostomy is decreased laryngeal injury, commonly found after intubation for more than 5 days. While a tracheostomy greatly facilitates handling of the airway and weaning from mechanical ventilation, the procedure itself has a small but well-defined morbidity when performed in critically ill patients [86–89]. Overall, timing of tracheostomy and the approach (conventional open versus percutaneous) is still debated in the surgical literature, but a conservative approach to airway management is always recommended when feasible. Medical personnel with expertise in management of conventional and alternative airway devices should be immediately available.

Exchanging the Endotracheal Tube

Exchange of the ETT may be required (cuff perforation, pilot balloon–valve failure, a damaged ETT, luminal narrowing, kinking) or be elective (change size or location). Some situations may be urgent/emergent as when oxygenation and ventilation suffer while temporary repairs to the pilot balloon–valve are made. Ineffective pulmonary toilet due to small ETT size, difficulty weaning, or inability to perform positive-pressure ventilation may warrant exchange. Tachypnea from increased imposed work of breathing due to small ETT size may be compensated for through the appropriate use of pressure support ventilation. However, one should differentiate this clinical picture from central hyperventilation due to neurological disease and luminal narrowing from biofilm accumulation.

The method of ETT exchange should be based on the particular airway status and its potential for difficulty, equipment choices, and the experience and judgment of the airway

Table 10.12 Advantages of continuous glottic viewing during ETT exchange (VL)

Pre-exchange airway evaluation to assist with management strategy
Assessment of glottic status to allow upsizing of replacement ETT
Confirmation of passing of AEC into trachea (via ETT)
Confirmation of ongoing AEC positioning within trachea (during exchange)
ETT manipulation to reduce arytenoid, vocal cord, and posterior structure hang-up
Observation/confirmation of reintubation of trachea with replacement ETT
Monitoring of depth of replacement ETT during intubation and following AEC removal
Observation of passive/active regurgitation and/or aspiration during exchange
Observation/evaluation of any laryngeal–glottic intubation trauma/damage/injury
Intubation adjunct for rescue if AEC or ETT becomes displaced or reintubation fails
Teaching/educational benefit for trainees and nursing and respiratory therapy staff

team. Maintaining continuous airway access during the exchange via an airway exchange catheter is recommended in all but the simplest, straightforward airway situations. While DL is recommended to assist with ETT exchange, viewing the periglottic anatomy is often restricted or impossible when using conventional methods. Alternatively, VL offers displacement of soft tissues coupled with improved glottic visualization (Table 10.12). Visualization offers the team to see the AEC advance into the trachea, removal of the old ETT, maintenance of the AEC within the trachea, reintubation of the trachea, troubleshoot difficulty advancing the new ETT, and confirmation that the new ETT is properly positioned within the trachea [90]. A strategy for exchanging an ETT is outlined in Table 10.13.

An alternative approach would be that the old ETT is backed out of the trachea over an AEC while an ETT-loaded FOB is advanced into the trachea. In case of accidental displacement of the tube exchanger, the second ETT-loaded FOB in place can be used for intubation of the trachea.

In summary, exchanging an ETT or extubating a difficult airway in the NeuroICU can be dangerous, even in expert hands, and the potential for secondary brain injury is great. The rate of complications is potentially high and specialized personnel equipped with an assortment of advanced airway rescue devices should be readily available.

Dislocation of ETT (Partial or Complete Extubation of the Trachea)

Partial or complete extubation of the trachea is typified by the tube being in one of three potential locations within the airway: cuff between vocal cords (partial extubation), ETT tip at level of vocal cords (complete extubation), and the ETT tip-cuff in hypopharynx (complete extubation) (Fig. 10.41a–c). A dislocated ETT may masquerade as a

Table 10.13 Strategy and preparation for ETT exchange

1. Review patient history, problem list, medications, ventilatory support
2. Assemble conventional/rescue airway equipment
3. Assemble personnel (nursing, respiratory therapy, surgeon, airway colleagues)
4. Sedation/analgesia ± neuromuscular blocking agents (minimize patient participation)
5. Optimal positioning, e.g., ramping for obese
6. Airway assessment (external/internal with VL assistance)
7. Discuss primary/rescue strategies and role of team members, choose new ETT
8. Suction out airway, advance lubricated large AEC via ETT to 22–26 cm depth
9. Elevate airway tissues with laryngoscope/hand, remove old ETT, pass new ETT (preferably VL assisted)
10. Remove AEC and check ETT with capnography/bronch with swivel adapter and check capnography with AEC in place (VL obviates these steps)

"cuff leak" and ETT exchange may be contemplated. It is imperative to *check the status* of the pilot balloon: if intact (holds insufflated air), then the ETT tip-cuff location is likely not "intratracheal." If the "cuff leak" is erroneously identified as a malfunctioning ETT cuff and the airway team passes an airway exchange catheter (AEC), the misplaced distal tip of the ETT may allow passage of the AEC to areas external to the trachea, e.g., esophagus and pyriform sinus.

Two methods we strongly recommend to diagnostically and therapeutically manage the possible ETT tip–cuff dislocation are as follows: first choice, flexible FOB to diagnose the tip location and therapeutically allow reintubation of the trachea, if possible (85 % likely at authors' institution), and second choice, laryngoscopy, preferably VL as opposed to DL so to allow improved visualization of the airway and possibly improve the margin of safety in this potentially life-threatening consequence of the intubated ICU patient.

An airway caveat: The level of the ETT at the dentition line has little correlation with ETT tip location in the ICU setting (based on a database of partial extubation at the author's institution). For example, with the ETT at less than 20 cm at the dentition line, 55 % of ETTs were above the glottis when evaluated by FOB. When the ETT is further than 20 cm, 73 % were at the level of glottis or above glottis, in the hypopharynx. Overall, 51 % of ETT tips were above the vocal cords, 32 % were at the level of the vocal cords, and in 17 % the cuff was located between the vocal cords on FOB examination [91].

The management of this clinical situation with DL alone is fraught with complications such as severe hypoxemia, esophageal intubation, loss of the airway, bradycardia, and cardiac arrest. Diagnostic and therapeutic management with FOB or VL is the authors' choice to deal with ETT dislocation. Nearly, 20 % had the ETT tip abutting the vocal cords, pharyngeal wall, or other tissues that made it very difficult to advance the FOB into the trachea. Thus, alternative airway

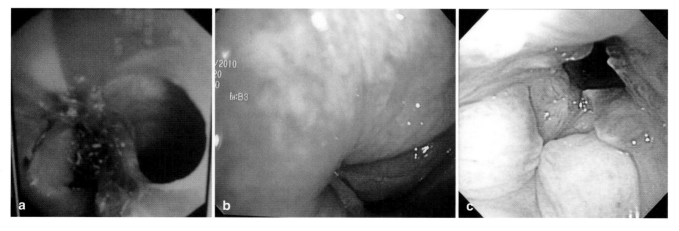

Fig. 10.41 (**a–c**) Partial and complete tracheal extubation. Cuff between vocal cords and tip of ETT impaled against thyroid cartilage (**a**), ETT tip impinged on thyroid cartilage with vocal cords seen distally (**b**), and ETT tip well above glottis offering a full view via FOB (**c**)

management schema beyond the FOB and VL must be available to rescue the airway in the event difficulty is encountered.

The Difficult Airway Cart (DAC)

It is absolutely imperative that the ICU has a stocked DAC. Even if staff members outside the ICU staff use the contents of the DAC, e.g., anesthesia airway team, the two departments need to coordinate the purchase of the DAC, its restocking, checking, maintenance, and upgrading for optimal care. Standard contents are suggested by various societies (Table 10.14) [2, 3, 7, 92]. Customization of the contents to the needs, experience, and skill level of the airway team is warranted. A carry tote bag to transport needed airway equipment to the patient's bedside is another warranted accessory for the ICU and the airway team (Table 10.15).

Table 10.14 Suggested content of the difficult airway cart

Adult
  A. Nasal:
    Nasopharyngeal airways: sizes 6, 7, 8
    Nasal endotracheal tubes: sizes 6.0, 7.0, 8.0
  B. Oral:
    Oropharyngeal airways: sizes S, M, L
    Stylets/intubating guides:
      (a) Endotracheal tube stylet
      (b) Gum elastic bougie: sizes 10 Fr, 15 Fr
    ETT: cuffed sizes 5.0–9.0 (Hi-Lo evacuation)
    ETT: Parker specialty ETT (FlexTip, 6.0–8.0)
    ETT: wire-reinforced ETT-6.0–9.0
    Fiber-optic laryngoscope blades:
      (a) Curved: Macintosh 3, 4
      (b) Straight: Miller 2, 3, 4
    Fiber-optic laryngoscope handles: regular, stubby, slender models
    Laryngeal masks: (LMA or variant)
      (a) Classic style: sizes 3, 4, 5
      (b) Fastrach® intubating laryngeal masks: sizes 3, 4, 5
      (c) Supreme® LMA (ProSeal®): sizes 3, 4, 5
    ETT for laryngeal masks: sizes 6.0–7.0 cuffed, Aintree catheter
    Combitube®: adult, small adult (alternative: King LT®, EZ® tube)
    Lung isolation:
      (a) Cook-Arndt bronchial blocker (various sizes) or
      (b) Univent ETT with blocker (various sizes)
      (c) Double-lumen endotracheal tubes: sizes 35, 37, 39, 41 Fr
  C. Cricothyroid membrane:
    Transcricothyroid membrane jet ventilation:
      (a) Intravenous catheters: #14, #12 gauge (length: 2 in.)
      (b) Jet ventilation hose with controller handle and pressure downregulator and Luer lock connector

Table 10.14 (continued)

    Retrograde transcricothyroid membrane kit
    Melker percutaneous dilational cricothyroidotomy set: sizes 3, 4, 6
    Patil cricothyroidotomy catheter
    Surgical cricothyroidotomy:
      (a) #3 scalper handle, #11 blade, trachea retraction hook, tissue spreader
      (b) Size 6.0 endotracheal tube
      (c) Cuffed tracheostomy tubes: sizes 4–8
  D. Accessory equipment
    Confirming position of endotracheal tube: ETCO$_2$ colorimetric detector
    Esophageal detector syringe or self-inflating bulb
    Endotracheal tube exchange catheters: with jet ventilation capability
    Patil-Syracuse mask or VBM mask (diaphragm/portal to allow FOB via masking)
    Bronchoscopic swivel adapter
    Oxygen delivery
      (a) Ambu manual resuscitation bag with masks
      (b) Mapleson D with pressure gauge
      (c) Oxygen tubing with nipple for connecting to oxygen wall outlet or tank
      (d) Stethoscope
    Suction:
      (a) Endotracheal suction
        Catheters: sizes #10, #12, #14
      (b) Yankauer oral suction
        Suction tubing
    Others:
      (a) Spare batteries and bulbs for laryngoscope
      (b) Bite blocks
      (c) Magill forceps
    Local anesthetic and nasal vasoconstrictor
      (a) Atomizer for spraying lidocaine 4 % solution
      (b) Benzocaine spray 20 % solution
      (c) 1 % phenylephrine spray
    Fiberoptic bronchoscope with intubating airway and defogger
    Dedicated NeuroICU adult rigid fiberoptic laryngoscope (your choice)
Pediatric
  A. Age-/size-appropriate straight/curved laryngoscope blades
  B. Masks: neonatal, infant, toddler, child
  C. Oral and nasal airway (variety of sizes)
  D. Flexible pediatric FOB
  E. LMA: 0–3 (SGA variants)
  F. Neonatal/pediatric VL (GlideScope®, Airtraq®, Storz®) choose one or more
  G. Pediatric retrograde intubation kit
  H. Size-/age-appropriate surgical access kit

Modified with kind permission of Springer Science+Business Media from McGuire and Wong [92]

Table 10.15 Portable travel bag

Carried to the bedside and assumes that a locked and secure tackle box containing standard airway management equipment/medications/suction is available throughout the institution:

A. Bougie (airway exchange catheters optional)

B. Classic LMA-SGA devices (various adult sizes)

C. Fastrach® LMA (sizes 3, 4, 5)

D. LMA Supreme® (sizes 3, 4, 5)

E. Combitube®/King LT®/EasyTube® (choose one, several sizes)

F. Airtraq® Optical Laryngoscope—various sizes (budget conscious)

G. Optional: GlideScope® Ranger, McGrath® Scope

H. Optional: optical stylet—Levitan, Shikani (Clarus® Medical)

I. Surgical access kit (hospital based or purchased commercially)

J. Transtracheal needle-jet equipment (do not carry it unless you understand its execution and use). 12, 14 g needles, alternative; Cook–Enk® System

Special Considerations for the Pediatric Difficult Airway

The airway anatomy of a child progressively approaches that of the adult over the first several years of life. A newborn's airway anatomy, however, substantially differs from the adult. Common findings include a large tongue and epiglottis, large tonsils and adenoids, and a relatively anterior position of the larynx. Neonatal or pediatric airway anatomy in children with neurological abnormalities and associated congenital craniofacial pathology represents a formidable challenge to the physician attempting to obtain tracheal access. Other clinical concerns are a small functional residual capacity and high oxygen consumption, leading to a faster rate of desaturation, and an immature autonomic nervous system exquisitely sensitive to hypoxemia and airway manipulation, which may lead to bradycardia.

Adequate topical anesthesia of the airway for fiber-optic intubation of the trachea may be impractical or impossible in children in the ICU scheduled for an elective neurosurgical procedure or radiological test. In these cases, the patient may be transported to an anesthetizing locale for the popular approach of maintaining spontaneous ventilation with inhalation anesthesia induction. Nevertheless, a difficult airway kit should be available and pediatric airway manipulation should be managed by personnel with appropriate pediatric airway skills. Currently, the advent of VL offers the operator access to pediatric- and neonatal-sized devices that have expanded the management armamentarium. The devices that we believe should be immediately available when dealing with pediatric difficult intubation in the pediatric or neonatal neurological or NeuroICU include:

1. Flexible pediatric/neonatal FOB
2. Small-size LMA's (sizes 1–3)
3. Pediatric retrograde endotracheal intubation kit (22 gauge catheter that will accommodate 0.018 in. guide wire)
4. Video laryngoscopy device—pediatric/neonatal models
5. Age-/size-appropriate surgical airway access

Training Issues in Managing Difficult Airways

The inability to successfully intubate the trachea in neurologically injured patients is a leading cause of morbidity and mortality. A dedicated intensivist physician in charge of the NeuroICU should be familiar with the evaluation and management of difficult airways in the critically ill patient. If not personally competent in airway management, then expert consultation with the anesthesiology airway team should be immediately available and provided in the NeuroICU 24 h a day, in order to avoid unnecessary patient risk. Training with mannequins and simulated drills of difficult airways in human cadavers are also recommended in order to improve and maintain skill levels [93–96]. Rehearsing the common airway management scenarios in the NeuroICU setting (extubation, difficult airway intubation, ETT exchange, partial extubation, self-extubation, displaced tracheostomy) may improve patient safety.

In summary, the management of the airway in the NeuroICU is an important skill that can dramatically impact the patient's outcome and survival. There is no easy answer to the question of how to rapidly acquire such skills. We recommend *constant presence in the unit* of specialized medical personnel with proven skill in the management of difficult airways and airway equipment as well as in-depth knowledge of unique problems of the neurologically injured patient.

References

1. Peterson GN, Domino KB, Caplan RA, et al. Management of the difficult airway: a closed claims analysis. Anesthesiology. 2005;105:33–9.
2. Crosby ET, Cooper RM, Douglas MJ, et al. The unanticipated difficult airway with recommendations for management. Can J Anaesth. 1998;45(7):757–76.
3. Practice Guidelines for Management of the Difficult Airway. An updated report by the American Society of Anesthesiologists Task Force on Management of the Difficult Airway. Anesthesiology. 2003;98:1269–77.
4. Metzner J, Posner KL, Lam MS, et al. Closed claims' analysis. Best Pract Res Clin Anaesthesiol. 2011;25(2):263–76.
5. Leach RM, Treacher DS. ABC of oxygen: oxygen transport – 2. Tissue hypoxia. BMJ. 1998;317:1370–3.
6. Kochanek PM. Bakken lecture: the brain, the heart, and therapeutic hypothermia. Cleve Clin J Med. 2009;76:8–12.
7. Henderson JJ, Popat MT, Latto IP, et al. Difficult Airway Society guidelines for management of the unanticipated difficult intubation. Anaesthesia. 2004;59(7):675–94.

8. Heidegger T, Gerig HJ, Henderson JJ. Strategies and algorithms for management of the difficult airway. Best Pract Res Clin Anaesthesiol. 2005;19(4):661–74.

9. Yentis SM. Predicting difficult intubation – worthwhile exercise or pointless ritual? Anaesthesia. 2002;57(2):105–9.

10. Rosenblatt W, Ianus AI, Sukhupragarn W, et al. Preoperative endoscopic airway examination (PEAE) provides superior airway information and may reduce the use of unnecessary awake intubation. Anesth Analg. 2011;112(3):602–7.

11. Cook TM. A new practical classification of laryngeal view. Anaesthesia. 2000;55:274–9.

12. Yentis SM. Laryngoscopy grades. Anaesthesia. 1999;54(12):1221–2.

13. Mort TC. Emergency tracheal intubation: complications associated with repeated laryngoscopic attempts. Anesth Analg. 2004;99(2):607–13.

14. Leibowitz AB. Persistent preoxygenation efforts before tracheal intubation in the intensive care unit are of no use: who would have guessed? Crit Care Med. 2009;37:335–6.

15. Mort TC, Waberski BH, Clive J. Extending the preoxygenation period from 4 to 8 mins in critically ill patients undergoing emergency intubation. Crit Care Med. 2009;37:68–71.

16. Langeron O, Masso E, Huraux C, et al. Prediction of difficult mask ventilation. Anesthesiology. 2000;92(5):1229–36.

17. Mort TC. The incidence and risk factors for cardiac arrest during emergency tracheal intubation: a justification for incorporating the ASA Guidelines in the remote location. J Clin Anesth. 2004;16:508–16.

18. Mort TC. Esophageal intubation with indirect clinical tests during emergency tracheal intubation: a report on patient morbidity. J Clin Anesth. 2005;17(4):255–62.

19. Warner MA, Warner ME, Weber JG. Clinical significance of pulmonary aspiration during the perioperative period. Anesthesiology. 1993;78(1):56–62.

20. Niederman MS. Distinguishing chemical pneumonitis from bacterial aspiration: still a clinical determination. Crit Care Med. 2011;39(6):1543–4.

21. Mort TC. Complications of emergency tracheal intubation: immediate airway-related consequences: part II. J Intensive Care Med. 2007;22:208–15.

22. Nishisaki A, Nguyen J, Colborn S, et al. Influence of residency training on multiple attempts at endotracheal intubation. Can J Anaesth. 2010;57:823–9.

23. Griesdale DE, Bosma TL, Kurth T, Isac G, Chittock DR. Complications of endotracheal intubation in the critically ill. Intensive Care Med. 2008;34:1835–42.

24. Mort TC. Complications of emergency tracheal intubation: hemodynamic alterations – part I. J Intensive Care Med. 2007;22:157–65.

25. Benumof JL, Dagg R, Benumof R. Critical hemoglobin desaturation will occur before return to an unparalyzed state following 1 mg/kg intravenous succinylcholine. Anesthesiology. 1997;87:979–82.

26. Takahata O, Kubota M, Mamiya K, et al. The efficacy of the "BURP" maneuver during a difficult laryngoscopy. Anesth Analg. 1997;84:419–21.

27. Saxena S. The ASA, difficult airway algorithm: is it time to include video laryngoscopy and discourage blind and multiple intubation attempts in the nonemergency pathway? Anesth Analg. 2009;108(3):1052.

28. Sakles JC, Mosier JM, Chiu S, et al. Tracheal intubation in the emergency department: a comparison of GlideScope(®) video laryngoscopy to direct laryngoscopy in 822 intubations. J Emerg Med. 2012;42(4):400–5.

29. Brown CA, Bair AE, Pallin DJ, National Emergency Airway Registry (NEAR) Investigators, et al. Improved glottic exposure with the Video Macintosh Laryngoscope in adult emergency department tracheal intubations. Ann Emerg Med. 2010;56(2):83–8.

30. Cooper RM, Pacey JA, Bishop MJ, McCluskey S. Early clinical experience with a new videolaryngoscope (GlideScope) in 728 patients. Can J Anaesth. 2005;52(2):191–8.

31. Mort TC. Tracheal tube exchange: feasibility of continuous glottic viewing with advanced laryngoscopy assistance. Anesth Analg. 2009;108(4):1228–31.

32. Rosenblatt WH. The Airway Approach Algorithm: a decision tree for organizing preoperative airway information. J Clin Anesth. 2004;16(4):312–6.

33. Cheney FW, Posner KL, Lee LA, et al. Trends in anesthesia-related death and brain damage: a closed claims analysis. Anesthesiology. 2006;105(6):1081–6.

34. Rosenblatt WH. Preoperative planning of airway management in critical care patients. Crit Care Med. 2004;32(4 Suppl):S186–92.

35. Andrew Z, John DD, Marc O. Use of the Aintree intubation catheter in a patient with an unexpected difficult airway. Can J Anaesth. 2005;52(6):646–9.

36. Pennant JH, Walker MB. Comparison of the endotracheal tube and the laryngeal mask in airway management by paramedical personnel. Anesth Analg. 1992;74:531–4.

37. Mort TC. Laryngeal mask airway and bougie intubation failures: the Combitube as a secondary rescue device for in-hospital emergency airway management. Anesth Analg. 2006;103(5):1264–6.

38. Vézina D, Lessard MR, Bussières J, et al. Complications associated with the use of the esophageal-tracheal Combitube™. Can J Anaesth. 1998;45(1):76–80.

39. Hubble MW, Wilfong DA, Brown LH, et al. A meta-analysis of prehospital airway control techniques part II: alternative airway devices and cricothyrotomy success rates. Prehosp Emerg Care. 2010;14(4):515–30.

40. Metterlein T, Frommer M, Ginzkey C, et al. Randomized trial comparing two cuffed emergency cricothyrotomy devices using a wire-guided and a catheter-over-needle technique. J Emerg Med. 2011;41(3):326–32.

41. Berkow LC, Greenberg RS, Kan KH, et al. Need for emergency surgical airway reduced by a comprehensive difficult airway program. Anesth Analg. 2009;109(6):1860–9.

42. Cardoso MMSC, Banner MJ, Melker RJ, et al. Portable devices used to detect endotracheal intubation during emergency situations: a review. Crit Care Med. 1998;26(5):957–64.

43. Rudraraju P, Eisen LA. Confirmation of endotracheal tube position: a narrative review. J Intensive Care Med. 2009;24(5):283–92.

44. Chou HC, Tseng WP, Wang CH, et al. Tracheal rapid ultrasound exam (T.R.U.E.) for confirming endotracheal tube placement during emergency intubation. Resuscitation. 2011;82(10):1279–84.

45. Rosenblatt WH, Wagner PJ, Ovassapian A, et al. Practice patterns in managing the difficult airway by anesthesiologists in the United States. Anesth Analg. 1998;87:153–7.

46. Ferson DZ, Rosenblatt WH, Johansen MJ, Osborn I, Ovassapian A. Use of the intubating LMA-Fastrach in 254 patients with difficult-to-manage airways. Anesthesiology. 2001;95(5):1175–81.

47. Tentillier E, Heydenreich C, Cros AM, Schmitt V, Dindart JM, Thicoipe M. Use of the intubating laryngeal mask airway in emergency pre-hospital difficult intubation. Resuscitation. 2008;77(1):30–4.

48. Timmermann A, Russo SG, Rosenblatt WH, Eich C, Barwing J, Roessler M, Graf BM. Intubating laryngeal mask airway for difficult out-of-hospital airway management: a prospective evaluation. Br J Anaesth. 2007;99(2):286–91.

49. Keller C, Brimacombe J, Kleinsasser A, Brimacombe L. The Laryngeal Mask Airway ProSeal(TM) as a temporary ventilatory device in grossly and morbidly obese patients before laryngoscope-guided tracheal intubation. Anesth Analg. 2002;94(3):737–40.

50. Brimacombe J, Keller C. The ProSeal Laryngeal Mask Airway. A randomized, crossover study with the standard laryngeal mask airway in paralyzed, anesthetized patients. Anesthesiology. 2000;93(1):104–9.

51. Reinhart DJ, Simmons G. Comparison of placement of the laryngeal mask airway with endotracheal tube by paramedics and respiratory therapists. Ann Emerg Med. 1994;24(2):260–3.

52. Davies PRF, Tighe SQM, Greenslade GL, et al. Laryngeal mask airway and tracheal tube insertion by unskilled personnel. Lancet. 1990;336:977–9.

53. Devitt JH, Wenstone R, Noel AG, et al. The laryngeal mask airway and positive-pressure ventilation. Anesthesiology. 1994;80:550–5.

54. Lim SL, Tay DHB, Thomas E. A comparison of three types of tracheal tube for use in laryngeal mask assisted blind orotracheal intubation. Anaesthesia. 1994;49:255–7.

55. Fukutome T, Amaha K, Nakazawa K, et al. Tracheal intubation through the intubating laryngeal mask airway in patients with difficult airways. Anaesth Intensive Care. 1998;26(4):387–91.

56. Baskett PJF, Parr MJA, Nolan JP. The intubating laryngeal mask: results of a multicentre trial with experience of 500 cases. Anaesthesia. 1998;53:1174–9.

57. Benumof JL, Scheller MS. The importance of transtracheal jet ventilation in the management of the difficult airway. Anesthesiology. 1989;71:769–78.

58. Leibovici D, Fredman B, Gofrit ON, et al. Prehospital cricothyroidotomy by physicians. Am J Emerg Med. 1997;15:91–3.

59. Chesnut RM. Secondary brain insults after head injury: clinical perspectives. New Horiz. 1995;3(3):366–75.

60. Jones GM, Murphy CV, Gerlach AT, et al. High-dose dexmedetomidine for sedation in the intensive care unit: an evaluation of clinical efficacy and safety. Ann Pharmacother. 2011;45(6):740–7.

61. Shatney CH, Brunner RD, Nguyen TQ. The safety of orotracheal intubation in patients with unstable cervical spine fracture or high spinal cord injury. Am J Surg. 1995;170:676–80.

62. Keller C, Brimacombe J, Keller K. Pressure exerted against the cervical vertebrae by this tender and intubating laryngeal mask airways: a randomized controlled crossover study in fresh cadavers. Anesth Analg. 1999;89:1296–300.

63. Shakespeare WA, Lanier WL, Perkins WJ, Pasternak JJ. Airway management in patients who develop neck hematomas after carotid endarterectomy. Anesth Analg. 2010;110(2):588–93.

64. Salins SR, Pothapragada KC, Korula G. Difficult oral intubation in acromegalic patients – a way out. J Neurosurg Anesthesiol. 2011;23(1):52.

65. Sharma D, Prabhakar H, Bithal PK, et al. Predicting difficult laryngoscopy in acromegaly: a comparison of upper lip bite test with modified Mallampati classification. J Neurosurg Anesthesiol. 2010;22(2):138–43.

66. Benditt JO. Management of pulmonary complications in neuromuscular disease. Phys Med Rehabil Clin N Am. 1998;9(1):167–85.

67. Miller KA, Harkin CP, Bailey PL. Postoperative tracheal extubation. Anesth Analg. 1995;80:149–72.

68. Mort TC. Continuous airway access for the difficult extubation: the efficacy of the airway exchange catheter. Anesth Analg. 2007;105(5):1357–62.

69. Cooper RM. Extubation of the difficult airway. Anesthesiology. 1997;87(2):460.

70. Cooper RM. Consider other extubation strategies to maintain difficult airways. Chest. 1995;108(4):1183.

71. Keck JP, Mort TC. Airway assessment in the known or suspected difficult airway ICU patient ready for extubation. Anesthesiology. 2010;A363.

72. Chung YH, Chao TY, Chiu CT, Lin MC. The cuff-leak test is a simple tool to verify severe laryngeal edema in patients undergoing long-term mechanical ventilation. Crit Care Med. 2006;34(2):409–14.

73. Mhanna MJ, Zamel YB, Tichy CM, Super DM. The "air leak" test around the endotracheal tube, as a predictor of postextubation stridor, is age dependent in children. Crit Care Med. 2002;30(12):2639–43.

74. Cheng KC, Hou CC, Huang HC, Lin SC, Zhang H. Intravenous injection of methylprednisolone reduces the incidence of postextubation stridor in intensive care unit patients. Crit Care Med. 2006;34(5):1345–50.

75. Loudermilk EP, Hartmanngruber M, Stoltfus DP, Langevin PB. A prospective study of the safety of tracheal extubation using a pediatric airway exchange catheter for patients with a known difficult airway. Chest. 1997;111:1660–5.

76. Hartmannsgruber MWB, Loudermilk EP, Stoltzfus DP. Prolonged use of a cook airway exchange catheter obviated the need for postoperative tracheostomy in an adult patient. J Clin Anesth. 1997;9:496–8.

77. Hagberg C. Chapter 16: Extubation of the difficult airway. In: Handbook of difficult airway management. Philadelphia: Churchill Livingstone; 2000.

78. Cooper RM. Extubation techniques. Anesthesiol Clin North Am. 1995;13(3).

79. Biro P, Priebe HJ. Staged extubation strategy: is an airway exchange catheter the answer? Anesth Analg. 2007;105(5):1182–5.

80. Epstein SK. Decision to extubate. Intensive Care Med. 2002;28:535–46.

81. Chang LC, Liu PF, Huang YL, et al. Risk factors associated with unplanned endotracheal self-extubation of hospitalized intubated patients. Appl Nurs Res. 2011;24(3):188–92.

82. Lucas da Silva PS, de Carvalho WB. Unplanned extubation in pediatric critically ill patients: a systematic review and best practice recommendations. Pediatr Crit Care Med. 2010;11(2):287–94.

83. Mort TC. Unplanned tracheal extubation outside the operating room: a quality improvement audit of hemodynamic and tracheal airway complications associated with emergency tracheal reintubation. Anesth Analg. 1998;86(6):1171–6.

84. Kirton O, Dehaven CB, Morgan J, et al. Elevated imposed work of breathing, masquerading as ventilator weaning intolerance. Chest. 1995;108:1021–5.

85. Shah C, Kollef MH. Endotracheal tube intraluminal volume loss among mechanically ventilated patients. Crit Care Med. 2004;32(1):120–5.

86. Skolarus LE, Morgenstern LB, Zahuranec DB, et al. Acute care and long-term mortality among elderly patients with intracerebral hemorrhage who undergo chronic life-sustaining procedures. J Stroke Cerebrovasc Dis. 2013;22(1):15–21.

87. Fernandez R, Tizon AI, Gonzalez J, et al. Intensive care unit discharge to the ward with a tracheostomy cannula as a risk factor for mortality: a prospective, multicenter propensity analysis. Crit Care Med. 2011;39(10):2240–5.

88. Kilic D, Fındıkcıoglu A, Akin S, et al. When is surgical tracheostomy indicated? Surgical "U-shaped" versus percutaneous tracheostomy. Ann Thorac Cardiovasc Surg. 2011;17(1):29–32.

89. Ganuza JR, Garcia FA, Gambarrutta C, et al. Effect of technique and timing of tracheostomy in patients with acute traumatic spinal cord injury undergoing mechanical ventilation. J Spinal Cord Med. 2011;34(1):76–84.

90. Benumof JL. Airway exchange catheters: simple concept, potentially great danger. Anesthesiology. 1999;91(2):342–4.

91. Shapiro AE, Mort TC. ETT displacement masquerading as a cuff leak in the ICU patient. In: Annual meeting of the American Society of Anesthesiologists, Oct 2009.

92. McGuire GP, Wong DT. Airway management: contents of a difficult intubation cart. Can J Anaesth. 1999;46(2):190–1.

93. Frengley RW, Weller J, Weller JM, et al. The effect of a simulation-based training intervention on the performance of established critical care unit teams. Crit Care Med. 2011;39(12):2605–11.

94. Pott LM, Randel GI, Straker T, et al. A survey of airway training among U.S. and Canadian anesthesiology residency programs. J Clin Anesth. 2011;23(1):15–26.

95. Blike G, Cravero J, Andeweg S, et al. Standardized simulated events for provocative testing of medical care system rescue capabilities. In: Henriksen K, Battles JB, Marks ES, Lewin DI, editors. Advances in patient safety: from research to implementation, Programs, tools, and products, vol. 4. Rockville: Agency for Healthcare Research and Quality (US); 2005.

96. Koppel JN, Reed AP. Formal instructions in difficult airway management: a survey of anesthesiology residency programs. Anesthesiology. 1995;83:1343–6.

97. Benumof JL. Airway management: principles and practice, chapter 7. St. Louis: Mosby Yearbook; 1996.

98. Gravenstein N, Kirby RR, editors. Clinical anesthesia practice. Philadelphia: WB Saunders Company; 1996.

99. Gabrielli AG, Layon AJ. Airway management in the neurointensive care unit. In: Layon AJ, Gabrielli AG, Friedman WA, editors. Textbook of neurointensive care. Philadelphia: WB Saunders; 2004.

100. Epstein NE, et al. Can airway complications following multilevel anterior cervical surgery be avoided? J Neurosurg. 2001; 94(2):185–8.

101. Manski TJ, et al. Bilateral vocal cord paralysis following anterior cervical discectomy and fusion. J Neurosurg. 1998;89: 839–43.

102. Kwon B, et al. Risk factors for delayed extubation after single-stage, multi-level anterior cervical decompression and posterior fusion. J Spinal Disord Tech. 2006;19(6):389–93.

103. Mazzon D, et al. Upper airway obstruction by retropharyngeal hematoma after cervical spine trauma with percutaneous tracheostomy. J Neurosurg Anesthesiol. 1998;10(4):237–40.

Neurologic Injury and Mechanical Ventilation

11

Kevin W. Hatton

Contents

K.W. Hatton, MD
Division of Critical Care Medicine, Department of Anesthesiology,
University of Kentucky, 800 Rose Street,
Lexington, KY 40502, USA
e-mail: kevin.hatton@uky.edu

Abstract

Patients with many different types of neurologic injury may develop respiratory system failure for a variety of reasons. In addition, the potential complications of respiratory system failure, including hypoxemia and acidosis, may cause significant additional injury to patients with neurologic disease. Mechanical ventilation (MV) is a supportive therapy that can be used to prevent these systemic complications of respiratory system failure in patients with and without neurologic injury.

While MV is generally delivered through one of several conventional modes of ventilation, several advanced modes of ventilation have also been recently developed to further increase the effectiveness of MV. Regardless of the mode of MV used, careful titration and monitoring of many different MV settings is needed to optimize oxygenation and ventilation. The use of one or more adjunctive therapies may be necessary to improve oxygenation in conditions associated with severe respiratory system dysfunction, such as acute respiratory distress syndrome (ARDS). Specific protocols have been described for MV in these patients to gain the maximum benefit to the patient while reducing the potential for complications.

Ventilator separation (typically through tracheal extubation) is an important consideration in MV therapy. The use of protocolized spontaneous breathing trials to determine the optimum timing for ventilator separation has not been validated in patients with neurologic disease; nevertheless, a daily evaluation for the appropriateness of extubation is probably warranted. Careful monitoring for recovery of neurologic dysfunction is an important facet to ventilator separation as many patients may have resolution of their respiratory system dysfunction but cannot be separated from MV due to their underlying neurologic injury.

A.J. Layon et al. (eds.), *Textbook of Neurointensive Care*,
DOI 10.1007/978-1-4471-5226-2_11, © Springer-Verlag London 2013

Keywords

Respiratory system physiology • Mechanical ventilation Treatment of hypoxemia • Positive end-expiratory pressure (PEEP) • Recruitment maneuver • Spontaneous breathing trial • Ventilator-induced lung injury • Lung protective ventilation strategies

Introduction

The respiratory system (RS) is a complicated organ system whose primary function is to facilitate respiration (commonly described as the movement of oxygen and carbon dioxide gas across the alveolocapillary membrane). The RS consists of the conducting airways (both inside and outside of the thorax), the lung parenchyma, the pulmonary vasculature, and the associated lymphatic channels. In addition, the RS is also responsible for immunologic defense from the external environment, for filtering the blood of unwanted toxins, and for providing a reservoir for blood during acute stress events. Because of the central role that the RS plays in the maintenance of internal homeostasis, through the continuous exchange of oxygen and carbon dioxide between the patient and the external environment, patient injuries or disease processes that result in a serious decrement in RS function may result in significant patient morbidity or death.

Non-respiratory system disease or injury (e.g., central or peripheral nervous system disease) can result in significant RS dysfunction. Additionally, many therapies for non-respiratory system disease or injury may directly interfere with normal RS function.

Basic Respiratory System Physiology

The gas movements that occur during inspiration and exhalation in the lung, collectively called ventilation, are passively dependent on a complicated interplay of three variables: driving pressure (ΔP), gas volume (V), and airflow (F). The driving pressure is the net pressure developed across the respiratory system during inspiration ($P_{alveolus} - P_{atmosphere}$). During the inspiratory phase of a spontaneous, unassisted breath, the muscles of respiration contract to create a slight negative intrathoracic pressure that is conveyed to the lungs and alveoli across the pleural space. The ΔP is therefore slightly negative during the inspiratory phase of spontaneous ventilation and gas flows from the higher pressure (atmospheric) to the lower pressure (alveoli). During the inspiratory phase of positive pressure ventilation (as will be discussed later in this chapter), the ventilator creates a slight positive pressure relative to the alveolar pressure, and again, gas flows from the higher pressure (ventilator) to the lower pressure (alveoli).

Table 11.1 Forces within the lung and respiratory tract that counteract the effect of the driving pressure during inspiration

Elastic resistance properties:
Elastic resistance of lung tissue and chest wall
Resistance at the alveolar gas–fluid interface from surface forces
Nonelastic (resistive) properties:
Frictional resistance to gas flow through airways
Viscoelastic tissue resistance from deformation of thoracic tissue
Inertia associated with gas and tissue movement

Data from Lumb [1]

Several important forces combine to counteract the inspiratory flow produced by the effect of ΔP on the lung (Table 11.1) [1]. These forces can be grouped into lung tissue and respiratory tract elastic properties (E), airflow and frictional resistance (R), and airflow inertia (I). The Equation of Motion describes this complex interplay:

$$\Delta P = E + R + I$$

The collective effect of the elastic and nonelastic (resistive) forces within the lung, if allowed to act independent of other forces, will tend to cause the lung to completely collapse and expel all the air from the respiratory tract. This occurs when the lungs are experimentally or clinically removed from the thorax and sources of ventilation. During inspiration, the diaphragm and other muscles perform work to overcome these elastic and resistive forces. This work is stored as potential energy or dissipated as heat within the lung and thoracic tissues. The stored energy is then used to passively expel air during the expiratory phase of respiration.

The balance of elastic forces applied to the lung during inspiration can be described by the measured lung compliance (its reciprocal is known as elastance) during mechanical ventilation. Lung compliance is physically defined as the change in lung volume (typically tidal volume (V_T)) divided by the change in transmural pressure gradient (in cm H_2O). There are two different ways to describe the lung compliance: the static lung compliance (C_{stat}) and the dynamic lung compliance (C_{dyn}). C_{stat} is measured when the lung is held at a constant (static) volume for a short period of time and is typically greater than 150 mL/cm H_2O. The short inspiratory pause creates the so-called plateau pressure (P_{plat}) (Fig. 11.1), which is used to derive the transmural pressure gradient for the C_{stat} calculation:

$$C_{stat} = Vt / (P_{plat} - PEEP)$$

Dynamic lung compliance (C_{dyn}) is used less frequently in clinical practice. When used, C_{dyn} is typically measured during normal tidal ventilation. For C_{dyn}, the transmural pressure is calculated using the peak inspiratory pressure (PIP):

$$C_{dyn} = Vt / (PIP - PEEP)$$

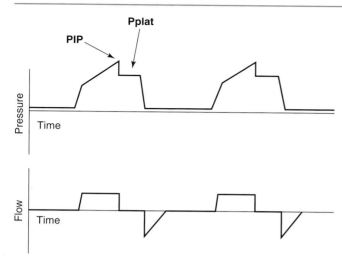

Fig. 11.1 Idealized pressure–time and flow–time graphs for mechanical ventilation. Note that the plateau pressure can be measured when flow returns to zero. *PIP* peak inspiratory pressure, *Pplat* plateau pressure

Table 11.2 Common lung volumes and capacities

	Abbreviation	Definition
Residual volume	RV	Volume in lung after maximal forced exhalation
Expiratory reserve volume	ERV	Volume expelled during maximal forced exhalation after tidal expiration
Tidal volume	V_T	Volume of gas inspired or exhaled during normal breathing
Inspiratory reserve volume	IRV	Volume inspired during maximal forced inspiration after tidal inspiration
Functional residual capacity	FRC	RV + ERV
Vital capacity	VC	ERV + V_T + IRV
Total lung capacity	TLC	RV + ERV + V_T + IRV

Lung Volumes

The anatomical lung volumes are somewhat artificial constructs used to describe the interplay between the various elastic and resistive forces within the thorax. Because these forces govern the amount of gas represented in each of the lung volumes, measured changes in any of the lung volumes or capacities indirectly reflect changes in the elastic or restrictive forces acting on the lungs.

Four specific lung volumes have been described, including the residual volume, expiratory reserve volume, tidal volume, and inspiratory reserve volume (Tables 11.2 and 11.3). Unfortunately, only the latter three lung volumes can be directly measured through direct spirometry. The residual volume requires special techniques such as

Table 11.3 Approximate normal values for the various lung volumes in men and women when breathing spontaneously

	Men (mL)	Women (mL)
Residual volume	1,250	1,000
Expiratory reserve volume	1,000	750
Tidal volume	500	500
Inspiratory reserve volume	3,500	2,000
Functional residual capacity	2,250	1,750
Vital capacity	5,000	3,250
Total lung capacity	6,250	4,250

Data from Stocks and Quanier [3]

plethysmography, dilutional, or washout techniques for evaluation [2, 3]. The most common lung capacities used clinically, the functional residual capacity, the vital capacity, and the total lung capacity (Table 11.2), are summations of more than one lung volume and can also be useful for understanding the interplay between the various elastic and resistive forces.

Minute Ventilation and Dead Space

The minute ventilation (V_E) is the product of the respiratory rate and the V_T. The inspired minute ventilation is slightly larger (but generally less than 1 % larger) than the exhaled minute ventilation because more oxygen is inspired than carbon dioxide is exhaled with each breath. The alveolar minute ventilation (V_A) is the amount of inspired gas that enters the alveolus per minute and is a fraction of the total V_E. The V_A is the only part of the minute ventilation capable of taking part in gas exchange.

The portion of V_E that is not involved in gas exchange is known as the dead space (V_D). In clinical settings, it is difficult and cumbersome to measure and is, therefore, rarely directly evaluated [4]. Despite this, V_D is an important component of ventilation with important physiologic and pathologic ramifications that can cause significant respiratory system dysfunction. Dead space arises from either anatomic or physiologic causes. Anatomic dead space is that portion of the respiratory tract that conducts air from the mouth or nose to the alveolus; there are no gas exchange surfaces in these conducting airways and this portion of the dead space volume is relatively fixed (approximately 2 mL/kg). On the other hand, gas in the physiologic dead space, also sometimes termed the alveolar dead space, is not involved in gas exchange due to a relative or absolute lack of pulmonary blood flow within that region of lung. When physiologic dead space occurs for pathologic or disease-specific reasons, it is sometimes termed pathologic dead space. Pathologic dead space occurs when alveoli are ventilated but are not perfused, as may occur with fat emboli or venous thromboemboli.

An increase in the dead space as a fraction of total ventilation (abbreviated as V_D/V_T) results in impaired ventilation and reduced carbon dioxide elimination. If carbon dioxide production does not simultaneously decrease, the arterial partial pressure of carbon dioxide ($PaCO_2$) will also rise and a respiratory acidosis will ensue. Additionally, significant increases in V_D/V_T may result in patient hypoventilation as will be discussed later in this chapter.

Distribution of Ventilation

Alveolar lung units receive different levels of ventilation depending on both gravitational and nongravitational forces that influence gas flow during inspiration and exhalation. For example, when patients are upright and spontaneously breathing, the majority of the inspiratory gas flows to the dependent base of the lungs. This flow becomes progressively less toward the nondependent apex. This effect is patient-position dependent, such that when patients are supine or lateral, the majority of the inspiratory gas continues to flow to the dependent areas of the lung; however, these areas may be very different from the areas ventilated while standing. At high flow rates (fast breathing), this distribution pattern is eliminated and inspiratory gas flow is uniform throughout the lung. At very high flow rates (very fast and deep breaths), the nondependent lung regions may even receive a majority of the ventilation.

The nongravitational forces that affect the distribution of ventilation are related to a host of factors that, when combined, cause individual lung units to fill and empty at different rates. These different rates can be described by a concept known as the "time constant (τ)." The τ is the time that it takes to fill approximately 63 % of the volume of any individual functional lung unit. At any given time, there are functional lung units with significant negative effect from nongravitational forces that cause the alveoli to fill relatively slowly (and therefore have long τ) mixed with functional lung units with negligible effect from these same forces that cause the alveoli to fill relatively quickly (and therefore have short τ). It is not possible to clinically measure the τ for any individual lung unit; instead, the τ_{RS} can be measured as it is a volume-weighted average of the time constants for each of the lung units ventilated during inspiration. The τ_{RS} can be calculated from the product of the respiratory system compliance and resistance and is frequently used to monitor changes in lung function as well as to set the inspiratory time during mechanical ventilation [5].

Distribution of Perfusion

Similar to the distribution of ventilation, each functional lung unit receives a different amount of pulmonary blood flow that is influenced by both gravitational and nongravitational forces. Gravitational forces play an even greater role in the distribution of perfusion than they do with regard to ventilation. The majority of blood flows to the gravity-dependent lung zones and only a small portion flows to the gravity-independent lung zones. Significant nongravitational factors that affect pulmonary perfusion have also been described but are somewhat difficult to elucidate due to the gravitational effect of Earth. While studies have been performed in the low gravitational environment of space to better understand these forces, it remains unclear how best to apply these principles in clinical practice.

To define the combined gravitational and nongravitational forces that affect the pulmonary blood flow, the calculated pulmonary vascular resistance (PVR) can be used. PVR is affected by lung volume, global and regional pulmonary disease, cardiac disease, and regional alveolar oxygen content. The latter is affected by hypoxic pulmonary vasoconstriction (HPV) and will also be discussed later in this chapter.

Ventilation and Perfusion Relationships

Because there are differences in the distribution of ventilation and perfusion, three generic states exist within the lung. These states have been idealized into three specific zones with each characterized by differences in ventilation and perfusion. In reality, there is a clinical continuum between the physiologic effects of Zone 1 (dead space) and Zone 3 (shunt) in all patients.

In Zone 1, lung units receive more ventilation than perfusion, which results in physiologic dead space. This occurs because the alveolar pressure (from ventilation) is somewhat less affected than the pulmonary arterial and venous pressures by the gravitational and nongravitational effects on the lungs. The pressure differential between the alveolus and vascular structures causes the collapse of pulmonary capillary beds with no resultant gas exchange across these alveoli. The primary physiologic effect of increased Zone 1 is an increase in V_D/V_T, a decrease in expired carbon dioxide, and an increase in $PaCO_2$. In mathematical terms, the ventilation to perfusion ratio (V/Q ratio) for Zone 1 lung units, therefore, approaches infinity.

In Zone 2, lung units receive a balance between ventilation and perfusion. The alveoli in these lung units are capable of adequate and appropriate gas exchange. Blood flow through these alveoli closely matches the alveolar ventilation, and in mathematical terms, the *V/Q* ratio for Zone 2 lung units approximates 1.

In Zone 3, lung units receive more perfusion than ventilation. This physiologic effect results in pulmonary shunt. Pulmonary blood continues to flow across the capillaries but the alveoli receive relatively less ventilation. Gas exchange, therefore, cannot occur across the thin membrane separating the gas within the alveolus and the blood within the pulmonary capillaries. The physiologic effect of increased Zone 3 is a decrease in the oxygen uptake from the inspired air with a resultant decrease in the arterial partial pressure of oxygen (PaO_2) and oxygen saturation (SaO_2). HPV, as previously stated, acts to decrease the degree of pulmonary shunt as a mechanism to reduce hypoxemia and desaturation. In mathematical terms, the *V/Q* ratio for Zone 3 lung units approximates 0.

Gas Exchange

Gas exchange occurs across a very thin membrane, the alveolocapillary membrane (ACM), by simple passive diffusion from high pressure to lower pressure areas. The ACM is an ideal surface for this function as it is very thin but encompasses an enormous surface area. During inspiration, fresh gas with a relatively high oxygen partial pressure (FiO_2) is brought to the ACM by the actions of ventilation as described previously. From this conceptual understanding, actual calculation of the alveolar partial pressure of oxygen (P_AO_2), an important determinant of systemic oxygen delivery, is possible from the formula found in Table 11.4.

At sea level, the calculated room air P_AO_2 approximates 100 mmHg. As is obvious from the equation in Table 11.4, the P_AO_2 can be affected by FiO_2, barometric pressure, $PaCO_2$, and the RQ. Also, it should be obvious that, in most clinical situations, changes in FiO_2 and barometric pressure have a significantly greater effect on P_AO_2 than do changes in $PaCO_2$ and respiratory quotient.

Ideally, complete exchange of the oxygen in inspired air would occur across the ACM and the arterial oxygen partial pressure (PaO_2) would, therefore, equal the inspired alveolar oxygen partial pressure (P_AO_2). Unfortunately, this exchange is not perfect and the PaO_2 is always less than the P_AO_2 due to abnormalities in diffusion and shunt (both cardiac and pulmonary shunt play a role in this setting). In normal patients under routine conditions, the small degree of physiologic shunt (approximately 5 % of the pulmonary blood flow) and the minimal diffusion abnormalities result in only a small reduction in the oxygen partial pressure between the alveolus and the pulmonary blood. This difference is not usually clinically significant; however, moderate to severe

Table 11.4 Important formulas to evaluate respiratory system function

CaO_2	$(1.34 \times Hgb \times SaO_2) + (0.003 \times PaO_2)$
CcO_2	$(1.34 \times Hgb \times 1) + (0.003 \times PAO_2)$
PAO_2	$FiO_2 \times (Pb - Pwv) - PaCO_2/RQ$
DaO_2	$10 \times CaO_2 \times CO$
Qsp/Qt	$(CcO_2 - CaO_2)/(CcO_2 - CvO_2)$

Abbreviations: *CaO_2* arterial oxygen content, *Hgb* the hemoglobin (g/dL), *SaO_2* the arterial hemoglobin saturation (%), *PaO_2* the partial pressure of oxygen in the arterial blood (mmHg), *CcO_2* capillary oxygen content, *PAO_2* the partial pressure of oxygen in the alveolus (mmHg), *FiO_2* fraction of oxygen in inspired gas, *Pb* barometric pressure, *Pwv* water vapor pressure, *PaCO_2* the partial pressure of carbon dioxide in the arterial blood, *RQ* respiratory quotient, *DaO_2* arterial oxygen delivery, *CO* cardiac output, *Qsp* the amount of blood flowing through the shunt, *Qt* the total blood flow (identical to CO), *CvO_2* mixed venous blood oxygen content

pulmonary disease can drastically increase the pulmonary shunt fraction and lead to a significant gap between the P_AO_2 and PaO_2.

Likewise, under normal conditions, the relatively high systemic carbon dioxide partial pressure passively diffuses across the ACM into the alveolar gas and is ultimately expelled from the body during the exhalation phase of respiration. Pulmonary shunt has little effect on carbon dioxide elimination (until the shunt fraction increases to 50 % or more) due to the relatively high diffusion rate of carbon dioxide (compared to oxygen) across the ACM. In contrast, hypoventilation, either from reduced V_E or increased V_D/V_T, will rapidly lead to increased systemic carbon dioxide levels ($PaCO_2$).

Mechanical Ventilation

As has been previously discussed, the RS is complex and has an important role in maintaining appropriate internal homeostasis. Abnormalities in RS function may quickly result in a series of catastrophic patient injuries that could lead to death. RS dysfunction is therefore generally treated rapidly and aggressively through a variety of therapies. With few exceptions, the RS must continue to function for the patient to continue to survive. To this end, mechanical ventilation (MV) is a therapy commonly utilized during periods of significant RS dysfunction. While MV can be used to improve systemic oxygenation, ventilation, or both, it is most often a temporary therapy until the underlying RS abnormality is reversed. Rarely, it can be part of a permanent therapy for patients with severe end-stage RS or neuromuscular disease (as in patients with spinal cord injury causing diaphragmatic paralysis). The use of any MV modality should be coupled with a constant attempt to optimize the balance between the potential benefits and the associated complications inherent in mechanical ventilatory support.

Negative Pressure Ventilation (NPV)

NPV provides mechanical ventilation by generating a driving pressure (ΔP) or pressure differential between the upper airway (usually, either the oropharynx or the extrathoracic trachea) and the lower airways (the intrathoracic trachea, bronchi, bronchioles, and alveoli). This pressure differential is most commonly created within the "iron lung." The iron lung is a historical type of MV using an external vacuum to decrease the pressure within the iron lung (but outside of the patient's body) to subatmospheric pressure. It is this subatmospheric pressure—applied to patient structures inside the iron lung, including the thoracic and abdominal cavities—that is transmitted through the chest wall to the intrathoracic airways. The patient's head and proximal airway, outside the iron lung, are at atmospheric pressure, so the negative pressure within the iron lung generates the driving pressure which causes air movement.

The iron lung was used most effectively during the polio epidemics of the first half of the twentieth century and led directly to the development of specific "respiratory care" units throughout Europe and North America. It has since been abandoned in favor of positive pressure ventilation (PPV) because of the difficulties related to the care of patients housed within the iron lung and the interval advancements in positive pressure ventilation.

Positive Pressure Ventilation (PPV)

With significant advancements in positive pressure ventilation (PPV) occurring over the last 50 years, including the development of cuffed endotracheal tubes and ventilators capable of delivering multiple ventilatory modes, PPV has largely supplanted NPV in patients with severe RS dysfunction.

PPV provides ventilation by generating a ΔP across the upper and lower airways. This ΔP arises when the airways are subjected to a positive airway pressure generated by the increased pressure of the gas within the ventilator. PPV can be provided either invasively (via endotracheal or tracheostomy tube) or noninvasively (via nasal cannula, face mask, face shield, or head enclosure). In addition, PPV can be provided in a number of conventional and advanced modes to facilitate oxygenation and ventilation.

Basic PPV Physiology

The basic physiology for both invasive and noninvasive PPV is similar. An explanation of this physiology is essential to understanding the potential benefits and complications associated with each modality. A number of settings or "variables" are frequently used to describe the various

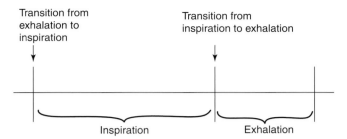

Fig. 11.2 The phases of ventilation

Table 11.5 Trigger and cycle variables for each of the most common types of conventional mechanical ventilation

Mode	Trigger variable	Cycle variable
Controlled mandatory ventilation (CMV)	Time	Time
Assist control ventilation (ACV)	Time or patient	Time
Pressure-control ventilation (PCV)	Time or patient	Time
Intermittent mandatory ventilation (IMV)	Time	Time
Synchronized intermittent mandatory ventilation (SIMV)	Time or patient	Time
Pressure support ventilation (PSV)	Patient	Flow

manipulations of mechanical ventilation. Some of these settings are quite easy to understand, while others may take significant consideration and education before their use becomes intuitive. The main settings used for most conventional modes of ventilation include the mode of ventilation, FiO_2, respiratory rate, tidal volume (or inspiratory pressure limit in a pressure "controlled" mode of ventilation), and PEEP/CPAP. Most of these settings will be described in detail in the discussion to follow.

The respiratory cycle consists of four distinct phases: the transition from exhalation to inspiration, the phase of inspiration, the transition from inspiration to exhalation, and the phase of exhalation. These four phases are graphically illustrated in Fig. 11.2. The operator-defined variable (setting) that is used to determine when the mechanical ventilator should transition from exhalation to inspiration is typically known as the "trigger" and the variable (setting) that determines the transition from inspiration to exhalation is typically known as the "cycle limit." Each of the conventional modes of ventilation has a slightly different way of defining these four phases (Table 11.5).

Volume Versus Pressure Control

The various modes of PPV differ significantly in the way that they provide the inspiratory phase of the respiratory cycle,

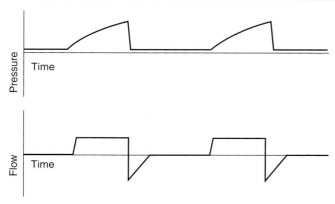

Fig. 11.3 Idealized pressure–time and flow–time graphs with PEEP set above zero for volume-controlled modes of ventilation

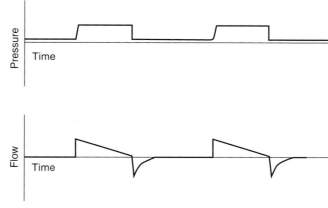

Fig. 11.4 Idealized pressure–time and flow–time graphs with PEEP set above zero for pressure-controlled modes of ventilation

and in general, all modes can be classified as either volume controlled or pressure controlled based on these differences.

In *volume-controlled* modes of ventilation, the tidal volume delivered by the ventilator during the inspiratory phase is held constant with each breath. Traditionally, this is accomplished through the delivery of a constant flow from the ventilator to the patient for a set time (Fig. 11.3). In this way, the ventilator operator can set the tidal volume (either directly or indirectly) and the ventilator will deliver this volume of gas without regard for the pressures that are generated.

In *pressure-controlled* modes of ventilation, the inspiratory pressure generated in the airway is held constant throughout the inspiratory phase and with each breath. This occurs through a more complex system whereby the ventilator delivers an initial very high gas flow rate into the patient with a decelerating (or decreasing) gas flow throughout the rest of the inspiratory phase (Fig. 11.4). In this way, the ventilator operator can set the maximum inspiratory pressure that can be generated regardless of the flow rate that is used or the tidal volume that is delivered. Because of this, the tidal volume may be highly variable from breath to breath and will be dependent on both the respiratory system compliance and resistance at the time of inspiration.

Positive End-Expiratory Pressure (PEEP)

Positive end-expiratory pressure is an important setting on all modern ventilators that adds a small but variable degree of resistance to expiratory flow and, therefore, maintains an operator-defined airway pressure throughout the expiratory phase of respiration. It is used to prevent de-recruitment of the lung, to reinforce an acceptable FRC, and to optimize static lung compliance by increasing the mean airway pressure (and by extension, the mean alveolar pressure) above the threshold where collapse of unstable alveoli occurs. Its major physiologic effect is to improve oxygenation; further

discussion of the positive and negative characteristics of the use of PEEP can be found later in this chapter. Physiologically, there are no differences between PEEP and continuous positive airway pressure (CPAP).

Conventional Ventilation

In general, conventional ventilation is provided through one of several modes designed to either control, assist, or support ventilation. In *control* modes of ventilation, the patient provides essentially none of the total inspiratory effort and the work of breathing should be very close to zero. In *assist* modes of ventilation, the patient provides some of the inspiratory effort but typically has to do little more than trigger the ventilator. The work of breathing should still be very close to zero. In *support* modes of ventilation, the patient must provide a variable portion of the inspiratory effort (depending on settings) and the patient's work of breathing will be highly variable and may even approximate (or be greater than) the work of breathing without mechanical ventilation.

Controlled Mandatory Ventilation

Controlled mandatory ventilation (CMV) is a control type of ventilation that is time triggered and time cycled. CMV provides either an operator-defined tidal volume or pressure to the patient during inspiration at an operator-defined set rate (Fig. 11.5). Because both the respiratory rate and the inspiratory–expiratory time (*I:E*) ratio are operator-defined settings in this mode, the ventilator is both triggered and cycled based on time (sometimes referred to as machine triggered and machine cycled, respectively). This set rate is always delivered and all mechanical ventilation is totally independent of patient effort. Because ventilation is completely controlled in this mode of ventilation, CMV is most frequently used for patients who cannot make spontaneous efforts and is an ideal

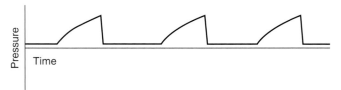

Fig. 11.5 Idealized pressure–time graph for controlled mandatory ventilation (CMV) with PEEP set above zero. In this mode of ventilation, each breath is triggered after a specified time has elapsed. The breaths can be delivered in either volume controlled (shown) or pressure controlled (not shown), depending on the ventilator settings

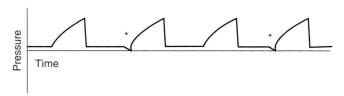

Fig. 11.6 Idealized pressure–time graph for assist control ventilation (ACV) with PEEP set above zero. In this mode of ventilation, each breath is triggered either due to patient initiation (*asterisks*) or after a specified time has elapsed (*no asterisks*). The breaths in ACV can be delivered in either volume controlled (shown) or pressure controlled (not shown), depending on the ventilator settings

mode for patients receiving neuromuscular blockade or general anesthesia. For this reason, it is the most widely used mode of MV in anesthesia machines; however, it is rarely used outside of the operating room due to the high risk of patient–ventilator asynchrony in spontaneously breathing patients.

Assist Control Ventilation

Assist control ventilation (ACV) is a time- or patient-triggered, time-cycled, assist, or control type of ventilation where the ventilator delivers either an operator-defined tidal volume or inspiratory pressure in response to the operator-defined rate or the patient's own respiratory drive (Fig. 11.6). In ACV, every breath that the patient attempts to take generates both a relative negative airway pressure and inspiratory flow from the ventilator to the patient. Depending on the settings used, either the pressure or the flow change will be detected by a sensor and will trigger the ventilator to deliver either a set volume or a set pressure—depending upon whether the mode is volume or pressure limited—and the minute ventilation will thus be greater than the operator-defined (controlled) settings. The trigger sensitivity can be set by the operator to achieve varying levels of patient ventilation assist. Every breath is delivered, regardless of whether the ventilator has been triggered by the patient or the machine, with the same operator-defined tidal volume or pressure. In this way, the set rate serves as a component of the minimum minute ventilation for the patient and additional breaths are completely assisted. If the patient is breathing

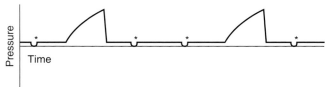

Fig. 11.7 Idealized pressure–time graph for intermittent mandatory ventilation (IMV) with PEEP set above zero. In this mode of ventilation, each set breath is triggered after a specified time has elapsed. In addition, the patient can breathe spontaneously between these machine-triggered breaths. The spontaneous breaths create a small relative negative pressure that are depicted in this graph and noted with *asterisks*. The machine-triggered breaths in IMV can be delivered in either volume controlled (shown) or pressure controlled (not shown), depending on the ventilator settings

spontaneously at a rate higher than the set rate, changing the set rate will not result in reductions to the minute ventilation. If the patient's spontaneous rate drops below the operator-set rate, then the set rate will function as a minimum rate delivered by the ventilator.

Intermittent Mandatory Ventilation

Intermittent mandatory ventilation (IMV) is a mode of ventilation similar to CMV in which the ventilator provides a number of operator-defined breaths delivered at a specified rate (Fig. 11.7). These breaths can be provided in either volume-targeted (most common) or pressure-targeted modes. Between these mandatory breaths, however, the patient may make spontaneous efforts and the ventilator will provide gas flow to facilitate these breaths. Most modern ventilators can, additionally, provide pressure support ventilation to reduce the work of breathing to patients during these spontaneous breaths.

IMV was developed as a weaning mode that allowed the clinician operator to wean patients from full ventilator control (as in CMV) to completely spontaneous ventilation. Weaning in IMV can be accomplished by gradually reducing the number of mandatory breaths provided by the ventilator. As the set rate is decreased, patients should increase the number and/or volume of their spontaneous breaths to maintain a stable minute ventilation. In that way, patients can be converted, over the course of hours to days, from complete ventilator control to simple ventilator support (or less) with relative safety and ease. Once the patient has been weaned to some minimal ventilator support level, most patients can be liberated (extubated) from the ventilator altogether.

Synchronized Intermittent Mandatory Ventilation

Synchronized intermittent mandatory ventilation (SIMV) is similar to IMV except the mandatory breaths provided by the ventilator are synchronized to the patient's spontaneous respiratory rate (Fig. 11.8). This is accomplished using a

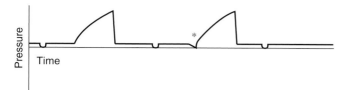

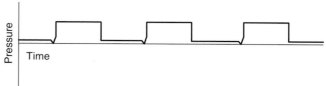

Fig. 11.8 Idealized pressure–time graph for synchronized intermittent mandatory ventilation (SIMV) with PEEP set above zero. In this mode of ventilation, each set breath (or mandatory breath) is synchronized to a patient trigger after a specified time has elapsed. In addition, the patient can breathe spontaneously between the mandatory breaths. The spontaneous breaths create a small relative negative pressure that are depicted in this graph and noted with *asterisks*. The mandatory breaths in SIMV can be delivered in either volume controlled (shown) or pressure controlled (not shown), depending on the ventilator settings

Fig. 11.10 Idealized pressure–time graph for pressure support ventilation (PSV) with PEEP set above zero. In this mode of ventilation, each breath is triggered by the patient

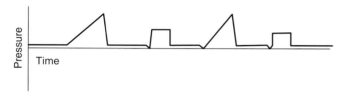

Fig. 11.9 Idealized pressure–time graph for synchronized intermittent mandatory ventilation (SIMV) with PEEP set above zero. In addition, pressure support is being applied to the additional patient-initiated breaths between the mandatory breaths

microprocessor-defined "lockout" period during which the ventilator will not respond to patient triggers. During this lockout period, the patient may take spontaneous breaths (similar to IMV). After the lockout period elapses, the ventilator will provide the next synchronized mandatory breath and attempts to deliver these breaths based on patient triggers to reduce the risk of patient–ventilator asynchrony.

As with IMV, SIMV was designed as a weaning mode that allows the clinician operator to gradually convert the patient from full ventilator control to very little or no support. Pressure support (as described in discussion that follows) may be applied to the spontaneous breaths in order to reduce the work of breathing (Fig. 11.9).

Pressure Support Ventilation

Pressure support ventilation (PSV) is a patient-triggered, pressure-targeted, flow-cycled mode of ventilation that provides an operator-defined level of partial inspiratory support for every patient-triggered breath (Fig. 11.10). In essence, every inspiratory effort made by the patient is supported or "boosted" by gas flow from the ventilator to the patient to achieve an operator-defined airway pressure (the pressure support). This provides several benefits to the patient, including a dramatic decrease in the work of breathing (when compared to unsupported spontaneous ventilation), an improvement in patient–ventilator synchrony, and a reduction in respiratory muscle disuse atrophy (when compared to controlled ventilation) [6–9].

In PSV, every breath is triggered by spontaneous respiratory efforts from the patient. The ventilator will deliver no additional breaths in the absence of patient effort, although modern ventilators have safety features that prevent prolonged apnea. Most ventilators have the ability to detect the negative pressure or flow bias that is generated by the patient during spontaneous respiratory efforts. Once the breath is initiated and the demand valve is opened, the ventilator delivers gas flow via a servo-controlled mechanism that maintains a set pressure level throughout the inspiratory period. To accomplish this, the ventilator delivers a very high initial flow rate that is continuously decreased through a servo control to maintain the operator-defined set pressure.

The pressure support level can be set in several ways and careful attention to this setting is critical for the success of this mode of ventilation. Although no guidelines for the use of PSV have been published, many experts advocate the use of the minimum pressure level that results in a comfortable, stable breathing pattern for the patient. When using this strategy, the pressure support level could be titrated to the respiratory rate (goal rate less than 30 breaths/min) as an indirect method of assessing the comfort and effectiveness of the inspiratory support. Other authors have suggested that the pressure support level could be titrated to a specific tidal volume, even though the best target tidal volume for this strategy has not yet been identified.

In this mode, the ventilator is cycled from inspiration to exhalation when the flow rate decreases to a set minimum (either an absolute flow rate 2–8 L/min) or to a preset percentage of maximum flow (typically 1–80 %). This allows the ventilator to "sense" when the muscles used for ventilation begin to relax or when the patient actively uses accessory exhalation muscles. Also, as a safety measure to prevent the patient from receiving inappropriate gas flow, some ventilators will cycle to exhalation if a small over-pressurization (typically 1–5 cm H_2O) occurs or after an operator-defined inspiratory time has elapsed.

PSV has been advocated because it maintains patient–ventilator synchrony, as well as playing a role in many weaning schemes. First and one of the major uses of PSV is its ability to be used as a weaning mode, either alone or in conjunction with IMV or SIMV ventilation. When PSV is used alone for weaning, the patient can be converted from a controlled or assisted MV mode to PSV as the patient demonstrates the ability to breathe spontaneously. At first, the pressure support level is set to provide substantial support for every breath. Gradually, and as tolerated by the patient, the pressure support level is reduced until it is at a level that the clinician operator may consider separating the patient from the ventilator (such as 10 cm H$_2$O). When used with IMV or SIMV ventilation, PSV is used to support the spontaneous breaths taken by the patient between the mandatory breaths in one of two ways. The pressure support is either set a specific level (typically 10 cm H$_2$O) and the mandatory rate is gradually reduced or the pressure support is set at a level that corresponds with patient support requirements. Over time, the mandatory rate and the pressure support should be reduced to the prescribed level that the clinician operator believes is an appropriate predictor for successful ventilator separation.

Dual Control Ventilation

One of the major limitations of the conventional modes of ventilation is the consideration that either the tidal volume (as in volume-controlled modes) or the inspiratory pressure level (as in pressure-controlled modes) can be held constant, but not both simultaneously. Several ventilator manufacturers have developed software-based algorithms using continuous feedback systems to provide an artificial means to control both the inspiratory pressure and the tidal volume. Although their respective companies have specifically trademarked most of these modalities, they are strikingly similar and likely have the same physiologic effect on the lungs and respiratory system.

In pressure-regulated volume-control (PRVC) ventilation, for example, the ventilator provides an initial "test breath" designed to measure the driving pressure (by measuring the plateau pressure during an inspiratory pause) that is necessary to deliver the set tidal volume (Fig. 11.11). Using this driving pressure, the ventilator then automatically provides pressure-controlled ventilation at that driving pressure. Using a software-based feedback system, the driving pressure is increased or decreased every third breath to target the operator-defined tidal volume. In essence, the delivered tidal volume is measured and compared against the desired (or set) tidal volume. If the delivered tidal volume is less than the desired tidal volume, the inspiratory pressure is automatically increased in a stepwise fashion until the target tidal volume is achieved. On the other hand, if the delivered tidal volume is greater than the desired tidal volume, the inspiratory pressure is automatically decreased in a similarly stepwise fashion until the target tidal volume is achieved (Fig. 11.11). In this way, PRVC ventilation attempts to target both a constant inspiratory pressure (pressure-control properties) and a constant tidal volume (volume-control properties).

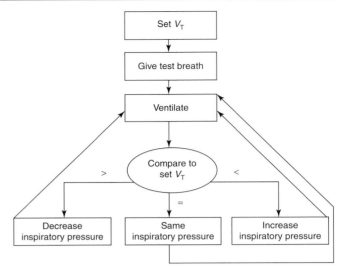

Fig. 11.11 Flow diagram of dual control ventilation. In these modes of ventilation, the ventilator attempts to provide the set tidal volume using a computer-based algorithm based on the depicted flow diagram

PRVC breaths can be delivered using ventilator modes similar to either ACV or SIMV (PRVC is delivered only during the mandatory breaths) to facilitate respiratory system support, providing a degree of flexibility to this dual-mode strategy. Because the effectiveness of the delivered inspiratory pressure is constantly being reassessed and adjusted automatically by the ventilator, rapid changes in airway resistance or lung tissue or chest wall compliance may dramatically affect how the ventilator functions. Frequent coughing or biting on the tube, for example, may result in inappropriately high inspiratory pressures (and tidal volumes) when these problems resolve. A degree of suspicion should be maintained for these problems and the mode of ventilation may have to be changed if these problems persist.

New and Emerging Modes of Ventilation

Airway Pressure Release Ventilation

Airway pressure release ventilation (APRV) is a mode of ventilation that is designed to provide a continuously elevated airway pressure combined with intermittent airway pressure "releases" to improve ventilation and carbon dioxide exhalation. APRV was initially developed as a modification to continuous positive airway pressure (CPAP) for the treatment of severe hypoxemia in patients with ARDS [10]. In addition, APRV provides significant benefit by allowing spontaneous ventilation during inspiration. Studies have shown that spontaneous ventilation improves alveolar recruitment, particularly in dependent zones near the diaphragm, which may contribute to improved oxygenation in these patients [11, 12].

Unfortunately, few studies have been able to demonstrate improvements in long-term patient outcomes, such as mortality or length of ICU stay, and APRV is, therefore, generally utilized as a mode of ventilation reserved for patients with severe hypoxemia that have not responded to conventional ventilation [13–15]. Nevertheless, there are some centers that provide routine MV with APRV in patients with and without ARDS. These centers have developed specific protocols to assist with the initiation, maintenance, and weaning of MV. Continued studies are warranted to assess the application of APRV in these populations.

High-Frequency Oscillatory Ventilation

High-frequency oscillatory ventilation (HFOV) is a mode of ventilation that uses a rapidly moving piston pump to create rapid but shallow oscillations in the gas within the airway. These oscillations (typically at a rate of 150–500/min) are able to achieve effective ventilation and carbon dioxide removal through a number of complicated mechanisms. The sustained airway pressures generated by the bias flow are capable of recruiting collapsed alveoli, particularly in conditions such as ARDS and ALI. In HFOV, the FiO_2 and mean pressure are the settings used to improve oxygenation while the amplitude and frequency are adjusted to improve ventilation.

Published studies using HFOV have described conflicting results, as most studies to date have demonstrated improved oxygenation in patients with severe ARDS/ALI with very little effect on mortality or ICU length of stay [16–18]. Additionally, HFOV is a complicated mode of MV due to the need for intense sedation and/or neuromuscular blockade, as well as the potential for hemodynamic instability due to an increase in the intrathoracic pressure. Similar to APRV, HFOV is generally considered to be a mode of MV that should be reserved for patients with severe hypoxemia that have not responded to conventional ventilation.

Neurally Adjusted Ventilatory Assist

Neurally adjusted ventilatory assist (NAVA) is a mode of ventilation that attempts to reduce the delay from the central nervous system initiation of ventilation to the delivery of fresh gas by the ventilator. With conventional modes of ventilation, a small delay occurs from the time the patient initiates a breath, due to the method whereby the ventilator detects that breath, to the time when the ventilator delivers fresh gas to the patient. NAVA, using continuous monitoring of respiratory muscle (diaphragm) electrical excitation rather

than changing gas flow or pressure within the ventilator circuit, more closely matches the ventilator gas flow to the exact time of patient demand. Additionally, NAVA uses diaphragmatic electrical excitation to determine the amount of pressure support to apply to the patient in direct proportion to the amount of electrical excitation that is detected.

NAVA has been successfully used in a wide range of patients with a number of RS and non-RS diseases [19–21]. NAVA appears to be particularly effective in patients with significant patient–ventilator asynchrony [22, 23]. Although NAVA shows great promise, there are few studies that demonstrate reduced length of ventilation or ICU stay in most patient populations. Additionally, the use of NAVA requires specialized ventilators and equipment that may not be available in all hospitals. Larger studies using NAVA are currently underway and their publication may substantially change the way MV is provided in the future.

Proportional Assist Ventilation

Proportional assist ventilation (PAV) is a mode of ventilation that attempts to match the degree of ventilator support to the patient's ventilator support need. PAV uses a number of measured variables and operator-defined settings to automatically adjust the MV pressure support generated for each breath. Using PAV, as the patient generates more spontaneous inspiratory force, the ventilator generates less pressure support to match the unique demand of the patient on a breath-by-breath basis. Similar to NAVA, PAV is associated with reduced patient–ventilator asynchrony and work of breathing [24, 25].

As with the other advanced modes of ventilation, few studies have been conducted to demonstrate improved long-term outcomes with PAV. In addition, there is a risk of patient injury with PAV due to a potential feedback circuit when the airway gas flow may trigger additional, unintended ventilation; careful monitoring is necessary to prevent this complication. At this time, PAV is used in specialized centers with variable success. Additional studies will be necessary before PAV can be recommended for widespread use.

Noninvasive Positive Pressure Ventilation

Although the use of noninvasive mechanical ventilation (NIV) is a relatively new technology for patients with respiratory failure, it has been championed as a major advancement in the care of patients with respiratory failure [26]. NIV encompasses a number of ventilator modalities and modes that involve the external application of positive airway pressure to the upper airway without the need of an invasive endotracheal tube or tracheostomy. In this way, NIV attempts to provide patients with a form of ventilation that simultaneously maximizes the benefits and minimizes the risks associated with invasive positive pressure ventilation.

Noninvasive mechanical ventilation has been evaluated in many different clinical situations and scenarios with variable effect on both short- and long-term outcomes. NIV has been shown to effectively reverse the systemic effects of respiratory failure in patients with COPD exacerbations and cardiogenic pulmonary edema [27–30]. In addition, the use of NIV in these patients may reduce the need for invasive mechanical ventilation, shorten the hospital and ICU length of stay, and reduce overall mortality in these patients. NIV has also been shown to improve outcomes in immunosuppressed patients with respiratory failure due to the increased risk of lower respiratory tract infections with invasive positive pressure ventilation [31]. Additional, but less well-validated, potential indications for NIV include patients with acute asthma attack, postoperative respiratory failure, and extubation failure [32–35]. Although controversial, some authors have also suggested that patients with respiratory failure and "Do Not Intubate" orders could be treated with NIV as a palliative measure for dyspnea at the end of life or during terminal extubation [36–38].

NIV is typically delivered through a tight-fitting nasal or facial mask. Although facial shields and helmets have also been developed for selected patients requiring NIV, they are used far less frequently [39, 40]. The most commonly used NIV modalities are biphasic positive airway pressure (BiPAP) and continuous positive airway pressure (CPAP). BiPAP is generally used for patients with an increased work of breathing and an associated hypoventilation component. In BiPAP ventilation, the airway pressure alternates between two different pressures during each respiratory cycle. The higher level (or inspiratory pressure [IPAP]) is typically set to reduce the work of breathing and to increase the delivered tidal volume, whereas the lower level (or expiratory pressure [EPAP]) is used to prevent de-recruitment and atelectasis. The level of IPAP is generally set between 5 and 15 cm H_2O, whereas the EPAP is generally set between 5 and 10 cm H_2O. Few patients tolerate more than approximately 15–20 cm H_2O of peak inspiratory pressure; this threshold can sometimes be a significant limitation for patients with severe pulmonary disease who might require somewhat higher ventilator pressures.

Continuous positive airway pressure (CPAP) is used for patients with hypoxemic respiratory insufficiency. Like PEEP, CPAP functionally increases the mean airway pressure to increase recruitment and prevent de-recruitment of unstable, collapsed, or fluid-filled alveoli. Physiologically, CPAP reduces the shunt fraction while increasing the dead space fraction.

Few studies have specifically evaluated the use of NIV (either BiPAP or CPAP) in patients with neurologic injury, as one of the most important limitations to the use of NIV includes the increased incidence of complications in patients with neurologic dysfunction. Unfortunately, the successful use of NIV requires a cooperative patient with intact protective airway reflexes, a somewhat rare population for patients with significant neurologic dysfunction. For this reason, NIV should be used with extreme caution in neurologic patients with respiratory failure, and when used in these patients, they should be monitored closely for signs and symptoms of worsening neurologic function, respiratory function, or aspiration.

Strategies to Improve Oxygenation

Oxygen is normally transported from the respiratory system to the rest of the body in two forms: either as O_2 dissolved in blood or as that bound to hemoglobin. The calculated arterial oxygen content (CaO_2) is used to describe the amount of oxygen within the arterial blood and can be determined from the formula in Table 11.4. Normal CaO_2 is approximately 20 mL O_2 per 100 mL of blood. Low CaO_2 is termed hypoxemia. Prolonged and/or severe hypoxemia will result in patient morbidity or mortality due to tissue hypoxia and organ system dysfunction.

Tissue hypoxia is caused by reduced cellular oxygen delivery and can be caused by a number of factors, including hypoxemia, low cardiac output, arterial vessel vasoconstriction, or arterial vessel obstruction, as might occur during acute ischemic stroke. The calculated global oxygen delivery (DaO_2) is frequently used to describe the amount of oxygen that is delivered by the cardiopulmonary system; the formula for DaO_2 can be found in Table 11.4.

Causes of Hypoxemia

Hypoxemia is caused by anemia (low hematocrit), hemoglobin desaturation, or a reduced amount of oxygen dissolved in blood (low PaO_2). A careful history and physical examination will usually reveal important clues for the cause(s) of hypoxemia. For example, information obtained regarding any history of significant respiratory disease, such as pneumonia, chronic obstructive pulmonary disease (COPD), or asthma, may be particularly useful in determining the cause(s) of hypoxemia. Likewise, physical examination may reveal lung abnormalities such as inspiratory rales, parenchymal consolidation, or pneumothorax. Physical examination of the heart, including a careful evaluation of the heart sounds, may also point to specific cardiac or pulmonary abnormalities for hypoxemia. Diagnostic testing, such as arterial blood gas analysis, chest x-ray, or echocardiography, may be used for either initial diagnosis or confirmatory testing.

Because hypoxemia is an important source of hypoxia, tissue ischemia, and organ system dysfunction, the application of therapies to prevent or reverse hypoxemia is an important part of respiratory care of patients regardless of the underlying systemic injury. Although many classifications and diagnostic schemes have been described, the easiest considers just three main causes of hypoxemia within hospitalized patients. These causes include the following:

- Pulmonary shunt/dead space
- Cardiac shunt
- Hypoventilation

Shunt is a condition where pulmonary blood flow bypasses ventilated portions of the lung, either by passing from the right side of the heart directly to the left side of the heart (a condition known as cardiac shunt) or by passing from the pulmonary arteries to the pulmonary veins through regions of the lung that are not well ventilated (a condition known as pulmonary shunt). The degree of shunt present in any individual patient (commonly known as the shunt fraction) can be calculated as a fraction of total blood flow based on blood gas measurements. The formula for the shunt fraction can be found in Table 11.4.

Pulmonary shunt is the most common cause of hypoxemia and results from a variety of conditions, such as pneumonia, pulmonary edema, atelectasis, acute respiratory distress syndrome (ARDS), acute lung injury (ALI), pulmonary contusion, and pneumothorax. Treatment of pulmonary shunt requires, in most cases, a reversal of the underlying pathology and recruitment of unstable or collapsed alveoli. To accomplish this, PEEP and other means to increase the mean airway pressure are frequently used, either with or without a recruitment maneuver (RM) to improve oxygenation due to pulmonary shunt.

Cardiac shunt results from the mixing of poorly oxygenated venous blood with oxygenated blood in the left atrium or left ventricle. This blood is then ejected systemically which results in arterial hypoxemia. Intracardiac shunt occurs either from congenital deformation (such as a patent foramen ovale (PFO), atrial septal defect (ASD), or ventricular septal defect (VSD)). Frequently, these congenital abnormalities are corrected early in life or are monitored closely by cardiologists for progression of symptoms. Other causes of cardiac shunt include septal rupture from myocardial infarction or blunt cardiac injury. Cardiac shunts can frequently be visualized using Doppler echocardiography of the heart. In cases where Doppler echocardiography is equivocal, a "bubble study" can be performed with echocardiographic visualization of the agitated saline across the shunt.

Hypoventilation is the third major cause of hypoxemia and is usually also associated with hypercarbia and respiratory acidosis. This constellation of findings can be associated with either absolute hypoventilation (defined by a reduced minute ventilation) or relative hypoventilation (defined by a normal minute ventilation). Absolute hypoventilation occurs when the patient has a slow (or absent) respiratory rate and/or a reduced tidal volume. Relative hypoventilation occurs due to an increase in the systemic carbon dioxide production (as might occur during fever, seizures, shivering, or specific disorders, such as neuromalignant syndrome) or an increase in the respiratory system dead space relative to the total minute ventilation.

Hypoventilation causes hypoxemia through the effect of increased $PaCO_2$ on the alveolar oxygen partial pressure as described in the equations in Table 11.4. In addition, hypoventilation may lead to atelectasis and pulmonary shunt. Hypoventilation can usually be reversed with an increase in the patient's respiratory rate and/or tidal volume. Additionally, the underlying etiology for hypoventilation should be sought and rapidly reversed, if possible. Continued hypoventilation despite reversal of the underlying pathology is an indication for mechanical support of ventilation in many chronic respiratory disease states, such as chronic obstructive pulmonary disease (COPD) and pulmonary fibrosis.

Therapies to Improve Oxygenation

Supplemental oxygen is a simple, rapid therapy to reverse hypoxemia in most patients. It can be lifesaving in patients and can be delivered to almost every patient, either at home or in the hospital setting. Supplemental oxygen can be applied through a nasal cannula, a face mask, or a face mask with reservoir. A nasal cannula can generally be used to apply supplemental oxygen to attain a FiO_2 of up to 28 %; a traditional face mask used to provide supplemental oxygen can deliver a FiO_2 up to 60 %, while a tight-fitting face mask with an oxygen reservoir can deliver a FiO_2 up to 90 %.

In patients with more severe hypoxemia, therapies utilizing continuous or intermittent positive airway pressure and mechanical ventilation may be necessary. These therapies can include PEEP with and without recruitment maneuvers (RM), as well as a number of adjunctive and rescue therapies.

The use of PEEP to improve oxygenation is well established through multiple previously published studies across many populations. PEEP has two major effects within the lung to improve oxygenation. First, PEEP sustains an increased mean airway pressure when used in conjunction with most MV modes. This increased mean airway pressure provides a distending force on collapsed alveoli that is able to change their geometric shape and push the alveolus beyond the lower inflection point on its pressure–volume curve. Secondly, PEEP prevents closure (or de-recruitment) of unstable alveoli. Both of these actions of PEEP are important in the reversal of hypoxemia caused by pulmonary shunt. Unfortunately, the improvement in alveolar collapse caused by PEEP is largely dependent on the specific lung areas that are to be reopened [41, 42]. Because the static compliance of alveoli is reduced at very low volumes, more airway pressure (and therefore PEEP) is required to open these collapsed alveoli than to perform tidal ventilation within those same alveoli (after opening) [43]; hence, it is more "efficient" to add PEEP to stabilize alveoli than it is to continuously reopen then after collapse. It is also less damaging to stabilize airways in this manner via the prevention of "shear trauma."

Increases in PEEP also frequently induce overdistention of normal or highly compliant lung regions with resultant additional lung injury and the potential for pneumothorax. Additionally, the sustained airway pressure typically causes increased intrathoracic pressure which, when transmitted to the intrathoracic vessels, may cause severe hypotension. This hypotension usually responds to mild fluid resuscitation or with reduction in PEEP settings.

Unfortunately, because several large-scale evaluations of PEEP titration strategies have failed to reduce VILI or improve long-term outcomes in patients, it remains unclear how best to determine the optimal PEEP setting in any individual patient [44–46]. Some authors have suggested that PEEP should be set at the level that is associated with the highest PaO_2/FiO_2 ratio, lowest static compliance, narrowest $PaCO_2$–$PetCO_2$ gradient, or least hemodynamic disturbance. An alternative approach that requires specific and complicated equipment utilizes the lower inflection point (LIP) of a patient-specific inspiratory pressure–volume curve. None of these approaches has been associated with significantly improved outcomes over any of the other approaches, and until additional research becomes available, it might be best to use the approach most easily applied within your own specific institution.

In patients with neurologic injury, the effect of PEEP on intracranial pressure has previously been an area of concern. Several recent publications, however, suggest that in volume-resuscitated patients, the use of low to moderate PEEP (typically less than 20 cm H_2O) has no significant negative impact on ICP [47–49]. In fact, improvements in systemic oxygenation may actually reduce and improve ICP in these patients when increased PEEP is applied.

Recruitment maneuvers (RM) are another modality used to improve oxygenation. RM are performed with the temporary increase in the sustained airway pressure. This pressure is transmitted to atelectatic lung segments similar to PEEP. Historically, RM have been performed with the use of continuous positive airway pressure (CPAP) accomplished either by the manual application of positive pressure through a ventilator bag within the inline circuit (as might happen with ventilators used by anesthesia personnel in the operating room) or through the use of a CPAP mode on the mechanical ventilator in nonoperating room environments. Recent research suggests, however, that the use of pressure-control

Table 11.6 Settings commonly used for recruitment maneuvers

Mode	PCV	CPAP
Inspiratory pressure (cm H_2O)	35	35
PEEP (cm H_2O)	15	NA
Respiratory rate	20	NA
Inspiratory time (seconds)	2	40

Abbreviations: *PCV* pressure-controlled ventilation, *CPAP* continuous positive pressure ventilation

ventilation recruitment maneuvers (PCV-RM) is as effective as the sustained CPAP recruitment maneuvers (CPAP-RM) in both cardiac and neurosurgical populations [50, 51]. Although small, these studies suggest that PCV-RM and CPAP-RM have similar efficacy (for reversing hypoxemia) while the PCV-RM is associated with less hemodynamic disturbances. Settings used for CPAP-RM and PCV-RM in these studies can be found in Table 11.6.

Adjunctive and Rescue Therapies for Hypoxemia

Adjunctive agents such as inhaled nitric oxide (iNO) and inhaled epoprostenol (iEpoprostenol) have also been described in the reversal of hypoxemia, particularly in patients with ARDS/ALI. Both of these agents function through an augmentation of the normal hypoxic vasoconstriction (HPV) physiology. Normally, HPV causes relative pulmonary vasoconstriction in vessels supplying blood flow to alveoli with reduced ventilation. HPV, therefore, shunts blood away from underventilated lung segments. iNO and iEpoprostenol augment this beneficial physiologic response by inducing vasodilation in pulmonary vessels that supply blood to normally ventilated lung segments. The combination of HPV (which moves blood flow away from hypoventilated segments) and iNO and iEpoprostenol (which move blood flow toward normally ventilated segments) can result in significant improvement in hypoxemia.

Unfortunately, while these therapies have been associated with improvements in physiology (oxygenation), multiple studies have failed to demonstrate significant benefit in clinically significant outcomes from these adjunctive therapies [52–54]. Additionally, they are associated with significant cost and may be complex and time consuming to initiate. For these reasons, many institutions have instituted specific protocols and requirements for the use of these adjunctive agents while other hospitals have ceased to provide these therapies.

Prone positioning has also been investigated as an adjunctive (or rescue) therapy for severe hypoxemia in patients with ARDS/ALI. Prone positioning can be accomplished either with the use of a specialized patient bed or by simply turning the patient prone in a normal ICU bed. Both methods require specialized nursing care to prevent inadvertent dislodgement of catheters and tubes, as well as to prevent decubitus ulcer formation across the weight-bearing ventral surfaces. No specific studies of this adjunctive therapy have been performed in patients with neurologic injury, and the effectiveness of this technique in general medical and surgical patients is still being debated. For these reasons, routine prone positioning cannot be recommended for patients with neurologic injury and severe hypoxemia.

Extracorporeal life support (ECLS) is a definitive mode for rescue in patients with severe hypoxemia. ECLS uses a mechanical pump to push blood through a porous membrane oxygenator to add oxygen directly to the blood without the need for respiratory system function. ECLS requires the intravascular placement of large-bore cannulae in either the arterial (venoarterial ECLS) or venous (venovenous ECLS) systems. While the use of ECLS was not historically associated with improved outcomes, recent advances in technology and the earlier deployment of this therapy in specialized, regional centers have been associated with improved mortality in patients with severe ARDS/ALI [55–57]. Additionally, a number of these specialized centers across the globe demonstrated significant improvements in patient outcomes with the early use of ECLS during the recent H1N1-variant influenza pandemic [58, 59]. Unfortunately, patients with ECLS require systemic anticoagulation to prevent thrombosis and thromboembolic complications and neurologic injury is frequently a contraindication for this lifesaving therapy. At current, ECLS should only be used as a rescue therapy in patients that can tolerate systemic anticoagulation.

Hypoxemia is a serious, life-threatening complication of respiratory system dysfunction. Hypoxemia is usually caused by pulmonary shunt, although cardiac shunt and hypoventilation can also play a role in select patients. Hypoxemia can generally be temporarily reversed with increased FiO_2. Definitive therapy usually requires the application of PEEP with or without an RM to reopen collapsed alveoli. Adjunctive and rescue therapies can be used in patients with severe hypoxemia, although their use should be based on a specific evaluation of the potential benefits and risks of each therapy for each individual patient.

Weaning from Mechanical Ventilation

The transition from full MV support of RS function to spontaneous, unassisted ventilation (generally termed weaning) is an important consideration throughout the period of ventilator therapy and, in most circumstances, should be anticipated from the start of MV (Fig. 11.12). Patients with neurologic injury, however, may be different from other critically ill populations because of the high incidence of central

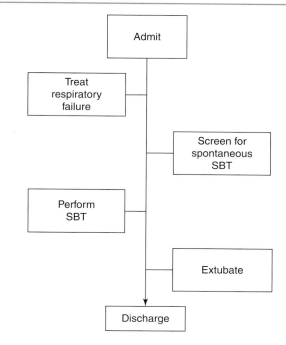

Fig. 11.12 Idealized flow of patient care from admission and initiation of mechanical ventilation to extubation and discharge

and peripheral nervous system dysfunction that exists independent of the underlying RS function. For this reason, weaning from MV may be both simpler and more complicated for these patient groups and lessons learned and strategies employed with other critically ill patient populations may not be completely generalizable to this patient population. Nevertheless, the development of a successful weaning strategy will play a pivotal role in the successful long-term outcome for many patients.

In this section, the phrase "weaning" will be used extensively. It is meant to convey the concept of transition from one end of an MV spectrum to another. Several different strategies for "weaning" have been described over the past few decades. These strategies have been employed in many different ways and have been bitterly debated, but have only been compared in a very few clinical trials.

Historically, weaning from MV has been accomplished through the use of any one of a number of ventilator modes designed to facilitate this transition from full mechanical ventilator support to spontaneous, unassisted ventilation. As previously described, the main goal of MV is to support RS function, including both oxygenation and ventilation; weaning from full MV to unassisted, spontaneous ventilation should only occur once the underlying RS abnormality and need for MV have been resolved (because, e.g., either sedation or paralysis has been removed or the severity of the lung disease has improved) and then only after the physiologic response to weaning has been monitored for its systemic effect [60].

Somewhat different from patients requiring mechanical ventilation in the general medical or surgical population, patients with neurologic injury who require mechanical ventilation have many overlapping and interrelated physiologic responses, and one of the most important determinants of the ability of any individual patient to wean from mechanical to spontaneous ventilation is the patient's underlying neurologic function. In general, the acute neurologic injury must be stabilized and the risk of additional neurologic injury from the potential physiologic stress of weaning must be minimized. Additionally, the patient's other organ systems must also be stabilized and ready for the stresses of ventilator weaning. For this reason, the process of ventilator weaning entails a careful coordination between the various patient care members, including the neurosurgeon, neurologist, critical care staff, nurses, and respiratory care specialists.

Weaning Predictors

Because ventilator separation failure is associated with increased morbidity and mortality, a number of predictors of successful weaning have been described and evaluated both in many different patient populations and scenarios. Unfortunately, most tests lack adequate positive or negative predictive value to be used clinically [61–63]. The most useful tests appear to include the minute ventilation, respiratory frequency, tidal volume, the negative inspiratory force (NIF), and the frequency–tidal volume ratio (f/V_T, RSBI) [60, 61, 64] (Table 11.7).

The f/V_T ratio is also sometimes referred to as the rapid shallow breathing index (RSBI) and is measured during the first few minutes of unassisted ventilation [64, 65]. When initially published, Yang and Tobin demonstrated a sensitivity of approximately 0.97, a specificity of 0.64, for weaning failure when the RSBI was less than 105 breaths/min/L [64]. Multiple follow-up studies have analyzed the data in a number of settings and of all weaning predictors, the RSBI appears to have the greatest utility in predicting the outcome of ventilator weaning, although the applicability of the published data cannot be easily translated to the bedside as the various methods of unassisted ventilation (PSV, CPAP, T-piece) used in the studies may have led to unanticipated confounding in the statistical analyses [60, 66].

Although weaning predictors have been extensively studied and defined, their overall utility in a strategy for ventilator weaning and discontinuation remains controversial and recent published guidelines do not support their routine or isolated use in the weaning process [67–69]. Despite this, many clinicians and respiratory therapists routinely employ them in their daily decision-making as it relates to ventilator weaning.

Table 11.7 Weaning parameter values typically used to predict weaning outcome

Parameter	Values to predict weaning outcome
Minute ventilation	≤15 L/min
Respiratory frequency	≤35 breaths/min
Tidal volume	≥5 mL/kg body weight
Negative inspiratory force (NIF)	≤−20 cm H_2O
Rapid shallow breathing index (RSBI)	≤105 breaths/min/L

Weaning Modes

Concerns related to ventilator-induced diaphragmatic weakness and dysfunction in critically ill patients led to the development of "progressive reduction" ventilation that is used in many clinical situations [70]. This strategy is designed to recondition and retrain the muscles of respiration through the gradual reduction in the amount of support provided by the ventilator to the patient [71]. The use of SIMV is typically used for this progressive reduction in ventilator support as an attempt to provide neuromuscular "rest" during mandatory breaths and neuromuscular "work" during spontaneous breaths (which can also be supported with PSV). Therefore, to increase the "work" performed during SIMV, the mandatory rate is reduced gradually until the patient has been weaned from high support (or low work) to low support (or high work). Unfortunately, recent work suggests that neuromuscular rest does not occur during the mandatory breaths due to a complex interaction within the brain's respiratory centers [72, 73]. In fact, studies indicate that weaning patients by a gradual reduction strategy with SIMV is associated with the longest duration of mechanical ventilation when compared to PSV and T-piece assessments [74, 75]. Although no studies have been published to support the idea, newer modes of ventilation, including PAV and NAVA, may provide improvements in progressive weaning by reducing the risk of patient–ventilator asynchrony during ventilation [76, 77].

Spontaneous Breathing Tests

The strategy of periodic spontaneous breathing tests (SBT) is based on an assessment of the ability of patients to wean from fully supported ventilation without a gradual reduction in the level of support provided to the patient. This strategy arose from the observation that many patients who experienced an unintentional extubation or ventilator separation were able to maintain acceptable levels of oxygenation and ventilation even though they had not fully completed the "weaning" process [60, 78]. This finding suggests that patients may be ready to transition to unassisted ventilation at a faster rate than was prescribed by the care team, and in fact, it suggests that many patients may not even require the

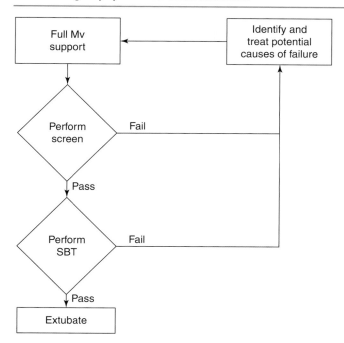

Fig. 11.13 Flow diagram of the two-step ventilator separation process. *Abbreviations*: *MV* mechanical ventilation, *SBT* spontaneous breathing trial

Table 11.8 Hemodynamic and respiratory parameters used to determine readiness for spontaneous breathing trial

Parameter	Threshold values for readiness
PaO_2/FiO_2	≥ 200
PEEP	≤ 5 cm H_2O
f/V_T (RSBI)	≤ 105 breaths/min/L
Airway reflexes	Intact reflexes (adequate cough during suctioning)
Vasopressor use	No vasopressor infusion except dopamine ≤ 5 mcg/kg/min
Sedation use	No sedation infusions

Data from Ely et al. [86]

Table 11.9 Hemodynamic and respiratory parameters used to determine an unsuccessful spontaneous breathing trial

Parameter	Values
Respiratory rate	≥ 35 breaths/min for at least 5 min
Tidal volume	≤ 5 mL/kg patient weight
Oxygen saturation (SpO_2)	$\leq 90\%$
Heart rate	≥ 140 beats per minute or sustained rate $\geq 20\%$ greater (or less) than baseline
Systolic blood pressure	≥ 180 mmHg or ≤ 90 mmHg
Additional clinical symptoms	Agitation, anxiety, diaphoresis, or chest pain

extensive progressive reduction in ventilator support used historically.

Practically, the SBT employs a two-step process to maximize patient safety and reduce the risk of unintended physiologic deterioration (Fig. 11.13). In the first step, patients are evaluated for the "appropriateness" of the SBT (often termed "readiness testing") [79, 80]. During this phase, patients are screened for a number of physiologic and pathologic conditions that would exclude them from the second phase of the test (Table 11.8). Patients who pass this initial screening phase (or readiness test) would then be given an SBT for 30–120 min [80–82]. When performing this SBT, either low-level pressure support ventilation (typically, pressure support ≤ 10 cm H_2O and PEEP ≤ 5 cm H_2O), CPAP (with pressure set ≤ 5 cm H_2O), or unassisted T-piece ventilation can be employed [83, 84]. Patients who have undergone tracheostomy can generally be placed on supplemental oxygen support only for their SBT. During the SBT, patients are monitored for hemodynamic and physiologic responses that would indicate that the patient is not yet ready for unassisted ventilation (Table 11.9). Patients who fail their SBT are returned to full mechanical ventilator support (Fig. 11.13) and the clinical team should engage in aggressive attempts to determine and correct the underlying source of SBT failure. Once the likely sources of failure have been corrected, the SBT process can be repeated. There does not seem to be benefit in attempting the SBT process more frequently than every 24 h, although if patients have failed for reasons related

to sedation or analgesia, these patients may pass their SBT once sedation and analgesia have been addressed [75, 79].

The use of protocol-driven daily SBT assessment is a natural extension of this strategy and has been extensively studied within multiple hospital settings and populations. Ely and colleagues, using the first published physician-driven protocol, were able to demonstrate reduced duration of mechanical ventilation and complication rates with no effect on ICU or hospital length of stay or mortality [85, 86]. Since then, additional studies, using both nurse-driven and respiratory therapist-driven protocols, have also demonstrated improved patient outcomes and reduced duration of mechanical ventilation with this strategy [87, 88].

Although patients with neurologic injury share many common characteristics with other critically ill patients, their specific central and peripheral nervous systems injuries may provide enough differences to make generalization from other populations difficult. Fortunately, several studies incorporating a daily SBT protocol in patients with neurologic injury have been published to date. In 2001, Naven and colleagues published the results of their prospective, randomized control trial of 100 patients based on the well-described and validated 2-step process described by Ely and colleagues [89]. Because of the specific patient population involved in this trial, patients with indwelling intracranial pressure (ICP) monitoring did not undergo SBT screening until the ICP monitor was removed. Additionally, because the neurologic evaluation in the screening process was very

Table 11.10 Hemodynamic and respiratory parameters used to determine readiness for spontaneous breathing trial in neurosurgical patients

Parameter	Threshold values for readiness
Glasgow Coma Scale	≥8
Airway reflexes	Intact reflexes (adequate cough during suctioning)
Tracheal suctioning	≤2 times/h
Serum sodium concentration	135–145 mEq/L
Core temperature	<38.5 °C during the previous 8 h
PaO_2/FiO_2	≥200
PEEP	≤5 cm H_2O
$PaCO_2$	≤50 mmHg
Heart rate	≤125 beats/min
Systolic blood pressure	≥90 mmHg
Vasopressor use	No vasopressor infusion except dopamine ≤5 mcg/kg/min

Data from Navalesi et al. [90]

crude and there was no specific protocol to reduce the time from successful completion of the SBT to extubation, most patients continued mechanical ventilation for at least 24 h after successful SBT due to concerns related to the patient's neurologic status and no significant reduction in any important outcome measure, including the duration of mechanical ventilation (6 days vs. 6 days [$p = 0.387$]), was seen [89]. In 2008, Navalesi and colleagues published the results of their study of 318 patients using a similar protocol with an improved screening process targeted toward neurosurgical patients [90] (Table 11.10). These investigators demonstrated a reduction in the need for reintubation (12.5 % vs. 5.0 % [$p = 0.047$]) but no significant difference in the length of ventilation (5.0 days vs. 5.0 days [$p = 0.942$]). Although these studies highlight the difficulty in applying treatment strategies from other critical care populations to the neuro-critical care population, they do suggest that a daily SBT (with appropriate screening) may improve care to these complex patients.

Complications of Mechanical Ventilation

Unfortunately, mechanical ventilation is a double-edged sword. On the one hand, MV can rapidly reverse the negative systemic effects of many respiratory system abnormalities. On the other hand, MV has also been associated with a number of significant short- and long-term complications. Of specific concern, ventilator-induced lung injury (VILI), ventilator-associated pneumonia (VAP), and ventilator-associated diaphragmatic dysfunction (VADD) are among the most important complications to consider during mechanical ventilation.

Ventilator-Induced Lung Injury

Ventilator-induced lung injury (VILI) is a serious complication of MV that results from diffuse injury of individual alveoli, resulting in a non-cardiogenic pulmonary edema clinically indistinguishable from ALI/ARDS. VILI is now known to arise from the disastrous consequences of one or more of several mechanisms related to stress injury to the lung parenchyma: volutrauma, atelectrauma, and pulmonary oxygen toxicity (POT). Increasingly, the importance of bio-trauma (the term used to describe the systemic effects of VILI) has also become an important topic for research and discussion. Also of note, barotrauma is sometimes described as a type of VILI because it is a lung injury that occurs during MV; however, it results in a different type of injury and will be discussed separately within this chapter.

Volutrauma

Volutrauma results from the unequal distribution of gas during inspiration in a lung with an underlying heterogeneous injury (as occurs due to ALI/ARDS) (Fig. 11.14). As previously described, during normal MV, fresh gas moves into the patient due to a positive pressure (relative to the patient) generated at the ventilator. This fresh gas then moves down the conducting airways to the terminal bronchioles and alveoli based on the specific resistive and elastic (the inverse of compliance) properties within the respiratory tracts and alveoli. In general, less air flows to highly resistive airways and highly elastic (poorly compliant) alveoli. For this reason, when tidal volume is kept constant, lung areas with low compliance and/or high resistance receive relatively lower proportions of the total volume, and lung areas with normal or increased compliance and/or reduced resistance receive relatively higher proportions of the total volume. This increased amount of gas flow into normal lung tissue results in alveolar overdistention and stretch-induced injury to the alveolocapillary membrane (ACM) resulting in diffuse alveolar damage similar to ARDS and the activation of an inflammatory-mediated cascade with systemic consequences.

Atelectrauma

Atelectrauma (also termed shear trauma) results from the cyclic opening and closing of unstable alveoli. During MV, the balance of forces that govern the stability of the alveolar volume may be negatively affected and tend toward collapse and atelectasis. In this way, unstable alveoli may completely collapse during exhalation only to be reopened during inspiration setting up a repeating cycle that leads to ACM disruption with resultant diffuse alveolar damage and systemic inflammation. The utilization of PEEP/CPAP to stabilize unstable alveoli may help prevent this.

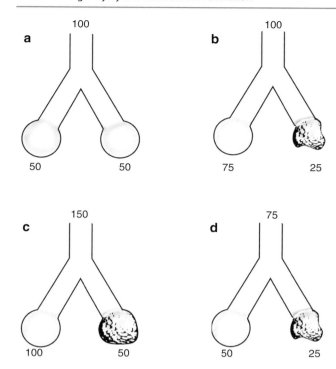

Fig. 11.14 (**a–d**) Idealized depictions of the effect of various ventilation strategies on alveoli with variable compliance, as occurs in conditions such as acute respiratory distress syndrome (ARDS). In (**a**), both alveoli have similar compliance and the delivered tidal volume (100 ml) is equally distributed between the alveoli. In (**b**), one of the alveoli has a decreased compliance and the volume delivered to that alveoli is substantially reduced. Concurrently, a small increase in the volume delivered to the normal alveoli can be seen. In (**c**), the delivered tidal volume has been increased to maintain a normal volume within the injured alveoli. Unfortunately, this results in a very large increase in tidal volume (overdistention) within the previously normal alveoli. In (**d**), the delivered tidal volume has been reduced to maintain a normal volume to the normal alveoli. To attain this, a small volume in the abnormal alveoli is tolerated

Pulmonary Oxygen Toxicity

Pulmonary oxygen toxicity (POT) is a controversial form of VILI whereby the exposure of alveoli to oxygen and high-inspired concentration (typically described as an $FiO_2 > 0.6$) may cause further injury to the alveoli and ACM as a result of the production of a number of highly reactive oxygen-free radical compounds [91, 92]. In laboratory animals, the prolonged delivery of oxygen during both hyperbaric and normobaric conditions has been shown to result in significant alveolar injury [92, 93]. No studies have been able to convincingly demonstrate the harmful effects of POT resulting in VILI during short-term oxygen exposure in humans [91, 92]. In addition, few studies have been conducted in humans during normocarbic conditions and the long-term consequences of this therapy are unknown [92, 93].

Table 11.11 The ARDSnet ventilation protocol

	Protocol for ARDSnet ventilation
Mechanical ventilation (MV) initiation	Use any MV mode
	Use IBW for all V_T settings
	Set initial V_T to 8 mL/kg
	Reduce V_T by 1 mL/kg every 2 h until $V_T = 6$ mL/kg
	Set respiratory rate (RR) <35 breaths/min
	Set I:E rate <1:1
MV titration for plateau pressure (Pplat)	Measure Pplat every 4 h
	If Pplat >30 cm H_2O, reduce V_T by 1 mL/kg (minimum $V_T = 4$ mL/kg)
	If Pplat <25 cm H_2O, increase V_T by 1 mL/kg (maximum $V_T = 6$ mL/kg)
MV titration for pH	If pH = 7.15–7.30, increase RR (maximum 35 bpm) until pH >7.30 or $PaCO_2 < 25$ mmHg
	If pH <7.15, increase RR to 35 and consider increase V_T

Data from The Acute Respiratory Distress Network [44]

Barotrauma

Barotrauma is a form of lung injury that occurs from the delivery of positive pressure ventilation using very high ventilating pressures delivered to the lung tissue. Barotrauma results in any of several related clinical conditions, such as pneumothorax and pneumomediastinum. These conditions result from gas escape from the conducting airways and alveoli due to mechanical disruption of the lung support tissues and structures [94]. Like other forms of VILI, barotrauma results from overdistention of alveoli. In barotrauma, however, overdistention results in rupture of the bronchiolar or alveolar walls with extension of gas into the pulmonary interstitium [95].

Prevention Strategies

Recently, studies involving a large number of patients have evaluated the development of "lung protective strategies" (LPS) to reduce the risk of VILI during MV. Most of this work has involved MV for patients with a diagnosis of ARDS and/or ALI. Additionally, a growing consensus suggests that these same strategies should also be used for patients who are at risk for the development of ALI or ARDS as well [96–98].

LPS are generally designed to reduce the risk of alveolar overdistention and lung injury from volutrauma, atelectrauma, and barotrauma with resultant decreases in biotrauma and other systemic effects [44, 99]. The most important LPS study to date targeted a combination of low tidal volumes and airway plateau pressure measurements to reduce the risk of volutrauma and barotrauma, respectively. This trial, known as ARMA, randomized patients to receive either a low tidal volume ventilation regimen (frequently called the ARDSnet protocol [Table 11.11]) compared to a significantly higher tidal volume ventilation regimen [44]. This study randomized 861 patients with ALI or ARDS and was stopped early because it conclusively demonstrated a significant reduction in mortality—39.8 % versus 31.0 %—corresponding to an absolute risk reduction of 22 % [44].

Multiple studies have attempted to reduce the harmful effects of atelectrauma using a strategy known as open lung ventilation. Using these open lung ventilation strategies, increased PEEP is used to recruit collapsed lung segments and maintain the lung in an open state. This serves to prevent the harmful effects of atelectasis during exhalation. Unfortunately, none of these studies have shown improvement in patients at highest risk for atelectrauma [45, 46, 100]. Additionally, a meta-analysis of this data failed to demonstrate an additional improvement of the open lung ventilation strategy when combined with low tidal volume ventilation [101].

Because of the findings in these studies, low tidal volume ventilation should be used in patients with ALI/ARDS. Patients with one or more risk factors for the development of ALI/ARDS should also be considered for low tidal volume ventilation. It is not clear whether lung protective strategies, including low tidal ventilation or open lung ventilation, might produce different outcomes in patients with head injuries. No specific studies of any LPS have been conducted in this population. It should be noted that several of the described short-term consequences of low tidal volume ventilation, including hypercarbia and hypoxemia, may have negative effects on patients with head injuries and an individualized risk–benefit analysis is warranted [44].

Ventilator-Associated Pneumonia

Ventilator-associated pneumonia (VAP) is a form of hospital-acquired lower respiratory tract infection in patients requiring MV. VAP is the most common hospital-acquired infection (HAI) in patients admitted to the ICU [102, 103]. Although controversial because of differences in definitions and confounding medical issues in these patients, the published incidence of VAP appears to be approximately 25 % [103, 104]. In patients with head injury, the incidence of VAP is significantly higher and may be as high as 50 % [105, 106]. Additionally, the development of VAP appears to be an independent contributor to morbidity and mortality in intubated patients, both with and without concomitant head injury [102, 103, 107].

VAP occurs when the normally sterile lower respiratory tract is infected with bacteria or other pathogens. Although some investigators have described the creation of a biofilm around the endotracheal tube as the cause of VAP, it is generally believed that VAP is mainly due to a breakdown in the normal host defenses [102]. During MV, endotracheal

Table 11.12 The Modified Clinical Pneumonia Infection Score

	0 points	1 point	2 points
Temperature	>36.5° and <38.4°	>38.5° and <38.9°	>39.0° or <36.0°
WBC count (1,000/mm³)	>4.0 and <11.0	<4.0 or >11.0	<4.0 or >11.0 and >500 band forms
P/F ratio	>240 or ARDS	–	<240 and no ARDS
Secretions	Rare	Copious	Copious and purulent
CXR results	No infiltrate	Diffuse infiltrates	Localized infiltrate
Micro results	Negative	–	Positive

Adapted with permission of the American Thoracic Society (Copyright © 2013) from Fartoukh et al. [109]

Abbreviations: *WBC* white blood cells, *P/F* PAO₂/FiO₂ ratio, *ARDS* acute respiratory distress syndrome, *CXR* chest x-ray, *Micro* microbiology

intubation allows microaspiration of pathogen-laden secretions to occur from the oropharynx into the lower respiratory tract. Early-onset VAP (EO-VAP) is defined as VAP that occurs in the first 4 days of MV and is generally associated with pathogens that are highly sensitive to antimicrobial therapy. Late-onset VAP (LO-VAP) is defined as VAP that occurs after the fifth day of MV and is associated with multidrug resistant pathogens and increased morbidity and mortality.

VAP is diagnosed when systemic evidence of infection occurs in the setting of a clinical suspicion for a pulmonary source. Although a clinical scoring system (the clinical pulmonary infection score [CPI]) has been described (Table 11.12), the widespread adoption of the CPIS has been limited by its somewhat-moderate sensitivity (65 %) and specificity (64 %) [108–110]. For many clinicians, the presence of a new or progressive infiltrate on chest radiography or purulent sputum production in the setting of two or more criteria for the systemic inflammatory response syndrome (SIRS) remains the best initial diagnostic criteria for many clinicians. The use of microbiologic analysis of fluid obtained from either broncheoalveolar lavage (BAL) or protected alveolar lavage (PAL) may also be performed to improve diagnostic accuracy and to aid in guiding appropriate antimicrobial therapy. Diagnostic strategies incorporating laboratory markers for systemic infection, including C-reactive protein and procalcitonin, have also been described [111, 112]. Validation of their diagnostic accuracy is ongoing.

Because the morbidity and mortality associated with VAP is substantial, a number of investigators and governmental regulators recommend the routine use of the so-called ventilator bundle (Table 11.13). Although controversial, this bundle has been associated with a significant improvement in VAP incidence (a reduction from 10.2 cases/1,000 ventilator days to 3.4 cases/1,000 ventilator days) within a surgical intensive care unit [113–115]. No specific studies in patients

Table 11.13 Ventilator bundle

Key components	Comments
Head of bed elevation	30–45° is the recommended elevation
Daily oral care	Oral care with 0.12 % chlorhexidine to decontaminate the oropharyngeal mucosa
Daily sedation interruption	Has been related to a decreased length of MV
Daily assessment for extubation readiness	Has been related to a decreased length of MV
Peptic ulcer prophylaxis	Has been related to reduced mortality in critically ill patients. Unclear direct effect on VAP
Deep venous thrombosis prophylaxis	Has been related to reduced mortality in critically ill patients. Unclear direct effect on VAP

with head injury have been performed; however, because the potential improvements in patient care far outweigh the negative consequences of most of the practices within the published ventilator bundles, the systematic implementation of a ventilator bundle should be a routine practice for all intubated patients.

The antimicrobial treatment of VAP depends on a number of factors including the length of time on MV and the potential for MDR pathogens. Consensus guidelines for the treatment of VAP have been published by multiple societies. The American Thoracic Society published their most recent guidelines in 2005 [102]. These guidelines recommend initial, empiric antibiotics that should be based on a number of additional factors such as cost, availability, and hospital formulary availability. After specific microbiology analysis, the initial antimicrobial therapy can be tailored to the specific resistance patterns on the individual pathogen. Although controversial, the duration of antimicrobial treatment should not exceed approximately 8 days (except in the case of *Pseudomonas aeruginosa*) if the patient exhibits an appropriate clinical response. Patients with *P. aeruginosa* VAP should be treated for at least 15 days [116, 117].

Ventilator-Induced Diaphragmatic Dysfunction

Because the diaphragm plays a central role in sustaining nonsupported ventilation after MV, diaphragmatic weakness and dysfunction can significantly reduce the risk of successful separation from MV. Increasing evidence suggests that ventilator-induced diaphragmatic dysfunction (VIDD) may occur rapidly after the institution of MV [118–120]. This dysfunction appears to affect both muscular strength and endurance and appears to be related to changes in the muscle fibers themselves, somewhat more than can be accounted for by muscle atrophy alone [121, 122]. In lab animals, these findings have been linked to reduced protein synthesis,

increased protein breakdown, muscle fiber remodeling, and direct and indirect muscle fiber injury [123–128].

Although controversial, it appears that VIDD may be at least partially prevented by MV strategies that allow the diaphragm to contract as normally as possible [129–131]. It is not yet clear whether specific ventilator modes or support levels provide the best prophylaxis against VIDD. The use of sedation and analgesic strategies that promote diaphragmatic activity may also be beneficial. Antioxidants therapy and vitamin supplementation (specifically vitamins E and C) may also prevent significant VIDD [132].

Conclusion

The respiratory system is a complex organ system. Its crucial role is in providing systemic oxygenation and eliminating carbon dioxide. Complex therapies, including conventional and advanced modes of ventilation, in conjunction with inhaled therapies and extracorporeal support systems, are utilized to support the respiratory system in many patients. These therapies require extensive training and continuous evaluation and reevaluation to ensure the maximum benefit with the least potential for harm is provided to the patients with and without neurologic injury. Future technologies offer the potential for significant benefit in many patients with both acute and chronic respiratory system dysfunction.

References

1. Lumb AB. Nunn's applied respiratory physiology. 6th ed. Philadelphia: Elsevier; 2005. p. 25–38.
2. Evans SE, Scanlon PD. Current practice in pulmonary function testing. Mayo Clin Proc. 2003;78(6):758–63.
3. Stocks J, Quanier PH. Reference values for residual volume, functional residual capacity and total lung capacity. ATS Workshop on Lung Volume Measurements. Official Statement of the European Respiratory Society. Eur Respir J. 1995;8(3):492–506.
4. Sinha P, Flower O, Soni N. Dead space ventilation: a waste of breath! Intensive Care Med. 2011;37(5):735–46.
5. Nicolai T. The physiological basis of respiratory support. Paediatr Respir Rev. 2006;7(2):97–102.
6. Brochard L, Harf A, Lorino H, Lemaire F. Inspiratory pressure supports prevents diaphragmatic fatigue during weaning from mechanical ventilation. Am Rev Respir Dis. 1989;139:513–21.
7. Ershowsky P, Krieger B. Changes in breathing pattern during pressure support ventilation. Respir Care. 1987;32:1011–6.
8. Tokioka H, Saito S, Kosaka F. Effect of pressure support ventilation on breathing pattern and respiratory work. Intensive Care Med. 1989;15:491–4.
9. Van de Graaff WB, Gordey K, Dornseif SE, et al. Pressure support: changes in ventilatory pattern and components of the work of breathing. Chest. 1991;100:1082–9.
10. Downs JB, Stock MC. Airway pressure release ventilation: a new concept in ventilator support. Crit Care Med. 1987;15:459–61.
11. Putensen C, Mutz N, Putensen-Himmer G, Zinserling J. Spontaneous breathing during ventilator support improves

ventilation-perfusion distributions in patients with acute respiratory distress syndrome. Am J Respir Crit Care Med. 1999;159:1241–8.

12. Yoshida T, Rinka A, Kaji A, et al. The impact of spontaneous ventilation on distribution of lung aeration in patients with acute respiratory distress syndrome: airway pressure release ventilation versus pressure support ventilation. Anesth Analg. 2009;109(6): 1892–900.

13. Putensen C, Zech S, Wrigge H, et al. Long-term effects of spontaneous breathing during ventilatory support in patients with acute lung injury. Am J Respir Crit Care Med. 2001;164(1):43–9.

14. Maxwell RA, Green JM, Waldrop J, et al. A randomized prospective trial of airway pressure release ventilation and low tidal volume ventilation in adult trauma patients with acute respiratory failure. J Trauma. 2010;69(3):501–10.

15. Gonzalez M, Arroliga AC, Frutos-Vivar F, et al. Airway pressure release ventilation versus assist-control ventilation: a comparative propensity score and international cohort study. Intensive Care Med. 2010;36(5):817–27.

16. Derdak S, Mehta S, Stewart TE, et al. High-frequency oscillatory ventilation for acute respiratory distress syndrome in adults: a randomized, controlled trial. Am J Respir Crit Care Med. 2002;166(6):801–8.

17. Bollen CW, van Well GT, Sherry T, et al. High frequency oscillatory ventilation compared with conventional mechanical ventilation in adult respiratory distress syndrome: a randomized controlled trial. Crit Care. 2005;9(4):R430–9.

18. Sud S, Sud M, Friedrich JO, et al. High frequency oscillation in patients with acute lung injury and acute respiratory distress syndrome (ARDS): systematic review and meta-analysis. BMJ. 2010;340:c2327.

19. Terzi N, Pelieu I, Guittet L, et al. Neurally adjusted ventilatory assist in patients recovering spontaneous breathing after acute respiratory distress syndrome: physiological evaluation. Crit Care Med. 2010;38(9):1830–7.

20. Coisel Y. Neurally adjusted ventilatory assist in critically ill postoperative patients: a crossover randomized study. Anesthesiology. 2010;113:925–35.

21. Colombo D, Cammarota G, Bergamaschi V, et al. Physiologic response to varying levels of pressure support and neutrally adjusted ventilatory assist in patients with acute respiratory failure. Intensive Care Med. 2008;34(11):2010–8.

22. Piquilloud L, Vignaux L, Bialais E, et al. Neurally adjusted ventilatory assist improves patients-ventilator interaction. Intensive Care Med. 2011;37(2):263–71.

23. Spahija J, de Marchie M, Albert M, et al. Patient-ventilator interaction during pressure support ventilation and neutrally adjusted ventilatory assist. Crit Care Med. 2010;38(2):518–26.

24. Passam F, Hoing S, Prinianakis G, et al. Effect of different levels of pressure support and proportional assist ventilation on breathing pattern, work of breathing and gas exchange in mechanically ventilated hypercapnic COPD patients with acute respiratory failure. Respiration. 2003;70(4):355–61.

25. Giannouli E, Webster K, Roberts D, Younes M. Response of ventilator-dependent patients to different levels of pressure support and proportional assist. Am J Respir Crit Care Med. 1999;159(6):1716–25.

26. Garpestad E, Brennan J, Hill NS. Noninvasive ventilation for critical care. Chest. 2007;132(2):711–20.

27. Bott J, Carroll MP, Conway JH, et al. Randomized controlled trial of nasal ventilation in acute ventilator failure due to chronic obstructive airways disease. Lancet. 1993;341(8860):1555–7.

28. Brochard L, Isabey D, Piquet J, et al. Reversal of acute exacerbations of chronic obstructive lung disease by inspiratory assistance with a face mask. N Engl J Med. 1990;323(22):1523–30.

29. Winck JC, Azevedo LF, Costa-Pereira A, et al. Efficacy and safety of non-invasive ventilation in the treatment of acute cardiogenic pulmonary edema – a systematic review and meta-analysis. Crit Care. 2006;10(2):R69.

30. Ho KM, Wong K. A comparison of continuous and bi-level positive airway pressure non-invasive ventilation in patients with acute cardiogenic pulmonary oedema: a meta-analysis. Crit Care. 2006; 10(2):R49.

31. Antonelli M, Conti G, Bufi M, et al. Noninvasive ventilation for treatment of acute respiratory failure in patients undergoing solid organ transplantation: a randomized trial. JAMA. 2000;283(2): 235–41.

32. Soroksky A, Klinowski E, Ilgyev E, et al. Noninvasive positive pressure ventilation in acute asthmatic attack. Eur Respir Rev. 2010;19(115):39–45.

33. Soroksky A, Stav D, Shpirer I. A pilot prospective, randomized, placebo-controlled trial of bi-level positive airway pressure in acute asthmatic attack. Chest. 2003;123(4):1018–25.

34. Squadrone V, Coha M, Cerutti E, et al. Continuous positive airway pressure for treatment of postoperative hypoxemia: a randomized controlled trial. JAMA. 2005;293(5):589–95.

35. Auriant I, Jallot A, Hervé P, et al. Noninvasive ventilation reduces mortality in acute respiratory failure following lung resection. Am J Respir Crit Care Med. 2001;164(7):1231–5.

36. Curtis JR, Cook DJ, Sinuff T, et al. Noninvasive positive pressure ventilation in critical and palliative care settings: understanding the goals of therapy. Crit Care Med. 2007;35(3):932–9.

37. Schettino G, Altobelli N, Kacmarek RM. Noninvasive positive pressure ventilation reverses acute respiratory failure in select "do-not-intubate" patients. Crit Care Med. 2005;33(9):1976–82.

38. Levy MM, Tanios MA, Nelson D, et al. Outcomes of patients with do-not-intubate orders treated with noninvasive ventilation. Crit Care Med. 2004;32(10):2002–7.

39. Kwok H, McCormack J, Cece R, et al. Controlled trial of oronasal versus nasal mask ventilation in the treatment of acute respiratory failure. Crit Care Med. 2003;31(2):468–73.

40. Antonelli M, Pennisi MA, Pelosi P, et al. Noninvasive positive pressure ventilation using a helmet in patients with acute exacerbation of chronic obstructive pulmonary disease: a feasibility study. Anesthesiology. 2004;100(1):16–24.

41. Albert SP, DiRocco J, Allen GB, et al. The role of time and pressure on alveolar recruitment. J Appl Physiol. 2009;106(3):757–65.

42. Gattinoni L, D'Andrea L, Pelosi P, et al. Regional effects and mechanism of positive end-expiratory pressure in early adult respiratory distress syndrome. JAMA. 1993;269(16):2122–7.

43. Gattinoni L, Carlesso E, Brazzi L, Caironi P. Positive end-expiratory pressure. Curr Opin Crit Care. 2010;16:39–44.

44. The Acute Respiratory Distress Syndrome Network. Ventilation with lower tidal volumes as compared with traditional tidal volumes for acute lung injury and the acute respiratory distress syndrome. N Engl J Med. 2000;342:1301–8.

45. Meade MO, Cook DJ, Guyatt GH, et al. Ventilation strategy using low tidal volumes, recruitment maneuvers, and high positive end-expiratory pressure for acute lung injury and acute respiratory distress syndrome. JAMA. 2008;299(6):637–45.

46. Mercat A, Richard JM, Vielle B, et al. Positive end-expiratory pressure setting in adults with acute lung injury and acute respiratory distress syndrome. JAMA. 2008;299(6):646–55.

47. McGuire G, Crossley D, Richards J, Wong D. Effects of varying levels of positive end-expiratory pressure on intracranial pressure and cerebral perfusion pressure. Crit Care Med. 1997;25:1059–62.

48. Huynh T, Messer M, Sing RF, et al. Positive end-expiratory pressure alters intracranial and cerebral perfusion pressure in severe traumatic brain injury. J Trauma. 2002;53(3):488–92.

49. Mascia L, Grasso S, Fiore T, et al. Cerebro-pulmonary interactions during the application of low levels of positive end-expiratory pressure. Intensive Care Med. 2005;31(3):373–9.

50. Celebi S, Koner O, Menda F, et al. The pulmonary and hemodynamic effects of two different recruitment maneuvers after cardiac surgery. Anesth Analg. 2007;104(2):384–90.

51. Nemer SN, Caldeira JB, Azeredo LM, et al. Alveolar recruitment maneuver in patients with subarachnoid hemorrhage and acute

respiratory distress syndrome: a comparison of 2 approaches. J Crit Care. 2011;26(1):22–7.

52. Afshari A, Brok J, Moller AM, Wetterslev J. Inhaled nitric oxide for acute respiratory distress syndrome and acute lung injury in adults and children: a systematic review with meta-analysis and trial sequential analysis. Anesth Analg. 2011;112(6):1411–21.

53. Afshari A, Brok J, Moller AM, Wetterslev J. Inhaled nitric oxide for acute respiratory distress syndrome and acute lung injury in adults and children. Cochrane Database Syst Rev. 2010;(7): CD002787.

54. Afshari A, Brok J, Moller AM, Wetterslev J. Aerosolized prostacyclin for acute lung injury (ALI) and acute respiratory distress syndrome (ARDS). Cochrane Database Syst Rev. 2010;(8): CD007733.

55. Hill DJ, O'Brien TG, Murray JJ. Prolonged extracorporeal oxygenation in severe acute respiratory failure (shock-lung-syndrome). N Engl J Med. 1972;286:629–34.

56. Zapol WM, Snider MT, Hill JD, et al. Extracorporeal membrane oxygenation in severe acute respiratory failure. A randomized prospective study. JAMA. 1979;242(20):2193–6.

57. Peek GJ, Mugford M, Tiruvoipati R, et al. Efficacy and economic assessment of conventional ventilatory support versus extracorporeal membrane oxygenation for severe adult respiratory failure (CESAR): a multicenter randomized controlled trial. Lancet. 2009;374(9698):1351–63.

58. Australia and New Zealand Extracorporeal Membrane Oxygenation (ANZ ECMO) Influenza Investigators. Extracorporeal membrane oxygenation for 2009 Influenza A (H1N1) acute respiratory distress syndrome. JAMA. 2009;302(17):1888–95.

59. Roch A, Lepaul-Ercole R, Grisoli D, et al. Extracorporeal membrane oxygenation for severe influenza A (H1N1) acute respiratory distress syndrome: a prospective observational comparative study. Intensive Care Med. 2010;36(11):1899–905.

60. Epstein SK. Weaning from ventilatory support. Curr Opin Crit Care. 2009;15(1):36–43.

61. Epstein SK. Weaning parameters. Respir Care Clin N Am. 2000;6:263–301.

62. Meade M, Guyatt G, Cook D, et al. Predicting success in weaning from mechanical ventilation. Chest. 2001;120(6 Suppl):400S–24.

63. Monaco F, Drummond GB, Ramsay P, et al. Do simple ventilation and gas exchange measurements predict early successful weaning from respiratory support in unselected general intensive care patients? Br J Anaesth. 2010;105(3):326–33.

64. Yang KL, Tobin MJ. A prospective study of indexes predicting the outcome of trials of weaning from mechanical ventilation. N Engl J Med. 1991;324(21):1445–50.

65. Epstein SK. Etiology of extubation failure and the predictive value of the rapid shallow breathing index. Am J Respir Crit Care Med. 1995;152(2):545–9.

66. El-Khatib MF, Zeineldine SM, Jamaleddine GW. Effect of pressure support ventilation and positive end expiratory pressure on the rapid shallow breathing index in intensive care unit patients. Intensive Care Med. 2008;34(3):505–10.

67. MacIntyre NR, Cook DJ, Ely Jr EW, et al. Evidence-based guidelines for weaning and discontinuing ventilatory support: a collective task force facilitated by the American College of Chest Physicians; the American Association for Respiratory Care; and the American College of Critical Care Medicine. Chest. 2001;120(6 Suppl):375S–95.

68. Boles JM, Bion J, Connors A, et al. Weaning from mechanical ventilation. Eur Respir J. 2007;29(5):1033–56.

69. Girad TD, Kress JP, Fuchs BD, et al. Efficacy and safety of a paired sedation and ventilator weaning protocol for mechanically ventilated patients in intensive care (Awakening and Breathing Controlled trial): a randomised controlled trial. Lancet. 2008; 371(9607):126–34.

70. Fitting JW. Respiratory muscles during ventilator support. Eur Respir J. 1994;7(12):2223–5.

71. Hess D. Ventilator modes used in weaning. Chest. 2001;120 (6 Suppl):474S–6.

72. Imsand C, Feihl F, Perret C, Fitting JW. Regulation of inspiratory neuromuscular output during synchronized intermittent mechanical ventilation. Anesthesiology. 1994;80(1):13–22.

73. Marini JJ, Smith TC, Lamb VJ. External work output and force generation during synchronized intermittent mandatory ventilation: effect of machine assistance on breathing effort. Am Rev Respir Dis. 1988;138(5):1169–79.

74. Brochard L, Rauss A, Benito S, et al. Comparison of three methods of gradual withdrawal from ventilatory support during weaning from mechanical ventilation. Am J Respir Crit Care Med. 1994;150(4):896–903.

75. Esteban A, Frutos F, Tobin MJ, et al. A comparison of four methods of weaning patients from mechanical ventilation. Spanish Lung Failure Collaborative Group. N Engl J Med. 1995;332(6):345–50.

76. Kacmarek RM. Proporational assist ventilation and neutrally adjusted ventilator assist. Respir Care. 2011;56(2):140–8.

77. Navalesi P, Costa R. New modes of mechanical ventilation: proportional assist ventilation, neutrally adjusted ventilator assist, and fractal ventilation. Curr Opin Crit Care. 2003;9(1):51–8.

78. Mion LC, Minnick AF, Leipzig R, et al. Patient-initiated device removal in intensive care units: a national prevalence study. Crit Care Med. 2007;35(12):2714–20.

79. Ely EW, Baker AM, Evans GW, Haponik EF. The prognostic significance of passing a daily screen of weaning parameters. Intensive Care Med. 1999;25(6):581–7.

80. Girard TD, Kress JP, Fuchs BD, et al. Efficacy and safety of a paired sedation and ventilator weaning protocol for mechanically ventilated patients in intensive care (Awakening and Breathing Controlled trial): a randomised controlled trial. Lancet. 2008; 371(9607):126–34.

81. Esteban A, Alía I, Tobin MJ, et al. Effect of spontaneous breathing trial duration on outcome of attempts to discontinue mechanical ventilation. Spanish Lung Failure Collaborative Group. Am J Respir Crit Care Med. 1999;159(2):512–8.

82. Perren A, Domenighetti G, Mauri S, et al. Protocol-directed weaning from mechanical ventilation: clinical outcome in patients randomized for a 30-min or 120-min trial with pressure support ventilation. Intensive Care Med. 2002;28(8):1058–63.

83. Jones DP, Byrne P, Morgan C, et al. Positive end-expiratory pressure vs T-piece. Extubation after mechanical ventilation. Chest. 1991;100(6):1655–9.

84. Esteban A, Alía I, Gordo F, et al. Extubation outcome after spontaneous breathing trials with T-tube or pressure support ventilation. The Spanish Lung Failure Collaborative Group. Am J Respir Crit Care Med. 1997;156(2 Pt 1):459–65.

85. Ely EW, Baker AM, Dunagan DP, et al. Effect on the duration of mechanical ventilation of identifying patients capable of breathing spontaneously. N Engl J Med. 1996;335(25):1864–9.

86. Ely EW, Bennett PA, Bowton DL, et al. Large-scale implementation of a respiratory therapist-driven protocol for ventilator weaning. Am J Respir Crit Care Med. 1999;159:439–46.

87. Kollef MH, Shapiro SD, Silver P, et al. A randomized, controlled trial of protocol-directed versus physician-directed weaning from mechanical ventilation. Crit Care Med. 1997;25(4):567–74.

88. Marelich GP, Murin S, Battistella F, et al. Protocol weaning of mechanical ventilation in medical and surgical patients by respiratory care practitioners and nurses: effect on weaning time and incidence of ventilator-associated pneumonia. Chest. 2000;118(2): 459–67.

89. Namen AM, Ely EW, Tatter SB, et al. Predictors of successful extubation in neurosurgical patients. Am J Respir Crit Care Med. 2001;163(3 Pt 1):658–64.

90. Navalesi P, Frigerio P, Moretti MP, et al. Rate of reintubation in mechanically ventilated neurosurgical and neurologic patients: evaluation of a systematic approach to weaning and extubation. Crit Care Med. 2008;36(11):2986–92.

91. Jackson RM. Pulmonary oxygen toxicity. Chest. 1985; 88(6):900–5.

92. Stogner SW, Payne DK. Oxygen toxicity. Ann Pharmacother. 1992;26(12):1554–62.

93. Bitterman H. Bench-to-bedside review: oxygen as a drug. Crit Care. 2009;13(1):205.

94. Pierson DJ. Alveolar rupture during mechanical ventilation: role of PEEP, peak airway pressure, and distending volume. Respir Care. 1988;33:472–84.

95. Maunder RJ, Pierson DJ, Hudson LD. Subcutaneous and mediastinal emphysema: pathophysiology, diagnosis, and management. Arch Intern Med. 1984;144:1447–53.

96. Gajic O, Dara SI, Mendez JL, et al. Ventilator-associated lung injury in patients without acute lung injury at the onset of mechanical ventilation. Crit Care Med. 2004;32:1817–24.

97. Wolthuis EK, Choi G, Dessing MC, et al. Mechanical ventilation with lower tidal volumes and positive end-expiratory pressure prevents pulmonary inflammation in patients without preexisting lung injury. Anesthesiology. 2008;108:46–54.

98. Schultz MJ, Haitsma JJ, Slutsky AS, Gajic O. What tidal volume should be used in patients without acute lung injury? Anesthesiology. 2007;106(6):1226–31.

99. Amato MB, Barbas CS, Medeiros DM, et al. Effect of a protective-ventilation strategy on mortality in the acute respiratory distress syndrome. N Engl J Med. 1998;338:347–54.

100. Brower RG, Lanken PN, MacIntyre N, et al. Higher vs. lower positive end-expiration pressures in patients with the acute respiratory distress syndrome. N Engl J Med. 2004;351(4):327–36.

101. Briel M, Meade M, Mercat A, et al. Higher vs. lower positive end-expiratory pressure in patients with acute lung injury and acute respiratory distress syndrome: systematic review and meta-analysis. JAMA. 2010;303(9):865–73.

102. American Thoracic Society. Guidelines for the management of adults with hospital-acquired, ventilator-associated, and healthcare-associated pneumonia. Am J Respir Crit Care Med. 2005;171(4):388–416.

103. Vincent JL, Bihari DJ, Suter PM, et al. The prevalence of nosocomial infection in intensive care units in Europe. Results of the European prevalence of infection in intensive care (EPIC) study. EPIC international advisory committee. JAMA. 1995;274(8):639–44.

104. Rello L, Ollendorf DA, Oster G, et al. Epidemiology and outcomes of ventilator-associated pneumonia in a large US database. Chest. 2002;122:2121.

105. Lepelletier D, Roquilly A, Demeure dit latte D, et al. Retrospective analysis of the risk factors and pathogens associated with early-onset ventilator-associated pneumonia in surgical-ICU head-trauma patients. J Neurosurg Anesthesiol. 2010;22:32–7.

106. Brochard R, Albaladejo P, Brezac G, et al. Early onset pneumonia: risk factors and consequences in head trauma patients. Anesthesiology. 2004;100(2):234–9.

107. Heyland DK, Cook DJ, et al. The attributable morbidity and mortality of ventilator-associated pneumonia in the critically ill patient. Am J Respir Crit Care Med. 1999;159:1249–56.

108. Pugin J, Ackenthaler R, Mili N, et al. Diagnosis of ventilator-associated pneumonia by bacteriologic analysis of bronchoscopic and nonbronchoscopic "blind" bronchoalveolar lavage fluid. Am Rev Respir Dis. 1991;143(5):1121–9.

109. Fartoukh M, Maitre B, Honore S, et al. Diagnosing pneumonia during mechanical ventilation: the clinical pulmonary infection score revisited. Am J Respir Crit Care Med. 2003;168:173–9.

110. Shan J, Chen HL, Zhu JH. Diagnostic accuracy of clinical pulmonary infection score for ventilator-associated pneumonia: a meta-analysis. Respir Care. 2011;56(8):1087–94.

111. Palazzo SJ, Simpson T, Schnapp L. Biomarkers for ventilator-associated pneumonia: review of the literature. Heart Lung. 2011;40(4):293–8.

112. Rea-Neto A, Youssef NC, Tuche F, et al. Diagnosis of ventilator-associated pneumonia: a systematic review of the literature. Crit Care. 2008;12(2):R56.

113. Bird D, Zambuto A, O'Donnell C, et al. Adherence to ventilator-associated pneumonia bundle and incidence of ventilator-associated pneumonia in the surgical intensive care unit. Arch Surg. 2010;145(5):465–70.

114. Lorente L, Blot S, Rello J. Evidence on measures for the prevention of ventilator-associated pneumonia. Eur Respir J. 2007;30(6):1193–207.

115. Zilberberg MD, Shorr AF, Kollef MH. Implementing quality improvements in the intensive care unit: ventilator bundle as an example. Crit Care Med. 2009;37(1):305–9.

116. Chastre J, Wolff M, Fagon JY, et al. Comparison of 8 vs 15 days of antibiotic therapy for ventilator-associated pneumonia in adults: a randomized trial. JAMA. 2003;290(19):2588–98.

117. Combes A, Luyt CE, Fagon JY, et al. Early predictors for infection recurrence and death in patients with ventilator-associated pneumonia. Crit Care Med. 2007;35(1):146–54.

118. Anzueto A, Peters JI, Tobin MJ, et al. Effects of prolonged mechanical ventilation on diaphragmatic function in healthy adult baboons. Crit Care Med. 1997;25(7):1187–90.

119. Sassoon CS, Caiozzo VJ, Manka A, Sieck CC. Altered diaphragm contractile properties with controlled mechanical ventilation. J Appl Physiol. 2002;92:2585–95.

120. Radell PJ, Remahl S, Nichols DG, Eriksson LI. Effects of prolonged mechanical ventilation and inactivity on piglet diaphragm function. Intensive Care Med. 2002;28:358–64.

121. Le Bourdelles G, Viires N, Boczkowski J, et al. Effects of mechanical ventilation on diaphragmatic contractile properties in rats. Am J Respir Crit Care Med. 1994;149(6):1539–44.

122. Powers SK, Shanely RA, Coobes JS, et al. Mechanical ventilation results in progressive contractile dysfunction in the diaphragm. J Appl Physiol. 2002;92(5):1851–8.

123. Bernard N, Matecki S, Py G, et al. Effects of prolonged mechanical ventilation on respiratory muscle ultrastructure and mitochondrial respiration in rabbits. Intensive Care Med. 2003;29(1):111–8.

124. Shanely RA, Van Gammeren D, DeRuisseau KC, et al. Am J Respir Crit Care Med. 2004;170(9):994–9.

125. Zergeroglu MA, McKenzie MJ, Shanely RA, et al. Mechanical ventilation-induced oxidative stress in the diaphragm. J Appl Physiol. 2003;95(3):1116–24.

126. DeRuisseau KC, Shanely RA, Akunuri N, et al. Am J Respir Crit Care Med. 2005;172(10):1267–75.

127. Radell P, Edstrom L, Stibler H, et al. Changes in diaphragm structure following prolonged mechanical ventilation in piglets. Acta Anaesthesiol Scand. 2004;48(4):430–7.

128. Powers SK, Kavazis AN, Levine S. Prolonged mechanical ventilation alters diaphragmatic structure and function. Crit Care Med. 2009;37(10 Suppl):S347–53.

129. Sassoon CS, Zhu E, Caiozzo VJ. Assist-control mechanical ventilation attenuates ventilator-induced diaphragmatic dysfunction. Am J Respir Crit Care Med. 2004;170(6):626–32.

130. Gayan-Ramirez G, Testelmans D, Maes K, et al. Intermittent spontaneous breathing protects the rat diaphragm from mechanical ventilation effects. Crit Care Med. 2005;33(12):2804–9.

131. Futier E, Constantin JM, Combaret L, et al. Pressure support ventilation attenuates ventilator-induced protein modifications in the diaphragm. Crit Care. 2008;12(5):R116.

132. Nathens AB, Neff MJ, Jurkovich GJ, et al. Randomized prospective trial of antioxidant supplementation in critically ill surgical patients. Ann Surg. 2002;236(6):814–22.

Blood Pressure Management After Central Nervous System Injury

12

Fred Rincon, Jack C. Rose, and Stephan A. Mayer

Contents

Abstract

Uncontrolled hypertension is often encountered after brain injury. The mechanisms surrounding this physiopathological response are related to autoregulatory responses aimed at preserving the cerebral blood flow in injured areas. The initial hypertensive response may precipitate further injury. Conversely, aggressive blood pressure reduction may be associated with ischemia. Despite the clear role of blood pressure as a modulator of acute brain injury, there is considerable controversy and a lack of high-quality data regarding the demographics, outcomes, and optimal management of high blood pressure in acute brain-injured patients. Recognition of the autoregulatory abnormalities seen after brain injury and careful control of blood pressure are necessary for the optimal management of these patients.

Keywords

Hypertensive emergency • Hypertension • Stroke • Cerebral edema

Introduction

Central nervous system (CNS) injury is a common precipitant of hypertensive crisis and a contributor to end-organ damage. Acute ischemic stroke (AIS), intracerebral hemorrhage (ICH), subarachnoid hemorrhage (SAH), traumatic brain injury (TBI), and several other CNS insults can precipitate a "pressor" response that may lead to aggravation of primary brain injury. Extremes of blood pressure, both high and low, are associated with higher morbidity and mortality in all subtypes of hemorrhagic and ischemic strokes [1–5], TBI [6], and other CNS insults such as cardiac arrest [7].

Because extreme levels of blood pressure may be detrimental to these patients, optimal practice involves admission to an intensive care unit (ICU) or at least to an intermediate level of care (IMC) where narrow targets of blood pressure can be maintained using intermittent or

F. Rincon, MD, MSc, MBE, FACP, FCCP, FCCM
Department of Neurosurgery, Thomas Jefferson University,
901 Walnut Street, Philadelphia, PA 19107, USA
e-mail: fred.rincon@jefferson.edu

J.C. Rose, MD
Department of Neurosciences, California Pacific Medical Center,
2100 Webster Street, #404, San Francisco, CA 94115, USA
e-mail: rosejc@sutterhealth.org

S.A. Mayer, MD, FCCM (✉)
Neurocritical Care Division, Columbia University Medical Center,
177 Fort Washington Ave, MHB Suite 8-300,
New York, NY 10032, USA
e-mail: sam14@columbia.edu

A.J. Layon et al. (eds.), *Textbook of Neurointensive Care*,
DOI 10.1007/978-1-4471-5226-2_12, © Springer-Verlag London 2013

continuous intravenous antihypertensive or vasoactive medications. However, there are no studies that have evaluated the effects on short- or long-term outcomes from this aggressive approach, particularly in hypertensive crisis.

Despite the clear role of blood pressure as a modulator of acute brain injury, there is considerable controversy and a lack of high-quality data regarding the demographics, outcomes, and optimal management of high blood pressure in acute brain-injured patients. Recent data from small epidemiological studies and the results of phase II clinical trials have helped us to understand the implication of the problem, implications of medical therapies, and the implementation of alternatives for the management of hypertension during neurological emergencies.

Epidemiology of Hypertensive Crisis

The majority of prehospital emergency medical services (EMS) are not permitted to deliver intravenous antihypertensive medications, and not all agencies that use intravenous medications use the same one for a similar indication. In some areas of the USA, advanced level EMS personnel are permitted to give intravenous antihypertensives under strict medical control orders. Most EMS systems are instructed to maintain infusions during transfers, but infusions must be initiated by a physician at the referring institution prior to transport and maintained under direct or telecommunicated physician supervision. In this environment, acute severe hypertension is seen frequently in the emergency department (ED) particularly in the context of life-threatening neurological conditions.

The incidence of hypertensive emergency is disproportionately higher in the elderly, male, and African American populations [8], and approximately 1–2 % of all patients with hypertension are estimated to have hypertensive emergencies [9, 10]. One study of ED admissions found that hypertensive crises accounted for 28 % of all medical emergencies and urgencies, with 77 % having history of chronic hypertension [11].

In the Study of Treatment of Acute Hypertension (STAT) [12], nearly 30 % of 1,566 patients presenting to an ED with acute hypertension had a CNS insult. The most common diagnoses were SAH (38 %), ICH (31 %), and AIS (18 %), followed by TBI (8 %), hypertensive encephalopathy (4 %), and status epilepticus (1 %). The mortality rate of patients with CNS insults was four times as higher than hypertensive patients with no CNS involvement (24 % vs. 6 %, $p<0.0001$). Among hypertensive neurological patients, median initial blood pressure was 183/95 mmHg and did not differ between survivors and non-survivors. There was also no difference in maximal levels of systolic or diastolic blood pressure. However, non-survivors had significantly *lower* minimum systolic and diastolic blood pressures during the course of treatment (103/45 vs. 118/55 mmHg, $p<0.0001$), with the highest risk of hypotension within the first 6 h of admission (Fig. 12.1). The most commonly used first antihypertensive was labetalol (48 %), followed by nicardipine (15 %), hydralazine (15 %), and sodium nitroprusside (13 %) (Table 12.1). Mortality was also associated with an increased risk of neurological deterioration (32 % vs. 10 %, $p<0.0001$).

The STAT registry suggests that blood pressure overtreatment may be a significant contributor to poor outcome in patients with stroke and other forms of severe brain injury. This may be due to secondary ischemic injury in the setting of impaired cerebral autoregulation. Strategies aimed at emphasizing rapid and precise blood pressure control while avoiding overtreatment are needed [12].

Physiology and Pathophysiology

Neural Mechanisms of Blood Pressure Control

The brain plays an important role in setting and modulating blood pressure. Results of experiments have demonstrated the importance of the baroreceptor reflex, brainstem pressor and depressor centers, and the interaction between bulbospinal pressor and medullary depressor pathways [13]. Activation or dysfunction of these structures during acute neurological disease is thought to be triggered by direct injury or by neurohumoral stimulation as a protective response against further cellular damage [14]. The peripheral mechanisms of blood pressure dynamics are better understood (Fig. 12.2). Blood pressure is equal to the product of cardiac output (CO itself is a product of stroke volume times heart rate) and the systemic vascular resistance (SVR, $BP=CO\times SVR$). Most significant blood pressure derangements in the setting of neurological injury reflect changes in SVR, with circulating and local factors acting on endothelium and vascular smooth muscle [14]. Triggers of acute changes in peripheral vasomotor tone include excess catecholamines, angiotensin II, vasopressin-ADH, aldosterone, thromboxane, endothelin, prostaglandins, and nitric oxide [15]. Vascular smooth muscle contraction is calcium dependent, involving L-type calcium channel opening and intracellular storage release.

Autoregulation

Cerebral perfusion pressure (CPP) is calculated from the mean arterial pressure (MAP) minus the intracranial pressure (ICP). In healthy individuals ICP is approximately 5 mmHg; CPP is therefore effectively equal to MAP. Cerebrovascular autoregulation refers to the brain's ability to

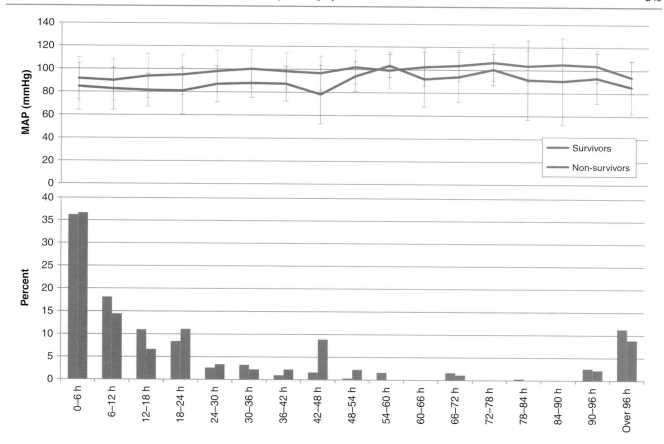

Fig. 12.1 Level and timing of lowest-recorded mean arterial blood pressure (*MAP*) in neurological patients with hypertensive crisis. Regardless of mortality status, lowest-recorded blood pressure occurred most frequently within 6 h of admission. "Percent" in *bottom* panel refers to timing of lowest-recorded BP among dead and alive patients (Reprinted with permission from Mayer et al. [12])

maintain a constant CBF despite large changes in CPP (see the extended plateau segment of Fig. 12.3) [14]. This typically holds for CPP levels between 50 and 150 mmHg [16] and is accomplished by neuro-myogenic modification of the diameter of precapillary arterioles—the key determinant of cerebral vascular resistance. Beyond the upper and lower limits of autoregulation, CBF passively follows changes in CPP in a linear fashion; these limits are shifted to the right in patients with chronic hypertension (Fig. 12.3) [16]. Acute neurological diseases such as ischemic stroke, severe TBI, and SAH associated with vasospasm can impair cerebrovascular autoregulation in zones of injury so that CBF becomes entirely pressure passive (Fig. 12.3).

Stage 1 cerebral hemodynamic failure refers to situations in which autoregulation and collateral recruitment adequately maintain CBF [14]. Normal CBF averages 50 ml/100 g/min; the human ischemic threshold is approximately 20 ml/100 g/min but varies with the degree of coexisting pathology and the location and duration of ischemia [17]. PET studies have shown that coupling of CBF to cerebral metabolic activity can be altered in cases of moderate ischemia so that metabolism is maintained by increasing the fraction of oxygen extracted (OEF) from the blood [17]. This process is called Stage 2 cerebral hemodynamic failure [14]. When both stages are exhausted, frank cerebral energy failure and cellular death ensue (Fig. 12.3).

CPP and ICP

When intracranial compliance is reduced as a result of an intracranial mass lesion or brain edema, autoregulation-triggered vasodilation increases cerebral blood volume (CBV) and can therefore raise ICP. Patients with increased ICP are especially vulnerable to decreases in MAP since CPP (by definition) is reduced when ICP is high, and vasodilatory compensation only aggravates the situation. Failure of autoregulation at the extremes of CPP and the relationship between ICP and CBF are shown in Fig. 12.3. Beyond the lower limit of autoregulation, passive vessel collapse occurs and ischemic damage predominates; above the upper limit, autoregulatory breakthrough leads to increased intravascular pressure and volume, hyperperfusion injury, and vasogenic edema [14].

Table 12.1 Parenteral vasoactive agents in neurological emergencies: preferred antihypertensives and vasopressors

Drug	Mechanism	Dose	Onset	Duration	Common adverse effects	Cautions
Antihypertensives						
Labetalol	α1, β1, β2 antagonist	20–80 mg bolus every 10 min, up to max 300 mg; 0.5–2 mg/min infusion	5–10 min	3–6 h	Bradycardia (heart block), dizziness, nausea, vomiting, scalp tingling, bronchospasm, orthostatic hypotension, hepatic injury	Asthma, COPD, LV failure, second or third degree AV block
Esmolol COPD	β1 antagonist	500 µg/kg bolus, 50–300 µg/kg/min infusion	1–2 min	10–30 min	Bradycardia (heart block), hypotension, nausea, bronchospasm	Asthma, LV failure, second or third degree AV block
Nicardipine	L-type CCB (dihydropyridine)	5–15 mg/h infusion	5–10 min	30 min–4 h	Reflex tachycardia, headache, nausea, flushing, local phlebitis	LV failure, severe AS, cardiac ischemia
Enalaprilat	ACE inhibitor	0.625 mg bolus, then 1.25–5 mg every 6 h	15–30 min	6–12 h	Variable response, precipitous fall in BP in high-renin states, headache, cough	Acute MI, h/o hypersensitivity
Fenoldopam	DA-1 agonist	0.1–0.3 µg/kg/min infusion	5–15 min	30 min–4 h	Tachycardia, headache, nausea, dizziness, flushing	Glaucoma, liver disease (cirrhosis with portal HTN)
Clevidipine	L-type CCB (dihydropyridine)	1–2 mg/h infusion	2–4 min	5–15 min	Headache, nausea, vomit	Soybean allergy
Nitroprusside[a]	Nitrovasodilator (arterial and venous)	0.25–10 µg/kg/min infusion	Immediate	1–4 min	Nausea, vomiting, muscle twitching, sweating, thiocyanate and cyanide intoxication	Coronary artery disease, elevated ICP
Vasopressors and inotropes						
Phenylephrine	α1 agonist	40–180 µg/min	Immediate	20–40 min	Headache, myocardial ischemia, tachycardia, nausea, dyspnea	Tachyarrhythmias, CAD, thyroid disease
Dopamine	DA-1 agonist / α1, DA-1 agonist / α1, β1, DA-1 agonist	1–2.5 µg/kg/min / 2.5–10 µg/kg/min / >10 µg/kg/min	1–2 min	<10 min	Headache, tachycardia, nausea, chest pain, dyspnea, ischemic limb necrosis	Tachyarrhythmias, CAD, sulfa hypersensitivity
Norepinephrine	α1, β1 agonist	2–40 µg/min	Immediate	<10 min	Tachycardia, infusion site necrosis, limb ischemia	Myocardial ischemia, sulfa hypersensitivity
Epinephrine	α1, β1 agonist	2–0 µg/min	Immediate	<10 min	Tachycardia, infusion site necrosis, limb ischemia	Myocardial ischemia, sulfa hypersensitivity
Dobutamine[b]	β1, β2 agonist	2–20 µg/kg/min	1–2 min	10–15 min	Headache, tachycardia, nausea, dyspnea, cardiac ectopy	Tachyarrhythmias, myocardial ischemia, severe hypotension, obstructive HCM
Vasopressin	V1a, V2 agonist	0.01–0.03 units/min	Immediate	10–15 min	Rebound hypotension	Ischemic skin intestinal ischemia Decreased cardiac output and hepato-splanchnic flow

Adapted with kind permission of Springer Science+Business Media from Rose and Mayer [14]

Abbreviations: COPD chronic obstructive pulmonary disease, LV left ventricle, AV atrioventricular, CCB calcium channel blocker, ACE angiotensin-converting enzyme, MI myocardial infarction, CAD coronary artery disease, PVC premature ventricular contraction, HCM hypertrophic cardiomyopathy

[a]Nitroprusside is becoming less favored for use in neurological emergencies (see text)

[b]Dobutamine primarily augments cardiac output and has a minimal pressor effect

Blood Pressure Management in Specific Neurological Emergencies

Severe hypertension without acute end-organ damage is referred to as a hypertensive urgency. These patients may be treated with an oral antihypertensive within 24 h to several days in a closely monitored inpatient or outpatient setting [18]. Hypertensive emergencies refer to conditions in which BP elevation occurs in the setting of acute end-organ damage involving the brain, heart, kidneys, or retina. In the case of neurological hypertensive emergencies, brain injury can both cause and result from blood pressure elevation. Hypertensive emergencies require intensive blood pressure control with intravenous antihypertensive agents, usually within 1 h of occurrence [19].

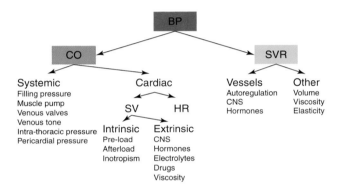

Fig. 12.2 Determinants of blood pressure (*BP* blood pressure, *CO* cardiac output, *SVR* systemic vascular resistances, *SV* stroke volume, *HR* heart rate, *CNS* central nervous system)

Choice of Agent

Intravenous antihypertensive agents available for the management of hypertensive crises fall into the broad categories of arterial vasodilators (hydralazine, fenoldopam, nicardipine, and enalaprilat), venous vasodilators (nitroglycerin), mixed venous and arterial vasodilators (sodium nitroprusside), negative inotropic/chronotropic agents with (labetalol) or without vasodilator properties (esmolol), and α-adrenergic receptor blockers for increased sympathetic activity (phentolamine) [20]. Intermittent intravenous labetalol is most often selected as the initial intravenous antihypertensive for stroke patients with acute severe hypertension (50 %), followed by nicardipine (15 %), hydralazine (15 %), and sodium nitroprusside (13 %) [12]. Nicardipine is more often administered initially for patients with acute hemorrhagic stroke than for patients with AIS [20]. Clevidipine, an ultrashort-acting dihydropyridine L-type calcium channel blocker with rapid onset and offset of action, has also recently been approved for the reduction of blood pressure [21]. Comparative studies have demonstrated that clevidipine is as safe and effective as nitroglycerin, sodium nitroprusside, or nicardipine for reducing blood pressure but has greater ability to maintain a given target range [22–24] (Table 12.1).

Intracerebral Hemorrhage

Blood pressure is frequently elevated in patients with acute ICH, and these elevations are often the highest encountered in the practice of medicine [25]. Causes of this extreme vasopressor response include upregulation of the sympathetic

Fig. 12.3 Cerebrovascular autoregulation and its failure, relationships between cerebral blood flow (*CBF*), cerebral vascular resistances (*CVR*), and oxygen extraction fraction (*OEF*) across different levels of cerebral perfusion pressure (*CPP*). The curve depicting intracranial pressure (*ICP*) applies only to pathological conditions of reduced intracranial compliance (Adapted with kind permission of Springer Science+Business Media from Rose and Mayer [14])

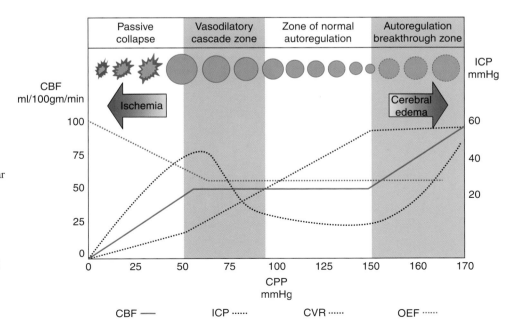

nervous system, renin-angiotensin axis, and pituitary-adrenal axis [14]. The presence or degree of acute hypertension may affect the outcome after ICH. Single-center studies and a systematic review have reported an increased risk of deterioration, death, or dependency with extremely high or low admission blood pressure after ICH [3–5, 26–28]. In the majority of cases, elevated admission blood pressure is the primary issue in acute ICH.

Uncontrolled hypertension could theoretically contribute to acute expansion of the hematoma within the first 3–4 h of onset and later aggravate peri-hematoma edema and ICP, both of which may translate into adverse outcomes after ICH. Hematoma size is an important determinant of mortality after ICH, and early hematoma growth (Fig. 12.4) has been consistently associated with poor clinical outcomes [29–33]. An expanding hematoma may result from persistent bleeding and or rebleeding from a single arteriolar rupture. Some studies have reported evidence of hematoma growth from bleeding into an ischemic penumbra zone surrounding the hematoma [34, 35], but other reports have not confirmed the existence of ischemia at the hypoperfused area in the periphery of the hematoma. In a classic study by Brott and colleagues [29], no association was demonstrated between hematoma growth and levels of blood pressure, but the use of antihypertensive agents may have negatively confounded this association. Similarly, initial blood pressure levels were not associated with hematoma growth in the Recombinant Activated Factor VII ICH Trial [36].

Despite the conflicting evidence, it is generally agreed that extreme hypertension after ICH should be carefully treated. Controversy exists regarding the optimal threshold for treatment and target level, however. Overly aggressive blood pressure reduction in setting of impaired autoregulation might predispose to ischemia in peri-hematoma brain tissue, whereas intact autoregulation might result in reflex vasodilation and increases in ICP. In a pilot trial of blood pressure reduction after ICH, 14 patients with supratentorial ICH were randomized to receive either labetalol or nicardipine within 22 h after ictus to lower the MAP by 15 %. Cerebral blood flow (CBF) studies were performed before and after treatment with positron emission tomography and [15O] water. No changes in global or peri-hematoma CBF were observed [37]. Two early studies demonstrated that a controlled, pharmacologically based reduction in blood pressure had no adverse effects on cerebral blood flow in humans or animals [38, 39].

The results of the Intensive Blood Pressure Reduction in Acute Cerebral Hemorrhage Trial (INTERACT) were published in 2008 [40]. This study was an open-label trial of 403 patients randomized to a target systolic blood pressure of <180 or <140 mmHg within 6 h of onset. The study showed a trend toward lower relative and absolute growth in hematoma from baseline to 24 h in the intensive treatment group compared with the control group. In addition, there was no excess of neurological deterioration or other adverse events related to intensive blood pressure lowering, nor were there any differences across several measures of clinical outcome, including disability and quality of life between groups, although the trial was not powered to detect such outcomes. INTERACT provides important preliminary data that early and intensive blood pressure reduction can reduce ongoing bleeding in acute ICH; the data are insufficient to recommend a definitive policy.

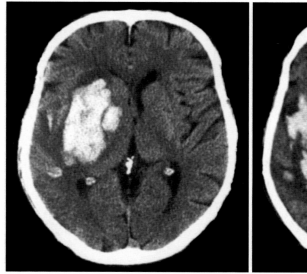

Fig. 12.4 Hematoma growth (Reprinted with permission from Mayer et al. [90])

2.0 h after onset   6.5 h after onset

The Antihypertensive Treatment in Acute Cerebral Hemorrhage (ATACH) trial [41, 42] also confirmed the feasibility and safety of early rapid blood pressure reduction in ICH. This study employed a dose escalation scheme using intravenous nicardipine for blood pressure reduction in 80 patients with ICH, with an eventual systolic target of <140 mmHg. No effect was seen on outcome or neurological worsening. Both INTERACT and ATACH have shown that while early and intensive blood pressure lowering is clinically feasible, whether such treatment improves clinical outcomes remains unclear.

Current ICH guidelines from the American Heart Association indicate systolic blood pressure should be maintained below 180 mmHg and mean arterial pressure below 130 mmHg with *continuous* infusion agent (Table 12.1) during the acute phase of ICH [43]. In addition, in patients who have larger hemorrhages (generally >30 ml) who are at risk for intracranial hypertension, ICP monitoring should be considered to ensure that CPP is maintained above 60 mmHg. A more recent study of 18 comatose ICH patients using brain multimodality monitoring showed that CPP levels >80 mmHg were associated with a reduced risk of critical brain tissue hypoxia, which in turn was associated with increased mortality [44]. Preferred agents are beta-blockers and calcium channel blockers (Table 12.1). The use of nitroprusside has drawbacks since this agent is associated with higher rate of medical complications [45] and may exacerbate cerebral edema and intracranial pressure [46]. Oral and sublingual agents are not preferred, because of the need for immediate and precise blood pressure control. Though no prospective study has addressed the timing of conversion from IV to oral antihypertensive management, this process can generally be started between 24 and 72 h, as long as the patient's critical condition has been stabilized [47].

Acute Ischemic Stroke

Much controversy exists regarding the management of blood pressure during the acute and subacute phases of ischemic stroke [48]. Current American Stroke Association (ASA) guidelines [49] recommend withholding antihypertensive therapy for AIS unless there is planned thrombolysis and evidence of concomitant non-cerebral hypertensive organ damage (e.g., acute myocardial ischemia, aortic dissection, pulmonary edema, or renal failure) or if the blood pressure is excessively high—arbitrarily chosen to be SBP >220 or DBP >120 mmHg based on the upper limit of normal cerebral autoregulation [49] (Table 12.2).

Some facts regarding blood pressure and AIS are undisputed. The vast majority (usually estimated at 80 %) of patients with cerebral ischemia present with acutely elevated blood pressure regardless of etiologic subtype or preexisting hypertension, and this dramatic blood pressure elevation spontaneously attenuates over time, starting within the first 24 h and continuing to decline steadily for the next 7–10 days [50, 51]. An ischemic penumbra exists for up to 3–6 h after the onset of ischemia and plays an important role in modifiable tissue injury [16]. Cerebral ischemia impairs autoregulation and probably leads to focal pressure-passive CBF [16, 52], which in turn may be aggravated by significant pharmacological lowering of the blood pressure [53]. Case reports and small series have shown short-term clinical improvement from pharmacological blood pressure *elevation* among certain AIS patients [54], but this intervention is not supported by improvements in long-term clinical outcomes and may be associated with more cardiac and pulmonary dysfunction at expense of temporal neurological improvement [49].

It remains unclear whether acute hypertension is causally associated with increased stroke morbidity and mortality. Retrospective studies have reported conflicting data: some reports have found an association between elevated admission blood pressure and both poor outcome [55, 56] and good outcome [57]. More recent studies have reported a U-shaped relationship where poor outcome was associated with especially low or high admission blood pressure [2, 53]. Some studies have found that a spontaneous decline in blood pressure within the first 4–48 h after stroke is associated with improved outcome [58], whereas others have found a higher risk of poor outcome with early and steep reductions in blood pressure [59]. These contradictions may be explained in part by active blood pressure lowering with antihypertensive medication, which was not carefully controlled for in these observational studies [48].

Subarachnoid Hemorrhage

Prevention of Rebleeding

Aneurysmal SAH carries a high rate of mortality and morbidity, much of which is related to the direct effects of hemorrhage and aneurysm rebleeding. Left untreated, the cumulative risk of rebleeding is 20 % at 2 weeks and 30 % at 1 month after initial rupture. However, there is little evidence that uncontrolled hypertension definitively increases the risk of rebleeding [60]. Nonetheless, most centers actively control elevated blood pressure to a SBP of ≤160 mmHg or lower prior to open surgical or endovascular treatment of the ruptured aneurysm. One recent study reported a positive linear correlation between very early rebleeding and increasing SBP ≥160 mmHg [61], but one could find fault with their criteria for rebleeding. A more recent study of 574 SAH patients found that admission Hunt and Hess grade and large aneurysm size, but not admission blood pressure, were independent risk factors for rebleeding, which occurred in nearly 7 % of

Table 12.2 Summary of BP management in selected neurological emergencies

Condition	Target (mmHg)	Recommended medications	Level of evidence[a]
Acute ischemic stroke			
Outside t-PA window			
Most cases[b]	BP ≤ 220/120	Labetalol, esmolol, or nicardipine IV	II
		Candesartan PO	I
Fluctuating deficit or large DWI-PWI mismatch	Consider induced hypertension up to 20–25 % baseline MAP elevation	Phenylephrine, Levophed, or dopamine IV, follow with midodrine or fludrocortisone PO	III
IV thrombolysis	BP ≤185/110 before and ≤180/105 after t-PA	Labetalol, esmolol, or nicardipine IV	II
Intracerebral hemorrhage			
Acute phase	MAP ≤ 130	Labetalol, esmolol, or nicardipine IV	III
Post-craniotomy	MAP ≤ 100	Labetalol, esmolol, or nicardipine IV	III
Comatose with ICP monitor	CPP > 80	Labetalol, esmolol, or nicardipine IV	III
Subarachnoid hemorrhage			
All cases for 21 days	Avoid SBP ≤100	Nimodipine 60 mg PO every 4 h	I
Pre-repair	SBP ≤ 160	Labetalol, esmolol, or nicardipine IV	III
Symptomatic vasospasm	Raise SBP to maximum 200–220	Phenylephrine, dopamine, or norepinephrine IV	II
Poor grade with ICP monitor	CPP > 70	Phenylephrine, dopamine, or norepinephrine IV	III
Severe traumatic brain injury			
Acute phase (pre-ICP monitor)	SBP ≥ 90	Phenylephrine, dopamine, or norepinephrine IV	II
ICU phase (post-ICP monitor)	CPP 50–70	Phenylephrine, dopamine, or norepinephrine IV	I
Traumatic spinal cord injury			
For the first 7 days	SBP ≥ 90	Phenylephrine, dopamine, or norepinephrine IV	II
Spinal cord infarction			
Within several hours of onset	MAP ≥95 and lumbar drain to maintain CSF pressure ≤10 cm	Phenylephrine, dopamine, or norepinephrine IV	III
Hypertensive encephalopathy			
Within 1 h	Lower MAP by 20–25 % or DBP to ≤110 (whichever is higher)	Labetalol, esmolol, or nicardipine IV	II
Eclampsia			
All cases	Maintain MAP 105–125	MgSO$_4$ 2 g/h IV	I
		Labetalol, esmolol, or nicardipine IV	III

Adapted with kind permission of Springer Science + Business Media from Rose and Mayer [14]
Abbreviations: *t-PA* tissue plasminogen activator, *DWI* diffusion weighted imaging, *PWI* perfusion weighted imaging
[a]*Class I* based on one or more high-quality randomized controlled trials, *Class II* based on two or more high-quality prospective or retrospective cohort studies, *Class III* case reports and series, expert opinion
[b]Requires absence of acute hypertensive non-cerebral organ injury

patients [62]. Extremes of blood pressure on admission (MAP >130 or <70 mmHg) have also been associated with poor outcome after SAH [63].

The specific blood pressure target and agents used to treat acute hypertension in acute SAH vary between centers and clinicians. Some experts advocate not treating unless the MAP is greater than 140 mmHg, whereas others aggressively maintain SBP less than or equal to 120 or 160 mmHg [64]. Current AHA management guidelines reflect the uncertainty that comes from the lack of definitive data, noting that while antihypertensive therapy alone is not recommended to prevent rebleeding, it is frequently used in combination with monitored bed rest [60]. If elevated blood pressure is treated, an arterial catheter is generally indicated, and a short-acting parenteral agent that has minimal adverse cardiovascular and

ICP effects is desirable; labetalol, esmolol, and nicardipine best meet these criteria (Table 12.1).

Poor-Grade SAH

In poor-grade SAH patients (Hunt-Hess grade 4 or 5), as in severe TBI, the overriding concern is the maintenance of adequate CPP in the face of ICP elevation [64, 65]. Aggressive volume resuscitation with isotonic crystalloid is also indicated to minimize hypovolemia from excessive natriuresis. Pain and agitation may also contribute to arterial hypertension, which may respond to analgesics and sedation with agents such as propofol, fentanyl, and dexmedetomidine. Nimodipine (60 mg PO every 6 h) can significantly lower blood pressure, leading some clinicians to give reduced doses on a sliding scale based on systolic blood pressure; we

Fig. 12.5 Risk of brain tissue hypoxia and metabolic crisis, reflecting energy failure and secondary ischemia, as a function of cerebral perfusion pressure (*CPP*) level in 30 poor-grade SAH patients. *LPR* lactate/pyruvate ratio, *bGlu* brain glucose concentration (Reprinted with permission from Schmidt et al. [66])

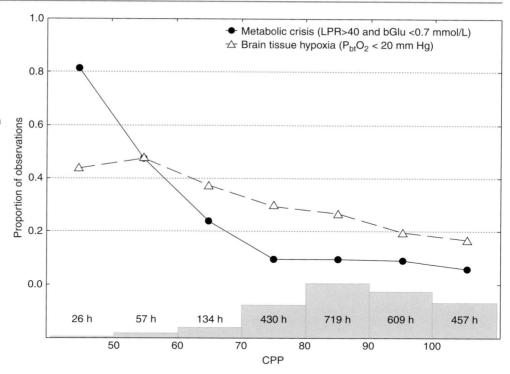

give 30 mg PO for SBP 120–140 mmHg and hold nimodipine for SBP <120 mmHg [64] (Table 12.2).

In poor-grade patients (Hunt-Hess 4 and 5), aggressive blood pressure reduction must be weighed against the risk of cerebral ischemia or reflex vasodilation and ICP elevation. A recent study in a cohort of poor-grade SAH patients studied with brain multimodality monitoring after aneurysm repair found that CPP >70 mmHg was associated with a lower risk of brain tissue hypoxia and oxidative metabolic crisis (Fig. 12.5) [66]. This study suggests that a CPP of 70 mmHg may be the low "safe threshold" for these patients and demonstrates the feasibility of using multimodality monitoring to optimize CPP targets in individual patients.

Hypertensive Normovolemic Therapy

Delayed cerebral ischemia (DCI) from vasospasm occurs in 20–30 % of SAH patients and causes significant morbidity and mortality. Untreated, nearly half of all poor outcomes are attributed to this complication [67, 68]. Historically, most institutions started rescue therapy for symptomatic vasospasm with "triple-H" therapy: hypervolemia, hypertension, and hemodilution achieved by aggressive colloid and crystalloid infusion (target central venous pressure ≥8 or pulmonary diastolic pressure >14 mmHg) and vasopressor administration (Tables 12.1 and 12.3). Triple-H therapy was recommended based on

uncontrolled case series demonstrating deficit resolution and improved outcomes; controlled trials demonstrating unequivocal safety and efficacy have not been reported [64]. Most intensivists elevate blood pressure until resolution of the neurological deficit, up to a maximal SBP of 200–220 mmHg. Prophylactic use of triple-H therapy following aneurysm treatment has not been shown to reduce the frequency DCI [69]. Inducing hypertension can be challenging, especially in patients with cardiac and renal dysfunction. Congestive heart failure and myocardial ischemia are the most common complications; aneurysm rebleeding was rare with triple-H therapy after surgical or endovascular aneurysm repair [69]. Hypertensive normovolemic therapy should be performed in an ICU with capabilities for arterial blood pressure and central venous or pulmonary artery catheter measurements and frequent chest x-ray, fluid balance, electrolyte, electrocardiogram, and cardiac enzyme assessments. Phenylephrine is used most often as a first-line agent because tachycardia often complicates the use of dopamine or norepinephrine. The inotropes dobutamine or milrinone can then be added to maintain for cardiac index augmentation (optimally >4.0 L/min/m²) in the face of medically refractory spasm [69] or when left ventricular performance is reduced [70]. Recent published guidelines from the Neurocritical Care Society warn against the induction of hypervolemia based on higher risk of pulmonary complications [71].

Table 12.3 Hemodynamic effects of vasopressors on cerebral circulation

Drug	CBF	ICP	CMRO$_2$	PbtO$_2$
Phenylephrine	⇑	⇑	⇔	⇔
Norepinephrine	⇑	⇔	⇔	⇑
Epinephrine	⇑	N/A	⇑	N/A
Dopamine	⇑	⇔	⇔	⇔
Vasopressin	⇑	N/A	⇔	⇑

Adapted with kind permission of Springer Science + Business Media from Muzevich and Voils [91]

CBF cerebral blood flow, *ICP* intracranial pressure, *CMRO$_2$* cerebral metabolic rate of oxygen, *PbtO$_2$* brain tissue oxygen tension

Traumatic Brain and Spinal Cord Injury

Hypertension is much less common than hypotension in trauma patients for a variety of reasons including exsanguination, vasodilation due to neurogenic mechanisms or the systemic inflammatory response syndrome, pneumothorax, and neurogenic stunned myocardium. In the Study of Treatment of Acute Hypertension (STAT) [12], only 8 % of 432 neurological patients presenting to an emergency department (ED) with acute hypertension had TBI. Conversely, acute hypotension (SBP < 90 mmHg) is an important factor associated with poor outcome in TBI [6, 65]. Multiple clinical studies of severe TBI have reported improved outcome versus historical controls with intensive resuscitation protocols focusing on including blood pressure or CPP support [65]. The goal of fluid resuscitation in the prehospital and hospital setting is to optimize cardiac output, cerebral blood flow, and brain tissue perfusion to prevent secondary ischemic brain injury. A landmark study by Cooper and colleagues [6] demonstrated that a regimen of hypertonic saline was not superior to conventional crystalloid therapy for resuscitation after in hypotensive TBI patients with Glasgow Coma Scale scores of 3–8.

The pathophysiology of traumatic CNS injury is thought to involve both primary and secondary insults: primary injury such as diffuse axonal damage is sustained immediately, whereas secondary injury begins shortly after the traumatic event and involves complex cellular and molecular processes. Ischemia has traditionally been considered a major component of the secondary injury process. This premise has led investigators to focus on CPP and ICP optimization after severe TBI to avoid or prevent irreversible ischemic CNS damage. Both regional and global hemispheric CBF reductions occur immediately after TBI [72, 73]. More recent studies suggest that concomitant early metabolic suppression (perhaps related to mitochondrial dysfunction) may mitigate the development of ischemia at low CBF levels [74]. The extent to which TBI impairs cerebrovascular autoregulation is another important area of uncertainty. Current opinion favors a spectrum of autoregulatory dysfunction—ranging from no clinical dysfunction in some patients to significant pressure passivity and/or rightward shifting of the curve in others. A triphasic hemodynamic response to severe TBI has been described, with an initial period of hypoperfusion on day 0, followed by hyperemia on days 1–3 and relative vasospasm from days 4–15 [75].

CPP Monitoring and Therapy

The traditional management approach to severe TBI has focused on treating reducing ICP and brain edema, as significant ICP elevations have been strongly associated with increased morbidity and mortality. Measures such as aggressive hyperventilation and osmodiuresis to maintain ICP below 20 mmHg at all times and at all costs were employed without attention to the potentially detrimental effects that these measures might have on CBF. More recently, two alternative strategies have more been articulated: CPP-targeted therapy and intracranial volume minimization. The first, sometimes described as "the Rosner approach" (based on the neurosurgeon who developed and popularized it) by maintaining relatively high CPP levels [76–78] at the expense of added cardiopulmonary stress.

This CPP augmentation strategy has been shown to minimize the frequency of ICP elevation and result in better outcomes versus historical controls treated with traditional ICP reduction strategies [78]. The only randomized trial comparing this approach to traditional ICP strategies found a reduction in the number of jugular venous desaturations with the higher CPP target [79]. At the same time, clinical outcomes were no different, and a significant increase in the risk of acute respiratory distress syndrome was found in the high CPP group. A recent study has found that norepinephrine is more predictable and effective than dopamine for raising blood pressure and transcranial Doppler flow velocities after severe TBI [80].

An alternate approach, developed by and named after investigators in Lund, Sweden, employs measures including the judicious use of antihypertensives to minimize intravascular hydrostatic pressure and cerebral blood volume. The "Lund concept" assumes a disruption of the blood–brain barrier and recommends manipulations to decrease the hydrostatic forces and increase osmotic pressures to minimize cerebral blood volume and vasogenic edema [81]. This is achieved in theory by maintaining relatively low CPP levels of 50–70 mmHg while ensuring a euvolemic state with normal hemoglobin, pCO_2, and plasma protein concentrations [82].

Invasive brain multimodality monitoring of CBF, brain tissue oxygen tension, jugular venous oxygen saturation, and microdialysis has shown promise as a means of which therapeutic strategy might be most useful in a particular patient. Computerized bedside graphical displays (ICU Pilot®, CMA Microdialysis, Solna, Sweden) can allow clinicians to identify whether ICP and MAP are positively correlated, in which a low CPP would be preferable, or negatively correlated, in which the a higher CPP would be desirable. Clinical trials are needed to determine whether goal-directed CPP therapy based on individualized multimodality monitoring targets can improve outcome after TBI [83, 84]. Until further data is available, the Brain Trauma Foundation guidelines recommending a CPP target 50–70 mmHg [65] (Table 12.2).

Spinal Cord Injury (SCI)

The management of BP in acute SCI is less complex than in severe TBI, despite the belief that the spinal cord has vascular autoregulation similar to the brain. There are two syndromes that can present with markedly abnormal blood pressure unique to SCI: neurogenic shock, due to acute inhibition of resting sympathetic peripheral vasomotor tone, and autonomic dysreflexia, in which blood pressure is labile and extreme hypertension can be triggered by minor physical stimulation below the level of injury [85]. Both syndromes occur primarily after cervical or upper thoracic cord injury.

Inferred from TBI and animal SCI data, systemic hypotension is thought to contribute to increased secondary CNS injury as well as to non-neurological (especially cardiac) morbidity and mortality. Consistent with this hypothesis are several small, uncontrolled series that report improved outcomes in SCI patients from aggressive medical intensive care with attention to maximizing physiological parameters, including blood pressure. Most of these studies deliberately maintained MAP >90 mmHg for 1 week with vasopressors and volume resuscitation. Current guidelines suggest that hypotension (SBP <90 mmHg) be scrupulously avoided after acute SCI and that MAP be maintained at or above 90 mmHg during the first week after injury (Table 12.2).

Spinal Cord Infarction

For the treatment of acute spinal cord infarction, induced hypertension combined with aggressive lumbar CSF drainage to maximize spinal perfusion pressure is a preferred treatment. Most experience with this technique has come from patients with delayed spinal ischemia after thoracoabdominal aortic aneurysm repair. Lumbar drainage to maintain CSF pressure <10 cm H_2O, with or without vasoactive drugs to maintain MAP >95 mmHg, has been reported to result in marked clinical improvement when instituted within several hours of the onset of symptoms [86] (Table 12.2). More experience with this type of intervention and the role of novel techniques for neuroprotection such as mild to moderate induced hypothermia is needed before it can be widely recommended.

Hypertensive Encephalopathy

Hypertensive encephalopathy (HE) arises from systemic blood pressure elevation sufficient to regionally overwhelm the upper limit of cerebrovascular autoregulation (Fig. 12.3). Pressure and volume overload of the cerebral circulation classically leads to endothelial dysfunction, blood–brain barrier disruption, hydrostatic vasogenic edema, petechial hemorrhages, and a characteristic pattern of edema on magnetic resonance imaging, which primarily involves the posterior circulation (posterior reversible encephalopathy syndrome). This anatomic predilection is felt to be due to the scarcity of sympathetic innervation of distal posterior circulation vessels. Papilledema and intracranial hypertension may be present, particularly when global brain edema is present. The blood pressure may be extremely high (exceeding 250/150 mmHg), but the rate of rise and the baseline blood pressure may be just as important determinants of disease severity than the peak blood pressure that is reached.

Untreated, hypertensive encephalopathy can lead to seizures, cortical blindness, frank hemorrhage, coma, and death. Despite a lack of randomized clinical trial data, treatment is generally directed toward decreasing the MAP by 20–25 % or the DBP to 100 mmHg (whichever is higher) within 1 h (Table 12.2). Comatose patients should have an ICP monitor placed; ICP should be maintained below 20 mmHg and CPP within a tight range of 70–90 mmHg. Short-acting parenteral antihypertensives (such as labetalol, nicardipine, or enalaprilat) should be given initially, and drugs such as nitroprusside that can cause cerebral vasodilation or increased ICP are best avoided. Fenoldopam may be the favored therapy in the setting of acute renal insufficiency.

Eclampsia

This condition refers to a particular form of hypertensive encephalopathy that occurs in the setting of pregnancy-induced hypertension. Because of its association with microvascular and endothelial damage, neurological manifestations of HE can occur at much lower blood pressures in eclamptic patients than in patients with essential hypertension [87]. Blood pressure management is significantly more complicated than essential hypertension-related encephalopathy. In eclampsia, the physiology of pregnancy can alter drug metabolism, there are two circulations to consider, and certain antihypertensives are strictly contraindicated based on adverse fetal effects (namely, ACE inhibitors and angiotensin receptor blockers). Based on consensus opinion and small numbers of randomized trials, MAP in eclampsia is targeted between 105 and 125 mmHg [87]. Magnesium sulfate (2 g/h IV) reduces the risk of recurrent seizures and lowers blood pressure [88]; it should be administered to all preeclamptic and eclamptic patients. As in other neurological emergencies, initial control of blood pressure with a fast-acting easily titratable agent such as labetalol or nicardipine is advised [87–89].

References

1. Carlberg B, Asplund K, Hagg E. The prognostic value of admission blood pressure in patients with acute stroke. Stroke. 1993; 24:1372–5.
2. Vemmos KN, Tsivgoulis G, Spengos K, et al. U-shaped relationship between mortality and admission blood pressure in patients with acute stroke. J Intern Med. 2004;255:257–65.
3. Willmot M, Leonardi-Bee J, Bath PM. High blood pressure in acute stroke and subsequent outcome: a systematic review. Hypertension. 2004;43:18–24.
4. Zhang Y, Reilly KH, Tong W, et al. Blood pressure and clinical outcome among patients with acute stroke in Inner Mongolia, China. J Hypertens. 2008;26:1446–52.
5. Dandapani BK, Suzuki S, Kelley RE, Reyes-Iglesias Y, Duncan RC. Relation between blood pressure and outcome in intracerebral hemorrhage. Stroke. 1995;26:21–4.
6. Cooper DJ, Myles PS, McDermott FT, et al. Prehospital hypertonic saline resuscitation of patients with hypotension and severe traumatic brain injury: a randomized controlled trial. JAMA. 2004;291:1350–7.
7. Kilgannon JH, Roberts BW, Reihl LR, et al. Early arterial hypotension is common in the post-cardiac arrest syndrome and associated with increased in-hospital mortality. Resuscitation. 2008;79:410–6.
8. Lip GY, Beevers M, Potter JF, Beevers DG. Malignant hypertension in the elderly. QJM. 1995;88:641–7.
9. Rosamond W, Flegal K, Friday G, et al. Heart disease and stroke statistics–2007 update: a report from the American Heart Association Statistics Committee and Stroke Statistics Subcommittee. Circulation. 2007;115:e69–171.
10. Hajjar I, Kotchen TA. Trends in prevalence, awareness, treatment, and control of hypertension in the United States, 1988–2000. JAMA. 2003;290:199–206.
11. Zampaglione B, Pascale C, Marchisio M, Cavallo-Perin P. Hypertensive urgencies and emergencies. Prevalence and clinical presentation. Hypertension. 1996;27:144–7.
12. Mayer SA, Kurtz P, Wyman A, et al. Clinical practices, complications, and mortality in neurological patients with acute severe hypertension: The Studying the Treatment of Acute hyperTension (STAT) registry. Crit Care Med. 2011;39(10):2330–6.
13. Chalmers J. Volhard lecture. Brain, blood pressure and stroke. J Hypertens. 1998;16:1849–58.
14. Rose JC, Mayer SA. Optimizing blood pressure in neurological emergencies. Neurocrit Care. 2004;1:287–99.
15. Vaughan CJ, Delanty N. Hypertensive emergencies. Lancet. 2000;356:411–7.
16. Powers WJ. Acute hypertension after stroke: the scientific basis for treatment decisions. Neurology. 1993;43:461–7.
17. Baron JC. Perfusion thresholds in human cerebral ischemia: historical perspective and therapeutic implications. Cerebrovasc Dis. 2001;11 Suppl 1:2–8.
18. Marik PE, Varon J. Hypertensive crises: challenges and management. Chest. 2007;131:1949–62.
19. Feldstein C. Management of hypertensive crises. Am J Ther. 2007;14:135–9.
20. Awad AS, Goldberg ME. Role of clevidipine butyrate in the treatment of acute hypertension in the critical care setting: a review. Vasc Health Risk Manag. 2010;6:457–64.
21. Pollack CV, Varon J, Garrison NA, Ebrahimi R, Dunbar L, Peacock 4th WF. Clevidipine, an intravenous dihydropyridine calcium channel blocker, is safe and effective for the treatment of patients with acute severe hypertension. Ann Emerg Med. 2009;53:329–38.
22. Aronson S, Dyke CM, Stierer KA, et al. The ECLIPSE trials: comparative studies of clevidipine to nitroglycerin, sodium nitroprusside, and nicardipine for acute hypertension treatment in cardiac surgery patients. Anesth Analg. 2008;107:1110–21.
23. Levy JH, Mancao MY, Gitter R, et al. Clevidipine effectively and rapidly controls blood pressure preoperatively in cardiac surgery patients: the results of the randomized, placebo-controlled efficacy study of clevidipine assessing its preoperative antihypertensive effect in cardiac surgery-1. Anesth Analg. 2007;105:918–25, table of contents.
24. Singla N, Warltier DC, Gandhi SD, et al. Treatment of acute postoperative hypertension in cardiac surgery patients: an efficacy study of clevidipine assessing its postoperative antihypertensive effect in cardiac surgery-2 (ESCAPE-2), a randomized, double-blind, placebo-controlled trial. Anesth Analg. 2008;107:59–67.
25. Qureshi AI, Ezzeddine MA, Nasar A, et al. Prevalence of elevated blood pressure in 563,704 adult patients with stroke presenting to the ED in the United States. Am J Emerg Med. 2007;25:32–8.
26. Fogelholm R, Avikainen S, Murros K. Prognostic value and determinants of first-day mean arterial pressure in spontaneous supratentorial intracerebral hemorrhage. Stroke. 1997;28:1396–400.
27. Terayama Y, Tanahashi N, Fukuuchi Y, Gotoh F. Prognostic value of admission blood pressure in patients with intracerebral hemorrhage. Keio Cooperative Stroke Study. Stroke. 1997;28:1185–8.
28. Hemphill 3rd JC, Bonovich DC, Besmertis L, Manley GT, Johnston SC. The ICH score: a simple, reliable grading scale for intracerebral hemorrhage. Stroke. 2001;32:891–7.
29. Brott T, Broderick J, Kothari R, et al. Early hemorrhage growth in patients with intracerebral hemorrhage. Stroke. 1997;28:1–5.
30. Fujii Y, Takeuchi S, Sasaki O, Minakawa T, Tanaka R. Multivariate analysis of predictors of hematoma enlargement in spontaneous intracerebral hemorrhage. Stroke. 1998;29:1160–6.
31. Fujii Y, Tanaka R, Takeuchi S, Koike T, Minakawa T, Sasaki O. Hematoma enlargement in spontaneous intracerebral hemorrhage. J Neurosurg. 1994;80:51–7.
32. Kazui S, Naritomi H, Yamamoto H, Sawada T, Yamaguchi T. Enlargement of spontaneous intracerebral hemorrhage. Incidence and time course. Stroke. 1996;27:1783–7.
33. Davis SM, Broderick J, Hennerici M, et al. Hematoma growth is a determinant of mortality and poor outcome after intracerebral hemorrhage. Neurology. 2006;66:1175–81.
34. Siddique MS, Fernandes HM, Wooldridge TD, Fenwick JD, Slomka P, Mendelow AD. Reversible ischemia around intracerebral hemorrhage: a single-photon emission computerized tomography study. J Neurosurg. 2002;96:736–41.

35. Rosand J, Eskey C, Chang Y, Gonzalez RG, Greenberg SM, Koroshetz WJ. Dynamic single-section CT demonstrates reduced cerebral blood flow in acute intracerebral hemorrhage. Cerebrovasc Dis. 2002;14:214–20.

36. Broderick JP, Diringer MN, Hill MD, et al. Determinants of intracerebral hemorrhage growth: an exploratory analysis. Stroke. 2007;38:1072–5.

37. Powers WJ, Zazulia AR, Videen TO, et al. Autoregulation of cerebral blood flow surrounding acute (6 to 22 hours) intracerebral hemorrhage. Neurology. 2001;57:18–24.

38. Powers WJ, Adams RE, Yundt KD. Acute pharmacological hypotension after intracerebral hemorrhage does not change cerebral blood flow. Stroke. 1999;30:242.

39. Qureshi AI, Wilson DA, Hanley DF, Traystman RJ. Pharmacologic reduction of mean arterial pressure does not adversely affect regional cerebral blood flow and intracranial pressure in experimental intracerebral hemorrhage. Crit Care Med. 1999;27:965–71.

40. Anderson CS, Huang Y, Wang JG, et al. Intensive blood pressure reduction in acute cerebral haemorrhage trial (INTERACT): a randomised pilot trial. Lancet Neurol. 2008;7:391–9.

41. Qureshi AI. Antihypertensive treatment of acute cerebral hemorrhage (ATACH): rationale and design. Neurocrit Care. 2007;6:56–66.

42. Qureshi AI, Palesch YY, Martin R, et al. Effect of systolic blood pressure reduction on hematoma expansion, perihematomal edema, and 3-month outcome among patients with intracerebral hemorrhage: results from the antihypertensive treatment of acute cerebral hemorrhage study. Arch Neurol. 2010;67:570–6.

43. Broderick J, Connolly S, Feldmann E, et al. Guidelines for the management of spontaneous intracerebral hemorrhage in adults: 2007 update: a guideline from the American Heart Association/American Stroke Association Stroke Council, High Blood Pressure Research Council, and the Quality of Care and Outcomes in Research Interdisciplinary Working Group. Stroke. 2007;38:2001–23.

44. Ko SB, Choi HA, Parikh G, et al. Multimodality monitoring for cerebral perfusion pressure optimization in comatose patients with intracerebral hemorrhage. Stroke. 2011;42(11):3087–92.

45. Halpern NA, Goldberg M, Neely C, et al. Postoperative hypertension: a multicenter, prospective, randomized comparison between intravenous nicardipine and sodium nitroprusside. Crit Care Med. 1992;20:1637–43.

46. Turner JM, Powell D, Gibson RM, McDowall DG. Intracranial pressure changes in neurosurgical patients during hypotension induced with sodium nitroprusside or trimetaphan. Br J Anaesth. 1977;49:419–25.

47. Qureshi AI, Tuhrim S, Broderick JP, Batjer HH, Hondo H, Hanley DF. Spontaneous intracerebral hemorrhage. N Engl J Med. 2001;344:1450–60.

48. Johnston KC, Mayer SA. Blood pressure reduction in ischemic stroke: a two-edged sword? Neurology. 2003;61:1030–1.

49. Adams Jr HP, del Zoppo G, Alberts MJ, et al. Guidelines for the early management of adults with ischemic stroke: a guideline from the American Heart Association/American Stroke Association Stroke Council, Clinical Cardiology Council, Cardiovascular Radiology and Intervention Council, and the Atherosclerotic Peripheral Vascular Disease and Quality of Care Outcomes in Research Interdisciplinary Working Groups: The American Academy of Neurology affirms the value of this guideline as an educational tool for neurologists. Circulation. 2007;115:e478–534.

50. Wallace JD, Levy LL. Blood pressure after stroke. JAMA. 1981;246:2177–80.

51. Britton M, Carlsson A, de Faire U. Blood pressure course in patients with acute stroke and matched controls. Stroke. 1986;17:861–4.

52. Novak V, Chowdhary A, Farrar B, et al. Altered cerebral vasoregulation in hypertension and stroke. Neurology. 2003;60:1657–63.

53. Castillo J, Leira R, Garcia MM, Serena J, Blanco M, Davalos A. Blood pressure decrease during the acute phase of ischemic stroke is associated with brain injury and poor stroke outcome. Stroke. 2004;35:520–6.

54. Hillis AE, Ulatowski JA, Barker PB, et al. A pilot randomized trial of induced blood pressure elevation: effects on function and focal perfusion in acute and subacute stroke. Cerebrovasc Dis. 2003;16:236–46.

55. Ahmed N, Wahlgren G. High initial blood pressure after acute stroke is associated with poor functional outcome. J Intern Med. 2001;249:467–73.

56. Aslanyan S, Fazekas F, Weir CJ, Horner S, Lees KR. Effect of blood pressure during the acute period of ischemic stroke on stroke outcome: a tertiary analysis of the GAIN International Trial. Stroke. 2003;34:2420–5.

57. Leonardi-Bee J, Bath PM, Phillips SJ, Sandercock PA. Blood pressure and clinical outcomes in the International Stroke Trial. Stroke. 2002;33:1315–20.

58. Semplicini A, Maresca A, Boscolo G, et al. Hypertension in acute ischemic stroke: a compensatory mechanism or an additional damaging factor? Arch Intern Med. 2003;163:211–6.

59. Oliveira-Filho J, Silva SC, Trabuco CC, Pedreira BB, Sousa EU, Bacellar A. Detrimental effect of blood pressure reduction in the first 24 hours of acute stroke onset. Neurology. 2003;61:1047–51.

60. Bederson JB, Connolly Jr ES, Batjer HH, et al. Guidelines for the management of aneurysmal subarachnoid hemorrhage: a statement for healthcare professionals from a special writing group of the Stroke Council, American Heart Association. Stroke. 2009;40:994–1025.

61. Ohkuma H, Tsurutani H, Suzuki S. Incidence and significance of early aneurysmal rebleeding before neurosurgical or neurological management. Stroke. 2001;32:1176–80.

62. Naidech AM, Janjua N, Kreiter KT, et al. Predictors and impact of aneurysm rebleeding after subarachnoid hemorrhage. Arch Neurol. 2005;62:410–6.

63. Claassen J, Vu A, Kreiter KT, et al. Effect of acute physiologic derangements on outcome after subarachnoid hemorrhage. Crit Care Med. 2004;32:832–8.

64. Komotar RJ, Schmidt JM, Starke RM, et al. Resuscitation and critical care of poor-grade subarachnoid hemorrhage. Neurosurgery. 2009;64:397–410, discussion −1.

65. Brain Trauma Foundation, American Association of Neurological Surgeons, Congress of Neurological Surgeons. Guidelines for the management of severe traumatic brain injury. J Neurotrauma. 2007;24 Suppl 1:S1–106.

66. Schmidt JM, Ko SB, Helbok R, et al. Cerebral perfusion pressure thresholds for brain tissue hypoxia and metabolic crisis after poor-grade subarachnoid hemorrhage. Stroke. 2011;42:1351–6.

67. Frontera JA, Fernandez A, Schmidt JM, et al. Clinical response to hypertensive hypervolemic therapy and outcome after subarachnoid hemorrhage. Neurosurgery. 2010;66:35–41; discussion.

68. Frontera JA, Fernandez A, Schmidt JM, et al. Defining vasospasm after subarachnoid hemorrhage: what is the most clinically relevant definition? Stroke. 2009;40:1963–8.

69. Treggiari MM, Walder B, Suter PM, Romand JA. Systematic review of the prevention of delayed ischemic neurological deficits with hypertension, hypervolemia, and hemodilution therapy following subarachnoid hemorrhage. J Neurosurg. 2003;98:978–84.

70. Naidech A, Du Y, Kreiter KT, et al. Dobutamine versus milrinone after subarachnoid hemorrhage. Neurosurgery. 2005;56:21–61; discussion 6–7.

71. Diringer MN, Bleck TP, Claude Hemphill 3rd J, et al. Critical care management of patients following aneurysmal subarachnoid hemorrhage: recommendations from the Neurocritical Care Society's Multidisciplinary Consensus Conference. Neurocrit Care. 2011;15:211–40.

72. Marion DW, Darby J, Yonas H. Acute regional cerebral blood flow changes caused by severe head injuries. J Neurosurg. 1991;74:407–14.

73. McLaughlin MR, Marion DW. Cerebral blood flow and vasoresponsivity within and around cerebral contusions. J Neurosurg. 1996;85:871–6.

74. Verweij BH, Muizelaar JP, Vinas FC, Peterson PL, Xiong Y, Lee CP. Impaired cerebral mitochondrial function after traumatic brain injury in humans. J Neurosurg. 2000;93:815–20.

75. Martin NA, Patwardhan RV, Alexander MJ, et al. Characterization of cerebral hemodynamic phases following severe head trauma: hypoperfusion, hyperemia, and vasospasm. J Neurosurg. 1997;87:9–19.

76. Chambers IR, Banister K, Mendelow AD. Intracranial pressure within a developing intracerebral haemorrhage. Br J Neurosurg. 2001;15:140–1.

77. Fernandes HM, Siddique S, Banister K, et al. Continuous monitoring of ICP and CPP following ICH and its relationship to clinical, radiological and surgical parameters. Acta Neurochir Suppl. 2000;76:463–6.

78. Rosner MJ, Rosner SD, Johnson AH. Cerebral perfusion pressure: management protocol and clinical results. J Neurosurg. 1995;83:949–62.

79. Robertson CS, Valadka AB, Hannay HJ, et al. Prevention of secondary ischemic insults after severe head injury. Crit Care Med. 1999;27:2086–95.

80. Steiner LA, Johnston AJ, Czosnyka M, et al. Direct comparison of cerebrovascular effects of norepinephrine and dopamine in head-injured patients. Crit Care Med. 2004;32:1049–54.

81. Lundberg N. Continuous recording and control of ventricular fluid pressure in neurosurgical practice. Acta Psychiatr Scand Suppl. 1960;36:1–193.

82. Eker C, Asgeirsson B, Grande PO, Schalen W, Nordstrom CH. Improved outcome after severe head injury with a new therapy based on principles for brain volume regulation and preserved microcirculation. Crit Care Med. 1998;26:1881–6.

83. Nordstrom CH, Reinstrup P, Xu W, Gardenfors A, Ungerstedt U. Assessment of the lower limit for cerebral perfusion pressure in severe head injuries by bedside monitoring of regional energy metabolism. Anesthesiology. 2003;98:809–14.

84. Steiner LA, Czosnyka M, Piechnik SK, et al. Continuous monitoring of cerebrovascular pressure reactivity allows determination of optimal cerebral perfusion pressure in patients with traumatic brain injury. Crit Care Med. 2002;30:733–8.

85. Stevens RD, Bhardwaj A, Kirsch JR, Mirski MA. Critical care and perioperative management in traumatic spinal cord injury. J Neurosurg Anesthesiol. 2003;15:215–29.

86. Sinha AC, Cheung AT. Spinal cord protection and thoracic aortic surgery. Curr Opin Anaesthesiol. 2010;23:95–102.

87. Sibai BM. Treatment of hypertension in pregnant women. N Engl J Med. 1996;335:257–65.

88. Lucas MJ, Leveno KJ, Cunningham FG. A comparison of magnesium sulfate with phenytoin for the prevention of eclampsia. N Engl J Med. 1995;333:201–5.

89. Carbonne B, Jannet D, Touboul C, Khelifati Y, Milliez J. Nicardipine treatment of hypertension during pregnancy. Obstet Gynecol. 1993;81:908–14.

90. Mayer SA, Rincon FR, Mohr JP. Intracerebral hemorrhage. In: Rowland D, Pedley TA, editors. Merritt's neurology. Philadelphia: Lippincott Williams & Wilkins; 2009. p. 276–80.

91. Muzevich KM, Voils SA. Role of vasopressor administration in patients with acute neurologic injury. Neurocrit Care. 2009;11:112–9.

Cardiac Implications of Neurological Disease

13

Cesare Iani, Ennio Montinaro, Novella Bonaffini, and Achille Gaspardone

Contents

C. Iani, MD • E. Montinaro, MD
Department of Neurology and Stroke Unit,
Ospedale S. Eugenio-ASL RMC,
P.le dell'Umanesimo 10, Rome 00144, Italy
e-mail: cesareiani@gmail.com; montinaro.ennio@aslrmc.it

N. Bonaffini, MD
Department of Neurology and Stroke Unit,
Ospedale S. Eugenio-ASL RMC,
Via Hugo Pratt 66, Rome 00144, Italy
e-mail: nbonaffini@yahoo.com

A. Gaspardone, MPhil, MD, FESC, FACC, EAPCI (✉)
Division of Cardiology, Department of Medicine,
Ospedale S. Eugenio-ASL RMC, P.le dell'Umanesimo 10,
Rome 00144, Italy
e-mail: a_gaspardone@yahoo.com

Abstract

For a long time, empirical observation and popular wisdom have suggested a tight link between neurological disease and cardiac complications, yet only in recent years has the improvement of knowledge supported by new technical approaches allowed a more detailed insight in the mechanisms underlying such connection. Both acute and chronic brain diseases may have relevant impacts on heart eliciting arrhythmias as well as myocardial ischemia, which might have catastrophic consequences. In this chapter, we will illustrate the most frequent acute and chronic neurological diseases in which clinical relevant cardiac complications manifest. In the first section, the physiological basis of the complex and intriguing relationship between heart and brain under physiological conditions will be discussed. Thereafter, we will focus on cerebrovascular accidents, along with traumatic brain and spinal cord injury, epilepsy, immune-mediated polyradiculoneuropathies, and myasthenia gravis, which represent the most frequent categories for acute neurocardiac complications. In the second part of this chapter, recent additions to our knowledge on dysautonomia and myocardial denervation observed in neurological degenerative disease will be illustrated. A better understanding of the intimate connections between brain and heart is the basis for a more affective prevention of cardiac complications in patients with neurological disease and customized therapeutical interventions of neurological diseases.

Keywords

Arrhythmias • Myocardial infarction • Sudden death • Stroke • Dysautonomia • Subarachnoid hemorrhage • Brain trauma • Epilepsy

A.J. Layon et al. (eds.), *Textbook of Neurointensive Care*,
DOI 10.1007/978-1-4471-5226-2_13, © Springer-Verlag London 2013

Introduction

Empirical observation long ago suggested a tight link between neurological disease and cardiac complications, yet only in recent years have new technical approaches allowed a more detailed insight in the mechanisms underlying such connections [1]. In this chapter, we will illustrate the most frequent neurological diseases in which relevant cardiac complications manifest either in the acute or chronic state. In our first section, the physiological basis of this complex and intriguing relationship between heart and brain under normal conditions will be discussed. Thereafter, we will focus on cerebrovascular accidents, traumatic brain (TBI) and spinal cord (SCI) injury, epilepsy, immune-mediated polyradiculoneuropathies, and myasthenia gravis, which represent the most frequent categories for acute neurocardiac complications. In the second part of this chapter, recent additions to our knowledge on dysautonomia and myocardial denervation observed in neurological degenerative disease will be illustrated (Table 13.1).

The Brain and the Heart

As often happens, folk wisdom and literature come to conclusions that science only much later is able to confirm. Shrouded in the mists of time, conditions referred to as "heartache," "broken heart," and sudden deaths occurring shortly after the loss of one's beloved or stressful emotions have been attributed to a close connection between heart and brain. Heart and brain have a close and bidirectional interaction. In Chinese traditional medicine, there is not a definite concept for mind or heart. Rather, a single concept, the *Xin* embraces both and could be translated as a unique word: heart-mind [2].

Physiologically, the brain may be considered one of the first vascular stations of the circulatory system after its origin in the heart. On the other hand, a wide network of selective innervation links deep brain structures to the heart, which is deeply permeated with a tiny neural network (intrinsic cardiac nerve) (Fig. 13.1a, b).

Sudden cardiac death—the "voodoo death" [3]—precipitated by psychological stress represents the extreme example of the interaction of brain activation on cardiac activity. Sudden cardiac death in people without any evidence of coronary artery disease or cardiomyopathy during earthquakes has been reported [4]. What is clear is that there is such a thing as being "scared to death" and, in recent years, scientific evolution has allowed a more concrete investigation of the mechanisms implied in such phenomena. Though the poetry of a "broken heart" is certainly missed as it gives way to science, many studies have focused on a condition known as "myocardial stunning" or "Takotsubo cardiomyopathy"

where emotions and stress lead to heart dysfunction. Indeed, it is well known that strong emotions and mental stress can precipitate cardiac dysrhythmias and sudden death in patients with heart disease.

To date, many cerebral areas are recognized as being involved in brain–heart regulation. We are still unsure if a discrete cerebral area influences cardiac activity or whether a more complex network interaction, resulting from stimulation/inhibition processes, is responsible for the final effect. Further, we are unsure whether conditioning activity—as in an ischemic cardiac insult—is able to modulate the internal cellular environment of the heart and later predispose the same subject to cerebromediated cardiac insult [5].

The anatomy and physiology of the neurocardiac axis suggests an interaction between the central nervous system (CNS), autonomic nervous system (ANS), and the heart and has been studied in the last four decades. Observation of animal models or human pathologic conditions, with or without pharmacological interventions, electrocardiography (ECG), electroencephalography (EEG) and evoked potential recordings, measurement of hormones, plasma and urine levels of catecholamines are some of the methods employed to investigate the neurocardiac axis. Recently, functional magnetic resonance imaging (fMRI) and positron emission tomography (PET), as well as other newer techniques, have allowed us to define a more complex neurocardiac network. Drawing on the anatomy and physiology studies of the last century, which identified autonomic cerebral control centers in the brainstem and hypothalamus, neuroimaging has expanded our knowledge from a static concept of central effectors to a more dynamic interaction of anatomical structures [6, 7].

Early scientific works identified the hypothalamus, brainstem, and spinal cord as the autonomic effectors of cardiocirculatory activity. Cortical areas such as the anterior cingulate cortex, insular cortex, amygdaloid nucleus, basal ganglia, and their connections with the brainstem and spinal cord situated below these structures have now been recognized as the anatomic link connecting emotions and cardiac activity [8–10] (Figs. 13.2 and 13.3).

Some authors have focused on stress as a possible key factor in cerebral-cardiac interactions. Toivonen, in particular, investigated arousal effects on the ambulatory ECG of 30 healthy physicians without known heart diseases. Recordings were compared just before and during emergency calls [11]. An inversion of the T wave was seen in 67 % subjects, and asymptomatic ST depression was recorded in 33 %, findings suggesting that arousal can significantly affect ventricular repolarization even in putatively normal hearts, presumably through sympathetic mechanisms [12].

Prodysrhythmic electrical instability of the myocardium can therefore be linked to psychological stress and is associated with abnormal activation of some cerebral areas, which lead to abnormal efferent autonomic drive to the heart.

Table 13.1 Cardiac implications of neurological diseases

Neurological diseases	Temporal profile: acute/chronic	Neuroanatomic involvement: cns/pns/ans Plaque/muscle	Cardiac manifestations	Diagnostic tools
Cerebrovascular disorders				
Ischemic stroke	Acute/chronic	CNS	Arrhythmias, myocardial infarct	EKG, Holter-EKG-loop recovery arteriography ding
Hemorrhagic stroke	Acute/chronic	CNS	Takotsubo-like syndrome	Echocardiography transthoracic (TTE)
Subarachnoid hemorrhage (SAH)	Acute/chronic	CNS	Sudden death	Echocardiography transesophageal (TEE)
PRES (posterior reversible encephalopathy syndrome)	Acute	CNS	Myocardial Ischemia	Coronary arteriography/ ventriculography
			Takotsubo-like syndrome	MRI-CT-cardiac SPECT-I^{123}MIBG-cardiac PET-cardiac
Traumatic injury				
Brain trauma	Acute/chronic	CNS	Arrhythmias, sudden death, dysautonomia	EKG, Holter-EKG
Spinal cord injury	Acute/chronic	CNS/PNS	Arrhythmias, sudden death, dysautonomia	TTE-TEE
Immune-mediated injury				
Acute polyradiculoneuropathy (GBS)	Acute	PNS	Arrhythmias, dysautonomia, Takotsubo-like syndrome	EKG, Holter-EKG, TTE-TEE
Myasthenia gravis crisis	Acute	PNS/muscle, plaque	Arrhythmias, Takotsubo-like syndrome	EKG, Holter-EKG, TTE-TEE
Polymyositis	Acute/chronic	Muscle	Arrhythmias	EKG, Holter-EKG
Epilepsy				
Epileptic status	Acute	CNS	Arrhythmias, sudden death	EKG, Holter-EKG, loop recording
			Takotsubo-like syndrome	TTE-TEE EEG-polysomnography
SUDEP	Acute/chronic		Sudden death	
Degenerative diseases				
Synucleinopathies				
Parkinson's disease	Chronic	CNS, ANS	Dysautonomia	SPECT I^{123}-MIBG
Multiple-system atrophy				PET-^{18}FD
Lewy body dementia				EKG, Holter-EKG, loop recording
PAF (pure autonomic failure)				Tilt test
Tauopathies				
Alzheimer disease	Chronic	CNS, ANS?	Dysautonomia?	SPECT I^{123}-MIBG
Progressive supranuclear palsy				PET-^{18}FD
Frontotemporal dementia				EKG, Holter-EKG, loop recording
Miscellanea				
Neurocardiogenic syncope (vasovagal, carotid sinus syndrome, situational)	Acute	CNS, ANS	Dysautonomia	EKG, Holter-EKG, loop recording Tilt test
Neurogenic orthostatic hypotension (hereditary amyloidosis, hereditary sensory and autonomic neuropathy (HSAN type III), immune-mediated autonomic neuropathy)	Chronic	PNS, ANS	Dysautonomia	EKG, Holter-EKG, loop recording Tilt test Genetic test, serum autoantibodies
Channelopathies	Chronic	CNS, PNS	QT prolongation, ventricular arrhythmias, sudden death	EKG, Holter-EKG, loop recording Genetic test

CNS central nervous system, *PNS* peripheral nervous system, *musc* muscle, *ANS* autonomic nervous system

Fig. 13.1 (**a**, **b**) Intrinsic cardiac nervous system. (**a**) Microphotograph of left mouse atrium preparation demonstrating simultaneous staining of choline acetyltransferase (ChAT-positive in *red*) and tyrosine hydroxylase (TH-positive in *green*) as different nerve pathways. (**b**) Photomicrograph of the dorsoposterior side of the 1-month-old canine heart illustrates the location, course, and extent (capacity) of the left dorsal neural ganglionated plexus revealed on the total heart employing histochemical staining for acetylcholinesterase. Note the high concentration of epicardial ganglionated nerves inside the Marschall ligament on the left atrium that massively proceed forward of the coronary sinus and to ventricular coronary blood vessels. Epicardial ganglia are seen as dark differently sized spots along the stained nerves. The *arrow points* to the site where the extrinsic cardiac nerves are reflected onto the heart and subsequently course epicardially as the left dorsal ganglionated nerve subplexus. *ICV* orifice of the inferior vena cava, *Lau* left auricle, *LIPV* root of the left inferior pulmonary vein, *LSPV* root of the left superior pulmonary vein, *LV* left ventricle, *RA* right atrium, *RIPV* root of the right inferior pulmonary vein, *RSPV* root of the right superior pulmonary vein, *RV* right ventricle, *SVC* root of the superior vena cava. Scale bar 2 mm (Figures from Professor Dainius Pauza with permission of BMJ Publishing Group Ltd from Taggart et al. [1])

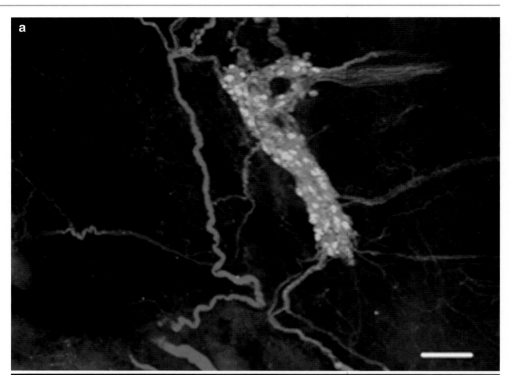

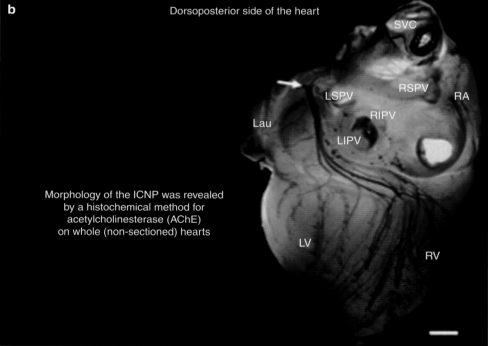

On the other hand, prodysrhythmic cerebral activity in autonomic centers may be amplified by afferent feedback from dysfunctional myocardial activity [6]. Moreover, a heartbeat-evoked potential (HEP), an index of afferent cardiac signal, has been described through EEG recording and is supposed to reflect individual differences in interoceptive sensitivity, or the awareness of one's own heartbeats. Patients subjected to stressors and studied by co-recorded EEG–fMRI techniques are able to express different functional responses of the myocardium through a cardio-cortical feedback of myocardial function during stress [6, 13].

Another relevant hypothesis regarding cardiac stress-induced dysrhythmias is based on the evidence that dysrhythmogenic myocardial substrate results from repolarization inhomogeneity, probably induced by asymmetrical cardiac autonomic drive, though an abnormal myocardium could, in a reverse manner, influence brain activity as well. Elucidation of the pathophysiologic mechanisms will require

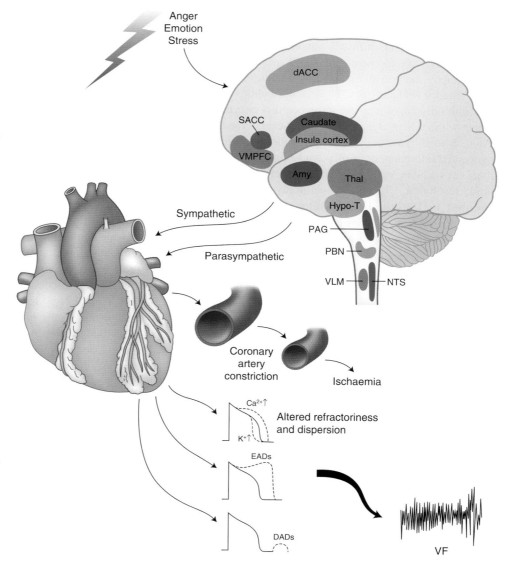

Fig. 13.2 Brain activity associated with sympathetic cardiac control. Significant changes in regional brain activity associated with increasing low-frequency (LF, sympathetic) power across derived from frequency analysis of interbeat interval (from ECG). Numbers illustrate laterality (mm) in normal space. This *t* contrast (a method to statistically extrapo-late signals of sympathetic activity), resulting from multiple regression *t*-test statistical analysis of specific signals, represents activity that is uniquely related to sympathetic influences on heart rate (Reprinted with permission of Oxford University Press in part from Critchley et al. [153])

Fig. 13.3 Schematic view of brain autonomic nerves and the heart as an interactive system. Brain and brainstem regions are shown concerned with processing mental stress and emotion and with autonomic nerves and reflexes and to the heart. Autonomically mediated effects modulate epicardial coronary artery and microvascular tone and thus myocardial perfusion. Both sympathetic and parasympathetic neural inputs to the heart influence a number of electrophysiological parameters, the result of which includes altered action potential duration and refractoriness and the generation of early and delayed after-depolarizations. *AMY* amygdala, *dACC* dorsal anterior cingulate cortex, *DAD* delayed after-depolarization, *EAD* early after-depolarization, *HYPO-T,* hypothalamus, *NTS* nucleus tractus solitarius, *PAG* periaqueductal grey, *PBN* parabrachial nucleus, *THAL* thalamus, *VF* ventricular fibrillation, *VLM* ventrolateral medulla, *VMPFC* ventromedial prefrontal cortex (Reprinted with permission of BMJ Publishing Group Ltd from Taggart et al. [1])

more work [14]. Other clues on the potential role of mental stress in predisposing to dysrhythmias, in the absence of coronary ischemia, derive from the observation, in patients with implantable cardiac defibrillators, of ventricular tachycardia when subjected to an effortful mental arithmetic task [15].

Original research conducted on late-stage Parkinson's disease or dystonia patients treated with deep brain stimulation (DBS) have shown—via recordings from the implantable cerebral electrodes in discrete areas of the brain—specific electrical activity in the studied areas that appear to be a relevant part of the neuro-circuitry controlling cardiovascular functions, thus confirming the dynamic heart-brain interaction [16]. An object of further research is the possibility of therapeutically controlling heart activity through stimulation of specific brain areas [17].

Psychological stress triggering cardiac alterations is the key feature of a novel clinical entity known as transient left ventricular apical ballooning (TLVAB), or Takotsubo-like cardiomyopathy. The name Takotsubo is a Japanese term referring to the distinctive ballooning appearance of the mid and apical left ventricle on angiogram resembling an octopus trap. The apical ballooning syndrome is characterized by sudden onset of chest pain and ECG alterations such as ST-segment elevation, diffuse T-wave inversions, and abnormal QS-wave development. Echocardiography or left ventriculography shows wall motion abnormalities involving the lower anterior wall and apex. These abnormalities are associated with only slight increase in myocardial enzymes in the patient without hemodynamically significant coronary artery lesion. Nonetheless, the clinical presentation mimics acute myocardial infarction, its onset often being preceded by emotional or psychological stress, and characterized by extremely rapid resolution. Takotsubo cardiomyopathy was first described in 1991 in Japanese literature with a dramatic female predominance. Originally considered a geographical or ethnic disorder, given its apparent predilection for Japanese patients in published literature, recent studies have described Takotsubo cardiomyopathy worldwide [18–20] (Fig. 13.4a–c). The pathophysiology of TLVAB is unknown, but most authors attribute TLVAB to a sudden enhanced sympathetic activity in the CNS, resulting in high catecholamine levels in the blood and/or high levels of norepinephrine released directly into the myocardium [21]. In a small, but very intriguing study conducted by Wittstein, reversible TLVAB was investigated in 19 previously healthy patients admitted to the coronary care unit for chest pain or symptomatic heart failure precipitated by acute emotional stress. Plasma levels of catecholamines, metabolites, and neuropeptides were measured on day one and throughout the patients' hospital stay and compared with a sample of patients with myocardial infarction [19]. On the first hospital days, plasma levels of catecholamines among patients with stress cardiomyopathy were 2–3 times the values of patients with myocardial infarction and 7–34 times normal values. These results led the authors to the

conclusion that an exaggerated sympathetic stimulation is probably central to the cause of stress cardiomyopathy. There are three suggested hypotheses to explain potential mechanisms. One is coronary arterial spasm which is thought to be unlikely given the absence of ST-segment elevation and nonsignificant increase of cardiac enzymes. An alternative hypothesis is a sympathetically mediated microcirculatory dysfunction. The third possible mechanism of catecholamine-mediated myocardial stunning is direct myocyte injury. The histological correlate of the latter is called *contraction band necrosis* and is a unique form of myocyte injury characterized by hypercontracted sarcomeres, dense eosinophilic transverse bands, and an interstitial mononuclear inflammatory response that is different from the polymorphonuclear inflammation seen in infarction. Contraction band necrosis (CBN) has been described in clinical states of catecholamine excess such as pheochromocytoma and SAH and is seen in the postmortem examination in people who died under terrifying circumstances, such as a fatal asthma attack or violent assault; this is consistent with the hypothesis of damage related to elevated levels of catecholamines [22, 23].

The peculiarity of stress-related myocardial stunning is that the contractile abnormalities are limited to the apex and midportion of the left ventricle, with relative sparing of the basal segments, which has been hypothesized as due to a greater density of sympathetic nerves at the base of the heart compared to the apex, as well as an enhanced responsiveness of apical myocardium to sympathetic stimulation. An alternative explanation of the different involvement of apex and base has been attributed to a base to apex perfusion gradient which would result in regional differences in myocardial blood flow in the setting of catecholamine-mediated epicardial or microvascular vasoconstriction. Yet to be explained is the female propensity of the condition, which is probably related to a different hormonal environment through mechanisms which remain to be identified [19].

The autonomic nervous system is likely a key link between brain activity and the heart in the genesis of dysrhythmias. Functional neuroimaging and advances in molecular cardiology have added important details in the comprehension of the precise mechanisms by which brain activity influences cardiac electrophysiology [1]. Focal stimulation of selected brain regions is able to produce changes in heart rate, blood pressure, ECG, and rhythm. In rats, stimulation of the left insular cortex may induce QT-segment prolongation, ST-segment depression, a decrease in heart rate, heart block, and asystole, suggesting the importance of hemispheric laterality in cardiac autonomic regulation [24]. In a related manner, in patients undergoing surgery for epilepsy, stimulation of the left insula induces bradycardia and a decrease in blood pressure, while stimulation of the opposite side increased both heart rate and BP.

Studies conducted in recent years with fMRI have added precious evidence to the analysis of the circuitry involved in

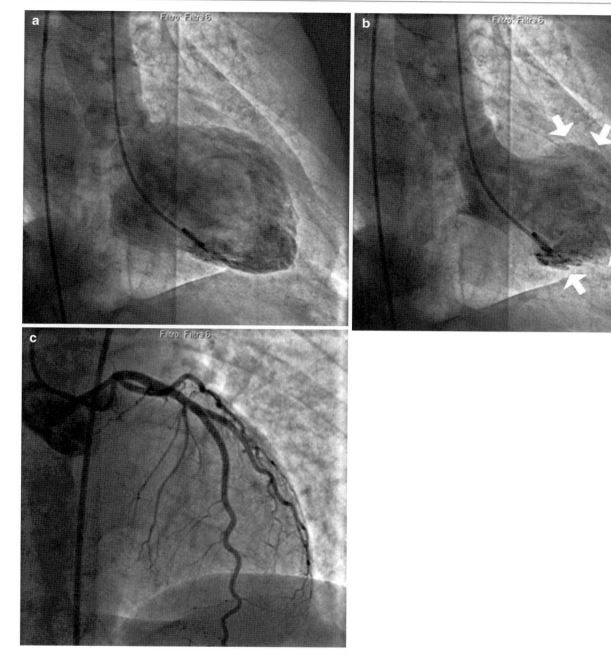

Fig. 13.4 (**a–c**) Left ventriculography in a young female patient with a Takotsubo syndrome occurring after an emotional stress. During diastole left ventricle appears moderately enlarged (**a**). During systole a large hypo-akinetic area involving the anterolateral, apical, and distal inferior segments of the left ventricle can be observed (**b**, *white arrows*). Left ventricular dysfunction occurs in the absence of epicardial left coronary artery abnormalities (**c**)

stress-induced dysrhythmias and have identified a specific group of cortical and subcortical brain regions (such as the anterior cingulated cortex, insular cortex, amygdala, basal ganglia) playing key roles in autonomic balance, the rupture of which, when sympathetic and parasympathetic activities are not balanced, seems to be responsible for stress-induced dysrhythmogenesis and sudden cardiac death [9, 14, 25].

Neurological Disease and the Heart

Relatively recently, the enhanced interest in cerebrovascular disease—the third leading cause of mortality and first for morbidity in western countries—has yielded evidence linking the brain and the cardiovascular systems. Data from both North American and European databases suggest that 25–30 % of ischemic strokes are of cardioembolic origin, while from 25 to 80 %, according to different data sets, of ischemic or hemorrhagic strokes induce cardiac complications such as acute myocardial ischemia, rhythm disturbances, myocardial stunning, and sudden death [26–32].

The pathophysiology of traumatic brain injury (TBI) occurs during the first 10 min post-injury, during which time apnea with consequent cerebral hypoxia and catecholamine surge or stress-related massive sympathetic discharge lead to a synergistic injury effect. Spinal cord injury (SCI) has taught us how the heart is dysregulated when it lacks spinal control with superior centers directly regulating the heart through chemical mediators and/or electrical stimuli. Besides neurovascular and TBI/SCI influence on cardiac activity, another pathologic process complicated by cardiac involvement is the immune-mediated dysautonomic failure observed during acute demyelinating polyradiculopathy or Guillain-Barré syndrome (GBS). Additionally, epilepsy can be complicated by sudden death, and, finally, cardiac derangement is a key feature of degenerative diseases such as Parkinson's disease. The latter disease highlights the concept that progressive degeneration of the autonomic nervous system parallels the motor and cognitive dysfunction normally thought of in this state.

Improved neurocritical care worldwide has led to the development of neurointensive care units committed to stroke, TBI/SCI care, and the care of other neurological illnesses with acute manifestations in which patients need to be monitored from the very early phase of the illness in the effort to improve outcome. While a large amount of data are extant regarding the effects of such conditions on the heart, from the acute through the chronic phase, more knowledge needs to be added to improve care and outcome.

Subarachnoid Hemorrhage

Subarachnoid hemorrhage (SAH), although generally occurring without focal brain involvement, was one of the first pathologic conditions in which cardiac involvement during acute neurological illnesses were noted. Subjects affected by SAH have a prevalence of cardiac injury ranging from 17 to 40 %. The alterations described in patients affected by SAH are elevated cardiac troponin I levels (cTnI), QTc prolongation, ST-segment depression or elevation, T-wave changes, and dysrhythmias. The main hypothesis formulated to explain the high incidence of cardiac injury in aneurysmal SAH (aSAH) suggests that aneurysmal rupture causes a catecholamine surge in cardiac nerve endings which results in subendocardial myocyte damage known as contraction band necrosis (CBN) [33]. Cardiac injury is relevant in such patients as it has been observed that elevated cTnI is associated with an increased risk of cardiopulmonary complications, delayed cerebral ischemia, and death or poor functional outcome at discharge [34]. Moreover, myocardial damage seems to be proportionately worse as aSAH severity increases; alterations in QTc prolongation and dysrhythmias are not only significantly more prevalent in patients with cTnI elevation but persist in a consistent percentage of patients on follow-up ECG performed 5–12 days after the acute event. Finally, regional wall motion abnormalities (RWMA) have been found to be more frequent in aSAH patients and fail to normalize on follow-up echocardiography [34].

In an attempt to better define the pathophysiology of left ventricular (LV) systolic dysfunction observed in aSAH, Banki and colleagues designed a study to simultaneously evaluate myocardial sympathetic innervation, myocardial perfusion (both by scintigraphic imaging), and LV systolic function in SAH patients. They noted that LV systolic dysfunction in SAH patients was associated with normal myocardial perfusion, but abnormal sympathetic innervation, suggesting an association between functional myocardial sympathetic denervation and cardiac injury and dysfunction. These findings support the hypothesis of excessive release of catecholamines from myocardial sympathetic nerves after aSAH resulting in cardiac dysfunction; this may be considered a form of neurocardiogenic injury [35] (Fig. 13.5). Further support to the neurocardiogenic injury hypothesis is given by an interesting study showing that genetic polymorphisms, which modulate the catecholamine sensitivity of the adrenoceptors, are associated with an increased risk of cardiac injury and dysfunction after aSAH. Patients with particular types of polymorphism showed a 10- to 15-fold increase in the odds ratio of developing myocardial injury and LV dysfunction [36]. In another study, plasma B-type natriuretic peptide (BNP), a substance released from the heart in patients with myocardial infarction and congestive heart failure, was measured in the acute phase of aSAH. The results showed an increase in BNP levels in aSAH patients and that high BNP levels were significantly associated with inpatient mortality, thus yielding additional evidence of cardiac injury and dysfunction occurring during aSAH and of its contribution to poor neurological outcome [37].

The theories formulated to explain the pathogenesis of aSAH-induced cardiac dysfunction are mainly three: (1) multivessel coronary artery spasm causing ischemia, (2) microvascular dysfunction, and (3) catecholamine toxicity. The first two hypothesis are not supported by clinical evidence; the rare cases in which coronary angiograms of aSAH patients were available have demonstrated normal coronary arteries even in presence of ongoing S-T segment elevation, and no alteration in myocardial perfusion of aSAH patients has been documented in support of the microvascular dysfunction hypothesis [35, 38]. Thus, the most widely accepted theory for SAH-induced myocardial injury is the "catecholamine hypothesis."

Fig. 13.5 Cardiac manifestations during acute SAH (Reprinted with kind permission of Springer Science + Business Media from Lee et al. [38])

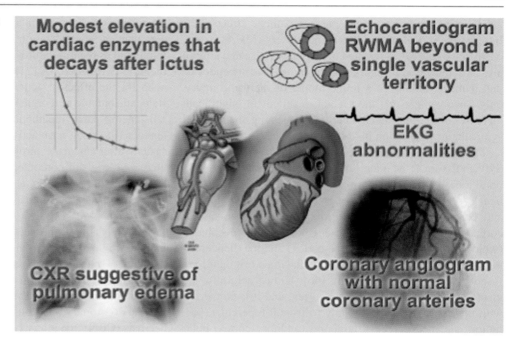

Clinical evidence has shown that patients affected by aSAH have an increase in plasma norepinephrine within 48 h of symptom onset, persisting in the first week [39]. The classic pathologic myocardial changes described in patients with aSAH are myocardial CBN which is a specific form of myocyte injury characterized by hypercontracted sarcomeres, dense eosinophilic transverse bands, and an interstitial mononuclear inflammatory response [19, 40]. Similar histological changes have been reported in a variety of conditions ranging from Takotsubo cardiomyopathy and pheochromocytoma to fatal status epilepticus and violent assault victims who died without sustaining internal injuries sufficient to explain their deaths [19, 41]. This observation suggests common features between aSAH-induced myocardial damage and stress-related cardiac dysfunction, possibly through sympathetic discharge which is shared by these conditions [9, 19, 39]. Suspected pathogenesis of Takotsubo cardiomyopathy includes the same three earlier mentioned theories formulated to explain aSAH-induced myocardial dysfunction, with the catecholamine hypothesis being the most widely accepted; this suggests an intriguing overlap between the two kinds of cardiac alteration which may both be interpreted as "neurogenic stress myocardium," as proposed by Lee and colleagues, where the catecholamine surge seems essential in producing this kind of cardiac damage [38].

Ischemic Stroke

Acute ischemic stroke, like other brain insults, may cause a wide spectrum of cardiac abnormalities from its very early phase including sudden death; cardiac dysrhythmias such as bradycardia, ectopic supraventricular or ventricular beats, supraventricular paroxysmal tachycardia, flutter, or atrial fibrillation; QT-segment prolongation; ischemic damage; left ventricular wall motion dysfunction; and cerebrogenic pulmonary edema.

Since first clinical reports of case series in the late 1960s, clinicians have noticed the close interaction between neurological insults and cardiac activity [29, 42]. Norris and colleagues collected prospective data on 312 consecutive patients with either ischemic or hemorrhagic stroke, or transient ischemic attack (TIA), observing a 50 % incidence of cardiac dysrhythmias after brain insult. These dysrhythmias were seen primarily with hemispheric involvement, rather than with involvement of the brainstem, as one might expect. Moreover, the investigators observed elevated plasma levels of the myocardial fraction of creatinine phosphokinase (CK-MB), suggesting clinically undetected myocardial lesions during acute neurological illness. Pathologic studies have revealed diffuse myocardial damage characterized by micro-islands of necrosis and subendocardial hemorrhages in stroke patients [29]. Acute cerebrovascular diseases are, therefore, a well-recognized cause of cardiac derangement. Ischemic stroke represents a good model to investigate neurocardiac influences through anatomo-topographical correlations of brain lesions, the onset of which may be determined with some accuracy [12].

Following experimental and clinical studies, the insular region was identified as the anatomical site linked most closely to cerebrogenic cardiac dysfunction after ischemic stroke. Stimulation of the right anterior insular cortex, in preoperative patients undergoing epilepsy surgery, generated sympathetic-derived cardiovascular responses, while left insular stimulation resulted in parasympathetic effects [43]. In a murine model of middle cerebral artery (MCA) stroke, occlusion of the MCA resulted in increased pulse and arterial pressure, increased plasma catecholamines, and subendocardial damage. While, in a feline model of the same injury, only involvement of the insula resulted in significant increases of plasma catecholamines, suggesting an abnormal sympathetic stimulation [44, 45].

The insula is a deep cortical region located inside the Sylvian fissure at the intersection of frontal-parietal and temporal lobes in the opercular region, formed by about six cortical gyri and subdivided by a central sulcus into an anterior and posterior insular cortex. Embryologically, the insular cortex overlies the cerebral site where the telencephalon (which gives origin to the whole cortex) and the diencephalon (from which thalamus and hypothalamus originate) are fused together developmentally [46]. Ultrastructurally, the insula belongs to the paralimbic cortex, and it is connected with the entire cortex, especially to frontal (opercular, premotor, and medial areas), temporal (auditory cortex, polar and superior temporal cortex), parietal (primary and secondary sensory areas), and limbic structures (amygdala, entorhinal cortex, and olfactory cortex) [47]. The insula is also connected to the basal ganglia and thalamus through the underlying claustrum and striatum [48]. The insula represents important somatosensory/interoceptive and vestibular cortical processing area [49]. The insular arterial supply emanates from the MCA—primarily the MCA-2 segment—whose origins are at the apex of the insula itself but also, to a lesser extent, the M1 and M3 segments [50]. Over the past 10–15 years, the insular cortex has been noted as a key region in the genesis of cerebromediated cardiac complications, resultant from its extensive autonomic and limbic connections. The right insula has generally been identified as the center for sympathetic autonomic modulation, whereas the left is thought to have a role in parasympathetic control [27]. In clinical studies, insular infarcts strongly correlate with sympathetic activation (high norepinephrine plasma concentration) and nighttime blood pressure increases [51]. Other recent clinical work with newer MRI techniques underscored the importance of right insula involvement for cerebrogenic cardiac effect, finding a strong correlation with raised plasma levels of cardiac troponin T (cTnT), a sensitive marker of myocardial injury [52]. In 208 ischemic stroke patients, reduced heart rate variability (HRV), a marker of cardiac autonomic derangement, and an increased 1-year mortality were noted among patients with right insular lesions [53]. Other relative small clinical studies supported the view of a right insular stroke lesion prevalence in patients with dysautonomic imbalance [54, 55]. An increased 1-year probability of adverse cardiac outcomes in patients without coronary artery disease has been noted when the left insula is involved in an ischemic stroke [56]. Thus, while there are some data

supporting the right insula as the main source of autonomic derangement, lateralization does not appear to be totally influential as regards cardiovascular outcome, and some clarification is required [57]. There may be a different mechanism for the effect of acute stroke and that in the chronic state, attributable to reorganization of neuronal circuitry and rebalancing parasympathetic and sympathetic nervous system activity. Long-term activation of the autonomic nervous system after an acute stroke event has been noted, with increased levels of norepinephrine and pathologic nighttime blood pressure increases, a combination that represents an independent risk for future cardiovascular and cerebrovascular events [27].

Pathophysiological aspects of cerebrogenic cardiac abnormalities are mainly due to the direct toxic effect on the myocardium of raised catecholamine plasma levels. Secondly, catecholamine autoxidation may cause damage via generation of free radicals. And finally, there may be sympathomediated coronary vasoconstriction [56]. Contraction band necrosis (CBN), the injury type seen, results from an intense sympathetic nervous system activation [52]; most of the described alterations share the common denominator of being secondary to intense sympathetic nervous system stimulation due both to direct intracardiac release of catecholamines and indirectly through the adrenomedullary gland [3].

While many mechanisms converge to determine cardiac dysfunction in the absence of any underlying cardiac disease, most patients suffering ischemic stroke have preexisting heart disease. The presence of CAD, or any other overt cardiomyopathy, can alter the feedback between cardiac function and cerebral structures determining an abnormal output to the heart. Nonetheless, there are few controlled studies looking at the incidence of dysrhythmias after stroke in those with coronary artery diseases (CAD), despite small series reporting that 20 % of stroke patients have nonsymptomatic CAD [58]. Perhaps to drive home this point, a recent autopsy study compared 803 consecutive patients having died secondary to stroke or other neurological disorders, most without a preexisting history of CAD [59]. Notwithstanding this lack of history, however, the presence of plaques and coronary artery stenosis greater than 50 % was noted in 72 and 38 % of subjects, respectively. Further, 40.8 % had evidence of previous myocardial infarct, of which about 66 % were clinically silent.

Comparing pre- and poststroke ECGs, Lavy found new cardiac dysrhythmias in 39 % of patients without a cardiac history [60]. In a similar study, Goldstein compared ECGs obtained within 24 h of stroke onset with those obtained 4 months earlier in 53 patients with stroke and in controls. Thirty-two percent of stroke patients had new QT-segment prolongation, compared to just 2 % of controls. T-wave inversion and U waves were present in 15 % of stroke patients but in none of the controls. New-onset cardiac dysrhythmias, of which atrial fibrillation (AF) was the most frequent, were noted in 25 % of stroke patients but only 3 % of controls [61]. The clinical paradigm which very often represents a challenge for the neurointensivist is a patient with acute stroke presenting with atrial fibrillation but with no past history of dysrhythmias. Is the dysrhythmia cause or consequence of the cerebral lesion? Very often a neurological disease uncovers an underlying cardiac condition (Fig. 13.6a–c).

Other studies evaluated the more dysrhythmia-sensitive ECG-Holter monitoring and found an incidence of ventricular dysrhythmias after stroke which varied from 25 to 75 %, but no statistical correlation with cardiac comorbidities or for preexistent conditions was noted [29, 62, 63]. AF is a common finding in ECG stroke studies, but the causal relationship between stroke and AF has been seldom discussed in detail [64]. About 20–25 % of ischemic strokes occur related to AF, the single most important risk factor [65]. Additionally, in about 25 % of elderly people with AF, the dysrhythmia is intermittent and termed paroxysmal atrial fibrillation (PAF); AF and PAF share essentially the same odds of developing ischemic stroke [66].

Thirty-six percent of stroke survivors have cryptogenic stroke, 19 % of which have been found to be of cardioembolic origin, underscoring the need of poststroke cardiac monitoring. In fact these patients are at high risk of stroke recurrence, so reaching an etiologic determination allows for better prevention therapy [67]. One consecutive series reported a 4.9 % rate of previously unknown AF at stroke presentation [68], while Holter monitoring in poststroke patients has yielded a detection range for AF/PAF of 3.8–6.1 % [69]. Reviewing autonomic function after ischemic stroke, one investigation analyzed heart rate variability (HRV) in 28 stroke patients and 21 matching controls for 18–43 months post event. These clinicians found impaired cardiovascular autonomic function expressed through lower parasympathetic tone and a tendency for right-sided strokes to present increased sympathetic cardiac activity, which puts patients at increased risk for cardiac dysrhythmias [70].

Beside dysrhythmias, myocardial infarct (MI) is another potential complication of ischemic stroke [59]. While somewhat difficult to recognize acutely due to a nonspecific cTnI elevation during the acute phase of stroke, it is a significant prognostic factor for in-hospital death or nonfatal cardiac event [71].

In a retrospective 6-year case series of 1,357 patients, an overall 0.9 % poststroke MI (12 patients) rate was observed, usually occurring during the initial 10 days poststroke. Half of these patients were noted to have an acute DWI lesion in the insular region on MRI. In 8 of the 12 poststroke MI patients, the cardiac event occurred as a painless infarction, mostly noted in those stroke patients with alterations of language or consciousness; this makes an argument for cardiac monitoring during the acute phase of stroke [72].

Another cardiac complication seldom looked for is the Takotsubo-like wall motion abnormalities or myocardial stunning following acute stroke; this process is thought due to massive catecholamine release secondary to a stress response. A recent study examined 569 consecutive patients within 24 h of stroke onset found seven patients, all female gendered, developing Takotsubo cardiomyopathy. The cardiac dysfunction developed most often within 10 h of stroke onset but was also seen 6–12 days after the index event [73]. In future, early investigation with transthoracic echocardiography will expand the recognition of Takotsubo in ischemic stroke patients.

Signs of (nonischemic) myocytolysis have been documented in 26 % of patients dying of nonischemic causes (pneumonia, sepsis), in 89 % of SAH, 71 % of intracerebral hemorrhage, and 52 % of ischemic stroke deaths. While important in directing attention to cardiac issues in stroke patients, these data come from a selected group of cases for whom postmortem data were available. Thus, despite well recognized, frequency and consequences of cerebrally induced cardiac dysfunction may still be underestimated due to confounding factors in its assessment linked to coincident—and often asymptomatic—cardiac disease [12].

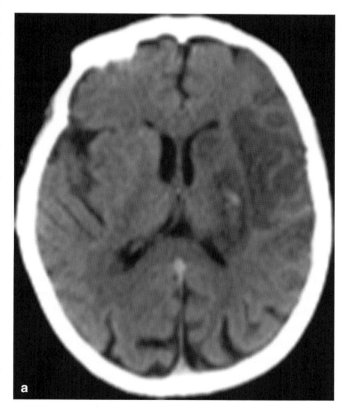

Fig. 13.6 (**a–c**) An 81-year-old woman with acute right-sided hemiparesis and aphasia with left insular involvement (**a**: brain CT at 24 h) developed 5 h after stroke, atrial fibrillation, and left bundle block on ECG with elevation of serum TnT and CK-MB. (**b**) ECG time 0. (**c**) ECG after 5 h from stroke

Fig. 13.6 (continued)

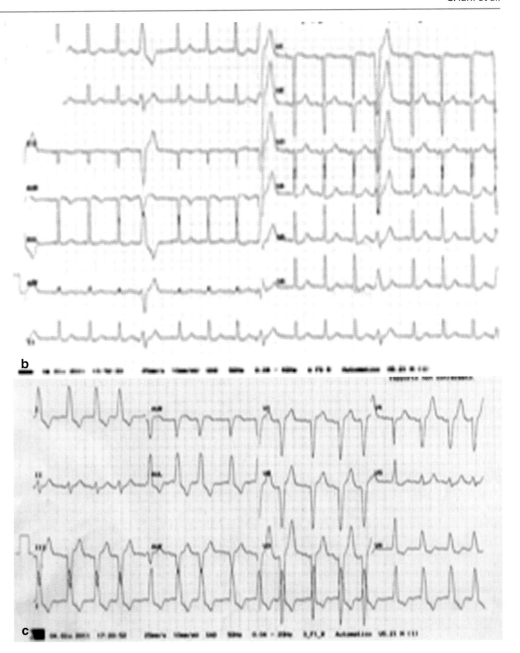

Prosser and colleagues retrospectively analyzed natural history in 846 acute stroke patients enrolled in a neuroprotective drug (lubeluzole) trial, describing the temporal profile and predictive factors for cardiac mortality and serious cardiac adverse events within the first 3 months after stroke. The 3 month mortality was 21.3 %, with cardiac etiology being the second most frequent cause, accounting for 19.4 % of all deaths, with a peak around day 14. Serious but nonfatal cardiac events occurred in 161/846 (19 %) stroke patients, 80 % of whom had a previous history of ischemic heart disease or chronic heart failure. Mortality was more frequent (46 %) in patients suffering from at least one serious cardiac adverse event, most of which occurred during the first 3 days poststroke; this temporal peak likely reflects the pathophysiology of the acute stress response. Investigators noted the usefulness of cardiac monitoring and beta-blockers for at least the first 72 h poststroke [74]. The incidence of early cardiac mortality in stroke patients has been reported at about 6 % in several studies [75, 76]. The annual cardiac mortality after stroke (5–10 %) represents the single most common cause of death in long-term follow-up as well [77]. Kaplan and coworkers reported on a prospective population-based cohort study of stroke in adults 65 years of age and older [78], that over a median follow-up of 3.2 years, 57 % of patients died, 22 % suffered from recurrence of ischemic stroke, while up to 17.4 % showed signs of ischemic coronary disease.

In summary, monitoring cardiac function during the acute phase of ischemic stroke is important for appropriate therapeutic intervention such as the use of beta-blockers for hypertension control and dysrhythmogenic activity prevention [79]. A more profound knowledge of brain areas related to cardiac complications in stroke patients and attention to their identification within the ischemic brain region may guide the stroke physician in choosing the most appropriate therapy to prevent secondary cardiac injury.

Intracerebral Hemorrhage

Spontaneous intracerebral hemorrhage (ICH) accounts for 15 % of cerebrovascular accidents and is burdened from a very high 30-day mortality (30–52 %) compared to ischemic stroke. Thus, cardiac derangement could account for a significant proportion of early mortality in this subset of patients despite the few systematic data that have been collected.

While there are data from investigations on the cardiac effects of ischemic stroke and subarachnoid hemorrhage, few studies have addressed cardiac abnormalities after ICH. A murine study first showed a direct link between ICH and cardiomyocyte pathology due to intracellular calcium metabolism dysregulation in the acute phase [80]. QTc-segment prolongation, ST-T segment morphologic changes, sinus bradycardia, and inverted T waves were the most frequent observed ECG abnormalities in the acute phase of a spontaneous ICH [32]. In a case series of 100 cerebrovascular accidents, 12 patients with ICH had 100 % of the ECG changes [42], and in the work of Norris and colleagues [29], 47 % of 30 patients with ICH, out of a total 312 patients with cerebrovascular accidents, had cardiac dysrhythmias with ventricular ectopic beats the most common rhythm disturbance. Neither of these series was controlled for the time interval between the index event and the time of observation.

Another two studies verified troponin levels as a marker of cardiac insult in ICH patients. In the Mayo series of 110 patients [81], 64 % had ECG abnormalities, whereas a positive TnT was detected only in about 20 % of subjects, although there were sampling problems. Hays and colleagues studied a population of 729 ICH patients [82]. While 18 % showed an increased TnI level, only 1.2 % died from cardiac causes.

Nonetheless, definitive data are lacking regarding ICH and cardiac complications. Use of beta-blockers in the acute setting seems an appropriate therapeutic intervention.

PRES and Cardiac Abnormalities

Posterior reversible encephalopathy syndrome (PRES), a recent clinical entity characterized by transient neurological features and provisional neuroimaging findings during hypertensive crisis, can lead to a reversible stunned myocardium. As there are few extant data, careful cardiac monitoring of these patients, possibly including transthoracic echocardiography, along with acute MRI is needed [83, 84].

Traumatic Brain Injury

Traumatic brain injury (TBI), a common condition in clinical practice, is frequently complicated by cardiac abnormalities, depending mainly on the severity of the head injury. The pathophysiology of blunt TBI consists of different types of cerebral lesions which vary, on a severity scale, from focal or diffuse axonal injury (DAI) at microscopic level to surface or deep tissue contusion, with focal or diffuse neuronal damage and intraparenchymal hemorrhagic lesions with or without subarachnoid bleeding. The lesions result from a mechanism of acceleration-deceleration where autonomic dysregulation derives from sudden damage to cerebral regulatory centers. The traumatic damage is usually accompanied by cerebral edema and elevation of intracranial pressure (ICP), which in turn compromises cerebral perfusion pressure (CPP) and may result in cerebral ischemia. A decrease in CPP to less than about 60 mmHg, especially when associated with hypoxemia—usually defined as a SpO_2 less than 90 %—and the sudden apnea provoked by the trauma itself may result in a measurable worsening in ultimate outcome [85].

The acute phase of trauma is known to produce ECG abnormalities in up of 40 % of TBI patients, the gravity of which depends upon the initial Glasgow Coma Scale (GCS) score, cardiac comorbidity of patients, and general conditions. Because of the young age prevalent in TBI, it is not frequent to run into cardiac comorbidities. While isolated brain trauma represents a "platform" to understand the cardiac effects of neurocardiac control and while there is general agreement that autonomic instability is the leading mechanism underlying the cardiac pathophysiology of TBI, detailed data are lacking [86–88]. The dysautonomia is noted in both the acute and the chronic phases and is thought to be related to paroxysmal autonomic nervous system over activity [86–90]. The clinical picture, in either acute or chronic phase, usually presents as signs of autonomic dysregulation, with blood pressure and cardiac rhythm abnormalities, elevated body temperature and diaphoresis, and muscle dystonia with hypercatabolic state. Cardiac abnormalities include rhythm alteration with both increase and decrease of heart rate, ST-segment depression, and abnormal ventricular wall motion function.

Early attempts to explain autonomic storm were first summated by Penfild who postulated a "diencephalic seizure" as responsible for the downstream autonomic dysregulation. Since then, clinical observations, experimental data, and deductions from pharmacology suggest that the dysautonomia following TBI results from "disconnection" of upper brainstem structures, causing a release of excitatory spinal cord activity. More recently the excitatory to inhibitory ratio (EIR) model has provided understanding of the mechanisms underlying the autonomic overdrive of medullary centers. According to this model, lack of inhibitory drive from diencephalic-mesencephalic centers determines the abnormal processing of afferent stimuli through the spinal cord which originate paroxysmal autonomic over activity [87]. Indeed non-painful stimuli, e.g., muscle stretching, touching the skin, as well as loud noise or emotional inputs, are able to trigger autonomic paroxysms. In TBI patients with dysautonomia, dissociation of normal sympathetic-parasympathetic balance between heart rate and parameters of heart rate variability (HRV) was found as compared to patients without dysautonomia and controls [91]. This model represents the rationale to administer gabapentin or baclofen as useful medications in head-injured patients beside the standard trauma medications.

Autonomic overactivity can develop as soon as trauma occurs and continue, or start later during the recovery phase, in the rehabilitation setting, as paroxysmal phenomena lasting for months after the initial trauma event, and continuing—after severe TBI—for up to about 1 year. In children with severe head injury, an increased incidence of cardiac dysrhythmias—in particular premature atrial contraction and a tendency to prolonged QTc interval—has been observed in therapeutic hypothermia subjects [92, 93].

Spinal Cord Injury

Traumatic spinal cord injury (SCI)—a major health problem—usually involves young people, with about 80 % male prevalence, a bimodal median age of 32 years of age for younger and 74 years of age for older victims, and a mortality rate of between 1 and 3 % and about 25 and 39 %, respectively [94], leaving a significant degree of disability, which leads to about 50 % complete or partial tetraplegia and 40 % complete or partial paraplegia [95]. Interruption of medullary pathways determines the acute sensorimotor deficits, which may be of variable degree, along with autonomic derangements which, themselves, depend upon the lesion level. Besides respiratory complications, recent data have highlighted how cardiovascular disturbances are the leading cause of death in the acute—as well as in the chronic—stages of SCI [96, 97].

Sympathetic intermediolateral nuclei in the lateral medulla extend from the level of T1 through the L2 segment of the spinal cord, giving rise to preganglionic sympathetic neurons which synapse with postganglionic neurons in the paravertebral sympathetic chain or in perivisceral gangliar

structures. At the T1–T6 level, postganglionic sympathetic fibers, known as cardiac sympathetic chain, originate and are directed to the heart and related vessels. The basic mechanism of cardiovascular derangement in the SCI patient is interruption of descending autonomic control pathways with consequent suppression of sympathetic and unbalanced vagal nerve-mediated parasympathetic activity. Analysis of heart rate variability (HRV) in acute SCI patients, compared with controls, showed marked alteration in low frequencies in SCI subjects, whereas high frequencies were comparable to controls, indicating a lack of sympathetic—and intact parasympathetic—tone in SCI [98]. As is known, sympathetic activity raises pulse rate and blood pressure, while parasympathetic activity via the right vagus nerve predisposes to bradydysrhythmias and, through the left vagus nerve, to atrioventricular block. Cardiac damage may arise from acute autonomic disruption as well as from massive adrenomedullary response consequent to the original trauma.

Heart disease accounts for about 30 % of the acute and long-term death rate in SCI patients. The period of peak mortality is within 6 weeks of injury, and older patients are more affected, for reasons not yet completely understood [96, 99, 100]. More to the long term, the most frequent causes of death related to the circulatory system—occurring at a median of 55 months post-SCI—were, in decreasing order of frequency, heart failure, atrial fibrillation, atherosclerosis and ischemic heart disease, ventricular tachycardia, abdominal aneurysm rupture, cerebrovascular disease, cardiac arrest, cardiomyopathy, and "ill-defined heart disease" [94, 100].

In the acute stage of SCI, the sudden lack of sympathetic drive exposes the patients to bradycardia, hypotension, and hypothermia: neurogenic shock. This must not to be confused with hypovolemic shock, in which hypotension occurs along with tachycardia; unfortunately, the two situations may coexist and are difficult to separate. Cardiac dysrhythmias are linked to the level, and hence severity, of SCI; the more cranial the lesion, the more severe the dysrhythmia. In the acute setting and for the first 4–6 weeks post-injury, the risk of dysrhythmias is very high and is not completely abolished even in the chronic stage [100]. The most common dysrhythmia is ventricular bradycardia causing hemodynamic instability, which may progress to asystole/cardiac arrest. In the chronic phase, bradydysrhythmias are more frequent in high cervical lesions and sometimes require pacemaker implantation.

Although less frequent, tachydysrhythmias may characterize the clinical picture of acute SCI and are represented by paroxysmal supraventricular tachycardia (PSVT), sinus tachycardia, and atrial flutter or fibrillation. Not infrequently seen are ST-segment elevation and other abnormalities such as premature atrial contractions (PACs), intraventricular conduction delay (IVCD), and bundle branch block (BBB).

Nonetheless, bradydysrhythmias represent the most frequent (64–77 %) rhythm disturbances seen in cervical spine injuries.

Autonomic dysreflexia, rare in the acute phase of SCI, usually is seen after the first month of injury and mainly in patients with T6 or higher-level lesions. It is due to the reorganization of an imbalanced sympathetic system. In particular, the aberrant sprouting of peptidergic fibers below the cord lesion may amplify disinhibited sympathetic spinal neurons along with hyper-responsiveness of peripheral alpha-adrenoceptors. Autonomic dysreflexia is characterized by sudden episodes of arterial hypertension, with systolic blood pressure values up to 300 mmHg, accompanied by bradycardia and signs of sympathetic hyperreactivity such as piloerection, sweating, facial flushing with headache, and blurred vision; the disorder is usually triggered by noxious stimuli such as endotracheal suctioning, bladder emptying, or bowel stimulation and is mediated by an unbalanced vaso-vagal reflex. The episodes may recur three to four times in a day and may precipitate post-event tachydysrhythmias or acute coronary syndrome in predisposed patients. Finally, one may see cardiovascular deconditioning, with resultant upregulation of nitric oxide synthase and increased levels of plasma nitric oxide, both of which contribute to prolonged hypotension [94, 100, 101].

Therapeutic interventions are limited and are directed toward sustaining blood pressure in case of neurogenic shock, controlling hypertensive emergencies with appropriate drugs, and preventing inappropriate stimuli, which may precipitate autonomic dysreflexia.

Guillain-Barrè Syndrome

Autonomic dysfunction is a well-recognized manifestation of Guillain-Barrè syndrome (GBS) and has been reported more commonly in the acute demyelinating subtype of the disease [102]. Dysautonomia is considered a distinctive feature of GBS in the differential diagnosis with chronic inflammatory demyelinating polyneuropathy (CIDP) [103]. Different degrees of autonomic nervous system involvement have been reported and can be seen in up to 70 % of patients with GBS.

Autonomic dysfunction manifests as increased heart rate and labile hypertension associated with elevated plasma noradrenaline concentrations. An impairment of catecholamine uptake by the diseased peripheral nerves is thought to be responsible for plasma catecholamine elevation [104]. Cardiovascular abnormalities attributed to autonomic neuropathy in GBS patients take different forms. Rhythm abnormalities range from sustained sinus tachycardia—the most common observed and usually not requiring treatment—to bradydysrhythmias, reported in 50 % of patients; a small

percentage of these cases present with potentially serious events necessitating administration of atropine or pacemaker placement [105, 106]. Blood pressure variability has been attributed to impaired baroreceptor reflex pathways and to altered catecholamine levels, causing postural hypotension and hypertensive episodes [104].

A wide spectrum of electrocardiographic changes, such as QT-segment prolongation, giant T waves, ST-T segment changes, and atrioventricular blocks, have been described in patients with GBS, suggesting myocardial involvement [104]. One reported fatal case of intractable cardiac dysrhythmias showed signs of severe myocarditis on postmortem evaluation [107].

Anecdotal reports of reversible left ventricular dysfunction during GBS are found in the literature, matching the characteristics described in neurogenic stunned myocardium (i.e., rapid onset and resolution of symptoms, ECG changes accompanied by mildly elevated cardiac enzymes, severe left ventricular systolic dysfunction, and segmental wall motion abnormalities). The actual incidence of this kind of myocardial involvement in GBS patients is unknown and may be underestimated because echocardiographic examinations are not routinely performed in such cases [108, 109].

Myasthenia Gravis

Myasthenia gravis (MG) is an autoimmune disorder leading to fluctuating muscle weakness and fatigability. Circulating antibodies are directed against acetylcholine receptors at the postsynaptic neuromuscular junction, inhibiting the stimulative effect of the acetylcholine. ICU admission of patients affected by myasthenia is mostly related to respiratory failure due to a myasthenic crisis. Different aspects must be taken in consideration when evaluating heart disease in myasthenic patients. The first is that hypoxia, hypercapnic acidosis, and associated respiratory infections which may occur in the myasthenic crisis could give rise to alterations in heart muscle; indeed bronchopneumonia is a common autopsy finding in patients with myasthenia gravis [110]. The second important issue is that many patients with myasthenia are in an age-group where coronary vascular disease is frequent and may cause pathologic changes to the myocardium. Patients with myasthenia gravis may develop MG-related heart disease in a minority of cases and, in particular, when a thymoma is present. Symptoms of myocardial involvement are mainly dysrhythmias; microscopic study of symptomatic patients has shown signs of focal myocarditis [111]. In a recent study on 924 myasthenic patients, only three were found to have myocarditis, manifesting with T-wave abnormalities, atrioventricular dissociation, and wide QRS; this suggests that myocarditis is a rare complication of MG [112].

Recent case reports have described the association of Takotsubo cardiomyopathy (transient left ventricular apical ballooning, TLVAB) with myasthenic crisis. In two of the cases, patients were admitted for MG crisis without any identified psychological stress and subsequently developed TLVAB, suggesting that the MG crisis itself and/or plasmapheresis treatments played a causative role in the development of TLVAB [113]. In a third case report, a personally significant stressful life event triggered cardiac symptoms consistent with TLVAB, and shortly after cardiac catheterization, the patient developed a myasthenic crisis [113].

Dermatomyositis and Polymyositis

Polymyositis and dermatomyositis are chronic inflammatory muscle diseases clinically characterized by muscle weakness and fatigue and histopathologically by inflammatory cell infiltrates in skeletal muscle. Extramuscular involvement is common, such as the skin in dermatomyositis, interstitial lung disease, arthritis, gastrointestinal involvement, and Raynaud's phenomenon, suggesting that myositis is a systemic inflammatory connective tissue disease. Annual incidence per 100,000 population is approximately 0.5 [114].

The frequency of heart involvement in patients with myositis varies between 6 and 75 %, depending on whether clinical manifestations or subclinical involvement is considered, on the criteria used to define heart involvement, and on the method used to assess cardiac involvement [115]. Cardiac involvement as a cause of death in polymyositis was reported in 10–20 % of cases, and congestive heart failure was observed in between 3 and 45 % of myositis patients. The lack of a matched control population makes it difficult to determine whether such figures are reliable [116]. Subclinical cardiac involvement is much more common than overtly manifest heart disease. ECG changes are the most commonly observed alterations and include atrial and ventricular dysrhythmias, atrioventricular block, BBB, prolongation of P-R intervals, nonspecific ST-T wave changes, and abnormal Q waves [117].

Dysrhythmias and conduction abnormalities are probably due to inflammatory involvement of the myocardium and the conduction system. Histopathological studies have documented mononuclear inflammatory cell infiltrates in the endomysium and in perivascular areas; these findings are suggestive of myocarditis in patients affected by polymyositis and dermatomyositis [118]. Myocarditis could be the cause of congestive heart failure, which is one of the most frequently reported clinical cardiac manifestations in polymyositis and dermatomyositis. Vascular alterations in the coronary arteries of these patients have also been described, manifesting as vasculitis, intimal proliferation, medial sclerosis, and microvascular disease, all potential causes of

clinical symptoms such as dysrhythmias and angina pectoris [116]. The assessment of cardiac involvement in muscular inflammatory disease has been made by echocardiographic studies, which have shown that left ventricular diastolic dysfunction is the most common alteration. Gadolinium-DTPA-enhanced MRI, which is able to detect myocardial inflammation, and, though rarely in clinical practice, endomyocardial biopsy have also been used to assess myocardial involvement. Troponin I remains the most specific laboratory test to detect myocardial involvement, especially in this group of patients in whom not only muscle-specific creatinine kinases (CK-MM) but also myocardial (MB) and brain (BB) isoenzymes are elevated even in the absence of cardiac involvement; the elevated CK values are thought to be due to an upregulation of the CK-B subunit during regeneration of damaged skeletal muscle fibers [116]. The low incidence of idiopathic inflammatory myopathies has allowed studies only on small groups of patients, leading to suggestive but not conclusive evidence of cardiac involvement. Clinically manifest cardiac involvement appears to be infrequent in polymyositis and dermatomyositis, but cardiovascular manifestations represent a major cause of death in these patients, indicating that significant cardiac involvement could be underestimated.

Epilepsy

Cardiac asystole induced by epileptic seizures is a rare complication (Fig. 13.7). In a recent retrospective study of 1,244 patients undergoing long-term video-EEG monitoring, only five patients with seizure-induced asystole were found. In these patients, eleven asystolic events during a total of 19 seizure episodes were recorded; the cardiac events appeared only in frontal and temporal focal epilepsies with a lateralization to the left side, proving to be a relatively uncommon complication [119]. Of the five cases described, three had pacemakers implanted and the remaining two required further cardiac evaluation.

Status epilepticus (SE), defined as a single seizure or multiple recurrent seizures lasting over 30 min, is a dramatic complication of epilepsy and a medical emergency carrying a mortality rate ranging between 20 and 30 %. Anoxia followed by cardiac arrest accounts for the highest mortality in older patients during SE; other conditions leading to an intermediate risk of mortality are stroke, metabolic alterations, drug overdose, tumors, and trauma. The chain of events leading from prolonged convulsive activity to death is the result of massive autonomic activation with consequent tachycardia, hyperthermia, increased plasma glucose, lactic acidosis, and hypertension. The previously mentioned conditions are a challenge in the acute setting; additionally, even after the acute responses subside, with some return to normality, the

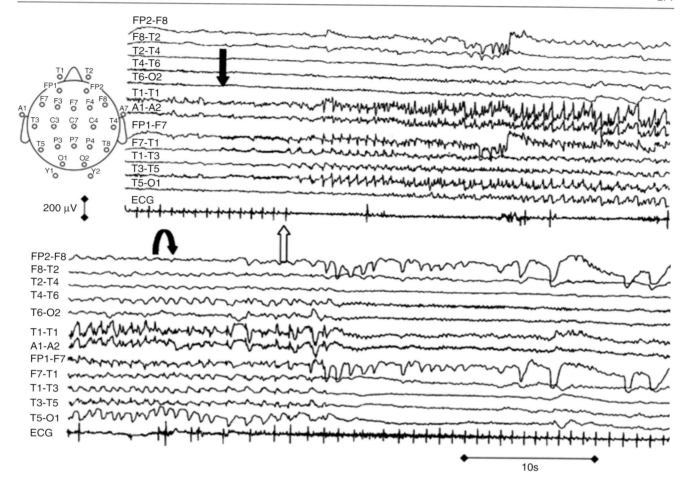

Fig. 13.7 Ictal asystole: simultaneous EEG and ECG show epileptiform discharges over the left anterior temporal region (*filled out arrow*) with subsequent asystole commencing about 10 s later (*unfilled arrow*).

Onset of tonic arm posturing is marked (*curved arrow*). Scalp electrode montage is according to the 10/20 system (Reprinted with permission of BMJ Publishing Group Ltd from Lim et al. [154])

danger of terminal damage to the nervous system remains a serious threat [120].

Studies in animal models have documented neuropathological damage in chemically paralyzed rats with prolonged SE, even when the metabolic variables are controlled, suggesting that the epileptic discharge itself contributes to neuronal damage [121]. Yet despite this observation, it has been noted that more than 90 % of SE-induced mortality does not occur during the seizures, or even within the initial 24 h of the events, but within the 30 days following seizure activity [122, 123]; there is clearly more to learn about this pathophysiology.

Boggs described two different patterns in hemodynamic changes prior to death in a group of patients studied in the weeks following SE [124]. One, characterized by a gradual decline in blood pressure and heart rate before death, documented clear myocardial injury in the postmortem examinations, while the second group, in which no change in cardiovascular parameters were recorded immediately before death, had autopsy studies showing no evidence of

cardiac damage. The investigators concluded that the second group of patients probably sustained very subtle cardiac damage leading to a latent dysrhythmogenicity which eventually resulted in a terminal cardiac event [120]. In order to shed some light on the mechanisms underlying an increased susceptibility to dysrhythmia in patients following SE, a recent murine study evaluated myocardial damage, alterations in cardiac electrical activity, and susceptibility to experimentally induced arrhythmias produced by SE [125]. The animal model showed that SE increased heart rate and blood pressure consistent with activation of the sympathetic nervous system and induced cardiac myofilament damage. Furthermore, 10–12 days following seizures, the electrical activity of the heart was altered such that there was increased susceptibility to lethal ventricular dysrhythmias, even though no evidence of anatomical or structural damage was noted [125].

It has been proposed that the cardiorespiratory effects of seizure activity are due to a seizure-induced excitation of the rostral brain areas projecting to the autonomic centers in the brainstem. Indeed, areas in the medulla such as the nucleus of the tractus solitarius, the dorsal motor nucleus of the vagus, and the ventrolateral medulla seem to be activated by seizures independently of the associated hypertension. These areas of the brain are critical in regulating peripheral sympathetic nervous system activity, and their stimulation results in sympathoexcitation. Consequently, it appears that an intense activation of the sympathoexcitatory centers throughout the brain during SE produces increased sympathetic nervous system activity and catecholamine release, inducing myocyte damage and altered ECG [125].

Catecholamine storm triggered by seizures may be the basis of Takotsubo cardiomyopathy described both in seizures and in convulsive status epilepticus [126–128]. Moreover, the incidence of this condition may be largely underestimated during the postictal period because patients are usually unable to complain of chest discomfort due to prolonged alteration of consciousness and, further, the increased creatinine phosphokinase levels may not be helpful since they generally reflect injury to the skeletal muscle. The monitoring of ECG activity to prevent serious cardiac complications is mandatory [128].

Patients affected by epilepsy are at increased risk of a sudden death condition termed sudden unexpected death in epilepsy (SUDEP) and described as the sudden, unexpected, nontraumatic, and non-drowning death of patients with epilepsy. The death may be witnessed or unwitnessed and may occur with or without evidence of a seizure, excluding documented SE. In cases of definite SUDEP, postmortem examination does not reveal a structural or toxicologic cause of death [129]. The incidence of SUDEP varies according to the criteria used to define the condition and ranges from 0.35 to 2.7 per 1,000 person-years; SUDEP accounts for up to 17 % of all deaths in patients with epilepsy [130, 131]. Risk factors for SUDEP include chronic epilepsy and, in particular, refractory seizures, as well as a history of primary or secondary generalized tonic-clonic seizures. As regards therapy-related risk factors, polytherapy with antiepileptic drugs and frequent dose changes appear associated with SUDEP, independent of seizure frequency [130]. The current consensus is that SUDEP is primarily a "seizure-related" event but the mechanisms underlying SUDEP are unknown. Proposed mechanisms are acute neurogenic pulmonary edema, which is well described in relation to severe head injury and SAH, and could explain the frequent finding of pulmonary edema in SUDEP patients at autopsy. Neurogenic pulmonary edema is caused by an intense generalized vasoconstriction with consequent increased pulmonary vascular resistance which may be induced by massive seizure-related sympathetic outburst. Another hypothesis of the origin of SUDEP is cardiac dysrhythmias precipitated by seizure discharges acting via the autonomic nervous system. This is suggested by the observation that ictal

dysrhythmias occurred in 42 % of hospitalized epilepsy patients in one study, and ictal asystole, atrial fibrillation, and repolarization abnormalities have been described in other works. Additionally, ECG abnormalities seem to have a higher occurrence in patients with generalized tonic-clonic seizures, and these are the types of seizures associated with higher risk of SUDEP. Studies involving epilepsy surgery programs suggest that successful epilepsy surgery reduces the risk of SUDEP, yet being seizure-free—rather than merely having a reduction of seizures—appears to be the real "protective" factor after surgery [131]. In summary, abundant evidence exists that autonomic dysfunction and cardiac dysrhythmias are associated with seizures. Chronic epilepsy with intractable seizures and tonic-clonic seizures, in particular, are associated with an increased risk of SUDEP. The data are not entirely clear, and further studies are required to elucidate the mechanism[s] of SUDEP.

Degenerative Neurological Diseases and the Heart

The key feature of cardiovascular dysfunction in Parkinson's disease (PD) and other disorders of the basal ganglia is dysautonomia. Much time has passed since motor and cognitive dysfunction represented the most common recognizable clinical element to guide a diagnosis toward neurodegenerative disorders such as Parkinson's disease (PD), multiple-system atrophy (MSA), and Alzheimer disease (AD). For about a decade, a more detailed characterization of what are thought to be minor clinical signs—such as hypotension or bladder dysfunction—has highlighted a considerable role for the autonomic nervous system in neurodegenerative diseases [132, 133]. This suggests a lack not only in dopamine neurotransmission but in noradrenergic sympatho-transmission as well. Studies of autonomic dysfunction in such diseases are providing new insights into their pathophysiological mechanism and potentials for therapies.

Orthostatic hypotension (OH), postprandial hypotension, and supine hypertension are well-recognized examples of cardiac autonomic dysfunctions seen in Parkinsonian syndromes. Besides these, other dysautonomic disturbances, such as urinary incontinence, constipation, heat/cold intolerance, and sweating and salivary gland dysfunction, have been noted.

The historic classification of neurodegenerative diseases based upon grouping of clinical characteristics has been recently altered by a different viewpoint based upon neuropathological features, for which common clinical manifestations underlie common cellular abnormalities. Parkinson's disease (PD), Lewy body dementia (LBD), multiple-system atrophy (MSA), and pure autonomic failure (PAF) represent the group of synucleinopathies where α-synuclein, a cytosolic protein, pathologically accumulates, leading to a progressive cellular degeneration. The link between cardiac sympathetic denervation and Lewy body neuronal cell deposits derives from the strong correlation observed in familial forms of PD with synuclein gene mutation or triplication [134]. Clinically, all these forms share the coexistence of autonomic disturbances, albeit to different degrees. On the other hand, another group with similar clinical features—like cognitive and motor disturbances—has been classified together, such as progressive supranuclear palsy (PSP), cortico-basal ganglionic degeneration (CBD), frontotemporal dementia (FTD), and Alzheimer disease (AD); these share the common finding at the cellular level of deposits of hyperphosphorylated tau protein and now represent the neurodegenerative group of tauopathies. In this group, autonomic disturbances, though present, are less well delineated than in synucleinopathies.

Synucleinopathies

Parkinson's Disease (PD), Multiple-System Atrophy (MSA), and Lewy Body Dementia (LBD)

Pathological observations have detected how synucleinopathies share the presence of Lewy body deposits, a hallmark of degeneration. In PD and LBD, there is postganglionic autonomic structure damage involving the heart and paravertebral sympathetic ganglia, whereas in MSA, there is predominant involvement of spinal and brainstem structures [135] (Fig. 13.8).

Cell loss or Lewy body formation has been documented in the locus coeruleus of PD patients, which is the main source of norepinephrine in the brain. The dorsal motor nucleus of the vagus nerve also shows cell loss or Lewy bodies in PD patients, yet the main source of vagal efferents mediating reflexive bradycardia is the nucleus ambiguus and seems to be intact in PD [136]. Interesting, then, is the finding of Papapetropoulos who demonstrated a higher density of Lewy bodies in the insular cortex of patients with PD + OH as compared to patients with PD and no orthostatic hypotension [137]. Despite a significant scientific literature, there is still unclarity as to the precise mechanisms of these disorders [134], and the peripheral versus central origin of OH in PD remains a debated topic.

Newer imaging techniques have confirmed "in vivo" pathologic findings. Goldstein and colleagues found, in PD, a significantly low myocardial concentration of 6[^{18}F] fluoro-dopamine with positron emission tomographic (PET) scanning and, accordingly, low plasma concentrations of norepinephrine and its metabolites directly collected from the coronary sinus outflow, with or without autonomic failure. This is an unequivocal sign of postganglionic cardiac noradrenergic denervation, seen in the early stages of the disease,

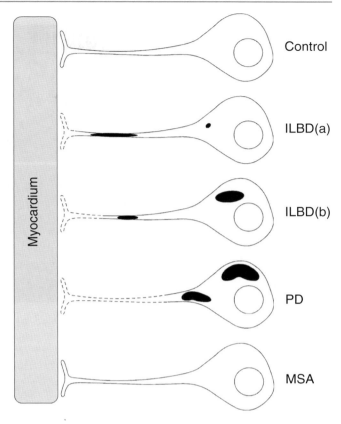

Fig. 13.8 Schematic illustration of the degenerative process of the cardiac sympathetic nervous system. In ILBD(a) α-synuclein aggregates abundantly accumulate in the distal axons in contrast to sparse α-synuclein aggregates in the paravertebral sympathetic ganglia. In ILBD(b), α-synuclein aggregates in the distal axons diminish, while they increase in number and quantity in the paravertebral sympathetic ganglia. In PD, α-synuclein aggregates in the distal axons disappear with regression of TH-ir axons, whereas α-synuclein aggregates accumulate much more abundantly in the paravertebral sympathetic ganglia. In MSA, α-synuclein aggregates are basically not observed as seen in controls, with a few exceptions. *Black shading* indicates α-synuclein aggregates. The *line* indicates the outline of TH-ir axons or their mother neurons. The *dotted line* indicates degeneration of TH-ir axons. *ILBD(a)* ILBD with preserved TH-ir axons, *ILBD(b)* ILBD with decreased TH-ir axons (Reprinted with permission of Oxford University Press from Orimo et al. [135])

as well. The investigators coined the term "sympathetic cardioneuropathy" for this observation. Interestingly, patients with MSA and autonomic failure (Shy-Drager syndrome) had increased 6[^{18}F]fluoro-dopamine cardiac concentrations and slightly increased norepinephrine spillover, suggesting intact cardiac sympathetic terminals, probably with hypersensitivity due to an abolished preganglionic sympathetic traffic (Fig. 13.9). Another nuclear medicine technique, cardiac scintigraphy using a tracer analogue of norepinephrine the [^{123}I] metaiodobenzylguanidine ([^{123}I] MIBG-SPECT) is usually applied to detect cardiac damage from different pathologic entities, from myocardial infarction to diabetic or amyloidotic polyneuropathy.

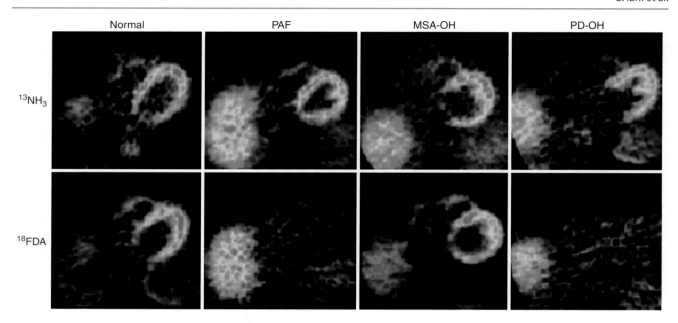

Fig. 13.9 Cardiac PET scans in a control subject and in patients with pure autonomic failure (*PAF*), multiple-system atrophy with orthostatic hypotension (*MSA–OH*), and PD with orthostatic hypotension (*PD–OH*). *Top*: nitrogen-13-labelled ammonia (*13NH3*) perfusion scans. *Bottom*: 18F-dopa 3 (*18FDA*) sympathoneural scans in each patient. Note absence of cardiac 18F-dopa imaging in PAF and PD–OH and normal radioactivity in MSA–OH (Reprinted with permission of Elsevier from Goldstein [136])

Many authors have demonstrated a reduction in cardiac innervation in PD patients with or without clinical evidence of dysautonomia, even in the early stages of the disease (Hoehn-Yahr stage I or II) and in patients with LBD, but not in MSA patients where a more centrally located dysfunction operates [138–142]. The peculiarity of this observation, apart from its high sensitivity to identify patients with PD (89.7 %), is that the decrease in MIBG uptake seems to have no direct relationship with cardiac functional deterioration. Patients with decreased MIBG uptake affected by PD, though showing abnormal autonomic function, had no alteration in left ventricular function on echocardiography and no serious dysrhythmia on 24-h Holter ECG [143]. OH, a common finding in PD and considered due to L-dopa treatment, has been demonstrated to be independent of the pharmacological side effects of the agent, but dependent upon the autonomic derangement linked to neurodegeneration, though it can be precipitated by therapy. Indeed, we generally ignore the contribution of parasympathetic degeneration in PD and OH [144]. Moreover, OH is characteristic of MSA, in which there is no cardiac denervation and where autonomic degeneration is mostly preganglionic with a different neuropathological pattern. In fact, synuclein deposits precipitate in the oligodendroglial—instead of neuronal—cells, as seen in PD or LBD. What is still unknown of degenerative diseases, like PD, are the cortical sites involved in autonomic derangement, while peripheral involvement has been characterized [135]. Sudden falls in blood pressure occurs even in the early phases, despite being more common in late phases of PD.

The incidence varies from 40 to 60 %, depending upon the clinical phase of disease [132, 133].

The arterial baroreflex is the main neurocirculatory reflex implicated in OH. Distortion of stretch sensitive cells in large artery walls, and in the heart itself, causes increased vagal outflow to the heart, resulting in bradycardia and, with decreased sympathetic outflow to the cardiovascular system, vasodilation. Baroreflex cardiovagal gain—calculated from the relation between the interval between heartbeats and systolic blood pressure after intravenous injection of a vasoconstrictor or vasodilator or estimated from the relation between interbeat interval and systolic blood pressure during phase II of the Valsalva maneuver—is used to understand OH. Patients with PD and no orthostatic hypotension demonstrated low baroreflex cardiovagal gain, as compared to normal age-matched controls, but patients with PD and orthostatic hypotension showed a very low baroreflex cardiovagal gain [136]. The site, or sites, of the central neural lesions that produce baroreflex failure in PD are largely unknown.

In another study, Goldstein and colleagues [136] looked at OH in PD patients. Analyzing plasma norepinephrine levels and baroreflex cardiovagal gain assessment in PD patients with and without symptoms of orthostatic hypotension, the investigators found that baroreflex failure, involving both cardiovagal and sympathoneural circuits (a presumably preganglionic lesion), associated with sympathetic denervation (a postganglionic lesion), produces OH in PD, while neither baroreflex failure nor cardiac sympathetic denervation does

[136]. Combined cardiac denervation and baroreflex hypofunction characterizes virtually all patients with PD and orthostatic hypotension, but it is unknown whether subclinical dysautonomia precedes symptomatic PD [132].

Some investigators found interesting results in a preliminary study evaluating heart rate variability (HRV) through polysomnography recordings in patients with idiopathic REM (rapid eye movement) behavior disorders (iRBD), a population known to be at risk to develop PD or LBD, with a reported risk of 45 % at 11.5 years [143, 145]. A significant reduction of HRV in study subjects compared to controls suggests both sympathetic and parasympathetic influences on cardiac function, highlighting a new and easy tool to apply in daily clinical practice by which to diagnose preclinical PD or to better categorize patients with synucleinopathies [143].

Knowledge of cardiac and autonomic derangement is particularly useful in degenerative disease for differential clinical diagnostic determination and, as well, for therapeutic implications. Limited data exist regarding the influence of degenerative disease-induced dysautonomia upon the QT-segment interval despite previous work on rate-corrected QT (QTc) that found QTc to be prolonged in PD and MSA, but not in PSP, patients as compared to healthy controls. This is an important issue in terms of using antipsychotic drugs for behavioral disturbance control in these patients, as these pharmacologic agents may further prolong the QTc, putting the patient at risk for dysrhythmias.

L-Dopa therapy in PD patients contributes to OH with its vasodilatory effect. Moreover, selegiline, amantadine, and dopamine agonists, common therapeutic tools, may potentiate OH in PD and MSA patients, as well [144, 146]. Fludrocortisone and midodrine therapy, to counteract OH, may sometimes exacerbate supine hypertension in PD patients, so they should be avoided at bedtime; calcium antagonists and nitrates may be used to treat the hypertension [133, 136].

Tauopathies

Alzheimer Disease (AD), Progressive Supranuclear Palsy (PSP), Cortico-Basal Degeneration (CBD), and Frontotemporal Dementia (FTD)

Clinical AD is associated with a wide range of dysautonomic phenomena, such as increased pupillary dilation, altered skin conductivity, blunted autonomic response to noxious stimuli, diminished HRV, depressed baroreflex sensitivity, and orthostasis. Among the brain regions implicated in autonomic control, the insula has been widely investigated as potential cause of autonomic dysfunction.

The insula appears to be involved in the degenerative process of AD very early in the disorder's course, to the point

that observational autopsy studies have noted that as many as 40 % of non-demented septuagenarians and octogenarians may have AD pathology sufficiently advanced to affect the insular cortex. A suggestion—not proven by any stretch of the imagination—is that many cardiac and noncardiac "age-related" changes may actually be secondary to AD. Twenty-four-hour ECG recordings of subjects older than 80 years of age have shown frequent unexplained tachydysrhythmias and bradydysrhythmias. Insular neurofibrillary tangles (NFT) have recently been evaluated in a pathology study, in relation to the QTc, yielding a non-statistically significant—but highly suggestive—association between QTc prolongation and right insular involvement [147]. As for differential diagnosis, myocardial scintigraphic studies with MIBG imaging are proving to be potentially very reliable in distinguishing AD from LBD, since marked reduction of MIBG uptake has been observed in most patients with LBD but not in AD [148].

Muscular Dystrophies

Muscular dystrophies (MD) are a group of hereditary muscle diseases in which a defect in muscle proteins leads to muscle cell death, with consequent progressive muscle weakness and wasting. The most common, and also the most severe, form of MD is Duchenne's type (DMD), an X-linked, very early-age onset, early dependency, and short life expectancy MD. Mortality in DMD patients is primarily related to cardiac and/or respiratory muscle failure. It is estimated that approximately 75 % of patients with DMD die of respiratory failure and 20 % die from heart failure. Cardiac involvement in DMD is characterized by cardiac muscle degeneration with fibrous tissue replacement and fatty infiltration, typically occurring late in the course of the disease [149]. Many studies have attempted to detect early myocardial damage, or to correlate left ventricular dysfunction with skeletal muscle or lung function tests, but have failed to find any useful relationship [52]. More recent studies have used MRI to evaluate heart involvement and have noted that T2 relaxation times of cardiac muscle in DMD patients free of cardiac complaints were decreased in comparison to healthy volunteers [150]. Another more recent MRI study has investigated myocardial inflammation in DMD as a precipitating factor for heart failure, documenting myocardial fibrosis in 6 of 20 patients, and evidence of active myocarditis on histological analysis in four of the six patients with fibrosis. Considering that abnormal dystrophin has also been identified as a potential susceptibility gene product for viral infection of the myocardium and that dystrophin deficiency seems to potentiate the unfavorable course of enterovirus-induced cardiomyopathy, inflammatory aspects of myocardial dysfunction in DMD could be an important object of future interest [150].

Miscellanea

A group of neurally mediated cardiocirculatory syndromes includes conditions such as neurocardiogenic syncope, neurogenic orthostatic hypotension syndromes, and channelopathies. Neurocardiogenic syncope is a rather frequent condition characterized by acute failure of the autonomic nervous system to maintain blood pressure in a predisposed subject. Carotid sinus syndrome and situational syncope, such as might occur after vagal stimulation with urination, defecation, and/or coughing, are other well-known conditions of this category. Vagal syncope usually occurs in adolescents and even late in life in some individuals and may be elicited by visual, olfactory, and/or situational stimuli—such as closed, crowded, hot, or smoky environments. For idiopathic vagal reactions, there is no specific treatment. Patient must be informed to avoid vagal stimuli; to recognize prodromal symptoms such as decreased heart rate, sweating, yawning, and/or nausea with epigastric heaviness; and how to manage syncopal episodes (lying down with legs uplifted). Drinking water and salting food can be useful to prevent vagal syncope.

Neurogenic orthostatic hypotension is actually more than one condition that operates through a common mechanism of reduced baroreflex responsiveness, decreased cardiac compliance, and attenuation of the vestibulosympathetic reflex. It is characterized by a reduction of at least 20 mmHg of systolic blood pressure or 10 mmHg of diastolic blood pressure during the first 3 min of standing after being in a supine position for a prolonged period. Primary causes of neurogenic orthostatic hypotension can be degenerative, such as hereditary amyloidosis, hereditary sensory and autonomic neuropathy (HSAN type III), and immune-mediated autonomic neuropathy [151, 152].

Channelopathies (ion channel disease) represent the most common cause of sudden arrhythmic death syndrome (SADS). This heterogeneous group includes Brugada syndrome, early repolarization syndrome, long QT syndrome, catecholaminergic polymorphic ventricular tachycardia, short QT syndrome, progressive cardiac conduction defect, and inherited atrial fibrillation. Common features of ion channel diseases are a structurally normal heart, a genetic basis, and predisposition to fatal dysrhythmias. A variety of genetic mutations have been identified, and the chance of a positive genetic test varies from 20 to 70 %. A history of sudden death can be obtained in up to 30 % of patients' families. A detailed description of specific channelopathies is beyond the scope of this chapter; however, it should be recognized that these predominantly cardiac syndromes may have neurologic-associated clinical manifestations, including epilepsy and familiar hemiplegic migraine.

References

1. Taggart P, Critchley H, Lambiase PD. Heart-brain interactions in cardiac arrhythmia. Heart. 2011;97(9):698–708.
2. Schwartz B. The world of thought in ancient China. Cambridge: Harvard University Press; 1985.
3. Samuels MA. 'Voodoo' death revisited: the modern lessons of neurocardiology. Cleve Clin J Med. 2007;74 Suppl 1:S8–16.
4. Leor J, Poole WK, Kloner RA. Sudden cardiac death triggered by an earthquake. N Engl J Med. 1996;334(7):413–9.
5. Hua F, et al. c-Fos expression in rat brain stem and spinal cord in response to activation of cardiac ischemia-sensitive afferent neurons and electrostimulatory modulation. Am J Physiol Heart Circ Physiol. 2004;287:H2728–38.
6. Gray MA, Taggart P, Sutton PM, Groves D, Holdright DR, Bradbury D, Brull D, Critchley HD. A cortical potential reflecting cardiac function. Proc Natl Acad Sci U S A. 2007;104(16):6818–23.
7. Hagemann D, Waldstein SR, Thayer JF. Central and autonomic nervous system integration in emotion. Brain Cogn. 2003; 52(1):79–87.
8. Natelson BH. Neurocardiology. An interdisciplinary area for the 80s. Arch Neurol. 1985;42(2):178–84. Review.
9. Davis AM, Natelson BH. Brain-heart interactions. The neurocardiology of arrhythmia and sudden cardiac death. Tex Heart Inst J. 1993;20(3):158–69. Review.
10. Benarroch E. Chapter 4. In: Robertson D, et al., editors. Primer on autonomic nervous system. 2nd ed. Philadelphia: Elsevier; 2004.
11. Toivonen L, Helenius K, Viitasalo M. Electrocardiographic repolarization during stress from awakening on alarm call. J Am Coll Cardiol. 1997;30:774–9.
12. Oppenheimer S. Cerebrogenic cardiac arrhythmias: cortical lateralization and clinical significance. Clin Auton Res. 2006;16:6–11.
13. Critchley HD, Wiens S, Rotshtein P, Ohman A, Dolan RJ. Neural systems supporting interoceptive awareness. Nat Neurosci. 2004;7(2):189–95.
14. Critchley HD, Taggart P, Sutton PM, Holdright DR, Batchvarov V, Hnatkova K, Malik M, Dolan RJ. Mental stress and sudden cardiac death: asymmetric midbrain activity as a linking mechanism. Brain. 2005;128(Pt 1):75–85.
15. Lampert R, Jain D, Burg MM, Batsford WP, McPherson CA. Destabilizing effects of mental stress on ventricular arrhythmias in patients with implantable cardioverter-defibrillators. Circulation. 2000;101(2):158–64.
16. Green AL, Paterson DJ. Identification of neurocircuitry controlling cardiovascular function in humans using functional neurosurgery: implications for exercise control. Exp Physiol. 2008;93(9):1022–8.
17. Green AL, Wang S, Owen SL, Paterson DJ, Xie K, Liu X, Bain PG, Stein JF, Aziz TZ. Functional Neurosurgery Resident Award: controlling the cardiovascular system with deep brain stimulation. Clin Neurosurg. 2006;53:316–23.
18. Dote K, Sato KT, et al. Myocardial stunning due to simultaneous multi vessel coronary spasms: a review of 5 cases. J Cardiol. 1991; 21:203–14.
19. Wittstein I, Thiemann DR, et al. Neurohumoral features of myocardial stunning due to sudden emotional stress. N Engl J Med. 2005;352:539–48.
20. Sharkey S, Lesser J, et al. Acute and reversible cardiomyopathy provoked by stress in women from the United States. Circulation. 2005;111:472–9.
21. Hessel E. The brain and the heart. Anesth Analg. 2006; 103(3):522–6.
22. Desmet W, Dynamic LV. Obstruction in apical ballooning syndrome: the chicken or the egg? Eur J Echocardiogr. 2006;7:1–3.

23. Merli E, Sutcliffe S, et al. TakoTako-Tsubo cardiomyopathy: new insights into the possible underlying pathophysiology. Eur J Echocardiogr. 2006;7:53.

24. Oppenheimer SM, Wilson JX, et al. Insular cortex stimulation produces lethal cardiac arrhythmias: a mechanism of sudden death? Brain Res. 1991;550:115–21.

25. Critchley HD, Corfield DR, et al. Cerebral correlates of autonomic cardiovascular arousal: a functional neuroimaging investigation in humans. J Physiol. 2000;523:259–70.

26. Kolominsky-Rabas PL, Weber M, et al. Epidemiology of ischemic stroke subtypes according to TOAST criteria: incidence, recurrence, and long-term survival in ischemic stroke subtypes: a population-based study. Stroke. 2001;32:2735–40.

27. Rincon F, Dhamoon M, et al. Stroke location and association with fatal cardiac outcomes. Northern Manhattan Study (NOMAS). Stroke. 2008;39:2425–51.

28. Grau AJ, Weimar C, et al. Risk factors, outcome, and treatment in subtypes of ischemic stroke: the German stroke data bank. Stroke. 2001;32(11):2559–66.

29. Norris JW, Froggatt GM, Hachinski VC. Cardiac arrhythmias in acute stroke. Stroke. 1978;9(4):392–6.

30. Cheung RTF, Hachinski W. The insula and cerebrogenic sudden death. Arch Neurol. 2000;57:1685–8.

31. Touzé E, Varenne O, et al. Risk of myocardial infarction and vascular death after transient ischemic attack and ischemic stroke: a systematic review and meta-analysis. Stroke. 2005;36(12):2748–55. Review.

32. van Bree MD, Roos YB, et al. Prevalence and characterization of ECG abnormalities after intracerebral hemorrhage. Neurocrit Care. 2010;12(1):50–5.

33. Hravanak M, Frangiskakis M, et al. Elevated cardiac troponin I and relationship to persistence of electrocardiographic and echocardiographic abnormalities after aneurysmal subarachnoid hemorrhage. Stroke. 2009;40:3478–84.

34. Naidech AN, Kreiter KT, et al. Cardiac troponin elevation, cardiovascular morbidity and outcome after subarachnoid hemorrhage. Circulation. 2005;112:2851–6.

35. Banki N, Kopelnik A, et al. Acute neurocardiogenic injury after subarachnoid hemorrhage. Circulation. 2005;112:3314–9.

36. Zaroff JG, Pawlikoska L, et al. Adrenoceptor polymorphisms and the risk of cardiac injury and dysfunction after subarachnoid hemorrhage. Stroke. 2006;37:1680–5.

37. Tung PP, Olmsted E, et al. Plasma B-type natriuretic peptide levels are associated with early cardiac dysfunction after subarachnoid hemorrhage. Stroke. 2005;36:1567–71.

38. Lee V, Oh JK, et al. Mechanisms in neurogenic stress cardiomyopathy after aneurismal subarachnoid hemorrhage. Neurocrit Care. 2006;05:243–9.

39. Naredi S, Lambert G, et al. Increased sympathetic nervous activity in patients with non-traumatic subarachnoid hemorrhage. Stroke. 2000;31:901–6.

40. Manno EM, Pfeifer EA, et al. Cardiac pathology in patients with status epilepticus. Neurocrit Care. 2005;2:231.

41. Cebelin MS, Hirsch CS. Human stress cardiomyopathy. Myocardial lesions in victims of homicidal assaults without internal injuries. Hum Pathol. 1980;11:123–32.

42. Dimant J, Grob D. Electrocardiographic changes and myocardial damage in patients with acute cerebrovascular accidents. Stroke. 1977;8(4):448–55.

43. Oppenheimer SM, Gelb A, Girvin JP, Hachinski VC. Cardiovascular effects of human insular cortex stimulation. Neurology. 1992;42(9):1727–32.

44. Cechetto DF, Wilson JX, Smith KE, Wolski D, Silver MD, Hachinski VC. Autonomic and myocardial changes in middle cerebral artery occlusion: stroke models in the rat. Brain Res. 1989;502(2):296–305.

45. Hachinski VC, Smith KE, Silver MD, Gibson CJ, Ciriello J. Acute myocardial and plasma catecholamine changes in experimental stroke. Stroke. 1986;17(3):387–90.

46. Nolte J. The human brain. 4th ed. St. Louis: Mosby; 1999.

47. Cereda C, Ghika J, Maeder P, Bogousslavsky J. Strokes restricted to the insular cortex. Neurology. 2002;59(12):1950–5.

48. Augustine JR. Circuitry and functional aspects of the insular lobe in primates including humans. Brain Res Brain Res Rev. 1996;22(3):229–44. Review.

49. Critchley HD. The human cortex responds to an interoceptive challenge. Proc Natl Acad Sci U S A. 2004;101(17):6333–4.

50. Türe U, Yasargil MG, Al-Mefty O, Yasargil DCH. Arteries of insula. J Neurosurg. 2000;92:676–87.

51. Sander D, Winbeck K, Klingelhöfer J, Etgen T, Conrad B. Prognostic relevance of pathological sympathetic activation after acute thromboembolic stroke. Neurology. 2001;57(5):833–8.

52. Ay H, Koroshetz WJ, et al. Neuroanatomic correlates of stroke-related myocardial injury. Neurology. 2006;66:1325–9.

53. Colivicchi F, Bassi A, Santini M, Caltagirone C. Prognostic implications of right-sided insular damage, cardiac autonomic derangement, and arrhythmias after acute ischemic stroke. Stroke. 2005;36(8):1710–5.

54. Tokgosoglu SL, Batur MK, et al. Effects of stroke localization on cardiac autonomic balance and sudden death. Stroke. 1999;30:1307–11.

55. Christensen H, Boysen G, Christensen AF, Johannesen HH. Insular lesions, ECG abnormalities, and outcome in acute stroke. J Neurol Neurosurg Psychiatry. 2005;76(2):269–71.

56. Laowattana S, Zeger SL, Lima JA, Goodman SN, Wittstein IS, Oppenheimer SM. Left insular stroke is associated with adverse cardiac outcome. Neurology. 2006;66(4):477–83.

57. Fink JN, Frampton CM, Lyden P, Lees KR, Virtual international stroke trials archive investigators. Does hemispheric lateralization influence functional and cardiovascular outcomes after stroke?: an analysis of placebo-treated patients from prospective acute stroke trials. Stroke. 2008;39(12):3335–40.

58. Urbinati S, Di Pasquale G, Andreoli A, Lusa AM, Ruffini M, Lanzino G, Pinelli G. Frequency and prognostic significance of silent coronary artery disease in patients with cerebral ischemia undergoing carotid endarterectomy. Am J Cardiol. 1992;69(14):1166–70.

59. Gongora-Rivera F, Labreuche J, Jaramillo A, Steg PG, Hauw JJ, Amarenco P. Autopsy prevalence of coronary atherosclerosis in patients with fatal stroke. Stroke. 2007;38(4):1203–10.

60. Lavy S, Yaar I, Melamed E, Stern S. The effect of acute stroke on cardiac functions as observed in an intensive stroke care unit. Stroke. 1974;5(6):775–80.

61. Goldstein D. The electrocardiogram in stroke: relationship to pathophysiological type and comparison with prior tracings. Stroke. 1979;10:253–9.

62. Rem JA, Hachinski VC, Boughner DR, Barnett HJ. Value of cardiac monitoring and echocardiography in TIA and stroke patients. Stroke. 1985;16(6):950–6.

63. Orlandi G, Fanucchi S, Strata G, Pataleo L, Landucci Pellegrini L, Prontera C, Martini A, Murri L. Transient autonomic nervous system dysfunction during hyperacute stroke. Acta Neurol Scand. 2000;102(5):317–21.

64. Lin HJ, Wolf PA, Benjamin EJ, Belanger AJ, D'Agostino RB. Newly diagnosed atrial fibrillation and acute stroke. The Framingham Study. Stroke. 1995;26(9):1527–30.

65. Hart RG. Atrial fibrillation and stroke prevention. N Engl J Med. 2003;349(11):1015–6.

66. Hart RG, Pearce LA, Rothbart RM, McAnulty JH, Asinger RW, Halperin JL. Stroke with intermittent atrial fibrillation: incidence and predictors during aspirin therapy. Stroke Prevention in Atrial Fibrillation Investigators. J Am Coll Cardiol. 2000;35(1):183–7.

67. Tayal AH, Tian M, Kelly KM, Jones SC, Wright DG, Singh D, Jarouse J, Brillman J, Murali S, Gupta R. Atrial fibrillation detected by mobile cardiac outpatient telemetry in cryptogenic TIA or stroke. Neurology. 2008;71(21):1696–701.

68. Paciaroni M, Agnelli G, Caso V, Venti M, Milia P, Silvestrelli G, Parnetti L, Biagini S. Atrial fibrillation in patients with first-ever stroke: frequency, antithrombotic treatment before the event and effect on clinical outcome. J Thromb Haemost. 2005; 3(6):1218–23.

69. Liao J, Khalid Z, Scallan C, Morillo C, O'Donnell M. Noninvasive cardiac monitoring for detecting paroxysmal atrial fibrillation or flutter after acute ischemic stroke: a systematic review. Stroke. 2007;38(11):2935–40.

70. Dütsch M, Burger M, Dörfler C, Schwab S, Hilz MJ. Cardiovascular autonomic function in poststroke patients. Neurology. 2007; 69(24):2249–55.

71. Di Angelantonio E, Fiorelli M, Toni D, Sacchetti ML, Lorenzano S, Falcou A, Ciarla MV, Suppa M, Bonanni L, Bertazzoni G, Aguglia F, Argentino C. Prognostic significance of admission levels of troponin I in patients with acute ischemic stroke. J Neurol Neurosurg Psychiatry. 2005;76(1):76–81.

72. Lee SJ, Lee KS, Kim YI, An JY, Kim W, Kim JS. Clinical features of patients with a myocardial infarction during acute management of an ischemic stroke. Neurocrit Care. 2008;9(3):332–7.

73. Yoshimura S, Toyoda K, Ohara T, Nagasawa H, Ohtani N, Kuwashiro T, Naritomi H, Minematsu K. Takotsubo cardiomyopathy in acute ischemic stroke. Ann Neurol. 2008;64(5):547–54.

74. Prosser J, MacGregor L, Lees KR, Diener HC, Hacke W, Davis S, VISTA Investigators. Predictors of early cardiac morbidity and mortality after ischemic stroke. Stroke. 2007;38(8):2295–302.

75. Silver FL, Norris JW, Lewis AJ, Hachinski VC. Early mortality following stroke: a prospective review. Stroke. 1984; 15(3):492–6.

76. Algra A, Gates PC, Fox AJ, Hachinski V, Barnett HJ, North American Symptomatic Carotid Endarterectomy Trial Group. Side of brain infarction and long-term risk of sudden death in patients with symptomatic carotid disease. Stroke. 2003;34(12):2871–5.

77. Beneficial effect of carotid endarterectomy in symptomatic patients with high-grade carotid stenosis. North American Symptomatic Carotid Endarterectomy Trial Collaborators. N Engl J Med. 1991;325(7):445–53.

78. Kaplan RC, Tirschwell DL, Longstreth Jr WT, Manolio TA, Heckbert SR, Lefkowitz D, El-Saed A, Psaty BM. Vascular events, mortality, and preventive therapy following ischemic stroke in the elderly. Neurology. 2005;65(6):835–42.

79. Adams Jr HP, del Zoppo G, Alberts MJ, Bhatt DL, Brass L, Furlan A, Grubb RL, Higashida RT, Jauch EC, Kidwell C, Lyden PD, Morgenstern LB, Qureshi AI, Rosenwasser RH, Scott PA, Wijdicks EF, American Heart Association, American Stroke Association Stroke Council, Clinical Cardiology Council, Cardiovascular Radiology and Intervention Council, Atherosclerotic Peripheral Vascular Disease and Quality of Care Outcomes in Research Interdisciplinary Working Groups. Guidelines for the early management of adults with ischemic stroke: a guideline from the American Heart Association/American Stroke Association Stroke Council, Clinical Cardiology Council, Cardiovascular Radiology and Intervention Council, and the Atherosclerotic Peripheral Vascular Disease and Quality of Care Outcomes in Research Interdisciplinary Working Groups: the American Academy of Neurology affirms the value of this guideline as an educational tool for neurologists. Stroke. 2007;38(5):1655–711; Stroke. 2007; 38(9):e96.

80. Fang CX, Wu S, Ren J. Intracerebral hemorrhage elicits aberration in cardiomyocyte contractile function and intracellular Ca2+ transients. Stroke. 2006;37(7):1875–82.

81. Maramattom BV, Manno EM, Fulgham JR, Jaffe AS, Wijdicks EF. Clinical importance of cardiac troponin release and cardiac abnormalities in patients with supratentorial cerebral hemorrhages. Mayo Clin Proc. 2006;81(2):192–6.

82. Hays A, Diringer MN. Elevated troponin levels are associated with higher mortality following intracerebral hemorrhage. Neurology. 2006;66(9):1330–4.

83. Banuelos PA, Temes R, Lee VH. Neurogenic stunned myocardium associated with reversible posterior leukoencephalopathy syndrome. Neurocrit Care. 2008;9(1):108–11.

84. Papanikolaou J, Tsirantonaki M, Koukoulitsios G, Papageorgiou D, Mandila C, Karakitsos D, Karabinis A. Reversible posterior leukoencephalopathy syndrome and tako-tsubo cardiomyopathy: the role of echocardiographic monitoring in the ICU. Hellenic J Cardiol. 2009;50(5):436–8.

85. Layon J, Friedman WA, Gabrielli A, editors. Textbook of neurointensive care. Philadelphia: WB Saunders; 2003. Chapter 8.

86. Blackman JA, Patrick PD, Buck ML, Rust Jr RS. Paroxysmal autonomic instability with dystonia after brain injury. Arch Neurol. 2004;61(3):321–8. Review.

87. Baguley IJ, Heriseanu RE, Cameron ID, Nott MT, Slewa-Younan S. A critical review of the pathophysiology of dysautonomia following traumatic brain injury. Neurocrit Care. 2008;8(2):293–300. Review.

88. Singleton RH, Adelson PD. Chapter 3: Diffuse axonal injury and dysautonomia. In: Bhardwa JA, Ellegala DB, Kirsch JR, editors. Acute brain and spinal cord injury: evolving paradigms and management. New York: Informa Healthcare; 2008.

89. Boeve BF, Wijdicks EF, Benarroch EE, Schmidt KD. Paroxysmal sympathetic storms ("diencephalic seizures") after severe diffuse axonal head injury. Mayo Clin Proc. 1998;73(2):148–52.

90. Kishner S, et al. Post head injury autonomic complications. 2008. http://emedicine.medscape.com/article/325994-overview#showall

91. Baguley IJ, Heriseanu RE, Felmingham KL, Cameron ID. Dysautonomia and heart rate variability following severe traumatic brain injury. Brain Inj. 2006;20(4):437–44 (Abstract).

92. Bourdages M, et al. Cardiac arrhythmias associated with severe traumatic brain injury and hypothermia therapy. Pediatr Crit Care Med. 2010;11(3):439–41.

93. Bourdages M, Bigras JL, Farrell CA, Hutchison JS, Lacroix J, Canadian Critical Care Trials Group. Cardiac arrhythmias associated with severe traumatic brain injury and hypothermia therapy. Pediatr Crit Care Med. 2010;11(3):408–14.

94. Furlan JC, Fehlings MG. Cardiovascular complications after acute spinal cord injury: pathophysiology, diagnosis, and management. Neurosurg Focus. 2008;25(5):E13. Review.

95. Rowland JW, Hawryluk GW, Kwon B, Fehlings MG. Current status of acute spinal cord injury pathophysiology and emerging therapies: promise on the horizon. Neurosurg Focus. 2008; 25(5):E2. Review.

96. Garshick E, Kelley A, Cohen SA, Garrison A, Tun CG, Gagnon D, Brown R. A prospective assessment of mortality in chronic spinal cord injury. Spinal Cord. 2005;43(7):408–16.

97. Stein DM, Menaker J, McQuillan K, Handley C, Aarabi B, Scalea TM. Risk factors for organ dysfunction and failure in patients with acute traumatic cervical spinal cord injury. Neurocrit Care. 2010;13(1):29–39.

98. Bunten DC, Warner AL, Brunnemann SR, Segal JL. Heart rate variability is altered following spinal cord injury. Clin Auton Res. 1998;8(6):329–34.

99. Furlan JC, Fehlings MG. The impact of age on mortality, impairment, and disability among adults with acute traumatic spinal cord injury. J Neurotrauma. 2009;26(10):1707–17.

100. Grigorean VT, Sandu AM, Popescu M, Iacobini MA, Stoian R, Neascu C, Strambu V, Popa F. Cardiac dysfunctions following spinal cord injury. J Med Life. 2009;2(2):133–45. Review.

101. Mathias CJ. Chapter 81: Autonomic disturbances in spinal cord injuries. In: Robertson D, editor. Primer on the autonomic nervous system. 2nd ed. Philadelphia: Elsevier; 2004.

102. Asahina M, Kuwabara S, et al. Autonomic function in demyelinating and axonal subtypes of Guillain Barrè syndrome. Acta Neurol Scand. 2002;105(1):44–50.

103. Dionne A, Nicolle MW, Hahn AF. Clinical and electrophysiological parameters distinguishing acute-onset chronic inflammatory demyelinating polyneuropathy from acute inflammatory demyelinating polyneuropathy. Muscle Nerve. 2010;41:202–7.

104. Mukerji S, Aloka F, et al. Cardiovascular complications of the Guillain-Barrè syndrome. Am J Cardiol. 2009;104:1452–5.

105. Pfeiffer G, Schiller H, et al. Indicators of dysautonomia in sever Guillain Barrè syndrome. J Neurol. 1999;246:1015–22.

106. Greenland P, Griggs RC. Arrhythmic complications in the Guillain Barrè syndrome. Arch Intern Med. 1980;40:1053–5.

107. Hodson AK, Hurwitz BJ, et al. Dysautonomia in Guillain-Barrè syndrome with dorsal root ganglioneuropathy, wallerian degeneration and fatal myocarditis. Ann Neurol. 1984;15(1):88–95.

108. Finkelstein JS, Melek BH. Guillain-Barrè syndrome as a cause of reversible cardiomyopathy. Tex Heart Inst J. 2006;33:57–9.

109. Iga K, Himura Y, et al. Reversible left ventricular dysfunction associated with Guillain Barrè syndrome-an expression of catecholamine cardiotoxicity? Jpn Circ J. 1995;59:236–40.

110. Gibson TC. The heart in myasthenia gravis. Am Heart J. 1975; 90(3):389–96.

111. Hofstad H, Ohm OJ, Mork SJ, Aarli JA. Heart disease in myasthenia gravis. Acta Neurol Scand. 1984;70(3):176–84.

112. Suzuki S, Utsugisawa K, et al. Autoimmune targets of heart and skeletal muscles in myasthenia gravis. Arch Neurol. 2009; 66(11):1334–8.

113. Beydoun SR, Wang JT, et al. Emotional stress as a trigger of myasthenic crisis and concomitant takotsubo cardiomyopathy: a case report. J Med Case Reports. 2010;4:393.

114. Bradley WG. Polymyositis: an overdiagnosed entity. Neurology. 2004;63(2):402.

115. Gottdiener JS, Sherber HS, et al. Cardiac manifestations in polymyositis. Am J Cardiol. 1978;41(7):1141–9.

116. Lundberg IE. The heart in dermatomyositis and polymyositis. Rheumatology. 2006;45:iv18–21.

117. Stern R, Godbold JH, et al. ECG abnormalities in polymyositis. Arch Intern Med. 1984;144:2185–9.

118. Haupt HM, Hutschins GM, et al. The heart and cardiac conduction system in polymyositis-dermatomyositis: a clinicopathologic study of 16 autopsied patients. Am J Cardiol. 1982;50:998–1006.

119. Rocamora R, Kurthen M, et al. Cardiac asystole in epilepsy: clinical and neurophysiologic features. Epilepsia. 2003;44(2):179–85.

120. Boggs JG. Mortality associated with status epilepticus. Epilepsy Curr. 2004;4(1):25–7.

121. Nevander G, Ingvar M, et al. Status epilepticus in well-oxygenated rats causes neuronal necrosis. Ann Neurol. 1985;18:281–90.

122. De Lorenzo RJ, Towne AR, et al. Status epilepticus in children, adults and the elderly. Epilepsia. 1992;33 suppl 4:S15–25.

123. Towne AR, Pellock JM, et al. Determinants of mortality in status epilepticus. Epilepsia. 1994;35:27–34.

124. Boggs JG, Maramarou A, et al. Hemodynamic monitoring prior to and at the time of death in status epilepticus. Epilepsy Res. 1998;31(3):199–209.

125. Metcalf C, Poelzing S, et al. Status epilepticus induces cardiac myofilament damage and increased susceptibility to arrhythmias in rats. Am J Physiol Heart Circ Physiol. 2009;297:H2120–7.

126. Lemke DM, Hussain SI, et al. Tako-tsubo cardiomyopathy associated with seizures. Neurocrit Care. 2008;9:112–7.

127. Legriel S, Bruneel F, et al. Recurrent takotsubo cardiomyopathy triggered by convulsive status epilepticus. Neurocrit Care. 2008; 9:118–21.

128. Shimutzu M, Kagawa A, et al. Neurogenic stunned myocardium associated with status epilepticus and postictal catecholamine surge. Intern Med. 2007;47:269–73.

129. Nashef L. Sudden unexpected death in epilepsy: terminology and definitions. Epilepsia. 1997;38(suppl11):S6–8.

130. Tomson T, Walczak T, et al. Sudden unexpected death in epilepsy: a review of incidence and risk factors. Epilepsia. 2005;46 suppl 11:54–61.

131. Jehi L, Najm IM. Sudden unexpected death in epilepsy: impact, mechanisms and prevention. Cleve Clin J Med. 2008;75 suppl 2:s66–70.

132. Goldstein DS. Cardiac denervation in patients with Parkinson disease. Cleve Clin J Med. 2007;74 Suppl 1:S91–4.

133. Walter BL. Cardiovascular autonomic dysfunction in patients with movement disorders. Cleve Clin J Med. 2008;75 Suppl 2:S54–8.

134. Goldstein DS. Neuroscience and heart-brain medicine: the year in review. Cleve Clin J Med. 2010;77 Suppl 3:S34–9.

135. Orimo S, Uchihara T, Nakamura A, Mori F, Kakita A, Wakabayashi K, Takohashi H. Axonal alpha-synuclein aggregates herald centripetal degeneration of cardiac sympathetic nerve in Parkinson's disease. Brain. 2008;131(Pt3):642–50.

136. Goldstein D. Dysautonomia in Parkinson's disease: neurocardiological abnormalities. Lancet Neurol. 2003;2:669–76.

137. Post S, Papetropulos KK. Chapter 5C. In: Halliday G, Barker R, Rowe D, editors. Non dopamine lesions in Parkinson Diseases. Cambridge: Oxford Press; 2010.

138. Orimo S, Ozawa E, Nakade S, Sugimoto T, Mizusawa H. (123) I-metaiodobenzylguanidine myocardial scintigraphy in Parkinson's disease. J Neurol Neurosurg Psychiatry. 1999;67(2):189–94.

139. Yoshita M, Taki J, Yamada M. A clinical role for [(123)I]MIBG myocardial scintigraphy in the distinction between dementia of the Alzheimer's-type and dementia with Lewy bodies. J Neurol Neurosurg Psychiatry. 2001;71(5):583–8.

140. Nagayama H, Hamamoto M, Ueda M, Nagashima J, Katayama Y. Reliability of MIBG myocardial scintigraphy in the diagnosis of Parkinson's disease. J Neurol Neurosurg Psychiatry. 2005; 76(2):249–51.

141. Marquié Sayagués M, Da Silva Alves L, Molina-Porcel L, Alcolea Rodríguez D, Sala Matavera I, Sánchez-Saudinós MB, Camacho Martí V, Estorch Cabrera M, Blesa González R, Blesa González R, Gómez-Isla T, Gómez-Isla T, Lleó Bisa A, Lleó Bisa A. (123) I-MIBG myocardial scintigraphy in the diagnosis of Lewy body dementia. Neurologia. 2010;25(7):414.

142. Camacho V, Marquié M, Lleó A, Alvés L, Artigas C, Flotats A, Duch J, Blesa R, Gómez-Isla T, Carrió I, Estorch M. Cardiac sympathetic impairment parallels nigrostriatal degeneration in probable dementia with Lewy bodies. Q J Nucl Med Mol Imaging. 2011;55(4):476–83.

143. Valappil RA, Black JE, Broderick MJ, Carrillo O, Frenette E, Sullivan SS, Goldman SM, Tanner CM, Langston JW. Exploring the electrocardiogram as a potential tool to screen for premotor Parkinson's disease. Mov Disord. 2010;25(14):2296–303.

144. Goldstein DS, Eldadah BA, Holmes C, Pechnik S, Moak J, Saleem A, Sharabi Y. Neurocirculatory abnormalities in Parkinson disease with orthostatic hypotension: independence from levodopa treatment. Hypertension. 2005;46(6):1333–9.

145. Iranzo A, Molinuevo JL, Santamaría J, Serradell M, Martí MJ, Valldeoriola F, Tolosa E. Rapid-eye-movement sleep behavior disorder as an early marker for a neurodegenerative disorder: a descriptive study. Lancet Neurol. 2006;5(7):572–7.

146. Wenning GK, Colosimo C, Geser F, Poewe W. Multiple system atrophy. Lancet Neurol. 2004;3(2):93–103. Erratum in: Lancet Neurol. 2004;3(3):137.

147. Royall DR. Insular Alzheimer disease pathology and the psycho-metric correlates of mortality. Cleve Clin J Med. 2008;75 suppl 2:S97–9.

148. Nakajima K, Yoshita M, et al. Ionidne-123-MIBG sympathetic imaging in Lewy-body diseases and related movement disorders. Q J Nucl Med Mol Imaging. 2008;52:378–87.

149. Sasaki K, Sakata K, et al. Sequential changes in cardiac structure and function in patients with Duchenne-type muscular dystrophy: a two-dimensional echocardiographic study. Am Heart J. 1998; 135:937–44.

150. Mavrogeni S, Tzelepis G, et al. Cardiac and sternocleidomastoid muscle involvement in Duchenne muscular dystrophy an MRI study. Chest. 2005;127:143–8.

151. Grubb BP. Clinical practice. Neurocardiogenic syncope. N Engl J Med. 2005;352(10):1004–10.

152. Freeman R. Clinical practice. Neurogenic orthostatic hypotension. N Engl J Med. 2008;358(6):615–24.

153. Critchley HD, Mathias CJ, Oliver J, et al. Human cingulated cortex and autonomic control: converging neuroimaging and clinical evidence. Brain. 2003;126:213–2152.

154. Lim ECH, Lim S-H, Wilder-smith E. Brain seizes, heart ceases: a case of ictal asystole. J Neurol Neurosurg Psychiatry. 2000; 69:557–9.

Sedation and Analgesia in Neurointensive Care

14

Federico A. Villa and Giuseppe Citerio

Contents

F.A. Villa, MD • G. Citerio, MD (✉)
Neuro-Anesthesia and Neuro-Intensive Care Unit,
Department of Anesthesia and Critical Care,
Ospedale San Gerardo, Via Pergolesi 33,
Monza 20052, Italy
e-mail: villa.federico@fastwebnet.it; gciterio@gmail.com

Abstract

In the neurointensive care setting, specific considerations of sedation are required; sedation may act as a therapeutic agent itself, when causing a reduction in cerebral metabolic rate of oxygen, cerebral blood flow, and intracranial pressure and in the incidence of seizures. However, the physician must be aware of the effects of every sedative agent on cerebral physiology, in order to obtain beneficial effects and avoid side effects. In this chapter, the effects of sedative agents on cerebral physiology are described in order to provide knowledge for an adequate sedative strategy.

Keywords

Sedation • Cerebral metabolic rate of oxygen • Cerebral blood flow • Intracranial pressure • Seizures • Propofol • Benzodiazepines • Delirium

Introduction

Sedation and analgesia (S&A) are fundamental in the management of the critically ill patient. Recent emphasis on weaning from the ventilator and reducing ventilator-associated pneumonia has produced improved S&A guidelines that assure comfort, has reduced time on the ventilator, has resulted in a decreased intensive care unit (ICU) length of stay (LOS), and has prevented neurologic deterioration [1, 2].

The neurointensive care unit (NICU), when compared to the general ICU, requires special considerations. S&A used in the general ICU limits the stress response to critical illness, provides anxiolysis, improves patient–ventilator synchrony, and facilitates care. However, when used in the NICU, S&A is fundamental as a therapeutic strategy. For example, extracted data from the published reports of two large, randomized, pharmacologic, clinical trials on traumatic brain injury show the use of S&A in more than 90 % of the patients [3]. Nevertheless, clinical practice varies

A.J. Layon et al. (eds.), *Textbook of Neurointensive Care*,
DOI 10.1007/978-1-4471-5226-2_14, © Springer-Verlag London 2013

widely as a result of institutional and national biases and because individual patient's response to S&A differs from patient to patient and from time to time [4, 5].

Table 14.1 shows the ideal properties of a sedative drug for the NICU. Pharmacokinetic and cost characteristics of common sedative and analgesics used in the NICU are reviewed in Table 14.2. Neurophysiology characteristics of common sedative and analgesics used in the NICU are reviewed in Table 14.3 [6].

The literature available on the use of S&A in the ICU includes a recent summary published by the American Society of Critical Care Medicine [7], and analyzed in detail [8–11], it does not specifically address the use of sedatives in the NICU. Specific logistics include intracranial pressure control, reduction of cerebral oxygen consumption, and seizure reduction, which are the focus of this chapter.

Specific Rationale for the Use of Sedation and Analgesia in the Neurointensive ICU

Reduction of Cerebral Metabolic Rate of Oxygen Consumption

To maintain adequate oxygen availability and energy balance at the neuronal level, treatment is directed at both increasing oxygen delivery by optimizing cerebral and systemic hemodynamics and reducing cerebral metabolic demand [12–19]. Selected sedatives used in NICU offer a protective effect by reducing oxygen demand and increasing oxygen delivery [20–22].

The γ-aminobutyric acid (GABA) type A receptor system, the main fast-acting inhibitory neurotransmitter system in the brain, is the pharmacological target for many drugs used clinically to treat, for example, anxiety disorders and epilepsy, and to induce and maintain sedation titrated to the desired effect. GABA type A receptor stimulation results in a reduction of cerebral metabolism of O_2 ($CMRO_2$). For example, in healthy

Table 14.1 Properties of an ideal agent for neurointensive care sedation

Rapid onset and rapid recovery, allowing prompt neurologic evaluation
Predictable clearance independent of end-organ function, avoiding the problem of drug accumulation
Easily titration to achieve adequate levels of sedation
Reduced intracranial pressure by cerebral blood volume reduction or cerebral vasoconstriction
Reduced cerebral blood flow and cerebral metabolic rate of oxygen consumption, maintaining their coupling
Maintenance of cerebral autoregulation and normal cerebral vascular reactivity to changes in arterial carbon dioxide tension
Minimal cardiovascular depressant effects
Inexpensive

Modified with permission from Citerio and Cormio [110]

Table 14.2 Pharmacokinetic parameters, dosing, and cost of sedative and analgesic agents presented in the text

	Intravenous bolus dose	Continuous intravenous infusion	Elimination half-time, h	Clearance, ml/min/kg	Metabolic pathway	Active metabolites	Cost
Lorazepam	0.02–0.06 mg/kg	0.01–0.10 mg/kg/h	10–20	0.75–1.00	Glucuronidation	None	Inexpensive
Midazolam	0.02–0.08 mg/kg	0.04–0.30 mg/kg/h	2.0–2.5	4–8	CYP3A4	Yes	Moderate
Fentanyl	25–125 µg	10–100 µg/h	3.7	13	CYP3A4	None	Inexpensive
Remifentanil	Not recommended	0.05–0.25 µg/kg/min	0.3	44	Plasma esterases	None	Expensive
Propofal	Not recommended	5–200 µg/kg/min	7.2	24	Hepatic	None	Expensive
Dexmedetomidine	1 µg/kg	0.2–0.7 µg/kg/h	2	8.2	Glucuronidation and CYP2D6	None	Expensive

Reprinted with permission from Citerio and Cormio [110]

Table 14.3 Cerebral and systemic characteristics of the available molecules

	Propofol	Midazolam	Lorazepam	Fentanyl	Remifentanil
Rapid onset	+++	+++	+	+++	+++
Fast recovery	+++	++	+	++	+++
Easily titrated	+++	++	+	++	+++
ICP reduction	$\downarrow\downarrow$	$\downarrow$	$\downarrow$	$\downarrow/\leftrightarrow$	$\downarrow/\leftrightarrow$
CBF reduction	$\downarrow\downarrow$	$\downarrow\downarrow$	$\downarrow$	$\leftrightarrow$	$\leftrightarrow$
$CMRO_2$ reduction	$\downarrow\downarrow$	$\downarrow$	$\downarrow$	$\downarrow$	$\downarrow$
MAP	$\downarrow\downarrow$	$\downarrow$	$\downarrow$	$\downarrow$	$\downarrow\downarrow$

Reprinted with permission from Citerio and Cormio [110]

$\uparrow$ modest increase, $\uparrow\uparrow$ pronounced increase, $\leftrightarrow$ no clear effect, $\downarrow$ modest decrease, $\downarrow\downarrow$ pronounced decrease, +++ very favorable, ++ favorable, + not favorable, *CBF* cerebral blood flow, *CMRO$_2$* cerebral metabolic rate of oxygen consumption, *ICP* intracranial pressure, *MAP* mean arterial pressure

subjects an infusion of propofol at 6 mg/kg/h for 40 min may result in a decrease of $CMRO_2$ up to 34 % [23].

Cerebral metabolism is globally decreased by one-third to one-half of normal in the severely head-injured patient, usually because of the lower metabolic expenditure associated with coma and/or superimposed hypoxia/ischemia, primarily due to secondary insults. Sedation strategies should be designed to depress either the basal or activation components of cerebral metabolism. Common agents used to achieve this goal include central nervous system depressants, such as propofol, benzodiazepines, barbiturates, and similar drugs.

The metabolic suppression of $CMRO_2$ is dose dependent until the electroencephalogram becomes isoelectric. Beyond this level, no further suppression of cerebral oxygen consumption occurs, and the minimal consumption for cellular homeostasis persists.

Effects on Cerebral Blood Flow

When selecting sedative drugs, the maintenance of sufficient cerebral blood flow and at the same time the provision of sedation are paramount and should be considered. For example, cerebral blood flow measured by positron emission tomography is reduced with propofol [24, 25].

Propofol further decreases cerebral blood volume and, in turn, intracranial pressure. This makes propofol most suitable for patients with reduced intracranial compliance [23–25].

The effects of intravenous sedatives on cerebral blood flow (CBF) have primarily been investigated for diazepam, midazolam, and propofol. All of these agents cause a dose-dependent decrease in $CMRO_2$ and CBF. However, the decrease of intracerebral vascular resistance results in a decrease in intracranial pressure (ICP).

Because of its pharmacokinetics, specific effects on cerebral hemodynamic variables, and at the same time preservation of autoregulation and vasoreactivity to carbon dioxide, propofol approximates the ideal sedative more than benzodiazepines. An intravenous bolus produces a dose-dependent, coupled decrease in CBF and $CMRO_2$, similar to that described using barbiturates. The effects on CBF are probably secondary to a reduction in $CMRO_2$. A strong linear correlation between CBF and $CMRO_2$ has been demonstrated [23] using propofol. In experimental studies, escalating propofol doses lead to burst suppression on the electroencephalogram with a decrease of CBF by 38–58 % and $CMRO_2$ by 22 to 43 %. Similar results may be achieved with the use of short-acting semisynthetic narcotics. In humans, EEG burst suppression ratios of 50 and 100 % can be obtained with propofol and remifentanil, respectively, with a proportional reduction of CBF velocity of 22 and 33 % and no changes in arteriovenous oxygen saturation difference, suggesting intact flow–metabolism coupling [23–27].

All sedative agents may cause a decrease in mean arterial blood pressure by inducing both cardiac depression and peripheral vasodilatation. The decrease in blood pressure can cause an increase in intracranial pressure as a result of autoregulatory compensation and, consequently, a reduction in CPP. The hemodynamic effects are usually dose dependent. Therefore, it is important to assess the preload status of the patient to predict the hemodynamic response of the sedative agent, in consideration of cardiac function, and the concurrent use of hyperosmotic agents. When compared with propofol, midazolam is associated with less hypotension but a more variable interval for recovery after the cessation of the infusion [28–34]. Propofol causes more cardiovascular depression when the patient needs to be rapidly induced for general anesthesia; the major cardiovascular effect of propofol is a profound decrease in mean arterial pressure, resulting from a decrease in systemic vascular resistance, cardiac contractility, and preload. A bolus of 2–2.5 mg/kg propofol results in a 25–40 % reduction in systolic blood pressure. This potent effect on mean arterial pressure may affect CPP by one of two mechanisms. If autoregulation is intact, a reduction in mean arterial pressure will produce reflex cerebral vasodilatation and a possible increase in intracranial pressure. Alternatively, if autoregulation is impaired, hypotension may produce a critical decrease in CPP and CBF. The risk of hypotension is greatest in the presence of hypovolemia [35] and should always be considered when this drug is used in bloused in the NICU.

Some additional concerns regarding the use of propofol in the NICU arise from case reports describing cardiac failure in head injury patients receiving long-term propofol infusions and propofol infusion syndrome (PRIS) [35–37]. The combination of anesthetic rather than sedative doses of propofol for controlling intracranial hypertension and the association of vasopressors to maintain CPP are the possible causes of the development of adverse fatal events. Based on these observations, long-term infusion of propofol at dosages higher than 5 mg/kg/h is discouraged in the ICU. Opioids, like benzodiazepines, have little hemodynamic effect on euvolemic patients. When opioids and benzodiazepines are administered concomitantly, they may exhibit a synergistic effect on hemodynamics. The reasons for this synergy are not entirely clear.

The cerebral physiologic effects of opioids are controversial. Morphine-related increases in CBF, described in early reports, were probably secondary to an increase in arterial carbon dioxide tension resulting from respiratory depression. In general, opioids slightly decrease $CMRO_2$, CBF, and intracranial pressure, as long as normocapnia is maintained by mechanical ventilation. Opioids can produce short-lasting, mild decreases in mean arterial pressure, followed by decreases in CPP. In particular, remifentanil may cause decreases in both cerebral metabolic rate and intracranial pressure, with minimal changes in CPP and cerebral blood flow [38]. Opioids lead to dose-dependent, centrally mediated respiratory depression, which may be profound. The carbon dioxide response curve is shifted to the right, and the ventilatory response to hypoxia is obliterated. For this reason, in intubated spontaneously ventilating NICU patients, if opioids are administered, strict end-tidal carbon dioxide trend monitoring or frequent blood gas analysis must be implemented to identify rapid onset of respiratory depression.

Intracranial Pressure Control

Adequate control of the intracranial pressure (ICP) is one of the main therapeutic goals of managing the critically ill neurologic patient: sedatives may reduce ICP by different mechanisms. In the injured brain, cerebral circulation autoregulation is frequently impaired. Therefore, agitation and associated blood pressure elevations may cause intracranial pressure surges; moreover, the severely agitated patient will have an enhanced cerebral metabolism.

Severe agitation and coughing as in the case of intolerance of the endotracheal tube may increase intrathoracic pressure, reducing jugular venous outflow. In this situation, cerebral metabolism and CBF are increased and venous return is decreased. The additive effect of these phenomena can lead to deleterious increases in intracranial pressure. As cerebral perfusion pressure (CPP) is reduced, additional cerebral vasodilator cascade can reduce it even further. Adequate sedation of an agitated NICU patient with a borderline CPP will block this cascade [7, 10, 11].

As previously described, most of the sedatives used in the NICU decrease the cerebral metabolic rate of oxygen consumption ($CMRO_2$), producing a reduction in CBF, a reduction of cerebral blood volume (CBV), and a decrease in intracranial pressure. The applicability of this concept is not only limited to traumatic brain injury patients but also can be extended to patients with stroke and subarachnoid hemorrhage [17].

Seizures Suppression

Seizures are a frequent event in neuroinjury patients [39–41]. Convulsive and nonconvulsive seizures occurred in 22 % of the traumatic brain injury cohort and in 15 % of patients with intracerebral hemorrhage or subarachnoid hemorrhage [17]. Seizures produce a massive increase in cerebral metabolism and possibly a mismatch between oxygen delivery and metabolism in the brain area affected. Together with antiepileptic drugs, sedation appears to be an attractive option in reducing seizures in the NICU.

Benzodiazepines increase the seizure threshold and are useful anticonvulsants [42, 43]. In fact, in all settings benzodiazepines are a first-line treatment of a new onset of seizures.

The ability of propofol to protect against seizures has provided conflicting data [29, 43]. More recent studies showed that standard or high-dose propofol infusion (2 mg/kg induction bolus followed by 150–200 μg/kg/min infusion) can be reliably used as an anticonvulsant, even for the control of status epilepticus [31–34]. Experimental data have shown propofol to have strong anticonvulsant properties, which have proved to be very effective in controlling refractory status epilepticus. A recent statement by the European Federation of Neurological Societies included the use of propofol as an antiepileptic for convulsive epileptic status in the ICU setting [33].

Current Use of Sedative and Analgesic Agents

Propofol

Propofol (2, 6-diisopropylphenol) is a potent intravenous hypnotic agent which is widely used for the induction and maintenance of anesthesia and for sedation in the ICU. At room temperature, propofol is an oil and insoluble in aqueous solution. Present formulations consist of 1 or 2 % propofol, 10 % soybean oil, 2.25 % glycerol, and 1.2 % egg phosphatide. Edetate disodium (EDTA) or metabisulfite is added to retard bacterial and fungal growth.

Propofol is a global central nervous system depressant. It directly activates GABA receptors. In addition, propofol inhibits the NMDA receptor and modulates calcium influx through slow calcium ion channels. Propofol has a rapid onset of action with a dose-related hypnotic effect.

Propofol is highly lipophilic with a large volume of distribution. This property results in rapid uptake and elimination from the CNS, resulting in rapid onset of action and rapid recovery when discontinued.

In a recent investigation, patients with a higher sequential organ failure assessment (SOFA) were more likely to show a deeper level of sedation when on propofol [38]. In another study, it was demonstrated that the offset of propofol activity can vary considerably and is related to the depth of sedation, the duration of the infusion, and patient size. In non-neuroinjured patients, the predicted emergence time (full awakening and normal orientation) from a deep sedation (Ramsay 4) averaged 25 h for a 24-h infusion but increased to nearly 3 days for propofol infusions lasting 7–14 days [44].

A recent prospective study showed that, in medical patients requiring >48 h of mechanical ventilation, sedation with propofol results in significantly fewer ventilator days compared with intermittent lorazepam when sedatives are interrupted daily [45], one possible explanation being the shorter half-life of propofol, relative to lorazepam.

Propofol, a pure sedative–hypnotic alkyl phenol, exhibits rapid onset and short duration of action once discontinued after lighter sedation. These characteristics make this agent particularly advantageous in the NICU because it is possible to reduce sedation rapidly to conduct a thorough neurologic examination of the patient. Because of rapid central nervous system penetration and subsequent redistribution after a single dose, the onset of action of propofol is rapid (1–2 min), and its effect is brief (10–15 min). For this reason, propofol must only be administered by continuous infusion when used for sedation. Propofol is very lipid soluble, has a large volume of distribution, and can be given for prolonged periods of time without significant changes in its pharmacokinetic profile. Because propofol has no active metabolites, the termination of its clinical effect is dependent solely on redistribution to peripheral fat tissue stores. When the infusion is discontinued, the fat tissue stores redistribute the drug back into the plasma but usually not reaching clinically significant levels. Emergence from light level of sedation with propofol in ICU patients varies with the duration of sedation, with a slightly longer recovery reported after more than 12 h of infusion; however, it is rare for the effect to last longer than 60 min after the infusion is stopped.

Opioids

Analgesia is required in almost all NICU patients, and morphine derivatives appear to be an appropriate choice. Morphine, fentanyl, and remifentanil are the opioids that are most frequently used in the ICU [46]. Opioids stimulate the μ-, κ-, and δ-opioid receptors, which are distributed within the central nervous system. The μ-receptor is the primary site of opioid activity and is subdivided into the μ1- and μ2-subreceptors. Stimulation of the μ1-subreceptor leads to inhibition of neuronal pain [25]. Morphine, with its prolonged duration of action, and meperidine and its metabolite, normeperidine, which can precipitate seizures, are not ideal analgesics in the NICU setting. Normeperidine use is also associated with neuroexcitatory effects including tremor, delirium, and seizures [26].

The intravenous route of administration is preferred because it allows a faster onset and better titrability [27]. Fentanyl, with high lipid solubility, has a very rapid onset and a short duration of action after a single dose because of redistribution into peripheral tissues. Caution must be exercised, however, as the pharmacokinetics are altered with prolonged administration. Moreover, fentanyl is a substrate CYP3A4 and is affected by CYP3A4 inducers, such as phenytoin, which is frequently used in the NICU [25]. Genetic factors have been shown to regulate both opioid pharmacokinetics and pharmacodynamics and could be the reason for the variability in response to opioids that is observed in clinical practice [47].

Remifentanil has unique pharmacokinetic properties that make it attractive for use in neurocritical care. It has an ester structure that makes it susceptible to very rapid hydrolysis by nonspecific esterases in blood and tissue, with lack of drug accumulation following repeated boluses or continuous infusion. Remifentanil has a rapid blood–brain equilibration time (1.0 and 1.5 min), and its context-sensitive half-time is also short, i.e., 3–5 min. This time is unaffected by the duration of the infusion. Remifentanil has potential for use as an analgesic agent and, because of its ultrashort duration of action, requires the use of a continuous infusion [35–37, 48, 49].

Remifentanil is metabolized directly in the plasma by nonspecific esterases. The primary metabolite is remifentanil acid, a compound with little pharmacologic activity. Remifentanil acid is eliminated by the kidneys, and the action of remifentanil is not prolonged by renal injury. In addition, dose adjustments are not required in patients with hepatic dysfunction. Because of its short half-life, remifentanil has unique pharmacokinetic properties that make it attractive for use in neurocritical care. It may facilitate frequent awakening to evaluate neurologic and respiratory parameters [50]. In a study of patients with traumatic brain injury who were mechanically ventilated, remifentanil was used for on-top analgesia in head trauma patients without adverse effects on cerebrovascular hemodynamics, cerebral perfusion pressure, or intracranial pressure [51].

Benzodiazepines

Benzodiazepines such as midazolam, lorazepam, and diazepam are sedatives widely used in the ICU. They have anxiolytic, sedative, and hypnotic properties. Benzodiazepines experimentally increase the frequency of opening of the GABA$_a$ chloride channel in response to binding of GABA [52]. These pharmacologic effects depend on the degree of the binding of benzodiazepines to the GABA receptor; effects include anxiolysis, sedation, muscle relaxation, anterograde amnesia, respiratory depression, and anticonvulsant activity.

Midazolam, with its high clearance and short half-life, is a useful alternative to propofol [29–31, 42, 53–55]. However, a continuous infusion of midazolam for more than 24 h will cause the loss of rapid recovery properties; the known explanation for this phenomenon is the accumulation of active metabolites. Therefore, midazolam, administered via titrated continuous infusions, is recommended only for short-term use, as it produces unpredictable awakening when infusions continue for longer than 48–72 h. Moreover, the pharmacokinetics of midazolam change considerably when it is administered via continuous infusion to critically ill patients for extended periods of time (>24 h). This lipid-soluble drug undergoes oxidation in the liver via the CYP450 enzyme system to form water-soluble hydroxylated metabolites, which are excreted in the urine. The primary metabolite of midazolam, 1-hydroxymidazolam glucuronide, has central nervous system (CNS) depressant effects and may accumulate in the patient who is critically ill, especially if kidney failure is present. Also, the drug accumulates in peripheral tissues, particularly in obese subjects, as well as in the bloodstream and is not metabolized. When the drug is stopped, peripheral tissue stores release midazolam back into the plasma, and the duration of clinical effect can be prolonged.

In one study in patients on prolonged sedation, elevated levels of 1-hydroxymidazolam glucuronide were detected an average of 67 h after the midazolam infusion was discontinued [56].

These properties are reflected in the 2002 recommendation of Society of Critical Care Medicine (SCCM) consensus guidelines, where it was stated that midazolam be used only for short-term (<48 h) therapy and that lorazepam should be used for patients in the ICU requiring long-term sedation [57]. A randomized controlled trial compared lorazepam with midazolam for long-term sedation and found no difference in the time to awakening between the groups [58].

Numerous factors affect the response to benzodiazepine and include age, concurrent pathology, prior alcohol use, and therapy with other sedative drugs. Also, recent studies suggested that there is a genetic variability in the response of patients to benzodiazepines [59].

Recent reports have alerted clinicians to the risks for toxicity related to propylene glycol (a diluent used to facilitate drug solubility) accumulation in patients receiving intravenous lorazepam [60]. Toxicity of propylene glycol may cause hyperosmolar states, cellular toxicity, metabolic acidosis, and acute tubular necrosis. It has been proposed to use the osmolar gap as a surrogate marker for serum propylene glycol concentration. In critically ill patients receiving lorazepam for sedation, an osmolar gap above 10 was associated with concentrations previously reported to cause toxicity [61].

Ketamine

Ketamine is nonbarbiturate phencyclidine that provides analgesia and anesthesia with relative hemodynamic stability and is frequently used during hemorrhagic shock [62]. However, due to the known effects on CBF and ICP, this drug has found very little application in the neurosurgical ICU setting [63, 64]. Potential side effects of ketamine are increase of $CMRO_2$, CBF, and ICP.

In other reports, ketamine was shown to decrease CBF and ICP in head trauma patients sedated using both ketamine and propofol or with a $PaCO_2$ maintained constant [65], and in an experimental setting ketamine even had neuroprotective properties [66]. The potential advantages of using ketamine in traumatic brain injury patients are maintenance of

hemodynamic status as well as CPP, with absence of withdrawal symptoms. One study investigated the cerebral hemodynamics of ketamine used for sedation of severe head injury patients. Ketamine was compared with sufentanil as an analgesic, either in combination with midazolam and showed comparable effects in maintaining intracranial pressure and cerebral perfusion pressure of severe head injury patients under controlled mechanical ventilation [67]. Larger clinical trials are needed to test the potential side effects of ketamine in the brain-injured patient before recommending the use in routine clinical practice.

Dexmedetomidine

Dexmedetomidine (DEX) is a new drug that has been recently introduced into clinical practice [68–71]. It is a selective α-2 agonist that provides anxiolysis and sedation without causing respiratory depression. Dexmedetomidine has analgesic, hypnotic, and anxiolytic effects.

Dexmedetomidine is the dextro enantiomer of medetomidine, with a specificity for the α-2 receptor, which is seven times that of clonidine, the agonist for the α-2 receptor subtypes that mediates the effects of dexmedetomidine.

Dexmedetomidine has an onset of action approximately 15 min after intravenous injection and reaches peak concentrations in 1 h after continuous IV infusion.

The pharmacokinetics of DEX is largely influenced by liver rather than renal function. DEX is metabolized in the liver through glucuronide conjugation in the cytochrome P450 enzyme system. There are no known active or toxic metabolites; hepatic clearance may be decreased in patients with severe liver disease, although it is less affected by renal disease [72].

Other studies investigated the immune, cardiovascular, and respiratory response of varying doses of dexmedetomidine in healthy, young human volunteers. Dexmedetomidine-induced dose-dependent decreases in systolic and diastolic blood pressure and in heart rate and plasma norepinephrine levels [73–77]. Some studies reported a transient hypertensive response after IV high-dosage boluses, because of activation of peripheral vascular alpha-2 receptors before the central sympatholytic effect. Only minimal effects of dexmedetomidine on the respiratory system were observed throughout a broad range of plasma concentrations [78].

At present time, the FDA-approved duration of infusion of dexmedetomidine remains 24 h.

In October 2008, dexmedetomidine was FDA-approved for procedural sedation in nonintubated patients.

The peculiarity of sedation with DEX in comparison to propofol and midazolam is the easy arousability of patients under sedation: it is possible to reach a "cooperative sedation" during which patients may still be arousable during procedures or respond to neurologic testing during craniotomies [79].

DEX has some concerning effects on cerebral circulation. DEX sedation in volunteers seems to cause a decrease in regional and global cerebral blood flow [80], but the ratio with CMRO2 and flow metabolism coupling is maintained [81]; MRI studies showed that the cerebral blood flow pattern is similar to what is observed in natural sleep [82]. Low-dose dexmedetomidine showed an additive effect with meperidine on lowering the shivering threshold [83]. The neuroprotective properties of DEX have been investigated, and animal studies showed a preconditioning effect and attenuation of ischemia–reperfusion injury [84].

Similarly to clonidine, DEX has been used in the treatment of withdrawal from drugs (cocaine, alcohol, opioids); the mechanism could be the counterbalance of the central hyperadrenergic states induced by the withdrawal; in one study DEX was used successfully to control withdrawal in patients with history of cocaine and opioid abuse undergoing cerebral angioplasty for cerebral vasospasm [85, 86].

Barbiturates

Currently, barbiturates are used in the NICU only in specific conditions.

Barbiturates are associated with high incidence of systemic complications (i.e., hemodynamic instability, immunosuppression, hyper-/hypokalemia, atelectasis) and an unfavorable pharmacodynamic profile given that they accumulate in peripheral tissues after long-term infusions, leading to prolonged recovery from sedation. Thus, they are recommended only as second-tier therapy for refractory intracranial hypertension [87]. The other indication for barbiturates is the treatment of refractory status epilepticus as described in the most recent guidelines issued by the European Federation of Neurological Societies (EFNS) [88].

Side Effects of Sedative Agents

Propofol

While propofol lacks analgesic properties, it holds many of the characteristics of an "ideal" sedative. For this reason it should not be used alone during sedation for painful procedures. Concerning its hemodynamic effect, propofol induces both vasodilatation and a negative inotropic effect and by these mechanisms may cause hypotension of various grades of severity. The hypotensive effect of propofol may be pronounced in hypovolemic patients or in patients with a reduced cardiac output (such as those on other cardiodepressant medications) and in the elderly. Thus, when used to sedate patients affected by acute neurological injuries, propofol may decrease cerebral perfusion pressure even if it

induces a decrease in ICP [89]. Moreover, propofol may potentiate the cardiodepressant effects of alcohol, opioids, benzodiazepines, barbiturates, antihypertensives, and antiarrhythmics. When used in the NICU at high doses (i.e., as a first-line therapy for intracranial hypertension or for EEG burst suppression), invasive blood pressure and even cardiac output monitoring may be necessary to monitor the hemodynamic adverse effects.

Propofol causes a dose-dependent respiratory depression: during bolus or continuous infusions, continuous monitoring of pulse oximetry, respiratory rate and depth of respiration, and blood pressure are recommended. Propofol is insoluble in water and is suspended in an emulsion of soy, glycerol, and egg phospholipids; these components are susceptible to bacterial contamination, regardless of the presence of disodium edetate or EDTA as bacteriostatic agents. The carrier solution frequently causes pain at the injection site. This effect can be lessened by administration through a central or larger vein or by premedication with IV lidocaine in the same vein.

The emulsion carrier contains egg and soy proteins and can be responsible for rare immunologic reactions in patients with severe allergic reactions to these food substances.

One common side effect, particularly after prolonged high-rate infusions in the ICU, is hypertriglyceridemia, which is caused by the lipid vehicle. Moreover, the lipid vehicle contains 1.1 kcal/mL, which should be taken in consideration when computing the nutritional metabolic requirement.

Recently, propofol-related infusion syndrome' (PRIS) has been described in pediatric and adult patients receiving doses greater than 80 mcg/kg/min for prolonged periods of time. The exact mechanism of PRIS is still unclear, but the clinical signs include metabolic acidosis, hyperkalemia, rhabdomyolysis, hypoxia, and progressive myocardial failure [90–92]. Monitoring for electrolytes and increases in lactic acid, creatinine kinase, and triglycerides is recommended in patients receiving high doses >50 mcg/kg/min for longer than 48 h. All these laboratory parameters should be checked at least once daily for patients at risk. A hospital policy limiting the use of propofol to a safe limit is recommended.

Benzodiazepines

Their anticonvulsant properties make benzodiazepines a first-line treatment option for acute management of seizures and status epilepticus. However, tolerance can occur rapidly leading to the need for increasing the dose to maintain efficacy. Benzodiazepines are pure sedative agents, with no analgesic properties; thus, analgesia should be added when pain is a concern. IV benzodiazepine may cause hypotension and increased heart rate at higher dose and, in susceptible patients, hypovolemia, low cardiac output state, or severe vasodilation. High doses of benzodiazepines may cause respiratory depression and apnea, leading to an elevation in ICP caused by hypercarbia.

Benzodiazepine sedation overdose is not uncommon in neuroinjury patients. Risk vs. benefit of benzodiazepine use in the neuroICU should be carefully evaluated after prolonged infusions (48–72 h) or in patients with altered renal function. Flumazenil can reverse the effects of benzodiazepines, but it should be used carefully because of the risk of lowering seizure threshold and an increase in ICP.

Another major side effect of benzodiazepines, delirium, is discussed later in this chapter.

Opioids

Opioids do not have a direct effect on ICP or cerebral blood flow. However, when they act as respiratory depressants may cause hypercarbia with consequent increase in ICP. For this reason, all patients receiving narcotics in the NICU should receive continuous monitoring of respiratory rate and pulse oximetry with lowest possible FiO_2 to avoid late unmasking of hypercarbia.

Other common adverse reactions to narcotics include histamine release causing urticaria and flushing, somnolence, respiratory depression, chest wall and other muscle rigidity (primarily with fentanyl and remifentanil), dysphoria or hallucinations (primarily with morphine), nausea and vomiting, GI dysmotility, and vasodilatation with hypotension. Full anaphylactic shock is extremely rare. Opioids can be reversed by their antagonist, naloxone, which should be titrated slowly and in low doses first to avoid an "overshoot" phenomenon that can result in a catecholamine peak leading to hypertension, tachycardia, and emergence agitation. This reaction can exacerbate intracranial hypertension.

Dexmedetomidine

The most common adverse effects of dexmedetomidine include dry mouth, bradycardia, hypotension, lightheadedness, and anxiety. Bradycardia and hypotension are frequently observed during the initial loading dose; thus, arterial pressure and cerebral perfusion pressure should be continuously monitored. DEX does not have a significant effect on ICP. Hypotension and bradycardia can be exacerbated by concomitant administration of antihypertensive and antidysrhythmic medications.

Monitoring Sedation in the NICU

Monitoring the level sedation in the NICU is crucial. The improper use of sedatives in dosages either too high or too low may affect the neurological examination and may lead to the wrong neurological diagnosis. Oversedation increases the risk of infections by delaying weaning from mechanical ventilation, and the increased length of stay is associated with increased costs. By contrast, an undersedated patient may be agitated, anxious, and at risk for self-extubation, recalling unpleasant events or simply desynchronizing with mechanical ventilation.

Sedation scales are used to evaluate arousal, depth of sedation, and response to stimuli [93]. The Ramsay Scale evaluates consciousness, while the Richmond Agitation–Sedation Scale (RASS) examines cognition; Sedation Agitation Scale (SAS) and the Motor Activity Assessment scale (MAAS) monitor sedation and arousal. The use of sedation scales can reduce the amount of sedatives given to achieve a specific sedation target, decreasing the number of days on mechanical ventilation and cost of hospital stay [94], but no validation is available in the neuroICU environment.

Recently, processed electroencephalogram (EEG) algorithms have been introduced into clinical practice as a method to monitor objectively and quantitatively the level of consciousness in ICU patients. One example is the determination of bispectral index (BIS) [95], which has been associated with a decrease in sedative use in intraoperative care [96], but never validated in neurocritically ill patients.

Delirium in the NICU

Delirium is an acute brain dysfunction, defined as an acute disturbance of consciousness accompanied by inattention, disorganized thinking, and perceptual disturbances that fluctuate over a short period of time [97]. Numerous risk factors have been described [98–101]:

- Host factors age, baseline comorbidities, baseline cognitive impairment, and genetic predisposition
- Factors related to the acute illness: sepsis, hypoxemia and metabolic disturbances, primary central nervous system disease, shock, liver disease, acute respiratory distress syndrome, postoperative status, kidney disease, heart failure, and anemia
- Iatrogenic and environmental factors, metabolic disturbances, anticholinergic medications, sedatives and analgesic medications, and sleep disturbances

The American Psychiatric Society has published its guidelines on delirium, which included a list of substances that can cause delirium through intoxication or withdrawal, including sedative agents and analgesics [102].

In trauma ICU, sedatives and analgesics were found to be risk factors for development of delirium [103, 104]. Midazolam was an independent risk factor for the development of delirium in both surgical and trauma patients; the association between opioids and delirium was inconsistent, with the use of fentanyl but not morphine as a risk factor for delirium in surgical ICU patients but not in trauma patients [105, 106]. Similar results were seen in a study performed in burn trauma patients [107]. Again, benzodiazepines were found to be an independent risk factor for the development of delirium.

A recently introduced evidence-based clinical bundle has been suggested as a way to improve patient outcome and recovery [108]. ABCDE stands for awakening and breathing trials, choice of appropriate sedation, delirium monitoring, and early mobility exercise.

Benzodiazepines are known to increase the risk of delirium in a dose-dependent manner. Multiple studies have shown that protocolized target-based sedation and daily spontaneous awakening trials reduce the number of days on mechanical ventilation. This strategy also exposes the patient to smaller cumulative doses of sedatives.

In the critically ill NICU patient, the interruption of sedation may have negative effects because it could also induce a stress response. ICP and the CPP levels can increase during interruption of sedation, when compared to baseline levels recorded during continuous sedation. In the majority of patients, these changes are transient and tolerable. However, in a subset of patients with very low cerebral compliance, the interruption of continuous sedation can induce marked ICP and CPP changes that can produce secondary injuries [109]. Those patients should be excluded from repeated evaluations, and information should instead be gathered from other multimodality monitoring methods in combination with neuroimaging [110].

NICU Sedation and Analgesia: A Suggested Approach

Because no single drug can achieve all of the requirements for sedation and analgesia in the ICU, the use of a combination of drugs, each titrated to specific end points, is usually a more effective approach. This strategy allows lower doses of individual drugs and reduces the problems of drug accumulation. At our institution, we implemented a simplified sedation protocol based on time of presentation of the neuroinjury or ICP:

- In the acute phase (i.e., first 48–72 h or until intracranial hypertension is controlled), a continuous infusion of a combination of propofol (1.5–6 mg/kg/h) and fentanyl (0.5–1.5 μg/kg/h) is used.

- In the subacute phase (i.e., after 72 h or when intracranial pressure is normalized), intermittent boluses of benzodiazepines (in our case, lorazepam 0.05 mg/kg every 2–6 h) follows.

We continue to sedate patients until no ventilatory support is required, and then we taper sedation slowly to prevent withdrawal symptoms in 24–48 h.

References

1. Kress JP, Pohlman AS, O'Connor MF, Hall JB. Daily interruption of sedative infusions in critically ill patients undergoing mechanical ventilation. N Engl J Med. 2000;342:1471–7.
2. Hogarth DK, Hall J. Management of sedation in mechanically ventilated patients. Curr Opin Crit Care. 2004;10(1):40–6.
3. Hukkelhoven CW, Steyerberg EW, Farace E, et al. Regional differences in patient characteristics, case management, and outcomes in traumatic brain injury: experience from the tirilazad trials. J Neurosurg. 2002;97:549–57.
4. Bertolini G, Melotti R, Romano P, et al. Use of sedative and analgesic drugs in the first week of ICU stay. A pharmacoepidemiological perspective. Minerva Anestesiol. 2001;67: 97–105.
5. Soliman HM, Melot C, Vincent JL. Sedative and analgesic practice in the intensive care unit: the results of a European survey. Br J Anaesth. 2001;87:186–92.
6. Rhoney DH, Parker D Jr. Use of sedative and analgesic agents in neurotrauma patients: effects on cerebral physiology. Neurol Res. 2001; 23:237–259.
7. Jacobi J, Fraser GL, Coursin DB, et al. Clinical practice guidelines for the sustained use of sedatives and analgesics in the critically ill adult. Crit Care Med. 2002;30:119–41.
8. Cohen IL, Abraham E, Dasta JF, et al. Management of the agitated intensive care unit patient. Crit Care Med. 2002;30(suppl): S116–7.
9. Blanchard AR. Sedation and analgesia in intensive care. Medications attenuate stress response in critical illness. Postgrad Med. 2002;111:59–60, 63–4, 67–70.
10. Gemma M, Tommasino C, Cerri M, et al. Intracranial effects of endotracheal suctioning in the acute phase of head injury. J Neurosurg Anesthesiol. 2002;14:50–4.
11. Hurford WE. Sedation and paralysis during mechanical ventilation. Respir Care. 2002;47:334–46.
12. Gehlbach BK, Kress JP. Sedation in the intensive care unit. Curr Opin Crit Care. 2002;8:290–8.
13. Kress JP, Pohlman AS, Hall JB. Sedation and analgesia in the intensive care unit. Am J Respir Crit Care Med. 2002;166: 1024–8.
14. Ostermann ME, Keenan SP, Seiferling RA, et al. Sedation in the intensive care unit: a systematic review. JAMA. 2000;283: 1451–9.
15. Mirski MA, Muffelman B, Ulatowski JA, et al. Sedation for the critically ill neurologic patient. Crit Care Med. 1995;23: 2038–53.
16. Prielipp RC, Coursin DB. Sedative and neuromuscular blocking drug use in critically ill patients with head injuries. New Horiz. 1995;3:458–68.
17. Kraus JJ, Metzler MD, Coplin WM. Critical care issues in stroke and subarachnoid hemorrhage. Neurol Res. 2002;24 suppl 1: S47–57.
18. Oertel M, Kelly DF, Lee JH, et al. Metabolic suppressive therapy as a treatment for intracranial hypertension—why it works and when it fails. Acta Neurochir Suppl. 2002;81:69–70.
19. Robertson CS, Cormio M. Cerebral metabolic management. New Horiz. 1995;3:410–22.
20. Clausen T, Bullock R. Medical treatment and neuroprotection in traumatic brain injury. Curr Pharm Des. 2001;7:1517–32.
21. Grasshoff C, Gillessen T. The effect of propofol on increased superoxide concentration in cultured rat cerebrocortical neurons after stimulation of N-methyl-d-aspartate receptors. Anesth Analg. 2002;95:920–2.
22. Starbuck VN, Kay GG, Platenberg RC, et al. Functional magnetic resonance imaging reflects changes in brain functioning with sedation. Hum Psychopharmacol. 2000;15:613–8.

23. Oshima T, Karasawa F, Satoh T. Effects of propofol on cerebral blood flow and the metabolic rate of oxygen in humans. Acta Anaesthesiol Scand. 2002;46(7):831–5.

24. Engelhard K, Werner C. Inhalational or intravenous anesthetics for craniotomies? Pro inhalational. Curr Opin Anaesthesiol. 2006;19:504–8.

25. Trescot AM, Datta S, Lee M, et al. Opioid pharmacology. Pain Physician. 2008;11(2 Suppl):S133–53.

26. Armstrong PJ, Bersten A. Normeperidine toxicity. Anesth Analg. 1986;65(5):536–8.

27. Barr J, Donner A. Optimal intravenous dosing strategies for sedatives and analgesics in the intensive care unit. Crit Care Clin. 1995;11(4):827–47.

28. Angelini G, Ketzler JT, Coursin DB. Use of propofol and other nonbenzodiazepine sedatives in the intensive care unit. Crit Care Clin. 2001;17:863–80.

29. Magarey JM. Propofol or midazolam – which is best for the sedation of adult ventilated patients in intensive care units? A systematic review. Aust Crit Care. 2001;14:147–54.

30. Walder B, Elia N, Henzi I, et al. A lack of evidence of superiority of propofol versus midazolam for sedation in mechanically ventilated critically ill patients: a qualitative and quantitative systematic review. Anesth Analg. 2001;92:975–83.

31. Weinbroum AA, Halpern P, Rudick V, et al. Midazolam versus propofol for long-term sedation in the ICU: a randomized prospective comparison. Intensive Care Med. 1997;23:1258–63.

32. Power KN, Flaatten H, Gilhus NE, Engelsen BA. Propofol treatment in adult refractory status epilepticus. Mortality risk and outcome. Epilepsy Res. 2011;94(1–2):53–60.

33. Meierkord H, Boon P, Engelsen B, Göcke K, Shorvon S, Tinuper P, Holtkamp M, European Federation of Neurological Societies. EFNS guideline on the management of status epilepticus in adults. Eur J Neurol. 2010;17(3):348–55.

34. Marik PE, Varon J. The management of status epilepticus. Chest. 2004;126(2):582–91.

35. Rosow C. Remifentanil: a unique opioid analgesic. Anesthesiology. 1993;79:875–6.

36. Pitsiu M, Wilmer A, Bodenham A, et al. Pharmacokinetics of remifentanil and its major metabolite, remifentanil acid, in ICU patients with renal impairment. Br J Anaesth. 2004;92:493–503.

37. Dumont L, Picard V, Marti RA, et al. Use of remifentanil in a patient with chronic hepatic failure. Br J Anaesth. 1998;81: 265–7.

38. Peeters MY, Bras LJ, DeJongh J, et al. Disease severity is a major determinant for the pharmacodynamics of propofol in critically ill patients. Clin Pharmacol Ther. 2008;83(3):443–51.

39. Bladin CF, Alexandrov AV, Bellavance A, et al. Seizure after stroke: a prospective multicenter study. Arch Neurol. 2000;57:1617–22.

40. Reith J, Jorgensen HS, Raaschou HO, et al. Seizure in acute stroke: predictors and prognostic significance. The Copenhagen Stroke Study. Stroke. 1997;28:1585–9.

41. Vespa PM, Nuwer MR, Nenov V, et al. Increased incidence and impact of nonconvulsive and convulsive seizures after traumatic brain injury as detected by continuous electroencephalographic monitoring. J Neurosurg. 1999;91:750–60.

42. Hanley DF, Pozo M. Treatment of status epilepticus with midazolam in the critical care setting. Int J Clin Pract. 2000;54:30–5.

43. Walder B, Tramer MR, Seeck M. Seizure-like phenomena and propofol: a systematic review. Neurology. 2002;58:1327–32.

44. Barr J, Egan TD, Sandoval NF, et al. Propofol dosing regimens for ICU sedation based upon an integrated pharmacokinetic-pharmacodynamic model. Anesthesiology. 2001;95(2):324–33.

45. Carson SS, Kress JP, Rodgers JE, et al. A randomized trial of intermittent lorazepam versus propofol with daily interruption in mechanically ventilated patients. Crit Care Med. 2006;34(5): 1326–32.

46. Mehta S, Burry L, Fischer S, et al. Canadian survey of the use of sedatives, analgesics, and neuromuscular blocking agents in critically ill patients. Crit Care Med. 2006;34(2):374–80.

47. Somogyi AA, Barratt DT, Coller JK. Pharmacogenetics of opioids. Clin Pharmacol Ther. 2007;81(3):429–44.

48. Egan TD, Lemmens HJ, Fiset P, et al. The pharmacokinetics of the new short- acting opioid remifentanil (GI87084B) in healthy adult male volunteers. Anesthesiology. 1993;79:881–92.

49. Delvaux B, Ryckwaert Y, Van Boven M, et al. Remifentanil in the intensive care unit: tolerance and acute withdrawal syndrome after prolonged sedation. Anesthesiology. 2005;102:1281–2.

50. Karabinis A, Mandragos K, Stergiopoulos S, et al. Safety and efficacy of analgesia-based sedation with remifentanil versus standard hypnotic-based regimens in intensive care unit patients with brain injuries: a randomised, controlled trial [ISRCTN50308308]. Crit Care. 2004;8:R268–80.

51. Engelhard K, Reeker W, Kochs E, et al. Effect of remifentanil on intracranial pres- sure and cerebral blood flow velocity in patients with head trauma. Acta Anaesthesiol Scand. 2004;48:396–9.

52. Charney DS, Mihic SJ, Harris RA. Hypnotics and sedatives. In: Hardman JG, Limbird LE, editors. Goodman and Gilman's the pharmacological basis of therapeutics. 10th ed. New York: McGraw-Hill; 2001. p. 399–427.

53. Shafer A. Complications of sedation with midazolam in the intensive care unit and a comparison with other sedative regimens. Crit Care Med. 1998;26:947–56.

54. Hanaoka K, Namiki A, Dohi S, et al. A dose-ranging study of midazolam for postoperative sedation of patients: a randomized, double-blind, placebo-controlled trial. Crit Care Med. 2002;30:1256–60.

55. Shelly MP, Mendel L, Park GR. Failure of critically ill patients to metabolise midazolam. Anaesthesia. 1987;42:619–26.

56. McKenzie CA, McKinnon W, Naughton DP, et al. Differentiating midazolam over sedation from neurological damage in the intensive care unit. Crit Care. 2005;9(1):R32–6.

57. Jacobi J, Fraser GL, Coursin DB, Riker RR, Fontaine D, Wittbrodt ET, Chalfin DB, Masica MF, Bjerke HS, Coplin WM, Crippen DW, Fuchs BD, Kelleher RM, Marik PE, Nasraway Jr SA, Murray MJ, Peruzzi WT, Lumb PD, Task Force of the American College of Critical Care Medicine (ACCM) of the Society of Critical Care Medicine (SCCM), American Society of Health-System Pharmacists (ASHP), American College of Chest Physicians. Clinical practice guidelines for the sustained use of sedatives and analgesics in the critically ill adult. Crit Care Med. 2002;30(1):119–41. No abstract available. Erratum in: Crit Care Med 2002 Mar;30(3):726.

58. Barr J, Zomorodi K, Bertaccini EJ, et al. A double-blind, randomized comparison of i.v. lorazepam versus midazolam for sedation of ICU patients via a pharmacologic model. Anesthesiology. 2001;95(2):286–98.

59. Fukasawa T, Suzuki A, Otani K. Effects of genetic polymorphism of cytochrome P450 enzymes on the pharmacokinetics of benzodiazepines. J Clin Pharm Ther. 2007;32(4):333–41.

60. Yahwak JA, Riker RR, Fraser GL, et al. Determination of a lorazepam dose threshold for using the osmol gap to monitor for propylene glycol toxicity. Pharmacotherapy. 2008;28(8):984–91.

61. Barnes BJ, Gerst C, Smith JR, et al. Osmol gap as a surrogate marker for serum propylene glycol concentrations in patients receiving lorazepam for sedation. Pharmacotherapy. 2006;26(1):23–33.

62. Tweed WA, Minuck MS, Mymin D. Circulatory responses to ketamine anesthesia. Anesthesiology. 1972;37:613–9.

63. Gardner AE, Dannemiller FJ, Dean D. Intracranial cerebrospinal fluid pressure in man during ketamine anesthesia. Anesth Analg. 1972;51:741–5.

64. Takeshita H, Okuda Y, Sari A. The effects of ketamine on cerebral circulation and metabolism in man. Anesthesiology. 1972;36:69–75.

65. Albanèse J, Arnaud S, Rey M, et al. Ketamine decreases intracranial pressure and electroencephalographic activity in traumatic

brain injury patients during propofol sedation. Anesthesiology. 1997;87(6):1328–34.

66. Shapira Y, Lam AM, Eng CC, et al. Therapeutic time window and dose response of the beneficial effects of ketamine in experimental head injury. Stroke. 1994;25:1637–43.

67. Bourgoin A, Albanèse J, Wereszczynski N, Charbit M, Vialet R, Martin C. Safety of sedation with ketamine in severe head injury patients: comparison with sufentanil. Crit Care Med. 2003;31:711–7.

68. Coursin DB, Coursin DB, Maccioli GA. Dexmedetomidine. Curr Opin Crit Care. 2001;7:221–6.

69. Drummond G. Dexmedetomidine may be effective, but is it safe? Br J Anaesth. 2002;88:454–5.

70. Maze M, Scarfini C, Cavaliere F. New agents for sedation in the intensive care unit. Crit Care Clin. 2001;17:881–97.

71. Shelly MP. Dexmedetomidine: a real innovation or more of the same? Br J Anaesth. 2001;87:677–8.

72. De Wolf AM, Fragen RJ, Avram MJ, Fitzgerald PC, Rahimi-Danesh F. The pharmacokinetics of dexmedetomidine in volunteers with severe renal impairment. Anesth Analg. 2001;93:1205–9.

73. Belleville JP. Effects of intravenous dexmedetomidine in humans: part I: sedation, ventilation, and metabolic rate. Anesthesiology. 1992;77:1125–33.

74. Bloor BC, Ward DS, Belleville JP, et al. Effects of intravenous dexmedetomidine in humans: part II: hemodynamic changes. Anesthesiology. 1992;77:1134–42.

75. Talke P, Richardson CA, Scheinin M, et al. Postoperative pharmacokinetics and sympatholytic effects of dexmedetomidine. Anesth Analg. 1997;85:1136–42.

76. Triltsch AE, Welte M, von Homeyer P, et al. Bispectral index–guided sedation with dexmedetomidine in intensive care: a prospective, randomized, double blind, placebo-controlled phase II study. Crit Care Med. 2002;30:1007–14.

77. Venn RM, Bryant A, Hall GM, et al. Effects of dexmedetomidine on adrenocortical function, and the cardiovascular, endocrine and inflammatory responses in postoperative patients needing sedation in the intensive care unit. Br J Anaesth. 2001;86:650–6.

78. Ebert TJ, Hall JE, Barney JA, et al. The effects of increasing plasma concentrations of dexmedetomidine in humans. Anesthesiology. 2000;93:382–94.

79. Bekker A, Sturaitis MK. Dexmedetomidine for neurological surgery. Neurosurgery. 2005;57(1 Suppl):1–10.

80. Stump DA, James RL, Bennett J. Dexmedetomidine-induced sedation in volunteers decreases regional and global cerebral blood flow. Anesth Analg. 2002;95:1052–9.

81. Drummond JC, Dao AV, Roth DM, et al. Effect of dexmedetomidine on cerebral blood flow velocity, cerebral metabolic rate, and carbon dioxide response in normal humans. Anesthesiology. 2008;108:225–32.

82. Coull JT, Jones ME, Egan TD, et al. Attentional effects of noradrenaline vary with arousal level: selective activation of thalamic pulvinar in humans. Neuroimage. 2004;22:315–22.

83. Doufas AG, Lin CM, Suleman MI, et al. Dexmedetomidine and meperidine additively reduce the shivering threshold in humans. Stroke. 2003;34:1218–23.

84. Dahmani S, Rouelle D, Gressens P, et al. Effects of dexmedetomidine on hippocampal focal adhesion kinase tyrosine phosphorylation in physiologic and ischemic conditions. Anesthesiology. 2005;103:969–77.

85. Maccioli GA. Dexmedetomidine to facilitate drug withdrawal. Anesthesiology. 2003;98:575–7.

86. Farag E, Chahlavi A, Argalious M, et al. Using dexmedetomidine to manage patients with cocaine and opioid withdrawal, who are undergoing cerebral angioplasty for cerebral vasospasm. Anesth Analg. 2006;103:1618–20.

87. Bratton SL, Chestnut RM, Ghajar J, et al. Guidelines for the management of severe traumatic brain injury XI. Anesthetics, analgesics, and sedatives. J Neurotrauma. 2007;24(1 Suppl):S71–6; Erratum in: J Neurotrauma. 2008;25(3):276–8.

88. Meierkord H, Boon P, Engelsen B, et al. EFNS guideline on the management of status epilepticus in adults. Eur J Neurol. 2010; 17(3):348–55.

89. Kelly DF, Goodale DB, Williams J, et al. Propofol in the treatment of moderate and severe head injury: a randomized, prospective, double-blinded pilot trial. J Neurosurg. 1999;90:1042–52.

90. Cannon ML, Glazier SS, Bauman LA. Metabolic acidosis, rhabdomyolysis, and cardiovascular collapse after prolonged propofol infusion. J Neurosurg. 2001;95:1053–6.

91. Kelly DF. Propofol-infusion syndrome. J Neurosurg. 2001;95:925–6.

92. Laham J. Propofol: risk vs. benefit. Clin Pediatr (Phila). 2002;41:5–7.

93. DeJonge B, Cook D, Appere-De-Vecchi C, et al. Using and understanding sedation scoring systems: a systematic review. Intensive Care Med. 2000;26:275–85.

94. Brook AD, Ahrens TS, Schaiff R, et al. Effect of a nursing-implemented sedation protocol on the duration of mechanical ventilation. Crit Care Med. 1999;27(12):2609–15.

95. Riess ML, Graefe UA, Goeters C, et al. Sedation assessment in critically ill patients with bispectral index. Eur J Anaesthesiol. 2002;19:18–22.

96. Klopman MA, Sebel PS. Cost-effectiveness of bispectral index monitoring. Curr Opin Anaesthesiol. 2011;24:177–81.

97. Sanchez-Izquierdo Riera JA, Caballero-Cubedo RE, Perez-Vela JL, et al. Propofol versus midazolam: safety and efficacy for sedating the severe trauma patient. Anesth Analg. 1998;86:1219–24.

98. Olson DM, Thoyre SM, Peterson ED, Graffagnino C. A randomized evaluation of bispectral index-augmented sedation assessment in neurological patients. Neurocrit Care. 2009;11(1):20–7.

99. American Psychiatric Association. Diagnostic and statistical manual of mental disorders. 4th ed. Washington, D.C.: American Psychiatric Association; 2000.

100. Dyer CB, Ashton CM, Teasdale TA. Postoperative delirium: a review of 80 primary data collection studies. Arch Intern Med. 1995;155:461–5.

101. Dubois MJ, Bergeron N, Dumont M, et al. Delirium in an intensive care unit: a study of risk factors. Intensive Care Med. 2001;27:1297–304.

102. Marcantonio E, Juarez G, Goldman L, et al. The relationship of postoperative delirium with psychoactive medications. J Am Med Assoc. 1994;272:1518.

103. Pandharipande P, Shintani A, Peterson J, et al. Lorazepam is an independent risk factor for transitioning to delirium in intensive care unit patients. Anesthesiology. 2006;104:21–6.

104. American Psychiatric Association. Practice guidelines for the treatment of patients with delirium. Am J Psychiatry. 1999;156 (5 suppl):1–20.

105. Pandharipande P, Cotton B, Shintani A, et al. Prevalence and risk factors for development of delirium in surgical and trauma intensive care unit patients. J Trauma. 2008;65:34–41.

106. Lat I, McMillian W, Taylor S, et al. The impact of delirium on clinical outcomes in mechanically ventilated surgical and trauma patients. Crit Care Med. 2009;37:1898–905.

107. Agarwal V, O'Neill P, Cotton B, et al. Prevalence and risk factors for development of delirium in burn intensive care unit patients. J Burn Care Res. 2010;31:706–15.

108. Morandi A, Brummel NE, Ely EW. Sedation, delirium and mechanical ventilation: the "ABCDE" approach. Curr Opin Crit Care. 2011;17(1):43–9.

109. Skoglund K, Enblad P, Marklund N. Effects of the neurological wake-up test on intracranial pressure and cerebral perfusion pressure in brain-injured patients. Neurocrit Care. 2009;11(2):135–42.

110. Citerio G, Cormio M. Sedation in neurointensive care: advances in understanding and practice. Curr Opin Crit Care. 2003;9(2): 120–6.

Endocrine Issues in Neurocritical Care

15

Steven B. Greenberg, Arthur J. Tokarczyk,
Cameron Zahed, and Douglas B. Coursin

Contents

S.B. Greenberg, MD (✉)
Department of Anesthesiology, NorthShore University HealthSystem,
University of Chicago, 2650 Ridge Ave,
Evanston, IL 60201, USA
e-mail: sbgreenb@gmail.com

A.J. Tokarczyk, MD
Department of Anesthesiology, NorthShore University HealthSystem,
University of Chicago Pritzker School of Medicine,
Evanston, IL 60201, USA
e-mail: atokarczyk@hotmail.com

C. Zahed, MD, MS
Department of Anesthesiology, Internal Medicine,
and Critical Care, University of Wisconsin Hospital and Clinics,
600 Highland Ave, Madison, WI 53792, USA
e-mail: czahed@wisc.edu

D.B. Coursin, MD
Department of Medicine, University of Wisconsin School of Medicine
and Public Health, Madison, WI 53792, USA

Department of Anesthesiology, University of Wisconsin School of
Medicine and Public Health, B6/319 UW CSC,
Madison, WI 53792-3272, USA
e-mail: dcoursin@wisc.edu

Abstract

The endocrine system is an integral organ system that maintains homeostasis in humans. Critical illness causes dysregulation of the endocrine system and threatens to disrupt human hormonal balance. Neurologically injured patients are at particularly high risk for various endocrinopathies depending on their individual insults and comorbidities. Hormonal imbalances seen in the neurocritically ill may vary depending on the acute or chronic phase of critical illness. Emerging therapeutic hormonal measures continue to be investigated in order to reverse the deleterious effects of hormonal dysregulation, particularly in the chronic phase of critical illness. Neurointensivists should be aware of the various perioperative endocrine abnormalities and the associated ICU polypharmacy that also causes endocrine disorders. Recognition of these causes may lead to earlier interventions.

Keywords

Endocrine • Critically ill • Hormonal imbalance •
Neurointensive care • Drug-induced endocrine disorders

A.J. Layon et al. (eds.), *Textbook of Neurointensive Care*,
DOI 10.1007/978-1-4471-5226-2_15, © Springer-Verlag London 2013

Introduction

The endocrine system is vital to the maintenance of homeostasis in the human body. This complex system is comprised of a variety of glands that secrete hormones into the bloodstream to regulate numerous body functions. Endocrine is derived from the Greek word "endo" meaning inside and "crinis" for secrete [1]. Hormones that are released from a plethora of glands are responsible for regulating metabolism, growth, mood, development, tissue integrity, and cardiovascular and immune function.

There are many similarities between the endocrine system and the nervous system. Both rely on the process of signaling and function through stimulus–response interactions. The term "neuroendocrine" system has been developed on the premise that hormones are similar to neurotransmitters (produced by the hypothalamus and stored in axons) in the brain, but they are secreted in the bloodstream and can act by stimulating or suppressing target cells that may be located far from their origin of secretion. The endocrine and nervous systems are intimately involved with one another. For example, neurotransmitters (i.e., dopamine, serotonin, endorphins, and enkephalins) along with the sympathetic/ parasympathetic systems may promote or suppress hormone secretion. Nervous system-derived stimuli (tactile, auditory, olfactory) also modulate the release or suppression of a multitude of hormones. Therefore, it is imperative to understand the close interactions between these two systems in order to identify and manage abnormalities that may occur in both systems [2].

This chapter will focus on endocrine abnormalities encountered in the Neurointensive Care Unit (NICU) both those related to premorbid endocrinopathies, most commonly diabetes and thyroid abnormalities, and those that develop secondary to the neurologic insult. Discussion of the physiology and pathophysiology of the hypothalamic-pituitary axis and the neuroendocrine stress response during critical illness will be featured.

As a result of the neurologic injury stress-induced response, dysglycemia, defined as hypo, hyper, or labile glucose levels, is one of the primary endocrine derangements seen in the NICU patient [3]. This chapter addresses the physiologic derangements of the brain during both hyper- and hypoglycemia and the potential deleterious effects of glucose variability on the brain. Monitoring glucose and achieving optimal glucose control will also be discussed as they pertain to the NICU population [3].

In addition to dysglycemia, other endocrine abnormalities are seen during development of specific neurologic pathologies or syndromes. The relationship between the following diseases and endocrine abnormalities will be discussed: traumatic brain injury (TBI), stroke, subarachnoid hemorrhage (SAH)/intracranial hemorrhage (ICH), meningitis/encephalitis, endocrine secreting tumors, and progressive neurologic diseases. Lastly, endocrine abnormality-induced mental status changes and drug-induced endocrine disorders seen in NICU patients and the endocrinopathy of brain death will be explored.

Anatomy/Physiology of the Hypothalamic-Pituitary Axis (HPA)

The hypothalamus and pituitary gland are closely integrated and are responsible for a majority of the responses of the endocrine system. The pituitary gland consists of two portions, the anterior (adenohypophysis) and posterior (neurohypophysis). Each component has its own unique connection to the hypothalamus as well as its own arsenal of secretory hormones [4].

The hypothalamus, a part of the diencephalon located below the thalamus, is responsible for releasing neuropeptides through the hypophyseal tract that activate or inhibit responses from both the posterior and anterior pituitary glands [4, 5]. Figure 15.1 depicts the anatomy of both the anterior and pituitary glands. There are two types of neurons that are primarily responsible for the endocrine activity of the hypothalamus, magnocellular and parvocellular neurons [2, 4]. The magnocellular neurons are located in the paraventricular and supraoptic nuclei of the hypothalamus. These neurons are primarily responsible for the production of the hormones oxytocin and arginine vasopressin (AVP) that are released from the posterior pituitary gland. Contrary to magnocellular neurons, the parvocellular neurons release both

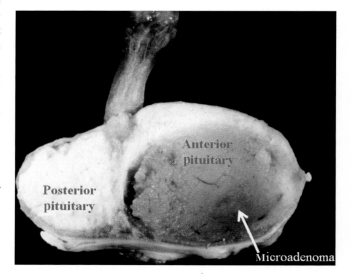

Fig. 15.1 Anatomic specimen of a pituitary gland with a microadenoma in the anterior pituitary. Note the cleft between the anterior and posterior pituitary (Courtesy of Ivan S. Ciric, M.D., FACS, Emeritus Professor of Neurosurgery, Feinberg School of Medicine, and Clinical Professor, Pritzker School of Medicine, University of Chicago)

inhibitory and releasing neurohormones [corticotropin-releasing hormone (CRH), luteinizing hormone-releasing hormone (LHRH), somatostatin (SS), dopamine (DA), thyroid-releasing hormone (TRH), growth hormone-releasing hormone (GHRH)] that interact with the anterior pituitary gland [2, 4].

An intricate capillary system allows for the transport of neurohormones from the hypothalamus to the anterior pituitary gland. The middle, inferior, and superior hypophyseal arteries are primarily responsible for providing blood supply to the posterior pituitary gland. There are venous connections between both the anterior and posterior glands that allow for neuropeptides to cross to the adjacent gland [4, 5].

The posterior pituitary gland is an extension of the hypothalamus and as previously stated secretes both AVP and oxytocin. Release of these hormones is caused by the influx of calcium through voltage-gated channels. AVP primarily targets the collecting ducts of the kidney as well as smooth muscle cells and is responsible for both increasing water permeability and vasoconstriction. Oxytocin acts on the uterus and mammary epithelial cells and is responsible for uterine contraction and breast milk release [4].

While the posterior pituitary gland releases only two primary hormones, the anterior pituitary gland releases several hormones to organs throughout the body. This gland is primarily responsible for the production and release of the following hormones: growth hormone (GH), adrenocorticotropic hormone (ACTH), thyroid-stimulating hormone (TSH), luteinizing hormone (LH), follicle-stimulating hormone (FSH), and prolactin (PRL). Growth hormone is primarily an anabolic hormone that participates in the growth of muscle and bone. Somatostatin inhibits its release, while GHRH allows for its secretion. ACTH targets the adrenal gland and is released in response to physical and emotional stress/starvation [6]. It promotes the production of adrenocortical hormones (glucocorticoids, mineralocorticoids, and androgens) and is involved in skin coloration. These hormones may contribute to hyperglycemia as well as suppression of the inflammatory response. Thyroid-stimulating hormone stimulates the release of triiodothyronine (T3) and thyroxine (T4) by the thyroid gland. These hormones play an integral role in modulation of energy use and metabolism. In addition, they are vital for promotion of regular growth and development. Negative feedback of both TRH and TSH is controlled by thyroid hormones produced by the thyroid gland [7].

Sex hormones produced by the anterior pituitary gland include LH, FSH, and PRL. Luteinizing hormone stimulates androgen production in men and mediates androgen production by the ovary in women. Follicle-stimulating hormone in combination with testosterone aids in the production of sperm in men, while FSH promotes aromatization of androgens to estrogens in women. Prolactin is released in a diurnal fashion and is a stress hormone. Prolactin may also have immune-boosting capabilities as evidenced by the presence of PRL receptors on human B and T lymphocyte [7] (Table 15.1).

Pathophysiology of the HPA

Indirect or direct injury to the central nervous system (CNS) can have profound effects on the integrity of the endocrine system. Central nervous system dysfunction may be responsible for inadequate release, production, or inhibition of secretory hormones. Hypopituitarism results in either partial or complete reduction in anterior pituitary hormone secretion resulting from either pituitary or hypothalamic dysfunction. In a systematic review, all-cause mortality from hypopituitarism was significantly increased by a factor of 1.3–2.2 times compared with age-/sex-matched controls [8]. A recent retrospective study suggested that hypopituitarism was associated with an increase in cardiovascular-, respiratory-, or cerebrovascular-related death by between 1.44 and 2.44 times in age-matched controls [9]. It remains very difficult to identify definitive risk factors for hypopituitarism due to the heterogenous causes involved. While the incidence (12–42 new cases per million per year) and prevalence (300–455 per million) are rare, hypopituitarism is likely underestimated, particularly in neurocritical care patients [10].

Etiology

There are multiple causes of hypopituitarism with some more frequently encountered in the NICU. Causes of hypopituitarism can be divided into the following categories: congenital (isolated vs. multiple pituitary hormone deficits), pituitary/peripituitary tumors (nonfunctioning and functioning pituitary adenomas), infiltrative conditions (sarcoid, histiocytosis X, lymphocytic hypophysitis, and primary hemochromatosis), infectious (tuberculosis, syphilis, mycoses), and head injury/vascular (pituitary apoplexy, aneurysms, SAH) [11].

Brain injury may account for upward of 70 % of cases of hypopituitarism with these cases frequently underreported and underrecognized [10]. Clinical features depend on the magnitude and type of hormone deficiency. Symptoms and signs such as fatigue, hypotension, cold intolerance, or infertility are often nonspecific and are likely to be missed by clinicians. Special consideration of hypopituitarism is recommended for those patients with severe TBI, severe SAH, basilar skull fractures, diffuse axonal injury, and increased intracranial pressure and those who have a prolonged length of stay in the NICU [12]. The amount of intracerebral blood and/or cerebral edema has been associated with an increased

Table 15.1 Endocrine glands and action of the primary hormones

Gland	Hormone	Action
Posterior pituitary	Oxytocin	Uterine smooth muscle contraction, milk expulsion (mammary glands)
	Antidiuretic hormone(ADH)	Vasoconstrictor
		Increases renal water reabsorption
Anterior pituitary	Thyroid-stimulating hormone (TSH)	Stimulates release of T3 and T4 by thyroid gland
	Adrenocorticotropic hormone (ACTH)	Involved in synthesis of glucocorticoids and mineralocorticoids and androgens, redistributes body energy in response to stress/starvation
	Prolactin	Growth of breasts
		Lactogenesis
	Luteinizing hormone (LH)	Promotes testosterone secretion and spermatogenesis in men
		Promotes ovulation and estrogen release in females
	Follicle-stimulating hormone (FH)	Spermatogenesis in men
		Promotes follicular growth/egg development in women
Thyroid gland	Thyroxine/triiodothyronine	Augments metabolic rate
		Temperature regulation
		Increases O_2 consumption
Adrenal cortex	Mineralocorticoids	Increases sodium/water renal reabsorption, facilitates renal potassium excretion
	Glucocorticoids	Increases blood glucose level
		Suppresses inflammation
	Androgens	Precursor to testosterone
		Secondary sexual characteristic development
Gland	Hormone	Action
Pancreatic islet cells	Insulin	Reduces serum glucose
		Drives glucose into cells
		Stimulates protein synthesis and storage of glycogen and fat
	Glucagon	Increases serum glucose
		Increases lipolysis
		Enhances hepatic glucose production and glycogenolysis
	Somatostatin	Inhibits release of insulin, glucagon, and some GI hormones
Ovary	Estrogen	Promotes growth/development of female sex organs
	Progesterone	Stimulates development/differentiation of sex organs

risk for hypopituitarism [12]. In addition, interruption of the hypothalamo-hypophyseal portal blood supply secondary to trauma may result in anterior pituitary dysfunction [12].

Symptomatology and Diagnosis

Clinical features of hypopituitarism depend on the underlying pathology, rapidity of onset, and severity. Compression lesions that are responsible for producing hypopituitarism usually cause visual abnormalities and headache. Less commonly, cerebrospinal rhinorrhea, temporal lobe epilepsy, and changes in personality can be seen with space occupying lesion-induced hypopituitarism [10].

Pituitary secreting tumors are often responsible for symptoms secondary to excessive production and/or profound deficiency in a variety of hormones. For instance, patients with PRL-secreting adenomas often present with hypogonadism because high levels of PRL inhibit FSH and LH. A patient with a GH-secreting tumor may develop both

acromegaly and hypogonadism, which is a combination of symptoms associated with hormone excess and deficiency. These mixed pictures make it challenging for clinicians to appropriately diagnose the underlying pathology [10].

Appropriate diagnosis of the cause of hypopituitarism may require a combination of a complete history, careful clinical examination, biochemical studies, and imaging. Physical examination should include a visual field assessment as pituitary adenomas may be associated with visual defects (i.e., double vision or field cuts) [10]. Magnetic resonance imaging (MRI) plays an important role in discovering any type of mass lesion in the hypothalamus or pituitary gland. Computer tomography with contrast is an adequate alternative in most cases when an MRI is unobtainable or contraindicated [10].

Basal serum hormonal measurements should include TSH, thyroxine (T4), triiodothyronine (T3), FSH, LH, estradiol, testosterone, PRL, insulin-like growth factor 1, and a 9:00 a.m. cortisol [10]. More advanced testing is required to assess GH secretion and ACTH-adrenal axis-related problems. Table 15.2

Table 15.2 Clinical features/tests for hypopituitarism

Hormone deficiency	Symptomatology	Testing
TSH	Fatigue, apathy, cold intolerance, weight gain, dry skin, psychomotor retardation, constipation	Decreased serum free/total T4+ inappropriately normal or low TSH
ACTH	Fatigue, weakness, anorexia, weight loss, nausea, vomiting, hypoglycemia, hemodynamic compromise	Basal 9 a.m. cortisol <100 nmol/ or >400–500 nmol/L
		Requires provocative test: insulin tolerance test (ITT): cortisol level >500 nmol/L with normal ACTH
GH	Decreased muscle mass, strength, energy	ITT (gold standard): severe deficiency when peak GH response <3 μg/L
	Increased central adiposity	Alternative tests: GHRH + arginine test
	Impaired thermogenesis	Glucagon stim. test
	Decreased sweating	
ADH	Polyuria, polydipsia, nocturia	Diabetes insipidus: large urine volumes >3 L/day or low osmolality <300 mOsmol/kg
		8-h water deprivation test with administration of desmopressin
Prolactin	Inability to breast-feed	NA
Gonadotropins	Men: decrease muscle mass, erythropoiesis, energy, vitality, erectile dysfunction, soft testes	Low serum testosterone with normal or low gonadotropin levels in men and low estradiol levels in premenopausal women without appropriate increased gonadotropins
	Females: dyspareunia, breast atrophy, amenorrhea/oligomenorrhea	Postmenopausal women: absence of normal increase in gonadotropins
	Both sexes: infertility, loss of libido, flushes	

depicts the clinical features and tests of the main hormone deficiencies seen in hypopituitarism. The following tests may lead to the diagnosis of other rare causes of hypopituitarism: serum and cerebrospinal fluid angiotensin-converting enzyme (sarcoid), serum ferritin (hemochromatosis), and serum human chorionic gonadotropin (germ cell tumors) [10].

Management

An in-depth discussion of the management of all hormone deficiencies is beyond the scope of this chapter. However, the general treatment of hypopituitarism is predicated on hormone replacement therapies and surgical interventions that target the underlying focused pathophysiology. For instance, while prolactinomas are usually medically treated with dopamine agonists, it may be preferable to remove a GH adenoma because of the high surgical cure rates [10]. Surgical resection is also preferred for most compression lesions [10].

The primary goal of hormone replacement therapy is to reestablish normal levels of secretory hormones that are deficient. An expedient return to hormonal homeostasis may reduce the likelihood of adverse effects associated with over- and undertreatment. For instance, patients with GH deficiency may be placed on a nighttime subcutaneous dose of GH [10]. Exogenous replacement of GH may improve bone and mineral density, exercise capabilities, strength, and hyperlipidemia [10]. Similarly, patients with ACTH deficiency may require hydrocortisone to prevent life-threatening effects of adrenal insufficiency. An 8-h serum daytime

cortisol curve can be obtained to diagnose over-/undertreatment [10]. Unlike ACTH deficiency, TSH deficiency is primarily monitored by clinical improvement. The treatment of choice is thyroxine. Coupled with clinical examination, a serum free T4 level is monitored to keep levels within the normal range. Overtreatment may result in atrial fibrillation or other tachydysrhythmias [10].

Gonadotropin deficiency requires sex hormone replacement specific to men and women. For example, testosterone replacement in men given by the intramuscular, buccal, or transdermal patch or gel route can have profound beneficial effects on body composition, behavior, and sexual function [10].Testosterone levels and resolving symptomatology are the primary monitoring modalities utilized to gauge the administration of appropriate therapy. In women, estrogen replacement mitigates the symptoms involved with this deficiency and aids in improving bone integrity. However, close monitoring for cardiovascular pathology and breast cancer is warranted in all patients who require long-term estrogen/progesterone therapy [10].

Neuroendocrine Stress Response in Critical Illness

Dysglycemia in the Neurointensive Care Unit

Almost 13 % of adult Americans have diabetes mellitus. Forty percent of these individuals are unaware that they have diabetes [13]. Further stress-induced glucose variability, hyperglycemia, and hypoglycemia occur frequently in the neurointensive care patient. Hypoglycemia occurs in the presence or absence of infused insulin or known diabetes. Glucose management in the ICU remains a controversial topic for various patient populations including those with or without diabetes, neurologic and trauma patients, and post-surgical and neurosurgical patients. Concerns about poor wound healing and infection were initially the major driving forces in the call for increasingly "tight" control of glucose and euglycemia. Recent studies including the multinational NICE-SUGAR Trial reported that aggressive insulin therapy may lead to increased morbidity and mortality [14]. A possible mechanism may be related in part to the increased incidence of hypoglycemia when tight glycemic control protocols are universally applied [14, 15].

The optimal level of glucose control in the neurologic or neurosurgical patient is even more concerning given the challenges in measuring glucose and glucose metabolites in the injured brain. Subarachnoid hemorrhage, TBI, or stroke may result in changes in the brain and blood–brain barrier (BBB) that alter normal glucose availability to neurons. After initial neurologic insult or neurosurgical intervention, the goal of neurointensive care is to salvage the area of brain tissue surrounding the injury that is still viable. Hypoglycemia is detrimental to neuronal survival and overall outcome after brain injury [16]. Injured brain tissue and the surrounding penumbra develop abnormal glucose transport through the damaged BBB. Hyperglycemia in ischemic brain tissue is also detrimental and results in increased anaerobic metabolism and increased lactate production with exacerbation of local acidosis.

Using arterial-jugular differences in oxygen and glucose in separate studies, Holbein and Vespa demonstrated that higher arterial blood glucose levels may be associated with a lower oxygen extraction ratio (OER) [16, 17]. However, Abate and colleagues, using positron electron transmission (PET), demonstrated that in some cases a higher glucose metabolism is associated with a higher OER [18].The mechanisms of these changes are unclear. Although high glucose metabolism with a high OER could be attributed to ischemic hyperglycolysis, other compensatory responses to injury could also be responsible. For example, upregulation in the neuronal cell glucose transporter 3 (GLUT3) protein, which occurs after severe TBI, facilitates increased neuronal uptake of glucose and may help explain Abate's findings. However, as Holbein and colleagues point out in their discussion, downregulation of the GLUT1 transporter in the damaged BBB after severe TBI has been shown to decrease endothelial flux of glucose even at higher arterial blood glucose levels, thereby leading to reduced cerebral glucose availability despite an adequate arterial supply [17]. This would result in an increase in lactate production and decrease in intracellular pH with cellular distress, which results in impaired metabolic

activity and possibly adverse outcome. Thus, peripheral arterial and venous glucose sampling do not accurately represent levels of glucose in the injured brain. The evolving use of brain microdialysis allows detection of glucose levels at the site of injury and in the future may guide therapeutic measures to adjust the supply of glucose delivery to the injured brain [16, 17].

The citric acid cycle (Krebs cycle) is the predominant glucose-mediated method to generate cellular energy. In aerobic conditions a fully metabolized glucose molecule results in 30–32 molecules of ATP. When oxygen levels are depleted, cells convert to anaerobic metabolism and glucose is metabolized to pyruvate generating only 2 molecules of ATP. During ischemia the levels of ATP decrease from the oxygen-dependent citric acid cycle. An increase in anaerobic metabolism occurs as brain cells attempt to compensate for the loss of ATP production from the citric acid cycle. During this process, it is necessary to generate NAD+ from NADH by converting pyruvate to lactate. This causes an increase in lactate and decrease in pyruvate leading to an increased lactate/pyruvate ratio (LPR).

Because of the importance of accurate glucose measurement in the brain and desire to maintain sufficient substrate to maintain aerobic metabolism, many neurointensive care centers are instituting microdialysis to repetitively sample the neuronal extracellular fluid via a microcatheter. Other metabolic products are measured including metabolites of energy failure such as glycerol, glutamate, lactate, and pyruvate.

The inefficiency of anaerobic glucose metabolism results in decreased blood glucose levels surrounding the area of damaged tissue. Microdialysis measurements should show further decrease of pyruvate, increased levels of lactate, and resultant increased LPR prior to the onset of ICP changes or resultant clinical symptoms. A LPR greater than 25 is considered an early warning sign of cerebral energy failure [19].

Glucose variability develops commonly in critically ill patients. The greater the degree of glucose variability, even when it develops within the normal range of peripheral glucose (70–110 mg/dL), the greater the morbidity and mortality [20]. Like the association of hypoglycemia with increased mortality, it remains open to investigation as to whether there is a cause and effect impact of hypoglycemia and glucose variability in the critically ill. Future studies are needed to determine the impact, if any, of improved CNS glucose levels and limitation in glucose variability. At present the recommendation of the American Association of Clinical Endocrinologists and American Diabetes Association is to initiate insulin therapy in critically ill patients who have a glucose >180 mg/dL with a goal of maintaining the peripheral glucose at 140–180 mg/dL [21].

Hormonal Changes During the Acute Phase of Critical Illness

Critical illness is associated with dysregulation of the hypothalamic-pituitary axis. It is important for critical care physicians to recognize the inherent hormonal changes that occur during the acute and chronic phases of critical illness in the NICU (Fig. 15.2). Table 15.3 depicts the changes in hormone levels depending on the time period during critical illness. Early diagnosis of these abnormalities may reduce associated morbidity and mortality [7].

The acute neuroendocrine changes associated with critical illness involving the somatotropic, thyroid, gonadal/lactotropic, and adrenal axes should be appreciated. The early hours to days of stress-induced injury are marked by significant GH resistance [7]. While the amount of circulating GH actually increases, the effector protein levels of insulin-like growth factor 1 (IGF-1) and GH-dependent IGF-binding proteins (IGFBPs) are markedly decreased [22]. There is also a reduction in hepatic and muscle GH receptor gene expression in the critically ill. From a survival viewpoint, inhibition of anabolism via a reduction in functional GH may be crucial in providing the body the necessary energy substrates [7].

Similar to GH, thyroid hormones are integral to the processes of metabolism and the body's use of energy. During the early phase of critical illness, plasma levels of T3 are reduced and rT3 levels are increased, due to the changed conversion of T4 [23]. This is now commonly referred to as nonthyroidal illness. Decreased levels of T3 during the first day of critical illness may indicate the severity of illness [23]. During most acute illnesses, TSH and T4 transiently rise and then return to normal levels (except in severe illness where T4 levels may be low). While TSH normalizes, low levels of T3 persist. The persistence of low T3 is referred to as the "low T3 syndrome" [22]. Other substrates such as cytokines, thyroid hormone-binding proteins, and elevated levels of free fatty acids and bilirubin may mimic the low T3 syndrome profile. The acute reduction in T3 levels may mimic the protective process that is seen during starvation. The goal of this mechanism is to reduce energy expenditure, which may also be useful during critical illness [24].

The gonadal and lactotropic axes are also affected during the acute phase of critical illness. Despite increased levels of LH, testosterone levels are reduced during acute injury [7]. The action of the body to reduce anabolism through reduction in testosterone levels may be viewed as a way to reduce the use of energy and divert energy expenditures to the most vital organ systems for survival [24]. During multiorgan failure, the body may go through a "metabolic shutdown" state where hormones contribute to a hibernation-like effect to promote subsequent recovery [25]. Unlike testosterone, PRL levels are elevated during acute critical illness. This process may be directed by cytokines, oxytocin, and/or vasoactive intestinal peptide. One hypothesis that may explain the increased levels of PRL is that it may help enhance immunity and mitigate infection [7].

Study results are variable when discussing levels of estradiol during the acute phase of critical illness. While some trials demonstrate a large increase in estrogen levels, others show that total estrogen levels are decreased [22]. Overall, estradiol levels are mostly maintained during the acute critical illness phase due to a reduction in sex hormone-binding globulin [22].

Lastly, the adrenal axis plays an integral role in the body's response to critical illness. Under normal circumstances, healthy individuals secrete cortisol via a diurnal pattern. Cortisol negatively feeds back on both CRH and ACTH [23]. However, in acute illness, the diurnal pattern of cortisol release disappears. Due to the increase release of both CRH

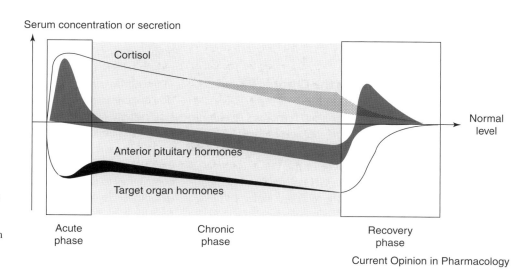

Fig. 15.2 Changes in hormones during acute and chronic phases of critical illness (Reprinted with permission of Elsevier from Vanhorebeek and Van den Berghe [22])

Serum concentration or secretion

Cortisol

Anterior pituitary hormones

Target organ hormones

Normal level

Acute phase

Chronic phase

Recovery phase

Current Opinion in Pharmacology

Table 15.3 Hormonal changes during the acute/chronic phases of critical illness

Hormone	Acute phase	Prolonged phase
Somatotropic axis		
Pulsatile GH release	↑	↓
GHBP	↓	↑
IGF-I	↓	↓↓
ALS	↓	↓↓
IGFBP-3	↓	↓↓
Thyroid axis		
Pulsatile TSH release	↑=	↓
T4	↑=	↓
T3	↓	↓↓
rT3	↑	↑=
Gonadal and lactotropic axis		
Pulsatile LH release	↑=	↓
Testosterone	↓	↓↓
Pulsatile prolactin release	↑	↓
Adrenal axis		
ACTH	↑	↓
Cortisol	↑↑	↑=↓

Reproduced with permission of Elsevier from Vanhorebeek and Van den Berghe [7]

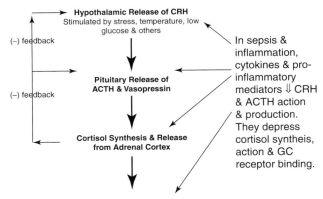

Fig. 15.3 Hypothalamic-pituitary adrenal axis. Depicts the HPA release of CRH, ACTH, and cortisol in certain patients with sepsis. *CRH* corticotropin releasing hormone, *ACTH* adrenocorticotropic hormone, *GC* glucocorticiod, *NF-KB* NF-kappaB factor, *AP-1* activator protien 1, *NO* nitric oxide, *PLA2* phospholipase A

and ACTH in acute illness, cortisol levels initially rise [22]. There is also a significant increase in free cortisol due to a reduction in the cortisol-binding globulin protein [23].While higher levels of cortisol reflect a more significant type of stress, low levels of cortisol may reflect the body's inadequate response to stress (such as in certain cases of sepsis or other inflammatory states; Fig. 15.3). Acute stress-related hypercortisolism is vital to protect critically ill patients from the inflammatory response, hemodynamic instability, and the lack of carbohydrates, fat, and protein necessary for survival during the high metabolic state of critical illness [24]. However, as discussed next, persistent hypercortisolism may be an indicator for an increase in mortality, especially among patient with septic shock [26].

Hormonal Changes During the Chronic Phase

In certain circumstances, the hormonal responses to chronic critical illness vastly differ from the acute phase [7]. For instance, the levels of IGF-1, IGFBP-3, and acid-labile subunit (ALS) are substantially lower in the chronic phase of critical illness [22]. However, the GH resistance of acute illness is somewhat reversed in the chronic state. Evidence from studies suggests that GH secretagogues can increase IGF-1 and IGFBP levels during the chronic phase of critical illness [7]. These data support the notion that GH resistance is partially corrected [7]. A deficiency originating from the

hypothalamus or an inactivity of endogenous GHRP-like GH secretagogues is the likely etiology of hyposomatotropism [7]. There may also be a reduction in somatostatin activity. Lack of pulsatile GH release may explain the development of the wasting syndrome during chronic critical illness [23]. Observational studies suggest that the GH axis is more suppressed in men than women. It remains to be proven, whether this hypothesis is a reasonable explanation for a higher risk of poor outcomes associated with endocrinologic abnormalities in men versus women [7].

Pulsatile TSH secretion is also markedly reduced during prolonged critical illness [7]. This reduction in TSH results in low serum levels of both T4 and T3 [22]. The following hypotheses may explain the reduction in TSH: changed set point for negative feedback, elevated somatostatin levels, reduced TRH-induced stimulation of TSH, and a reduction in the ability of thyrotropes to produce TSH [7]. The reduction of gene expression of TRH seen in studies of chronically sick patients who subsequently died may account for the primary mechanism of reduced TSH levels [22].

The chronic phase of critical illness also alters the peripheral metabolism of the thyroid hormone. This phenomenon contributes to the low T3 syndrome [22]. The enzyme type 1 deiodinase is also reduced and, therefore, contributes to a reduction in peripheral conversion of T4 to T3, the most active form of circulating thyroid hormone [7]. The combination of TRH with GHRP-2 may facilitate increases in serum levels of TSH, T4, and T3 [24]. This demonstrates the interrelationship between the thyroid and somatotropic axes. Low levels of TSH, T4, and T3 coupled with higher rT3 levels may indicate a poor overall prognosis in critically ill patients with prolonged illness [24].

Similar to the thyroid axis, the gonadal and lactotropic axes are also profoundly depressed during chronic illness [7]. Serum levels of testosterone become nearly undetectable due to suppressed LH levels and release [22].While total estradiol concentrations are low, free estradiol levels are relatively maintained due to a reduction in sex hormone-binding globulin [22]. Prolactin secretion is reduced to a greater degree during chronic illness versus the acute phase [7]. Reduced PRL secretion may contribute to an increased risk of infection or other morbidities. Drugs, such as dopamine, may further suppress PRL secretion and, therefore, contribute to further immunosuppression [7]. Unlike sex hormones, cortisol levels remain elevated in the chronically ill [7, 24]. Cortisol-binding globulin also returns to near-normal levels during chronic illness [22]. Hypercortisolism may be responsible for an increased risk of infection during the chronic phase of critical illness. Therefore, elevation in cortisol does not seem to be universally helpful in maintaining survival [22].

Endocrine Issues in Specific Neuropathologies

Stroke

Globally, stroke is a leading cause of morbidity and mortality. Stroke or cerebral vascular accidents (CVAs) are the number three cause of death in the United States. Eighty to eight five percent of CVAs are thrombotic or embolic events that disrupt cerebral blood flow to affected areas of the brain and cause ischemic damage to neural tissue. The remaining fifteen to twenty percent of CVAs are hemorrhagic strokes from either intracerebral hemorrhage (ICH), usually due to uncontrolled hypertension, or SAH. The incidence of hemorrhagic strokes is evenly divided between ICH and SAH [27]. Embolic/thrombotic strokes and hemorrhagic strokes each have associated neuroendocrine pathology [27].

Subarachnoid Hemorrhage

Subarachnoid hemorrhages can arise from trauma, arteriovascular malformations, illicit drug use such as cocaine and amphetamines, vasculitides, and abnormal bleeding disorders. The most common cause of SAH is due to ruptured saccular aneurysms (aSAH) from weakened cerebral arterial vasculature [28].

The prevalence of aSAH is five percent, or 10–15 million Americans [29]. Most SAHs occur between the ages of 40 and 60 years. Approximately ten percent of patients with SAH die before reaching the hospital [29]. Over sixty percent

of the remaining SAH patients have high morbidity and disablement [30, 31]. Mortality of treated patients is approximately 50 % in the first 30 days. The high mortality and morbidity associated with a SAH is due to complications in the 15 days after the aneurysm has been secured by either surgery or angiography. The most dreaded complications of a SAH are continued bleeding and vasospasm [32, 33].

Aneurysms occur in weakened cerebral arteries due to risk factors including cigarette smoking, hypertension, moderate to heavy alcohol use, family history of aneurysms, and genetic factors including autosomal dominant polycystic kidney disease, glucocorticoid-remediable aldosteronism, and Ehlers-Danlos syndrome. Other etiologies include over-the-counter sympathomimetic drugs, estrogen deficiency, antithrombotic therapy, and prior to antithrombotic [34].

Subarachnoid hemorrhage is a known risk factor for neuroendocrine dysfunction acutely as well as in long-term survivors. The most common endocrine abnormality following SAH is hypopituitarism particularly resulting in deficiency of growth hormone (GH) and corticotropin (CRF). One study of 60 patients with spontaneous SAH found that 56.9 % of patients developed at least one anterior pituitary hormone deficiency within 72 h of insult. Gonadotropin and GH secretion failure were the most prominent at 33.3 and 22.0 %, respectively. ACTH and TSH deficiencies were less frequent at 7.1 and 1.8 %, respectively [34].

Ischemic Stroke

Endocrine dysfunction can occur in all types of CVAs in both the acute and chronic phase of the disease process. Pituitary and hypothalamic strokes, although rare, obviously cause the greatest dysfunction. In these cases, panhypopituitarism is common with minimal recovery [35]. Elevated levels of primarily endothelin-1, AVP, and cortisol seen in acute stroke patients may be implicated in exacerbating neurologic deficits and may contribute to worse outcomes. The possible mechanisms that have been proposed include direct neural toxicity, vasoconstriction of blood vessels thereby reducing blood flow, and promotion of brain edema. Lastly, the abnormal leptin secretion observed during stroke may lead to the poor nutritional status among stroke patients. Further studies are required to elucidate the importance of endocrine dysfunction in overall outcome of patients suffering from stroke [35].

Traumatic Brain Injury and Adrenal Insufficiency

Although TBI most often causes growth hormone and/or gonadotropin deficiency, acute symptomatic and asymptomatic ACTH deficiency have been reported to occur in 8 % of patients with severe TBI. Common clinical symptoms consistent with adrenal insufficiency include nausea, vomiting, hyperpigmentation, fever, abdominal pain, hypo-volemia, hypotension, and shock. In neurointensive care patients in shock, adrenal crisis usually presents with hypotension refractory to vasopressors or volume resuscitation. Laboratory findings consistent with adrenal insufficiency include hypoglycemia, hyponatremia, hyperkalemia, azotemia, hypercalcemia, and eosinophilia. Although high-dose methylprednisolone treatment in TBI has been shown to be detrimental to outcome (CRASH), in patients with hemodynamic instability, treatment with low-dose (physiologic replacement, based on degree of stress) glucocorticoid supplementation may be necessary for the first few days after TBI [36]. Prior assessment of adrenal function by cosyntropin stimulation testing would be prudent [37, 38].

Chronic hypopituitarism requiring hormone replacement occurs in 20 % of TBI patients, while mild hormonal deficits occur in 30 % of patients after mild, moderate, or severe TBI. These data suggest the importance of long-term follow-up testing for hormonal deficiencies in patients 6 months after recovering from TBI [39]. Finally, even though TBI-associated pituitary dysfunction is most often suspected after automobile crashes or falls, recent studies show repeated concussions such as in explosions and aggressive sports activity can lead to panhypopituitarism [40].

Progressive Neurologic Disease: Guillain-Barré Syndrome

Guillain-Barré syndrome (GBS) or Landry-Guillain-Barré syndrome is a peripheral nerve disease that is one of the most common causes of acute, progressive weakness. Guillain, Barré, and Strohl described this syndrome in 1916, and it was traditionally viewed as an acute inflammatory demyelinating polyradiculoneuropathy (AIDP). The onset of GBS is commonly preceded by a viral illness by about 2 weeks, although it has also been associated with *Campylobacter jejuni* enteritis [41], surgery, immunization, Hodgkin's disease, and systemic lupus erythematosus [42].

Patients with GBS may present with weakness and paresthesias located in the fingers or toes, which may progress proximally into the limbs within a few days. Additional symptoms may include weakness of facial and pharyngeal muscles and pain in the lower half of the body. The height of severe pain occurs within the first 1–3 weeks of presentation and persists for a few weeks before resolution over the next few months. Less severe GBS forms may only present with mild weakness, but the duration may extend for several months [42].

Autonomic dysfunction may affect 50 % of all patients who suffer from GBS [42]. Autonomic dysfunction may present as sympathetic and parasympathetic nervous system escalation or deficiency, arrhythmias, hypertension, ileus, and/or incontinence [42].

The diagnostic work-up of AIDP may include analysis of cerebral spinal fluid (CSF), nerve conduction studies, a complete blood count (CBC), and an electrolyte panel. Cerebrospinal fluid analysis typically reveals elevated protein in the absence of pleocytosis, termed albuminocytological dissociation. CSF abnormalities may not appear for up to 1 week after onset. Evaluation of nerve conduction shows slowing of nerve conduction velocity, even blockage of conduction, while evaluation of axonal variants will reveal low amplitudes and normal velocities [43]. The CBC is usually unchanged, while serum electrolytes may demonstrate hyponatremia from SIADH [44, 45].

The management of patients with GBS will involve the evaluation of respiratory function, the need for intubation, anticipation and treatment of autonomic dysfunction, and consideration for specific treatment, including intravenous immunoglobulin (IVIG) and plasmapheresis/plasma exchange. Patients with progressive weakness will require close respiratory monitoring and pulmonary toilet, with the need for intubation determined by the ability to protect the airway, adequacy of self-management of secretions, and/or risk for hypoventilation. Factors that may be associated with the need for mechanical ventilation include less than 7 days from onset of symptoms to admission, inability to lift the head, and a vital capacity less than 1–1.5 L coupled with the rapidity at which the vital capacity drops [46]. Clinicians should evaluate patient respiratory muscle strength and pulmonary function prior to weaning these patients from the ventilator. Duration of intubation is variable, and tracheostomy may not be required in a small percentage of patients [47]. Typical ICU care should be performed on patients with GBS including prophylaxis for deep vein thrombosis, monitoring for pressure sores, and providing appropriate pain relief.

The standard treatment for progressive GBS is either pheresis/exchange or IVIG. Plasmapheresis is recommended in patients with severe symptoms, including inability to walk, respiratory failure or distress, or bulbar muscle weakness [48, 49]. It may also be utilized for patients with milder symptoms. Although pheresis/exchange is the gold standard for treatment, IVIG has been demonstrated as being at least as equally effective in treatment of GBS [50]. Corticosteroids are neither effective nor recommended in reversal of weakness in GBS.

Endocrine Abnormalities and Guillain-Barré Syndrome

GBS has been associated with numerous endocrine disturbances, specifically the syndrome of inappropriate antidiuretic hormone secretion (SIADH), diabetes insipidus (DI), Hashimoto's thyroiditis, and elevated serum cortisol levels. There are no specific associations between GBS and the somatotropic or gonadal axis.

Albeit rare, GBS has been associated with other autoimmune disorders, including Hashimoto's thyroiditis (HT). HT is an autoimmune disorder characterized by antibodies against thyroid peroxidase and thyroglobulin resulting in antibody-mediated destruction of the thyroid gland follicles. This results in hypothyroidism due to depletion of the thyroid gland follicles. The association with GBS has been described in case reports since 1975 [51, 52]. The mechanism of association is poorly understood but may be due to a common autoimmune pathway [51, 52]. Often times, serum cortisol concentrations are elevated during acute stress. Stress-induced hypercortisolism may be the mechanism by which GBS patients are observed to have elevated cortisol levels. However, while elevated cortisol and catecholamine levels have been discussed in the literature for decades [53], the exact mechanism remains unclear. Even in the early description of elevated cortisol levels during GBS, it was appreciated that cortisol levels increased as the disease progressed and then normalized as the symptoms of GBS improved [53, 54]. Elevated cortisol levels at presentation can be predictive of requiring mechanical ventilation and developing dysautonomia [55]. One proposed mechanism of cortisol escalation implicates cytokines promoting steroidogenesis [54]. Serum levels of transforming growth factor beta 1 (TGF-β1) and tumor necrosis factor alpha (TNF-α) may be related to the severity of GBS in patients (i.e., TGF-β1 levels decrease and TNF-α increases as motor strength worsens, while TGF-β1 levels increase and TNF-α levels decrease as the weakness improves) [54]. Since TGF-β1 inhibits and TNF-α activates steroidogenesis, cortisol levels may correlate with the severity of weakness during GBS [54]. Some of the early approaches to treatment and immunomodulation of GBS included corticotropin and cortisol injections [53]. While these treatment modalities initially demonstrated favorable results in case reports, a recent meta-analysis of six trials showed no benefit of corticosteroid therapy in the management of GBS [50]. Therefore, specific treatment for hypercortisolism may not be necessary, as levels appear to quickly improve with resolution of the underlying illness [53, 54].

Disturbances in AVP may also be seen in patients with GBS. Inappropriately elevated activity of AVP, as it occurs in various disease states, is termed SIADH and results from excessive free water retention and hyponatremia. On the other hand, diabetes insipidus (DI) results from insufficient levels or response to AVP and may lead to hypernatremia and hypovolemia. The incidence of SIADH in patients with GBS is 26–48 % [44, 56, 57]. Contrary to SIADH, DI rarely occurs in patients with GBS [58, 59]. Symptoms of moderate hyponatremia (serum sodium <130 mEq/L) include confusion, mental status changes, cramping, and weakness, whereas more severe hyponatremia (Na <115 mEq/L) may result in seizures or even coma. Without recognizing that acute rapid development of hyponatremia associated with

SIADH can occur in conjunction with GBS, clinicians may fail to make a timely diagnosis of GBS [44].

The mechanism for hyponatremia and SIADH in GBS is poorly understood but likely multifactorial. In one case report, suppression of AVP release did not result in an expected diuretic response, suggesting that the cause of SIADH may not be directly due to excessive secretion of AVP [60]. In this case, a source of AVP may be located outside the hypothalamus or pituitary glands, a mechanism independent of AVP, or due to aberrant renal sensitivity to AVP. SIADH may develop at any point in the course of GBS. In one case series of patients, hyponatremia occurred in 46 % of patients *after* initiation of IVIG therapy [56]. This suggests that pseudohyponatremia associated with IVIG therapy may be an additional cause of hyponatremia in GBS. The mechanism for the hyponatremia associated with IVIG administration is likely due to increased serum viscosity due to hyperproteinemia and pseudohyponatremia, rather than direct AVP activity [61].

Concomitant SIADH with GBS may complicate the diagnosis and delay treatment of GBS and has been associated with a higher mortality in patients with GBS [57]. Initial symptoms of weakness may be attributed to hyponatremia and may delay appreciation of an independent cause of weakness. Specific risks for SIADH in GBS include the need for mechanical ventilation and bulbar weakness [57]. Furthermore, IVIG therapy may worsen an already present hyponatremia [61]. Therefore, the intensivist needs to anticipate and remain vigilant for changes in serum sodium levels throughout the course of GBS.

SIADH is often secondary to an underlying process, and reversal of the cause will eventually allow resolution of the SIADH and associated hyponatremia. With mild to moderate hyponatremia (Na >120 mEq/L), appropriate therapy may be limited to treatment of the underlying causative disorder and fluid restriction. Worsening or symptomatic hyponatremia often can be treated with hypertonic saline or a vasopressin receptor antagonist, such as conivaptan or tolvaptan, in order to reduce the retention of water from the renal collecting ducts. These drugs target the V2 vasopressin receptor in the kidneys in order to reduce fluid retention and correct hyponatremia. With symptomatic hyponatremia, sodium correction needs to be corrected deliberately, albeit slowly and in a controlled manner. The rate of correction may be limited to 10–12 mEq/L per 24 h, as an excessively rapid correction may result in central pontine myelinolysis [62].

Endocrine Abnormalities in Meningitis/Encephalitis

While relatively uncommon, CNS infections may be associated with endocrine abnormalities both independent of and in conjunction with critical illness. Some of the major central nervous system (CNS) infections include meningitis and encephalitis. Meningitis refers to leptomeningeal inflammation with symptoms of neck stiffness, headache, and photophobia. Diagnosis of meningitis is largely dependent on a combination of suspicious symptomatology and CSF analysis. Purulent CSF due to bacterial meningitis is usually associated with an elevated white blood cell count (WBC), a depressed glucose concentration, and an elevated protein concentration. Encephalitis may also be diagnosed by utilizing a combination of existing neurologic deficits and abnormalities in CSF analysis. Viral encephalitis may present with a similar CSF analysis as aseptic meningitis (i.e., mildly elevated WBC, mildly depressed glucose concentration, and normal to mildly elevated protein concentration).

Several pathogens that cause meningitis and encephalitis may cause endocrine abnormalities. Some of the more common pathogens that are associated with adult bacterial meningitis are *Streptococcus pneumoniae* and *Neisseria meningitidis*. *Mycobacterium tuberculosis* is an uncommon cause of bacterial meningitis but is classically associated with inducing hypopituitarism [63].

As opposed to bacterial meningitis, encephalitis is a less common infection associated with inflammation. The severity of encephalitis can be mild and self-limiting or even life threatening. Computer tomography scanning and an MRI may demonstrate temporal lobe encephalitis associated with herpes simplex encephalitis (HSE) [64]. CSF analysis with PCR evaluation for herpes simplex virus (HSV) DNA can confirm the diagnosis. Nonviral causes of encephalitis, such as Lyme disease, neurosyphilis, Rocky Mountain spotted fever, or toxoplasmic encephalitis, require specific diagnostic testing.

Management of these infectious processes as discussed elsewhere in this book (Chap. 22) requires prompt initiation of antimicrobial therapy. CSF gram stain and culture results can help guide therapy, although antibiotics and steroids, if indicated, should not be delayed in order to perform a timely lumbar puncture. Initial antimicrobial therapy needs to include agents that cross the blood–brain barrier and provide adequate coverage of likely pathogens, typically third-generation cephalosporins or meropenem, and the addition of vancomycin in the case of resistant pneumococci. Ampicillin should be included in the regimen if *Listeria* is a potential causative agent. A 2007 Cochrane review of adjuvant corticosteroids in patients with acute bacterial meningitis suggested that corticosteroids reduce the risk of death and short-term neurologic deficits in adults and severe hearing loss in children [65]. Additional supportive measures, such as anticonvulsant therapy, prevention of aspiration and protection of the airway, and control of the source of the infection, should also be considered for the management of these patients.

The specific endocrine derangements associated with CNS infections are poorly studied. CNS infection-related endocrine abnormalities may be coincidental during the presence or treatment of a primary intracranial mass or hormone-secreting tumor. A small prospective study of sixteen noncritically ill adults with acute meningitis suggested that 31.25 % of patients analyzed had acute pituitary abnormalities within the first 24 h of admission, and 44 % of the patients demonstrated low T3 syndrome [66]. Additionally, chronic pituitary sequelae at 12 months were observed in 31.25 % of the same patient population [66]. Concurrent head CT or MRI of patients with bacterial or viral infections do not demonstrate consistent anatomic abnormalities of the hypothalamus or pituitary gland [67, 68]. In a retrospective study of 49 patients with tuberculous meningitis, an MRI was performed in 10 patients with endocrine abnormalities and enhancing tissue was discovered in 2 patients with GH deficiency [48, 63]. One patient was found to have nodular lesions in the suprasellar, basal, and interhemispheric cisterns, but the MRI of the other patient demonstrated only enhancing tissue in the hypothalamus [68].

After resolution of acute meningitis, and up to 4 years after infection, GH deficiency can also be observed in approximately 28 % of patients [68]. In another study of noncritically ill patients with meningitis, acute somatotropic deficiency occurred in approximately 20 % of patients, while chronic deficiency of GH was less common [66]. One retrospective study that included patients who developed tuberculous meningitis during childhood suggested that the most common endocrine abnormality was GH deficiency [67]. Short stature occurred in those patients who developed GH deficiency prior to a growth spurt, without appropriate administration of hormonal therapy. The mechanism of GH deficiency is not well understood, although the presence of enhancing tissue on MRI in the area of the hypothalamus in two patients with a history of tuberculous meningitis may suggest a hypothalamic cause of GH deficiency [4].

Thyroid hormone abnormalities can also be seen in patients with CNS infections. In patients with acute meningitis that are not critically ill, low T3 syndrome has been demonstrated in a significant portion of patients on admission [66]. Fortunately, low T3 syndrome resolves over time and does not appear to lead to chronic thyroid hormone deficiency. Abnormal TSH and free T4 levels are not easily demonstrated in patients with meningitis, suggesting a primary lack of pituitary or thyroid gland dysfunction in meningitis [63].

Deficiencies in sex hormones secondary to abnormal pituitary function are also observed in patients with meningitis [63, 66]. While these gonadotropic derangements are seen in the acute phase of meningitis, gonadotropic dysfunction appears to resolve over time or results in mild deficiency [67]. In patients with chronic gonadotropin deficiency due to childhood tuberculous meningitis, the cause of gonadotropic deficiency may originate in the pituitary gland or hypothalamus, rather than from a peripheral insensitivity to GH [63]. Abnormal (PRL) levels sporadically occur in the acute phase of meningitis but chronic hyperprolactinemia after meningitis has not been described [66, 69, 70].

Adrenal insufficiency (AI) has received significant attention in the setting of critical illness. ACTH deficiency appears later after resolution of meningitis in 21–25 % of patients [66, 67]. The decrease in ACTH may be due to decreased corticotropin-releasing hormone from the hypothalamus, which may result in AI [63].

The reversibility of endocrine abnormalities due to CNS infection depends on the underlying endocrine abnormality and concomitant control and treatment of the underlying infection. Some endocrine sequelae, such as low T3, are self-limited and should not require treatment except in extreme circumstances with symptoms due to hypothyroidism. On the other hand, acute symptoms of growth hormone deficiency may not be apparent, and so replacement therapy, especially in those patients with tuberculous meningitis, may be initiated to prevent growth retardation [71]. Gonadotropin deficiencies observed in patients with CNS infections may be treated with administration and monitoring of testosterone in men and estradiol and progesterone in women. CNS infection associated ACTH deficiency may be treated with initial doses of hydrocortisone and then longer-acting steroids for chronic administration. These patients may be prone to Addisonian crisis. Therefore, they may require additional steroids during periods of physiologic stress, due to an inability to increase cortisol or other stress hormones.

Endocrine Response in CNS and Endocrine Secreting Tumors

Pituitary Tumors

Pituitary tumors are relatively common in the general population and are a diverse group of tumors, with a frequency in the general population as high as 17–20 % [72, 73]. They are typically classified by size, as either microadenomas if less than 1 cm or macroadenomas if greater than 1 cm. Macroadenomas are less common, with an incidence of 0.16–0.2 % in the general population [72, 74]. The size may not correlate with secretory function; 40 % of patients with active Cushing's disease have normal MRI scans. Adenomas can also be differentiated by their hormonal activity (i.e., PRL-secreting tumors causing hyperprolactinemia, GH-secreting tumors causing acromegaly or gigantism, ACTH-secreting tumors causing Cushing's syndrome, and TSH-secreting tumors causing hyperthyroidism) [72]. The treatment of choice for symptomatic tumors is surgical resection, with the exception of PRL-secreting tumors. The intensivist will primarily encounter the patient with a pituitary

adenoma postoperatively, and the perioperative management involves both endocrinologic and nonendocrinologic assessment and interventions. Rarely, a pituitary adenoma may lead to hemorrhage or necrosis, leading to pituitary apoplexy. This results in a sudden increase in sellar pressure and pituitary impairment that may require immediate supportive therapy, hormone replacement, and surgical evaluation [72].

The physiology, associated symptoms, and management of a pituitary adenoma depend on its classification. A significant proportion of pituitary adenomas are hormonally active, with PRL-secreting adenomas being the most common, accounting for 26–43 % of tumors [72, 74]. Other active adenomas include GH adenomas at 3–13 % [72, 74], ACTH adenomas at 5–12 % [72, 74], LH/FSH adenomas at 1–9 %, and TSH adenomas at 0.7 % [75]. More aggressive forms of PRL-secreting tumors are typically associated with multiple endocrine neoplasia-1 (MEN-1) syndrome [62]. Men tend to present with larger tumors and associated clinical symptoms as compared to women [76]. Patients can demonstrate amenorrhea, infertility, hypogonadism, impotence, decreased libido, osteoporosis, obesity [77], and galactorrhea [78].

Evaluation of patients with PRL-secreting tumors includes a morning serum PRL level coupled with TSH and thyroid hormone levels, IGF-1 levels, serum electrolytes, and a pregnancy test [79]. Contrast-enhanced MRI is 55–90 % sensitive [80], while PRL levels may correlate with tumor size [81]. Visual acuity testing should be done with any symptomatic patient or presence of a macroadenoma. Dopamine agonists have been shown to normalize PRL levels, restore gonadal function, and reduce pituitary adenoma size [82–84]. Surgery and radiation therapy are reserved for patients unresponsive or intolerant of dopamine agonist therapy [84].

GH-secreting somatotropinomas are the next most common hormonally active pituitary adenoma [85] with 75 % occurring as macroadenomas. Signs and symptoms in adults include the following: acromegaly, tachycardia, hypertension, left ventricular hypertrophy, dysrhythmias [86, 87], obstructive sleep apnea (OSA), airway obstruction, insulin resistance, diabetes [88], polyneuropathy, and myalgias. Hypopituitarism, hyperthyroidism, and hyperprolactinemia [89] may also be seen in patients with GH-secreting tumors [90]. An evaluation of these patients consists of an oral glucose tolerance test [91], serum IGF-1 levels, thyroid hormone levels, serum PRL, and serum electrolytes [90]. An MRI can be used to detect a pituitary source of acromegaly and tumor size often correlates with GH elevation [79]. A thorough cardiac evaluation prior to surgery is essential due to an increased incidence of atherosclerosis, hypertension, and dysrhythmias. Respiratory evaluation for OSA should include a sleep study, while patients over the age of 55 years should undergo colonoscopy due to increased incidence of colorectal neoplasms with acromegaly [86–90].

Surgical therapy is the first-line treatment for GH-secreting adenomas, achieving normalization of IGF-1 and glucose tolerance in 50–60 % of patients [92, 93]. As GH-secreting adenomas may go undiagnosed for several years, there is a high likelihood of a macroadenoma that is not amenable to complete resection, and additional therapy may be necessary. Somatostatin analogue therapy is able to lower serum IGF-1 and GH levels in most patients [94], although medical therapy can reduce tumor size slightly in only about 30 % of patients [95]. Octreotide, Sandostatin LARTM (long-acting octreotide), and lanreotide have been used and typically are associated with cholelithiasis, gallbladder sludge, and diarrhea. GH receptor antagonism with pegvisomant has been demonstrated to normalize serum IGF-1 levels [96], with little evidence of increasing tumor size despite escalation of an increase in serum GH levels [96, 97]. Medical therapy is typically continued during radiation therapy in order to control serum GH and PRL levels [93–98].

Patients with ACTH-secreting tumors can initially present with symptoms of Cushing's syndrome, which include central obesity, cutaneous thinning, hypertension, osteopenia, acne, purple striae, thinning of the hair, oligomenorrhea, amenorrhea, decreased libido, impotence, muscle weakness, depression, anxiety, hyperglycemia, and headache [99]. These patients may also develop hyperglycemia, leukocytosis, and hypokalemic metabolic alkalosis [100].

Initial evaluation of patients with ACTH-secreting adenomas may include a CBC, serum electrolytes, and a 24-h urine cortisol. The urine cortisol will be significantly elevated in Cushing's syndrome [101, 102]. Coupled with an elevated urine cortisol level, an elevated ACTH level further suggests a pituitary ACTH-secreting adenoma, although ectopic foci are still possible [103]. A high-dose dexamethasone or CRH test may be performed to further delineate the source of the hormonal abnormality [79]. Inferior petrosal sinus sampling for cortisol can detect the pituitary source of ACTH [99]. MRI has been observed to detect a tumor in 62 % of patients [104]. There is no specific medical therapy to counteract ACTH hypersecretion. Therefore, control of excessive cortisol production is typically reserved for patients that do not achieve normal cortisol levels after therapy or are unable to undergo surgery or radiation. Ketoconazole has been shown to inhibit steroid synthesis [101] and has been demonstrated to control excessive cortisol levels in patients with pituitary adenomas [105]. Metyrapone and mitotane are also able to inhibit steroid synthesis [100]. Although ketoconazole is often chosen as initial medical therapy because it is well tolerated, it may cause serious hepatic side effects. Serum transaminase levels usually resolve with discontinuation of ketoconazole, but excessive doses or unrecognized toxicities have been associated with hepatic failure in rare instances. Additionally, ketoconazole can cause excessive inhibition of steroid synthesis. Therefore, serum cortisol levels should be monitored closely and the dose of ketoconazole should be titrated accordingly [100, 105].

If excessive cortisol secretion continues despite institution of medical therapies, bilateral adrenalectomy is an option for persistent symptomatic Cushing's disease [105, 106]. Laparoscopic adrenalectomy is becoming a more accepted option due to its associated reduced morbidity. With surgical resection, these patients are still at risk for Nelson's syndrome, an escalation of ACTH production and resultant hyperpigmentation [105].

Luteinizing hormone and FSH-secreting adenomas typically do not present with specific syndromes, and hypersecretion of gonadotropins occurs in a minority of patients [107]. As a result, presenting symptoms of a gonadotropic pituitary adenoma are mostly associated with mass effect, such as visual changes, hypopituitarism, and headaches. Signs of hypogonadism may be present, such as loss of libido, low testosterone, impotence, infertility, oligomenorrhea, and amenorrhea. Evaluation of these patients includes measuring serum LH, FSH, PRL, testosterone, estradiol, TSH, thyroid hormone, ACTH, cortisol, and IGF-1. Contrast-enhanced MRI may also be helpful in characterizing nonsecreting adenomas.

Surgery is the first line of therapy for gonadotropin-secreting adenomas, with radiation therapy as an option for recurrent or unresectable tumors. A few case reports have demonstrated that bromocriptine [108] and cabergoline [108, 109] may achieve some symptomatic relief and reduction in tumor size. Further evidence must validate these findings for other patients with these types of tumors [110].

One of least common pituitary adenomas is the TSH-secreting neoplasm. Up to a third of TSH-secreting adenomas also secrete additional pituitary hormones and are associated with macroadenomas in 90 % of patients [111]. There is an equal distribution between males and females [112]. Clinicians should anticipate signs and symptoms of hyperthyroidism in these patients. Patients with these tumors can also present with headaches, visual field defects, acromegaly, gynecomastia, oligomenorrhea, amenorrhea, infertility, and impotence [111, 113].

Clinicians may order a CBC, serum electrolytes, TSH, free T3, free T4, PRL, GH, and an MRI to evaluate these patients. Ultrasound of the thyroid may detect a goiter or nodules that may be present from chronic stimulation [113]. If an adenoma is not identified on contrast-enhanced MRI, bilateral petrosal sampling may allow identification of tumor location [114]. Additionally, the cause of TSH secretion may be due to resistance to thyroid hormone [115].

TRH administration will result in little or no response in 90 % of patients with TSH-secreting tumors [111], due to a paucity of TRH receptors on thyrotropic adenomas [116]. Management of TSH-secreting adenomas is primarily surgical. However, somatostatin analogues have been shown in select reports to control TSH secretion, normalize thyroid hormone levels, and shrink tumor size [117, 118].

Perioperative Management of Pituitary Adenomas

The neurointensivist will most commonly encounter patients with pituitary adenomas in the postoperative period. These patients will require routine postoperative critical care and endocrine management. Postoperative complications can include intracranial bleeding, wound infection, meningitis, vision changes, CSF leakage, airway obstruction, obtundation, epistaxis, electrolyte disturbances, and delirium. Endocrine complications that are observed in the postoperative period such as DI, SIADH, adrenal insufficiency, and hyper- and hypoglycemia will be discussed.

Diabetes insipidus is the most common endocrine abnormality after resection of pituitary tumors [119]. One large series of 1,571 patients observed that approximately one-third of patients developed DI within 24 h after undergoing transsphenoidal resection of pituitary tumors [119]. Diabetes insipidus may persist for over a week in a small portion of patients. Patients generate large amounts of dilute urine, with urine osmolality values less than serum osmolality. The mechanism of AVP deficiency is likely due to injury to the posterior pituitary gland or neurohypophyseal system from surgical manipulation. It typically presents with thirst and acute onset of polyuria of approximately 3–6 L/day in mild AVP deficiency and can reach 18 L/day with the absence of AVP [120]. Diagnosis of DI can be made with demonstration of serum sodium above 145 mEq/L and low urine osmolality below 200 mOsm/kg. If patients are not closely monitored, volume depletion, hypernatremia, and hyperosmolality can develop, with associated hemodynamic instability and mental status changes [121].

With mild polyuria of less than 6 L/day, patients with DI should be able to maintain adequate oral intake. As polyuria worsens or continues without resolution, AVP replacement therapy should be provided [120]. Desmopressin (DDAVP), a synthetic analogue of AVP, is currently used due to its rapid onset and ease of use in the postoperative setting. During the acute postoperative phase while DDAVP is administered, close monitoring of urine output and serum sodium is necessary to avoid excessive water retention and hyponatremia from overtreatment [122, 123].

The syndrome of inappropriate secretion of ADH is caused by excessive AVP secretion and results in fluid retention and hyponatremia. This may be due to primary secretion of AVP or secondary to hypocortisolism or hypothyroidism [124, 125]. Laboratory evaluation reveals hyponatremia, a urine sodium greater than 20 mEq/L, and a urine osmolality greater than 300 mOsm/kg. Serum uric acid will also be decreased. If the patient is hypotensive, serum cortisol levels should be checked, or a cosyntropin stimulation test may be performed. If the patient exhibits signs of severe hypothyroidism, serum

thyroid hormone levels should be obtained because of the association with SIADH mentioned earlier.

With mild to moderate hyponatremia (Na >120 mEq/L), appropriate therapy may be limited to treatment of the underlying causative disorder and fluid restriction. Worsening or symptomatic hyponatremia often can be treated with hypertonic saline or a vasopressin receptor antagonist, such as conivaptan or tolvaptan, in order to reduce the retention of water from the renal collecting ducts. The rate of correction needs to be monitored closely, as an excessively rapid correction may result in central pontine myelinolysis [126].

Patients with pituitary adenomas may also develop new hypopituitarism after surgery. Low serum cortisol levels may prompt immediate glucocorticoid replacement therapy. Dexamethasone can be administered initially, since hydrocortisone can interfere with interpretation of a cosyntropin stimulation test. However, the lack of salt-retaining (mineralocorticoid) activity with dexamethasone warrants conversion to hydrocortisone [125].

Patients with GH-secreting tumors may develop fluid retention and edema through renal sodium retention [127]. A postoperative decline in GH can induce mobilization of fluid on the first postoperative day. Although the patient is at risk for DI, the intensivist should be careful not to mistake this diuresis for cerebral salt wasting or DI, as evidenced by normal serum sodium levels [120].

Postoperative management of patients after surgery for PRL-secreting tumors typically only requires routine postoperative care. A serum PRL level is measured on the first or second postoperative day in order to assess the likelihood of surgical cure [122]. The acute management of patients with TSH-secreting tumors mirrors that of those patients with PRL-secreting tumors. However, these patients may have a serum TSH level checked on the first or second postoperative day. These patients will continue to require monitoring for hypo- or hyperthyroidism, depending on the success of surgical cure. Acute hypothyroidism is unlikely due to the long half-life of thyroxine [122].

Craniopharyngiomas

Craniopharyngiomas are rare, sellar or parasellar epithelial tumors that can occur along the path of the craniopharyngeal duct. The overall incidence of craniopharyngiomas is 0.14 cases per 100,000 person-years, accounting for approximately 0.7 % of primary intracranial tumors in adults, increasing to 2.5–3.4 % in children [123]. They can be discovered at any age, although there tends to be a bimodal distribution at ages 5–14 years and 50–74 years [128]. No gender differences have been appreciated in population studies in the United States, but there is an increased incidence in African-Americans, as compared to Caucasians [123].

Histologic analysis of craniopharyngiomas reveals two primary tumor subtypes, adamantinomatous and papillary

[129, 130]. Although craniopharyngiomas are generally benign, malignant forms can also occur [129, 131]. These tumors have been found to express pituitary hormones such as TSH, ACTH [132], estrogen receptors [133], progesterone receptors [134], and IGF-1 receptors [135]. Specific endocrine abnormalities occur in a majority of patients with craniopharyngiomas [132].

Initial symptoms of patients with craniopharyngiomas are dependent on the location and size of the mass and can include neurologic, visual, or endocrine abnormalities. These patients can present with a variety of symptoms that include headache, nausea, vomiting, visual changes, growth failure in children, and hypogonadism in adults [136]. One of the more severe symptoms is a decrease or loss of consciousness in 3–29 % of patients [137, 138].

These patients may also develop DI or, in rare circumstances, SIADH [139]. Growth failure can occur in 7–93 % of patients [140, 141], while sexual development abnormalities can occur in 4–24 % of patients [130, 142]. Patients with craniopharyngiomas may present with GH, FSH, LH, ACTH, TSH, and vasopressin deficiencies [136, 143]. Therefore, a neurointensivist may want to be familiar with the constellation of signs and symptoms of patients with craniopharyngiomas [137].

There is significant variability regarding the management and treatment of craniopharyngiomas owing to a lack of prospective, randomized studies, and the variability of the presentation and location of craniopharyngiomas. The primary treatment option is surgical resection followed by external beam radiation [138–141]. The surgical options include either craniotomy through various approaches or the transsphenoidal route for infrasellar or infradiaphragmatic tumors [141]. Radiation therapy may induce enlargement of cystic tumors in 14 % of cases [144] and could potentially worsen symptoms before eventual improvement. As a result, aspiration prior to surgery or radiation therapy may prevent further decompensation with treatment [145]. Overall surgical mortality has improved significantly in the last several decades [130, 142, 146]. Acute complications from the classic transsphenoidal approach include meningitis, DI, and recurrence of prior or new hypothalamic-pituitary axis abnormalities [136].

Although some aspects of hypopituitarism can exist in a majority of patients with craniopharyngioma preoperatively, new deficiencies can present postoperatively. The most common deficiencies include GH, FSH/LH, ACTH [142, 147], TSH, and vasopressin [142], with three or more hormonal abnormalities occurring in 54–100 % patients [137]. Furthermore, little evidence supports return of preoperative pituitary deficiencies [142, 148, 149]. As a result, perioperative monitoring requires evaluation of all potential hormonal derangements and appropriate treatment or hormone replacement therapy.

As mentioned earlier, acute replacement of GH is often deferred until the patient has returned to baseline [150]. Sex hormone replacement is also deferred in the acute perioperative period. Urine output can be profound, due to DI caused by a primary deficiency of AVP. The associated hypovolemia and hypernatremia can be significant, and patients may not be able to maintain adequate oral intake to match urine output. DDAVP may be required to treat DI. Additionally, patients with DI appear to be at risk for thrombotic events, presumably due to volume contraction, and pharmacologic thromboprophylaxis is encouraged when appropriate [151].

Hypothyroidism due to TRH or TSH deficiency from hypothalamic-pituitary compression or injury may require preoperative or postoperative treatment. If a patient exhibited signs of hypothyroidism requiring treatment prior to surgery, thyroid replacement should be continued postoperatively. Intravenous levothyroxine at a reduced dose can be initiated for the patient unable to take oral medication for several days. If the patient exhibits signs of myxedema coma such as obtundation, seizures, hypothermia, hypoglycemia, or unexplained heart failure, additional supportive measures and consideration of acute hormone replacement must be considered [149, 150].

Patients with craniopharyngiomas may also develop hypoadrenal crisis perioperatively. Initially, adrenal insufficiency may be treated with dexamethasone to avoid effects of hydrocortisone therapy on the cosyntropin stimulation test. Because dexamethasone lacks salt-retaining activity, therapy should eventually be converted to hydrocortisone. These patients may be prone to Addisonian crisis and require additional steroids during periods of physiologic stress, due to the inability to increase cortisol or other stress hormones [148].

Meningiomas

Meningiomas are one of the most common primary intracranial tumors, typically discovered in middle to late adult life, and account for 20 % of all intracranial tumors [152]. The cellular origin of meningiomas has been shown to be the arachnoid cap cells near the arachnoid villi [153]. Symptoms caused by the presence of a meningioma are due to the location and size of the mass. They occur more often in females and African-Americans and are more commonly benign than malignant [153, 154].

The increased incidence of meningiomas in females may be due to the presence of sex hormone receptors (both estrogen and progesterone) on these tumors [155–158]. Meningiomas have also been found to express additional cell-surface hormone receptors (i.e., androgen, glucocorticoid, somatostatin, PRL, IGF-1, IGF-2 [151], thyroid hormone [159], and GnRH [160]). The importance of most of these surface hormone receptors remains poorly defined [155, 156, 161].

However, the presence of sex hormone receptors on meningiomas may have prognostic implications. Manipulation of estrogen or progesterone levels could theoretically alter the risk of developing meningiomas. In the Nurses' Health Study, the relative risk (RR) for diagnosis of meningioma for premenopausal women was 2.48, while for postmenopausal women on hormone replacement therapy (HRT), it was 1.86. There was no increased risk for those women on oral contraceptive pills [162]. However, the association between HRT and the development of meningiomas in women is not readily reproducible in other studies [163]. Further studies are warranted to more clearly delineate which women may be at highest risk to develop meningiomas [155–158, 161–163].

As mentioned earlier, GH and IGF-1 may be involved in meningioma occurrence and growth. Blockade of GH receptors on meningioma cells in cell culture and in mice models with a GH receptor antagonist, pegvisomant, reduced DNA synthesis in meningioma cells and reduced tumor size [164], while administration of IGF-1 seemed to have the opposite effect [165]. Since the decrease in tumor size also correlated with a decrease in serum IGF-1 levels, the cause of tumor shrinkage could be due to GH receptor blockade or decreased IGF-1 levels, or both. To date, no in vitro studies have been done involving GH receptor blockade in patients with meningiomas [164–166].

The standard first-line therapy for meningiomas is surgery, with or without radiation therapy. In a minority of cases, the meningioma recurs or is only partially resected. As a result, chemotherapy and hormonal therapy is considered.

Hormonal therapy may have a role in recurrent meningiomas not appropriate for surgery or radiation therapy. Since estrogen receptors are only present in 8–40 % of meningiomas [166, 167], hormonal therapy has initially targeted progesterone activity. A small trial [167] of 14 patients with unresectable meningiomas used the progesterone antagonist mifepristone (RU486) and demonstrated objective improvement in 5 patients with mild side effects [168]. Aside from endometrial hyperplasia, mifepristone appears to be well tolerated on a long-term basis [169]. These positive findings were not supported in a later double-blind, randomized, placebo-controlled trial involving 198 patients with unresectable meningiomas [170]. The lack of response with progesterone antagonism in this larger trial may be explained by the low incidence of progesterone receptors in recurrent or aggressive meningiomas, as described earlier. Small case reports and nonrandomized trials have observed that tamoxifen, an estrogen receptor antagonist, may partially reduce tumor size in some patients with non-resectable refractory meningiomas [171]. The true efficacy of hormone therapy involving progesterone or estrogen receptors still remains unclear and requires further large population-based studies.

Hormonal Therapy for Critical Illness

Hormone replacement therapy during critical illness is controversial [22]. It is challenging for clinicians to determine which neuroendocrine response to illness is helpful or harmful. As mentioned previously, the acute illness phase is marked by energy conservation, while the chronic phase is signified by further catabolism which results in weakness and prolonged recovery. Targeted interventions that slow or reverse the deterioration that occurs in the chronic phase may be advantageous to human survival [7].

One large multicenter study attempted to determine the effects of GH administration during the chronic phase of critical illness. The results demonstrated an increase in morbidity and mortality associated with exogenous GH use [172]. This may have been due in part to the partial recovery of GH sensitivity during the chronic phase of critical illness and the high potentially toxic doses of GH administered to the study patients [172]. While GH has anabolic effects, it also may have the following deleterious effects on patients with critical illness: promotes edema formation, causes insulin resistance, and alters immune system activity [173]. IGF-1 may be a suitable alternative in the future as it has been shown to inhibit protein breakdown. However, further studies are required to investigate its waning efficacy with prolonged use [22].

Similar to GH administration, thyroid hormone replacement during critical illness has not been shown to be definitively beneficial. While these hormones play an integral role in protein synthesis, lipolysis, and muscle energy use, exogenous administration (particularly T3 administration) has been shown to increase mortality in animals with sepsis [22]. Thyroxine supplementation may also produce negative side effects that can prolong ICU length of stay [22]. Preliminary studies indicate that combination therapy of GH-releasing peptide-2 with TRH may appropriately activate the somatotropic and thyroid axes during the chronic phase of critical illness. This activation may be associated with reduced catabolism. Therefore, future studies must further investigate the potential positive effects of hypothalamic releasing hormones on outcomes in critically ill patients [7, 22].

Unlike the previously mentioned hormones, low-dose, prolonged glucocorticoid administration during severe, refractory septic shock has been shown to improve overall survival [174]. However, a subsequent larger multicenter randomized controlled trial did not show a similar benefit in reducing mortality [175]. The discrepancy in the findings of these studies is most likely due to different patient populations (medical ICU vs. surgical ICU), etiology of sepsis (respiratory vs. abdominal), and different control group mortality (sicker patients in the first study) [21]. Full stress dose replacement steroids (200–300 mg/day of hydrocortisone) are still used frequently in critically ill patients with severe refractory septic shock [21]. However, there is no clinical indication for larger doses of steroids (pharmacologic as opposed to maximal physiologic) in such a setting.

Testosterone may be another hormone that has beneficial effects in critically ill patients. Testosterone when administered to burn-injured patients may reduce catabolism [176]. Other androgens may facilitate faster functional recovery and wound healing while reducing weight loss in burn-injured patients [173]. However, other studies suggest supplemental administration of testosterone may suppress the immune system [22]. Further studies are required in order to identify which critically ill patient population could benefit from androgen administration [22].

Altered Mental Status and Endocrine Abnormalities

Altered mental status may occur as the presenting symptom of an endocrine abnormality and describes a condition in which there exists a change in mentation, cognition, consciousness, and/or awareness [177, 178]. One study reported that endocrine abnormalities accounted for approximately 5 % of all cases of altered mental status changes presenting to an emergency room [178]. Derangements in thyroid hormones, glucose, and endogenous cortisol levels account for most of the endocrine-related mental status changes that occur in the NICU [179].

Hyper- or hypothyroidism develops in roughly 2 % of adults [177]. Changes in mental status may occur in approximately 50 % of patients suffering from thyroid dysfunction [177]. This may be due to the important role of the thyroid axis in metabolism and its relationship with neurotransmission. Patients with hyperthyroidism may present with extreme fatigue. These patients may also develop hyperthyroidism-associated anxiety and emotional lability. These nonspecific symptoms may lead to the underdiagnosis of hyperthyroidism in the NICU. Lastly, dementia, delirium, and disorientation can all be presenting symptoms of hyperthyroidism. Therefore, clinicians should order thyroid indices (i.e., TSH, free T4) upon recognition of these symptoms and have a suspicion for endocrine abnormalities [177].

Hypothyroidism is also associated with mental status changes. A decrease in cerebral blood flow, glucose utilization, and a desensitization of neuroreceptors are primarily responsible for the presenting symptomatology [177]. Weakness, depression, and even coma are all symptoms associated with hypothyroidism [177]. Due to the nonspecific nature of all of these symptoms, thyroid indices may be measured during the initial work-up of the patient with altered mental status.

Both hyper- and hypoglycemia can cause profound mental status changes. Lethargy, weakness, confusion, fatigue, emotional lability, seizures, and even coma are all associated with dysglycemia [177]. These symptoms usually mark impending neurologic injury without prompt reversal in the glucose abnormality. It is imperative that glucose is checked in anyone who has developed acute mental status changes in the NICU. In patients who are intubated and sedated, symptoms of autonomic system activation (tachycardia, sweating, tremors, and hypertension) may be the only recognized ones to prompt clinicians to identify a dysglycemic state, which may be life threatening [177].

Adrenal dysfunction may also present in patients with altered mental status. Approximately 20 % of patients with Cushing's syndrome can present with psychosis that may be difficult to distinguish from schizophrenia [177]. Cushing's syndrome and Addison's disease can also present as severe depression, which is often seen prior to the typical physical exam findings [177]. While none of the tests for adrenal dysfunction are 100 % specific and/or sensitive, a 9:00 a.m. cortisol level and a subsequent ITT (insulin tolerance test) are initial tests that may be helpful to heighten clinician suspicion for adrenal dysfunction [177].

Drug-Induced Endocrine Abnormalities in the NICU

A national campaign continues to promote reductions in the number of iatrogenic medication errors. Polypharmacy is a commonality in neurointensive care. Therefore, NICU patients are at an increased risk for drug-induced endocrine disorders. Table 15.4 illustrates some of the drugs used in the NICU that cause endocrine abnormalities. This section will focus on the primary drug-induced endocrine disorders seen in the NICU.

Drug-Induced Adrenal Abnormalities

Two drugs used frequently in the ICU are associated with adrenal dysfunction, etomidate and glucocorticoids [180]. Etomidate, an anesthetic/sedative drug, suppresses the adrenal axis. This drug blocks 11β-hydroxylase, which is an enzyme that converts cholesterol into cortisol. Nearly 30 years ago, etomidate infusions in the ICU were shown to significantly increase mortality [180]. Therefore, use of ICU etomidate infusions was abandoned [180].

Few clinicians in the 1980s thought that one dose of etomidate could have a similar effect as ICU etomidate infusions. In the late 1990s, many emergency medicine departments were utilizing etomidate in over 80 % of patients requiring rapid sequence tracheal intubations [181]. Anesthesiologists still

Table 15.4 Drug-induced endocrine disorders in the ICU

Hormone	Drugs	Proposed mechanism
CRH and ACTH	Glucocorticoids, opioids, and benzodiazepines	Negative feedback suppression
Cortisol	Phenobarbital	Induces cortisol metabolism
	Phenytoin	
	Rifampin	
	Etomidate	Inhibits cortisol production
	Azole antifungals	Chronic use inhibits cortisol synthesis
	Opioids	Decreases cortisol secretion
		Decreases free fraction cortisol
TSH	Dobutamine	Decrease TSH concentration
	Dopamine	
	Corticosteroids	Direct inhibition of TSH release
Thyroid hormone	Phenobarbital	Increases clearance of thyroxine
	Phenytoin	Same
	Rifampin	Same
	Carbamazepine	Same
	Amiodarone	Increases thyroid hormone synthesis
		Inhibits type I 5-deiodinase
	Iodinated contrast dye	Increases thyroid hormone through iodine administration
	Heparin	Increases free fraction of thyroid hormone
	Furosemide	Increase free fraction by displacement from protein binding sites
	Lithium	Decrease thyroid hormone secretion
	Atypical antipsychotics	Unknown—decreases free and total T4
Insulin	ACE inhibitors	Hypoglycemia—increases peripheral insulin sensitivity
	Fluoroquinolones	Hypoglycemia—promotes insulin secretion
	Pentamidine	Hypoglycemia—increases insulin secretion
	Sulfonylureas	Same
	Salicylates	Hypoglycemia—increase insulin secretion, glucose utilization, decreases gluconeogenesis
Hormone	Drug	Mechanism
Insulin	Glucocorticoids	Hyperglycemia—increases gluconeogenesis, decreases insulin secretion, increases insulin resistance
	Pentamidine	Hyperglycemia—impairs insulin release
	Calcineurin inhibitors	Hyperglycemia—decreases insulin production and release
	Vasopressors (epinephrine)	Hyperglycemia—promotes glycogenolysis, gluconeogenesis
	Atypical antipsychotics	Unknown

Reproduced with permission from Thomas et al. [180]

use etomidate in and outside of the operating room to intubate hemodynamically unstable patients.

Recent studies suggest that a single dose of etomidate in critically ill patients may lead to refractory hypotension, increased cytokine release, and increased mortality [182]. Etomidate-induced adrenal dysfunction in septic shock patients may be mitigated by the administration of hydrocortisone. A recent retrospective study investigated the effects of etomidate on adrenal suppression in patients with sepsis [182]. This study analyzed the use of etomidate in patients enrolled in the multicenter randomized controlled trial CORTICUS. The results revealed that etomidate administration was associated with a trend toward or even an independent risk factor for mortality depending on the characteristics included in the multivariate analysis [182]. In this study,

patient administration of hydrocortisone did not reverse mortality risk [182]. These data suggest that etomidate should not be utilized routinely in patients with sepsis or septic shock [182].

A recent prospective randomized trial attempted to address the potential use of alternatives to etomidate during rapid sequence tracheal intubation [181]. This study demonstrated that ketamine, a neuroleptic anesthetic agent, was safe and associated with a reduced risk of adrenal insufficiency [181]. However, there was no mortality difference between the groups who received etomidate or ketamine [181]. Less than 20 % of this study's patient population was septic [181]. Therefore, further studies are required to investigate other suitable alternatives to etomidate in septic patients and also define in which patients etomidate absolutely is contraindicated.

Many patients presenting to the NICU are or have taken glucocorticoids (hydrocortisone, prednisone, methylprednisolone, or dexamethasone) in the past. Controversy continues regarding the institution of "stress dose steroids" in this patient population. Many clinicians administer supplemental steroids based on the premise of avoiding distributive shock. However, studies suggest that the dose and duration of previous steroid therapy does not predict the development of adrenal insufficiency. In fact, some transplant units have eliminated "stress dose steroids" in patients who previously received steroids without adrenal compromise [180]. Avoiding steroid replacement therapy may reduce immunosuppression and other deleterious effects induced by steroids. Patients with significant hypotension who have been on steroids recently should be considered for replacement therapy [180].

Other drugs utilized in the NICU may induce metabolism of cortisol and thus cause adrenal insufficiency. Two antiseizure agents used in the NICU, phenytoin and phenobarbital, are often mentioned as inducers of the P450 (CYP-450) system that may increase metabolism of cortisol. These drugs may exacerbate adrenal insufficiency in critically ill patients with existing adrenal dysfunction [179, 183].

Phenytoin is a first-line medication for prevention of seizures in patients with TBI [180]. However, this drug facilitates an increase in the urinary excretion ratio of 6β-hydroxycortisol/cortisol within 1 week of initiation. Some studies have suggested that phenytoin use is associated with adrenal suppression in patients with TBI [180]. However, the frequency in which this occurs remains ill defined [180]. An alternative agent for seizure prophylaxis may be levetiracetam, but further studies are required to address its efficacy.

Phenobarbital has also been implicated in suppressing the adrenal axis [179]. It has been suggested that both phenobarbital and phenytoin may reduce the effect of exogenous steroids by increasing its metabolism. Patients requiring chronic steroids who have been placed on these agents may experience symptoms of adrenal insufficiency [184]. Therefore, it is imperative to monitor these patients closely for hemodynamic compromise and other adrenal suppression symptoms. Some experts recommend doubling or even tripling the dose of steroids in the setting of phenytoin or phenobarbital use [180]. Although it is conceivable that patients with neurologic injury (i.e., traumatic brain injury) are more susceptible to drug-induced deficits of steroid production, further studies are warranted regarding the exact effect of phenobarbital in patients with TBI who subsequently develop hypopituitarism [183].

Antibiotic-antifungal agents ("the azoles") have also been implicated in causing adrenal suppression [180]. These medications inhibit CYP-450 enzymes that are integral in endogenous steroid production. The most potent inhibitor appears to be ketoconazole. Mixed results are available regarding the steroid inhibitory effect of both fluconazole and itraconazole [180]. Those patients who are on both exogenous steroid replacement and azole antifungals are more susceptible to steroid-induced adverse effects due to the azole agents' inhibition of the CYP-450 metabolism of steroids. Clinicians must be cognizant of "azole" induced effects on steroidogenesis [180].

Benzodiazepines and opioids may also suppress the adrenal axis [183]. Benzodiazepine administration may result in a dose-dependent reduction in serum cortisol levels [183]. Opioids may also reduce cortisol secretion. In addition, opioids may increase cortisol-binding globulin, which can result in a reduction of free cortisol [183]. Critically ill patients may be especially susceptible to these agents' adrenal suppressive effects [183]. Further investigation is required to ascertain these agents' true clinical effects on the adrenal axis [183].

Drug-Induced Thyroid Hormone Abnormalities

While there are several ICU medications that may affect the thyroid axis, the following three specific drugs deserve mention: amiodarone, lithium, and dopamine [180].

Amiodarone is a common antiarrhythmic agent utilized for both ventricular and supraventricular arrhythmias in the NICU. Amiodarone appears very similar in structure to thyroxine and is composed of approximately 40 % iodine [180]. The iodine moiety may contribute to a condition referred to as "amiodarone-induced thyrotoxicosis (AIT)" [185]. Amiodarone-induced thyrotoxicosis I (an iodine-induced form) is most commonly seen in patients with established thyroid disease, while AIT II is a form of thyroiditis that actually causes release of thyroid hormone from the dysfunctional thyroid gland. It can be seen both during and after amiodarone treatment due to amiodarone's long half-life [185]. Amiodarone-induced thyrotoxicosis has been associated with nearly a three-time increase risk of stroke, myocardial infarction, and mortality [186]. Treatment includes the institution of antithyroid agents, methimazole and/or propylthiouracil [184]. Concomitant steroid therapy is also recommended, especially in AIT II [184]. Unfortunately, it is very difficult to distinguish AIT I from AIT II, and therefore, patients with either type usually receive steroid therapy, in the lowest dose possible, starting at 30–40 mg of prednisone (or another glucocorticoid equivalent) [184].

Amiodarone is also associated with the development of hypothyroidism [180]. The mechanism is not clearly elucidated in the literature. However, it may be due to abnormalities in iodine organification and thyroid production [184]. Fortunately for patients, this type of hypothyroidism is readily treated with levothyroxine and usually creates mild symptoms of hypothyroidism [184]. Dronedarone, a new oral antiarrhythmic agent in the same class as amiodarone, may reduce thyroid-induced abnormalities due to its lack of the iodine moiety. Ongoing trials will attempt to validate this notion [180].

Dopamine may also impair the thyroid axis [180]. It can decrease TSH and thyroxine production [180]. This effect may occur within 24 h of administration and is usually reversed after 24 h of discontinuing dopamine [180]. While it has been suggested that dopamine be used in patients with septic shock, recent data indicate a potential for increased mortality associated with patients who receive dopamine for shock [187, 188]. Thyroid inhibition may be implicated in the future as an associated cause of increased mortality in critically ill patients with shock who receive dopamine [189].

Lithium, primarily used in patients with bipolar disease, also inhibits thyroid function. It reduces thyroxine release and thyroid hormone synthesis. Lithium-related thyroid hormone inhibition is more common among chronic users of lithium. Although rare, lithium may be responsible for causing myxedema coma, and therefore, critical care physicians must closely monitor these patients for symptoms [190].

Other notable drugs that may cause thyroid hormone abnormalities include phenobarbital, phenytoin, carbamazepine (increased thyroid hormone metabolism), heparins (increased free fraction of thyroid hormone), iodinated contrast dye (increased thyroid hormone synthesis), and furosemide (displacement from protein binding). All of these agents may be used in the NICU, and therefore, clinicians should be cognizant of these hormone-altering effects [180].

Drug-Induced Glucose Abnormalities

There are several drugs that may cause hypoglycemia and hyperglycemia. This review will focus on agents that are more commonly used in the ICU. ACE inhibitor use may lead to hypoglycemia by increasing peripheral insulin sensitivity [180]. A recent report noted that ACE inhibitor use may be responsible for approximately 15 % of hypoglycemia-related admissions of patients with diabetes. Another systematic review suggested that ACE inhibitor administration was associated with a threefold increased risk for hypoglycemia. However, evidence supporting this notion is of poor quality. Better designed trials should validate the presence of ACE inhibitor-induced hypoglycemia in critically ill patients [180, 191, 192].

Fluoroquinolones and sulfonylureas are other drugs taken by critically ill patients that may cause hypoglycemia [180]. The fluoroquinolone antibiotics may stimulate pancreatic insulin secretion. Both levofloxacin and gatifloxacin are associated with the most frequent reports of hypoglycemia, while ciprofloxacin does not seem to induce low glucose levels. Risk factors for fluoroquinolone-induced hypoglycemia

include renal failure, sepsis, and simultaneous hypoglycemic agent administration [193].

Sulfonylureas, especially the older generation of sulfonylureas, may be associated with severe hypoglycemia in patients with sulfonylurea overdose and in those who receive concomitant use of drugs that inhibit the CYP2C9 enzyme system. Octreotide may reverse this hypoglycemic effect. However, these drugs are not easily reversible due to their long duration of action. Intensivists should have a heightened awareness for hypoglycemia in patients presenting with mental status changes who are on chronic sulfonylurea use [180, 194].

While hypoglycemia has been shown to be an independent predictor of mortality, most clinicians still agree that significant (>180–200 mg/dL) hyperglycemia is also deleterious. The polypharmacy so often seen in patients who are in the ICU contributes to an increased risk for hyperglycemia. A few agents are worth discussing for their effect on glucose levels [180].

Glucocorticoids are often administered to NICU patients to reduce swelling and inflammation (patients with reactive airway diseases, bacterial meningitis, brain tumors) and treat autoimmune diseases (lupus cerebritis) and in some patients with refractory shock (severe sepsis). However, glucocorticoids increase gluconeogenesis and insulin resistance and decrease pancreatic insulin secretion [195]. Clinicians should be aware of these effects and treat the expected hyperglycemia accordingly. Recently, a study suggested that administering hydrocortisone by continuous infusion rather than by bolus allows for better glycemic control [196]. Further studies are warranted on how to best approach this iatrogenic cause of hyperglycemia.

Other drugs that have been associated with hyperglycemia include pentamidine, calcineurin inhibitors (immunosuppressive agents), adrenergic agents (i.e., epinephrine, norepinephrine, and albuterol), and atypical antipsychotics [180]. Pentamidine, an anti-pneumocystis agent, may cause impaired insulin release. However, pentamidine seems to have a biphasic effect on glucose levels. At first, pentamidine may increase insulin secretion and, therefore, cause hypoglycemia. However, with chronic therapy, pancreatic β-cell destruction may occur, which leads to hyperglycemia [180]. The calcineurin inhibitors (cyclosporine and tacrolimus) can cause posttransplant diabetes. The proposed mechanism is a reduction in insulin synthesis and release. This phenomenon usually occurs early on in the administration of these drugs to transplant patients [197]. Epinephrine, through its profound β2-adrenergic activation, has the most profound effect on raising glucose levels among the adrenergic vasopressor class. This vasopressor activates glycogenolysis, increases hepatic gluconeogenesis, and stimulates glucagon and cortisol [198]. Lastly, atypical antipsychotics can also cause profound hyperglycemia. It is not clear by which mechanism this occurs. The risk seems to be highest with clozapine and olanzapine. Patients on these medications can present with life-threatening diabetic ketoacidosis or hyperosmolar non-ketotic coma [199]. Therefore, clinicians should have a heightened awareness for the development of hyperglycemia in patients on atypical antipsychotics [180].

The Endocrinopathy of Brain Death

Hormonal changes do occur after brain death secondary to both posterior and anterior pituitary dysfunction. The primary derangement among brain-dead donors is in the posterior pituitary that results in diabetes insipidus, which is discussed elsewhere [200]. Nearly 80 % of patients with brain death develop a significant decrease in ADH, which creates hypernatremia, hypovolemia, hyperosmolality, and inappropriate diuresis [200]. These abnormalities can lead to hypovolemia and tissue hypoperfusion and, therefore, need to be aggressively treated in brain-dead organ donors.

Although less affected than the posterior pituitary, the anterior pituitary gland may also become dysfunctional upon brain death [200]. Brain death can be signified by abnormalities in thyroid function, adrenal function, and dysglycemia. One study involving 22 brain-dead donors demonstrated that TSH, T4, and T3 were all reduced to below normal values in the majority of patients. However, other studies suggest that brain-dead donors really suffer from a euthyroid sick syndrome (nonthyroidal illness)-like state rather than an absolute TSH deficiency [200]. An expedient decrease in T3 as a result of reduced secretion of TSH by the anterior pituitary can be also seen in brain-dead patients [200]. Clinicians involved in organ transplant procurement have attempted to infuse T3 with mixed efficacy. The most robust evidence supporting its use is derived from an analysis of the UNOS database. Analyses of this database suggest that utilizing triple hormonal therapy (T3, cortisol, and insulin) improves survival of heart grafts and reduces the overall odds of death [201]. Further studies are required to determine whether exogenous thyroid administration consistently thwarts thyroid dysfunction in brain-dead organ donors and improves organ function and successful transplantation.

Hyperglycemia is also commonly seen in brain-dead organ donors. The primary reason for this is insulin resistance [202]. However, there are also trials that suggest that insulin levels are decreased in brain-dead patients. A decrease in insulin and/or resistance to insulin leads to a lack of cellular glucose utilization. This phenomenon can result in the development of anaerobic metabolism and acidemia. High levels of intravenous insulin are often administered to brain-dead organ donors in order to minimize severe hyperglycemia-induced hypovolemia and hypoperfusion [202].

Cortisol levels may also be decreased in the brain-dead patient. One study suggested that 50 % of brain-dead organ donors develop adrenal insufficiency as indicated by a serum cortisol <11,527 ng/dL [200]. This may be due to a reduction in the secretion of ACTH from the anterior pituitary. A reduction in cortisol levels coupled with decreased T3 levels may contribute to hemodynamic instability. Therefore, steroids are often administered to brain-dead organ donors to restore cardiovascular homeostasis [202].

Recent practice suggests that there is a benefit to a combination hormone replacement approach. Specifically, methylprednisolone (15 mg/kg bolus), triiodothyronine (4 mcg bolus followed by infusion of 3 mcg/h), and arginine vasopressin (1 U bolus followed by 0.5–4 mU/kg/h) administration to brain-dead organ donors has been associated with an increased rate of successful organ donations [203]. This combination may also reduce the odds of organ recipient death within 30 days by 46 % [203]. Beneficial effects may also be seen in brain-dead organ donors who receive corticosteroids alone or with T3/T4. In addition to the hemodynamic effects of corticosteroids, they may also reduce cytokine release, which may improve graft survival [203].

Thyroid administration continues to be controversial in brain-dead organ donors. Those experts who continue to use T3 administration during brain-dead organ donor resuscitation believe that T3 increases arterial pressure and improves tissue perfusion. However, others believe that the expensive cost of T3 does not outweigh its proposed sporadic benefits. T4 has been used as a cheaper alternative. However, the conversion of T4 to T3 may take several hours and is often unpredictable. In addition, T4 may be converted into rT3 which does not have the proposed beneficial effects of T3. Further prospective studies should elucidate whether T3 administration can consistently improve graft survival in recipients [203, 204].

Summary

The endocrine system is a complex organ system that secretes hormones, which play a primary role in both catabolism and anabolism. Various hormones are crucial to homeostasis, help modulate immune response, and regulate cardiovascular function. During critical illness, certain hormones may mitigate the catabolic response, while others may exacerbate it. Clinicians should be aware of hormonal changes that occur during the acute and chronic phases of critical illness. It has yet to be determined which hormones are effective in reversing the catabolic effect of critical illness. Future studies should elucidate which hormone replacement therapies during critical illness may improve outcomes.

Dysglycemia is one of the responses to catabolism in critically ill patients. It is often seen in patients with neurologic injuries. Newer monitoring techniques may aid clinicians in minimizing glucose derangements. The impact of this on outcome in NICU patients remains open to investigation. Avoiding both hypo- and hyperglycemia, however, is a goal that continues to be a priority for neurointensive care patients.

Several disease processes have been discussed in this chapter relating to their effect on the endocrine system. Often times, the somatotropic, thyroid, gonadal, lactotropic, and adrenal axes are dysfunctional during neurocritical illness. However, these changes in the hormonal milieu are under-recognized and underreported due to heterogeneous etiologies and concurrent pathologies. Therefore, intensivists should be cognizant of these changes so they may be able to anticipate the pathophysiologic effects and manage the symptoms accordingly.

Some important points to keep in mind are:

- The endocrine system is vital to maintaining homeostasis in humans.
- The hypothalamic-pituitary hormone axis is universally dysregulated during critical illness.
- Neurologic patients are at particular risk for various endocrinopathies depending on their original neurologic insult, associated comorbidities, and evolution of their ICU course.
- Dysglycemia in the neurocritically ill is common. The relationship of peripheral glucose to CNS glucose levels remains under intense investigation. Optimal glucose measurement and management remains open to debate.
- Hormonal abnormalities vary depending on the acute or chronic phase of critical illness.
- New therapeutic hormonal interventions continue to be investigated in critically ill patients in an attempt to curb and/or reverse the catabolic state seen in the chronic phase of critical illness.
- Recognition of endocrine dysfunction during Guillain-Barré syndrome is important in the overall management of this syndrome.
- Meningitis and encephalitis have also been shown to cause derangements in hormonal homeostasis. Failure to recognize these abnormalities may result in worse patient outcomes.
- Neurointensivists should be aware of the perioperative endocrine abnormalities associated with pituitary adenomas, craniopharyngiomas, and meningiomas.
- The polypharmacy seen in the ICU can result in drug-induced endocrine disorders.
- Physicians should recognize medications used commonly in the NICU that are associated with endocrine abnormalities: dopamine, phenytoin, phenobarbital, fluoroquinolones, lithium, ACE inhibitors, glucocorticoids, vasopressors, benzodiazepines, and opioids, among others.

References

1. http://en.wikipedia.org/wiki/Endocrinology.
2. Kreiger DT. Brain peptides, part 1. N Engl J Med. 1981;304:876.
3. Smith FG, Sheehy AM, Vincent JL, Coursin DB. Critical illness-induced dysglycaemia: diabetes and beyond. Crit Care. 2010; 14:327.
4. Amar AP, Weiss MH. Pituitary anatomy and physiology. Neurosurg Clin N Am. 2003;13:11–23.
5. Gimpl G, Fahrenholz F. The oxytocin receptor system: structure, function, and regulation. Physiol Rev. 2001;81:629.
6. Eikermann M, Schimidt U. Does adrenal size matter? Anesthesiology. 2011;115:223–4.
7. Vanhorebeek I, Van den Berge G. The neuroendocrine response to critical illness is a dynamic process. Crit Care Clin. 2006;22:1–15.
8. Clayton RN. Mortality, cardiovascular events and risk factors in hypopituitarism. Growth Horm IGF Res. 1998;8:69–76.
9. Monson JP, Besser GM. Premature mortality and hypopituitarism. Lancet. 2001;357:1972–3.
10. Ascoli P, Cavagnini F. Hypopituitarism. Pituitary. 2006;9:335–42.
11. Prabhakar VK, Shalet SM. Aetiology, diagnosis, and management of hypopituitarism in adult life. Postgrad Med. 2006;82:259–66.
12. Schneider HJ, Kreitschmann-Andermahr I, Ghigo E, et al. Hypothalamopituitary dysfunction following traumatic brain injury and aneurysmal subarachnoid hemorrhage. A systematic review. JAMA. 2007;298:1429–38.
13. Cowie CC, Rust KF, Ford ES, et al. Full accounting of diabetes and pre-diabetes in the U.S. population in 1988–1994 and 2005–2006. Diabetes Care. 2009;32:287–94.
14. Finfer S, Chittock DR, Su SY, NICE-SUGAR Study Investigators, et al. Intensive versus conventional glucose control in critically ill patients. N Engl J Med. 2009;360:1283–97.
15. Van den Berghe G, Wouters P, et al. Intensive insulin therapy in critically ill patients. N Engl J Med. 2001;345:1359–67.
16. Vespa PM, Boonyaputthikul R, McArthur DL, et al. Intensive insulin therapy reduces microdialysis glucose values without altering glucose utilization or improving lactate/pyruvate ratio after traumatic brain injury. Crit Care Med. 2006;34:850–6.
17. Holbein M, Bechir M, Ludwig S, et al. Differential influence of arterial blood glucose on cerebral metabolism following severe traumatic brain injury. Crit Care. 2009;13:R13.
18. Abate MG, Trivedi M, Fryer TD, et al. Early derangements in oxygen and glucose metabolism following head injury: the ischemic penumbra and pathophysiological heterogeneity. Neurocrit Care. 2008;9:319–25.
19. Timofeev I, Carpenter KL, Nortje J, et al. Cerebral extracellular chemistry and outcome following traumatic brain injury: a microdialysis study of 223 patients. Brain. 2011;134:484–94.
20. Krinsley JS. Glycemic variability: a strong independent predictor of mortality in critically ill patients. Crit Care Med. 2008;36: 3008–13.
21. Moghissi ES, Korytkowski MT, DiNardo M, et al. American Association of Clinical Endocrinologists and American Diabetes Association consensus statement on inpatient glycemic control. Diabetes Care. 2009;32:1119–31.
22. Vanhorebeek I, Van den Berghe G. Hormonal and metabolic strategies to attenuate catabolism in critically ill patients. Curr Opin Pharmacol. 2004;4:621–62.
23. Sakharova OV, Inzucchi SE. Endocrine assessments during critical illness. Crit Care Clin. 2007;23:467–90.
24. Nylen ES, Muller B. Endocrine changes in critical illness. J Intensive Care Med. 2004;19:67–82.
25. Mongardon N, Dyson A, Singer M, et al. Is MOF an outcome parameter or a transient adaptive state in critical illness? Curr Opin Crit Care. 2009;15:431–6.

26. Annane D, Sébille V, Troché G, et al. A 3-level prognostic classification in septic shock based on cortisol levels and cortisol response to corticotrophin. JAMA. 2000;283:1038–45.

27. Sudlow CL, Warlow CP. For the international stroke incidence collaboration. Stroke. 1997;28:491–9.

28. Kase CS. Intracerebral hemorrhage. Baillieres Clin Neurol. 1995;4:247–78.

29. Stebhens WE. Aneurysm and anatomical variations of cerebral arteries. Arch Pathol. 1963;75:45.

30. Jordan LC, Johnston SC, Wu YW, Sidney S, Fullerton HJ. The importance of cerebral aneurysms in childhood hemorrhagic stroke: a population-based study. Stroke. 2009;40(2):400.

31. Rinkel GJ, Djibuti M, Algra A, et al. Prevalence and risk of rupture of intracranial aneurysms: a systematic review. Stroke. 1998;29:251.

32. Broderick JP, Brott TG, et al. Initial and recurrent bleeding are the major causes of death following subarachnoid hemorrhage. Stroke. 1994;25(7):1342.

33. Kale SP, Edgell RC, Alshekhlee A, et al. Age-associated vasospasm in aneurysmal subarachnoid hemorrhage. J Stroke Cerebrovasc Dis. 2013;22:22–7.

34. Parenti G, Cecchi PC, Ragghianti B, et al. Evaluation of the anterior pituitary function in the acute phase after spontaneous subarachnoid hemorrhage. J Endocrinol Invest. 2001;34:361–5.

35. Franceschini R, Tenconi GL, Zoppoli F, et al. Endocrine abnormalities and outcomes of ischemic stroke. Biomed Pharmacother. 2001;55:458–65.

36. Roberts I, Yates D, Sandercock P, et al. Effect of intravenous corticosteroids on death within 14 days in 10008 adults with clinically significant head injury (MRC CRASH trial): randomized placebo-controlled trial. Lancet. 2004;364:1321–8.

37. Rothman MS, Arciniegas DB, Filley CM, et al. The neuroendocrine effects of traumatic brain injury. J Neuropsychiatry Clin Neurosci. 2007;19:363–72.

38. Edwards P, Arango M, Balica L, et al. Final results of MRC CRASH, a randomized placebo-controlled trial of intravenous corticosteroid in adults with head injury-outcomes at 6 months. Lancet. 2005;365:1957–9.

39. Bavisetty S, Bavisetty S, McArthur DL, et al. Chronic hypopituitarism after traumatic brain injury: risk assessment and relationship to outcome. Neurosurgery. 2008;62:1080–93.

40. Ives JC, Alderman M, Stred SE. Hypopituitarism after multiple concussions: a retrospective case study in an adolescent male. J Athl Train. 2007;42:431–9.

41. Rees JH, Soudain SE, Gregson NA, et al. Campylobacter jejuni infection and Guillain-Barré syndrome. N Engl J Med. 1995;333:1374–9.

42. Ropper AH. The Guillain-Barré syndrome. N Engl J Med. 1992;326:1130–6.

43. Asbury AK, Cornblath DR. Assessment of current diagnostic criteria for Guillain-Barré syndrome. Ann Neurol. 1990;27:S21.

44. Hoffmann O, Reuter U, Schielke E, et al. SIADH as the first symptom of Guillain-Barré syndrome. Neurology. 1999;53:1365.

45. Ramanathan S, McMeniman J, Cabela R, Holmes-Walker DJ, et al. SIADH and dysautonomia as the initial presentation of Guillain-Barré syndrome. J Neurol Neurosurg Psychiatry. 2012;83:344–5. doi:10.1136/jnnp.2010.233767.

46. Sharshar T, Chevret S, Bourdain F, et al. Early predictors of mechanical ventilation in Guillain-Barré syndrome. Crit Care Med. 2003;31:278–83.

47. Hughes RAC, Wijdicks EFM, Benson E, et al. Supportive care for patients with Guillain-Barré syndrome. Arch Neurol. 2005;62:1194–8.

48. McKhann GM, Griffin JW. Plasmapheresis and the Guillain-Barré syndrome. Ann Neurol. 1987;22:762–3.

49. Cortese I, Chaudhry V, So YT, et al. Evidence-based guideline update: plasmapheresis in neurologic disorders. Neurology. 2011;76:294–300.

50. Hughes RAC, Swan AV, Raphael JC, et al. Immunotherapy for Guillain-Barré syndrome: a systematic review. Brain. 2007;130:2245–57.

51. Potz G, Neundorfer B. Polyradiculoneuritis and Hashimoto's thyroiditis. J Neurol. 1975;210:283–9.

52. Behar R, Penny R, Powell HC. Guillain-Barré syndrome associated with Hashimoto's thyroiditis. J Neurol. 1986;233:233–6.

53. Davies AG, Dingle HR. Observations on cardiovascular and neuroendocrine disturbance in the Guillain-Barré syndrome. J Neurol Neurosurg Psychiatry. 1972;35:176–9.

54. Créange A, Bélec L, Clair B, et al. Circulating transforming growth factor beta 1 (TGF- β1) in Guillain-Barré syndrome: decreased concentrations in the early course and increase with motor function. J Neurol Neurosurg Psychiatry. 1998;64:162–5.

55. Strauss J, Aboab J, Rottman M, et al. Plasma cortisol levels in Guillain-Barré syndrome. Crit Care Med. 2009;37:2436–40.

56. Colls BM. Guillain-Barré syndrome and hyponatremia. Intern Med J. 2003;33:5–9.

57. Saifudheen K, Jose J, Gafoor VA, et al. Guillain-Barré syndrome and SIADH. Neurology. 2011;76:701–4.

58. Pessin MS. Transient diabetes insipidus in the Landry-Guillain-Barré syndrome. Arch Neurol. 1972;27:85–6.

59. Berteau P, Morvan J, Bernard AM, et al. The association of acute polyradiculoneuritis, transitory diabetes insipidus and pregnancy. Apropos of a case and review of the literature. J Gynecol Obstet Biol Reprod. 1990;19:793–802.

60. Cooke CR, Latif KA, Huch KM, et al. Inappropriate antidiuresis and hyponatremia with suppressible vasopressin in Guillain-Barré syndrome. Am J Nephrol. 1998;18:71–6.

61. Steinberger B, Ford SM, Coleman TA. Intravenous immunoglobulin therapy results in post-infusional hyperproteinemia, increased serum viscosity, and pseudohyponatremia. Am J Hematol. 2003;73:97–100.

62. Burgess JR, Sheperd JJ, Parameswaran V, et al. Spectrum of pituitary disease in multiple endocrine neoplasia type 1 (MEN 1): clinical, biochemical, and radiological features of pituitary disease in a large MEN 1 kindred. J Clin Endocrinol Metab. 1996;81:2642–6.

63. Lam KSL, Sham MMK, Tam SCF, et al. Hypopituitarism after tuberculous meningitis in childhood. Ann Intern Med. 1993;118:701–6.

64. Tien RD, Felsberg GJ, Osumi AK. Herpes virus infections of the CNS. MR findings. AJR Am J Roentgenol. 1993;161:167–76.

65. Van de Beek D, de Gans J, McIntyre P, et al. Corticosteroids for acute bacterial meningitis. Cochrane Database Syst Rev. 2007;(1):CD004405.

66. Tsiakalos A, Xynos I, Sipsas NV, et al. Pituitary insufficiency after infectious meningitis: a prospective study. J Clin Endocrinol Metab. 2010;95:3277–81.

67. Schaefer S, Boegershausen N, Meyer S, et al. Hypothalamic-pituitary insufficiency following infectious diseases of the central nervous system. Eur J Endocrinol. 2008;158:3–9.

68. Tanriverdi F, Alp E, Demiraslan H, et al. Investigation of pituitary functions in patients with acute meningitis: a pilot study. J Endocrinol Invest. 2008;31:489–91.

69. Ickenstein GW, Klotz JM, Langohr HD. Virus encephalitis with symptomatic Parkinson syndrome, diabetes insipidus and panhypopituitarism. Fortschr Neurol Psychiatr. 1999;67:476–81.

70. Lichtenstein MJ, Tilley WS, Sandler MP. The syndrome of hypothalamic hypopituitarism complicating viral meningoencephalitis. J Endocrinol Invest. 1982;5:111–5.

71. Bartsocas CS, Pantelakis SN. Human growth hormone therapy in hypopituitarism due to tuberculous meningitis. Acta Paediatr Scand. 1973;62:304–6.

72. Ezzat S, Asa SL, Couldwell WT, et al. The prevalence of pituitary adenomas: systematic review. Cancer. 2004;101:613–9.

73. Chambers EF, Turski PA, LaMasters D, et al. Regions of low density in the contrast-enhanced pituitary gland: normal and pathologic processes. Radiology. 1982;144:109–13.

74. Terada T, Kovacs K, Stefaneanu L, et al. Incidence, pathology, and recurrence of pituitary adenomas: study of 647 unselected surgical cases. Endocr Pathol. 1995;6:301–10.

75. Watson JC, Shawker TH, Nieman LK, et al. Localization of pituitary adenomas by using intraoperative ultrasound in patients with Cushing's disease and no demonstrable pituitary tumor on magnetic resonance imaging. J Neurosurg. 1998;89:927–32.

76. Jeffcoat WJ, Pound N, Sturrock ND, et al. Long term follow-up of patients with hyperprolactinaemia. Clin Endocrinol. 1996;45:299–303.

77. Greenman Y, Tordjman K, Stern N. Increased body weight associated with prolactin secreting pituitary adenomas: weight loss with normalization of prolactin. Clin Endocrinol. 1998;48:547–53.

78. Faglia G. Prolactinomas and hyperprolactinemic syndrome. In: DeGroot LJ, Jameson JL, editors. Endocrinology. 4th ed. Philadelphia: WB Saunders; 2001.

79. Simard MF. Pituitary tumor endocrinopathies and their endocrine evaluation. Neurosurg Clin N Am. 2003;14:41–54.

80. Rand T, Kink E, Sator M, et al. MRI of microadenomas in patients with hyperprolactinaemia. Neuroradiology. 1996;38:744–6.

81. Molitch ME. Disorders of prolactin secretion. Endocrinol Metab Clin North Am. 2001;30:585–609.

82. Molitch ME, Elton RL, Blackwell RE, et al. Bromocriptine as primary therapy for prolactin-secreting macroadenomas: results of a prospective multicenter study. J Clin Endocrinol Metab. 1985;60:698–705.

83. Biller BM, Molitch ME, Vance ML, et al. Treatment of prolactin-secreting macroadenomas with the once-weekly dopamine agonist cabergoline. J Clin Endocrinol Metab. 1996;81:2338–43.

84. Thorner MO, Schran HF, Evans WS, et al. A broad spectrum of prolactin suppression by bromocriptine in hyperprolactinemic women: a study of serum prolactin and bromocriptine levels after acute and chronic administration of bromocriptine. J Clin Endocrinol Metab. 1980;50:1026–33.

85. Wenig BM, Heffess CS, Adair CF. Neoplasms of the pituitary gland. In: Wenig BM, Heffess CS, Adair CF, editors. Atlas of endocrine pathology. 1st ed. Philadelphia: WB Saunders; 1997.

86. Colao A, Cuocolo A, Marzullo P. Impact of patient's age and disease duration on cardiac performance in acromegaly: a radionuclide angiography study. J Clin Endocrinol Metab. 1999;84:1518–23.

87. Minniti G, Jaffrain-Rea ML, Moroni C, et al. Echocardiographic evidence for a direct effect of GH/IGF-1 hypersecretion on cardiac mass and function in young acromegalics. Clin Endocrinol. 1998;49:101–6.

88. Quabbe H-J, Plockinger U. Metabolic aspects of acromegaly and its treatment. Metabolism. 1996;45:61–2.

89. Cannavo S, Squadrito S, Finocchiaro MD, et al. Goiter and impairment of thyroid function in acromegalic patients: basal evaluation and follow-up. Horm Metab Res. 2000;32:190–5.

90. Jenkins PJ, Frajese V, Jones AM, et al. Insulin like growth factor I and the development of colorectal neoplasia in acromegaly. J Clin Endocrinol Metab. 2000;85:3218–21.

91. Vance ML. Endocrinological evaluation of acromegaly. J Neurosurg. 1998;89:499–500.

92. Lissett CA, Peacey SR, Laing I, et al. The outcome of surgery for acromegaly: the need for a specialist pituitary surgeon for all types of growth hormone (GH) secreting adenomas. Clin Endocrinol. 1998;49:653–7.

93. Kreutzer J, Vance ML, Lopes MBS, Laws ER. Surgical management of growth hormone secreting pituitary adenomas. An outcome study using modern remission criteria. J Clin Endocrinol Metab. 2001;86:4072–7.

94. Vance ML. Medical treatment of functional pituitary tumors. Neurosurg Clin N Am. 2003;14:81–7.

95. Barkan AL. Acromegaly: diagnosis and therapy. Endocrinol Metab Clin North Am. 1989;18:277–310.

96. Trainer PJ, Drake WM, Katznelson L, et al. Treatment of acromegaly with the growth hormone-receptor antagonist pegvisomant. N Engl J Med. 2000;342:1171–7.

97. Van der Lely AJ, Hutson RK, Trainer PJ, et al. Long-term treatment of acromegaly with pegvisomant, a growth hormone receptor antagonist. Lancet. 2001;358:1754–9.

98. Landolt AM, Haller D, Lomax N, et al. Octreotide may act as a radioprotective agent in acromegaly. J Clin Endocrinol Metab. 2000;85:1287–9.

99. Bonelli FS, Huston J, Carpenter PC, et al. Adrenocorticotropic hormone-dependent Cushing's syndrome: sensitivity and specificity of inferior petrosal sinus sampling. AJNR Am J Neuroradiol. 2000;21:690–6.

100. Nieman LK. Medical therapy of Cushing's disease. Pituitary. 2002;5:77–82.

101. Tucker WS, Snell BB, Island DP, et al. Reversible adrenal insufficiency induced by ketoconazole. JAMA. 1985;253:2413–4.

102. Nieman LK. Cushing's syndrome. In: DeGroot LJ, Jameson JL, editors. Endocrinology. 4th ed. Philadelphia: WB Saunders; 2001.

103. Belsky JL, Cuello B, Swanson LW, Simmons DM, Jarrett RM, Braza F. Cushing's syndrome due to ectopic production of corticotropin-releasing factor. J Clin Endocrinol Metab. 1985;60:496–500.

104. Doppman JL, Frank JA, Dwyer AJ, et al. Gadolinium DTPA enhanced imaging of ACTH secreting microadenomas of the pituitary gland. J Comput Assist Tomogr. 1988;12:728–35.

105. Shimon I, Melmed S. Management of pituitary tumors. Ann Intern Med. 1998;129:472–83.

106. Newell-Price J, Bertagna X, Grossman AB, Nieman LK. Cushing's syndrome. Lancet. 2006;367:1605–7.

107. Young Jr WF, Scheithauer BW, Kovacs KT, Horvath E, Davis DH, Randall RV. Gonadotroph adenoma of the pituitary gland: a clinicopathologic analysis of 100 cases. Mayo Clin Proc. 1996;71:649–56.

108. Vance ML, Ridgway EC, Thorner MO. Follicle stimulating hormone and alpha subunit secreting pituitary tumor treated with bromocriptine. J Clin Endocrinol Metab. 1985;61:580–4.

109. Verhelst J, Berwaerts J, Abs R, et al. Obstructive hydrocephalus as complication of a giant nonfunctioning pituitary adenoma: therapeutical approach. Acta Clin Belg. 1998;53:47–52.

110. Leese G, Jeffreys R, Vora J. Effects of cabergoline in a pituitary adenoma secreting follicle-stimulating hormone. Postgrad Med J. 1997;73:507–8.

111. Beck-Peccoz P, Bruckner-Davis F, Persani L, Smallridge RC, Weintraub BD. Thyrotropin-secreting pituitary tumors. Endocr Rev. 1996;17:610–38.

112. Burgess JR, Shepherd JJ, Greenaway TM. Thyrotropinomas in multiple endocrine neoplasia type 1 (MEN-1). Aust N Z J Med. 1994;24:740–1.

113. Bruckner-Davis F, Oldfield EH, Skarulis MC, et al. Thyrotropin-secreting pituitary tumors: diagnostic criteria, thyroid hormone sensitivity, and treatment outcome in 25 patients followed at the National Institutes of Health. J Clin Endocrinol Metab. 1999;84:476–86.

114. Frank SJ, Gesundheit N, Doppman JL, et al. Preoperative lateralization of pituitary microadenomas by petrosal sinus sampling: utility in two patients with non-ACTH-secreting tumors. Am J Med. 1989;87:679–82.

115. Faglia G, Beck-Peccoz P, Piscitelli G, et al. Inappropriate secretion of thyrotropin by the pituitary. Horm Res. 1987;26:79–99.

116. Spada A, Bassetti M, Martino E, et al. In vitro studies on TSH secretion and adenylate cyclase activity in a human TSH-secreting pituitary adenoma. Effects of somatostatin and dopamine. J Endocrinol Invest. 1985;8:193–8.

117. Beck-Peccoz P, Persani L. Medical management of thyrotropin secreting pituitary adenomas. Pituitary. 2002;5:83–8.

118. Ness-Abramof R, Ishay A, Harel G, et al. TSH-secreting pituitary adenomas: follow-up of 11 cases and review of the literature. Pituitary. 2007;10:307–10.

119. Blumberg DL, Sklar CA, Wisoff J, et al. Abnormalities of water metabolism in c children and adolescents following craniotomy for a brain tumor. Childs Nerv Syst. 1994;10:505–8.

120. Singer I, Oster JR, Fishman LM. The management of diabetes insipidus in adults. Arch Intern Med. 1997;157:1293–301.

121. Seckl JR, Dunger DB. Postoperative diabetes insipidus. Correct interpretation of water balance and electrolyte data essential. BMJ. 1989;298:2–3.

122. Turner HE, Adams CB, Wass JA. Transsphenoidal surgery for microprolactinoma: an acceptable alternative to dopamine agonists? Eur J Endocrinol. 1999;140:43–7.

123. Central Brain Tumor Registry of the United States (CBTRUS). Available at: http://www.cbtrus.org/2011-NPCR-SEER/WEB-0407-Report-3-3-2011.pdf. Accessed 8 Aug 2011.

124. Raff H. Glucocorticoid inhibition of neurohypophyseal vasopressin secretion. Am J Physiol. 1987;252:635–44.

125. Chinitz A, Turner FL. The association of primary hypothyroidism and inappropriate secretion of the antidiuretic hormone. Arch Intern Med. 1965;116:871–4.

126. Laureno R, Karp BI. Myelinolysis after correction of hyponatremia. Ann Intern Med. 1997;126:57–62.

127. Hirschberg R, Adler S. Insulin like growth factor system and the kidney physiology, pathophysiology and therapeutic implications. Am J Kidney Dis. 1998;31:901–19.

128. Bunin GR, Surawicz TS, Witman PA, et al. The descriptive epidemiology of craniopharyngioma. J Neurosurg. 1998;89:547–51.

129. Kristopaitis T, Thomas C, Petruzzelli G, et al. Malignant craniopharyngioma. Arch Pathol Lab Med. 2000;124:1356–60.

130. Weiner HL, Wisoff JH, Rosenberg ME, et al. Craniopharyngiomas: a clinicopathological analysis of factors predictive of recurrence and functional outcome. Neurosurgery. 1994;35:1001–11.

131. Nelson GA, Bastian FO, Schlitt M, et al. Malignant transformation of craniopharyngioma. Neurosurgery. 1988;22:427–9.

132. Szeifert GT, Pasztor E. Could craniopharyngiomas produce pituitary hormones? Neurol Res. 1993;15:68–9.

133. Thapar K, Stefaneanu L, Kovacs K, et al. Estrogen receptor gene expression in craniopharyngiomas: an in situ hybridization study. Neurosurgery. 1994;35:1012–7.

134. Honegger J, Renner C, Fahlbusch R, et al. Progesterone receptor gene expression in craniopharyngiomas and evidence for biological activity. Neurosurgery. 1997;41:1359–64.

135. Ulfarsson E, Karstrom A, Yin S, et al. Expression and growth dependency of the insulin-like growth factor I receptor in craniopharyngioma cells: a novel therapeutic approach. Clin Cancer Res. 2005;11:4674–80.

136. Karavitaki N, Cudlip S, Adams CBT, et al. Craniopharyngiomas. Endocr Rev. 2006;27:371–97.

137. Hetelekidis S, Barnes PD, Tao ML, et al. 20-year experience in childhood craniopharyngioma. Int J Radiat Oncol Biol Phys. 1993;27:189–95.

138. Duff JM, Meyer FB, Ilstrup DM, et al. Long-term outcomes for surgically resected craniopharyngiomas. Neurosurgery. 2000;46:291–305.

139. Gonzales-Portillo G, Tomita T. The syndrome of inappropriate secretion of antidiuretic hormone: an unusual presentation for childhood craniopharyngioma: report of three cases. Neurosurgery. 1998;42:917–21.

140. Banna M, Hoare RD, Stanley P, et al. Craniopharyngioma in children. J Pediatr. 1973;83:781–5.

141. Baskin DS, Wilson CB. Surgical management of craniopharyngiomas. J Neurosurg. 1986;65:22–7.

142. Karavitaki N, Brufani C, Warner JT, et al. Craniopharyngiomas in children and adults: systematic analysis of 121 cases with long-term follow-up. Clin Endocrinol. 2005;62:397–409.

143. Van Effenterre R, Boch AL. Craniopharyngioma in adults and children; a study of 122 surgical cases. J Neurosurg. 2002;97:3–11.

144. Rajan B, Ashley S, Thomas DGT, et al. Craniopharyngioma: improving outcome by early recognition and treatment of acute complications. Int J Radiat Oncol Biol Phys. 1997;37:517–21.

145. Fahlbusch R, Honegger J, Paulus W, et al. Surgical treatment of craniopharyngiomas: experience with 168 patients. J Neurosurg. 1999;90:237–50.

146. Hoffman HJ, DeSilva M, Humphreys RP, et al. Aggressive surgical management of craniopharyngiomas in children. J Neurosurg. 1992;76:47–52.

147. DeVile CJ. Craniopharyngioma. In: Wass JAH, Shalet SM, editors. Oxford textbook of endocrinology and diabetes. 1st ed. Oxford: Oxford University Press; 2002.

148. Paja M, Lucas T, Garcia-Uria F, et al. Hypothalamic-pituitary dysfunction in patients with craniopharyngioma. Clin Endocrinol. 1995;42:467–73.

149. Dusick JR, Fatemi N, Mattozo C, et al. Pituitary function after endonasal surgery for nonadenomatous parasellar tumors: Rathke's cysts, craniopharyngiomas, and meningiomas. Surg Neurol. 2008;70:482–90.

150. De Vile CJ, Grant DB, Hayward RD, et al. Growth and endocrine sequelae of craniopharyngioma. Arch Dis Child. 1996;75:108–14.

151. Crowley RK, Sherlock M, Agha A, et al. Clinical insights into adipsic diabetes insipidus: a large case series. Clin Endocrinol. 2007;66:475–82.

152. Bondy M, Ligon BL. Epidemiology and etiology of intracranial meningiomas: a review. J Neurooncol. 1996;29:197–205.

153. Rockhill J, Mrugala M, Chamberlain MC. Intracranial meningiomas: and overview of diagnosis and treatment. Neurosurg Focus. 2007;23:1–7.

154. Nakasu S, Hirano A, Shimura T, et al. Incidental meningiomas in autopsy study. Surg Neurol. 1987;27:319–22.

155. Donnell MS, Meyer GA, Donegan WL. Estrogen-receptor protein in intracranial meningioma. J Neurosurg. 1979;50:499–502.

156. Black PM, Carroll R, Zhang J. The molecular biology of hormone and growth factor receptors in meningiomas. Acta Neurochir Suppl. 1996;65:50–3.

157. Carroll RS, Zhang J, Black PM. Expression of estrogen receptors alpha and beta in human meningiomas. J Neurooncol. 1999;42:109–16.

158. Pravdenkova S, Al-Mefty O, Sawyer J, et al. Progesterone and estrogen receptors: opposing prognostic indicators in meningioma. J Neurosurg. 2006;105:163–73.

159. Wang CJ, Lin PC, Howng SL. Expression of thyroid hormone receptors in intracranial meningiomas. Kaohsiung J Med Sci. 2003;19:334–8.

160. Hirota Y, Tachibana O, Uchiyama N, Hayashi Y, Nakada M, Kita D, Watanabe T, Higashi R, Hamada J, Hayashi Y. Gonadotropin-releasing hormone (GnRH) and its receptor in human meningiomas. Clin Neurol Neurosurg. 2009;111:127–33.

161. Lee E, Grutsch J, Persky V, et al. Association of meningioma with reproductive factors. Int J Cancer. 2006;119:1152–7.

162. Jhawar BS, Fuchs CS, Colditz GA, et al. Sex steroid hormone exposures and risk for meningioma. J Neurosurg. 2003;99:848–53.

163. Custer B, Longstreth Jr WT, Phillips LE, et al. Hormonal exposures and the risk of intracranial meningioma in women: a population-based case–control study. BMC Cancer. 2006;6:152.

164. McCutcheon IE, Flyvbjerg A, Hill H, et al. Antitumor activity of the growth hormone receptor antagonist pegvisomant against human meningiomas in nude mice. J Neurosurg. 2001;94:487–92.

165. Friend KE, Radinsky R, McCutcheon IE. Growth hormone receptor expression and function in meningiomas: effect of a specific receptor antagonist. J Neurosurg. 1999;91:93–9.

166. Hsu DW, Efird JT, Hedley-Whyte ET. Progesterone and estrogen receptors in meningiomas: prognostic considerations. J Neurosurg. 1997;86:113–20.

167. Korhonen K, Salminen T, Raitanen J, et al. Female predominance in meningiomas cannot be explained by differences in progesterone, estrogen, or androgen receptor expression. J Neurooncol. 2006;80:1–7.

168. Grunberg SM, Weiss MH, Spitz IM, et al. Treatment of unresectable meningiomas with the anti-progesterone agent mifepristone. J Neurosurg. 1991;74:861–6.

169. Grunberg SM, Weiss MH, Russell CA, Spitz IM, Ahmadi J, Sadun A, Sitruk-Ware R. Long-term administration of mifepristone (RU486): clinical tolerance during extended treatment of meningioma. Cancer Invest. 2006;24:727–33.

170. Grunberg SM, Rankin C, Townsend C, et al. Phase III double-blind randomized placebo controlled study of mifepristone (RU-486) for the treatment of unresectable meningioma. Proc Am Soc Clin Oncol. 2001;20:222 (abstract).

171. Goodwin JW, Crowley J, Eyre HJ, et al. A phase II evaluation of tamoxifen unresectable or refractory meningiomas: a Southwest Oncology Group Study. J Neurooncol. 1993;15:73–7.

172. Takala J, Ruokonen E, Webster NR, et al. Increased mortality associated with growth hormone treatment in critically ill adults. N Engl J Med. 1999;34:785–92.

173. Angele MK, Ayala A, Cioffi WG, et al. Comparison of the anabolic effects and complications of human growth hormone and the testosterone analog, oxandrolone, after severe burn injury. Burns. 1999;25:215–21.

174. Annane D, Sebille V, Charpentier C, et al. Effect of low doses of hydrocortisone and fludrocortisone on mortality in patients with septic shock. JAMA. 2002;288:862–71.

175. Sprung CL, Annane D, Keh D, et al. Hydrocortisone therapy for patients with septic shock. N Engl J Med. 2008;358:111–24.

176. Ferrando AA, Sheffield-Moore M, Wolf SE, et al. Testosterone administration in severe burns ameliorates muscle catabolism. Crit Care Med. 2001;29:1936–42.

177. Basakis AM, Kunzler C. Altered mental status due to metabolic or endocrine disorders. Emerg Med Clin North Am. 2005;23:901–8.

178. Kanich W, Brady WJ, Huff S. Altered mental status: evaluation and etiology in the ED. Am J Emerg Med. 2002;20:613–7.

179. Brooks SM, Werk EE, Ackerman SJ, et al. Adverse effects of phenobarbital on corticosteroid metabolism in patients with bronchial asthma. N Engl J Med. 1972;286:1125–8.

180. Thomas Z, Bandali F, McCowen K, et al. Drug-induced endocrine disorders in the intensive care unit. Crit Care Med. 2010;38:S219–30.

181. Jabre P, Combes X, Lapostolle F, et al. Etomidate versus ketamine for rapid sequence intubation in acutely ill patients: a multicenter randomized controlled trial. Lancet. 2009;374:293–300.

182. Lipiner-Friedman D, Sprung CL, Laterre PF, et al. Adrenal function in sepsis: the retrospective Corticus cohort study. Crit Care Med. 2007;35:1012–8.

183. Mistraletti G, Donatelli F, Carli F. Metabolic and endocrine effects of sedative agents. Curr Opin Crit Care. 2005;11:312–7.

184. Cohen-Lehman J, Dahl P, Danzi S, et al. Effects of amiodarone therapy on thyroid function. Nat Rev Endocrinol. 2010;6:34–41.

185. Tanda ML, Bogazzi F, Martino E, et al. Amiodarone-induced thyrotoxicosis: something new to refine the initial diagnosis? Eur J Endocrinol. 2008;159:359–61.

186. Yiu KH, Jim MH, Siu CM, et al. Amiodarone-induced thyrotoxicosis is a predictor of adverse cardiovascular outcome. J Clin Endocrinol Metab. 2009;94:109–14.

187. Sakr Y, Reinhart K, Vincent JL, et al. Does dopamine administration in shock influence outcome? Results of the Sepsis Occurrence in Acutely Ill Patients (SOAP) Study. Crit Care Med. 2006;34:589–97.

188. De Backer D, Biston P, Devriendt J, et al. Comparison of dopamine and norepinephrine in the treatment of shock. N Engl J Med. 2010;362:779–89.

189. Kaptein EM, Spencer CA, Kamiel MB, et al. Prolonged dopamine administration and thyroid hormone economy in normal and critically ill subjects. J Clin Endocrinol Metab. 1980;51:387–93.

190. Oakley PW, Dawson AH, Whyte IM. Lithium: thyroid effect and altered renal handling. J Toxicol Clin Toxicol. 2000;38:333–7.

191. Herings RM, de Boer A, Stricker BH, et al. Hypoglycaemia associated with use of inhibitors of angiotensin converting enzyme. Lancet. 1995;345:1195–8.

192. Murad MH, Coto-Yglesias F, Wang AT, et al. Clinical review: drug-induced hypoglycemia: a systematic review. J Clin Endocrinol Metab. 2009;94:741–5.

193. Singh M, Jacob JJ, Kapoor R, et al. Fatal hypoglycemia associated with levofloxacin use in an elderly patient in the postoperative period. Langenbecks Arch Surg. 2008;393:235–8.

194. Carr R, Zed PJ. Octreotide for sulfonylurea-induced hypoglycemia following overdose. Ann Pharmacother. 2002;36:1727–32.

195. Clore JN, Thurby-Hay L. Glucocorticoid-induced hyperglycemia. Endocr Pract. 2009;15:469–74.

196. Loisa P, Parviainen I, Tenhunen J, et al. Effect of mode of hydrocortisone administration on glycemic control in patients with septic shock: a prospective randomized trial. Crit Care. 2007;11:R21.

197. Romagnoli J, Citterio F, Violi P, et al. Post-transplant diabetes mellitus after kidney transplantation with different immunosuppressive agents. Transplant Proc. 2004;36:690–1.

198. Barth E, Albuszies G, Baumgart K, et al. Glucose metabolism and catecholamines. Crit Care Med. 2007;35:S508–18.

199. Yood MU, DeLorenze G, Quesenberry Jr CP, et al. The incidence of diabetes in atypical antipsychotics users differs according to agent – results from a multisite epidemiologic study. Pharmacoepidemiol Drug Saf. 2009;18:791–9.

200. Sazontseva IE, Kozlov IA, Moisuc YG, et al. Hormonal response to brain death. Transplant Proc. 1991;23:2467.

201. Rosendale JD, Kauffman HM, McBride MA, et al. Hormonal resuscitation yields more transplanted hearts, with improved early function. Transplantation. 2003;75:1336–41.

202. Howlett TA, Keogh AM, Perry L, et al. Anterior and posterior pituitary dysfunction in brain dead donors. Transplantation. 1989;47:828–34.

203. Rosengard BR, Feng S, Alfrey EJ, et al. Report of the Crystal City meeting to maximize the use of organs recovered from the cadaver donor. Am J Transplant. 2002;2:701–11.

204. Smith M. Physiologic changes during brain stem death—lessons for management of the organ donor. J Heart Lung Transplant. 2004;23:S217–24.

Hematologic and Coagulation Implications of Neurologic Disease

Jan S. Moreb

Contents

Abstract

The incidence of hematologic disorders in any intensive care unit (ICU), including a neurointensive care unit (NeuroICU), could be high. In this chapter, we will cover three major topics that include decreased blood counts, increased blood counts, and spontaneous and induced coagulopathies. Anemia—defined as hemoglobin less than 12 g/dL—can be found in up to 95 % of patients admitted to ICU, while acute neurologic emergencies often involve bleeding into the central nervous system (CNS) or clotting of blood vessels and ischemia. Some of the hematologic diseases could present primarily with CNS symptoms, while others may just be encountered in patients admitted to the NeuroICU. Spontaneous and induced coagulopathies can be associated with strokes, and optimal treatment requires early involvement of the consultant hematologist. The use of anticoagulants can be life saving but almost never an easy decision.

Keywords

NeuroICU • Strokes • Anemia • Thrombocytopenia • Coagulopathy • Anticoagulation

Introduction

The interface between hematology and neurology is broad, and neurological complications in the course of hematological diseases are frequent and varied. The incidence of hematologic disorders in any intensive care unit (ICU), including a neurointensive care unit (NeuroICU), could be high. For example, anemia—defined as hemoglobin less than 12 g/dL—can be found in up to 95 % of patients admitted to ICU, while acute neurologic emergencies often involve bleeding into the central nervous system (CNS) or clotting of blood vessels and ischemia. In approximately 1 % of all patients with ischemic stroke and in up to 4 % of young adults with stroke, the major precipitant of brain ischemia is a hematologic disorder or coagulopathy predisposing to thrombosis

J.S. Moreb, MD
Division of Hematology and Oncology, Department of Medicine,
University of Florida College of Medicine,
1600 SW Archer Rd, Gainesville, FL 32610, USA
e-mail: morebjs@medicine.ufl.edu

A.J. Layon et al. (eds.), *Textbook of Neurointensive Care*,
DOI 10.1007/978-1-4471-5226-2_16, © Springer-Verlag London 2013

[1–5]. Early hematologic intervention could be critical in these instances.

On the other hand, patients with a spontaneous stroke or post a serious motor vehicle accident in which injuries to the brain and spinal cord are sustained may be at risk for venous thromboembolism (VTE). Prevention and treatment of VTE in neurologic and neurosurgical patients could be complex with multiple aspects to be considered. This subject will be covered by Chap. 17.

In this chapter, we will cover three major topics that include decreased blood counts, increased blood counts, and spontaneous and induced coagulopathies. Some of these topics were summarized and discussed before in the 4th edition of *Civetta, Taylor, Kirby's Critical Care* textbook, Chap. 173 [6]. Thus, more neurological perspectives and updates will be provided here.

Decreased Blood Counts

Anemias

Anemia (hemoglobin concentration less than 12 g/dL) is present in 95 % of patients in the ICU, with about one-third of those having, upon admission, a concentration of less than 10 g/dL. In the assessment, particular attention should be paid to the time of onset, the patient's ethnic origin, concurrent illness, procedures the patient has undergone, drugs the patient is receiving, and a history of transfusions. One practical approach is to classify anemia into two major categories: anemia resulting from under-production versus anemia due to increased destruction of red blood cells (RBC) (Table 16.1). These considerations will affect the type of laboratory tests and the need for transfusions.

Every effort should be exerted to obtain diagnostic tests prior to any transfusions. These should include a complete blood count, including hematocrit, hemoglobin, mean corpuscular volume (MCV) and hemoglobin (MCH), a reticulocyte count, and a stained blood smear. In addition, serum bilirubin and lactate dehydrogenase (LDH) are useful to determine the presence of hemolysis. If immune hemolysis is suspected, direct and indirect Coombs tests should be ordered; if hemoglobinopathy is suspected, hemoglobin electrophoresis should be obtained before transfusion.

The physician in the ICU may be faced with the immediate decision of whether the patient requires transfusion with packed red blood cells (PRBC). For years, many physicians firmly believed that hemoglobin of 10 g/dL or hematocrit of 30 % was desirable in anemic patients, especially those undergoing surgical procedures and/or with critical illness [7]. This approach of using fixed transfusion triggers has been recognized as the main reason for high

Table 16.1 Anemia classification

Anemias secondary to marrow underproduction
Decreased erythropoietin production
Renal disease
Endocrine deficiency
Starvation
Inadequate response to erythropoietin
Iron deficiency
B_{12} deficiency
Folic acid deficiency
Anemia of chronic disease
Marrow infiltration
Sideroblastic anemia
Myelodysplastic syndrome
Marrow failure
Congenital dyserythropoietic anemia
Aplastic anemia
Pure red cell aplasia
Toxic marrow damage
Anemias secondary to increased destruction
Acquired
Immune-mediated hemolytic anemia
Paroxysmal nocturnal hemoglobinuria
Hemolytic anemia due to red cell fragmentation (TTP, DIC)
Hemolytic anemia due to chemical or physical agents
Infections
Acquired hemoglobinopathies (methemoglobinemia)
Hereditary
Congenital hemoglobinopathies (sickle cell disease)
Enzyme deficiency (G6PD, pyruvate kinase)
Red cell membrane defects (spherocytosis, elliptocytosis)

Adapted with permission from Moreb [6]
TTP thrombotic thrombocytopenic purpura, *DIC* disseminated intravascular coagulation

transfusion rates in ICU patients and is finally being replaced by a more physiologic approach in which the patient's intravascular volume and tissue oxygen needs are considered. A restrictive transfusion policy, in which hemoglobin concentration is maintained between 7 and 9 g/dL, has proved to be effective and yields decreased death rates in comparison to the liberal strategy [7–9]. Indeed, in young traumatized patients, the hemoglobin is sometimes allowed to drift to as low as 5 g/dL, as long as there are no signs of oxygen delivery deficit such as elevated lactate levels, an unacceptable heart rate, or other symptoms. These patients are most often started on recombinant erythropoietin and have iron stores repleted, if necessary, to keep from undergoing transfusion.

Patients with acute myocardial infarction or unstable angina [7], and some cancer patients, may benefit from a higher hemoglobin level. Patients with a hemoglobin greater than or equal to 10 g/dL are unlikely to benefit from blood transfusion.

Anemia in Critical Illness

Anemia with a hemoglobin less than or equal to about 8.5 g/dL is the most frequent type of anemia encountered in the ICU. As a result, more than 50 % of these patients receive RBC transfusions (RBCT) during their ICU stay, as do more than 85 % of patients with an ICU length of stay longer than 7 days. This trend was confirmed by two large studies: the CRIT study in the United States [10] and the ABC trial in Europe [11]. Both studies also showed that the number of RBCT a patient received were *independently* associated with longer ICU stay and increase in mortality. These and other similar epidemiologic studies have revealed some similarities. First, the vast majority of critically ill patients have anemia on admission to the ICU. Second, the most common indication for RBCT in the ICU was treatment of the anemia. Third, the transfusion trigger in all these studies was hemoglobin of about 8.5 g/dL. Finally, RBCT were increased in patients with prolonged ICU length of stay and increased age.

Possible mechanisms involved in anemia of acute critically ill patients include a blunted erythropoietin (EPO) response to anemia, with blood concentrations being inappropriately low in these patients; suppression of erythropoiesis by proinflammatory cytokines; possible blood loss from frequent phlebotomies; and blood loss from gastrointestinal bleeding as a result of gastric tubes, stress-induced mucosal ulcerations, acute renal failure, and the frequent coagulation problems often seen in ICU patients. This anemia shares characteristics with anemia of chronic inflammation such as high ferritin concentrations and low-to-normal transferrin saturation with functional iron deficiency [9].

Until recently, we understood little about the pathogenesis of anemia of chronic inflammation. It now appears that the inflammatory cytokine interleukin-6 (IL-6) induces the production of hepcidin, an iron-regulatory hormone that may be responsible for the hypoferremia and suppressed erythropoiesis [12]. This discovery should lead to studies focused on the role of hepcidin in the anemia of the critically ill patient and better understanding of its pathogenesis.

The approach to treatment of this type of anemia should include measures to reduce blood loss, a restrictive blood transfusion policy, and possibly the use of recombinant human EPO (rh-EPO). Recent Cochrane-sponsored systematic review of the literature (17 trials involving 3,746 patients), comparing the clinical outcomes in patients randomized to restrictive versus liberal transfusion thresholds or triggers [13], has revealed that the restrictive transfusion strategies reduced the risk of receiving an RBCT by a relative 37 %. The restrictive transfusion strategies did not appear to impact the rate of adverse events and did not impact the length of stay in ICU or hospital, but there was statistically significant reduction in the rates of infection (RR = 0.76; 95 % CI 0.6–0.97). Thus, the existing evidence supports the use of restrictive transfusion triggers in patients who are free of serious cardiac disease and those without acute bleeding.

Multiple studies have shown that the subcutaneous administration of rh-EPO at 40,000 units weekly, starting between days 3 and 7 of the ICU stay, resulted in a significant reduction in RBCT and a higher hemoglobin level [14, 15]. Since iron is locked up in the phagocytic system and hardly available, the administration of intravenous iron together with rh-EPO may result in an enhanced rh-EPO effect. As only about 10 % of oral iron is bioavailable, this route may not be appropriate in ICU patients. Additionally, because there have been anaphylactoid reactions reported with iron dextran, iron gluconate is the preferred formulation. Iron gluconate is administered at a dose of 125 mg diluted in 100 mL saline over 1 h infusion or undiluted at a rate of 12.5 mg/min daily for eight sessions, to a total cumulative dose of 1,000 mg; iron administered in this fashion has been shown not to be a risk factor for infections [16].

Anemia in Neurologically Critically Ill Patients

Because reduced oxygen delivery contributes to "secondary" cerebral injury, anemia may not be as well tolerated among neurocritical care patients. Therefore, special considerations may be needed in certain neurological critical illnesses such as traumatic brain injury (TBI), subarachnoid hemorrhage (SAH), ischemic stroke, and intracerebral hemorrhage (ICH). Reviewing the literature always leads to the conclusion that clear guidance for transfusing neurocritical patients has been lacking [17–21]. Multiple studies have shown that anemia of Hgb < 7 g/dL is associated with worse outcomes in nontraumatic SAH [22, 23], ICH [24], severe TBI [25], and ischemic stroke [26–30].

Whether the outcome can be improved by more frequent use of blood transfusions remains unclear [21, 31]. As mentioned earlier, major randomized studies showed worse outcome with the liberal approach of blood transfusions. However, there are ample data from animal studies as well as human physiologic studies and observational studies to suggest that such severe anemia can have detrimental effect in the brain-injured patient [17]. Furthermore, the coexistence of other physiologic stressors, such as low blood pressure, may make anemia less tolerable. Thus, physiologically, there is strong evidence that in severe anemia, a Hgb < 7 g/dL, risk may be increased in the neurocritical care patient. On the other hand, there are risks associated with RBCT including infections, immunosuppression, impairment of microcirculatory blood flow, 2,3-diphosphoglycerate deficiency, and an array of biochemical and physiological derangements including hypocalcemia, coagulopathy, hyperkalemia, and hypothermia. Transfusion-related acute lung injury (TRALI) is the most common cause of transfusion-related mortality reported to the Food and Drugs Administration [32]. Some of the complications are a result of inherent properties of the

Table 16.2 Anemia and transfusions in neurocritical care patients

Although the relation has not been proven with certainty to be causative, anemia is consistently associated with worse outcomes among neurocritical care patients (NCP)
Although a transfusion threshold of 7 g/dL is safe in many general critical care patients, it remains unclear if this is also true in NCP
Both severe anemia and RBCT are associated with poor clinical outcome in the NCP and, conversely, high hemoglobin levels result in improved clinical outcome
Risks associated with RBCT include infections, immunosuppression, impairment of microcirculatory blood flow, 2,3-diphosphoglycerate deficiency, hypocalcemia, coagulopathy, hyperkalemia, and hypothermia
Transfusion-related acute lung injury (TRALI) is the most common cause of transfusion-related mortality
The implementation of strategies to increase hemoglobin concentration while concurrently avoiding RBCT is warranted in this patient population
Selected NCP may benefit from RBCT if Hgb is <8–9 g/dL; however, because of the risks of transfusions, the number of transfusions should be kept to minimum
The duration of red blood cell storage may have implications on the cerebral consequences of transfusion
There is little guidance to clinicians in deciding when to transfuse anemic stroke and neurocritical care patients; clearly, randomized clinical trials are needed

blood products being transfused; others are a consequence of the storage of the red blood cells.

In summary (Table 16.2), there is no evidence that anemia seen in the NeuroICU patient should be treated differently than the anemia of general critically ill patients. Both severe anemia and RBCT are associated with poor clinical outcome in neurocritically ill patients, and, conversely, high hemoglobin levels result in improved clinical outcome. Thus, the implementation of strategies to increase hemoglobin concentration while concurrently avoiding RBCT is warranted in this patient population [33]. It is also true that selected NCP may benefit from RBCT if Hgb is <8–9 g/dL; however, because of the risks of transfusions, the number of transfusions should be kept to minimum.

Sickle Cell Anemia

Patients with sickle cell anemia may be seen in NeuroICU due to cerebrovascular symptoms or for other unrelated reasons. Cerebral ischemia can be seen in up to 25–29 % [34, 35] of patients with sickle cell disease (SCD). Thus, it will be important to be familiar with the pathophysiology of the disease, its manifestations, and treatments available.

Sickle cell hemoglobin (hemoglobin S) is the result of a single nucleotide mutation in the sixth codon of the β-globin gene (β^s). Heterozygous inheritance of hemoglobin S does not usually cause disease or symptoms but is detectable as sickle cell trait [36]. Homozygous inheritance or compound heterozygous inheritance with another β-globin gene results in disease. The discussion here is directed primarily toward homozygous sickle cell disease which includes those genotypes associated with chronic hemolytic anemia and vaso-occlusive pain: homozygous sickle cell disease (hemoglobin SS), hemoglobin SC disease (hemoglobin SC), sickle-β^0 thalassemia (hemoglobin $S\beta^0$), and sickle-β^+ thalassemia (hemoglobin $S\beta^+$), and other less common hemoglobin mutants. The clinical manifestations are related to the degree of intracellular polymerization of deoxyhemoglobin S, and it is different among the various genotypes.

The clinical symptoms of SCD affect multiple organs and may vary widely among patients. Chief among the clinical features are episodes of severe pain—namely, crises—in the chest, back, abdomen, or extremities. The acute chest syndrome, a frequent—and sometimes fatal—complication, affects more than 40 % of patients with SCD and can lead to acute and chronic respiratory insufficiency, including pulmonary hypertension. Its cardinal features are fever, pleuritic chest pain, referred abdominal pain, cough, lung infiltrates, and hypoxia.

Undoubtedly, the etiologic source of pain in SCD early in life is vaso-occlusion, which is ubiquitous. Cerebral arterial thrombosis occurs in about 25 % of patients with hemoglobin SS [34]. The mean age for ischemic stroke is about 10 years, but in young adults hemorrhagic strokes are more frequent [34]. This is the result of a chronic process referred to as the sickle cell vasculopathy [37] caused by repeated episodes of adhesion of sickled red blood cells to the endothelium leading to intimal hyperplasia and stenosis, arterial dissection, and small vessel vasculitis. The intracranial segment of the internal carotid artery (ICA) is most commonly affected [38]. The lenticulostriate arteries may provide collateral blood supply and enlarge, giving rise to a moyamoya pattern (stenosis/occlusion of supraclinoid ICA with dilated lenticulostriate vessels) [39]. Other complications of SCD are summarized in Table 16.3.

The goals of the SCD treatment are either to relieve symptoms of the complications or to prevent complications by using some of the new treatments targeting disease mechanisms. The treatment of the painful crisis is supportive. Dehydration, acidosis, infection, and hypoxemia all promote red cell sickling and should be prevented or corrected. Adequate relief of pain in the hospitalized patient usually requires parenteral administration of opioid analgesics at frequent fixed intervals. Sufficient analgesics should be used to

Table 16.3 Complications of sickle cell disease

Recurrent strokes in young adults
Parvovirus B19-induced aplastic crisis
Hyperbilirubinemia from cholestatic syndrome or cholecystitis and liver disease
Splenic infarctions
Autosplenectomy with increased risk of fulminant septicemia caused by encapsulated organisms such as *Streptococcus pneumoniae* and *Haemophilus influenzae*
Hematuria
Priapism
Bone infarctions with the risk of avascular necrosis, osteomyelitis, and other musculoskeletal manifestations
Leg ulcers
Spontaneous abortions

relieve pain without worrying about addiction or side effects of opiates; patients can be given oral analgesics to take at home. Oxygen is often administered in sickle cell crisis, although its benefits are uncertain. Antibiotics that cover major pulmonary pathogens should be administered to patients with acute chest syndrome. Because there is no clear evidence that transfusion therapy shortens a simple painful crisis and because the crisis is unpredictable and self-limited, transfusion is not a treatment for the uncomplicated painful crisis.

Transfusions are not needed for the usual anemia or episodes of pain. Urgent transfusions are needed when there is a severe sudden drop in hemoglobin, especially in children in whom splenic sequestration or aplastic crises present in this manner and in severe acute chest syndrome with hypoxia. Chronic red cell transfusions have been shown to prevent strokes in patients with SCD, although the optimal duration of transfusion is unknown. However, the risks of transfusions must be weighed against the benefits. These risks include alloimmunization, infections, and iron overload. For patients undergoing general anesthesia, preoperative transfusion to a hematocrit above 30 % has been shown to reduce postoperative complications. Leukocyte-depleted red cells that are phenotypically matched for the antigens most frequently associated with immune response are preferred for transfusion. Exchange transfusion is the most rapid method to reduce the hemoglobin S concentration to less than 30 % in urgent situations that arise from complications of SCD, such as stroke and severe acute chest syndrome, and in patients with striking cholestatic syndrome and signs of liver failure.

Hydroxyurea Treatment to Prevent Complications

In a double-blind, placebo-controlled trial, hydroxyurea was shown to reduce the pain episodes, acute chest syndrome, blood transfusions, and hospitalizations [40], with decades of accumulated experience and documented efficacy since then [41]. The improvements noted with hydroxyurea treatment correlate to increases in hemoglobin F levels and a decrease in granulocytes, monocytes, and reticulocytes [42]. Hydroxyurea treatment should be reserved for patients with SCD who have severe complications. Other experimental treatments aimed at interrupting the disease mechanisms are in progress [43].

Other Specific Anemias

Other types of anemia can be in the differential diagnosis of anemia in NeuroICU, and some may be associated with CNS involvement.

Autoimmune Hemolytic Anemia

When a patient is critically ill from autoimmune hemolytic anemia (AIHA), the presenting signs and symptoms are those of normovolemic anemia, unless massive hemolysis is associated with hypotension, significant hemoglobinuria, and acute renal failure. Variable levels of jaundice may also be present in the nonmassive AIHA. Initial laboratory data may show an elevated reticulocyte index (greater than 2)—identifying the mechanism of the anemia as hemolytic—an elevated indirect bilirubinemia, and LDH; the blood smear shows increased numbers of diffusely basophilic red cells, reflecting the increased reticulocytes, and variable numbers of microspherocytes and fragmented cells, indicative of the hemolysis. In some instances, the urine may be discolored red, brown, or black if there has been sufficient intravascular hemolysis to produce hemoglobinuria. A positive result on direct antiglobulin (Coombs) test, indicating that immunoglobulin or complement is on the surface of the circulating red cells, identifies the immune etiology of the hemolysis. In the absence of recent transfusion, the diagnosis of AIHA is confirmed. This information may first become available when the blood bank attempts to crossmatch the patient's blood for transfusion.

It is important to determine, by history and appropriate laboratory studies, whether the hemolysis could be related to a drug the patient is taking and whether it is caused by warm-reacting (usually IgG) or cold-reacting (usually IgM) antibodies. The mechanisms whereby drugs produce immune hemolysis are not absolutely clear, but evidence suggests an alteration of red cell surface antigens by the drug and production of antibodies that lead to hemolysis [44, 45].

The mainstay of treatment of AIHA caused by warm-reacting antibodies is the administration of corticosteroids, usually given in dosages equivalent to 60–80 mg/day of prednisone or its equivalent. In patients who do not respond to steroids, splenectomy, high-dose intravenous gamma globulin, rituximab chimeric anti-CD20 antibody, alemtuzumab humanized anti-CD52 antibody, or treatment with other immunosuppressive drugs may be useful.

Steroids are usually ineffective in AIHA caused by cold-reactive antibodies (cold agglutinin disease), but responses have been observed using larger doses. Patients with cold agglutinins may have symptoms related to impaired blood flow in acral parts where the blood temperature is low enough to permit agglutination of red blood cells by antibodies. Warming usually prevents or alleviates such symptoms; however, in a small percentage of cases, plasmapheresis to reduce the concentration of the offending IgM antibodies may be required. In drug-induced immune hemolysis, discontinuing the drug is usually the only treatment needed.

In the patient with AIHA with a critical degree of anemia, transfusion must be considered [46, 47]. It may be impossible to find compatible red blood cells by the usual cross-matching procedures, and transfused cells may be subject to rapid antibody-mediated destruction. On the other hand, the patient must not be allowed to die because of undue caution regarding the transfusion of incompatible red cells. The key to optimal care in this critical situation is close communication between the intensivist and the blood bank physician. When an AIHA patient is transfused, the patient must be observed closely for signs of accelerated hemolysis, such as visible hemoglobin in the plasma or urine.

Certain special considerations pertain to transfusion of patients with cold-reacting antibodies. Administered blood should be warmed to body temperature. Transfusion of plasma, which contains complement, should be avoided because hemolysis is complement mediated and may be limited by depletion of complement in vivo.

In massive hemolysis, therapeutic efforts should be directed at maintenance of blood pressure, renal blood flow, and urinary output. Intravenous fluids and diuretics such as furosemide should be used to maintain a urine flow of 100 mL/h.

Hemolytic Anemia from G6PD Deficiency

Red blood cell glucose-6-phosphate dehydrogenase (G6PD) deficiency is inherited as an X-linked recessive disorder, affecting various population groups around the world. In the United States, African Americans are the group most often affected, with a gene frequency of about 11 %. They have the G6PD A—variant of the enzyme and a mild to moderate deficiency. A recent study by the US Army found that 2.5 % of males and 1.6 % of females were deficient. Clinically significant hemolysis occurs when red cells are subjected to an oxidative metabolic challenge, as may occur with exposure to certain drugs or with certain illnesses. Among drugs producing hemolysis are some sulfonamides, nitrofurantoins, and antimalarials such as primaquine. Illnesses most likely to trigger hemolysis are acute infections. Infectious hepatitis, in particular, has been associated with severe hemolytic episodes in G6PD-deficient patients.

Hemolysis in the G6PD-deficient patient may be sudden and massive, usually becoming apparent 1–3 days after the inciting stress, such as administration of an oxidant drug; hemoglobinemia and hemoglobinuria may occur. The blood smear shows polychromatophilia within a few days, reflecting the developing reticulocytosis. Early in the course of the hemolytic episode, Heinz bodies may be identified in red cells by special staining methods. The red cell enzyme deficiency may be readily detected by laboratory assay when the patient is in a stable state but may be more difficult to demonstrate during a hemolytic episode. This is because the enzyme deficiency is greatest in the oldest red cells. These cells are the first destroyed in a hemolytic episode, and, as they are replaced by newly produced young cells, the overall red cell enzyme level may rise to the normal range. This replacement of susceptible erythrocytes by more resistant cells also tends to ameliorate the hemolysis with time.

If the diagnosis is suspected, any potentially offending drugs should be stopped. Otherwise, supportive care is usually all that is necessary. Although the deficiency is an X-linked trait, female heterozygotes may have hemolytic episodes.

Hemolytic Anemia from Red Cell Injury in the Circulation

Fragmentation and destruction of red cells in the circulation may result from increased shear stresses caused by turbulent blood flow. The two major categories of disease in which this kind of hemolysis occurs are malfunctioning intravascular prosthetic devices—for example, heart valves, vascular grafts, and shunts—and disorders affecting blood vessels that result in microangiopathic hemolytic disease, such as disseminated intravascular coagulation or thrombotic microangiopathy (TMA).

TMA encompasses the spectrum of thrombotic thrombocytopenic purpura (TTP) and hemolytic uremic syndrome. These forms of hemolytic disease are rarely of sufficient severity to require critical care. However, they can be seen in critically ill patients admitted to the ICU and have been associated with various initiating factors such as severe infections, drug intake, malignancies, connective tissue diseases, allogeneic stem cell transplantation, and pregnancy [48]. Because hemolysis is intravascular, hemoglobinemia and hemoglobinuria may be present. Characteristically, the blood smear shows red cell fragmentation producing micropoikilocytes (schistocytes). Typically, the TMA patients will also have thrombocytopenia, fever, and possibly neurologic and renal involvement.

Specific treatment is directed at the underlying disorder. Supportive measures may be required for the effects of hemolysis itself and to minimize any adverse renal consequences of hypotension and hemoglobinuria. These may include blood transfusion and hydration to ensure adequate urine flow. Occasionally, a badly malfunctioning prosthesis, such as an artificial heart valve, may require replacement, but this is more often necessary to correct a life-threatening hemodynamic abnormality than to alleviate severe hemolysis. The treatment of TMA with plasma administration, either infusion or plasmapheresis, is the only effective therapy that has dramatically improved the prognosis of these patients.

Aplastic Crisis in Hemolytic Anemia

Sudden intensification of anemia in hemolytic disease resulting from a precipitous reduction in the rate of red cell production is known as *aplastic crisis*. It may occur in the course of any hemolytic disease but has been most commonly reported in congenital hemolytic disorders such as hereditary spherocytosis and sickle cell anemia. It is most common in children, but may also be seen in adults. Patients characteristically have fever, anorexia, nausea, and vomiting; abdominal pain and headache are common. Their anemia is usually severe and may be life-threatening; mild leukopenia and thrombocytopenia are often present. The aplastic nature of the anemia is demonstrated by an extremely low reticulocyte count and marked reduction in erythroid precursors in the bone marrow. The episode is self-limited, and recovery usually begins by 2 weeks. In the recovery phase, there is a return of vigorous erythropoiesis and often an outpouring of nucleated red cells and reticulocytes into the blood, frequently accompanied by leukocytosis and immature white blood cells. There is convincing evidence that parvovirus B19 is the cause of most aplastic crises.

Treatment is via transfusion with red blood cells. The volume given should be sufficient to alleviate signs or symptoms of inadequate tissue oxygenation; that amount need not be exceeded, as episodes are self-limited, and the patient's hematocrit will return rapidly to its baseline level.

Paroxysmal Nocturnal Hemoglobinuria (PNH)

PNH is a rare, acquired stem cell disorder in which abnormal erythrocyte cell membranes are sensitive to lysis by complement. The molecular event is a somatic mutation in a gene called phosphatidylinositol glycan anchor biosynthesis, class A (PIG-A). The PIG-A gene is required for the first step in glycosylphosphatidylinositol (GPI) anchor biosynthesis. Failure to synthesize GPI anchors leads to an absence of all proteins that utilize GPI to attach to the plasma membrane. Two GPI-anchor proteins, CD55 and CD59, are complement regulatory proteins; their absence on the surface of PNH cells leads to complement-mediated hemolysis [49]. This disorder primarily affects young adults, presenting with chronic hemolytic anemia often coupled with mild granulocytopenia and thrombocytopenia. Episodes of nocturnal hemolysis with morning hemoglobinuria occur in only a minority of patients. Venous thrombosis, particularly of the hepatic and cortical veins, is common. Stroke due to arterial occlusion has not been clearly documented. Diagnosis is based on flow cytometric analysis of CD58 and CD59 and other parameters [50].

Eculizumab, a monoclonal antibody to complement factor C5, effectively reduces intravascular hemolysis and also thrombotic risk [51, 52].

Leukopenias

The term *leukopenia* refers to a total white blood cell (WBC) count of less than 4,000 cells/μL, whereas granulocytopenia or neutropenia refers to a circulating granulocyte count below 1,500 cells/μL. WBC and granulocyte levels are lower in some ethnic groups, e.g., Africans, African Americans, and Yemenite Jews, without any clinical significance. The clinical importance of granulocytopenia relates to the associated increased risk of bacterial infection, especially with absolute neutrophil count of <500 cells/μL. Agranulocytosis implies severe neutropenia or a complete absence of granulocytes. Three patient groups may be encountered in critical care situations: (a) patients with neutropenia from primary bone marrow diseases or cytotoxic treatment, (b) patients in whom neutropenia exists alone or in combination with other cytopenias as an aplastic process, and (c) patients with neutropenia or agranulocytosis caused by immunologic mechanisms.

Primary Bone Marrow Diseases and Cytotoxic Treatment

This is the largest and most frequent entity that causes neutropenia. Bone marrow diseases such as leukemias, myelodysplastic syndrome, and marrow fibrosis frequently present with neutropenia. Chemotherapy-induced neutropenia is a common complication of the treatment of cancer. The risk of life-threatening infections increases with the increased severity of neutropenia and its duration, and many of these patients, whether inpatient or outpatient, end up in the ICU due to a rapid onset of septic shock. In current practice, the occurrence of neutropenic fever is an indication for hospitalization and prompt institution of intravenous wide-spectrum antibiotics. Before starting antibiotics, cultures of blood, sputum, and urine should be obtained in all patients, and other sites should be cultured as indicated in individual patients. All patients should have chest radiographs taken as well. The common effects of bacterial infections—purulent sputum in pneumonia, pyuria in urinary tract infection, or abscess formation—are usually absent because of lack of granulocytes.

Many antibiotic regimens have been tested, and guidelines for a rational approach to therapy have been formulated [53]. The choice of an antibiotic regimen should take into account any findings in the individual patient that suggest a specific site of infection and any knowledge of patterns of infection in a given institution. If cultures are positive, the antibiotic treatment should be adjusted accordingly. If cultures are negative, as is frequently the case, empirical therapy should be continued if the patient remains neutropenic and until counts recover. If, on the other hand, fever continues and the patient's general condition deteriorates with persistent neutropenia, it is appropriate in selected patients to prescribe empirical treatment with an antifungal agent because of the frequency of fungal infections in patients with prolonged neutropenia. At this point, involving an infectious disease specialist is recommended. Patients should be screened by obtaining a CT scan of the sinuses, chest, abdomen, and pelvis for possible foci of invasive fungal infections. The galactomannan antigen test for aspergillus should be done routinely on blood and sputum (usually obtained by bronchoalveolar lavage) of immunosuppressed patients with neutropenia. If patients have central venous catheter, fungal and bacterial blood cultures should be obtained, and removal of catheters should be considered if blood cultures are positive for fungal infection or certain bacterial infections that are difficult to eradicate.

Various regimens of prophylactic antibiotics have been investigated for their efficacy in preventing infection in the neutropenic patient. The results have been too variable to justify blanket recommendations [54, 55]. The routine therapeutic use of colony-stimulating factors (such as G-CSF and GM-CSF) in febrile neutropenia to stimulate the proliferation and maturation of neutrophil progenitor cells was not recommended by the American Society of Clinical Oncology (ASCO). However, these stimulating factors should be considered in such patients at high risk for infection-related complications or who have prognostic factors that are predictive of poor clinical outcomes. High-risk features include expected prolonged (greater than 10 days) and profound (less than 0.1×10^3 cells/μL) neutropenia, age older than 65 years, uncontrolled primary disease, pneumonia, hypotension, multiorgan dysfunction, invasive fungal infection, or being hospitalized at the time of the development of the fever [56]. On the other hand, colony-stimulating factors are recommended for primary and secondary prophylaxis used to prevent chemotherapy-induced neutropenia [57].

ICU physicians should be aware of respiratory status deterioration or acute respiratory distress syndrome (ARDS) during neutropenia recovery with or without the use of G-CSF [57, 58]. This could be related to the release of inflammatory cytokines by resident alveolar neutrophils and macrophages. Mortality can be as high as 62 % in these patients, and, therefore, immediate evaluation by bronchoscopy to rule out infection and early use of high-dose steroids could be critical for their survival.

Bone Marrow Aplasia

Neutropenia is part of the pancytopenia commonly present in aplastic anemia. Some cases of aplastic anemia seem to have an autoimmune basis; in others, a drug or chemical exposure may be suspected as a cause. No tests are available to prove an association in individual cases. Many medications have been linked with aplastic anemia, which occurs as an idiosyncratic reaction in a small percentage of patients exposed to a given drug. Drugs for which an etiologic role seems likely include chloramphenicol, phenylbutazone, indomethacin, diphenylhydantoin, sulfonamides, and gold preparations. In at least half the cases of aplastic anemia, no cause is found or suspected.

The principles of treating infectious complications resulting from neutropenia in aplastic states are the same as those outlined earlier for neutropenia in malignant diseases. The treatment of aplastic anemia includes allogeneic bone marrow transplantation in suitable patients, immunosuppressive therapy including antithymocyte globulin, and other supportive care measures such as antibiotic prophylaxis and colony-stimulating factors.

Immune and Drug-Related Granulocytopenia

Neutropenia in adults often occurs as an isolated finding or in association with autoimmune disease such as rheumatoid arthritis, systemic lupus erythematosus, and other similar conditions. The evaluation should include the following: peripheral blood smear to seek out large granular lymphocytes (LGL); measurement of antinuclear antibodies, rheumatoid factor, and other autoantibodies; and possibly a bone marrow examination. Patients with chronic neutropenia, either idiopathic or autoimmune, usually do not require treatment.

Drug-induced agranulocytosis is a serious medical problem and occurs in 1–3 % of patients treated with certain medications. Drug-induced granulocytopenia should always be suspected in an ICU patient developing the situation while being exposed to multiple medications and antibiotics. The characteristic clinical syndrome includes high fever, chills, and severe sore throat (agranulocytic angina) caused by bacterial infection. Oral and pharyngeal ulcers, necrotizing tonsillitis, pharyngeal abscesses, and bacteremia may occur. The blood will demonstrate a virtual absence of granulocytes. Bone marrow examination is not usually indicated except for special cases, and it will show absence of all granulocyte precursors or only the mature cells. The picture may superficially resemble acute leukemia or a state of maturation arrest; the disease mechanism is often unclear. In some cases, it is an antibody against the drug acting as a hapten in association with endogenous antigen on neutrophil surface. Other drugs may impair production of neutrophils by direct toxic mechanism.

Serial blood counts are now recommended for patients on some drugs such as phenothiazines, clozapine, sulfasalazine, and antithyroid drugs because of the relatively high frequency of drug-induced neutropenia. Otherwise, management should include prompt withdrawal of all potentially

Table 16.4 Thrombocytopenia in ICU: mechanisms and causes

Six possible mechanisms

Hemodilution

Increased consumption

Increased destruction

Decreased production

Increased sequestration

Laboratory artifact (pseudothrombocytopenia)

Specific causes

Sepsis, multiorgan failure

Trauma or major surgery

Bone marrow failure (leukemia, aplastic anemia)

Immune-mediated platelet consumption (ITP, passive alloimmune thrombocytopenia, and posttransfusion purpura)

Drug induced (heparin, *GPIIb/GPIIIa inhibitors, antibiotics*)

TTP and related disorders (HUS, TMA, and peripartum HELLP syndrome)

offending drugs and the use of broad-spectrum antibiotics. The time to recovery may be proportional to the severity but is usually within about a week after withdrawal of the offending drug.

Thrombocytopenias

Thrombocytopenia is a common laboratory abnormality in ICU patients that has been associated with adverse outcomes. The incidence of thrombocytopenia—defined as a platelet count of less than 150×10^3 cells/µL—has been reported to be 23–41.3 %, with mortality rates up to 54 % [59]. The incidence of more severe thrombocytopenia—less than 50×10^3 cells/µL—is lower, about 10–17 %, but is associated with greater mortality [59]. The relationship between the time course of platelet counts and mortality in 1,449 critically ill patients was examined in a prospective multicenter observational study in 40 ICUs from Europe, the United States, and Australia [60]. There was a documented increase in mortality in patients who had thrombocytopenia on day 4 of admission to the ICU and even higher mortality in those patients with documented thrombocytopenia by day 14.

Systematic evaluation of thrombocytopenia is essential to the identification of and management of the causes [59]. There are numerous potential causes of thrombocytopenia in the ICU (Table 16.4). While sepsis is the most common cause, accounting for more than 48 % of thrombocytopenia cases in the ICU, more than 25 % of ICU patients have more than one cause [61]. Drug-induced thrombocytopenia presents a diagnostic challenge inasmuch as many medications can cause thrombocytopenia, and critically ill patients often receive multiple drugs. One such drug is heparin, the most common cause of drug-induced thrombocytopenia due to immune mechanisms [59].

The first step in the diagnosis of true thrombocytopenia is to consider the mechanism [62]. Thrombocytopenia has six major mechanisms: hemodilution, increased consumption (both are common in ICU after tissue trauma, bleeding, and disseminated intravascular coagulopathy [DIC]), increased destruction (immune mechanism), decreased production, increased sequestration, and by laboratory artifact of pseudo-thrombocytopenia (Table 16.4) [63]. Several laboratory findings and clinical signs can help in determining the mechanism and making the diagnosis. As noted earlier, the presence of large platelets on the blood smear or by mean platelet volume (MPV) suggests active thrombopoiesis, though this finding may be equivocal. Therefore, examination of the bone marrow for the presence of megakaryocytes is often necessary to distinguish between increased destruction (presence of megakaryocytes) and decreased production (absence of megakaryocytes). The presence of splenomegaly raises the possibility of sequestration. Other laboratory tests are not necessary to evaluate the thrombocytopenia itself. The bleeding time is not useful in assessing thrombocytopenia. There is also the possibility of platelet clumping induced by the commonly used anticoagulant EDTA; platelet cold agglutinins; partial clotting of the blood sample; and platelet satellitosis, a disorder in which platelets cluster around white blood cells. When pseudothrombocytopenia is suspected, examining the peripheral blood smear and close communication with the laboratory are necessary.

On the other hand, the dynamics of platelet counts can also be helpful. Many ICU patients show significant decrease in platelet counts during the first days in ICU [60, 64]. A typical cause for a decrease in platelet counts is major surgery (cardiopulmonary bypass, major trauma, vascular surgery) with initial decrease in platelet count by day 4 post surgery followed by an increase above the baseline level. Blunted or absent of such physiologic compensation mechanism after the initial decrease is associated with adverse outcomes and increase mortality [60, 63–65]. Persistent low platelet count beyond day 4 post surgery is most likely caused by severe consumption due to early sepsis, circulatory shock, multiorgan failure, and rarely TTP [66, 67]. A new and rapid decrease in platelet counts that begins after day 4 and after platelet count has already started to increase again is typical for immune-mediated causes such as heparin-induced thrombocytopenia (HIT), but also other drugs and posttransfusion purpura (PTP, rare) and transfusion-induced passive alloimmune thrombocytopenia (rare).

Patients Admitted to ICU with Thrombocytopenia

Platelet counts between 50 and 100×10^3 cells/µL after major surgery without bleeding at admission to ICU could be normal and require only monitoring. On the other hand, if bleeding is present due to trauma or surgery, then loss or consumption of platelets is ongoing, and platelet counts should be monitored frequently and maintained at $80–100 \times 10^3$ cells/µL. In trauma patients, tranexamic acid (loading dose of 1 g intravenous bolus followed by infusion of 1 g over 8 h) reduced mortality and risk of death due to bleeding [68].

If moderate thrombocytopenia is associated with an acute thromboembolic complication, severe pulmonary embolism, diabetic ketoacidosis, catastrophic antiphospholipid syndrome, and if the patient received heparin within the last 10 days, HIT has to be considered [63].

A frequent clinical challenge is the ICU patient with moderate thrombocytopenia who also requires treatment with antiplatelet drugs after recent ischemic stroke or stent placement. No management guidelines exist except for withholding the drugs in case of bleeding symptoms and transfusion of platelets in case of severe bleeding.

Severe thrombocytopenia of $<20 \times 10^3$ cells/µL on admission to ICU could be due to bone marrow failure (such as acute leukemia), severe coagulopathy (sepsis, meningococcemia, and, in endemic areas, malaria), and immune-mediated platelet consumption. ITP and TTP need to be differentiated early due to the available specific treatments.

There is often the need for intervention in patients with severe thrombocytopenia and bleeding and before confirming specific diagnosis. In this situation, transfusion of two units of platelet concentrates often controls the bleeding and is diagnostic at the same time. Platelet count determination within 1 h after the transfusion can distinguish between bone marrow failure (platelet counts increase) versus immune-mediated thrombocytopenia (platelet counts stay low). This approach should be avoided in patients with TTP because of the increased risk of thrombosis. Thus, blood smear should be reviewed before platelet transfusion is ordered.

Thrombocytopenia in ICU That Requires Special Management

Pseudothrombocytopenia is relatively common and should be considered in the differential diagnosis. This is especially important because of the antiplatelet agents, GPIIb/IIIa inhibitors, which induce pseudothrombocytopenia almost as frequently as true thrombocytopenia [63]. The exclusion of platelets clumps by microscopic examination of blood smear is essential.

Posttransfusion purpura should be considered if patient received transfusion within the last 2 weeks. Typically, it is severe thrombocytopenia seen in females who were immunized against this platelet alloantigen during previous pregnancy. Treatment is symptomatic by IVIg 1 g/kg for two consecutive days.

Passive alloimmune thrombocytopenia is caused by the transmission of platelet anti-human platelet antigen 1a allo-antibodies found in transfused plasma or red blood cells

immediately before severe thrombocytopenia occurs; this effect will be transient.

GPIIb/GPIIIa inhibitor-induced thrombocytopenia typically manifests within 24 h of treatment with one of these inhibitors, such as abciximab, tirofiban, or eptifibatide [69]. The risk for thrombocytopenia is higher during the second exposure with more severe thrombocytopenia $<20 \times 10^3$ cells/µL. After ruling out pseudothrombocytopenia, the offending drug should be stopped, and the platelet counts recover within 2–3 days. Platelet transfusions can be effective in case of significant bleeding.

Thrombotic thrombocytopenic purpura (TTP) and its closely related disorders—hemolytic uremic syndrome (HUS), thrombotic microangiopathy (TMA), and peripartum HELLP (hemolysis, elevated liver enzymes, and low platelets) syndrome—may be catastrophic and rapidly fatal. This disease entity was discussed in the first section of this chapter in regard to microangiopathic hemolytic anemia. TTP was defined by a pentad of abnormalities: thrombocytopenia from increased platelet destruction, microangiopathic hemolytic anemia caused by mechanical damage to red cells as a result of the vascular lesions, neurologic abnormalities, renal abnormalities, and fever. With the advent of curative plasma exchange in the 1970s, the urgency to establish a diagnosis and start treatment has resulted in using limited diagnostic criteria. Now only thrombocytopenia and microangiopathic hemolytic anemia are sufficient to begin plasmapheresis.

The clinical presentation is variable, but the thrombocytopenia and hemolytic anemia are often severe. A wide variety of fluctuating neurologic abnormalities may be present, including seizures, altered consciousness, delirium, and paresis. Renal abnormalities may include uremia, hematuria, and proteinuria. The reasons for fever are unclear. Besides thrombocytopenia, laboratory abnormalities include an increase in lactate dehydrogenase, absent or very low levels of haptoglobin, fragmented red blood cells, and reticulocytosis.

The basic pathogenic mechanism behind these syndromes is most likely related to the vascular endothelial cells. A role for ultra-large von Willebrand factor (vWF) multimers has been identified and is linked to endothelial damage and the occurrence of disseminated platelet thrombi in the microcirculation. TTP is often caused by low levels of a specific metalloprotease (ADAMTS13) that rapidly cleaves these multimers [70, 71]. Deficiency of this metalloprotease activity can be inherited or acquired due to autoantibodies [72]. In a small subset of TTP patients, these antibodies can be triggered by drugs: ticlopidine, clopidogrel, mitomycin C, quinine, cyclosporine, FK506 (tacrolimus), and some chemotherapeutic drugs.

Plasma exchange has dramatically changed TTP-HUS prognosis and outcome. Plasma infusion is less effective in adults, but it could be adequate in congenital TTP caused by ADAMTS13 deficiency. The duration of plasma exchange is unpredictable. Long durations, up to several months, may be required in patients with repeated relapses. Patients with auto-antibodies may also require immunosuppressive therapy.

Heparin-induced thrombocytopenia (*HIT*) is an anticoagulant-induced prothrombotic disorder caused by platelet activation of heparin-dependent antibodies of the immunoglobulin G class [59]. HIT is very frequently considered as a potential cause for thrombocytopenia in ICU patients, although it is relatively rare, with an incidence of 0.3–0.5 %. The diagnosis of HIT should be considered when the platelet count falls to less than 150×10^3 cells/µL, or a more than 50 % decrease of the platelet count from baseline, between days 5 and 14 from start of heparin therapy. A high index of suspicion on the physician's part is key in making the diagnosis. Patients with early-onset severe thrombocytopenia $<20 \times 10^3$ cells/L usually do not have HIT. The thrombocytopenia is usually moderate and resolves within a few days of discontinuing heparin. Rapid onset HIT can be observed in preimmunized patients who had received heparin within the past 30 days. HIT without thrombosis is called *isolated HIT*, whereas *HIT thrombotic syndrome* (HITTS) denotes HIT complicated with thrombosis.

HIT is an immune-mediated hypersensitivity reaction to platelet factor 4 (PF4)/heparin complex. PF4 is a heparin-binding protein found naturally in platelet α granules, which undergoes conformational changes once bound to heparin. Anti-PF4/heparin antibodies are produced by many patients taking heparin, but only a few will develop thrombocytopenia [73]. Anti-PF4/heparin antibodies are transient and usually become undetectable within a median of 50–85 days. If heparin is readministered to a patient with high levels of HIT antibodies, abrupt thrombocytopenia can occur. However, this likely will be more than 100 days after the last exposure to heparin [59]. It is important to note that seroconversion can be found by ELISA (enzyme-linked immunosorbent assay) in up to 15 % of patients on heparin; however, this does not constitute a diagnosis of HIT. In general, surgical patients, individuals exposed to higher doses of heparin for a longer time, and patients receiving unfractionated heparin (UFH), as opposed to low-molecular-weight heparin (LMWH), are more likely to develop HIT.

The frequency of HIT in ICU patients was examined in two major studies [73, 74]. The results suggested that only a small minority of ICU patients with thrombocytopenia receiving UFH have HIT, and that the PF4/heparin-reactive antibodies are more likely to be detected by ELISA assay than serotonin release assay (SRA), suggesting a possible overdiagnosis—due to a high false-positive rate by ELISA—of HIT. The Complications After Thrombocytopenia Caused by Heparin (CATCH) registry is a recent attempt to achieve better understanding of the prevalence, consequences, and temporal relationship of HIT and thrombocytopenia among patients treated with anticoagulants. The thrombotic sequelae

of HIT carry significant morbidity and may even be lethal. Some of the morbid events include deep venous thrombosis (DVT), pulmonary embolism, skin necrosis, limb ischemia, thrombotic stroke, and myocardial infarction [59]. The mortality rate associated with HIT ranges between 10 and 20 % [59]. Venous thrombosis is the most common manifestation, with lower limb DVT predominating.

All strategies should be used to prevent HIT in ICU patients. Heparin locks for central venous catheters and hemodialysis catheters are commonly used in the ICU setting and may need to be reconsidered. Hemodialysis without heparin has been shown to be safe and effective. However, once the diagnosis of HIT is recognized, heparin should promptly be substituted with a direct thrombin inhibitor, such as argatroban or lepirudin, or the heparinoid danaparoid (not available in the United States) to reduce the risk of life-threatening thromboembolic events. Because warfarin can temporarily reduce the synthesis of protein C and S, causing a hypercoagulable state, it should never be used alone in the initial treatment of HIT, and its use should be postponed until substantial platelet recovery has occurred. Consultation with a hematologist in these situations should be considered in all critically ill patients. The argatroban dose is 2 µg/kg/min in continuous infusion and dilution of 1 mg/mL. Dose adjustment is needed for hepatic impairment (use 25 % of the dose), with the aim of a 1.5–3 times prolongation of activated prothrombin time (aPTT) in comparison to baseline. On the other hand, lepirudin treatment consists of a bolus 0.4 mg/kg (maximum of 44 mg), given over 10–15 s and followed by continuous infusion at 0.15 mg/kg/h, with the goal of a 1.5–3 times prolongation of aPTT over baseline. The dose should be modified if creatinine is >1.5 mg/dL or clearance is <60 mL/min. If given with Coumadin, discontinue lepirudin when an international normalized ratio (INR) of 2.0 is obtained.

In summary, the approach to patients with suspected or confirmed HIT includes the following:

1. Discontinuation of all heparin
2. Administration of alternative nonheparin anticoagulation, such as argatroban or lepirudin
3. Testing for anti-PF4/heparin antibodies, followed, if positive, by a serotonin release assay
4. Avoiding prophylactic platelet transfusions
5. Allowing platelet recovery before starting warfarin
6. Assessing for lower extremity DVT

Patients with previous HIT who are antibody negative and require cardiac surgery should receive UFH in preference to other anticoagulants, which are less validated for this purpose. Preoperative and postoperative anticoagulation should be handled with an anticoagulant other than UFH or LMWH. Patients with recent or active HIT should have surgery delayed until antibody is negative, if possible; otherwise, an alternative anticoagulant should be used [75].

Bleeding Risk and Platelet Transfusions

Treatment of thrombocytopenia depends on the cause and is discussed later in this chapter under the specific entities. Thrombocytopenia usually increases the risk of bleeding, and the risk is not restricted to very low platelet counts. Additional factors contribute to the risk of bleeding even with moderate thrombocytopenia, such as DIC, platelet function defects, hyperfibrinolysis, and invasive interventions. Bleeding in ICU patients with platelet counts $>30 \times 10^3$ cells/μL is more likely to be indicator of disturbed hemostasis. Low hematocrit increases the risk of bleeding, and transfusion of RBCs up to HCT of 30–35 % might be an additional therapeutic option in patients with microvascular hemorrhage.

Even low platelet counts that are not associated with bleeding often influence management and treatment decisions. They often prompt physicians to withhold or delay necessary invasive procedures and can lead to a reduction in the intensity of anticoagulation and prophylactic platelet transfusions. Platelet transfusion triggers in ICU patients are not very well studied. Retrospective studies indicate that liberal platelet transfusion in ICU is associated with increased risk for infection, prolonged ICU stay, and even mortality [76]. Evidence is weak for safe cutoff values in ICU patients with thrombocytopenia and when transfusions are indicated. There are some consensus guidelines put out by expert panels with the aim of optimizing platelet transfusion therapy.

Several factors should be considered in deciding whether platelet transfusion is likely beneficial. When thrombocytopenia is caused by destruction or sequestration of the patient's own platelets, transfused platelets are subject to the same fate. Thus, platelet transfusions most often are of little benefit and are reserved for treatment of severe bleeding. When thrombocytopenia is caused by decreased platelet production, as in hematologic malignancies or during recovery from stem cell transplantation, serious hemorrhage can be prevented by regular transfusion of platelets. It is generally acceptable to use prophylactic transfusion to keep the platelet count greater than 10,000–20,000 cells/μL. Transfusion of one random-donor platelet unit per 10 kg of recipient weight, or single-donor unit from apheresis, is usually used to achieve that goal, which can be confirmed by a repeat platelet count within an hour posttransfusion. The effectiveness of platelet transfusions is diminished in febrile, infected patients who may require larger and more frequent transfusions. Actively bleeding patients require more frequent transfusion and a higher target of platelet count, usually above 50,000 cells/μL. Patients with intracranial hemorrhage, high risk for bleeding, or candidates for intracranial surgery may require even higher target of platelet count above 100,000 cells/μL. Chronically transfused patients may become refractory to platelet transfusions from random donors because of alloimmunization. Single-donor platelets limit exposure to foreign antigens and may delay immunization. Platelets obtained from family members by platelet apheresis may be considered in patients who are at risk for bleeding and refractory to random-donor platelets.

Increased Blood Counts

As with decreased blood counts, increased blood counts can lead to neurological complications requiring admission to the NeuroICU. Myeloproliferative disorders (MPD) are the main entity associated with increase in one or more of the cellular blood components. In young patients with cerebral infarction, hematologic disorders including thrombocytosis were the cause in 8.1 % of cases [77]. Cerebral venous thrombosis could be the presenting symptom of MPD [78]. A substantial proportion of patients with splanchnic venous thrombosis and a small, but significant, number of patients with cerebral vein thrombosis (CVT) can be recognized as carriers of the JAK2 V617F mutation, closely related to MPD diagnosis, in the absence of overt signs of MPD. The clinical significance of such findings deserves further investigation [79].

Erythrocytosis

Erythrocytosis, defined as an abnormally increased red cell mass, may require critical care due to complications of blood hyperviscosity or because of hemorrhagic or thromboembolic complications that threaten some of these patients. The initial clue to the presence of erythrocytosis is usually a high value for hematocrit or hemoglobin concentration. Such values may be present without true erythrocytosis—that is to say, in the presence of a normal red cell mass—if the plasma volume is contracted. This circumstance is usually apparent, although it is often advisable to quantify the red cell mass (RCM) by direct measurement using radioisotopic red cell labels. The RCM is usually increased when the hematocrit is above 60 % in a man or 57 % in a woman.

True erythrocytosis results from one of two general mechanisms:

1. Polycythemia vera (PV) is a clonal abnormality of bone marrow stem cells resulting in autonomous overproduction of red cells and often of granulocytes and platelets.
2. Secondary erythrocytosis results from excess erythropoietin production in response to hypoxemia, abnormalities of oxygen release from hemoglobin, or autonomous hormone production (e.g., by renal or other tumors).

When the RCM is expanded and the hematocrit increased, blood viscosity is increased, and diminished blood flow, stasis, thrombosis, and tissue hypoxia may ensue. On the other hand, hemorrhagic tendency is also increased, particularly in

Table 16.5 2008 World Health Organization diagnostic criteria for polycythemia vera (PV)

Major criteria

1. Hgb > 18.5 g/dL (men) > 16.5 g/dL (women)

   or Hgb or Hct > 99th percentile of reference range for age, sex, or altitude of residence

   or red cell mass > 25 % above mean normal predicted

   or Hgb > 17 g/dL (men)/> 15 g/dL (women) if associated with a sustained increase of 2 g/dL from baseline that cannot be attributed to correction of iron deficiency

2. Presence of JAK2V617F or JAK2 exon 12 mutation

Minor criteria

1. Bone marrow trilineage myeloproliferation
2. Subnormal serum erythropoietin level
3. Endogenous erythroid colony growth

Adapted with permission from Tefferi [80]

PV diagnosis requires meeting either both major criteria and one minor criterion or the first major criterion and two minor criteria

PV, where elevated platelet counts and abnormalities of platelet function may also be present.

Polycythemia Vera

The current criteria for the diagnosis of PV are according to the 2008 World Health Organization diagnostic criteria summarized in Table 16.5 [80]. The detection by PCR of Janus kinase 2 (JAK2) tyrosine kinase in up to 97 % of patients with PV increases the sensitivity and specificity of early diagnosis. The JAK2 V617F point mutation makes hematopoietic progenitors hypersensitive to the different growth factors, resulting in proliferation of all lineages. Risks in uncontrolled PV are primarily hyperviscosity and thromboembolic or hemorrhagic events.

Neurological manifestations are frequent in uncontrolled PV. Cerebral thrombosis is reported in 32–38 % during the course of the disease. Erythrocytosis can lead to small vessel intravascular thrombosis and lacunar infarcts. Symptoms resulting from decreased cerebral flow, such as headache, dizziness, and changes in vision are the most common manifestations of hyperviscosity due to erythrocytosis.

Patients with uncontrolled PV may present as medical emergencies requiring ICU care and urgent therapy. The mainstay of such therapy is phlebotomy to reduce hematocrit to less than 45 %. This may be done as rapidly as 1 unit of blood every other day in young adults. Electrolyte solutions or plasma expanders should be administered with phlebotomy, as necessary, to avoid circulatory instability from sudden changes in blood volume. Elderly patients may tolerate phlebotomy less well, so that removal of volumes of 200–300 mL at less frequent intervals may be necessary. Because of the clinical observations of increased thrombosis with aggressive phlebotomy, the simultaneous use of cytotoxic chemotherapy is recommended as part of the initial therapy

of patients older than 60 years of age, as well as in younger patients with thrombotic risk factors or a history of thrombosis. Hydroxyurea is often used for this purpose in an initial dose of 15–30 mg/kg/day. Emergency plateletpheresis may also be considered in such emergencies to lower an elevated platelet count.

Other treatment options include low-dose aspirin (81 mg/day), interferon-α (IFN-α), and anagrelide; these may be used together with phlebotomy as needed. In general, patients with PV should avoid practices and habits that augment hypercoagulability such as smoking, use of oral contraceptives, or hormone replacement therapy. Aggressive antithrombotic prophylaxis should be given postoperatively in addition to maintaining normal hematocrit and platelet counts.

Secondary Erythrocytosis or Polycythemia

The diagnosis of secondary erythrocytosis is made in a patient with an increased RCM in whom the criteria for PV are not met. These patients could either have physiologically appropriate increased RCM (for example, secondary to tissue hypoxemia) or inappropriately increased RCM (for example, secondary to increased erythropoietin production). Additional studies are needed to differentiate the diverse causes of polycythemia. Indications for phlebotomy in secondary erythrocytosis are less clear than in PV. The best current advice is to individualize therapy so as to maximize the patient's exercise tolerance and overall sense of well-being.

Thrombocytoses

With the availability of a platelet (PLT) count as part of a routine blood count, an elevated platelet count or thrombocytosis has become an important clinical problem in hospitalized patients. Unlike thrombocytopenia, the literature dealing with thrombocytosis in ICU patients is very scant. Furthermore, unlike thrombocytopenia, the presence of thrombocytosis predicts a favorable outcome in ICU patients, whereas a blunted rise in platelet count may be associated with worse outcome. Thrombocytosis in hospitalized patients is classified according to its origin into primary (or clonal) and secondary (or reactive) forms.

Primary thrombocytosis refers to a persistent elevation of platelet count due to clonal thrombopoiesis, as it occurs in myeloproliferative disorders including essential thrombocythemia (ET), PV, myelodysplastic syndrome, chronic myelogenous leukemia, and myelofibrosis. ET has been associated with small and large vessel ischemic stroke as well as microvessel vascular occlusive events [81] and even moyamoya syndrome [82] like that seen in sickle cell disease. Its natural history encompasses both vascular occlusive and hemorrhagic complications. Patients with extreme PLT counts >$1,500 \times 10^3$ cells/μL may experience hemorrhagic complications due to the acquired von Willebrand disease [83]. Patients with lower PLT counts are more likely to have thrombotic complications, and risk factors have been identified including age, previous history of thrombotic events, JAK2 V617F allele burden, and leukocytosis [84].

Secondary thrombocytosis is due to various conditions, some of them short-lived, such as acute bleeding, infection, trauma or other tissue injury, and surgery; other causes, such as malignancy, postsplenectomy, chronic infection, iron deficiency, or chronic inflammatory disease, may persist for a longer time. Multiple studies have been conducted on adult and pediatric hospitalized patients with an elevated platelet count (more than 500×10^3 cells/μL), and the main conclusions suggest that, whereas most patients have secondary thrombocytosis, a higher platelet count and increased thromboembolic complications are significantly associated with primary thrombocytosis [85, 86]. In one study, even when using greater than or equal to $1,000 \times 10^3$ cells/μL as the basis for defining extreme thrombocytosis, 82 % of 231 patients analyzed were found to have an elevated platelet count due to reactive (secondary) thrombocytosis [87]. In this study, the risk of bleeding and/or thrombosis was 56 % in primary thrombocytosis, but only 4 % in the secondary type. Unless additional risk factors are present, secondary thrombocytosis is not associated with an increased risk of thromboembolic events.

The treatment for primary thrombocytosis, such as ET, is based on risks for thrombosis or bleeding in the presence of vasomotor symptoms. Patients at increased risk—age older than 60 years, history of thromboembolism, and a platelet count greater than $1,500 \times 10^3$ cells/μL—should receive platelet-lowering agents such as hydroxyurea, anagrelide, or IFN-α. Low-dose aspirin can be used for the relief of vasomotor symptoms, but if there is no relief, platelet-lowering agents should be added. Hydroxyurea is the recommended drug in patients 60 years of age or older, whereas IFN-α is the cytoreductive agent of choice for childbearing women. The aim should be to lower the platelet count to less than 400×10^3 cells/μL. Arterial or venous thrombosis should be treated with heparin and, possibly, thrombolysis in some arterial events; plateletpheresis may be indicated in both types of events. Low-dose aspirin may be useful in arterial thrombosis. In hemorrhage, it is appropriate to stop antiplatelet agents and transfuse platelets if the bleeding is persistent. Some patients with uncontrolled thrombocytosis (greater than $1,500 \times 10^3$ cells/μL) were found to have an acquired defect of von Willebrand factor, which contributes to the risk of bleeding. Thus, DDAVP, cryoprecipitate, or factor VIII concentrate may be indicated to treat hemorrhage in these patients [88].

Leukocytosis

As in thrombocytosis, leukocytosis can be due to primary bone marrow disorders or secondary disorders in response to acute infection or inflammation. Secondary leukocytosis is physiologic and transient, resolving after treating the underlying cause. *Leukemoid reaction* refers to a persistent leukocytosis of more than 50×10^3 cells/μL, with shift to the left. The major causes for such a reaction include severe infections, severe hemorrhage, acute hemolysis, hypersensitivity, and malignancies (paraneoplastic syndrome) [89].

Leukocytosis due to a primary bone marrow disorder with uncontrolled clonal growth of immature cells can result in an emergency situation known as the hyperleukocytosis syndrome. This occurs in leukemic states when the white blood cell count is high. Signs and symptoms are most commonly related to the central nervous system, eyes, and lungs. They include stupor, altered mentation, dizziness, visual blurring, retinal abnormalities, dyspnea, tachypnea, and hypoxia. Intracranial and pulmonary infarction or hemorrhage and sudden death may occur. Priapism and peripheral vascular insufficiency have also been linked with the syndrome. Although the pathogenesis is incompletely understood, autopsies have shown white cell aggregates, microthrombi, and microvascular invasion (leukostatic tumors). The syndrome occurs more commonly in acute (AML) and chronic myelogenous leukemia (CML) than in acute lymphoblastic leukemia, and occurs rarely, if ever, in chronic lymphocytic leukemia. The level of the white blood cell count at which the syndrome appears is variable, depending perhaps on the maturity and size of the white blood cells present and the degree of coexisting anemia. A white count exceeding 100×10^3 cells/μL in acute myelogenous leukemia or the accelerated phase of CML is usually an alarming sign and an indication for prompt treatment. If there are signs or symptoms attributable to the hyperleukocytosis syndrome, then leukopheresis is indicated to rapidly and safely decrease the white count. At the same time, chemotherapy should be initiated, and treatment with allopurinol and intravenous hydration with urine alkalinization should be started in anticipation of the hyperuricemia. Hydroxyurea (6 g by mouth) is frequently used initially to produce rapid leukemic cell kill [89].

Spontaneous and Induced Coagulopathies in NeuroICU

Coagulopathy Stroke

Each year, about 790,000 people experience a new or recurrent stroke in the United States [90]. Approximately 610,000 are new attacks; most are ischemic (87 %), while 10 % are intracerebral hemorrhage (ICH), and 3 % are subarachnoid hemorrhage stroke. Although there are known risk factors for stroke, many of the ischemic strokes are cryptogenic and happen in patients younger than 55 years of age. In such patients, there is frequently an association with atrial septal abnormalities such as patent foramen ovale (PFO) or atrial septal aneurysm (ASA). Overall, both ischemic and hemorrhagic strokes are associated with either hypercoagulable state or de novo and iatrogenic coagulopathies that lead to ICH and require hematology consultation.

Cryptogenic Stroke

There is a strong association between ischemic stroke and PFO in young adults, with PFO being demonstrated in 40–50 % of the cases [91]. There are 50,000–100,000 new cases of cryptogenic strokes with PFO in the United States each year [92]. A metanalysis of nine case–control studies showed fivefold increase in risk of stroke in patients with ASA, and the strongest correlation was noted with the combination of both PFO and ASA in patients <55 years of age [93]. The cause of stroke in these patients could be paradoxical embolization of thrombus, air, or fat from the venous system through the PFO and into the arterial circulation. However, this is debatable because some studies showed no association between stroke recurrence and degree of shunting across the PFO. Thus, other venous and arterial hypercoagulable states may exist that can favor the formation of local thrombosis for which these patients should be screened for.

Diagnosis of cryptogenic stroke requires excluding the other etiologies. Neuroimaging is focused on the identification of an acute thrombus or stenotic lesions within the cerebral or carotid vasculature by using appropriate combinations of CT, MRI, CT or MR angiography, and carotid or transcranial ultrasonography. Cardiac evaluation is performed with either transthoracic (TTE) or transesophageal echocardiography (TEE). The most sensitive test for the diagnosis of PFO is the TEE with a "bubble" study using intravenous injection of agitated saline. The appearance of air bubbles in the left atrium or cerebral circulation identifies PFO with right-to-left shunting. Further studies to rule out other potential causes of stroke or factors that might contribute to thromboembolism should be performed. Full workup requires a complete blood count, lipid levels, and a hypercoagulable panel (protein C and protein S, antithrombin III deficiency, factor V Leiden mutation, prothrombin G20210A mutation, antiphospholipid and anticardiolipin antibodies, and lupus anticoagulant). The results of these studies have implications to the overall treatment of these patients.

The best strategy for secondary prevention in patients with cryptogenic stroke is yet to be determined [94]. The overall rate of stroke recurrence ranges from 0 to 12 % according to different publications, with average annual rate of 2 %. Some patients are considered at higher risk, such as those with ASA and other features suggestive of hypercoagulability. Percutaneous PFO closure is usually technically very successful and can reduce the risk of recurrent strokes, transient ischemic attacks, and peripheral emboli. Combining that with antiplatelet (mainly aspirin) or warfarin therapy (target INR 2–3), can reduce the risk further, especially if there is any laboratory or clinical evidence (such as developing deep vein thrombosis while recovering from cryptogenic stroke) for hypercoagulability. Patients with other evidence of hypercoagulability may need to stay on warfarin for life. Medical therapy only without PFO closure is an alternative approach, and ongoing trials will determine which strategy is more effective.

Ischemic Stroke with Hemorrhagic Transformation

Hemorrhagic transformation occurs due to damage of blood vessel walls compromised by ischemia with blood extravasation into the brain parenchyma. Older age, large infarct size, sustained high blood pressure, and early administration of anticoagulants are among the risk factors for such complication. Prompt discontinuation of antiplatelet agents or anticoagulation is indicated. Otherwise, the treatment could follow the same approach used for ICH.

Anticoagulation-Associated Versus Spontaneous ICH

Nontraumatic forms of IHC account for about 10–30 % of all stroke hospital admissions [95] leading to catastrophic disability, morbidity, and mortality in about 30–50 % of patients. Depending on the underlying cause of hemorrhage, IHC can be primary (85 % of cases) with spontaneous rupture of blood vessels damaged by hypertension or amyloid vasculopathy, or secondary due to ischemic stroke, tumor, trauma, or coagulopathy. Hematologists may have a role in the treatment of both types of ICH.

Evidence-based medical therapies are limited to guidelines or options regarding reduction of blood pressure, intracranial pressure monitoring, osmotherapy, fever and glycemic control, seizure prophylaxis, and care in NeuroICU.

Hemostatic therapy is important to control the size of the bleeding early as a strategy to improve survival and outcome of ICH [96], which is also true for intraventricular bleeding and acute subdural hematoma [97]. Recombinant factor VII in its activated form (rFVIIa, Novoseven®, Novo Nordisk, Bagsvaerd, Denmark) has been used in several randomized studies to treat patients with spontaneous ICH, and, although some studies showed reduction in the size of the hematoma, there was no improvement in survival and an increase of arterial thromboembolic adverse events was noticed [95, 98, 99]. A pilot clinical trial with epsilon aminocaproic acid, an antifibrinolytic agent, had similarly negative results. On the basis of these studies, the routine use of hemostatic therapy in spontaneous ICH cannot be recommended.

For the anticoagulation-associated ICH, the primary aim of the treatment should be the rapid restoration of normal coagulation parameters. Warfarin treatment is the drug most frequently associated with ICH. These patients should be reversed immediately and without waiting for the laboratory results. Fresh frozen plasma (FFP, 15 mL/kg) and vitamin K (10 mg orally when possible, otherwise 2–5 mg intravenously over 60 min) should be given in order to rapidly normalize the international normalized ratio (INR) to <1.4. Unfortunately, this process may take hours to normalize INR, and the clinical outcome is often poor. An alternative to FFP is prothrombin complex concentrate (15–30 Units/kg), which carries low risk of thrombotic complications and very low incidence of transfusion-related infections and can be better tolerated in patients at risk of volume overload. A single dose of rVIIa can normalize INR within minutes and speed the reversal of warfarin effect in ICH patients [95]. This approach has been used to expedite neurosurgical interventions with good clinical results [100]. When this approach is used, rVIIa should be used in adjunct with coagulation factor replacements and vitamin K, since its effect can last only few hours.

The risk of bleeding with antiplatelet therapy (APT) was evaluated in a meta-analysis involving 338,191 patients [101]. Low-dose aspirin (<100 mg) and dipyridamole resulted in the lowest hemorrhagic complications with total bleeding rates of 3.6 and 6.7 %, respectively. This included stroke as well as other sites of bleeding. The use of aspirin in combination with other APT, such as clopidogrel (Plavix®, Bristol-Myers Squibb, New York, NY) or ticlopidine (Ticlid®, Basel, Switzerland), leads to higher risk of postoperative bleeding, particularly if higher doses of aspirin are used (200 mg to 325 mg/day). The incidence of hemorrhagic complications was the highest among patients receiving intravenous and oral platelet surface glycoprotein IIb/IIIa inhibitors, with total bleeding rates of 49 and 44.6 %, respectively [101]. Patients on APT presenting with ICH have higher mortality rate [102], although this remains controversial [103, 104]. Whether the increased mortality can be ameliorated by therapies designed to restore normal platelet function is uncertain. Studies using platelet infusion to reverse the APT effect did not show improved mortality or outcome [105, 106]. Desmopressin (DDAVP) has been shown to be effective in reversing the effects of several APT. For patients with CNS bleeding, the APT drugs should be stopped, and possibly PLT transfusion and DDAVP should be given.

Patients with ICH who have been anticoagulated with unfractionated (half-life of 2 h) or low-molecular-weight heparin (LMWH, inhibition of factor Xa can last 4–12 h) should be reversed with protamine sulfate. Protamine dose is usually 1 mg per 100 units of unfractionated heparin or per 1 mg of LMWH. Patients with thrombocytopenia or platelet dysfunction can be treated with a single dose of DDAVP (0.3 µg/kg intravenously over 30 min), platelet transfusions until PLT count >100,000 cells/µL, or both.

The use of newer anticoagulants such as thrombin inhibitors, lepirudin (Refludan™, Baxter Healthcare, Deerfield, IL), argatroban, and bivalirudin (Angiomax™, The Medicines Company, Parsippany, NJ) may be associated with lower incidence of ICH [107], but these newer drugs do not have a specific antidote or reversal therapy. Also, factor Xa inhibitors (fondaparinux, idraparinux, and idrabiotaparinux), which are being developed for the treatment of VTE, have no specific antidotes. The ability of rFVIIa to reverse the coagulopathy of these drugs in emergency situations remains untested, except for case reports [108].

Bleeding due to the use of thrombolytic therapy such as recombinant tissue plasminogen activator (tPA) and others [109] also has no demonstrated effective treatments to reverse their effects. Combination of thrombolytic therapy with other anticoagulant therapy increases the risk of bleeding. Treatment includes the immediate discontinuation of these drugs, obtaining coagulation profile, and use of cryoprecipitate, FFP, platelet, and RBC transfusions as indicated.

Restarting anticoagulation in patients with a strong indication, such as a mechanical heart valve or atrial fibrillation with a history of cardioembolic stroke, can be safely implemented after 10 days [110]. However, the decision to restart anticoagulation can be complex, and specific clinical considerations may need to be taken into account [111]. Patients who developed DVT or just had recent pulmonary embolism should be considered for prophylactic retrievable inferior vena cava filter placement until anticoagulation can be resumed.

Intraventricular Hemorrhage

Once intraventricular hemorrhage (IVH) develops, the prognosis of ICH is much worse due to hydrocephalus and high intracerebral pressure caused by the development of intraventricular thrombosis. Other than an external ventricular drain to evacuate the bleeding, thrombolysis has become part of the treatment, using urokinase or tissue plasminogen activator (tPA), in order to help clear the forming clot and reduce the risk of hydrocephalus. Such treatment has been in practice for IVH of the newborn. Low doses of tPA, such as 1 mg every 8 h given through the drain until blood has cleared, are recommended. Complications of this approach include infection and possible rebleeding. Clinical studies have demonstrated 30 to 35 % decrease in mortality, but results of randomized placebo-controlled studies are not available [112, 113].

Cerebral Sinus Venous Thrombosis

Acute thrombosis of the cerebral draining venous system can result in venous stroke with a subacute presentation that includes headaches, blurry vision, confusion, and seizures. The treatment depends on the precipitating factors which include inherited or acquired hypercoagulable disorders, sepsis, dehydration, head trauma, and medications such as oral contraceptives. Anticoagulation is usually used as soon as the diagnosis is established. Both retrospective and randomized prospective studies have demonstrated the benefit and safety of the practice. Long-term anticoagulation is also indicated for 3–6 months if the predisposing factor was transient and longer if it is a case of sustained hypercoagulability.

Coagulopathy in Traumatic Brain Injury

Traumatic brain injury (TBI) is the leading cause of death and disability after trauma [114, 115]. Approximately 1.4 million people in the United States experience TBI yearly and 50,000 die from it (The National Institute of Neurological Disorders and Stroke website: www.nidds.nih.gov).

Various levels of coagulopathy develop in these patients with severe TBI [116]. A meta-analysis showed the incidence of coagulopathy to be 32.7 % [117]. The definition of coagulopathy in these instances is often short of the usual definition of disseminated intravascular coagulopathy (DIC) as outlined by the International Society of Thrombosis and Hemostasis [116, 117]. Often, prolonged PT/elevated INR with or without low PLT count or prolonged aPTT will be used to define TBI-related coagulopathy, although full-blown DIC can definitely be seen in these patients. TBI-related coagulopathy should be differentiated from the dilutional coagulopathy seen after large volumes of crystalloid are administered and the coagulopathy caused by taking preinjury anticoagulants such as warfarin. This de novo coagulopathy is thought to be caused from release of tissue thromboplastin and activation of fibrinolysis [114] and carries a significant impact on the ultimate outcome of these severe TBI patients. Independent risk factors for this coagulopathy in isolated TBI include Glasgow Coma Scale of ≤8, Injury Severity Scale ≥16, hypotension on admission, cerebral edema, subarachnoid hemorrhage, and midline shift [115]. These patients end up in NeuroICU for treatment and often need surgical interventions.

Because of its prognostic significance, it is important to identify and treat the TBI-related coagulopathy early. There are no guidelines for the treatment of the coagulopathy, and no randomized studies have been performed to determine the impact of available therapeutic interventions. In general, FFP and vitamin K are used to reverse the coagulopathy, but this approach results in slow correction times and can be restricted by the volume required in patients at risk for pulmonary edema. FFP and PLT transfusions should be used in patients with active bleeding. Heparin administration followed by aggressive replacement of PLTs and FFP is indicated in the treatment of patients with DIC in general; however, most clinicians treating patients with TBI will be reluctant to use heparin because of risk of bleeding and lack of clinical evidence. Administration of protein C, antithrombin III, or antifibrinolytic therapy can potentially be used to treat TBI-related coagulopathy, but, again, clinical evidence is lacking. Recombinant factor VIIa (30–90 µg/kg) provides rapid and successful correction of TBI-related coagulopathy and has been shown to be cost-effective and safe in some case series and retrospective studies [114]. However, rFVIIa should be administered with caution due to increased risk of thromboembolic complications. To date, there has been only one small randomized placebo-controlled prospective study on the use of rFVIIa in trauma [118], which showed significant decrease in RBCT in patients with severe blunt trauma treated with rFVIIa.

Coagulopathy in Emergent Neurosurgery

Many patients in the NeuroICU will be admitted after neurosurgical procedures or will require invasive procedures during their stay. The management of CNS hemorrhage usually requires rapid surgical intervention. Hematologists are frequently consulted by surgeons to evaluate patients with different induced or inherited coagulopathies, hemorrhagic or thromboembolic, prior to surgery or invasive procedure. These include congenital hemostatic defects, anticoagulation therapy, known hypercoagulability condition, and drug-induced, cardiac-related (mechanical prosthetic heart valve or atrial fibrillation), or disease-/surgery-induced defects. Most of these conditions are chronic and can be handled in a timely manner in consultation with the hematologist. In each situation, assessment of the perioperative thromboembolic risk, the bleeding risk, and the risk benefit ratio for the intervention should be taken into account.

Prolonged INR (>1.4) before neurosurgical intervention will usually prompt a hematology consult. This, again, could be due to warfarin treatment, liver failure, TBI, DIC, or inherited deficiency of factor VII. The conventional approach of vitamin K and FFP administration is usually limited by the length of time it takes to achieve normalization of INR.

Multiple reports have documented the usefulness and safety of rFVIIa (40–90 µg/kg) in these situations which can correct INR in as early as 20 min and a thus allow the prompt surgical intervention.

In liver failure coagulopathy, the hemostatic defects can be complex and include deficiency of clotting factors, excessive fibrinolysis, thrombocytopenia, platelet dysfunction, and lack of adequate response to platelet transfusion due to splenomegaly. The treatment should include the administration of FFP, cryoprecipitate, and platelet transfusions. Whether treatment with rFVIIa infusions has a role in this coagulopathy has not been established, but some report on using it to reverse coagulopathy in patients undergoing liver transplant [119, 120].

Brain Tumor-Associated Coagulopathy

Secondary ICH and VTE are known complications of brain tumors. VTE prophylaxis and treatment in these neurosurgical patients are discussed in Chap. 17. Hemorrhage from brain tumor can be seen both with primary brain tumor, such as glioblastomas, schwannomas, and hemangioblastomas, as well as secondary metastatic solid tumors and hematologic malignancies. DIC caused by malignancies, such as acute promyelocytic leukemia, can result in bleeding into the brain parenchyma and subdural or subarachnoid spaces. One should be vigilant with a high index of suspicion for ICH in oncologic patients complaining about headaches or sudden onset of neurologic symptoms. ICH in cancer patients is often viewed as a catastrophic and terminal event, although limited data on outcome exist [121]. In recent years, the advances in cancer therapy and the availability of NeuroICUs may have changed the demographics, pathophysiology, and prognosis of this complication [121]. In a recent review by Navi and colleagues [121], 208 cancer patients with CNS hemorrhage were identified between 2000 and 2007. The analysis showed that 181 patients (87 %) had ICH, 46 (22 %) had SAH, and 28 (14 %) had IVH. Some patients had more than one hemorrhage, 18 (9 %) had coexistent subdural hemorrhage, and none had epidural hemorrhage. Forty patients (19 %) were on therapeutic anticoagulation, but only 6 (3 %) were supratherapeutic; 27 (13 %) patients were on antiplatelet agents at the time of hemorrhage. The cancer contributing to hemorrhage was a solid tumor in 141 patients (68 %), a primary brain tumor in 34 (16 %), and a hematologic tumor in 33 (16 %). Melanoma (15 %), lung (14 %), glioma (12 %), breast (7 %), and leukemia (6 %) were the most common primary malignancies. Renal cell (4 %), testicular (2 %), hepatocellular (1 %), and thyroid (1 %) cancers were infrequent despite their known propensity to bleed. Earlier reports showed primary brain tumors to be the major reason for cerebral bleeding in cancer patients. In one series of 110 patients with bleeding cerebral neoplasms, 77 % had primary brain tumors and 23 % had metastatic solid tumors [122]. Similarly, 62 % of patients with intratumoral hemorrhage (ITH) in a different cohort of 58 cases had primary brain tumors [123]. This changing demographic may represent longer survival of patients with solid tumors, use of new drugs such the antiangiogenic therapy, or the higher likelihood of primary brain tumors with ICH to be clinically silent and thus not lead to acute neuroimaging.

Furthermore, in Navi's study [120], the majority of patients were symptomatic (94 %) from the hemorrhage. Hemiparesis (48 %), headache (41 %), and impaired consciousness (34 %) were the most common symptoms or signs; few patients had seizures (17 %) or coma (6 %). DIC was documented in 4 patients, 2 of whom had acute promyelocytic leukemia. Overall, ITH (61 %) and coagulopathy (46 %) were the most common causes of ICH in this population.

The treatment for ICH in these patients should follow the approach discussed previously, although the prognosis of the underlying malignant process is always taken into consideration. Prognosis is generally poor; however, many patients retain independence after ICH, ultimately succumbing to their underlying malignancy rather than the hemorrhage itself. Poor prognostic indicators were impaired consciousness, hemiparesis, multiple hemorrhagic foci, hydrocephalus, and treatment for increased intracerebral pressure. Recent chemotherapy, not having a primary brain tumor, and lack of ventriculostomy also predicted poor outcome [121].

References

1. Bogousslavsky J, Van Melle G, Regli F. The Lausanne Stroke Registry: analysis of 1,000 consecutive patients with first stroke. Stroke. 1988;19:1083–92.
2. Hart RG, Sherman DG, Miller VT, Easton JD. Diagnosis and management of ischemic stroke: selected controversies. Curr Probl Cardiol. 1983;8:43–53.
3. Adams HP, Butler MJ, Biller J, Toffal GJ. Nonhemorrhagic cerebral infarction in young adults. Arch Neurol. 1986;43:793–6.
4. Klein GM, Seland TP. Occlusive cerebrovascular disease in young adults. Can J Neurol Sci. 1984;11:302–4.
5. Hart RG, Kanter MC. Hematologic disorders and ischemic stroke. A selective review. Stroke. 1990;21:1111–21.
6. Moreb JS. Hematologic conditions in the ICU, chapter 173. In: Gabrielli A, Layon AJ, Yu M, editors. Civetta, Taylor, and Kirby's critical care. 4th ed. Philadelphia: Lippincott Williams &Wilkins; 2009. p. 2561–75.
7. Fakhry SM, Fata P. How low is too low? Cardiac risks with anemia. Crit Care. 2004;8 Suppl 2:S11.
8. Napolitano LM. Scope of the problem: epidemiology of anemia and use of blood transfusions in critical care. Crit Care. 2004;8 Suppl 2:S1.
9. van de Wiel A. Anemia in critically ill patients. Eur J Intern Med. 2004;15:481.
10. Corwin HL, Gettinger A, Pearl RG, et al. The CRIT study: anemia and blood transfusion in the critically ill–current clinical practice in the United States. Crit Care Med. 2004;32:39.

11. Vincent JL, Baron JF, Reinhart K, et al. Anemia and blood transfusion in critically ill patients. JAMA. 2002;288:1499.

12. Andrews NC. Anemia of inflammation: the cytokine-hepcidin link. J Clin Invest. 2004;113:1251.

13. Carless PA, Henry DA, Carson JL, Hebert PP, McClelland B, Ker K. Transfusion thresholds and other strategies for guiding allogeneic red blood cell transfusion. Cochrane Database Syst Rev. 2010;10, CD002042.

14. Corwin HL, Gettinger A, Pearl RG, et al. Efficacy of recombinant human erythropoietin in critically ill patients: a randomized controlled trial. JAMA. 2002;288:2827.

15. Silver M, Corwin MJ, Bazan A, et al. Efficacy of recombinant human erythropoietin in critically ill patients admitted to a long-term acute care facility: a randomized, double-blind, placebo-controlled trial. Crit Care Med. 2006;34:2310.

16. Moore AR, et al. Meta-analysis of efficacy and safety of intravenous ferric carboxymaltose (Ferinject) from clinical trial reports and published trial data. BMC Blood Disord. 2011;11:4.

17. Kramer AH, Zygun DA. Anemia and red blood cell transfusion in neurocritical care. Crit Care. 2009;13:R89.

18. Leal-Novala SR, Múñoz-Gómezb M, Murillo-Cabezasa F. Optimal hemoglobin concentration in patients with subarachnoid hemorrhage, acute ischemic stroke and traumatic brain injury. Curr Opin Crit Care. 2008;14:156–62.

19. Pendem S, Rana S, Manno EM, Gajic O. A review of red cell transfusion in the neurological intensive care unit. Neurocrit Care. 2006;4:63–7.

20. Gould S, Cimino MJ, Gerber DR. Packed red blood cell transfusion in the intensive care unit: limitations and consequences. Am J Crit Care. 2007;16:39–49.

21. Naidech AM. Anaemia and its treatment in neurologically critically ill patients: being reasonable is easy without prospective trials. Crit Care. 2010;14:149–50.

22. Kramer AH, Zygun DA, Bleck TP, Dumont AS, Kassell NF, Nathan B. Relationship between hemoglobin concentrations and outcomes across subgroups of patients with aneurysmal subarachnoid hemorrhage. Neurocrit Care. 2009;10:157–65.

23. Naidech AM, Jovanovic B, Wartenberg KE, Parra A, Ostapkovich N, Connolly ES, Mayer SA, Commichau C. Higher hemoglobin is associated with improved outcome after subarachnoid hemorrhage. Crit Care Med. 2007;35:2383–9.

24. Diedler J, Sykora M, Hahn P, Heerlein K, Schölzke MN, Kellert L, Bösel J, Poli S, Steiner T. Low hemoglobin is associated with poor functional outcome after non-traumatic, supratentorial intracerebral hemorrhage. Crit Care. 2010;14:R63.

25. Zygun DA, Nortje J, Hutchinson PJ, Timofeev I, Menon DK, Gupta AK. The effect of red blood cell transfusion on cerebral oxygenation and metabolism after severe traumatic brain injury. Crit Care Med. 2009;37:1074–8.

26. Sacco S, Marini C, Olivieri L, Pistoia F, Carolei A. Contribution of hematocrit to early mortality after ischemic stroke. Eur Neurol. 2007;58:233–8.

27. Diamond PT, Gale SD, Evans BA. Relationship of initial hematocrit level to discharge destination and resource utilization after ischemic stroke: a pilot study. Arch Phys Med Rehabil. 2003;84:964–7.

28. Harrison MJ, Pollock S, Kendall BE, Marshall J. Effect of hematocrit on carotid stenosis and cerebral infarction. Lancet. 1981;2:114–5.

29. Lowe GDO, Jaap AJ, Forbes CD. Relation of atrial fibrillation and high hematocrit to mortality in acute stroke. Lancet. 1983;1:784–6.

30. Allport LE, Parsons MW, Butcher KS, MacGregor L, Desmond PM, Tress BM, Davis S. Elevated hematocrit is associated with reduced reperfusion and tissue survival in acute stroke. Neurology. 2005;65:1382–7.

31. Timmons SD. The life-saving properties of blood: mitigating cerebral insult after traumatic brain injury. Neurocrit Care. 2006;5:1–3.

32. Goldman M, Webert KE, Arnold DM, Freedman J, Hannon J, Blajchman MA. TRALI consensus panel. Transfus Med Rev. 2005;19:2–31.

33. Leal-Noval SR, Muñoz M, Páramo JA, García-Erce JA. Spanish consensus statement on alternatives to allogeneic transfusions: the 'Seville document'. Transfus Altern Transfus Med. 2006;8:178–202.

34. Ohene-Frempong K, Weiner SJ, Sleeper LA, Miller ST, Embury S, Moohr JW, et al. Cerebrovascular accidents in sickle cell disease: rates and risk factors. Blood. 1998;91:288–94.

35. Pegelow CH, Macklin EA, Moser FG, Wang WC, Bello JA, Miller ST, et al. Longitudinal changes in brain magnetic resonance imaging findings in children with sickle cell disease. Blood. 2002;99:3014–8.

36. Sears DA, et al. Sickle cell trait. In: Embury SH, Hebbel RP, Mohandas N, editors. Sickle cell disease: basic principles and clinical practice. New York: Raven Press; 1994. p. 381.

37. Hebbel RP, Vercellotti G, Nath KA. A systems biology consideration of the vasculopathy of sickle cell anemia: the need for multimodality chemo-prophylaxis. Cardiovasc Hematol Disord Drug Targets. 2009;9:271–92.

38. Moritani T, Numaguchi Y, Lemer NB, Rozans MK, Robinson AE, Hiwatashi A, et al. Sickle cell cerebrovascular disease usual and unusual findings on MR imaging and MR angiography. J Clin Imaging. 2004;28:173–86.

39. Kirkham FJ. Therapy insight: stroke risk and its management in patients with sickle cell disease. Nat Clin Pract Neurol. 2007;3:264–78.

40. Charache S, Terrin ML, Moore RD, et al. Effect of hydroxyurea on the frequency of painful crises in sickle cell anemia. N Engl J Med. 1995;332:1317.

41. McGann PT, Ware RE. Hydroxyurea for sickle cell anemia: what have we learned and what questions still remain? Curr Opin Hematol. 2011;18:158–65.

42. Charache S. Mechanism of action of hydroxyurea in the management of sickle cell anemia in adults. Semin Hematol. 1997; 34 Suppl 3:15.

43. Buchanan GR, DeBaun MR, Quinn CT, et al. Sickle cell disease. Hematology Am Soc Hematol Educ Program 2004:35.

44. Garratty G. Drug-induced immune hemolytic anemia. Hematology Am Soc Hematol Educ Program 2009:73–9.

45. Salama A. Drug-induced immune hemolytic anemia. Expert Opin Drug Saf. 2009;8:73–9.

46. Jeffries LC. Transfusion therapy in autoimmune hemolytic anemia. Hematol Oncol Clin North Am. 1994;8:1087.

47. Reardon JE, Marquea MB. Laboratory evaluation and transfusion support of patients with autoimmune hemolytic anemia. Am J Clin Pathol. 2006;125 Suppl 1:S71.

48. Coppo P, Adrie C, Azoulay E, et al. Infectious diseases as a trigger in thrombotic microangiopathies in intensive care unit (ICU) patients? Intensive Care Med. 2003;29:564.

49. Pu JJ, Brodsky RA. Paroxysmal nocturnal hemoglobinuria from bench to bedside. Clin Transl Sci. 2011;4:219–24.

50. Höchsmann B, Rojewski M, Schrezenmeier H. Paroxysmal nocturnal hemoglobinuria (PNH): higher sensitivity and validity in diagnosis and serial monitoring by flow cytometric analysis of reticulocytes. Ann Hematol. 2011;90:887–99.

51. McKeage K. Eculizumab: a review of its use in paroxysmal nocturnal haemoglobinuria. Drugs. 2011;71:2327–45.

52. van Bijnen ST, van Heerde WL, Muus P. Mechanisms and clinical implications of thrombosis in paroxysmal nocturnal hemoglobinuria. J Thromb Haemost. 2012;10(1):1–10.

53. Hughes WT, Armstrong D, Bodey GP, et al. 2002 Guidelines for the use of antimicrobial agents in neutropenic patients with cancer. Clin Infect Dis. 2002;34:730.

54. van de Wetering MD, de Witte MA, Kremer LC, et al. Efficacy of oral prophylactic antibiotics in neutropenic afebrile oncology

patients: a systematic review of randomised controlled trials. Eur J Cancer. 2005;41:1372.

55. Gafter-Gvili A, Fraser A, Paul M, et al. Meta-analysis: antibiotic prophylaxis reduces mortality in neutropenic patients. Ann Intern Med. 2005;142:979.

56. Smith TJ, Khatcheressian J, Lyman GH, et al. 2006 Update of recommendations for the use of white blood cell growth factors: an evidence-based clinical practice guideline. J Clin Oncol. 2006;24:3187.

57. Azoulay E, Darmon M, Delclaux C, et al. Deterioration of previous acute lung injury during neutropenia recovery. Crit Care Med. 2002;30:781.

58. Karlin L, Darmon M, Thiery G, et al. Respiratory status deterioration during G-CSF-induced neutropenia recovery. Bone Marrow Transplant. 2005;36:245.

59. Napolitano LM, Warkentin TE, Almahameed A, et al. Heparin-induced thrombocytopenia in the critical care setting: diagnosis and management. Crit Care Med. 2006;34:1.

60. Akca S, Haji-Michael P, de Mendonca A, et al. Time course of platelet counts in critically ill patients. Crit Care Med. 2002;30:753.

61. Vanderschueren S, De Weerdt A, Malbrain M, et al. Thrombocytopenia and prognosis in intensive care. Crit Care Med. 2000;28:1871.

62. Rutherford CJ, Frenkel EP. Thrombocytopenia. Issues in diagnosis and therapy. Med Clin North Am. 1994;78:555.

63. Greinacher A, Selleng K. Thrombocytopenia in the intensive care unit patient. Hematology Am Soc Hematol Educ Program. 2010;30:135–43.

64. Nijsten MW, ten Duis HJ, Zijlstra JG, Porte RJ, Zwaveling JH, Paling JC, The TH. Blunted rise in platelet count in critically ill patients is associated with worse outcome. Crit Care Med. 2000;28:3843–6.

65. Vandijck DM, Blot SI, De Waele JJ, Hoste EA, Vandewoude KH, Decruyenaere JM. Thrombocytopenia and outcome in critically ill patients with bloodstream infection. Heart Lung. 2010; 39:21–6.

66. Chang JC. Review: postoperative thrombocytopenia: with etiologic, diagnostic, and therapeutic consideration. Am J Med Sci. 1996;311:96–105.

67. Chang JC, Aly ES. Acute respiratory distress syndrome as a major clinical manifestation of thrombotic thrombocytopenic purpura. Am J Med Sci. 2001;321:124–8.

68. CRASH-2 trial collaborators, Shakur H, Roberts I, Bautista R, Caballero J, Coats T, Dewan Y, El-Sayed H, Gogichaishvili T, Gupta S, Herrera J, Hunt B, Iribhogbe P, Izurieta M, Khamis H, Komolafe E, Marrero MA, Mejía-Mantilla J, Miranda J, Morales C, Olaomi O, Olldashi F, Perel P, Peto R, Ramana PV, Ravi RR, Yutthakasemsunt S. Effects of tranexamic acid on death, vascular occlusive events, and blood transfusion in trauma patients with significant haemorrhage (CRASH-2): a randomised, placebo-controlled trial. Lancet. 2010;376:23–32.

69. Aster RH, Curtis BR, Bougie DW, Dunkley S, Greinacher A, Warkentin TE, Chong BH, Scientific and Standardization Committee of The International Society On Thrombosis and Haemostasis. Thrombocytopenia associated with the use of GPIIb/IIIa inhibitors: position paper of the ISTH working group on thrombocytopenia and GPIIb/IIIa inhibitors. J Thromb Haemost. 2006;4:678–9.

70. Tsai HM. Physiologic cleavage of von Willebrand factor by a plasma protease is dependent on its conformation and requires calcium ion. Blood. 1996;87:4235.

71. Furlan M, Robles R, Galbusera M, et al. von Willebrand factor-cleaving protease in thrombotic thrombocytopenic purpura and the hemolytic-uremic syndrome. N Engl J Med. 1998;339:1578.

72. George JN. The thrombotic thrombocytopenic purpura and hemolytic uremic syndromes: overview of pathogenesis (Experience of The Oklahoma TTP-HUS Registry, 1989–2007). Kidney Int Suppl. 2009;112:S8–10.

73. Verma AK, Levine M, Shalansky SJ, et al. Frequency of heparin-induced thrombocytopenia in critical care patients. Pharmacotherapy. 2003;23:745.

74. Crowther MA, Cook DJ, Meade MO, et al. Thrombocytopenia in medical-surgical critically ill patients: prevalence, incidence, and risk factors. J Crit Care. 2005;20:348.

75. Keeling D, Davidson S, Watson H. Haemostasis and thrombosis task force of the British committee for standards in haematology. The management of heparin-induced thrombocytopenia. Br J Haematol. 2006;133:259.

76. Arnold DM, Crowther MA, Cook RJ, Sigouin C, Heddle NM, Molnar L, Cook DJ. Utilization of platelet transfusions in the intensive care unit: indications, transfusion triggers, and platelet count responses. Transfusion. 2006;46:1286–91.

77. Lisovoski F, Rousseaux P. Cerebral infarction in young people. A study of 148 patients with early cerebral angiography. J Neurol Neurosurg Psychiatry. 1991;54:576–9.

78. Haan J, Caekebeke JF, van der Meer FJ, Wintzen AR. Cerebral venous thrombosis as presenting sign of myeloproliferative disorders. J Neurol Neurosurg Psychiatry. 1988;51:1219–20.

79. De Stefano V, Fiorini A, Rossi E, Za T, Farina G, Chiusolo P, Sica S, Leone G. Incidence of the JAK2 V617F mutation among patients with splanchnic or cerebral venous thrombosis and without overt chronic myeloproliferative disorders. J Thromb Haemost. 2007;5:708–14.

80. Tefferi A. Annual Clinical Updates in Hematological Malignancies: a continuing medical education series: polycythemia vera and essential thrombocythemia: 2011 update on diagnosis, risk-stratification, and management. Am J Hematol. 2011;86:292–301.

81. Miller TD, Farquharson MH. Essential thrombocythaemia and its neurological complications. Pract Neurol. 2010;10:195–201.

82. Lazzaro MA, Cochran EJ, Lopes DK, Prabhakaran S. Moyamoya syndrome in an adult with essential thrombocythemia. Neurol Int. 2011;3:e3.

83. Schafer AI. Molecular basis of the diagnosis and treatment of polycythemia vera and essential thrombocythemia. Blood. 2006;107:4214–22.

84. Carobbio A, Finazzi G, Antonioli E, Guglielmelli P, Vannucchi AM, Delaini F, Guerini V, Ruggeri M, Rodeghiero F, Rambaldi A, Barbui T. Thrombocytosis and leukocytosis interaction in vascular complications of essential thrombocythemia. Blood. 2008;112:3135–7.

85. Gurung AM, Carr B, Smith I. Thrombocytosis in intensive care. Br J Anaesth. 2001;87:926.

86. Valade N, Decailliot F, Rebufat Y, et al. Thrombocytosis after trauma: incidence, aetiology, and clinical significance. Br J Anaesth. 2005;94:18.

87. Buss DH, Cashell AW, O'Connor ML, et al. Occurrence, etiology, and clinical significance of extreme thrombocytosis: a study of 280 cases. Am J Med. 1994;96:247.

88. Barbui T, Finazzi G. When and how to treat essential thrombocythemia. N Engl J Med. 2005;353:85–6.

89. Heit JA, Ho PM, Howard VJ, Kissela BM, Kittner SJ, Lackland DT, Lichtman JH, Lisabeth LD, Makuc DM, Marcus GM, Marelli A, Matchar DB, McDermott MM, Meigs JB, Moy CS, Mozaffarian D, Mussolino ME, Nichol G, Paynter NP, Rosamond WD, Sorlie PD, Stafford RS, Turan TN, Turner MB, Wong ND, Wylie-Rosett J, American Heart Association Statistics Committee and Stroke Statistics Subcommittee. Heart disease and stroke statistics – 2011 update: a report from the American Heart Association. Circulation. 2011;123:e18–209.

90. Lloyd-Jones D, Adams R, Carnethon M, et al. Heart disease and stroke statistics—2009 update: a report from the American Heart

Association Statistics Committee and Stroke Statistics Subcommittee. Circulation. 2009;119:e21–181.

91. Homma S, Di Tullio MR. Patent foramen ovale and stroke. J Cardiol. 2010;56:134–41.

92. Saver JL. Emerging risk factors for stroke: patent foramen ovale, aortic arch atherosclerosis, antiphospholipid antibodies, and activated protein C resistance. J Stroke Cerebrovasc Dis. 1997;6:167–72.

93. Overell JR, Bone I, Lees KR. Interatrial septal abnormalities and stroke: a meta-analysis of case–control studies. Neurology. 2000;55:1172–9.

94. Di Tullio MR, Homma S. Patent foramen ovale and stroke: what should be done? Curr Opin Hematol. 2009;16:391–6.

95. Rincon F, Mayer SA. Clinical review: critical care management of spontaneous intracerebral hemorrhage. Crit Care. 2008;12:237.

96. Masotti L, Di Napoli M, Godoy DA, Rafanelli D, Liumbruno G, Koumpouros N, Landini G, Pampana A, Cappelli R, Poli D, Prisco D. The practical management of intracerebral hemorrhage associated with oral anticoagulant therapy. Int J Stroke. 2011;6:228–40.

97. Bershad EM, Farhadi S, Suri MF, Feen ES, Hernandez OH, Selman WR, Suarez JI. Coagulopathy and inhospital deaths in patients with acute subdural hematoma. J Neurosurg. 2008;109:664–9.

98. Yuan ZH, Jiang JK, Huang WD, Pan J, Zhu JY, Wang JZ. A meta-analysis of the efficacy and safety of recombinant activated factor VII for patients with acute intracerebral hemorrhage without hemophilia. J Clin Neurosci. 2010;17:685–93.

99. Mayer SA, Brun NC, Begtrup K, et al. Recombinant activated factor VII for acute intracerebral hemorrhage. N Engl J Med. 2005;352:777–85.

100. Freeman WD, Brott TG, Barrett KM, Castillo PR, Deen Jr HG, Czervionke LF, Meschia JF. Recombinant factor VIIa for rapid reversal of warfarin anticoagulation in acute intracranial hemorrhage. Mayo Clin Proc. 2004;79:1495–500.

101. Serebruany VL, Malinin AI, Eisert RM, Sane DC. Risk of bleeding complications with antiplatelet agents: meta-analysis of 338,191 patients enrolled in 50 randomized controlled trials. Am J Hematol. 2004;75:40–7.

102. Thompson BB, Béjot Y, Caso V, Castillo J, Christensen H, Flaherty ML, Foerch C, Ghandehari K, Giroud M, Greenberg SM, Hallevi H, Hemphill 3rd JC, Heuschmann P, Juvela S, Kimura K, Myint PK, Nagakane Y, Naritomi H, Passero S, Rodríguez-Yáñez MR, Roquer J, Rosand J, Rost NS, Saloheimo P, Salomaa V, Sivenius J, Sorimachi T, Togha M, Toyoda K, Turaj W, Vemmos KN, Wolfe CD, Woo D, Smith EE. Prior antiplatelet therapy and outcome following intracerebral hemorrhage: a systematic review. Neurology. 2010;75:1333–42.

103. Moussouttas M, Malhotra R, Fernandez L, Maltenfort M, Holowecki M, Delgado J, Lawson N, Badjatia N. Role of antiplatelet agents in hematoma expansion during the acute period of intracerebral hemorrhage. Neurocrit Care. 2010;12:24–9.

104. Sansing LH, Messe SR, Cucchiara BL, Cohen SN, Lyden PD, Kasner SE, CHANT Investigators. Prior antiplatelet use does not affect hemorrhage growth or outcome after ICH. Neurology. 2009;72:1397–402.

105. Creutzfeldt CJ, Weinstein JR, Longstreth Jr WT, Becker KJ, McPharlin TO, Tirschwell DL. Prior antiplatelet therapy, platelet infusion therapy, and outcome after intracerebral hemorrhage. J Stroke Cerebrovasc Dis. 2009;18:221–8.

106. Campbell PG, Sen A, Yadla S, Jabbour P, Jallo J. Emergency reversal of antiplatelet agents in patients presenting with an intracranial hemorrhage: a clinical review. World Neurosurg. 2010;74:279–85.

107. McRae SJ, Ginsberg JS. New anticoagulants for the prevention and treatment of venous thromboembolism. Vasc Health Risk Manag. 2005;1:41–53.

108. Zalpour A, Kroll MH, Afshar-Kharghan V, Yusuf SW, Escalante C. Role of factor xa inhibitors in cancer-associated thrombosis: any new data? Adv Hematol. 2011;2011:196135.

109. Singer OC, Berkefeld J, Lorenz MW, Fiehler J, Albers GW, Lansberg MG, Kastrup A, Rovira A, Liebeskind DS, Gass A, Rosso C, Derex L, Kim JS, Neumann-Haefelin T, MR Stroke Study Group Investigators. Risk of symptomatic intracerebral hemorrhage in patients treated with intra-arterial thrombolysis. Cerebrovasc Dis. 2009;27:368–74.

110. Ananthasubramaniam K, Beattie JN, Rosman HS, Jayam V, Borzak S. How safely and for how long can warfarin therapy be withheld in prosthetic heart valve patients hospitalized with a major hemorrhage? Chest. 2001;119:478–84.

111. Eckman MH, Rosand J, Knudsen KA, Singer DE, Greenberg SM. Can patients be anticoagulated after intracerebral hemorrhage? A decision analysis. Stroke. 2003;34:1710–6.

112. Andrews CO, Engelhard HH. Fibrinolytic therapy in intraventricular hemorrhage. Ann Pharmacother. 2001;35:1435–48.

113. Bartek Jr J, Hansen-Schwartz J, Bergdal O, Degn J, Romner B, Welling KL, Fischer W. Alteplase (rtPA) treatment of intraventricular hematoma (IVH): safety of an efficient methodological approach for rapid clot removal. Acta Neurochir Suppl. 2011;111:409–13.

114. Stein DM, Dutton RP, Kramer ME, Scalea TM. Reversal of coagulopathy in critically ill patients with traumatic brain injury: recombinant factor VIIa is more cost-effective than plasma. J Trauma. 2009;66:63–72.

115. Talving P, Benfield R, Hadjizacharia P, Inaba K, Chan LS, Demetriades D. Coagulopathy in severe traumatic brain injury: a prospective study. J Trauma. 2009;66:55–61.

116. Harhangi BS, Kompanje EJ, Leebeek FW, Maas AI. Coagulation disorders after traumatic brain injury. Acta Neurochir (Wien). 2008;150:165–75.

117. Taylor Jr FB, Toh CH, Hoots WK, Wada H, Levi M. Towards definition, clinical and laboratory criteria, and a scoring system for disseminated intravascular coagulation. Thromb Haemost. 2001;86:1327–30.

118. Boffard KD, Riou B, Warren B, Choong PI, Rizoli S, Rossaint R, Axelsen M. Recombinant factor VIIa as adjunctive therapy for bleeding control in severely injured trauma patients: two parallel randomized, placebo-controlled, doubleblind clinical trials. J Trauma. 2005;59:8–15.

119. Gala B, Quintela J, Aguirrezabalaga J, Fernández C, Fraguela J, Suárez F, Gómez M. Benefits of recombinant activated factor VII in complicated liver transplantation. Transplant Proc. 2005;37:3919–21.

120. Lodge JP, Jonas S, Jones RM, Olausson M, Mir-Pallardo J, Soefelt S, Garcia-Valdecasas JC, McAlister V. Efficacy and safety of repeated perioperative doses of recombinant factor VIIa in liver transplantation. Liver Transpl. 2005;11:973–9.

121. Navi BB, Reichman JS, Berlin D, Reiner AS, Panageas KS, Segal AZ, DeAngelis LM. Intracerebral and subarachnoid hemorrhage in patients with cancer. Neurology. 2010;74:494–501.

122. Licata C, Turazzi S. Bleeding cerebral neoplasms with symptomatic hematoma. J Neurosurg Sci. 2003;47:201–10.

123. Yuguang L, Meng L, Shugan Z, et al. Intracranial tumoural haemorrhage: a report of 58 cases. J Clin Neurosci. 2002;9:637–9.

Venous Thromboembolism in the Neurologic Intensive Care Unit

17

Chamisa MacIndoe and David Garcia

Contents

Abstract

Venous thromboembolism (VTE) is a particular risk to the critically ill neurology or neurosurgical patient, regardless of inciting event. The clinical consequences of VTE have a significant impact on morbidity and mortality, yet there remains a significant variability of clinical practice, for both detection and prophylaxis. This is in part due to the paucity of data from randomized clinical trials that has resulted in a lack of clear clinical guidelines. Additionally, the risk of both prophylactic and therapeutic anticoagulation is more substantial in this particular patient population. This chapter discusses current data regarding risk assessment, prevention, and treatment of VTE. Ultimately, until further higher level evidence is available, the safest approach may be to individualize each patient's care and subsequently choose VTE prophylaxis or treatment based on that patient's particular risk/benefit assessment.

Keywords

Venous thromboembolism • Pulmonary embolism • Deep venous embolism • Anticoagulation • Prophylaxis

Introduction

Venous thromboembolism (VTE) is a relatively common process that encompasses both deep venous thrombosis (DVT) and pulmonary embolism (PE) [1]. In general, approximately two-thirds of cases present as isolated DVT and one-third present as PE with or without DVT. The significant clinical consequences of VTE may include recurrence, death, postthrombotic syndrome, subsequent bleeding after anticoagulation [2], persistent right ventricular failure, and pulmonary hypertension [3]. There is an increased likelihood for VTE in the neurologically injured patient population, but it is difficult to estimate risk precisely because of a lack of a standard definition for VTE (clinically symptomatic or asymptomatic) and variation in detection methods [4].

C. MacIndoe, DO
Department of Neurosurgery,
University of New Mexico,
Albuquerque, NM 87113, USA
e-mail: chamisa.macindoe@gmail.com

D. Garcia, MD (✉)
Department of Hematology,
University of New Mexico,
1924 Avenida Las Campanas,
Albuquerque, NM 87107, USA
e-mail: davidg99@um.edu

A.J. Layon et al. (eds.), *Textbook of Neurointensive Care*,
DOI 10.1007/978-1-4471-5226-2_17, © Springer-Verlag London 2013

Table 17.1 Risk factors for VTE

	Endothelial injury	Hemodynamics-stasis/turbulent flow	Hypercoagulability
Patient-specific risks	Prior history of VTE Age >40 (risk doubles each decade beyond 40) Tobacco use	Obesity	Inherited thrombophilia (e.g., antiphospholipid syndrome)
Disease-specific risks	Central venous catheters	Venous compression – tumor, hematoma, arterial abnormality	Hyperestrogenic states – pregnancy, postpartum, oral contraceptives, selective estrogen modulators
	Associated traumatic injuries	Cardiovascular disease – congestive heart failure	Cancer and cancer therapy
		Immobilization – weakness, paralysis, sedation, bed rest	CNS trauma or surgery

Although often asymptomatic, proximal DVT and PE are relevant in the NeuroICU because they impact morbidity, mortality, and resource utilization.

The most feared complication of VTE is death due to pulmonary embolism (PE); 5–10 % of hospitalized patients who suffer PE will die prior to discharge [5]. For patients who survive pulmonary embolism, 5–10 % will be left with echocardiographic evidence of chronic thromboembolic pulmonary artery hypertension [6]. Although deep vein thrombosis (DVT) is not lethal, it puts patients at risk for PE. In up to 10 % of cases, DVT causes a symptom constellation of chronic pain, edema, and skin ulcers known as the post-thrombotic syndrome [7]. VTE in the NeuroICU has unique implications compared to other settings. In the setting of both ischemic and hemorrhagic CNS lesions, the otherwise routine treatment with anticoagulation takes on an entirely different risk/benefit balance. This chapter will inform clinicians about estimating the risk for, preventing, and treating VTE specifically in the NeuroICU.

Pathogenesis

Normal, physiologic hemostasis is a complex process that involves numerous steps. Thrombosis (or pathologic clot formation) is typically the result of more than one insult or perturbation of normal physiology. Rudolf Virchow theorized in the 1800s that thrombosis was the result of at least one of three derangements: endothelial injury or dysfunction, hemodynamic changes (stasis or turbulent blood flow), and/or hypercoagulability [8]. This triad still forms the basis for understanding the development of VTE. Most hospitalized patients have at least one risk factor for VTE, and it has been reported that as many as 40 % of inpatients have three or more risk factors [9].

In the setting of serious neurologic illness (stroke, trauma, surgery, malignancy, etc.), patients may experience endothelial dysfunction as a consequence of catheter placement, trauma, or operative vascular compromise. Venous stasis may occur in the NeuroICU because of underlying pathology

(traumatic brain injury, stroke-related paresis or plegia) or as a result of therapeutic ICU sedation and neuromuscular blockade. Patients with neurologic illness, especially traumatic brain injury (TBI), have increased levels/activation of tissue factor (TF) and von Willebrand factor (vWF), two procoagulant proteins that have important roles in normal hemostasis [10]. This excess circulating TF and vWF likely induce a hypercoagulable state that also promotes pathologic clot formation and, in some cases, disseminated intravascular coagulation (DIC) [11].

In one review of 1,231 patients treated for VTE, 96 % had one or more preexisting recognized risk factors for VTE. The strongest risk factors that were found to correlate with VTE were increasing age, prolonged immobility, major surgery, malignancy, prior VTE, multisystem trauma, and chronic heart failure [8]. Neurologically injured patients are generally considered to have a much higher risk than the general surgical population due to prolonged intraoperative periods, perioperative lower extremity paresis and paralysis, and prolonged recovery time [12]. Cancer and sepsis are not uncommon in the NeuroICU; both conditions promote thrombosis through a variety of mechanisms [13, 14]. Specifically, patients with malignant brain tumors, partly related to their medical management with steroids and chemotherapy, have higher rates of VTE [12, 15]. Additionally, many studies have noted that TBI itself may be an independent risk factor for VTE due to the lengthy period of immobility, the delay in initiating prophylaxis in the setting of intracranial hemorrhage (ICH) [16], and the previously discussed hypercoagulability that frequently results from trauma. Other characteristics (e.g., obesity, prior history of VTE) not specific to the NeuroICU may also affect VTE risk. Table 17.1 lists a number of risk factors pertinent to many NeuroICU patients [2]. While inherited hypercoagulability, referred to as thrombophilia, is associated with an increased risk for VTE, and although several inherited forms of thrombophilia have been described, these conditions are relatively uncommon. Therefore, unless previously documented in a patient's medical history, these hypercoagulable conditions

Table 17.2 Disease-specific estimated risk of symptomatic VTE without prophylaxis

Population	Estimated risk (%)	Factors that might increase the risk
Ischemic stroke	5–10 [19]	Risk is higher in those with a National Institutes of Health Stroke Scale (NIHSS) of >14 [20]
Intracranial hemorrhage Subarachnoid hemorrhage	5–10 [21–23][a]	
Spinal cord injury	10–20 [24–27]	Associated traumatic injuries
Craniotomy	5–10 [4, 28, 29]	Surgery for malignant disease: increased hypercoagulable state secondary to malignant brain tumors associated treatment with steroids and chemotherapy [12]
Spinal surgery	2–5 [30–35]	
TBI	5–20 [36, 37][b]	Age >40 years, lower extremity fracture, major head injury, more than 3 ventilator days, venous injury, and major surgical procedure
		Other traumatic injuries, such as pelvic fractures, spinal cord injury, and shock are associated with an increased risk [37]

[a]We presume this number to be similar to the rate of symptomatic events in ischemic stroke
[b]The percentage of VTE in the trauma population is extremely variable, and the actual rate is highly dependent on the nature and severity of associated traumatic injuries. However, patients with multisystem and/or major trauma have the highest risk for VTE [9]

do not influence management for the neurologically injured patient, who usually has more than one acquired risk factor for VTE.

Estimating Baseline VTE Risk

In order to decide whether (or how aggressively) to prescribe thromboprophylaxis for a particular patient in the NeuroICU, the clinician must first estimate the patient's risk of developing VTE without prophylaxis. The relative incidence of first-time VTE in the general population is approximately 70–113 cases per 100,000 population annually, with the incidence of clinically diagnosed DVT being twice that of PE [17]. VTE is thought to be a multifactorial disease [18], and VTE risk increases with the number of risk factors. While most clinicians are aware of such risk factors, assigning quantitative risk at the bedside is difficult. The vast majority of NeuroICU patients fall into one of three risk categories: moderate, high, or very high. While almost all NeuroICU patients will benefit from some form of VTE prophylaxis, clinicians must identify those patients for whom the risks and costs of pharmacologic strategies are justified.

Patients admitted to the NeuroICU often fall into one of several common disease categories; in Table 17.2, estimates of the disease-specific VTE risk are presented. Estimates of VTE risk within subgroups of NeuroICU patients are limited by multiple factors: individual study design, the nature of other traumatic injuries, patient-specific factors, and the specific technique for detecting VTE. Perhaps the most important limitation of the available evidence about VTE risk is that most studies use routine surveillance (with venography, ultrasound, or fibrinogen uptake) of lower extremity veins and report all observed clots. In such studies, the vast majority of observed cots occur in asymptomatic patients, and the clinical relevance of such clots is unknown. Since not all of these asymptomatic clots would go on to cause symptomatic disease, we have, in

Table 17.2, made our best approximation (using available evidence) about the expected rate of VTE in patients who receive no prophylaxis. In some cases, we have slightly adjusted the reported rate of symptomatic events upward to account for the fact that some, or all, patients from the supporting studies received VTE prophylaxis.

Overall, due to the wide variability of patient-specific factors and an increased overall incidence of VTE within the NeuroICU population, risk assessment must be individualized [38].

Prophylaxis for VTE

Several options are available for the prevention of VTE in the NeuroICU: intermittent pneumatic compression devices (IPC), graduated compression stockings (GCS) [39], low-dose unfractionated heparin (UFH), low-molecular-weight heparin (LMWH), and fondaparinux [28]. Selecting a VTE prevention strategy is complicated not only because it can be difficult to precisely define a patient's baseline VTE risk but also because the relative efficacy of different strategies is not well defined for most comparisons. In addition, the risk of potentially devastating bleeding complications is especially high in the NeuroICU.

Mechanical Prophylaxis

GCS

Recent high-quality evidence has raised serious doubts about the utility of GCS in patients with acute stroke [40]. The CLOTS 1 trial enrolled 2,518 patients and randomly assigned them to routine care plus thigh-length GCS or routine care and the avoidance of GCS. The use of thigh-length GCS in patients with stroke did not reduce the rate of proximal (symptomatic and asymptomatic) DVT and was associated with an increased risk of skin breakdown [19]. However, in contrast to patients with stroke, there is some evidence that patients in the postoperative period, including neurosurgical patients, have a reduced VTE rate with the use of GCS [39, 40]. Therefore, GCS may be beneficial in the surgical patient, but more high-quality evidence is needed. Currently available evidence suggests that if GCS are to be used for VTE prevention, thigh-high stockings may be more effective than their below-knee counterparts [41].

IPC

Medium-quality evidence indicates that, compared to no treatment, IPCs will reduce the risk of VTE for most patients in the NeuroICU. In a pooled analysis of multiple neurosurgical patients, IPCs were found to be statistically better than no treatment; in a comparison of ICDs versus GCS, there was a slight benefit from IPCs over GCS [21, 28]. The CLOTS 3 trial is currently determining whether IPCs are beneficial in the prevention of DVT after acute stroke [40]. Further trials are needed to determine the true benefit of IPCs in all patient groups because the number of published high-quality clinical studies is low.

Interpreting the evidence for VTE prevention with mechanical methods of prophylaxis is further complicated by the heterogeneity of device type, size, and pressure across different studies. Finally, the evidence of efficacy for mechanical devices can only be applied to clinical practice if the devices are used appropriately and kept on the patient at all times. These caveats notwithstanding, mechanical VTE prevention methods remain the preferred option for NeuroICU patients with a high risk of bleeding [9].

Inferior Vena Cava Filters

Vena cava filters are designed to mechanically trap emboli and are typically placed in the inferior vena cava, thus are generally referred to as inferior vena cava (IVC) filters. However, occasionally, these filters may be placed in the superior vena cava as well. Many of these are temporary and may be removed after up to approximately 12 weeks, depending on the manufacturer. Historically, IVC interruption devices have been utilized in patients who have proximal DVT or PE and are unable to receive anticoagulation or in patients who have objective evidence of PE recurrence despite adequate therapeutic anticoagulation. However, the use of these filters has increased (especially in the United States). In some centers, IVC filters are placed in all, or most, patients with multi-trauma and no established VTE; free-floating thrombus; and massive PE. The Cochrane Collaboration reviewed IVC filters for efficacy and safety and, out of hundreds of reports, was only able to find two RCTs, as most others had major methodological deficits. The authors of the Cochrane review concluded that there is currently inadequate evidence to recommended filters for patients other than those with a failure of – or a contraindication to – anticoagulation [42].

The American College of Chest Physicians (ACCP) guidelines do not recommend IVC filters for primary VTE prevention, citing inadequate evidence of benefit and a known risk of complications such as caval thrombosis, malpositioning of the device, and failure to remove a temporary filter [9]. The evidence for IVC filters as a primary VTE prevention strategy has been reviewed elsewhere. There are some small, methodologically poor studies that suggest benefit [43–46]. However, IVC filters can have serious complications, and, pending better evidence, IVC filters should not be routinely used as a VTE prophylaxis strategy.

Pharmacologic Prophylaxis

Provided that IPCs can be applied optimally, further studies are needed to define the marginal benefit of pharmacologic or combination strategies. Current evidence does not definitively answer the question: "How many patients would need to receive combination (pharmacologic + mechanical) prophylaxis instead of mechanical methods in order to prevent 1 symptomatic DVT or PE?" The corollary question "How many serious bleeds caused by VTE prophylaxis will be prevented by combination prophylaxis?" also remains unanswered. Current evidence has several limitations: (1) the number of head-to-head comparisons of mechanical versus combination prophylaxis is small; (2) none of the trials is definitive; (3) endpoints (i.e., DVT detected by ultrasound surveillance) of questionable clinical relevance have been used for many studies.

Combination Versus Mechanical

Combined methods of prophylaxis are currently recommended for the patients at very high risk of VTE [9]. Studies in selected neurosurgical patients have shown that the combination of mechanical methods (GCS in the largest studies) plus pharmacologic prophylaxis significantly reduced the risk of DVT compared to mechanical measures alone [9]. In a population of particularly high-risk patients in a single-center trial, Goldhaber and colleagues combined GCS and IPCs with either LMWH or UFH and demonstrated a significantly reduced rate of both asymptomatic and symptomatic DVT in both the LMWH and UFH groups [47]. The findings of this study are consistent with data from a larger trial that found a significant reduction in DVT when enoxaparin combined with GCS was compared to GCS alone [48]. Based on this evidence, we suggest that combination prophylaxis should be considered for those neurologically injured patients with numerous VTE risk factors (e.g., obesity, prior VTE, advanced age, active cancer). In cases where the risk of devastating hemorrhage is prohibitive, pharmacologic interventions should be withheld until the bleeding risk subsides.

Bleeding Risks with Prophylaxis

Limitations of currently available evidence preclude precise estimates of the degree to which low-dose anticoagulants increase the absolute risk of major bleeding in the NeuroICU. In a pooled analysis of neurosurgical patients, ICH rates were 2.1 % for postoperative LMWH and 1.1 % for nonpharmacologic methods [49]. Similarly, a meta-analysis in 2010 of 6 cranial neurosurgery RCTs that evaluated the impact of UFH or LMWH (versus no pharmacologic prophylaxis) noted that heparin use confers an increased risk of bleeding: minor bleeding was statistically more common in the patients who received an anticoagulant (absolute risk increase, 2.8 %). Intracranial hemorrhage was numerically more common (absolute risk increase, 0.7 %) in the patients who received UFH/LMWH, but the difference was not statistically significant, possibly because of a low overall number of events [50]. Finally, an analysis of several studies comparing UFH/LMWH versus no heparin suggests that the risk of ICH doubles with pharmacologic prophylaxis, but low total number of events precludes a precise estimate of relative risk [28].

Accounting for the heterogeneity of patients in the NeuroICU, prophylaxis should be tailored to the type of neurologic insult. For example, Danish and colleagues suggest that mechanical prophylaxis may be superior to heparin products in craniotomy patients who have a high bleeding risk [4], but the patient with an ischemic stroke at low risk for hemorrhagic transformation would be a good candidate for early pharmacologic prophylaxis. Likewise, the patient with intracerebral malignancy is at an increased risk for VTE and may often derive net benefit from combination methods of prophylaxis.

LMWH Versus UFH

The PROphylaxis for ThromboEmbolism in Critical Care Trial (PROTECT) studied dalteparin (LMWH) versus low-dose UFH in critically ill medical and general surgical patients (excluding major trauma and neurosurgical patients) and found that the rate of VTE and major bleeding was similar between both groups. However, the dalteparin-treated patients had a lower risk of PE (1.3 % versus 2.3 %; $p = 0.01$) compared to the patients who received UFH [51]. Although PE was a secondary endpoint in the PROTECT study, the finding that an LMWH was more effective than UFH is consistent with results from PREVAIL, an RCT that evaluated enoxaparin daily versus UFH every 12 h for the prevention of VTE after acute ischemic stroke; the PREVAIL study found enoxaparin to be more effective than UFH in prevention of VTE with no significant difference in symptomatic ICH [20]. A subgroup analysis of this study reports that the use of LMWH in these patients was not followed by any

Table 17.3 Agents utilized in the United States for VTE *prophylaxis*

Agent	Usual prophylactic dose
Unfractionated heparin	5,000 U subcutaneously every 8–12 h
Low-molecular-weight heparins	
Enoxaparin	30 mg subcutaneously twice daily or 40 mg subcutaneously once daily
Dalteparin	5,000 U subcutaneously daily
Fondaparinux	2.5 mg subcutaneously daily

Data from Nutescu [58]

negative neurologic outcomes and suggests that LMWH is a safe option for VTE prevention in the patient with ischemic stroke [52]. In summary, current evidence indicates LMWH is more effective than UFH for patients with critical illness, but in patients whose thrombosis risk is moderate or low, the efficacy difference between LMWH and UFH may be clinically unimportant.

Timing of Administration

Although some studies suggest an increased risk of bleeding complications when heparin products are administered preoperatively or in the early postoperative period [9, 53], the ideal timing for perioperative pharmacologic prophylaxis is not known. Despite a lack of specific guidelines, the general range of postoperative prophylaxis is usually 12–48 h after surgery (select institutions do not initiate pharmacologic prophylaxis within 72 h of the procedure [54]).

Additional Pharmacologic Considerations

Other considerations for pharmacologic prophylaxis are the specific agent, physiologic clearance, and appropriate dosage (Table 17.3). The current agents utilized in the United States are generally low-dose UFH, low-dose LMWH (such as enoxaparin, dalteparin, or tinzaparin), and fondaparinux (selective inhibitor of factor Xa). We do not discuss fondaparinux because it has not been studied as a VTE prevention strategy for patients with critical neurologic illness and its long half-life makes it problematic for NeuroICU patients who may require multiple invasive procedures.

In addition to being slightly more effective than UFH, LMWHs probably cause heparin-induced thrombocytopenia less often than UFH. The LMWHs are cleared (to differing degrees) by the kidneys. When given in prophylactic doses, dalteparin and tinzaparin do not appear to accumulate or increase the risk of bleeding, even in patients with significant renal insufficiency; on the other hand, enoxaparin should be dose-adjusted or avoided in patients with an estimated

Table 17.4 American College of Chest Physicians (ACCP) recommendations for VTE prevention

Patient population	Recommendations (2008 guidelines)
Neurosurgery patients	Optimally placed IPCs (with or without GCS)
	In patients who are at particularly high risk for VTE, the addition of either postoperative LMWH or UFH is recommended (when feasible from a hemostasis standpoint)
Traumatic brain injury, major trauma	Optimally placed IPCs (with or without GCS)
	When high bleeding risk decreases, the addition of low-dose LMWH is recommended
Acute spinal cord injury	Optimally placed IPCs (with or without GCS)
	Once primary hemostasis is evident and further bleeding risk is decreased, LMWH is recommended
	Alternatives to this are the combination of IPCs (with or without GCS) plus UFH or LMWH
	Recommend against the use of IVC filter for primary thromboprophylaxis
Acute neurologic disease, other medical conditions	Routine VTE risk assessment
	Optimally placed IPCs (with or without GCS)
	Once any bleeding risk decreased, the addition of either LMWH or UFH is recommended

Data from Geerts et al. [9]

Table 17.5 Signs/symptoms of DVT and PE

DVT	PE
Pain on palpation, especially posterior calf tenderness	Dyspnea
Unilateral edema	Tachypnea
Diameter difference between affected calf and opposite side	Pleuritic chest pain
Dilated superficial veins (occasionally)	Cough
Warmth	Hemoptysis
	Tachycardia
	Hypoxemia
	Hypocapnia
	Low-grade fever
	Syncope
	Hypotension or cyanosis if severe
	Clinical DVT signs

Data from Bounameaux et al. [60]

GFR < 30 mL/min [55]. For patients treated with UFH, the choice between BID and TID regimens remains controversial. One meta-analysis indicates that TID regimens have better efficacy with slightly increased bleeding [56], while a more recent pooling of 16 trials failed to show important differences in clinical event rates between these two regimens [57].

Overall, despite multiple studies, there is no specific data that clearly delineates the risk versus benefit of anticoagulants for prophylaxis. Additional studies are warranted to further establish a more definite risk of hemorrhagic complications, as the current literature may be difficult to interpret due to the inevitable confounding factors related to patient and surgery-specific factors, the timing of prophylaxis, etc. Until further studies provide data to support more specific guidelines, decisions about timing and type of pharmacologic prophylaxis must be left to the discretion of the individual practitioner, who is best able to weigh the individual patient's risks and benefits (Table 17.4).

Diagnosis of Thromboembolism

Even when patients are able to interact with the medical team, VTE diagnosis can be difficult because the disease can manifest in many different ways and with a wide range of clinical severity (Table 17.5). The spectrum includes a trivial calf vein thrombus on one hand and a large PE with cardiogenic shock on the other. In the critical care setting, the diagnosis of VTE can be especially challenging because many patients are unable to communicate because of intubation, sedation, or coma. Thus, the clinician cannot rely on complaints of common symptoms like dyspnea and pleuritic chest pain, leg swelling, and discomfort. Instead, the healthcare team must be vigilant for signs like unilateral extremity edema, unexplained hypoxemia, respiratory alkalosis, tachycardia, or tachypnea [58–60].

Pulmonary Embolism

Although clinical studies such as chest x-ray, electrocardiography, and arterial blood gas sampling can provide clues that PE may be present, these sorts of evaluations have a limited role once PE has been considered, because none can confirm or exclude the diagnosis with certainty.

Computed tomographic angiography (CTA) of the chest has the highest positive and negative predictive values of any test used to exclude or objectively confirm the diagnosis of PE. High-quality evidence indicates that a "negative" technically adequate CTA, performed with a modern, multidetector scanner eliminates PE as a diagnostic possibility [61]. Unfortunately, CTA is sometimes not feasible for a critically ill patient because the study requires transport to the radiology department. CTA also requires the administration of IV contrast, something that may be contraindicated in a critically ill patient with marginal renal function. Finally, CTA has the potential to identify small vascular filling defects of unknown clinical significance. There is some evidence [62] that these isolated subsegmental "clots" carry a more benign clinical prognosis than traditional PE. As such, CTA may also lead to harm by prompting the unnecessary use of inferior vena cava (IVC) filters or anticoagulation.

Ventilation-perfusion (V/Q) scintigraphy (scanning) is an alternative to CTA. V/Q scans are helpful when interpreted as "normal" (PE is excluded) or "high probability," but V/Q scans are often interpreted as "low probability" or "indeterminate." In such cases, the posttest probability of disease is often too high to withhold treatment, but further confirmatory testing is still necessary. For outpatients with a relatively low pretest probability of PE, negative bilateral lower extremity ultrasound *combined with* a low-probability V/Q scan may represent sufficient evidence to withhold treatment [63]. One practical advantage of the V/Q scanner (a nuclear camera) is that, in some institutions, it may be portable; finally, V/Q scanning is not contraindicated in patients with renal insufficiency.

A low plasma D-dimer concentration can exclude the diagnosis of PE (and DVT), but there are some important considerations associated with D-dimer measurement. First, D-dimer levels can increase for many reasons other than acute thrombosis (recent surgery, infection, cancer, pregnancy, and others). Thus, this test will often be elevated (and therefore not helpful) when measured in NeuroICU patients. Secondly, the clinician must be familiar with the characteristics of the particular D-dimer assay at his or her institution;

they should confirm that there are specific studies of how that assay (and its chosen "cutoff value") performs as a test to exclude VTE [64].

Deep Vein Thrombosis

For symptomatic patients, compression ultrasonography (CUS) is a sensitive and specific way to look for DVT. Normally, because they have pliable walls, the deep veins can be easily compressed with an ultrasound probe. When a clot is present, the lumen cannot be obliterated with the probe and the vein segment is referred to as noncompressible. Because it is relatively inexpensive, technically straightforward, and portable, CUS is usually the best initial diagnostic study for NeuroICU patients with suspected DVT. In patients whose clot may be confined to the pelvic veins, CUS may not be able to evaluate the vessel of interest. In such cases, CT venography (when available) is the best alternative. As with PE, D-dimer (when its concentration is low) can be used to exclude DVT. However, the utility of this test is limited in the NeuroICU for the reasons discussed previously. Patients with suspected upper extremity DVT are usually evaluated with CUS, although there is less evidence documenting the accuracy of this technique to detect upper extremity clot [65].

Treatment of VTE

Once the diagnosis has been established, the appropriate management of PE or DVT must be tailored to the individual patient.

Pulmonary Embolism

PE can be categorized into massive, submassive, or low-risk PE. Massive PE may be defined by an acute PE with sustained hypotension (systolic BP<90 mmHg) unrelated to another cause, pulselessness, or profound bradycardia with signs of shock. For patients with submassive PE, several factors can help identify those at risk for adverse short term outcomes, including clinical scores that address comorbidities and age [66, 67]. Worsening respiratory insufficiency, right ventricular (RV) dysfunction on echocardiography, RV dilation on CT scan, and elevated troponins and natriuretic peptides all indicate increased severity [67].

Since 1960, the mainstay of treatment for PE has been (and remains) therapeutic anticoagulation (Table 17.6) [68]. Patients with confirmed PE and no contraindications should be treated immediately with therapeutic anticoagulation (LMWH, UFH, or fondaparinux) [67, 69]. Some literature

Table 17.6 ACCP 2008 recommendations for PE treatment in selected circumstances

Selected treatment	Recommended patient selection
Initial anticoagulation	All patients without contraindications
	UFH is specifically recommended initially in those with massive PE who may need thrombolysis or surgical intervention
IVC filters	Only for patients who fail anticoagulation or with high risk of bleeding
	Not recommended for routine use
Thrombolytics	Only patients with evidence of hemodynamic compromise *without* bleeding risk
	Consider in normotensive patients at high risk for death (severe RV strain, elevated troponin, etc.)
Interventional catheter-based techniques	Only in select patients who are hemodynamically compromised and unable to receive thrombolytic therapy
	Requires special institutional expertise and support
Surgical embolectomy	Patients who specifically require surgical excision of a right atrial thrombus or impending paradoxical arterial embolism or closure of a patent foramen ovale
	Only select patients who are hemodynamically compromised who are unable to receive thrombolytic therapy or who fail therapy
	Requires special institutional expertise and support

Data from Kearon et al. [69]

suggests treatment based on the patient's severity and risk of death as discussed earlier. Based on this data, the general recommended treatment would be the following: low-risk PE, therapeutic anticoagulation; intermediate-risk or submassive PE, therapeutic anticoagulation and close monitoring of clinical status and RV function; high-risk or massive PE, therapeutic anticoagulation plus consideration of thrombolysis or embolectomy for selected patients [70].

Thrombolysis with an agent such as alteplase can be considered in addition to anticoagulation in certain individualized circumstances, but the possible benefit must be weighed against the potential risks (both massive and minor hemorrhage). Absolute contraindications to thrombolysis include the following: any prior ICH, known structural cerebrovascular disease (e.g., arteriovenous malformation), intracerebral malignancy, ischemic stroke within 3 months, suspected aortic dissection, active bleeding or bleeding diatheses, recent spinal or cranial surgery, or significant closed-head injury or facial trauma within 3 months. Therefore, many NeuroICU patients are unlikely to qualify for thrombolysis, but guidelines recommend consideration of this treatment if the patient has PE with hemodynamic compromise and low risk of bleeding complications. Significant controversy exists about whether patients with hemodynamically stable submassive PE derive net clinical benefit from thrombolysis [67]. Kostantinides and coworkers performed a PRCT that compared alteplase plus heparin versus heparin only for submassive PE in patients with a low risk of bleeding and found no difference in mortality [71]. For most patients with submassive PE in the NeuroICU, the risks of thrombolysis will outweigh any potential benefit.

Catheter-based interventions can recanalize occlusions in the pulmonary arterial system in patients with massive PE [72]; however, further evidence is needed related to the risks and benefits of these interventions. The proposed benefits of catheter-based therapy include a reduction in RV pressure and

strain, increased systemic perfusion, and improved RV recovery. The risks are rare but serious, including pulmonary and cerebral hemorrhage and right atrial or ventricular perforation [67]. Presently, therefore, this technique should be only be done at a center with physicians having significant experience and in patients who are unstable with massive PE that have failed, or who have contraindications to, systemic thrombolysis [69, 70].

Surgical embolectomy is performed with cardiopulmonary bypass and allows right atrial thrombus extraction and the prevention of paradoxical embolism. The decision to perform surgical embolectomy for patients with imminently life-threatening massive PE is influenced by several considerations, most importantly the expertise and capabilities of the local institution. Similar to catheter-based interventions, surgical embolectomy is only recommended for patients with massive PE and hemodynamic instability or with respiratory insufficiency not responding to other measures (e.g., anticoagulation or thrombolysis) [67, 69].

IVC filters are recommended for (1) patients with confirmed PE (or proximal DVT) with contraindications to anticoagulation or (2) patients who have recurrent PE despite therapeutic anticoagulation. These patients should be started on anticoagulation when possible, and retrievable filters should be removed as soon as this can be practically and safely be done. Pending high-quality, prospective evidence of net benefit, we recommend against the routine use of IVC filters as an adjuvant to standard anticoagulant therapy [67, 69].

DVT

Unless there is specific contraindication, patients with DVT should receive therapy with therapeutic doses of LMWH, UFH, or fondaparinux (Table 17.7). Long-term anticoagulation generally can be achieved with warfarin overlapped with

Table 17.7 Common agents utilized in the United States for VTE *treatment*

Agent	Usual therapeutic dose
Unfractionated heparin	80 units/kg IV bolus, followed by 18 units/kg/h to keep aPTT 1.5–2 times control or plasma heparin levels of 0.3–0.7 IU/mL anti-factor Xa activity
Low-molecular-weight heparins	
Enoxaparin	1 mg/kg subcutaneously twice daily or 1.5 mg/kg subcutaneously once daily
Dalteparin	100 IU/kg subcutaneously twice daily or 200 IU/kg subcutaneously once daily
Tinzaparin	175 IU/kg subcutaneously once daily
Fondaparinux	5–10 mg subcutaneously daily – depending on the patient weight range: 5 mg for <50 kg, 7.5 mg for 50–100 kg, 10 mg for >100 kg
Direct thrombin inhibitors	*(Indicated for patients with suspected or proven heparin-induced thrombocytopenia)*
Argatroban	2 mcg/kg/min (normal liver function)
Lepirudin	0.1 mg/kg/h (normal renal function)
Bivalirudin	0.75 mg/kg IV bolus, then 1.75 mg/kg/h
Warfarin	5–10 mg orally on day 1 of heparin. Overlap with heparin until INR becomes therapeutic (2.5–3) for two consecutive days

Data from Nutescu [58], Jaff et al. [67], Emadi and Streiff [73]

initial anticoagulation for a minimum of 5 days and until the INR is above 2.0. IVC filters should only be used in patients with acute proximal DVT and contraindications to anticoagulation. Pharmacomechanical thrombolysis should be reserved for patients who have an extensive clot burden in a proximal (e.g., iliac or femoral) vein and who are at low risk for bleeding [58, 67, 69, 73].

Superficial Vein Thrombosis and Upper Extremity Thrombosis

Superficial VTE commonly affects the lower limbs and is associated with previously discussed risk factors for VTE but also may be associated with chronic venous insufficiency. Most clinicians treat *symptomatic* superficial leg or deep calf vein thrombosis. Current guidelines suggest anticoagulation with either LMWH or UFH. However, if anticoagulation is contraindicated, follow-up ultrasound may help to ensure there is no further propagation to the deep/proximal system [69].

DVT of the upper extremities accounts for approximately 1–4 % of all DVT and may lead to PE in up to one-third of cases. Common causes are malignancy, thrombophilia, or – often – indwelling catheters. Symptoms may include pain, edema, or functional impairment, but some patients are completely asymptomatic [69, 74]. Generally, thromboses in the axillary, subclavian, and internal jugular veins are usually treated with full-dose anticoagulation. However, thromboses in the basilic and cephalic veins are usually monitored without full-dose therapy. In such situations, it is reasonable either to use low-dose anticoagulation or to treat more conservatively with warm compresses and anti-inflammatory agents; patient-specific risk factors must be taken into account when determining who will need anticoagulation. If an upper extremity clot occurs in the vicinity of a central

venous catheter (CVC), we suggest that the catheter should be removed if it is feasible to do so. That notwithstanding, one small study of outpatients suggests that, in situations where continued use of a CVC is necessary, many ambulatory patients can be safely treated without immediate removal of the device [75].

References

1. Middeldorp S. Duration of anticoagulation for venous thromboembolism. BMJ. 2011;342:d2758.
2. Cushman M. Epidemiology and risk factors for venous thrombosis. Semin Hematol. 2007;44(2):62–9.
3. Ribeiro A, et al. Pulmonary embolism: one-year follow-up with echocardiography Doppler and five-year survival analysis. Circulation. 1999;99(10):1325–30.
4. Danish SF, et al. Prophylaxis for deep venous thrombosis in craniotomy patients: a decision analysis. Neurosurgery. 2005;56(6):1286–94.
5. Cohen AT, et al. Venous thromboembolism risk and prophylaxis in the acute hospital care setting (ENDORSE study): a multinational cross-sectional study. Lancet. 2008;371(9610):387–94.
6. Pengo V, et al. Incidence of chronic thromboembolic pulmonary hypertension after pulmonary embolism. N Engl J Med. 2004;350(22):2257–64.
7. Kahn SR, Ginsberg JS. Relationship between deep venous thrombosis and the postthrombotic syndrome. Arch Intern Med. 2004;164(1):17–26.
8. Anderson Jr FA, Spencer FA. Risk factors for venous thromboembolism. Circulation. 2003;107(23 Suppl 1):I9–16.
9. Geerts WH, et al. Prevention of venous thromboembolism: American College of Chest Physicians Evidence-Based Clinical Practice Guidelines (8th Edition). Chest. 2008;133(6 suppl):381S–453.
10. Reiff DA, et al. Traumatic brain injury is associated with the development of deep vein thrombosis independent of pharmacological prophylaxis. J Trauma. 2009;66(5):1436–40.
11. Harhangi BS, et al. Coagulation disorders after traumatic brain injury. Acta Neurochir (Wien). 2008;150(2):165–75; discussion 175.
12. Bauman JA, et al. Subcutaneous heparin for prophylaxis of venous thromboembolism in deep brain stimulation surgery. Neurosurgery. 2009;65(2):276–80.

13. Kessler CM. The link between cancer and venous thromboembolism: a review. Am J Clin Oncol. 2009;32(4 Suppl):S3–7.

14. Prandoni P. Acquired risk factors of venous thromboembolism in medical patients. Pathophysiol Haemost Thromb. 2006;35(1–2):128–32.

15. Farray D, Carman T, Fernandezjr B. The treatment and prevention of deep vein thrombosis in the preoperative management of patients who have neurologic diseases. Neurol Clin. 2004;22(2):423–39.

16. Dudley RR, et al. Early venous thromboembolic event prophylaxis in traumatic brain injury with low-molecular-weight heparin: risks and benefits. J Neurotrauma. 2010;27(12):2165–72.

17. White RH. The epidemiology of venous thromboembolism. Circulation. 2003;107(23 Suppl 1):I4–8.

18. Rosendaal FR. Venous thrombosis: a multicausal disease. Lancet. 1999;353(9159):1167–73.

19. Dennis M, et al. Effectiveness of thigh-length graduated compression stockings to reduce the risk of deep vein thrombosis after stroke (CLOTS trial 1): a multicentre, randomised controlled trial. Lancet. 2009;373(9679):1958–65.

20. Sherman DG, et al. The efficacy and safety of enoxaparin versus unfractionated heparin for the prevention of venous thromboembolism after acute ischaemic stroke (PREVAIL Study): an open-label randomised comparison. Lancet. 2007;369(9570):1347–55.

21. Lacut K, et al. Prevention of venous thrombosis in patients with acute intracerebral hemorrhage. Neurology. 2005;65(6):865–9.

22. Ray WZ, et al. Incidence of deep venous thrombosis after subarachnoid hemorrhage. J Neurosurg. 2009;110(5):1010–4.

23. Goldstein JN, et al. Risk of thromboembolism following acute intracerebral hemorrhage. Neurocrit Care. 2009;10(1):28–34.

24. Chen D, et al. Medical complications during acute rehabilitation following spinal cord injury – current experience of the Model Systems. Arch Phys Med Rehabil. 1999;80(11):1397–401.

25. Waring WP, Karunas RS. Acute spinal cord injuries and the incidence of clinically occurring thromboembolic disease. Paraplegia. 1991;29(1):8–16.

26. Green D, et al. Spinal Cord Injury Risk Assessment for Thromboembolism (SPIRATE Study). Am J Phys Med Rehabil. 2003;82(12):950–6.

27. Jones T, et al. Venous thromboembolism after spinal cord injury: incidence, time course, and associated risk factors in 16,240 adults and children. Arch Phys Med Rehabil. 2005;86(12):2240–7.

28. Collen JF, et al. Prevention of venous thromboembolism in neurosurgery: a metaanalysis. Chest. 2008;134(2):237–49.

29. Chan AT, et al. Venous thromboembolism occurs frequently in patients undergoing brain tumor surgery despite prophylaxis. J Thromb Thrombolysis. 1999;8(2):139–42.

30. Collins R, et al. Reduction in fatal pulmonary embolism and venous thrombosis by perioperative administration of subcutaneous heparin. Overview of results of randomized trials in general, orthopedic, and urologic surgery. N Engl J Med. 1988;318(18):1162–73.

31. Prevention of fatal postoperative pulmonary embolism by low doses of heparin. An international multicentre trial. Lancet. 1975; 2(7924):45–51.

32. White RH, Zhou H, Romano PS. Incidence of symptomatic venous thromboembolism after different elective or urgent surgical procedures. Thromb Haemost. 2003;90(3):446–55.

33. Cheng JS, et al. Anticoagulation risk in spine surgery. Spine (Phila Pa 1976). 2010;35(9 Suppl):S117–24.

34. Sansone JM, del Rio AM, Anderson PA. The prevalence of and specific risk factors for venous thromboembolic disease following elective spine surgery. J Bone Joint Surg Am. 2010;92(2):304–13.

35. Gerlach R, et al. Risk of postoperative hemorrhage after intracranial surgery after early nadroparin administration: results of a prospective study. Neurosurgery. 2003;53(5):1028–34; discussion 1034–5.

36. Bratton SL, et al. Guidelines for the management of severe traumatic brain injury. V. Deep vein thrombosis prophylaxis. J Neurotrauma. 2007;24 Suppl 1:S32–6.

37. Knudson MM, et al. Thromboembolism after trauma: an analysis of 1602 episodes from the American College of Surgeons National Trauma Data Bank. Ann Surg. 2004;240(3):490–6; discussion 496–8.

38. Caprini JA. Risk assessment as a guide for the prevention of the many faces of venous thromboembolism. Am J Surg. 2010;199 (1 Suppl):S3–10.

39. Sachdeva A et al. Elastic compression stockings for prevention of deep vein thrombosis. Cochrane Database Syst Rev. 2010;(7): CD001484.

40. Naccarato M et al. Physical methods for preventing deep vein thrombosis in stroke. Cochrane Database Syst Rev. 2010:(8): CD001922.

41. CLOTS (Clots in Legs Or sTockings after Stroke) Trial Collaboration. Thigh-length versus below-knee stockings for deep venous thrombosis prophylaxis after stroke a randomized trial. Ann Intern Med. 2010;153:553–62.

42. Young T, Tang H, Hughes R. Vena caval filters for the prevention of pulmonary embolism. Cochrane Database Syst Rev. 2010;(2): CD006212.

43. Carlin AM, et al. Prophylactic and therapeutic inferior vena cava filters to prevent pulmonary emboli in trauma patients. Arch Surg. 2002;137(5):521–5; discussion 525–7.

44. Rodriguez JL, et al. Early placement of prophylactic vena caval filters in injured patients at high risk for pulmonary embolism. J Trauma. 1996;40(5):797–802; discussion 802–4.

45. Rogers FB, et al. Routine prophylactic vena cava filter insertion in severely injured trauma patients decreases the incidence of pulmonary embolism. J Am Coll Surg. 1995;180(6):641–7.

46. Wilson JT, et al. Prophylactic vena cava filter insertion in patients with traumatic spinal cord injury: preliminary results. Neurosurgery. 1994;35(2):234–9; discussion 239.

47. Goldhaber SZ, et al. Low rate of venous thromboembolism after craniotomy for brain tumor using multimodality prophylaxis. Chest. 2002;122(6):1933–7.

48. Agnelli G, et al. Enoxaparin plus compression stockings compared with compression stockings alone in the prevention of venous thromboembolism after elective neurosurgery. N Engl J Med. 1998; 339(2):80–5.

49. Agnelli G. Prevention of venous thromboembolism in surgical patients. Circulation. 2004;110(24 Suppl 1):IV4–12.

50. Hamilton MG, et al. Venous thromboembolism prophylaxis in patients undergoing cranial neurosurgery: a systematic review and meta-analysis. Neurosurgery. 2011;68(3):571–81.

51. Cook D, et al. Dalteparin versus unfractionated heparin in critically ill patients. N Engl J Med. 2011;364(14):1305–14.

52. Kase CS, et al. Neurological outcomes in patients with ischemic stroke receiving enoxaparin or heparin for venous thromboembolism prophylaxis: subanalysis of the prevention of VTE after acute ischemic stroke with LMWH (PREVAIL) study. Stroke. 2009; 40(11):3532–40.

53. Dickinson LD, et al. Enoxaparin increases the incidence of postoperative intracranial hemorrhage when initiated preoperatively for deep venous thrombosis prophylaxis in patients with brain tumors. Neurosurgery. 1998;43(5):1074–81.

54. Scudday T, et al. Safety and efficacy of prophylactic anticoagulation in patients with traumatic brain injury. J Am Coll Surg. 2011; 213(1):148–53; discussion 153–4.

55. Lim W, et al. Meta-analysis: low-molecular-weight heparin and bleeding in patients with severe renal insufficiency. Ann Intern Med. 2006;144(9):673–84.

56. King CS, et al. Twice vs three times daily heparin dosing for thromboembolism prophylaxis in the general medical population: a meta-analysis. Chest. 2007;131(2):507–16.

57. Phung OJ, et al. Dosing frequency of unfractionated heparin thromboprophylaxis: a meta-analysis. Chest. 2011;140(2):374–81.

58. Nutescu EA. Assessing, preventing, and treating venous thromboembolism: evidence-based approaches. Am J Health Syst Pharm. 2007;64(11 Suppl 7):S5–13.

59. Stein PD, Henry JW. Clinical characteristics of patients with acute pulmonary embolism stratified according to their presenting syndromes. Chest. 1997;112(4):974–9.

60. Bounameaux H, Perrier A, Righini M. Diagnosis of venous thromboembolism: an update. Vasc Med. 2010;15(5):399–406.

61. Stein PD, et al. Multidetector computed tomography for acute pulmonary embolism. N Engl J Med. 2006;354(22):2317–27.

62. Carrier M, et al. Subsegmental pulmonary embolism diagnosed by computed tomography: incidence and clinical implications. A systematic review and meta-analysis of the management outcome studies. J Thromb Haemost. 2010;8(8):1716–22.

63. Wells PS, et al. Use of a clinical model for safe management of patients with suspected pulmonary embolism. Ann Intern Med. 1998;129(12):997–1005.

64. Ceriani E, et al. Clinical prediction rules for pulmonary embolism: a systematic review and meta-analysis. J Thromb Haemost. 2010; 8(5):957–70.

65. Spiezia L, Simioni P. Upper extremity deep vein thrombosis. Intern Emerg Med. 2010;5(2):103–9.

66. Jimenez D, Aujesky D, Yusen RD. Risk stratification of normotensive patients with acute symptomatic pulmonary embolism. Br J Haematol. 2010;151(5):415–24.

67. Jaff MR, et al. Management of massive and submassive pulmonary embolism, iliofemoral deep vein thrombosis, and chronic thromboembolic pulmonary hypertension: a scientific statement from the American Heart Association. Circulation. 2011;123(16): 1788–830.

68. Barritt DW, Jordan SC. Anticoagulant drugs in the treatment of pulmonary embolism. A controlled trial. Lancet. 1960;1(7138):1309–12.

69. Kearon C, et al. Antithrombotic therapy for venous thromboembolic disease: American College of Chest Physicians Evidence-Based Clinical Practice Guidelines (8th Edition). Chest. 2008;133 (6 Suppl):454S–545.

70. Konstantinides S. Clinical practice. Acute pulmonary embolism. N Engl J Med. 2008;359(26):2804–13.

71. Konstantinides S, et al. Heparin plus alteplase compared with heparin alone in patients with submassive pulmonary embolism. N Engl J Med. 2002;347(15):1143–50.

72. Kuo WT, et al. Catheter-directed therapy for the treatment of massive pulmonary embolism: systematic review and meta-analysis of modern techniques. J Vasc Interv Radiol. 2009;20(11):1431–40.

73. Emadi A, Streiff M. Diagnosis and management of venous thromboembolism: an update a decade into the new millennium. Arch Iran Med. 2011;14(5):341–51.

74. Prandoni P, Bernardi E. Upper extremity deep vein thrombosis. Curr Opin Pulm Med. 1999;5(4):222–6.

75. Kovacs MJ, et al. A pilot study of central venous catheter survival in cancer patients using low-molecular-weight heparin (dalteparin) and warfarin without catheter removal for the treatment of upper extremity deep vein thrombosis (The Catheter Study). J Thromb Haemost. 2007;5(8):1650–3.

Water and Electrolyte Management in Neurological Disease

18

Maryam Rahman, Nathan Kohler, and Azra Bihorac

Contents

M. Rahman, MD, MS (✉)
Department of Neurological Surgery,
University of Florida College of Medicine,
100265, Gainesville, FL 32610, USA
e-mail: mrahman@ufl.edu

N. Kohler, MD, PhD
Department of Radiology, Florida Hospital,
601 E. Rollins Street, Orlando, FL 32803, USA
e-mail: nathan.kohler.md@flhosp.org

A. Bihorac, MD, PhD
Division of Critical Care Medicine, Department of Anesthesiology,
University of Florida College of Medicine, 1600 SW Archer Road,
100254, Gainesville, FL 32608, USA
e-mail: abihorac@anest.ufl.edu

Abstract

Water and electrolyte disturbance can significantly impact the medical course of patients with neurological diseases. Specifically, hypo- and hypernatremia are common in neuro-patients and are associated with significant morbidity and mortality. The diagnosis and treatment algorithms for management of sodium disturbance in neuro-patients are discussed in this chapter. Disorders of potassium, calcium, phosphorus, and magnesium homeostasis are also discussed, as are their treatments.

Keywords

Dysnatremia • Hyponatremia • Hypernatremia • Electrolyte disturbance • Cerebral salt wasting • Syndrome of inappropriate antidiuretic hormone • Diabetes insipidus • Hypomagnesemia • Hypermagnesemia • Hypophosphatemia • Hyperphosphatemia • Hypercalcemia • Hypocalcemia

A.J. Layon et al. (eds.), *Textbook of Neurointensive Care*,
DOI 10.1007/978-1-4471-5226-2_18, © Springer-Verlag London 2013

Introduction

Electrolyte disorders may develop rapidly in patients in the neurointensive care unit and can significantly impact their disease course. The controlling mechanisms of electrolyte homeostasis may become disturbed by acute brain injury due to trauma or craniotomy or in the setting of primary or secondary central nervous system (CNS) disease. Sodium and water homeostasis abnormalities especially can have grave consequences for patients with neurological problems. In this chapter, we will discuss the basic elements that maintain homeostasis and then address specific electrolyte derangements, their management, and potential outcomes. Clinical scenarios will be used to emphasize certain clinical points.

Sodium and Water Balance

Disorders of the sodium plasma concentration are among the most common and potentially clinically dangerous electrolyte abnormalities among neurological and neurosurgical patients. Water balance is major determinant of plasma sodium concentration, and understanding of mechanisms that regulate water homeostasis is critical for understanding of sodium disorders. Water constitutes between 50 and 60 % of total body weight depending on age and gender. Total body water (TBW) is divided into two major compartments within the body: 2/3 in the intracellular space and 1/3 in the extracellular space. The extracellular fluid is further divided into the vascular compartment (1/3) and the interstitial space (2/3) (Fig. 18.1a).

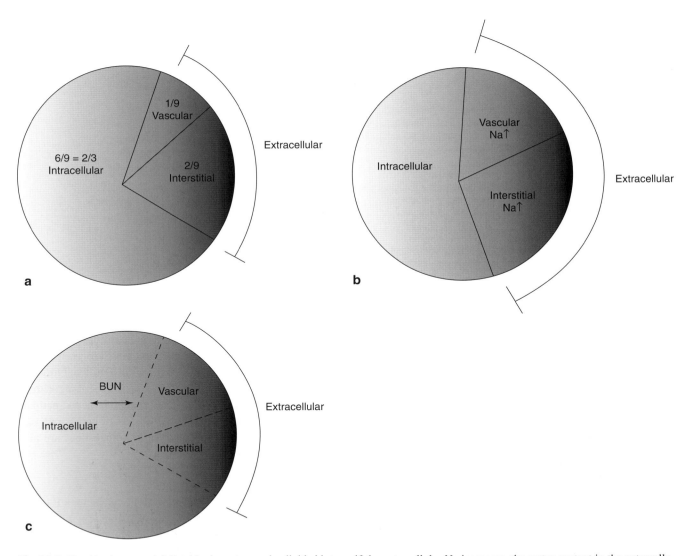

Fig. 18.1 Total body water. (**a**) Total body water can be divided into the intracellular and extracellular fluid compartments. The extracellular fluid compartment can be further divided into the vascular and interstitial compartments. Sodium cannot freely diffuse across the cell membrane and is a major determinant of tonicity (**b**). Therefore, if the extracellular Na increases, the water content in the extracellular space increases as well. (**c**) Because BUN diffuses easily through the cell membrane, it allows for equilibration between the intracellular and extracellular compartments if the extracellular Na increases or decreases

The water moves between the intracellular and the extracellular fluid compartments in response to osmotic forces exerted across the semipermeable cellular membrane and determined by the concentration of solute particles in the fluid. The osmotic activity of the solutes in body fluids is usually measured as serum osmolality defined as the number of osmoles of solute per kilogram of water (mOsm/kg H_2O). The major solutes determining plasma osmolality are sodium (mMol/L), blood urea nitrogen (BUN) (mg/dL), and glucose (mg/dL). The calculated serum osmolality can differ from the actual osmolality due to other osmotically active exogenous solutes, such as alcohol, resulting in an "osmolar gap." The equation to calculate estimated serum osmolality is:

$$Serum\ Osmolality\left(mOsm / kg\ H_2O\right) = 2\left(Na\right) + BUN / 2.8 + glucose / 18$$

The differences in osmolality between the intracellular and the extracellular compartments separated by semipermeable cell membrane create an osmotic gradient. This *osmotic gradient* contributes to effective osmolality or tonicity and dictates fluid shifts between compartments. S*odium* in the intracellular and extracellular compartments (Fig. 18.1b) is major determinant of tonicity since it cannot freely diffuse across the cellular membrane. Conversely, BUN diffuses easily through the cell membrane and will rapidly equilibrate between the intracellular and extracellular compartments even in the face of azotemia (Fig. 18.1c). Since total plasma sodium content is the principal determinant of the relative volumes of the intracellular and extracellular fluids, mechanisms aimed at regulating effective circulating volumes are involved in the maintenance of stable plasma sodium concentration. On the other hand, mechanisms aimed at regulation of water balance maintain a relatively constant plasma tonicity. Water and sodium balance are regulated through two different regulatory systems: osmoreceptors and hypothalamic–pituitary axis control plasma tonicity, while baroreceptors, in conjunction with multiple vasopressors, hormones, vascular system, and kidneys, constitute short- and long-term response to changes in effective circulating volumes through sodium conservation and excretion. *Hyper- and hypovolemia* are *disorders of sodium balance*. On the other hand, osmoreceptors sense plasma tonicity and regulate water intake and loss. Therefore, *hyper- and hypotonic states* are *disorders* of *water balance*.

Regulation of Water Balance and Plasma Osmolality

Plasma tonicity is regulated strictly by water intake and loss primarily by thirst and the ability of renal tubules to conserve or excrete water. Water loss that cannot be controlled physiologically includes "insensible losses" through the skin and lungs as well as some loss through the gastrointestinal tract. These losses can add up; a normal 70-kg person loses approximately 1.5 L/day of water. If this volume is not offset by an intake of at least the same volume of water, plasma tonicity increases. Osmolality of ECF, including plasma, is tightly regulated between 280 and 290 mOsm/kg. Changes in ECF osmolality can cause water to flow across cell membranes to equilibrate the osmolality of the cytoplasm with that of the ECF leading potentially through the alteration of cell volume and intracellular ionic strength to cell death. Hence, in response to change in plasma osmolality, humans engage promptly a myriad of physiological responses that actively oppose osmotic perturbations and serve to restore ECF osmolality towards a seemingly fixed osmotic "set point" near 300 mOsm/kg [1]. Increase in ECF osmolality stimulates the sensation of thirst, to promote water intake, and release of vasopressin (VP, also known as antidiuretic hormone [ADH]), to enhance water reabsorption in the kidney. In contrast, ECF hypo-osmolality suppresses basal VP secretion in humans [2, 3]. Because renal water reabsorption is partly stimulated by VP levels at rest [2], this inhibition of VP release effectively stimulates diuresis. This osmoregulatory response is initiated by the peripheral and central osmoreceptors that provide a sensory mechanism that can detect osmotic perturbations in the ECF. Peripheral osmoreceptors exist along the upper regions of the alimentary tract and in the blood vessels that collect solutes absorbed from the intestines, including the oropharyngeal cavity [4], the gastrointestinal tract [5], the splanchnic mesentery [6], the hepatic portal vein, and the liver [7]. The primary central osmoreceptors that modulate thirst and VP release are located in regions of the brain that are devoid of a blood–brain barrier, such as the hypothalamus and circumventricular organs [8, 9], and the neurons in the organum vasculosum laminae terminalis (OVLT) and subfornical organ, as well as magnocellular neurosecretory cells (MNCs) in the hypothalamic supraoptic nucleus (SON) [10, 11], have been proposed to serve as primary osmoreceptors in humans [12, 13]. Osmoreceptor neurons are specialized neurons whose basal electrical activity effectively encodes the osmotic set point. Their intrinsic ability to transduce osmotic perturbations into changes in the rate or pattern of action-potential discharge allows them to become proportionally excited by hypertonic stimuli and inhibited by hypo-osmotic stimuli [1]. Recent studies have suggested that osmosensory transduction in osmoreceptor neurons is a mechanical process associated with an osmotically evoked change in cell volume [1, 11]. Although the exact molecular composition of the mammalian central osmoreceptor transduction channel remains unknown, members of the transient receptor potential vanilloid (TRPV) family of cation channels seem to have important roles in osmosensation and osmoregulation [14].

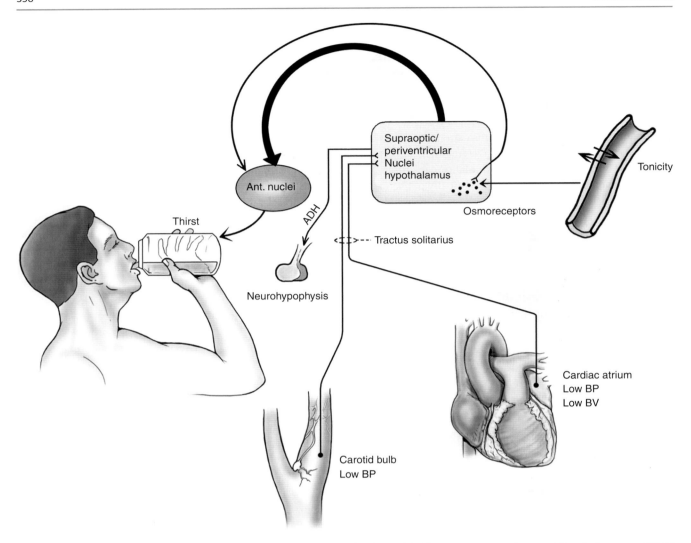

Fig. 18.2 Sodium physiology. Osmoreceptors in the hypothalamus and circumventricular organs sense increases in plasma tonicity as well as decreases in circulating volume either because of true volume loss or low perfusion state such as cardiac failure. These osmoreceptors induce thirst via the anterior nucleus of the thalamus to increase water intake. They also send efferents to the supraoptic and paraventricular hypotha- lamic nuclei. These neurons produce antidiuretic hormone (*ADH*) which is transported to the neurohypophysis and secreted to take its effect in the kidney for water retention. *Ant nuclei* anterior nucleus of the thalamus, *BP* blood pressure, *BV* blood volume (Used with permis- sion of David Peace, Medical Illustrator, University of Florida School of Medicine, Department of Neurosurgery)

Information derived from peripheral and cerebral osmore- ceptors is transmitted to a subset of MNCs located in the paraventricular nucleus (PVN) and SON of the hypothala- mus involved in the synthesis of a nine amino acid peptide hormone arginine vasopressin (AVP), a major regulator of free water excretion by the kidney (Fig. 18.2). The firing rate of MNCs that prevails under resting conditions (~1–3 Hz) mediates basal VP secretion, whereas decreases and increases in firing frequency inhibit and enhance hormone release dur- ing ECF hypotonicity and hypertonicity, respectively [15]. The synthesized peptide is enzymatically cleaved from its prohormone and is transported to the posterior pituitary where it is stored within neurosecretory granules. The increase in plasma osmolality causes secretion of AVP into

the bloodstream, leading to the activation of AVP V2 recep- tors in the kidney and insertion of aquaporin-2 water chan- nels into the apical membranes of collecting tubule principal cells [16]. As a result, the increase in water permeability of the collecting duct allows free water conservation and restores plasma osmolality set point towards normal limits.

Regulation of Sodium Balance and Effective Plasma Volume

Although maintenance of sodium homeostasis requires a balance between intake and excretion of Na$^+$, the lack of tight regulation of sodium intake places emphasis on the renal excretion of sodium as the main mechanism for sodium regulation [17]. Since Na$^+$ ensures maintenance of the ECF volume and directly supports blood pressure, the mechanisms for renal excretion of sodium are numerous and substantially more complex than those involved in the regulation of water balance. Renal Na$^+$ excretion varies directly with the effective circulating volume from urine Na$^+$ concentration as low as 1 mMol/L in the presence of volume depletion to over 100 mMol/L with effective volume expansion [18]. The changes in renal Na$^+$ excretion can result from alterations in the filtered load, determined by the glomerular filtration rate (GFR), and in tubular reabsorption, which is affected by multiple factors, including the renin–angiotensin–aldosterone system and natriuretic hormones, atrial natriuretic peptide (ANP), and urodilatin [18]. Low effective circulating volume also induces release of renin and norepinephrine. Renin leads to conversion of angiotensin I to angiotensin II which increases sodium reabsorption at the proximal tubule. The resulting aldosterone release causes reabsorption of sodium by the distal tubule and collecting duct. The norepinephrine causes decreased glomerular filtration rate and stimulates sodium reabsorption at the proximal tubule. These mechanisms all lead to increased sodium and water retention to increase circulating volume. In contrast, expansion of the ECF volume results in an appropriate increase in urinary sodium excretion induced by suppression of the renin–angiotensin–aldosterone system, a small elevation in GFR, and effect of natriuretic hormones. ANP is primarily released from the atria in response to volume expansion, which appears to be sensed as an increase in atrial stretch [19]. It causes increases in the glomerular filtration rate (GFR) without raising renal blood flow, directly reduces sodium reabsorption in the inner medullary collecting duct by closing the Na channels, and also diminishes sodium reabsorption in the proximal tubule through the local release of dopamine.

Hyponatremia

Hyponatremia is the most common electrolyte disorder encountered in clinical medicine [20]. Approximately one million hospitalizations per year in the USA have a principal or secondary diagnosis of hyponatremia. The annual cost of managing patients with hyponatremia has been estimated at $3.6 billion [20]. In addition to monetary costs, hyponatremia is associated with adverse outcomes for patients. Specifically, the mortality rates are significantly higher in hyponatremic patients across a broad range of primary disorders [21]. In some disease states, such as congestive heart failure, hyponatremia is an independent risk factor for increased mortality [22, 23].

The prevalence of hyponatremia in the neurosurgical population has been reported as high as 50 % [24–26]. Because of the cerebral effects of hyponatremia, neurosurgical patients are at increased risk for complications. Such complications include severe cerebral edema, mental status changes, seizures, vasospasm, and death. Unfortunately, these complications may also arise from the inappropriate treatment of hyponatremia. Correction of hyponatremia that is too slow or fast can lead to cerebral edema, seizures, osmotic demyelinating syndrome, or death [27, 28].

Despite the costs and complications associated with hyponatremia in the neurosurgical population, few randomized studies have been completed, describing when hyponatremia becomes clinically significant and how it should be treated. The evaluation and treatment of hyponatremia are left to the discretion of the individual healthcare provider or treatment team. This lack of a standardized treatment approach contributes to variable outcomes. A diagnostic and treatment protocol is proposed here.

Evaluation of Hyponatremia

Although hyponatremia is classically defined as serum sodium (Na) of less than 135 mMol/L, clinically significant hyponatremia has not been clearly defined [20, 29]. Hyponatremia is associated with increased mortality [30, 31]. In a prospective study of patients hospitalized for medical illnesses other than dysnatremia, a serum Na less than 130 mMol/L was associated with a 60-fold increase in fatality (11.2 % versus 0.19 %). Patients with a serum Na less than 120 mMol/L had a mortality rate of 25 % compared to 9.3 % in patients with a serum Na greater than 120 mMol/L [21]. Another prospective study showed that hyponatremic patients (mean Na 125.3 mMol/L) were seven times more likely to die in the hospital and more than twice as likely to die after discharge compared to normonatremic patients even when controlling for underlying diagnoses ($p < 0.0001$) [32]. In another study, hyponatremic patients with a serum Na improvement (greater than or equal to 2 mMol/L) had a mortality rate of 11.1 % at 60 days post discharge compared to with a 21.7 % mortality rate in those showing no improvement [33]. Change in serum Na was a significant predictor of 60-day mortality (hazard ratio [HR] 0.736, 95 % confidence interval (CI) 0.569–0.952 for each 1 mMol/L increase from baseline).

Additional morbidity is associated with a serum Na of less than 130 mMol/L [20, 29, 34]. A case–control study of emergency department (ED) patients found 21 % (26 of 122) of hyponatremic (Na less than 135 mMol/L) patients presented with falls compared to 5 % (13 of 244) of normonatremic patients matched in multiple comorbidities. The mean serum Na of hyponatremic patients was 126 mMol/L (range 115–132). The severity of the hyponatremia did not correlate with likelihood of presenting with falls [35]. A frequently cited study by Arieff and colleagues prospectively evaluated 65 patients with a serum Na less than 128 mMol/L. The patients who developed hyponatremia over 48 h or less were all symptomatic and had a mean serum Na of 114 mMol/L. The mean serum Na of chronic (longer than 48 h) hyponatremic patients was 115 mMol/L in symptomatic patients and 122 mMol/L in asymptomatic patients. All patients who developed seizures had a serum Na less than 121 mMol/L [36].

In SAH patients in particular, hyponatremia has a clear association with increased morbidity. Hyponatremia in SAH patients is associated with increased rates of cerebral ischemia [37, 38]. In one study, patients who were not fluid restricted demonstrated cerebral ischemia in 24 % of normonatremic and 12 % of hyponatremic (Na less than 135 mMol/L) patients [39]. Another prospective study of SAH patients demonstrated that hyponatremia was significantly (odds ratio 2.7, 95 % confidence interval 1.2–6.1) associated with poor outcomes at 3 months. Poor outcomes were classified according to the Glasgow Outcome Scale (GOS) of death, vegetative state, or severe disability [40].

The serum Na value indicating *clinically significant hyponatremia* varies in the literature; therefore, we recommend commencing diagnostic workup for a *serum Na less than 131 mMol/L*.

Diagnostic Workup for Hyponatremia

Causes of hyponatremia have traditionally been categorized by body fluid status. No standard reference test exists for the evaluation of hyponatremia. The lack of standard tests for the evaluation of hyponatremia often leads to inadequate evaluations of hyponatremic patients, such as failure to check plasma osmolality (P_{osm}), urine Na, and urine osmolality (U_{osm}). In a retrospective study of 104 patients with a serum Na of less than 125 mMol/L, osmolality was measured in only 26 % of patients. Mortality was higher in the group with inadequate workup and management (41 % versus 20 %, $p = 0.002$) [39]. Therefore, most experts have proposed a *combination of physical exam (PE) findings and laboratory tests to distinguish between the etiologies of hyponatremia* [25, 27, 29, 41–43]. This approach is especially important to distinguish between SIADH and CSW.

Neurosurgery patients often develop hyponatremia in the setting of natriuresis. *Hyponatremia with natriuresis is caused by either SIADH or CSW once diuretic use has been excluded.* Criteria for SIADH proposed by Janicic and colleagues include P_{osm} less than 275 mOsm/kg, inappropriate urinary concentration (U_{osm} greater than 100 mOsml/kg), clinical euvolemia (absence of orthostasis, tachycardia,

decreased skin turgor, dry mucous membranes, or edema and ascites), elevated urinary Na excretion with normal salt and water intake, and absence of other causes of euvolemic hypo-osmolality (hypothyroidism, hypocortisolism) [29]. However, these criteria have proven to be inadequate in distinguishing between SIADH and CSW. Ten of 12 neurosurgery patients in a prospective study who met the lab criteria for SIADH (serum Na less than 135 mMol/L, P_{osm} less than 280 mOsm/kg, urine Na greater than 25 mMol/L, and U_{osm} greater than P_{osm}) had low blood cell mass, plasma volume, and total blood volume compared to controls [44]. Extracellular fluid status is the key to distinguishing between SIADH and CSW [41, 44–47]. Determination of extracellular fluid (ECF) status using physical exam (PE) alone has been shown to be inaccurate [46]. A prospective study of 35 patients with a serum Na less than 130 mMol/L divided the patients into four groups (those who had received diuretics, polydipsic patients, saline responders, and saline nonresponders). Saline responders were patients who had a sustained increase in plasma Na of at least 5 mMol/L. All patients were initially determined to be hypo- or normovolemic based on PE findings (mucosal hydration, skin turgor, jugular vein distension), orthostatic changes in pulse (increase of 10 % upright compared to supine), and systolic blood pressure (decrease of 10 % upright compared to supine). The saline responders and those who had received diuretics were considered the true hypovolemic patients. Clinical determination of ECF status using PE finding parameters had a sensitivity of 41.1 % and a specificity of 80 %. Based on several studies about the evaluation of hyponatremia, a urinary Na of less than 30 mMol/L has a positive predictive value of 71–100 % for an infusion of 0.9 % saline to increase the serum Na level [47, 48]. Uric acid has also been used to distinguish SIADH from other etiologies of hyponatremia. In the study of saline responsiveness in hyponatremic patients, the polydipsic and saline nonresponsive patients tended to have lower plasma urea and uric acid compared to the other two groups [48]. A serum uric acid level of less than 4 mg/dL (in the presence of hyponatremia) has been calculated to have a positive predictive value for SIADH of 73–100 %. However, the definitions for SIADH used in these studies were broad and most likely included patients with CSW [49].

To distinguish between SIADH and CSW, central venous pressure (CVP) can be used to determine intravascular volume status. Damaraju and coworkers treated hyponatremia based on CVP values (less than 5 cm H_2O, 6–10 cm H_2O, greater than 10 cm H_2O). Hypovolemic patients (CVP less than 5 cm H_2O) were given normal saline (50 mL/kg/day) and salt (12 g/d). Normovolemic patients (CVP 6–10 cm H_2O) were given normal saline with 12 g of salt per day. In addition, patients with anemia (hematocrit less than 27 %) were administered whole blood. No patients were found to be hypervolemic (CVP greater than 10 cm H_2O). Seventy-three percent of patients corrected their serum Na within 72 h, and 12 % more within the following 24–48 h. The patients included three nonresponders, and two of these patients were found to have severe dehydration on blood volume measurements [46]. Another prospective study used CVP to categorize seven hyponatremic patients as SIADH (CVP 6–10 cm H_2O) and four patients as CSW (CVP less than 6 cm H_2O). The SIADH patients were treated with less than 800 mL/day of fluid restriction, and the CSW patients were treated with fluid replacement (50–100 mL/kg/day). Four patients achieved a normal serum Na within 36 h, and the other seven patients within 72 h [50].

Treatment of hyponatremia in SAH has generated controversy given the association of fluid restriction or dehydration with symptomatic vasospasm [38, 39]. Traditionally, hyponatremia in SAH patients has been attributed to SIADH [25]. However, more recent studies show that hyponatremic SAH patients often demonstrate a negative Na balance (loss of Na in urine greater than Na intake per day) and lower ECF [37]. Peptides such as atrial natriuretic peptide (ANP), brain natriuretic peptide (BNP), C-type natriuretic peptide (CNP), and digoxin-like substance have been found in SAH patients. Some have suggested a correlation between the presence of these peptides and CSW causing a delayed hyponatremia [37, 51]. In a prospective study of eight SAH patients that met criteria for SIADH proposed by Janicic, a linear relationship was found between ANP levels and urinary Na excretion [29]. ANP was found to be elevated in 14 SAH patients compared to controls in a study by Widjicks and coworkers [52]. Eight patients had a twofold increase in ANP above baseline and demonstrated natriuresis and a negative Na balance. Three of these patients had infarcts. Another study showed cerebrospinal fluid (CSF) adrenomedullin concentrations were significantly elevated in hyponatremic patients (Na less than 135 mMol/L) and patients who developed delayed ischemic neurological deficits [53]. Natriuretic peptides are associated with natriuresis but not always hyponatremia. In a study of 21 SAH patients, elevated ANP was present in all SAH patients compared to controls, regardless of serum Na level [54].

ADH has been shown to have limited diagnostic value in hyponatremia. The "appropriateness" of an ADH level has not been defined. SIADH has been documented in patients with no detectable ADH [55]. A prospective study of severe head injury patients found that patients who developed hyponatremia within 3 days of injury had higher ADH levels compared to patients who developed hyponatremia a week after the injury. However, ADH was detectable in all patients [43].

A general approach to the evaluation of hyponatremia is shown (Fig. 18.3 and Table 18.1). Using the evaluation paradigm, a *serum Na value of less than 131 mMol/L* should prompt a workup that includes measuring *serum and urine* *osmolarity and urine electrolytes and an evaluation of extracellular fluid (ECF) volume status.* A normal or high serum osmolality may result from lab error or pseudohyponatremia from hyperglycemia or hypertriglyceridemia. Hypotonic hyponatremia is categorized by ECF volume status. Volume status can be determined based on criteria listed in Table 18.1. Hypovolemia results from extrarenal loss or intrarenal loss such as CSW, diuretics, or adrenal insufficiency. In normovolemic patients, thyroid disease, hypocortisolism, and polydipsia should be ruled out before a diagnosis of SIADH is given. Moreover, hypervolemic hyponatremia is less common in neurosurgical patients, and the treatment team should rule out cirrhosis, congestive heart failure, and renal failure.

Treatment of Hyponatremia

Generally, the rate of correction of hyponatremia is determined by the severity of symptoms and rapidity of onset. Studies have shown that the severity of hyponatremia symptoms correlate with the magnitude of hyponatremia and the rate of onset [21, 36]. Given the significant morbidity/mortality associated with severely symptomatic hyponatremia, evidence exists to correct symptomatic severe hyponatremia aggressively with hypertonic saline. This approach is based loosely on the idea that acute hyponatremia tends to be more symptomatic and that treatment complications happen in the setting of chronic hyponatremia [36, 56].

Central pontine myelinolysis or osmotic demyelinating syndrome (ODS) is the most frequently cited complication in the treatment of hyponatremia. This entity was first described in the 1970s [57]. ODS is more likely to occur with correction of serum Na greater than 12 mMol/day and in the setting of chronic hyponatremia (greater than 48 h) [28]. In a retrospective study of patients with ODS, all patients had chronic hyponatremia (prior to admission) and a serum Na less than 110 mMol/L. All of the patients had their Na corrected faster than 12 mMol/day [58]. A review of the literature found that all of the patients with severe hyponatremia (Na less than 106 mMol/L) and a Na correction greater than 12 mMol/L/day developed some type of neurological complication. No neurological complications developed in those who were corrected more slowly [58].

A prospective study of 33 medical patients with symptomatic hyponatremia (mean serum Na 108 mMol/L) showed no episodes of ODS despite an increase of mean serum Na to 126 mMol/L within 48 h [59]. The authors evaluated a group of 12 patients retrospectively who all had evidence of cerebral demyelinating lesions at autopsy. The rate of correction of their hyponatremia was similar to the prospectively evaluated patients. However, they all had one of four characteristics: an increase in serum Na to normal or hypernatremic levels within 48 h, a serum Na change of more than

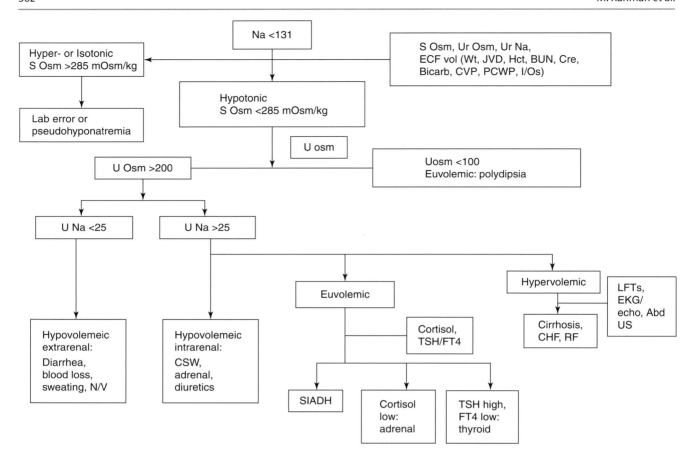

Fig. 18.3 Hyponatremia diagnostic protocol. Hyponatremic patients should undergo a workup including lab values and physical exam findings. Hypotonic hyponatremia can be categorized by volume status. *S* serum, *Osm* osmolarity, *Ur* urine, *ECF* extracellular fluid, *vol* volume, *Wt* weight, *JVD* jugular venous distension, *Hct* hematocrit, *BUN* blood urea nitrogen, *Cre* creatinine, *bicarb* bicarbonate, *CVP* central venous pressure, *PCWP* pulmonary catheter wedge pressure, *I/Os* in and out, *N/V* nausea and vomiting, *CSW* cerebral salt wasting, *adrenal* adrenal insufficiency, *TSH* thyroid stimulating hormone, *FT4* free T4, *LFTs* liver function tests, *EKG* electrocardiogram, *echo* echocardiogram, *Abd US* abdominal ultrasound, *CHF* congestive heart failure, *RF* renal failure

Table 18.1 Diagnostic criteria for CSW versus SIADH

	CSW	SIADH
S Na (mmol/L*)	<135	<135
S Osm (mOsm/kg*)	<285	<285
U Osm (mOsm/kg*)	>200	>200
U Na (mmol/L)	>25	>25
Weight	↓	↑
Fluid balance	↓	↑
JVD	−	+
Hct	↑	↓
BUN	↑	↓
Cre	↑	↓
Uric acid	− ↓	↓
Bicarb	↑	↓
CVP cm H$_2$O	<6	≥6
Pulm wedge pressure mmHg	<8	≥8

*Must have starred criteria and at least three of the non-starred criteria for diagnosis

S Na serum sodium, *S Osm* serum osmolality, *U Osm* urine osmolality, *U Na* urine sodium, *JVD* jugular venous distension, *Hct* hematocrit, *BUN* blood urea nitrogen, *Cre* creatinine, *Bicarb* bicarbonate, *CVP* central venous pressure, *pulm* pulmonary

25 mMol/L within 48 h, a hypoxic episode, and/or hepatic encephalopathy [59]. Based on case reports and animal data, the development of ODS is associated with the rate and magnitude of Na correction in chronic hyponatremia (greater than 48 h), with hypokalemia, and with malnourished states (alcoholism, cirrhosis, burns) [57]. Chronic hyponatremia should not be rapidly corrected. Generally, rapid correction at a rate over 1 mMol/L/h should be reserved for severely symptomatic and/or acute hyponatremia (less than 48 h). Severe symptoms (e.g., seizures, coma) indicate cerebral edema and should trigger prompt treatment [57, 58]. A retrospective study of inpatients with serum Na greater than 115 mMol/L demonstrated an increase in mortality in patients who had slower correction of their hyponatremia. The serum Na after 48 h of treatment was 127.1 mMol/L in survivors versus 118.8 mMol/L in patients who died ($p = 0.0016$) [23].

Syndrome of Inappropriate Secretion of Antidiuretic Hormone (SIADH)

The treatment of SIADH has been based on fluid restriction unless patients are severely symptomatic, in which case hypertonic saline is used [17]. In a study of 55 hyponatremic patients after transsphenoidal pituitary tumor resection, all 44 asymptomatic patients (80 %) were treated as outpatients with fluid restriction and a high-salt diet. Six of these patients had follow-up and showed improvement in serum Na. The 11 symptomatic patients were hospitalized. Three of these patients responded to fluid restriction and salt tablets, and eight patients required hypertonic saline [60]. The reasoning for treatment with fluid restriction versus hypertonic saline was not given.

Other treatments for SIADH include diuretics and urea. A prospective study described use of Lasix and ethacrynic acid in 11 of 12 SIADH patients and two volunteers. Na supplements were necessary in nine of 11 patients, and treatment of hypokalemia was required in seven patients. Two of the patients required higher doses of diuretics [61]. In a retrospective study of hyponatremia in neurosurgical patients, 40 g of urea in 100–150 mL of normal saline (NS) was given every 8 h in addition to a continuous infusion of NS at 60–100 mL/h for 1–2 days. Patients were not categorized as SIADH or CSW as these data were unavailable. The pretreatment mean Na was 130 mMol/L (range 119–134), and posttreatment mean was 138 mMol/L (range 129–148) ($p < 0.001$). In 85 % of cases, only 1 day of treatment was necessary [62].

The new ADH receptor blocker conivaptan has been approved for use in euvolemic hyponatremia based on improvement in hyponatremia in randomized controlled trials [63]. Since this class of drug can cause volume depletion, further human studies are necessary to determine their role in treatment of hyponatremia in the neurosurgical population [64].

Cerebral Salt Wasting

Treatment for cerebral salt wasting (CSW) has been studied mostly in the setting of subarachnoid hemorrhage (SAH). A retrospective analysis of 134 SAH patients demonstrated the risks associated with fluid restriction in the treatment of hyponatremia [38]. Twenty-six of the 44 hyponatremic patients (Na less than 135 mMol/L) were treated with fluid restriction (less than 1 L/24 h in normothermic patients). Cerebral infarction developed in 21 of the 26 fluid-restricted patients and in 27 of the 44 patients with a Na less than 135 mMol/L compared to 19 of the 90 normonatremic patients [38]. Another study of SAH patients demonstrated a negative Na balance in all patients regardless of serum Na between days 2 and 3 following SAH [37]. Repletion of volume has become the standard treatment. A case report of a patient with CSW described a recurrence of hyponatremia when the intravenous (IV) fluids were stopped [65]. A study of 21 hyponatremic (Na less than 130 mMol/L) neurosurgical patients and three controls categorized patients into groups based on hematocrit, CVP, and total blood volume. Group A (hypovolemic and anemic) and group B (hypovolemic without anemia) were treated with isotonic saline and oral salt. Group A patients also received blood transfusions. No patients demonstrated hypervolemic hyponatremia. The end points were 72 h after entry or two consecutive serum Na values of greater than 130 mMol/L. All of the patients had correction of their hyponatremia (Na greater than 130 mMol/L) within 72 h [66]. This study demonstrates that many neurosurgical patients develop hyponatremia in the setting of volume depletion and respond to fluid and Na replacement.

The loss of fluid and Na can also be treated with fludrocortisone. Fludrocortisone is a synthetic adrenocortical steroid with mineralocorticoid properties. Mineralocorticoids act on the distal tubules of the kidney to enhance Na reabsorption. In the neurosurgical literature, this medication has mostly been studied in SAH patients [67]. A randomized controlled trial in SAH patients showed that fludrocortisone reduced the frequency of a negative Na balance (63 % versus 38 %, $p = 0.041$). The treatment group did tend to have a higher plasma volume compared to controls, although this was not statistically significant. More patients in the control group developed cerebral ischemia (31 % versus 22 %, $p = 0.349$). Consequently, more control patients were treated with volume expanders which may have masked the volume expanding benefits of fludrocortisones [68]. Another randomized controlled trial in SAH patients showed that 0.1 mg of fludrocortisone three times a day reduced the mean Na and water intake, urinary Na excretion, and urine volume ($p<0.01$). The patients demonstrated a decrease in serum potassium that was easily corrected [69].

Similar studies have demonstrated a benefit from hydrocortisone in SAH patients. One study randomized 28 SAH patients to no hydrocortisone or 1,200 mg/day of hydrocortisone for 10 days [70]. All patients were treated with replacement of water and Na to prevent vasospasm. The treatment group never experienced a serum Na less than 135 mMol/L compared to 43 % of the control group that developed hyponatremia. The treatment group also had

lower urine volume and lower infusion volume to maintain CVP 8–12 cm H$_2$O. Both were statistically significant. Failure to maintain an adequate CVP was observed in 12 control patients (86 %) compared to three treatment patients (21 %) ($p<0.05$). A randomized controlled trial of hydrocortisone in 71 SAH patients failed to show a statistically significant difference in outcome between patients randomized to placebo versus those receiving 1,200 mg/day of hydrocortisone for 10 days after surgery. Nevertheless, hydrocortisone did prevent excess Na excretion and urine volume. It also maintained the targeted Na level throughout the 14 days [71]. A general protocol for the treatment of SIADH and CSW in acute hyponatremia is provided (Figs. 18.4 and 18.5).

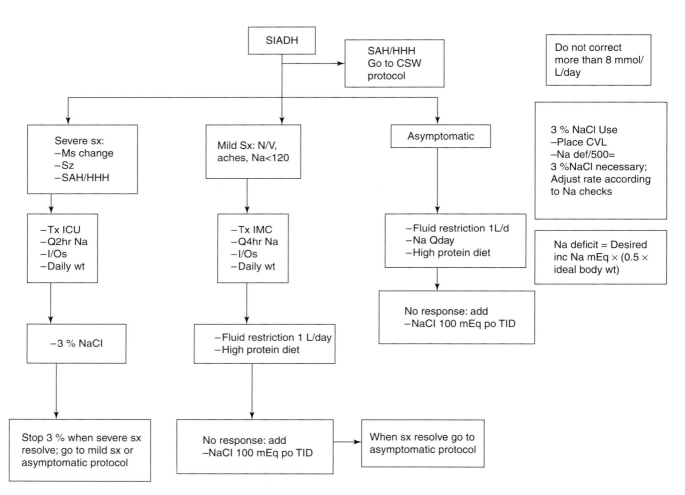

Fig. 18.4 Treatment of SIADH. Symptoms are used to guide the treatment of SIADH. Patients with severe symptoms or SAH at risk for vasospasm will receive hypertonic saline; otherwise the cornerstone of treatment for SIADH is fluid restriction. Acute hyponatremia and/or severe symptoms should have 6 mmol/L corrected over 6 h or until severe symptoms improve. The total correction of Na should not exceed 8 mmol/L over 24 h. Therefore, if 6 mmol/L is corrected in 6 h, the Na should not be increased more than 2 mmol/L in the following 18 h. The

total correction of Na is based on the Na deficit which is calculated conservatively with the formula depicted. With improvement of symptoms, the patients can be moved to the less aggressive treatments in the algorithm, until Na reaches 131 mmol/L. *MS* mental status, *sx* symptoms, *sz* seizure, *tx* transfer, *ICU* intensive care unit, *I/Os* in and out, *wt* weight, *N/V* nausea and vomiting, *IMC* intermediate care unit, *CVL* central venous line, *def* deficit, *inc* increase

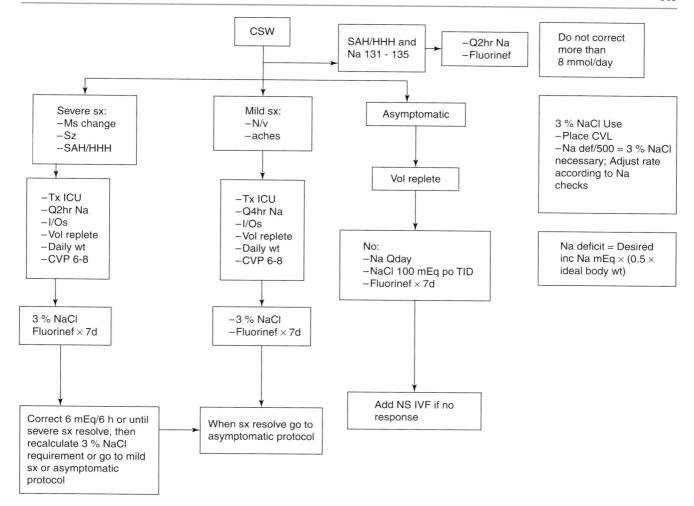

Fig. 18.5 Treatment of CSW. Once a diagnosis of CSW is confirmed, treatment is based on symptoms. Patients with severe symptoms should be treated in the ICU with hypertonic saline and fludrocortisone. Acute hyponatremia and/or severe symptoms should have 6 mmol/L corrected over 6 h or until severe symptoms improve. The total correction of Na should not exceed 8 mmol/L over 24 h. Therefore, if 6 mmol/L is corrected in 6 h, the Na should not be increased more than 2 mmol/L in the following 18 h. The total correction of Na is based on the Na deficit which is calculated conservatively with the formula depicted. With improvement of symptoms, the patients can be moved to the less aggressive treatments in the algorithm, until Na reaches 131 mmol/L. SAH patients are an exception and receive treatment even for a serum Na of 131–135 mmol/L. *HHH* hypervolemia, hypertension, hemodilution, *sx* symptoms, *MS* mental status, *sz* seizure, *Tx* transfer, *ICU* intensive care unit, *IMC* intermediate care unit, *hr* hour, *I/Os* in and out, *vol* volume, *wt* weight, *N/V* nausea and vomiting, *U* urine, *CVL* central venous line, *def* deficit, *inc* increase, *NS* normal saline, *IVF* intravenous fluids

Hypernatremia

Hypernatremia, defined as a rise in the serum sodium concentration above 145 mMol/L, is a common electrolyte disorder that almost always results from a deficit of water in relation to total body sodium stores [72]. The water deficit occurs as a consequence of net water loss or a hypertonic sodium gain. The presence of hypernatremia does not signify that there is an excess of sodium content in the body as sodium stores may be either normal (in cases of pure water loss) or decreased (in cases of hypotonic fluids losses such as vomiting or diarrhea) [72]. Hypertonic sodium gain usually results from clinical interventions or accidental sodium loading. Because sodium is a functionally impermeable solute and a major determinant of effective plasma osmolality, hypernatremia invariably denotes hypertonic hyperosmolality and always causes cellular dehydration, at least transiently.

Hypernatremia frequently develops in hospitalized patients as an iatrogenic condition, and some of its most serious complications result not from the disorder itself but from inappropriate treatment of it. In a multicenter cohort study of

8,441 patients with ICU-acquired hypernatremia, 11 % experienced mild to moderate hypernatremia (Na greater than 145 mMol/L), while 4 % had severe (Na greater than 150 mMol/L) hypernatremia, and hospital mortality was increased in both groups. While patients without hypernatremia had a mortality of 15.2 %, patients with mild to moderate hypernatremia had a mortality of 29.5 %, and patients with severe hypernatremia had a mortality of 46.2 % [73].

Since sustained severe hypernatremia can only occur when thirst mechanisms or access to water are impaired, patients with altered mental status, intubated patients, infants, and elderly persons are at the highest risk for hypernatremia. Critically ill patients in general and patients in neurocritical care units particularly frequently meet these conditions and are at the highest risk. Additionally, problems encountered with the patients' thirst mechanism including hypodipsia may be a part of neurological impairment. Furthermore, these patients may have excessive diaphoresis from agitation or fever, which can further exacerbate hypotonic fluid losses.

The effects of hypernatremia on brain tissue cause induction of a series of compensatory responses aimed at restoring brain volume. These involve the generation of osmotically active substances known as idiogenic osmoles or organic brain osmoles [74, 75]; this process is not immediate but occurs over hours to days [76]. Through the generation of idiogenic osmoles, the brain is capable of maintaining volume at hyperosmolar states. Rapid overcorrection of hypernatremia, greater than 12 mMol/dL/day, especially in the presence of chronic hyperosmolality, can render the brain incapable of eliminating the accumulated osmoles promptly enough, resulting in cerebral edema, generalized tonic–clonic seizures, coma, and death [77].

Assessment of the patient with hypernatremia should begin with evaluation of the extracellular fluid volume. Attention should be focused on recent changes in body weight, presence of peripheral edema, pulse rate, access to free water, hourly intake and output, intraoperative fluids, colloids or blood products given, orthostatic changes in blood pressure, and jugular venous distension. Initial assessment of hypernatremia should be evaluated with basic laboratory analysis, including serum sodium and osmolality, as well as urine sodium, osmolality, and specific gravity.

Low urine sodium concentration of less than 10 mMol/L, in addition to other clinical signs of hypervolemia, would suggest decreased extracellular fluid volume. The fractional excretion of sodium (Fe_{Na}) lower than 1 % is suggestive of volume depletion in non-edematous patients.

Hypernatremia with low extracellular fluid volume implies a loss of hypotonic fluids and usually implies that major route of water loss is extrarenal. Excessive diuresis, vomiting, and diarrhea are the usual suspects in those situations. Hypernatremia with normal extracellular fluid volume indicates a loss of free water. Diabetes insipidus should be excluded and the appropriateness of the tonicity of fluids for ongoing replacement reassessed [78]. Hypernatremia with high extracellular fluid volume results from a gain of hypertonic fluids. It is usually iatrogenic, secondary to the use of hypertonic NaCl and NaHCO$_3$ solutions or hypertonic feeding associated with osmotic diuresis, but it can also occur in cases of mineralocorticoid excess.

Clinical Manifestations of Hypernatremia

Hypernatremia usually becomes symptomatic only when the serum sodium concentration exceeds 160 mMol/L [79]. However, the rapidity of the elevation of serum sodium levels is equally important. With rapid elevation, stupor emerges more frequently. The signs and symptoms of hypernatremia mostly reflect central nervous system dysfunction caused by the reduction of intracellular fluid volume in the brain. These symptoms may remain undetected in patients with other, more obvious causes for the neurological symptoms, such as extensive and prolonged brain injuries. Decreased level of consciousness and confusion are the most common manifestations, with the level of consciousness correlating with the severity of the hypernatremia. Generalized tonic–clonic seizures can occur, but rapid progression to deep levels of coma is rare and should prompt additional tests for other possible causes [36]. Hypernatremia may initially present as intense thirst but may disappear with progression of the disorder. Absence of thirst in a patient with pronounced hypernatremia and preserved level of consciousness should raise suspicion for hypothalamic dysfunction. Finally, neuromuscular manifestations are uncommon, but rhabdomyolysis has been reported in a series of anecdotal cases [80].

Common Causes of Hypernatremia in the Neurointensive Care Unit

Hypernatremia in the neurointensive care unit is most commonly due to net free water loss, often related to a defective central release of vasopressin (VP) or antidiuretic hormone (ADH), or induced osmotic diuresis. Acute severe hypernatremia is most often iatrogenic produced by the administration of hypertonic saline solutions (e.g., 2, 3, or 23 % NaCl) given as a treatment for increased intracranial pressure, or as hypervolemic therapy in patients with subarachnoid hemorrhage diagnosed with symptomatic vasospasm, or sodium bicarbonate solutions for correction of lactic acidosis [81]. Less commonly, acute hypernatremia can be caused by nutritional formulas or repeated use of hypertonic saline enemas.

Hyperosmolal therapy is often utilized in the treatment of critically ill neurological and neurosurgical patients presenting with cerebral edema. Although to a lesser degree than hypertonic saline infusion, mannitol is expected to cause hypernatremia from free water loss. Serum osmolality must be monitored and should not exceed 320 mOsm/kg because the dehydrated state correlates with the risk of renal failure [82]. Tromethamine (THAM), an alkalinizing agent, can represent a useful therapeutic alternative to mannitol in patients with increased intracranial pressure and hypernatremia [83, 84].

Diabetes Insipidus

Diabetes insipidus (DI) is most commonly encountered among patients undergoing pituitary surgery or with craniopharyngiomas [85]. However, DI is theoretically a risk factor for patients with head injuries, primary or metastatic brain neoplasms, global anoxic brain damage, meningitis or encephalitis, massive cerebral edema, and diencephalic herniation syndromes [86]. It is almost obligatory for patients fulfilling brain death criteria.

DI is classically diagnosed in patients with an elevated sodium level (serum sodium greater than 145 mMol/L), an elevated urine output (greater than 30 mL/kg/day), and a low urine specific gravity (less than 1.003) [87]. DI in the neurointensive care unit is most often secondary to hypothalamic/pituitary dysfunction leading to ADH deficiency (central or hypothalamic diabetes insipidus). Clinically, significant free water loss and polyuria do not occur until more than three fourths of the ADH-producing neurons are destroyed. DI may also be encountered as a consequence of renal unresponsiveness to ADH. Nephrogenic DI occurs in critically ill patients most commonly secondary to acute kidney injury (e.g., iodinated contrast dye or the polyuric phase of tubular necrosis); however, it may be encountered in patients with preexisting conditions (lithium use, aminoglycosides, or amphotericin B) [88].

The clinical hallmarks of DI are polyuria and polydipsia especially in patients with intact thirst mechanisms; nocturia is normally present. DI in the neurointensive care unit frequently shows an abrupt onset. In patients with reduced level of consciousness, impaired access to water, or without intact thirst mechanisms, hypernatremia may ensue. In fact, patients with intact thirst mechanisms who have central or nephrogenic DI may be able to regulate their own osmolality through oral intake of free water. In addition to hypertonic encephalopathy and circulatory collapse, the "washout" effect induced by polyuria leads to hypomagnesemia, hypocalcemia, hypokalemia, and hypophosphatemia [89].

Unless the hypothalamic damage is severe and irreversible, the disruption of ADH secretion may be partial and temporary. This often is the case in patients following pituitary surgery or head trauma. In more than half of those cases, normal osmoregulation returns after 3–5 days. A study of 881 patients undergoing transsphenoidal microneurosurgery found that persistent DI was only present in 12.4 % of cases. In addition, independent risk factors included CSF leak (33.3 % transient, 4.4 % persistent), Rathke cleft cyst (38.7 %), Cushing's disease (22.2 %), and craniopharyngioma (62.1 %) [85]. In such patients, the return of normal hypothalamic function needs to be anticipated and monitored to avoid excessive treatment with fluids or overcorrection with free water leading to hyponatremia and central pontine myelinolysis.

Brain death is a common cause of DI in the neurointensive care unit. Occasionally, it may precede the diagnosis of brain death in patients with severe diencephalic herniation causing the compression of the pituitary stalk against the diaphragma sellae. In patients who are clinically "brain dead," the death of the neurosecretory neurons of the hypothalamus is rapidly followed by a sudden decrease in blood pressure often preceded by massive diuresis. In cases where organ donation may be considered, this situation calls for a very aggressive treatment with intravenous fluid replacement and intravenous vasopressin to avoid hypoperfusion to those organs [86, 90].

The Approach to the Hypernatremia Patient

When treating the hypernatremic patient, the first priority it is to assess the patient's volume status and to treat the hypovolemia [91, 92]. Volume replacement with crystalloids (0.9 % NaCl) normally suffices to maintain cardiac output and adequate perfusion pressures. However, severe cases may require the use of colloids such as hetastarch or 5 % albumin solutions.

Following stabilization of hemodynamic status, attention should be focused on correcting the patient's free water deficit. The calculation relies on the assumption that the total body water (TBW) and serum sodium concentration (sNa) are always constant. Hence,

$$Current\ TBW \times Current\ sNa = Normal\ TBW \times Normal\ sNa$$

Therefore, assuming that a normal sNa is 140 mMol/L, the current TBW may be calculated as follows:

$$Current\ TBW = Normal\ TBW \times (140 / Current\ sNa)$$

Normal TBW in liters usually accounts for 60 % of lean body weight in kilograms for men and 50 % in women. The proportion of TBW decreases with age, representing 50 % in elderly men and 45 % in elderly women [93]. The free water deficit can then be calculated through the difference between normal TBW and current TBW:

$$Free\ water\ deficit = Normal\ TBW - Current\ TBW$$

Thus, in an elderly man with a lean body weight of 68 kg and a sNa of 168 mMol/L deemed to be caused by free water depletion, the calculation of water deficit will proceed as follows:

$$\text{Normal TBW} = 0.5 \times 68 = 34 \text{ L}$$

$$\text{Current TBW} = 34 \times (140 / 168) = 28 \text{ L}$$

$$\text{Water deficit} = 34 - 28 = 6 \text{ L}$$

The actual volume of replacement fluid needed to correct the free water deficit will depend on the sodium concentration present in the replacement fluid chosen. Hypotonic solutions are preferred in these situations. The volume of the replacement fluid can be calculated using the following formula:

$$\text{Replacement fluid volume (Liters)} = \text{Free Water Deficit} \times (1 / 1 - X)$$

where X = replacement fluid Na divided by the isotonic fluid Na.

Thus, for our previous example, if we choose to replace the deficit with 0.45 % NaCl solution, the calculation would continue as follows:

$$\text{Replacement fluid volume (Liters)} = 6 \times (1 / 1 - 0.5) = 12 \text{ L}$$

When hypernatremia develops over a period of hours, rapid correction of water deficit is safe, because the accumulated electrolytes can be rapidly eliminated from brain cells [75]. A reduction of sNa by 1 mMol/h is appropriate for these patients.

However, the approach to correcting hypernatremia in patients with hypernatremia of longer or unknown duration must be exercised with caution. In these cases, it is prudent to assume that accumulated organic brai.n osmoles (idiogenic osmoles) have already occurred. This creates equilibrium between the osmolality of brain cells and the surrounding interstitial fluid. The process of eradication of these osmoles will take several days to be completed. Therefore, the rate of correction of hypernatremia in these patients needs to be slower to avoid the risk of cerebral edema. A maximal rate of 0.5 mMol/L/h or 10 mMol/L/day is usually recommended [75, 94].

Traditionally, half of the total volume is given over the first 24 h while carefully monitoring the decline in serum sodium level. However, an alternative formula that estimates the change in sNa caused by the retention of 1 L of any replacement fluid can be used to estimate the rate of infusion. This formula

$$\text{Change in serum Na} = \text{replacement fluid Na} - \text{sNa} / \text{TBW} + 1$$

does not focus on the calculation of free water deficit and should be used in place of the traditional formulas described previously.

The required volume of replacement fluid is then obtained by dividing the change in sNa targeted for a given treatment period (usually 10 mMol/L/day) by the result obtained from this formula. Once more, back to our previous example,

$$\text{Change in serum Na} = 77 - 168 / 34 + 1 = -2.6$$

This result means that the retention of 1 L of half normal (0.45 % NaCl) will reduce the sNa by 2.6 mMol/L. Thus, assuming to reduce the sNa by 10 mMol/L over 24 h, we would need to provide approximately 3.8 L (10/2.6) of the solution, hence nearly 160 mL of 0.45 % NaCl/h.

It is always necessary to compensate for ongoing fluid losses (obligatory or incidental, measureable, and insensible) while correcting the existing water deficit. Therefore, an average of 1.5 L/day will be required in addition to the volume given to correct the deficit. This amount may vary according to individual cases, and it may be much greater in patients with profuse continuous losses (e.g., diabetes insipidus, gastric suctioning, excessive sweating). Close monitoring of electrolyte concentrations (2–6 h) and fluid balance (hourly) is the best way to ensure safe and adequate correction of hypernatremia.

Obviously, the underlying cause for the hypernatremia needs to be addressed. Often, the hypernatremia cannot be fully corrected until its cause is identified and treated. Furthermore, mild cases of hypernatremia can be fully reversed by managing the underlying cause, such as stopping gastrointestinal fluid losses, controlling fever, avoiding glucosuria, and changing a nutritional formula. Management is particularly essential in the polyuric patient with possible diabetes insipidus.

Management of the Polyuric Patient (Fig. 18.6)

Polyuria is common in the neurointensive care unit, and free water loss through diabetes insipidus is a common cause of hypernatremia. At our institution, we have identified patients with a urine output greater than 200 mL/h as necessitating further workup for polyuria and possible diabetes insipidus [87]. Again, the initial workup of these patients includes evaluation of fluid balance, body weight, intraoperative and current fluids given, volume status, vital signs, and current mental status. Volume status is crucial in the assessment of the polyuric patient. Those patients who received several liters of fluid intraoperatively may be fluid overloaded, and postoperative diuresis may be appropriate.

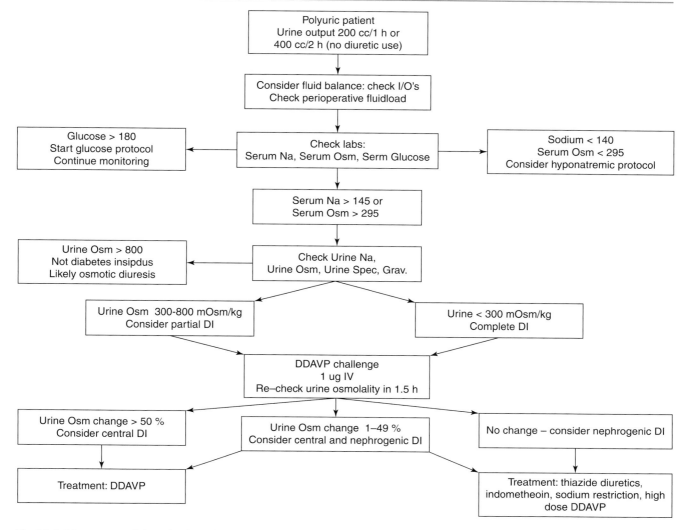

Fig. 18.6 Management of the polyuric patient

Following this initial evaluation, a simple set of labs are drawn, namely, serum sodium, urine sodium, serum osmolarity, urine osmolarity, and a STAT glucose [95]. A urine specific gravity may be drawn, in conjunction with the urine osmolarity. Some groups have found that this value, urine specific gravity, has better correlation with the urine concentration in response to DDAVP than does the urine osmolarity. However, it must be noted that the urine specific gravity may be falsely elevated when there are large concentrations of large molecules in the urine, namely, glucose, radiocontrast media, or the antibiotic carbenicillin. In these situations, the specific gravity should be correlated with the urine osmolarity. If the glucose is greater than 180 mg/dL, the diagnosis of DI cannot be established, as the polyuria may be related to elevated glucose, and an insulin protocol should be started promptly. Alternatively, if the urine osmolarity is greater than 800 mOsm/kg H_2O, the patient may be undergoing osmotic diuresis secondary to osmotic therapy (mannitol), and the diuresis may be appropriate for that patient. If the sodium is less than 140 mMol/L, the practitioner should consider evaluation and treatment with a hyponatremic protocol (discussed in the next section).

Those patients identified with urine osmolarity less than 800 mOsm/kg H_2O should be considered as possibly having diabetes insipidus. DI can be partial or complete, depending on the number of ADH-producing and ADH-releasing cells within the hypothalamic pituitary axis. Those patients with a urine osmolarity between 300 and 800 mOsm/kg H_2O should be considered as possibly having partial DI. Patients with urine osmolarity less than 300 mOsm/kg H_2O should be considered as having complete DI. Both sets of patients should prompt a standard desmopressin (DDAVP) challenge [96].

DDAVP has several preparations including intravenous, intramuscular, nasal, and oral. In the critically ill patient, the practitioner should use the intravenous form of DDAVP for the initial challenge to diagnose the type of DI (central of nephrogenic) as this has a bioavailability of 1. At this point, the practitioner must manage the intake and output expectantly, namely, hourly intake and output documentation with serum sodium and osmolarity checks every 2–4 h. This is will help to avoid over correction of hypernatremia.

Central and nephrogenic DI is diagnosed based on the kidney's response to DDAVP. If the response to DDAVP results in a urine osmolarity change greater than 50 %, the practitioner should consider central DI and treat with DDAVP alone and the patient may be treated with DDAVP. In patients with a urine osmolarity which does not change in response to DDAVP, nephrogenic DI should be considered with treatments including thiazide diuretics, indomethacin, sodium restriction, and high-dose DDAVP [97]. To those patients who have a urine osmolarity change between 1 and 49 %, central and nephrogenic DI must be considered with a treatment that includes both modalities.

As discussed previously, DI in the neurointensive care unit is a largely transient diagnosis. Patients undergoing pituitary surgery commonly have a transient period of DI secondary to traction on the pituitary or pituitary stalk during surgery. In addition, patients diagnosed with permanent DI may undergo a triple-phase response characterized by an initial phase of DI, followed by SIADH, and ultimately DI [98]. The pathology of the triple-phase response has been well documented in the literature and arises initially due to shock on ADH-releasing cells in the posterior pituitary leading to a lack of ADH. Those cells ultimately die, resulting in release of stored ADH causing SIADH and transient hyponatremia. Ultimately, when the posterior pituitary no longer has functional cells capable of releasing ADH, the body undergoes complete DI. The triple-phase response may take several days to complete. In each of these situations, the management of sodium and total body water must be monitored closely as to avoid rapid swings in osmolality. Those patients with underlying hypothalamic tumors such as craniopharyngiomas may have no functional ADH-releasing cells at the time of diagnosis and therefore may be managed expectantly for DI. A fundamental understanding of the underlying pathology is key to the management of free water in the neurointensive care unit.

Following the administration of the DDAVP challenge, it is important to monitor ongoing fluid losses. There may be a rapid correction in urinary output. As a result, if fluids are continued which account for urinary output, the patient may become hyponatremic from a hypernatremic state within hours. The half-life of the IV formulation of DDAVP is approximately 12 h; however, patients may have different responses to the IV formulation. Therefore, it is appropriate in the initial management of patients with DI to not schedule doses of DDAVP. Rather, DDAVP should be dosed initially on the urinary output of the patient. In patients undergoing evaluation for DI, some authors have suggested that specific gravity is the most sensitive indicator for trends in urine sodium output.

Patients considered at high risk for DI, namely, those patients undergoing pituitary or hypothalamic surgery, should be monitored, at least initially, in the neurointensive care unit. The most widely published protocol for the evaluation of patients undergoing pituitary surgery involves serum sodium and urine specific gravity evaluation every 4 hours, with serum glucose checks every 6 h and with intake and output monitored every 2–4 h [99].

As DI may be transient, initial dosing of DDAVP should be given such that the urinary output is less than 200 mL/h. In those patients in whom central DI has been established and is not transient, the patients may be transitioned from IV formulation DDAVP to alternative treatments. Common chronic treatment for DI includes nasal and oral formulations. The approximate equivalency for DDAVP is 1 mg IV, approximately 10 mg nasally, which approximates 100 mg orally; however, the dosage must be tailored to the individual patient.

Patients diagnosed with nephrogenic DI may also have transient elevated urinary output, especially in the acute tubular necrosis phase should their DI be secondary to acute kidney injury. Treatment for nephrogenic DI includes thiazide diuretics, indomethacin, sodium restriction, and high-dose DDAVP. Thiazide diuretics act on the distal convoluted tubule and inhibit the sodium chloride cotransporter. This leads to an elevated concentration of sodium in the distal convoluted tubule and collecting duct. The proposed mechanism reaction includes an extracellular volume contraction secondary to the excretion of sodium caused by the thiazide diuretic. As a result, the glomerular filtration rate decreases in the proximal convoluted tubule and sodium and water absorption are increased. The decreased glomerular filtration rate causes less water and sodium to be delivered to the collecting tubules and, thus, less water is excreted [100]. Indomethacin is commonly used in nephrogenic DI due to its inhibition of prostaglandins. Prostaglandins inhibit the hydro-osmotic effect of antidiuretic hormone in the collecting duct. Therefore, by blocking the action of prostaglandins in the renal medullary collecting duct, indomethacin can enhance the action of DDAVP [97]. In addition, nonsteroidal anti-inflammatory drugs cause an unopposed constriction of the afferent arteriole in the kidney, decreasing renal perfusion and urine output.

Disorders of Potassium Homeostasis

As sodium is the predominant extracellular cation, potassium is the major intracellular cation and a sodium–potassium exchange pump conserves potassium while extruding sodium. Only 2 % of the total pool of body potassium is present in the extracellular compartment and approximately 0.4 % in plasma. Thus, serum potassium concentrations are poor indicators of the status of total body potassium stores.

This marked difference in potassium content between the intracellular and extracellular compartments has an important practical implication. The abundant pool of intracellular potassium is very effective in replenishing extracellular stores when potassium is lost. Therefore, potassium depletion must be twice as great as potassium accumulation to produce degree of change in serum potassium concentration [58, 101].

Nearly 90 % of the potassium ingested is absorbed by the small intestine and this absorption is fairly constant. Increased dietary loads are rapidly accommodated inside the cells; increased transcellular movement of potassium prevents dangerous swings in serum potassium concentration. Renal excretion is tightly regulated through the mechanisms of tubular reabsorption (proximal tubules) and secretion (distal tubules), but changes in urine potassium concentration in response to different dietary loads occur more slowly.

Factors Affecting Internal Potassium Balance (Transcellular Shift)

1. *Acid–base changes*: Acidosis (in particular that induced by inorganic acids) promotes potassium exit from the cells, while alkalosis or even increased serum bicarbonate concentration in the absence of alkalemia stimulates potassium movement into the cells. These effects are explained by changes in the electrical gradient.
2. *Insulin*: It stimulates cellular uptake of potassium by enhancing Na-K ATPase activity.
3. *Catecholamines*: Beta$_2$-adrenergic agonists increase potassium uptake by peripheral muscle, and beta$_1$-adrenergic agonists have the same effect in the heart. These actions would also be mediated by modulation of the Na-K ATPase pump. Conversely, alpha-adrenergic agonists can promote cellular potassium loss.
4. *Tonicity*: Serum hypertonicity and cellular dehydration favor movement of potassium out of cells by exacerbating the chemical gradient.

Factors Affecting External Potassium Balance (Renal Excretion)

1. *Distal tubular flow rate and sodium delivery:* Potassium is secreted into the distal tubular lumen in exchange for sodium. Increased tubular flow rate (secondary to increased glomerular filtration rate) and distal sodium delivery favor potassium secretion and subsequent urinary excretion.

2. *Mineralocorticoids:* Aldosterone stimulates potassium secretion in the distal nephron. In turn, serum potassium levels regulate adrenal secretion of aldosterone (hyperkalemia stimulates and hypokalemia suppresses aldosterone secretion). The effect of aldosterone on tubular potassium excretion can be estimated by calculating the *transtubular potassium gradient*:

$$\text{Transtubular } K^+ \text{gradient} = \left[U\left(K^+\right) / \left(U_{osm} / P_{osm}\right) \right] \div P\left(K^+\right)$$

where $U(K^+)$ is the urinary concentration of potassium (U_{osm}/P_{osm}), is the ratio between urine and plasma osmolalities, and $P(K^+)$ is the serum potassium concentration. This index is useful in cases of hypokalemia to document if potassium is being inappropriately lost in the urine. A result greater than five indicates an aldosterone effect, while a result of less than three indicates lack of effect.

3. *Antidiuretic hormone:* ADH also stimulates potassium secretion independently of other factors. Thus, ADH compensates for the effects of changes in distal tubular flow on potassium secretion (e.g., water ingestion would induce potassium loss in the urine by increasing distal tubular flow if it did not concomitantly inhibit the secretion of AHD).

4. *Acid–base effects:* Acute systemic acidosis increases hydrogen ion concentrations and decreases potassium concentration inside renal epithelial cells. These effects lead to a decline in potassium secretion. Opposite changes occur with acute systemic alkalosis. These effects are mitigated or reversed in chronic acid–base disorders. In addition, potassium depletion stimulates renal acid excretion and renal ammoniagenesis; in turn, these changes have a sparing effect on the bicarbonate pool.

5. *Dietary potassium*: Renal adaptation to changes in dietary potassium intake can be profound (urinary potassium concentration can range from 20 to 150 mmol/L), but full expression of this response only occurs after days.

Hyperkalemia

Hyperkalemia is not particularly common in the NeuroICU, but it deserves attention because, when severe, it can be life-threatening [102]. Hyperkalemia is usually defined as a serum potassium concentration exceeding 5.5 mMol/L. However, serious complications are typically not observed until levels are greater than 7.0 mMol/L. In addition, spurious elevations of serum potassium concentrations (pseudohyperkalemia) are quite common, and the unexpected finding of hyperkalemia in an asymptomatic patient should always prompt a repeat confirmatory measurement before any

Table 18.2 Common causes of hyperkalemia in the NeuroICU

Pseudohyperkalemia
Renal insufficiency
Hypoadrenalism
Diabetes ketoacidosis
Drugs
ACE inhibitors
Beta blockers
Digoxin
Heparin
Nonsteroidal anti-inflammatory drugs
Potassium-sparing diuretics
Antibiotics (such as trimethoprim–sulfamethoxazole, potassium penicillin)
THAM
Succinylcholine
In trauma patients
Rhabdomyolysis
Rewarming after (induced) hypothermia
Massive blood transfusions

Reproduced with permission from Rabinstein and Wijdicks [119]
ACE angiotensin-converting enzyme, *THAM* tromethamine

therapeutic measures are taken. Pseudohyperkalemia can occur secondary to hemolysis during venipuncture and in patients with severe thrombocytosis or leukocytosis.

Causes of true hyperkalemia in the ICU are listed in Table 18.2. Cases of hyperkalemia in the NeuroICU usually share the same causes with those in any other ICU. However, trauma patients are particularly at risk due to myonecrosis and higher incidence of prerenal insufficiency and blood transfusions. In addition, when hypothermia is induced in patients with head trauma and increased intracranial pressure, hyperkalemia can occur during the rewarming phase and exacerbate the risk of cardiac arrhythmia. Several drugs have been associated with the development of hyperkalemia, but more pertinent to the NeuroICU are THAM (alkalinizing agent used for control of raised intracranial pressure) and succinylcholine, the latter being especially dangerous in patients with spinal cord injuries and prolonged immobilization.

Clinical Manifestations of Hyperkalemia

The most dangerous consequences of hyperkalemia are cardiac conduction abnormalities due to changes in the electrical excitability of cellular membranes. Initial "peaking" of the T waves (tall, tented T waves best seen in precordial leads) is followed by diminished amplitude of P waves and progressive widening of the PR interval and QRS complexes. Eventually, ventricular fibrillation and asystole ensue [103].

Neurological manifestations may include proximal limb weakness and burning dysesthesias. Progression to generalized paralysis with respiratory compromise has been reported but is rare [104, 105]. Patients may exhibit myotonia that can be elicited by muscle percussion. Weakness should recover within hours of reversal of the hyperkalemia; failure to recover shortly after treatment should suggest other causes are responsible for the weakness.

Management of Hyperkalemia

Acute management of hyperkalemia should be focused on avoiding life-threatening cardiac arrhythmias. The effect of the therapeutic maneuvers can be monitored using the electrocardiogram. In cases of severe hyperkalemia, calcium carbonate should be administered immediately (calcium carbonate 10 %, 10 mL over 3 min; can repeat once after 5 min if needed) to antagonize the actions of potassium on the cellular membrane. The response to calcium will last for approximately 20–30 min and will allow time for the administration of other therapies aimed at enhancing potassium clearance. A combination of insulin and dextrose can be administered to promote a shift of potassium into cells (10 units of regular insulin added to 500 mL of 10 % dextrose infused over 10 min). Bicarbonate infusion can also stimulate this transcellular shift, but its use is not advisable because it can bind calcium, rendering it ineffective. Removal of potassium from the organism can be achieved by using cation-exchange resins such as polystyrene sulfonate (Kayexalate, 50–100 g mixed with 200 mL 20 % dextrose and water in a retention enema) that increase gastrointestinal clearance of potassium, or furosemide (20–80 mg) to increase its urinary excretion. Hemodialysis may be indispensable in patients with renal failure [103].

Hypokalemia

Hypokalemia is defined as a serum potassium concentration below 3.5 mMol/L. Although most commonly mild and well tolerated, it may represent considerable danger in patients with underlying heart disease as it can trigger cardiac arrhythmias, or advanced liver failure as it can precipitate hepatic coma [106]. Hypokalemia generally occurs as a result of insufficient intake, excessive gastrointestinal or renal losses, or increased cellular sequestration. In many ICU patients, hypokalemia is multifactorial in origin.

For the most part, the causes of hypokalemia in the NeuroICU also resemble those in other intensive care settings (Table 18.3). However, certain elements specific to neurological and neurosurgical patients can contribute to the decline in serum potassium concentration. Potassium depletion can result from the use of osmotic diuretics in patients with raised intracranial pressure or high doses of corticosteroids in acute spinal cord injury. It can also occur in cases of diabetes insipidus, severe trauma (due to the catabolic state and high levels of catecholamines), and hypovolemia (which leads to increased secretion of aldosterone). Finally, induced

Table 18.3 Common causes of hypokalemia in the NeuroICU

Decreased potassium intake
Potassium shift into cells
Alkalosis
Beta-adrenergic agonists
Insulin
(Induced) hypothermia
Total parenteral nutrition
Increased potassium losses (potassium depletion)
Vomiting or nasogastric suctioning
Diarrhea
Excessive sweating
Potassium-wasting diuretics (loop diuretics, thiazides)
Hypomagnesemia
Other drugs (amphotericin B, penicillin derivatives)

Reproduced with permission from Rabinstein and Wijdicks [119]

hypothermia can produce hypokalemia by promoting the transcellular shift of potassium into the cells (the caveat is that severe hypothermia typically produces hyperkalemia secondary to massive cell death).

Clinical Manifestations of Hypokalemia

Severe hypokalemia (serum potassium concentration below 2.5 mMol/L) can be complicated with diffuse muscle weakness and mental status changes. Cardiac arrhythmias (especially in patients with preexisting heart disease, or concomitant hypomagnesemia, and those taking digoxin) and paralytic ileus are also possible. It can precipitate coma in patients with advanced liver cirrhosis and lower the threshold for multifocal atrial tachycardia in patients with obstructive lung disease. Electrocardiographic abnormalities include prominent U waves, flattening and inversion of T waves, and prolongation of the QT interval. Ventricular arrhythmias constitute the ultimate danger [107].

The muscle weakness induced by hypokalemia can be profound and, in the extreme form, can result in flaccid quadriplegia and neuromuscular respiratory failure. Cramps, myalgias, and occasional myoclonus can accompany the weakness. In addition, patients with severe hypokalemia frequently have some degree of rhabdomyolysis; although usually mild, hypokalemic rhabdomyolysis can be severe and result in acute renal failure [108, 109].

Management of Hypokalemia

Treatment of hypokalemia consists of providing adequate potassium supplementation to replenish body stores and eliminating or treating all potential causes of increased transcellular shift (such as alkalosis) or excessive loss (such as diuretics). The standard method of intravenous potassium replacement is adding 20 mMol of potassium chloride (KCl) to 100 mL of isotonic saline and infusing this mixed solution over 1 h [110]. When rapid administration of higher concentrations of potassium is necessary, it is safer to use a central venous access or two peripheral lines because of the irritating properties of the hyperosmotic potassium solutions. Dose rates as high as 80 mMol/h have been used safely in cases of severe hypokalemia [106].

Since the redistribution of potassium is difficult to predict in critically ill patients, monitoring the response to treatment by serially measuring serum potassium concentrations becomes essential. Ongoing potassium losses must be considered when calculating daily replacement rates. Measuring serum magnesium level is always recommended in patients with refractory hypokalemia since hypomagnesemia promotes excessive urinary potassium losses.

Disorders of Calcium, Phosphorus, and Magnesium Homeostasis

Calcium

Calcium is a predominantly extracellular cation that is primarily stored in bones. Calcium circulating levels are tightly regulated by parathyroid hormone (PTH) and vitamin D. PTH is primarily responsible for mediating the responses to acute changes in serum calcium concentration; its secretion is stimulated by ionized hypocalcemia – calcium is heavily protein bound in the circulation and only the free fraction is physiologically active – and leads to release of calcium from bone, absorption from the gastrointestinal tract (through vitamin D), and reabsorption by the renal tubules. Conversely, PTH secretion is inhibited by ionized hypercalcemia and elevated 1,25-dihydroxyvitamin D levels. Meanwhile, vitamin D is synthesized in the skin (requires ultraviolet light exposure) or absorbed from the diet, and it then undergoes two steps of hydroxylation in the liver (25-hydroxylase) and the kidney (1-hydroxylase, stimulated by PTH, hypophosphatemia, acidemia, and calcitonin) to reach its active form as 1,25-dihydroxyvitamin D. Vitamin D increases renal calcium reabsorption and intestinal tract absorption. Calcitonin, another calciotropic hormone, also plays a role in maintaining calcium homeostasis by inhibiting bone resorption and increasing calcium urinary excretion.

Phosphorus

Phosphorus is predominantly an intracellular anion; thus, serum levels are poor indicators of total body stores (most phosphorus is deposited in bone). Circulating phosphorus binds to protein less avidly than calcium or magnesium. Its homeostasis is primarily maintained by regulation in the kidney, where urinary phosphorus excretion is increased in the presence of PTH and calcitonin and decreased by the actions of vitamin D. In addition, PTH induces phosphorus release from bone, while calcitonin secretion has the opposite effect. Intestinal absorption of phosphorus is enhanced by vitamin D.

Magnesium

Magnesium is the second most abundant intracellular cation in the organism after potassium. More than half of the total body stores is located in bone, whereas less than 1 % is present in plasma. Hence, there is poor correlation between serum magnesium levels and total body magnesium pool. Magnesium depletion is usually prominent when a patient presents with hypomagnesemia. Only 55 % of the total serum magnesium concentration circulates in the ionized (physiologically active) form, while the rest is either protein bound or chelated (by phosphate or sulfate in general). Techniques to measure the free fraction are not routinely available for clinical use [111].

Hypercalcemia

Ionized hypercalcemia is defined as ionized serum calcium concentration exceeding 1.3 mMol/L (or 5.1 mg/dL). Common causes include malignancies, hyperparathyroidism, renal failure, prolonged immobilization, granulomatous diseases, phosphorus depletion, and drugs (calcium itself, lithium, thiazides, vitamin D) (Table 18.4). Severe hypercalcemia is very rarely encountered in the NeuroICU. The clinical manifestations of hypercalcemia involve the gastrointestinal (nausea, vomiting, peptic ulcers, ileus, and pancreatitis in the most severe cases), cardiovascular (hypercalcemia increases vascular resistance, but blood pressure may be low secondary to volume depletion, increased resistance to catecholamines, lower threshold for digitalis toxicity, QT interval shortening, and occasional arrhythmias) [112], renal (polyuria, nephrolithiasis, nephrocalcinosis), and neurologic. Typical neuropsychiatric features include confusion, lethargy, depression, and memory impairment. Neuromuscular manifestations such as weakness, hypotonia, and hyporeflexia may also be present. The most severe cases can lead to psychosis, obtundation, and even coma [113]. Management should begin with the use of saline solution for volume repletion and then concentrate on correcting the hypercalcemia per se. Reduction of serum calcium concentration can be achieved using furosemide, calcitonin, steroids, pamidronate, plicamycin, or, in patients with renal failure, hemodialysis. Mobilization of the patient and correction of concomitant electrolyte abnormalities are also important.

Table 18.4 Common causes calcium imbalance of in the NeuroICU

| *Hypercalcemia* |
| Renal failure |
| Prolonged immobilization |
| Disseminated malignancy |
| Phosphorus depletion |
| Drugs (especially calcium supplements) |
| *Hypocalcemia* |
| Sepsis |
| Rhabdomyolysis |
| Renal insufficiency |
| Neck surgery (transient or permanent hypoparathyroidism) |
| Hypomagnesemia |
| Alkalosis |
| Drugs (phenytoin, phenobarbital, cimetidine, aminoglycosides) |

Reproduced with permission from Rabinstein and Wijdicks [119]

Hypocalcemia

Ionized hypocalcemia is defined as ionized serum calcium concentration below 1.1 mMol/L (or 4.5 mg/dL). It is often encountered in critically ill patients [114] but not especially frequent in the NeuroICU. Common causes include renal dysfunction, sepsis, rhabdomyolysis, hypoparathyroidism (always a risk after neck surgery), blood transfusions, hypomagnesemia, fat embolism, alkalosis, and drugs such as phenytoin, phenobarbital, cimetidine, theophylline, and aminoglycosides (Table 18.4). Clinical manifestations are mainly related to enhanced cardiac and neuromuscular excitability and depressed myocardial contractility. Thus, patients with hypercalcemia may present with hypotension, decreased cardiac output, bradycardia, QT and ST prolongation, and, in advanced stages, ventricular arrhythmias and cardiac arrest [114, 115]. Neuromuscular manifestations include tetany, paresthesias, weakness, and seizures. Patients are often confused and irritable and occasionally they may be frankly psychotic [116]. Laryngeal spasm is a rare but dreadful complication. Management of symptomatic hypocalcemia consists of appropriate intravenous calcium replacement therapy (calcium chloride 10 % contains three times more elemental calcium than calcium gluconate 10 %), correction of coexistent electrolyte imbalances, and treatment of the underlying cause [114].

Hyperphosphatemia

Hyperphosphatemia is defined as serum phosphorus concentration exceeding 1.45 mMol/L (4.5 mg/dL). Most cases are the result of renal insufficiency or widespread cell necrosis, as seen in sepsis, rhabdomyolysis, multiple trauma, fulminant hepatitis, tumor lysis, and other conditions (Table 18.5). When symptoms are present, they are usually related to the

Table 18.5 Common causes phosphorus imbalance of in the NeuroICU

Hyperphosphatemia

Renal insufficiency

Sepsis

Rhabdomyolysis

Multiple trauma with widespread cell necrosis

Hypophosphatemia

Head trauma (especially after fluid resuscitation)

Sepsis

Nasogastric suctioning

Sucralfate

Hypercalcemia

Hypomagnesemia

Refeeding syndrome

Chronic alcoholism

Drugs (diuretics, steroids, beta-adrenergic agonists)

Reproduced with permission from Rabinstein and Wijdicks [119]

Table 18.6 Common causes magnesium imbalance of in the NeuroICU

Hypermagnesemia

Renal failure

Excessive magnesium intake (supplements, parenteral nutrition)

Adrenal insufficiency

Hypomagnesemia

Head trauma (especially after fluid resuscitation)

Nasogastric suctioning

Chronic alcoholism

Refeeding syndrome

Hypercalcemia

Hypophosphatemia

Drugs (diuretics, aminoglycosides, amphotericin B)

Reproduced with permission from Rabinstein and Wijdicks [119]

associated hypocalcemia. Deposits of ectopic calcification can result from the formation of insoluble calcium–phosphorus complexes. Treatment is based on eliminating the underlying cause and promoting phosphorus clearance by using saline plus furosemide or hemodialysis. In addition, aluminum oxide and calcium acetate or carbonate can bind phosphorus in the lumen of the gastrointestinal tract and prevent its absorption.

Hypophosphatemia

Hypophosphatemia is defined as a serum phosphorus concentration below 0.8 mMol/L (or 2.5 mg/dL). It may be caused by nasogastric suctioning, use of phosphorus-binding antiacids (aluminum salts, sucralfate), renal tubular defects, hypercalcemia (especially if due to hyperparathyroidism), hypomagnesemia, carbohydrate loading, refeeding syndrome, sepsis, chronic alcoholism, and drugs such as diuretics, insulin, salicylates, beta-adrenergic agonists, or steroids (Table 18.5). Although clinically silent when mild to moderate, severe hypophosphatemia can impair cellular energy production and produce cardiac failure, hemolytic anemia (by reducing deformability of erythrocytes), tissue hypoxia (by depletion of 2,3-diphosphoglycerate), and extreme muscle weakness that may result in respiratory insufficiency [117] as well as weaning failure in ventilated patients. Other neurological symptoms may include ataxia, tremor, confusion, irritability, and seizures. Appropriate management of hypophosphatemia requires treating the underlying cause, correcting other electrolyte derangements, and replacing phosphorus sufficiently. When administering phosphorus intravenously (usually as potassium phosphate), it is necessary to be cautious because it may induce hypocalcemia and calcium phosphate precipitation in the blood [114].

Hypermagnesemia

Hypermagnesemia is defined as a serum magnesium concentration exceeding 1.1 mMol/L (or 2.0 mEq/L or 2.4 mg/dL). Frequent causes are renal failure, excessive magnesium intake (antacids, parenteral nutrition, supplements), and adrenal insufficiency (Table 18.6). It is usually well tolerated, but extreme levels of hypermagnesemia can impair neuromuscular transmission leading to areflexic paralysis and respiratory failure. It can also produce vasodilatation, hypotension, heart block, and even cardiac arrest. Acute treatment must focus in antagonizing the neuromuscular and cardiac effects by administering intravenous calcium (1 g of calcium chloride 10 % over 5–10 min). Reduction of magnesium levels can be accomplished by infusing saline and furosemide to increase urinary excretion or prescribing phosphate-containing chelators to prevent intestinal absorption.

Hypomagnesemia

Hypomagnesemia is defined as serum magnesium concentration below 0.65 mMol/L (or 1.3 mEq/L or 1.7 mg/dL). It is a very prevalent derangement in any ICU and it frequently complicates other electrolyte imbalances, particularly hypokalemia and hypophosphatemia. Often undiagnosed, magnesium depletion can exist even in the absence of hypomagnesemia. It is usually due to exaggerated gastrointestinal or renal losses. Among its multiple causes, some of the more common are nasogastric suction, malnutrition, diarrhea, hyperalimentation, refeeding syndrome, various renal disorders, hypercalcemia, hypophosphatemia, diabetic ketoacidosis, excessive sweating, and drugs such as diuretics, laxatives, aminoglycosides, amphotericin B, ethanol, digoxin, and calcium supplementation (Table 18.6). Hypomagnesemia, as well as hypokalemia and hypophosphatemia, are very often present at admission in patients with head trauma [118]. The most conspicuous clinical presentations are related to cardiac abnormalities, typically torsades de pointes and QT prolongation, but it also can produce coronary artery spasm and exacerbate digitalis toxicity and neurological dysfunction including altered cognition, apathy, delirium, seizures, tremors, ataxia, nystagmus, hyperreflexia, muscle weakness, spasms, paresthesias, and, rarely, tetany. As previously mentioned, hypomagnesemia can have metabolic effects leading to hypokalemia, hypocalcemia, and hypophosphatemia. Intravenous magnesium sulfate should be administered immediately in severely symptomatic patients (2 g over 2 min followed by 10 g in 500 mL of isotonic saline over the next 12 h). It is essential to correct all associated electrolyte disorders and eliminate all potential causes while ensuring adequate replacement.

Acknowledgments Dr. Alejandro A. Rabinstein and Dr. Eelco F. M. Wijdicks authored this chapter in the first edition of this work. We thank them for allowing us to incorporate material from that first edition chapter into this new second edition chapter.

References

1. Bourque CW. Central mechanisms of osmosensation and systemic osmoregulation. Nat Rev Neurosci. 2008;9(7):519–31.
2. Robertson GL, Shelton RL, Athar S. The osmoregulation of vasopressin. Kidney Int. 1976;10(1):25–37.
3. Claybaugh JR, Sato AK, Crosswhite LK, Hassell LH. Effects of time of day, gender, and menstrual cycle phase on the human response to a water load. Am J Physiol Regul Integr Comp Physiol. 2000;279(3):R966–73.
4. Kuramochi G, Kobayashi I. Regulation of the urine concentration mechanism by the oropharyngeal afferent pathway in man. Am J Nephrol. 2000;20(1):42–7.
5. Andersen LJ, Jensen TU, Bestle MH, Bie P. Gastrointestinal osmoreceptors and renal sodium excretion in humans. Am J Physiol Regul Integr Comp Physiol. 2000;278(2):R287–94.
6. Choi-Kwon S, Baertschi AJ. Splanchnic osmosensation and vasopressin: mechanisms and neural pathways. Am J Physiol. 1991;261(1 Pt 1):E18–25.
7. Adachi A. Thermosensitive and osmoreceptive afferent fibers in the hepatic branch of the vagus nerve. J Auton Nerv Syst. 1984;10(3–4):269–73.
8. McKinley MJ. The sensory circumventricular organs of the mammalian brain : subfornical organ, OVLT and area postrema. New York: Springer; 2003.
9. Thrasher TN, Brown CJ, Keil LC, Ramsay DJ. Thirst and vasopressin release in the dog: an osmoreceptor or sodium receptor mechanism? Am J Physiol. 1980;238(5):R333–9.
10. Oliet SH, Bourque CW. Properties of supraoptic magnocellular neurones isolated from the adult rat. J Physiol. 1992;455:291–306.
11. Oliet SH, Bourque CW. Mechanosensitive channels transduce osmosensitivity in supraoptic neurons. Nature. 1993;364(6435):341–3.
12. Ciura S, Bourque CW. Transient receptor potential vanilloid 1 is required for intrinsic osmoreception in organum vasculosum lamina terminalis neurons and for normal thirst responses to systemic hyperosmolality. J Neurosci. 2006;26(35):9069–75.
13. Morita H, Ogino T, Fujiki N, et al. Sequence of forebrain activation induced by intraventricular injection of hypertonic NaCl detected by Mn2+ contrasted T1-weighted MRI. Auton Neurosci. 2004;113(1–2):43–54.
14. Colbert HA, Smith TL, Bargmann CI. OSM-9, a novel protein with structural similarity to channels, is required for olfaction, mechanosensation, and olfactory adaptation in Caenorhabditis elegans. J Neurosci. 1997;17(21):8259–69.
15. Bourque CW. Osmoregulation of vasopressin neurons: a synergy of intrinsic and synaptic processes. Prog Brain Res. 1998;119:59–76.
16. Knepper MA. Molecular physiology of urinary concentrating mechanism: regulation of aquaporin water channels by vasopressin. Am J Physiol. 1997;272(1 Pt 2):F3–12.
17. Verbalis JG. Disorders of body water homeostasis. Best Pract Res Clin Endocrinol Metab. 2003;17(4):471–503.
18. Rose BD, Post TW. Clinical physiology of acid base and electrolyte disorders. 6th ed. New York: McGraw-Hill; 2006.
19. Weidmann P, Hasler L, Gnadinger MP, et al. Blood levels and renal effects of atrial natriuretic peptide in normal man. J Clin Invest. 1986;77(3):734–42.
20. Boscoe A, Paramore C, Verbalis JG. Cost of illness of hyponatremia in the United States. Cost Eff Resour Alloc. 2006;4:10.
21. Anderson RJ, Chung HM, Kluge R, Schrier RW. Hyponatremia: a prospective analysis of its epidemiology and the pathogenetic role of vasopressin. Ann Intern Med. 1985;102(2):164–8.
22. Bennani SL, Abouqal R, Zeggwagh AA, et al. Incidence, causes and prognostic factors of hyponatremia in intensive care. Rev Med Interne. 2003;24(4):224–9.
23. Nzerue CM, Baffoe-Bonnie H, You W, Falana B, Dai S. Predictors of outcome in hospitalized patients with severe hyponatremia. J Natl Med Assoc. 2003;95(5):335–43.
24. Peruzzi WTM, Shapiro BAMF, Meyer PRJMM, Krumlovsky FM, Seo B-WB. Hyponatremia in acute spinal cord injury. [Article]. Crit Care Med. 1994;22(2):252–8.
25. Sherlock M, O'Sullivan E, Agha A, et al. The incidence and pathophysiology of hyponatraemia after subarachnoid haemorrhage. Clin Endocrinol (Oxf). 2006;64(3):250–4.
26. Sata A, Hizuka N, Kawamata T, Hori T, Takano K. Hyponatremia after transsphenoidal surgery for hypothalamo-pituitary tumors. Neuroendocrinology. 2006;83(2):117–22.
27. Diringer MN, Zazulia AR. Hyponatremia in neurologic patients: consequences and approaches to treatment. Neurologist. 2006;12(3):117–26.
28. Adrogue HJ. Consequences of inadequate management of hyponatremia. Am J Nephrol. 2005;25(3):240–9.
29. Janicic N, Verbalis JG. Evaluation and management of hypo-osmolality in hospitalized patients. Endocrinol Metab Clin North Am. 2003;32(2):459–81, vii.
30. Beukhof CM, Hoorn EJ, Lindemans J, Zietse R. Novel risk factors for hospital-acquired hyponatraemia: a matched case–control study. [Article]. Clin Endocrinol. 2007;66(3):367–72.
31. Gill G, Huda B, Boyd A, et al. Characteristics and mortality of severe hyponatraemia – a hospital-based study. [Article]. Clin Endocrinol. 2006;65(2):246–9.
32. Tierney WM, Martin DK, Greenlee MC, Zerbe RL, McDonald CJ. The prognosis of hyponatremia at hospital admission. J Gen Intern Med. 1986;1(6):380–5.
33. Rossi J, Bayram M, Udelson JE, et al. Improvement in hyponatremia during hospitalization for worsening heart failure is associated with improved outcomes: insights from the Acute and Chronic Therapeutic Impact of a Vasopressin Antagonist in Chronic Heart Failure (ACTIV in CHF) trial. Acute Card Care. 2007;9(2):82–6.
34. Fraser CL, Arieff AI. Epidemiology, pathophysiology, and management of hyponatremic encephalopathy. Am J Med. 1997;102(1):67–77.

35. Renneboog B, Musch W, Vandemergel X, Manto MU, Decaux G. Mild chronic hyponatremia is associated with falls, unsteadiness, and attention deficits. Am J Med. 2006;119(1):71 e1–8.

36. Arieff AI, Llach F, Massry SG. Neurological manifestations and morbidity of hyponatremia: correlation with brain water and electrolytes. Medicine (Baltimore). 1976;55(2):121–9.

37. Kurokawa Y, Uede T, Ishiguro M, et al. Pathogenesis of hyponatremia following subarachnoid hemorrhage due to ruptured cerebral aneurysm. Surg Neurol. 1996;46(5):500–7; discussion 507–8.

38. Wijdicks EF, Vermeulen M, Hijdra A, van Gijn J. Hyponatremia and cerebral infarction in patients with ruptured intracranial aneurysms: is fluid restriction harmful? Ann Neurol. 1985;17(2):137–40.

39. Hasan D, Wijdicks EF, Vermeulen M. Hyponatremia is associated with cerebral ischemia in patients with aneurysmal subarachnoid hemorrhage. Ann Neurol. 1990;27(1):106–8.

40. Qureshi AI, Suri MF, Sung GY, et al. Prognostic significance of hypernatremia and hyponatremia among patients with aneurysmal subarachnoid hemorrhage. Neurosurgery. 2002;50(4):749–55; discussion 755–6.

41. Palmer BF. Hyponatremia in patients with central nervous system disease: SIADH versus CSW. Trends Endocrinol Metab. 2003;14(4):182–7.

42. Maesaka JK, Gupta S, Fishbane S. Cerebral salt-wasting syndrome: does it exist? Nephron. 1999;82(2):100–9.

43. Vingerhoets F, de Tribolet N. Hyponatremia hypo-osmolarity in neurosurgical patients. "Appropriate secretion of ADH" and "cerebral salt wasting syndrome". Acta Neurochir (Wien). 1988;91(1–2):50–4.

44. Nelson PB, Seif SM, Maroon JC, Robinson AG. Hyponatremia in intracranial disease: perhaps not the syndrome of inappropriate secretion of antidiuretic hormone (SIADH). J Neurosurg. 1981;55(6):938–41.

45. Betjes MG. Hyponatremia in acute brain disease: the cerebral salt wasting syndrome. Eur J Intern Med. 2002;13(1):9–14.

46. Damaraju SC, Rajshekhar V, Chandy MJ. Validation study of a central venous pressure-based protocol for the management of neurosurgical patients with hyponatremia and natriuresis. Neurosurgery. 1997;40(2):312–6; discussion 316–7.

47. Chung HM, Kluge R, Schrier RW, Anderson RJ. Clinical assessment of extracellular fluid volume in hyponatremia. Am J Med. 1987;83(5):905–8.

48. Musch W, Thimpont J, Vandervelde D, Verhaeverbeke I, Berghmans T, Decaux G. Combined fractional excretion of sodium and urea better predicts response to saline in hyponatremia than do usual clinical and biochemical parameters. Am J Med. 1995;99(4):348–55.

49. Beck LH. Hypouricemia in the syndrome of inappropriate secretion of antidiuretic hormone. N Engl J Med. 1979;301(10):528–30.

50. Docci D, Cremonini AM, Nasi MT, et al. Hyponatraemia with natriuresis in neurosurgical patients. Nephrol Dial Transplant. 2000;15(10):1707–8.

51. Wijdicks EF, Vermeulen M, van Brummelen P, den Boer NC, van Gijn J. Digoxin-like immunoreactive substance in patients with aneurysmal subarachnoid haemorrhage. Br Med J (Clin Res Ed). 1987;294(6574):729–32.

52. Wijdicks EF, Ropper AH, Hunnicutt EJ, Richardson GS, Nathanson JA. Atrial natriuretic factor and salt wasting after aneurysmal subarachnoid hemorrhage. Stroke. 1991;22(12):1519–24.

53. Kubo Y, Ogasawara K, Kakino S, Kashimura H, Yoshida K, Ogawa A. Cerebrospinal fluid adrenomedullin concentration correlates with hyponatremia and delayed ischemic neurological deficits after subarachnoid hemorrhage. [Article]. Cerebrovasc Dis. 2008;25(1–2):164–9.

54. Diringer M, Ladenson PW, Stern BJ, Schleimer J, Hanley DF. Plasma atrial natriuretic factor and subarachnoid hemorrhage. Stroke. 1988;19(9):1119–24.

55. Kern PA, Robbins RJ, Bichet D, Berl T, Verbalis JG. Syndrome of inappropriate antidiuresis in the absence of arginine vasopressin. J Clin Endocrinol Metab. 1986;62(1):148–52.

56. Fraser JF, Stieg PE. Hyponatremia in the neurosurgical patient: epidemiology, pathophysiology, diagnosis, and management. Neurosurgery. 2006;59(2):222–9; discussion 222–9.

57. Decaux G, Soupart A. Treatment of symptomatic hyponatremia. Am J Med Sci. 2003;326(1):25–30.

58. Sterns RH, Riggs JE, Schochet Jr SS. Osmotic demyelination syndrome following correction of hyponatremia. N Engl J Med. 1986;314(24):1535–42.

59. Ayus JC, Krothapalli RK, Arieff AI. Treatment of symptomatic hyponatremia and its relation to brain damage. A prospective study. N Engl J Med. 1987;317(19):1190–5.

60. Zada G, Liu CY, Fishback D, Singer PA, Weiss MH. Recognition and management of delayed hyponatremia following transsphenoidal pituitary surgery. J Neurosurg. 2007;106(1):66–71.

61. Decaux G. Treatment of the syndrome of inappropriate secretion of antidiuretic hormone by long loop diuretics. Nephron. 1983;35(2):82–8.

62. Reeder RF, Harbaugh RE. Administration of intravenous urea and normal saline for the treatment of hyponatremia in neurosurgical patients. J Neurosurg. 1989;70(2):201–6.

63. Ghali J, Koren MJ, Taylor JR, Brooks-Asplund E, Fan K, Long WA, Smith N. Efficacy and safety of oral conivaptan: a V1A/V2 vasopressin receptor antagonist, assessed in a randomized, placebo-controlled trial in patients with euvolemic or hypervolemic hyponatremia. J Clin Endocrinol Metabol. 2006;91(6):2145–52.

64. Schrier RW, Schrier RW, Gross P, Gheorghiade M, Berl T, Verbalis JG, Czerwiec FS, Orlandi C. Tolvaptan, a selective oral vasopressin V2-receptor antagonist, for hyponatremia. N Engl J Med. 2006;355(20):2099–112.

65. Diringer M, Ladenson PW, Borel C, Hart GK, Kirsch JR, Hanley DF. Sodium and water regulation in a patient with cerebral salt wasting. Arch Neurol. 1989;46(8):928–30.

66. Sivakumar V, Rajshekhar V, Chandy MJ. Management of neurosurgical patients with hyponatremia and natriuresis. Neurosurgery. 1994;34(2):269–74; discussion 274.

67. Wijdicks EF, Vermeulen M, van Brummelen P, van Gijn J. The effect of fludrocortisone acetate on plasma volume and natriuresis in patients with aneurysmal subarachnoid hemorrhage. Clin Neurol Neurosurg. 1988;90(3):209–14.

68. Hasan D, Lindsay KW, Wijdicks EF, et al. Effect of fludrocortisone acetate in patients with subarachnoid hemorrhage. Stroke. 1989;20(9):1156–61.

69. Mori T, Katayama Y, Kawamata T, Hirayama T. Improved efficiency of hypervolemic therapy with inhibition of natriuresis by fludrocortisone in patients with aneurysmal subarachnoid hemorrhage. J Neurosurg. 1999;91(6):947–52.

70. Moro N, Katayama Y, Kojima J, Mori T, Kawamata T. Prophylactic management of excessive natriuresis with hydrocortisone for efficient hypervolemic therapy after subarachnoid hemorrhage. Stroke. 2003;34(12):2807–11.

71. Katayama Y, Haraoka J, Hirabayashi H, et al. A randomized controlled trial of hydrocortisone against hyponatremia in patients with aneurysmal subarachnoid hemorrhage. Stroke. 2007;38(8):2373–5.

72. Adrogue HJ, Madias NE. Hypernatremia. N Engl J Med. 2000;342(20):1493–9.

73. Darmon M, Timsit JF, Francais A, et al. Association between hypernatraemia acquired in the ICU and mortality: a cohort study. Nephrol Dial Transplant. 2010;25(8):2510–5.

74. Lien YH, Shapiro JI, Chan L. Effects of hypernatremia on organic brain osmoles. J Clin Invest. 1990;85(5):1427–35.

75. Gullans SR, Verbalis JG. Control of brain volume during hyperosmolar and hypoosmolar conditions. Annu Rev Med. 1993;44:289–301.

76. Pollock AS, Arieff AI. Abnormalities of cell volume regulation and their functional consequences. Am J Physiol. 1980;239(3):F195–205.

77. Mohmand HK, Issa D, Ahmad Z, Cappuccio JD, Kouides RW, Sterns RH. Hypertonic saline for hyponatremia: risk of inadvertent overcorrection. Clin J Am Soc Nephrol. 2007;2(6):1110–7.

78. Tisdall M, Crocker M, Watkiss J, Smith M. Disturbances of sodium in critically ill adult neurologic patients: a clinical review. J Neurosurg Anesthesiol. 2006;18(1):57–63.

79. Riggs JE. Neurologic manifestations of fluid and electrolyte disturbances. Neurol Clin. 1989;7(3):509–23.

80. Abramovici MI, Singhal PC, Trachtman H. Hypernatremia and rhabdomyolysis. J Med. 1992;23(1):17–28.

81. Gipstein RM, Boyle JD. Hypernatremia complicating prolonged mannitol diuresis. N Engl J Med. 1965;272:1116–7.

82. Rosner MJ, Coley I. Cerebral perfusion pressure: a hemodynamic mechanism of mannitol and the postmannitol hemogram. Neurosurgery. 1987;21(2):147–56.

83. Yoshida K, Corwin F, Marmarou A. Effect of THAM on brain oedema in experimental brain injury. Acta Neurochir Suppl (Wien). 1990;51:317–9.

84. Wolf AL, Levi L, Marmarou A, et al. Effect of THAM upon outcome in severe head injury: a randomized prospective clinical trial. J Neurosurg. 1993;78(1):54–9.

85. Nemergut EC, Zuo Z, Jane Jr JA, Laws Jr ER. Predictors of diabetes insipidus after transsphenoidal surgery: a review of 881 patients. J Neurosurg. 2005;103(3):448–54.

86. Wijdicks E. Acid–base disorders, hypertonic and hypotonic states. In: The clinical practice of critical care neurology. Philadelphia: Lippincott-Raven; 1997. p. 363–76.

87. Dumont AS, Nemergut 2nd EC, Jane Jr JA, Laws Jr ER. Postoperative care following pituitary surgery. J Intensive Care Med. 2005;20(3):127–40.

88. Sands JM, Bichet DG. Nephrogenic diabetes insipidus. Ann Intern Med. 2006;144(3):186–94.

89. Power BM, Van Heerden PV. The physiological changes associated with brain death – current concepts and implications for treatment of the brain dead organ donor. Anaesth Intensive Care. 1995;23(1):26–36.

90. Wijdicks E, Atkinson J. Pathophysiologic responses to brain death. In: Wijdicks E, editor. Brain death. Philadelphia: Lippincot, Williams & Wilkins; 2001. p. 29–43.

91. Marino P. Hypertonic and hypotonic syndromes. In: Marino P, editor. The ICU book. Baltimore: Williams & Wilkins; 1998. p. 631–46.

92. Ayus J, Carmelo C. Sodium and potassium disorders. In: Shoemaker W, Ayres S, Grenvik A, Holbrook P, editors. Textbook of critical care. Philadelphia: WB Saunders; 2000. p. 853–61.

93. Oh M, Carroll H. Regulation of intracellular and extracellular volume. In: Arieff A, DeFronzo R, editors. Fluid and electrolyte, and acid–base disorders. 2nd ed. New York: Churchill Livingstone; 1995. p. 1–28.

94. Bagshaw SM, Townsend DR, McDermid RC. Disorders of sodium and water balance in hospitalized patients. Can J Anaesth. 2009;56(2):151–67.

95. Fukuda I, Hizuka N, Takano K. Oral DDAVP is a good alternative therapy for patients with central diabetes insipidus: experience of five-year treatment. Endocr J. 2003;50(4):437–43.

96. Miller M, Dalakos T, Moses AM, Fellerman H, Streeten DH. Recognition of partial defects in antidiuretic hormone secretion. Ann Intern Med. 1970;73(5):721–9.

97. Stasior DS, Kikeri D, Duel B, Seifter JL. Nephrogenic diabetes insipidus responsive to indomethacin plus dDAVP. N Engl J Med. 1991;324(12):850–1.

98. Lindsay RS, Seckl JR, Padfield PL. The triple-phase response – problems of water balance after pituitary surgery. Postgrad Med J. 1995;71(837):439–41.

99. Vance ML. Perioperative management of patients undergoing pituitary surgery. Endocrinol Metab Clin North Am. 2003;32(2):355–65.

100. Magaldi AJ. New insights into the paradoxical effect of thiazides in diabetes insipidus therapy. Nephrol Dial Transplant. 2000;15(12):1903–5.

101. Brown RS. Extrarenal potassium homeostasis. Kidney Int. 1986;30:116.

102. Williams ME. Endocrine crises. Hyperkalemia. Crit Care Clin. 1991;7:155–74.

103. Ayus JC, Caramelo C. Sodium and potassium disorders. In: Shoemaker WC, Ayres SM, Grenvik A, Holbrook PR, editors. Textbook of critical care. 4th ed. Philadelphia: W. B. Saunders Company; 2000. p. 853–61.

104. Dutta D, Fischler M, McClung A. Angiotensin converting enzyme inhibitor induced hyperkalaemic paralysis. Postgrad Med J. 2001;77:114–5.

105. Evers S, Engelien A, Karsch V, Hund M. Secondary hyperkalaemic paralysis. J Neurol Neurosurg Psychiatry. 1998;64:249–52.

106. Freedman BI, Burkart JM. Endocrine crises. Hypokalemia. Crit Care Clin. 1991;7:143–53.

107. Weiner ID, Wingo CS. Hypokalemia – consequences, causes, and correction. J Am Soc Nephrol. 1997;8:1179–88.

108. Lucatello A, Sturani A, Di Nardo A, Fusaroli M. Acute renal failure in rhabdomyolysis associated with hypokalemia. Nephron. 1994;67:115–6.

109. Nishihara G, Higashi H, Matsuo S, Yasunaga C, Sakemi T, Nakamoto M. Acute renal failure due to hypokalemic rhabdomyolysis in Gitelman's syndrome. Clin Nephrol. 1998;50:330–2.

110. Kruse JA, Carlson RW. Rapid correction of hypokalemia using concentrated intravenous potassium chloride infusions. Arch Intern Med. 1990;150:613–7.

111. Elin RJ. Magnesium: the fifth but forgotten electrolyte. Am J Clin Pathol. 1994;102:616–22.

112. Chang CJ, Chen SA, Tai CT, et al. Ventricular tachycardia in a patient with primary hyperparathyroidism. Pacing Clin Electrophysiol. 2000;23:534–7.

113. Kleeman CR. Metabolic coma. Kidney Int. 1989;36:1142–58.

114. Zaloga GP, Roberts PR. Calcium, magnesium, and phosphorus disorders. In: Shoemaker WC, Ayres SM, Grenvik A, Holbrook PR, editors. Textbook of critical care. Philadelphia: WB Saunders Company; 2000. p. 853–61.

115. Zaloga GP. Hypocalcemia in critically ill patients. Crit Care Med. 1992;20:251–62.

116. Snowdon JA, Macfie AC, Pearce JB. Hypocalcaemic myopathy with paranoid psychosis. J Neurol Neurosurg Psychiatry. 1976;39:48–52.

117. Newman JH, Neff TA, Ziporin P. Acute respiratory failure associated with hypophosphatemia. N Engl J Med. 1977;296:1101–3.

118. Polderman KH, Bloemers FW, Peerdeman SM, Girbes AR. Hypomagnesemia and hypophosphatemia at admission in patients with severe head injury. Crit Care Med. 2000;28:2022–5.

119. Rabinstein AA, Wijdicks EFM. Body water and electrolytes. In: Layon AJ, Gabrielli A, Friedman WA, editors. Textbook of neuro-intensive care. Philadelphia: WB Saunders; 2004.

Acute Kidney Injury and Renal Replacement Therapy in the Neurologically Injured Patient

19

Abdo Asmar, Mourad M. Alsabbagh, Michiko Shimada, Azra Bihorac, and A. Ahsan Ejaz

Contents

A. Asmar, MD
Department of Clinical Science,
University of Central Florida, Orlando, FL 32608, USA

M.M. Alsabbagh, MD • A.A. Ejaz, MD, FASN (✉)
Division of Nephrology, Hypertension, and Transplantation,
University of Florida College of Medicine, 100224,
Gainesville, FL 32608, USA
e-mail: ejazaa@gmail.com; ejazaa@medicine.ufl.edu

M. Shimada, MD, PhD
Division of Cardiology, Respiratory Medicine, and Nephrology,
Hirosaki University Graduate School of Medicine,
Hirosaki City, Japan

A. Bihorac, MD, PhD
Division of Critical Care Medicine, Department of Anesthesiology,
University of Florida College of Medicine, 1600 SW Archer Road,
100254, Gainesville, FL 32608, USA
e-mail: abihorac@anest.ufl.edu

Abstract

Lexicography, epidemiology, pathomechanisms, risk factors, and treatment options for AKI are discussed, with specific emphasis on patients in the neurocritical care units.

Keywords

Acute kidney injury • Neurocritical unit

Introduction

Acute kidney injury (AKI) is a clinical-biochemical syndrome that is characterized by sudden (i.e., hours to days) deterioration in renal function resulting in diminished ability of the kidneys to eliminate nitrogenous waste products and other uremic toxins. AKI has been associated with increased short- and long-term all-cause mortality, progression of chronic kidney disease, and resource utilization. Understanding the true scope of the problem has been hampered by the lack of a standardized definition of AKI. Nevertheless, AKI is common among hospitalized patients, especially in those who are critically ill.

Despite advances in medical sciences, the mortality associated with AKI remains high in critically ill patients. Data are scarce on the incidences, risk factors, mechanisms, optimal management strategies, and outcomes of the patients in the neurointensive care unit (neuroICU). The complex neurocritical issues confound the management of AKI in this setting and require special attention to avoid further brain injury. This chapter discusses the issues in the diagnosis, prevention, and treatment of AKI, especially as they relate to the patients in the neuroICU.

Issues in the Diagnosis of Acute Kidney Injury

Evolution of the Terminology of Acute Kidney Injury

The lexicography of what is now universally accepted as AKI is related to many key historical figures and events. "Ischuria Renalis" by William Heberden in 1802 is believed to be the first ever description of the entity of AKI [1]. At the beginning of the twentieth century, AKI related to pregnancy, burns, toxic agents, trauma, or renal surgery was described as "acute Bright's disease" in William Osler's *Textbook of Medicine* [1]. During World War I, AKI received much attention in several publications but yet again under a different name: "war nephritis" [2]. The entity was disregarded until World War II, when the classical paper on crush syndrome was published [3]. Homer W. Smith is credited for the introduction of the term "acute renal failure" in a chapter titled "Acute Renal Failure Related to Traumatic Injuries" in his textbook *The Kidney: Structure and Function in Health and Disease* [1]. In an effort to standardize the terminology and definition, the Acute Dialysis Quality Initiative consortium of nephrologists and intensivists from around the world published a consensus definition of acute kidney injury in 2004, known as the RIFLE criteria [4]. The RIFLE criteria, as we will discuss later, were modified in 2007 to Acute Kidney Injury Network (AKIN) criteria for AKI [5]. The term AKI was proposed to reflect the entire spectrum of acute renal failure, recognizing that an acute decline in kidney function is often secondary to an injury that causes functional or structural changes in the kidneys.

AKIN Criteria for Acute Kidney Injury

The RIFLE criteria comprise the following categories: at risk is the least severe category of AKI, followed by injury, failure, loss, and end-stage renal disease (Table 19.1). This definition was intended to establish the presence or absence of clinical AKI in a given patient or situation and to describe its severity. RIFLE uses two criteria: change in blood creatinine or GFR from a baseline value and urine flow rates per body weight over a specified time period of 7 days. RIFLE was validated in several studies including a systemic review of more than 70,000 patients that demonstrated a stepwise increase in the relative risk of mortality as AKI progressed through the RIFLE stages (risk: RR 2.4, failure: RR 6.37) [6].

The modification of the RIFLE to AKIN criteria in 2007 was necessitated to accommodate emerging data indicating that small changes in serum creatinine from baseline were also associated with increased mortality [7, 8]. AKIN differs from RIFLE criteria in that risk, injury, and failure have been replaced with stages 1, 2 and, 3 respectively; the change in GFR has been eliminated; the use of an absolute increase in creatinine of at least 0.3 mg/dL has been added to stage 1; and patients starting renal replacement therapies are automatically classified as stage 3, regardless of their creatinine and urine output. Another noteworthy difference between RIFLE and AKIN is the time needed to diagnose AKI. In the RIFLE criteria, the proposed time frame for making a diagnosis of AKI is 1 week. In AKIN, this time frame is changed to change in creatinine values within a 48-h period. It is imperative that the AKIN diagnostic criteria be used only after an optimal state of hydration has been achieved and a urinary obstruction has been excluded when clinically indicated [5].

Table 19.1 The RIFLE and the acute kidney injury criteria for acute kidney injury

System	Serum creatinine criteria	Urine output criteria
RIFLE class[a]		
Risk	Serum creatinine increase to 1.5-fold or GFR decrease >25 % from baseline	<0.5 mL/kg/h for 6 h
Injury	Serum creatinine increase to 2.0-fold or GFR decrease >50 % from baseline	<0.5 mL/kg/h for 12 h
Failure	Serum creatinine increase to 3.0-fold or GFR decrease >75 % from baseline or serum creatinine ≥354 μmol/L (≥4 mg/dL) with an acute increase of at least 44 μmol/L (0.5 mg/dL)	Anuria for 12 h
Loss	Persistent ARF=complete loss of kidney function >4 weeks	
ESKD	End-stage kidney disease (>3 months)	
AKIN stage[b]		
1.	Serum creatinine increase ≥26.5 μmol/L (≥0.3 mg/dL) or increase to 1.5–2.0-fold from baseline	<0.5 mL/kg/h for 6 h
2.	Serum creatinine increase >2.0–3.0-fold from baseline	<0.5 mL/kg/h for 12 h
3.	Serum creatinine increase >3.0-fold from baseline or serum creatinine ≥354 μmol/L (≥4.0 mg/dL) with an acute increase of at least 44 μmol/L (0.5 mg/dL) or need for RRT	<0.3 mL/kg/h for 24 h or anuria for 12 h or need for RRT

[a]Data from Mehta and Chertow [4]
[b]Data from Mehta et al. [5]

Limitations of the AKIN Criteria for Acute Kidney Injury

It is important to note that while these criteria have allowed the description, epidemiology, and natural history of AKI in patients presenting to the intensive care unit, there are constraints to their application outside epidemiological research as they do not address the timing of kidney injury nor do they yield any information about the etiology of AKI. The use of serum creatinine to detect and assess the severity of AKI in the definitions of AKI is limited by its biologic variability, bias, and nonspecificity affecting creatinine measurement, medications and other interfering agents, nutrition, and alterations in circulating serum creatinine produced by nonrenal disease states. Therefore, the absolute level does not always reflect the severity of the underlying kidney damage. Rises in serum creatinine occur 12–24 h following tissue injury and therefore do not detect early stage kidney injury. Furthermore, creatinine kinetic studies have shown that the time to reach a 50 % increase in serum creatinine is directly related to baseline kidney function and ranges from 4 h with normal kidney function to 27 h with stage 4 chronic renal failure [9]. None of the current classification accounts for the presence of chronic kidney disease in the definition of AKI. Serum creatinine is a functional measure of renal function but not a very good marker for structural renal damage. Another issue with the AKIN criteria is its use of 6- and 12-h urine output measurements; while critical in our day-to-day clinical practice, it is, again, information retrospectively collected, perhaps after a significant amount of renal damage has occurred.

AKIN criteria suffer from dependency on knowing the patient's baseline serum creatinine. The baseline serum creatinine value, which is reflective of the patient's premorbid kidney function, should be known, and this is the value to which we compare subsequent creatinine values to diagnose AKI. However, in many cases baseline serum creatinine values might not be readily available to practicing physicians. The introduction of novel biomarkers of AKI into clinical practice such as neutrophil gelatinase-associated lipocalin (NGAL), interleukin-18, and kidney injury molecule-1 may bypass this issue and allow for detection of molecular- and cellular-level injury 12–24 h earlier than with serum creatinine measurements.

Epidemiology of Acute Kidney Injury in the NeuroICU

The period prevalence of AKI in the general ICU population has been reported to be 5.7 % in a multinational, multicenter study, where AKI was defined as urine output <200 mL per 12-h period and/or blood urea nitrogen >84 mg/dL [10]. In another European multicenter study, the incidence of AKI using the RIFLE criteria was 42.7 % [11]. For comparison, AKI accounts for 1 % of all hospital admissions in the USA [12]. Despite the abundance of data on the epidemiology of AKI in the general intensive care unit, there is limited information on patients specifically admitted to the neuroICU. In a single-center cohort of 787 consecutive patients with subarachnoid hemorrhage admitted to the neuroICU, the incidence of AKI using RIFLE criteria was 23.1 % [13]. In a prospective study, the incidence of AKI by AKIN criteria after acute stroke was 27 % [14]. By the same criteria, 23 % of patients with traumatic brain injury (TBI) admitted to the neurosurgical unit had AKI [15]. AKI has been reported in 12.5 % of patients with posterior reversible encephalopathy syndrome [16]. In a European study, the second-most common diagnostic reason (17 %) for admission to the intensive care unit was neurological [11]. These data suggest that the incidence rates for AKI in the general and neuroICUs are comparable. This is probably predictable based on the heavy burden of comorbid conditions present in these patients, lengthy ICU stays, operative interventions, and potentially aggressive and unique fluid management strategies, such as the administration of hyperosmolar solutions to prevent and treat delayed neurological deficits. Moreover, these patients undergo a significant number of contrast-utilizing radiographic studies, all of which may contribute to the development of AKI.

AKI is associated with significantly increased short- and long-term mortality, lengths of hospital stay, and resource utilization, the magnitude of which increases with worsening severity of AKI [8, 17]. Two-thirds of patients with AKI require dialysis therapies [18, 19], and hospital mortality associated with AKI exceeds 40 % in most studies, although newer evidence suggests that there may be some improvement in outcomes. In stroke patients, AKI is an independent predictor of 10-year mortality with 24 % higher probability of death compared with those without AKI [11]. In patients with subarachnoid hemorrhage, mild increase in serum creatinine was associated with fourfold risk for in-hospital death, worse discharge and 3-month outcome, and a trend toward worse 12-month outcome [13]. In TBI patients, AKI was associated with higher incidence of poor outcome (74 %) when compared with patients without renal dysfunction [15]. These data provide evidence that AKI is common in neuroICU patients, is associated with high mortality, and is a novel independent predictor for adverse outcomes.

Risk Factors for Acute Kidney Injury in the NeuroICU

Epidemiological data have suggested a progressive increase in the incidence of AKI over the past few decades. Given the rising incidence, the high mortality and morbidity associated

Table 19.2 Risk factors for acute kidney injury in the neuroICU

General risk factors	
Demographics	Age
	Black race
	Male gender
Comorbid conditions	Diabetes mellitus
	Hypertension
	Poor cardiac function/coronary artery disease
	Peripheral vascular disease
	Chronic kidney disease
	Advance liver disease
	HIV + status
	Malnutrition (hypoalbuminemia)
	Generalized debilitating conditions
Medications	NSAIDs
	IVIG (sucrose containing)
	Hyperosmolar solutions
	Antibiotics (aminoglycosides, vancomycin)
Diagnostic studies	Radiocontrast
Neuro-specific risk factors	Acute stroke
	TTP
	PRES syndrome
	Guillain-Barre
	Status epilepticus
	Chronic neurodegenerative diseases
	Neurogenic bladder
	Critical illness polyneuropathy

with AKI, as well as the paucity of available interventions to improve clinical end points such as need for dialysis or mortality, tremendous efforts need to be applied for early recognition and prevention of the development of this disorder. The general and neuroICU-specific risk factors are summarized in Table 19.2. It is evident from the table that a decrease or loss in functional capacity of an organ, whether due to demographic reasons, comorbid conditions or natural progression of chronic conditions, increases the risk for AKI, and adverse outcomes. Data from the US Medicare database report average AKI rates of 18.5, 20.8, 25.8, and 28.6 cases per 1,000 discharges for age groups 64 years or younger, 65–74, 75–84, and 85 years, respectively [20]. The average AKI rates during the 10-year follow-up were 28.3 for men and 20.0 cases per 1,000 discharges for women and 22.3, 34.4, and 24.3 cases per 1,000 discharges for white, black, and patients of other races, respectively. Chronic kidney disease is a strong predictor of AKI [21–23]. In a nested case–control study of 602,584 hospitalized patients, 74 % of the dialysis-requiring AKI occurred among those with preexisting chronic kidney disease with an estimated GFR less than 60 mL/min/1.73 m^2. Compared with the control group, patients with baseline estimated GFR 45–59 mL/min/1.73 m^2 and estimated GFR 15–9 mL/min/1.73 m^2 had

nearly twofold increase and 29-fold increase in adjusted odds ratio of dialysis-requiring AKI, respectively, even after adjusting for age, sex, race, ethnicity, and other baseline conditions. One other finding of this study is that even within the same estimated GFR category, patients with diabetes had a much higher likelihood of developing dialysis-requiring AKI than those without diabetes. Chronic kidney diseases also predispose to adverse neurological events. The occurrence rate of subdural hematoma in long-term dialysis patients has been reported to be ten times higher than that of the general population [24].

Over the last few years, there have been multiple studies demonstrating the strong association between the presence of proteinuria and the risk of developing AKI [22, 23, 25]. The risk of AKI increases along with the severity of baseline proteinuria. A study of nearly one million Canadian adults demonstrated increased rates of hospital admission with AKI and AKI requiring dialysis for patients with heavy proteinuria across all values of baseline renal function [25]. In patients with acute ischemic stroke not treated with thrombolytic agents, decreased eGFR and presence of dipstick proteinuria have been reported to be strong negative predictors of 30-day survival [26]. While clinicians might easily recognize that patients already have a deranged baseline renal function by simply observing an abnormal laboratory values, the presence of proteinuria can be easily overlooked. This is either most likely because urinalysis is not routinely obtained or simply because most non-nephrologists do not recognize the multiple risks associated with proteinuria, including AKI. Radiology centers require measurement of the baseline renal function prior to the administration of contrast material. One could easily argue that the recent convincing data about proteinuria and AKI should prompt clinical identification of existing proteinuria or albuminuria. This should be a part of the kidney-risk profile so that an individual at increased risk of AKI can receive aggressive preventive measures.

Proposed Mechanisms of Acute Kidney Injury

The mechanisms of AKI in the neuroICU involve those that are common for all ICUs and those that are characteristic for the neuroICU. More often than not, there is more than one mechanism at play in any given patient. In general, AKI is classified into prerenal, intrarenal, and postrenal AKI (Table 19.3).

Prerenal AKI

Prerenal azotemia is defined as diminished glomerular filtration rate (GFR) secondary to renal hypoperfusion in an

Table 19.3 Classifications and some of the proposed mechanisms of acute kidney injury

Prerenal azotemia	Diminished GFR secondary to renal hypoperfusion
	Imbalance between the amount of solute presented to the kidneys for clearance and the kidneys' ability to clear them
Intrarenal acute kidney injury	
Acute tubular necrosis	Intrarenal vasoconstriction
	Impaired renal autoregulation
	Impaired tubuloglomerular feedback
	Tubular obstruction
	Tubular backleak
	Direct tubular toxicity by medications, pigments
Acute interstitial nephritis	Hypersensitivity reaction
	Cell-/antibody-mediated immune reaction to renal or extrarenal antigens
	Immune complex
Acute glomerulonephritis	Genetic mutations
	Immune dysregulation
	Antibody formation
	Complement activation
Postrenal	Structural obstruction
	Functional obstruction

otherwise structurally intact kidney or an imbalance between the amounts of solute that needs to be cleared versus the kidney's ability to clear them; prerenal azotemia is reversible when the underlying cause is corrected. In patients with renal hypoperfusion, compensatory mechanisms to maintain GFR become active. These compensatory mechanisms include afferent arteriolar dilation, efferent arteriolar constriction, and neurohormonal effects to increase tubular reabsorption of fluid and maintenance of cardiac output. This means that patients with renal hypoperfusion may have AKI according to oliguria criteria without change in serum creatinine. Moreover, this is a retrospective diagnosis because reversibility can only be determined by the response to fluid administration over time. Prerenal AKI can be considered as volume-responsive AKI, i.e., organ perfusion and renal function will improve with volume infusion. Other causes need to be explored for volume-unresponsive AKI.

Acute Tubular Necrosis

Intrarenal causes of AKI can be divided into acute tubular necrosis (ATN), acute tubulointerstitial nephritis (AIN), and acute glomerulonephritis depending on the anatomical site of injury. Acute glomerulonephritis is relatively uncommon in the hospital setting and will not be discussed further. Acute tubular injury is the most common cause of AKI. The initiating event is thought to be the loss of renal blood flow autoregulation related to the loss of balance between

vasoconstrictors (angiotensin, endothelin, thromboxane A2, adenosine, sympathetic nerve activity) and vasodilators (nitric oxide, prostaglandin E2). This results in renal hypoperfusion, oxidative stress, activation of the inflammatory cascade, and further renal vasoconstriction and cellular damage [27]. The general mechanisms whereby prolonged hypotension, contrast agents, pigments, inotropic agents with vasoconstrictive properties, medications, and multiple other factors cause AKI are listed in Table 19.3.

Neurological Injury as the Cause of AKI

Multiple factors are commonly present in the neuroICU patient, making them vulnerable to AKI. There are provocative data that AKI may also be secondary to the neurological injury itself. Elevated cerebral spinal fluid cytokine levels have been identified in patients following subarachnoid hemorrhage. One study showed that the release of IL-1β, IL-6, and TNF-α in the subarachnoidal space of patients with SAH was markedly increased [28]. Importantly, there appears to be delivery of these cytokines to the systemic circulation [29]. Such inflammatory cytokines could potentially be responsible for the non-neurological organ dysfunction seen with neurological injury, including renal disease. AKI may develop due to renal ischemia following hypoperfusion as a complication of TBI. There is evidence that posterior hypothalamic lesions trigger renal vasoconstriction by activation of the renin-angiotensin system that results in reduced renal blood flow [30].

Acute Tubulointerstitial Nephritis

Acute tubulointerstitial nephritis (AIN) defines a pattern of renal injury usually associated with an abrupt deterioration in renal function characterized histopathologically by inflammation and edema of the renal interstitium. Medications, infectious agents, and underlying systemic diseases that are prevalent in most neurocritical unit patients are also the most common causes of AIN, the removal or management of which often leads to renal improvement. Severe and prolonged AIN can lead to severe AKI requiring renal replacement therapies with adverse renal outcomes [31, 32].

Postrenal AKI

Postrenal AKI is an easily reversible condition. The prognosis depends on the interval from onset to diagnosis and relief of obstruction, unilateral versus bilateral obstruction, and the etiology of the obstruction. Functional changes associated with acute obstruction are reversible; however, chronic obstruction leads to renal parenchymal fibrosis and progression to chronic kidney disease. Careful attention is warranted for neuroICU patients with neurogenic bladder due to spinal cord defects or trauma, multiple sclerosis, Parkinson disease, stroke, diabetes, and conditions that can cause autonomic dysfunction.

NeuroICU-Specific AKI

Causes of AKI in patients admitted to the neuroICU may include rhabdomyolysis, especially in patients admitted with TBI and those with status epilepticus. Another major contributor to AKI, mortality, and morbidity is infection. There is evidence that severe head injury causes suppression of cellular immune function, resulting in higher rate of infection [33]. Sepsis occurs commonly in patients admitted to the neuroICU and is considered to be the most common cause of AKI in critically ill patients [18]. ICU patients with septic AKI are generally much sicker, have greater risk of mortality, and have longer stays in hospital than patients with nonseptic AKI [34]. Exposure to different types of nephrotoxins is a very common cause for AKI. Medication use is a known risk factor for AKI including acute interstitial nephritis and toxic tubular necrosis. Propofol is a sedative agent widely used in the neuroICU and operating room settings. Propofol-related infusion syndrome (PRIS), though rare, is an often fatal syndrome that has been observed in critically ill patients receiving propofol for sedation; it should be quickly recognized and treated. PRIS is characterized by severe unexplained metabolic acidosis, dysrhythmias, AKI, rhabdomyolysis, hyperkalemia, and cardiovascular collapse [35]. Patients admitted to the neuroICU are often repeatedly exposed to radiocontrast agents. Intravascular radiocontrast agents are a known risk for the development of AKI in high-risk patients. Mechanisms of radiocontrast media-induced nephrotoxicity include alterations in intrarenal blood flow causing vasoconstriction, direct tubular toxicity, and generation of reactive oxygen species. Hyperosmotic therapy using mannitol or hypertonic saline has become one of the first-line treatments for cerebral edema and raised intracranial pressure in the neurocritical care. Mannitol use has been associated with the development of AKI, a condition referred to as osmotic nephrosis. This term describes a morphological pattern with vacuolization and swelling of the renal proximal tubular cells. The risk of mannitol-induced AKI in patients with normal kidney function usually increases when the total mannitol dose exceeds 1,100 g. The dose required to cause AKI in patients with CKD is much smaller about 300 g. Daily dose exceeding 200 g or an osmolal gap greater than 60 mOsm/kg is a risk factor for developing AKI. Independent risk factors for the development of AKI in the setting of mannitol use are chronic kidney disease and concomitant diuretic use [36].

Hypertonic saline has become increasingly popular in the neuroICU for the management of cerebral edema. Hypertonic saline use can lead to hypernatremia, a known risk factor for the development of AKI. With increasing degrees of hypernatremia, the incidence of renal failure tends to also increase [37]. The mechanism of hypernatremia-induced AKI is not clearly understood. One possible mechanism is that hypernatremia can lead to renal dysfunction through intravascular dehydration and vasoconstriction either directly or through a tubuloglomerular feedback mechanism. Hypertonic saline use can also lead to worsening hypertension control, a particularly important aspect in a group of critically ill patients that require careful titration of blood pressure to a desired therapeutic target. It is also important to remember that renal failure itself can lead to hypernatremia especially when the kidneys are unable to maximally concentrate urine.

Aggressive reduction of high blood pressure is a critical aspect of care of the neuroICU patient [38]. There is emerging evidence for more intensive blood pressure reduction (MAP < 110 mmHg or systolic blood pressure <140 mmHg) within the first few hours of hospital admission for patients with acute cerebral hemorrhage to reduce hematoma and perihematoma volume [39]. Frank hypotension is avoided, but in patients with underlying impaired renal blood flow autoregulation, the reduction in blood pressure could result in renal hypoperfusion, a condition known as normotensive ischemic AKI [40].

Prevention of Acute Kidney Injury

There are multiple risk factors, most often in combinations, that predispose patients to the development of AKI. The initial care of patients admitted to the neuroICU is risk stratification focusing on the identification and, if possible, modification of patient risk factors for developing AKI. Early recognition of AKI and initiation of therapy are the key to successful outcomes. Novel biomarkers of AKI such as NGAL and IL-18 may help in the early detection of AKI before a fall in GFR occurs and may facilitate interventions to prevent or manage AKI. However, the lack of approved and sensitive markers of early structural injury and the difficulty in assessing renal function in a non-steady state make this a challenging proposition. General strategies that help diminish renal damage in hospitalized patients are maintaining adequate hydration, avoiding hypotension, maintaining optimal mean arterial pressure, and minimizing nephrotoxic exposure (Table 19.4).

Irrespective of the insult leading to AKI and the associated risk factors, particular attention should be focused on optimizing cardiac output and blood pressure. Both true and relative hypovolemias, as seen in cases of decreased effective circulating volume, are significant risk factors for the

Table 19.4   Prevention of acute kidney injury

General measures

Identify risk factors

Maintain adequate blood pressure

Optimize fluid balance

Adjust medication dosage to renal function

Avoid NSAIDS

Avoid contrast exposure, utilize prophylactic measures when appropriate

Prophylaxis recommendations

Acetylcysteine 1,200 mg orally on the day before and on the day of administration of the contrast agent, for a total of 2 days [71], plus

Saline (0.45 %) IV at a rate of 1 mL/kg-body weight/h for 12 h before and 12 h after administration of the contrast agent [72]

For emergency procedures [73], 154 mEq/L of sodium bicarbonate bolus of 3 mL/kg/h for 1 h before iopamidol contrast, followed by an infusion of 1 mL/kg/h for 6 h after the procedure [74]

Reduced contrast load

development of AKI. Therefore, timely recognition and restoration of the circulating blood volume are generally effective in preventing AKI, especially when it is induced by drugs and contrast media. Moreover, the administration of fluids is most beneficial if it is started early in the phase of AKI. Once the injury is advanced, particularly if there is no positive response initially, further fluid should be balanced against the potential risk of developing volume overload.

Treatment of Acute Kidney Injury in the NeuroICU

Conservative Management

The management of the neuroICU patient is discussed elsewhere in this textbook; here we will discuss only a few aspects of the care of the AKI patient. The supportive care of the patient with AKI involves the optimization of fluid balance, avoiding hypotension, maintaining optimal mean arterial pressure, and minimizing exposure to nephrotoxic agents; correction of potassium, phosphorus, and magnesium by restricting their intake or at times removal of potassium by synthetic ion-exchange resins; correction of acid–base disorder; adequate nutrition; and dose adjustment of antibiotics and other medications.

Fluid resuscitation remains the most controversial aspect of the management of AKI. While fluid administration is beneficial and rapidly reverses prerenal AKI in hypovolemic patients and in those in early phase of AKI, it must be balanced against the potential risk of developing volume overload in more severe AKI. Fluid therapy is effective in the prevention of AKI, but has not been shown to be beneficial in established AKI where there is persistent renal

vasoconstriction and other intrarenal causes for hypoperfusion. These patients develop acute AKI despite further fluid loading [41]. Persistent fluid challenges should be avoided if they do not lead to an improvement in renal function or if oxygenation deteriorates, as positive fluid balance can have a negative impact on clinical outcomes.

The choice of resuscitation fluid and the method of administration are also important determinants of outcomes. In a multicentered, randomized, double-blinded trial to compare the effect of fluid resuscitation with albumin or saline on mortality in a heterogeneous population of patients in the ICU, no differences in 28-day mortality were demonstrated [42]. Patients with severe sepsis had a favorable response to resuscitation with albumin. In contrast, patients with TBI resuscitated with albumin had a higher mortality rate (relative risk 1.88) [43]. Resuscitation with fluid boluses has been recently reported to be associated with increased 48-h mortality in critically ill children [44], while conservative strategy of fluid management in patients with acute lung injury has been shown to improve lung function and shorten the duration of mechanical ventilation and ICU stay without increasing nonpulmonary-organ failure [45]. These studies suggest the link between fluid balance, AKI, and adverse outcome. Diuretics are also frequently utilized in the ICU setting for volume management, but their use has been associated with increased risk of death and *nonrecovery* of renal function [46]. High-dose diuretics can help maintain urinary output, but do not have an impact on the survival and renal recovery rate of patients with established AKI [47]. It is important to note that diuretics in the recovery phase of renal replacement therapy-dependent AKI can increase urinary volume and sodium excretion but do not lead to a shorter duration of kidney injury or more frequent renal recovery [48].

Renal Replacement Therapies

Indications for Renal Replacement Therapies

One of the most vexing issues in the critically ill patient is the timing of the initiation of renal replacement therapies (dialysis). The classical indications for renal replacement therapies include volume overload, refractory hyperkalemia, severe metabolic acidosis, and acute uremic end-organ damage such as pericarditis or encephalopathy. There is growing consensus that these findings are late sequelae of AKI and that initiation of renal replacement therapies should precede their occurrence. In the absence of these urgent indications, there is no consensus on the level of severity of AKI and the optimal timing for initiation of renal replacement therapies. In a prospective multicenter observational study conducted at 54 intensive care units in 23 countries enrolling 1,238 patients, early (less than 2 days of admission to ICU or serum creatinine less than 3.5 mg/dL) initiation of renal replacement therapies was associated with lower mortality, duration of hospital stay, and dialysis dependence [49]. The early initiation of renal replacement therapies was also associated with lower mortality in patients with AKI following cardiac surgery [50, 51]. However, no benefits of early initiation of renal replacement therapies were demonstrated in patients with AKI due to sepsis [52]. Another emerging issue is that of fluid balance in patients with AKI. Fluid balance is a predictor of AKI and increases the mortality in patients with AKI [53]. In a multicenter study, fluid overload at the time of diagnosis of AKI was not associated with recovery of kidney function. However, patients with fluid overload when their serum creatinine reached its peak were significantly less likely to recover kidney function [54]. These findings suggest that volume overload may be an important and independent indication to start early renal replacement therapies in critically ill patients with AKI.

Modalities of Renal Replacement Therapies

There are four main modalities of acute renal replacement therapies: acute intermittent hemodialysis (IHD), continuous renal replacement therapies (CRRT), sustained low-efficiency dialysis (SLED), or prolonged intermittent dialysis and acute peritoneal dialysis. The major differences between intermittent and continuous therapies are the speed and the mechanism that removes fluid and toxic wastes. CRRT was developed as therapy for patients unable to tolerate standard IHD, and this remains its primary indication. IHD is capable of removing large amounts of fluids and wastes in a short period of time using diffusion, while continuous renal replacement therapies remove water and wastes at a slow, or more physiological and steady, rate using diffusion, convection, or combination of both. While the goals of renal replacement therapies are to manage fluids and electrolytes, remove toxic uremic products, and manage fluid balance, patients with acute brain injury who are in need of renal support require careful consideration. In this subset of patients, an already affected brain (primary injury) is greatly influenced by systemic alterations that may adversely affect its function (secondary injury).

Care must be taken during dialytic therapy not to cause or exacerbate secondary brain injury related to the replacement therapy itself. The medical care of the critically ill neurological patient requires special knowledge and training in the physiology of intracranial pressure, cerebral blood flow, postoperative care, neuromonitoring, and on how extracorporeal therapies impact these. Renal replacement therapies including CRRT remain the primary responsibility of the nephrologists in most centers. However, neurointensivists are also involved in the adjustment and continuous monitoring of hemodynamic parameters. Therefore, a basic understanding of the issues in renal replacement therapy and care of the acute brain injury patients is critical for physicians taking care of these patients. It needs to be emphasized that there was no survival benefit using intermittent versus continuous therapies [55] or lower- versus higher-intensity CRRT to reduce mortality in the general ICU [56].

Critical Aspects of Renal Replacement Therapies in Acute Brain Injury Patients

The use of renal replacement therapy in the neuroICU is complicated by the issue of intracranial compliance, an important concept in the management of acute brain injury patients. The volume inside the cranium is fixed, and the pressure-volume relationship between intracranial pressure; volume of cerebrospinal fluid, blood, and brain tissue; and cerebral perfusion pressure – known as the Monro-Kellie doctrine – is in a state of volume equilibrium, such that any increase in volume of one of the cranial constituents must be compensated by a decrease in volume of another. Increased intracranial pressure can cause a decrease in cerebral perfusion pressure which can then elicit strong systemic hypertensive response, dilatation of cerebral blood vessels, and further lowering of cerebral perfusion pressure and worsening ischemic brain injury. Renal replacement therapies can contribute to increased intracranial pressures in acute brain injury patients. The exact mechanisms are not known; however, several hypotheses have been postulated. The *reverse urea hypothesis* suggests that the slower removal of urea from the brain compared to the plasma creates an osmotic gradient that results in cerebral edema [57]. The *idiogenic osmole hypothesis* suggests that the osmotic gradient between brain and plasma develops during rapid dialysis because of newly formed brain osmoles [58]. Others have suggested that the *rapid infusion of bicarbonate* in high doses during hemodialysis can cause a paradoxical intracellular acidosis that leads to a compensatory production of intracellular osmoles and water movement into the brain along a concentration gradient resulting in worsening cerebral edema [59]. Another important mechanism may be the *intradialytic hypotension* whereby even the resultant minor change in cerebral blood flow can result in significant increases in intracranial pressures [60]. In TBI patients with low or decreased intracranial compliance (monitored or anticipated), the dialysate temperature may also affect existing body temperatures (hyperthermia) and worsen intracranial hypertension [61]. However, the effect of low dialysate temperatures in this setting has not been studied in randomized clinical trials.

Intermittent Versus Continuous Renal Replacement Therapies in the Acute Brain Injury Patients

Intradialytic hypotension during intermittent hemodialysis therapy is not a major problem in most ICU patients who are able to maintain mean arterial pressure; it is managed by fluid resuscitation, decreasing the ultrafiltration rate and blood flow rate. However, it is a very serious issue in patients with altered intracranial compliance where even a small drop in mean arterial pressure during dialysis can lead to surges in intracranial pressure and worsening cerebral edema [62]. In fact, significant pre- and postprocedure changes in the density of white and gray matter consistent with cerebral edema were observed by CT scans in all patients after IHD but none in those with CRRT [63].

In patients with acute hepatic failure, cranial and mean arterial blood pressures were demonstrated to remain stable during CRRT but decreased significantly with IHD [64]. Rapid shifts in fluid and solute concentrations during intermittent renal replacement therapies may be poorly tolerated and increase cerebral edema and intracranial pressure. On the other hand, CRRT has been shown to lower or stabilize intracranial pressures in patients with or without renal dysfunction [65, 66]. Preference should be given to the utilization of continuous versus intermittent renal replacement therapy, whenever available, in the care of the neuroICU patient with decreased intracranial compliance.

The requirement for anticoagulation is not a barrier to the initiation of CRRT. Systemic anticoagulation with heparin has now been replaced with regional citrate-based anticoagulation in most renal replacement therapy protocols. Regional citrate anticoagulation provides longer circuit patency and less bleeding than heparin [67]. CRRT may also be performed without anticoagulation, using frequent saline flushes and regional anticoagulation with heparin [68].

The choice of modality is often restricted by practice patterns due to cost, availability of technology, and reimbursement policies. If continuous modalities of therapy are not available, IHD can be used successfully, if carefully prescribed and monitored [69]. The prescription should include a dialyzer membrane with small surface area, low blood flow rate (100–150 mL/min) and dialysate flow rate, high dialysate sodium concentrate, low bicarbonate and cooler dialysate temperature (35 °C), low rate of urea removal, and low rate of ultrafiltration, so as to diminish changes in effective blood volume to maintain cardiovascular stability [70]. Intermittent mannitol infusion may help to maintain plasma osmolality and prevent acute elevations in intracranial pressure. Another form of continuous renal replacement therapy that can be utilized when intermittent or continuous therapies are not available is peritoneal dialysis (PD). Although primarily used in end-stage renal disease patients, it remains relevant in the setting of AKI in many parts of the world because of its lower cost and ease of use. It is therefore important for physicians to understand potential ways to optimize PD since, despite the much lower rate of urea clearance than intermittent renal replacement therapies, dialysis disequilibrium syndrome may still occur with

aggressive ultrafiltration prescriptions that can decrease cardiac output and cerebral perfusion pressures.

References

1. Eknoyan G. Emergence of the concept of acute renal failure. Am J Nephrol. 2002;22:225–30.
2. Davies FC, Weldon RP. A contribution to the study of 'war nephritis'. Lancet. 1917;ii:118–20.
3. Bywaters EG, Beall D. Crush injuries with impairment of renal function. Br Med J. 1941;1:427–32.
4. Mehta RL, Chertow GM. Acute renal failure definitions and classification: time for change? J Am Soc Nephrol. 2003;14:2178–87.
5. Mehta RL, Kellum JA, Shah SV, Molitoris BA, Ronco C, Warnock DG, et al. Acute Kidney Injury Network (AKIN): report of an initiative to improve outcomes in acute kidney injury. Crit Care. 2007; 11:R31.
6. Cruz D, Ricci Z, Ronco C. Clinical review: RIFLE and AKIN – time for reappraisal. Crit Care. 2009;13:211.
7. Coca SG, Peixoto AJ, Garg AX, Krumholz HM, Parikh CR. The prognostic importance of a small acute decrement in kidney function in hospitalized patients: a systematic review and meta-analysis. Am J Kidney Dis. 2007;50:712–20.
8. Chertow GM, Burdick E, Honour M, Bonventre JV, Bates DW. Acute kidney injury, mortality, length of stay, and costs in hospitalized patients. J Am Soc Nephrol. 2005;16:3365–70.
9. Waikar SS, Bonventre JV. Creatinine kinetics and the definition of acute kidney injury. J Am Soc Nephrol. 2009;20:672–9.
10. Uchino S, Bellomo R, Goldsmith D, et al. An assessment of the RIFLE criteria for acute renal failure in hospitalized patients. Crit Care Med. 2006;34:1913–7.
11. Piccinni P, Cruz DN, Gramaticopolo S, Garzotto F, Dal Santo M, Aneloni G, Rocco M, Alessandri E, Giunta F, Michetti V, Iannuzzi M, Belluomo Anello C, Brienza N, Carlini M, Pelaia P, Gabbanelli V, Ronco C. Prospective multicenter study on epidemiology of acute kidney injury in the ICU: a critical care nephrology Italian collaborative effort (NEFROINT). Minerva Anestesiol. 2011;77(11):1072–83.
12. Kaufman J, Dhakal M, Patel B, Hamburger R. Community-acquired acute renal failure. Am J Kidney Dis. 1991;17:191–8.
13. Zacharia BE, Ducruet AF, Hickman ZL, et al. Renal dysfunction as an independent predictor of outcome after aneurysmal subarachnoid hemorrhage: a single-center cohort study. Stroke. 2009;40:2375–81.
14. Tsagalis G, Akrivos T, Alevizaki M, et al. Long-term prognosis of acute kidney injury after first acute stroke. Clin J Am Soc Nephrol. 2009;4:616–22.
15. Li N, Zhao W-G, Zhang W-F. Acute kidney injury in patients with severe traumatic brain injury: implementation of the acute kidney injury network stage system. Neurocrit Care. 2011;14:377–81.
16. Ni J, Zhou LX, Hao HL, Liu Q, Yao M, Li ML, Peng B, Cui LY. The clinical and radiological spectrum of posterior reversible encephalopathy syndrome: a retrospective series of 24 patients. J Neuroimaging. 2011;21(3):219–24.
17. Hobson CE, Yavas S, Segal MS, Schold JD, Tribble CG, Layon AJ, Bihorac A. Acute kidney injury is associated with increased long-term mortality after cardiothoracic surgery. Circulation. 2009;119(18):2444–53.
18. Uchino S, Kellum JA, Bellomo R, Doig GS, Morimatsu H, Morgera S, Schetz M, Tan I, Bouman C, Macedo E, Gibney N, Tolwani A, Ronco C, Beginning and Ending Supportive Therapy for the Kidney (BEST Kidney) Investigators. Acute renal failure in critically ill patients: a multinational, multicenter study. JAMA. 2005;17(294):813–8.
19. Mehta RL, Pascual MT, Soroko S, Savage BR, Himmelfarb J, Ikizler TA, Paganini EP, Chertow GM, Program to Improve Care in Acute

Renal Disease. Spectrum of acute renal failure in the intensive care unit: the PICARD experience. Kidney Int. 2004;66:1613–21.

20. Xue JL, Daniels F, Star RA, et al. Incidence and mortality of acute renal failure in Medicare beneficiaries, 1992 to 2001. J Am Soc Nephrol. 2006;17:1135–42.

21. Hou SH, Bushinsky DA, Wish JB, Cohen JJ, Harrington JT. Hospital-acquired renal insufficiency: a prospective study. Am J Med. 1983;74:243–8.

22. Hsu CY, Ordoñez JD, Chertow GM, et al. The risk of acute renal failure in patients with chronic kidney disease. Kidney Int. 2008;74:101–7.

23. Huang TM, Wu VC, Young GH, et al. Preoperative proteinuria predicts adverse renal outcomes after coronary artery bypass grafting. J Am Soc Nephrol. 2010;22:156–63.

24. Sood P, Sinson GP, Cohen EP. Subdural hematomas in chronic dialysis patients: significant and increasing. Clin J Am Soc Nephrol. 2007;2:956–9.

25. James MT, Hemmelgarn BR, Wiebe N, et al. Glomerular filtration rate, proteinuria, and the incidence and consequences of acute kidney injury: a cohort study. Lancet. 2010;376:2096–103.

26. Brzosko S, Szkolka T, Mysliwiec M. Kidney disease is a negative predictor of 30-day survival after acute ischaemic stroke. Nephron Clin Pract. 2009;112:c79–85.

27. Devarajan P. Update on mechanisms of ischemic acute kidney injury. J Am Soc Nephrol. 2006;17:1503–20.

28. Fassbender K, Hodapp B, Rossol S, et al. Inflammatory cytokines in subarachnoid haemorrhage: association with abnormal blood flow velocities in basal cerebral arteries. J Neurol Neurosurg Psychiatry. 2001;70:534–7.

29. McKeating EG, Andrews PJ, Signorini DF, et al. Transcranial cytokine gradients in patients requiring intensive care after acute brain injury. Br J Anaesth. 1997;78:520–3.

30. Gruber A, Reinprecht A, Illievich UM, et al. Extracerebral organ dysfunction and neurologic outcome after aneurysmal subarachnoid hemorrhage. Crit Care Med. 1999;27:505–14.

31. Ejaz AA, Fitzpatrick PM, Haley WE, Wasiluk A, Durkin AJ, Zachariah PK. Amlodipine besylate induced acute interstitial nephritis. Nephron. 2000;85:354–6.

32. Rastegar A, Kashgarian M. The clinical spectrum of tubulointerstitial nephritis. Kidney Int. 1998;54:313–27.

33. Quattrocchi KB, Frank EH, Miller CH, et al. Suppression of cellular immune activity following severe head injury. J Neurotrauma. 1990;7:77–87.

34. Bagshaw SM, George C, Bellomo R, ANZICS Database Management Committee. Changes in the incidence and outcome for early acute injury in a cohort of Australian intensive care units. Crit Care. 2007;11:R68.

35. Casserly B, O'Mahony E, Timm EG, Haqqie S, Eisele G, Urizar R. Propofol infusion syndrome: an unusual cause of renal failure. Am J Kidney Dis. 2004;44:e98–101.

36. Dickenmann M, Oettl T, Mihatsch MJ. Osmotic nephrosis: acute kidney injury with accumulation of proximal tubular lysosomes due to administration of exogenous solutes. Am J Kidney Dis. 2008; 51:491–503.

37. Aiyagari V, Deibert E, Diringer MN. Hypernatremia in the neurologic intensive care unit: how high is too high? J Crit Care. 2006;21:163–72.

38. Broderick J, Connolly S, Feldmann E, Hanley D, Kase C, Krieger D, Mayberg M, Morgenstern L, Ogilvy CS, Vespa P, Zuccarello M, American Heart Association/American Stroke Association Stroke Council; American Heart Association/American Stroke Association High Blood Pressure Research Council; Quality of Care and Outcomes in Research Interdisciplinary Working Group. Guidelines for the management of spontaneous intracerebral hemorrhage in adults: 2007 update: a guideline from the American Heart Association/American Stroke Association Stroke Council, High Blood Pressure Research Council, and the Quality of Care and Outcomes in Research Interdisciplinary Working Group. Circulation. 2007;116:e391–413.

39. Anderson CS, Huang Y, Arima H, Heeley E, Skulina C, Parsons MW, Peng B, Li Q, Su S, Tao QL, Li YC, Jiang JD, Tai LW, Zhang JL, Xu E, Cheng Y, Morgenstern LB, Chalmers J, Wang JG, INTERACT Investigators. Effects of early intensive blood pressure-lowering treatment on the growth of hematoma and perihematomal edema in acute intracerebral hemorrhage: the Intensive Blood Pressure Reduction in Acute Cerebral Haemorrhage Trial (INTERACT). Stroke. 2010;41:307–12.

40. Abuelo JG. Normotensive ischemic acute renal failure. N Engl J Med. 2007;357:797–805.

41. Van Biesen W, Yegenaga I, Vanholder R, Verbeke F, Hoste E, Colardyn F, Lameire N. Relationship between fluid status and its management on acute renal failure (ARF) in intensive care unit (ICU) patients with sepsis: a prospective analysis. J Nephrol. 2005; 18:54–60.

42. The SAFE Study Investigators. A comparison of albumin and saline for fluid resuscitation in the intensive care unit. N Engl J Med. 2004;350:2247–56.

43. SAFE Study Investigators; Australian and New Zealand Intensive Care Society Clinical Trials Group; Australian Red Cross Blood Service; George Institute for International Health, Myburgh J, Cooper DJ, Finfer S, Bellomo R, Norton R, Bishop N, Kai Lo S, Vallance S. Saline or albumin for fluid resuscitation in patients with traumatic brain injury. N Engl J Med. 2007;357:874–84.

44. Maitland K, Kiguli S, Opoka RO, Ignore C, Olupot-Olupot P, Akech SO, Nyeko R, Mtove G, Reyburn H, Lang T, Brent B, Evans JA, Tibenderana JK, Crawley J, Russell EC, Levin M, Babiker AG, Gibb DM, The FEAST Trial Group. Mortality after fluid bolus in African children with severe infection. N Engl J Med. 2011; 364(26):2483–95.

45. National Heart, Lung, and Blood Institute Acute Respiratory Distress Syndrome (ARDS) Clinical Trials Network, Wiedemann HP, Wheeler AP, Bernard GR, Thompson BT, Hayden D, de Boisblanc B, Connors Jr AF, Hite RD, Harabin AL. Comparison of two fluid-management strategies in acute lung injury. N Engl J Med. 2006;354:2564–75.

46. Mehta RL, Pascual MT, Soroko S, Chertow GM, PICARD Study Group. Diuretics, mortality, and nonrecovery of renal function in acute renal failure. JAMA. 2002;288(20):2547–53.

47. Cantarovich F, Rangoonwala B, Lorenz H, Verho M, Esnault VL, High-Dose Furosemide in Acute Renal Failure Study Group. High-dose furosemide for established ARF: a prospective, randomized, double-blind, placebo-controlled, multicenter trial. Am J Kidney Dis. 2004;44:402–9.

48. van der Voort PH, Boerma EC, Koopmans M, Zandberg M, de Ruiter J, Gerritsen RT, Egbers PH, Kingma WP, Kuiper MA. Furosemide does not improve renal recovery after hemofiltration for acute renal failure in critically ill patients: a double blind randomized controlled trial. Crit Care Med. 2009;37:533–8.

49. Bagshaw SM, Uchino S, Bellomo R, Morimatsu H, Morgera S, Schetz M, Tan I, Bouman C, Macedo E, Gibney N, Tolwani A, Oudemans-van Straaten HM, Ronco C, Kellum JA. Timing of renal replacement therapy and clinical outcomes in critically ill patients with severe acute kidney injury. J Crit Care. 2009;24: 129–40.

50. Demirkiliç U, Kuralay E, Yenicesu M, Cağlar K, Oz B, Cingöz F, Günay C, Yildirim V, Ceylan S, Arslan M, Vural A, Tatar H. Timing of replacement therapy for acute renal failure after cardiac surgery. J Card Surg. 2004;19:17–20.

51. Elahi MM, Lim MY, Joseph RN, Dhannapuneni RR, Spyt TJ. Early hemofiltration improves survival in post-cardiotomy patients with acute renal failure. Eur J Cardiothorac Surg. 2004;26:1027–31.

52. Bouchard J, Soroko SB, Chertow GM, Himmelfarb J, Ikizler TA, Paganini EP, Mehta RL, Program to Improve Care in Acute Renal Disease (PICARD) Study Group. Fluid accumulation, survival and recovery of kidney function in critically ill patients with acute kidney injury. Kidney Int. 2009;76:422–7.

53. Kambhampati G, Ross EA, Alsabbagh MM, Asmar A, Pakkivenkata U, Ejaz NI, Arif AA, Ejaz AA. Fluid balance and AKI: a prospective observational study. Clin Exp Nephrol. 2012;16(5):730–8.

54. Chou YH, Huang TM, Wu VC, Wang CY, Shiao CC, Lai CF, Tsai HB, Chao CT, Young GH, Wang WJ, Kao TW, Lin SL, Han YY, Chou A, Lin TH, Yang YW, Chen YM, Tsai PR, Lin YF, Huang JW, Chiang WC, Chou NK, Ko WJ, Wu KD, Tsai TJ, NSARF Study Group. Impact of timing of renal replacement therapy initiation on outcome of septic acute kidney injury. Crit Care. 2011;15:R134.

55. Mehta RL, McDonald B, Gabbai FB, Pahl M, Pascual MT, Farkas A, Kaplan RM, Collaborative Group for Treatment of ARF in the ICU. A randomized clinical trial of continuous versus intermittent dialysis for acute renal failure. Kidney Int. 2001;60:1154–63.

56. The RENAL Replacement Therapy Study Investigators. Intensity of continuous renal-replacement therapy in critically ill patients. N Engl J Med. 2009;361:1627–38.

57. Silver SM, DeSimone Jr JA, Smith DA, Sterns RH. Dialysis disequilibrium syndrome (DDS) in the rat: role of the "reverse urea effect". Kidney Int. 1992;42:161–6.

58. Silver SM, Sterns RH, Halperin ML. Brain swelling after dialysis: old urea or new osmoles? Am J Kidney Dis. 1996;28:1–13.

59. Arieff AI, Guisado R, Massry SG, Lazarowitz VC. Central nervous system PH in uremia and the effects of hemodialysis. J Clin Invest. 1976;58:306–11.

60. Sulowicz W, Radziszewski A. Pathogenesis and treatment of dialysis hypotension. Kidney Int. 2006;70:S36–9.

61. Salci K, Nilsson P, Howells T, Ronne-Engström E, Piper I, Contant Jr CF, Enblad P. Intracerebral microdialysis and intracranial compliance monitoring of patients with traumatic brain injury. J Clin Monit Comput. 2006;20:25–31.

62. Davenport A. Practical guidance for dialyzing a hemodialysis patient following acute brain injury. Hemodial Int. 2008; 12:307–12.

63. Ronco C, Bellomo R, Brendolan A, Pinna V, La Greca G. Brain density changes during renal replacement in critically ill patients with acute renal failure. Continuous hemofiltration versus intermittent hemodialysis. J Nephrol. 1999;12:173–8.

64. Davenport A, Will E, Davison A. Effect of renal replacement therapy on patients with combined acute renal and fulminant hepatic failure. Kidney Int. 1993;43:S245–51.

65. Fletcher JJ, Bergman K, Feucht EC, Blostein P. Continuous renal replacement therapy for refractory intracranial hypertension. Neurocrit Care. 2009;11:101–5.

66. Fletcher JJ, Bergman K, Carlson G, Feucht EC, Blostein PA. Continuous renal replacement therapy for refractory intracranial hypertension? J Trauma. 2010;68:1506–9.

67. Davenport A, Tolwani A. Citrate anticoagulation for continuous renal replacement therapy (CRRT) in patients with acute kidney injury admitted to the intensive care unit. Nephrol Dial Transplant Plus. 2009;2:439–47.

68. Tan HK, Baldwin I, Bellomo R. Continuous veno-venous hemofiltration without anticoagulation in high-risk patients. Intensive Care Med. 2000;26:1652–7.

69. Davenport A. Renal replacement therapy in the patient with acute brain injury. Am J Kidney Dis. 2001;37:457–66.

70. Jost CM, Agarwal R, Khair-el-din T, Graybum PA, Victor RG, Henrich WL. Effects of cooler temperature dialysate on hemodynamics stability in 'problem' patients. Kidney Int. 1993;41: 961–4.

71. Briguori C, Colombo A, Violante A, Balestrieri P, Manganelli F, Paolo Elia P, Golia B, Lepore S, Riviezzo G, Scarpato P, Focaccio A, Librera M, Bonizzoni E, Ricciardelli B. Standard vs double dose of N-acetylcysteine to prevent contrast agent associated nephrotoxicity. Eur Heart J. 2004;25:206–11.

72. Tepel M, van Der Giet M, Schwarzfeld C, et al. Prevention of radiographic-contrast-agent-induced reductions in renal function by acetylcysteine. N Engl J Med. 2000;343:180–4.

73. Joannidis M, Druml W, Forni LG, Groeneveld AB, Honore P, Oudemans-van Straaten HM, Ronco C, Schetz MR, Woittiez AJ, Critical Care Nephrology Working Group of the European Society of Intensive Care Medicine. Prevention of acute kidney injury and protection of renal function in the intensive care unit. Expert opinion of the Working Group for Nephrology, ESICM. Intensive Care Med. 2010;36:392–411.

74. Merten GJ, Burgess WP, Gray LV, Holleman JH, Roush TS, Kowalchuk GJ, Bersin RM, Van Moore A, Simonton 3rd CA, Rittase RA, Norton HJ, Kennedy TP. Prevention of contrast-induced nephropathy with sodium bicarbonate: a randomized controlled trial. JAMA. 2004;291:2328–34.

Nutrition in the Neurointensive Care Unit

20

Larissa D. Whitney, Lawrence J. Caruso, Peggy White, and A. Joseph Layon

Contents

L.D. Whitney, PA-C, BS, MS
Department of Critical Care Medicine, Geisinger Medical Center,
Danville, PA 17821, USA
e-mail: ldwhitney@geisinger.edu

L.J. Caruso, MD
Department of Anesthesiology, University of Florida
College of Medicine, 100254, Gainesville, FL 32610, USA
e-mail: lcaruso@anest.ufl.edu

P. White, MD
Department of Anesthesiology,
University of Florida College of Medicine,
1600 Archer Road, Gainesville, FL 32610-0254, USA
e-mail: pmann@anest.ufl.edu

A.J. Layon, MD, FACP (✉)
Critical Care Medicine, Pulmonary and Critical Care Medicine,
The Geisinger Health System, 100 North Academy Way,
Danville, PA 17822, USA

Temple University School of Medicine,
Philadelphia, PA, USA
e-mail: ajlayon@geisinger.edu

Abstract

Approximately 30–50 % of hospitalized patients worldwide suffer from malnutrition, making the importance of maintaining adequate nutritional support crucial to critically ill patients. Achieving an adequate level of nutritional support revolves around counteracting hypermetabolic effects of injury or illness by reducing the severity of malnutrition and preventing complications such as overfeeding. Early recognition, prevention, and appropriate initiation of supplemental nutrition will aid in optimizing nutritional status. Patients able to reach and maintain an optimal level of nutritional status will benefit from faster recovery, improved wound healing, and an increase in rehabilitative efforts. Likewise, a decrease in hospital length of stay, complication rates, morbidity, and mortality will occur.

Keywords

Malnutrition • Hypermetabolism • Immunonutrition • Antioxidants • Starvation • Refeeding syndrome

A.J. Layon et al. (eds.), *Textbook of Neurointensive Care*,
DOI 10.1007/978-1-4471-5226-2_20, © Springer-Verlag London 2013

Introduction

Nutritional support is a routine adjunctive therapy to the management of critically ill patients, as worldwide studies have shown that approximately 30–50 % of hospitalized patients are malnourished. The main goal of nutritional support therapy is to attenuate the level of malnutrition and prevent overfeeding. Maximizing a patient's nutritional status will not only improve length of stay but will decrease morbidity and mortality rates by improving wound healing and rehabilitative efforts. Prolonged starvation syndrome, or underfeeding, can lead to severe complications such as "autocannibalism," a metabolic state characterized by the breakdown of visceral protein and skeletal muscle to meet metabolic requirements necessary for sustaining life. Such metabolic compromise can rapidly progress to weight loss, organ dysfunction, and immune system impairment. This chapter will review basic concepts of nutritional support in critically ill patients and highlight key issues in special populations. Additionally, daily nutritional requirements, formulations, and routes of feeding will be discussed.

Malnutrition and Starvation

Malnutrition

As defined by the World Health Organization, malnutrition is "the cellular imbalance between supply of nutrients and energy and the body's demand for them to ensure growth, maintenance, and specific functions." Virtually every organ system is affected by malnutrition, and it is globally noted to be one of the most important risk factors for illness and death [1]. Depending on the specific nature of nutritional imbalance, malnutrition can be described as primary, secondary, or both. Primary malnutrition is defined as inadequate energy intake, most often secondary to insufficient food supply and poor appetite secondary to illness or eating disorders. Secondary malnutrition is described when a patient has sufficient dietary intake without adequate energy absorption, typically a result of infection (i.e., measles), diarrhea, or medical conditions affecting the digestive tract [2].

Starvation

Starvation, as defined by the World Health Organization, is a "severe deficiency in caloric energy, nutrient, and vitamin intake" [1]. It is recognized as the most extreme form of malnutrition, posing one of the greatest threats to public health worldwide. Common symptoms and effects of starvation include a loss of muscle mass, catabolysis, vitamin deficiency, diarrhea, edema, heart failure, dehydration, and the progression to multiorgan system failure [1]. Starvation can be a consequence of numerous causes, from prolonged fasting to severe disease, but regardless of cause the course remains consistent.

The unstressed individual handles short periods of starvation fairly well. The fall in glucose and insulin levels during fasting results in lipolysis and utilization of fat as the primary source of energy. Cells that require glucose (brain, red blood cells, and white blood cells) rely on glycogen reserves in the liver and muscle to supply approximately 180 g/day of glucose. After 1–2 days, however, these glycogen reserves are depleted, and muscle breakdown provides amino acids for gluconeogenesis. During this phase, approximately 75 g/day of protein are catabolized [2, 3].

After 1 week of starvation, the brain begins to shift its energy substrate from glucose to ketones, while the blood cells remain dependent on glucose. By the fifth week of starvation, this shift reduces the glucose requirement from 180 g/day to approximately 80 g/day. The decreased need for glucose results in less muscle protein breakdown (20 g/day vs. 75 g/day) [3].

Effects of Starvation

Metabolic Response

Malnutrition in critically ill patients occurs secondary to hypermetabolism and accelerated catabolism. Multi-trauma patients rapidly develop significant negative nitrogen balance as metabolic processes converge, and a hypermetabolic state arises. Subsequent development of hypermetabolic organ failure is one of the most serious conditions affecting postsurgical and critically ill patients as malnutrition is rapidly progressive to a hypercatabolic state that results in protein and muscle mass loss that is two to three times that seen during starvation of noncritically ill individuals [4]. Insulin resistance in peripheral tissues and gluconeogenesis shifts glucose toward tissues that are solely dependent on it to meet energy consumption requirements. Commonly, hypermetabolism peaks after 2–4 days from time of insult and abates between days 7 and 10. A persistent hypermetabolic state is detrimental, leading to increased oxygen consumption, excessive nitrogen excretion, and increase in lactate production; this may progress to multiorgan system failure [5].

Within days of onset of starvation, reduced catecholamine levels and peripheral conversion of thyroxine (T_4) to triiodothyronine (T_3) lead to a decrease in resting metabolic expenditure (RME) [6]. As the loss of lean tissue mass increases, there is further decrease in RME [7]. Sodium-potassium pump activity decreases, which also results in a decrement in RME [8]. Keys and coworkers conducted a study of 36 college-aged men who had consumed a normal diet for 3 months before initiation of the investigation and were then placed on diets containing two-thirds their energy requirements; this continued for a 6-month period. After 24 weeks of diet restriction, data showed that the RME in these participants had decreased by approximately 40 % [9].

Skeletal muscle is the body's largest protein reservoir and thus the best indicator for measuring protein homeostasis. The unintentional loss of 5–10 % of body weight as a result of protein degradation (muscle wasting) and decreased protein synthesis is a significant complication of many disease processes [10]. Protein metabolism in trauma and surgical patients may be roughly estimated by measurement of nitrogen balance and turnover rates of whole-body protein [11]. In the hypermetabolic state, up to 1 % of whole-body protein may be lost per day [4]. In studies of elective surgical patients, protein synthesis falls as breakdown remains unchanged. Contrasting results are noted in septic, trauma, and burn patients as protein synthesis and degradation rates increase [11]. Although the physiology of muscle wasting is poorly understood, there is an association between the onset of muscle wasting in relation to disease outcome, quality of life, length of stay, debilitation, and rehabilitative efforts [10].

Effects on Organ Function

The underlying mechanisms of malnutrition and starvation on organ function in humans remain poorly understood. The evidence base for nutritional support relies primarily on information from military detention camps, poverty-stricken individuals, famine records, and information from studies in human volunteers, hospitalized patients, and animals [12]. Controlling specific nutrient deficiencies and preventing the progression from malnutrition to starvation have been effective with current nutritional support regimens and therefore have become factors in decreasing morbidity and mortality [13].

In a malnourished state, skeletal muscle mass decreases to a greater proportion than body weight. A decrease in muscle mass should not be confused with muscle function, as muscle function may decrease prior to any recognizable fall in muscle mass and correlates more closely with serum transferrin and prealbumin than with actual muscle mass [12]. Similarly, malnutrition and starvation alter function and decrease the mass of visceral organs. A reflection of decreasing metabolic demands is demonstrated by altered cardiac function as cardiac mass, cardiac output, and stroke volume decline in proportion to body weight [14].

Enteral starvation is associated with a lack of gut stimulation, which promotes the development of intestinal atrophy and leads to a decreased absorption of glucose, fat, and protein [14–16]. There is some evidence that trickle feeds at 10–30 mL/h may, among other things, prevent mucosal atrophy and promote faster return of cognitive function in neurologically critically ill patients [17].

Alterations in pulmonary function include decreased respiratory muscle function and blunted ventilatory response to hypercarbia and hypoxia. Additionally, anemia, impaired wound healing, and altered immune function place the malnourished patient at increased risk for developing complications such as atelectasis, bronchopneumonia, intestinal malabsorption, and sepsis [18, 19].

Multiple system organ failure (MSOF) is one of the most serious conditions seen in critical illness [5]. Characterized by a persistent hypermetabolic state, it is a clinical syndrome associated with severe infection in the presence of dead or injured tissue or severe inflammatory states. Lundholm termed this hypermetabolism-multiple organ failure (HOF) complex [5].

The typical metabolic response peaks around day 3 and dissipates between days 7 and 10, post-insult. In hypermetabolic states, this response persists for up to 21 days and is commonly associated with acute lung injury. High cardiac output, low systemic vascular resistance, and increased oxygen consumption depict the physiologic changes associated with HOF [20]. Reported occurrence of HOF in surgical patients is 10–20 % following emergent operations and 30–50 % in patients with intra-abdominal abscesses. Mortality rates vary from 30 to 100 %, depending on the number of organs affected. The development of septic shock increases mortality rates to 70 %. In patients with three or more organ systems in failure, mortality has been reported to be near 100 %, although in recent years this has seemed to decrease. Tissue destruction, infection, and acute hemorrhage and shock are the most common inciting factors for HOF (also known as MSOF: multiple system organ failure) [5].

Immune Effects and Infection Rates

Although the effects of malnutrition in relation to discrete components of immune response are difficult to integrate into clinical practice (see the section in this chapter on Immunonutrition), these concepts have been studied. In malnourished and critically ill patients, energy consumption increases to sustain activated immune responses, which may result in severe protein-energy malnutrition. Alterations in cellular immunity, complement activity, cytokine production, and antibody affinity have all been demonstrated in animal or human studies. The synergistic relationship between infection and malnutrition has been described as malnutrition inhibits immune responses and infection exacerbates malnutrition by causing further anorexia and malabsorption [21].

Inadequate dietary intake can weaken immunologic responsiveness through changes in mucous membranes. Mucosal linings are essential defenses against infection and damage while decreasing the susceptibility to infection, at least if they are intact and healthy. Malnutrition affects infection incidence, increases severity of illness, and may do the same to length of stay. Malnutrition is an independent risk factor for the development of nosocomial infections, which are associated with increased mortality, increased ICU stay, increased cost, and increased readmission rates. Additionally, malnutrition is highly associated with respiratory complications and development of pressure ulcers.

None of this is new. In 1936, Studley reported a correlation between preoperative weight loss and postoperative mortality and infectious complications between patients undergoing surgery for gastric ulcer. In this retrospective analysis of 46 patients with chronic peptic ulcer disease, patients who lost more than 20 % of their baseline weight prior to surgery had a perioperative mortality rate of 33.3 %, with all deaths being infection associated. Patients who had lost less than 20 % of their baseline weight suffered a mortality of only 3.5 %. Furthermore, weight loss was a better predictor of mortality than the age of the patient, preoperative cardiorespiratory status, and the type and duration of the operation. Incidence of infection unassociated with mortality was not reported in this study [22].

Rhoads and Alexander reported a higher infection rate in a group of general surgery patients with hypoproteinemia, defined as a serum less than 6.3 g/dL. The infections were grouped as wound, urinary tract, respiratory, and miscellaneous. Patients with hypoproteinemia had an increase in infection rates both as a whole and within each group than those with serum protein greater than 6.3 g/dL. However, the authors of this study were unable to differentiate causality from association [23].

In a prospective study of patients with severe head injury, Grahm and coworkers randomized 32 patients to receive either early or delayed enteral feeding following injury. Early feeding was initiated within 36 h of injury and delayed feeding 3–5 days following injury. Patients in the early feeding group had improved caloric and nitrogen intake, as well as a more positive nitrogen balance. In addition, patients with early initiation of nutrition had significantly lower rates of early infection within a 7-day post-injury period than those who received delayed feeding. Length of ICU stay was also decreased in the early feeding group [24].

In contrast to the benefits of early enteral nutrition as described in the Grahm study, a large, multicenter Veterans Affairs study identified an increased risk of infection in patients receiving perioperative intravenous nutrition. In this prospective, randomized study of 395 malnourished patients undergoing major abdominal or thoracic procedures, patients were randomly assigned either to receive total parenteral nutrition(TPN) for 7–15 days preoperatively and 3 days postoperatively or to receive no perioperative TPN. The group receiving TPN had a higher rate of infection, particularly pulmonary infections, than the control group. In subgroup analysis, the higher risk of infection with TPN held true for those who were classified as mildly malnourished but not those classified as borderline malnourished or severely malnourished. In the latter two groups, there was no difference in infection rates between TPN and control patients [25].

In summary, critical illness is often associated with protein-energy malnutrition and increased consumption of fat and lean tissue, leading to a reduction in immune function, impaired intestinal barrier, and bacterial translocation resulting in systemic inflammatory response syndrome and infection. Malnutrition puts patients at increased risk for anemia, impaired wound healing, and altered immune function and subsequent development of atelectasis, bronchopneumonia, intestinal translocation, and sepsis [26]. There are suggestions that malnutrition compromises discrete components of the immune system, but it remains difficult to determine whether malnutrition in itself increases the rate of infection, based on available data. More importantly, it remains unclear whether aggressive attempts at intravenous feeding to correct the nutritional deficit will reduce the risk of infection and, if so, which patient populations will benefit most.

Wound Healing

In healthy individuals, wound healing is divided into three phases: inflammation, proliferation, and maturation. Wound healing requires increased consumption of proteins and calories and can be described as the body's process of replacing injured tissue with healthy tissue. Adequate nutritional support is a fundamental part of wound management. Hypermetabolism will cause a loss of total body water resulting in increased collagen and cell turnover rates adversely affecting the healing process. In malnourished states, fibroblast proliferation and neovascularization are impaired due to a decrease in cellular and humeral immunity associated with tissue collagen loss, impaired collagen synthesis, and impaired wound healing.

Essential nutrients for adequate wound healing include trace elements and antioxidants for cell metabolism, fatty acids to maintain cell membrane integrity, and amino acids to regulate normal cell function and wound repair. Monitoring protein levels can prove of some benefit, as highly exudative wounds will have increased insensible loss. Fluid status also remains essential in wound healing as dehydration reduces efficiency of blood circulation and impairs the supply of oxygen and nutrients to the wound. While malnutrition has clearly been identified as detrimental to wound healing, the ability of nutritional support to reverse this impairment has not conclusively been demonstrated.

Wound healing models using implanted fine-bore polytetrafluoroethylene (PTFE) tubing provide some insight on wound healing. This tubing can be inserted subcutaneously and removed after 7–10 days. Measurement of hydroxyproline accumulation provides a measure of collagen deposition. In these studies, malnutrition was associated with decreased hydroxyproline accumulation, suggesting reduced collagen deposition and impaired wound healing [27, 28]. Animal studies have demonstrated the adverse effects of protein-calorie malnutrition on the strength of colonic anastomoses and on abdominal wall wounds. The effects of these changes on clinical outcomes such as wound infection or dehiscence are not well-defined. Human studies have primarily described the correlation between hypoalbuminemia and wound complications, although low albumin levels may occur independent of malnutrition [29–31].

In summary, malnutrition leads to decreased collagen synthesis and likely increases the risk of wound complications. Some studies show that optimizing nutrition with adequate caloric intake and nutrient supplementation will prevent protein-energy malnutrition and promote wound healing; however, this remains unconfirmed. The ability to reverse these changes and the best method of doing so remain in question.

Immunity and Critical Illness: Hinting at Immunonutrition

In critical illness, the release of inflammatory mediators and the production of counter-regulatory hormones increase, leading to a cascade of metabolic events. Providing adequate nutrition is essential to support anabolism, restructure uninhibited catabolism, preserve a functional immune system, and maximize patient outcome. Patients with severe sepsis and organ dysfunction or septic shock may have increased energy expenditure of approximately 20 % greater than expected based on calculation using the Harris-Benedict formula due to the metabolic derangements seen with these disorders [32]. In patients who have undergone major surgical procedures, a period of immunosuppression may be precipitated by arginine deficiency. During catabolic/hypermetabolic states, arginase activity increases, therefore decreasing the level of circulating arginine within the body and decreasing a patient's immune response [33]. Patients with a severe neurologic insult are noted to have excessive urinary nitrogen losses that can exceed 25 g/day in combination with a 40–50 % increase in their basal energy expenditure. Resultant from the severity of the insult, it may take weeks from the time of neurologic injury to regain a neutral to positive nitrogen balance [32].

Protein-calorie malnutrition—in addition to increased energy consumption and resultant fat and lean tissue loss—is often present in high catabolic states such as severe traumatic injury, major surgery, and disorders with a significant inflammatory response. This leads to impaired immune function, compromise of the intestinal barrier, and, potentially, bacterial translocation resulting in systemic inflammatory response syndrome (SIRS) and infection [26].

Immunonutrition is a form of nutritional support focusing on the ability of nutrients to influence the cellular immune activity. It is thought that improving cellular-mediated immune response will improve gut barrier function, immune function, and the ability to heal while simultaneously decreasing hyperinflammation. Nutritional formulae contain both macronutrients, such as lipids, carbohydrates, peptides, and/or proteins, and micronutrients, such as vitamins and minerals. The difference between immune-modulating nutritional formulations and those that are not so considered is that the former contain specific immune-enhancing nutrients including glutamine, arginine, n-acetyl cysteine, branched-chain amino acids, nucleotides, omega-3 fatty acids, antioxidants, and taurine. The immunosuppressive effects of nutrient imbalance are most easily identified in a malnourished state; glutamine and arginine are, perhaps, the most studied immune-enhancing nutrients [33, 34].

Glutamine is the most abundant amino acid in the body and acts an essential oxidative force necessary for rapid cell replication [4]. Glutamine is intimately involved in reducing bacterial overgrowth and translocation by maintaining gut integrity, providing for nitrogen transport, visceral protein synthesis, and ammonia production. Glutamine is utilized most by lymphocytes, macrophages, and cells of the gastrointestinal mucosa. During stressed states, an increase in exogenous glutamine requirements occurs to prevent muscle depletion and catabolism. Supplementing glutamine during metabolic stress has proven beneficial as glutamine is needed substrate for glutathione synthesis, required for the generation of arginine. The use of glutamine may be an effective alternative for arginine administration in critically ill patients, but it is unclear whether arginine metabolism is affected by the route of glutamine administration [35].

Arginine is considered semi-essential as it is indispensable in times of metabolic stress when the body becomes dependent on additional exogenous arginine [35]. Essential during episodes of critical illness, arginine bioavailability decreases in traumatic and septic states. Arginine is synthesized in the kidney via the citrulline pathway and assists in ammonia clearance and enhancing the excretion of nitrogen [36]. Arginine is an essential component of protein and necessary for synthesis of creatine, proline, polyamines, and ornithine [34], as well as for the production of nitric oxide [35, 36]. It is also key in wound healing, growth and proliferation of cells, collagen synthesis, and immune function and plays a role in stimulating the secretion of insulin, prolactin, glucagon, and growth hormone. In the healthy adult, arginine supplementation has been shown to promote wound healing and improve proliferation of blood lymphocytes in response to mitogens [34].

Data in the severely ill are of interest. One meta-analysis combined nutritional data from 17 randomized trials in 2,305 surgical patients who had undergone elective surgery for gastrointestinal or head and neck cancer and cardiac surgery to compare IMPACT supplementation and standard control formulations. Results from the study showed a 39–61 % reduction in postoperative infectious complications and an average reduction in length of stay by 2 days ($p<0.0001$) in the immune-nutrition group [37].

A review focusing on the effects of immunonutrition in critically ill patients with shock, sepsis, and organ failure noted that treatment with arginine-rich formulae did not impact mortality or infection rates but did decrease length of stay secondary to better rehabilitative potential. While there are concerns related to high arginine concentration formulae, nonstatistically significant data show that mortality in patients receiving this formula has been noted to be lower than those receiving other nutritional formulae [36].

The inflammatory state results in oxidative stress. Antioxidants, including vitamin C, vitamin E, zinc, copper, n-acetyl cysteine, and selenium, are utilized in the prevention of oxidative stress and are essential in maintaining adequate defenses against such oxidative activity. Specifically, vitamin E appears to improve T-cell and cell-mediated immunity. The antioxidant enzyme systems require the trace elements zinc, copper, and selenium, responsible for some of the functionality of antioxidants. Trace element levels tend to decline in the postoperative period, possibly contributing to an increased susceptibility to infection. In immunosuppressed and critically ill patients, supplementation with copper, selenium, and zinc has been shown to improve immune function [34].

Limited animal data support administration of branched-chain amino acid precursors to glutamine to improve immune function and prevent infection [34]. In response to oxidative stress, glutamine plays a significant role in intracellular redox regulation through conversion to glutathione. Glutathione is protective against oxidative injury, decreasing free radicals and providing cell membrane protection [35]. Glutamine is also thought to regulate plasma levels of taurine, an osmoregulator and nonessential amino acid that functions to protect cells from "self-destruction." Taurine is present in high concentration in immune-enhancing cells and constitutes approximately 50 % of free amino acids within lymphocytes. In health, taurine is abundant in the cytosol of inflammatory cells and is involved in free radical inactivation. In trauma, surgical, septic, and other critically ill stressed-state patients, taurine levels may decline [35].

N-acetyl cysteine, a precursor of glutathione, is an antioxidant responsible for enhancing T-cell activity, improving cell-mediated immune function, and decreasing the production of inflammatory cytokines. Preserving N-acetyl cysteine can prevent depletion of glutathione in the lung, liver, immune cells, and small intestine during inflammatory states. The use of N-acetyl cysteine has not shown statistically significant effect on mortality rates [34].

Omega-3 fatty acids, or fish oil, have been shown to modulate immune response by enhancing lymphocyte function and minimizing inflammatory response. A meta-analysis [34] showed that for surgical patients with gastrointestinal, head, or neck malignancy, major benefit related to immune function occurred with a combination of fish oil and arginine supplementation. The arginine-omega-3-nucleotide formulation showed a much more significant impact on infection than arginine-only supplemented formulae ($p<0.0001$). The primary outcome of this study, a decrease in infectious complications, was observed in that they were reduced by 41 % ($p<0.00001$); there was no change in mortality. Recommendations are to start supplementation at least 5 days preoperatively and continue postoperatively as feasible [34].

Activation of lymphocytes during stressed states initially causes an increase in energy requirements, followed by a need for ribonucleic acid (RNA) and deoxyribonucleic acid (DNA) synthesis for protein production and cell division. Dietary RNA is thought to be necessary in maintaining adequate immune function. Nucleotides are essential in the regulation of T-cell-mediated immune responses and increased protein synthesis [38]. Animal studies have shown improvement in antibody and T-cell responses with nucleotide supplementation [34].

To conclude the discussion on immunonutrition, it is important to note that current literature widely supports the use of immune-enhancing nutrients in trauma patients and in those after major surgery; there is a suggestion that complication and infection rates are reduced. However, overwhelming sepsis accompanied by prolonged mechanical ventilation carries a poor prognosis that is not likely altered by nutritional formulations. Immunonutrition may improve outcome in malnourished patients with less life-threatening illness, but the literature remains controversial [39].

Assessment of Nutritional Needs

Screening

When screening critically ill patients for nutritional support, severity of disease, organ system functions, metabolic abnormalities, gastrointestinal function, and projected impact of therapeutic interventions must be considered. The primary goals of adequate nutritional support in the critically ill include providing adequate protein and caloric intake, promoting immune response, enhancing wound healing capabilities, and preventing or replacing essential nutrient deficiencies [40]. As noted previously, many patients are malnourished prior to hospitalization; this may be unrecognized and lead to inadequate nutritional treatment [41]. The use of nutritional screening tools will identify patients who are at risk for malnutrition and who need a more detailed assessment.

Malnutrition has been measured in terms of change in body composition and structure, change in organ and tissue function, and laboratory measurements of immunological and biochemical variables. The initial step in determining nutritional needs is to thoroughly evaluate the patient's present nutritional status, preadmission dietary history, recent weight loss, alcohol intake, body mass index, and functional status to recognize the presence of, or risk of, developing malnutrition. In the critical care setting, a change in body weight likely represents fluid imbalances and is not a reliable predictor of outcome [4].

A detailed, yet nutritionally focused, physical examination should be performed on all critically ill patients. Body habitus, oral health, edema, skin turgor, muscle bulk, and loss of muscle mass should be assessed [41]. Objective, noninvasive, and inexpensive evaluation through anthropometric measurements of skinfold thickness, triceps, and mid-arm muscle circumference can be done quickly at bedside but offer little clinical benefit as the measurements vary with size and are affected by fluid shifts [4]. Additionally, these measurements overestimate body fat in malnourished individuals while underestimating body fat in obese patients. As noted by Bistrian and colleagues approximately 40 years ago, anthropometry is not an accurate tool for critically ill patients [41].

A basic metabolic profile, complete blood count, liver function panel, magnesium, and phosphorus level should be considered with the initial laboratory assessment of critically ill patients [40]. Despite low sensitivity and specificity, plasma albumin and prealbumin levels are often measured. These levels reflect alterations in protein degradation, protein synthesis, and distributive losses indicative of critical illness, not nutritional status. Furthermore, these levels are easily altered by a host of factors including corticosteroids insulin, dehydration, thyroid hormone, inflammation, hepatic and renal dysfunction, volume overload, and malabsorption. Some literature supports the use of albumin as an effective tool for predicting mortality, sepsis, and severe infection [4]. Bioelectrical impedance analysis (BIA) is a noninvasive method of assessment which depends on the difference in electrical conductivity between the fat and fat-free mass. However, the technique assumes a normal hydration state that may not be the case in many patients hospitalized in the ICU. Further validation is needed before this technique can be accepted into routine clinical practice in the NeuroICU [42, 43].

Because there appears to be no good answer to the question of how to clinically evaluate nutritional status in the critically ill, we follow a baseline and then weekly serum prealbumin levels, tracking whether or not the values increase over time with nutritional support.

Effects of Stress or Injury on Response to Starvation

As we noted earlier, the metabolic response to illness and injury differs significantly from the effects of starvation. The hormonal milieu following stress or injury is characterized by an increase in catecholamine, glucocorticoid, glucagon, and growth hormone levels. Given the level of hyperglycemia and insulin resistance that develops at the cellular level, insulin levels are relatively low. Muscle breakdown provides amino acids used for wound healing, visceral protein, and acute-phase reactant synthesis and used to provide substrate for gluconeogenesis. This increase in protein catabolism continues until the levels of catecholamines and glucocorticoids decrease, as the inciting insult is controlled or reversed. Continued starvation with persistent stress state leads to rapid depletion of skeletal and visceral protein, resulting in weakness, impaired immune response, organ dysfunction, and, potentially, death. The hypermetabolic state seen in critical illness is characterized by a significantly negative nitrogen balance [4]. Nutritional support decreases net nitrogen loss, but positive nitrogen balance is not achieved until the hormonal milieu is restored toward normal levels.

Nutritional Requirements

The resting energy expenditure is a useful tool for preventing underfeeding or overfeeding in the acute care setting, either of which can have unfavorable effects on patient outcome. Once determined that a patient requires nutritional support, caloric needs must be calculated. There are several formulae available to estimate caloric requirements based on age, gender, weight, and height. A standard weight-based estimate of caloric needs is 25–30 kcal/kg of ideal body weight; ideal body weight is calculable (Devine formula) based upon the patient's height and gender [44]:

$$\text{Male IBW}(\text{kg}) = 50 + 2.3 \times [(\text{TH in cm} / 2.54) - 60]$$

$$\text{Female IBW}(\text{kg}) = 45 + 2.3 \times [(\text{TH in cm} / 2.54) - 60]$$

where TH = true height. If true height is not available, the patient's representation of their height is the next closest measure for the calculation [44].

A variation on the theme of Weir—the metabolic cart—allows the measurement of oxygen consumption and carbon dioxide production to determine caloric needs for a patient [45, 46]. The formulae for Weir's equation and the Harris-Benedict equation are shown herewith:

Harris-Benedict equation:

$$Male : (66.5 + 13.8 \times weight) + (5.0 \times height) - (6.8 \times age)$$

$$Female : (665.1 + 9.6 \times weight) + (1.8 \times height) - (4.7 \times age)$$

Weir equation:

$$REE = \left[3.9\left(VO_2\right) + 1.1\left(VCO_2\right)\right] \times 1.44$$

$$VO_2 = oxygen\ uptake\left(mL\ /\ min\right)$$

$$VCO_2 = \left(carbon\ dioxide\ output\right) mL\ /\ min$$

Modified Weir equation:

$$REE = 3.9 \times oxygen\ consumption + 1.1 \times carbon\ dioxide\ production$$

$$TEE = REE \times activity\ factor$$

Activity factor = 1.15 for bedbound patients, 1.25 for ambulatory patients

As utilized with the initial evaluation of the Harris-Benedict equation, caloric needs can also be measured precisely using indirect calorimetry. The Harris-Benedict equations have been shown to overestimate the actual energy expenditure measurements performed by indirect calorimetry by 6–15 % [47, 48]. By measuring the patient's oxygen consumption and carbon dioxide production, the respiratory quotient and caloric expenditure can be calculated. The resulting resting energy expenditure must then be multiplied by an activity factor ranging from 1.0 to 1.25, depending on how active the patient is during the remainder of the day [49, 50]. Indirect calorimetry is most frequently identified as the gold standard for caloric measuring [47, 48].

Simpler estimates of metabolic requirements are based solely on weight and the severity of injury. An adequate estimate of caloric needs is typically provided with more precise estimates or direct measurement recommended for patients who will require long-term support by using approximately 25–30 kcal/kg ideal body weight. Ideally, more than 55–60 % of goal caloric needs should be met by the first 7 days of hospitalization.

Our best sense of this literature is that while the Harris-Benedict equation is the most widely accepted formula utilized for determining resting energy requirements in humans [51, 52], indirect calorimetry is the gold standard

to determine caloric needs [53]. Where that cannot be obtained, the Penn State University modification of the Mifflin St. Jeor equation is the most consistent across patient subgroups and statistical measures [54]. These two equations are detailed herewith:

Mifflin St. Jeor equation:

$$Men : 10\left(wt\right) + 6.25\left(ht\right) - 5\left(age\right) + 5$$

$$Women : 10\left(wt\right) + 6.25\left(ht\right) - 5\left(age\right) - 161$$

Pennsylvania State University modification of the Mifflin equation:

$$PSU\left(m\right) = Mifflin\left(0.96\right) + T_{max}\left(167\right) + Ve(31) - 6212$$

T_{max} is maximum body temperature in the previous 24 h, and Ve is minute ventilation at the time of measurement, read from the ventilator, not the calorimeter.

Source of Calories

Carbohydrates

Polysaccharides, or carbohydrates, are polymers of simple sugars, in various combinations including glucose, galactose, and fructose. Carbohydrates are typically used to provide the majority of nonprotein calories during nutritional support and are the main source of cellular energy. Patients can usually metabolize 5 g/kg/day of carbohydrate. With enteral nutrition, disaccharide and polysaccharides are used and provide 4 kcal of energy per gram of carbohydrate. Intravenous formulations contain dextrose, which provides only 3.4 kcal/g due to water content. As a result of high energy requirements, patients with neurologic injury, particularly traumatic brain injury, may require higher levels of carbohydrate intake. This increased carbohydrate load, together with the insulin resistance typically seen in these stressed patients, often leads to hyperglycemia. The use of steroids potentiates the insulin resistance, and patients may require large doses of insulin to maintain normoglycemia [4, 17].

Hyperglycemia seems to be more problematic with the use of parenteral nutrition as compared to enteral nutrition. One approach to this problem is to use a tight intravenous sliding scale for regular insulin administration to maintain the glucose level between 120 and 150 mg/dL. Each day, the amount of insulin administered by sliding scale during the previous 24 h is tabulated, and one-third to one-half of that amount is added to the TPN. We do not add more than 50–80 units of regular insulin to each bag of 1.5–2 L TPN solution. The rationale for this decision is that if more insulin is added and the patient becomes hypoglycemic, the entire bag of TPN will have to be stopped. If the patient requires—as many do—further amounts of insulin to maintain glycemic control, we avoid longer-acting subcutaneous insulin preparations due to erratic absorption in critically ill patients and the risk of hypoglycemia if feedings are stopped, as frequently happens with enteral nutrition. If hyperglycemia remains a problem despite appropriate insulin supplementation, the amount of carbohydrate can be decreased, and the calories can be provided with lipids [4, 17, 55, 56].

Lipids

Lipids as an energy source for cells provide additional calories and prevent fatty acid deficiency. There are several advantages to using fat as a calorie source. First, fewer glucose calories are needed, reducing the risk of hyperglycemia. Second, because fat has higher caloric density than dextrose, fluids can be more easily restricted if necessary. Finally, metabolism of lipids, with a respiratory quotient (RQ) of 0.7, generates less carbon dioxide than the metabolism of dextrose, which has an RQ of 1.0. This difference may be significant in a patient with marginal respiratory status. Typically, lipid is administered to provide 30–40 % of non-protein calories [4, 17].

The type of lipid administered may have important implications in the critically ill patient. The omega-6 fatty acids, primarily linoleic acid, are precursors of arachidonic acid, giving rise to potent inflammatory mediators, which may have a pathologic role in sepsis and multiorgan failure. Omega-3 fatty acids give rise to less potent inflammatory mediators and may be beneficial in controlling the inflammatory response. In fact, some studies have shown improved outcome when enteral feedings were supplemented with omega-3 fatty acids in addition to RNA and glutamine [57, 58]. However, decreasing the production of inflammatory mediators may impair the host response to infection, and these supplements should be used with caution until more data are available. Intravenous lipid formulations currently contain large amounts of linoleic acid with very little omega-3 fatty acids.

We recommend the provision of a lipid source with 50–70 % medium-chain triglycerides and an omega-6 to omega-3 ratio of 2:1–8:1 to minimize negative effects of omega-6 fatty acids on the immune system and to provide an easily absorbed and utilized source of lipids.

Protein

Proteins are essential molecules utilized in all cell activity and are the most important macronutrients for supporting immune function and maintaining lean body mass. Nitrogen requirements will vary depending on the severity of the patient's stress response. Healthy, unstressed individuals will typically require roughly 0.5 g of protein (0.08 g nitrogen) per kilogram ideal body weight per day to maintain nitrogen balance. During periods of physiologic stress, however, protein catabolism significantly increases, leading to increased nitrogen excretion and negative nitrogen balance. In most patients, this net nitrogen loss can be attenuated or even eliminated by administering large amounts of calories and protein. In patients undergoing gastrectomy, Holden and colleagues showed that 40 kcal/kg/day and 0.34 g nitrogen per kg per day significantly decreased nitrogen loss compared to lower levels of calorie and protein intake. Some of these patients achieved nitrogen equilibrium. Effects on clinical outcome were not reported in this study [57, 58].

Protein needs should be continually assessed throughout the hospital stay. We recommend the provision of 2–2.3 g protein per kg ideal body weight per day if renal function is normal. If the gut is utilized, protein should be administered as small peptides to improve tolerance, absorption, utilization, and gut integrity.

Micronutrients

Micronutrients are substances present in relatively small amounts in serum and tissue and include vitamins (organic) and trace elements (inorganic). These substances play important roles in various metabolic pathways, including macronutrient utilization, wound healing, antioxidant defense, nucleic acid synthesis, oxygen transport, and control of metabolic rate. The role of specific micronutrients and the effects of deficiency states have been reviewed elsewhere [59, 60]. Measurement of serum levels of specific micronutrients is difficult; deficiencies are best prevented by beginning supplementation early in the course of illness. Provision of 1–2 L/day of enteral nutrition will typically contain adequate doses of micronutrients. For patients receiving TPN, micronutrients should be added as commercial preparations of vitamins and trace elements.

Timing of Initiating Nutritional Support

Prolonged starvation will clearly lead to death, but conflicting data on how soon one must initiate nutritional support remain. The use of early feeding in critically ill patients with a greater than 10 % weight loss in the 6 months prior to admission or severe prehospital malnutrition with BMI less than 18.5 is widely supported. Some studies have suggested that initiation of enteral feeling within 48 h will lower infection rates and improve wound healing [40]. However, adequately nourished patients can withstand several days of postoperative semi-starvation without adverse effects [61]. Guidelines published by the American Society of Parenteral and Enteral Nutrition (ASPEN) suggest that supplemental nutrition may be beneficial to mildly malnourished patients if they are not expected to resume feeding within 7 days. Severely malnourished patients should receive some form of nutrition within 1–3 days [61, 62].

The argument for delaying feeds in metabolically stressed patients is twofold. First, anorexia following injury may be an adaptive response. During an inflammatory response, tumor necrosis factor (TNF-α) and interleukin-1 (IL-1) cause appetite suppression, which may provide some survival benefit. For example, elimination of the energy expenditure required to acquire food conserves energy for other processes such as wound healing, particularly if the individual failed to obtain food due to inability to effectively compete while injured. Also, diversion of blood flow to the gut after eating might be harmful in times of hemodynamic instability. Second, ingestion of specific substrates, such as omega-6 fatty acids, may potentiate the inflammatory response and possibly contribute to MSOF [61, 62].

The clinical decision to start nutrition is based upon the patient's pre-injury nutritional status, the nature of their injury, and the expectation of when they will be able to resume normal oral intake. Initiation of nutritional support is a matter of both art and science. Most previously well-nourished patients can tolerate several days of minimal nutritional support with protein-sparing levels of carbohydrates without developing deleterious effects, while malnourished patients typically benefit from earlier initiation of nutritional support [61, 62].

Route of Nutrient Administration

Intestinal Barrier Function

The intestinal lumen contains the largest number of bacteria and toxins in the body, including a wide variety of anaerobic and aerobic bacteria [5]. The gut serves as an immunologic and metabolic organ responsible for digesting and excreting food as well maintaining a barrier against bacteria and antigens [63]. Physical stressors including trauma and major surgery have been associated with increased intestinal permeability, though no studies have actually evaluated the influence of physiologic strain on intestinal permeability in humans. In most patients, bacterial concentration distal to the ileocecal valve is 102 colony-forming units per mL with anaerobic bacteria outnumbering aerobes by 1,000-fold. Stress stimulates the secretion of water, mucus, and ions. Defects in the intestinal barrier related to stress commonly result in enhanced passage of molecules through the mucosal barrier [64]. Enteral starvation is associated with alterations in intestinal villous morphology and permeability. The main concern with intestinal barrier function is translocation of bacteria and endotoxins becoming a trigger for MSOF.

Bacterial translocation can be described as "the passage of viable resident bacteria from the gastrointestinal tract to normally sterile tissues" [63].

Impairment of the intestinal wall is thought to result in an uncontrolled and continuous release of antigens and over-stimulated macrophages, resulting in translocation. The combination of malnutrition with intestinal hypoperfusion and metabolic stress increases the risk for bacterial translocation, impairs the functionality of the intestinal wall, and precipitates infection [5]. Critically ill patients are at increased risk of developing significant proximal gut overgrowth of enteric organisms. Bacterial translocation is thought to occur on a frequent basis in the human population but is not fully understood. Increased septic morbidity is associated with bacterial translocation in surgical, trauma, critically ill, and immunosuppressed patients [65].

Enteral Feeding

The majority of emerging literature surrounding nutrition in the critically ill supports the implementation of early post-operative nutritional support in high-risk surgical and multiple trauma patients. The implementation of early nutritional support is associated with decreasing septic morbidity, improving wound healing, and maintaining adequate immune functioning. It is generally accepted that using the enteral route is the preferred method of nutritional support in patients with a functional gastrointestinal tract; however, the optimal route of delivery remains debated. Enteral nutrition is felt to prevent gastrointestinal atrophy, maintain a competent immune system, attenuate stress response to injury, and preserve the normal gut flora. Unfortunately, current studies lack adequate sample sizes to determine whether enteral nutrition improves clinical outcome by maintaining normal intestinal barrier function [66–68]. To receive maximum benefit from enteral nutrition, clinicians should minimize nothing by mouth orders for procedures and avoid holding enteral feeds for gastric volumes less than 500 mL [17]. If the hypermetabolic state associated with major surgical procedure and multiple traumatic injuries is not supported by exogenous substrate administration, proteolysis of skeletal muscle occurs followed by exhaustion of crucial proteins [66].

The small bowel and colon harbor large numbers of potentially pathogenic bacteria, and many clinicians believe translocation of bacteria and/or toxins contributes to multi-organ failure. By preventing villous atrophy and maintaining normal permeability, enteral nutrition could theoretically prevent bacterial translocation. However, this theory has yet to be proven. Current research has shown that enteral nutrition maintains gut function by preserving tight junctions, stimulating blood flow, and causing the release of cholecystokinin, gastrin, bombesin, and bile salts [17]. While animal studies show intestinal atrophy with total parenteral nutrition (TPN), gut atrophy and bacterial translocation are not necessarily related. Illig and colleagues examined histologic intestinal structure and intestinal permeability to lactulose and mannitol in rats fed parenterally or enterally [69]. Parenteral feeding alone led to significant intestinal atrophy, cecal bacterial overgrowth, and increased lactulose permeability. However, bacterial translocation, as measured by cultures of mesenteric lymph nodes, blood, and peritoneal fluid, was not significantly increased. Additionally, although TPN can be more rapidly advanced, the use of TPN is accompanied by increased nitrogen excretion [66]. Conversely, Helton and Garcia demonstrated in a murine model that prevention of the intestinal atrophy associated with parenteral feeding does not prevent bacterial translocation. By orally administering 16,16-dimethyl-PGE2, a synthetic prostaglandin with trophic effects on the gut, these investigators were able to prevent intestinal atrophy in rats receiving parenteral nutrition. However, the rate of bacterial translocation was similar with and without prostaglandin and was much higher than the rate in animals receiving enteral feeds [59, 70]. Longer-term (7–14 days) studies in rats show that total parenteral nutrition, as compared to enteral feeding, may increase bacterial translocation to mesenteric lymph nodes, but the effects on distal bacterial spread and mortality are not clear [67, 71–73].

Several human studies have reported positive mesenteric lymph nodes in patients undergoing abdominal surgery. Presumably, the source of bacteria was the gut [44, 46, 74, 75]. In the largest study, involving 267 patients, bacterial translocation occurred in 10 % of patients, but there was no correlation between bacterial translocation and nutritional status or intestinal villous height [52, 76]. Others have been unable to demonstrate either gut atrophy [60, 74] or increased permeability [77, 78] following short periods (5–21 days) without enteral feeding, though there are decreases in enzyme activities of the brush border [62, 79]. While several studies suggest lower septic morbidity with enteral nutrition compared to TPN (see the section on Parenteral Nutrition in this chapter) [66, 80], there are no studies directly relating enteral nutrition and bacterial translocation in humans.

In summary, bacterial translocation likely does occur in humans and could potentially lead to infection. However, short-term absence of enteral nutrition in humans causes neither gut atrophy nor increased permeability. At this time, the relationship between bacterial translocation and enteral nutrition remains unclear.

Reaching full nutritional goals by enteral feeding alone remains difficult in patients with poor appetites or inability to eat. Placement and maintenance of a post-pyloric feeding tube is often time-consuming and labor intensive. While some studies have shown no difference in aspiration risk between gastric and intestinal feeding [73, 74, 81, 82], these studies involved relatively small numbers of patients. Thus, it is our practice to feed into the small bowel whenever possible. More recent studies have shown a reduction in hospital-acquired pneumonia in patients who received small intestine feeds as opposed to gastric feeds [83]. For further prevention of pneumonia, consider the institution of a respiratory bundle including head of bed above 30°, subglottic suction, and chlorhexidine mouth care for intubated patients. The rationale for this approach is supported by the findings of delayed gastric emptying [42, 75] and lower esophageal sphincter dysfunction in patients with traumatic brain injury [76, 84]. Furthermore, post-pyloric feeding is often better tolerated, allowing increased caloric intake and improved nitrogen balance [24].

Other commonly encountered complications of enteral feeding include diarrhea and abdominal distention. These can typically be treated by reducing the volume of feeding. It is important to first determine the cause of the diarrhea. Review current medications and look for possible infectious cause of diarrhea. Infectious causes of diarrhea, such as *C. difficile* toxin, should be ruled out. Once infection is ruled out, adding fiber to the formula or adding anti-motility agents may be helpful.

Parenteral

Total parenteral nutrition (TPN), or hyperalimentation (HAL), is often used for nutritional support when the enteral route cannot be utilized. TPN has the advantage of being relatively well tolerated, often making it easier to achieve full nutritional support when compared to enteral feeding. In addition, the amounts of carbohydrate, fat, protein, and electrolytes can be easily adjusted on a daily basis. Disadvantages of TPN include the need for central venous access, risk of refeeding syndrome if nutrition is advanced too rapidly, relatively high risk of hyperglycemia, and possibly an increased risk of infection. Our colleague and mentor, Edward M. Copeland, III, has recently very nicely reviewed the history of TPN use on malignancy [85].

Peripheral parenteral nutrition (PPN) is less hypertonic and can be given through a peripheral vein. While full caloric support is not possible, PPN may be useful to supplement enteral feeding when complete enteral nutrition cannot be achieved. Regardless of whether central or peripheral parenteral nutrition is used, continued attempts to initiate enteral nutrition should be made and advanced as tolerated. Once 60 % of goal enteral nutrition is met, the parenteral nutrition can be stopped to avoid overfeeding. The Canadian Clinical Practice Guideline for nutritional support in mechanically ventilated critically ill patients notes that there is reduced mortality in patients receiving intravenous glutamine with parental nutrition [83].

Enteral versus Parenteral Nutrition

Given the preceding considerations, the preferred route of nutrient administration remains controversial. Parenteral nutrition is typically easier to administer and may allow full nutritional goals to be reached earlier, possibly improving outcome. However, several studies in critically ill trauma victims have demonstrated reduced morbidity in patients receiving enteral nutrition as compared to parenteral nutrition [41, 45, 66, 78–80]. In a meta-analysis of 230 high-risk surgical patients, those administered early enteral nutrition had lower rates of infection than those receiving early parenteral nutrition [66]. The difference was most evident in blunt trauma patients. When catheter sepsis was factored out, the difference in infection rates remained. Based on the available data, we recommend starting early enteral feeding in patients with neurologic injury. If full nutrition cannot be tolerated within 24–48 h, parenteral nutrition can be added as a supplemental or complete source of nutrition.

Special Formulations

In recent years, enteral feeding formulae have been supplemented with nutrients designed to enhance immune function and improve outcome. These additives include arginine, nucleotides, omega-3 fatty acids, and glutamine. While these specialized formulae are touted as immune enhancing, their benefits have only been demonstrated in select groups of patients, and many of the studies in humans have been limited by design flaws or small sample size. In a meta-analysis of immune-enhancing diets (IEDs) in critically ill patients, supplementation of enteral feeds with arginine, omega-3 fatty acids, and nucleotides, with or without glutamine, significantly reduced infection rates, ventilator days, and hospital length of stay. Mortality rates were not affected [55, 56]. According to the ASPEN guidelines, diets supplemented with glutamine have been shown to reduce the rate of infection complications, ICU length of stay, and mortality. However, the studies supporting these data were done with a glutamine preparation that is not available in North America. Antioxidant vitamins (vitamin E, ascorbic acid), trace minerals (selenium, zinc, copper), and parental selenium may also improve outcomes. These results were found in critically ill septic, burn, and trauma patients requiring mechanical ventilation, and the correlation with the critically ill neurologically impaired patient is unknown. While these findings are not insignificant, as of yet, these specialized enteral formulae have not been well studied in patients with severe neurologic injury, and clinical information is inadequate to recommend routine use of these products.

It is relatively clear that, at least as far as arginine goes, its use in the medically critically ill patient either leads to no better or even worse outcome; by way of contrast, in critically ill surgical or trauma patients, it seems to improve outcome [86].

Monitoring Nutritional Status

Just as assessing initial nutritional status is difficult in critically ill patients, monitoring the response to nutritional support is also somewhat challenging. Weight gain is often unreliable due to large fluid shifts. Nitrogen balance can be measured at intervals of 2–3 days to assess trends, with the understanding that positive nitrogen balance is difficult or impossible to achieve in the early days following acute injury. Albumin levels are not useful due to the long half-life (about 20 days), but prealbumin, an acute-phase reactant with a half-life of two to three days, can provide a measure of protein synthesis. Serial measurements of resting energy expenditure will allow fine-tuning of caloric intake, since the metabolic rate may decrease as the acute response to injury abates [51, 80].

Nitrogen balance studies assess the adequacy of the present treatment more than an identification of past deficits:

$$\text{Nitrogen balance} = \frac{\text{Dietary protein}}{6.25} - \left(\frac{\text{Urine urea nitrogen}}{0.8} + 4 \right)$$

A positive nitrogen balance in the range of 2–4 g/day is desired but can be difficult to achieve in the critically ill patient. Furthermore, if a patient is having increased stool losses and the number 4 in the previous equation, otherwise known as the "fudge factor," is utilized, the patient in positive nitrogen balance may actually have a negative balance.

Clinicians should use caution when using these equations to predict caloric needs as they are much less reliable in critically ill patients and those in extremes of weight.

Special Populations

The NeuroICU Patient

In the neurologically injured patient, the hypermetabolic state is characterized by a marked negative nitrogen balance, diminished lipolysis, and the development of relative glucose intolerance. In addition to elevated catecholamine, glucocorticoid, glucagon, and growth hormone levels, the hyperdynamic state associated with severe neurologic injury is accompanied by increased cardiac output and cardiac work, tachycardia, and mild hypertension. Increased pulmonary shunting and increased oxygen delivery and use correlate with arterial levels of epinephrine and norepinephrine. The result is a potentially significant prolonged increase in oxygen consumption and caloric requirements that can persist for up to 1 year. Biochemical consequences of stressed states include hyperglycemia, impaired wound healing, and decreased serum levels of proteins including albumin, transferrin, retinol-binding protein, and prealbumin. A simultaneous decrease in C-reactive protein, interleukin-1, and interleukin-6 as well as depressed cell-mediated immune function occurs. In addition, serum zinc levels are depressed, and urinary zinc losses increase dramatically, therefore decreasing protein and collagen synthesis. Physiologic consequences of metabolic stress include delayed upper gastrointestinal function resulting in delayed gastric emptying and increased gastric residuals, sepsis, altered vascular permeability, and intestinal edema with mucosal damage, malabsorption, and bacterial translocation. Increased energy requirements are an adaptive modification in individuals with neurologic insult.

Patients with head injury typically have higher energy expenditure than other critically ill patients, with resting energy expenditure as much as 60 % higher than predicted [49, 87–89]. The cause of this elevated energy expenditure is not completely understood but is at least partly due to increased muscle tone. Patient temperature and barbiturate use also influence energy expenditure. Due to significant variation in resting energy expenditure between patients, this population is likely to benefit from direct measurement of resting energy expenditure using indirect calorimetry. In the head-injured patient, the goal of nutritional support is maintenance rather than repletion. Attempting to fully replete nutritional status can be harmful, leading to increased carbon dioxide production, deposition of fat and glycogen in the liver, and hyperglycemia.

Studies in patients with severe head injury suggest that early nutritional support may improve outcome. Rapp and colleagues prospectively randomized head injury patients to receive either TPN or enteral feeding. Because gastric feedings were poorly tolerated, patients in the TPN group received significantly more calories and protein as compared to those in the enteral feeding group. Over the 18-day study period, mortality was significantly lower in the TPN group with eight deaths in the enteral group as compared to no deaths in the TPN group ($p < 0.001$) [50, 77]. In another prospective study, Young and colleagues also compared enteral feeding and TPN feeding. Again, the TPN patients achieved higher caloric and protein intake compared to those receiving

enteral nutrition, and this translated to better neurologic outcomes at 3 months post-injury. At 6 and 12 months post-injury, the difference in neurologic outcome was no longer statistically significant [48].

Avoidance of hyperglycemia is of particular concern in the patient with neurologic injury, as several studies suggest that elevated glucose levels may worsen neurologic outcome. The exact goal for glucose management in critically ill patients remains unclear as data differ between studies. The American Diabetes Association currently recommends keeping blood glucose levels between 110 and 140 mg/dL in critically ill patients [90]. In animals, administration of intravenous glucose before or during resuscitation from cardiac arrest worsens neurologic outcome as compared to controls receiving no glucose [88, 89, 91, 92]. Observational studies in humans reveal that hyperglycemia is associated with worse neurologic outcome following traumatic brain injury (TBI). Young and colleagues followed glucose levels in 59 brain-injured patients and found that patients with peak glucose levels greater than 200 mg/dL within 24 h of admission had worse neurologic outcome at 3–12 months [56, 91]. Similarly, Rovlias and Kotsuo prospectively studied 267 patients with TBI who underwent general anesthesia for hematoma evacuation or placement of intracranial pressure monitoring. In patients with severe head injury and GCS of eight or below, postoperative glucose levels greater than 200 mg/dL were associated with worse outcome [58, 92]. Multivariate analysis confirmed that glucose levels were an independent predictor of outcome.

There are no prospective, randomized studies to date comparing tight versus loose glucose control, and it is unlikely that such a study will be performed secondary to associated risks. Based on the available data, it is recommended that carbohydrate intake be monitored closely with supplemental insulin administered as needed to maintain a serum glucose level greater than 110 mg/dL but less than 140 mg/dL in nondiabetic patients to avoid worsening of neurologic outcome following brain injury; insulin therapy should be initiated for serum glucose greater than 180 mg/dL [90]. The same approach seems reasonable for other forms of neurologic insult including spinal cord injury. Given these data, our practice is to keep the serum glucose levels between 120 and 150 mg/dL—recognizing that hypoglycemia is also a potential problem—and to use an intravenous insulin infusion to maintain the glucose values in this range.

Patients with spinal cord injury are particularly at high risk for developing hyperglycemia as large doses of corticosteroids are frequently administered for 24–48 h post-injury. The patient with spinal cord injury represents a special situation with regard to nitrogen balance. In this group, it may be impossible to achieve positive nitrogen balance despite administration of large amounts of calories and protein. Rodriguez and colleagues compared ten patients with spinal cord injury with 20 control patients matched for time, gender, age, and injury severity score (ISS) [55, 60]. Despite receiving 120 % of predicted caloric needs and 2.4 g protein per kilogram per day, patients with spinal cord injury did not achieve positive nitrogen balance until 2 months after injury, while 85 % of those without spinal cord injury achieved positive nitrogen balance by the third week after injury. Indirect calorimetry confirmed that the delivered calories were adequate, providing an average of 110 % of measured energy needs. The mechanism of persistent negative nitrogen balance in patients with spinal cord injury is not fully understood but may be related to muscle breakdown from immobilization and denervation atrophy. Following the period of acute injury, energy expenditure may be significantly less than that predicted by standard formulae [57, 66]. In patients who cannot regulate their own intake, indirect calorimetry may be useful to determine caloric requirements.

The Obese Patient

In obese patients, estimations of caloric needs are less accurate, and a more direct measurement of caloric need should be used for accuracy [17]. Current ASPEN guidelines recommend permissive underfeeding for obese patients. If the patient's BMI is above 30, the goal feeds should be 60–70 % of the targeted energy requirements. Protein requirements should be 2 or 2.5 g/kg of ideal body weight for a BMI between 30 and 40 and for BMI greater than 40, respectively. However, underfeeding should be performed with extreme caution in neurologically impaired critically ill patients. A study by Bolinger and colleagues in 1966 analyzed lean body mass and energy expenditure in an obese woman who received a very-low-calorie diet for 3 weeks. This study showed an increase in metabolic efficacy with normalized nitrogen balance and increase in lean body mass energy efficiency [93]. Nonetheless, we have successful clinical experience utilizing the ASPEN guidelines for the morbidly obese patient, albeit in a non-published series of multidisciplinary ICU patients.

Complications

The efficacy of artificial nutrition in critically ill patients remains unclear, but complications associated with feeding have been identified. Serious and even fatal metabolic complications are associated with overfeeding patients and with the initiation of feeding after a prolonged period of starvation known as refeeding. Patients in the extremes of size and age are highly vulnerable to developing overfeeding

syndrome. Excessive protein intake has been associated with hypertonic dehydration, metabolic acidosis, and azotemia. Hyperglycemia, hepatic steatosis, and hypertriglyceridemia have been associated with high quantities of carbohydrate infusions. Disproportionately high-fat infusions have led to the development of fat overload syndrome and hypertriglyceridemia. Aggressive forms of overfeeding can potentiate hypercapnia and increase the risk of refeeding syndrome.

Azotemia develops when the rate of urea production surpasses the rate of excretion causing a surplus of nitrogen-rich compounds in the blood stream often resulting in renal failure. Accelerated proteolysis in conjunction with excessive protein delivery will frequently precipitate azotemia. Excessive protein intake also causes an acid–base imbalance within the blood stream resulting in metabolic acidosis. Lastly, extraordinarily high protein infusion can lead to hypertonic dehydration. This condition is characterized by cellular dehydration and shrinkage as a result of extracellular water losses being greater than electrolyte losses. The fluid shift causes a subsequent increase in plasma osmolarity creating a hypertonic volume deficit [4].

Excessive infusion of carbohydrates associated with overfeeding syndrome can lead to a myriad of complications including hyperglycemia, hypertriglyceridemia, and hepatic steatosis. Regardless of overfeeding, hyperglycemia is a common complication in critically ill patients due to increased catecholamine levels and decreased insulin resistance, which has been associated with increased infection and higher mortality rates in the critically ill population. Hyperglycemia in neurology patients is associated with worse neurologic outcomes. Overfeeding with excessive carbohydrate and fat often leads to the development of hypertriglyceridemia. For patients receiving a propofol infusion, a lipid-based medication shown to decrease tissue oxidation and carbon dioxide production, a lipid infusion rate greater than 2 g/kg/day has been associated with rapid onset hypertriglyceridemia [4]. Exogenous lipid administration associated with overfeeding or fat redistribution from adipose tissue results in hepatic steatosis, defined as an accumulation of hepatic fat and triglyceride concentration greater than 5 % of the total liver weight. As a result, hepatocytes develop a decreased sensitivity to insulin precipitating insulin resistance. Although typically a reversible process, if the inciting agent is not removed or controlled, hepatic steatosis can progress to steatohepatitis, cirrhosis, and/or hepatocellular carcinoma [94].

Fat overload syndrome is a life-threatening complication of overfeeding coupled with high-fat-concentration infusions. This condition is manifested by respiratory distress, coagulopathies, and abnormal liver function tests. In severe cases, renal failure, fever, rash, thrombocytopenia, anemia, hypertension, and tachycardia develop. Another complication of overfeeding in critically ill patients is the development of hypercapnia. As the ratio of carbohydrates to fat increases in overfeeding, substrate oxidation and intracellular carbon dioxide increase simultaneously, leading to cellular breakdown and increased adenosine triphosphate production [4].

One of the most severe complications in critically ill patients during the initiation of artificial feeding is refeeding syndrome, which often occurs following periods of starvation or in the early stages of overfeeding. While the body remains in a catabolic state, intracellular phosphate is released and excreted through urine. Refeeding syndrome is characterized by a massive shift in essential electrolytes such as magnesium, phosphorus, and potassium from the extracellular to intracellular space. Body cell mass is depleted slowly leading to an increase in sodium retention with extracellular expansion. With extracellular expansion, an instantaneous increase in morbidity and mortality rates occurs. The initiation of aggressive nutritional support is linked to an increase in cardiovascular demand. However, starvation and overall catabolism associated with critical illness lead to a depletion of cardiac muscle mass, putting the patient at increased risk for complications.

Lastly, patients receiving long TPN often require central venous access, putting them at greater risk for central line-associated infection and procedural complications. Complications associated with placement of a central venous catheter include bleeding, hematoma formation, catheter occlusion, pneumothorax, malposition, air embolism, and arterial puncture [4].

Summary

Nutritional support plays an essential role in the care of critically ill patients and those with severe neurologic injury based on the known metabolic reactions associated with malnutrition and hypermetabolic states. The basis of nutritional support focuses on improving physiologic impairments in cardiac function, acid–base balance, respiratory muscle function, renal function and electrolyte balance, and the coagulation cascade. Benefits include attenuation of protein catabolism, improved respiratory function, immune response, and decreased length of stay. Whenever possible, literature suggests that enteral feeding is preferred over parenteral nutrition. Rapid identification of malnourished patients and those at high risk of developing malnutrition remains crucial to patient outcome in the intensive care unit. Delivery of 25–30 kcal/kg ideal body weight per day and 1.5 g of protein per kilogram ideal body weight per day is a reasonable starting point, with modification based—preferably—on measured energy expenditure and measurement of nitrogen balance and/or prealbumin levels. The primary goal of therapy in malnourished patients during a catabolic state is to meet energy requirements and supplement hypermetabolism to prevent protein catabolism. Clinicians should actively work to supplement essential vitamins and minerals while slowly reaching nutritional goals and preventing the development of detrimental complications. Nutritional support guidelines will need constant monitoring and may need to be modified to promote recovery from critical illness and aid in maintaining a sense of metabolic stability. Proficient nutritional support is best reached with repeated evaluation and close monitoring of feeding tolerance.

Acknowledgment We want to acknowledge that Dr. Ricardo Laramendi was a coauthor with Dr. Caruso on the previous edition of this chapter. The first edition chapter served as inspiration for the second edition chapter.

References

1. World Health Organization. Management of severe malnutrition: a manual for physicians and other senior health workers. Geneva: World Health Organization; 1999. p. 4–39.
2. Saladin KS. Anatomy and physiology: the unity of form and function. New York: McGraw-Hill; 2001.
3. Cahill Jr GF. Starvation in man. N Engl J Med. 1970;282:668–75.
4. Slone DS. Nutritional support of the critically ill and injured patient. Crit Care Clin. 2004;20:135–57.
5. Lundholm K, Hytlander A, Sandstrom R. Nutrition and multiple organ failure. Nutr Res Rev. 1992;5:97–115.
6. Danforth E, Burger AG. The impact of nutrition on thyroid hormone physiology and action. Annu Rev Nutr. 1989;9:201–27.
7. Ravussin E, Lillioja S, Anderson TE, et al. Determinants of 24-hour energy expenditure in man: methods and results using a respiratory chamber. J Clin Invest. 1986;78:1568–78.
8. Patrick J, Golden MHN. Leukocyte electrolytes and sodium transport in protein energy malnutrition. Am J Clin Nutr. 1977;30:1478–81.
9. Keys A, Brozek J, Henschel A, et al. The biology of human starvation. Minneapolis: University of Minnesota Press; 1950.
10. Castaneda C. Muscle wasting and protein metabolism. J Anim Sci. 2002;80:E98–105.
11. Gadisseux P, Ward JD, Young HF, Becker DP. Nutrition and the neurosurgical patient. J Neurosurg. 1984;60:219–32.
12. Moran L, Custer P, Murphy G, Grant J. Nutritional assessment of lean body mass. JPEN J Parenter Enteral Nutr. 1980;4:595.
13. Muller JM, Brenner U, Dienst C, Pichlmaier N. Preoperative parenteral feeding in patients with gastrointestinal carcinoma. Lancet. 1982;9(8263):68–71.
14. Grant JP. Clinical impact of protein malnutrition on organ mass and function. In: Blackburn GL, Grant JP, Young VR, editors. Amino acids: metabolism and medical applications. Boston: John Wright; 1983. p. 347–58.
15. Viteri FE, Schneider RE. Gastrointestinal alterations in protein-calorie malnutrition. Med Clin North Am. 1974;58:1487–505.
16. Adibi SA, Allen ER. Impaired jejunal absorption rates of essential amino acids induced by either dietary, calorie, or protein deprivation in man. Gastroenterology. 1970;54:404–13.
17. McClave SA, Matrindale RG, Vanek VW, et al. Guidelines for the provision and assessment of nutritional support therapy in the adult critically ill patient: society of critical care medicine and American society for parenteral and enteral nutrition. JPEN J Parenter Enteral Nutr. 2009;33:277–316.
18. Weissman C, Askanazi J, Rosenbaum S, et al. Amino acids and respiration. Ann Intern Med. 1983;98:41–4.

19. Doekel RC, Zwilich CW, Scoggin CH, et al. Clinical semi-starvation: depression of the hypoxic ventilatory response. N Engl J Med. 1976;295:358–61.

20. Cerra FB, Alden PA, Negro F, et al. Sepsis and exogenous lipid modulation. JPEN J Parenter Enteral Nutr. 1988;12:63S–8.

21. Chandra RK, Kumari S. Nutrition and immunity: an overview. J Nutr. 1994;124(suppl):1433S–5.

22. Studley H. Percentage weight loss, a basic indicator of surgical risk in patients with chronic peptic ulcer. Nutr Hosp. 2001;16(4):141–3.

23. Rhoads JE, Alexander CE. Nutritional problems of surgical patients. Ann N Y Acad Sci. 1955;63:268–75.

24. Grahm TW, Zadrozny DB, Harrington T. The benefits of early jejunal hyperalimentation in the head-injured patient. Neurosurgery. 1989;25:729–35.

25. Buzby GP. The veterans affairs total parenteral nutrition cooperative study group: perioperative total parenteral nutrition in surgical patients. N Engl J Med. 1991;325:525–32.

26. Li S, Xu Y, Xi W, et al. Effects of enteral immunonutrition on immune function in patients with multiple trauma. World J Emerg Med. 2011;2:206–9.

27. Haydock DA, Hill GL. Improved wound healing response in surgical patients receiving intravenous nutrition. Br J Surg. 1987;74:320–3.

28. Schroeder D, Gillanders L, Mahr K, et al. Effects of immediate postoperative enteral nutrition on body composition, muscle function, and wound healing. JPEN J Parenter Enteral Nutr. 1991;15:376–83.

29. Daly JM, Vars HM, Dudrick SJ. Effects of protein depletion on strength of colonic anastomoses. Surg Gynecol Obstet. 1972;134:15–21.

30. Irvin TT, Hunt TK. Effect of malnutrition on colonic healing. Ann Surg. 1974;180:765–72.

31. Irvin TT. Effects of malnutrition and hyperalimentation on wound healing. Surg Gynecol Obstet. 1978;146:33–7.

32. Btaiche IF, Marik PE, Ochoa J, et al. Nutrition in critical illness, including immunonutrition. In: Merritt R et al., editors. The A.S.P.E.N. nutrition support practice manual. 2nd ed. Silver Springs: American Society for Parenteral and Enteral Nutrition; 2005.

33. Calder P. Immunonutrition. Br Med J. 2003;327:117–8.

34. Calder P. Immunonutrition in surgical and critically ill patients. Br J Nutr. 2007;98:S133–9.

35. Vermeulen M. Specific amino acids in the critically ill patient-exogenous glutamine/arginine: a common denominator? Crit Care Med. 2007;35:S568–76.

36. Stechmiller JK, Childress B, Porter T. Arginine immunonutrition in critically ill patients: a clinical dilemma. J Crit Care. 2004;13:17–23.

37. Waitzberg DL, Saito H, Plank LD, et al. Postsurgical infections are reduced with specialized nutrition support. World J Surg. 2006;30:1592–604.

38. O'Leary MJ, Coakley JH. Nutrition and immunonutrition. Br J Anaesth. 1996;77:118–27.

39. McCowen KC, Bistrian BR. Immunonutrition: problematic or problem solving? Am J Clin Nutr. 2003;77:764–70.

40. Taylor BE, Collins GL. Nutrition in the intensive care unit. In: The Washington manual of critical care. Philadelphia: Lippincott, Williams, and Wilkins; 2008. p. 463–72.

41. Bistrian BR, Blackburn GL, Vitale J, Cochran D, Naylor J. Prevalence of malnutrition in general medical patients. JAMA. 1976;235:1567–70.

42. Pennington CR. Disease and malnutrition in British hospitals. Proc Nutr Soc. 1997;56:393–407.

43. Dietch EA. Simple intestinal obstruction causes bacterial translocation in man. Arch Surg. 1989;124:699–701.

44. Stehman CR, Buckley RG, Dos Santos FL, et al. Bedside estimation of patient height for calculating ideal body weight in the emergency department. J Emerg Med. 2011;41:97–101.

45. Weir JB. New method for calculating metabolic rate with special reference to protein metabolism. J Physiol (London). 1949;109:1–6.

46. Brooks SG, May J, Sedman P, et al. Translocation of enteric bacteria in humans. Br J Surg. 1993;80:901–2.

47. Garrel DR, Jobin N, de Jonge LH. Should we still use the Harris-Benedict equations? Nutr Clin Pract. 1996;11:99–103.

48. Young B, Ott L, Twyman D, et al. The effect of nutritional support on outcome from severe head injury. J Neurosurg. 1987;67:668–76.

49. Van Way III CW. Nutritional support in the injured patient. Surg Clin North Am. 1991;71:537–48.

50. Rapp RP, Young B, Twyman D, et al. The favorable effect of early parenteral feeding on survival in head-injured patients. J Neurosurg. 1983;58:906–12.

51. Harris JA, Benedict FG. Standard basal metabolism constants for physiologists and clinicians. In: A biometric study of basal metabolism in man. Philadelphia: JP Lippincott Publisher; 1919.

52. Sedman PC, Macfie J, Sagar P, et al. The prevalence of gut translocation in humans. Gastroenterology. 1994;107:643–9.

53. Lev S, Cohen J, Singer P. Indirect calorimetry measurements in the ventilated critically ill patient: facts and controversies – the heat is on. Crit Care Clin. 2010;26:e1–9.

54. Frankenfield DC, Coleman A, Alam A, Cooney RN. Analysis of estimation methods for resting metabolic rate in critically ill adults. J Parenter Enteral Nutr. 2009;33:27–36.

55. Beale RJ, Bryg DJ, Bihari DJ. Immunonutrition in the critically ill: a systematic review of clinical outcome. Crit Care Med. 1999;27:2799–805.

56. Young B, Ott L, Dempsey R, et al. Relationship between admission hyperglycemia and neurologic outcome of severely brain-injured patients. Ann Surg. 1989;221:466–72.

57. Holden WD, Krieger H, Levey S, Abbott WE. The effect of nutrition on nitrogen metabolism in the surgical patient. Ann Surg. 1957;146:563–79.

58. Rovlias A, Kotsou S. The influence of hyperglycemia on neurological outcome in patients with severe head injury. Neurosurgery. 2000;46:335–42.

59. Demling RH, DeBiasse MA. Micronutrients in critical illness. In: Lang CH, Abumrad NN, editors. Critical care clinics: nutrition in the critically ill patient. Philadelphia: WB Saunders Company; 1995.

60. Rodriguez DJ, Clevenger FW, Osler TM, et al. Obligatory negative nitrogen balance following spinal cord injury. JPEN J Parenter Enteral Nutr. 1991;15:319–22.

61. ASPEN Board of Directors and the Clinical Guidelines Task Force. Guidelines for the use of parenteral and enteral nutrition in adult and pediatric patients. JPEN J Parenter Enteral Nutr. 2002;26:1SA–38.

62. Guedon C, Schmitz J, Lerebours E, et al. Decreased brush border hydrolase activities without gross morphologic changes in human intestinal mucosa after prolonged total parenteral nutrition of adults. Gastroenterology. 1986;90:373–8.

63. MacFie J. Current status of bacterial translocation as cause of surgical sepsis. Br Med Bull. 2004;71:1–11.

64. Soderholm JD, Perdue MH. Stress and intestinal barrier function. Am J Physiol Gastrointest Liver Physiol. 2001;28:G7–13.

65. O'Boyle CJ. Microbiology of bacterial translocation in humans. Gut. 1998;42:29–35.

66. Moore FA, Feliciano DV, Adrassy RJ, et al. Early enteral feeding, compared with parenteral, reduces postoperative septic complications: the results of a meta-analysis. Ann Surg. 1992;216:172–83.

67. Li L, Kudsk K, Gocinski B, et al. Effects of parenteral and enteral nutrition on gut-associated lymphoid tissue. J Trauma. 1995;39:44–51.

68. Cox SA, Weiss SM, Posuniak EA, et al. Energy expenditure after spinal cord injury: an evaluation of stable rehabilitation patients. J Trauma. 1985;25:419–23.

69. Illig KA, Ryan CK, Hardy DJ, et al. Total parenteral nutrition-induced changes in gut mucosal function: atrophy alone is not the issue. Surgery. 1992;112:631–7.

70. Helton WS, Garcia R. Oral prostaglandin E₂ prevents gut atrophy during intravenous feeding but not bacterial translocation. Arch Surg. 1993;128:178–84.

71. Alverdy JC, Aoys E, Moss GS. Total parenteral nutrition promotes bacterial translocation from the gut. Surgery. 1988;104:185–90.

72. Shou J, Lappin J, Minnard EA, et al. Total parenteral nutrition, bacterial translocation, and host immune function. Am J Surg. 1994;167:145–50.

73. Strong RM, Condon SC, Solinger MR, et al. Equal aspiration rates from postpyloric and intragastric-placed small-bore nasoenteric feeding tubes: a randomized, prospective study. JPEN J Parenter Enteral Nutr. 1992;16:59–63.

74. Spain DA, DeWeese RC, Reynolds MA, Richardson JD. Transpyloric passage of feeding tubes in patients with head injuries does not decrease complications. J Trauma. 1995;39:1100–2.

75. Ott L, Young B, Phillips R, et al. Altered gastric emptying in the head-injured patient: relationship to feeding intolerance. J Neurosurg. 1991;74:738–42.

76. Saxe JM, Ledgerwood AM, Lucas CE, Lucas WF. Lower esophageal sphincter dysfunction precludes safe gastric feeding after head injury. J Trauma. 1994;37:581–6.

77. Elia M, Goren A, Behrens R, et al. Effect of total starvation and very low calorie diets on intestinal permeability in man. Clin Sci. 1987;73:205–10.

78. Moore FA, Moore EE, Jones TN, et al. TEN versus TPN following major abdominal trauma-reduced septic morbidity. J Trauma. 1989;29:916–23.

79. Kudsk KA, Croce MA, Fabian TC, et al. Enteral versus parenteral feeding: effects on septic morbidity after blunt and penetrating abdominal trauma. Ann Surg. 1992;215:503–13.

80. Socolow EL, Woeber KA, Purdy RH, et al. Preparation of I-131-labeled human serum prealbumin and its metabolism in normal and sick patients. J Clin Invest. 1965;44:1600–9.

81. Twyman D. Nutritional management of the critically ill neurologic patient. Crit Care Clin. 1997;13:39–49.

82. Dabrowski GP, Rombeau JL. Practical nutritional management in the trauma intensive care. Surg Clin North Am. 2000;80:921–32.

83. Heyland DK. Nutritional support in the critically ill patients. A critical review of the evidence. Crit Care Clin. 1998;14:423–40.

84. Celaya-Pérez S. Soportenutricional en situacionesespeciales. En: Guíapráctica de nutrición artificial. Zaragoza: Venus IndustriasGráficas; 1992. p. 216–21.

85. Copeland III EM, Pimiento JM, Dudrick SJ. Total parenteral nutrition and cancer – from the beginning. Surg Clin North Am. 2011;91:727–36.

86. Popovic PJ, Zeh III HJ, Ochoa JB. Arginine and immunity. J Nutr. 2007;137:1681S–6.

87. Hadley MN, Grahm TW, Harrington T, et al. Nutritional support and neurotrauma: a critical review of early nutrition in fort five acute head injury patients. Neurosurgery. 1986;19:367–73.

88. Moore R, Najarian MP, Konvolinka CW. Measured energy expenditure in severe head trauma. J Trauma. 1989;29:1633–6.

89. Clifton GL, Robertson CS, Grossman RG, et al. The metabolic response to severe head injury. J Neurosurg. 1984;60:687–96.

90. Moghissi E, Kortytkowski M, Dianrdo M, et al. American association of clinical endocrinologists and American diabetes association consensus statement on inpatient glycemic control. Diabetes Care. 2009;6:1119–31.

91. D'Alecy LG, Lundy EF, Barton KH, et al. Dextrose containing intravenous fluid impairs outcome and increases death after eight minutes of cardiac arrest and resuscitation in dogs. Surgery. 1986;100:505–11.

92. Lundy EF, Kuhn JE, Kwon JM. Infusion of 5% dextrose increases mortality and morbidity following six minutes of cardiac arrest in resuscitated dogs. J Crit Care. 1987;2:4–14.

93. Fricker J, Rozen R, Melchior JC, et al. Energy-metabolism adaptation in obese adults on a very-low-calorie diet. Am J Clin Nutr. 1991;53:826–30.

94. Garg A, Misra A. Hepatic steatosis, insulin resistance and adipose tissue disorders. J Clin Endocrinol Metab. 2002;87:3019–22.

Neurologic Implications of Critical Illness and Organ Dysfunction

21

Aaron N. LacKamp and Robert D. Stevens

Contents

A.N. LacKamp, MD (✉)
Department of Anesthesiology and Critical Care Medicine,
Johns Hopkins University School of Medicine,
4940 Eastern Avenue, Baltimore, MD 21224, USA
e-mail: alackam1@jhmi.edu

R.D. Stevens, MD
Department of Anesthesiology, Critical Care Medicine,
Neurology, and Neurosurgery, Johns Hopkins University
School of Medicine, Meyer 8-140, 600 N Wolfe Street,
Baltimore, MD 21287, USA
e-mail: rstevens@jhmi.edu

Abstract

Critical illness has consequences for the nervous system. Patients experiencing critical illness are at risk for common global neurologic disturbances, such as delirium, long-term cognitive dysfunction, ICU-acquired weakness, sleep disturbances, recurrent seizures, and coma. In addition, complications related to specific organ dysfunction may be anticipated. Cardiovascular disease presents the possibility for CNS injury after cardiac arrest, sequelae of endocarditis, aberrancies of blood flow autoregulation, and malperfusion. Respiratory disease is known to cause short-term effects of hypoxia and long-term effects after ARDS. Sepsis encephalopathy and sickness behavior syndrome are early signs of infection in patients. In addition, commonly encountered organ dysfunction including uremia, hepatic failure, endocrine, and metabolic disturbances present with neurologic findings which may manifest in the critically ill patient as well.

Keywords

Delirium • Cognitive dysfunction • Coma • Posterior reversible encephalopathy syndrome • PRES • ICU-acquired weakness • ICU-AW • Critical illness polyneuropathy • Critical illness myopathy • Critical illness polyneuromyopathy • CIPNM • Sleep deprivation • Cerebral autoregulation • Hypertensive crisis • ARDS • Hepatic encephalopathy • Uremia • Dialysis disequilibrium syndrome • Septic encephalopathy • Sickness behavior syndrome

Introduction

Life-threatening alterations in central and peripheral nerve function are a central manifestation of systemic critical illness. Neurologic failure is an important sign which may herald a treatable underlying disease. It is related to many factors: changes in inflammatory and immune signaling, hypoxia, circulatory shock, infection, endocrine changes,

A.J. Layon et al. (eds.), *Textbook of Neurointensive Care*,
DOI 10.1007/978-1-4471-5226-2_21, © Springer-Verlag London 2013

metabolic changes, and medications. Acquired neurologic disorders such as delirium and ICU-acquired weakness are independently associated with adverse short-term outcome. Cognitive impairment and neuromuscular weakness are prevalent in survivors of critical illnesses in particular ARDS and sepsis. Given this chronicity, neurologic expressions of critical illness may be viewed as distinct disorders with self-sustaining biological mechanisms rather than dependent processes which resolve with remission of the inciting illness. Management should be directed to underlying mechanisms as well as symptoms.

Neurologic Disorders Acquired During Critical Illness

Altered Mental Status

The term "altered mental status" refers broadly to any change in the overall level of conscious awareness. The level of consciousness is described as a clinical spectrum ranging from hyperalert to unresponsive, with intermediate states that include delirium, lethargy, obtundation, stupor, and coma. Severe brain injury may evolve toward chronic disorders such as the vegetative and minimally conscious states. Consciousness may be viewed in terms of two separate dimensions: the level of wakefulness and the level of awareness. Wakefulness and awareness are often covariable but may be unlinked as in the vegetative state.

Delirium

Delirium is an acute confusional state developing in the setting of systemic disease. Cardinal features are an acute alteration in mental status with inattention, disorganized thinking, and a fluctuating course. Delirium presents in two motoric subtypes, the more prevalent hypoactive delirium and the more easily recognized hyperactive form. Hyperactive delirium is readily identified, while the hypoactive form may be overlooked and untreated. The incidence of delirium is very high, up to 80 % of mechanically ventilated patients [1] and 30–40 % of less severe patients in the ICU [2]. In recent years, the significance of delirium has been recognized beyond the immediate safety of the patient, as delirium in the ICU has been shown to be predictive of mortality [1, 3, 4], prolonged ICU stay [5], increased cost [6], and long-term cognitive impairment [7, 8].

Different screening and assessment tools have been developed for identifying and rating patients with delirium in the ICU. The Confusion Assessment Method for the ICU (CAM-ICU) [9, 10] generates a binary result with patients categorized as either having or not having delirium; the tool may be implemented by the bedside nurse along with other routine clinical assessments. When compared with standard identifiers, the sensitivity and specificity of CAM-ICU is good (81 and 96 %), and the inter-rater reliability is high (kappa 0.79) [11]. CAM-ICU does not assess the type or severity of delirium; however, the burden of delirium can be quantified by estimating the time a patient is in delirium (Fig. 21.1) [12]. The Intensive Care Delirium Screening Checklist (ICDSC) [13] assigns a numerical score based on the presence or absence of eight characteristics. The ICSDC can be used to identify patients with incomplete presentations who may be at risk for delirium (subsyndromal delirium).

The pathogenesis of delirium in the ICU is believed to reflect a multifactorial process. Patients receive sedative and pain medication and may have sepsis or fever, sleep deprivation, weakness, lethargy, and a host of metabolic derangements [14]. Risk factors for delirium in the ICU include hypertension [2, 15], alcoholism [2, 15], dementia, isolation from social contact [14], and environmental factors such as the absence of a window [15]. Dementia is both a predisposing factor [14, 16] and a differential diagnosis. Age, a risk factor in the general medical population, is not associated with delirium in the ICU [2, 14]. Delirium must also be differentiated from alcohol and substance withdrawal states which have distinct biological mechanisms and treatment implications.

The management of delirium should be driven by a methodical consideration of inciting mechanisms. Specific strategies include pharmacologic and non-pharmacologic interventions and should target all psychomotor types of delirium. Medications that could worsen delirium should be minimized. Benzodiazepines should be avoided whenever possible as they have been shown to increase the likelihood of delirium [17, 18]. Medications with anticholinergic side effects, and especially any anticholinergic drug known to cross the blood–brain barrier such as atropine, should be avoided. Sedation protocols and daily interruptions of sedation should be implemented to decrease the exposure to deliriogenic medications and lessen the impact of delirium. Pharmacologic treatment centers on the use of antipsychotic medication both for confusional states and as a mild sedative. Neuroleptic medications such as haloperidol and more recently atypical antipsychotics such as quetiapine and olanzapine have found frequent use in ICU-associated delirium [19–23]. These medications work particularly well against agitated symptoms of delirium, but may also be theoretically beneficial in hypoactive delirium analogously to their benefits against the negative symptoms of schizophrenia. A randomized controlled trial may help determine if antipsychotics are in fact efficacious for hypoactive delirium [20].

Non-pharmacologic management includes removal of unnecessary catheters and devices, noise reduction, measures to promote sleep [24] (see section on sleep disorders in this chapter), and reorientation strategies. Patients benefit from the presence of calendars and clocks and from reassuring contact with family and ICU staff. Familiar items from

CAM-ICU Worksheet

Feature 1: Acute Onset or Fluctuating Course	Score	Check here if Present
Is the pt different than his/her baseline mental status? OR Has the patient had any fluctuation in mental status in the past 24 hours as evidenced by fluctuation on a sedation scale (i.e., RASS), GCS, or previous delirium assessment?	Either question Yes →	☐
Feature 2: Inattention		
Letters Attention Test (See training manual for alternate **Pictures**) Directions: Say to the patient, *"I am going to read you a series of 10 letters. Whenever you hear the letter 'A, , indicate by squeezing my hand."* Read letters from the following letter list in a normal tone 3 seconds apart. **S A V E A H A A R T** **Errors are counted when patient fails to squeeze on the letter "A" and when the patient squeezes on any letter other than "A."**	Number of Errors >2 →	☐
Feature 3: Altered Level of Consciousness		
Present if the Actual RASS score is anything other than alert and calm (zero)	RASS anything other than zero →	☐
Feature 4:Disorganized Thinking		
Yes/No Questions (See training manual for alternate set of questions) 1. Will a stone float on water? 2. Are there fish in the sea? 3. Does one pound weigh more than two pounds? 4. Can you use a hammer to pound a nail? **Errors are counted when the patient incorrectly answers a question.** **Command** Say to patient: "Hold up this many fingers" (Hold 2 fingers in front of patient) "Now do the same thing with the other hand" (Do not repeat number of fingers) *If pt is unable to move both arms, for 2nd part of command ask patient to "Add one more finger" **An error is counted if patient is unable to complete the entire command.**	Combined number of errors >1 →	☐

Overall CAM-ICU Feature 1 **plus** 2 **and** either 3 **or** 4 present = CAM-ICU positive	Criteria Met →	☐ **CAM-ICU Positive (Delirium Present)**
	Criteria Not Met →	☐ **CAM-ICU Negative (No Delirium)**

Fig. 21.1 CAM-ICU Worksheet (Copyright © 2002, E. Wesley Ely, MD, MPH, and Vanderbilt University. All Rights Reserved. Used with permission)

home and pictures may also be beneficial. Continuing routines from daily life such as reading newspapers, morning and evening routines, engaging in conversation, and being able to see outside a window are other examples of non-pharmacologic interventions.

Coma

Coma is characterized by loss of alertness and awareness and is demonstrated by unresponsiveness to stimuli. Historical gradations of decreasing arousal include hypersomnolence, lethargy (patient is difficult to arouse), obtundation (incomplete arousal), stupor (no sustained arousal from sleeplike state), and finally coma (lack of arousal). Coma may occur secondary to any number of neurologic injuries, but it may also develop in the setting of a severe metabolic or physiologic disturbance.

The biological origin of coma is understood by the study of (1) ascending brainstem arousal systems and their projections in the diencephalon, basal forebrain, and neocortex (Fig. 21.2) [25], and (2) thalamocortical integrative systems responsible for higher-order awareness and cognition. The arousal system maintains alertness (wakefulness, vigilance) and serves as a gating mechanism for sensory inputs. It originates from the tegmental sections of the rostral pons and the midbrain. Two large branches ascend: one through the lateral hypothalamus and another through the thalamus. Neurotransmitters involved in these pathways are predominantly:

Table 21.1 Etiologic categories of coma

Hemispheric lesion with brain shift
Diffuse bihemispheric structural lesion
Diencephalon lesion involving both thalami
Cerebellar lesion with brainstem compression or ischemia
Primary brainstem (mesencephalon–pons) lesion
Diffuse physiologic brain dysfunction from acute metabolic derangement, drugs, or intoxication
Psychogenic unresponsiveness

Reproduced with permission of Oxford University Press, USA, from Wijdicks [26]

1. Noradrenergic neurons from the locus coeruleus with diffuse cortical projections
2. Histaminergic neurons prominent in the lateral hypothalamus
3. Cholinergic neurons in the dorsal pons with diffuse ascending and descending projections, but notably connections to the thalamus that are thought to regulate sleep and wakefulness
4. A more recently characterized orexin system located in the hypothalamus and responsible for modulating arousal pathways

Coma may result from injury or impairment at all levels of the arousal/awareness system (Table 21.1) [26]. Discrete lesions in the dorsal and paramedian midbrain or pons may cause coma. Injury to either of the main branches through the lateral hypothalamus or through the thalamus will independently cause coma, just as a bihemispheric or diffuse cortical process. Drugs, toxins, or metabolic factors that interfere with these pathways may cause coma (Table 21.2) [27].

Coma caused by brainstem lesions are generally neurologic emergencies requiring swift decisive intervention (Table 21.3) [26]. Diffuse cortical causes of coma may be more slowly evolving, although they should be met with prompt initiation of treatment as well. Localization is aided by the testing of cranial nerves whose nuclei are in proximity to arousal systems. Pupillary findings may be characteristic, such as the pinpoint pupils seen in pontine lesions. Extraocular movements are controlled by pathways adjacent to the ascending arousal system, and vestibuloocular and oculocephalic reflexes may be helpful. Well-defined respiratory patterns may be associated with injury at different levels of the brainstem. Cheyne–Stokes respirations are linked with lesions above the midbrain, tachypnea with midbrain lesions, apneusis (breath holding at full inspiration) with rostral pontine lesions, and irregular ataxic breathing with lesions in the lower pons and upper medulla.

Coma is assessed by evaluating the response to graded stimulus. The Glasgow Coma Scale (GCS) assesses motor, verbal, and eye responses and is a powerful predictor of outcome in critically ill patients. The Full Outline of Unresponsiveness (FOUR) score [28] provides a quantitative

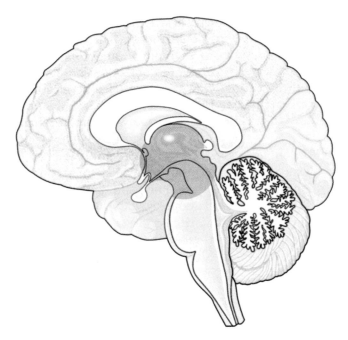

Fig. 21.2 Ascending arousal centers. Injuries to the ascending arousal system, from the rostral pons through the thalamus and hypothalamus (purple region), can cause loss of consciousness (Reprinted with permission of The McGraw-Hill Company from Saper [25])

Table 21.2 Common causes of metabolic encephalopathy presenting as coma

Loss of substrate of cerebral metabolism
Hypoxia
Hypoglycemia
Global ischemia
Multifocal ischemia resulting from emboli or diffuse intravascular coagulation
Multifocal ischemia resulting from cerebral vasculitis
Derangement of normal physiology
Hyponatremia or hypernatremia
Hyperglycemia/hyperosmolar
Hypercalcemia
Hypermagnesemia
Ongoing seizures
Postseizure state
Postconcussive state
Hypothyroidism
Hypocortisolism
Toxins
Drugs
Hypercarbia
Liver failure
Renal failure
Sepsis
Meningitis/encephalitis
Subarachnoid blood

Reproduced with permission of The McGraw-Hill Company from Saper [27]

Table 21.3 Physical signs in patients with impaired consciousness

Eyelid edema
Myxedema
Trauma
Cavernous sinus thrombophlebitis
Fever
Meningoencephalitis
Epidural abscess
Sympathetic storms
Hypertension
Subarachnoid hemorrhage
Intracerebral hematoma (with intraventricular extension)
Eclampsia or PRES
Hypotension
Brain death
Spinal cord injury

Reproduced with permission of Oxford University Press, USA, from Wijdicks [26]

measure of breathing patterns, pupillary responses, and the response to stimulus by motor response and eye opening (Table 21.4). The FOUR score provides more detailed information on brainstem function than the GCS; however, its prognostic value has not been shown to be superior.

Table 21.4 The FOUR score

Eye response
4 = eyelids open or opened, tracking, or blinking to command
3 = eyelids open but not tracking
2 = eyelids closed but open to loud voice
1 = eyelids closed but open to pain
0 = eyelids remain closed with pain
Motor response
4 = thumbs-up, fist, or peace sign
3 = localizing to pain
2 = flexion response to pain
1 = extension response to pain
0 = no response to pain or generalized myoclonus status
Brain stem reflexes
4 = pupil and corneal reflexes present
3 = one pupil wide and fixed
2 = pupil or corneal reflexes absent
1 = pupil and corneal reflexes absent
0 = absent pupil, corneal, and cough reflex
Respiration
4 = not intubated, regular breathing pattern
3 = not intubated, Cheyne–Stokes breathing pattern
2 = not intubated, irregular breathing
1 = breathes above the ventilator
0 = breathes at ventilator rate or apnea

Reproduced with permission from Wijdicks et al. [28]

Resolution of coma does not always result in return to consciousness. The persistent vegetative state is seen when signs of arousal (e.g., spontaneous eye opening) return, but there is no awareness of self or of the environment. The minimally conscious state is a state of severely impaired consciousness characterized by inconsistently appearing, but unequivocal, signs of conscious awareness (e.g., tracking of objects, simple phonation or speech, but without evidence of reliable communication).

Seizures and Status Epilepticus

New-onset seizures are uncommon but can occur due to alcohol or substance withdrawal or severe metabolic disturbance (Table 21.5) [29]. Nonconvulsive status seizures or status epilepticus may produce alteration of mental status and coma. Studies indicate that as many as 20 % of critically ill patients with coma have nonconvulsive status epilepticus (NCSE) [30]. Nonconvulsive status most often follows a clearly defined seizure and usually occurs in the setting of anoxic–ischemic damage, traumatic brain injury, withdrawal from sedatives or antiepileptics, or sepsis. In patients at risk (i.e., history of seizures, known primary brain injury, sepsis), continuous EEG monitoring for at least 24 h should be considered. Treatment is the same as for convulsive seizures or status.

Table 21.5 Causes of new-onset seizures in critical illness

Causes	Patients (n)
Drug withdrawal	18
Morphine	11
Propoxyphene	5
Midazolam	1
Meperidine	1
Metabolic abnormalities	18
Hyponatremia	10
Hypocalcemia	4
Acute uremia	2
Hyperglycemia	1
Hypoglycemia	1
Drug toxicity	8
Antibiotics	5
Antiarrhythmics	3
Stroke	5
Unknown	6
Total	55

Reproduced with permission from Wijdicks and Sharbrough [29]

Posterior Reversible Encephalopathy Syndrome

Posterior reversible encephalopathy syndrome (PRES), also known as posterior reversible leukoencephalopathy syndrome, is characterized by headache, altered mental status, seizures, and visual disturbances (even cortical blindness) associated with CT or MRI evidence of vasogenic edema usually in the parietal and occipital lobes. This condition is associated with severe hypertension, immunosuppressive drugs, and hypertensive disorders of pregnancy (eclampsia or preeclampsia). Though the exact pathophysiology is unknown, prevailing theories point toward a disturbance of autoregulatory mechanisms in the cerebral vasculature leading to endothelial injury, blood–brain barrier breakdown, and vasogenic edema [31, 32]. MRI is more sensitive and specific for making this diagnosis than CT. Treatment should be targeted toward the underlying cause, blood pressure management, and seizure prophylaxis. Long-term prognosis with this condition is generally very good. Resolution of clinical and radiologic findings occurs over days to weeks in the majority of cases.

Sleep Disorders and Sleep Deprivation

Normal patterns of sleep and wakefulness are compromised in the ICU setting. The sickness behavior linked to acute infection (discussion to come) induces daytime hypersomnolence and disruptions in sleep. Pain is common among various critical illness states and may prevent rest at night. Delirium is common in the critically ill, and agitated delirium may keep patients in an animated state, initiating a vicious cycle of sleep deprivation

and agitated delirium. Critical illness and the ICU environment are associated with a high likelihood of sleep disruption and deprivation [33–38]. Patients are subject to procedures and assessments around the clock, and persistent lighting and noise may remove important cues driving circadian regulation. Noise is a major contributor to sleep impairment in the ICU due to physiologic alarms, overhead paging systems, staff conversations, and radio or television. Mechanical ventilation and patient-ventilator dyssynchrony in particular may disrupt sleep. Assist-control ventilation has been shown to be superior to pressure-support modes if nocturnal hyperventilation results in central apneas and arousals [39]. Further, proportional assist ventilation (PAV) may be superior to pressure support at night, an effect attributed to improved ventilator tolerance and synchrony [40]; additionally, PAV also avoids nocturnal hyperventilation. Medications, including stimulants and catecholamine agents, may decrease sleep. Benzodiazepine sedation may decrease REM sleep and the restorative effect of sleep.

Continuous polysomnography [41] studies have documented the marked fragmentation of sleep in the intensive care setting; patients with fragmented sleep spend less time in deeper stages of sleep. With frequent interruptions, the efficiency of sleep decreases, resulting in lower quality of sleep, although the total time spent in sleep over a 24-h period may be similar to controls.

Sleep deprivation has many detrimental consequences. Cognitive function declines, and eventually delirium is induced. Agitation and irritability are common, eventually hallucinosis may occur. Animal studies of prolonged sleep deprivation and of selective REM deprivation seem to indicate that, if carried out indefinitely; total sleep deprivation will be uniformly fatal. The cause for the mortality related to sleep deprivation is not clear. Sleep deprivation alters immune function, but not in a predictable way. Animals may be more likely to survive influenza when sleep deprived, but bacterial sepsis becomes increasingly fatal. Sleep deprivation alters metabolism, animals markedly increase caloric intake, but still experience cachexia over time. There is negative nitrogen balance and an overall catabolic state. Sleep deprivation is a stressor, but the effects of sleep deprivation can be distinguished from stress [42].

Management of sleep disturbance in the ICU should target environmental modification. Sedative agents may be helpful in the short term but are unlikely to have the restorative properties of natural sleep [43–47].

Long-Term Cognitive Impairment Following Critical Illness

Long-term impairments in cognition occur with significant frequency among the survivors of critical illness [48–50]. Memory and executive function, attention, processing speed, intellectual function, and visual-spatial testing are frequently affected [49]. Reported rates of cognitive dysfunction at the time of discharge are similar to the rates of ICU delirium. One recent cohort by Girard showed evidence of cognitive impairment in 79 % of ICU survivors at 3 months and 71 % at 1 year, with severe cognitive impairment at 1 year in 36 % of subjects [8]. The rate of cognitive impairment was higher than in other reports perhaps because it included an older sample (median age 61 years), which is consistent with the adult ICU population in the United States.

Acute delirium in hospitalized patients is linked to long-term neurocognitive dysfunction [51]. It has been observed that the natural history of dementia may be accelerated by an intervening period of critical illness [52]. Surprisingly, the severity of critical illness does not appear to correlate with the likelihood of long-term cognitive dysfunction [53–55], although length of stay did correlate with cognitive dysfunction in non-delirious patients immediately following the acute illness [56]. The normal decline with aging may not have been fully accounted for in all longitudinal cohort studies involving the elderly after ICU admission [57].

Cognitive assessments may be confounded by covariables present in survivors of critical illness: sleep deprivation and recovery can have persisting effects months after ICU discharge. Generalized weakness and fatigue are common in the survivors of critical illness, and the methods of testing in these studies were often modified in order to accommodate the fatigue commonly present in the ICU survivors. Depression and post-traumatic stress disorder are common in ICU survivors and can confound neuropsychological performance.

Long-term cognitive outcomes are important in that they can predict functional outcome after the illness. Older, previously high-functioning patients may need institutionalization or other costly care [49]. Younger patients have a low return to full employment rate (49 and 65 % of previously employed returned to their previous employment at 1 and 2 years, respectively) and lower quality-of-life scores after critical illness [58]. These factors represent an increased personal and societal burden of critical illness whose magnitude is only beginning to be appreciated.

ICU-Acquired Weakness

There are many causes of severe muscle weakness that can occur in critically ill patients (Table 21.6) [59]. Preexisting conditions that cause weakness may be exacerbated in the critically ill. The etiologies may be broken down anatomically: cortical lesions, brainstem lesions, myelopathies, anterior horn disease, polyneuropathies, neuromuscular junction disorders, and intrinsic myopathies.

If there is no plausible etiology for severe weakness other than the underlying critical illness, then a diagnosis of ICU-acquired weakness (ICU-AW) should be considered [60–75].

Table 21.6 Acute generalized weakness syndromes in critically ill patients

Bilateral or paramedian brain or brainstem lesions[a]
  Trauma
  Infarction
  Hemorrhage
  Infectious and noninfectious encephalitides
  Abscess
  Central pontine myelinolysis
Spinal cord disorders[a]
  Trauma
  Nontraumatic compressive myelopathies
  Spinal cord infarction
  Immune-mediated myelopathies (transverse myelitis, neuromyelitis optica)
  Infective myelopathies (e.g., HIV, West Nile virus)
Anterior horn cell disorders
  Motor neuron disease
  Poliomyelitis
  West Nile virus infection
  Hopkins syndrome (acute postasthmatic amyotrophy)
Polyradiculopathies
  Carcinomatous
  HIV-associated
Peripheral nervous disorders
  Guillain-Barré syndrome[b]
  Diphteric neuropathy
  Lymphoma-associated neuropathy
  Vasculitic neuropathy
  Porphyric neuropathy
  Paraneoplastic neuropathy
  Critical illness polyneuropathy
Neuromuscular junction disorders
  Myasthenia gravis
  Lambert–Eaton myasthenic syndrome
  Neuromuscular-blocking drugs
  Botulism
Muscle disorders
  Rhabdomyolysis
  Disuse myopathy
  Cachexia
  Infectious and inflammatory myopathies[c]
  Mitochondrial myopathies
  Drug-induced and toxic myopathies
  Critical illness myopathy
  Decompensation of congenital myopathies (e.g., myotonic dystrophy, Duchenne muscular dystrophy, adult-onset acid maltase deficiency)

Reproduced with permission from Stevens et al. [59]
HIV human immunodeficiency virus
[a]Upper motor neuron signs (increased tone, hyperreflexia) may be absent in the acute setting
[b]Includes acute inflammatory demyelinating polyneuropathy, acute motor axonal neuropathy, and acute motor and sensory axonal neuropathy
[c]Includes polymyositis, dermatomyositis, and pyomyositis

ICU-AW is an umbrella term which includes critical illness polyneuropathy (CIP), critical illness myopathy (CIM), and

Table 21.7 MRC score

Grade	Description
0	No contraction
1	Flicker or trace of contraction
2	Active movement with gravity eliminated
3	Active movement against gravity
4	Active movement against gravity and resistance
5	Normal power

For MRC sum score, grade 4 limbs, 3 muscle groups in each limb

the overlap condition critical illness neuromyopathy (CINM). As many as 50 % of patients with sepsis, multiorgan failure, or prolonged mechanical ventilation demonstrate evidence of ICU-AW [76]. Factors associated with ICU-AW include sepsis, systemic inflammatory response syndrome (SIRS), multiple-system organ failure, renal replacement therapy, mechanical ventilation, catecholamine administration, and poor glycemic control. Exposure to glucocorticoids and the use of neuromuscular blockers (NMBA) in the ICU were implicated in ICU-AW, but have shown inconsistent association with ICU-AW in recent systematic review [75].

The weakness of ICU-AW is generalized and symmetric. Distal extremity strength such as grip strength may be affected earlier than proximal muscles. Decreased tone is common, and deep tendon reflexes are generally normal to decreased. Weakness may affect the diaphragm leading to prolonged respiratory failure, but facial involvement is rare, as facial grimace is generally preserved. Quantification of the degree of impairment should be done for initial diagnosis and following the progress of disease. The recommended measure of global weakness is the Medical Research Council (MRC) sum score (Table 21.7). The MRC score grades strength in a functional muscle group from 0 to 5. The sum score is generated when three muscle groups are tested from each extremity giving a maximum score of 60. ICU-AW is considered with MRC sum score < 48, severe weakness < 36. The test is repeatable and not costly to perform. Patients must be awake and cooperative for this assessment, and distal extremity strength is not tested.

ICU-AW was initially described by comparison to Guillain–Barré syndrome. Guillain-Barré remains an important differential diagnosis because it can be treated with plasma exchange and intravenous immunoglobulin. Distinguishing features of GBS, in addition to a consistent history and clinical onset, are the greater involvement of cranial nerves (generally absent in ICU-AW), the existence of dysautonomia, and elevated cerebrospinal fluid protein.

EMG and nerve conduction studies are recommended in cases of diagnostic uncertainty, if weakness is severe or if there is no improvement in neuromuscular function over the course of hospitalization. In cooperative patients capable of voluntary muscle contraction, nerve conduction studies and electromyography can distinguish CIP from CIM. When

voluntary contraction cannot be obtained, direct muscle stimulation and muscle biopsy may be helpful if a severe underlying myopathy is suspected. Prolonged paralysis after neuromuscular-blocking agents (NMBA) may exist as another subcategory of ICU-AW, generally occurring in the setting of concurrent multiorgan failure [76].

ICU-AW is associated with prolongation of mechanical ventilation [62, 65] and higher in-hospital mortality [64, 69], longer ICU stays, longer hospital stays, and greater associated costs. Long-term effects of ICU-AW include persistent weakness up to 1 year after ICU discharge [67]. While specific therapies for ICU-AW do not exist, efforts to mitigate or prevent it are centered on early physical therapy and occupational therapy [74]. The solution often involves culture change in the intensive care environment to allow early mobilization of patients.

Neurobiologic Effects of Medications Commonly Used in the ICU

Sedatives

Benzodiazepines and other GABA-ergic agents such as propofol are commonly used in critically ill patients needing sedation for mechanical ventilation or other procedures. Benzodiazepines are, however, associated with a significant risk of developing delirium, and there is interest in alternative sedative regimens. Dexmedetomidine in particular has been associated with a lower likelihood of delirium than benzodiazepines [77, 78].

Antibiotics

Several broad-spectrum antibiotics including fluoroquinolones, cefepime, and piperacillin have been linked with encephalopathy, while imipenem has been associated with seizures and metronidazole with peripheral neuropathy. The aminoglycosides induce ototoxicity and impair synaptic transmission at the neuromuscular junction. Vancomycin also has an association with ototoxicity. The determination of whether an encephalopathy is related to an infection or the drug used to treat it may be difficult to make and may complicate management of CNS infections. Ascribing neurologic effects to antibiotic therapy should be a diagnosis of exclusion.

Immune Suppressants

The deleterious effects of steroids on central and peripheral neurologic function are well known and include agitation, delirium and psychosis, and ICU-AW. There is a sizable body of information on the neurologic side effects of immunosuppressive medications used in the setting of solid organ or hematological transplantation [79–86]. Neurologic complications after liver transplantation are particularly common [79, 86], exacerbated by the requirement of many metabolites to be cleared via hepatic metabolism. Following liver transplantation, encephalopathy has been noted in up to 47 % of patients and seizures in 10 % [84].

The calcineurin inhibitors are a significant cause of neurotoxicity. The choice of calcineurin inhibitor (cyclosporine versus tacrolimus) has no significant impact on neurologic complication rates (17 versus 19 %) [84]. Cyclosporine neurotoxicity may appear in up to 60 % of patients receiving the drug and includes headache, amnesia, paresthesias, agitation, anxiety, insomnia, and tremor; more significant findings include decreased responsiveness, hallucinations, delusions, ataxia, aphasia, stroke-like findings, cortical blindness, and seizures. Tacrolimus-associated neurologic manifestations are similarly varied. Symptoms include headache, confusion, myoclonus, seizures, visual disturbances, encephalopathy, and memory loss; hypertension is often induced. Toxicity can occur even with low trough levels, and the time to onset averages 15 days. Drug levels must be monitored closely immediately posttransplant as changes in renal function or volume of distribution can increase drug levels into neurotoxic range. The development of nephrotoxicity further elevates levels. Mycophenolate mofetil has a neurologic side effect profile that is milder than the calcineurin inhibitors.

Neurological Implications of Organ Dysfunction

Cardiovascular

Cardiac and vascular causes of encephalopathy characteristically have an abrupt onset. Intracranial hemorrhages (aneurysmal subarachnoid hemorrhage or primary intracerebral hemorrhage) or ischemic stroke may result in coma if lesions involve bilateral cerebral hemispheres, bilateral thalami, or if they are located in reticular activating system in the rostral brainstem. Focal strokes affecting the right parietal lobe and the basal ganglia have been associated with delirium. When a cerebrovascular etiology is likely, brain CT and/or MRI should be obtained emergently; consultation with neurology and/or neurosurgery is recommended.

A probe-patent foramen ovale is present on 30 % of postmortem subjects but rarely has clinical significance as normal left atrial pressures exceed right atrial pressures. This situation can be reversed in mechanically ventilated patients due to positive pressure ventilation and coughing secondary to airway stimulation, increasing the risk of paradoxical emboli. Neurosurgical patients in the seated operative position are theoretically at increased risk of paradoxical embolism, but the evidence is conflicting whether this occurs any more frequently in practice.

Endocarditis

Manifestations of infective endocarditis (IE) are protean. The diagnosis is based upon evidence of cardiac vegetations and the presence of positive blood cultures [87]. Stroke risk correlates with the size of the vegetation and occurs in 30 % of patients with mitral valve endocarditis and in 10 % of patients with aortic valve endocarditis [88–94]. The risk of cerebral embolism diminishes rapidly after initiation of intravenous antibiotic therapy. Neurologic sequelae are not infrequent after cerebral embolism, with meningitis occurring in 10.7 %, followed by intracranial hemorrhage (9.2 %) and intracranial abscess (7.7 %). Infective aneurysms may occur as a result of microemboli. Reported sites of aneurysms include the aorta, mesentery, and distal MCA. The cerebral aneurysms are usually silent and can, occasionally, regress; delayed rupture after 6 months is very rare. Rupture of an infective cerebral aneurysm may be seen in 0.6–4 %.

The cornerstone of IE therapy is appropriately targeted antimicrobial therapy continued for 4–6 weeks. Early surgery [95–97] should be considered if the patient develops heart failure or if there is severe or rapid degeneration of the infected valve, recurrent emboli, or development of a perivalvular abscess. Cardiac surgery may need to be deferred in patients with large-volume ischemic strokes or those with intracranial hemorrhage. Overall, the mortality is lower after high-risk valve surgery than with conservative management alone when a restrictive surgical selection is employed.

Cardiac Arrest

Anoxic–ischemic encephalopathy (AIE) is the most devastating consequence of cardiac arrest, with historically few survivors returning to their previous levels of neurologic functioning. The use of therapeutic moderate hypothermia has been associated with significantly improved outcome following out-of-hospital ventricular fibrillation arrest [98, 99], and a recent prospective series indicates that a little more than one quarter of cardiac arrest survivors may gain functional independence in the long term [100, 101]. Currently, it appears reasonable to extrapolate these findings to comatose survivors of cardiac arrest in the inpatient setting. With greater implementation of hypothermia, existing prognostic models for post-cardiac arrest AIE [102] (anoxic–ischemic encephalopathy) have been seriously challenged [103, 104]. Hypothermia has multiple side effects including cardiac dysrhythmias, decreased cardiac output, pneumonia, atelectasis, decreased clearance of sedatives, shivering if paralytic agents are not used, hyperglycemia and decreased insulin secretion, and cold diuresis and hypovolemia.

Hypertensive Crisis

In a hypertensive emergency, the end organs most acutely affected are brain, heart, kidney, and large arteries. The most common complications are intracranial hemorrhage and pulmonary edema. Neurologic manifestations of hypertensive emergency are headache, nausea and vomiting, visual disturbances, confusion, and loss of consciousness. Hypertensive encephalopathy without hemorrhage may develop due to vasogenic edema and may be appreciable on neuroimaging as a specific subtype of PRES.

Altered Cerebral Autoregulation in Chronic Hypertension

Autoregulation of the cerebral vasculature allows vascular tone to correct for fluctuations in arterial blood pressure. Cerebral autoregulation is most protective of hypertensive fluctuations, but will also allow maintenance of adequate cerebral blood flow (CBF) at low blood pressures, provided mean arterial pressures (MAP) exists between 50 and 150 mmHg. In chronic hypertension, the CBF–MAP relationship is shifted to accommodate for the elevated blood pressures, hence increasing the risk of cerebral ischemia at the arterial blood pressure which would be tolerated in normal subjects. It is therefore reasonable to target higher blood pressures in patients with chronic hypertension.

Respiratory Failure

Hypoxia and Hypercapnia

Neurologic manifestations of acute hypoxemia include agitation and delirium, progressing to seizures, myoclonus, obtundation, and coma when hypoxemia is of sufficient magnitude or duration. After sudden prolonged or severe hypoxia, a global encephalopathy analogous to AIE may be seen. Incremental decreases in PaO_2 may be better tolerated, as seen in high-altitude mountaineers. Myoclonus is a nonspecific finding, but is common in hypoxic encephalopathy. Myoclonic status (persistent myoclonus for the majority of the day post-event) portends poor outcome in comatose patients [105]. Coma survivors with intermittent myoclonus may occasionally develop Lance-Adams intention myoclonus on awakening, which itself may be a debilitating chronic condition [100, 106].

Neurologic manifestations of acute hypercapnia include somnolence, lethargy, and coma. Patients with chronic lung disease will have metabolically compensated hypercapnia with minimal neurologic expression. The cognitive impairment observed in patients with advanced COPD is likely reflective of both hypoxia and hypercapnia. Cognitive impairment with hypercapnia appears to correlate most with the change in $PaCO_2$ from baseline, rather than the absolute value. In patients with baseline $PaCO_2$ of 40 mmHg, significant neurological impairment occurs with a $PaCO_2$ in the range of 60–80 mmHg; in COPD patients, the noticeable effect will occur at a similar delta from their baseline. The effect of $PaCO_2$ of 90–100 mmHg in a baseline normocapnic patient may be equivalent to 1 MAC of anesthesia (roughly a normalized unit of full general anesthesia due to any agent).

ALI/ARDS

Nearly half of acute lung injury (ALI) survivors will have demonstrable long-term functional impairments [53, 67, 101, 107–110]. Survivors of ALI are at risk for significant long-term neurocognitive impairments [53, 107]. Cognitive sequelae in this population can derive from prolonged hypoxemia, hypotension, sepsis, and inflammation; however, the exact underlying pathophysiology is not certain. Delirium may be an epiphenomenon indicating neurologically significant critical illness, as delirium correlates with long-term cognitive sequelae in the critically ill [8] and with mortality at 6 months [1].

Impaired neurocognitive performance following ALI has been documented in several studies by Hopkins and colleagues. Global cognitive impairment was noted in 30 % of patients who were assessed 1 year after acute respiratory distress syndrome (ARDS), and significant impairment was noted in at least one domain of cognition in 55 % of study subjects [107]. In a follow-up study, significant residual impairment in at least one domain of testing was observed in 47 % of patients at 2 years [53]. At 6 year follow-up, the incidence of neurocognitive defect may be decreased to 25 % of patients [110].

Studies using head CT have shown that ALI survivors may be at increased risk for brain atrophy when compared to age-matched controls [111]. Although CTs in many ALI patients were normal, there was a significant increase in averaged brain atrophy as measured by volumetric ventricle-to-brain ratio compared to controls. In the study, there was no control for the timing of the imaging, and many CTs were performed early in the course of illness (within the first 2 weeks); the study failed to show correlation between degree of hypoxia and atrophy, although the pattern was similar to atrophy seen following AIE.

Sickness Behavior Syndrome

The sickness behavior syndrome (SBS) is an adaptive and evolutionarily advantageous physiologic and behavioral response to a systemic inflammatory state. Presenting signs include anorexia, fatigue, somnolence, social withdrawal, aching joints, fever, and chills. SBS is prominent in autoimmune disease and in sepsis, but may also play a role in malaise of other chronic conditions including heart failure, obesity, Alzheimer's, stroke, and depression [112].

There may be several signaling pathways involved in SBS, both humoral and neural. IL-1, IL-6, and TNF-alpha play a prominent role. Pro-inflammatory cytokines activate vagal afferents to the brainstem, with input to the hypothalamus and limbic system. By interacting with the hypothalamic–pituitary axis, IL-1 can cause fever via induction of prostaglandin E2 and cortisol release. Autoimmune diseases activate a pathway involving anti-self T lymphocytes, in which the T-cells bind to CD40+ on B-cells, dendritic cells, and macrophages to produce pro-inflammatory cytokines that are independent of the pathway for SBS induced by bacterial lipopolysaccharide [113]. Although SBS is adaptive in mammals to learn to avoid poisons in the wild and to recuperate during illness, in the ICU the effect is maladaptive and may delay resolution of illness and recovery.

Sepsis-Associated Encephalopathy

Sepsis-associated encephalopathy (SAE) [114–122] is a disturbance of brain function arising in the setting of sepsis arising from a non-CNS source. It is characterized by alteration in mental status, diffuse slowing on EEG, typically a normal head CT, and normal CSF indicating absence of meningitis, all in the presence of systemic sepsis. In patients with bacteremia, 87 % had abnormal EEG and 70 % had neurologic symptoms ranging from lethargy to coma [114]. SAE is commonly viewed as a reversible condition; however, patients may develop long-lasting deficits. Often, patients emerging from SAE are noted to have ICU-AW which may take longer to resolve. ICU-AW is noted in up to 70 % of patients with SAE [65].

Clinical presentation may be subtle. CNS dysfunction may be one of the earliest signs of infection and may allow for timely diagnostic evaluation and therapy. Early presenting signs of SAE include inattention and fluctuating mental status consistent with acute delirium [114]. More severe SAE presents as coma. Motor manifestations may include velocity-dependent resistance to passive movement that diminishes as the limb is moved slowly (gegenhalten or paratonic rigidity) [114] but also asterixis, tremor, or myoclonus. The electroencephalogram (EEG) is very sensitive for sepsis-associated encephalopathy, even before clinically evident neurologic findings appear. Routine use of EEG in septic patients has been suggested as a means of categorizing patients with SAE [115]. The EEG change follows a progression with severity of encephalopathy and correlates with mortality. Early changes include slowing of the dominant rhythm: the thetas (19 % mortality), deltas (36 % mortality), the appearance of generalized triphasic waves (50 % mortality), and burst suppression (67 % mortality) [115]. While CT findings are generally unremarkable, MRI may reveal ischemic stroke or a pattern of leukoencephalopathy, which may represent breakdown of the blood–brain barrier [116]; these findings on MRI correlate with poor outcome [116]. CSF analysis is negative for infection, but elevated protein may be present. Serum biomarker S100B may be elevated in some patients but does not correlate with severity of illness [117].

The pathophysiology of SAE is not well understood. Elevated cytokine levels inhibit endothelial nitric oxide synthase (eNOS) resulting in vasoconstriction and impaired microcirculatory flow. Cerebral autoregulation is impaired in septic shock patients; thus, hypotension during septic shock may result in significant decreases in CBF [120]. The endothelial dysfunction in sepsis also produces a procoagulant state, potentially contributing to microvascular infarcts [116]. Endotoxemia may cause impairment of blood–brain barrier, leading to vasogenic edema and altering brain homeostasis. There may also be an alteration in the ratio of amino acids transported across the BBB, as aromatic amino acids are more readily transported than branch-chained amino acids. There is some indication that addition of branch-chained amino acids may be of benefit in the treatment of SAE [123].

Management of SAE is predicated on treatment of the underlying infection. Antibiotic therapy may not reverse the encephalopathy in all cases as more endotoxin may be initially released with antibiotic therapy, or a severe or irreversible injury may have already occurred. In addition to management of organ failure and metabolic disturbances, avoidance of neurotoxic drugs is recommended.

Liver Failure

The liver contributes importantly to normal CNS function. The brain is dependent on glucose homeostasis, which is maintained with the aid of the liver. In addition, the liver is involved in intermediate steps of metabolism for many substrates used in the brain. Most importantly, the liver is essential in eliminating toxic metabolites that would modulate CNS function.

Acute Liver Failure

Acute liver failure (ALF) is defined as the rapid development of encephalopathy and impaired synthetic function in a patient with previously normal liver function. The etiology is most commonly a toxic ingestion or viral hepatitis. Presenting symptoms are neurologic, often preceding any clinically evident jaundice. Mania, agitation, and delirium are common early findings, along with nausea, vomiting, and abdominal pain; the neurologic features evolve rapidly to coma. Generalized seizures are common. Cerebral edema [124, 125] is the principal consequence of ALF and has both cytotoxic and vasogenic components.

Table 21.8 Stages of hepatic encephalopathy (West Haven Criteria)

Stage 0: Lack of detectable personality changes. No asterixis
Stage 1: Trivial lack of awareness. Impaired attention span. Altered sleep, euphoria, or depression. Mild asterixis may be present
Stage 2: Lethargy or apathy. Disorientation. Inappropriate behavior. Slurred speech. Asterixis
Stage 3: Gross disorientation. Bizarre behavior. Semi-stupor. Asterixis absent
Stage 4: Coma

Reproduced with permission from Ferenci et al. [130]

Table 21.9 Neurologic findings in malabsorptive syndromes

Vitamin deficiency	Neurological disease
Thiamine	Polyneuropathy, beriberi, Wernicke-Korsakoff syndrome, cortical cerebellar degeneration, nutritional amblyopia
Pyridoxine	Peripheral neuropathy Associated with INH therapy
Niacin	Pellagra (dermatitis, diarrhea, dementia)
Vitamin B12	Myelopathy, axonal peripheral neuropathy, dementia, optic neuropathy. Subacute combined degeneration of the spinal cord. Deficiency may be caused by pernicious anemia, celiac disease, or ileal resection
Vitamin D	Osteomalacic myopathy. May be caused by partial gastrectomy or celiac disease
Vitamin E	Spinocerebellar degeneration, ophthalmoplegia, myopathy, peripheral neuropathy

Reproduced with permission from Mancall [133]

The cornerstone of management is to identify liver transplant candidates and preserve neurologic function. Transplantation may increase ALF survival from 15–20 % to 60–80 % [126, 127]. Admission to the ICU for aggressive management and rapid evaluation for transplantation are essential. ICP monitoring and ICP management with hypertonic saline or mannitol may allow treatment or prevention of brain herniation and irreversible neurologic injury. Medical management should include interventions to reduce serum ammonia, seizure prophylaxis, sedation, and induced hypothermia [124, 128].

Hepatic Encephalopathy

Chronic liver disease may produce encephalopathy with intermittent exacerbation. The encephalopathy is initiated by impaired clearance of metabolites from portosytemic shunting of blood in the setting of portal hypertension and, in late disease, loss of sustainable synthetic function due to cirrhosis; hepatic encephalopathy (HE) is a clinical diagnosis [129, 130]. The diagnosis can be supported by hyperammonemia, but severity does not always correlate well with blood ammonia levels. Clinical findings include short-term memory loss, hypersomnia, insomnia, lethargy, asterixis, slurred speech, erratic behavior, and coma (Table 21.8). Sensitive neuropsychiatric testing may be required to evaluate milder disease. Some patients may be functional in society at baseline.

Acute decompensation is associated with gastrointestinal bleeding events, due to the concomitant esophageal varices seen with portal hypertension. Infections commonly precipitate deterioration as well, notably subacute bacterial peritonitis, pneumonia, and urinary tract infection. Renal failure, malnutrition from cachexia, overaggressive diuresis and hypoperfusion, and exogenous narcotics or benzodiazepines may contribute a second cause of encephalopathy and make the disease clinically evident. There may be worsening of portosystemic shunt as after portal vein thrombosis or after TIPS procedure. Lastly, there may be an additional hepatic insult such as superimposed viral hepatitis, alcoholic hepatitis, or drug-induced liver injury.

EEG abnormalities in HE include – in order of worsening severity – theta rhythms, generalized triphasic waves, and predominant delta rhythm. The EEG may have characteristic high-amplitude low-frequency bursts. The most consistent laboratory finding is hypoalbuminemia and clotting factor deficiency. Other laboratory findings are inconsistent, but in general elevated serum ammonia levels are expected. Ammonia levels should be taken fasting and preferably from arterial samples. Elevated ammonia levels may exert its effect indirectly by inducing astrocyte dysfunction, thus explaining the occasional unlinking of hyperammonemia and neurologic effects [124]. HE is associated with loss of regulation of cerebral blood flow, impaired oxygen metabolism, and conversion of astrocytes to Alzheimer type 2 cells [131, 132]. A head CT should be performed to evaluate for brain edema and to rule out structural lesions. MRI is more sensitive and specific for cerebral edema and may demonstrate increased signal in bilateral basal ganglia on T1-weighted imaging.

The treatment of acute exacerbations should identify and remove precipitating factors. Lactulose or other cathartics may aid in the elimination of protein metabolites. Enteral neomycin, metronidazole, or rifaximin can be very helpful in reducing the bacterial flora of the gut. Long-term management requires limitation of enteral protein to 0.5 g/kg/day and titration of lactulose to adequate stool frequency and abatement of neurologic symptoms.

Nutritional and Malabsorptive Disorders in the Critically Ill

Nutritional disorders and malabsorptive disorders may occasionally produce neurologic symptoms in the ICU (Table 21.9). When present, deficiency of water-soluble vitamins such as thiamine, riboflavin, niacin, and pyridoxine is usually due to insufficient nutritional intake [133]. Deficiency of fat-soluble vitamins, such as vitamin A, D, E, and K, can occur in the ICU in the setting of postsurgical short gut syndrome, pancreatic insufficiency, hepatic disease with bile acid deficiency, colchicine, laxatives, Zollinger–Ellison syndrome, or poorly controlled celiac disease [134] or Crohn's disease.

Wernicke's Encephalopathy

Wernicke's encephalopathy is a rare and preventable condition caused by thiamine deficiency. It is most commonly seen in patients with chronic alcoholism, cancer, and in late-stage AIDS. Clinical presentation includes ophthalmoplegia, nystagmus, gait ataxia, and altered mental status. MRI may reveal T2-hyperintense lesions surrounding the cerebral aqueduct and third ventricle and in the mamillary bodies and medial thalami. Treatment is with intravenous thiamine. The administration of glucose to susceptible patients without prior thiamine supplementation can precipitate Wernicke's encephalopathy or worsen existing disease. In any patient who is potentially at risk for Wernicke's encephalopathy, thiamine should be administered prior to giving any glucose containing solutions.

Encephalopathy of Renal Failure

Uremic Encephalopathy

Uremic encephalopathy can develop with both acute and chronic renal failure. Presenting symptoms include headache, tremor, myoclonus, obtundation, and coma. The cause of the neurologic dysfunction is thought to be due to accumulation of dialyzable toxins including urea, guanidino compounds, uric acid, hippuric acid, atypical amino acids, polyamines, phenols, acetone, glucuronic acid, carnitine, myoinositol, and phosphates. Uremic encephalopathy resolves with renal replacement therapy, yet a delay of 1–2 days is common before clinical improvement is seen.

Dialysis Disequilibrium Syndrome

An acute neurologic complication that may occur with hemodialysis is dialysis disequilibrium syndrome (DDS). Symptoms include headache, nausea, confusion, and ataxia. Severely affected patients may develop seizures, obtundation, and coma. This condition usually develops during or immediately after hemodialysis and is thought to be caused by rapid changes in serum osmolality leading to brain edema. DDS is self-limiting and symptoms generally resolve over several hours.

Encephalopathy Associated with Endocrine Disorders

Severe hypothyroidism and hyperthyroidism can cause an acute encephalopathy. Myxedema coma is the severest form of hypothyroidism and manifests with lethargy or coma in association with bradycardia, hypothermia, hyponatremia, and hypercapnic/hypoxemic respiratory failure. Thyrotoxicosis may present with a range of neurologic symptoms from psychosis and agitation to delirium, somnolence, and even coma. Acute adrenal insufficiency typically presents with circulatory shock and electrolyte abnormalities, yet it can also be associated with lethargy and coma. Hashimoto's encephalopathy – also known as steroid-responsive encephalopathy with autoimmune thyroiditis – is a heterogenous syndrome of neurologic symptoms associated with anti-thyroid antibodies and/or autoimmune thyroid dysfunction. Its presentation can range from subacute, recurrent episodes of focal neurologic deficits to a rapidly progressive dementia or coma. Treatment is with corticosteroids.

Metabolic Encephalopathy

Common electrolyte disturbances that result in encephalopathy are hyponatremia, hypernatremia, hypoglycemia, and hyperglycemic crises. Acute hyponatremia may cause brain edema with clinical signs ranging from confusion to coma and death [135–140]. The severity of clinical presentation depends on the rate of decrease and the absolute serum sodium level. Correction of hyponatremia should be achieved in a controlled manner to avoid the development of an osmotic demyelination syndrome. Hypernatremia leads to neurologic dysfunction through a hyperosmolar state that effectively dehydrates the brain. The rate of correction of hypernatremia should also be cautious to prevent the development of cerebral edema.

Hypoglycemia can present with encephalopathy or occasionally as focal neurologic deficits, especially in patients with prior strokes or other brain lesions. Correction of hypoglycemia should be performed rapidly with intravenous dextrose to prevent permanent brain injury. Depending on the severity and duration of hypoglycemia, the clinical response to treatment may lag significantly behind the return to normoglycemia. Severe hyperglycemia resulting from decompensated diabetes mellitus is another important cause of encephalopathy. Brain dysfunction results from serum hyperosmolarity associated with acidosis and electrolyte depletion. Treatment priorities are intravascular volume resuscitation, intravenous insulin, and electrolyte repletion.

Summary

The neurologic expression of critical illness is prevalent and associated with adverse outcome. Both the central and the peripheral nervous system may be affected. Recognition may be delayed due to sedation and emphasis on systemic resuscitation. Intensive care providers must work systematically to identify and treat supervening neurologic disorders. Research is needed to discover biological mechanisms and implement preventive and therapeutic interventions.

References

1. Ely EW, Shintani A, Truman B, et al. Delirium as a predictor of mortality in mechanically ventilated patients in the intensive care unit. JAMA. 2004;291:1753–62.

2. Ouimet S, Kavanaugh BP, Gottfried SB, Skrobik Y. Incidence, risk factors and consequences of ICU delirium. Intensive Care Med. 2007;33:66–73.

3. Pisani MA, Kong SY, Kasl SV, et al. Days of delirium are associated with 1-year mortality in an older intensive care unit population. Am J Respir Crit Care Med. 2009;180:1092–7.

4. van den Boogaard M, Peters SAE, van der Hoeven JG, et al. The impact of delirium on the prediction of in-hospital mortality in intensive care patients. Crit Care. 2010;14:R146.

5. Ely EW, Gautam S, Margolin R, et al. The impact of delirium in the intensive care unit on hospital length of stay. Intensive Care Med. 2001;27:1892–900.

6. Milbrandt EB, Deppen S, Harrison PL, et al. Costs associated with delirium in mechanically ventilated patients. Crit Care Med. 2004;32:955–62.

7. van den Boogaard M, Schoonhoven L, Evers AW, et al. Delirium in critically ill patients: impact on long-term health related quality of life and cognitive functioning. Crit Care Med. 2012;40:112–8.

8. Girard TD, Jackson JC, Pandharipande PP, et al. Delirium as a predictor of long-term cognitive impairment in survivors of critical illness. Crit Care Med. 2010;38:1513–20.

9. Ely EW, Margolin R, Francis J, et al. Evaluation of delirium in critically ill patients: validation of the Confusion Assessment Method for the Intensive Care Unit (CAM-ICU). Crit Care Med. 2001;29:1370–9.

10. Ely WE, Inouye SK, Bernard GR, et al. Delirium in mechanically ventilated patients – validity and reliability of the confusion assessment method for the intensive care unit (CAM-ICU). JAMA. 2001;286:2703–10.

11. Luetz A, Heymann A, Radtke FM, et al. Different assessment tools for the intensive care unit delirium: which score to use? Crit Care Med. 2010;38:409–18.

12. CAM-ICU Worksheet 2010. http://www.mc.vanderbilt.edu/icudelirium/docs/CAM_ICU_worksheet.pdf. Accessed 16 May 2012.

13. Bergeron N, Dubois MJ, Dumont M, Dial S, Skrobik Y. Intensive care delirium screening checklist: evaluation of a new screening tool. Intensive Care Med. 2001;27:859–64.

14. Van Rompaey B, Elseviers MM, Schuurmans MJ, Shortridge-Baggett LM, Truijen S, Bossaert L. Risk factors for delirium in intensive care patients: a prospective cohort study. Crit Care. 2009;13(3):R77.

15. Dubois MJ, Bergeron N, Dumont M, Dial S, Skrobik Y. Delirium in an intensive care unit: a study of risk factors. Intensive Care Med. 2001;27:1297–304.

16. Pisani MA, Murphy TE, Van Ness PH, Araujo KL, Inouye SK. Characteristics associated with delirium in older patients in a medical intensive care unit. Arch Intern Med. 2007;167:1629–34.

17. Pandharipande P, Shintani A, Peterson J, et al. Lorazepam is an independent risk factor for transitioning to delirium in intensive care unit patients. Anesthesiology. 2006;104:21–6.

18. Pandharipande P, Cotton BA, Shintani A, et al. Prevalence and risk factors for development of delirium in surgical and trauma intensive care unit patients. J Trauma. 2008;65(1):34–41.

19. Hipp DM, Ely EW. Pharmacological and nonpharmacological management of delirium in critically ill patients. Neurotherapeutics. 2012;9:158–75.

20. Girard TD, Panharipande PP, Carson SS. Feasibility, efficacy, and safety of antipsychotics for intensive care unit delirium: the MIND randomized, placebo-controlled trial. Crit Care Med. 2010;38: 428–37.

21. Lonergan E, Britton AM, Luxenberg J. Antipsychotics for delirium. Cochrane Database Syst Rev. 2007;(2):CD005594.

22. Devlin JW, Skrobik Y, Riker RR. Impact of quetiapine on resolution of individual delirium symptoms in critically ill patients with delirium: a post-hoc analysis of a double-blind, randomized, placebo-controlled study. Crit Care. 2011;15(5):R215.

23. Devlin JW, Roberts RJ, Fong JJ. Efficacy and safety of quetiapine in critically ill patients with delirium: a prospective, multicenter, randomized, double-blind, placebo-controlled pilot study. Crit Care Med. 2010;38:419–27.

24. Figueroa-Ramos MI, Arroyo-Novoa CM, Lee KA, Padilla G, Puntillo KA. Sleep and delirium in ICU patients: a review of mechanisms and manifestations. Intensive Care Med. 2009;35:781–95.

25. Saper CB. Brainstem modulation of sensation, movement, and consciousness. In: Kandel ER, Schwartz JH, Jessel TM, editors. Principles of neural science. 4th ed. New York: McGraw-Hill; 2000. p. 897.

26. Wijdicks EFM. Coma and other states of altered awareness in the intensive care unit. In: Neurologic complications of critical illness. 3rd ed. New York: Oxford University Press; 2009.

27. Saper CB. Brainstem modulation of sensation, movement, and consciousness. In: Kandel ER, Schwartz JH, Jessel TM, editors. Principles of neural science. 4th ed. New York: McGraw-Hill; 2000.

28. Wijdicks EFM, Bamlet WR, Maramattom BV, Manno EM, McClelland RL. Validation of a new coma scale: the FOUR score. Ann Neurol. 2005;58:585–93.

29. Wijdicks EFM, Sharbrough FW. New-onset seizures in critically ill patients. Neurology. 1993;43:1042–4.

30. Towne AR, Waterhouse EJ, Boggs JG, et al. Prevalence of non-convulsive status epilepticus in comatose patients. Neurology. 2000;54:340–5.

31. Bartynski WS, Tan HP, Boadman JF, Shapiro R, Marsh JW. Posterior reversible encephalopathy syndrome after solid organ transplantation. AJNR Am J Neuroradiol. 2008;29:924–30.

32. Bartynksi WS. Posterior reversible encephalopathy syndrome, part 2: controversies surrounding pathophysiology of vasogenic edema. AJNR AM J Neuroradiol. 2008;29:1043–9.

33. Friese R. Sleep and recovery from critical illness and injury: a review of theory, current practice, and future directions. Crit Care Med. 2008;36:697–705.

34. Hardin KA. Sleep in the ICU potential mechanisms and clinical implications. Chest. 2009;136:284–94.

35. Stanchina ML, Abu-Hijleh M, Chaudhry BK, Carlisle CC, Millman RP. The influence of white noise on sleep in subject exposed to ICU noise. Sleep Med. 2005;6:423–8.

36. Bijwadia JS, Ejaz MS. Sleep and critical care. Curr Opin Crit Care. 2009;15:25–9.

37. Marzano C, Ferrara M, Curcio G, De Gennaro L. The effects of sleep deprivation in humans: topographical electroencephalogram changes in non-rapid eye movement (NREM) sleep versus REM sleep. J Sleep Res. 2010;19:260–8.

38. Weinhouse GL, Schwab RJ, Watson PL, Patil N, Vaccaro B, Pandharipande P. Review bench-to-bedside review: delirium in ICU patients – importance of sleep deprivation. Crit Care. 2009;13:234–42.

39. Parthasarathy S, Tobin MJ. Effect of ventilator mode on sleep quality in critically ill patients. Am J Respir Crit Care Med. 2002;166:1423–9.

40. Bosma K, Ferreyra G, Ambrogio C, et al. Patient-ventilator interaction and sleep in mechanically ventilated patients: pressure support versus proportional assist ventilation. Crit Care Med. 2007;35:1048–54.

41. Watson P. Measuring sleep in critically ill patients: beware the pitfalls. Crit Care. 2007;11:159–60.

42. Rechtschaffen A, Bergmann BM. Sleep deprivation in the rat by the disk-over-water method. Behav Brain Res. 1995;69:55–63.

43. Nelson AB, Faraguna U, Tononi G, Cirelli C. Effects of anesthesia on the response to sleep deprivation. Sleep. 2010;33(112):1659–67, S1–S2.

44. Pal D, Lipinski WJ, Walker AJ, Turner AM, Mashour GA. State-specific effects of anesthesia on sleep homeostasis. Selective recovery of slow wave but not rapid eye movement sleep. Anesthesiology. 2011;114:302–10.

45. Mashour GA, Lipinski WJ, Matlen LB, Walker AJ, Turner AM, Schoen W, Lee U, Poe GR. Isoflurane anesthesia does not satisfy the homeostatic need for rapid eye movement sleep. Anesth Analg. 2010;110:1283–9.

46. Trompeo AC, Vidi Y, Locane MD, Braghiroli A, Mascia L, Bosma K, Ranieri VM. Sleep disturbances in the critically ill patients: role of delirium and sedative agents. Minerva Anestesiol. 2011;77:1–2.

47. Tung A, Bergmann BM, Herrera S, Cao D, Mendelson WB. Recovery from sleep deprivation occurs during propofol anesthesia. Anesthesiology. 2004;100:1419–26.

48. Hopkins RO, Jackson JC. Long-term neurocognitive function after critical illness. Chest. 2006;130:869–78.

49. Iwashyna TJ, Ely EW, Smith DM, Langa KM. Long-term cognitive impairment and functional disability among survivors of severe sepsis. JAMA. 2010;304(16):1787–94.

50. Myhren H, Ekeberg O, Stokland O. Health-related quality of life and return to work after critical illness in general intensive care unit patients: a 1-year follow-up study. Crit Care Med. 2010;38(7):1554–61.

51. Witlox J, Eurelings LS, de Jonghe JF, Kalisvaart KJ, Eikelenboom P, van Gool WA. Delirium in elderly patients and the risk of post-discharge mortality, institutionalization, and dementia: a meta-analysis. JAMA. 2010;304:443–51.

52. Fong TG, Jones RN, Shi P, et al. Delirium accelerates cognitive decline in Alzheimer disease. Neurology. 2009;72:1570–5.

53. Hopkins RO, Weaver LK, Collingridge D, et al. Two-year cognitive, emotional, and quality-of-life outcomes in acute respiratory distress syndrome. Am J Respir Crit Care Med. 2005;171:340–7.

54. Jackson JC, Gordon SM, Burger C, et al. Acute respiratory distress syndrome and long-term cognitive impairment: a case study [abstract]. Arch Clin Neuropsychol. 2003;18:688.

55. Rothenhäusler HB, Ehrentraut S, Stoll C, Schelling G, Kapfhammer HP. The relationship between cognitive performance and employment and health status in long-term survivors of the acute respiratory distress syndrome: results of an exploratory study. Gen Hosp Psychiatry. 2001;23:90–6.

56. Jones C, Griffiths RD, Slater T, Benjamin KS, Wilson S. Significant cognitive dysfunction in non-delirious patients identified during and persisting following critical illness. Intensive Care Med. 2006;32:923–6.

57. Iwashyna TJ, Netzer G, Langa KM, Cigolle C. Spurious inferences about long-term outcomes: the case of severe sepsis and geriatric conditions. Am J Respir Crit Care Med. 2012;185:835–41.

58. Cheung AM, Tansey CM, Tomlinson G, et al. Two-year outcomes, health care use, and costs of survivors of acute respiratory distress syndrome. Am J Respir Crit Care Med. 2006;174:538–44.

59. Stevens RD, Marshall SA, Cornblath DR, Hoke A, Needham DM, de Jonghe B, Ali NA, Sharshar T. A framework for diagnosing and classifying intensive care unit-acquired weakness. Crit Care Med. 2009;37(10 suppl):S299–308.

60. Howard RS, Tan V, Z'Graggen WJ. Weakness on the intensive care unit. Pract Neurol. 2008;8:280–95.

61. Bednarik J, Lukas Z, Vondracek P. Critical illness polyneuromyopathy: the electrophysiological components of a complex entity. Intensive Care Med. 2003;29:1505–14.

62. DeJonghe B, Sharshar T, Lefaucheur JP, Authier FJ, Durand-Zaleski I, Boussarsar M, Cerf C, Renaud E, Mesrati F, Carlet J, Raphael JC, Outin H, Bastuji-Garin S. Paresis acquired in the intensive care unit a prospective multicenter study. JAMA. 2002;288(22):2859–67.

63. De Seze M, petit H, Wiart L, Cardinaud JP, Gaujard E, Joseph PA, Mazaux JM, Barat M. Critical illness polyneuropathy a 2-year follow-up study in 19 severe cases. Eur Neurol. 2000;43:61–9.

64. Garnacho-Montero J, Madrazo-Osuna J, Garcia-Garmendia JL, Ortiz-Leyba C, Jimenez-Jimenez FJ, Barrero-Almodovar A, Garnacho-Montero MC, Moyano-Del Estad MR. Critical illness polyneuropathy: risk factors and clinical consequences. A cohort study in septic patients. Intensive Care Med. 2001;27:1288–96.

65. Garnacho-Montero J, Amaya-Villar R, Garcia-Garmendia JL, Madrazo-Osuna J, Ortiz-Leyba C. Effect of critical illness polyneuropathy on the withdrawal from mechanical ventilation and the length of stay in septic patients. Crit Care Med. 2005;33(2):349–54.

66. Guarneri B, Bertolini G, Latronico N. Long-term outcome in patients with critical illness myopathy or neuropathy: the Italian multicentre CRIMYNE study. J Neurol Neurosurg Psychiatry. 2008;79:838–41.

67. Herridge MS, Cheung AM, Tansey CM, Matte-Martyn A, Diaz-Granados N, Al-Saidi F, Cooper AB, Guest CB, Mazer CD, Mehta S, Stewart TE, Barr A, Cook D, Slutsky AS. One-year outcomes in survivors of the acute respiratory distress syndrome. N Engl J Med. 2003;348(8):683–93.

68. Latronico N, Peli E, Botteri M. Critical illness myopathy and neuropathy. Curr Opin Crit Care. 2005;11:126–32.

69. Leitjen FSS, Harinck-de Weerd JE, Poortvliet DCJ, de Weerd AW. The role of polyneuropathy in motor convalescence after prolonged mechanical ventilation. JAMA. 1995;274:1221–5.

70. Maramattom BV, Wijdicks EFM. Acute neuromuscular weakness in the intensive care unit. Crit Care Med. 2006;34(11):2835–41.

71. Maramattom B, Wijdicks EFM, Sundt TM, Cassivi SD. Flaccid quadriplegia due to necrotizing myopathy following lung transplantation. Transplant Proc. 2004;36:2830–3.

72. Niskanen M, Karl A, Halonen P. Five-year survival after intensive care- comparison of 12,180 patients with the general population. Crit Care Med. 1996;24(2):1962–7.

73. Schweickert WD, Hall J. ICU-acquired weakness. Chest. 2007;131:1541–9.

74. Schweickert WD, Pohlman MC, Nigos C, Pawlik AJ, Esbrook CL, Spears L, Miller M, Franczyk M, Deprizio D, Schmidt GA, Bowman A, Barr R, McCallister KE, Hall JB, Kress JP. Early physical and occupational therapy in mechanically ventilated, critically ill patients: a randomized controlled trial. Lancet. 2009;373:1874–82.

75. Stevens RD, Dowdy DW, Michaels RK, Mendez-Tellez PA, Pronovost PJ, Needham DM. Neuromuscular dysfunction acquired in critical illness: a systematic review. Intensive Care Med. 2007;33:1876–91.

76. Watling SM, Dasta JF. Prolonged paralysis in intensive care unit patients after the use of neuromuscular blocking agents: a review of the literature. Crit Care Med. 1994;22:884–93.

77. Riker RR, Shehabi Y, Bokesch PM, et al. SEDCOM (Safety and Efficacy of Dexmedetomidine Compared With Midazolam) Study Group. Dexmedetomidine vs midazolam for sedation of critically ill patients: a randomized trial. JAMA. 2009;301:489–99.

78. Pandharipande PP, Pun BT, Herr D, et al. Effect of sedation with dexmedetomidine vs lorazepam on acute brain dysfunction in mechanically ventilated patients: the MENDS randomized controlled trial. JAMA. 2007;298:2644–53.

79. Braakman HMH, Lodder J, Postma AA, Span LFR, Mess WH. Vasospasm is a significant factor in cyclosporine-induced neurotoxicity: case report. BMC Neurol. 2010;10:30.

80. Jain A, Kashyp R, Dodson F, Kramer D, Hamad I, Khan A, Eghestad B, Starzl TE, Fung JJ. A prospective randomized trial of tacrolimus and prednisone versus tacrolimus, prednisone, and

mycophenolate mofetil in primary adult liver transplantation: a single center report. Transplantation. 2001;72:1091–7.

81. McDiarmid SV, Busuttil RW, Ascher NL, Burdick J, D'alessandro AM, Esquivel C, Kalayoglu M, Klein AS, Marsh JW, Miller CW, Schwartz ME, Shaw BW, SO SK. FK506 (tacrolimus) compared with cyclosporine for primary immunosuppression after pediatric liver transplantation. Transplantation. 1995;59:530–6.

82. Mueller AR, Platz KP, Bechstein WO, Schattenfroh N, Stoltenburg-Didinger G, Blumhardt G, Christe W, Neuhaus P. Neurotoxicity after orthotopic liver transplantation a comparison between cyclosporine and FK506. Transplantation. 1994;58:155–69.

83. Pfitzmann R, Klupp J, Langrehr JM, Uhl M, Neuhaus R, Settmacher U, Steinmueller T, Neuhaus P. Mycophenolatemofetil for immunosuppression after liver transplantation: a follow-up study of 191 patients. Transplantation. 2003;76:130–6.

84. Saner FH, Gensicke J, Olde Damink SWM, Pavlakovic G, Treckmann J, Dammann M, Kaiser GM, Sotiropoulos GC, Radtke A, Koeppen S, Beckebaum S, Cicinnati V, Nadalin S, Malago M, Paul A, Broelsch CE. Neurologic complications in adult living donor liver transplant patients: an underestimated factor? J Neurol. 2010;257:253–8.

85. Selzner N, Durand F, Bernuau J, Heneghan MA, Tuttle-Newhal JE, Belghiti J, Clavien PA. Conversion from cyclosporine to FK506 in adult liver transplant recipients: a combined north American and European experience. Transplantation. 2001;76:1061–5.

86. Umeda Y, Matsuda H, Sadamori H, Shinoura S, Yoshida R, Sato D, Utsumi M, Yagi T, Fujiwara T. Leukoencephalopathy syndrome after living-donor liver transplantation. Exp Clin Transplant. 2011;9:139–44.

87. Li JS, Sexton DJ, Mick N, et al. Proposed modifications to the Duke criteria for the diagnosis of infectious endocarditis. Clin Infect Dis. 2000;30:633–8.

88. Cabell CH, Pond KK, Peterson GE, et al. The risk of stroke and death in patients with aortic and mitral valve endocarditis. Am Heart J. 2001;142:75–80.

89. Derex L, Bonnefoy E, Delahaye F. Impact of stroke on therapeutic decision making in infective endocarditis. J Neurol. 2010;257:315–21.

90. Ruttmann E, Willeit J, Ulmer H, et al. Neurological outcome of septic cardioembolic stroke after infective endocarditis. Stroke. 2006;37:2094–9.

91. Rostagno C, Rosso G, Puggelli F, et al. Active infective endocarditis: clinical characteristics and factors related to hospital mortality. Cardiol J. 2010;16:566–73.

92. Amodeo MR, Clulow T, Lainchbury J, et al. Outpatient intravenous treatment for infective endocarditis: safety, effectiveness, and one-year outcomes. J Infect. 2009;59:387–93.

93. Bishara J, Leibovici L, Gartman-Israel D, et al. Long-term outcome of infective endocarditis: the impact of early surgical intervention. Clin Infect Dis. 2001;33:1636–43.

94. Murdoch DR, Corey GR, Hoen B, et al. Clinical presentation, etiology, and outcome of infective endocarditis in the 21st century. Arch Intern Med. 2009;169(5):463–73.

95. Denk K, Vahl CF. Endokarditis: entscheidungshilfen fur den optimalen zeitpunkt zur operativen sanierung. Herz. 2009;34:198–205.

96. Wang A, Pappas P, Anstrom KJ, et al. The use and effect of surgical therapy for prosthetic valve infective endocarditis: a propensity analysis of a multicenter international cohort. Am Heart J. 2005;150:1086–91.

97. Perrotta S, Aljassim O, Jeppsson A, Bech-Hanssen O, Svensson G. Survival and quality of life after aortic root replacement with homografts in acute endocarditis. Ann Thorac Surg. 2010;90:1862–8.

98. Bernard SA, Gray TW, Buist MD, et al. Treatment of comatose survivors of out-of-hospital cardiac arrest with induced hypothermia. N Engl J Med. 2002;346:557–63.

99. Hypothermia After Cardiac Arrest Study Group. Mild therapeutic hypothermia to improve the neurologic outcome after cardiac arrest. N Engl J Med. 2002;346:549–56.

100. Lance JW, Adams RD. The syndrome of intention or action myoclonus as a sequel to hypoxic encephalopathy. Brain. 1963;86:111–36.

101. Herridge MS, Tansey CM, Matté A, Tomlinson G, Diaz-Granados N, Cooper A, et al. Canadian Critical Care Trials Group. Functional disability 5 years after acute respiratory distress syndrome. N Engl J Med. 2011;364:1293–304.

102. Wijdicks EF, Hijdra A, Young GB, Bassetti CL, Wiebe S, Quality Standards Subcommittee of the American Academy of Neurology. Practice parameter: prediction of outcome in comatose survivors after cardiopulmonary resuscitation (an evidence-based review): report of the Quality Standards Subcommittee of the American Academy of Neurology. Neurology. 2006;67:203–10.

103. Bouwes A, Binnekade JM, Kuiper MA, et al. Prognosis of coma after therapeutic hypothermia: a prospective cohort study. Ann Neurol. 2012;71:206–12.

104. Rossetti AO, Oddo M, Logroscino G, Kaplan PW. Prognostication after cardiac arrest and hypothermia: a prospective study. Ann Neurol. 2010;67:301–7.

105. Wijdicks EFM, Parisi JE, Sharbrough FW. Prognostic value of myoclonus status in comatose survivors of cardiac arrest. Ann Neurol. 1994;35:239–43.

106. English WA, Griffin NJ, Nolan JP. Myoclonus after cardiac arrest: pitfalls in diagnosis and prognosis. Anaesthesia. 2009;64:908–11.

107. Hopkins RO, Weaver LK, Pope D, Orme JF, Bigler ED, Larson-Lohr V. Neuropsychological sequelae and impaired health status in survivors of severe acute respiratory distress syndrome. Am J Respir Crit Care Med. 1999;160:50–6.

108. Hopkins RO, Weaver LK, Chan KJ, Orme JF. Quality of life, emotional, and cognitive function following acute respiratory distress syndrome. J Int Neuropsychol Soc. 2004;10:1005–17.

109. Jackson JC, Hart RP, Gordon SM, et al. Six-month neuropsychological outcome of medical intensive care unit patients. Crit Care Med. 2003;31:1226–34.

110. Rothenhausler HB, Ehrentraut S, Stoll C, Schelling G, Kapfhammer HP. The relationship between cognitive performance and employment and health status in long-term survivors of the acute respiratory distress syndrome: results of an exploratory study. Gen Hosp Psychiatry. 2001;23:90–6.

111. Hopkins RO, Gale SD, Weaver LK. Brain atrophy and cognitive impairment in survivors of acute respiratory distress syndrome. Brain Inj. 2006;20(3):263–71.

112. Dantzer R, Kelley KW. Twenty years of research on cytokine-induced sickness behavior. Brain Behav Immun. 2007;21:153–60.

113. Taraborrelli C, Palchykova S, Tobler I, Gast H, Birchler T, Fontana A. TNFR1 is essential for CD40, but not for lipopolysaccharide-induced sickness behavior and clock gene dysregulation. Brain Behav Immun. 2011;25:434–42.

114. Wilson JX, Young GB. Sepsis-associated encephalopathy: evolving concepts. Can J Neurol Sci. 2003;30:98–105.

115. Young GB, Bolton CF, Archibald YM, Austin TW, Wells GA. The electroencephalogram in sepsis-associated encephalopathy. J Clin Neurophysiol. 1992;9:145–52.

116. Sharshar T, Carlier R, Bernard F, et al. Brain lesions in septic shock: a magnetic resonance imaging study. Intensive Care Med. 2007;33:798–806.

117. Piazza O, Russo E, Cotena S, Esposito G, Tufano R. Elevated S100B levels do not correlate with severity of encephalopathy during sepsis. Br J Anaesth. 2007;99:518–21.

118. Iacobone E, Bailly-Salin J, Polito A, Friedman D, Stevens RD, Sharshar T. Sepsis-associated encephalopathy and its differential diagnosis. Crit Care Med. 2009;37(10 Supp.):S331–6.

119. Siami S, Annane D, Sharshar T. The encephalopathy in sepsis. Crit Care Clin. 2008;24:67–82.

120. Taccone FS, Castanares-Zapatero D, Peres-Bota D, Vincent JL, Berre J, Melot C. Cerebral autoregulation is influenced by carbon dioxide levels in patients with septic shock. Neurocrit Care. 2010;12:35–42.

121. Jackson AC, Gilbert JJ, Young B, Bolton CF. The encephalopathy of sepsis. Can J Neurol Sci. 1985;12:303–7.

122. Nauwynck M, Huyghens L. Neurological complications in critically ill patients; septic encephalopathy, critical illness polyneuropathy. Acta Clin Belg. 1998;53:92–7.

123. Freund HR, Ryan JA, Fischer JE. Amino acid derangements in patients with sepsis: treatment with branched chain amino acid rich infusions. Ann Surg. 1978;188:423–30.

124. Raghavan M, Marik PE. Therapy of intracranial hypertension in patients with fulminant hepatic failure. Neurocrit Care. 2006;4: 179–89.

125. Gottlieb A, DeBoer KR. Brain preservation during orthotopic liver transplantation in a patient with acute liver failure and severe elevation in intracranial pressure. J Gastrointest Surg. 2005;9(7):888–90.

126. Lockwood AH. Hepatic encephalopathy. In: Aminoff MJ, editor. Neurology and general medicine. 3rd ed. Philadelphia: Churchill Livingstone; 2001.

127. Gotthardt D, Riediger C, Heinz Weiss K, Encke J, Schemmer P, Schmidt J, Sauer P. Fulminant hepatic failure: etiology and indications for liver transplantation. Nephrol Dial Transplant. 2007;22 suppl 8:viii5–8.

128. Jalan R, Olde Damink SWM, Deutz NEP, Hayes PC, Lee A. Moderate hypothermia in patients with acute liver failure and uncontrolled intracranial hypertension. Gastroenterology. 2004;127: 1338–46.

129. Blei A, Cordoba J, et al. Hepatic encephalopathy. Am J Gastroenterol. 2001;96:1968–76.

130. Ferenci P, Lockwood A, Mullen K, et al. Hepatic encephalopathy-definition, nomenclature, diagnosis, and quantification: final report of the working party at the 11th world congress of gastroenterology, Vienna, 1998. Hepatology. 2002;35:716–21.

131. Jalan R. Pathophysiological basis of therapy of raised intracranial pressure in acute liver failure. Neurochem Int. 2005;47:78–83.

132. Norenberg MD. A light and electron microscopic study of experimental portal-systemic (ammonia) encephalopathy: progression and reversal of the disorder. Lab Invest. 1977;36:618.

133. Mancall EL. Nutritional disorders of the nervous system. In: Aminoff MJ, editor. Neurology and general medicine. 3rd ed. New York: Churchill Livingstone; 2001.

134. Chin RL, Latov N, Green PHR, et al. Neurologic complications of celiac disease. J Clin Neuromusc Dis. 2004;5:129–37.

135. Androgue HJ, Madias NE. Hypernatremia. N Engl J Med. 2000; 342:1493–9.

136. Androgue HJ, Madias NE. Hyponatremia. N Engl J Med. 2000; 342:1581–9.

137. Elhassan EA, Schrier RW. Hyponatremia: diagnosis, complications, and management including V2 receptor antagonists. Curr Opin Nephrol Hypertens. 2011;20:161–8.

138. Halawa I, Andersson T, Tomson T. Hyponatremia and risk of seizures: a retrospective cross-sectional study. Epilepsia. 2011;52(2):410–3.

139. Samuels MA, Seifter JL. Encephalopathies caused by electrolyte disorders. Semin Neurol. 2011;31:135–8.

140. Sterns RH. Severe symptomatic hyponatremia: treatment and outcome. A study of 64 cases. Ann Intern Med. 1987;107:656–64.

Central Nervous System Infections

22

Lennox K. Archibald and Ronald G. Quisling

Contents

L.K. Archibald, MD, PhD, FRCP (✉)
Department of Medicine, College of Medicine,
University of Florida College of Medicine and
the Malcom Randall VA Medical Center,
Gainesville, FL 32610, USA
e-mail: lennox.archibald@medicine.ufl.edu

R.G. Quisling, MD
Department of Radiology, Neuroradiology Section,
University of Florida College of Medicine, JHMHC, 100374,
Gainesville, FL 32610, USA
e-mail: quislr@radiology.ufl.edu

A.J. Layon et al. (eds.), *Textbook of Neurointensive Care*,
DOI 10.1007/978-1-4471-5226-2_22, © Springer-Verlag London 2013

Abstract

Central nervous system (CNS) infections—i.e., infections involving the brain (cerebrum and cerebellum), spinal cord, optic nerves, and their covering membranes—are medical emergencies that are associated with substantial morbidity, mortality, or long-term sequelae that may have catastrophic implications for the quality of life of affected individuals. Acute CNS infections that warrant neurointensive care (ICU) admission fall broadly into three categories—meningitis, encephalitis, and abscesses—and generally result from blood-borne spread of the respective microorganisms. Other causes of CNS infections include head trauma resulting in fractures at the base of the skull or the cribriform plate that can lead to an opening between the CNS and the sinuses, mastoid, the middle ear, or the nasopharynx. Extrinsic contamination of the CNS can occur intraoperatively during neurosurgical procedures. Also, implanted medical devices or adjunct hardware (e.g., shunts, ventriculostomies, or external drainage tubes) and congenital malformations (e.g., spina bifida or sinus tracts) can become colonized and serve as sources or foci of infection. Viruses, such as rabies, herpes simplex virus, or polioviruses, can spread to the CNS via intraneural pathways resulting in encephalitis. If infection occurs at sites (e.g., middle ear or mastoid) contiguous with the CNS, infection may spread directly into the CNS causing brain abscesses; alternatively, the organism may reach the CNS indirectly via venous drainage or the sheaths of cranial and spinal nerves. Abscesses also may become localized in the subdural or epidural spaces. Meningitis results if bacteria spread directly from an abscess to the subarachnoid space. CNS abscesses may be a result of pyogenic meningitis or from septic emboli associated with endocarditis, lung abscess, or other serious purulent infections. Breaches of the blood–brain barrier (BBB) can result in CNS infections. Causes of such breaches include damage (e.g., microhemorrhage or necrosis of surrounding tissue) to the BBB; mechanical obstruction of microvessels by parasitized red blood cells, leukocytes, or platelets; overproduction of cytokines that degrade tight junction proteins; or microbe-specific interactions with the BBB that facilitate transcellular passage of the microorganism. The microorganisms that cause CNS infections include a wide range of bacteria, mycobacteria, yeasts, fungi, viruses, spirochaetes (e.g., neurosyphilis), and parasites (e.g., cerebral malaria and strongyloidiasis). The clinical picture of the various infections can be nonspecific or characterized by distinct, recognizable clinical syndromes. At some juncture, individuals with severe acute CNS infections require critical care management that warrants neuro-ICU admission. The implications for CNS infections are serious and complex and include the increased human and material resources necessary to manage very sick patients, the difficulties in triaging patients with vague or mild symptoms, and ascertaining the precise cause and degree of CNS involvement at the time of admission to the neuro-ICU. This chapter addresses a wide range of severe CNS infections that are better managed in the neuro-ICU. Topics covered include the medical epidemiology of the respective CNS infection; discussions of the relevant neuroanatomy and blood supply (essential for understanding the pathogenesis of CNS infections) and pathophysiology; symptoms and signs; diagnostic procedures, including essential neuroimaging studies; therapeutic options, including empirical therapy where indicated; and the perennial issue of the utility and effectiveness of steroid therapy for certain CNS infections. Finally, therapeutic options and alternatives are discussed, including the choices of antimicrobial agents best able to cross the BBB, supportive therapy, and prognosis.

Keywords

Acute bacterial meningitis • Amoebic meningoencephalitis • Aseptic meningitis • Aspergillus infections of the CNS • Bartonella (cat-scratch disease) CNS infection • Blastomycosis of the CNS • Brain abscess • Candida CNS infections • Cat-scratch fever • Cerebral malaria • Cerebritis • CNS complications of strongyloidiasis • CNS infections caused by rapidly growing mycobacteria • CNS complications of Rocky Mountain spotted fever • CNS mucormycosis • CNS mycoses • CNS zygomycosis • Coccidioidal meningitis • Cryptococcus meningitis • Cytomegalovirus encephalitis • Dengue • Echinococcus involvement of the CNS • External ventricular drainage infections • Fungal CNS infections • Fungal meningitis • Histoplasma CNS infections • HIV encephalopathy • Ehrlichiosis of the CNS • Lyme disease • Mycobacterium tuberculosis infections of the CNS • Neurocysticercosis • Neurosyphilis • Parasitic infections of the CNS • Progressive multifocal leukoencephalopathy • Pyogenic bacterial abscesses of the CNS • Rhinocerebral mucormycosis • Rickettsial diseases of the CNS • Spinal epidural abscess • Spinal tuberculosis • Steroids use in CNS infections • Therapy of CNS infections • Vertebral osteomyelitis • Viral meningitis • Whipple's disease of the CNS

Introduction

Acute infections of the central nervous system (CNS) are medical emergencies that if not addressed promptly result in significant mortality or long-term sequelae that have catastrophic implications for the quality of life of affected individuals. To fully understand the pathogenesis, clinical implications, and management of CNS infections, some knowledge of applied neuroanatomy is essential.

The CNS is defined by the brain (cerebrum and cerebellum), spinal cord, optic nerves, and their covering membranes. These structures are protected within the rigid confines of the skull and spinal canal of the vertebral column. The cerebral cortex (the outermost, gray tissue layer of the cerebrum) and the spinal cord are covered by three layers of continuous protective tissue called the meninges. The innermost meningeal layer that directly overlies the cerebral cortex is called the pia mater. The middle and outermost layers are known as the arachnoid and dura mater, respectively. The dura mater forms several intracranial compartments, including sinuses for venous drainage. Parts of the arachnoid—the arachnoid villi—project into these sinuses. The subpial space is continuous with the Virchow-Robin spaces. These two spaces transmit penetrating vessels to and from the brain parenchyma and do not connect with the subarachnoid space. The subarachnoid space lies between the pia mater and the arachnoid and is continuous in nature; the subdural space lies between the arachnoid and the dura mater. The epidural space lies between the dura and the skull. Certain infections can access the subpial and Virchow-Robin spaces, while most do not. Infections within the epidural spaces are usually caused by direct extension from adjacent infections and the infection remains in close proximity to the inciting source. Subdural infections are often associated with an extracerebral source, but these infections can spread widely within the subdural compartment well away from the inciting source. It is not uncommon to develop serous subdural effusions in bacterial meningitis. Subarachnoid infections are most often caused by hematogenous dissemination of organisms or viruses.

Cerebrospinal fluid (CSF) is continuously produced by the choroid plexuses within the four ventricles of the brain. CSF fills the lateral and third ventricles and circulates to the fourth ventricle, which lies between the cerebellum and the midbrain. CSF flows from the fourth ventricle into the subarachnoid space, where it bathes the entire CNS, and drains via the arachnoid villi into the superior sagittal sinus in the dura mater, where it is resorbed into the bloodstream.

A working knowledge of the blood supply is also essential for understanding the pathogenesis of CNS infections. The capillary supply to the brain and spinal cord is unique—the outermost layers of endothelial cells are fused together. These specialized brain microvascular endothelial cells constitute the blood–brain barrier, which separates the brain and the meninges from the circulating blood and impedes the influx of microorganisms, toxic agents, and most other compounds, while regulating the flow of essential nutrients and molecules for normal neural function. Thus, pathogens that breach the blood–brain barrier can cause CNS infections. Causes of such breaches include damage (e.g., microhemorrhage or necrosis of surrounding tissue) to the barrier; mechanical obstruction of microvessels by parasitized red blood cells, leukocytes, or platelets; overproduction of cytokines that degrade tight junction proteins; or microbe-specific interactions with the blood–brain barrier that facilitate transcellular passage of the microorganism (e.g., Escherichia coli, mycobacteria, and spirochaetes). The therapeutic implications are obvious—to be effective, antimicrobials prescribed for CNS infections must be able to cross the blood–brain barrier.

Routes of Infection

Acute CNS infections fall broadly into three categories—meningitis, encephalitis, and abscesses—and generally result from blood-borne spread of the respective microorganisms. Bacteremia or viremia can result from infection at sites adjacent or contiguous to the CNS, such as the mastoid, sinuses, or middle ear, or from primary infections at more remote anatomic sites (e.g., lungs, heart, skin, gastrointestinal tract, or kidney). In children the most common predisposing conditions are sinus or middle ear infection, which lead to transient bacteremia and hematogenous seeding of the CNS [1–3]. Bacterial infections of the paranasal and otomastoid sinuses often produce phlebothrombosis of adjacent draining cortical (cerebral) veins. This thrombotic process can extend into regional dural sinuses. The phlebothrombosis becomes thrombophlebitis offering a direct route of transmission from the infected sinus to the adjacent extra axial spaces or to the brain along cortical venous drainage pathways. Recognition of the venous involvement is essential, since the venous obstruction can produce intra axial brain swelling which may obscure the extra axial infection source contributing to misleading interpretations on brain and spinal imaging studies. The common relationship between paranasal sinus and otomastoid causes of intracranial infection reinforces the need for the clinician and radiologic imager to be well versed in both head and neck and paraspinous anatomy.

In patients with bacteremia or viremia, the organism, upon entering the venous sinuses, may cross the blood–brain barrier, penetrate the dura and arachnoid, and gain access to the subarachnoid space, thereby causing infection of the CSF and further dissemination of the infection throughout this anatomic space. Fractures at the base of the skull or the cribriform plate can lead to an opening between the CNS and the sinuses, mastoid, the middle ear, or the nasopharynx. Since

Table 22.1 Causes of bacterial meningitis and overall case fatality rate according to organism

Organism	% of total cases	Incidence	Predisposing conditions	Case fatality rate (%)
Streptococcus pneumoniae	47	1.1	Otitis media; sinusitis; alcoholism; cirrhosis; pneumococcal pneumonia; immunosuppression; skull fracture; CSF leak; myeloma; sickle cell disease	21
Neisseria meningitidis	25	0.6	"Closed" institutional setting; lack of specific antibody; complement deficiencies	3
Group B Streptococcus	12	0.3	Neonatal period; colonized mothers; preterm labor; prolonged rupture of membranes; intrapartum fever	7
Listeria monocytogenes	8	0.2	Neonatal period; immunosuppression; age; alcoholism/cirrhosis	15
Haemophilus influenzae	7	0.2	Lack of antibody to polysaccharide capsule; preceding otitis media	6

Adapted with permission of the Massachusetts Medical Society from Schuchat et al. [1]

these sites are all contiguous with the upper respiratory tract, CSF leaks occurring at any of these sites may enable respiratory flora to track back up into the subarachnoid space. Extrinsic contamination of the CNS can occur intraoperatively during neurosurgical procedures and, further, implanted medical devices or adjunct hardware (e.g., shunts, ventriculostomies, or external drainage tubes) can become colonized and serve as foci of infection. Congenital malformations, such as spina bifida or sinus tracts, can become colonized and serve as sources of infection. Viruses, such as rabies, herpes simplex virus (HSV), or polioviruses, can spread to the CNS via intraneural pathways resulting in encephalitis.

If infection occurs at sites (e.g., middle ear or mastoid) contiguous with the CNS, infection may spread directly into the CNS causing brain abscesses; alternatively, the organism may reach the CNS indirectly via venous drainage or the sheaths of cranial and spinal nerves. Abscesses also may become localized in the subdural or epidural spaces. Meningitis results if bacteria spread directly from an abscess to the subarachnoid space. CNS abscesses may be a result of pyogenic meningitis or from septic emboli associated with endocarditis, lung abscess, or other serious purulent infections, such as those caused by the *Streptococcus milleri* group.

Acute Bacterial Meningitis

Bacterial meningitis, a serious brain infection, can develop rapidly into a life-threatening infection even in previously healthy children or adults. Bacteria that cause meningitis enter the bloodstream, are carried toward the brain, and somehow manage to cross the defensive line of the blood–brain barrier outlined previously.

Definition

Bacterial meningitis can be defined as an inflammatory response to pyogenic bacterial invasion of the pia mater, the arachnoid membranes, and surrounding the CNS. This infection typically involves the entire length of the neuraxis including the brain (cerebrum, cerebellum), spinal cord, optic nerves, and their covering membranes because of the continuous nature of the subarachnoid space. Pyogenic meningitis is associated with a marked, acute inflammatory exudate; non-pyogenic microorganisms (e.g., mycobacteria or spirochetes like *Leptospira* spp.) are less commonly implicated. Clinically, onset is acute with development of headache, fever, irritability, and stiff neck with or without focal neurological signs over hours to a few days. Although the overall annual incidence of pyogenic bacterial meningitis in the United States is decreasing, the outcome is invariably fatal if left untreated [1, 4].

Epidemiology

The common causes of bacterial meningitis in the United States include *Streptococcus pneumoniae*, *Neisseria meningitidis*, group B *Streptococcus* spp., *Listeria monocytogenes*, and *Haemophilus influenzae*. Collectively, these agents account for over 95 % of cases (Table 22.1). The age distribution, predisposing conditions, and fatality rates for the most common agents are summarized in Fig. 22.1 and Table 22.1.

Streptococcus pneumoniae

Of the three predominant organisms (*S. pneumoniae*, *N. meningitidis*, and *H. influenzae*) most often implicated in community-associated meningitis in the United States, *S. pneumoniae* is the most common and affects all age groups, except infants in the immediate neonatal period. The risk of pneumococcal meningitis varies with age but is significantly higher in infants than in young children and adults. Over the age of 70 years, the incidence rises again to approximately double the average incidence for young and middle-aged adults. In adults the major predisposing factors for infection include alcoholism, splenectomy, human immunodeficiency virus (HIV) infection, other acquired immunodeficiency

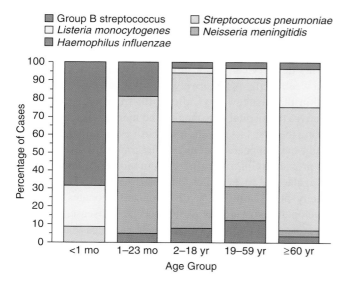

Fig. 22.1 Pathogenic agents of bacterial meningitis according to age group (Used with permission of the Massachusetts Medical Society from Schuchat et al. [1])

conditions, diabetes, other underlying chronic conditions (e.g., chronic renal disease), and prior viral respiratory infection. Pneumococcal meningitis is the most common form of recurrent meningitis in patients who have CSF leaks. *S. pneumoniae* is spread by respiratory transmission in the general population and results in colonization of the nasopharynx with rates commonly in the range of 5–10 % of healthy adults. During the wintertime, carriage rates can rise to 20–30 % in certain populations depending on age and other factors. Overcrowding in day-care centers, military barracks, and prisons is often implicated in the transmission.

N. meningitidis

This is an aerobic, gram-negative diplococcus that colonizes the mucosal surface of the nasopharynx. The main mode of transmission is via direct contact with large droplet respiratory secretions from patients or asymptomatic carriers; humans are the only host. Invasive disease caused by this organism occurs in three clinical forms: meningitis (50 % of cases), blood infection (30 %), and pneumonia (10 %); other forms account for the remainder (10 %) of the cases. *N. meningitidis* has now become the leading cause of bacterial meningitis in the United States with an estimated annual incidence of approximately 0.5–1.5 cases per 100,000 population and at least tenfold higher in less-developed countries [1]. Persons at risk include household contacts of infected patients, military recruits, college freshmen who live in dormitories, microbiologists who work with isolates of *N. meningitidis*, persons traveling to a country where meningococcal disease is epidemic or highly endemic, and patients without spleens or with terminal complement component deficiencies. Infants less than 1 year of age and adolescents ages

16–21 years have higher rates of disease than other age groups, although infection can occur in all age groups including the elderly.

Strains of *N. meningitidis* are characterized according to the serologic recognition of polysaccharide epitopes on their capsule and outer membrane and are classified into serogroups A, B, C, W135, and Y. In the United States, strains from serogroups B, C, and Y cause the majority (45 %) of infections, whereas in less-developed countries serogroups A and C predominate; serogroup A has also been implicated in epidemics in sub-Saharan Africa.

H. influenzae

This is a small, pleomorphic, aerobic or facultative anaerobic gram-negative coccobacilli that is classified according to six serologically distinct antigenic types based on capsular polysaccharides a–f. Of these, only *H. influenzae* type b (Hib) is pathogenic. Although the nonencapsulated form of *H. influenzae* is a common inhabitant of the upper respiratory tract of healthy humans and causes localized infection (e.g., conjunctivitis or otitis media in children) without bacteremia, the more virulent encapsulated Hib serotype causes more invasive disease and is an important cause of meningitis or epiglottitis. Hib meningitis is relatively uncommon during the first 2 months of life probably because of the presence of passively transferred maternal antibodies. But by the fourth month of life, children lose these antibodies and become at risk of Hib meningitis. The occurrence of *H. influenzae* meningitis is directly associated with the presence and development of type-specific anticapsular antibodies to polyribosylribitol phosphate. Whether vaccine-induced or occurring naturally, presence of these antibodies is directly related to protection from invasive *H. influenzae* infection [5]. Various clinical studies have shown these antibodies to be opsonic and bactericidal against *H. influenzae* in vitro and protective in vivo. In the pre-vaccine era, colonization with nontypable strains of *H. influenzae* led to the development of cross-reacting antibodies that were largely protective against infection caused by type b strains. Before the introduction of the Hib conjugate polysaccharide capsular vaccine in 1986, *H. influenzae* was the most common cause of acute bacterial meningitis in children under the age of 5, with as many as 1 in 200 children acquiring invasive *H. influenzae* infection, including epiglottitis, septicemia, arthritis, and soft tissue infections in addition to meningitis. However, by 1995, the prevalence of meningitis caused by Hib had fallen 55 % [6]. Risk factors for Hib meningitis include malignancy, chronic renal disease, sickle cell disease, immunoglobulin dyscrasias, HIV infections, and cystic fibrosis.

Listeria monocytogenes

This is a facultative anaerobic, intracellular gram-positive bacillus that remains a significant cause of neonatal meningitis in the USA. Although the mode of transmission to humans is generally fecal-oral, transmission of the pathogen to the neonate generally occurs at the time of birth in mothers who had asymptomatic colonization of the genital or gastrointestinal tract prior to delivery. Domestic and wild animals are the main reservoirs for *L. monocytogenes*, but as the prevalence of stool carriage of this organism among asymptomatic adults is about 1 %, humans remain a small but still significant reservoir.

Generally, healthy adults exposed to the organism do not become ill, unless exposed to high numbers of infectious organisms, such as during an outbreak. *L. monocytogenes* causes meningitis most often in adults with depressed cell-mediated immunity, patients on steroids or other immunosuppressive agents, HIV-infected individuals, transplant recipients, and other vulnerable populations, such as persons with diabetes, alcohol abuse, chronic liver disease, renal disease requiring hemodialysis, or persons greater than 60 years of age. Outbreaks of *L. monocytogenes* meningitis in the United States and elsewhere have been associated with unpasteurized milk products, such as Swiss or feta cheese, undercooked chicken or hot dogs, seafood, vegetables, or coleslaw.

Other Microorganisms

Gram-negative microorganisms are important causes of acute bacterial meningitis. Persons with diabetes, a history of alcohol abuse, hepatic cirrhosis, or chronic urinary tract infections are particularly susceptible. *E. coli* with the K1 capsular polysaccharide antigen accounts for a majority of the cases of gram-negative meningitis in the newborn [7]. Carriage rates of the *E. coli* K1 serotypes vary in different populations but range from 7 to 38 % in women of childbearing age and may be as high as 50 % in nursing personnel [8–10]. In a study of 231 children presenting with bacterial meningitis to the emergency department during the era of widespread heptavalent conjugate pneumococcal vaccination, *E. coli* was implicated in 4 % and other gram-negative bacilli in 3.0 % [11, 12]. Other gram-negative organisms such as *Klebsiella* spp., *Enterobacter* spp., *Pseudomonas* spp., *Citrobacter* spp., and *Salmonella* spp. may also cause meningitis in the neonatal period, with an epidemiology similar to that of the *E. coli* K1 strains. Gram-negative bacillary meningitis still carries a worse prognosis than meningitis with a gram-positive organism [13]. Beyond the neonatal period, the vast majority of cases of gram-negative meningitis occur in the inpatient setting, especially following neurosurgery (e.g., craniotomy) and during placement of devices, such as ventriculostomy tubes, spinal surgery, or in patients who have suffered head trauma [14].

Group B Streptococcus (*Streptococcus agalactiae*) is the single most frequent cause of neonatal meningitis. This organism has been cultured from vaginal secretions in 30–40 % of women prior to delivery. During pregnancy, labor, and delivery, the microorganism can be transmitted to amniotic fluid or the newborn may become colonized as it passes through the birth canal. Transmission to the infant during delivery can result in neonatal meningitis within the first week of life. Alternatively, the organism may be acquired within the first few days after birth from adult contacts—relatives or hospital personnel—and meningitis may develop during the first 1–2 months after birth even though the infant might have appeared healthy at the time of delivery. While the probability of transmission from mothers colonized with *S. agalactiae* to neonates delivered vaginally is approximately 50 %, only 2 % of colonized neonates go on to develop invasive group B streptococcal disease. Group B streptococci produce polysaccharide capsules that manifest nine antigenic serotypes (types Ia–VIII). The type III group is responsible for the vast majority of neonatal meningitis; virulence factors (e.g., those causing production of higher levels of neuraminidase) have been described as an explanation for this.

Almost any microorganism that crosses the blood–brain barrier can cause acute meningitis. Other bacterial agents include group A streptococci, non-pneumococcal alpha hemolytic streptococci, *Neisseria gonorrhea*, *Salmonella* species, *Flavobacterium meningosepticum*, non-influenzae *Haemophilus* species, and even *Bacillus anthracis* (anthrax). Although *S. aureus* and *Staphylococcus epidermidis* are rarely implicated as causes of primary bacterial meningitis, these organisms are relatively common causes of bacterial meningitis following trauma, in situ CSF shunts, or neurosurgical procedures. Other microorganisms, such as *Mycobacterium* spp., *Nocardia* spp., yeasts and fungi (e.g., *Coccidioides immitis*, *Histoplasma capsulatum*, or *Cryptococcus neoformans*), *Treponema* spp., *Brucella* spp., *Leptospira* spp., or *Toxoplasma gondii*, can also produce meningitis. However, with the exception of *Leptospira* spp., these microorganisms tend to produce a more chronic form of meningitis and would not be considered agents of acute bacterial meningitis in the first instance [15]. For example, *Mycobacterium* spp., *C. immitis*, *H. capsulatum*, or *C. neoformans* would more likely produce chronic granulomatous inflammatory changes rather than acute pyogenic infections.

Pathogenesis of Meningeal Invasion

Colonization of the respiratory tract or nasopharynx is the critical first step preceding infection caused by the three microorganisms (*S. pneumoniae*, *N. meningitides*, and *H. influenzae*) most commonly associated with community-acquired meningitis. Biologically, colonization is mediated by affinity of these organisms for the nasopharyngeal mucosa. Colonization is facilitated by attachment and adherence of the microorganisms to cell surface receptors on nasopharyngeal epithelial cells, enabling them to replicate in the upper airway for prolonged periods. All three pathogens, typically, may colonize the upper airway without producing symptoms. Both host susceptibility and pathogen-specific factors (e.g., virulence and pathogenicity) are critical in the development of invasive disease. Many of these factors, though identified and characterized, are still not fully understood. For example, splenectomy definitely predisposes the affected person to invasive disease by *S. pneumoniae*, while it appears to have relatively little effect on the occurrence of invasive *N. meningitidis* disease, despite the fact that both are encapsulated organisms.

Adherence to nasopharyngeal mucosa is mediated by fimbriae or pili, in the case of gram-negative organisms. The pili of *N. meningitidis* are filamentous glycoproteins attached to the bacterial surface, traverse the polysaccharide capsule, and extend beyond the surface of the bacterium, where they can bind to specific receptors on nasopharyngeal cells, in this instance the CD4+ receptor [16, 17]. After receptor binding, further interaction with the host cell is established by certain outer membrane proteins on *N. meningitidis*, designated Opa and Opc [18]. Binding of the outer membrane proteins to specific receptors promotes engulfment of the *N. meningitidis* by the epithelial cells followed by transportation of the bacteria across the cell in membrane-bound vacuoles to the intravascular space; organisms also gain access to the intravascular space by creating separations in the tight junctions of columnar epithelial cells. *N. meningitidis* also possess other outer membrane proteins that function as IgA proteases, which can specifically degrade the surface IgA antibodies on epithelial cells, further enhancing the probability of invasive disease [19]. Once the mucosal barrier has been breached, the development of meningococcal disease is dependent upon the survival of the organism in the bloodstream.

Here, the most important virulence factor for survival of meningococci is the polysaccharide capsule that protects the organism against complement-mediated phagocytosis by neutrophils in the reticular endothelial system [20, 21]. Host defense is clearly determined by the existing humoral antibody to specific polysaccharide capsular types and the cellular responses of the innate immune system.

Protective IgG antibody for meningococcal disease is acquired through maternal transmission and is protective for the first few months after birth. Colonization by nonpathogenic *Neisseria* species and a possibly cross-reacting gram-negative organism such as *E. coli* K1 induces protective antibodies. Antibodies protect by promoting optimization of phagocytosis through opsonization and specific lysis via complement activation. For this reason, patients who are deficient in complement factor C5 are particularly susceptible to repeated invasive infections by *N. meningitidis*. In fact, individuals with an inherited deficiency of any of the terminal components of complement C5, C6, C7, and C8 have a greater risk of invasive disease [22].

Virulence factors for the invasion of *S. pneumoniae* seem to be primarily a function of the capsular polysaccharide type. There are at least 93 known capsular serotypes of *S. pneumoniae* with the various serotypes having different propensities for producing disease or developing antibiotic resistance [23, 24].

Colonization of the upper airway by *H. influenzae* is also mediated by fimbrial attachment to epithelial cells. Alpha fimbriae enhance the binding to the anterior nasopharynx and β fimbriae facilitate binding to the posterior ciliated nasopharyngeal cells [25]. Although *H. influenzae* type b strains that lack fimbriae generally are unable to colonize the nasopharynx, isolates from CSF do not express fimbria, suggesting that while the presence of fimbriae on *H. influenzae* is important for colonization of and attachment to nasopharyngeal mucosa, it does not appear play a significant role in the pathogenesis of meningitis [26, 27].

N. meningitis, *S. pneumoniae*, *H. influenzae* type b and other pathogens are capable of invading the CNS and infecting the meninges due to the incorporation of virulence factors [28]. The chain of events that ultimately lead to invasion of the subarachnoid space by these pathogens includes a cascade of events involving nasopharyngeal or middle ear colonization, bloodstream dissemination of the respective pathogen, crossing of the blood–brain and blood-CSF barriers, and finally entrance and survival of the implicated pathogen into the subarachnoid space and subsequent infection [28]. Bacteria migrate through the brain microvascular endothelial cells in enclosed vacuoles via a mechanism that is dependent on F-actin. Thus, transport through the cell appears to be dependent on cytoskeletal rearrangement involving both microfilaments and microtubules. Because of the blood–brain barrier, immunoglobulin and complement protein levels and leukocytes are significantly lower in CSF than in serum and interstitial fluid. Thus, in the early phase of infection involving the subarachnoid space, bacterial replication proceeds virtually unchecked by host defense mechanisms. Although the major host response to the invasion of the subarachnoid space by pathogenic microorganisms is a rapid influx of polymorphonuclear leukocytes, opsonization of bacteria and subsequent phagocytosis by neutrophils are hindered by the relative paucity of complement and immunoglobulins and the intrinsic fluid nature of CSF which is less facilitating to phagocytosis as compared to solid tissues. In addition, leukocyte proteases derived from the initial influx of leukocytes degrade whatever complement components are present in the CSF [29–31].

Lipopolysaccharide (LPS) molecules from gram-negative bacteria are known to be extremely potent in the development of inflammation, and intracisternal injection of purified LPS from *H. influenzae* also elicits a strong inflammatory

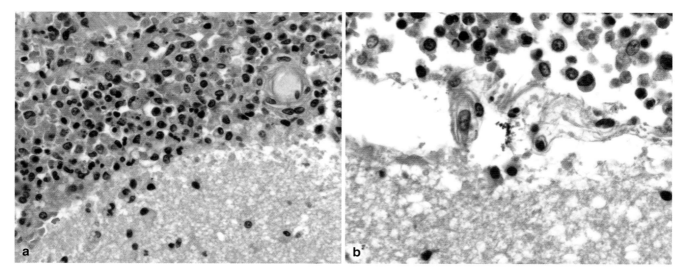

Fig. 22.2 (a) Acute purulent meningitis caused by the *Streptococcus pneumoniae*. Leptomeninges expanded by a dense necroinflammatory infiltrate with neutrophils, lymphocytes, and macrophages (H&E 40×). (b) Gram stain of exudate specimens showing gram-positive diplococci (Both courtesy of Anthony Yachnis, MD, and Kelly Devers, MD, University of Florida College of Medicine)

response [31, 32]. The mechanism by which LPS and other bacterial cell wall components (e.g., teichoic acid and peptidoglycans from *S. pneumoniae*) act to stimulate inflammation is probably through the induction of inflammatory cytokines such as Interleukin 1 (IL-1) or tumor necrosis factor (TNF) [29, 32]. In vitro studies with LPS and with IL-1 and TNF show that incubation with endothelial cell monolayers leads to a rapid, transient increase in the expression of the intercellular adhesion molecules (ICAM-1 and ICAM-2) as well as the selectin molecules such as ELAM-1. As a result, neutrophils are able to bind to CNS vascular endothelial cells at vastly increased rates and then subsequently migrate by diapedesis into the subarachnoid space. At the same time, adherence of neutrophils to the capillary endothelium increases the permeability of the blood vessels enabling more protein leakage into the CSF and subarachnoid space, adding to the inflammatory exudate. Figure 22.2a, b shows the dense inflammatory infiltrate with neutrophils, lymphocytes, and macrophages seen in a patient with purulent meningitis caused by *S. pneumoniae*. IL-1 and TNF, in turn, stimulate leukocytes and other categories of inflammatory cells to produce and secrete a host of other proinflammatory cytokines, proteolytic enzymes, free radicals, and nitric oxide. The end result is edema of the surrounding tissues, cell injury, and tissue necrosis. Infiltration of the walls of small arteries and cortical veins also leads to a vasculitis with intimal thickening, narrowing and occlusion of small arteries, thrombophlebitis of the cortical veins, and thrombosis of the major venous sinuses, leading to ischemia and infarction of brain tissues.

Inflammation of the pia mater and arachnoid affects glucose transport into the CSF resulting in a net lowering of CSF glucose levels. The pathophysiologic consequences of this intense neutrophil response in the subarachnoid space, tissue edema, and vasculitis account for most, if not all, of the serious clinical and pathologic consequences of meningitis, such as the increased permeability of the blood–brain barrier, increased intracranial pressure (ICP), hydrocephalus, and reduced cerebral blood flow, leading to cerebral hypoxia and death [32].

The ICP is raised via several mechanisms. First, vasogenic cerebral edema is caused by the increased permeability of the blood–brain barrier, which is a direct result of inflammatory bacterial products or the inflammatory cytokines released in response to these products. Second, the alterations in brain cellular membranes lead to cytotoxic cerebral edema resulting from increased intracellular water content, potassium leakage, and a shift in brain metabolism to anaerobic glycolysis with increased lactate production. And third, as a result of the inflammation in the subarachnoid space, there is decreased ability to reabsorb CSF, which leads to interstitial edema in brain parenchyma. All three mechanisms contribute to increased ICP pressure, which in turn may precipitate transtentorial brain herniation.

Clinical Manifestations

In the typical clinical presentation of meningitis in adults, fever, headache, and stiff neck predominate although there might be varying degrees of altered consciousness. Though vomiting is a common symptom generally attributed to raised ICP, it is also a well-recognized manifestation of the effects of the inflammatory process on the midbrain. The nature of the presentation of meningitis depends on the underlying microorganism responsible for the infection. For example, in pneumococcal meningitis (S. pneumoniae is the most common etiologic agent implicated in adult bacterial meningitis cases), the patient might have had pneumonia and bloodstream dissemination before progression to meningitis. Thus, the patient might have presented with chills and rigors or symptoms of upper respiratory tract infection, bronchitis, or pneumonia several days before the actual onset of meningitis symptoms. In the classic series by Carpenter and Petersdorf, approximately 27 % of patients had a sudden onset of headache, confusion, lethargy, and alteration of consciousness within the first 24 h before admission to hospital [33]. In contrast, 53 % presented with a more slowly progressive course over 1–7 days.

In a review of 493 episodes of meningitis, Durand and colleagues found that 95 % of the patients with acquired meningitis had a temperature greater than 37.7 °C on admission, while neck stiffness was present in 88 %. Only 22 % were alert, 51 % were confused or lethargic, and 22 % were responsive only to pain. Within the first 24–48 h of onset, 29 % had suffered focal seizures or had exhibited focal neurologic signs [34]. The most common predisposing factors for acute meningitis included pneumonia, sinusitis, otitis media, alcoholism, diabetes, or immunosuppression associated with conditions, such as malignancy, connective tissue diseases, sickle cell disease, diabetes, organ transplantation, splenectomy, dialysis, or steroids and other immunosuppressive therapy. For patients with some of these underlying conditions, the clinical presentation of meningitis may not be classic because of alteration of the immune response, with the diagnosis only being made upon further investigation of altered sensorium, persistent headache, or new onset seizures or neurological symptoms or signs. The presentation of patients with meningococcal meningitis may be similar to those with pneumococcal meningitis; clinically, one might not be able to distinguish between the two. However, meningococcal meningitis is part of the spectrum of N. meningitidis sepsis and the manifestations of meningococcal septicemia may precede the meningitis by 12–24 h. Signs indicative of underlying sepsis may dominate the clinical presentation. The initial presentation in meningococcemia may be completely nonspecific, with the patient simply complaining of feeling unwell but without overt symptoms or signs of meningitis. The clinical condition of these patients may progress to irreversible shock and death before the development or obvious manifestation of meningitis.

Early in meningococcemia, the patient may exhibit a subtle petechial rash (Fig. 22.3) that precedes progression to fulminant disseminated intravascular coagulation (DIC) and development of a more severe, prodigious purpuric rash leading to necrosis of the fingers and toes (Fig. 22.3). Purpura fulminans in the patient with meningococcemia is classically associated with hemorrhagic necrosis of the adrenal gland— the Waterhouse-Friderichsen syndrome. Thus, the clinical manifestation of meningococcal meningitis depends on the relative degree of meningococcemia and shock, as well as the severity of meningitis.

It is important to recognize that the presentation of meningitis in the elderly and the very young may be subtler or more insidious compared with young adults and children. For example, in a review of 54 cases, Gorse and coworkers found that confusion was a predominating symptom in presentation among the elderly compared with the younger age group, and pneumonia was also more likely to be present in the older age group [35]. Typical symptoms and signs are also less commonly reported in the elderly since these patients often have cervical rigidity due to osteoarthritis, cervical spondylosis, or existing cerebrovascular disease. In addition, there may be hypertonicity of the neck muscles in conditions like Parkinson's disease. Among the elderly, the meningitis itself may progress more rapidly, and patients are more likely to present in coma when compared with younger patient populations. With the development of coma, nuchal rigidity may be markedly less pronounced. Thus, when meningitis is suspected in the elderly, true nuchal rigidity has to be distinguished by careful physical examination. The absence of fever does not rule out the diagnosis of meningitis in the elderly patient.

In children, the presentation of meningitis is fundamentally similar to that in young and middle-aged adults, although nonspecific symptoms, such as irritability, nausea and vomiting, respiratory symptoms, and photophobia are more common in children. In neonates and infants, meningitis may present simply as fever or irritability; generally, there is a tendency for fever to be higher in children as compared to that in adults. The classic physical signs of meningeal inflammation or irritation described in medical textbooks are the Brudzinski's and Kernig's signs [36, 37]. Although Brudzinski originally described several signs of inflammation of the meninges, the best known of these is the so-called "nape of the neck" sign—the classic Brudzinski's sign. This sign is elicited by flexing the neck forward. The stretching of the meninges induced by this movement results in involuntary flexion of the hips and knees. Kernig's sign is elicited with the patient in the supine position and the thigh flexed on the abdomen with the knee flexed at a 45° angle. Upon passive extension of the leg in the presence of meningeal irritation, the patient resists extension with complaints of lower back and hamstring pain. Kernig's and Brudzinski's signs are neither sensitive nor specific indicators of meningitis and are potentially elicited in only about 50 % of children and only 5 % of adults with acute bacterial meningitis.

Fig. 22.3 Petechial rash associated with meningococcal meningitis

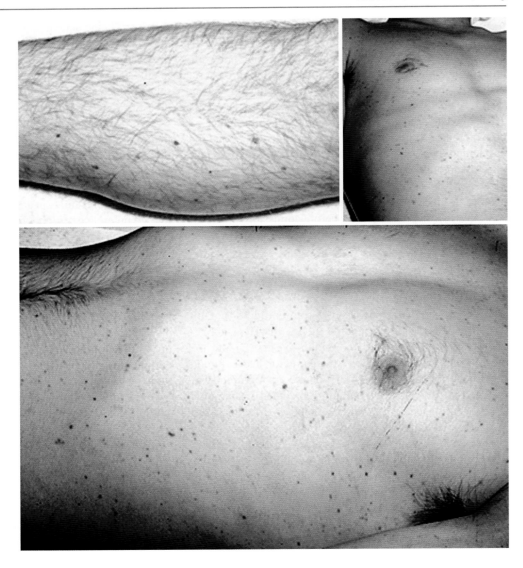

Diagnosis

An acute CNS infection is a medical emergency and bacterial meningitis may have to be differentiated from aseptic meningitis, encephalitis, brain abscess, subdural empyema, or noninfectious conditions affecting the CNS. Differentiation from encephalitis can be difficult and initially is made on clinical grounds. The classic features of meningitis (headache, neck stiffness, photophobia, fever, and vomiting) are often absent in neonates, patients who are immunocompromised—including persons with HIV infection—alcoholics, or the elderly. In encephalitis, altered state of consciousness, confusion, convulsions, and obtundation predominate. As the level of consciousness declines in patients with meningitis or encephalitis, differentiation between the two may only be possible through laboratory and radiographic findings. Because acute bacterial meningitis is a medical emergency, therapy should be implemented

on clinical grounds without waiting for proof by laboratory or radiographic studies.

Fever and altered mental status with or without meningismus may occur in a variety of systemic infections as well as noninfectious conditions. For example, Rocky Mountain spotted fever (RMSF) can present with fever, shock, and a petechial rash (Fig. 22.4a–c), which must be differentiated from the rash associated with early meningococcemia (Fig. 22.3). Meningococcal disease may initially present simply as meningococcemia with shock and skin rash with minimal or absent meningeal signs. Other infections that present with headache and fever include brain abscess, influenza, leptospirosis, dengue, typhoid, parameningeal infections, or Q fever. Noninfectious, organic conditions, such as subarachnoid hemorrhage, acute hemorrhagic or ischemic strokes, cerebral venous sinus thrombosis, autoimmune disorders (e.g., temporal arteritis), neuroleptic malignant syndrome, status epilepticus, or toxic encephalopathies of

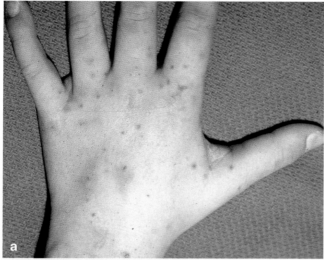

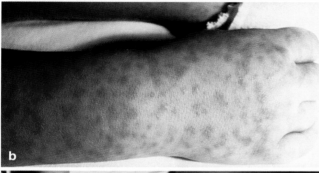

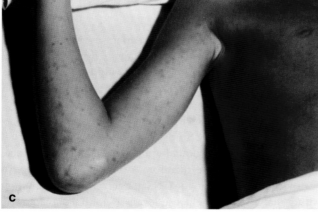

Fig. 22.4 (**a–c**) Rocky Mountain spotted fever rash (**a**: Courtesy of Daniel J. Sexton, MD, Duke University Medical Center; **b**, **c**: Courtesy of the Centers for Disease Control and Prevention)

various causes, can present precipitously with severe headache and fever, or nuchal rigidity.

Lumbar Puncture and CSF Analysis

A lumbar puncture and analysis of the CSF facilitate the diagnosis of meningitis and other conditions affecting the CNS.

However, the decision to perform a lumbar puncture on a patient with meningitis at presentation is precluded by the presence of raised ICP, which increases the risk of uncal, midbrain, medullary, or cerebellar tonsillar herniation after the procedure, leading to irreversible brain injury or death. Cerebral herniation occurs in about 5 % of patients with acute bacterial meningitis, accounting for about 30 % of the mortality [38]. Of note, the role of a CT scan is primarily to ascertain whether a space-occupying lesion is present; a CT scan cannot rule out the presence of increased ICP. Clinical signs suggestive of impending herniation include deteriorating level of consciousness, brainstem signs (including pupillary changes, decorticate posturing, or irregular respirations), a very recent seizure, absent oculocephalic reflexes, or papilledema. Lumbar puncture should be delayed in such patients, even for those with a normal CT scan, until preventive measures can be implemented to decrease ICP [38–42]. Other contraindications to immediate lumbar puncture include septic or hemodynamic shock, cardiorespiratory failure, presence of predisposing conditions for parameningeal abscesses (e.g., sinusitis, chronic ear discharge, or suppurative lung disease), bleeding disorders, and infection or loss of skin (e.g., burns) over the lumbar spine.

If the clinical picture is suggestive of bacterial meningitis or other intracranial infection and the patient is critically ill, especially if there is a rash or altered mental status, blood cultures should be drawn immediately and intravenous antimicrobial therapy initiated without delay. If the patient is not critically ill, one is certainly justified in withholding antimicrobial therapy until radiographic studies and lumbar puncture can be performed. If raised ICP is suspected and no focal lesions are defined by radiographic studies, one might consider intravenous infusion of mannitol (1 g/kg body weight) to reduce cerebral edema followed by a lumbar puncture after an interval of about 20 min. In addition to mannitol infusion, elective intubation and mechanical ventilation of the patient may be considered prior to the lumbar puncture procedure. Under these conditions, and using a 22-gauge needle, lumbar puncture can be performed without a significantly increased risk of herniation.

After insertion of the needle, the opening CSF pressure should be measured with the patient in the supine position. Normal opening pressure ranges from 1 to 10 cm H_2O in young children, 6–20 cm H_2O after 8 years of age, and up to 25 cm H_2O in obese patients [43]. The level should fluctuate with respiration and can be elevated by the Valsalva maneuver. If the CSF pressure is measured again at the end of the procedure after appropriate volumes of CSF have been obtained and has dropped to zero, the possibility of a complete CSF block should be considered. CSF is normally crystal clear and colorless, not unlike a fine gin. A minimum of 200 white blood cells or 400 red blood cells/mm³ is necessary to impart turbidity to the fluid. CSF will appear reddish if more than 6,000 red blood cells/mm³ are present [43].

Table 22.2 CSF findings in acute and chronic meningitis and other CNS infectious conditions

Type of infection	Macroscopic appearance	Cells	Protein (mg/dL)	Glucose (mg/dL)	Other tests
Normal	Clear	<5 lymphocytes/mm³	15–45	50–75	Negative test results
Bacterial meningitis (*S. pneumoniae*; *N. meningitides*; *L. monocytogenes*)	Cloudy or turbid	*Increased (commonly > 200)* *Typically >90 % PMNs* Can be normal in meningococcemia	>100	Reduced (<40)	Gram stain, bacterial culture, and antigen tests may be positive
Viral meningitis (enteroviruses; herpes simplex; arboviral encephalitis)	Clear or rarely opalescent	Increased May have PMN predominance early in the course of infection; converts to lymphocytic predominance within 12–24 h	Usually <100	Normal	Gram stain, bacterial culture, and antigen tests negative PCR for HSV, VZV, arboviruses, and enteroviruses may be positive
Fungal meningitis (cryptococcus; histoplasmosis; coccidioidomycosis)	Cloudy or turbid	>100 (<50 %) Usual range 100–400 usually lymphocytic predominance May be normal in cryptococcal meningitis	100–900	< 40	Cryptococcus can be diagnosed from India ink preps, antigen tests, or culture; PCR
Tuberculous meningitis	Cloudy or turbid	Increased Typically >100 Usual range 100–400 PMN early but converts to lymphocytic predominance	100–900	<40	Acid-fast bacilli occasionally seen on CSF smear stained with Kinyoun or Ziehl-Neelsen stains
Parameningeal infections (sinusitis; epidural abscess; paraspinous abscess)	Clear	<100 (<50 %) Occasionally PMN predominance If rupture into CSF, like acute meningitis	Increased	Normal	

Adapted with permission from Rand et al. [521]

Xanthochromia is a yellow, orange, or pink discoloration of the CSF and is caused by the lysis of red blood cells resulting in hemoglobin breakdown to oxyhemoglobin, methemoglobin, and bilirubin. Discoloration begins after RBCs have been in spinal fluid for about 2 h. In cases of subarachnoid hemorrhage, xanthochromia occurs within 2–4 h after the initial cerebral bleed; xanthochromia may develop in vitro if the CSF specimen contains increased numbers of red blood cells and is not centrifuged immediately upon arrival in the laboratory. Xanthochromia also occurs when CSF protein concentrations are greater than 150 mg/dL. The macroscopic appearance of CSF only enables a diagnostic path for purulent versus aseptic meningitis; however, appearance alone is not sufficient to make a specific diagnosis of bacterial or viral meningitis.

In adults and children older than the neonatal age group, normal CSF generally contains less than 5 white cells/mm³, usually small lymphocytes. In neonates, CSF may contain up to 25–30 white cells/mm³ with up to 60 % neutrophils; this falls after a few days to the range of 8–9 white cells/mm³ [8]. Because red cells may be present in spinal fluid as a result of subarachnoid hemorrhage or through a traumatic tap, it is important to note whether red tinged or bloody CSF clears as sequential specimen tubes of CSF are obtained. Such clearing suggests a traumatic tap and can be documented in the laboratory by counting the red cells in successive tubes. CSF cells should be counted in the laboratory within 1–2 h of collection; further delays may result in a false low cell count because of cell lysis or adherence of cells to the walls of the specimen tube.

Glucose enters the CSF by transport through the choroid plexus and capillary endothelium in the subarachnoid space. CSF glucose levels are therefore a function of both active transport of glucose into the CNS and its rate of consumption within the CNS. CSF glucose levels in normal subjects are, on average, 60–70 % of the blood glucose levels. However, a study by Skipper and Davis showed the CSF to serum glucose ratio was accurate when the serum glucose was between 89 and 115 mg/dL [44]. For blood glucose levels greater than 125 mg/dL, the ratio was less than 60 %; for blood glucose levels greater than 192 mg/dL, the ratio fell to 50 % even among normal patients with no evidence of meningitis.

CSF protein levels are generally less than 40 mg/dL due to the exclusion of larger proteins by the blood–brain barrier. When the barrier breaks down during meningitis, CSF protein tends to rise and increases with duration of disease prior to initiation of therapy. Protein levels in newborn infants are significantly higher compared to older children and adults, averaging 90 mg/dL with normal levels up to 170 mg/dL. Extremely high levels (more than 1 g/dL) of CSF protein are suggestive of a CSF spinal block. Elevation of CSF protein on its own, however, is not specific for any specific type of meningitis.

Table 22.2 summarizes the CSF characteristics (macroscopic appearance, white cell count range and differential, protein and glucose levels) typically encountered in meningitis caused by various classes of organisms. In general, high CSF white cell counts are found in bacterial meningitis, where levels may be greater than 10,000 cells/mm^3 with 95 % polymorphonuclear leukocytes (PMNs). Typically, WBC count in bacterial meningitis ranges between 500 and 5,000 cells/mm^3, CSF glucose less than 40 mg/dL, and protein levels in the 100–500 mg/dL range. It is important to recognize that a predominance of PMNs may occur early in viral meningitis, within the first 24–48 h, but this gradually shifts to a mononuclear predominance over the next 8 h if the lumbar puncture is repeated [45, 46]. In patients with meningitis caused by *L. monocytogenes*, the organism grows and survives within the host cell cytoplasm, thereby stimulating a monocytic CSF response; in infants there may be a monocytic predominance.

Once CSF specimens are obtained, a gram stain should be performed immediately in patients with suspected bacterial meningitis followed by plating on solid culture media. Centrifugation of CSF improves the yield for both gram stain smears and culture. In general, a CSF concentration greater than 10^3 organisms/mL is required in order for organisms to be identified on light microscopy of the gram stain. With lower concentrations, there are simply too few organisms to detect by direct microscopy. Approximately 75 % of patients with acute bacterial meningitis will have a positive gram stain, and this percentage may drop to about 50 % among patients who have received significant doses of prior antimicrobial therapy. Generally, the gram stain is positive in 90 % of untreated patients with pneumococcal meningitis, 86 % of patients with meningitis due to *H. influenzae*, and approximately 75 % of cases due to *N. meningitidis* [47]. Among children, the overall sensitivity of gram stain to detect bacterial meningitis is 67 %. Moreover, most children without bacterial meningitis have negative gram stain with a negative predictive value of 99.9 %. Thus, CSF gram stain is useful in evaluating children for empiric therapy of bacterial meningitis [48].

In addition to gram stain, a number of other rapid diagnostic tests have been developed over the past 20 years for diagnosis of acute bacterial meningitis. In the 1970s counter immunoelectrophoresis (CIE) was used for direct detection of bacterial polysaccharide antigens; this test is quite insensitive and is no longer in use. Agglutination tests are commercially available for *H. influenza*, *S. pneumoniae*, and five serotypes of *N. meningitidis*. However, the sensitivity and specificity of these tests are no better than that of the gram stain, and they provide no additional diagnostic yield above and beyond the gram stain and the clinical picture and rarely influence the decision to treat empirically [49, 50]. Therefore, they are not currently recommended in the diagnosis of acute bacterial meningitis upon initial presentation. The underlying problem with these tests is that they are not sensitive and specific enough to establish a diagnosis upon which to initiate appropriate therapy. For example, if a patient is sick enough to be admitted to the hospital, and found to have a low CSF glucose level and raised CSF white blood count, one would still initiate empiric antimicrobial and supportive therapy even if the agglutination tests are negative.

Miscellaneous Testing

C-reactive protein (CRP) can be measured in CSF and, when greater than 100 μg/mL, may be useful in differentiating bacterial from viral meningitis [51]. Extensive literature exists describing the application of real-time polymerase chain reaction (PCR) for detection and quantification of various bacterial and viral pathogens in CSF of patients with a putative diagnosis of bacterial meningitis. Real-time PCR is faster and more sensitive than previous technologies. However, this technique is expensive and not readily available in most hospital laboratories. Moreover, in clinical practice, physicians are likely to initiate empirical antimicrobial therapy anyway after requesting testing by conventional methods, especially for patients with typical CNS symptoms and signs. In this case, rapid diagnostic testing using PCR assays is likely to not make a difference in the clinical the clinical decision making and medical management of the patient.

Imaging Studies

Neuroimaging plays little role in the diagnosis of acute bacterial meningitis except as indicated earlier to rule out the presence of mass lesions and raised ICP, which might increase the risk of herniation when lumbar puncture is performed. The major value of CT and MRI scans in patients with acute bacterial meningitis is in the investigation of complications, such as cerebral infarction, vasculitis, abscess, or hydrocephalus. Figure 22.5a–d shows the typical neuroradiological appearances of the brain in patients with meningitis caused by *L. monocytogenes*, *N. meningitidis*, *S. pneumoniae*, and *M. tuberculosis*. In patients with prolonged fever of 10 days duration or longer, up to 25 % may have a subdural effusion

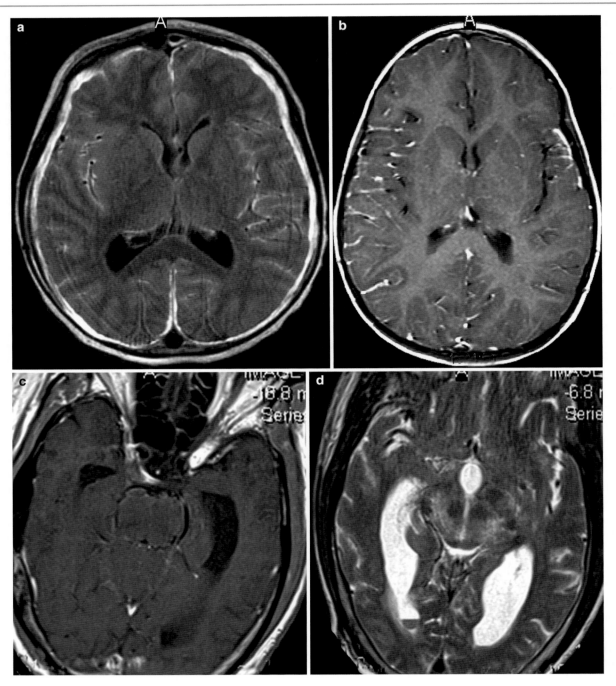

Fig. 22.5 (**a**, **b**) Acute meningitis; images include fluid-sensitive, FLAIR T2-w sequence (**a**) and post-contrast T1-w (**b**) axial sequences. Findings in acute meningitis are frequently subtle especially viral meningitis. The FLAIR sequence. A presents normal CSF within the ventricles and sulci as hypointense (dark) relative to brain. With pial inflammation there is leak of proteinaceous fluid into the subpial and subdural spaces. This highly proteinaceous fluid is hyperintense (bright relative to brain) and thus becomes visualized on fluid-sensitive MRI sequences. Serous subdural effusions are often present as well, which are imaged as high-intensity fluid outside the brain, as in this case, but without contrast enhancement along their surfaces. These types of fluid collections are considered noninfective and they typically clear spontaneously after medical treatment. The contrasted MRI (**b**) demonstrates pial hyperemia along the right lateral cerebral convexity (compare to

left side). On the left there is thickening of the pia probably early subpial empyema. (**c**, **d**) Listeria rhombencephalitis; images include post-contrast T1-w section (**c**) and a T2-w sequence (**d**). When the distribution of the inflammatory process involves mainly the upper brain stem, as in this instance, it is described as rhombencephalitis. Rhombencephalitis is uncommon but is one the manifestations of Listeria-based meningitis, as in this case. Note there is relatively little abnormal enhancement in this case of Listeria infection. If there is thick obvious enhancement in a similar distribution, findings would be more consistent with a granulomatous infection, as in fungal or tuberculous meningitis. Similar findings can also be part of noninfectious granulomatous pial disease, as in neurosarcoidosis and non-Langerhans histiocytosis; thus, tissue confirmation is usually necessary

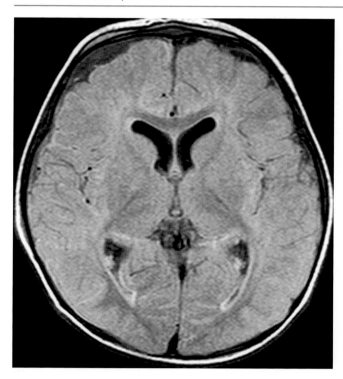

Fig. 22.6 Active meningitis and secondary subdural effusions. This FLAIR sequence, which emphasizes tissue edema, but deemphasizes bulk CSF signal, shows increased signal along the trigones of the lateral ventricular surfaces indicative of ependymitis, plus increased signal along the pial surfaces indicative of meningitis, plus minimal ventriculomegaly. All of these findings commonly occur in acute meningitis. Additionally, there are small bifrontal extra axial fluid collections without any signal along their margins which are consistent with likely sterile subdural effusions. The fluid signal is minimally higher than CSF within the lateral ventricles indicating elevated CSF protein, a feature common to reactive subdural effusions

(Fig. 22.6). In some cases this may progress to a subdural empyema, which may account for the prolonged fever (Fig. 22.7). Cortical infarction is a common complication of bacterial meningitis and usually results from vasospasm of cerebral vasculature or vasculitis associated with the meningitis itself. The MRI scan is more sensitive than CT imaging in detecting cerebritis and cortical infarction. Cerebritis is an early complication that may occur during the first 4 days (Fig. 22.8). Early necrotic regions filled with polymorphonuclear cells, lymphocytes, and plasma cells and with ill-defined parenchymal swelling characterize cerebritis. In late cerebritis (4–8 days), central necrosis increases, there is vascular proliferation and more inflammatory cells, and suppurative foci begin to breakdown and become encapsulated.

Treatment

The pathophysiology of the blood–brain barrier is of critical importance in determining the choice of antimicrobials for the treatment of acute bacterial meningitis. The penetration of the blood–brain barrier is a function of both the properties (e.g., lipid solubility, molecular size, and molecular structure) of the antimicrobial itself and the degree or extent of the inflammation of the meninges. For example, chloramphenicol, which is highly lipid soluble, will readily penetrate uninflamed meninges. Fortunately, in inflamed meninges therapeutic concentrations of penicillins, cephalosporins, and vancomycin can be achieved for treatment of the vast majority of cases of bacterial meningitis. Because only the free, unbound portion of an antimicrobial agent is capable of crossing the blood–brain barrier, the degree of protein binding of the antimicrobial in the patient serum is critical in determining how much of the agent eventually gets through to the CSF. With increased concentrations of protein in the CSF, protein binding becomes a significant factor in the effectiveness those antimicrobials that are highly protein bound.

The penetration of aminoglycosides is generally so poor that they are of little value in the treatment of acute meningitis when given intravenously, although they may be useful intrathecally. The penetration of the third-generation cephalosporins (e.g., ceftriaxone and cefotaxime) is significantly better than that of the first- and second-generation cephalosporins. Quinolones, tetracyclines, and macrolides do not penetrate the blood–brain barrier sufficiently to be useful first-line agents in the treatment of meningitis, whereas sulfa agents (e.g., trimethoprim-sulfa) and vancomycin, in the presence of inflamed meninges, may reach sufficient concentrations to be of therapeutic value.

Treatment regimens for acute bacterial meningitis in children above the age of 3 months and in adults up to the age of 50 is geared to treating the most common pathogens: *N. meningitides*, *S. pneumoniae*, and, less commonly, *H. influenzae*. The prevalence of penicillin-resistant *S. pneumoniae* has risen so that more than 50 % of strains may be resistant or exhibit intermediate resistance to penicillin in some parts of the United States and other countries. By definition, fully susceptible pneumococci are susceptible to penicillin at less than 0.1 μg/mL; intermediate susceptibility is defined by an MIC less than or equal to 2 μg/mL, whereas fully resistant *S. pneumoniae* are defined by MICs greater than or equal to 4 μg/mL. Among penicillin-resistant strains, resistance to the third-generation cephalosporins, including cefotaxime and ceftriaxone, has been increasing; resistance to ceftriaxone as high as 35 % has been documented for *S. pneumoniae* isolates in some areas [52–55].

Once a clinical diagnosis of acute bacterial meningitis is suspected or made, institution of antimicrobial therapy should be immediate. If clinical evaluation raises a suspicion of raised intracranial pressure, or if the patient manifests signs of papilledema or focal neurological deficits, blood should be drawn for culture and baseline testing (e.g., white

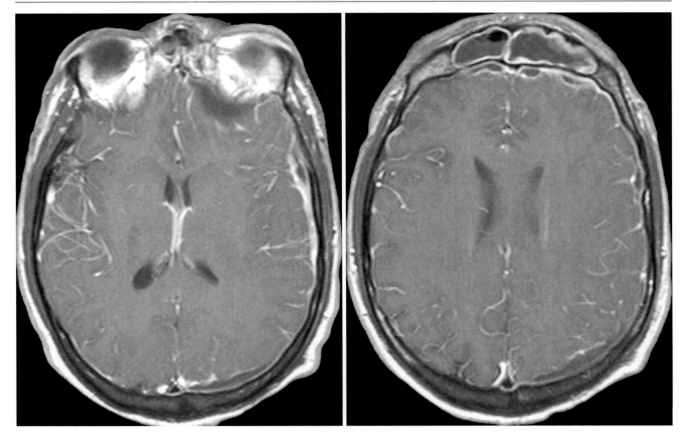

Fig. 22.7 Acute frontal sinusitis with secondary subdural empyema; images include contiguous post-contrast mid-convexity axial MRI sections. This case illustrates the spread pattern of subdural empyema. The source of the infection is the frontal sinus. Once the infection accesses the subdural space it can spread widely within the intracranial compart-

ment. In this instance, it continues all the way to the occipital region. These multicentric pockets of subdural empyema are often sequestered requiring multiple surgical drains. Thus, it is imperative that the full extent of the subdural empyema is appreciated

blood count and glucose), and empiric antimicrobial therapy initiated before the patient is sent off for imaging studies of the brain. Choice of empirical antimicrobial therapy is dictated by the age of the patient, vaccine status, and whether bacterial meningitis was acquired in the community or within the healthcare setting.

For community-associated meningitis, the microorganisms most commonly implicated *are S. pneumoniae, N. meningitidis, Listeria* spp., other *Streptococcus* spp., *S. aureus,* and *H. influenzae.* Healthcare-associated meningitis usually follows neurosurgical procedures, such as craniotomy, placement of ventriculostomy tubes, or deep brain stimulation of the brain for Parkinson's disease; pathogens most commonly implicated in healthcare settings include gram-negative microorganisms (e.g., *Enterobacteriaceae* and non-fermenters), *S. aureus,* and *Streptococcus* spp.

Initial empirical therapy for community-acquired meningitis: for adult and children 3 months–50 years, ceftriaxone or cefotaxime can be given, especially if risk factors (e.g., CSF leak, pneumonia, or sinusitis) for *S. pneumoniae* meningitis are present. If the patient is very sick or if gram-positive

cocci are seen on CSF microscopy, vancomycin should be added to the therapeutic regimen to cover for penicillin-resistant *S. pneumoniae* in a dose of 2–3 g/day given every 8–12 h in adults and at 60 mg/kg for children in four divided doses, until it is known that the penicillin MIC is less than 0.1 mg/mL For patients with a history of idiosyncratic reactions to penicillin or cephalosporins, vancomycin is recommended, although chloramphenicol may be used in adults. For patients with a history of severe penicillin allergy, chloramphenicol at a dose of 4–6 g/day in four divided doses for adults should be given in place of the third-generation cephalosporin together with vancomycin. In adults more than 60 years of age, patients with chronic alcoholism, immunosuppression, or other debilitating conditions, the possibility of *L. monocytogenes* meningitis should be considered. Empirical therapy to cover *L. monocytogenes* includes addition of maximal doses of ampicillin (12 g daily dosed every 4 h) to the cephalosporin or vancomycin regimen until culture results for blood or CSF become available. For patients with penicillin allergy, the use of chloramphenicol, imipenem, or trimethoprim/sulfamethoxazole can be considered as an

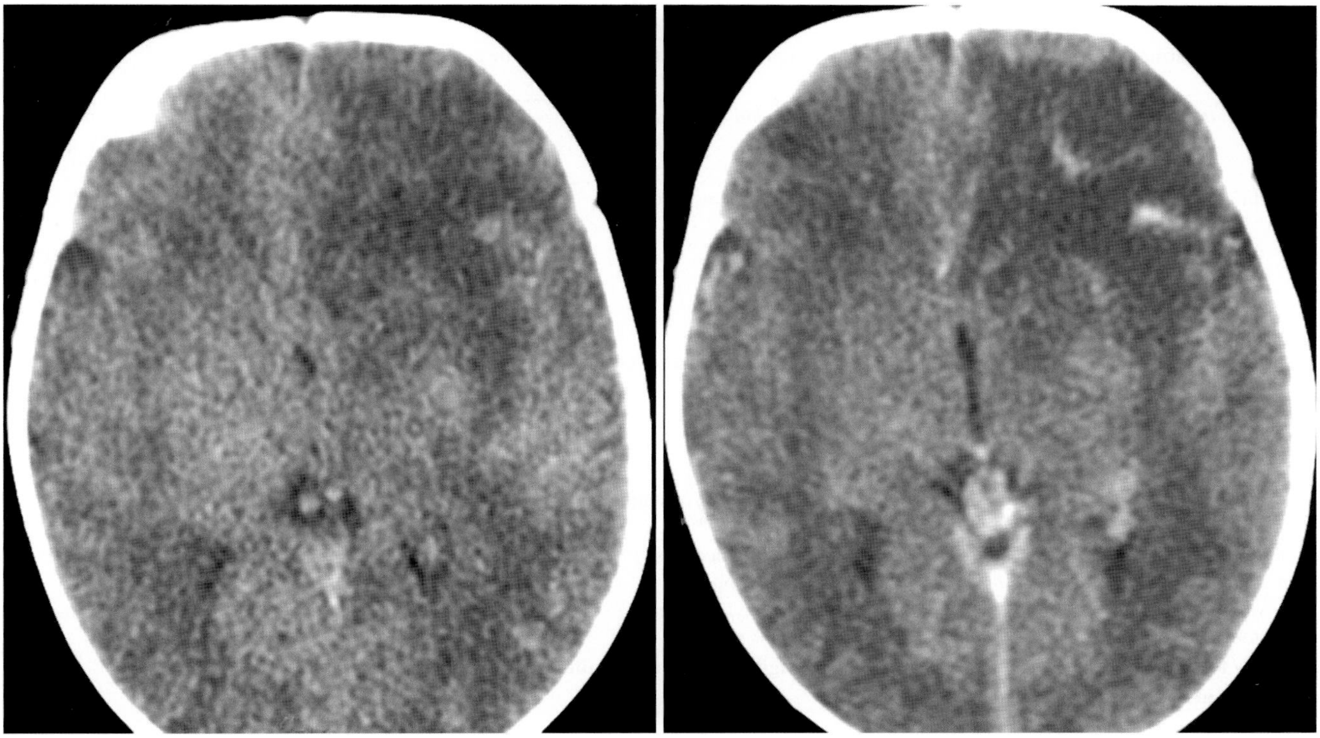

Fig. 22.8 Acute left frontal lobe bacterial cerebritis; images include pre and post-contrast CT sections sagittal projection lower thoracic area. The early phase of brain infection (early cerebritis) demonstrates nonspecific cerebral edema and poorly defined contrast enhancement. There is frequently reactive pial hyperemia. In later stages the cerebritis will organize into early then mature stages of brain abscess

alternative to cover for Listeria until culture results are available. Therapy may need to be broadened depending on the results of the gram stain. In cases where gram-negative diplococci are seen, it is probably prudent to wait until culture results confirm *N. meningitidis* before narrowing the bacterial coverage to penicillin because of the possibility that the gram stain might have been misinterpreted. Treatment of the most common etiologic agents of acute bacterial meningitis is summarized in Table 22.3.

The utility of adjunctive therapy with dexamethasone in the treatment of acute bacterial meningitis remains controversial. The use of dexamethasone as an adjunct to therapy in acute bacterial meningitis is complex. It has been shown clearly in animal models and in patient studies that dexamethasone reduces the level of inflammation and reduces the levels of the inflammatory cytokines IL1 beta and tumor necrosis factor alpha [56]. However, in an animal model, administration of dexamethasone together with vancomycin reduced the penetration of vancomycin into the CSF by 29 % and lowered the rate of bacterial clearance during the first 6 h in animals who received an intermediate dose of vancomycin. Animals that received a higher dose had therapeutic peaks maintained despite steroid use, suggesting that the anti-inflammatory effect of the steroids, which reduce entry of antibiotics into the CSF, may be overcome to some extent by increasing the dose [57]. In animal studies of experimental pneumococcal meningitis, an antibiotic-induced secondary inflammatory response in the CSF was demonstrated only in animals with high initial CSF bacterial concentrations; these effects were modulated by dexamethasone therapy [58].

Human studies of the use of dexamethasone have clearly shown that there is a reduction in severe hearing loss in patients who have *H. influenza* type b meningitis and there is a similar reduction in overall neurologic complications although perhaps not as significant. In children with meningitis due to *S. pneumoniae*, there also appears to be a significant reduction in long-term hearing loss [59]. Major side effects from dexamethasone include secondary fever and a small incidence of gastrointestinal bleeding which is probably negligible if treatment is limited to 2 days but increases up to 3 % in patients who received 4 or more days of treatment or more.

In summary, dexamethasone probably should be used as an adjunct in children at a dose of 0.4 mg/kg IV every 12 h for no more than 2 days and probably should be given just before, or at the time of, the first antibiotic dose to block any increase in any inflammatory cytokine production following initial bacterial lysis. A more recent study has shown that adjunctive dexamethasone in the treatment of acute bacterial

Table 22.3 Therapy of acute bacterial meningitis

Empirical treatment for patients with suspected meningitis but negative gram stain or culture

Age group	Likely organisms	Empiric regimen
Preterm to <1 month	Group B Streptococcus; *Escherichia coli*; *Listeria* sp.	Ampicillin 100 mg/kg IV q6h *plus* cefotaxime 50 mg/kg IV q6h or ampicillin 100 mg/kg IV q6h *plus* gentamicin 2.5 mg/kg IV q8h
1 month–50 years	*Streptococcus pneumoniae*; *Neisseria meningitidis*; *Haemophilus influenzae*; *Listeria* sp.	Adult: ceftriaxone 2 g IV q12h or cefotaxime 2 g IV q4-6 h *plus* vancomycin 15 mg/kg q6–8 h Child: ceftriaxone 100 mg/kg/day IV (doses given q12h) or cefotaxime 200–300 mg/kg/day IV (doses given q6h) *plus* vancomycin 60 mg/kg/day IV (doses given q6h)
>50 years	*S. pneumoniae*; *N. meningitidis*; *H. influenzae*; *Listeria* sp.; aerobic gram-negative microorganisms	Ampicillin 2 g IV q4h *plus* ceftriaxone 2 g IV q12h or cefotaxime 2 g IV q6h *plus* vancomycin 15 mg. kg IV q8–12 h
Trauma: skull fracture	*S. pneumoniae*; *H. influenzae*; Group B Streptococcus	Vancomycin 15 mg.kg IV q8–12 h *plus* ceftriaxone 2 g IV q12h
Trauma: penetrating	*Staphylococcus aureus*, coagulase-negative staphylococcus, *Enterobacteriaceae*, *Pseudomonas* spp.	Vancomycin 15 mg.kg IV q8–12 h *plus* cefepime 2 g IV q8h
Meningitis associated with shunts	*S. aureus*, coagulase-negative staphylococcus, *Enterobacteriaceae*, *Pseudomonas* spp.	Vancomycin 15 mg.kg IV q8–12 h *plus* cefepime 2 g IV q8h
Neurosurgery (e.g., craniotomy)	*S. aureus*, coagulase-negative staphylococcus, *Enterobacteriaceae*, *Pseudomonas* spp.	Vancomycin 15 mg.kg IV q8–12 h *plus* cefepime 2 g IV q8h

Therapy for patients with acute bacterial meningitis (suggested by gram stain or culture)—by microorganism

Microorganism	Treatment	Duration of therapy (days)
Streptococcus pneumoniae		
Penicillin-susceptible isolate (MIC <0.1 μg/mL)	Adults: penicillin G 4 million units IV q4h or ampicillin 2 g IV q4–6 h Children: 250,000–400,000 U/kg IV q4–6 h Severe penicillin allergy: substitute cephalosporin agent with chloramphenicol 75–100 mg/kg/day in 4 divided doses	10–14
Isolate with intermediate (MIC = 0.1–1 μg/mL) susceptibility to penicillin	Ceftriaxone 2 g IV q12h or cefotaxime 2 g IV q4–6 h	
Isolate resistant (≥2 μg/ mL) to penicillin	Ceftriaxone 2 g IV q12h or cefotaxime 2 g IV q4–6 h *plus* vancomycin 15 mg/kg q6–8 h	
Neisseria meningitidis	Adults: penicillin G 4 million units IV q4h or ampicillin 2 g IV q4–6 h or ceftriaxone 2 g IV q12h or cefotaxime 2 g IV q4–6 h. Penicillin allergy: as for *S. pneumoniae* above Children: penicillin G 250,000–400,000 U/kg IV q4–6 h. Penicillin allergy: substitute with chloramphenicol 75–100 mg/kg/day in 4 divided doses	7
Haemophilus influenzae		
Beta-lactamase positive	*Ceftriaxone 2 g IV q12h or cefotaxime 2 g IV q6h*	**7**
Beta-lactamase negative	*Ampicillin 2 g IV q q4–6 h*	
Group B Streptococcus (Streptococcus agalactiae)		
Suspected/empiric	Preterm: ampicillin 200–300 mg/kg/day IV in 3 divided doses *plus* cefotaxime Infants ≤7 days: ampicillin 200–300 mg/kg/day IV in 3 divided doses *plus* an aminoglycoside, adjusted for age and birth weight (BW), i.e., gentamicin 2.5 mg/kg IV q12h; 2.5 mg/kg IV q8–12 h if BW <2,000 g; 2.5 mg/kg IV q8h if BW >2,000 g Infants >7 days: ampicillin 300 mg/kg/day iv in 4–6 doses/ day *plus* an aminoglycoside, adjusted for age and BW, i.e., gentamicin 2.5 mg/kg IV q8–12 h if BW <2,000 g; 2.5 mg/ kg IV q8h if BW >2,000 g Intraventricular treatment not recommended	14–21

Table 22.3 (continued)

Known	Adults: penicillin G 4 million units IV q4h *plus* gentamicin 3–5 mg/kg IV daily, divided q8h	14–21
	Infants ≤7 days: penicillin G 250,000–450,000 U/kg/day IV in 3 divided doses	
	Infants >7 days: penicillin G 450,000 U/kg/day IV	
Listeria monocytogenes		
	Infants ≤7 days: ampicillin 200–300 mg/kg/day IV in 3 divided doses *plus* an aminoglycoside, adjusted for age and BW, i.e., gentamicin 2.5 mg/kg IV q12h if BW <2,000 g; 2.5 mg/kg IVq12h if BW >2,000 g	21 or longer
	Infants >7 days: ampicillin 300 mg/kg/day IV in 4–6 doses/day plus an aminoglycoside, adjusted for age and BW, i.e., gentamicin 2.5 mg/kg IV q8–12 h if BW <2,000 g; 2.5 mg/kg IV q8h if BW >2,000 g	
	Adults >50, alcoholism, or other risk factors: ampicillin 2 g IV q4h *plus* ceftriaxone 2 g IV q12h or cefotaxime 2 g IV q6h *plus* gentamicin 2 mg IV loading dose, then 1.7 mg/kg q8h *plus* dexamethasone 0.4 mg/kg IV q12 h x 2	
	Penicillin allergy: trimethoprim/sulfamethoxazole	
	Consider stopping gentamicin after 1 week	
	Where ampicillin is suggested, amoxicillin may be used	
Pseudomonas aeruginosa	Ceftazidime 1 g IV q8h or cefepime 2 g IV q8h *plus* gentamicin 3–5 mg/kg IV daily divided q8h	21
Enterobacteriaceae (e.g., *Escherichia coli*)	Ceftriaxone 2 g IV q12h or cefotaxime 2 g IV q4–6 h *plus* gentamicin 3–5mh/kg IV daily divided q8h	21

meningitis in adults does not appear to significantly reduce death or neurological disability and concludes that the benefit of adjunctive dexamethasone for all or any subgroup of patients with bacterial meningitis remains unproven [60].

The duration of treatment of bacterial meningitis is based on empiric observation. In general, the minimum duration treatment is 7 days as long as the patient is afebrile for the last 4–5 days. Treatment of *S. pneumoniae* generally takes longer than *H. influenzae* and *N. meningitidis* and may be extended to 10–14 days, depending on the patient's response. Meningitis following trauma and neurosurgical procedures is discussed elsewhere.

Complications

Elevated ICP is a result of cerebral edema due to acute bacterial meningitis and should be anticipated. Clinical manifestations of raised ICP include bradycardia, hypertension, altered mental status, drowsiness, obtundation and coma, third cranial nerve palsies, including unilateral or bilateral dilated, poorly reactive or nonreactive pupils, abnormal ocular movement, abnormal respiration, or decerebrate posturing. Papilledema is relatively uncommon and as such is an unreliable sign of raised ICP as it may take several hours to develop after the ICP has increased. Signs of herniation may supersede those of increased pressure and include unequal, dilated, or nonreactive pupils, dysconjugate eye movements, decorticate and decerebrate posturing, and bradycardia with abnormal respiratory patterns.

Patients who are awake and alert can be monitored closely. Patients who are obtunded or comatose, or who manifest other signs of increased ICP may well benefit from ICP monitoring. Pressures exceeding 20 mmHg should be treated and some studies suggest that even pressures greater than 15 mmHg may benefit from treatment [61]. An indication for treating at lower pressure levels is the phenomenon of "plateau waves" (Fig. 22.9), which are large elevations in pressure that occur spontaneously, or due to changes in cerebral blood flow, small shifts in intracranial blood volume resulting from hypoxia, fever, or otherwise innocuous events like tracheal suctioning. When these waves develop on a background of already increased ICP, herniation and irreversible brain stem injury may ensue [61, 62].

The treatment of increased ICP includes elevation of the head of the bed to 30° above the horizontal to facilitate venous drainage, intubation, and hyperventilation to reduce and maintain the arterial $PaCO_2$ concentrations to levels between 27 and 30 mmHg. Hypertonic osmotic agents, such as mannitol or hypertonic saline infusions, play a vital role in the reduction of elevated intracranial pressure and treatment of cerebral edema in patients with CNS infections [63–68]. Both mannitol and hypertonic saline reduce cerebral edema in many clinical syndromes [63–67]. However, recent data suggest that hypertonic saline appears to achieve a greater reduction in ICP than other osmotic agents [63, 65].

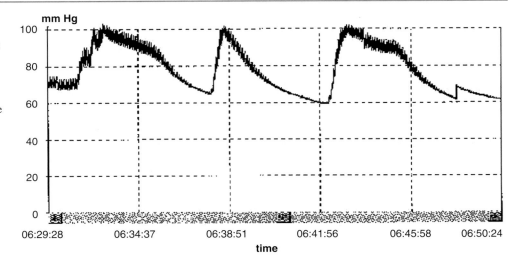

Fig. 22.9 Plateau waves: characterized by a sudden rapid elevation of intracranial pressure to 50–100 mmHg for 5–20 min. After a sustained period of elevation, the termination of the wave is characterized by a rapid decrease of ICP. These waves are thought to be caused by changes in cerebral blood flow

The object in using osmotic agents is to achieve a sustained reduction in intracranial pressure by modifying the modes and rates of administration of the respective osmotic agent [63–67].

Phenobarbital therapy may be considered if raised ICP remains uncontrolled by the foregoing interventions. Caution is advised in the use of hyperventilation to lower arterial PaCO$_2$ concentrations because overly vigorous treatment may cause these values to fall below 25 mmHg, running the risk of further reductions in cerebral blood flow causing cerebral ischemia. The dose of mannitol in children is 0.5–2.0 g/kg infused over 30 min and repeated as necessary; in adults the usual dose is 0.25–1 g/kg bolus injection and 0.25 g/kg every 2–3 h as needed. Mannitol and hypertonic saline act as hyperosmolar agents and remain almost entirely within the intravascular space, producing an osmotic gradient that shifts intracranial fluid into this space. Serum osmolality should be frequently checked and kept between 315 and 320 mOsm/L [61–63, 67–71].

Dexamethasone has been used to reduce intracranial swelling in other settings primarily because of its effectiveness in vasogenic cerebral edema. Various clinical studies support the use of adjunctive dexamethasone in infants or children with *H. influenza* type b meningitis to reduce the risk of neurologic and audiologic complications, especially in those with raised ICP or coma. High-dose barbiturates may be helpful when other methods have failed to control increased ICP. Barbiturates decrease the CNS metabolic demand for oxygen thereby decreasing cerebral blood flow which, in turn, causes a fall in ICP. Phenobarbital is given at an initial dose of 5–10 mg/kg, at a rate of 1 mg/kg per minute followed by 1–3 mg/kg/h [61, 62]. Such therapies require regular ICP measurements and monitoring of cerebral electrical activity with electroencephalography. Phenobarbital is given until the ICP falls to levels 20 mmHg or until approximately 90 % burst suppression on the EEG (i.e., nine

out of the ten screens of the EEG are flat) has been achieved. Serum phenobarbital concentrations should be kept within the range of 20–40 µg/mL. Pentobarbital is preferred because of its relatively short half-life (24 h) versus phenobarbital with a relatively longer half-life. Side effects of high-dose barbiturate therapy include cardiac depression with arrhythmias and hypotension, thus mandating invasive hemodynamic monitoring in these patients.

Seizures

Seizures occur in approximately 30–40 % of children and adults with acute bacterial meningitis within the first few days of illness. If not treated, seizures may progress to status epilepticus, which in turn can lead to anoxic damage of the temporal lobe, cerebellum, and thalamus. The principles of therapy are to control seizure activity quickly and definitively. To initiate therapy, short-acting anticonvulsants, such as lorazepam or diazepam, are administered followed by a long-acting agent like phenytoin. Lorazepam is given IV in doses of 1–4 mg in adults, and 0.05 mg/kg in children. Phenytoin is given IV at a dose of 18–20 mg/kg and at a rate of no more than 50 mg/min. The rate should be decreased if signs of toxicity, such as hypotension or a prolonged QT interval, develop. If phenytoin is not successful in controlling seizure activity, intubation and treatment with IV phenobarbital may be necessary. Patients must be watched and monitored carefully for signs of toxicity, such as hypotension and respiratory depression. Phenobarbital should be given IV at a rate of 100 mg/min until seizure activity stops, up to an initial dose of 20 mg/kg.

In children, the rate should be decreased to 30 mg/min. Should these measures fail to control seizures, general anesthesia and additional phenobarbital therapy may have to be considered.

Vaccination for Meningitis

N. meningitidis became a leading cause of bacterial meningitis in the United States after dramatic reductions in the incidence of *S. pneumoniae* and *H. influenzae* type b infections had been achieved as a result of using conjugate vaccines [1, 72, 73]. However, since 2000, meningococcal disease incidence has decreased and incidence for serogroups C and Y, which represent the majority of cases of vaccine-preventable meningococcal disease, is at historic lows. In 2005, a quadrivalent meningococcal polysaccharide-protein conjugate vaccine (MCV4) was licensed for use among persons aged 11–55 years, and during the same year, the Advisory Committee on Immunization Practices (ACIP) recommended routine vaccination with 1 dose of MCV4 for persons aged 11–12 years, persons entering high school (i.e., at approximately age 15 years) if not previously vaccinated with MCV4, and other persons at increased risk for meningococcal disease, including college freshmen living in dormitories [74]. In 2010, ACIP approved updated recommendations for the use of quadrivalent (serogroups A, C, Y, and W-135) meningococcal conjugate vaccines in adolescents and persons at high risk for meningococcal disease [75, 76]. The vaccine contains immunogenic polysaccharide capsular material from serogroups A, C, Y, and W-135. The vaccine has few side effects and is believed to be protective for at least 3–5 years.

Persons at increased risk for severe pneumococcal disease include those who are immunocompromised, asplenic or splenectomized, or patients with chronic illness such as chronic cardiovascular disease (e.g., congestive heart failure or cardiomyopathies), chronic pulmonary disease, diabetes mellitus, alcoholism, chronic liver disease (cirrhosis), or CSF leaks. CDC has updated recommendations from ACIP for prevention of invasive pneumococcal disease (i.e., bacteremia, meningitis, or infection of other normally sterile sites) through use of the 23-valent pneumococcal polysaccharide vaccine among all adults aged greater than or equal to 65 years and those adults aged 19–64 years with underlying medical conditions that put them at greater risk for serious pneumococcal infection [77].

Viral Meningitis and Encephalitis

Viral CNS infections may be classified as exogenous due to infection with a viral agent acquired outside the host or endogenous due to reactivation of viruses that have remained latent in the host. The majority of viral CNS infections are caused by exogenously acquired enteroviruses (Coxsackie virus A and B, echovirus, polio virus), arboviruses, and, less commonly, by HSV, mumps virus, varicella-zoster virus (VZV), cytomegalovirus (CMV), Epstein-Barr virus (EBV), adenovirus, human immunodeficiency virus (HIV), West Nile virus (WNV), rabies virus, or lymphocytic choriomeningitis virus. HSV encephalitis is unique in that it may occur as part of the primary infection or be seen in patients in whom the infection has been latent for many years. CNS infections due to the other herpes viruses, such as EBV, VZV, or CMV occasionally may be seen as part of the primary infection but may also occur as reactivated infections in patients who are immunosuppressed or HIV-infected.

Epidemiology

Meningitis and meningoencephalitis are the most common viral CNS infections encountered in the United States. The overwhelming majority of these infections are caused by enteroviruses, which produce disease in outbreaks occurring mainly during the summer months, but may occur during May to October in warmer parts of the United States. While virtually all of the various serotypes of echovirus and Coxsackie virus can produce meningitis and meningoencephalitis, in addition to other syndromes, the 15 most commonly noted enteroviruses in the United States during 1970–2005 accounted for 83.5 % of CDC reports with known serotype [78]. The five most commonly reported serotypes (echoviruses 9, 11, 30, and 6 and Coxsackie virus B5) in descending order of frequency accounted for approximately half (48 %) of all reports [78]. CSF was the most common specimen type. The epidemiologic pattern is one in which certain strains, such as echovirus 30 or echovirus 9, cause disease endemically, while other strains occur in sporadic outbreaks varying from year to year in different regions. Enteroviruses are transmitted from person to person by the fecal-oral route and their activity tends to be increased in areas of overcrowding, poverty, and generally poor hygienic conditions.

Arboviruses account for the majority of epidemic cases of encephalitis. Their occurrence follows an identical seasonal distribution to that of viral meningitis and meningoencephalitis associated with enteroviruses. However, the mode of transmission is completely different. Arboviruses are spread by the bite of infected mosquitoes, which are part of a complex cycle of enzootic transmission between birds, mosquitoes, and small mammals. The epidemiology of these diseases may be affected in part by prevention efforts from the public health authorities. For example, many states maintain surveillance systems that include testing of mosquitoes for the presence of virus, as well as sentinel chicken flocks to determine arbovirus activity. Such efforts lead to early recognition of an outbreak and warnings by public health authorities for the population to take precautions such as insect repellants, wearing long sleeve shirts, and avoiding outdoor activity in the early evening hours when transmission is most likely to occur. In addition, mosquito control activities may contribute to reduction in rates of infection.

In August of 1999, an outbreak of encephalitis was detected in the borough of Queens, New York City: 62 patients were confirmed infected with an agent identified as the arbovirus West Nile virus (WNV); seven eventually died. This followed a massive die-off among birds, particularly crows that had been observed during the month before the outbreak. Most of those affected with serious illness were elderly, although one patient was 29 years old [79–81]. In 2003, there were over 8,000 cases of WNV infections reported to the CDC with 199 deaths; most of these cases involved the CNS. During the ensuing decade, WNV occurrence started to spread westward across the continental United States, and by the end of 2004 approximately 1 in 400 blood donors were thought to be infected with WNV (CDC data).

Although rabies is rare among humans in the United States, potential exposures to rabid animals lead to between 16,000 and 39,000 persons receiving post rabies exposure prophylaxis each year [82]. Since the 1950s, the incidence of rabies in domestic animals has declined dramatically because of immunization of dogs and other domestic animals. Unlike the situation in developing countries, wild animals are the most important potential source of rabies for both humans and domestic animals in the United States; most reported cases of rabies occur among raccoons, skunks, and foxes and various species of bats [82]. During 2010, the number of rabies cases—both in animals and humans—reported in the United States fell 8 % compared with the previous year [83].

Pathogenesis

Viral infection of the CNS occurs via two distinct routes: hematogenous and neuronal. Enteroviruses and arboviruses are carried to the CNS via the blood stream, while HSV and the rabies virus are carried to the CNS via nerve cells themselves. Because viruses must replicate intracellularly, the ability to cause disease is largely determined by whether viral surface proteins can attach to specific receptors on specific cells in affected tissues—i.e., tissue trophism. An example of viral tissue tropism being determined by the combination of viral surface proteins and specific tissue receptors is that of the binding of the HIV GP120 to the CD4+ receptor on T4 lymphocytes. Other tissues with HIV tropism include monocytes and derived cells (macrophages), Langerhans cells, glial cells, and dendritic cells, all of which express the CD4+ receptor. Cells that do not express this receptor generally do not become infected with HIV [84]. So important are these surface binding sites for their respective cellular receptors that several viruses such as rhinovirus, influenza virus, and poliovirus have evolved "sophisticated" molecular mechanisms to protect these sites from the host immune response.

Enteroviruses are transmitted in human populations largely through fecal-oral transmission. These viruses survive stomach acid, replicate in the intestine, and an initial viremia leads to infection of multiple organs within the body. A secondary viremia from these sources can lead to CNS involvement. The prompt production of antibody disrupts this second viremia and prevents invasion of the CNS. In the case of arboviruses, humans typically become infected when an infectious mosquito pierces the host epidermis to take a blood meal, depositing virus principally in the extravascular tissue although direct inoculation into the bloodstream can occur. Local replication is followed by viremia, and brain involvement is probably determined by viral tropism and the rapidity of the host immune response.

For CNS infections that occur following a viremia, invasion of the brain involves attachment of the virus to the endothelial cells, presumably via specific receptors. Following invasion, an acute inflammatory reaction occurs with a perivascular distribution within the brain parenchyma and varying degrees of involvement of the meninges, depending on the infecting viral agent. The perivascular inflammatory response is predominately mononuclear although polymorphonuclear leukocytes may be seen. Infection of neural cells results in degenerative changes and phagocytosis by tissue macrophages or microglial cells. Some pathologic features are unique to certain viruses: for example, cerebral atrophy and production of multinucleated giant cells and multiple nodules of infected microglia are seen in the white matter in patients with HIV encephalitis (Fig. 22.10), or the characteristic features of multinucleation, nuclear molding, chromatin margination, ground glass nuclei, and Cowdry

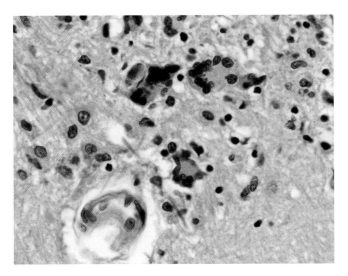

Fig. 22.10 Primary HIV infection of the CNS. The pathology specimen is from the brain of a 25-year-old male with recently diagnosed HIV. The patient developed pneumonia and died of respiratory failure. The figure shows perivascular inflammation with multiple giant cells involving a small vessel in the pons (H&E, 40×) (Courtesy of Anthony Yachnis, MD, and Kelly Devers, MD, University of Florida College of Medicine)

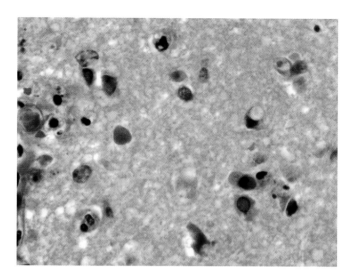

Fig. 22.11 Herpes encephalitis (autopsy case: 32-year-old male patient with end-stage AIDS). Figure shows herpesvirus-infected neurons with marginated chromatin and glassy, smudged nuclei. H&E 60× (Courtesy of Anthony Yachnis, MD, and Kelly Devers, MD, University of Florida College of Medicine)

type A intranuclear inclusion bodies seen in HSV infections (Fig. 22.11), with extensive asymmetrical necrosis in the temporal lobes, in the insulae, and in the cingulate gyri, typically seen in neuroimaging studies (Fig. 22.12a, b) [85]. In the case of rabies, histopathologic evidence of rabies encephalomyelitis (inflammation) in brain tissue and meninges includes mononuclear infiltration, perivascular cuffing of lymphocytes or polymorphonuclear cells, lymphocytic foci, Babes nodules consisting of glial cells, and the pathognomonic Negri body—an intracytoplasmic inclusion body within which the virus can be identified (Fig. 22.13a, b).

Some viral infections, most notably HSV and rabies, spread to the CNS via a neuronal route. In the case of HSV, the distribution involves the medial part of the temporal lobe bilaterally with one temporal lobe generally much more involved than the other. Autopsy studies carried out on patients who died during active HSV encephalitis show the presence of virus in the olfactory bulbs, olfactory tracts, and the tracts of the limbic system which end in the hippocampus, amygdala, insula, cingulate gyrus, and olfactory cortex [86]. Thus, the virus appears to gain access to the CNS from the nasal mucosa to the olfactory bulbs and olfactory tracts,

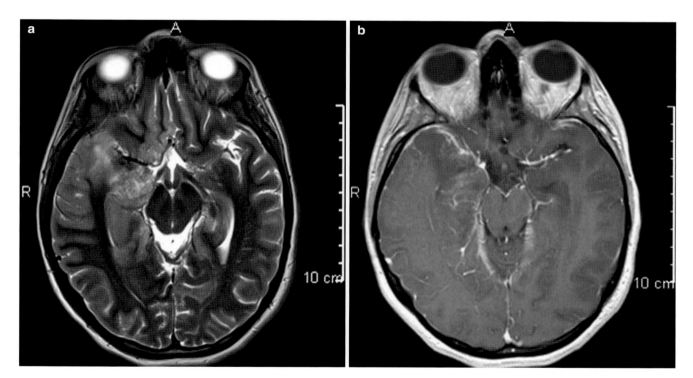

Fig. 22.12 (a, b) Herpes (HSV-1) encephalitis; images include low convexity axial T2-w sequence (a) and post-contrast T1-w sequence in the same brain section level. The T2-w image (a) illustrates cytogenic edema distributed not only within the anterior and mesial right temporal lobe but also within the frontotemporal association bundle and basifrontal cortex. It involves gray and white matter. There is less obvious change on the left. This pattern, in the right clinical context, is typical of HSV-1 cerebritis. It has a differential of tumoral gliomatosis, but the latter typically has a more prolonged presenting clinical course. The post-contrast T1-w image (b) demonstrates pial and perivascular enhancement. HSV-1 is an angiophilic organism which can produce a necrotizing intrinsic angiitis which can cause subarachnoid hemorrhage, although not in this case

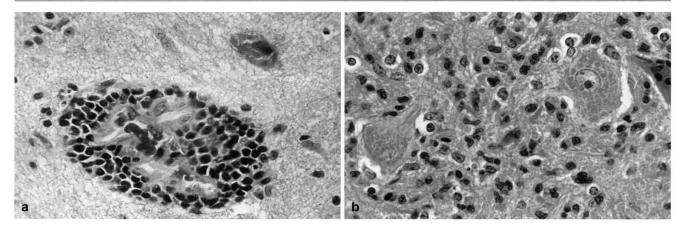

Fig. 22.13 (**a**) This micrograph depicts the histopathologic changes associated with rabies encephalitis prepared using an H&E stain. Note the perivascular cuffing due to the perivascular accumulation of inflammatory cell infiltrates (i.e., lymphocytes and polymorphonuclear leuko- cytes). Figure (**b**) is a photomicrograph of H&E stained brain tissue from a rabies encephalitis patient displaying the pathognomonic finding of Negri bodies within the neuronal cytoplasm (Both: Courtesy of the Centers for Disease Control and Prevention)

although the mechanism by which the virus does this remains unknown. About two-thirds of cases of HSV encephalitis in adults and older children occur in patients who have antibody to the virus at the time of infection. Many of these patients have a history of cold sores dating back 20–30 years. In the other one-third of patients, antibody to HSV is lacking at the time of onset of symptoms indicating that the encephalitis is likely part of the primary infection. Approximately 90–95 % of the cases of HSV encephalitis in older children and adults are due to HSV type I, with the remaining 5–10 % due to HSV type II. Neonatal herpes appears to be different, in that 90–95 % of these cases are due to HSV type II acquired from maternal or other sources at the time of birth. Infection of the CNS in neonates generally follows systemic viremic spread; however, there is no temporal lobe localization.

Rabies infection may result from contact with saliva or other secretions from infected animals as well as the animal bite itself. Rabies replicates initially at the local site of inoculation, and for this reason emergency preventive measures, such as thorough cleansing of the wound and infiltration with human rabies immunoglobulin, can be effective in preventing infection with this viral agent. In the process of local replication, the rabies virus invades the nerve sheaths and is transported via nerve cells to the CNS. The rapidity of the rabies virus in reaching the CNS is a function of the distance of the nerve endings from the CNS. Thus, bites on the lower extremities may take months to produce symptoms in the CNS, whereas bites in the face may reach the CNS within weeks. It is also important to recognize that the initial incident may be forgotten because of the length of time of the onset of CNS symptoms after the initial infecting event or because the inoculation may be unapparent as has been reported for bats [87]. Therefore, a high index of suspicion

for rabies is essential when managing patients with encephalitis of unknown cause, especially in patients who exhibit signs of hyperirritability.

Clinical Manifestations

Viral meningitis is an acute illness characterized by fever, headache, stiff neck, photophobia, and varying degrees of nonspecific symptoms such as malaise, myalgia, nausea, vomiting, abdominal pain, or diarrhea. Generally, neither disturbance of mental status nor abnormal neurological signs are characteristic of viral meningitis. The presence of obtundation, disorientation, seizures, or localized neurologic signs should suggest brain parenchymal involvement and a diagnosis of encephalitis or meningoencephalitis. Neck stiffness is generally less severe compared with bacterial meningitis. Clinical clues to an enteroviral etiology include presence of a viral exanthem, pleuropericarditis, pleurodynia, painful oropharyngeal ulcers, or peripheral vesicular lesions suggestive of hand, foot, and mouth disease. The CSF in patients with viral meningitis is usually clear with an elevated white cell count; polymorphonuclear leukocytes may predominate within the first 24–48 h, although this number rarely exceeds 80 % of total CSF white cells. CSF protein is generally mildly elevated, and the glucose is normal with the occasional exception in about 10–20 % of patients with mumps and less often in patients with enterovirus or HSV infection. In viral meningitis, the CSF gram stain will be negative and routine CSF cultures will not yield bacterial growth. When the initial CSF analysis shows over 50 % polymorphonuclear leukocytes, it is not uncommon for clinicians to repeat the lumbar puncture over the next 12–24 h to determine whether there is a shift towards a lymphocytic predominance, as one would expect in viral meningitis.

A parameningeal infectious focus (e.g., brain abscess) will characteristically be associated with a CSF pleocytosis, a likely elevated protein, and a normal glucose. Thus, a patient with an epidural abscess or a brain abscess could present with mild headache, fever, and a CSF picture identical to that of viral meningitis. Some cases of sphenoid or frontal sinusitis may feature a CSF pleocytosis. Patients with fungal and tuberculous meningitis may also present with headache, fever, and stiff neck, but in general the clinical course is longer than an acute viral meningitis. The CSF in patients with fungal or tuberculous meningitis generally has a relatively low glucose level, usually less than 40 mg/dL.

The CSF in patients with cryptococcal meningitis may be completely normal. Fever, headache, and nonspecific CSF findings can also be seen in other infections, such as syphilis, ehrlichiosis, and noninfectious conditions, such as sarcoidosis, Behcet's disease, systemic lupus erythematosus, vasculitis, or uveoparotitis.

Viruses other than enteroviruses can also produce aseptic meningitis. For example, HSV type II produces very typical aseptic meningitis with low-grade fever, headache, stiff neck, and photophobia as part of primary genital herpes infection. Therefore, it is important to question the sexually active patient about a history of genital herpetic lesions and to perform a pelvic examination in women where indicated. Aseptic meningitis can also be seen as part of the syndrome of primary HIV infection. Certain strains of leptospirosis will typically present with aseptic meningitis; however, most cases present in conjunction with systemic disease and severe involvement of other organs such as lung, liver, and kidney. Lymphocytic choriomeningitis virus (LCMV) belongs to the family *Arenavirus* and is found globally [88]. LCMV meningitis is typically associated with exposure to rodents, such as common house mouse (*Mus musculus* and *M. domesticus*), hamsters, and guinea pigs. Transmission occurs by inhalation (aerosol and droplet), fomites, or direct contact with excreta or blood from infected rodents. The incubation period is 1–2 weeks; symptoms are nonspecific and include fever, chills, myalgia, headache, photophobia, anorexia, pharyngitis, and cough. CNS invasion is seen only in a few patients either after an initial febrile illness. During the neurologic phase, patients acquire aseptic meningitis and peripheral leukocytosis. CSF leukocyte cell counts are often greater than 1,000 cells /μL, and glucose levels are low. LCMV meningitis may be associated with an ascending paralysis, transverse myelitis, or encephalitis; overall case fatality is less than 1 % [88].

The laboratory diagnosis of viral meningitis is generally one of exclusion. Viral cultures of CSF that yield growth of enteroviruses are diagnostic. However, these are positive in only 30–50 % of cases. PCR has become available for the diagnosis of enteroviral meningitis and these PCR platforms correlate very well with the results of viral culture. Unfortunately, PCR testing may not be routinely available at clinical microbiology laboratories for various reasons, including cost cutting measures and lack of trained personnel. Sending specimens to reference laboratories or highly specialized research laboratories is an alternative, but results generally will not be available during the acute phase of the patient's illness. In the case of HSV meningitis, the diagnosis is confirmed if HSV is cultured from CSF or detected by PCR. For aseptic meningitis associated with systemic infections, such as leptospirosis, syphilis, or ehrlichiosis, diagnosis can be confirmed through standard serologic testing generally available at state public health laboratories or reference laboratories.

Because there are over 75 different enterovirus serotypes, testing is only possible for a subset of these. In addition there is tremendous overlap in the serologic response between the different serotypes such that seroconversion to one or more enterovirus serotype can occur. Moreover, since there is no specific therapy, expensive laboratory testing is unlikely to affect patient outcome. For these reasons, serologic studies for the diagnosis of enterovirus infections are generally not indicated.

A common diagnostic misconception is the usefulness of CSF antibodies. With the exception of the venereal disease research laboratory (VDRL) test, which indicates active CNS syphilis, and the ratio of measles antibodies in CSF to serum levels in extremely rare cases of subacute sclerosing panencephalitis (SSPE), routine CSF antibody testing does not affect patient outcomes. In general, infectious viral agents can more readily be diagnosed from serum rather than CSF studies. Tests for common viral infections and preferred diagnostic methods are outlined in Table 22.4.

Finally, certain drugs such as sulfa and nonsteroidal antiinflammatory agents can produce acute syndromes of aseptic meningitis (Table 22.5). Other noninfectious factors have been associated with an aseptic meningitis picture, including intravenous immunoglobulin, intrathecal administration of drugs, receipt of certain vaccines, malignancies, autoimmune conditions, and connective tissue disorders (Table 22.5) [89].

The hallmark of the presentation of viral encephalitis is fever, headache, confusion, drowsiness, and convulsions. Prominent signs include an altered level of consciousness with or without focal neurologic signs or meningism (i.e., the triad of neck stiffness, photophobia, and headache) in the setting of an acute febrile illness. By and large, the differential diagnosis is the same as for acute bacterial or viral meningitis. Varying degrees of nuchal rigidity can be present in patients with encephalitis. Lumbar puncture yields CSF with a picture similar to that of viral meningitis. HSV, VZV, arboviruses, and enteroviruses can now be diagnosed by PCR analyses of CSF specimens. MRI imaging is a useful test for

Table 22.4 Laboratory diagnosis of selected viral diseases

Virus	CNS disease	Serology	Viral culture	Direct antigen	PCR/other
Herpes viruses					
Herpes simplex	Temporal lobe encephalitis	About 2/3 seropositive on admission, not helpful in Dx	Almost always negative in CSF, throat, etc.	None for CSF FA can be done on brain biopsy	≥ 90 % sensitive on CSF—reference labs and some academic medical centers only
Varicella	Encephalitis in HIV patients	Not helpful diagnostically	Usually negative in CSF, throat, etc.	None for CSF FA can be done on brain biopsy	Reference labs only MRI may be suggestive
Cytomegalovirus	Encephalitis in HIV patients	Almost always positive	Urine, throat, blood may be positive—consistent with but not proof of encephalitis	Antigenemia test on blood, positive test consistent with but not proof of encephalitis	If CSF positive, encephalitis likely, but asymptomatic HIV patients may also be positive MRI may be suggestive
Epstein-Barr Virus	Rare encephalitis in mononucleosis	Monospot test good presumptive test, may be negative in up to 20 % in 1st week VCA-IgG and IgM, positive IgM virtually diagnostic	Not available	Not available	Reference labs only, not needed for diagnosis
Human herpes virus 6 and 7 (HHV 6 and 7)	Seizures, encephalitis in 1–3 year olds	Reference labs only	Reference labs only	Not available	Reference labs only
Respiratory viruses					
Influenza A and B Parainfluenza 1–3 Adenovirus Respiratory syncytial virus (RSV)	Parainfluenza occasionally, others rarely cause encephalitis	Not useful	NP swabs; throat washings Cultures via bronchoscopy Excellent sensitivity, diagnostic if positive	Direct antigen ELISA available for RSV (excellent sensitivity), and Influenza (moderately sensitive)	Not available
Enterovirus					
Coxsackie Echovirus	Summertime outbreaks of meningitis, meningoencephalitis	Not useful: too many serotypes and too much cross-reactivity	Send stool, throat, CSF If throat or CSF culture positive—diagnostically definitive If stool culture positive—presumptive (enteroviruses may be shed in stool for weeks)	None	Available in reference labs, picks up most serotypes, may take a week to get results
Arboviruses					
St. Louis encephalitis California encephalitis	Summertime outbreaks of encephalitis	Diagnostic, if positive Serum is preferred specimen; CSF not helpful	Generally not available	Not available	Not available
Western equine Eastern equine La Crosse West Nile virus		Done in reference laboratory and public health labs			

		ELISA Confirm with Western Blot	Research labs only	P 24 antigen in serum	
HIV	Encephalopathy	ELISA Confirm with Western Blot	Research labs only	P 24 antigen in serum	Reference labs, many tertiary medical centers, used for following treatment
Lymphocytic choriomeningitis virus	Meningitis	Reference laboratory	Not available	Not available	Not available
JC virus	Progressive multifocal leukoencephalopathy. Mostly in HIV & other immunocompromised patients	Reference laboratory	Not available	Not available	Available in reference laboratories. Diagnostic if positive on CSF. MRI highly suggestive. Brain biopsy definitive
Rabies	Encephalitis	Reference or state public health labs. Antibody is generally undetectable before day 6, 50 % by day 8, and 100 % by day 15	Research labs only	Direct fluorescent antibody staining of hair follicles in skin biopsy from nape of the neck above the hairline—50 % positive in 1st week, higher later	RT-PCR may be available in reference labs, state public health labs. Send saliva, CSF, or tissue

Adapted with permission from Rand et al. [521]

Table 22.5 Nonviral causes of aseptic meningitis and encephalomyelitis

Infective causes

Ehrlichia spp.	Rocky Mountain spotted fever
Bacterial endocarditis	Brain abscess/cerebritis
Staphylococcus aureus	*Treponema pallidum* meningitis
Lyme disease	Leptospirosis
Mycoplasma pneumoniae	*Listeria monocytogenes* (rhomboid encephalitis)
Typhus	*Legionella* spp.
Cat-scratch disease	*Nocardia* spp.
Mycobacterium tuberculosis meningitis	*Cryptococcus neoformans meningitis*
Histoplasmosis	Coccidioidomycosis
Cerebral amebiasis	Cerebral malaria
Trypanosomiasis	Cerebral abscess and other parameningeal infections
Partially treated bacterial meningitis	CNS cysts (e.g., craniopharyngioma, dermoid/epidermoid)

Noninfective medical conditions

Malignancy, especially lymphoma	Behçet's disease
Still's Disease	Systemic lupus erythematosus
Chronic subdural hematoma	Vasculitis
Intrathecal injections	Neurosurgery-related procedures

Drugs

Certain nonsteroidal anti-inflammatory drugs

Antimicrobial agents, including trimethoprim, cephalosporins, penicillin, amoxicillin, isoniazid, ciprofloxacin, metronidazole, and sulfonamides

Carbamazepine

Ranitidine, famotidine

Azathioprine

Sulfasalazine

Indinavir

Vaccines: measles, mumps, rubella (MMR), alone or in combination

Monoclonal antibodies (e.g., muromonab-CD3) [OKT3] that targets the CD3 receptor

Intravenous immunoglobulin

Adapted with permission from Rand et al. [521]

ascertaining HSV encephalitis and for differentiating post infectious encephalomyelitis from viral encephalitis. It is important to recognize that some patients with arbovirus encephalitis, particularly Eastern equine encephalitis and West Nile virus encephalitis, may have focal lesions by MRI (Fig. 22.14). However, the distribution of these lesions is not consistent and differs from the pattern seen on neuroimaging studies of HSV encephalitis (Fig. 22.12a, b). Diagnosis of arbovirus encephalitis can almost always be made by serological testing as antibody titers to all of the common arboviruses are generally present by the time the patient presents with symptoms. Because there is only a very low background frequency of these antibodies in the general healthy population, a positive arbovirus serology can be accepted as clinically definitive of exposure or infection.

The diagnosis of HSV encephalitis is of critical importance because of the effectiveness of acyclovir in improving patient outcomes. HSV is the most common cause of sporadic encephalitis. Patients with HSV type I encephalitis generally present with a 3- to 5-day history of fever, headache, and focal signs, including dysphasia and personality changes that may progress to obtundation and coma; the latter can occur abruptly and may be associated with the onset of seizures. HSV encephalitis can occur in any age group from childhood through old age at any time of the year—i.e., there is no characteristic seasonal variation pattern in occurrence. The incidence is estimated at 1 in 250,000 to 1 in 500,000 people per year; HSV encephalitis accounts for approximately 10–20 % of viral encephalitides in the United States.

A diagnosis of HSV encephalitis is supported by MRI findings showing bilateral temporal lobe involvement that is generally asymmetrical (Fig. 22.12a, b). CT imaging may reveal frontotemporal changes in HSV encephalitis. In untreated patients, this may progress to hemorrhagic lesions; swelling of the more severely affected temporal lobe may result in a mass effect sufficient to produce a shift of the midline structures and tentorial herniation. PCR for HSV in the spinal fluid is almost uniformly positive in patients with HSV encephalitis, despite the fact that in 1–4 % of cases, one cannot grow the virus from CSF or specimens from other anatomic sites in patients [90, 91]. The use of PCR in combination

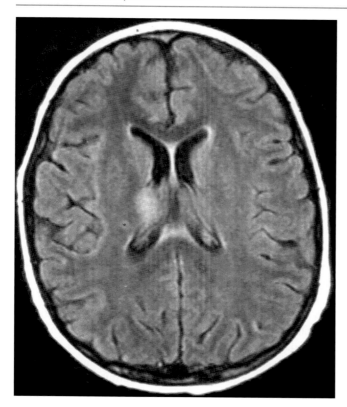

Fig. 22.14 West Nile viral thalamic encephalitis T2-w mid-convexity brain section. Arbovirus (West Nile virus in this example) encephalitis typically has multicentric areas of cytogenic edema, which typically involve gray matter both in the cortex and in the central nuclear structures. The lesions are usually multicentric but not symmetric between hemispheres. In this example cytogenic edema is evident in the right thalamus and in the splenium of the corpus callosum. The splenial abnormality can be from the virus but may also occur following recent seizure activity

with the detection of a specific intrathecal antibody response to HSV currently represents the most reliable strategy for the diagnosis and monitoring of the treatment of adult patients with HSV encephalitis [90–93]. Serologic diagnosis is not particularly helpful early on, although, in general, all patients with HSV encephalitis will show a significant rise in HSV titer both in the spinal fluid and serum; seroconversion can be ascertained in patients with primary HSV infection. EEG studies may reveal focal features.

Conditions that mimic encephalitis include brain abscess, subdural empyema, cerebritis due to *Listeria* spp., mycoplasma, fungal infections, tuberculosis, cryptococcus, rickettsia, toxoplasmosis, mucor, and agents frequently associated with bacterial meningitis, such as pneumococcus and meningococcus (Fig. 22.5c, d) [94, 95]. Influenza A virus can cause encephalitis during epidemics; children are particularly affected. Tumors, subdural hematomas, CNS lupus, adrenal leukodystrophy, acute strokes, neuroleptic malignant syndrome, or Reye's syndrome can mimic the symptoms and signs of encephalitis.

Encephalitis can sometimes occur as part of systemic infection with common viruses that do not normally produce encephalitis. For example, EBV infection can, on occasion, present with seizures and even coma; these patients generally recover completely. CNS involvement with toxoplasmosis, lymphoma, VZV, and CMV in HIV-infected patients can also mimic the features of encephalitis. Table 22.5 lists nonviral infections that may resemble viral encephalitis.

Although rare, rabies should be considered in atypical cases of encephalitis or in cases where results of all investigations are negative. Because affected patients often do not have a history of having been bitten by an animal, a history of close contact with potentially infected animals, including bats, should be sought. Infection is almost always from inoculation but occasionally by inhalation. Rabies has been transmitted by corneal and solid organ allografts [96, 97]. The virus is transmitted to the CNS via nerve trunks. Proliferation in nerve cells in the brain and peripheral ganglia leads to an invariably fatal meningoencephalitis. The incubation period varies anywhere from 2 weeks more than year. Proximal bites with a relatively large inoculum of virus tend to be associated with shorter incubation periods. The onset is rapid with fever, anxiety, insomnia, headache, malaise, myalgia, fatigue, anorexia, nausea, vomiting, sore throat, and cough. The patient may complain of symptoms suggestive of paresthesia or fasciculation at the site of the original animal bite due to viral replication at the site of inoculation or in the dorsal ganglia of the sensory nerve supplying that area. The disease quickly progresses to an encephalitic phase consisting of agitation, excitation, and excessive motor activity. Patients may experience hallucinations, become combative, and develop muscle spasms with opisthotonus and involvement of the respiratory muscles. Painful spasms of the throat muscles, precipitated by attempts to swallow, may follow—this explains why patients tend to avoid drinking or swallowing. Spasms may be precipitated by mere air blowing onto the face; seizures are frequent. Periods of hallucinations and aberrant mentation may alternate with lucid periods that get progressively shorter as the disease progresses. Hyperesthesias with excessive reactivity to normal stimulation of light, sound, and touch are very common; autonomic nervous system changes such as dilated pupils, increased salivation, lacrimation, perspiration, and postural hypotension occur. Ultimately, brain stem function is affected with cranial nerve palsies, optic neuritis, and the characteristic hydrophobia due to the painful, violent involuntary contractions of the muscles of respiration and those in the pharynx and the larynx, initiated by attempts to swallow. Eventually the disease progresses to cardiorespiratory depression, coma, and death. Occasionally, rabies may present as an ascending paralysis clinically similar to the Guillain-Barré syndrome; corneal transplants from two patients presumed to have died from Guillain-Barré actually transmitted clinical rabies, resulting in the death of the recipients [98, 99]. The laboratory diagnosis of rabies requires viral isolation, positive serology (assuming the patient has not been immunized), or demonstration of the characteristic Negri bodies in brain tissue. Laboratory diagnostic evaluation for rabies includes serological testing plus demonstration of viral antigen by IFA in infected tissue, including corneal scrapings, skin biopsies or brain biopsies, and analysis of CSF or saliva specimens for rabies virus antigen or RNA [100]. Survival of patients with rabies is rare; most of the few who have survived received the rabies vaccine prior to the onset of illness.

In patients who have traveled overseas, encephalitis may be caused by various other infectious diseases, including Japanese B encephalitis, Murray Valley encephalitis, Omsk hemorrhagic fever, Kyasanur forest disease complex, Powassan virus, *louping ill*, Russian spring-summer encephalitis, Rift Valley fever, yellow fever, dengue, chikungunya, Hantaan virus, Puumala virus (a species of hantavirus), and the highly fatal hemorrhagic fevers caused by the Marburg, Ebola, and Lassa fever viruses.

B virus infection is caused by Macacine herpesvirus 1 (formerly Cercopithecine herpesvirus 1 (CHV-1)), an alphaherpesvirus closely related to herpes simplex virus. B virus is also commonly referred to as herpes B, monkey B virus, herpesvirus simiae, and herpesvirus B. The virus is commonly found among macaque monkeys, including rhesus macaques, pig-tailed macaques, and cynomolgus monkeys (also called crab-eating or long-tailed macaques), any of which can harbor latent B virus infection and appear to be natural hosts for the virus. Monkeys infected with B virus usually have no or only mild symptoms. In addition, rabbits, guinea pigs, and mice can be experimentally infected with B virus. The virus is related to human HSV but humans have little native ability to contain it in contrast to its natural host in whom it produces "cold sores." Human infection usually results from bites or scratches from macaques or mucocutaneous exposure to monkey saliva; laboratory personnel who work with ostensibly healthy monkeys or their tissues are particularly at risk. Indirect contact transmission, such as a needlestick injury with a contaminated needle has been documented. B virus is transmitted to humans from saliva in monkeys and reaches the brain via nerves at the site of the monkey bite. Patients acquire an ascending myelitis and fulminant meningoencephalitis, which leads to death. Infection is diagnosed by a rise in antibody titer or by isolating the virus from the CNS. There are seven different exposures for which postexposure prophylaxis is recommended: if postexposure prophylaxis is administered, it should be started soon (within hours) after the exposure. Neurologic tests should include lumbar puncture and MRI of the brain; electroencephalography (EEG) should also be considered. CSF samples should be sent for culture, PCR detection of viral DNA, and

serologic testing. While use of intravenous acyclovir and ganciclovir therapy for patients with the early stages of B virus disease, including patients with early signs of CNS disease has been associated with increased survival for some patients, antiviral therapy has not been effective in patients with advanced encephalomyelitis [101].

Treatment

No specific drug or serologic therapy is currently available for enterovirus or arbovirus infections. In general, viral meningitis due to enteroviruses is clinically mild, and most patients can be treated without admission to the hospital unless bacterial meningitis is a possibility in the differential diagnosis and needs to be ruled out. Patients with enteroviral meningitis usually recover within 7–10 days without antiviral therapy.

Intravenous acyclovir is indicated for patients with HSV or VZV meningitis. In patients with symptoms suggestive of encephalitis or brain parenchymal involvement, and in whom appropriate radiologic imaging studies have ruled out other pathology, such as brain abscess or subdural empyema, initiation of empiric intravenous acyclovir intravenously in doses appropriate for HSV encephalitis is indicated. Complications from acyclovir are relatively uncommon; timely diagnosis is of paramount importance since a successful outcome is largely associated with early institution of acyclovir therapy. Brain biopsy is not justified to prove the presence of herpes encephalitis prior to therapy. Before antiviral agents became available for the treatment of HSV encephalitis, the disease was fatal in approximately 70 % of patients, with an additional 20–25 % surviving with severe disabilities. The dose of acyclovir is 10 mg/kg IV every 8 h for 14–21 days.

Brain Abscess

Brain abscesses have been recognized since the days of Hippocrates in 460 BC. By definition, a brain abscess is a localized suppurative infection of the brain parenchyma [102]. The incidence in the general population has been estimated at 1.3–100,000 person-years, with the rates slightly higher in children between 5 and 9 years of age and after the age of 60 years. Most series document a male preponderance of between 2:1 and 3:1, and the age distribution is somewhat dependent on the associated underlying etiologies [103, 104]. While the etiology and distribution of associated diseases has remained essentially unchanged over the years for pyogenic brain abscesses, the AIDS epidemic has led to the occurrence of a large group of patients with brain abscess due to toxoplasmosis. Highly active antiretroviral therapy (HAART) has resulted in a reduction of morbidity and mortality in HIV-associated cerebral opportunistic infections.

Pathogenesis

Brain abscesses develop as localized areas of cerebritis (i.e., poorly demarcated areas of encephalitis), initially consisting of bacteria in the brain parenchyma together with inflammation and edema. Over the ensuing days this area of cerebritis becomes more localized with the development of necrosis in the middle and a ring-enhancing capsule. Ultimately, host defenses lead to the development of a well-formed fibrous capsule. The most common predisposing conditions for the development of a brain abscess are infections in the middle ear, paranasal sinuses, mastoids, and teeth (dental abscess). It is believed that bacteria reach the brain through valveless emissary veins, which traverse the cranium into the venous drainage system of the brain, or retrograde spread through the venous system. Alternatively, direct extension through an area of osteitis or osteomyelitis adjacent to the sinus or middle ear infection provides access to the CNS; chronic otitis media is a common predisposing factor with the abscesses most frequently forming in the temporal lobe or cerebellum. The other major mechanism by which the brain parenchyma becomes seeded is via metastatic transmission through the cerebral arteries from an extracranial focus of infection. Approximately 20 % of brain abscesses arise from a contiguous focus; 25 % are associated with hematogenous spread from a distant focus, such as a pyogenic lung abscess or bronchiectasis, and 25 % occur following trauma [105–107].

Hematogenous brain abscesses generally tend to be multiple and be located at the gray white matter junction; they also tend to follow a vascular distribution within the brain. Hematogenous dissemination from a contiguous focus of infection has also been described. Other distant foci that have been associated with brain abscess include wound infections, osteomyelitis, pelvic infection, cholecystitis, and other intra-abdominal foci. In fact, any procedure that results in a transient bacteremia can on occasion be associated with the subsequent development of a brain abscess. Despite its chronicity and relatively high frequency of bacteremia, and involvement of the brain in 20–40 % of cases, endocarditis accounts for only 1–5 % of cases of brain abscess [108, 109]. Patients with cyanotic congenital heart disease are at increased risk of acquiring brain abscesses. A significant number of brain abscesses are associated with penetrating trauma such as gunshot wounds, depressed skull fractures with retained with bone fragments, cranial penetration from objects such as pencils, animal bites, or even as a complication of cervical traction associated with pin-site infection. In patients with HIV infection, reactivation of toxoplasmosis can lead to brain abscesses. In approximately 25 % of cases no underlying etiology can be established.

Microbiology

The bacterial etiology of brain abscess is to a great extent dependent on the location of the abscess and the predisposing factors. Thus, aerobic, anaerobic, and microaerophilic streptococci are the most frequently isolated bacterial species. *Staphylococcus aureus* is the underlying cause of 25 % of brain abscesses and often associated with trauma, endocarditis, or following a neurosurgical procedure. In addition to streptococci, brain abscess associated with paranasal sinus or chronic otitis media infection may be caused by *Haemophilus* species, *Bacteroides* species, other anaerobes, and *Pseudomonas aeruginosa* in the case of chronic otitis media. If the source of bacteremia is intra-abdominal, *Enterobacteriaceae*, enterococci, and anaerobes are likely to be implicated; a urinary tract source is more likely associated with *Pseudomonas* spp. or *Enterobacteriaceae*, but not anaerobes. Brain abscess caused by anaerobes, including actinomyces, may be associated with spread from a lung abscess [110].

Although *S. aureus* is the most common organism complicating penetrating trauma, *Clostridium* species and *Enterobacteriaceae* are also commonly implicated. The nature of the precipitating trauma is important: for example, if trauma occurs in a water environment, *Pseudomonas* spp. and *Aeromonas* spp. would have to be among the organisms considered. Microorganisms associated with postoperative infections include *S. aureus*, *Staphylococcus epidermidis* and *Enterobacteriaceae*, and *Pseudomonas* spp.

Nocardia species are uncommon but important causes of brain abscesses (Fig. 22.15a, b), especially in immunocompromised populations [111–113]. The clinical presentation of Nocardia infections in the CNS is the same in normal and compromised hosts, although more frequent in compromised hosts. In a series of 11 cases and review of 120 cases of nocardial brain abscess in the literature, concomitant pulmonary disease was present in 34 %. Most of the brain abscesses were single; about one-third were multiple, and, overall, 38 % of the cases occurred in patients who were immunocompromised by virtue of HIV or other causes [113]. Rarely, *Mycobacterium tuberculosis* may produce a space-occupying lesion (tuberculoma), and while uncommon in the United States, tuberculomas are relatively common causes of brain abscesses in some less-developed countries [114, 115].

Yeasts and fungi are important causes of brain abscess. *Candida albicans* almost never causes isolated brain abscesses but may cause microabscesses in association with disseminated candidiasis. Although cryptococcal infection of the CNS typically affects patients with HIV infection, cryptococcomas are rarely observed [116]. Agents of phaeohyphomycosis, such as *Cladosporium, Bipolaris, Curvularia,* and *Wangiella*, as well as the agents of chromoblastomycosis have all been reported as causes of brain abscesses.

Aspergillus spp. are well-recognized causes of brain abscess but are almost always limited to immunocompromised patient

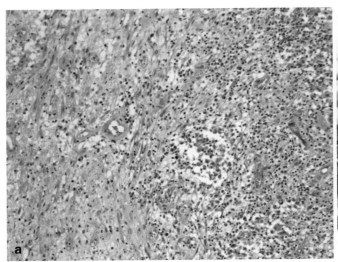
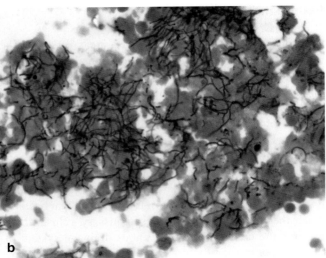

Fig. 22.15 (**a, b**) A 52-year-old female with a left frontal lobe intraparenchymal abscess caused by *Nocardia* sp. Figure (**a**) shows the thickened collagenous abscess wall with neovascularization adjacent to acute inflammatory infiltrate. H&E, 10×. In figure (**b**), Gomori methenamine silver (GMS) stain highlights numerous branching, filamentous bacteria. GMS, 60× (Both courtesy of Anthony Yachnis, MD, and Kelly Devers, MD, University of Florida College of Medicine)

populations, transplant patients in particular. *Aspergillus fumigatus* is the most common species affecting humans; maxillary sinusitis of dental origin or the lungs are the most common sites of primary *Aspergillus* spp. infection [117]. Infection reaches the brain directly from the nasal sinuses via vascular channels or is blood-borne from the lungs and gastrointestinal tract [117]. Zygomycoses such as Mucor Rhizopus and Rhizomucor produce brain infection by direct extension from the paranasal sinuses in poorly controlled diabetics. Cerebral mucormycosis without rhino-orbital or systemic involvement is an extremely rare condition mostly associated with parenteral drug abuse [118].

Protozoa and other parasites are important causes of brain abscess. The incidence of protozoal and helminthic infestations of the CNS is less than 1 %, but these infestations tend to follow a fatal course and are more common among children, the elderly, and immunocompromised individuals. *Toxoplasma gondii* is probably the most frequent protozoal cause of brain abscess in the United States and is almost entirely associated with HIV infection. Strongyloides, entamoeba, echinococcus, paragonimus, trichinosis, sparganosis, and angiostrongylus have all been reported, particularly in less-developed nations. Rarely, brain abscess due to naegleria and acanthamoeba occur in the United States.

Clinical Manifestations

Presentation, generally, is that of an intracranial mass lesion: subacute onset, headache, and focal neurological deficits [106, 109]. However, the classic triad of focal neurological signs, fever, and headache is present in less than 50 % of cases; nuchal rigidity is not prominent in patients with brain abscess. Similarly, patients with subdural empyema seem to present with a more localized headache and focal neurologic symptoms and altered level of consciousness. Other common signs and symptoms include fever, chills, seizures, nausea, vomiting, and altered sensorium [119]. Depending on the location of the lesion, fever and stiff neck may be present. Headache of varying degree of severity is the most consistent symptom among patients with brain abscess. The headache is generally not well localized and may be mild and difficult to differentiate from ordinary headaches. Fever is present in 40–50 % of cases, and focal neurologic symptoms and signs, such as hemiparesis, aphasia, ataxia, and sensory deficits, may be present in one-third to one-half of cases. Papilledema as a reflection of increased ICP is present in only a minority of cases [112, 119]. Likewise, seizures are observed in approximately 25–45 % of patients by the time they present. The seizures are most often generalized and associated with frontal lobe lesions. Other frequent CNS findings include altered mental states—confusion, aberrant behavior, and somnolence. To some extent, the presenting signs and symptoms are dependent on the location of the abscess. For example, cerebellar abscesses often present with nystagmus, ataxia in the ipsilateral extremities, vomiting, and dysmetria [120, 121]. Frontal lobe abscesses generally present with headache, drowsiness, and deterioration of mental status or aphasia together with hemiparesis and unilateral motor signs. Temporal lobe abscesses may present with or without aphasia or dysphasia, depending on whether the abscess is in the dominant hemisphere. Patients with occipital lobe abscesses may present

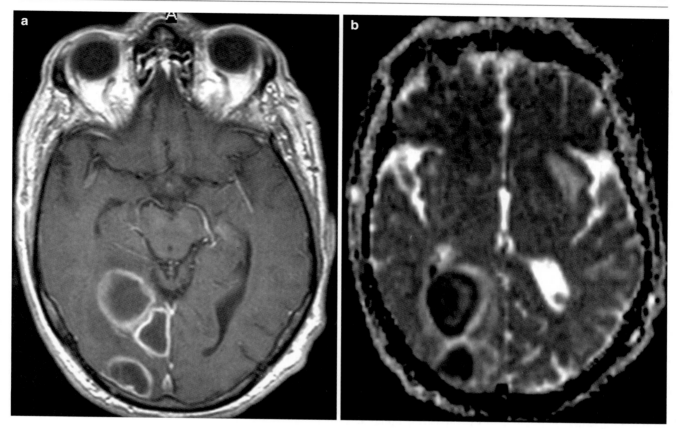

Fig. 22.16 (**a, b**) Occipital abscess with daughter abscesses; images include two MRI images in the low convexity region of brain. Figure (**a**) is a post-contrast T1-w sequence and the left image is an ADC map (apparent diffusion coefficient) sequence, which provides information as to the diffusibility of the free water in the area of abnormality. The post-contrast TD1-w sequence (**b**) demonstrates contiguous ring-enhancing lesions in the right occipital brain. These findings do not distinguish between tumors versus tumefactive lesions, especially

abscess. The diffusion sensitive imaging demonstrates free motion restriction within the central portions of the lesion. This in tandem with enhanced images is typical of brain abscess. The purulent material within the abscess contains increased water content (hyper intense of T2-w sequences), but it does not allow the water molecule to diffuse as well as fluid with the ventricles for instance. Hence, this ADC map shows the central water-restriction, often seen in pyogenic brain abscess

with homonymous hemianopia, while typical features in parietal lobe abscesses include hemianesthesia, homonymous hemianopia, neglect of one-half of the body, alexia, or impaired spatial perception. Pituitary abscesses may simulate a tumor and can present with visual field defects and endocrine abnormalities. Brain stem abscesses typically exhibit facial weakness, fever, headache, hemiparesis, dysphasia, and vomiting.

The differential diagnosis includes a wide range of other CNS infections, such as meningitis, subdural empyema, epidural abscess, viral encephalitis, and noninfectious causes, such as migraine, intracerebral and subarachnoid hemorrhage, venous sinus thrombosis, or malignancy.

Diagnosis

The diagnosis of a brain abscess is best established by neuroimaging [122, 123]. MRI is more sensitive than CT scans and provides information on the size, location, and stage of

the abscess together with the extent of surrounding edema and presence or absence of mass effect, such as midline shift, hydrocephalus, and impending herniation. The time line for bacterial brain abscess evolution is reasonably predictable and is divided into early cerebritis, late cerebritis, early abscess, mature abscess, and hopefully resolution (Fig. 22.8). Each of these stages takes place in roughly 4 days, hence the rule of 4 s for intra-axial brain abscess. This evolution of brain abscess is predicated on a normal immune system and does not apply in the immunocompromised host. Success of treatment is measured by progressively diminishing cross-sectional diameter of the abscess cavity. Radiologic changes in the abscess wall (i.e., thickness and contrast enhancement), surrounding edema, or status of internal contents are not reliable predictors of treatment success. Characteristic findings of a brain abscess are a ring-enhancing lesion in the contrast CT or MRI studies with a hypodense center reflecting the necrotic center of the abscess surrounded by a variable zone of edema [124] (Fig. 22.16a, b).

CT imaging studies are especially useful in defining contiguous head and neck pathology, which can be the source of infection. High detail CT imaging can detect the bone lysis of aggressive sinusitis and otomastoiditis better than MRI. CT is also better at defining bone dehiscence associated with prior trauma, which can also be the source for intracranial infection. MRI and CT are comparable in defining retropharyngeal abscess and chronic fungal sinus and skull base infections. CT is less sensitive than MRI for characterizing the stages of cerebritis and abscess formation and for excluding other causes of intra axial necrotic masses in the brain [125, 126]. MRI especially with diffusion brain imaging sequences maintains a high degree of sensitivity and specificity; see following discussion. However, some abscess remain in a chronic sequestered state and are difficult to differentiate from tumor; these are included in the category of tumefactive lesions along with others such as sequestered infarcts, thrombosed giant aneurysms, and Balo variant of multiple sclerosis, to name three.

The major difficulty with neuroimaging studies, especially CT imaging, is their sensitivity in differentiating an abscess from a tumor, including neuroblastomas and metastatic lesions. In one study, 8 out of 26 patients with a brain abscess were initially diagnosed as having a tumor [125]. Another study noted that in 18 % of CT scans from 100 patients with confirmed brain abscesses, the initial findings could not be radiographically distinguished from those typical of a malignancy [126].

MRI scanning provides soft tissue resolution and detail that is superior to that achieved with CT scanning [127]. In addition, there is no exposure to ionizing radiation, although the cost is substantially higher. On T1-weighted MRI scans, brain abscesses appear hypointense and show ring enhancement following administration of the contrast agent gadolinium. On T2-weighted sequences the central area of necrosis appears hyperintense and is surrounded by a well-defined hypointense capsule and readily discernible surrounding area of low density, representing cerebral edema. Another major advantage of MRI imaging studies is their ability to detect the cerebritis stage before the formation of the abscess with a fully developed capsule. The most helpful MR sequence is the diffusion techniques. This technique, most applicable once central necrosis has occurred, demonstrates the restriction of water movement within the forming fibrous abscess capsule. Other methods, such as magnetic resonance spectroscopy (MRS), can detect products of bacterial metabolism, such as lactate, acetate, or pyruvate, and may improve our ability to differentiate brain abscesses from malignancy [128–130].

Radionuclide brain scans using Indium-111-labeled leukocytes do not provide any advantage over conventional neuroimaging techniques. During the past several years, positron emission tomography (PET) with 18F-fluorodeoxyglucose (FDG) imaging have been playing larger roles in the diagnosis and management of patients with suspected brain abscesses [124, 131–134].

Routine laboratory studies are not particularly useful in the diagnosis of brain abscess. The white count is normal in 40 % of patients; the erythrocyte sedimentation rate is elevated in about 60 % while C-reactive protein levels are usually, but not invariably elevated. If the sedimentation rate is elevated, it may be useful to follow this over time to document a therapeutic response. Lumbar puncture in a patient with a space-occupying lesion is absolutely contraindicated unless an MRI or CT scan has indicated that herniation is unlikely to occur following an LP and there is a clear clinical suspicion of meningitis or meningeal carcinomatosis to justify taking the risk. The CSF in patients with brain abscess generally shows findings similar to any other parameningeal focus of infection, i.e., a pleocytosis with mixed neutrophils and lymphocytes, elevated protein levels, normal glucose levels, and a negative gram stain. CSF cultures are generally sterile, unless there is some anatomic connection between the abscess and the spinal fluid as may occur in cases in which the brain abscess is secondary to trauma or to a postoperative complication; blood cultures are positive in 10–20 % of patients. While reasonable empiric therapy can be devised for most common brain abscesses, culture of the material and transport to the laboratory under strictly anaerobic conditions is essential for optimal identification of the causative microorganism(s). In addition, a biopsy can be obtained and sent for pathologic evaluation to rule out malignancy, fungal invasion, and for detection of unusual microorganisms using special stains.

Treatment

Therapy for brain abscesses requires a combined medical and surgical approach [135]. Stereotactic-guided needle aspiration of pus drains the collection and enables procurement of specimens for gram stain, culture, and histology. Open craniotomy may be considered in cases where response to antimicrobial therapy is poor or the organism isolated from culture is antimicrobial-resistant. Antimicrobial therapy alone may be considered for patients with numerous abscesses that are not amenable to surgical drainage or for patients with small abscesses who have stable neurologic function. The choice of antimicrobials is determined both by the spectrum of microbiological agents known to cause brain abscess and the degree to which individual antimicrobials penetrate the blood–brain barrier and enter into the abscess cavity itself. For brain abscesses that develop in contiguity with frontal sinus infection, mixed aerobic and anaerobic flora may be assumed to be present. In this situation, even if anaerobic bacteria are not recovered, treatment should be given with high-dose penicillin 10–20 million units per day together with metronidazole 7.5 mg/kg IV every 6 h or

15 mg/kg IV every 12 h. If there is any suspicion that the abscess may have arisen from a dental focus, anaerobic cultures should be held for 7–14 days to enable detection of *Actinomyces* spp. growth. However, actinomycosis should respond to standard therapy with penicillin. Brain abscesses that are related to chronic otitis media and mastoiditis should be treated with a combination of antimicrobials that will cover anaerobes, *Enterobacteriaceae*, and *Pseudomonas* spp. Thus, a combination of cefotaxime, ceftazidime, or ceftriaxone plus metronidazole would work well in this clinical scenario. Although bacterial cultures may not always yield growth of anaerobes, particularly if the organisms are fastidious, the absence of growth of *Enterobacteriaceae* or *Pseudomonas* spp. on culturing abscess material from a patient who has not received prior intravenous antimicrobial therapy can be relied upon to rule out these particular organisms as the cause of infection. Similarly, the absence of *S. aureus* from culture of abscess matter would also be very good evidence that this agent is not involved in the pathogenesis of the abscess. In general, *S. aureus* is much more likely to be implicated in endocarditis, metastatic infection to the CNS, or in the setting of trauma or postsurgical wound infection. If a brain abscess is associated with a neurosurgical procedure, vancomycin should be included in the empirical therapeutic regimen to cover both methicillin-resistant *S. aureus* (MRSA) and coagulase-negative *Staphylococcus* spp.

A 6- to 8-week course of parenteral antimicrobial therapy plus regular follow-up computed tomography scans or MRI for at least 3 months to evaluate the therapeutic response is recommended. The antimicrobial regimen can be modified once antimicrobial susceptibility testing results become available. The dosage of third-generation cephalosporins is 2 g IV every 4 h for ceftazidime and 2 g IV every 12 h for ceftriaxone. Therapy is required for a minimum of 6 weeks. Patients with a brain abscess caused by *Nocardia* spp. should be treated with higher doses of trimethoprim/sulfamethoxazole (15 mg/kg/day of the trimethoprim component) in three to five divided doses until the infection is controlled; thereafter, the dose can be reduced to one double-strength trimethoprim/sulfamethoxazole tablet orally twice daily for 3–6 months in non-immunocompromised patients and up to a year in the immunocompromised person. In severely immunocompromised patients due to advanced AIDS lifelong treatment for Nocardia CNS infections may be required. The method of surgical intervention depends on the patient's clinical status and the neuroradiographic characteristics of the abscess.

Spinal Epidural Abscess

The epidural space is defined by an area posterolateral to the spinal cord between the dura and the vertebral column. It extends from the foramen magnum to the sacrum; the space is largest in the midthoracic and lumbar regions. The epidural space contains lymphatics, spinal nerve roots, loose fatty tissue, and small arteries. An epidural abscess is a collection of pus between the dura and the vertebral column. A spinal epidural abscess is a medical emergency because of the risk of spinal cord compression and potential progression to irreversible paraplegia or quadriplegia.

Spinal epidural abscess is more common in the elderly with a peak incidence during the 6th and 7th decades [136]. The disease is rare among children and typically affects patients whose comorbid conditions predispose them to immunocompromised states [136–140]. Other populations at risk include the aged, IV drug abusers, immunosuppression due to HIV infection, and spinal surgical procedures [141].

Pathophysiology

The formation of spinal epidural abscesses can be spontaneous or secondary to direct inoculation of a pathogen into the epidural space. The most common cause of the spontaneous infection in the epidural space is hematogenous spread from distant foci (50 %), such as infections of the skin and oral cavity, pneumonia and other respiratory tract infections, endocarditis, intra-abdominal and pelvic sepsis, and urinary tract infections [136]. Other causes of spontaneous abscess formation include direct extension (i.e., contiguous spread) from preexisting discitis or osteomyelitis in an adjacent vertebral body, extension of a decubitus ulcer or paraspinal abscess, blunt spinal trauma, or penetrating injuries. Secondary causes include postoperative infections (16 % of all spinal epidural abscesses) and infections associated with epidural anesthesia catheters [141–143]. An epidural hematoma resulting from trauma can also become secondarily infected and progress to an epidural abscess [136].

The location of an epidural abscess within the spinal canal is determined largely by the underlying cause of the epidural abscess [104, 136, 140, 141]. The majority of spontaneous spinal epidural abscesses that result from hematogenous spread of bacteria are usually located posteriorly within the spinal canal; epidural abscesses secondary to preexisting vertebral osteomyelitis are usually confined to the anterior spinal canal [140–145]. The segregation and isolation of abscesses to the anterior or posterior spinal canal is thought to be secondary to septations within the epidural fat [140]. These septations not only divide the epidural space into anterior and posterior compartments but also divide the space longitudinally. The longitudinal septations usually limit the extent of epidural abscess formation to up to four vertebral levels [140]. Postsurgical spinal epidural abscesses often involve multiple compartments, extending several levels and circumferentially around the spinal cord, secondary to disruption of the epidural septations [144]. In addition to causing compression of the spinal cord, pus and granulation tissue in the epidural space can cause ischemia of the spinal cord by compromising and reducing arterial blood flow. The neurologic sequelae of epidural abscess formation can be slowly progressive or dramatically acute in nature; in the latter scenario, complete paralysis could occur within a matter of hours [141]. The neurological injury is thought to be secondary to both compression of the neural elements vascular thrombosis and ischemia [140, 141, 146, 147].

Risk Factors

The majority of patients who develop a spinal epidural abscess have one or more identifiable risk factors [141, 143]. Implicated comorbid conditions include osteomyelitis, discitis, diabetes, degenerative joint disease of the spine, IV drug abuse, alcoholism, chronic renal failure, immunodeficiency states, and cancer [148]. The spectrum of risk factors is fairly consistent between reports of other large case series [136, 137, 140, 144]. Certain comorbid states such as diabetes and alcoholism result in an immunodeficient state that predisposes a patient to the development of a spinal abscess [144, 146]. Other risk factors have a more direct role in the development of spinal epidural abscesses. Discitis and the bacteremia associated with IV drug abuse, directly seed the epidural space with pathogens responsible for the epidural infection [141].

Microbiology of Spinal Epidural Abscess Formation

S. aureus is the microorganism most commonly isolated from spinal epidural abscesses followed by gram-negative organisms particularly *E. coli* and *Pseudomonas* spp. (18 %), other gram-positive organisms including *Streptococcus* spp. (10 %), or anaerobes (2 %); polymicrobial growth is observed in 5–10 % of cases. *Mycobacterium tuberculosis* has been implicated in various cases, especially in economically less-developed countries. Pathogens less frequently implicated as causes of spinal epidural abscesses include *Brucella* spp., *Actinomyces*, *Cryptococcus* spp., and *Aspergillus* spp. [136, 142, 143].

Clinical Features and Diagnostic Considerations

The classic clinical presentation of a patient with spinal epidural abscess is back pain and fever; nerve root pain often ensues—a result of nerve root compression caused by a ruptured intervertebral disc. Further progression to spinal cord compression may lead to motor weakness, bowel and bladder dysfunction, limb weakness, and paralysis [141]. In reality, the presentation is highly variable; other common clinical findings include fever (61 %), paresis (53 %), bowel or bladder dysfunction (36 %), sepsis (17 %), radiculopathy (12 %), and plegia (14 %) [149, 150]. Because of the general and nonspecificity of symptoms and signs, patients, not infrequently, may be misdiagnosed initially [148]. Point tenderness over the involved vertebral levels is present in about one-quarter of patients and is associated with underlying bony involvement [148]. The most common location of spinal epidural abscess formation is in the lumbar region, but thoracic and cervical involvement is not uncommon [136].

Time between symptom onset and presentation is highly variable and does not correlate well with intraoperative findings [151]. Neurological deficits are present on physical examination in the majority of patients at the time of presentation [136, 137, 139, 141, 143, 148]. Neurological decline can occur chronically over months or precipitously over a few hours [137, 139, 141, 143–146, 149].

The most consistent laboratory abnormality is an elevated erythrocyte sedimentation rate (ESR), which is almost always present; ESR and C-reactive protein have been found to be highly sensitive and moderately specific in identifying patients in the emergency room with spinal epidural abscess [152, 153]. Leukocytosis is found in roughly 75 % of patients [141, 148]. Results of CSF analysis are variable, ranging from normal to frank pus [144]. Blood cultures have been reported to be positive in up to 60 % of cases [140]. Contrast-enhanced MRI scans give superior resolution of soft tissue, the spinal cord, and epidural space when compared to CT myelography and are the diagnostic procedure of choice in many facilities. An epidural abscess appears as a low-intensity image on T1-weighted MRI scans (Fig. 22.17). Gadolinium-enhanced magnetic resonance imaging remains one of the most sensitive, specific, and accurate imaging methods for confirming and defining the presence of a spinal epidural abscess and determining its location [54, 137–139]. If MRI services are not available, myelography should be carried out. Lumbar puncture to determine CSF protein concentrations is not needed for diagnosis and may introduce bacteria into the subarachnoid space with consequent meningitis and, therefore, should not be performed [154].

Treatment

Surgical intervention for removal of pus and granulation tissue forms the basis of therapy, followed by a prolonged course of parenteral antimicrobials. If the patient has neurological signs at presentation, immediate surgical decompression of the spinal cord is absolutely essential. During the time that culture results are not available, and because

Fig. 22.17 Acute discitis with secondary osteomyelitis and anterior epidural empyema; images include post-contrast T1-w (on *left*) and T2-w (on *right*) sequences. In this instance there is a central disc infection with adjacent osteomyelitis in vertebral bodies above and below the disc infection. This is the pattern usually associated with primary disc infection with secondary bone involvement and is usually of pyogenic causative agent. Additionally, there is an anterior epidural abscess that bridges the infected motion segment

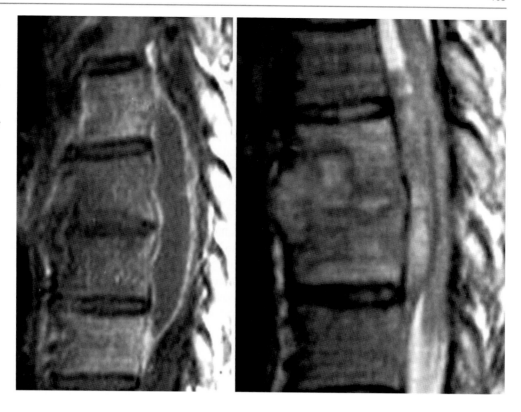

S. aureus is a commonly implicated pathogen in spinal epidural abscesses, an antistaphylococcal penicillin, a first-generation cephalosporin, or vancomycin should be included in the treatment regimen together with an agent that is active against gram-negative organisms, such as a third-generation cephalosporin. If MRSA is suspected or implicated, vancomycin should be used. If the infection follows a neurosurgical procedure, an antistaphylococcal penicillin, a third-generation cephalosporin, and an aminoglycoside are prescribed in combination. Spinal epidural abscess carries with it a high mortality rate and significant long-term sequelae, including paralysis. The mortality rate is estimated to be 14 %, and 35–40 % of patients will have neurological sequelae, such as residual weakness or permanent paralysis [136, 138, 140, 148]. Prognosis depends upon the clinical and neurological condition of the patient at the time of presentation [136, 141, 146, 149]. Patients presenting with sepsis or plegia have higher mortality and long-term morbidity rates [137, 138, 142, 144, 145, 148, 150, 154].

Spinal epidural abscesses have been treated with medical therapy alone [147]. However, the majority of these patients fell into one of three categories: (1) panspinal infections not amendable to drainage; (2) operative candidates with a history of poor health and comorbid conditions, such as chronic cardiac or pulmonary disease; or (3) complete paralysis for greater than 24 h [155]. In order to treat patients nonoperatively the clinician must obtain the organism by another means, such as blood culture or needle aspirate, and be willing to perform serial neurological exams and monitor the response to therapy with serial MRI scans [155]. However, caution is warranted in treating spinal epidural abscesses nonoperatively [147].

Vertebral Osteomyelitis

Pyogenic spinal infections, including vertebral osteomyelitis, account for approximately 2–4 % of all cases of osteomyelitis, ranking third behind infections of the femur and tibia in adults [156–159]. Over the past two decades, the incidence of vertebral osteomyelitis appears to have been increasing; this increase is thought to be associated with a parallel increase in the number of immunocompromised patients [156, 157, 160–163]. With an incidence ranging between 0.3 cases per 100,000 among persons less than or equal to 20 years of age and 6.5 per 100,000 among persons greater than 70 years of age, vertebral osteomyelitis is the most common type of hematogenously acquired osteomyelitis [156, 157, 159, 161]. The condition occurs more frequently in men, especially those aged 50 years or older [157, 162, 164, 165]. Risk factors associated with spontaneous, acute vertebral osteomyelitis include diabetes mellitus, systemic steroid use, history of a genital or urinary infection, urinary tract procedures, bacteremia, protein calorie malnutrition, IV drug abuse, malignancy, various immunodeficient states, or advanced age [156, 157, 165–168].

Vertebral osteomyelitis in younger populations is frequently associated with IV drug abuse [166]. In fact, drug abusers account for over half the cases of pyogenic spinal osteomyelitis in some large series [157, 162, 169]. The overall incidence of diabetes in patients with vertebral osteomyelitis is between 18 % and 25 % [156]. However, in one series, 43 % of adult patients with hematogenous vertebral osteomyelitis at a tertiary care hospital had diabetes [158].

Prolonged steroid use is a risk factor for vertebral osteomyelitis caused by bacteria and atypical mycobacteria [166, 170]. The common denominator in each of these predisposing conditions appears to be a deficiency in some aspect of cellular or humoral immunity [166]. Postsurgical vertebral osteomyelitis accounts for approximately 2.5 % of all spinal osteomyelitis and occurs more frequently in malnourished patients, diabetics, and patients on steroid therapy [165, 167, 169, 171]. As the prevalence of AIDS increased, there has been resurgence in the incidence of spinal tuberculosis and the emergence of other fungal causes of vertebral osteomyelitis in this population [159, 163, 166, 168].

Pathogenesis

Spontaneous vertebral osteomyelitis usually results from hematogenous spread of organisms through the segmental spinal arteries to the subchondral plate region of the vertebral body adjacent to the disc space [167, 168]. In adults, the nidus of infection begins in the vertebral bodies at the level of the end arteriolar arcades and, after endplate destruction, spreads secondarily into the avascular disc space [156, 168]. In children, the disc space contains vascular channels that allow primary seeding of the intervertebral disc [156, 168, 169]. Segmental spinal arteries typically bifurcate to supply adjacent vertebral segments, this bifurcation is thought to account for the fact that vertebral osteomyelitis typically involves two adjacent vertebrae and the intervening disc space [168]. Postoperative vertebral osteomyelitis usually occurs due to direct inoculation of the microorganism at the time of surgery [156, 157, 161, 164, 167, 169]. The principal sources of wound contamination are surgery personnel or the patient's own skin flora [167]. Unlike spontaneous vertebral osteomyelitis, the disc space is often the nidus of infection in patients who have undergone a surgical procedure [156, 167, 169]. Other sources or risk factors for vertebral osteomyelitis include inoculation via decubitus ulcers and trauma or IV drug abuse [165, 172–174].

Microbiology of Vertebral Osteomyelitis

Of the various microorganisms known to be associated with culture-positive, pyogenic vertebral osteomyelitis, gram-positive aerobic cocci are implicated 68 % of the time with *S. aureus* isolated in up to 60 % of cases, gram-negative aerobic bacilli in 29 % of the patients, and anaerobic bacteria in 3 % [156, 158, 163, 165–167, 175–181]. Radiological imaging is often unable to differentiate between vertebral osteomyelitis caused by mycobacteria and bacteria; thus, initial clinical assessment of a patient with spinal osteomyelitis should include tuberculosis in the differential diagnosis, especially in high-risk patients or in regions or countries with a high prevalence of mycobacterial infections or in countries where tuberculosis and HIV infection are endemic [163, 165, 166]. *Coccidioides immitis*, *Blastomyces dermatitidis*, *Cryptococcus neoformans*, *Aspergillus* species, and other less common fungi have all been implicated as causes of vertebral osteomyelitis [165, 182]. *Pseudomonas aeruginosa* and *S. aureus* are the most commonly implicated pathogens in vertebral osteomyelitis in IV drug abusers and occur at roughly equal rates [175, 183].

In elderly males with urinary tract infections or following invasive urological procedures, the most common causes of vertebral osteomyelitis are *E. coli* and *Proteus* species [165]. Postoperative spinal infections are usually caused by *S. aureus* [163, 165, 167, 168, 183]. Patients on long-term steroid treatment are susceptible to infections caused by atypical mycobacteria and *Aspergillus* spp. [117, 166, 170, 184–190]. Although vertebral osteomyelitis is generally caused by a single microorganism, contiguous sources of infection, such as a decubitus pressure ulcer or intra-abdominal abscess (e.g., psoas abscess), can lead to polymicrobial infection involving both aerobic and anaerobic microorganisms [165, 166].

Clinical Presentation and Diagnostic Considerations

Back pain is the most common (greater than 90 %) presentation of vertebral osteomyelitis [161, 166]. The pain is localized, continuous, and generally unrelated to movement or position [157]. Vertebral osteomyelitis acquired by the hematogenous mode tends to involve the lower dorsal and lumbar spine. Nearly all spine infections are associated with tenderness on palpation over the involved level: vertebral osteomyelitis tends to be localized to the lumbar and dorsal vertebrae in 58 and 30 % of cases, respectively [156, 157, 161, 166]. Involvement of the cervical vertebrae (11 %) has been noted among IV drug abusers and patients with pulmonary tuberculous [156]. Neurologic impairment, such as sensory loss, weakness, or radiculopathy, is reported in one-third of cases. The presence of radiculopathy, positive straight leg raise, and neurological deficit (4–16 %) is less reliable and often indicates the presence of epidural involvement [157, 166]. Fever is found in approximately half of patients with pyogenic spinal osteomyelitis, and constitutional symptoms, including malaise, night sweats, and anorexia, have been reported [157, 161, 167, 191].

Fig. 22.18 Spinal vertebral osteomyelitis with relative sparing of the disc space; images include T2-w sagittal image (*left*) and a post-contrast T1-w image (*right*). In this instance the spinal infection has virtually destroyed the L1 vertebral body. There is prominent residual contrast enhancement in the affected vertebral body. There is only minimal edema in the L1–2 disc space and relatively little enhancement. This complex would be consistent with hematogenous seeding the vascularized vertebral body rather than a primary disc infection with secondary osteomyelitis

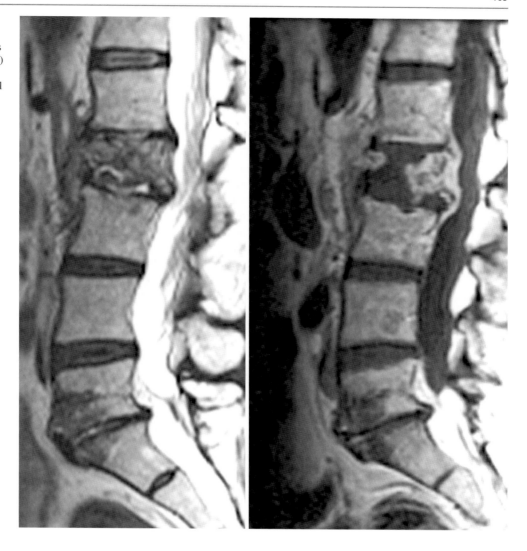

Vertebral osteomyelitis has an insidious onset and may prove to be a diagnostic challenge because of the nonspecific nature of the symptoms and signs. For example, the differential diagnosis of back pain in a patient with fever includes various viral syndromes, aortitis, pyelonephritis, and pancreatitis [161]. In the absence of fever, other causes of back pain, such as an osteoporotic fracture, spondylarthritis, degenerative disc disease, or spinal stenosis, might have to be ruled out [161, 168]. In several large patient series, the delay between the onset of symptoms and eventual diagnosis has ranged from 3 weeks to 3 months [157, 162, 168, 192]. These delays in diagnosis can result in significant neurological morbidity [168]. Other complications arising from vertebral osteomyelitis include paraspinal abscesses, soft tissue extension, and spinal cord compression.

A leukocytosis is found in less than half of patients with vertebral osteomyelitis [157]. The most common laboratory abnormality is an elevated ESR. Blood cultures are critical in the workup of a patient with a putative diagnosis of vertebral

osteomyelitis and, if positive (up to 78 % of blood cultures are positive), might obviate the need for an invasive diagnostic procedure to procure a biopsy specimen [157, 165, 178]. Plain X-ray findings include disc space narrowing and vertebral end plate changes that usually become apparent 2–4 weeks after symptom onset in approximately 80 % of patients [156, 157, 167, 191]. Technetium 99 m bone scanning combined with gallium scanning has a 90 % sensitivity and specificity for vertebral osteomyelitis [193]. MRI imaging is the most sensitive and specific imaging modality for vertebral osteomyelitis and has the added benefit of providing details regarding the presence of an epidural or paraspinal abscess and various other complications [156, 161, 194–196]. Characteristic MRI changes include decreased T1 signal and increased T2 signal of the involved vertebral endplates and disc space [156, 196] (Fig. 22.18). Positron emission tomographic (PET) scanning with 18F-fluorodeoxyglucose has a diagnostic accuracy similar to that of MRI and might be considered if the patient has metallic implants [195].

Optimal pharmacologic treatment requires that the infecting microbe be identified and antimicrobial susceptibility profile be determined [157]. If imaging is suggestive of vertebral osteomyelitis but blood cultures are negative for bacterial growth, then a biopsy of the infected vertebra is mandatory [156, 157, 167, 191]. The procedure of choice would depend on the presence of underlying intrinsic patient risk factors with input from surgical and interventional radiology personnel regarding CT-guided versus open biopsy [161]. When blood cultures are negative, a CT-guided needle biopsy can be used to make a definitive microbiological diagnosis 60–90 % of the time [157]. An open biopsy should be considered when both blood cultures and CT-guided aspirates are negative [167]. A skin test for tuberculosis should be placed in all patients and CT aspirates or biopsy material should be sent for routine fungal stains and cultures [167, 192]. If polymicrobial osteomyelitis is suspected (e.g., a patient with concomitant intra-abdominal sepsis), a biopsy should be performed whether or not blood cultures are positive for bacterial growth [181].

Treatment

Targeted antimicrobial therapy, spinal immobilization, and, when necessary, surgical interventions are the mainstays of treatment of vertebral osteomyelitis [156, 157, 161, 165]. Seventy-five percent of patients with spinal osteomyelitis can be managed without surgical intervention [156]. Prolonged courses of parental antimicrobials directed by specific culture results and antimicrobial susceptibilities are the rule [161, 165, 191]. Although there are no data from controlled trials that suggest the optimal duration of therapy, 4–6 weeks of antimicrobial therapy is usually recommended [176, 197, 198]. One large review suggested that 4 weeks therapy with high-dose IV antimicrobials is sufficient to treat pyogenic spinal osteomyelitis as long as the following criteria are met: (1) there are no undrained abscesses, (2) the patient is clinically stable, and (3) the ESR has decreased to one-half its original value [165].

For methicillin-susceptible *S. aureus* (MSSA), high-dose oxacillin (2 g every 6 h or cefazolin, 1–2 g every 8 h) is recommended. Alternatively, levofloxacin 750 mg orally once daily plus rifampin 300 mg taken orally every 12 h may be considered. MRSA or coagulase-negative staphylococci can be treated with IV vancomycin (1 g every 12 h) or daptomycin (greater than or equal to 6 mg/kg of body weight once daily). Streptococcal species can be treated with IV penicillin G (5 million units every 6 h) or IV ceftriaxone (2 g once daily). *Enterobacteriaceae* can be treated with ciprofloxacin (750 mg taken orally every 12 h) or IV ceftriaxone (2 g once daily). Infections caused by quinolone-resistant *Enterobacteriaceae* (including extended-spectrum β-lactamase-producing *E. coli*), can be treated effectively with IV imipenem (500 mg every 6

h). For *P. aeruginosa* infections, cefepime or ceftazidime, or piperacillin/tazobactam every 6 h, followed by ciprofloxacin (750 mg taken orally every 12 h). Anaerobes can be treated with IV clindamycin (300–600 mg administered intravenously every 6–8 h), IV penicillin G (five million units every 6 h), or IV ceftriaxone (2 g once daily) with metronidazole (500 mg taken orally every 8 h.) Tuberculous vertebral osteomyelitis requires an average of 12 months treatment with a combination of isoniazid, rifampin, ethambutol, and pyrazinamide, depending on regional susceptibility [156, 199]. Treatment of other less common bacterial and fungal causes of vertebral osteomyelitis should be tailored to the individual pathogen and to regional antimicrobial susceptibility profiles. Therapy is guided by clinical response and the ESR as outlined previously. Continued elevation of the ESR may necessitate more prolonged therapy.

The indications for surgical intervention in spinal osteomyelitis are the presence of a neurological deficit, spinal instability, unresponsiveness to medical therapy, or a non-diagnostic CT-guided biopsy [161, 162]. In addition, surgery is recommended for the drainage of epidural or paraspinal abscesses that often accompany vertebral osteomyelitis [165] The goals of surgery are decompression of the neural elements, correction of spinal deformity, debridement of necrotic tissue, and the promotion of long-term stability [156, 162, 168, 192]. A variety of surgical approaches have been described in the literature, each with its own advantages and disadvantages [156, 162, 192]. The basic principles of surgical intervention include early instrumentation and fusion at the time of the initial operation in order to facilitate ambulation and avoid the complications associated with prolonged bed rest [156, 162, 192].

External Ventricular Drainage

Infectious Considerations

A ventriculostomy is an external ventricular drainage (EVD) device or ventricular catheter that is placed into the cerebral ventricles enabling drainage of CSF externally. It is typically connected by tubing to a CSF collection device that can be elevated or lowered at the bedside to vary the amount of CSF that is drained. EVD devices are an integral aspect of the intensive care management of neurosurgical patients [200–202]. Common indications for their use include management of hydrocephalus, elevated intracranial pressure, or intracranial hemorrhage and the administration of intrathecal medications [200–205]. EVD devices provide diagnostic information and also facilitate therapeutic CSF drainage [206–208]. The most common complication involving the use of EVDs is infection; rates of infection up to 27 % have been reported [203, 204, 209–215].

Risk factors for the development of EVD-associated ventriculomeningitis include EVD duration greater than 11 days, frequency of CSF sampling, intraventricular hemorrhage, surgical technique (subcutaneously tunneled EVD, Rickham reservoir with percutaneous CSF drainage), neurosurgical operative procedure, and irrigation or manipulation of the drainage system [204, 210–214]. Conflicting data exist regarding the association between duration of ventricular drainage and the rate of EVD-associated infections [205, 210, 216, 217]. Some clinical series have shown a linear relationship between infection and duration of ventricular drainage [218, 219]. Various authors have advocated the routine changing of ventricular catheters after day 5 in order to lower the risk of infection, while others have suggested that the duration of monitoring is not a risk factor associated with infection. In fact, later studies have shown that a constant daily rate of infection actually decreases after day 10 or 11 of drainage [217, 219].

Diagnostic clues for EVD-related ventriculomeningitis may stem from clinical signs, such as fever, meningism, reduced level of consciousness, photophobia, phonophobia, and abnormal laboratory parameters (e.g., reduced CSF glucose, increased CSF protein, CSF pleocytosis, positive CSF culture, or gram's stain) [220]. Because the results of the CSF leukocyte count may be confounded by intraventricular hemorrhage, Pfausler and colleagues introduced the "cell index" as a new parameter for the diagnosis of EVD-related ventriculomeningitis [221]. They showed that a significant increase of this index is highly indicative of EVD-related ventriculitis in patients with hemorrhagic CSF and that calculation of the "cell index" on a daily basis allows the timely diagnosis and hence initiation of antimicrobial therapy of catheter-related ventriculomeningitis [221]. Coagulase-negative *Staphylococcus* (70 %), *S. aureus* (10 %), and gram-negative bacteria (15 %), including *P. aeruginosa*, *Acinetobacter* spp., *Klebsiella* spp., and *E. coli*, remain the most common microorganisms associated with ventriculomeningitis [220–224].

The role of perioperative and prophylactic antimicrobials in the prevention of EVD-associated infections has been extensively discussed and debated. Alleyne and colleagues reviewed over 300 patients who received either daily prophylactic antimicrobials or perioperative antimicrobials alone and found no significant difference in the infection rate between the two groups [225]. The benefit of systemic prophylactic antimicrobials for the first 24 h postoperatively to prevent shunt infection, regardless of the patient's age or the type of internal shunt being used, has been demonstrated although the benefit of its use after this period remains uncertain [226–229].

Current evidence suggests that antibiotic-impregnated catheters reduce the incidence of shunt infection [226, 229–235]. Other factors thought to be important in preventing infection include perioperative antimicrobial administration prior to skin incision, tunneling of the ventricular catheter, proper surgical skin prep, strict adherence to aseptic technique, use of a closed ventricular drainage system, and meticulous sterile nursing care [210, 211, 218, 225, 236–243]. Antimicrobial impregnated catheters have been manufactured for a variety of applications and have been shown to be effective in preventing EVD-associated infections [225, 230, 231, 235–239, 244, 245]. Beer and colleagues suggest that the management of EVD-related ventriculitis should involve decisions related to catheter exchange, the type and route of administration (intravenous versus intrathecal) of antimicrobial therapy, based on the type of suspected organism and its resistance pattern, and the duration of antimicrobial therapy [220]. Once the diagnosis is made, broad-spectrum antimicrobials should be administered, followed by diagnostic testing, and targeted antibiotic therapy as soon as antimicrobial susceptibility testing results become available.

Mycobacterium Tuberculous Infections

Tuberculous Meningitis

Tuberculosis has been known to humankind since antiquity, having been demonstrated relatively recently by molecular methods in mummies from both the new and the old world dating to 1,000–1,500 years BC [246, 247]. Tuberculosis was recognized on clinical grounds in the eighteenth century, and with the isolation of the organism by Robert Koch in 1882, its ability to produce CNS disease was quickly recognized. Before the HIV pandemic, *M. tuberculosis* infection and disease was already endemic in many economically less-developed countries, though not at pandemic proportions. With the onset of the HIV pandemic, there has been a dramatic, parallel increase in rates of tuberculosis among HIV-infected patients in many of these countries, especially sub-Saharan Africa, Southeast Asia, and increasingly the Indian subcontinent. At the end of the first decade of the new millennium, tuberculosis remains the second leading cause of death from an infectious disease worldwide after HIV, despite the availability of highly efficacious treatment for decades. In 2010, there were an estimated 8.5–9.2 million cases and 1.2–1.5 million deaths attributable to tuberculosis [248]. Indeed, *M. tuberculosis* has now been established as the first or second most common cause of bloodstream infections in febrile adults who present to emergency rooms in sentinel hospitals in East Africa and Thailand [249–253].

Although comparative rates of *M. tuberculosis* infections are relatively lower among HIV-infected patients in North America and Western Europe, the World Health Organization generally considers *M. tuberculosis* infections a true pandemic that is unequivocally linked with immuno-suppression resulting from HIV infection, though the problem has certainly been compounded by other factors associated with poverty, such as overcrowding, malnutrition, lack of access to healthcare, and poor sanitation, made particularly worse in refugee camps resulting from natural and man-made disasters and war [248]. The fact remains that at the end of the first decade of the twenty-first century, tuberculosis is the leading cause of death among HIV-infected patients worldwide, and tuberculosis meningitis remains the most rapidly progressive form of the disease.

Perhaps the most insidious occurrence resulting from the tuberculosis pandemic, with negative implications for effective therapy, is the emergence of multidrug-resistant (MDR) tuberculosis, defined as resistance to at least both isoniazid and rifampin, and extensively drug-resistant (XDR) strains of *M. tuberculosis* (i.e., strains resistant to practically all second-line agents) [248, 254–257]. Emerging resistance has made the management of pulmonary and extrapulmonary tuberculosis, including tuberculous meningitis, all the more difficult to manage.

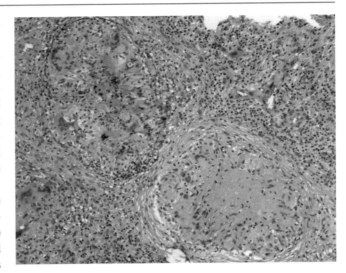

Fig. 22.19 A 40-year-old female with chronic headaches, anosmia, and blurred vision. Biopsy revealed chronic granulomatous meningitis with giant cells and non-caseating and focal caseating (necrotizing) granulomas. Special stains for acid-fast bacilli demonstrated only rare acid-fast organisms (Courtesy of Anthony Yachnis, MD, and Kelly Devers, MD, University of Florida College of Medicine)

Pathogenesis

Tuberculous meningitis can occur as a result of hematogenous seeding of the meninges; reactivation of metastatic *M. tuberculosis* foci in the meninges and brain parenchyma, which have been present asymptomatically for months to years following primary infection; or due to breakdown of an old tuberculous parameningeal granuloma with rupture into the subarachnoid space. In addition to HIV infection, other predisposing risk factors in adults include alcohol abuse, IV drug abuse, immunosuppression due to steroid and other immunosuppressive therapies, and chronic disorders, such as connective tissue diseases and chronic cardiopulmonary disease.

Pathologically, tuberculous meningitis leads to prodigious inflammation with production of a thick exudate at the base of the brain, particularly involving the optic nerves at the optic chiasm, the pons, and cerebellum. The histologic appearance depends on the stage of the disease. Initially it consists of polymorphonuclear leukocytes, macrophages, and lymphocytes. But later, after a phase of lymphocytic proliferation, granulomata with caseating centers become a prominent feature (Fig. 22.19). Another feature of tuberculous infection of the meninges is involvement of the blood vessels traversing the meninges: small- and medium-sized arteries are most often involved, although capillaries and veins may be similarly affected. The changes include granuloma formation and inflammation of the adventitia, which causes a reactive cellular proliferation of the intima, which in turn may lead to occlusion of the vessel and infarction of the areas supplied by the vessel. Clinically, this vasculitis is frequently found in the distribution of the middle cerebral artery

due to its anatomic location at the base of the brain, where the inflammatory response is most intense. This profound inflammatory response with vasculitis causes compression of neural tissues and compromises cerebral blood flow leading to cerebral ischemia and infarction, obstruction of CSF free flow, resulting in hydrocephalus and cerebral edema.

Hydrocephalus is one of the most frequent complications of tuberculous meningitis, commonly accompanying symptomatic primary infection in children. Hydrocephalus occurs either by mechanical blockage of the spinal aqueduct or the foramina of Luschka due to the exudate at the base of the brain or to edema of the surrounding brain parenchyma. Hydrocephalus may also be caused by blockage of CSF reabsorption at the base of the brain due to the intense infiltrate. The former mechanism leads to noncommunicating hydrocephalus and the latter mechanism to communicating hydrocephalus.

Clinical Presentation

The classical clinical presentation of tuberculous meningitis in adults is that of fever and headache, together with meningismus that becomes progressively more severe over a period of 2–3 weeks. However, the duration of prodromal symptoms can be quite variable and some patients have reported symptoms for several months before they actually sought medical attention. None of these symptoms or signs is universally present in all patients with tuberculous meningitis. Other frequently observed clinical features include lethargy and behavioral changes in 30–70 % of patients, seizures in 10–15 %, and cranial nerve palsies in up to 20–30 % of adults. Occasionally, abnormal movements such as chorea, hemiballismus, athetosis, myoclonus, and cerebellar signs and symptoms are observed. Localizing neurologic symptoms due to a tuberculoma depend on the size and location of the mass lesion. Strokes due to tuberculous vasculitis described previously usually involve the distribution of the middle cerebral artery and produce symptoms related to that vascular distribution. The most common cranial nerve abnormalities involve the sixth cranial nerve followed by the third, fourth, and the seventh but may involve the second, eighth, tenth, eleventh, and twelfth cranial nerves [258]. Coma is present or can develop in up to 30 % of adults and children. In some series as many as 50 % of children have a past history of tuberculosis whereas only 8–12 % of adults have such a history. Hydrocephalus is a serious and potentially devastating complication that may develop in up to 40 % and is associated with a variety of focal neurologic signs, including hemiparesis and blindness.

The differential diagnosis is quite wide and includes bacterial, viral, and fungal infections of the CNS as well as malignancies and noninfectious conditions such as CNS lupus (Table 22.5).

Diagnosis

Routine laboratory tests are not particularly helpful. The single most useful diagnostic procedure is CSF examination. The classic findings of elevated protein, depressed CSF glucose relative to serum, and pleocytosis with a lymphocytic predominance, together with a history of chronic illness over a matter of weeks as opposed to days as in acute bacterial meningitis, is strongly suggestive of a tuberculous or fungal etiology. Median CSF protein levels generally range between 100 and 400 mg/dL but may go as high 2 g/dL, although levels of that magnitude usually suggest mechanical blockage of CSF flow. The median white count generally runs between 100 and 200 WBC/mm³. The CSF glucose is less than 45 mg/dL in 70–80 % of patients. The glucose level tends to become progressively lower and the protein progressively higher as the duration of illness progresses without appropriate therapy; when treatment is successful, the glucose level tends to return towards normal. Although any one of these CSF parameters may be completely normal, it is extremely unusual for all three parameters to be completely normal in a patient with true tuberculous meningitis. If CSF analysis is completely normal and the laboratory reports *M. tuberculosis*, the report should be considered suspect until proven otherwise. Acid-fast smears of CSF are positive in less than 25 % of patients who ultimately have culture proven tuberculous meningitis, although CSF cultures may ultimately yield *M. tuberculous* growth in up to 70 % of patients.

The ESR varies considerably in series of patients with proven *M. tuberculous* meningitis, ranging from normal to more than 100 mm/h. Similarly, the syndrome of inappropriate antidiuretic hormone (SIADH), manifest by hyponatremia and hypochloremia, is not uncommon but is by no means diagnostic since the results are confounded by a variety of other events (e.g., vomiting and anorexia) that may accompany *M. tuberculosis* disease.

Chest radiographs are non-diagnostic although 25–50 % of adults may show radiographic evidence consistent with current or remote tuberculous infection [259]. In children who develop tuberculous meningitis on the heels of primary tuberculosis infection, chest radiographic evidence of *M. tuberculosis* infection has been observed in 50–80 % of cases. Miliary disease was commonly associated with tuberculous meningitis in the pre-antimicrobial era and remains common in HIV-endemic regions of the world; at the present time, though, it remains relatively uncommon in the United States.

Admission tuberculin skin testing as a diagnostic aid for the diagnosis of tuberculous meningitis is of limited utility: the performance of the test varies with age, BCG vaccination and nutritional status, HIV status (HIV-infected patients are often anergic to PPD skin testing), and technique of administration [260–262]. Thus, although skin testing may provide information regarding previous tuberculosis exposure or infection and might be useful in the diagnosis of meningitis in young children, it is not sufficiently sensitivity or specific for routine diagnosis of active *M. tuberculosis* meningitis [260, 263]. Similarly, interferon-gamma release assays (e.g., T-SPOT.TB), which are superior to tuberculin skin testing at diagnosing latent tuberculosis, are neither sufficiently sensitive nor specific for routine diagnosis of *M. tuberculosis* meningitis [264, 265].

Thus, in a patient with a nonspecific history that is suggestive of possible tuberculosis disease but with a CSF profile typical of aseptic meningitis, other causes of aseptic meningitis will have to be considered and ruled out if deemed necessary. Such infective causes include cryptococcal and other forms of fungal meningitis, early or partially treated bacterial meningitis, cerebral abscess and other parameningeal infections, *Listeria* spp. meningitis, leptospirosis, and syphilis. Noninfective causes that need to be considered in the differential diagnosis include carcinomatous meningitis, including lymphoma, connective tissue diseases, chronic subdural hematoma, and chemical- or drug-induced causes.

Modern radiographic techniques such as CT scan, MRI with gadolinium enhancement, and magnetic resonance angiography (MRA) are extremely sensitive in delineating CNS involvement, readily demonstrating meningeal inflammation and entrapment of cranial nerves in the basilar tuberculous exudate (Fig. 22.5c, d and 22.20) [266]. In addition, MRA can detect characteristic vascular narrowing which accompanies tuberculous meningitis but is less commonly seen with other pathologies. High-field MRA with contrast is more sensitive than conventional MRA in the

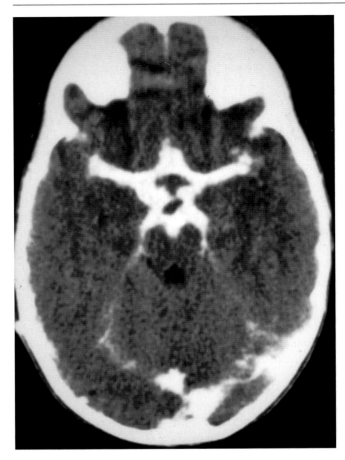

Fig. 22.20 Basilar tuberculous exudate in a patient with tuberculous meningitis

detection of occlusion of smaller vessels, which are more commonly involved in the pathogenesis of tuberculous meningitis [267].

Culture remains the gold standard for laboratory confirmation of tuberculosis and is required for isolating the organism, for drug-susceptibility testing and genotyping. Mycobacteria isolated from cultures are identified using standard biochemical analyses, nucleic acid probes, or 16S rRNA gene sequencing [268]. Real-time PCR assays that rapidly and specifically detect *M. tuberculosis* complex directly from acid-fast, smear-positive specimens and from broth cultures are now routinely conducted in various reference laboratories across the USA and now offer the potential to detect gene mutations responsible for drug resistance within hours of patient specimen collection compared with the average of 2 weeks required for traditional susceptibility testing methods. Real-time PCR assays used in the diagnosis of tuberculous meningitis have reported sensitivities ranging from 25 to 100 % and specificities of about 95 %. Thus, direct nucleic acid amplification tests should always be performed in conjunction with microscopy and culture, and each test result must be interpreted within the overall clinical

setting in which it is used. To date, there is still no *single* diagnostic method that is both sufficiently rapid and sensitive for detecting *M. tuberculosis* infection [269].

Treatment

Treatment of tuberculous meningitis consists of at least three, and usually four, drugs until the susceptibilities are established: isoniazid (INH), rifampin, ethambutol, and pyrazinamide are the standard, together with pyridoxine at 25–50 mg daily to prevent depletion by INH; many authors recommend dexamethasone for the first month to improve outcome. Treatment must be continued for at least 12 months. INH is generally used at a dose of 300 mg/day in adults or 10 mg/kg/day in children. The most serious side effect is hepatitis, which ranges from asymptomatic enzyme elevations to fulminant hepatic necrosis. The true risk of INH side effects is approximately 0.1 % among those receiving INH alone for prophylaxis and greater than 1 % for those receiving INH as part of a treatment regimen for tuberculosis [270]. The incidence of hepatotoxicity is higher in persons over 35 years of age, as well as those with other conditions affecting liver function such as alcoholism and viral hepatitis. The dose of rifampin is 600 mg/day and is only infrequently associated with side effects such as a flu-like syndrome and a hypersensitivity reaction with renal, hepatic, and hematologic toxicity. Pyrazinamide is given in a dose of 25 mg/kg/day and has a relatively low incidence of side effects; there is little added toxicity when combined with INH and rifampin. INH, rifampin, ethambutol, and pyrazinamide all have good penetration of the CSF. Ethambutol is generally administered at a dose of 25 mg/kg for the first 1–2months of treatment with a reduction in dose to approximately 15 mg/kg/day because of the risk of optic neuritis, seen in approximately 25 % of patients. The first clue to the development of this complication is loss of red-green vision or diminished visual acuity; ophthalmologic consultation is suggested in these situations. Streptomycin was one of the first drugs found to be active against tuberculosis and is commonly administered in a dose of 20–40 mg/kg/day for children and 1 g/day for adults. Unfortunately, the irreversible ototoxicity is so frequent that it is not advisable to use this agent unless absolutely necessary. Second-line antituberculous drugs such as para-aminosalicylic (PAS), cycloserine, ethionamide, kanamycin, and amikacin should only be used based on treatment failure with primary agents and antimicrobial susceptibility studies. Of these agents, ethionamide and cycloserine penetrate well into the CNS.

Because one cannot rule out tuberculosis based on all of the immediately available diagnostic modalities, empiric therapy often has to be given while awaiting the results of cultures. A negative test for cryptococcal antigen, absence of encapsulated yeast forms on microscopy of an India ink smear, and no growth of the microorganism within 10–14 days of CSF culture essentially rules out cryptococcal meningitis. However, other fungal meningitides cannot be totally ruled out, and some patients may have to be placed on empirical therapy with both antituberculous medications and amphotericin B. Occasionally, CNS symptomatology in patients treated in this fashion turn out to have a noninfectious etiology; in these patients, further radiographic or invasive diagnostic studies may be indicated. In patients who show no signs of improvement within the first week or so, and particularly in the setting where the patient is known to have a malignancy, cytological analysis of the CSF should be requested to rule out meningeal carcinomatosis.

Case reports and various studies have demonstrated the immediate effects of steroids in terms of defervescence and clearing of the sensorium, even after a few doses. While there seems to be general agreement that survival from tuberculous meningitis is improved with the use of steroids, survivors often do so with severe sequelae [259]. However, most authorities currently recommend using steroids in all patients with *M. tuberculosis* meningitis, regardless of severity of disease at presentation, with a reducing course over 6–8 weeks [60, 260, 271]. The dose of prednisone is 60 mg/day or 1 mg/kg/day, or dexamethasone may also be used at a dose of 8–16 mg/day in divided doses. Steroids are given for 3–6 weeks and then tapered over the ensuing 2–4 weeks. If results of susceptibility testing implicate multidrug-resistant strains of *M. tuberculosis*, intrathecal therapy might have to be considered [272].

For HIV-infected patients, antiretroviral therapy and antituberculosis treatment should be initiated at the same time, regardless of CD4 cell counts. Of note, tuberculous meningitis may be a manifestation of paradoxical tuberculosis-associated immune reconstitution inflammatory syndrome. The mortality rate among HIV-infected patients with multidrug-resistant tuberculous meningitis is significantly higher than the comparable rate for meningitis caused by susceptible strains. In short, the best way to prevent HIV-associated tuberculous meningitis is to diagnose and isolate infectious cases of tuberculosis promptly and administer appropriate treatment promptly in all patients in whom the diagnosis of tuberculous meningitis is suspected or ascertained [273].

Prognosis and Sequelae

Prior to the availability of antituberculous therapy, survival from tuberculous meningitis was exceedingly rare; survival rates currently are 70–80 % in most recent series. Perhaps the most significant prognostic factor for survival is the degree to which the disease has advanced at the time of initial presentation. Other factors correlating with poor response to therapy include age and coexistent miliary disease. The earliest sign of response to therapy in most cases is reduction in peak daily temperatures within the first 1–2 weeks and subjective improvement in fatigue and malaise over the same period. However, early studies pointed out that it was not uncommon for some markers of disease, such as the presence of bacilli in a smear of the CSF or a rise in CSF protein, to occur shortly after the initiation of treatment. In general, the glucose level in the CSF rises with successful treatment while the protein returns to normal more slowly, a process that may take as long as 6 months.

Up to 50 % of survivors have a variety of neurologic deficits. As with survival itself, the more seriously ill the patient is upon presentation, the more likely complications or sequelae are to occur. Among children, the most common of these are seizure disorders, ataxia, incoordination, persistent cranial nerve abnormalities, and spastic hemiparesis. Adults are most frequently left with chronic organic brain syndrome, often with cranial nerve palsies, paraplegia, and hemiparesis. Optic atrophy can lead to varying degrees of visual impairment or blindness in both children and adults.

Tuberculoma

Tuberculomas are space-occupying mass lesions within the brain parenchyma ranging in size from less than 1 mm to greater than 10 cm. The pathogenesis of tuberculomas is similar to that of tuberculous meningitis in that a tuberculous granuloma, seeded during the phase of acquiring the primary infection, breaks down and, because of its location within the brain parenchyma, produces a mass lesion rather than meningitis. Patients may present with fever, headache, focal or generalized seizure, or change in mental status and may manifest signs of proptosis, papilledema, or transient neurologic deficits. Clinical features are related to the anatomic location of the tuberculoma. Generally, patients have a single lesion on presentation. However autopsy series and sophisticated radiologic studies have shown that in up to 70 % of patients, multiple lesions are present. The duration of symptoms prior to presentation is somewhat longer than in tuberculous meningitis, averaging weeks to months with occasional patients having symptoms for years prior to diagnosis. In fact, 30 % of patients with tuberculomas may remain asymptomatic throughout their life. Neuroimaging CT scan and MRI have a 100 % diagnostic sensitivity (Fig. 22.21); however, tissue confirmation is essential in order to rule out malignancies or other ring-enhancing, space-occupying lesions, such as pyogenic bacterial abscesses, neurocysticercosis, or toxoplasmosis [124, 260].

Approximately 60 % of the specimens from tuberculomas stain positive for acid-fast bacilli on smear, and approximately the same number ultimately grow in culture. Caseating granulomata are invariably seen histologically. Treatment is essentially the same as for tuberculous meningitis, i.e., antituberculous therapy with adjunct

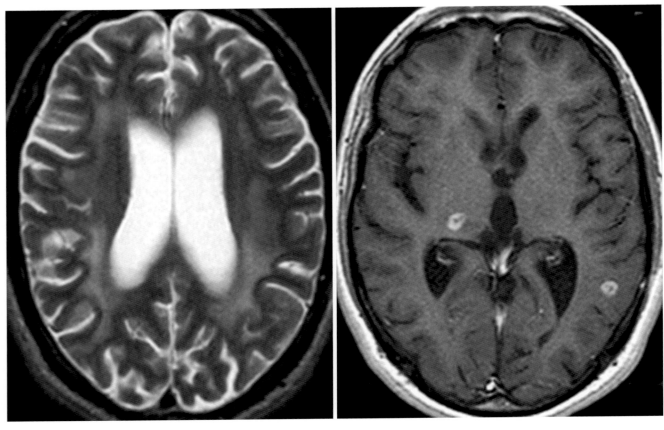

Fig. 22.21 AIDS-related complex and tuberculomas; images include T2-w spine echo (*left*) and post-contrast T1-w sequence (*right*). The T2-w sequence demonstrates features of AIDS-related complex with global pronounced atrophy and diffuse bilateral loss of myelin within the centrum semiovale. The *right* image demonstrates multicentric brain nodules. Their distribution is consistent with a hematogenous-type of disease dissemination. These nodules were found to be tuberculomas, but evidence of small nodular enhancing lesion s has a wide differential diagnosis

corticosteroids if cerebral edema is present, rather than surgery. The utility of adjunct steroids for patients with intracranial tuberculomas without meningitis has not been fully characterized by randomized controlled trials However, current published data suggest that for this patient population, steroid therapy should be considered because it mitigates symptoms and reduces the frequency of seizure attacks, tuberculoma size, and perilesional edema [260, 274, 275]. The indications for surgical intervention include development of hydrocephalus or coalescence of multiple tuberculomas to form a tuberculous cerebral abscess [260, 276].

Spinal Tuberculosis

Spinal tuberculosis is a destructive form of tuberculosis and accounts for approximately half of all cases of musculoskeletal tuberculosis and is more common in children and young adults [277]. Tuberculous spinal meningitis may accompany tuberculous meningitis or may occur as an isolated entity. While tuberculous meningitis is essentially a disease of childhood, tuberculomas and spinal tuberculosis invariably are adult manifestations [275]. The pathogenesis and pathologic findings consist of characteristic exudate surrounding many parts of the spinal cord with symptoms due to compression and vasculitic changes in the arterial supply. Common clinical manifestations include constitutional symptoms (e.g., fever, malaise, weight loss), back pain, spinal tenderness, paraplegia, and spinal deformities [277]. Symptoms consistent with transverse myelitis (i.e., paraparesis, loss or disturbance of sensation with a sensory level on the trunk, bowel and bladder dysfunction) and spinal block, as well as nerve root pain, paresthesia, and motor weakness, may be seen [163].

The thoracic region of vertebral column is most frequently affected and formation of a "cold" abscess around the lesion is another characteristic feature [277]. The onset can be sudden or present as a slow ascending paralysis over several months to years. MRI is a more sensitive imaging technique than radiographs and more specific than computed tomography and is generally required for accurate diagnosis of spinal tuberculosis and to rule out intramedullary lesions

[260, 277]. Neuroimaging-guided needle biopsy from the affected site in the center of the vertebral body remains the gold standard technique to establish a histopathologic diagnosis and underlying etiology [263, 277]. Antituberculous therapy remains the cornerstone of treatment and essentially is the same as for tuberculous meningitis. Indications for surgical intervention include development of compressive symptoms, large abscess formation, severe kyphosis, an evolving neurological deficit, or lack of response to medical treatment [163, 175, 277].

CNS Infections Caused by Rapidly Growing Mycobacteria

CNS infections associated with rapidly growing mycobacteria are rare. One of the few published reports has implicated *Mycobacterium mucogenicum*, which was isolated in pure culture and detected by PCR sequencing of CSF specimens from two immunocompetent patients who eventually died [278]. *M. mucogenicum* is frequently isolated from tap water or from respiratory specimens and is usually without clinical significance. Other case reports have described CNS infections caused by *Mycobacterium fortuitum*, another rapidly growing mycobacteria found in soil, dust, and water; these infections were all device-associated—a contaminated epidural catheter [279] and manipulation of ventriculoperitoneal shunt [280].

Patients with rapidly growing mycobacterial CNS infection usually present with subacute to chronic meningitis and neutrophilic pleocytosis and usually have a history of trauma or having undergone a neurosurgical procedure or manipulation of a device. CSF smears are often negative for acid-fast organisms but may show gram-positive rods [279–281]. Treatment requires a long course of two or more antimicrobial agents that have the ability to penetrate the blood–brain barrier, with adjunct immunomodulatory therapy with steroids, similar to that used in tuberculous meningitis [279–281].

Fungal CNS Infections

Fungal Meningitis

The most common causes of CNS mycoses include *Cryptococcus* spp. and the dimorphic fungi—*Histoplasma* spp., *Coccidioides* spp., and *Blastomyces* spp. In immunocompromised persons, *Aspergillus* spp., *Candida* spp., and the Mucorales are often implicated. Antifungal therapies that are useful in CNS infections include polyenes (e.g., amphotericin B and its lipid formulations) and azoles (e.g., fluconazole and itraconazole, voriconazole, and posaconazole).

Antifungal agents that lack CNS penetration include echinocandins (e.g., caspofungin, micafungin, and anidulafungin). Amphotericin B and flucytosine are used to initiate treatment for CNS yeast infections caused by *Candida* and *Cryptococcus neoformans*. Amphotericin B particularly in lipid formulation and voriconazole are preferred for aspergillus infections.

Cryptococcus Meningitis

Cryptococcus spp. are perhaps the most common fungus implicated in CNS infections. *C. neoformans* has a worldwide distribution and is commonly found in soil that has been contaminated with bird droppings. There are two varieties of *C. neoformans*: *C. neoformans* var *neoformans* and *C. neoformans* var gattii. These two species differ in their ecology, distribution in nature, epidemiology, presentation, clinical course, and therapy. *C. neoformans* var *neoformans* is found worldwide and produces most of the infections in patients in the United States, while *C. neoformans* var gattii is a more commonly found in Southeast Asia, Africa, Australia, and parts of Southern California. The most important determinant of CNS infection caused by *Cryptococcus* spp. is the immune status of the host. This can be most easily demonstrated by the marked increase in the number of cases associated with HIV infection and the fact that as the CD4+ count decreases the incidence of cryptococcal infection increases markedly, particularly at CD4+ counts less than 200 cells/mm^3. Although a variety of virulence factors have been described in *Cryptococcus* spp. infections, such as the production of the pigment melanin, its thick polysaccharide capsule is probably the most important virulence factor that protects the fungus from phagocytosis by the host.

The initial infection with *Cryptococcus* spp. is due to inhalation and the production of a pneumonitis, which is generally asymptomatic even in immunosuppressed patients. Symptomatic patients usually present with fever and cough and a variety of chest radiographic findings, such as nodular, pleural-based lesions and lobar infiltrates. The initial pneumonia generally clears without treatment, even in immunosuppressed patients. Dissemination from the pneumonitis results in seeding of various organs in the body; the CNS is particularly vulnerable (Fig. 22.22a–c). The organism may remain latent in the lung and at other sites indefinitely. Thus, most patients presenting with cryptococcal meningitis have no evidence of a concurrent pulmonary disease.

C. neoformans is the most common cause of fungal meningitis worldwide. Clinically, the presentation of cryptococcal meningitis is indistinguishable from that seen in chronic meningitis, associated with coccidioidomycosis, histoplasmosis, or tuberculous meningitis. Patients generally describe a history of 1–3 weeks of headache, fever, and stiff neck together

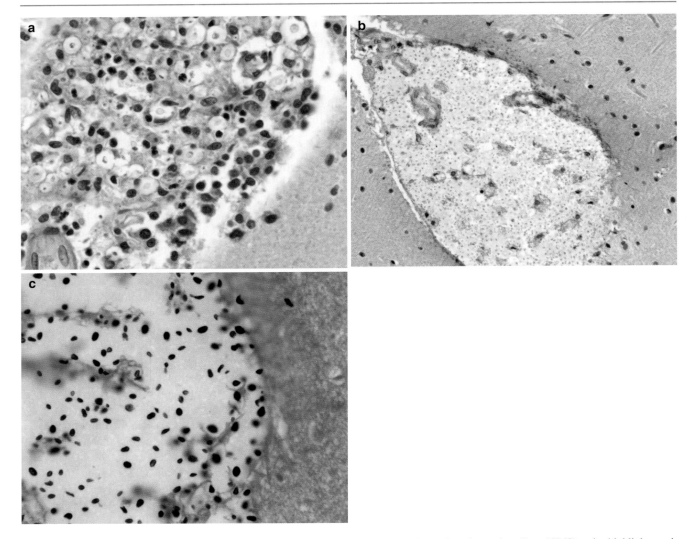

Fig. 22.22 (a–c) CNS cryptococcosis in a patient with HIV infection. Figure (a) shows a distended cerebellar subarachnoid space containing numerous encapsulated *Cryptococcus neoformans* yeast forms with pericapsular clearing (H&E, 40×). Figure (b) shows how mucicarmine stains the yeast capsules pink to magenta (Mucicarmine, 20×). Figure (c) shows a Gomori methenamine silver (GMS) stain, highlights variably sized yeast forms, with a few yeasts exhibiting "teardrop" budding (GMS, 60×) (All courtesy of Anthony Yachnis, MD, and Kelly Devers, MD, University of Florida College of Medicine)

with a variety of nonspecific symptoms, such as lethargy, confusion, nausea, vomiting, or rarely, symptoms suggestive of focal neurologic deficits. Patients may develop raised ICP with papilledema (33 %), cranial nerve palsies (20 %), and seizures; if left untreated, the condition progresses to obtundation and, ultimately, death. Occasionally, total visual loss develops secondary to fungal involvement of the optic tracts, as well as from adhesive arachnoiditis, chorioretinitis, or elevated ICP. Hydrocephalus is a frequent complication even in patients who responded to therapy. Neuroimaging can reveal the extent of CNS involvement: Figure 22.23 shows *C. neoformans* involvement of the basal ganglia.

The diagnosis of cryptococcal meningitis is usually not difficult. The classical and time-honored method for diagnosis is demonstration of the yeast in spinal fluid by India ink stain. Microscopically the India ink particles serve to outline the very large clear polysaccharide capsule surrounding the yeast. The test is positive in over 90 % of HIV-infected patients, but in only 50 % of patients with normal immunity. Several latex agglutination tests have been developed that detect the excess polysaccharide capsule produced in the spinal fluid of patients with cryptococcal meningitis. This test is positive in over 95 % of patients with the condition. While the test is highly reliable, it is important to recognize that there can be both false-negative and false-positive reactions. For example, HIV-infected patients with overwhelming cryptococcal meningitis may have so much polysaccharide capsule in their CSF that a "prozone" effect occurs, resulting in the finding that undiluted CSF or CSF tested at a 1:2 dilution may appear negative. Generally, upon dilution of the spinal fluid to 1:10 or greater, a positive

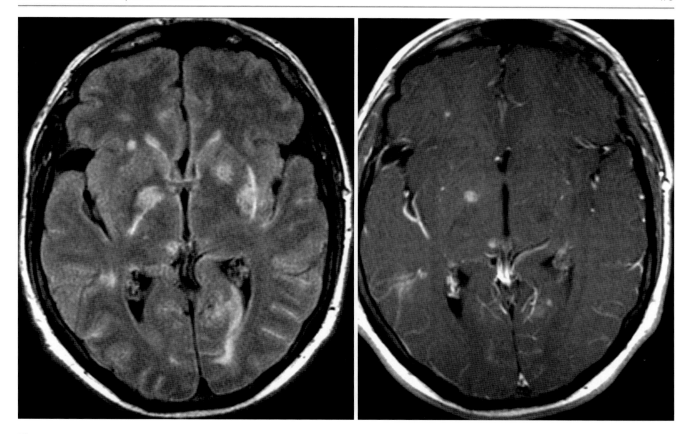

Fig. 22.23 MRI showing *Cryptococcus neoformans* involvement of the basal ganglia

reaction will be observed. Laboratories must be aware of this prozone effect and physicians who suspect cryptococcal meningitis in HIV-infected patients should alert the laboratory to ensure that this possibility is not overlooked. In addition, cross-reactions with *Trichosporon beigelii* or Capnocytophaga may occasionally produce false-positive latex agglutination tests. The latex agglutination should be confirmed by growth of cryptococci in culture. If a positive cryptococcal antigen titer is found in the CSF from a patient for whom CSF culture did not yielded growth of *Cryptococcus* spp., the antigen test cannot be assumed to be false-positive—a large volume (10–20 mL) of CSF should be obtained for repeating the cryptococcal antigen test and reculturing for cryptococcus. The higher the cryptococcal antigen titer, the less likely it is to be a false-positive result. CSF changes in cryptococcal meningitis generally parallel those of chronic tuberculous meningitis and other chronic meningitides (Table 22.2). CSF analysis is typically abnormal as follows: glucose is generally less than 40 mg/dL, protein is elevated in the large majority of patients, and the white count is usually elevated with a lymphocytic predominance.

Treatment of cryptococcal meningitis depends in part on host susceptibility factors. In patients with no underlying chronic illness or history of HIV infection, IV amphotericin B at a dose of 0.5–0.8 mg/kg/day together with oral flucytosine

37.5 mg/kg every 8 h should be administered until the patient becomes afebrile and culture-negative; generally, this takes approximately 6 weeks. This should probably be followed by a course of fluconazole 400 mg/day for an additional 2–3 months. Flucytosine may cause severe leukopenia and thrombocytopenia, particularly in patients with impaired renal function, which, in turn, may develop as a result of amphotericin therapy. Therefore, patients need to be monitored carefully for these particular toxic side effects. Some authorities recommend measuring flucytosine levels and adjusting the dose to give a peak of 70–80 mcg/L and a trough of 30–40 mcg/L. However, services for routine measurement of these levels may not be readily available at many hospitals. Alternative therapeutic regimens include various lipid-soluble amphotericin B preparations, which may be used for patients who develop nephrotoxicity. If the patient is intolerant to flucytosine, therapy with amphotericin B at a higher dose of 0.7–1 mg/kg/day for 6–8 weeks may be considered. Fluconazole 400 mg/day orally for 8–10 weeks may be curative, particularly in non-immunocompromised patients who are less ill. However, it should be recognized that fluconazole alone is less effective than the combination of amphotericin B plus flucytosine: the length of time that CSF cultures remain positive is longer and rates of treatment failure tend to be higher for fluconazole-only therapeutic regimens.

Histoplasmosis

Histoplasma spp. are dimorphic fungi (i.e., they change their characteristic morphology depending on temperature.) Along with *Coccidioides immitis* and *Blastomyces dermatitidis*, *H. capsulatum* exists as a mold at room temperature (greater than 23 °C) and converts to a yeast form at body temperature of 37 °C. The organism is widely disseminated in nature in the soil and may reach high levels in areas where birds roost and in caves inhabited by large numbers of bats. In vitro, the mold phase is characterized by both macro- and microconidia. The microconidia are small, smooth oval bodies ranging in diameter from 2 to 5 μm and are believed to be the infective phase because their small size enables them to be readily carried down to the terminal bronchioles and alveoli. Although found worldwide, histoplasmosis has a very distinct geographical distribution in the United States. Most cases occur in the Ohio and Mississippi River valleys in the Central Midwestern part of the United States with extension as far eastward as Maryland, Delaware, and some parts of Georgia and Florida. The disease is rarely seen west of Texas, Oklahoma, and Kansas.

Once inhaled, the microconidia are ingested by alveolar macrophages and rapidly undergo conversion to the yeast phase. From the initial pulmonary foci, the yeast rapidly migrates to hilar lymph nodes from which they can disseminate to multiple foci in the body. As is the case with cryptococcus and tuberculosis, an asymptomatic pulmonary infection frequently develops approximately 2–3 weeks after exposure. The development of the cellular immune response limits the spread of the organism and generally clears the initial, early, pulmonary focus, leaving minimal to no calcifications in hilar lymph nodes and lung tissue. The disseminated lesions are most commonly manifest by widespread calcific lesions in the spleen and liver after they heal.

Although the vast majority of primary infections in immunologically normal hosts resolve spontaneously, leaving the patient with a positive histoplasma skin test, there are a number of unfavorable outcomes. Dormant infections may reactivate following severe immunosuppression—HIV infection, post transplantation, or after therapy with TNF blockers. Pulmonary disease may go on to produce chronic cavitary histoplasmosis that is radiographically identical to pulmonary tuberculosis. The initial pulmonary infection may result in an acute progressive disseminated infection that characteristically presents with fever, chills, weight loss, hepatosplenomegaly, and pancytopenia from bone marrow involvement. This form of disseminated histoplasmosis most often affects those who are highly immunosuppressed due to AIDS, lymphoma, or iatrogenic therapy.

CNS involvement in this syndrome includes encephalitis, acute meningitis, and encephalopathy. Occasionally, histoplasmomas or mass lesions in the CNS are observed [282–286]. A similar syndrome of disseminated histoplasmosis may also be observed in patients with normal immunity who present with more of a low-grade chronic illness, rather than the acute presentation of disseminated histoplasmosis typically seen in immunosuppressed patients. Symptoms of CNS involvement are secondary to intracranial mass lesions, isolated chronic meningitis with or without other manifestations of disseminated histoplasmosis or meningitis. Some patients may have CNS disease secondary to emboli from histoplasma endocarditis. Wheat and colleagues found that approximately 40 % of patients with histoplasma meningitis had chronic meningitis as part of their disseminated disease [284]; 25–30 % had isolated chronic meningitis, and the remainder presented with various forms of mass lesions and encephalitis. In general, the duration of symptoms of histoplasma meningitis prior to diagnosis tends to be somewhat longer than the duration of symptoms for cryptococcal or tuberculous meningitis. In Wheat's series, approximately 30 % of patients had duration of symptoms less than 1 month; 44 % had symptoms for 2–6 months, and 27 % had symptoms lasting greater than 6 months before the diagnosis was made. Patients who present with localizing CNS signs and symptoms should have neuroimaging (CT scans or MRI) to rule out mass lesions. Those with systemic manifestations may have the diagnosis made by culture or biopsy of an enlarged lymph node, liver, or bone marrow. Diagnosis is best made by visualization of yeast in tissue or by culture. CSF findings are typical for chronic fungal and tuberculous meningitis, with 90 % of patients having a CSF pleocytosis with lymphocytic predominance (Table 22.2). At least 80 % of patients have an elevated CSF protein level and a glucose level less than 40 mg/dL. CSF white blood cells usually number between 50 and 500 cells/μl and are predominantly mononuclear.

Serologic testing for antibodies to *H. capsulatum* in blood is generally positive in 60–90 % of patients with CNS histoplasmosis. The standard assays are the complement fixation test that uses two separate antigens, yeast and mycelial (or histoplasmin), and the immunodiffusion assay [283]. Diagnosis is based on a fourfold rise in antibody titer; a single titer of ≥1:32 is suggestive but not diagnostic. However, in an endemic area, serological tests are often difficult to interpret because patients may have antibodies from prior exposure rather than active infection; likewise, skin testing in an endemic area is probably of no diagnostic value. In the series described by Wheat, CSF cultures were positive in only 26.7 % of patients [284].

Treatment

Histoplasmosis involving the CNS is difficult to treat. Amphotericin B given as a lipid formulation should be used for initial therapy in all patients at a dosage of 3–5 mg/kg daily for 3–4 months. Therapy can be assessed with serial weekly or biweekly lumbar punctures for CSF *Histoplasma* antigen levels, white blood cell counts, and complement fixation antibody titers. A rise in the CSF glucose and fall in the CSF cell count and protein levels would suggest successful response to treatment. Resolution of abnormal findings can help determine the duration of therapy [283]. Approximately 80 % of patients will respond to amphotericin, but at least half of those initial responders will relapse and approximately 20 % will die from the disease. Treatment with Amphotericin B should be followed by an oral azole agent for an undetermined period of time. Primary therapy with itraconazole or fluconazole is not useful in the treatment of CNS histoplasmosis—they do not cross the blood–brain barrier particularly well, and failure rates are remarkably high. Kauffman has categorically stated that primary azole therapy of CNS histoplasmosis should be discouraged [283]. Both azoles have been used successfully for secondary treatment following induction therapy with amphotericin B [283]. The dosage suggested for itraconazole is 200 mg twice or thrice daily, and that for fluconazole is 800 mg daily. In HIV-infected patients, suppressive treatment with itraconazole 200 mg orally daily should begin after the initial course of amphotericin.

Coccidioidal Meningitis

Infections with *Coccidioides immitis* have been recognized for over 100 years and were originally believed to be a nearly uniformly fatal. Like the other dimorphic fungi (*Histoplasma capsulatum* and *Blastomyces dermatitidis*), the natural habitat of *C. immitis* is soil. But unlike the other dimorphic fungi, *C. immitis* is not distributed worldwide but is limited to the lower Sonoran life zone, found primarily in the desert in the Southwest part of the United States, Mexico, and parts of South and Central America. The characteristics of this particular zone are an arid climate with a yearly rainfall of 5–20 in., hot summers, warm winters, and an alkaline soil. In the mold phase of the fungus, which is the form found in soil and other environmental sources, the hyphae fragment into specific structures known as arthrospores which are highly infectious and readily aerosolized when dust is produced. Thus, on occasion, dust storms have blown infectious spores of *C. immitis* as far north as Sacramento and beyond to produce outbreaks well outside the endemic area of the San Joaquin Valley. Transmission of the organism on fomites as far as the East Coast has been implicated in documented cases. The narrow environmental requirements of this fungus account for its endemic distribution within the United States. Epidemiologic studies of people who migrate into the Central Valley of California suggest that the annual risk of infection is approximately 15 %.

Pathogenesis
As is the case with the other dimorphic fungi, the initial route of infection is inhalation with an early focus of infection in lung tissue. The outcome of this infection is highly variable. Approximately one-half to two-thirds of patients demonstrated to be infected with this agent show little or absolutely no initial pulmonary infection. The majority of patients who become symptomatic develop a mild self-limited respiratory infection manifest by fever, cough, malaise, arthralgias, weight loss, and in some patients, a striking clinical syndrome of erythema nodosum and erythema multiforme. The vast majority of these symptomatic cases resolve within 2–4 weeks, occasionally taking up to several months, without treatment. Complications occur in no more than about 10 % of all patients with clinically symptomatic primary infections. Occasional patients will present with fulminant pneumonia and shock-like syndrome, possibly resulting from a particularly high inoculum or perhaps as a result of fungemia and miliary dissemination of the disease. Such a presentation is not uncommon among HIV patients with severe depression of the CD4+ count. Other manifestations include pulmonary nodules, cavities, and chronic lung disease indistinguishable from chronic tuberculosis. The most common site of disseminated lesions is the skin where maculopapular lesions may be progress to keratotic and verrucous ulcers with subcutaneous fluctuant abscesses.

The most serious form of disseminated disease following initial pulmonary infection is coccidioidal meningitis which is a result of lymphohematogenous spread from lungs to meninges [287]. Without treatment it is nearly uniformly fatal within 2 years of diagnosis [287–290]. Observational studies suggest about 80 % of patients who develop meningitis become symptomatic within 6 months of the initial infection [291]. The signs and symptoms of coccidioidal meningitis are very similar to those of other chronic fungal and tuberculous meningitides. Patients generally present with headache, fever, varying degrees of nuchal rigidity, nausea, vomiting, seizures, and altered mental status [287–291]. Factors that predispose to *C. immitis* dissemination and the development of meningitis include immunosuppression due to HIV infection, diabetes mellitus, alcohol abuse, pregnancy, steroids or other immunosuppressive drugs, and non-Caucasian race [289].

Diagnosis of coccidioidal meningitis is based on analysis of the CSF, which shows typical findings of elevated opening pressure (greater than 25 cm H_2O), elevated leukocyte count with a predominance of lymphocytes, elevated protein, and depressed glucose (Table 22.2). Occasionally, patients may have a significant CSF eosinophilia [292]. Thus, in a patient who presents with a history suggestive of chronic meningitis together with typical CSF findings, a history of travel to or having lived in an endemic area must be carefully sought after. Complications, such as meningitis, may occur as late as 2 years after the initial exposure, which may be exceedingly brief, such as a mere drive through the California's Central Valley [286, 288–291].

Although *C. immitis* grows well on typical fungal media, only about one-third of CSF cultures yield growth of the pathogen [289]. The most reliable method of diagnosis is the detection of complement fixing antibodies in the CSF. Although this testing may be negative in a few patients during the early phase of the disease, they eventually become positive over the ensuing months. In patients with pulmonary disease or extrapulmonary manifestations, biopsy with culture and histopathologic examination of involved tissue may give positive results. The demonstration of a spherule in tissue or a positive culture is diagnostic. MRI scans of the brain invariably are abnormal with evidence of basilar meningitis, hydrocephalus, or cerebral infarcts [289].

Treatment

Fluconazole at 400 mg/day is currently recommended as the treatment of choice for coccidioidal meningitis because the response rate of approximately 70 % is very close to that achieved with intrathecal amphotericin B, which was used in the past. In patients who do not respond to the 400 mg/day dose of fluconazole, higher doses may be used, otherwise options are limited. If there is no response to azole therapy, amphotericin B at a dose of 0.1–0.3 mg/kg/day may be given intrathecally, optimally through an Ommaya reservoir. Intravenous amphotericin B has poor CSF penetration and has a limited role in the management of coccidioidal meningitis [289]. Recent studies on rabbit models suggest that lipid preparations of amphotericin B tend to have better penetration of brain parenchyma and meninges and might be effective in treating coccidioidal meningitis. However, such studies have yet to be duplicated in humans [293, 294]. With the demonstration of rising CSF glucose and falling white cell count and protein, this schedule of amphotericin B administration may be decreased to three times a week after 2–3 weeks of daily treatment, and maintenance may be achieved with twice weekly or once weekly injections. Treatment with either oral fluconazole or intrathecal amphotericin B must be prolonged for at least 2 years after the spinal fluid becomes completely normal. In patients with HIV infection, therapy is continued for life. Patients who have disseminated extrapulmonary disease in addition to meningitis should also receive systemic amphotericin at 0.6–1.0 mg/kg/day for 7 days followed by 0.8 mg/kg every other day, to a total dose of 2.5–3 g. The amphotericin should then be followed by oral fluconazole 400 mg/day for up to a year after the course of amphotericin. It should be noted that the response rate is by no means 100 % in either meningitis or disseminated disease, and that relapses are not uncommon even in patients who respond initially.

As is the case with other fungi and tuberculosis, patients occasionally present with mass lesions in brain parenchyma caused by *C. immitis*. These lesions invariably require surgical drainage or excision. In addition, hydrocephalus is relatively common in patients with *C. immitis* meningitis, particularly in children, and must be managed with ventricular shunting. On occasion, *C. immitis* may actually grow in the shunt and cause obstruction. Patients who have a ventricular shunt in place cannot be administered intrathecal amphotericin B in an Ommaya reservoir. Rather, Amphotericin B must be administered intrathecally via intracisternal puncture or lateral neck injection under radiographic guidance. Although intrathecal therapy can be given via the lumbar route, this inevitably leads to varying degrees of potentially severe and debilitating arachnoiditis after several weeks.

Blastomycosis

Blastomycosis is a systemic pyogranulomatous disease caused by *Blastomyces dermatitidis*, another dimorphic fungus that grows as a yeast form at 37 °C and in a hyphal form at room temperature. *B. dermatitidis* exists in nature in the warm moist soils of wooded areas rich in organic debris, such as decaying vegetation. However, the reports of isolation of the organism in nature have been relatively few and somewhat inconsistent. *B. dermatitidis* occurrence follows the distribution of the Mississippi River and is most commonly reported in states such as Louisiana, Western Alabama, Central Arkansas, Missouri, Kentucky, Western Tennessee, and as far north as Minnesota. Outbreaks have occurred along the St. Lawrence River in Canada and in many parts of North and South Carolina [295].

Pathogenesis

Pulmonary infection occurs by the inhalation of conidia, which convert to the yeast form after deposition in the airways. Pulmonary manifestations vary from asymptomatic to overwhelming multilobar infection with involvement of hilar lymph nodes. From there, dissemination to skin and other organs may occur via lymphohematogenous spread. Normal host responses generate a characteristic pyogranulomatous reaction. Extrapulmonary involvement in descending order of frequency include skin (25 %), osteoarticular (25 %), genitourinary (17 %), and CNS (5 %) disease [295–299]. CNS disease is more common in immunocompromised patients, for example, 40 % of patients with AIDS who have blastomycosis also have CNS involvement as meningitis or mass lesions [295, 300, 301]. Less common metastatic sites include the liver, spleen, and naso-/oropharynx. Chronic pulmonary infection resembling tuberculosis or other chronic fungal disease may develop. Dissemination to the skin produces a variety of clinical manifestations, such as chronic verrucous lesions with crusting and purulent drainage, giant keratoacanthoma, and lesions mimicking pyoderma gangrenosum or squamous cell carcinoma. Suppurative granulomatous lesions of the skin and bone may develop and become chronic.

Pathologically, the histological response is that of neutrophils and non-caseating granulomata with epithelioid and giant cells. Because of a vigorous proliferative response, the pseudoepitheliomatous changes seen on skin and mucosal surfaces in response to *B. dermatitidis* may resemble squamous cell carcinoma.

Clinical Manifestations

Most acutely infected patients are asymptomatic or develop a self-limited respiratory illness. The vast majority of patients present with symptoms of pneumonia after an incubation period of 30–45 days. Symptoms are nonspecific, with fever, cough, myalgias, arthralgias, and pleuritic chest pain. Chest examination may reveal lobar or segmental consolidation, including mass lesions mimicking carcinoma with hilar lymphadenopathy. Involvement of the CNS is unusual, with cases generally presenting with meningitis, and rarely as intracranial mass lesion or abscesses that might be solitary or multiple [296, 300, 302].

Clinical involvement of the CNS accounts for 5–10 % of extrapulmonary blastomycosis in clinical reviews [299, 303, 304]. Although CNS blastomycosis may develop in patients without evidence of disseminated disease, most reported cases involving the CNS also have evidence of systemic infection. In addition to meningitis, patients with blastomycosis may present with blastomycomas or mass lesions in the CNS more frequently than is seen with other fungal CNS infections [296, 302]. While steroids and immunosuppressive treatment do not predispose to meningitis per se, they may predispose to dissemination of pulmonary blastomycosis and, hence, increase the probability of neurologic involvement.

Diagnosis

Because there is no highly specific serologic or diagnostic skin test material available, the diagnosis rests upon culture of the organism from pulmonary secretions, skin biopsy material, or direct visualization of round, multinucleated yeast forms that produce daughter cells from a single broad-based bud [305]. Histopathologic analysis of tissue specimens stained with methenamine silver or periodic acid-Schiff (PAS) reagents is the standard diagnostic method for extrapulmonary infection [295]. A urinary antigen is available to aid in diagnosis, but it is not particularly specific (79 %) and shows cross-reactivity by testing positive (96.3 %) in patients with histoplasmosis [306, 307]. Antibody assays by complement fixation or immunodiffusion remain nonspecific and insensitive, and the confirmatory diagnostic test at present remains growth of the organism in culture [308].

Treatment

Prior to the availability of amphotericin B and itraconazole, the disease was progressive and was associated with mortality rates greater than 60 %. Some patients with pulmonary disease have a self-limited infection, but it remains unclear whether the initial primary pulmonary infection should be treated. However, because of the inherent limited ability to predict which cases will disseminate, it certainly seems reasonable to treat most cases of pulmonary infection caused by *Blastomyces* spp. In mild to moderate cases of pulmonary disease, the treatment of choice is itraconazole 200 mg once or twice daily for 6–12 months. In moderately severe to severe disseminated blastomycosis, lipid amphotericin B 3–5 mg/kg/day or deoxycholate amphotericin B 0.3–1.0 mg/kg/day for 1–2 weeks should be used followed itraconazole, 200 mg twice daily for 12 months [295]. Mild to moderate disseminated CNS disease should be treated with high-dose lipid amphotericin B 5 mg/kg/day for 1–2 weeks followed itraconazole 200 mg twice daily for 12 months. If the patient is immunosuppressed or is HIV-infected, the recommended therapeutic regimen is lipid amphotericin B 3–5 mg/kg/day or deoxycholate amphotericin B 0.7–1.0 mg/kg/day for 1–2 weeks followed by itraconazole 200 mg twice daily for 12 months; lifelong suppressive therapy may be indicated in some patients, especially if immunosuppression cannot be reversed [295]. In patients with life-threatening disease, the total dose of amphotericin B may have to be increased.

Candida CNS Infections

Candida species are a part of the normal human enteric flora and rarely produce CNS disease. Meningitis is uncommon except as a complication of an operation or ventricular shunt. Neonates and premature infants seem to be at higher risk than adults. CNS infections caused by *C. albicans* account for a majority of the infections; infections caused by non-albicans species (e.g., *C. parapsilosis*, *C. tropicalis*, *C. glabrata*, *C. pseudotropicalis*, *C. guilliermondii*, *C. krusei*, or *C. lusitaniae*) are relatively less common. In general, CNS disease due to *Candida* species occurs as part of disseminated infection in hospitalized patients who have predisposing risk factors, such as prematurity, intravenous hyperalimentation, indwelling catheters, treatment with corticosteroids, neutropenia, diabetes, HIV infection, patients with leukemia, post neurosurgery, broad-spectrum antimicrobial use, or and indwelling bladder and intravenous catheters [309–313].

Four clinicopathologic disease groups of neurocandidiasis have been identified: (1) cerebral microabscesses that cause a diffuse encephalopathy. Patients with microabscesses are generally diagnosed with systemic candidiasis before death, and the neurologic involvement is usually only detected at autopsy [311, 313, 314]. (2) *Candida* meningitis that occurs together with disseminated microabscesses or alone as chronic meningitis with a dense exudate at the base of the brain and brain stem. Microscopic examination reveals changes consistent with granulomatous meningitis,

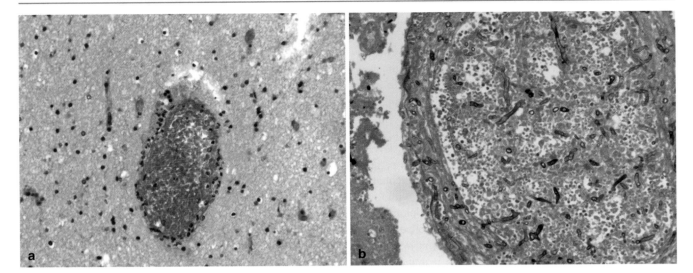

Fig. 22.24 (a) A 63-year-old male with disseminated mucor infection. Shows CNS vasculitis with neutrophils invading CNS parenchymal vessels with early vessel wall destruction (H&E, 20×). (b) Same patient. Features a Gomori methenamine silver (GMS)-stained speci- men demonstrating angioinvasion by fungi with broad aseptate hyphae and right-angle branching (GMS, 20×) (Both courtesy of Anthony Yachnis, MD, and Kelly Devers, MD, University of Florida College of Medicine)

sometimes with yeasts and hyphae; the onset is usually sub-acute with fever and headache [313, 315]. A cerebral CT scan might reveal hydrocephalus and CSF culture invariably yields the microorganism. (3) Cerebral macroabscesses are less frequent and may result in seizures and focal neurological signs; diagnosis is based on neuroimaging studies and biopsy [316]. And (4) vasculitis and mycotic aneurysms vascular complications lead to cerebral infarction and subarachnoid hemorrhage [317].

Zygomycetes and Zygomycosis

Zygomycosis is the term used to describe infection caused any of the zygomycetes—*Absidia*, *Rhizopus*, and *Mucor*. These saprophytic organisms are ubiquitous in the environment, especially soil and commonly found on bread. The genuses *Absidia*, *Rhizopus*, and *Mucor* can invade the CNS by direct extension or from hematogenous spread. Disseminated disease occurring via the hematogenous route may produce CNS mucormycosis resulting in infarction and abscess formation. The Zygomycetes tend to invade the paranasal sinuses or palate with subsequent progression through tissue, nerves, blood vessels, and fascial planes, followed by the vital structures at the base of the brain (Fig. 22.24a, b). In patients with diabetes, this disease typically presents as rhinocerebral mucor (Fig. 22.25). Patients are generally predisposed to this complication if their serum glucose has remained uncontrolled, and the patient has been acidotic for several weeks. Initial symptoms usually include sinus pain, headache, fever, and nasal stuffiness and discharge, which quickly

progresses to facial cellulitis, swelling, proptosis, carotid artery occlusion, cavernous sinus thrombosis, CNS infarction due to fungal thrombosis, CNS hemorrhage, abscess, cerebritis, blindness, and airway obstruction caused by head and neck infections. Death ensues if the condition is not treated. Other at-risk populations include persons who have been neutropenic for more than 2–3 weeks, iron overload, burns, HIV infection and AIDS, blood dyscrasias, transplantation, immunosuppression, chemotherapy, IV drug abuse, and high-dose steroids. Patients with rhinocerebral mucormycosis may manifest hyperglycemia and a metabolic acidosis. Lumbar puncture and CSF analysis invariably reveal a raised opening pressure, a neutrophilic pleocytosis, normal or slightly elevated protein levels, and low glucose levels. In most cases, however, CSF study findings are normal [318]. Neuroimaging studies help to support the diagnosis of rhinocerebral mucormycosis and to precisely determine the extent of disease. CT scanning and MRI reveal soft tissue extent of infection, mucosal thickening, and bony destruction of the sinuses and orbit, presence of cavernous sinus thrombosis, cerebritis, and cerebral edema (Fig. 22.25). Tissue biopsy is necessary to demonstrate the invasive hyphae. The Zygomycetes all appear as ribbon-like nonseptate hyphae in tissue with right- or obtuse-angle branching (Fig. 22.24b). Treatment of the condition is based on three main principles: rapid reversal of underlying predisposing factors, antifungal therapy with amphotericin B, and timely surgical intervention. Treatment includes control of the underlying predisposing condition (e.g., control of diabetic ketoacidosis, hypoxia, and electrolyte abnormalities), IV amphotericin B in a dose of at least 1 mg/kg/day, together with vigorous surgical debridement of

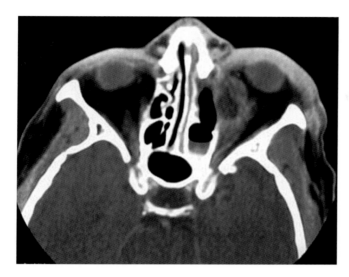

Fig. 22.25 Orbital mucormycosis. Image is a post-contrast axial CT section through the ethmoidal bridge. This case illustrates changes of a left subperiosteal, mesial, orbital abscess. There is little evidence of ethmoid sinusitis. However, it is not uncommon, as in this case, that invasive fungal infections arising either from sinusitis or rhinitis may have only subtle mucosal thickening on imaging, yet still can permeate bone creating soft tissue abscesses in the skull base

all involved tissue. Dexamethasone has been used to treat brain edema. Rhinocerebral mucormycosis carries a prognosis of high morbidity and mortality. Survival depends on the reversibility of underlying risk factors and early surgical intervention [319].

CNS Infections Caused by *Aspergillus* Species

Aspergillus fumigatus and *Aspergillus flavus* can produce CNS disease very similar to that described earlier for mucormycosis. Invasive aspergillosis can occur in patients with preexisting bronchiectasis, chronic bronchitis, asthma, tuberculosis, or in persons who are immunosuppressed (e.g., solid organ transplant recipients). Patients with prolonged and profound neutropenia (less than 100 cells /μL) are at high risk for invasive aspergillosis. Colonization with *Aspergillus* spp. can lead to tissue invasion with branching septate hyphae that are best visualized in tissue with silver stains and histologically distinct from other fungi—i.e., *Aspergillus* spp. have frequent septae that branch at 45° angles. Lung invasion can involve blood vessels leading to hematogenous spread. The majority of invasive CNS infections occur in immunosuppressed transplant patients in the hospital who had pulmonary disease that progressed to brain involvement via hematogenous dissemination. Compared with persons with uncontrolled diabetes who are more susceptible to infections caused by mucor, patients with prolonged neutropenia appear to be more susceptible to invasive *Aspergillus*

spp. sinus infection with direct extension from the maxillary and ethmoid sinuses with progression to cavernous sinus thrombosis. Voriconazole which has good CNS tissue penetration is usually first-line therapy with surgical debridement of all infected tissue. High-dose amphotericin B may be considered in treatment failure [320].

Opportunistic Infections Associated with HIV Infection

Despite the marked improvement in outcomes and outlook for HIV-infected patients with the introduction of highly active antiretroviral therapy (HAART) in 1995, there are still approximately 50,000 new cases of HIV infection per year in the United States [321]. HIV infection predisposes individuals to a variety of opportunistic infections of the brain, including infections caused by *Cryptococcus* spp., *Toxoplasma gondii*, CMV, or the polyomavirus (JC virus) that causes progressive multifocal leukoencephalopathy (PML). In addition, the virus itself is associated with a variety of neuropathologic manifestations.

Toxoplasma Gondii

Toxoplasmic encephalitis is caused by the protozoan *T. gondii*. Disease appears to occur almost exclusively because of reactivation of latent tissue cysts. Primary infection occasionally is associated with acute cerebral or disseminated disease. *T. gondii* causes latent infection in a significant proportion (10–90 %) of the world's population but uncommonly causes clinically significant disease [322]. In addition, *T. gondii* infects numerous wild and domestic animals. Human infection generally occurs through the ingestion of raw or undercooked meat that contains cysts, or by the ingestion of food or water contaminated by the oocysts shed in the stool of infected animals. In the United States, the major animal reservoir for this infection is the domestic cat. The life cycle is complex. The sexual phase of the cycle takes place in the cat with formation of oocysts in the mucosal lining of the intestine for approximately 3 weeks after initial infection. During this time, as many as ten million oocysts may be shed daily. Oocysts require 1–5 days to become infectious after being shed by the cat, a process that depends on temperature and availability of oxygen. During intestinal infection, the tachyzoite form of the organism, a 2–4 μm wide by 4–8 μm long crescent-like structure, is produced and disseminates to many different areas in the host. Wide ranges of intermediate hosts ingest the oocysts, which form latest cysts in many tissues, including muscle. In humans, as in many domestic and wild animals, this dissemination is asymptomatic and results in the formation of cysts in brain parenchyma as well as muscle and numerous other organs. Transmission to humans is a result of exposure to excreta from cats, ingestion of undercooked infected meat, or from contaminated water supplies.

Serologic surveys in the United States show that approximately 15 % of the general population have been infected with toxoplasmosis at some time in the past [323]. In contrast, the prevalence is much higher in economically underdeveloped countries and in certain parts of Europe where rates may range as high as 75 %. Although reactivation of toxoplasmosis in the brain generally leads to local replication with the production of single or multiple abscesses, hematogenous dissemination and infection in the lung and in other parts of the body have been documented. The incidence and attributable mortality in Europe and the United States have decreased substantially since the introduction of antiretroviral therapy and the broad use of prophylaxis regimens active against *T. gondii*.

Clinical Manifestations

In humans, primary infection with toxoplasma may, on occasion, produce a mononucleosis-like illness characterized by lymphadenopathy, fever, malaise, liver function abnormalities, and, occasionally, myocarditis. However, in the large majority of cases, primary infection is asymptomatic and only becomes recognized under conditions of extreme immunosuppression, such as occurs when CD4+ counts in HIV-infected individuals fall to levels less than 100 cells/mm^3, when the cysts break down and initiate symptomatic infection. In immunocompromised patients, reactivation of latent disease can cause life-threatening encephalitis. Patients with toxoplasmic encephalitis generally present with a syndrome of fever, headache and varying degrees of confusion, lethargy, obtundation, focal neurologic signs developing over a period of 1–3 weeks, lymphadenopathy, and splenomegaly. In some patients, the presentation can be abrupt, with seizures or cerebral hemorrhage. Hemiparesis and abnormalities of speech are quite common. Less commonly, brain stem involvement may result in cranial nerve deficits, while dyskinesias such as Parkinsonism, dystonia, tremor, and hemiballismus may also accompany the presenting syndromes. Patients occasionally present with endocrine abnormalities due to involvement of the pituitary axis as well as psychiatric manifestations, such as psychoses and dementia.

Diagnosis

The diagnosis is made by a combination of clinical, imaging, morphological, and serological investigations. In an HIV-infected patient, the finding of single or multiple ring-enhancing lesions by CT or MRI scanning strongly suggests toxoplasma encephalitis (Fig. 22.26a–c). If the patient is also known to be, or is found to be, serologically positive for antibodies to toxoplasma, the combination is virtually diagnostic. In patients with a single lesion, the major differential is lymphoma, and a brain biopsy may be required to make a definitive diagnosis. MRI has superior sensitivity when compared with CT scanning and should therefore be used as the initial diagnostic procedure when feasible. Toxoplasmic encephalitis lesions on MRI appear as high-signal abnormalities on T2-weighted studies and have a rim of enhancement surrounding the edema on T1-weighted, contrast-enhanced images. Other imaging techniques, such as PET, radionuclide (e.g., Thallium 201) scanning, and magnetic resonance techniques have been used to evaluate patients with AIDS who have focal CNS lesions and to specifically differentiate between toxoplasmosis and primary CNS lymphoma. Grossly, the acute lesions are hemorrhagic, necrotic, space-occupying lesions with surrounding edema. Histologically, there are cysts, free parasites, necrosis, and vasculitis (Fig. 22.27a, b). These lesions regress with treatment.

Laboratory studies, such as complete blood cell count (CBC), chemistries, and liver function tests, are typically normal. Affected patients may have a lymphocytosis. CSF analysis shows nonspecific abnormalities, such as elevated white count and protein levels. Attempts to improve the sensitivity by the detection of toxoplasma oligoclonal antibody bands have been reported but do not add any more diagnostic value than a positive serum antibody test. PCR for toxoplasmosis in CSF has been reported to have a sensitivity of 81 % in untreated patients with acute disease; the drawback is that many "in-house" PCR assays suffer from lack of standardization and variable performance according to the laboratory performing the assays [324].

Although a wide variety of antibody tests are available, including the original Sabin Feldman Dye Test, current

Fig. 22.26 (**a–c**) Toxoplasmosis in the right basal ganglia with a T2-w sequence (**a**), a diffusion-weighted image (**b**) and a post gadolinium image (**c**). Toxoplasmosis has a propensity for basal ganglia involvement. It has features which are often very similar to glioblastoma and primary CNS lymphoma and often different from pyogenic abscess. Note in this case that despite the marginal enhancement (similar to pyogenic abscess) the central portion of the abscess forms neither a distinct suppurative cavity nor exhibits water in its center as usually occurs in a pyogenic abscess cavity. In the context of an immunocompromised host, toxoplasmosis should be included as a potential tumefactive entity in the differential of any central nuclear mass

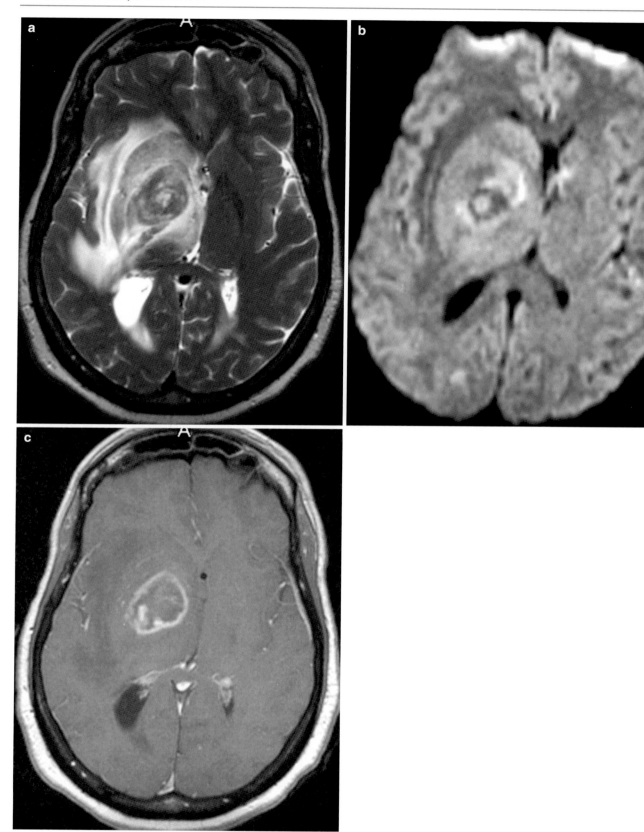

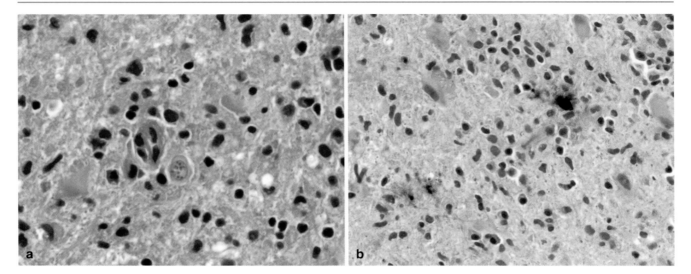

Fig. 22.27 (a) CNS toxoplasmosis. This figure features cysts (brady-zoites) of *Toxoplasma gondii* in brain tissue (H&E, 60×). (b) Shows an anti-Toxoplasma *gondii* antibody immunohistochemical study that is immunoreactive for both bradyzoites and trophozoites (Both courtesy of Anthony Yachnis, MD, and Kelly Devers, MD, University of Florida College of Medicine)

commercial ELISA (enzyme-linked immunosorbent assay), IgG, and IgM tests, along with the indirect fluorescent antibody test, are readily available and highly specific. Because the disease in HIV patients is almost always due to reactivation of an old focus, the IgG test should be positive and the IgM test should be negative in these individuals. However, diagnosis based on classical serological testing is often inconclusive as immunodeficient individuals often fail to produce significant titers of specific antibodies [324].

Treatment

Treatment should be instituted empirically for HIV-infected patients with compatible clinical and imaging studies. The standard drug regimens include 6 weeks of therapy with pyrimethamine 200 mg as a loading dose followed by 75–100 mg daily together with either sulfadiazine 1–1.5 g every 6 h or clindamycin 600–1,200 mg IV every 6 h. Folinic acid (leucovorin), 10–20 mg/day, is given to reduce bone marrow toxicity. If the patient is intolerant of sulfadiazine or clindamycin, the following may be given in addition to pyrimethamine and folinic acid: clarithromycin 1 g orally every 12 h, atovaquone 700 mg orally every 6 h, azithromycin 1,200–1,500 mg/day orally, or dapsone 100 mg/day.

A systematic review of therapeutic regimens for the management of toxoplasmic encephalitis in HIV-infected adults concluded that pyrimethamine + sulfadiazine and pyrimethamine + clindamycin were equivalent in effectiveness in the treatment of acute toxoplasmic encephalitis in HIV-infected individuals [324, 325]. The review also found that trimethoprim/sulfamethoxazole, which is cheap and readily available in developing countries, may be suitable first-line therapy for acute toxoplasmic encephalitis in HIV-infected

individuals and, in fact, was not found to be inferior compared with pyrimethamine + sulfadiazine [325]. More recent studies indicate that trimethoprim/sulfamethoxazole is indeed an alternative treatment for toxoplasmic encephalitis because it is inexpensive, well tolerated, and as effective as pyrimethamine-sulfadiazine [326]. Trimethoprim/sulfamethoxazole may be given 3–5 mg/kg of the trimethoprim component orally or IV every 12 h for 4–6 weeks. Other potential advantages of trimethoprim/sulfamethoxazole include less adverse events, ease of dosing, parenteral formulation, cost, and accessibility [326–328]. Pereira-Chioccola and colleagues recommend that complications, such as expansive brain lesions with a mass effect (e.g., deviation of the middle line structures or imminent risk of cerebral herniation) and cases with diffuse encephalitis should be administered adjunctive corticosteroid therapy. Seizures should be treated with appropriate anticonvulsant agents [327].

Signs of improvement are generally seen in the level of consciousness and in a decrease of fever within 5–7 days, with over 90 % generally responding by day 14 [329]. If there is no clinical or radiographic response within 10 days, alternative diagnoses and brain biopsy must be considered. Reactivation of latent infection in the CNS is a common HIV/AIDS-related complication. Thus, current guidelines recommend that patients with toxoplasmic encephalitis should be treated with the initial regimen for 4–6 weeks, depending upon the degree and rapidity of improvement, and then receive lifelong suppression with sulfadiazine 500–1,000 mg orally four times daily and with pyrimethamine 25–75 mg and folinic acid 10–20 mg both by mouth daily. Patients on long-term maintenance treatment for cerebral toxoplasmosis have a low risk for subsequently developing

Pneumocystis carinii pneumonia. This decreased risk is thought to be the result of chronic suppressive treatment with pyrimethamine and sulfonamides [330]. More recent data suggest that discontinuation of maintenance therapy against toxoplasmic encephalitis for individuals infected with HIV/AIDS, who are receiving successful antiretroviral therapy, might be safe and that patients who remain clinically and radiologically free of relapse at 6 months after discontinuation are unlikely to experience a relapse of toxoplasmic encephalitis [331, 332]. However, the overall body of published data in support of a policy that recommends discontinuing secondary prophylaxis remains relatively limited at the present time.

Cytomegalovirus (CMV)

CMV is a DNA herpes virus. CMV is similar to HSV and VZV in its ability to establish latent infection. CMV tends to infect epithelial cells and leukocytes. In HIV-infected adults, serologic evidence of prior CMV infection is present in over 90 % of individuals. Serologic surveys in the general adult population show a seroprevalence rate ranging between 50 and 80 %, depending upon the socioeconomic status and the particular group studied; the seroprevalence of CMV rises with age. Approximately 10 % of all infants born in the United States either have CMV infection at birth or acquire it within the neonatal period. The vast majority of these infections is asymptomatic and result from exposure to reactivated virus that is transmitted transplacentally in seropositive mothers. Subsequently, both children and adults may become infected through exposure to infected urine often from infants in day care; the virus may also be acquired from sexual contact, generally during the late teens and twenties, or by respiratory droplet infection. In non-immunocompromised adults, primary CMV infection is clinically identical to that of infectious mononucleosis and runs a self-limited course of 2–3 weeks characterized by fever, fatigue, malaise, lymphadenopathy, sore throat, and elevated liver enzymes, together with atypical lymphocytes in the blood smear.

In HIV-infected individuals, as long as cell-mediated immunity remains intact, symptomatic reactivation of CMV is not generally seen. However, as the disease progresses and the CD4+ count falls to less than 50 cells/mm³, reactivation of CMV becomes more frequent. CMV retinitis is the most common form recognized clinically, and in the pre-HAART era, up to 30 % of HIV-infected patients showed clinical evidence of CMV retinitis. The diagnosis of CMV retinitis is a based on the puffy white retinal infiltrates seen together with retinal hemorrhage. It may or may not be associated with systemic or other manifestations of CMV. Either one or both eyes may be involved at a given time.

There are several forms of CNS involvement with CMV and the pathogenesis appears to follow two different routes: (1) via the ependymal cells in the ventricles and (2) via the blood through capillary endothelial cells. Infection via the ependymal cells and CSF is manifest as necrotizing encephalitis limited to the periventricular areas, with numerous cytomegalic inclusions in and around the lesions. In contrast, infection acquired via hematogenous dissemination results in microglial nodular encephalitis, which is manifest pathologically as glial nodules formed by rod cells, few lymphocytes, and macrophages. Very little tissue damage is associated with these lesions [333]. The microglial nodular disease may involve multiple parts of the brain including the periventricular areas. As with CMV retinitis, these CNS complications occur very late in HIV infection and almost always in patients with CD4+ counts less than 50 cells/mm³. In the series reported by Grassi and coworkers, the mean CD4+ count for patients with microglial nodular encephalitis was 21 cells/mm³, while the average CD4+ count of patients with ventriculoencephalitis was 11 cells/mm³ [333].

Although there is considerable overlap of symptomatology between these two pathologic conditions, microglial nodular encephalitis is characterized by the onset of acute confusion associated with delirium and psychomotor agitation, whereas the onset of ventriculoencephalitis is insidious and generally characterized by cognitive disturbances, memory deficits, and mental sluggishness. Patients with either type of encephalopathy may complain of headaches and have seizures. CSF examination in these conditions reveals a slightly elevated protein, which tends to be lower in microglial nodular encephalitis, averaging approximately 60 mg/dL as compared with 172 mg/dL in ventriculoencephalitis. Glucose levels are normal and cells are generally, although not always, absent. Although MRI is more sensitive than CT scan in the diagnosis of these conditions, the MRI may be normal or show nonspecific changes [334, 335]. In patients with ventriculoencephalitis, typical MRI findings include a hyperintense ventricular rim on T2-weighted imaging or enhancements with gadolinium. Almost all cases show nonspecific cerebral atrophy. Systemic involvement with CMV is more frequently associated with microglial nodular encephalitis, which may be documented with CMV antigenemia testing or viral culture. Patients with ventriculoencephalitis are more likely to have the clinical syndrome of CMV radiculopathy [333, 335–338]. CMV infection in HIV patients may also involve the spinal cord. A syndrome characterized by ascending weakness of the lower extremities associated with loss of deep tendon reflexes progressing to loss of bowel and bladder control has been described [339]. The syndrome may begin with low back pain with radiation down to the legs or into the groin or anal area, followed over 1–3 weeks by the development of progressive weakness.

Laboratory diagnosis is carried out in several ways: (1) seroconversion, (2) DNA detection in infected tissues using PCR, (3) antigen detection in tissues, (4) cytopathology, (5) isolation of virus from tissue or secretions, or (vi) CMV cytopathology. Pathologically, the CMV radiculopathy is characterized by mononuclear infiltration of the cauda equina and lumbar sacral nerve roots together with CMV inclusions seen in the Schwann's cells and epithelial cells, leading to axonal destruction. Untreated, this condition generally progresses to irreversible paralysis. Analysis of CSF in patients with this syndrome characteristically shows elevation of neutrophils, sometimes as high as 5,000 cells/mm^3. Although the CSF protein is only mildly elevated and the glucose generally normal, some patients may have marked hypoglycorrhachia with glucose levels as low as 5–10 mg/dL.

Treatment

Ganciclovir 5 mg/kg IV every 12 h should be given for 14–21 days followed by maintenance with oral or IV doses that must be continued indefinitely to avoid or delay relapses, unless CD4+ recovery occurs. Valganciclovir, a prodrug of ganciclovir, possessing excellent oral bioavailability and antiviral activity is effective in both the induction phase and the maintenance phase of CMV retinitis therapy [340, 341]. Ganciclovir blocks CMV replication by inhibiting CMV DNA polymerase. Alternatively, foscarnet 90 mg/kg, adjusted for renal function, can be given IV twice daily for 2–3 weeks. Following induction with ganciclovir or foscarnet, HAART therapy can then be given in the hope of sustained improvement in CD4+ count and maintenance of a response to therapy. In the pre-HAART era, CMV encephalitis responded relatively poorly to ganciclovir, with survival generally in the 3–4 month range. The suppression of HIV replication and elevation in CD4 cells observed during HAART may allow AIDS patients to undergo immune reconstitution. Discontinuation of maintenance CMV therapy for these patients may be considered in these patients [332, 342, 343]. The drawback to withdrawing maintenance therapy is the risk of acquiring sight-threatening inflammatory conditions, including immune recovery uveitis [344].

HIV Encephalopathy and Dementia

HIV is a neurotropic virus that appears to enter the brain via infected macrophages early in the course of infection. HIV infection itself causes CNS complications, including encephalitis and dementia. Encephalopathy usually develops as part of the acute HIV syndrome during the seroconversion phase. Two pathogenic mechanisms are thought to underlie these CNS conditions. In the first mechanism, HIV and its fragments induce damage directly or indirectly through the accumulation of infected or activated macrophage and microglia cells that release neurotoxic mediators including both cellular activation products and viral proteins [345, 346]. The accumulation of these activated macrophage/microglia cells, some of which are infected, release a number of cytokines and small molecule mediators and viral proteins that act on bystander cells. These viral proteins and cellular products have neurotoxic properties and act directly and through induction of astrocyte dysfunction, leading to neuronal injury [346–348]. The second, less predominant, pathogenic mechanism is the ability of HIV to impair neurogenesis [349, 350]. Kaul suggests that both proposed pathogenic mechanisms occur side by side with other host-virus interactions [345].

Pathologically, the most frequent findings in persons with HIV encephalopathy are brain atrophy characterized by sulcal widening and ventricular dilatation together with varying degrees of meningeal fibrosis. The most distinctive histologic feature of this condition is white matter pallor, chiefly seen in a periventricular distribution together with microglial nodules, diffuse astrocytosis, and perivascular mononuclear inflammation. HIV can be readily demonstrated in these nodules by immunohistochemical techniques. HIV-associated dementia is a late phenomenon caused by cortical neuronal loss and abnormalities of the dendritic connections; cerebral atrophy in these patients invariably is confirmed on gross necropsy. Histologically, the brain of a person with HIV encephalitis is characterized by multiple nodules of infected microglia and microglial giant cells in the white matter (Fig. 22.10). These lesions also affect neural function by secreting toxic cytokines.

Clinically, HIV encephalopathy presents with altered mental status characterized by mental slowing frequently accompanied by clinical evidence of subcortical dementia, such as bradykinesia, postural instability, slow and clumsy gait, and altered muscle tone. Radiographically, the most common features are generalized cerebral atrophy together with widespread symmetric hyperintense white matter abnormalities seen on T2 imaging, which generally have a periventricular distribution. Examples are shown in Fig. 22.28. CSF studies are non-diagnostic: the CSF is commonly acellular and a mononuclear pleocytosis is seen in about 25 % of patients with cell counts generally less than 50 cells/mm^3 [351, 352]. CSF protein levels are elevated (usually less than 200 mg/dL) in 60 % of patients, while CSF immunoglobulin G levels are raised in about 80 %. Glucose levels in the CSF of HIV-infected patients are usually within normal limits.

HIV may be detected in CSF by a variety of techniques, including PCR, during all the clinical stages of infection, i.e., HIV is present in the CSF in the absence of neurologic abnormalities. Thus, the presence of HIV in the CSF is not diagnostic for HIV encephalopathy and HIV RNA levels in the CSF do not necessarily correlate with the corresponding plasma levels. Neuroimaging studies can support a diagnosis

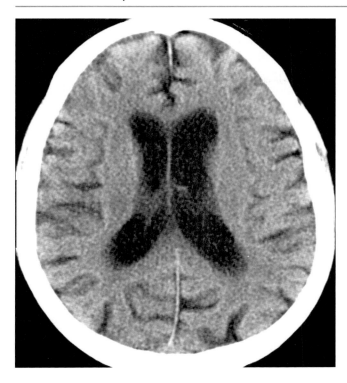

Fig. 22.28 Primary HIV infection of the CNS. Ventriculomegaly and sulcal dilatation (indicating cortical brain atrophy). There is no transependymal fluid to suggest elevated CSF pressure. These findings are indicative of both central and cortical brain atrophy which, in this case, is out of proportion to chronological age. Generalized atrophy is one of the features of primary HIV involvement of brain (Reproduced with permission from Rand et al. [521])

of AIDS dementia complex by revealing cortical atrophy and ventricular enlargement and hyperintense lesions in the periventricular white matter on MRI. HAART remains the main mode of medical treatment for HIV encephalopathy and other HIV-related cognitive disorders.

Parasitic Infections of the Central Nervous System

Cerebral Malaria

Despite its eradication from North America and Europe, it is estimated that malaria infects over 2.5 billion people worldwide and causes between one and three million deaths each year. The disease is caused by one of five different *Plasmodium* species: *P. vivax*, *P. ovale*, *P. malariae*, *P. knowlesi*, and *P. falciparum*. Most of the deaths and serious complications of malaria, especially CNS involvement, are caused by *P. falciparum*. Malaria sporozoites are transmitted from the female Anopheles mosquito to the patient at the time the mosquito bites a person for its blood meal. Sporozoites are carried rapidly to the liver where they

multiply in approximately 1 week to become tissue schizonts or the dormant hypnozoites produced by *P. vivax* and *P. ovale*. Infected liver cells then burst, releasing thousands of merozoites, each of which in turn infects red blood cells in the blood stream. Continued asexual replication in the bloodstream through repeated cycles of maturation and rupture of red cells with release of merozoites eventually results in symptomatic infection. During this process, some of the parasites develop into sexual forms called gametocytes which produce no symptoms themselves but which may circulate for a prolonged period of time. It is the ingestion of these gametocytes that leads to the sexual reproduction cycle in the Anopheles mosquito resulting in the motile sporozoites which invade the mosquito salivary glands and can be transmitted back to humans at the time of the next feeding.

Malaria is widely distributed in economically lessdeveloped countries, particularly sub-Saharan Africa, Central America and the Caribbean, South America, the Middle East, Far East, and Indonesia. The reader is strongly urged to access the CDC's website for the most up-to-date availability on the distribution and drug resistance among *Plasmodium* spp. on a country-by-country basis.

Pathogenesis

P. falciparum is the cause of the most malignant form of malaria and is associated with almost all serious complications associated with the infection. Cerebral malaria, in particular, is the most prominent and serious of these complications. Attributable mortality remains relatively high (20 %) and is often associated with delays in diagnosis and treatment. As *P. falciparum* trophozoites mature in the red blood cells, they induce the formation of small knobs on the surface of the red cell. These knobs bind to adhesion molecules (also known as intercellular adhesion molecule-1) on the microvascular endothelial cells, leading to sequestration. Sequestration is the process whereby erythrocytes containing mature forms of *P. falciparum* adhere to microvascular endothelial cells resulting in marked reduction or disappearance of these cells from the circulation. Sequestration of erythrocytes in small blood vessels and consequent obstruction of microcirculatory flow is a specific property of *P falciparum* and an important mechanism causing coma and death in cerebral malaria. *The second important factor in the pathogenesis of cerebral malaria is the increase in cytokine production.* In an attempt to control the infection, the host immune system produces a potent proinflammatory response in which cells of the macrophage-monocyte series are induced to release various cytokines, including tumor necrosis factor (TNF)-α, interleukin (IL)-1, IL-6, and IL-8 [353]. However, this response may also induce complications, such as severe anemia, hypoglycemia, and cerebral malaria.

The adhesion molecules are upregulated in malaria as a result of cytokine productions, TNF-α in particular.

Furthermore, parasitized erythrocytes tend to adhere to adjacent uninfected cells leading to rosetting. In addition, as the parasite matures inside the erythrocyte, the normally flexible cell becomes more spherical and rigid. Because of the rosetting and increased rigidity of parasitized erythrocytes, the erythrocytes become trapped in the capillaries. The end result of cytoadherence, rosetting, and rigidity is the enhancement of sequestration of *P. falciparum*-parasitized erythrocytes in the cerebral vasculature, stagnation of the cerebral blood flow, and secondary ischemia leading to tissue hypoxia, lactic acidosis, hypoglycemia, and prevention of delivery of nutrients to the tissues. High concentrations of TNF-α can precipitate cerebral malaria by increasing the sequestration of parasitized erythrocytes. Although all tissues potentially can become involved, the brain is the most profoundly affected [354–362].

In the CNS, this process results in delirium, impaired consciousness, convulsions, paralysis, coma, and, ultimately, rapid death if not treated. Systemic manifestations of severe falciparum malaria include anemia, lactic acidosis, hypoglycemia, pulmonary edema, adult respiratory distress syndrome, and disseminated intravascular coagulation. Of note, the pathophysiology of malaria does not include vasculitis or inflammatory cellular infiltration in or around the cerebral vasculature, and most patients have no evidence of cerebral edema. Raised intracranial pressure likely arises from an increase in the overall cerebral blood volume rather than brain swelling arising from cerebral edema and capillary leakage. Coma in malaria is generally not associated with raised intracranial pressure. Clinical features of *P. falciparum* malaria include fever and chills (83 %), altered sensorium (48 %), jaundice (27 %), anemia (75 %), cerebral involvement (45 %), thrombocytopenia (41 %), and renal failure (25 %).

The diagnosis should be considered in a person with altered consciousness, fever, and a relevant travel history, which is critically important to elicit, as is the history of whether the patient took or was compliant with prophylaxis for malaria. The location of the travel is particularly critical as *P. falciparum* is typically resistant to chloroquine. Resistance to trimethoprim/sulfamethoxazole, mefloquine, and other agents has been documented in many parts of the world, particularly Southeast Asia and sub-Saharan Africa. Because there is no latent form of *P. falciparum* in the liver, as there is for *P. vivax* and *P. ovale*, cases of *P. falciparum* malaria should become clinically evident within a month after leaving an endemic area.

The laboratory diagnosis of malaria is made from examination of the blood smear. Although delay is common because of the time needed for their preparation and reading, thick and thin blood smears remain the cornerstone of laboratory diagnosis of malaria in current practice. Despite the availability of rapid diagnostic testing for the detection of malaria based on lateral-flow immunochromatography in which clinicians can detect malaria parasite antigens from finger-prick blood specimens within 10–15 min, microscopic examination of blood smears remains the most cost-effective methodology for diagnosis of malaria, provided the results reach those who need to know in a timely manner.

Rapid diagnostic testing kits based on molecular platforms with high sensitivity and high negative predictive value for *P. falciparum* would be of particular use in acute care settings in regions of low malaria endemicity, where the diagnosis is suspected but lack of laboratory expertise precludes the diagnosis and reading of blood smears. Lastly, rapid diagnostic testing may benefit severely ill patients by confirming or excluding a malaria diagnosis rapidly and facilitating prompt intervention. Rapid test kits for malaria have limitations that preclude replacing microscopy of blood smears any time soon. These limitations include inability to ascertain parasitemia quantitatively or to differentiate between the four plasmodium species.

Treatment

Untreated, cerebral malaria is fatal. In cases of severe malaria with CNS involvement, the patient must be treated as though they have falciparum malaria regardless of the preliminary interpretation of the blood smear. According to CDC, if severe malaria is strongly suspected but a laboratory diagnosis cannot be made at that time, blood should be collected for diagnostic testing as soon as it is available and parenteral antimalarial drugs started empirically. Once the diagnosis is considered likely, parenteral quinidine gluconate should be started. The recommended therapeutic regimen includes a loading dose of 6.25 mg base/kg (=10 mg salt/kg) infused intravenously over 1–2 h followed by a continuous infusion of 0.0125 mg base/kg/min (=0.02 mg salt/kg/min). An alternative regimen is an intravenous loading dose of 15 mg base/kg (=24 mg salt/kg) of quinidine gluconate infused intravenously over 4 h, followed by 7.5 mg base/kg (=12 mg/kg salt) infused over 4 h every 8 h, starting 8 h after the loading dose. Quinidine gluconate therapy should be combined with doxycycline, tetracycline, or clindamycin. If the patient is unable to tolerate oral therapy, doxycycline (100 mg every 12 h) or clindamycin (5 mg base/kg every 8 h) may be given intravenously until the patient can be switched to oral therapy [354, 356, 359]. More recently, artemisinin derivatives, such as parenteral artesunate, have been shown to substantially reduce mortality in African children with severe malaria; the authors go on to suggest that parenteral artesunate should replace quinine as the treatment of choice for severe falciparum malaria worldwide [363].

Parenteral quinidine gluconate is cardiotoxic and can induce hyperinsulinemic hypoglycemia. Thus, a baseline EKG should be obtained before initiating therapy and glucose levels must be monitored closely. Critical care management includes continuous cardiac and blood pressure monitoring with appropriate supportive management of coexisting medical complications often associated with severe malaria: convulsions, renal failure, adult respiratory distress syndrome, disseminated intravascular coagulation, lactic acidosis, hypoglycemia, fluid and electrolyte abnormalities, circulatory collapse, acute renal failure, secondary bacterial infections, and severe anemia.

Intravenous corticosteroids are associated with poor outcomes and are absolutely contraindicated [361]. Brain swelling on CT scan is a common finding in adult patients with cerebral malaria but is not related to coma depth or survival. Mannitol therapy as adjunctive treatment for brain swelling in adult cerebral malaria prolongs coma duration and may be harmful [364]. Results of studies of antipyretics, anticonvulsants (phenobarbitone), anticytokine/anti-inflammatory agents (anti-TNF antibodies, pentoxifylline, dexamethasone), iron chelators, and hyperimmune sera have not proven beneficial in improving patient outcomes [359].

With treatment, almost all patients with CNS malaria recover completely if they survive the acute episode. However, globally, overall mortality in children and adults remains unacceptably high. Approximately 12 % of patients with cerebral malaria may have lasting neurologic sequelae, including cortical blindness, tremor, cranial nerve palsies, and sensory and motor deficits, although approximately 50 % of these sequelae resolve with time.

Amoebic Meningoencephalitis

A dramatic and almost uniformly fatal primary meningoencephalitis can be seen with infection caused by the free-living amoeba *Naegleria fowleri* and *Acanthamoeba* species. Free-living N. fowleri are found widespread in nature, particularly in the upper surface layers of lakes or shallow fresh water in warm climates. Acanthamoeba spp. are usually found in soil and in fresh and brackish water. Most cases in the United States, typically children or young adults, occur in the southeastern states. Clinically, patients present with sudden onset of high fever, photophobia, and headaches; progression to obtundation occurs relatively quickly. There is usually a classic history of swimming or waterskiing in warm, freshwater lakes. The amoebae invade the nasal cavity along the blood vessels associated with the olfactory nerves and traverse the cribriform plate to reach the frontal lobes and the surrounding meninges, where they rapidly produce a highly necrotizing, purulent, and destructive encephalitis. Because of the olfactory involvement, there may be alterations of smell or taste. Otherwise, nonspecific symptoms such as confusion, irritability, restlessness, and seizures with rapid progression to delirium, stupor, and coma ensue. The CSF is usually bloody, shows a leukocytosis with neutrophil

predominance, low glucose levels, and elevated protein. If the diagnosis is strongly suspected, one can examine the unstained CSF with a slide warmer to look for the typical, mobile, amoeboid motion of the trophozoites; gram stain and culture are usually negative. A PCR assay for *Naegleria*, *Acanthamoeba*, and *Balamuthia* has been developed by CDC [365, 366].

Frontal lobe involvement is readily seen on MRI but the diagnosis is often delayed because of the rarity of the condition and paucity of immediately diagnostic signs. Only a small number of patients have been reported to have survived and all received amphotericin B to which the pathogens are susceptible in vitro [367–370]. The optimal treatment regimen is not known for this condition and some authors recommend maximal systemic doses of amphotericin B with intracisternal amphotericin B adjunctive rifampin and doxycycline [371]. Surgical intervention usually involves placement of a reservoir for intrathecal amphotericin B and shunting to alleviate hydrocephalus.

Neurocysticercosis

Neurocysticercosis is the most common helminthic infection of the nervous system, and a leading cause of acquired epilepsy worldwide [372–374]. Cysticercosis is widespread in areas such as Mexico, Central America, South America, Africa, Southeast Asia, India, the Philippines, and Southern Europe. More recent data indicated that it is an increasing problem in Europe [372]. Neurocysticercosis in adults results from infection of the brain with the larval cysts of the cestode, *Taenia solium*, the pork tapeworm. Human infection occurs by two different mechanisms: [1] ingestion of the eggs leading to embryonation of the eggs and penetration of the intestinal wall with hematogenous transport of cysticerci to many different tissues, primarily muscle and brain, where they encyst and remain potentially infectious for long period of time. Alternatively, ingestion of undercooked pork can result in ingestion of the cysticerci by humans. In the latter instance the cysticerci mature into the typical tapeworm which attaches to the intestine and may grow to lengths of up to 3 m and live for up to 25 years. During this time it produces egg-filled segments, called proglottids, which are excreted in the feces. Ingestion of the eggs from these proglottids leads to neurocysticercosis, occasionally even by autoinfection from the patient's own intestinal tapeworm.

Symptomatic neurocysticercosis results from the enlargement of the cysticercal cysts in the brain parenchyma over a period of months to years. In the United States, patients may present with seizures due to neurocysticercosis that was acquired after a visit to an endemic part of the world 30 years previously. The clinical manifestations are nonspecific and varied depending on the number, size, and anatomic location of the cystic lesions. Seizures and headaches are common presenting symptoms. If the cysts block the flow of CSF, symptoms associated with raised ICP, such as headache, nausea, vomiting, changes in vision, dizziness, ataxia, and confusion, may result. When the cysts are located in the meninges, chronic meningitis may occur. An unusual form called "racemes" cysticercosis is caused by the proliferation of cysts at the base of the brain and can result in severe disease, including mental deterioration and death. Intraspinal cysts are common and may produce symptoms of cord compression; severity again depends on location and size of cysts.

The most frequent clinical presentations are seizures (64.8 %), symptoms associated with raised intracranial hypertension, and meningism [375]. Radiological studies of the skull show intracranial calcifications suggestive of cysticercosis in up to 50 % of patients [375]. Analysis of CSF invariably shows increased pressure, elevated lymphocyte and eosinophil counts, elevated protein levels, and reduced glucose levels. Neurocysticercosis is readily diagnosed by neuroimaging (CT scanning or MRI) studies in which mul-

tiple cysts of varying sizes and stages are demonstrated (Fig. 22.29a, b). MRI may show the parasites as well as the changes they induce in the nervous system [374, 376, 377]. Figure 22.29c, d shows the histology of the cyst wall with outer, middle, and inner layers. Serological testing is available with sensitivities as high as 94 % in patients with multiple cysts but significantly lower in those with single cysts [378]. Older cysts are often calcified. PCR assays have the highest sensitivity (95.9 %) but variable specificity (80 % or 100 %) depending on the controls used [378]. Serology is generally available through the CDC or at specific national commercial laboratories. However, the identification of specific antibodies and antigens is currently used only to support the diagnosis because of the limited specificity and sensitivity of current tests.

Treatment

Based on neuroimaging studies, CNS lesions can be classified into active and inactive neurocysticercosis (Fig. 22.29a). Patients with inactive parenchymal neurocysticercosis

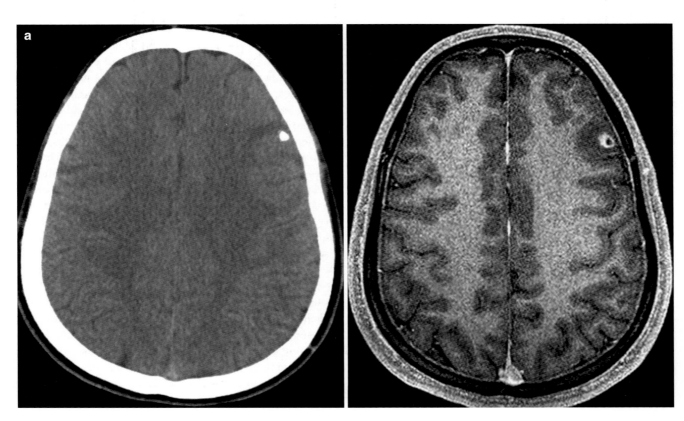

Fig. 22.29 (**a**) Neurocysticercosis. Images include non-contrast CT (*left*) and post-gadolinium-enhanced T1-w MRI (*right*). These images demonstrate the features of chronic neurocysticercosis. The frontal lesion is calcified as evident on the CT. However, it also produces local inflammation evident on the enhanced MR image. This local inflammatory reaction frequently can produce seizure activity. Hence, late state neurocysticercosis can be a mimic for cortical oligodendroglioma. (**b**) Neurocysticercosis; images include a panorama of the MRI sequences in the mid-convexity level of the brain including pre and post-contrast DT1-w sequences and T2-w spin echo sequences which illustrate typi-

cal findings of neurocysticercosis. The findings in this case are those of cystic nodules scattered in brain and in the depths of the sulci. The margins of the lesion show reactive hyperemia. Within some of the lesions an organism scolex is evident confirming the basis for the nodules. (**c**) Neurocysticercosis. A 25-year-old male from Latin America with a lateral ventricular cyst. The figure shows the cyst wall with outer cuticular layer, middle cellular layer, and inner reticular layer (H&E 20×). (**d**) Features a high-power view of a portion of the scolex (H&E 60×) (**d**: Courtesy of Anthony Yachnis, MD, and Kelly Devers, MD, University of Florida College of Medicine)

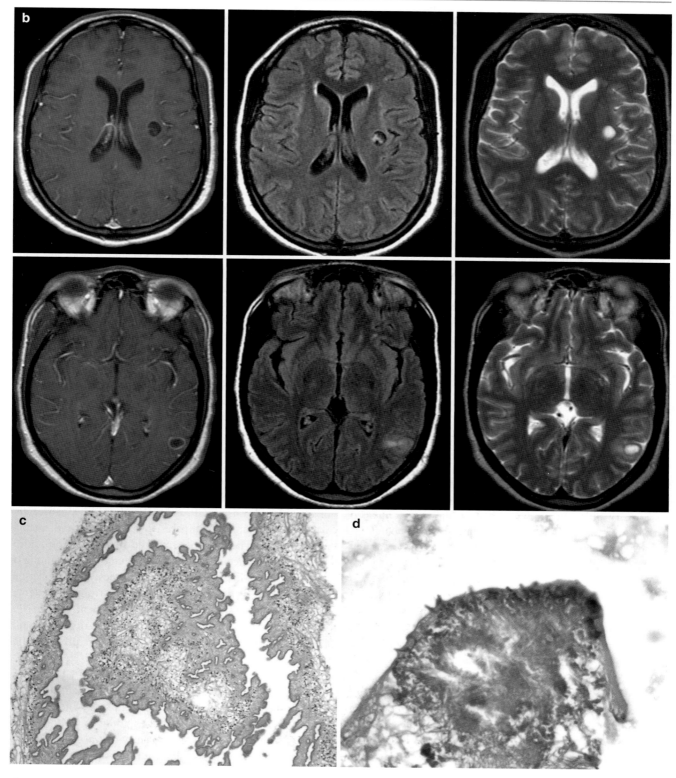

Fig. 22.29 (continued)

generally have no evidence of viable or degenerating parasites; the utility of antiparasitic drugs in these patients remains limited. However, these patients are at increased risk of developing seizures, and standard anticonvulsive therapy with phenytoin, phenobarbital, or carbamazepine is indicated. Patients who develop hydrocephalus need to be treated with ventricular peritoneal shunting. Virtually all patients with active neurocysticercosis have seizures, which must be treated with anticonvulsants. Probably the majority of these patients can be treated symptomatically and followed by MRI because the cysticerci typically undergo complete degeneration over a 1- to 2-year period. This process results in either calcified inactive cysticerci that continue to induce seizures thereby requiring continued therapy with anticonvulsants or, in a majority, a normal MRI in which case anticonvulsants may be tapered as long as the patients remain seizure free.

Cysticidal drugs (albendazole and praziquantel) have improved the prognosis of this condition and can be given with praziquantel at doses of 50–100 mg/kg/day for 15–30 days or albendazole 10–15 mg/kg/day for 8 days. Albendazole has been superior to praziquantel in trials comparing the efficacy of these drugs [376, 377, 379]. Another advantage of albendazole is that it also destroys subarachnoid and ventricular cysts [380, 381]. In some of these cases, particularly in patients with large subarachnoid cysts, higher doses (up to 30 mg/kg/day) or more prolonged, or even repeated, courses of albendazole may be needed. Although these agents kill the cysticerci, some controlled trials have not shown any clinical benefit over symptomatic treatment alone [382–384]. The main adverse side effect of praziquantel is worsening neurologic function, i.e., headaches, dizziness, seizures, and increased ICP probably as a result of an increase in the host inflammatory response and cerebral edema due to the larval death. There is a strong consensus that there is no role for anti-cysticidal drugs in patients with only calcified lesions and those patients with single enhancing lesions will do well regardless of antiparasitic therapy [385]. Riley and White point out that while antiparasitic therapy is indicated in patients with multiple subarachnoid cysticerci or giant cysticerci they are contraindicated in patients with cerebral edema (cysticercal encephalitis) [385].

Surgery plays an important role in the management of some forms of the disease, particularly hydrocephalus and intraventricular cysts. Standard treatment of ventricular neurocysticercosis has been the surgical removal of cysts that block CSF flow; in patients with ventricular cysticerci, endoscopic removal remains the preferred therapy [385]. Recent studies have found fewer shunt failures when such patients are treated with antiparasitic drugs [386–388]. Cysticercosis involving the basilar cisterns is associated with a prominent inflammatory arachnoiditis and can be complicated by both vasculitis, resulting in lacunar infarctions, and invasion of the cysticerci into larger vessels, resulting in strokes. Thus, some authors have recommended the addition of corticosteroids in the treatment of patients with cisternal cysticercosis [387–390].

A consensus guideline panel headed by Garcia and coworkers underscored four major tenets of managing neurocysticercosis [391, 392]: (1) individualize therapeutic decisions, including whether to use antiparasitic drugs, based on the number, location, and viability of the parasites within the CNS; (2) actively manage growing cysticerci either with antiparasitic drugs or surgical excision; (3) prioritize the management of intracranial hypertension secondary to neurocysticercosis before considering any other form of therapy; and (4) manage seizures as done for seizures due to other causes of secondary seizures because they are due to an organic focus that has been present for a long time [391].

Echinococcus

Echinococcal disease is caused by tapeworms that commonly infect dogs, cats, wolves, and other carnivores. It is found worldwide but is particularly common in countries surrounding the Mediterranean, parts of East Africa, Russia and South America. There is very little echinococcal disease in the United States, but it is important to recognize that bears, foxes, and wolves in Canada and Alaska are commonly infected with this parasite. Disease is produced when an egg from an infected animal is ingested and the oncosphere within is activated, penetrates the gut wall, and travels via veins or lymphatics to various tissues in the body where they form hydatid cysts. Up to 80 % of cysts occur in the liver and about 10 % in the lungs. CNS involvement is uncommon and occurs in only about 2 % of cases. At all anatomic sites, cysts may be single or multiple.

Of the four species that infect humans, *Echinococcus granulosus* and *E. multilocularis* account for the vast majority of cases. CNS disease is commonly characterized by slowly enlarging solitary cysts in the brain. Depending on the size and location of the cyst, the patient may remain asymptomatic. However, as the CNS lesion enlarges in size, symptoms may arise from the local effects of the lesion itself or secondary to raised ICP, resulting in headache, nausea and vomiting, seizures, hemiparesis, dysarthria, and cranial nerve palsies. The diagnosis may be suspected from radiographic appearance of the cyst itself seen on CT scanning or MRI. Classic radiographic features include a sharp, spherical border lacking a rim of enhancement or surrounding edema, although a fine rim of peripheral enhancement with perilesional edema may be seen if active inflammation is present. CT is superior for the detection of extrahepatic disease; MRI does not appear to add any diagnostic benefit.

Immunodiagnostic testing is available from CDC; sensitivity of these tests varies from 60 to 90 % and they are highly sensitive for liver cysts although less so for cysts in the brain. Thus, a negative test does not absolutely rule out cerebral echinococcal disease. History of travel to or living in an endemic area especially with exposure to sheep also increases the likelihood of the diagnosis of echinococcus. Patients with intracranial hydatid cysts usually present with focal neurological deficit and features of raised intracranial pressure due to interference with CSF flow. The treatment of hydatid cyst is surgical and the aim of the surgery is to excise the cyst in toto without rupture to prevent recurrence and anaphylactic reaction. Albendazole therapy is given in a daily dose of 10 mg/kg, taken three times for 4 months. It is a broad-spectrum oral antihelminthic drug, which acts by blocking glucose uptake of the larva and adult worm. The glycogen stores are thus depleted thereby decreasing the ATP formation resulting in death of the parasite. Albendazole can decrease the size of large cysts and cause smaller ones to disappear.

Strongyloidiasis

Strongyloides stercoralis is a small nematode with free-living forms found in soil, while parasitic forms (i.e., the adult female) live within intestinal crypts in the duodenum, the jejunal mucosal villi, or in the submucosa; the male does not enter the intestinal mucosa but are passed in stool. Normally, the adult worms bore into the mucosa and produce eggs, which pass out with stool. The eggs deposited by the female may hatch the rhabditiform larvae that enter the lumen of the intestine to be passed out in stool. Eggs released from these organisms normally mature in the soil to produce more rhabditiform larvae. In the environment, these larvae transform to the filariform infective larvae that can directly penetrate intact skin of humans and other mammals. For reasons not fully understood, in some patients the transformation from rhabditiform to the filariform infective larvae can also occur while still in the lower bowel or perianal area, before being passed out in the stool. The filariform larvae burrow through the intestinal wall and perianal skin to reinfect the patient, a phenomenon known as autoinfection. After burrowing through the skin, the filariform larvae enter the lymphatics and, ultimately, the venous system where they are carried to the pulmonary capillaries. Here, they migrate out of the blood vessels into alveoli, up the airways and then down through the esophagus to reach the small bowel. Symptoms include ground itch, urticarial, and pulmonary symptoms. A worm burden in the intestines might lead to a malabsorption syndrome. Chronic strongyloidiasis and autoinfection have been observed in World War II veterans who were in POW camps on the Pacific front up to 30 years after their return to the United States and the United Kingdom.

The most serious consequence of *S. stercoralis* infection occurs as a result of massive autoinfection caused by immunosuppression (e.g., persons on steroid therapy, organ transplant, HTLV-1 coinfection, cancer, or malnutrition) or following treatment of lymphoma, leukemia, or leprosy with corticosteroids or cytotoxic drugs. In this condition, known as the hyperinfection syndrome, the autoinfection cycle escalates to generate massive infection with millions of parasites throughout the whole intestine and hematogenous dissemination of the invasive form of the filariform larvae to all organs, including the liver, lungs, and brain.

As part of this hyperinfection syndrome in immunocompromised patients, CNS involvement may be manifest by headache, altered mentation, meningismus, focal or generalized seizures, or motor weakness. Encephalopathy is common and pyogenic meningitis caused by strongyloides larvae in the meninges can occur. A unique aspect of the hyperinfection syndrome is the likelihood that meningitis and septic shock due to *E. coli* and other gram-negative enteric organisms can occur. These gram-negative infections are thought to be caused by the enteric organisms being carried either on the larvae or within the gut of the larvae as they migrate through the tissues, resulting in bacterial meningitis once the CNS is invaded. Although an eosinophilia is common in strongyloidiasis, it is almost never seen in patients with the hyperinfection syndrome because of existing immunosuppression (usually corticosteroids) and is an indication of poor prognosis—the lower the eosinophil count, the worse the prognosis. The diagnosis can be made by identifying the larvae in stool, duodenal aspirate, or sputum. For massive strongyloidiasis, treatment with thiabendazole 25 mg/kg twice daily for 10 days has been effective. Ivermectin therapy has also proven effective in the treatment of the hyperinfection syndrome.

Toxocariasis

Toxocara canis and *Toxocara cati* are nematodes that infect the intestines of dogs and cats, respectively. As a result of this infection in domestic animals, the eggs of these organisms are distributed widely in the soil to which humans may be exposed. Human infection occurs when eggs are ingested and hatch in the small intestine. Larvae then migrate through the intestinal wall and into various tissues of the body, and most often manifest as visceral larvae migrans (VLM). Symptoms include abdominal pain, hepatomegaly, anorexia, nausea, vomiting, lethargy, behavioral changes, pneumonia, cough, wheezing, lymphadenopathy, or fever. The hallmark of the disease is striking eosinophilia. Older children, adolescents, or young adults may develop unilateral loss of vision; ophthalmoscopy reveals a lesion not unlike a retinoblastoma. When eosinophilia is seen in small children between the ages of 2 and 4, it readily suggests a clinical diagnosis of VLM. Though very uncommon, CNS involvement can manifest as dementia, meningoencephalitis, myelitis, cerebral vasculitis, epilepsy, or optic neuritis [393–396]. CNS involvement in patients with VLM may also present as encephalopathy with seizures. Other manifestations include meningoencephalitis, transverse myelitis, and psychiatric disturbances.

Treatment is diethylcarbamazine 2 mg/kg orally three times daily for 10 days or albendazole 400 mg orally twice a day for 5 days. Steroids are indicated for ocular disease and may be necessary for severe lung, heart, or CNS involvement. The differential diagnosis of parasitic eosinophilic meningitis includes infections caused by *Angiostrongylus cantonensis* and *Gnathostoma* species; meningitis caused by these organisms is caused by their random migration into the CNS.

Syphilis

Syphilis is caused by the spirochete *Treponema pallidum*, belonging to the family Spirochaetaceae. The organisms are thin, tightly coiled bacteria that exhibit a characteristic undulating movement under direct dark-field observation. Syphilis is categorized as early (primary, secondary, and tertiary) or late (late latent, late benign, and late clinical infection). Before penicillin became available, the prevalence of primary and secondary syphilis was high but fell rapidly with the introduction of antimicrobials after the Second World War. Syphilis is transmitted primarily through sexual contact between infected and uninfected persons. Less common modes of transmission include nonsexual contact with infectious lesions, such as breaks in the skin or mucous membrane that come into contact with infectious lesions containing spirochetes, transplacentally from mother to fetus in utero, transfusion of contaminated blood products, or laboratory accidents.

Pathogenesis

The initial manifestation is the primary chancre, which begins at the site of inoculation as a painless papule and rapidly ulcerates into a relatively painless and indurated ulcer that is dark-field positive. The primary chancre is frequently associated with regional, nonsuppurative, nontender lymphadenopathy. The chancre generally heals spontaneously within 3–6 weeks. The incubation period from exposure to clinical disease can range anywhere from 3 weeks to 3 months. Spirochetemia occurs at the onset of the primary chancre. For a period of 2–8 weeks following the primary chancre, the treponemes migrate to the lymphatics and gain access to the circulation to cause a systemic illness (the secondary syphilis phase) in approximately 30 % of untreated patients. Systemic manifestations of secondary syphilis include fever, malaise, headache, pharyngitis, anorexia, weight loss, and arthralgias. The classic manifestations are maculopapular, papular, or pustular skin lesions, which are distributed over the entire body, including the palms and soles and patients may develop patchy alopecia. Genital ulcerations, such as condylomata lata and mucous patches, develop in about 20–35 % of those with clinically evident secondary syphilis.

During the secondary syphilis phase, between 8 and 40 % of affected persons develop some evidence of CNS involvement, including meningitis and cranial nerve involvement; patients may complain of headache, decreased vision, tinnitus, and vertigo. During the secondary stage, spirochetes can be found in the blood, CNS, and aqueous humor of the eye. However, direct dark-field examination of the CSF in these patients rarely reveals spirochetes. Using rabbit inoculation to test CSF for viable *T. pallidum*, Lukehart and coworkers found that 30 % of 40 patients with primary and secondary syphilis had viable treponemes in CSF and that CNS invasion by the spirochete is common in early syphilis and is apparently independent of HIV infection [397].

The clinical manifestations of secondary syphilis resolve spontaneously, without antimicrobial therapy after a period of weeks to several months to enter the latent stage. Patients, however, remain seroreactive. During the secondary syphilis phase, patients generally remain asymptomatic until manifestations of tertiary syphilis appear years later in one-third of untreated patients. Clinically, tertiary syphilis is divided into three general categories: neurosyphilis, cardiovascular syphilis, and gummatous syphilis.

Neurosyphilis

Neurosyphilis is due to damage produced by meningovasculitis and degenerative parenchymal changes in the entire CNS. Since spirochete invasion of the CNS occurs during the primary stage, a small population of patients has continuing CNS involvement. Syphilitic meningitis is an early manifestation, usually occurring within the first 2 years of the primary infection and resulting from small vessel arteritis in the meninges, which accounts for the typical symptoms of headache, nausea, and vomiting seen in approximately 90 % of patients. In addition, up to 45 % of patients with syphilitic meningitis may have cranial nerve palsies. Seizures have been reported in 17 % and fever occurs in less than 50 %. The CSF white count is almost invariably abnormal, but there is only a mild decrease in CSF glucose.

Although there is some overlap of symptomatology, meningovascular syphilis presents with findings of meningitis together with focal neurologic findings due to syphilitic arteritis. The peak incidence of this condition is approximately 7 years after acquisition of syphilis and accounts for approximately 12 % of patients with CNS involvement [398–401]. Patients with meningovascular syphilis generally present with a history of several weeks to months of prodromal symptoms and signs, such as headache, vertigo, personality changes, behavioral changes, insomnia or seizures, and stroke-like neurologic deficits, most frequently involving the distribution of vessels in the territory of the middle cerebral artery followed by that of the basilar artery. Thus, while the distribution of strokes in such patients may be similar to that of the patient with atherosclerotic disease, the occlusive symptoms develop gradually over a period of time in meningeal vascular syphilis as opposed to sudden onset in patients with atherosclerotic strokes [401]. In contrast to the findings from the preantibiotic era, neurosyphilis is now most often identified in young patients with HIV coinfection [402, 403].

The majority of neurologic manifestations of tertiary syphilis involves the CNS parenchyma and is classified as parenchymatous neurosyphilis. This category includes two classical syndromes: general paresis and tabes dorsalis. In contradistinction to the pathogenesis of syphilitic meningitis or meningovascular syphilis, these syndromes result from progressive neuronal destruction with fibrosis and atrophy rather than ischemic damage from vasculitis. General paresis, also known as general paralysis of the insane, is a chronic progressive meningoencephalitis with a peak incidence 10–20 years after acquisition of syphilis. Patients generally present with gradual deterioration of mental functioning characterized by difficulties in concentration, irritability, and deficits of higher cognitive function. As the condition progresses, these manifestations become more obvious and symptoms may mimic psychiatric disease, including delusions, paranoia, emotional lability, memory loss, or dementia. Difficulties with motor control then develop with a loss of facial muscle and extremity tone, loss of fine motor control, and the development of tremors and dysarthria. Subsequently, patients may have seizures, loss of bowel and bladder control, and paralysis; the pupils become unresponsive to light and painful stimuli and may be constricted and unequal in size (the Argyll Robertson pupil). Untreated, the disease follows a progressive or subacute course over 3–4 years. Pathologically there is diffuse cortical atrophy, dilatation of the ventricles, and neuronal dropout with accompanying gliosis. Spirochetes can be demonstrated in 25–40 % of patients with silver stain. The diagnosis is established by a combination of the clinical presentation, positive serology, and elevated CSF white count and protein.

Tabes dorsalis results from progressive neuronal degeneration, especially the dorsal roots and the posterior column of the spinal cord. It has a peak incidence that is generally later than that of paresis, approximately 15–20 years after infection, and the progression of this condition is somewhat slower than that of paresis. The classical early symptomatology is "lightning pains" in the distribution of nerve roots. These pains are described as lancinating, lasting for minutes to hours, and most often involve the lower extremities. Ten percent to 20 % of patients with tabes may also present with episodic attacks of abdominal pain. In addition to pain, some patients experience episodic paresthesias. Ultimately, patients experience progressive loss of vibration and pro-prioceptive sensation, particularly in the lower extremities. As a result, the patients exhibit a characteristic broad-based, shuffling gait and may develop Charcot joints. Muscular atrophy develops in approximately 20 % of patients. The Argyll Robertson pupil, in which one or both pupils constrict with accommodation but do not react directly to light, is a characteristic feature of both general paresis and tabes dorsalis. Pathologically there is atrophy of the posterior columns of the spinal cord with inflammatory infiltrates and loss of neurons. In contrast to paresis, it is unusual to be able to stain the spirochete in nerve tissue. The diagnosis is readily made from the characteristic neurologic findings together with positive serology. However, CSF leukocytosis is observed in only 50 % of patients, and protein elevation is seen in approximately 53 % of patients.

Syphilitic gummas are progressive granulomatous tumor-like lesions primarily involving skin, mucous membranes, and bone but which can develop in any organ in the body including the brain. Gummas may arise in almost any part of the CNS but are most often associated with the pia mater and consist of rubbery masses varying in size from several millimeters to centimeters [404, 405]. Localized findings range from small superficial nodules to large radiating lesions. CNS symptoms depend on the anatomic location of the lesions.

Serologic Testing

Laboratory diagnosis of syphilis depends on the stage of the disease and clinical manifestations. Patients with lesions on moist skin or mucous membranes during either primary or secondary syphilis can usually be diagnosed by the demonstration of treponemes on dark-field microscopy. While treponemes can be demonstrated in dry lesions or lymph nodes by biopsy or saline aspiration, the yield is considerably lower. Serologic tests for syphilis are generally divided into two different types: nontreponemal and treponemal tests. Nontreponemal tests measure IgG or IgM antibodies directed at cardiolipin, which is released when the treponeme damages cells during an infection. Thus, a positive nontreponemal test is indicative of an active infection, but a confirmatory test with a treponemal test is required to verify that it is indeed a syphilis infection that is causing elevated cardiolipin levels. Currently, a standardized mixture of cardiolipin, cholesterol, and lecithin which has fewer false-positive reactions is used and forms the basis of today's standardized tests. The most common of these are the classic venereal disease research laboratory (VDRL), in which agglutination of the cardiolipin, cholesterol, and lecithin antigen is carried out on a slide using heated serum; the rapid plasma reagin (RPR) card test; the automated reagin test (ART); or the toluidine red unheated test (TRUST). Because of the stringency of the technical requirements for the test, the VDRL is generally performed only on CSF and serum screening tests are generally done with the RPR and its variants. Specific treponemal tests for syphilis include the *T. pallidum* hemagglutination (TPHA) test, the microhemagglutination test with *T. pallidum* antigen, the fluorescent treponemal antibody-absorption test (FTA-abs), the enzyme-linked immunosorbent assay (ELISA), and the hemagglutination treponemal test for syphilis (HATTS).

Nontreponemal tests (RPR and VDRL) rise during primary syphilis and reach their peak in secondary syphilis. They slowly decline with advancing age. With treatment, they revert to normal over a few weeks. It is important to note that the serologic response to syphilis increases gradually over the course of the primary infection, so that when the chancre is first observed no more than 10–20 % of patients may be seropositive by any method. However, this will increase with the duration of the chancre during primary infection to approximately 70 % for both the treponemal and nontreponemal tests by the time the chancre heals. During secondary syphilis, serologic tests, whether treponemal or nontreponemal, are positive in almost 100 % of patients.

Early treatment of the primary infection should render the patient seronegative within a year. Treatment of syphilis during the secondary and latent stages will generally result in a significant fall in the titer of the nontreponemal tests. These tests should be negative within 1 year in a patient treated for primary syphilis or within 2 years for a patient treated for secondary syphilis. Patients who remain seropositive by nontreponemal tests after treatment probably have either persistent infection or the so-called biologic false-positive sometimes seen in patients with HIV infection [406, 407].

In general, once the treponemal tests become positive, they remain so for life even if the patient has been successfully treated. Serologic tests can be used to diagnose neurosyphilis during the latent and late latent stages by testing CSF for VDRL antibodies. With the exception of rare false-positive results, possibly resulting from blood contamination, a reactive CSF-VDRL in the absence of substantial contamination of CSF with blood is diagnostic of neurosyphilis.

Although the specificity of the CSF-VDRL in diagnosing likely active neurosyphilis is 100 %, the sensitivity is only about 27 % and, in early syphilis, is of unknown prognostic significance [408, 409]. The insensitivity of the CSF-VDRL test limits its usefulness as a screening test for neurosyphilis. The CSF-FTA-abs test appears more sensitive for screening CSF but is less specific than the CSF-VDRL test in distinguishing currently active neurosyphilis from past syphilis. These findings imply that clinical judgment remains the sine qua non for establishing the diagnosis of active neurosyphilis. Most other tests are both insensitive and nonspecific and must be interpreted in relation to other test results and the

clinical assessment. Furthermore, one cannot use the more sensitive treponemal antibody tests with CSF to diagnose neurosyphilis as these antibodies cross the blood–brain barrier and are therefore likely to be present in the CSF of all patients who have positive serum treponemal tests for syphilis. Thus, a positive CSF treponemal test does not provide any additional information to that obtained by testing serum alone. For example, in one study the CSF-FTA-abs test was positive in 48 patients of whom only 15 had clinical neurosyphilis [408].

While one can resort to sophisticated methods of CSF analysis, such as levels of CSF treponemal antibody compared with serum levels adjusted for changes in the blood–brain barrier by using serum/CSF albumin ratios, and demonstrating a significantly higher than expected CSF level of specific treponemal antibody, it is probably safer to treat patients who have a reactive serum testing if they have any clinical signs of neurosyphilis. If the patient has no clinical manifestations of neurosyphilis and preventive treatment for latent neurosyphilis is being considered, treatment should be based on the presence of an abnormal number of white blood cells in the CSF rather than trying to fine tune the serologic diagnosis. Various studies using PCR have shown that DNA from *T. pallidum* can be detected in the CSF of patients with neurosyphilis. However, it remains unclear whether a positive PCR assay means that the patient has to be treated for latent neurosyphilis or that a negative test excludes the diagnosis of neurosyphilis. Neuroimaging using CT scanning or MRI can be used to document CNS gummas or other complications of tertiary syphilis.

In a recent review, Ghanem underscored the point that there is no gold standard for the diagnosis of neurosyphilis [403]. He also made the point that CDC's criteria for the diagnosis of neurosyphilis are based on surveillance definitions used mainly for epidemiologic purposes. He rendered two clinical categories of neurosyphilis: (1) "confirmed" neurosyphilis, which is defined as any stage of syphilis plus a reactive CSF-VDRL, and (2) presumptive neurosyphilis defined as any stage of syphilis, a nonreactive CSF-VDRL, a CSF pleocytosis, or elevated protein, with clinical signs or symptoms consistent with syphilis without an alternate diagnosis to account for these clinical features [403].

Asymptomatic neurosyphilis is defined by the presence of CSF abnormalities consistent with neurosyphilis in persons with serological evidence of syphilis and no neurological symptoms or signs [403]. Also, asymptomatic neurosyphilis can occur in both early and latent stages of syphilis. For example, among a large population with defined latent syphilis and no evidence of symptomatic neurological disease, 13.5 % were found to have asymptomatic neurosyphilis [410]. Moreover, patients with latent syphilis and asymptomatic neurosyphilis are more likely to have syphilitic involvement of the skin [410].

Treatment

The CSF is always abnormal in active disease, and only active disease responds to treatment. The preferred treatment for all manifestations of neurosyphilis is intravenous aqueous crystalline penicillin G 12–24 million units/day given in six divided doses for 10–14 days. Alternatively, 2.4 million units of procaine penicillin G can be given intramuscularly together with 500 mg/day of probenecid four times a day for 10–14 days. In penicillin-allergic patients, doxycycline 200 mg orally each day for 21 days or ceftriaxone 1 g IM or IV for 14 days has been recommended. However, treatment failures have been documented with ceftriaxone, especially in HIV-infected patients. Patients with syphilitic meningitis or meningovascular syphilis generally respond to treatment with the exception of cases in which the patient has focal cranial nerve abnormalities associated with syphilitic meningitis or larger ischemic defects caused by the arteritis associated with meningovascular syphilis.

For patients with tabes dorsalis or general paresis, improvement approaching cure is relatively uncommon and, in fact, for a majority of patients, disease progression continues despite "adequate" penicillin treatment [411]. Penicillin remains the drug of choice for all forms of neurosyphilis, but disease progression has been frequently reported following the use of penicillin G benzathine [398]. Thus, documentation of CSF resolution over the months following penicillin therapy is required to confirm curative treatment.

Patients with asymptomatic neurosyphilis appear to respond very well to treatment. In one study, 89 % of 454 patients who initially had ≥10 leukocytes/mm^3 of CSF had normalized their cell counts at a 1-year follow-up, as had 69 % of those with abnormal protein prior to treatment [412]. Because patients with primary and secondary syphilis are curable with standard treatment of benzathine penicillin G 2.4 million units IM weekly for three weekly doses, the question of proper treatment always arises when an asymptomatic patient is found to have a positive VDRL, RPR, or other screening test for syphilis. The problem is that this regimen does not reliably provide CSF levels in excess of 0.018 μg/mL of CSF in all patients, which is believed to be necessary to kill spirochetes within the CNS [413–415]. The treatment of cerebral gummas is IV penicillin G with neuroimaging follow-up recommended for most patients [416]. Surgery should be reserved for those unresponsive to antibiotics or those with acutely elevated intracranial pressure [416]. All patients found to have serologic evidence of syphilis, assuming that false-positive tests such as those due to pregnancy and other intercurrent illness can be ruled out, should have serologic testing for HIV because the ability to eradicate syphilis is considerably lower in HIV-infected patients and re-treatment may be necessary.

Lyme Disease

Lyme disease is due to systemic infection with the *microaerophilic* spirochete *Borrelia burgdorferi* and the body's immune response to the infection. Lyme disease was first recognized in the United States in the early 1970s when Dr. Allen Steere at Yale University investigated an outbreak of juvenile rheumatoid arthritis in the small towns of Lyme, Old Lyme, and East Haddam, Connecticut. In the initial report, they identified and ascertained 39 children and 12 adults who presented with a classic, characteristic, remitting, relapsing oligoarticular arthritis with onset in the summer or early fall. All of these patients lived in rural areas and half of the patients lived on two adjacent country roads. In addition, 13 of these patients had noted an unusual skin lesion an average of 4 months before the onset of the arthritis [417]. Subsequent prospective studies then defined neurologic abnormalities such as Bell's palsy, sensory radiculoneuritis, lymphocytic meningitis, and cardiac conduction abnormalities also associated with Lyme disease. These studies showed that at least a quarter of the patients remembered a tick bite at the site of the initial skin lesion, and based on examination of the actual tick from one of these patients, the vector was identified as *Ixodes scapularis* [418–420]. The agent of Lyme disease was finally isolated by Dr. Willy Burgdorfer from the Rocky Mountain Laboratory in Hamilton, Montana, when he was searching for evidence of Rocky Mountain spotted fever in ticks isolated from New York State. No rickettsia were found; however, spirochetes were seen in stains of the insect's digestive tract [421, 422].

Pathogenesis

The clinical manifestations fall broadly into three stages: early localized, early disseminated, and chronic disseminated. Approximately 50 % of untreated patients progress to disseminated disease. During the first stage, the earliest manifestations of Lyme disease occur at the site of the tick bite beginning as a red macule or papule that may expand to an area 10–15 cm with red outer borders and partial central clearing—the so-called "bull's eye" skin rash. The lesion develops as early as 3 days and as late as 30 days following the initial bite and generally lasts 3–4 weeks. It is most commonly located on the thigh or groin and develops in approximately 80 % of patients [419, 423, 424]. Following the entry of the spirochete into the patient via the tick bite, dissemination of the spirochete occurs during the development of this initial lesion, and while some patients may develop multiple secondary annular lesions that are similar to the primary site lesion, others may clear the infection without developing symptoms. All patients largely remain seropositive. In the second stage, the organism produces symptoms by direct invasion. Systemic symptoms of fatigue, lethargy, and malaise along with generalized lymphadenopathy, meningismus, encephalopathy, migratory musculoskeletal pain, splenomegaly, sore throat, and cough may develop in varying degrees during this early disseminated phase [423, 424]. For the most part, the systemic manifestations as well the erythema chronicum migrans lesions themselves usually resolve without treatment in 3–4 weeks. Untreated, however, the Lyme disease spirochete becomes sequestered and persists in various tissues, particularly the CNS, joints, heart, and the skin.

In some patients with meningitis, particularly in Europe, where the disease is caused by a different species of spirochete, significant neurologic abnormalities develop, including cranial neuritis which can present as an isolated facial palsy (motor and sensory), radicular mononeuritis multiplex, or myelitis alone or in varying combinations. Although these patients may have some neck stiffness on extreme flexion, typical Kernig's and Brudzinski's signs are not present. Patients may complain of excruciating headache as well as severe musculoskeletal pain. Early on, examination of the CSF may be normal, but patients may develop a lymphocytic pleocytosis with a normal glucose level.

During this early dissemination stage, cardiac symptoms and signs manifest, usually atrioventricular block with varying degrees of other forms occasionally noted including complete heart block, which rarely persists for more than a week and generally does not require the insertion of a pacemaker [425, 426]. Occasional patients have been described with osteomyelitis, myositis, panniculitis, eosinophilic fasciitis, conjunctivitis, or even deeper involvement of the orbital structures including panophthalmitis and choroid retinitis with exudative retinal detachment or interstitial keratitis.

The third stage of Lyme disease is characterized by arthritis, which develops in about 60 % of untreated patients. Symptoms include intermittent attacks of pain particularly involving the large joints (e.g., the knee), in an asymmetric pattern. Attacks of acute arthritis generally last weeks to months followed by periods of remission. Joint fluid counts range from 500 to 100,000 cells/mm³ with a high percentage of polymorphonuclear leukocytes. Even untreated, this condition resolves gradually over a period of years.

The late manifestations of CNS involvement of Lyme disease generally develop a year or more after the onset of illness and generally do not improve spontaneously. In both North American and European forms of this disease, persistence of the *B. burgdorferi* spirochete has been demonstrated in CSF and in brain parenchyma up to 9 years after the onset of illness [425–429]. The most common neurologic symptoms are speech abnormalities, limb weakness, gait difficulties, ataxia, bladder dysfunction, visual changes, hearing loss, mood changes, sleep disorders, and deteriorating memory and concentration. Symptoms of late progressive Lyme encephalomyelitis may develop either acutely or gradually and then worsen progressively over the ensuing months to years [427, 429–438]. Progression may be gradual or stepwise, characterized by sudden deterioration and only partial improvement between episodes. Headaches, nausea, vomiting, and neck stiffness have been reported but occur less often, while mental deficits such as behavioral changes, poor memory, and concentration are common. More severe changes including confusion, disorientation, dementia, delirium, and somnolence can occur. Symptoms such as apraxia, myoclonus, hemiparesthesia, and visual field abnormalities have been reported. Spinal cord involvement is common and myelitis may present as a progressive paraparesis or quadriparesis that can become very severe. Approximately 45 % of patients have cranial nerve palsies; involvement of the optic, facial, oculomotor, and vestibulocochlear cranial nerves have all been reported [426, 431, 439]. Peripheral radiculoneuritis occurs in less than 10 % of patients.

The CSF is abnormal in almost all cases of CNS involvement in Lyme disease. Generally, there is CSF pleocytosis, predominantly monocytic in the range of 100–200 cells/mm³, although levels as high as 2,300 cells/mm³ have been reported. CSF protein concentrations are usually greater than 50 mg/dL, usually in the range of 100–200 mg/dL, although concentrations levels as high as 1,800 mg/dL have been reported; glucose is generally normal to low. Oligoclonal bands specific for *B. burgdorferi* may be present.

EEG and CT abnormalities, including infarcts in the internal capsule, thalamus, lentiform nucleus, hydrocephalus, and cerebral atrophy, have been reported [430, 432, 440–443]. MRI shows additional lesions such as multifocal white matter abnormalities, infarcts, periventricular and sub-insular cavities, as well as atrophy of the pons and medulla [432, 440, 442–445]. MRI imaging in patients with myelitis have shown diffuse or focal signal abnormalities in relevant parts of the spinal cord [432, 446–449].

In contrast to the dramatic and objectively documented neurologic abnormalities and syndromes seen in a small number of patients with Lyme encephalopathy, a certain number of North American patients have reported the development of a less dramatic but nonetheless disabling CNS symptom complex. These patients complain of overwhelming fatigue, accompanied by loss of memory and concentration, and almost always without physical neurologic abnormalities. Psychological testing shows abnormalities or dysfunction in memory, ability to learn or acquire new information, attention span, concentration, problem solving, perceptual motor performance, and verbal fluency. Although depression and irritability are frequently reported, general fatigue appears to be the overriding complaint. Many of these patients fit the definition of the chronic fatigue syndrome as defined by the CDC. Objective laboratory and radiographic signs of infection are generally absent. CSF pleocytosis is present in less than 5 % of the cases, and CSF protein is elevated in only a minority of patients. Oligoclonal bands for *B. burgdorferi* are absent and patients with these complaints may or may not have antibodies to Lyme disease in the serum. Some of these patients have been reported to have MRI abnormalities, such as focal areas of increased signal in deep cerebral white matter [441, 450–452]. In general, symptoms in these patients do not improve spontaneously. A variable number of persons with this condition apparently do respond to courses of antimicrobial therapy, sometimes for 6 months or more [441, 450–453].

A number of North American patients have developed a mild multifocal polyneuropathy distinct from the meningopolyneuritis of early disseminated Lyme disease as a manifestation of late Lyme disease. Intermittent tingling and paresthesia of the extremities are the most common symptoms, occurring in approximately 50 % of patients with this form of late Lyme disease. The onset is generally 8 months to several years after the initial infection. The symptoms are usually distal, may be symmetric or asymmetric, and can involve both arms and legs. About 25 % of patients present with carpal tunnel syndrome or develop it at some point. Radicular pain occurs in 25–50 % of those with this syndrome; this pain is intermittent, asymmetric, and multifocal, typically radiating from the spine into the limbs or trunk [441, 452, 454–457]. Sensory changes such as mild stocking and glove distal sensory loss, as well as distal asymmetrical or truncal sensory loss also occur [441, 452, 454, 455, 458, 459].

Objective evidence of organic disease is much more common in these patients than in those reporting symptoms of chronic fatigue, with up to 83 % of patients having electromyographic abnormalities demonstrable particularly among those with distal paresthesia. In addition, CSF abnormalities, mostly in the form of increased protein concentration and intrathecal antibody synthesis specific for *B. burgdorferi* are found in up to 70 % of patients with these symptoms [441, 458]. Treatment with antimicrobials may improve the paresthesia and electrophysiologic conduction abnormalities but may require prolonged regimens from 3 to 7 months [441, 450, 454–456, 458]. Improvement among patients with radicular pain is less frequent and is only seen in about 50 %.

The diagnosis of Lyme disease can be made with reasonable assurance by a well-documented history of a tick bite and together with clinical evidence of typical skin lesions (erythema chronicum migrans). However, during this early stage of the disease, only 30–40 % of patients will have a serologic test positive for Lyme disease in an acute serum specimen, and only 60–70 % of these patients will be positive in the convalescent sera 2–4 weeks later. CDC recommends a two-step approach for serological testing: the first step in the workup of patients with putative Lyme symptoms is to obtain an antibody titer using an ELISA test to screen for the presence of antibody; the second step is confirmation of positive titers with a Western blot assay; both IgG and IgM antibodies are formed. However, persistence of the IgM antibody alone in the absence of an IgG response after the first month of illness may signal a false-positive reaction. After the first 1–2 months of infection, over 90 % of patients will have a specific IgG antibody response to the spirochete. It has been noted that patients treated effectively early in the course of erythema chronicum migrans may never develop a humoral immune response, although cellular immunity may be demonstrated and persist for years.

Treatment

Treatment of early dissemination and localized erythema chronicum migrans consists of doxycycline 100 mg twice a day for 20–30 days or amoxicillin 500 mg three times daily for 20–30 days, with some experts recommending the addition of probenecid 500 mg three times daily to the amoxicillin regimen. Cefuroxime axetil 500 mg orally three times daily for 2–3 weeks has also been recommended as has erythromycin 400 kg/mg/day in four divided doses for 2–4 weeks in children. For patients with arthritis, treatment with doxycycline or amoxicillin is extended to 1–2 months, and intravenous ceftriaxone 2 g a day for 14–30 days is also recommended.

For patients with early or late neurologic abnormalities, ceftriaxone 2 g IV daily for 2–4 weeks is generally recommended. Alternatives include penicillin G 20 million units IV in four divided doses daily for up to 30 days, as well as doxycycline 100 mg orally three times per day for 14–30 days. Treatment failures have been reported for all of these regimens and treatment may need to be repeated.

Cardiac abnormalities are treated as for early infection in those patients with first-degree AV block; IV ceftriaxone or penicillin is used for higher degrees of AV block. In patients with neurologic manifestations of early disseminated Lyme disease, IV therapy with penicillin or ceftriaxone can lead to a mild Herxheimer-like reaction with worsening of pain and fever during the first 18–20 h [425, 460]. In general, meningismus, radicular pain, and systemic symptoms improve within days although residual fatigue, arthralgias, and muscular skeletal pain can persist for some time thereafter. Motor deficits improve more slowly, over 2–3 months, and sometimes never fully recover. CNS abnormalities usually stop progressing and begin to improve slowly, but residual deficits may remain [428, 460–464]. CSF cell counts respond over the course of treatment but may not return to normal for several months, and the protein concentration falls even more slowly and may remain elevated for up to 1 year in some patients. If the patient does not respond by the end of the second week, treatment should be extended for at least another 2 weeks.

The severe abnormalities of late Lyme disease generally respond well to high-dose penicillin, doxycycline, or ceftriaxone [430, 432, 439, 442, 443, 449, 451, 452, 462–467]. Altogether 80–90 % of patients improve with IV cephalosporins, but recovery is slow and often incomplete, with little change occurring during the treatment itself and only developing over the subsequent weeks after treatment has stopped. At this time, there are no published data that support the routine use of steroid therapy in the management of CNS complications of Lyme disease. Finally, although a controversial issue, there are no convincing data that show prolonged antimicrobial therapy is effective for patients in whom symptoms persist after completing the recommended antimicrobial therapy for acute Lyme disease [468].

Miscellaneous Infections with CNS Complications

Rickettsial Disease

Rickettsiae are small gram-negative, obligate intracellular coccobacilli that are transmitted by tick bites. Rickettsiae grow freely in the cytoplasm of eukaryotic host cells on which they are dependent for nucleotide cofactors and ATP; they do not grow well outside the host cell. They can only be grown in living host cells, such as cell cultures and embryonated eggs. Most rickettsiae have animal reservoirs and are spread by infected arthropod vectors. Infections generally follow the distribution of the main vectors: *Dermacentor andersoni* (the wood tick) is the primary vector in the Western United States; *Dermacentor variabilis* (dog tick) is the principal vector in the Eastern United States. Infections are limited to warmer months.

Following the tick bite, Rickettsiae infect the vascular endothelium lining the small blood vessels causing a vasculitis—the primary pathologic feature of rickettsial infection, particularly RMSF. A combination of endothelial proliferation, necrosis, and perivascular inflammation, predominantly with a mononuclear cell infiltrate, leads to thrombosis and leakage of erythrocytes into surrounding tissues resulting in petechial lesions. Should systemic infection ensue, these vascular lesions occur throughout the body. This is in contrast to the infiltrate of polymorphonuclear leukocytes seen in typical immunocomplex vasculitis.

Rickettsial disease is characterized by fever, headache, rash, myalgias, and myositis. The most important rickettsiosis in the United States is Rocky Mountain spotted fever (RMSF), which is an acute febrile illness caused by *Rickettsia rickettsii*. As the name implies, the disease is seen in the Rocky Mountain States, such as Colorado and Wyoming, but also occurs in the inland parts of North Carolina, Virginia, and other Southeastern States. For RMSF, the incubation period between tick bite and onset of illness is 2–6 days. Fever, headache, rash, mental confusion, and myalgia are the predominant clinical features [469–471]. The rash usually develops on the second or third day of illness, initially on the wrists and ankles followed by spread to the trunk within hours. In contrast with a viral exanthem, the RMSF rash can appear on the palms and soles. About 25 % of patients may have an encephalitis at presentation with lethargy, confusion, or delirium. This may deteriorate to seizures and coma. As a result of the variability of the vessels involved in the CNS, a wide range of clinical neurologic features are associated with RMSF, including seizures, deafness, facial diplegia, gaze palsies, nystagmus, ataxia, dysphasia, transverse myelitis, neurogenic bladder, hemiplegia, and paraplegia or quadriplegia.

The diagnosis of RMSF is fundamentally a clinical diagnosis and depends on the history of a tick bite together with a compatible systemic illness with or without a rash [471]. The diagnosis of RMSF must be considered in all febrile patients who have known or possible exposure to ticks, especially if they live in or have traveled to endemic regions during warmer months [471]. Because culture of rickettsiae is difficult, serological testing remains the mainstay of confirming the diagnosis. However, though serologic diagnosis is highly accurate, it is not readily available in most institutions or as a routine service in the acute setting, and therefore treatment must be started empirically; patients with RMSF who received antirickettsial therapy within 5 days of the onset of symptoms are significantly less likely to die than those in whom therapy, for whatever reasons, was delayed [472].

The basic tenet of RMSF management, then, is the commencement of appropriate antimicrobial therapy without delay in conjunction with supportive therapy where indicated, i.e., IV hydration for hypovolemia or circulatory collapse, mechanical ventilatory support especially if the patient has developed ARDS, blood transfusion, and management of DIC. In adults and children, the recommended dose is doxycycline 100 mg per dose administered twice daily (orally or intravenously) for adults or 2.2 mg/kg body weight per dose administered twice daily (orally or intravenously) for children weighing less than 100 lbs (45.4 kg) [470]. Previously, for children under the age of 8 years, chloramphenicol was recommended because of the tooth discoloration associated with tetracyclines. However, in 1997, the American Academy of Pediatrics Committee on Infectious Diseases revised its recommendations and identified doxycycline as the drug of choice for treating presumed or confirmed RMSF in children of any age, because of the effectiveness of this antimicrobial in reducing attributable morbidity and potential mortality. Sulfonamides may worsen the disease and are therefore contraindicated.

Most patients show improvement within 2 days but may require up 7–10 days in severe cases. Despite modern therapeutic modalities, the fatality rate of RMSF is still in the range of 5–10 % [470]. Even after recovery, CNS abnormalities may persist in a significant number of patients with RMSF, including intellectual defects, impaired fine motor skills, aphasia, and EEG changes. Long-term neurological sequelae includes paraparesis; hearing loss; peripheral neuropathy; bladder and bowel incontinence; cerebellar, vestibular, and motor dysfunction; and language disorders [473]. Sexton and colleague made the point that the mechanism of such abnormalities is rickettsia-induced vasculitis with subsequent infarction of neural tissue and that although early treatment may prevent many, but not all, such complications, other factors, such as age and race, might be playing a role in the pathogenesis of severe disease [474].

Human Ehrlichiosis

Ehrlichia species are tiny, obligate, leukocyte-associated, gram-negative bacteria that replicate in membrane-bound compartments inside the host white blood cells to cause human disease. *Anaplasma phagocytophilum* causes human granulocytotropic anaplasmosis (HGA), previously known as human granulocytotropic ehrlichiosis (HGE). *A. phagocytophilum* is transmitted by *Ixodes scapularis*, which also transmits the agents that cause Lyme disease and babesiosis. *Ehrlichia chaffeensis*, the cause of human monocytic ehrlichiosis (HME), is transmitted by the Lone Star tick found on the whitetail deer and prefers to invade mononuclear leukocytes (e.g., macrophages). Both diseases are transmitted by deer or dog tick bites—HME is relatively common in the South and Southeast United States, while most cases of human HGA so far have been recorded from the upper Midwest, Northeast, and some parts of the South. HGA is the predominant form of ehrlichiosis in the United States and runs second only to Lyme disease as a tick-borne transmitted infection in the United States. More than 2,900 cases of HGA have been reported to the CDC between 1994 and 2005, with the annual number of cases of HGA exceeding that of HME at an estimated annual incidence of 1.6 cases per million in the US [475]. Ehrlichiosis is a seasonal disease with highest rates of occurrence from April to September. DNA studies of the agent that causes HGA show that it is mostly related to *Ehrlichia canis* but probably represents a different subspecies.

Both HGA and HME have incubation periods of about 7 (range 5–14) days after the tick bite. Symptoms of ehrlichiosis include high fever, chills, rigors, malaise, severe headache, myalgias, nausea, and vomiting and may include confusion, disorientation, obtundation, and ataxia in some patients [475]. Presentation may be abrupt or subacute in nature. Compared with RMSF, rashes are relatively uncommon (36 % of HME and 2 % of HGA) and are characteristically maculopapular with a distribution on the upper and lower limbs, trunk, or face. The petechial rash of RMSF is absent in ehrlichiosis. Patients with HME can develop aseptic meningitis and meningoencephalitis or progress to respiratory and renal insufficiency. Patients may develop

hepatosplenomegaly. Although respiratory insufficiency can also occur in HGA, meningoencephalitis is uncommon in this type of human ehrlichiosis.

CSF is frequently normal; other laboratory studies are non-diagnostic or nonspecific; thrombocytopenia is common in both types of ehrlichiosis. Wright stain of a peripheral blood and buffy coat smear might reveal the characteristic intracellular inclusions known as morulae; these inclusions are present in the cytoplasm of neutrophils and monocytes of HGA and HME, respectively. However, presence of morulae in smears is variable. Serologic confirmation of illness is the usual method of diagnosis and is highly accurate but available only from state and other reference laboratories; a fourfold rise of titers is considered diagnostic. The differential diagnosis includes RMSF, Lyme disease, and babesiosis. As with RMSF, treatment with doxycycline (100 mg twice daily) for 14 days or chloramphenicol must be given empirically [470, 475]. Untreated, mortality of all patients with human ehrlichiosis ranges remains significant, ranging from 2 to 10 %.

Human Bartonellosis (Cat-Scratch Disease)

Cat-scratch disease is caused by *Bartonella henselae*, a pleomorphic gram-negative bacillus that binds silver and can be identified by Warthin-Starry stains. The condition develops predominantly in persons under the age of 21 years after receiving a scratch from a kitten or feral cat; the organism is transmitted less commonly by cat fleas. The organism proliferates at the site of the injury and, following an incubation period of 3–21 days, one or more papules develop at the site of the bite or scratch. Regional lymphadenitis ensues with enlargement of epitrochlear, axillary, and cervical lymph nodes, along with fever and malaise. In the typical case of cat-scratch disease, a single enlarged, fluctuant lymph node is the most common occurrence; generalized lymphadenopathy is relatively uncommon. About one-third of patients will develop systemic symptoms, such as fever and malaise. Other clinical manifestations include endocarditis and granulomatous or suppurative hepatosplenic and osseous lesions.

B. henselae involvement of the CNS is not uncommon: patients may actually have a variety of CNS symptoms, including encephalopathy, retinitis, or Parinaud's ocular glandular syndrome (i.e., ocular granuloma or conjunctivitis with preauricular lymphadenopathy). In a large series of 130 seropositive patients with cat-scratch disease, the occurrence of neuroretinitis and encephalopathy was approximately 22 and 15 %, respectively.

Bartonella grows slowly on solid and liquid media and, if suspected, the medical microbiology laboratory should be contacted to hold the cultures for an extended period. Histological features of lymph nodes generally are nonspecific, showing features of chronic granulomatous and acute inflammatory changes. Diagnosis can be made serologically using an indirect immunofluorescence assay or enzyme immunosorbent assay to detect *B. henselae* antibodies; PCR assays have proven are more sensitive and specific at detecting *B. henselae*. Although most cases of cat-scratch disease in the normal host are self-limited and resolve over a period of 3–8 weeks, treatment is recommended. A 5-day course of azithromycin is the treatment of choice. Alternatives are clarithromycin, doxycycline, or ciprofloxacin for 10–14 days [476]. In severe cases, including patients with encephalopathy, IV azithromycin or gentamicin plus rifampin is recommended. Although there are reports of the effectiveness of adjunct steroid therapy in the management of patients with cat-scratch encephalitis, no randomized controlled trials have been carried out to determine whether steroids actually improve patient outcomes [477, 478].

Whipple's Disease

Whipple's disease is a slowly progressive systemic disease caused by *Tropheryma whippelii*, a gram-positive rod-shaped bacterium. The disease primarily affects Caucasian men over the age of 40 years. Whipple's disease is relatively uncommon with most reported cases from North America and Western Europe. The typical clinical manifestations are arthralgias (67 %), diarrhea (76 %), weight loss (92 %), abdominal pain (55 %), and other features of malabsorption [479]. Less commonly, patients may present with fever, chills, CNS abnormalities, seizures, cardiovascular symptoms, endocarditis, or darkening of the skin. CNS involvement is the most serious complication of Whipple's disease with neurological signs documented in 10–40 % of affected patients [479, 480]; damage to the CNS may be irreversible. *T. whippelii* is an unusual bacterium capable of intracellular survival. Left untreated, Whipple's disease is invariably fatal [481]. Although humans are the only known host for *T. whippelii*, a natural source has not been defined. The organism itself is ubiquitous in the environment and has been isolated from the stool of sewage workers suggesting that a possible mode of transmission might be fecal-oral [482]. It appears that the genetic predisposition of the host rather than the genotype of the bacterium is the key risk factor for infection [483, 484].

CNS involvement is one of the more frequent complications of this disease and can, on occasion, occur in the absence of recognized gastrointestinal or systemic involvement. The most frequent neurologic manifestations of Whipple's disease are dementia, decreasing levels of consciousness, progressive supranuclear ophthalmoplegia, myoclonus, and hypothalamic dysfunction. The dementia progresses slowly and is characterized by memory impairment, confusion, personality change, paranoia, emotional instability, and depression [479, 480, 485–491]. An unusual syndrome of synchronized ocular movements and contractions of the jaw, known as oculomasticatory myorhythmia, is sometimes seen and is unique to Whipple's disease [487–489].

The disease is most often diagnosed through upper gastrointestinal endoscopy with biopsy of the small bowel or a mesenteric lymph node. Macroscopically, the duodenal mucosa is pale yellow with dilated villi and ecstatic lymph vessels [479]. Periodic acid-Schiff (PAS) stains will reveal the presence of PAS positive material (e.g., mucin and carbohydrate) with occasional bacilliform organisms. Pathologic involvement of the brain is most often manifest by chalky, yellowish white, 1–2 mm nodules distributed diffusely throughout the cortical and subcortical gray matter of both the cerebrum and the cerebellum. The most frequently involved sites are the temporal, periventricular, and periaqueductal gray matter as well as the hippocampus, hypothalamus, and basal ganglia. Histologically, the nodules are made up of microglia that stain strongly positive with PAS. Although neuroimaging studies with CT or MRI may reveal cerebral atrophy, ring-enhancing lesions, hydrocephalus, or changes consistent with demyelination, these findings are nonspecific for Whipple's disease.

Although PCR diagnosis of Whipple's disease is possible, healthy carriers can have positive PCR even if they do not have Whipple's disease. Thus, PCR is better used when there is clinical suspicion of Whipple's disease rather than for screening [479]. Moreover, because of the wide range of conditions in the differential diagnosis of degenerative CNS diseases, tissue biopsy is generally required for diagnosis. For CNS disease, immunohistochemistry testing using specific antibodies is more sensitive than PAS staining by being able to identify *T. whipplei* in tissues, including those with negative PAS staining [479, 492]. CNS involvement, consistent with the characteristic clinical syndromes of Whipple's disease, and occurring in the setting of neuroimaging studies, biopsy proven systemic Whipple's disease, or PCR are also sufficiently diagnostic [493, 494].

Untreated, Whipple's disease is associated with high mortality rates. And because of the risk of CNS relapse, even while the patient is on oral trimethoprim/sulfamethoxazole, a regimen that includes antimicrobial agents (e.g., a third-generation cephalosporin) that penetrate the CNS is indicated [495, 496]. The initial treatment of CNS involvement in Whipple's disease is ceftriaxone 2 g IV once daily *or* procaine penicillin G 1–2 million units IM once daily, with streptomycin 1 g IM daily and trimethoprim/sulfamethoxazole one DS tablet three times daily for 14 days, followed by trimethoprim/sulfamethoxazole one DS tablet twice daily for at least 1 year [479, 484]. Some clinicians continue therapy for 2 years to life. For severe CNS disease with cerebral lesions, Schneider and colleagues recommend consideration of adjunct corticosteroid therapy as outlined in the guidelines for tuberculous meningitis [271, 479]. Unfortunately, the overall prognosis of CNS Whipple's disease is not good. With antimicrobial therapy, disease progression can be halted, but significant clinical improvement is limited, relapses are frequent, and established neurological defects are difficult to reverse.

Subacute Sclerosing Panencephalitis (SSPE)

This rare, progressive encephalitis usually occurs 2–10 years after an uncomplicated bout of measles. It occurs most frequently between the ages of 4 and 20 years and has a prolonged clinical course. It is thought to be due to reactivation of latent measles virus with high levels of IgM and IgG in the blood and CSF. Most of the pathologic features of the disease are localized to the CNS and retina. Histological findings include those of a subacute meningoencephalitis. Neuronophagia (neuronal degeneration) is common and residual neurons may contain intranuclear or cytoplasmic inclusion bodies. Progressive neurologic disease is characterized by seizures, behavioral abnormalities, and by gradual deterioration in intellectual, motor, and autonomic nervous system function. Management of the disease includes medical control of seizures. Although some authors have advocated the use of antiviral and immunomodulatory therapies (e.g., interferon, ribavirin, and Isoprinosine) to slow the progression of the disease and improve life expectancy in patients, the results are conflicting—the condition continues to show relentless progression. Only 5 % of individuals with SSPE undergo spontaneous remission; the remaining 95 % invariably die within 5 years of diagnosis [497].

Progressive Multifocal Leukoencephalopathy

Progressive multifocal leukoencephalopathy (PML) is an intractable, severe, usually fatal demyelinating disease that is caused by the JC virus, a small double-stranded, nonenveloped DNA virus, closely related to two other polyomavirus: BK virus and the simian virus SV 40 of monkeys. PML is primarily seen in highly immunosuppressed patients, especially those with AIDS and reticuloendothelial malignancies and in patients on immunosuppressive therapy [498]. In the latter case, the immunomodulatory agent most often implicated in the development of PML is the monoclonal antibody natalizumab [499]. It is believed that under conditions of immunosuppression, replication of JC virus in the CNS increases.

Polyomaviruses are not thought to cause disease in immunocompetent individuals. In the pre-AIDS era, it was recognized that the main risk factor for PML was reduced resistance in persons of any age. The typical

clinical features in these patients were impaired vision, motor weakness, and change in mentation, including personality changes [500]. It is estimated that the seroprevalence of the JC virus is 50 % in the 20–29 years age group; this rises to about 68 % in older persons [501]. Even normal brain tissue from immunocompetent individuals with no evidence of PML or demyelinating lesions has been found to harbor JC virus DNA sequences by PCR methodology, suggesting that the JC virus remains latent in the brain before immunosuppression [502–506]. The JC virus has also been detected in the blood of up to 22 % of immunosuppressed patients in the absence of PML [505, 507].

During 1979–1987, deaths related to PML increased fourfold from 1.5/10,000,000 persons in 1979 to 6.1/10,000,000 persons in 1987; this increase was largely attributed to the parallel increase in the incidence of HIV infection in the United States during this period [508]. PML-associated death rates peaked in the mid-1990s and have been decreasing since. For example, death rates have decreased from 2.7 deaths per one million persons during 1992–1995 to 0.6 per one million during 2002–2005 [509]. This significant decrease has been attributed to HAART which became the standard of care in the United States in 1996 [509].

CNS symptoms associated with PML reflect the anatomic location of pathologic brain lesions. PML characteristically presents with progressive focal neurologic defects, primarily hemiparesis, visual field defects, and cognitive deterioration [504, 509–514]. As the disease progresses, aphasia, ataxia, and cranial nerve defects may occur, ultimately resulting in cortical blindness, quadriparesis, profound dementia, seizures, and coma. The average duration of survival is approximately 4 months, although a subset of 5–10 % of patients, including some persons with HIV infection, survives for over a year following diagnosis.

The diagnosis is made from a combination of clinical features with characteristic findings on CT or MRI (Fig. 22.30a, b). The combination of a characteristic clinical picture and typical imaging findings supports a confident presumptive diagnosis of PML [323]. Definitive diagnosis requires brain biopsy and histologic examination, which should demonstrate characteristic cytopathic changes in the oligodendrocytes (Fig. 22.31a, b). These cells typically contain a homogeneous basophilic nuclear inclusion, and virus can be demonstrated by in situ hybridization. Viral damage to the oligodendrocytes, which synthesize and maintain myelin, ultimately leads to widespread, but patchy, multifocal demyelination, surrounded by giant, bizarre astrocytes containing intranuclear inclusions. The pathologic changes generally correlate with the patient's clinical status. Virus particles can be demonstrated in the inclusions by electron microscopy [515].

The CSF is invariably normal in the majority of patients with PML, although slight increases in protein levels and leukocyte counts have been documented for some. JC virus

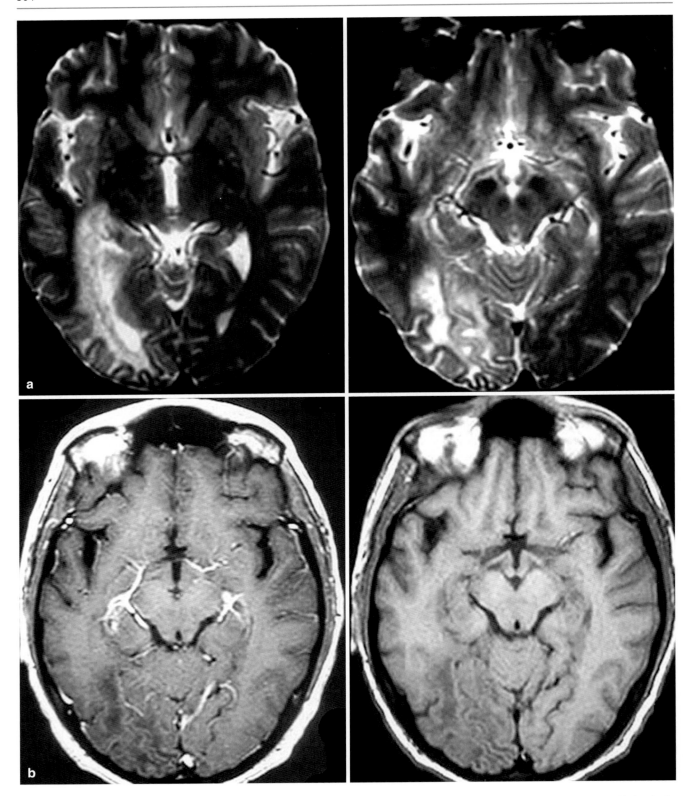

Fig. 22.30 (**a**, **b**) Progressive multifocal leukoencephalopathy (JC virus). Figure (**a**) includes two adjacent T2-w sections. Figure (**b**) includes a post-contrast (*left*) and pre contrast (*right*) images of the same area. These images demonstrate the features of PML with a focal area of abnormality affecting mainly white matter with no appreciable internal contrast enhancement. These findings are nonspecific but in the context of an immune compromised host, PML is an important consideration. PML can cross the midline through the corpus callosum in which case it simulates both lymphoma and diffusely infiltrating astrocytoma

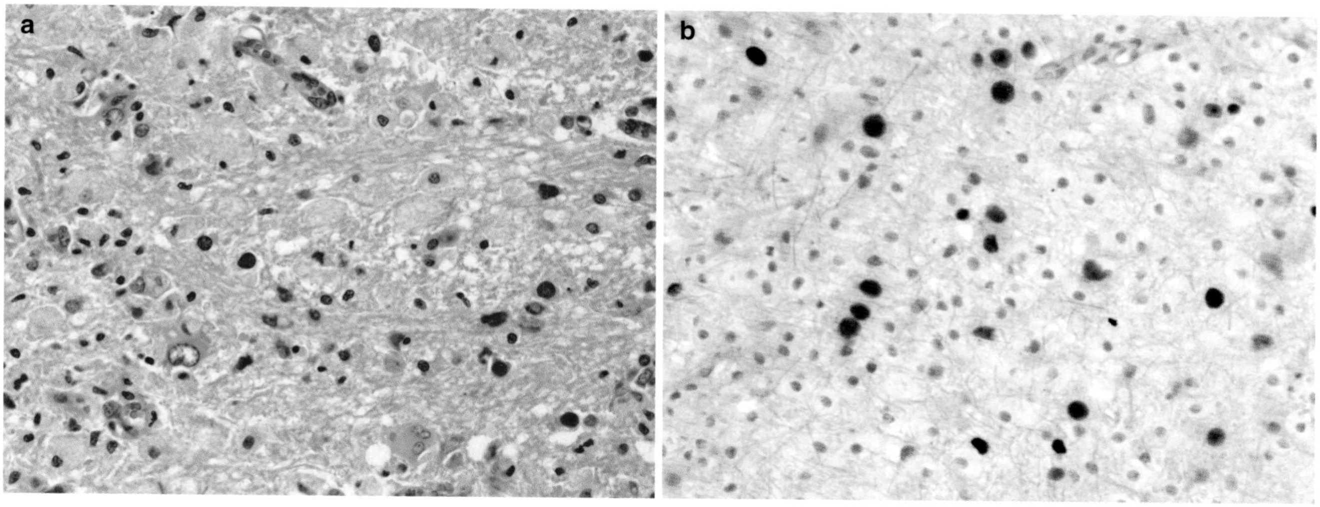

Fig. 22.31 (**a**) Progressive multifocal leukoencephalopathy (JC virus). Numerous foamy macrophages infiltrating CNS white matter and bizarre reactive astrocytes. Scattered oligodendroglia exhibit smudged glassy nuclei (H&E 40×). (**b**) Progressive multifocal leukoencepha- lopathy (JC virus) Immunohistochemical study for JC virus antibody is immunoreactive in infected glial cells (Both courtesy of Anthony Yachnis, MD, and Kelly Devers, MD, University of Florida College of Medicine)

can be detected in the CSF of most patients with PML, whether immunosuppressed or not [503, 516, 517]. In general, however, patients with PML are highly likely to have JC virus DNA in their CSF as compared with normal or immunosuppressed patients without PML. Despite the sensitivity of PCR testing for JC virus, occasional cases of PML have been observed in which no JC virus can be found even in brain tissue at autopsy [518].

Immune reconstitution represents the mainstay of treatment for PML. Thus, for HIV-infected persons with PML, the basis of therapy remains the initiation of antiretroviral therapy for persons who are not on therapy and optimizing the antiretroviral regimen to achieve virologic suppression in patients who are already receiving antiretroviral therapy [323]. With rapid reversal of immunosuppression followed by immunologic recovery, patients may suffer a paradoxical clinical deterioration termed immune reconstitution inflammatory syndrome (IRIS) [499]. High-dose corticosteroids are often recommended if a clinical and imaging syndrome resembling IRIS develops after immune restoration. The JC virus DNA detection in CSF by nucleic acid amplification techniques and the CD4+ cell count are the most promising prognostic marker; higher levels of CD4+ cell counts are associated with improved survival [512].

Cidofovir, an agent used in the treatment of CMV infection, does have activity against polyomaviruses in vitro and in animal models. In a non-blinded, multicenter trial, the 1-year survival among patients with PML was 61 % in HIV-1-infected patients who received HAART with cidofovir compared with 29 % in those who received HAART without cidofovir [519]. Thus, although blinded studies are needed to confirm this observation and treatment guidelines do not rec-

ommend its use, cidofovir should be strongly considered in the empiric treatment of PML, keeping in mind the risk of renal toxicity associated with its use. Initial reports of success with cytosine arabinoside (ara-C) have not been supported by a formal clinical trial [520].

Acknowledgment The first edition of this chapter on central nervous system (CNS) infections was authored by the following individuals: Dr. Kenneth H. Rand (Division of Infectious Diseases, Department of Medicine, University of Florida College of Medicine) and Drs. Arthur J. Ulm and David W. Pincus (Department of Neurological Surgery, University of Florida College of Medicine). Their chapter served as an inspiration and guideline for the organization and content of the second edition chapter on central nervous system (CNS) infections. For that, we are grateful.

References

1. Schuchat A, Robinson K, Wenger JD, et al. Bacterial meningitis in the United States in 1995. Active Surveillance Team. N Engl J Med. 1997;337:970–6.
2. Kim KS. Acute bacterial meningitis in infants and children. Lancet Infect Dis. 2010;10:32–42.
3. Prevention CfDCa. Prevention and control of meningococcal disease. Recommendations of the Advisory Committee on Immunization Practices (ACIP). MMWR Recomm Rep. 2005;54:1–21.
4. Hsu HE, Shutt KA, Moore MR, et al. Effect of pneumococcal conjugate vaccine on pneumococcal meningitis. N Engl J Med. 2009;360:244–56.
5. Fothergill LD, Wright J. Influenzal meningitis: relation of age incidence to bacterial power of blood against causal organism. J Immunol. 1933;24:273–84.
6. Thigpen MC, Whitney CG, Messonnier NE, et al. Bacterial meningitis in the United States, 1998–2007. N Engl J Med. 2011; 364:2016–25.

7. Unhanand M, Mustafa MM, McCracken Jr GH, Nelson JD. Gram-negative enteric bacillary meningitis: a twenty-one-year experience. J Pediatr. 1993;122:15–21.

8. Sarff LD, Platt LH, McCracken Jr GH. Cerebrospinal fluid evaluation in neonates: comparison of high-risk infants with and without meningitis. J Pediatr. 1976;88:473–7.

9. Sarff LD, McCracken GH, Schiffer MS, et al. Epidemiology of Escherichia coli K1 in healthy and diseased newborns. Lancet. 1975;1:1099–104.

10. Schiffer MS, Oliveira E, Glode MP, McCracken Jr GH, Sarff LM, Robbins JB. A review: relation between invasiveness and the K1 capsular polysaccharide of Escherichia coli. Pediatr Res. 1976;10:82–7.

11. Nigrovic LE, Kuppermann N, Malley R. Children with bacterial meningitis presenting to the emergency department during the pneumococcal conjugate vaccine era. Acad Emerg Med. 2008; 15:522–8.

12. Nigrovic LE, Kuppermann N, Macias CG, et al. Clinical prediction rule for identifying children with cerebrospinal fluid pleocytosis at very low risk of bacterial meningitis. JAMA. 2007;297:52–60.

13. May M, Daley AJ, Donath S, Isaacs D. Early onset neonatal meningitis in Australia and New Zealand, 1992–2002. Arch Dis Child Fetal Neonatal Ed. 2005;90:F324–7.

14. Weisfelt M, van de Beek D, Spanjaard L, de Gans J. Nosocomial bacterial meningitis in adults: a prospective series of 50 cases. J Hosp Infect. 2007;66:71–8.

15. Helbok R, Broessner G, Pfausler B, Schmutzhard E. Chronic meningitis. J Neurol. 2009;256:168–75.

16. Kallstrom H, Blackmer Gill D, Albiger B, Liszewski MK, Atkinson JP, Jonsson AB. Attachment of Neisseria gonorrhoeae to the cellular pilus receptor CD46: identification of domains important for bacterial adherence. Cell Microbiol. 2001;3:133–43.

17. Kallstrom H, Liszewski MK, Atkinson JP, Jonsson AB. Membrane cofactor protein (MCP or CD46) is a cellular pilus receptor for pathogenic Neisseria. Mol Microbiol. 1997;25:639–47.

18. Toleman M, Aho E, Virji M. Expression of pathogen-like Opa adhesins in commensal Neisseria: genetic and functional analysis. Cell Microbiol. 2001;3:33–44.

19. Mulks MH, Plaut AG. IgA protease production as a characteristic distinguishing pathogenic from harmless neisseriaceae. N Engl J Med. 1978;299:973–6.

20. Hill DJ, Griffiths NJ, Borodina E, Virji M. Cellular and molecular biology of Neisseria meningitidis colonization and invasive disease. Clin Sci (Lond). 2010;118:547–64.

21. Rouphael NG, Stephens DS. Neisseria meningitidis: biology, microbiology, and epidemiology. Methods Mol Biol. 2012;799: 1–20.

22. Wurzner R, Orren A, Lachmann PJ. Inherited deficiencies of the terminal components of human complement. Immunodefic Rev. 1992;3:123–47.

23. Song JH, Dagan R, Klugman KP, Fritzell B. The relationship between pneumococcal serotypes and antibiotic resistance. Vaccine. 2012;30(17):2728–37.

24. Hausdorff WP, Feikin DR, Klugman KP. Epidemiological differences among pneumococcal serotypes. Lancet Infect Dis. 2005;5:83–93.

25. Pfister HW, Fontana A, Tauber MG, Tomasz A, Scheld WM. Mechanisms of brain injury in bacterial meningitis: workshop summary. Clin Infect Dis. 1994;19:463–79.

26. Pichichero ME, Loeb M, Anderson, Smith DH. Do pili play a role in pathogenicity of Haemophilus influenzae type B? Lancet. 1982;2:960–2.

27. Mason Jr EO, Kaplan SL, Wiedermann BL, Norrod EP, Stenback WA. Frequency and properties of naturally occurring adherent piliated strains of Haemophilus influenzae type b. Infect Immun. 1985;49:98–103.

28. Filippidis A, Fountas KN. Nasal lymphatics as a novel invasion and dissemination route of bacterial meningitis. Med Hypotheses. 2009;72:694–7.

29. Mook-Kanamori BB, Geldhoff M, van der Poll T, van de Beek D. Pathogenesis and pathophysiology of pneumococcal meningitis. Clin Microbiol Rev. 2011;24:557–91.

30. Join-Lambert O, Morand PC, Carbonnelle E, et al. Mechanisms of meningeal invasion by a bacterial extracellular pathogen, the example of Neisseria meningitidis. Prog Neurobiol. 2010;91: 130–9.

31. Flierl MA, Rittirsch D, Huber-Lang MS, Stahel PF. Pathophysiology of septic encephalopathy – an unsolved puzzle. Crit Care. 2010;14:165.

32. Tunkel AR, Scheld WM. Pathogenesis and pathophysiology of bacterial meningitis. Clin Microbiol Rev. 1993;6:118–36.

33. Carpenter RR, Petersdorf RG. The clinical spectrum of bacterial meningitis. Am J Med. 1962;33:262–75.

34. Durand ML, Calderwood SB, Weber DJ, et al. Acute bacterial meningitis in adults. A review of 493 episodes. N Engl J Med. 1993;328:21–8.

35. Gorse GJ, Thrupp LD, Nudleman KL, Wyle FA, Hawkins B, Cesario TC. Bacterial meningitis in the elderly. Arch Intern Med. 1984;144:1603–7.

36. Verghese A, Gallemore G. Kernig's and Brudzinski's signs revisited. Rev Infect Dis. 1987;9:1187–92.

37. Ward MA, Greenwood TM, Kumar DR, Mazza JJ, Yale SH. Josef Brudzinski and Vladimir Mikhailovich Kernig: signs for diagnosing meningitis. Clin Med Res. 2010;8:13–7.

38. Joffe AR. Lumbar puncture and brain herniation in acute bacterial meningitis: a review. J Intensive Care Med. 2007;22:194–207.

39. Joffe AR. Prognostic factors in adults with bacterial meningitis. N Engl J Med. 2005;352:512–5; author reply 5.

40. Oliver WJ, Shope TC, Kuhns LR. Fatal lumbar puncture: fact versus fiction – an approach to a clinical dilemma. Pediatrics. 2003;112:e174–6.

41. Tattevin P, Bruneel F, Regnier B. Cranial CT before lumbar puncture in suspected meningitis. N Engl J Med. 2002;346:1248–51; author reply 51.

42. van Crevel H, Hijdra A, de Gans J. Lumbar puncture and the risk of herniation: when should we first perform CT? J Neurol. 2002;249:129–37.

43. Fishman RA. Cerebrospinal fluid in diseases of the nervous system. Philadelphia: WB Saunders Co; 1992.

44. Skipper BJ, Davis LE. Ascertaining hypoglycorrhachia in an acute patient. Am J Emerg Med. 1997;15:378–80.

45. Negrini B, Kelleher KJ, Wald ER. Cerebrospinal fluid findings in aseptic versus bacterial meningitis. Pediatrics. 2000;105:316–9.

46. Feigin RD, Shackelford PG. Value of repeat lumbar puncture in the differential diagnosis of meningitis. N Engl J Med. 1973;289: 571–4.

47. Herndon RM, Brumback RA. The cerebrospinal spinal fluid. Boston: Kluwer Academic Publishers; 1989.

48. Neuman MI, Tolford S, Harper MB. Test characteristics and interpretation of cerebrospinal fluid gram stain in children. Pediatr Infect Dis J. 2008;27:309–13.

49. Hayden RT, Frenkel LD. More laboratory testing: greater cost but not necessarily better. Pediatr Infect Dis J. 2000;19:290–2.

50. Mein J, Lum G. CSF bacterial antigen detection tests offer no advantage over Gram's stain in the diagnosis of bacterial meningitis. Pathology. 1999;31:67–9.

51. Gray BM, Simmons DR, Mason H, Barnum S, Volanakis JE. Quantitative levels of C-reactive protein in cerebrospinal fluid in patients with bacterial meningitis and other conditions. J Pediatr. 1986;108:665–70.

52. Skull SA, Leach AJ, Currie BJ. Streptococcus pneumoniae carriage and penicillin/ceftriaxone resistance in hospitalised children in Darwin. Aust N Z J Med. 1996;26:391–5.

53. Jones ME, Draghi DC, Karlowsky JA, Sahm DF, Bradley JS. Prevalence of antimicrobial resistance in bacteria isolated from central nervous system specimens as reported by U.S. hospital laboratories from 2000 to 2002. Ann Clin Microbiol Antimicrob. 2004;3:3.

54. Gouveia EL, Reis JN, Flannery B, et al. Clinical outcome of pneumococcal meningitis during the emergence of penicillin-resistant Streptococcus pneumoniae: an observational study. BMC Infect Dis. 2011;11:323.

55. Deghmane AE, Alonso JM, Taha MK. Emerging drugs for acute bacterial meningitis. Expert Opin Emerg Drugs. 2009;14: 381–93.

56. Ohga S, Okada K, Ueda K, et al. Cerebrospinal fluid cytokine levels and dexamethasone therapy in bacterial meningitis. J Infect. 1999;39:55–60.

57. Ahmed A, Jafri H, Lutsar I, et al. Pharmacodynamics of vancomycin for the treatment of experimental penicillin- and cephalosporin-resistant pneumococcal meningitis. Antimicrob Agents Chemother. 1999;43:876–81.

58. Lutsar I, Friedland IR, Jafri HS, et al. Factors influencing the anti-inflammatory effect of dexamethasone therapy in experimental pneumococcal meningitis. J Antimicrob Chemother. 2003;52: 651–5.

59. McIntyre PB, Berkey CS, King SM, et al. Dexamethasone as adjunctive therapy in bacterial meningitis. A meta-analysis of randomized clinical trials since 1988. JAMA. 1997;278:925–31.

60. van de Beek D, Farrar JJ, de Gans J, et al. Adjunctive dexamethasone in bacterial meningitis: a meta-analysis of individual patient data. Lancet Neurol. 2010;9:254–63.

61. Roos KL, Scheld WM. The management of fulminant meningitis in the intensive care unit. Infect Dis Clin North Am. 1989;3: 137–54.

62. Roos KL, van de Beek D. Bacterial meningitis. In: Vinken PJ, Bruyn GW, editors. Handbook of clinical neurology. Elsevier: vol. 96. 2010. p. 51–63.

63. Gwer S, Gatakaa H, Mwai L, Idro R, Newton CR. The role for osmotic agents in children with acute encephalopathies: a systematic review. BMC Pediatr. 2010;10:23.

64. Hinson HE, Stein D, Sheth KN. Hypertonic saline and mannitol therapy in critical care neurology. J Intensive Care Med. 2013;28(1):3–11.

65. Liu S, Li L, Luo Z, et al. Superior effect of hypertonic saline over mannitol to attenuate cerebral edema in a rabbit bacterial meningitis model. Crit Care Med. 2011;39:1467–73.

66. Murthy JM. Management of intracranial pressure in tuberculous meningitis. Neurocrit Care. 2005;2:306–12.

67. Qureshi AI, Suarez JI. Use of hypertonic saline solutions in treatment of cerebral edema and intracranial hypertension. Crit Care Med. 2000;28:3301–13.

68. Singhi S, Singhi P, Baranwal AK. Bacterial meningitis in children: critical care needs. Indian J Pediatr. 2001;68:737–47.

69. Czosnyka M, Pickard JD. Monitoring and interpretation of intracranial pressure. J Neurol Neurosurg Psychiatry. 2004;75:813–21.

70. Kumar G, Kalita J, Misra UK. Raised intracranial pressure in acute viral encephalitis. Clin Neurol Neurosurg. 2009;111:399–406.

71. Sala F, Abbruzzese C, Galli D, et al. Intracranial pressure monitoring in pediatric bacterial meningitis: a fancy or useful tool? A case report. Minerva Anestesiol. 2009;75:746–9.

72. Whitney CG, Farley MM, Hadler J, et al. Decline in invasive pneumococcal disease after the introduction of protein-polysaccharide conjugate vaccine. N Engl J Med. 2003;348:1737–46.

73. Pilishvili T, Lexau C, Farley MM, et al. Sustained reductions in invasive pneumococcal disease in the era of conjugate vaccine. J Infect Dis. 2010;201:32–41.

74. CDC. Prevention and control of meningococcal disease. Recommendations of the Advisory Committee on Immunization Practices (ACIP). MMWR Recomm Rep. 2005;54:1–21.

75. CDC. Updated recommendations for use of meningococcal conjugate vaccines – Advisory Committee on Immunization Practices (ACIP), 2010. MMWR Morb Mortal Wkly Rep. 2011;60:72–6.

76. CDC. Meningococcal conjugate vaccines policy update: booster dose recommendations. Pediatrics. 2011;128:1213–8.

77. CDC. Updated recommendations for prevention of invasive pneumococcal disease among adults using the 23-valent pneumococcal polysaccharide vaccine (PPSV23). MMWR Morb Mortal Wkly Rep. 2010;59:1102–6.

78. CDC. Enterovirus surveillance – United States, 1970–2005. MMWR Surveill Summ. 2006;55:1–20.

79. Asnis DS, Conetta R, Teixeira AA, Waldman G, Sampson BA. The West Nile Virus outbreak of 1999 in New York: the Flushing Hospital experience. Clin Infect Dis. 2000;30:413–8.

80. Rappole JH, Derrickson SR, Hubalek Z. Migratory birds and spread of West Nile virus in the Western Hemisphere. Emerg Infect Dis. 2000;6:319–28.

81. Rappole JH, Hubalek Z. Migratory birds and West Nile virus. J Appl Microbiol. 2003;94(Suppl):47S–58.

82. CDC. Human rabies prevention – United States, 2008: recommendations of the Advisory Committee on Immunization Practices. MMWR Recomm Rep. 2008;57:1–28.

83. Blanton JD, Palmer D, Dyer J, Rupprecht CE. Rabies surveillance in the United States during 2010. J Am Vet Med Assoc. 2011;239:773–83.

84. Sharpe AH, Fields BN. Pathogenesis of viral infections. Basic concepts derived from the reovirus model. N Engl J Med. 1985;312:486–97.

85. Iwasaka T, Kidera Y, Tsugitomi H, Sugimori H. The cellular changes in primary and recurrent infection with herpes simplex virus type 2 in an in vitro model. Acta Cytol. 1987;31:935–40.

86. Esiri MM. Herpes simplex encephalitis. An immunohistological study of the distribution of viral antigen within the brain. J Neurol Sci. 1982;54:209–26.

87. Pleasure SJ, Fischbein NJ. Correlation of clinical and neuroimaging findings in a case of rabies encephalitis. Arch Neurol. 2000;57:1765–9.

88. Peters CJ. Arenaviruses. In: Richman DD, Whitley RJ, Hayden FG, editors. Clinical virology. Washington, D.C.: American Society of Microbiology Press; 2009. p. 1009–29.

89. Jolles S, Sewell WA, Leighton C. Drug-induced aseptic meningitis: diagnosis and management. Drug Saf. 2000;22:215–26.

90. Dupuis M, Hull R, Wang H, et al. Molecular detection of viral causes of encephalitis and meningitis in New York State. J Med Virol. 2011;83:2172–81.

91. Murphy RF, Caliendo AM. Relative quantity of cerebrospinal fluid herpes simplex virus DNA in adult cases of encephalitis and meningitis. Am J Clin Pathol. 2009;132:687–90.

92. Cinque P, Cleator GM, Weber T, Monteyne P, Sindic CJ, van Loon AM. The role of laboratory investigation in the diagnosis and management of patients with suspected herpes simplex encephalitis: a consensus report. The EU Concerted Action on Virus Meningitis and Encephalitis. J Neurol Neurosurg Psychiatry. 1996;61:339–45.

93. Espy MJ, Uhl JR, Mitchell PS, et al. Diagnosis of herpes simplex virus infections in the clinical laboratory by LightCycler PCR. J Clin Microbiol. 2000;38:795–9.

94. Whitley RJ, Alford CA, Hirsch MS, et al. Vidarabine versus acyclovir therapy in herpes simplex encephalitis. N Engl J Med. 1986;314:144–9.

95. Whitley RJ, Cobbs CG, Alford Jr CA, et al. Diseases that mimic herpes simplex encephalitis. Diagnosis, presentation, and outcome. NIAD Collaborative Antiviral Study Group. JAMA. 1989;262:234–9.

96. CDC. Investigation of rabies infections in organ donor and transplant recipients – Alabama, Arkansas, Oklahoma, and Texas, 2004. MMWR Morb Mortal Wkly Rep. 2004;53:586–9.

97. CDC. Human-to-human transmission of rabies via corneal transplant – Thailand. MMWR Morb Mortal Wkly Rep. 1981;30: 473–4.

98. CDC. Human-to-human transmission of rabies by a corneal transplant-Idaho. MMWR. 1979;28:109–11.

99. Houff SA, Burton RC, Wilson RW, et al. Human-to-human transmission of rabies virus by corneal transplant. N Engl J Med. 1979;300:603–4.

100. Jackson AC. Rabies in the critical care unit: diagnostic and therapeutic approaches. Can J Neurol Sci. 2011;38:689–95.

101. Cohen JI, Davenport DS, Stewart JA, Deitchman S, Hilliard JK, Chapman LE. Recommendations for prevention of and therapy for exposure to B virus (cercopithecine herpesvirus 1). Clin Infect Dis. 2002;35:1191–203.

102. Canale DJ. William Macewen and the treatment of brain abscesses: revisited after one hundred years. J Neurosurg. 1996;84: 133–42.

103. Carpenter J, Stapleton S, Holliman R. Retrospective analysis of 49 cases of brain abscess and review of the literature. Eur J Clin Microbiol Infect Dis. 2007;26:1–11.

104. Nicolosi A, Hauser WA, Musicco M, Kurland LT. Incidence and prognosis of brain abscess in a defined population: Olmsted County, Minnesota, 1935–1981. Neuroepidemiology. 1991;10: 122–31.

105. Nielsen H, Harmsen A, Gyldensted C. Cerebral abscess. A long-term follow-up. Acta Neurol Scand. 1983;67:330–7.

106. Nielsen H, Gyldensted C, Harmsen A. Cerebral abscess. Aetiology and pathogenesis, symptoms, diagnosis and treatment. A review of 200 cases from 1935–1976. Acta Neurol Scand. 1982;65: 609–22.

107. Honda H, Warren DK. Central nervous system infections: meningitis and brain abscess. Infect Dis Clin North Am. 2009;23:609–23.

108. Harris PS, Cobbs CG. Cardiac, cerebral, and vascular complications of infective endocarditis. Cardiol Clin. 1996;14:437–50.

109. Muzumdar D, Jhawar S, Goel A. Brain abscess: an overview. Int J Surg. 2011;9:136–44.

110. Le Moal G, Landron C, Grollier G, et al. Characteristics of brain abscess with isolation of anaerobic bacteria. Scand J Infect Dis. 2003;35:318–21.

111. Cunha BA. Central nervous system infections in the compromised host: a diagnostic approach. Infect Dis Clin North Am. 2001;15:567–90.

112. Mathisen GE, Johnson JP. Brain abscess. Clin Infect Dis. 1997;25:763–79; quiz 80–1.

113. Mamelak AN, Obana WG, Flaherty JF, Rosenblum ML. Nocardial brain abscess: treatment strategies and factors influencing outcome. Neurosurgery. 1994;35:622–31.

114. Bartzatt R. Tuberculosis infections of the central nervous system. Cent Nerv Syst Agents Med Chem. 2011;11:321–7.

115. Bathla G, Khandelwal G, Maller VG, Gupta A. Manifestations of cerebral tuberculosis. Singapore Med J. 2011;52:124–30; quiz 31.

116. Jung A, Korsukewitz C, Kuhlmann T, et al. Intracerebral mass lesion diagnosed as cryptococcoma in a patient with sarcoidosis, a rare opportunistic manifestation induced by immunosuppression with corticosteroids. J Neurol. 2012;259(10):2147–50.

117. Nadkarni T, Goel A. Aspergilloma of the brain: an overview. J Postgrad Med. 2005;51 Suppl 1:S37–41.

118. Metellus P, Laghmari M, Fuentes S, et al. Successful treatment of a giant isolated cerebral mucormycotic (zygomycotic) abscess using endoscopic debridement: case report and therapeutic considerations. Surg Neurol. 2008;69:510–5; discussion 5.

119. Chun CH, Johnson JD, Hofstetter M, Raff MJ. Brain abscess. A study of 45 consecutive cases. Medicine. 1986;65:415–31.

120. Arseni C, Ciurea AV. Cerebellar abscesses. A report on 119 cases. Zentralbl Neurochir. 1982;43:359–70.

121. Turner RC, Dodson SC, Rosen CL. Medical management of cerebellar abscess: a case report and review of the literature. W V Med J. 2011;107:21–3.

122. Kastrup O, Wanke I, Maschke M. Neuroimaging of infections of the central nervous system. Semin Neurol. 2008;28:511–22.

123. Nathoo N, Nadvi SS, Narotam PK, van Dellen JR. Brain abscess: management and outcome analysis of a computed tomography era experience with 973 patients. World Neurosurg. 2011;75:716–26; discussion 612–7.

124. Garg RK, Sinha MK. Multiple ring-enhancing lesions of the brain. J Postgrad Med. 2010;56:307–16.

125. Holtas S, Tornquist C, Cronqvist S. Diagnostic difficulties in computed tomography of brain abscesses. J Comput Assist Tomogr. 1982;6:683–8.

126. Miller ES, Dias PS, Uttley D. CT scanning in the management of intracranial abscess: a review of 100 cases. Br J Neurosurg. 1988;2:439–46.

127. Nguyen JB, Black BR, Leimkuehler MM, Halder V, Nguyen JV, Ahktar N. Intracranial pyogenic abscess: imaging diagnosis utilizing recent advances in computed tomography and magnetic resonance imaging. Crit Rev Comput Tomogr. 2004;45:181–224.

128. Lai PH, Hsu SS, Ding SW, et al. Proton magnetic resonance spectroscopy and diffusion-weighted imaging in intracranial cystic mass lesions. Surg Neurol. 2007;68 Suppl 1:S25–36.

129. Lai PH, Hsu SS, Lo YK, Ding SW. Role of diffusion-weighted imaging and proton MR spectroscopy in distinguishing between pyogenic brain abscess and necrotic brain tumor. Acta Neurol Taiwan. 2004;13:107–13.

130. Desprechins B, Stadnik T, Koerts G, Shabana W, Breucq C, Osteaux M. Use of diffusion-weighted MR imaging in differential diagnosis between intracerebral necrotic tumors and cerebral abscesses. AJNR Am J Neuroradiol. 1999;20:1252–7.

131. Omuro AM, Leite CC, Mokhtari K, Delattre JY. Pitfalls in the diagnosis of brain tumours. Lancet Neurol. 2006;5:937–48.

132. Kang K, Lim I, Roh JK. Positron emission tomographic findings in a tuberculous brain abscess. Ann Nucl Med. 2007;21:303–6.

133. Kosterink JG. Positron emission tomography in the diagnosis and treatment management of tuberculosis. Curr Pharm Des. 2011;17:2875–80.

134. Kumar R, Basu S, Torigian D, Anand V, Zhuang H, Alavi A. Role of modern imaging techniques for diagnosis of infection in the era of 18F-fluorodeoxyglucose positron emission tomography. Clin Microbiol Rev. 2008;21:209–24.

135. Lu CH, Chang WN, Lui CC. Strategies for the management of bacterial brain abscess. J Clin Neurosci. 2006;13:979–85.

136. Mackenzie AR, Laing RB, Smith CC, Kaar GF, Smith FW. Spinal epidural abscess: the importance of early diagnosis and treatment. J Neurol Neurosurg Psychiatry. 1998;65:209–12.

137. Bluman EM, Palumbo MA, Lucas PR. Spinal epidural abscess in adults. J Am Acad Orthop Surg. 2004;12:155–63.

138. Tompkins M, Panuncialman I, Lucas P, Palumbo M. Spinal epidural abscess. J Emerg Med. 2010;39:384–90.

139. Sendi P, Bregenzer T, Zimmerli W. Spinal epidural abscess in clinical practice. QJM. 2008;101:1–12.

140. Martin RJ, Yuan HA. Neurosurgical care of spinal epidural, subdural, and intramedullary abscesses and arachnoiditis. Orthop Clin North Am. 1996;27:125–36.

141. Pradilla G, Ardila GP, Hsu W, Rigamonti D. Epidural abscesses of the CNS. Lancet Neurol. 2009;8:292–300.

142. Soehle M, Wallenfang T. Spinal epidural abscesses: clinical manifestations, prognostic factors, and outcomes. Neurosurgery. 2002;51:79–85; discussion 6–7.

143. Curry Jr WT, Hoh BL, Amin-Hanjani S, Eskandar EN. Spinal epidural abscess: clinical presentation, management, and outcome. Surg Neurol. 2005;63:364–71; discussion 71.

144. Hlavin ML, Kaminski HJ, Ross JS, Ganz E. Spinal epidural abscess: a ten-year perspective. Neurosurgery. 1990;27:177–84.

145. Nussbaum ES, Rigamonti D, Standiford H, Numaguchi Y, Wolf AL, Robinson WL. Spinal epidural abscess: a report of 40 cases and review. Surg Neurol. 1992;38:225–31.

146. Huang PY, Chen SF, Chang WN, et al. Spinal epidural abscess in adults caused by Staphylococcus aureus: clinical characteristics and prognostic factors. Clin Neurol Neurosurg. 2012;114(6): 572–6.

147. Wheeler D, Keiser P, Rigamonti D, Keay S. Medical management of spinal epidural abscesses: case report and review. Clin Infect Dis. 1992;15:22–7.

148. Maslen DR, Jones SR, Crislip MA, Bracis R, Dworkin RJ, Flemming JE. Spinal epidural abscess. Optimizing patient care. Arch Intern Med. 1993;153:1713–21.

149. Khanna RK, Malik GM, Rock JP, Rosenblum ML. Spinal epidural abscess: evaluation of factors influencing outcome. Neurosurgery. 1996;39:958–64.

150. Tang HJ, Lin HJ, Liu YC, Li CM. Spinal epidural abscess – experience with 46 patients and evaluation of prognostic factors. J Infect. 2002;45:76–81.

151. Del Curling Jr O, Gower DJ, McWhorter JM. Changing concepts in spinal epidural abscess: a report of 29 cases. Neurosurgery. 1990;27:185–92.

152. Davis DP, Salazar A, Chan TC, Vilke GM. Prospective evaluation of a clinical decision guideline to diagnose spinal epidural abscess in patients who present to the emergency department with spine pain. J Neurosurg Spine. 2011;14:765–70.

153. Davis DP, Wold RM, Patel RJ, et al. The clinical presentation and impact of diagnostic delays on emergency department patients with spinal epidural abscess. J Emerg Med. 2004;26:285–91.

154. Reihsaus E, Waldbaur H, Seeling W. Spinal epidural abscess: a meta-analysis of 915 patients. Neurosurg Rev. 2000;23:175–204; discussion 5.

155. Obrador GT, Levenson DJ. Spinal epidural abscess in hemodialysis patients: report of three cases and review of the literature. Am J Kidney Dis. 1996;27:75–83.

156. Khan IA, Vaccaro AR, Zlotolow DA. Management of vertebral diskitis and osteomyelitis. Orthopedics. 1999;22:758–65.

157. Strausbaugh LJ. Vertebral osteomyelitis. How to differentiate it from other causes of back and neck pain. Postgrad Med. 1995;97(147–8):51–4.

158. Bhavan KP, Marschall J, Olsen MA, Fraser VJ, Wright NM, Warren DK. The epidemiology of hematogenous vertebral osteomyelitis: a cohort study in a tertiary care hospital. BMC Infect Dis. 2010;10:158.

159. Grammatico L, Baron S, Rusch E, et al. Epidemiology of vertebral osteomyelitis (VO) in France: analysis of hospital-discharge data 2002–2003. Epidemiol Infect. 2008;136:653–60.

160. Digby JM, Kersley JB. Pyogenic non-tuberculous spinal infection: an analysis of thirty cases. J Bone Joint Surg Br. 1979;61:47–55.

161. Zimmerli W. Clinical practice. Vertebral osteomyelitis. N Engl J Med. 2010;362:1022–9.

162. Rezai AR, Woo HH, Errico TJ, Cooper PR. Contemporary management of spinal osteomyelitis. Neurosurgery. 1999;44:1018–25; discussion 25–6.

163. Nussbaum ES, Rockswold GL, Bergman TA, Erickson DL, Seljeskog EL. Spinal tuberculosis: a diagnostic and management challenge. J Neurosurg. 1995;83:243–7.

164. Priest DH, Peacock Jr JE. Hematogenous vertebral osteomyelitis due to Staphylococcus aureus in the adult: clinical features and therapeutic outcomes. South Med J. 2005;98:854–62.

165. Sapico FL. Microbiology and antimicrobial therapy of spinal infections. Orthop Clin North Am. 1996;27:9–13.

166. Broner FA, Garland DE, Zigler JE. Spinal infections in the immunocompromised host. Orthop Clin North Am. 1996;27:37–46.

167. Ozuna RM, Delamarter RB. Pyogenic vertebral osteomyelitis and postsurgical disc space infections. Orthop Clin North Am. 1996;27:87–94.

168. Cahill DW, Love LC, Rechtine GR. Pyogenic osteomyelitis of the spine in the elderly. J Neurosurg. 1991;74:878–86.

169. Acosta Jr FL, Chin CT, Quinones-Hinojosa A, Ames CP, Weinstein PR, Chou D. Diagnosis and management of adult pyogenic osteomyelitis of the cervical spine. Neurosurg Focus. 2004;17:E2.

170. Sarria JC, Chutkan NB, Figueroa JE, Hull A. Atypical mycobacterial vertebral osteomyelitis: case report and review. Clin Infect Dis. 1998;26:503–5.

171. Klein JD, Garfin SR. Nutritional status in the patient with spinal infection. Orthop Clin North Am. 1996;27:33–6.

172. Endress C, Guyot DR, Fata J, Salciccioli G. Cervical osteomyelitis due to i.v. heroin use: radiologic findings in 14 patients. AJR Am J Roentgenol. 1990;155:333–5.

173. Lafont A, Olive A, Gelman M, Roca-Burniols J, Cots R, Carbonell J. Candida albicans spondylodiscitis and vertebral osteomyelitis in patients with intravenous heroin drug addiction. Report of 3 new cases. J Rheumatol. 1994;21:953–6.

174. Rahman I, Bhatt H, Chillag S, Duffus W. Mycobacterium chelonae vertebral osteomyelitis. South Med J. 2009;102:1167–9.

175. Colmenero JD, Jimenez-Mejias ME, Sanchez-Lora FJ, et al. Pyogenic, tuberculous, and brucellar vertebral osteomyelitis: a descriptive and comparative study of 219 cases. Ann Rheum Dis. 1997;56:709–15.

176. Livorsi DJ, Daver NG, Atmar RL, Shelburne SA, White Jr AC, Musher DM. Outcomes of treatment for hematogenous Staphylococcus aureus vertebral osteomyelitis in the MRSA ERA. J Infect. 2008;57:128–31.

177. Lora-Tamayo J, Euba G, Narvaez JA, et al. Changing trends in the epidemiology of pyogenic vertebral osteomyelitis: the impact of cases with no microbiologic diagnosis. Semin Arthritis Rheum. 2011;41:247–55.

178. Mylona E, Samarkos M, Kakalou E, Fanourgiakis P, Skoutelis A. Pyogenic vertebral osteomyelitis: a systematic review of clinical characteristics. Semin Arthritis Rheum. 2009;39:10–7.

179. Nolla JM, Ariza J, Gomez-Vaquero C, et al. Spontaneous pyogenic vertebral osteomyelitis in nondrug users. Semin Arthritis Rheum. 2002;31:271–8.

180. Osenbach RK, Hitchon PW, Menezes AH. Diagnosis and management of pyogenic vertebral osteomyelitis in adults. Surg Neurol. 1990;33:266–75.

181. Patzakis MJ, Rao S, Wilkins J, Moore TM, Harvey PJ. Analysis of 61 cases of vertebral osteomyelitis. Clin Orthop Relat Res. 1991;(264):178–83.

182. Mete B, Kurt C, Yilmaz MH, et al. Vertebral osteomyelitis: eight years' experience of 100 cases. Rheumatol Int. 2012;32(11): 3591–7.

183. Barnes B, Alexander JT, Branch Jr CL. Cervical osteomyelitis: a brief review. Neurosurg Focus. 2004;17:E11.

184. Beluffi G, Bernardo ME, Meloni G, Spinazzola A, Locatelli F. Spinal osteomyelitis due to Aspergillus flavus in a child: a rare complication after haematopoietic stem cell transplantation. Pediatr Radiol. 2008;38:709–12.

185. Chang HM, Yu HH, Yang YH, et al. Successful treatment of Aspergillus flavus spondylodiscitis with epidural abscess in a patient with chronic granulomatous disease. Pediatr Infect Dis J. 2012;31:100–1.

186. Ranjan R, Mishra S, Ranjan S. Aspergillus vertebral osteomyelitis in an immunocompetent person. Neurol India. 2010;58:806–8.

187. Sethi S, Siraj F, Kalra K, Chopra P. Aspergillus vertebral osteomyelitis in immunocompetent patients. Ind J Orthop. 2012;46: 246–50.

188. Studemeister A, Stevens DA. Aspergillus vertebral osteomyelitis in immunocompetent hosts: role of triazole antifungal therapy. Clin Infect Dis. 2011;52:e1–6.

189. Tew CW, Han FC, Jureen R, Tey BH. Aspergillus vertebral osteomyelitis and epidural abscess. Singapore Med J. 2009; 50:e151–4.

190. Zhu LP, Chen XS, Wu JQ, Yang FF, Weng XH. Aspergillus vertebral osteomyelitis and ureteral obstruction after liver transplantation. Transpl Infect Dis. 2011;13:192–9.

191. An HS, Seldomridge JA. Spinal infections: diagnostic tests and imaging studies. Clin Orthop Relat Res. 2006;444:27–33.

192. Rath SA, Neff U, Schneider O, Richter HP. Neurosurgical management of thoracic and lumbar vertebral osteomyelitis and discitis in adults: a review of 43 consecutive surgically treated patients. Neurosurgery. 1996;38:926–33.

193. Turpin S, Lambert R. Role of scintigraphy in musculoskeletal and spinal infections. Radiol Clin North Am. 2001;39:169–89.

194. Palestro CJ, Love C, Miller TT. Diagnostic imaging tests and microbial infections. Cell Microbiol. 2007;9:2323–33.

195. Palestro CJ, Love C, Miller TT. Infection and musculoskeletal conditions: Imaging of musculoskeletal infections. Best Pract Res Clin Rheumatol. 2006;20:1197–218.

196. Vaccaro AR, Shah SH, Schweitzer ME, Rosenfeld JF, Cotler JM. MRI description of vertebral osteomyelitis, neoplasm, and compression fracture. Orthopedics. 1999;22:67–73; quiz 4–5.

197. Roblot F, Besnier JM, Juhel L, et al. Optimal duration of antibiotic therapy in vertebral osteomyelitis. Semin Arthritis Rheum. 2007;36:269–77.

198. Hadjipavlou AG, Mader JT, Necessary JT, Muffoletto AJ. Hematogenous pyogenic spinal infections and their surgical management. Spine. 2000;25:1668–79.

199. Perronne C, Saba J, Behloul Z, et al. Pyogenic and tuberculous spondylodiskitis (vertebral osteomyelitis) in 80 adult patients. Clin Infect Dis. 1994;19:746–50.

200. Dey M, Jaffe J, Stadnik A, Awad IA. External ventricular drainage for intraventricular hemorrhage. Curr Neurol Neurosci Rep. 2012;12:24–33.

201. Li LM, Timofeev I, Czosnyka M, Hutchinson PJ. Review article: the surgical approach to the management of increased intracranial pressure after traumatic brain injury. Anesth Analg. 2010;111:736–48.

202. Gigante P, Hwang BY, Appelboom G, Kellner CP, Kellner MA, Connolly ES. External ventricular drainage following aneurysmal subarachnoid haemorrhage. Br J Neurosurg. 2010;24:625–32.

203. The Brain Trauma Foundation. The American Association of Neurological Surgeons. The Joint Section on Neurotrauma and Critical Care. Recommendations for intracranial pressure monitoring technology. J Neurotrauma. 2000;17:497–506.

204. Gutierrez-Gonzalez R, Boto GR, Perez-Zamarron A. Cerebrospinal fluid diversion devices and infection. A comprehensive review. Eur J Clin Microbiol Infect Dis. 2012;31(6):889–97.

205. Ngo QN, Ranger A, Singh RN, Kornecki A, Seabrook JA, Fraser DD. External ventricular drains in pediatric patients. Pediatr Crit Care Med. 2009;10:346–51.

206. Speck V, Staykov D, Huttner HB, Sauer R, Schwab S, Bardutzky J. Lumbar catheter for monitoring of intracranial pressure in patients with post-hemorrhagic communicating hydrocephalus. Neurocrit Care. 2011;14:208–15.

207. Zhong J, Dujovny M, Park HK, Perez E, Perlin AR, Diaz FG. Advances in ICP monitoring techniques. Neurol Res. 2003;25:339–50.

208. Ghajar J. Intracranial pressure monitoring techniques. New Horiz. 1995;3:395–9.

209. Dasic D, Hanna SJ, Bojanic S, Kerr RS. External ventricular drain infection: the effect of a strict protocol on infection rates and a review of the literature. Br J Neurosurg. 2006;20:296–300.

210. Hoefnagel D, Dammers R, Ter Laak-Poort MP, Avezaat CJ. Risk factors for infections related to external ventricular drainage. Acta Neurochir. 2008;150:209–14; discussion 14.

211. Kitchen WJ, Singh N, Hulme S, Galea J, Patel HC, King AT. External ventricular drain infection: improved technique can reduce infection rates. Br J Neurosurg. 2011;25:632–5.

212. Kourbeti IS, Jacobs AV, Koslow M, Karabetsos D, Holzman RS. Risk factors associated with postcraniotomy meningitis. Neurosurgery. 2007;60:317–25; discussion 25–6.

213. O'Brien D, Stevens NT, Lim CH, et al. Candida infection of the central nervous system following neurosurgery: a 12-year review. Acta Neurochir. 2011;153:1347–50.

214. Schade RP, Schinkel J, Visser LG, Van Dijk JM, Voormolen JH, Kuijper EJ. Bacterial meningitis caused by the use of ventricular or lumbar cerebrospinal fluid catheters. J Neurosurg. 2005;102:229–34.

215. von der Brelie C, Simon A, Groner A, Molitor E, Simon M. Evaluation of an institutional guideline for the treatment of cerebrospinal fluid shunt-associated infections. Acta Neurochir (Wien). 2012;154(9):1691–7.

216. Korinek AM, Reina M, Boch AL, Rivera AO, De Bels D, Puybasset L. Prevention of external ventricular drain – related ventriculitis. Acta Neurochir. 2005;147:39–45; discussion 45–6.

217. Lo CH, Spelman D, Bailey M, Cooper DJ, Rosenfeld JV, Brecknell JE. External ventricular drain infections are independent of drain duration: an argument against elective revision. J Neurosurg. 2007;106:378–83.

218. Mayhall CG, Archer NH, Lamb VA, et al. Ventriculostomy-related infections. A prospective epidemiologic study. N Engl J Med. 1984;310:553–9.

219. Winfield JA, Rosenthal P, Kanter RK, Casella G. Duration of intracranial pressure monitoring does not predict daily risk of infectious complications. Neurosurgery. 1993;33:424–30; discussion 30–1.

220. Beer R, Pfausler B, Schmutzhard E. Management of nosocomial external ventricular drain-related ventriculomeningitis. Neurocrit Care. 2009;10:363–7.

221. Pfausler B, Beer R, Engelhardt K, Kemmler G, Mohsenipour I, Schmutzhard E. Cell index – a new parameter for the early diagnosis of ventriculostomy (external ventricular drainage)-related ventriculitis in patients with intraventricular hemorrhage? Acta Neurochir. 2004;146:477–81.

222. Kim JH, Desai NS, Ricci J, et al. Factors contributing to ventriculostomy infection. World Neurosurg. 2012;77:135–40.

223. Chi H, Chang KY, Chang HC, Chiu NC, Huang FY. Infections associated with indwelling ventriculostomy catheters in a teaching hospital. Int J Infect Dis. 2010;14:e216–9.

224. Stenehjem E, Armstrong WS. Central nervous system device infections. Infect Dis Clin North Am. 2012;26:89–110.

225. Alleyne Jr CH, Hassan M, Zabramski JM. The efficacy and cost of prophylactic and perioprocedural antibiotics in patients with external ventricular drains. Neurosurgery. 2000;47:1124–7; discussion 7–9.

226. Ratilal B, Costa J, Sampaio C. Antibiotic prophylaxis for surgical introduction of intracranial ventricular shunts. Cochrane Database Syst Rev. 2006;(3):CD005365.

227. Munch TN, Juhler M. Antibiotic prophylaxis in insertion of intracranial ventricular shunts. A survey of a Cochrane review. Ugeskr Laeger. 2008;170:131–5.

228. Ratilal B, Sampaio C. Prophylactic antibiotics and anticonvulsants in neurosurgery. Adv Tech Stand Neurosurg. 2011;36: 139–85.

229. Ratilal B, Costa J, Sampaio C. Antibiotic prophylaxis for surgical introduction of intracranial ventricular shunts: a systematic review. J Neurosurg Pediatr. 2008;1:48–56.

230. Muttaiyah S, Ritchie S, John S, Mee E, Roberts S. Efficacy of antibiotic-impregnated external ventricular drain catheters. J Clin Neurosci. 2010;17:296–8.

231. Abla AA, Zabramski JM, Jahnke HK, Fusco D, Nakaji P. Comparison of two antibiotic-impregnated ventricular catheters: a prospective sequential series trial. Neurosurgery. 2011;68:437–42; discussion 42.

232. Eymann R, Chehab S, Strowitzki M, Steudel WI, Kiefer M. Clinical and economic consequences of antibiotic-impregnated cerebrospinal fluid shunt catheters. J Neurosurg Pediatr. 2008;1:444–50.

233. Gutierrez-Gonzalez R, Boto GR. Do antibiotic-impregnated catheters prevent infection in CSF diversion procedures? Review of the literature. J Infect. 2010;61:9–20.

234. Lemcke J, Depner F, Meier U. The impact of silver nanoparticle-coated and antibiotic-impregnated external ventricular drainage catheters on the risk of infections: a clinical comparison of 95 patients. Acta Neurochir Suppl. 2012;114:347–50.

235. Soleman J, Marbacher S, Fandino J, Fathi AR. Is the use of antibiotic-impregnated external ventricular drainage beneficial in the management of iatrogenic ventriculitis? Acta Neurochir. 2012;154:161–4; discussion 4.

236. Zingale A, Ippolito S, Pappalardo P, Chibbaro S, Amoroso R. Infections and re-infections in long-term external ventricular drainage. A variation upon a theme. J Neurosurg Sci. 1999;43:125–32; discussion 33.

237. Babu MA, Patel R, Marsh WR, Wijdicks EF. Strategies to decrease the risk of ventricular catheter infections: a review of the evidence. Neurocrit Care. 2012;16:194–202.

238. Fichtner J, Guresir E, Seifert V, Raabe A. Efficacy of silver-bearing external ventricular drainage catheters: a retrospective analysis. J Neurosurg. 2010;112:840–6.

239. McCarthy PJ, Patil S, Conrad SA, Scott LK. International and specialty trends in the use of prophylactic antibiotics to prevent infectious complications after insertion of external ventricular drainage devices. Neurocrit Care. 2010;12:220–4.

240. Razmkon A, Bakhtazad A. Maintaining CSF drainage at external ventricular drains may help prevent catheter-related infections. Acta Neurochir. 2009;151:985.

241. Rivero-Garvia M, Marquez-Rivas J, Jimenez-Mejias ME, Neth O, Rueda-Torres AB. Reduction in external ventricular drain infection rate. Impact of a minimal handling protocol and antibiotic-impregnated catheters. Acta Neurochir. 2011;153:647–51.

242. Cummings R. Understanding external ventricular drainage. J Neurosci Nurs. 1992;24:84–7.

243. Narayan RK, Kishore PR, Becker DP, et al. Intracranial pressure: to monitor or not to monitor? A review of our experience with severe head injury. J Neurosurg. 1982;56:650–9.

244. Tamburrini G, Massimi L, Caldarelli M, Di Rocco C. Antibiotic impregnated external ventricular drainage and third ventriculostomy in the management of hydrocephalus associated with posterior cranial fossa tumours. Acta Neurochir. 2008;150:1049–55; discussion 55–6.

245. Lopez-Alvarez B, Martin-Laez R, Farinas MC, Paternina-Vidal B, Garcia-Palomo JD, Vazquez-Barquero A. Multidrug-resistant Acinetobacter baumannii ventriculitis: successful treatment with intraventricular colistin. Acta Neurochir. 2009;151:1465–72.

246. Nerlich AG, Haas CJ, Zink A, Szeimies U, Hagedorn HG. Molecular evidence for tuberculosis in an ancient Egyptian mummy. Lancet. 1997;350:1404.

247. Salo WL, Aufderheide AC, Buikstra J, Holcomb TA. Identification of Mycobacterium tuberculosis DNA in a pre-Columbian Peruvian mummy. Proc Natl Acad Sci U S A. 1994;91:2091–4.

248. Organization WH. WHO Report 2011: Global Tuberculosis Control. Geneva: World Health Organization; 2011.

249. Archibald LK, den Dulk MO, Pallangyo KJ, Reller LB. Fatal Mycobacterium tuberculosis bloodstream infections in febrile hospitalized adults in Dar es Salaam, Tanzania. Clin Infect Dis. 1998;26:290–6.

250. Archibald LK, McDonald LC, Nwanyanwu O, et al. A hospital-based prevalence survey of bloodstream infections in febrile patients in Malawi: implications for diagnosis and therapy. J Infect Dis. 2000;181:1414–20.

251. Archibald LK, McDonald LC, Rheanpumikankit S, et al. Fever and human immunodeficiency virus infection as sentinels for emerging mycobacterial and fungal bloodstream infections in hospitalized patients greater than /=15 years old, Bangkok. J Infect Dis. 1999;180:87–92.

252. Bell M, Archibald LK, Nwanyanwu O, et al. Seasonal variation in the etiology of bloodstream infections in a febrile inpatient population in a developing country. Int J Infect Dis. 2001;5:63–9.

253. McDonald LC, Archibald LK, Rheanpumikankit S, et al. Unrecognised Mycobacterium tuberculosis bacteraemia among hospital inpatients in less developed countries. Lancet. 1999;354:1159–63.

254. CDC. Emergence of Mycobacterium tuberculosis with extensive resistance to second-line drugs – worldwide, 2000–2004. MMWR Morb Mortal Wkly Rep. 2006;55:301–5.

255. CDC. Two simultaneous outbreaks of multidrug-resistant tuberculosis – Federated States of Micronesia, 2007–2009. MMWR Morb Mortal Wkly Rep. 2009;58:253–6.

256. Cegielski JP. Extensively drug-resistant tuberculosis: "there must be some kind of way out of here". Clin Infect Dis. 2010;50 Suppl 3:S195–200.

257. Shah NS, Wright A, Bai GH, et al. Worldwide emergence of extensively drug-resistant tuberculosis. Emerg Infect Dis. 2007;13:380–7.

258. Kent SJ, Crowe SM, Yung A, Lucas CR, Mijch AM. Tuberculous meningitis: a 30-year review. Clin Infect Dis. 1993;17:987–94.

259. Thwaites GE, Tran TH. Tuberculous meningitis: many questions, too few answers. Lancet Neurol. 2005;4:160–70.

260. Thwaites G, Fisher M, Hemingway C, Scott G, Solomon T, Innes J. British Infection Society guidelines for the diagnosis and treatment of tuberculosis of the central nervous system in adults and children. J Infect. 2009;59:167–87.

261. Joos TJ, Miller WC, Murdoch DM. Tuberculin reactivity in bacille Calmette-Guerin vaccinated populations: a compilation of international data. Int J Tuberc Lung Dis. 2006;10:883–91.

262. Kilpatrick ME, Girgis NI, Tribble D, Farid Z. The value of the tuberculin skin test in patients with tuberculous meningitis. J Egypt Public Health Assoc. 1996;71:1–8.

263. Thwaites GE, Schoeman JF. Update on tuberculosis of the central nervous system: pathogenesis, diagnosis, and treatment. Clin Chest Med. 2009;30:745–54, ix.

264. Ferrara G, Losi M, D'Amico R, et al. Use in routine clinical practice of two commercial blood tests for diagnosis of infection with Mycobacterium tuberculosis: a prospective study. Lancet. 2006;367:1328–34.

265. Ferrara G, Losi M, Meacci M, et al. Routine hospital use of a new commercial whole blood interferon-gamma assay for the diagnosis of tuberculosis infection. Am J Respir Crit Care Med. 2005;172:631–5.

266. Foerster BR, Thurnher MM, Malani PN, Petrou M, Carets-Zumelzu F, Sundgren PC. Intracranial infections: clinical and imaging characteristics. Acta Radiol. 2007;48:875–93.

267. Trivedi R, Saksena S, Gupta RK. Magnetic resonance imaging in central nervous system tuberculosis. Indian J Radiol Imaging. 2009;19:256–65.

268. Parsons LM, Somoskovi A, Gutierrez C, et al. Laboratory diagnosis of tuberculosis in resource-poor countries: challenges and opportunities. Clin Microbiol Rev. 2011;24:314–50.

269. Murthy JM. Tuberculous meningitis: the challenges. Neurol India. 2010;58:716–22.

270. Nolan CM, Goldberg SV, Buskin SE. Hepatotoxicity associated with isoniazid preventive therapy: a 7-year survey from a public health tuberculosis clinic. JAMA. 1999;281:1014–8.

271. Thwaites GE, Nguyen DB, Nguyen HD, et al. Dexamethasone for the treatment of tuberculous meningitis in adolescents and adults. N Engl J Med. 2004;351:1741–51.

272. Berning SE, Cherry TA, Iseman MD. Novel treatment of meningitis caused by multidrug-resistant Mycobacterium tuberculosis with intrathecal levofloxacin and amikacin: case report. Clin Infect Dis. 2001;32:643–6.

273. Garg RK, Sinha MK. Tuberculous meningitis in patients infected with human immunodeficiency virus. J Neurol. 2011;258:3–13.

274. Afghani B, Lieberman JM. Paradoxical enlargement or development of intracranial tuberculomas during therapy: case report and review. Clin Infect Dis. 1994;19:1092–9.

275. Galimi R. Extrapulmonary tuberculosis: tuberculous meningitis new developments. Eur Rev Med Pharmacol Sci. 2011;15:365–86.

276. Hall WA, Truwit CL. The surgical management of infections involving the cerebrum. Neurosurgery. 2008;62 Suppl 2:519–30; discussion 30–1.

277. Garg RK, Somvanshi DS. Spinal tuberculosis: a review. J Spinal Cord Med. 2011;34:440–54.

278. Adekambi T, Foucault C, La Scola B, Drancourt M. Report of two fatal cases of Mycobacterium mucogenicum central nervous system infection in immunocompetent patients. J Clin Microbiol. 2006;44:837–40.

279. Madaras-Kelly KJ, DeMasters TA, Stevens DL. Mycobacterium fortuitum meningitis associated with an epidural catheter: case report and a review of the literature. Pharmacotherapy. 1999;19:661–6.

280. Midani S, Rathore MH. Mycobacterium fortuitum infection of ventriculoperitoneal shunt. South Med J. 1999;92:705–7.

281. Talati NJ, Rouphael N, Kuppalli K, Franco-Paredes C. Spectrum of CNS disease caused by rapidly growing mycobacteria. Lancet Infect Dis. 2008;8:390–8.

282. Bradsher RW. Histoplasmosis and blastomycosis. Clin Infect Dis. 1996;22 Suppl 2:S102–11.

283. Kauffman CA. Histoplasmosis: a clinical and laboratory update. Clin Microbiol Rev. 2007;20:115–32.

284. Wheat LJ, Batteiger BE, Sathapatayavongs B. Histoplasma capsulatum infections of the central nervous system. A clinical review. Medicine. 1990;69:244–60.

285. Gottfredsson M, Perfect JR. Fungal meningitis. Semin Neurol. 2000;20:307–22.

286. Chakrabarti A. Epidemiology of central nervous system mycoses. Neurol India. 2007;55:191–7.

287. Williams PL. Coccidioidal meningitis. Ann N Y Acad Sci. 2007;1111:377–84.

288. Johnson RH, Einstein HE. Coccidioidal meningitis. Clin Infect Dis. 2006;42:103–7.

289. Mathisen G, Shelub A, Truong J, Wigen C. Coccidioidal meningitis: clinical presentation and management in the fluconazole era. Medicine. 2010;89:251–84.

290. Bouza E, Dreyer JS, Hewitt WL, Meyer RD. Coccidioidal meningitis. An analysis of thirty-one cases and review of the literature. Medicine. 1981;60:139–72.

291. Vincent T, Galgiani JN, Huppert M, Salkin D. The natural history of coccidioidal meningitis: VA-Armed Forces cooperative studies, 1955–1958. Clin Infect Dis. 1993;16:247–54.

292. Ragland AS, Arsura E, Ismail Y, Johnson R. Eosinophilic pleocytosis in coccidioidal meningitis: frequency and significance. Am J Med. 1993;95:254–7.

293. Capilla J, Clemons KV, Sobel RA, Stevens DA. Efficacy of amphotericin B lipid complex in a rabbit model of coccidioidal meningitis. J Antimicrob Chemother. 2007;60:673–6.

294. Clemons KV, Capilla J, Sobel RA, Martinez M, Tong AJ, Stevens DA. Comparative efficacies of lipid-complexed amphotericin B and liposomal amphotericin B against coccidioidal meningitis in rabbits. Antimicrob Agents Chemother. 2009;53:1858–62.

295. Chapman SW, Dismukes WE, Proia LA, et al. Clinical practice guidelines for the management of blastomycosis: 2008 update by the Infectious Diseases Society of America. Clin Infect Dis. 2008;46:1801–12.

296. Bariola JR, Perry P, Pappas PG, et al. Blastomycosis of the central nervous system: a multicenter review of diagnosis and treatment in the modern era. Clin Infect Dis. 2010;50:797–804.

297. Borgia SM, Fuller JD, Sarabia A, El-Helou P. Cerebral blastomycosis: a case series incorporating voriconazole in the treatment regimen. Med Mycol. 2006;44:659–64.

298. Chowfin A, Tight R, Mitchell S. Recurrent blastomycosis of the central nervous system: case report and review. Clin Infect Dis. 2000;30:969–71.

299. Gonyea EF. The spectrum of primary blastomycotic meningitis: a review of central nervous system blastomycosis. Ann Neurol. 1978;3:26–39.

300. Bakleh M, Aksamit AJ, Tleyjeh IM, Marshall WF. Successful treatment of cerebral blastomycosis with voriconazole. Clin Infect Dis. 2005;40:e69–71.

301. Pappas PG, Pottage JC, Powderly WG, et al. Blastomycosis in patients with the acquired immunodeficiency syndrome. Ann Intern Med. 1992;116:847–53.

302. Chander B, Deb P, Sarkar C, Garg A, Mehta VS, Sharma MC. Cerebral blastomycosis: a case report. Indian J Pathol Microbiol. 2007;50:821–4.

303. Bradsher RW, Chapman SW, Pappas PG. Blastomycosis. Infect Dis Clin North Am. 2003;17:21–40, vii.

304. Pappas PG. Blastomycosis. Semin Respir Crit Care Med. 2004; 25:113–21.

305. Saccente M, Woods GL. Clinical and laboratory update on blastomycosis. Clin Microbiol Rev. 2010;23:367–81.

306. Durkin M, Witt J, Lemonte A, Wheat B, Connolly P. Antigen assay with the potential to aid in diagnosis of blastomycosis. J Clin Microbiol. 2004;42:4873–5.

307. Smith JA, Kauffman CA. Blastomycosis. Proc Am Thorac Soc. 2010;7:173–80.

308. Martynowicz MA, Prakash UB. Pulmonary blastomycosis: an appraisal of diagnostic techniques. Chest. 2002;121:768–73.

309. Casado JL, Quereda C, Corral I. Candidal meningitis in HIV-infected patients. AIDS Patient Care STDS. 1998;12:681–6.

310. Goldani LZ, Santos RP. Candida tropicalis as an emerging pathogen in Candida meningitis: case report and review. Braz J Infect Dis. 2010;14:631–3.

311. Montero A, Romero J, Vargas JA, et al. Candida infection of cerebrospinal fluid shunt devices: report of two cases and review of the literature. Acta Neurochir. 2000;142:67–74.

312. Rodriguez-Arrondo F, Aguirrebengoa K, De Arce A, et al. Candidal meningitis in HIV-infected patients: treatment with fluconazole. Scand J Infect Dis. 1998;30:417–8.

313. Sanchez-Portocarrero J, Perez-Cecilia E, Corral O, Romero-Vivas J, Picazo JJ. The central nervous system and infection by Candida species. Diagn Microbiol Infect Dis. 2000;37:169–79.

314. Parker Jr JC, McCloskey JJ, Lee RS. Human cerebral candidosis – a postmortem evaluation of 19 patients. Hum Pathol. 1981;12: 23–8.

315. Bayer AS, Edwards Jr JE, Seidel JS, Guze LB. Candida meningitis. Report of seven cases and review of the english literature. Medicine. 1976;55:477–86.

316. Black JT. Cerebral candidiasis: case report of brain abscess secondary to Candida albicans, and review of literature. J Neurol Neurosurg Psychiatry. 1970;33:864–70.

317. Lipton SA, Hickey WF, Morris JH, Loscalzo J. Candidal infection in the central nervous system. Am J Med. 1984;76:101–8.

318. Bengel D, Susa M, Schreiber H, Ludolph AC, Tumani H. Early diagnosis of rhinocerebral mucormycosis by cerebrospinal fluid analysis and determination of 16s rRNA gene sequence. Eur J Neurol. 2007;14:1067–70.

319. Mallis A, Mastronikolis SN, Naxakis SS, Papadas AT. Rhinocerebral mucormycosis: an update. Eur Rev Med Pharmacol Sci. 2010;14:987–92.

320. Schwartz S, Thiel E. Cerebral aspergillosis: tissue penetration is the key. Medical mycology. 2009;47 Suppl 1:S387–93.

321. Prejean J, Song R, Hernandez A, et al. Estimated HIV incidence in the United States, 2006–2009. PLoS One. 2011;6:e17502.

322. Montoya JG, Liesenfeld O. Toxoplasmosis. Lancet. 2004;363: 1965–76.

323. Kaplan JE, Benson C, Holmes KH, Brooks JT, Pau A, Masur H. Guidelines for prevention and treatment of opportunistic infections in HIV-infected adults and adolescents: recommendations from CDC, the National Institutes of Health, and the HIV Medicine Association of the Infectious Diseases Society of America. MMWR Recomm Rep. 2009;58:1–207; quiz CE1–4.

324. Contini C. Clinical and diagnostic management of toxoplasmosis in the immunocompromised patient. Parassitologia. 2008;50: 45–50.

325. Dedicoat M, Livesley N. Management of toxoplasmic encephalitis in HIV-infected adults – a review. S Afr Med J. 2008;98:31–2.

326. Beraud G, Pierre-Francois S, Foltzer A, et al. Cotrimoxazole for treatment of cerebral toxoplasmosis: an observational cohort study during 1994–2006. Am J Trop Med Hyg. 2009;80:583–7.

327. Pereira-Chioccola VL, Vidal JE, Su C. Toxoplasma gondii infection and cerebral toxoplasmosis in HIV-infected patients. Future Microbiol. 2009;4:1363–79.

328. Portegies P, Solod L, Cinque P, et al. Guidelines for the diagnosis and management of neurological complications of HIV infection. Eur J Neurol. 2004;11:297–304.

329. Luft BJ, Hafner R, Korzun AH, et al. Toxoplasmic encephalitis in patients with the acquired immunodeficiency syndrome. Members of the ACTG 077p/ANRS 009 Study Team. N Engl J Med. 1993;329:995–1000.

330. Heald A, Flepp M, Chave JP, et al. Treatment for cerebral toxoplasmosis protects against Pneumocystis carinii pneumonia in patients with AIDS. The Swiss HIV Cohort Study. Ann Intern Med. 1991;115:760–3.

331. Bertschy S, Opravil M, Cavassini M, et al. Discontinuation of maintenance therapy against toxoplasma encephalitis in AIDS patients with sustained response to anti-retroviral therapy. Clin Microbiol Infect. 2006;12:666–71.

332. Soriano V, Dona C, Rodriguez-Rosado R, Barreiro P, Gonzalez-Lahoz J. Discontinuation of secondary prophylaxis for opportunistic infections in HIV-infected patients receiving highly active antiretroviral therapy. AIDS. 2000;14:383–6.

333. Grassi MP, Clerici F, Perin C, et al. Microglial nodular encephalitis and ventriculoencephalitis due to cytomegalovirus infection in patients with AIDS: two distinct clinical patterns. Clin Infect Dis. 1998;27:504–8.

334. Clifford DB, Arribas JR, Storch GA, Tourtellote W, Wippold FJ. Magnetic resonance brain imaging lacks sensitivity for AIDS associated cytomegalovirus encephalitis. J Neurovirol. 1996;2: 397–403.

335. Arribas JR, Storch GA, Clifford DB, Tselis AC. Cytomegalovirus encephalitis. Ann Intern Med. 1996;125:577–87.

336. Anders HJ, Goebel FD. Neurological manifestations of cytomegalovirus infection in the acquired immunodeficiency syndrome. Int J STD AIDS. 1999;10:151–9; quiz 60–1.

337. Cinque P, Cleator GM, Weber T, et al. Diagnosis and clinical management of neurological disorders caused by cytomegalovirus in AIDS patients. European Union Concerted Action on Virus Meningitis and Encephalitis. J Neurovirol. 1998;4:120–32.

338. Silva CA, Oliveira AC, Vilas-Boas L, Fink MC, Pannuti CS, Vidal JE. Neurologic cytomegalovirus complications in patients with AIDS: retrospective review of 13 cases and review of the literature. Rev Inst Med Trop São Paulo. 2010;52:305–10.

339. Eidelberg D, Sotrel A, Vogel H, Walker P, Kleefield J, Crumpacker 3rd CS. Progressive polyradiculopathy in acquired immune deficiency syndrome. Neurology. 1986;36:912–6.

340. Kurup A, Torriani FJ. Therapy and prevention of cytomegalovirus retinitis. Curr Infect Dis Rep. 2001;3:371–7.

341. Spector SA, McKinley GF, Lalezari JP, et al. Oral ganciclovir for the prevention of cytomegalovirus disease in persons with AIDS.

Roche Cooperative Oral Ganciclovir Study Group. N Engl J Med. 1996;334:1491–7.

342. Waib LF, Bonon SH, Salles AC, et al. Withdrawal of maintenance therapy for cytomegalovirus retinitis in AIDS patients exhibiting immunological response to HAART. Rev Inst Med Trop São Paulo. 2007;49:215–9.

343. Macdonald JC, Torriani FJ, Morse LS, Karavellas MP, Reed JB, Freeman WR. Lack of reactivation of cytomegalovirus (CMV) retinitis after stopping CMV maintenance therapy in AIDS patients with sustained elevations in CD4 T cells in response to highly active antiretroviral therapy. J Infect Dis. 1998;177: 1182–7.

344. Wohl DA, Kendall MA, Owens S, et al. The safety of discontinuation of maintenance therapy for cytomegalovirus (CMV) retinitis and incidence of immune recovery uveitis following potent antiretroviral therapy. HIV Clin Trials. 2005;6:136–46.

345. Kaul M. HIV-1 associated dementia: update on pathological mechanisms and therapeutic approaches. Curr Opin Neurol. 2009;22:315–20.

346. Yadav A, Collman RG. CNS inflammation and macrophage/microglial biology associated with HIV-1 infection. J Neuroimmune Pharmacol. 2009;4:430–47.

347. Giulian D, Vaca K, Noonan CA. Secretion of neurotoxins by mononuclear phagocytes infected with HIV-1. Science. 1990;250:1593–6.

348. Giulian D, Wendt E, Vaca K, Noonan CA. The envelope glycoprotein of human immunodeficiency virus type 1 stimulates release of neurotoxins from monocytes. Proc Natl Acad Sci U S A. 1993;90:2769–73.

349. Krathwohl MD, Kaiser JL. HIV-1 promotes quiescence in human neural progenitor cells. J Infect Dis. 2004;190:216–26.

350. Okamoto S, Kang YJ, Brechtel CW, et al. HIV/gp120 decreases adult neural progenitor cell proliferation via checkpoint kinase-mediated cell-cycle withdrawal and G1 arrest. Cell Stem Cell. 2007;1:230–6.

351. Nogales-Gaete J, Syndulko K, Tourtellotte WW. Cerebrospinal fluid (CSF) analyses in HIV-1 primary neurological disease. Ital J Neurol Sci. 1992;13:667–83.

352. Navia BA, Jordan BD, Price RW. The AIDS dementia complex: I. Clinical features. Ann Neurol. 1986;19:517–24.

353. Freitas do Rosario AP, Langhorne J. T cell-derived IL-10 and its impact on the regulation of host responses during malaria. Int J Parasitol. 2012;42(6):549–55.

354. Garg RK. Cerebral malaria. J Assoc Physicians India. 2000;48: 1004–13.

355. Higgins SJ, Kain KC, Liles WC. Immunopathogenesis of falciparum malaria: implications for adjunctive therapy in the management of severe and cerebral malaria. Expert Rev Anti Infect Ther. 2011;9:803–19.

356. Mackintosh CL, Beeson JG, Marsh K. Clinical features and pathogenesis of severe malaria. Trends Parasitol. 2004;20:597–603.

357. Medana IM, Day NP, Sachanonta N, et al. Coma in fatal adult human malaria is not caused by cerebral oedema. Malar J. 2011;10:267.

358. Ponsford MJ, Medana IM, Prapansilp P, et al. Sequestration and microvascular congestion are associated with coma in human cerebral malaria. J Infect Dis. 2012;205:663–71.

359. Warrell DA. Management of severe malaria. Parassitologia. 1999;41:287–94.

360. Warrell DA, Looareesuwan S, Phillips RE, et al. Function of the blood-cerebrospinal fluid barrier in human cerebral malaria: rejection of the permeability hypothesis. Am J Trop Med Hyg. 1986;35:882–9.

361. Warrell DA, Looareesuwan S, Warrell MJ, et al. Dexamethasone proves deleterious in cerebral malaria. A double-blind trial in 100 comatose patients. N Engl J Med. 1982;306:313–9.

362. Warrell DA, White NJ, Warrell MJ. Dexamethasone deleterious in cerebral malaria. Br Med J (Clin Res Ed). 1982;285:1652.

363. Dondorp AM, Fanello CI, Hendriksen IC, et al. Artesunate versus quinine in the treatment of severe falciparum malaria in African children (AQUAMAT): an open-label, randomised trial. Lancet. 2010;376:1647–57.

364. Mohanty S, Mishra SK, Patnaik R, et al. Brain swelling and mannitol therapy in adult cerebral malaria: a randomized trial. Clin Infect Dis. 2011;53:349–55.

365. Qvarnstrom Y, James C, Xayavong M, et al. Comparison of real-time PCR protocols for differential laboratory diagnosis of amebiasis. J Clin Microbiol. 2005;43:5491–7.

366. Qvarnstrom Y, Visvesvara GS, Sriram R, da Silva AJ. Multiplex real-time PCR assay for simultaneous detection of Acanthamoeba spp., Balamuthia mandrillaris, and Naegleria fowleri. J Clin Microbiol. 2006;44:3589–95.

367. Seidel JS, Harmatz P, Visvesvara GS, Cohen A, Edwards J, Turner J. Successful treatment of primary amebic meningoencephalitis. N Engl J Med. 1982;306:346–8.

368. CDC. Primary amebic meningoencephalitis – Arizona, Florida, and Texas, 2007. MMWR Morb Mortal Wkly Rep. 2008;57:573–7.

369. Lopez C, Budge P, Chen J, et al. Primary amebic meningoencephalitis: a case report and literature review. Pediatr Emerg Care. 2012;28:272–6.

370. Soltow SM, Brenner GM. Synergistic activities of azithromycin and amphotericin B against Naegleria fowleri in vitro and in a mouse model of primary amebic meningoencephalitis. Antimicrob Agents Chemother. 2007;51:23–7.

371. Visvesvara GS. Amebic meningoencephalitides and keratitis: challenges in diagnosis and treatment. Curr Opin Infect Dis. 2010;23:590–4.

372. Del Brutto OH. Neurocysticercosis in Western Europe: a re-emerging disease? Acta Neurol Belg. 2012;112(4):335–43.

373. Del Brutto OH. Neurocysticercosis among international travelers to disease-endemic areas. J Travel Med. 2012;19:112–7.

374. Del Brutto OH. Neurocysticercosis: a review. ScientificWorld Journal. 2012;2012:159821.

375. Takayanagui OM, Jardim E. Clinical aspects of neurocysticercosis: analysis of 500 cases. Arq Neuropsiquiatr. 1983;41:50–63.

376. Sotelo J, Del Brutto OH. Review of neurocysticercosis. Neurosurg Focus. 2002;12:e1.

377. Sotelo J, Del Brutto OH. Brain cysticercosis. Arch Med Res. 2000;31:3–14.

378. Michelet L, Fleury A, Sciutto E, et al. Human neurocysticercosis: comparison of different diagnostic tests using cerebrospinal fluid. J Clin Microbiol. 2011;49:195–200.

379. Sotelo J, del Brutto OH, Penagos P, et al. Comparison of therapeutic regimen of anticysticercal drugs for parenchymal brain cysticercosis. J Neurol. 1990;237:69–72.

380. Del Brutto OH. Albendazole therapy for subarachnoid cysticerci: clinical and neuroimaging analysis of 17 patients. J Neurol Neurosurg Psychiatry. 1997;62:659–61.

381. Takayanagui OM, Jardim E. Therapy for neurocysticercosis. Comparison between albendazole and praziquantel. Arch Neurol. 1992;49:290–4.

382. Padma MV, Behari M, Misra NK, Ahuja GK. Albendazole in neurocysticercosis. Natl Med J India. 1995;8:255–8.

383. Carpio A, Santillan F, Leon P, Flores C, Hauser WA. Is the course of neurocysticercosis modified by treatment with antihelminthic agents? Arch Intern Med. 1995;155:1982–8.

384. Padma MV, Behari M, Misra NK, Ahuja GK. Albendazole in single CT ring lesions in epilepsy. Neurology. 1994;44:1344–6.

385. Riley T, White Jr AC. Management of neurocysticercosis. CNS Drugs. 2003;17:577–91.

386. Shandera WX, White Jr AC, Chen JC, Diaz P, Armstrong R. Neurocysticercosis in Houston, Texas. A report of 112 cases. Medicine. 1994;73:37–52.

387. White AC, Garcia HH. Recent developments in the epidemiology, diagnosis, treatment, and prevention of neurocysticercosis. Current infectious disease reports. 1999;1:434–40.

388. White Jr AC. Neurocysticercosis: a major cause of neurological disease worldwide. Clin Infect Dis. 1997;24:101–13; quiz 14–5.

389. Jimenez-Vazquez OH, Nagore N. Cisternal neurocysticercosis. Br J Neurosurg. 2008;22:774–5.

390. Sotelo J. Clinical manifestations, diagnosis, and treatment of neurocysticercosis. Curr Neurol Neurosci Rep. 2011;11:529–35.

391. Garcia HH, Evans CA, Nash TE, et al. Current consensus guidelines for treatment of neurocysticercosis. Clin Microbiol Rev. 2002;15:747–56.

392. Garcia HH, Del Brutto OH, Nash TE, White Jr AC, Tsang VC, Gilman RH. New concepts in the diagnosis and management of neurocysticercosis (Taenia solium). Am J Trop Med Hyg. 2005;72:3–9.

393. Sommer C, Ringelstein EB, Biniek R, Glockner WM. Adult Toxocara canis encephalitis. J Neurol Neurosurg Psychiatry. 1994;57:229–31.

394. Moreira-Silva SF, Rodrigues MG, Pimenta JL, Gomes CP, Freire LH, Pereira FE. Toxocariasis of the central nervous system: with report of two cases. Rev Soc Bras Med Trop. 2004;37:169–74.

395. Maiga Y, Wiertlewski S, Desal H, Marjolet M, Damier P. Presentation of cerebral toxocariasis with mental confusion in an adult: case report and review of the literature. Bull Soc Pathol Exot. 2007;100:101–4.

396. Finsterer J, Auer H. Neurotoxocarosis. Rev Inst Med Trop São Paulo. 2007;49:279–87.

397. Lukehart SA, Hook 3rd EW, Baker-Zander SA, Collier AC, Critchlow CW, Handsfield HH. Invasion of the central nervous system by Treponema pallidum: implications for diagnosis and treatment. Ann Intern Med. 1988;109:855–62.

398. Simon RP. Neurosyphilis. Arch Neurol. 1985;42:606–13.

399. Hotson JR. Modern neurosyphilis: a partially treated chronic meningitis. West J Med. 1981;135:191–200.

400. Hooshmand H, Escobar MR, Kopf SW. Neurosyphilis. A study of 241 patients. JAMA. 1972;219:726–9.

401. Holmes MD, Brant-Zawadzki MM, Simon RP. Clinical features of meningovascular syphilis. Neurology. 1984;34:553–6.

402. Flood JM, Weinstock HS, Guroy ME, Bayne L, Simon RP, Bolan G. Neurosyphilis during the AIDS epidemic, San Francisco, 1985–1992. J Infect Dis. 1998;177:931–40.

403. Ghanem KG. REVIEW: neurosyphilis: a historical perspective and review. CNS Neurosci Ther. 2010;16:e157–68.

404. Weinert LS, Scheffel RS, Zoratto G, et al. Cerebral syphilitic gumma in HIV-infected patients: case report and review. Int J STD AIDS. 2008;19:62–4.

405. Horowitz HW, Valsamis MP, Wicher V, et al. Brief report: cerebral syphilitic gumma confirmed by the polymerase chain reaction in a man with human immunodeficiency virus infection. N Engl J Med. 1994;331:1488–91.

406. Fiumara NJ. Treatment of primary and secondary syphilis. Serological response. JAMA. 1980;243:2500–2.

407. Brown ST, Zaidi A, Larsen SA, Reynolds GH. Serological response to syphilis treatment. A new analysis of old data. JAMA. 1985;253:1296–9.

408. Davis LE, Schmitt JW. Clinical significance of cerebrospinal fluid tests for neurosyphilis. Ann Neurol. 1989;25:50–5.

409. Workowski KA, Berman S. Sexually transmitted diseases treatment guidelines, 2010. MMWR Recomm Rep. 2010;59:1–110.

410. Moore JE. Asymptomatic neurosyphilis V: a comparison of early and late asymptomatic neurosyphilis. Arch Derm Syphilol. 1928;18:99–108.

411. Wilner E, Brody JA. Prognosis of general paresis after treatment. Lancet. 1968;2:1370–1.

412. Curtis AC, Cutler JC, Gammon G, et al. Penicillin treatment of asymptomatic central nervous system syphilis. I. Probability of

progression to symptomatic neurosyphilis. AMA Arch Dermatol. 1956;74:355–66.

413. Dunlop EM, Al-Egaily SS, Houang ET. Penicillin levels in blood and CSF achieved by treatment of syphilis. JAMA. 1979;241:2538–40.

414. Mohr JA, Griffiths W, Jackson R, Saadah H, Bird P, Riddle J. Neurosyphilis and penicillin levels in cerebrospinal fluid. JAMA. 1976;236:2208–9.

415. Schoth PE, Wolters EC. Penicillin concentrations in serum and CSF during high-dose intravenous treatment for neurosyphilis. Neurology. 1987;37:1214–6.

416. Fargen KM, Alvernia JE, Lin CS, Melgar M. Cerebral syphilitic gummata: a case presentation and analysis of 156 reported cases. Neurosurgery. 2009;64:568–75; discussion 75–6.

417. Steere AC, Malawista SE, Snydman DR, et al. Lyme arthritis: an epidemic of oligoarticular arthritis in children and adults in three connecticut communities. Arthritis Rheum. 1977;20:7–17.

418. Steere AC, Malawista SE, Hardin JA, Ruddy S, Askenase W, Andiman WA. Erythema chronicum migrans and Lyme arthritis. The enlarging clinical spectrum. Ann Intern Med. 1977;86:685–98.

419. Steere AC, Broderick TF, Malawista SE. Erythema chronicum migrans and Lyme arthritis: epidemiologic evidence for a tick vector. Am J Epidemiol. 1978;108:312–21.

420. Wallis RC, Brown SE, Kloter KO, Main Jr AJ. Erythema chronicum migrans and lyme arthritis: field study of ticks. Am J Epidemiol. 1978;108:322–7.

421. Burgdorfer W. Discovery of the Lyme disease spirochete and its relation to tick vectors. Yale J Biol Med. 1984;57:515–20.

422. Burgdorfer W. The enlarging spectrum of tick-borne spirochetoses: R. R. Parker Memorial Address. Rev Infect Dis. 1986;8: 932–40.

423. Steere AC, Bartenhagen NH, Craft JE, et al. Clinical manifestations of Lyme disease. Zentralbl Bakteriol Mikrobiol Hyg A. 1986;263:201–5.

424. Steere AC, Bartenhagen NH, Craft JE, et al. The early clinical manifestations of Lyme disease. Ann Intern Med. 1983;99:76–82.

425. Steere AC. Lyme disease. N Engl J Med. 1989;321:586–96.

426. Yoshinari NH, Steere AC, Cossermelli W. A review of Lyme disease. Rev Assoc Med Bras. 1989;35:34–8.

427. Keller TL, Halperin JJ, Whitman M. PCR detection of Borrelia burgdorferi DNA in cerebrospinal fluid of Lyme neuroborreliosis patients. Neurology. 1992;42:32–42.

428. Preac-Mursic V, Weber K, Pfister HW, et al. Survival of Borrelia burgdorferi in antibiotically treated patients with Lyme borreliosis. Infection. 1989;17:355–9.

429. Shadick NA, Phillips CB, Logigian EL, et al. The long-term clinical outcomes of Lyme disease. A population-based retrospective cohort study. Ann Intern Med. 1994;121:560–7.

430. Ackermann R, Rehse-Kupper B, Gollmer E, Schmidt R. Chronic neurologic manifestations of erythema migrans borreliosis. Ann N Y Acad Sci. 1988;539:16–23.

431. Hanny PE, Hauselmann HJ. Lyme disease from the neurologist's viewpoint. Schweiz Med Wochenschr. 1987;117:901–15.

432. Kohler J, Kern U, Kasper J, Rhese-Kupper B, Thoden U. Chronic central nervous system involvement in Lyme borreliosis. Neurology. 1988;38:863–7.

433. Kuntzer T, Bogousslavsky J, Miklossy J, Steck AJ, Janzer R, Regli F. Borrelia rhombencephalomyelopathy. Arch Neurol. 1991;48: 832–6.

434. Meurers B, Kohlhepp W, Gold R, Rohrbach E, Mertens HG. Histopathological findings in the central and peripheral nervous systems in neuroborreliosis. A report of three cases. J Neurol. 1990;237:113–6.

435. Mokry M, Flaschka G, Kleinert G, Kleinert R, Fazekas F, Kopp W. Chronic Lyme disease with an expansive granulomatous lesion in the cerebellopontine angle. Neurosurgery. 1990;27:446–51.

436. Pachner AR. Borrelia burgdorferi in the nervous system: the new "great imitator". Ann N Y Acad Sci. 1988;539:56–64.

437. Rafto SE, Milton WJ, Galetta SL, Grossman RI. Biopsy-confirmed CNS Lyme disease: MR appearance at 1.5 T. AJNR Am J Neuroradiol. 1990;11:482–4.

438. Crisp D, Ashby P. Lyme radiculoneuritis treated with intravenous immunoglobulin. Neurology. 1996;46:1174–5.

439. O'Connell S. Lyme borreliosis: current issues in diagnosis and management. Curr Opin Infect Dis. 2010;23:231–5.

440. Mertens HG, Martin R, Kohlhepp W. Clinical and neuroimmunological findings in chronic Borrelia burgdorferi radiculomyelitis (Lyme disease). J Neuroimmunol. 1988;20:309–14.

441. Logigian EL, Kaplan RF, Steere AC. Chronic neurologic manifestations of Lyme disease. N Engl J Med. 1990;323:1438–44.

442. Reik Jr L. Stroke due to Lyme disease. Neurology. 1993;43: 2705–7.

443. Weder B, Wiedersheim P, Matter L, Steck A, Otto F. Chronic progressive neurological involvement in Borrelia burgdorferi infection. J Neurol. 1987;234:40–3.

444. Agarwal R, Sze G. Neuro-lyme disease: MR imaging findings. Radiology. 2009;253:167–73.

445. Hildenbrand P, Craven DE, Jones R, Nemeskal P. Lyme neuroborreliosis: manifestations of a rapidly emerging zoonosis. AJNR Am J Neuroradiol. 2009;30:1079–87.

446. Kohler J, Kasper J, Kern U, Thoden U, Rehse-Kupper B. Borrelia encephalomyelitis. Lancet. 1986;2:35.

447. Agosta F, Rocca MA, Benedetti B, Capra R, Cordioli C, Filippi M. MR imaging assessment of brain and cervical cord damage in patients with neuroborreliosis. AJNR Am J Neuroradiol. 2006;27: 892–4.

448. Bigi S, Aebi C, Nauer C, Bigler S, Steinlin M. Acute transverse myelitis in Lyme neuroborreliosis. Infection. 2010;38:413–6.

449. Chang BL, Shih CM, Ro LS, et al. Acute neuroborreliosis with involvement of the central nervous system. J Neurol Sci. 2010;295: 10–5.

450. Halperin JJ, Luft BJ, Anand AK, et al. Lyme neuroborreliosis: central nervous system manifestations. Neurology. 1989;39:753–9.

451. Halperin JJ. Nervous system lyme disease: diagnosis and treatment. Rev Neurol Dis. 2009;6:4–12.

452. Halperin JJ. Nervous system Lyme disease. J R Coll Physicians Edinb. 2010;40:248–55.

453. Halperin JJ. Central nervous system Lyme disease. Curr Neurol Neurosci Rep. 2005;5:446–52.

454. Halperin JJ, Pass HL, Anand AK, Luft BJ, Volkman DJ, Dattwyler RJ. Nervous system abnormalities in Lyme disease. Ann N Y Acad Sci. 1988;539:24–34.

455. Halperin J, Luft BJ, Volkman DJ, Dattwyler RJ. Lyme neuroborreliosis. Peripheral nervous system manifestations. Brain. 1990;113(Pt 4):1207–21.

456. Halperin JJ. Neuroborreliosis: central nervous system involvement. Semin Neurol. 1997;17:19–24.

457. Halperin JJ. Neuroborreliosis (nervous system Lyme disease). Curr Treat Options Neurol. 1999;1:139–46.

458. Logigian EL, Steere AC. Clinical and electrophysiologic findings in chronic neuropathy of Lyme disease. Neurology. 1992;42:303–11.

459. Halperin JJ. North American Lyme neuroborreliosis. Scand J Infect Dis Suppl. 1991;77:74–80.

460. Steere AC, Pachner AR, Malawista SE. Neurologic abnormalities of Lyme disease: successful treatment with high-dose intravenous penicillin. Ann Intern Med. 1983;99:767–72.

461. Kalish RA, Kaplan RF, Taylor E, Jones-Woodward L, Workman K, Steere AC. Evaluation of study patients with Lyme disease, 10-20-year follow-up. J Infect Dis. 2001;183:453–60.

462. Pfister HW, Preac-Mursic V, Wilske B, Einhaupl KM. Cefotaxime vs penicillin G for acute neurologic manifestations in Lyme borreliosis. A prospective randomized study. Arch Neurol. 1989;46:1190–4.

463. Pfister HW, Preac-Mursic V, Wilske B, Schielke E, Sorgel F, Einhaupl KM. Randomized comparison of ceftriaxone and cefotaxime in Lyme neuroborreliosis. J Infect Dis. 1991;163: 311–8.

464. Pfister HW, Rupprecht TA. Clinical aspects of neuroborreliosis and post-Lyme disease syndrome in adult patients. Int J Med Microbiol. 2006;296 Suppl 40:11–6.

465. Halperin JJ. Diagnosis and treatment of the neuromuscular manifestations of lyme disease. Curr Treat Options Neurol. 2007;9:93–100.

466. Logigian EL, Kaplan RF, Steere AC. Successful treatment of Lyme encephalopathy with intravenous ceftriaxone. J Infect Dis. 1999;180:377–83.

467. Halperin JJ, Shapiro ED, Logigian E, et al. Practice parameter: treatment of nervous system Lyme disease (an evidence-based review): report of the Quality Standards Subcommittee of the American Academy of Neurology. Neurology. 2007;69:91–102.

468. Klempner MS, Hu LT, Evans J, et al. Two controlled trials of antibiotic treatment in patients with persistent symptoms and a history of Lyme disease. N Engl J Med. 2001;345:85–92.

469. Sexton DJ, Kaye KS. Rocky mountain spotted fever. Med Clin North Am. 2002;86:351–60, vii–viii.

470. Chapman AS, Bakken JS, Folk SM, et al. Diagnosis and management of tickborne rickettsial diseases: Rocky Mountain spotted fever, ehrlichioses, and anaplasmosis – United States: a practical guide for physicians and other health-care and public health professionals. MMWR Recomm Rep. 2006;55:1–27.

471. Chen LF, Sexton DJ. What's new in Rocky Mountain spotted fever? Infect Dis Clin North Am. 2008;22:415–32, vii–viii.

472. Kirkland KB, Wilkinson WE, Sexton DJ. Therapeutic delay and mortality in cases of Rocky Mountain spotted fever. Clin Infect Dis. 1995;20:1118–21.

473. Archibald LK, Sexton DJ. Long-term sequelae of Rocky Mountain spotted fever. Clin Infect Dis. 1995;20:1122–5.

474. Sexton DJ, Kirkland KB. Rickettsial infections and the central nervous system. Clin Infect Dis. 1998;26:247–8.

475. Ismail N, Bloch KC, McBride JW. Human ehrlichiosis and anaplasmosis. Clin Lab Med. 2010;30:261–92.

476. Windsor JJ. Cat-scratch disease: epidemiology, aetiology and treatment. Br J Biomed Sci. 2001;58:101–10.

477. Weston KD, Tran T, Kimmel KN, Maria BL. Possible role of high-dose corticosteroids in the treatment of cat-scratch disease encephalopathy. J Child Neurol. 2001;16:762–3.

478. Genizi J, Kasis I, Schif A, Shahar E. Effect of high-dose methyl-prednisolone on brainstem encephalopathy and basal ganglia impairment complicating cat scratch disease. Brain Dev. 2007;29:377–9.

479. Schneider T, Moos V, Loddenkemper C, Marth T, Fenollar F, Raoult D. Whipple's disease: new aspects of pathogenesis and treatment. Lancet Infect Dis. 2008;8:179–90.

480. Slowik A, Szczudlik A. Whipple's disease – a rare cause of neurological symptoms and disorders. Neurol Neurochir Pol. 2002; 36:959–70.

481. Relman DA, Schmidt TM, MacDermott RP, Falkow S. Identification of the uncultured bacillus of Whipple's disease. N Engl J Med. 1992;327:293–301.

482. Schoniger-Hekele M, Petermann D, Weber B, Muller C. Tropheryma whipplei in the environment: survey of sewage plant influxes and sewage plant workers. Appl Environ Microbiol. 2007;73:2033–5.

483. Moos V, Loddenkemper C, Schneider T. Tropheryma whipplei infection. Colonization, self-limiting infection and Whipple's disease. Pathologe. 2011;32:362–70.

484. Moos V, Schneider T. Changing paradigms in Whipple's disease and infection with Tropheryma whipplei. Eur J Clin Microbiol Infect Dis. 2011;30:1151–8.

485. Abreu P, Azevedo E, Lobo L, Moura CS, Pontes C. Whipple disease and central nervous system. Acta Med Port. 2005;18: 199–208.

486. Bermejo P, Burgos A. Whipple's disease and central nervous system. Med Clin (Barc). 2006;127:379–85.

487. Durand DV, Lecomte C, Cathebras P, Rousset H, Godeau P. Whipple disease. Clinical review of 52 cases. The SNFMI Research Group on Whipple Disease. Societe Nationale Francaise de Medecine Interne. Medicine. 1997;76:170–84.

488. Louis ED. Whipple disease. Curr Neurol Neurosci Rep. 2003;3:470–5.

489. Louis ED, Lynch T, Kaufmann P, Fahn S, Odel J. Diagnostic guidelines in central nervous system Whipple's disease. Ann Neurol. 1996;40:561–8.

490. Scheld WM. Whipple disease of the central nervous system. J Infect Dis. 2003;188:797–800.

491. Vital Durand D, Gerard A, Rousset H. Neurological manifestations of Whipple disease. Rev Neurol. 2002;158:988–92.

492. Baisden BL, Lepidi H, Raoult D, Argani P, Yardley JH, Dumler JS. Diagnosis of Whipple disease by immunohistochemical analysis: a sensitive and specific method for the detection of Tropheryma whipplei (the Whipple bacillus) in paraffin-embedded tissue. Am J Clin Pathol. 2002;118:742–8.

493. Gerard A, Sarrot-Reynauld F, Liozon E, et al. Neurologic presentation of Whipple disease: report of 12 cases and review of the literature. Medicine. 2002;81:443–57.

494. Panegyres PK, Edis R, Beaman M, Fallon M. Primary Whipple's disease of the brain: characterization of the clinical syndrome and molecular diagnosis. QJM. 2006;99:609–23.

495. Schnider PJ, Reisinger EC, Berger T, Krejs GJ, Auff E. Treatment guidelines in central nervous system Whipple's disease. Ann Neurol. 1997;41:561–2.

496. Schnider PJ, Reisinger EC, Gerschlager W, et al. Long-term follow-up in cerebral Whipple's disease. Eur J Gastroenterol Hepatol. 1996;8:899–903.

497. Gutierrez J, Issacson RS, Koppel BS. Subacute sclerosing panencephalitis: an update. Dev Med Child Neurol. 2010;52:901–7.

498. Weissert R. Progressive multifocal leukoencephalopathy. J Neuroimmunol. 2011;231:73–7.

499. Fox R. Advances in the management of PML: focus on natalizumab. Cleve Clin J Med. 2011;78 Suppl 2:S33–7.

500. Brooks BR, Walker DL. Progressive multifocal leukoencephalopathy. Neurol Clin. 1984;2:299–313.

501. Egli A, Infanti L, Dumoulin A, et al. Prevalence of polyomavirus BK and JC infection and replication in 400 healthy blood donors. J Infect Dis. 2009;199:837–46.

502. White 3rd FA, Ishaq M, Stoner GL, Frisque RJ. JC virus DNA is present in many human brain samples from patients without progressive multifocal leukoencephalopathy. J Virol. 1992;66:5726–34.

503. Vago L, Cinque P, Sala E, et al. JCV-DNA and BKV-DNA in the CNS tissue and CSF of AIDS patients and normal subjects. Study of 41 cases and review of the literature. J Acquir Immune Defic Syndr. 1996;12:139–46.

504. Quinlivan EB, Norris M, Bouldin TW, et al. Subclinical central nervous system infection with JC virus in patients with AIDS. J Infect Dis. 1992;166:80–5.

505. Koralnik IJ, Boden D, Mai VX, Lord CI, Letvin NL. JC virus DNA load in patients with and without progressive multifocal leukoencephalopathy. Neurology. 1999;52:253–60.

506. Ferrante P, Caldarelli-Stefano R, Omodeo-Zorini E, Vago L, Boldorini R, Costanzi G. PCR detection of JC virus DNA in brain tissue from patients with and without progressive multifocal leukoencephalopathy. J Med Virol. 1995;47:219–25.

507. Dubois V, Dutronc H, Lafon ME, et al. Latency and reactivation of JC virus in peripheral blood of human immunodeficiency virus type 1-infected patients. J Clin Microbiol. 1997;35:2288–92.

508. Holman RC, Janssen RS, Buehler JW, Zelasky MT, Hooper WC. Epidemiology of progressive multifocal leukoencephalopathy in the United States: analysis of national mortality and AIDS surveillance data. Neurology. 1991;41:1733–6.

509. Christensen KL, Holman RC, Hammett TA, Belay ED, Schonberger LB. Progressive multifocal leukoencephalopathy deaths in the USA, 1979–2005. Neuroepidemiology. 2010;35:178–84.

510. Amend KL, Turnbull B, Foskett N, Napalkov P, Kurth T, Seeger J. Incidence of progressive multifocal leukoencephalopathy in patients without HIV. Neurology. 2010;75:1326–32.

511. Focosi D, Marco T, Kast RE, Maggi F, Ceccherini-Nelli L, Petrini M. Progressive multifocal leukoencephalopathy: what's new? Neuroscientist. 2010;16:308–23.

512. Hernandez B, Dronda F, Moreno S. Treatment options for AIDS patients with progressive multifocal leukoencephalopathy. Expert Opin Pharmacother. 2009;10:403–16.

513. Lima MA, Bernal-Cano F, Clifford DB, Gandhi RT, Koralnik IJ. Clinical outcome of long-term survivors of progressive multifocal leukoencephalopathy. J Neurol Neurosurg Psychiatry. 2010;81:1288–91.

514. Tavazzi E, White MK, Khalili K. Progressive multifocal leukoencephalopathy: clinical and molecular aspects. Rev Med Virol. 2012;22:18–32.

515. Silverman L, Rubinstein LJ. Electron microscopic observations on a case of progressive multifocal leukoencephalopathy. Acta Neuropathol. 1965;5:215–24.

516. McGuire D, Barhite S, Hollander H, Miles M. JC virus DNA in cerebrospinal fluid of human immunodeficiency virus-infected patients: predictive value for progressive multifocal leukoencephalopathy. Ann Neurol. 1995;37:395–9.

517. Hammarin AL, Bogdanovic G, Svedhem V, Pirskanen R, Morfeldt L, Grandien M. Analysis of PCR as a tool for detection of JC virus DNA in cerebrospinal fluid for diagnosis of progressive multifocal leukoencephalopathy. J Clin Microbiol. 1996; 34:2929–32.

518. Dorries K, Arendt G, Eggers C, Roggendorf W, Dorries R. Nucleic acid detection as a diagnostic tool in polyomavirus JC induced progressive multifocal leukoencephalopathy. J Med Virol. 1998; 54:196–203.

519. De Luca A, Giancola ML, Ammassari A, et al. Potent antiretroviral therapy with or without cidofovir for AIDS-associated progressive multifocal leukoencephalopathy: extended follow-up of an observational study. J Neurovirol. 2001;7:364–8.

520. Hall CD, Dafni U, Simpson D, et al. Failure of cytarabine in progressive multifocal leukoencephalopathy associated with human immunodeficiency virus infection. AIDS Clinical Trials Group 243 Team. N Engl J Med. 1998;338:1345–51.

521. Rand KH, Ulm AJ, Pincus DW. Central nervous system infections. In: Layon AJ, Gabrielli A, Friedman WA, editors. Textbook of neurointensive care. Philadelphia: WB Saunders; 2004.

Part V

Special Situations

Diagnosis and Treatment of Altered Mental Status

23

Bryan D. Riggeal, Candice S. Waked, and Michael S. Okun

Contents

B.D. Riggeal, MD
Rockdale Neurology Associates, 1301 Sigman Rd, NE,
Conyers, GA 30306, USA
e-mail: riggeal@gmail.com

C.S. Waked, DO
Department of Neurology, Emory University,
Atlanta, GA 32608, USA
e-mail: candice.waked@gmail.com

M.S. Okun, MD (✉)
Department of Neurology, University of Florida College of Medicine,
3450 Hull Rd, Gainesville, FL 32607, USA
e-mail: okun@neurology.ufl.edu

Abstract

Altered mental status is commonly encountered in the Neurological Intensive Care Unit, and the differential diagnosis is broad. The general and neurological examinations can give many clues both to the neurological and non-neurological causes. Neuroimaging, neurophysiological tests, and laboratory studies are often helpful in identifying the etiology, which can run the entire gamut of disease processes including vascular, neoplastic, metabolic, or infectious. In cases of brain death, it is essential to understand the diagnostic criteria as well as adjunctive studies.

Keywords

Delirium • Confusion • Encephalopathy • Brain death
Coma

Introduction

Altered mental status is a commonly encountered phenomenon in the Neurological Intensive Care Unit (NICU), but the reported range can be quite broad (13–70 %) [1]. It may occur secondary to a variety of neurological and non-neurological etiologies. The differential diagnosis of altered mental status in the NICU is dauntingly large. It is important to narrow the differential by employing an understanding of the mechanisms underpinning arousal, by acquiring a careful

A.J. Layon et al. (eds.), *Textbook of Neurointensive Care*,
DOI 10.1007/978-1-4471-5226-2_23, © Springer-Verlag London 2013

history and physical examination, and by running carefully through the list of potential medical and neurological causes of an alteration of mental status.

Presentations and Descriptions of the Level of Arousal

The grades for the degree of altered mental status [2] can be helpful when communicating with other health-care providers and also helpful in determining the severity of illness. They may or may not help in discerning a possible diagnosis and/or prognosis. There are many ways to grade the degree of altered mentation. None of these are localizing, but all are helpful in understanding the clinical picture. Next, we will review common terms used by ICU practitioners. It is important to use the terms with consistency.

Clouding of consciousness refers to a patient that is inattentive without frank confusion and without disorientation. These individuals are usually not anosognosic—they are aware of their deficit—which differs from other forms of altered mentation. This term is commonly used to describe individuals who use certain medications or have mild metabolic disturbances [3].

A *confusional state* is similar to clouding of consciousness but has the additional feature of added confusion and/or disorientation. These individuals can be hypervigilant and can be combative. This state may result from medication use but more commonly is associated with infections or is encountered in individuals with very little cognitive reserve. When seen in those with poor cognitive reserve, these individuals usually have baseline physical, medical, or environmental stressors that contribute to the confusional state [3].

Lethargy refers to individuals who spontaneously sleep most of the day. These individuals will wake with only mild stimulation but may also be confused. They may easily drift back to sleep if left unstimulated. During a bedside interview, they may require repeated stimuli to maintain appropriate attention and wakefulness. Often, these patients will be incomprehensible to a bedside examiner's ear, but they may occasionally provide useful historical and examination clues, especially if continuously stimulated. Lethargy is commonly associated with metabolic disturbances as well as other toxic etiologies [3].

Obtundation is a state when an individual is less responsive to stimuli than is seen in a somnolent state. These patients are usually not interested in their environment when they are aroused. Obtunded patients may be difficult to arouse and may require deep pain to assess appropriate responses. Obtunded patients are slowed in their responsiveness and may stop interacting with their environment if not constantly stimulated. This state can be caused by a multitude of etiologies including metabolic disturbances,

intoxications, brain lesions (with mild to moderate mass effect), CNS infections, seizures, and other etiologies [3].

Stupor is considered one level worse than obtundation. These individuals may react to deep pain but do not interact with their environment. They may only grimace or draw (their body or an extremity) away from the pain. A stuporous patient may otherwise not perform purposeful actions. This state results from similar etiologies as are encountered in obtundation [3].

Coma describes a patient who has no response to their environment and who frequently also has impaired brainstem reflexes (described in detail later in this chapter). Coma patients do not respond to deep pain and commonly have no corneal or gag reflex. Coma is usually due to severe impairment of the ascending reticular activating system (ARAS) and is indicative of a severe pathological process. Common causes of coma include anoxic brain injury, brainstem lesions, severe stroke or hemorrhage (usually with significant mass effect), and severe intoxications [3].

Neurocircuitry Underpinning the Level of Arousal

The level of arousal and the circuits that modulate consciousness have not been fully elicited. It is believed that the reticular activating system plays a very important role in mediating wakefulness. The reticular formation (throughout the brainstem), particularly in the periventricular region, gives rise to the ARAS. This system is thought to play a key role in activating the thalamocortical unit and in attentional processes. Once ascending to the level of the thalamus, the ARAS has a bilateral representation and continues to ascend to the ipsilateral hemisphere, respectively [4]. A depressed level of arousal can be induced by bilateral disruption of this system. At the level of the brainstem, discrete lesions will commonly include or compromise a significant portion of the reticular formation or even the ARAS, whereas lesions more rostral may only affect the ARAS on the ipsilateral side and therefore rarely produce alterations of consciousness (due to the preserved contralateral ARAS). This explains why supratentorial lesions rarely depress the level of arousal. One exception is significant mass effect that displaces brain tissue, resulting in compromise of the contralateral ARAS [5]. Initially, Plum and Posner wrote that supratentorial mass lesions resulting in a depressed level of arousal could cause a downward force that impinged upon the brainstem reticular formation [2]. However, this notion has now been expanded to include lateral forces that can (in the case of mass effect) also contribute to arousal issues [5–7]. These arousal systems have a fair amount of redundancy, and it is this redundancy that may account for the relatively short-lived attentional problems in many patients, regardless of the etiology [8].

CNS insults other than focal lesions can also disturb the level of arousal. Toxic or metabolic derangements that disturb the ARAS and/or the cortex more diffusely may result in clinical issues. It is not uncommon for toxic substances associated with systemic disease such as urea or ammonia to impair the function of the cerebral cortex more diffusely and therefore impair the terminal connections of the ARAS. This diffuse dysfunction of the cerebral cortex and ARAS may result in a depressed level of arousal and can be manifested by diffuse slowing on the electroencephalogram (EEG) [9].

Physical Examination and Evaluation in the ICU Setting

General

The importance of a complete general physical examination in the ICU setting cannot be overemphasized. Many people mistakenly believe an ICU patient cannot be examined neurologically. This is false. Much information can be gained from observing the level of arousal prior to stimulation, as well as by observing the individual's reaction to verbal and tactile stimulation [2]. It is important to observe if an individual appears to be responding to internal-based stimuli, if they exhibit any abnormal movements, or if they are manifesting a normal or alternatively abnormal breathing pattern. All of these observations can aid in narrowing the differential diagnosis for an altered mental status. Examining specific systems can also reveal signs that may be directly or indirectly related to the cause of the altered mental status. Some of the issues uncovered may necessitate treatment, but the patient themselves cannot relay symptoms as a result of their state of diminished cognition. Examining specific organ systems can be helpful in both determining organ specific conditions that could cause or contribute to an altered mental status or contribute to the manifestations of the process underlying the altered state [10].

Cardiac and Carotid Examination

Auscultation of the chest could reveal evidence of a murmur, distant heart sounds, or a pericardial rub, all of which may be clues to underlying hypoxemia or other causes that may have contributed to the altered mental status. It is important to keep in mind that aortic stenosis may present with syncope and a systolic ejection murmur radiating to the carotid artery region. The sound heard with aortic stenosis that radiates to the carotid artery region can sometimes be distinguished from that of carotid stenosis simply by auscultating over the ipsilateral eye (utilizing the bell of the stethoscope) [11]. If a sound is heard over the eye, it could be a referred sound

emanating through the ophthalmic artery (the first branch off of the internal carotid artery) or secondary to reversal of flow from a completely occluded contralateral carotid artery [12]. In aortic stenosis, the pulse may also be appreciated as late and as weak (a pulsus parvus et tardus). A pericardial rub may be a clue to underlying pericarditis or a cardiac tamponade, both of which may contribute to, or be associated with, an altered mental status (presumably due to a decreased cardiac outflow and hypoxemia). Listening for carotid bruits proximally and/or distally may clue the examiner in to the potential stroke and arterial dissection risk [13].

Heart failure and acute myocardial infarction can result in an altered mental status [14], potentially by the mechanism of hypoxemia. In the ICU setting a cardiac examination should always be used to evaluate for a S3/S4 heart sound, a Kussmaul sign or hepatojugular reflux—all of which may offer clues to an underlying etiology that may contribute to an altered mental status.

Pulmonary Examination and Respiratory Patterns

The pulmonary examination focuses on both the auscultation of the chest and also the overall breathing patterns. Abnormal breath sounds can be indicative of pulmonary issues such as pneumonia, pneumothorax, and foreign bodies—all of which may result in an altered mental status (presumably by hypoxemia).

Abnormal respiratory patterns may offer clues to the underlying etiology of a mental status change [15]. Occasionally, an abnormal respiratory pattern can be indicative of brainstem damage [16]. A summary of abnormal breathing patterns has been provided in Table 23.1.

Persistent hyperventilation can be seen in many conditions such as intoxication with acidifying compounds (e.g., aspirin), hepatic coma, metabolic acidosis, and fever. In cases of central nervous system (CNS) lesions, there may be *central neurogenic hyperventilation*. This condition is often precipitated by processes affecting the function of the midbrain and the pons. Neurogenic hyperventilation may be associated with primary CNS lymphoma [17].

Apneustic breathing has been described as a sudden, prolonged, gasping inspiration followed by a pause and then followed by an inadequate expiration. This breathing pattern should raise concern in the examiner, as it is commonly a clue that there is damage in the pneumotaxic centers located in the pons and in the medulla [18]. Other findings on physical examination that may be associated with apneustic breathing include absent brainstem reflexes (e.g., corneal and doll's eye reflexes, stupor, coma, decerebrate posturing). Occasionally, apneustic breathing can result from an acute intoxication.

Table 23.1 Summary of abnormal breathing patterns

Respiratory pattern	Description	Localization	Etiologies
Persistent hyperventilation	Hyperpnea	Midbrain, pons	Acidosis, hepatic coma, fever, CNS lymphoma
Apneustic breathing	Sudden, prolonged, gasping inspiration followed by a pause and then followed by an inadequate expiration	Pons, medulla	Lower brainstem lesion, acute intoxication
Kussmaul respirations	Slow, deep, labored, almost gasping respirations	Not CNS, usually metabolic	Acidosis, particularly diabetic ketoacidosis
Cheyne-Stokes respirations	Crescendo-decrescendo breathing pattern with irregular periods of apnea	Rarely pons and/or medulla	Metabolic encephalopathy, heart failure, intoxication, and carbon monoxide poisoning. Can rarely be caused by pontine/medullary lesions
Biot's respirations	Periods of alternating hyperpnea and hyperventilation with regular periods of apnea and constant tidal volumes	Medulla	Medullary lesions, narcotic overdose
Ataxic breathing	Completely disordered breathing pattern intermixed with irregular periods of apnea progressing to agonal respirations and eventually apnea	Medulla	Medullary lesions

Kussmaul respirations have been described as slow, deep, labored, almost gasping respirations. They have been associated with severe metabolic acidosis and have been classically described in diabetics and in ketoacidosis. Kussmaul respirations represent the later stages of acidosis. Earlier in acidosis, respirations are shallow and rapid as the brain attempts to compensate by hyperventilating and reducing the blood pH to near normal. Therefore, when the breathing pattern truly becomes slow and laborious, it is an ominous sign.

Cheyne-Stokes respirations have been classically described as a crescendo-decrescendo breathing pattern. Periodically, they alternate every 30–120 s, and the breathing pattern slowly shifts back and forth from that of rapid and deep to slow and shallow and eventually to a period of apnea. The slower and shallower breathing results in ineffective oxygen exchange, due to the increase in alveolar dead space. Cheyne-Stokes can be the respiratory pattern indicating imminent death; however, it may be encountered in reversible conditions. Cheyne-Stokes has been described in metabolic encephalopathy, heart failure, intoxication, and carbon monoxide poisoning. It has been encountered in conditions that damage the pontine/medullary respiratory centers [2].

Biot's respirations are similar to Cheyne-Stokes breathing with the important exception that the tidal volume usually does not fluctuate, and there are regular periods of apnea. This type of breathing may be indicative of a CNS lesion and usually localizes to the medullary region [19]. Biot's respirations have also been described in narcotic overdose [20].

Ataxic breathing has been described as a completely disordered breathing pattern intermixed with irregular periods of apnea. This breathing pattern may progress to agonal respirations, apnea, and death. Like Biot's respirations, the localization is usually medullary [21].

Abdominal Examination

The abdominal examination, when considering an altered mental status, should focus on a search for stigmata of liver disease. These stigmata can include spider angiomata, ascites, hepatomegaly, or caput medusa. The abdomen should be auscultated and palpated to evaluate for signs of intussusception, small bowel obstruction, bowel ischemia, bowel perforation, or appendicitis. The clinician should look for scars revealing prior surgeries, as these may offer important clues to etiology and especially prior history of organ transplantation [13].

Skin/Nail Examination

The skin and nails should be examined as they may reveal evidence of systemic diseases that could contribute to altering the mental status. The skin and nail examination may include evidence of yellowing (e.g., jaundice), other liver dysfunction, petechiae, signs of infection, microangiopathic hemolytic anemia, and splinter hemorrhages (a sign of systemic embolization). A clinician can also evaluate for stigmata of intravenous drug use such as track marks [13].

Neurological Examination

Glasgow Coma Scale (GCS)

The GCS, although simplistic and criticized for its lack of specificity, is the most commonly used scale to assess level of consciousness in clinical medicine. It is comprised of the summation of three scores: one each for motor, verbal, and

Table 23.2 Glasgow Coma Scale responses and scores

Score	Eye response	Verbal response	Motor response
1	No eye opening	No sounds	No response to pain
2	Opens eyes to pain	Incomprehensible noises	Decerebrate posturing (extension) in response to pain
3	Opens eyes to voice	Uses inappropriate words	Decorticate posturing (flexion) in response to pain
4	Opens eyes spontaneously	Confused or disoriented	Withdrawal to pain
5		Carries out normal conversation	Localizes to pain
6			Able to follow commands appropriately

Modified with permission of Elsevier from Teasdale and Jennett [124]

eye opening. Table 23.2 shows these responses and the corresponding scores for each. The sum of these three scores gives the GCS which lies with the range of 3–15 points, 3 being the worst and 15 being normal. This scale has less meaning than the levels of consciousness described previously, but is commonly used to communicate with other practitioners, and should therefore be thoroughly understood.

Higher Cortical Function

Often, a detailed higher cortical function examination is difficult to perform when altered mental status in the ICU is encountered. This should not stop an examiner from attempting this examination each day, especially as there may be fluctuations in the level of consciousness. Also, importantly in some conditions, there may be cognitive fluctuations at certain hours, so careful monitoring of the cortical examination and changes in mental status throughout the day and night can be critical.

Attention is tested by asking the patient to spell a word backward (e.g., WORLD), perform digit span [22], or count backward by sevens (which can also be used to test acalculia) [23]. Delirium and focal CNS lesions can sometimes be separated by the absence or presence of normal attention, as focal CNS lesions will rarely cause inattentiveness. It is also important to note that if a patient has poor attention, this may also affect their ability to participate in other portions of the neurological examination.

Other aspects of the higher cortical function examination that may be of particular value include noting abnormalities in language and in hemispatial/hemibody attention. These tests are likely to be disrupted in large hemispheric lesions; these lesions would typically depress consciousness, and they may show lateralization of the dysfunction to one or another brain hemisphere [24, 25].

Language is usually represented in the left hemisphere, and in many cases it is perisylvian in location [26]. Some general principles that may be helpful include examining fluency (e.g., getting words or letters out of the mouth), which may reflect more anterior lesions, and problems the patient has with comprehension, as this may reflect relatively more posterior lesions or dysfunction. Also, the more dorsal the lesion, the more likely the patient is to have spared repetition (e.g., transcortical aphasia), but if the lesion is causing dysfunction of the perisylvian cortex, especially caudally, they may be less likely to be able to repeat a phrase.

In the patient with right hemispheric damage, there may be hemispatial or hemibody neglect, especially if the lesion compromises the junction of the parietal, temporal, and occipital lobes. Hemispatial neglect is a syndrome where the individual manifests decreased spatial attention to people, objects, or any other stimuli in the environment, but this syndrome must be in the left of their plane of orientation. This is due to damage of the systems primarily in the right parietal lobe that may be responsible for spatial attention (e.g., although frontal and thalamic lesions may also result in these deficits) [24]. Lesions of the left parietal lobe rarely cause neglect, as the right parietal lobe services human attention to both hemispaces, while the left side gives only weak attention to the right hemispace [27].

Cranial Nerves

The cranial nerve examination is critical in a patient with an altered mental status, especially in the ICU setting. The ARAS originates in the pons and medulla and is condensed into a relatively small space running along with the corticobulbar tract, the cranial nerve nuclei, and the fascicles that interconnect these nuclei [4]. By these simple anatomical connections, a CNS lesion that is relatively localized within the brainstem can result in a disruption of a significant proportion of these ARAS fibers which may in turn result in an alteration of the level of consciousness. CNS lesions in the brainstem can result in deficits of cranial nerve function and level of arousal. It should be noted that many patients with altered mental status cannot fully participate in cranial nerve testing.

The pupillary response can be examined by shining a bright light into one eye and then observing the response in both eyes (i.e., the direct response) and then by examining the contralateral eye (e.g., a consensual response) [13]. The pupil should constrict briskly and equally in both eyes and with both responses. It is not uncommon for a patient in the ICU to be on multiple medications, especially sedatives and also paralytics. These medications may slow, dampen, or abolish a pupillary reaction, so medications must be considered as a factor when examining the eyes and recording abnormal responses (i.e., the benzodiazepine falsely dilated pupil) [28].

The neuroanatomy of the pupillary response is important. The light response begins with the photosensitive retinal ganglion cells which project via the optic nerve to the optic chiasm. At this point, 53 % of these fibers decussate, and 47 % stay ipsilateral. The optic tract terminates in the pretectal nucleus ipsilaterally, and this termination is located in the dorsal midbrain. The pretectal nuclei project bilaterally to the Edinger-Westphal nuclei, which are the parasympathetic subnuclei of the oculomotor nerve. The fibers decussate to synapse in the contralateral Edinger-Westphal nucleus and then travel through the posterior commissure [29]. The Edinger-Westphal nucleus has cholinergic neurons that project to the ipsilateral ciliary ganglion, which in turn projects to the pupillary constrictor muscles in an ipsilateral fashion. Understanding the neuroanatomy of this pathway can help to localize a neurological deficit. If for example, the pupillary reaction is brisk and equal to direct and consensual response bilaterally, the entire system—including the optic pathways, the dorsal midbrain, the posterior commissure, the third nerve nuclear complex, the third nerve, and the pupillary constrictor muscles—are likely intact.

A frequently encountered examination finding in the NICU is that of asymmetric pupils. The first step in approaching this patient is to determine which pupil is abnormal, the larger or smaller. If a pupil is abnormally large because it fails to constrict, this usually is due to an intrinsic problem within the eye such as iris tears or synechiae or alternatively parasympathetic dysfunction. If the smaller pupil is abnormal, this usually reflects sympathetic dysfunction such as a Horner's syndrome. This can be determined most easily by examining the patient in both brightly and dimly lit rooms. In a brightly lit room, both pupils would be expected to constrict, so if the failure is that of pupillary constriction, the size difference between the two eyes would increase. This would indicate that the larger pupil is the abnormal one. In a dimly lit room, both eyes would be expected to dilate, so if the failure is that of dilation, the difference between the two eyes would be greater in this scenario. This would indicate that the smaller pupil is abnormal [29]. An alternative scenario is that of physiological anisocoria, which is usually less than 0.5 mm difference between pupils and the difference is equal in light and dark.

A frequently encountered examination finding is a dilated pupil that reacts poorly to direct or to a consensual response. In some cases, however, whenever light is directed into a single-dilated pupil, the contralateral consensual response is normal. This situation may be encountered when there is a compromised third nerve, which carries the efferent parasympathetic fibers from the Edinger-Westphal nucleus to the pupillary constrictor muscles. The contralateral eye constricts to a consensual response, because the afferent limb made up of the optic nerve and tract remains intact [30].

A "blown pupil" that is dilated and poorly reactive to light, especially when more severe than the oculomotor deficits encountered, indicates an extrinsic compression of the nerve.

This manifestation results because the parasympathetic fibers travel peripherally in the nerve and are usually more susceptible to compressive forces when compared to the oculomotor fibers that are located more centrally within the nerve. The immediate concerns when faced with such an exam finding include an aneurysm, particularly of the posterior communicating artery, or alternatively a transtentorial herniation syndrome. The motor function of the oculomotor nerve may be lost as the compression worsens and may involve the inner portions of the nerve, so as the patient has increasing dysfunction of the oculomotor functions; it can then be inferred that the intracranial process is worsening. A compressive oculomotor nerve palsy can be caused by a few very important pathological processes including an aneurysm, particularly of the posterior communicating artery, as well as a transtentorial herniation syndrome [31]. Because this is an emergent situation, it is important to obtain CNS imaging as quickly as possible. A CT scan of the brain is usually adequate to rule out a transtentorial herniation, and a CT angiogram is required to evaluate properly for an aneurysm. It has been shown that it is very important to have a properly trained neuroradiologist who understands the indication(s) for the study and laterality of the findings [32, 33].

If the smaller pupil is abnormal, this usually indicates a failure of the sympathetic system in dilating the pupil. Several conditions can account for this issue, but the one of particular concern is a Horner's syndrome. The Horner's syndrome is characterized by the triad of miosis, anhidrosis, and ptosis. This can be caused by a lesion anywhere along the central or peripheral pathways containing axons related to the oculosympathetic system. If caused by a brainstem lesion, which is the main situation in which altered mental status can be associated with a Horner's syndrome, there will often be a contralateral loss of pain and temperature sensation because the descending sympathetics travel in close proximity to the spinothalamic tract. An ipsilateral ataxia and vertigo can be seen in cases of a lateral medullary syndrome. A Horner's syndrome can also be caused by lesions of the stellate ganglion as in the case of a pancoast tumor, or within the cavernous sinus, and/or as a result of a carotid dissection. Pharmacological testing can confirm a Horner's syndrome [34, 35]. One to two drops of 0.5 % apraclonidine in each eye will result in a reversal of anisocoria in the case of a Horner's syndrome. This reversal is due to the weak alpha-1 agonist properties of this medication which cause a significant mydriasis in the Horner's eye because of denervation hypersensitivity, and the strong alpha-2 properties that result in miosis in the unaffected eye [29, 36].

If the pupils both react briskly to light and then both constrict weakly to contralateral stimulation, it is likely that the ipsilateral optic nerve is damaged [29]. There may be a large differential diagnosis for an acute or subacute optic neuropathy, but the immediate primary concern when associated with an altered mental status in the ICU would be preexisting damage to the optic nerve, demyelinating disease, or acute disseminated encephalomyelitis. In the patient with HIV, the commonest optic neuropathy is caused by syphilis.

The corneal reflex is a monosynaptic connection comprised of two cranial nerves and connections within the pons. The afferent limb is the nasociliary branch of cranial nerve V1. When the cornea is touched with a sterile cotton swab, this signal travels into the brainstem at the level of the pons, descends to the caudal pons, and terminates in the bilateral facial nerve motor nuclei. The motor nucleus of VII projects ipsilaterally to the muscles of facial expression resulting in contraction of the orbicularis oculi bilaterally when either cornea is touched. If only one side of the face blinks when either cornea is touched, this indicates a peripheral facial nerve lesion on the side of decreased orbicularis oculi contraction. If both sides of the face manifest a decreased blink when one cornea is touched, but both contract normally when the other is touched, it is likely that there is either damage to the peripheral trigeminal nerve or to the fascicle that contains the fibers descending to the bilateral motor nuclei of VII. If the fascicle is damaged, it is common to have an exaggerated jaw jerk reflex (often evidence of a pontine issue and corticobulbar dysfunction) [37]. A patient may hold their jaw loosely open while an examiner places their finger on the chin and lightly strikes their own finger with a reflex hammer. The patient's jaw should normally gently recoil, but with an exaggerated jaw jerk, this becomes hyperactive and the patient may in some cases click their teeth together.

The brainstem connections in the lower pons and upper medulla can be tested by using the vestibulo-ocular reflex. The vestibulo-ocular reflex can be tested by performing a rapid head movement test, effectively turning the patient's head from side to side and observing for contralateral eye movement as well as nystagmus. This examination maneuver has been famously called a "doll's eyes" maneuver because the eye movements resemble that of an old fashioned doll that would move with head turning. In this circuit [38, 39], the vestibular systems project to the vestibular nuclei, which in turn stimulate the abducens nucleus on the side opposite the direction of head rotation and in turn inhibit the abducens nucleus on the side in which the head is turning. The abducens nucleus then projects via the abducens nerve to the ipsilateral lateral rectus and also, via the median longitudinal fasciculus, to the contralateral medial rectus subnucleus of the oculomotor complex. These eventually stimulate the medial rectus on the homolateral side. The connections result in both eyes moving in the direction opposite of head rotation. A diagram of these important eye movements is shown in Fig. 23.1. If the patient is awake, the vestibulo-ocular reflex is usually suppressed due to cortical projections overriding the internuclear mechanisms. If the patient is comatose and these systems remain intact, the eyes

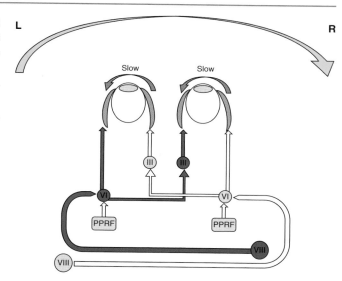

Fig. 23.1 Diagram of important eye movements in an examination maneuver that has been famously called a "doll's eyes" maneuver

should move conjugately in the direction opposite the head rotation [40]. Prior to performing this test, particularly in cases of trauma, it should be confirmed that the cervical spine is stable.

An alternative method, by which these systems can be tested, especially when the cervical spine is unstable, is to employ caloric testing [30, 41]. This can be performed with either warm or cold water, but cold water is usually utilized as it provides a more potent stimulus. After ensuring that the tympanic membrane is intact, the ear canal is irrigated with cold water. The typical response is for both eyes to slowly move in the direction toward irrigation. In a conscious patient, or in one with intact cerebral hemispheres, a fast corrective eye movement back toward primary position should manifest. The repetitive slow eye movements toward the irrigated ear and the fast movements away result in a phenomenon referred to as nystagmus. Since nystagmus is named for the fast phase, cold-water calorics result in nystagmus beating in the opposite direction of the irrigated ear. This can be easily remembered by the mnemonic "COWS." This stands for cold-opposite, warm-same.

An internuclear ophthalmoplegia, which is a disruption of the medial longitudinal fasciculus, can also be identified by a careful eye exam when the adducting eye does not move fully medially, and the abducting eye either does not move past midline or has slowed saccades such that the eyes are dysconjugate [39]. This maneuver can also aid in localizing the lesion to the dorsal pons/midbrain. In a comatose patient, the vestibulo-ocular reflex can be utilized to evaluate for this phenomenon.

Obtaining the gag reflex is accomplished by pressing a sterile tongue blade or cotton swab against the oropharynx region and by observing for symmetric palatal elevation without uvula deviation. The afferent limb of this reflex is largely mediated by cranial nerve nine, which terminates in the nucleus solitaries and the efferent limb, which is largely cranial nerve X originating in the nucleus ambiguus. This reflex indicates cranial nerve ten dysfunction, especially if the palate elevates asymmetrically and/or if the uvula deviates away from the side of weaker palate elevation. A weak gag reflex without asymmetric palate elevation or uvula deviation can indicate a cranial nerve nine lesion, but it can also be seen in perfectly normal individuals since up to one third of healthy people have an absent gag reflex [42].

Funduscopic Examination

The funduscopic examination is an often overlooked portion of the physical examination in a patient with altered mental status, yet it can provide some important clues to the diagnosis or clues to associated conditions. The funduscopic examination is accomplished with either an indirect or more commonly a direct ophthalmoscope. Commonly in the ICU setting, the pupils can be quite small, making the fundus difficult to visualize. A better examination can be achieved by applying mydriatic eye drops, either using a sympathomimetic like phenylephrine or an anticholinergic such as tropicamide. It is extremely important, especially in patients with alteration of consciousness, to document in the chart what kind of dilation you have performed, what time the dilation was performed, and to ensure that you dilate both eyes equally. Failure to do so could result in the inappropriate assumption that the patient could have a compressive third nerve palsy, and this could lead to unnecessary imaging studies and/or possibly even interventions, both of which could pose potential harm to the patient.

To perform the direct funduscopic examination, the direct ophthalmoscope is held next to the examiners eye, and light is directed into the patient's eye. A red reflex is found, and this represents the reflection of light bouncing off of the choroidal membrane. This red reflex is followed, while the examiner advances the ophthalmoscope closer to the patient's pupil until vessels are observed. Once the vessels are found, they are followed back to the optic disk to observe for any abnormalities, particularly optic disk edema. Once the optic disk is visualized, the remainder of the retina and vasculature is visualized. If the margins of the optic disk are indistinct, optic disk edema could be present but must be distinguished from the pseudoedema caused by a tilted disk, optic disk drusen, and other potential causes. If optic disk edema is present, it could be the result of increased intracranial pressure, in which case the edema observed is called papilledema. True optic disk edema that is not caused by increased intracranial pressure includes: optic neuritis associated with demyelinating disease, certain infectious etiologies, or some vascular causes. Papilledema, caused by increased intracranial pressure, can be a result of multiple etiologies including

brain neoplasm, infections such as meningitis or abscess, cerebral sinus thrombosis, idiopathic intracranial hypertension, or any other intracranial space occupying lesion. Optic disk edema uncommonly results from an acute process other than increased intracranial pressure such as a subarachnoid hemorrhage. The retinal vessels should also be inspected for attenuation, embolus, or evidence of cuffing, which can indicate CNS vasculitis. Hollenhorst plaques are bright, yellow, refractile plaques made of cholesterol in the retinal arterioles [43]. These indicate embolic disease, possibly from the internal carotid artery, which would corroborate carotid disease in cases of anterior circulation ischemic events.

Motor

The motor examination should include descriptions of bulk, tone, and strength, as well as observations of any abnormal hypo- or hyperkinetic movements. In a patient manifesting an altered mental status, this examination may prove to be a challenge. Patients may not follow commands, or alternatively they may be intubated, sedated, or paralyzed. When it is not possible to grade strength formally, tone and asymmetry of spontaneous movements can be observed, as well as potentially abnormal postures (such as external rotation of a weak lower extremity). Typically, with a peripheral nervous system lesion, tone is decreased, and with a central nervous system lesion, tone is increased. An exception to this is in cases of spinal pathology, when in the acute setting, the patient may have a flaccid paralysis, the so-called "spinal shock" syndrome [44].

Another portion of the motor examination is observation of the response to a painful stimulus. One example is when the trapezius is squeezed with enough force to result in pain, and the pain elicits a movement. A response to pain that would indicate at least partial preservation of neurological function would be for the patient to reach toward the source of the noxious stimulus, which would be a localizing and an appropriate response [30].

If there is a significant disruption of the motor systems above the level of the midbrain, the inhibition of the rubrospinal tract by the corticospinal systems is released, and the patient will usually exhibit decorticate posturing, which is elbow flexion, forearm supination, and wrist and finger flexion. If there is significant damage to the motor systems below the red nucleus, the rubrospinal tract is also affected, and therefore the tract that provides the dominant tone is the vestibulospinal tract, and this response results in decerebrate posturing, which is extension at the elbow, pronation of the forearm, and extension of the wrist [3].

Basal Ganglia Examination

Hyperkinetic movements (e.g., tremor, chorea) or hypokinetic movements (e.g., parkinsonism) should clue the clinician to the possibility of basal ganglia dysfunction. An MRI study and possibly follow-up laboratory analysis may be necessary. Clinicians should be aware of the chorea syndrome that may appear during diabetic ketoacidosis and also the chorea and other movement disorders that may appear as a result of liver, thyroid, or metabolic dysfunction. Finally, abrupt withdrawal of dopamine (Sinemet) can result in the neuroleptic malignant syndrome and should be avoided. The use of neuroleptic medications can exacerbate or unmask basal ganglia features and should be avoided if possible in ICU patients.

Reflex Examination

Abnormal reflexes are an important adjunct to the motor examination, particularly when accompanied by weakness. The reflexes may help to determine if the weakness is central or peripheral in origin. If a central nervous system lesion is present, the inhibition on the alpha motor neuron in the anterior horn cells of the spinal cord will be released, and there would be hyperexcitablity of the myotatic stretch reflex. When the tendon is tapped with a reflex hammer, the primary afferent fibers directly synapse on the motor neuron that supplies the attached muscles. Given that the descending inhibition on these neurons is released, the resulting contraction of the muscles is exaggerated. If a peripheral lesion is present, the reflex may be decreased, although the afferent limb of the stretch reflex is intact. If the motor neuron is damaged, the muscle cannot contract with full force, resulting in hyporeflexia [45].

The Babinski response is also a useful part of the motor examination. In testing the Babinski response, the lateral aspect of the plantar surface of the foot is scratched hard enough to produce a noxious stimulus. If the first movement of the great toe is upward, this is a Babinski sign. Experimental data in mice and humans indicate that this response results from damage to the medullary reticulospinal tract; however, in clinical practice, it is used to identify individuals simply with potential CNS damage [30, 46, 47].

Cerebellar Examination

The cerebellar examination is often difficult to test in an ICU setting and especially with an altered mental status. When present, cerebellar findings may be clues to posterior fossa lesions that may progress to include compromise of the ARAS in the brainstem and eventually cause depressed consciousness. Cerebellar findings include appendicular ataxia, dysmetria, rebound, dysdiadochokinesia, rhythm problems, and, in select cases, associated tremor. In the more mobile patient truncal titubation, wide-based gait, and eye movement abnormalities may be present with more midline and anterior cerebellar lesions [13, 30, 45].

Sensation

The sensory examination can be tricky in the ICU and even trickier in the setting of AMS. It is extremely subjective. A crude way of testing sensation in this setting is to provide a painful stimulus to each extremity, and if the patient responds to this pain, it is inferred that, grossly, the anterolateral system known as the spinothalamic tract may be intact. Testing for neuropathy, radiculopathy, plexopathy, or other issues may require a more intact mental status.

Laboratory Workup

Complete Blood Count (CBC)

The CBC can be helpful in cases of altered mental status for several reasons. A leukocytosis can indicate an infectious or neoplastic process, either of which can cause confusion, particularly in patients with decreased functional cognitive reserve. This does not exclude a CNS structural process as the cause, but it can be useful in pointing a clinician in a different direction. A low hemoglobin and hematocrit, indicating anemia, either may be completely unrelated to the altered mental status or can be symptoms of a systemic process causing the altered mental status such as a microangiopathic hemolytic anemia or can worsen cognition in patient with decreased cognition at baseline such as encountered in dementing illnesses [48, 49]. Thrombocytosis can either indicate a neoplastic process or could be reactive and support an infectious/inflammatory diagnosis. Thrombocytopenia can be seen in multiple conditions but particularly in microangiopathic hemolytic anemias [50] and disseminated intravascular coagulopathy, both of which can cause altered mental status.

Chemistries

Patients manifesting an acute confusional state/delirium or coma should at a minimum have a complete metabolic panel performed. Often, hyponatremia, diabetic ketoacidosis, acute uremia, and hepatic encephalopathy can be quickly uncovered. Also, certain treatable issues such as hypercapnia due to pulmonary insufficiency may result in an impairment of consciousness that requires ICU monitoring. Early treatment aids in prevention of complications and potentially death. Further workup is usually warranted to find the underlying etiology causing any metabolic disturbance.

Elevated ammonia levels can be encountered in the setting of severe liver damage and also as a result of medications such as valproate, which can also be associated with encephalopathy [51]. Often, if you treat the underlying etiology of the hyperammonemia, the encephalopathy can resolve. An example of this is decreasing the dosage of valproate or discontinuing it may be indicated if this is found to be the underlying cause. Treatment with lactulose, which is the mainstay of treatment, can increase the gastrointestinal excretion of ammonia and may speed the reversal of alterations in mental status, but the evidence here is lacking [52].

Neuroimaging

The history and examination should guide the clinician to a localization and, subsequently, an appropriately limited differential diagnosis. Based on this, imaging of the central nervous system may be warranted. Several modalities are available, each having advantages and disadvantages. The most pertinent imaging studies in most cases include CT and MRI of the brain. The advantage of CT is that it is fast, readily available, and less susceptible to movement artifact, while with MRI, the images are usually better quality, more sensitive in detecting pathology, and will usually give more information about a specific etiology. Selecting which study to utilize should vary depending on the clinical scenario encountered.

CT

Computed tomography (CT) of the brain is a fast and extremely efficient way to evaluate for structural abnormalities in a patient with an AMS. Especially in cases of an acute stroke, intracerebral hemorrhage, subdural hematoma, or epidural hematoma, the brain CT is very useful to quickly ascertain an underlying cause for an AMS. CT has an excellent spatial resolution [53, 54] but lacks the contrast resolution of MRI, which often makes it an inferior modality if searching for lesions within the CNS.

MRI

Magnetic resonance imaging (MRI) of the brain can be particularly useful for the evaluation and further characterization of lesions that may cause AMS (stroke, hemorrhage, venous issues, intracranial hypotension). The evaluation of posterior fossa lesions causing alterations in mental status is particularly useful as some of these etiologies may not be adequately imaged on CT. MRI is particularly important to fully characterize lesions, their appearance, involvement of adjacent structures (or lack thereof), and patterns of appearance on the various sequences, all of which aid in making a diagnosis. The excellent contrast resolution is quite useful in MRI given that many lesions within the CNS are often of similar density, resulting in similar contrast, and thus may be missed by CT scan. In acute stroke, the diffusion-weighted MRI is quite useful. In this condition, the brain CT may be normal early, and the diffusion-weighted MRI will show an acute brainstem infarct that may require close observation in the ICU setting or potentially warrant a surgical or endovascular intervention. Acute thalamic infarcts interrupting the reticular activating system may result in an alteration in mental status, which may not be seen on CT imaging; these also sometimes respond to dopamine or dopamine agonist therapy and manifest with fluctuating levels of consciousness.

The clinician should never hesitate to use a brain CT, MRI, or potentially both tests to uncover the etiology of any case of AMS, especially when the history and examination do not point clearly to the etiology.

Neurodiagnostics

Lumbar Puncture

The lumbar puncture is particularly important in the altered mental status workup, especially if an infectious etiology is suspected, if the patient is immunocompromised, or if a diagnosis remains elusive after an initial workup. Sampling of the CSF allows for evaluation of the chemical composition, quantification of the number of erythrocytes and leukocytes, culture of the fluid, polymerase chain reaction for DNA of infectious organisms, evaluation of abnormal cells, and detection of the presence of abnormal proteins such as specific antibodies. The spinal needle can also be attached to a manometer so that the CSF pressure can be measured. A normal CSF constitution is less than five leukocytes without any polymorphonuclear cells, no erythrocytes, 15–50 mg/dL of protein, and a glucose concentration that is about 2/3 that of the serum glucose; it is important to get a peripheral blood stick at the exact time of the LP [55]. A description of the commonly found values in some infectious CSF processes is depicted in Table 23.3.

EEG

The electroencephalogram (EEG) is commonly performed in the critical care setting, especially in patients with nonconvulsive status, where clinical presentation may prove hard to decipher. Continuous EEG monitoring in the ICU allows the physician to monitor the progress of antiepileptic treatment and to decide whether or not the patient will require more aggressive management. EEG is commonly abnormal in the setting of an alteration of consciousness and can offer clues as to elusive diagnoses [56]. EEG is particularly useful in situations in the ICU when the patient is delirious or having an AMS, and the history is unable to be obtained. It is common that patients with delirium from a metabolic disturbance, hypoglycemia, diabetic coma, or excess use of sedatives will have a slowing of the posterior dominant rhythm which is normally in the alpha frequency. In patients with hepatic

Table 23.3 Commonly found values in some infectious CSF processes in lumbar punctures

Component	Viral	Bacterial	Tuberculous	Fungal
WBC	<300	>1,000	50–500	50–500
Cell-type predominance	Mostly lymphocytes	Mostly neutrophils	Mostly lymphocytes and monocytes	Mostly lymphocytes
Glucose	>40	<40	<40	<40
Protein	Often normal or mildly elevated	Elevated (sometimes markedly so)	Elevated	Elevated

encephalopathy or uremic states, the EEG may show triphasic waves [57]. When there has been a benzodiazepine overdose, excessive beta activity may be seen. In the setting of CNS infections, such as herpes encephalitis, the EEG may show focal abnormalities as well as periodic lateralized discharges [58]. In the setting of severe anoxic brain injury where the patient is unresponsive and lacks brainstem reflexes, the EEG may reveal diffuse slowing or even a flat line. In the setting of a rapidly progressive dementia (e.g., CJD), the EEG may show periodic sharp wave complexes [59].

A flat line seen on EEG with no electrical potential of more than 2 mV during 30 min of recording is usually indicative of brain death [60]. Thus, EEG may aid in further treatment of underlying infection, seizures, metabolic disturbances, and brain death.

Evoked Potentials

Evoked potentials are obtained by providing a sensory stimulus—whether it is auditory, visual, or somatosensory—and recording the electroencephalographic potentials associated with them. These are typically not very useful in the diagnosis of altered mental status, but in cases of coma, brainstem auditory evoked responses and somatosensory evoked potentials may have some utility in prognosis, especially when other aspects of clinical evaluation are limited by conditions such as paralytics, intubation, and sedation [61].

Diseases and Disease-Specific Treatments

Delirium

Delirium is an extremely common phenomenon in ICU patients and is reported as high as 82 % [62, 63]. Development of delirium can be associated with a worse prognosis [62], and delay in treating delirium has been associated with increased mortality, increased nosocomial infections, a longer length of stay [64], and an increased rate of mechanical ventilation [65]. Delirium is defined as an acute fluctuating change in consciousness and cognition that develops over a brief period of time [66]. A hallmark of

delirium is waxing and waning alteration of consciousness along with profound inattentiveness. Interestingly, patients with delirium usually have a sense of heightened awareness to their surroundings.

Causes of delirium may include infection, metabolic disturbances, medications, alcohol withdrawal, and postoperative states, especially in the elderly population. This could be due to a lack of cognitive functional reserve leading to a state of confusion. If treatment of the underlying cause of delirium is found early, it may be resolved more expeditiously.

There is no specific treatment for delirium but rather an approach to minimize physical, medical, and emotional stresses should be undertaken in addition to treating the underlying cause(s).

Intoxications

Sedatives

Sedative hypnotic medications as well as ethanol cause depressed level of arousal by modulation of the $GABA_A$ (gamma-amino butyric acid) chloride channel. Benzodiazepines increase the frequency of channel opening by increasing the channel affinity for GABA [67]. Barbiturates increase the duration of channel opening when stimulated by GABA [68]. This mechanism explains why barbiturates are inherently more dangerous than benzodiazepines in overdose due to the fact that the chloride channel could potentially remain open nearly constantly with a barbiturate, but it still closes periodically with a benzodiazepine overdose. With the channel being open for a greater percentage of the time, the chloride will continue to influx and hyperpolarize the neuron, making it more resistant to depolarization, thus slowing signal propagation within the CNS. Flumazenil is an antagonist at the benzodiazepine binding site on the $GABA_A$ receptor. It reverses the action of benzodiazepines.

Cocaine and Other Sympathomimetics

Intoxication with cocaine leads to increased sympathetic stimulation by blocking reuptake of monoamines into the presynaptic nerve terminal [69]. This produces an excessive "fight or flight" response and produces a hyperdynamic state with patients usually having hypertension, tachypnea, tachycardia, diaphoresis, mydriasis, hyperthermia, and occasionally paranoia [70]. Individuals suffering from sympathomimetic intoxication may appear to be altered in the sense that they are hypervigilant, but will not often have frank confusion. However, excessive alpha stimulation, especially in the setting of beta blockade, can cause vasospasm, which can produce ischemia throughout the body, but if it occurs in the brain, it can cause stroke. If the stroke affects the ARAS as mentioned in the stroke section earlier, depressed level of consciousness can occur.

LSD

Lysergic acid diethylamide (LSD) is a hallucinogen that can cause inattentiveness, lethargy, hallucinations, and illusions. Patients will usually only present with "bad trips" that are prolonged and comprised of worrisome hallucinations or illusions and profound anxiety as well as gastrointestinal upset. It is commonly ingested by saturated pieces of paper. LSD has no specific antidote, but rather supportive care such as benzodiazepines and a calm, soothing environment are mainstays of treatment until the intoxication wears off [70].

GHB

Gamma-hydroxybutyric acid (GHB) is a commonly abused drug that acts on GABA receptors [71, 72] and likely a novel GHB receptor in the central nervous system to produce a syndrome of CNS depression. This drug has the effect of producing a very short-lived coma in overdoses but can also produce confusion, ataxia, nystagmus, and occasionally seizures if taken in smaller amounts [70]. Along with CNS depression effects, it can cause respiratory suppression and patients may require intubation. The drug can also have a withdrawal syndrome that can be quite similar to alcohol in that it features tremors, anxiety, tachycardia, visual and auditory hallucinations, and can even cause a Wernicke-Korsakoff syndrome [73]. One of the most worrisome effects of GHB is the sudden awakening phenomenon that can lead to self-extubation and aspiration [74].

Narcotics

Opioids are synthetic and semisynthetic derivatives of the poppy plant. They have long been used for therapeutic and recreational effects. In fact, heroin was once marketed by Bayer pharmaceuticals for its antitussive properties [11]. These compounds typically cause depressed consciousness, the degree of which is dependent on the dose, the route of administration, and the tolerance of the individual. In addition to depressed consciousness, decreased respiratory drive, miosis, and a host of idiosyncratic reactions can result from opioids [70]. By definition, the effects of an opioid can be reversed by naloxone, and this can be used as an antidote as it is a pure (mu) antagonist and will reverse the mental status changes and respiratory depression if given in an appropriate

dose. Some opioids have a very long half-life which may outlast the effects of naloxone, so observation for repeated worsening of the initial symptoms should be considered.

Ischemic Disease

Stroke

Ischemic stroke is discussed elsewhere in this book. It is quite rare for ischemic stroke to present with an isolated alteration of consciousness due to the unilaterality of the blood supply to many regions of the brain and the preservation of the contralateral ARAS in the majority of cases. In a study by Benbadis, only 4 % of patients had altered mental status due to a unilateral stroke, and the neurological exam is helpful in detecting those patients who need neuroimaging, with a 97 % negative predictive value [75]. In particular, strokes that cause depression of consciousness and altered mental status tend to be caused by thrombosis or by embolus of the basilar artery. This artery has penetrating branches that supply both sides of the brainstem in the area where the ARAS is confined to a small region. The majority of brainstem strokes are caused by small vessel lacunar strokes which are unilateral and do not usually cause altered mental status. However, in many cases of strokes caused by the basilar artery, the brainstem may be damaged bilaterally, and consciousness and mentation can be affected. In many of these cases, there is acute onset of cranial nerve deficits, and these are often associated with contralateral motor deficits. If extensive bilateral damage to the brainstem occurs, the patient will often manifest with significant bilateral weakness, cranial nerve palsies, dysarthria, dizziness, depressed consciousness, and in arguably the worst case scenario, a locked-in syndrome [76]. The paramedian thalamic arteries normally arise from the P1 to supply the mesial thalamus ipsilaterally through which the ARAS travels. Occasionally, a common trunk, called the artery of Percheron [77], arises from one PCA to supply both mesial thalami. In such a situation, a stroke of this artery can result in coma due to bilateral disruption of the ARAS [78]. Another cause of depressed consciousness is a posterior cerebral artery stroke or a large hemispheric stroke. Both of these clinical conditions can result in these findings, due to shifting of the intracranial contents and compromise of the contralateral ARAS [2].

Hemorrhagic Disease

Intraparenchymal Hemorrhage

Intraparenchymal hemorrhage can result from many causes but is usually associated with uncontrolled hypertension, amyloid angiopathy, underlying neoplasm, or alternatively vascular lesions. The location of these hemorrhages can often be a clue to the underlying etiology [79]. Hypertensive bleeds are usually located in the basal ganglia, pons, cerebellum, and thalamus. Those caused by amyloid angiopathy are commonly lobar in location. The location of the bleed will determine the resulting deficits. The sudden expansion of the intracranial contents and the resulting increased intracranial pressure can cause profound mass effect and compromise the ARAS bilaterally, especially when blood products are located within or near the more internal structures where the bilateral ARAS is confined to a relatively small space. This phenomenon may explain why patients with intraparenchymal bleeds have focal neurological deficits and also manifest with a state of stupor. Patients with increased intracranial bleeds will often present with nausea and vomiting from the increased intracranial pressure.

Subarachnoid Hemorrhage

Subarachnoid hemorrhage (SAH) is a potentially life-threatening condition usually caused by either trauma or a ruptured aneurysm. Patients with SAH often present with the "worst headache of their life," nuchal rigidity, cranial neuropathies, motor deficit, and altered mental status. The mortality rate of aneurysmal SAH is 7 % in those patients who are admitted to neurointensive care units. Therefore, it is paramount that this diagnosis does not get missed. Careful monitoring in the ICU can help prevent cerebral vasospasm and aneurysmal rupture. Complications of vasospasm include hydrocephalus and hyponatremia. Subarachnoid hemorrhage in the ICU setting can also result in seizures due to cortical irritability from the collection of blood: iron on the cortex is irritating and can cause seizures. This may result in more complications not only from a medical standpoint but also from the need of an antiepileptic medication. Antiepileptic medications can in some cases result in more complications.

Cerebral angiography remains the gold standard for diagnosis of cerebral vasospasm. Transcranial dopplers can also be performed to diagnose vasospasm, and these are becoming a more popular method of assessing vasospasm. The treatment of SAH consists of a triad of hypervolemia, hypertension, and hemodilution. Early treatment of subarachnoid hemorrhage can prevent further future complications. Around 70 % of patients who receive the treatment can reverse neurological complications from SAH [80]. In patients who have already undergone permanent neurological deficits from SAH, steroids and calcium channel blockers can be used.

Neoplasm

As described previously, mass lesions of any etiology can cause increased pressure on other parts of the ARAS and,

if significant enough, can cause depressed level of consciousness. Any neoplasm that either compromises the brainstem or has a significant mass effect such that both cerebral hemispheres are affected can cause an alteration of consciousness. In addition to this phenomenon, cerebral neoplasms, especially when cortically based, can cause cortical irritation and result in seizures. If a patient with a cerebral neoplasm presents with an altered mental status, the main considerations are increasing cerebral edema, decreased mental status, and seizures. As discussed earlier, neuroimaging and EEG are both useful in correctly diagnosing this potential etiology.

Posterior Reversible Encephalopathy Syndrome (PRES)

PRES can potentially be life threatening if not diagnosed and recognized early. Often, if this condition goes unrecognized and causes seizures, the patient may slip into status epilepticus. Treatment of HTN is crucial especially early as it can reverse fatal complications [81]. Clinical symptoms of PRES include headache, seizures, alteration in mental status, and visual changes. Imaging, particularly MRI in PRES, shows a parietal and occipital-predominant leukoencephalopathy. It is rare to have DWI positivity, but when present, this may indicate that the damage is irreversible. Etiologies include uncontrolled HTN, eclampsia, preeclampsia, collagen vascular diseases, infections, and shock [82, 83].

Demyelinating Disease

Rarely can demyelinating disease cause an alteration of consciousness as rarely does it cause bilateral dysfunction of the ARAS. Typically, demyelinating disease will affect discrete areas of the CNS and cause focal deficits that do not influence consciousness, such as weakness, sensory loss, ataxia, central vision loss, and diplopia. Two examples of demyelinating disease that can cause alterations of consciousness are acute demyelinating encephalomyelitis (ADEM) and tumefactive multiple sclerosis (MS).

ADEM is an acute, usually monophasic demyelinating illness that is typically considered to be postinfectious or postvaccination and/or autoimmune in etiology. It is much more common in children, and typically children have a worse prognosis. Almost universally, these patients present with fever, altered mental status, headache, and focal or multifocal exam findings. Due to the presentation, it is prudent to include encephalitis and meningitis in the differential diagnosis. Imaging will often show large "fluffy" areas of increased T2 signal in various areas of the deep cerebral white matter, but unlike MS, these lesions are usually not well circumscribed or ovoid, not periventricular in location, and can often involve areas of gray matter such as the basal ganglia [84]. Treatment for ADEM is supportive and many individuals use pulse steroids although the data for this are limited in adults. There is a particularly severe variant of ADEM called hemorrhagic leukoencephalopathy in which there is a particularly aggressive amount of edema as well as hemorrhage. This disorder can have a mortality rate as high as 70 %, but evidence points toward less residual deficits with aggressive therapies with corticosteroids [84, 85], intravenous immunoglobulins (IVIG), and plasma exchange [86].

Tumefactive MS is a disorder in which a patient either with undiagnosed MS or with longstanding disease develops a lesion that is particularly large, with significant cerebral edema to the point that there could be a potential herniation syndrome [87]. There is breakdown of the blood brain barrier, and the lesion enhances with contrast material, so many times this can be indistinguishable from a brain tumor or cerebral abscess [88]. If there are no other radiographic lesions that will help make a diagnosis of MS, a brain biopsy might be necessary to confirm this. There have been reports of mitoxantrone, rituximab, and alemtuzumab having beneficial results as well as autologous stem cell transplantation, but it is usually a fatal disease and often challenging to diagnose and treat [89].

Infections

Meningitis

Meningitis commonly presents with photophobia, altered mental status, headache, neck pain, seizures, and fevers. This condition can be caused by bacteria and viruses but can also be caused by fungi. Meningitis results from pathology of the meninges, if the brain parenchyma is affected and is evidenced by seizures, cortical dysfunction, or memory disturbances. Meningitis can be diagnosed by CSF analysis showing a pleocytosis. Bacterial causes tend to show a neutrophil-predominant CSF leukocytosis, whereas viral and tuberculous meningitis have a lymphocyte-predominant pleocytosis [90, 91].

Bacterial and fungal meningitis, if left untreated, can lead to fatal outcomes. The common causes of bacterial meningitis include *Streptococcus pneumoniae*, *Neisseria meningitidus*, and (in individuals over the age of 50) *Listeria monocytogenes*. Commonly, because of the broad spectrum of action and the good CNS coverage, a third- or fourth-generation cephalosporin such as ceftriaxone or cefepime is usually used [92]. Due to the rise of multidrug resistant *S. pneumoniae*, vancomycin is also commonly used. In elderly patients, ampicillin is usually added as a third drug to cover for *L. monocytogenes*. *Mycobacterium tuberculosis* can cause a monocyte and lymphocyte-predominant basilar meningitis that can present like other bacterial meningitis but can

also have cranial nerve palsies. This condition is particularly prevalent in individuals with the human immunodeficiency virus (HIV) and in patients from areas where *M. tuberculosis* is endemic. Recent trauma can also introduce atypical organisms into the CSF and result in meningitis. These organisms commonly include Staphylococci species and gram negative organisms such as *Pseudomonas aeruginosa* [93].

Fungal meningitis is usually seen in patients with immunodeficiencies or immunosuppressed states. The common cause of fungal meningitis is *Cryptococcus neoformans*. Viral meningitis typically has similar but milder symptoms and is usually self-limiting [94]. The causes of viral meningitis are multiple and include many enteroviruses and arboviruses. Other causes of viral meningitis include organisms such as cytomegalovirus, Epstein-Barr virus, and varicella zoster virus.

Encephalitis

Encephalitis can present similarly to meningitis but has additional features of parenchymal involvement including seizures, alterations in consciousness, memory loss, and headache. Nearly all cases of encephalitis are caused by viruses. The most frequent and treatable cause of encephalitis that always must be considered is *Herpes simplex*. This virus causes an encephalitis that is fatal in 70 % of untreated patients [95]. HSV encephalitis can be treated using acyclovir, but most patients with this disorder will have some sequelae and will not regain full function—although most regain meaningful function [96]. The CSF analysis will show a lymphocytic pleocytosis in cases of encephalitis. In encephalitis caused by HSV, there is often hemorrhagic necrosis, particularly of the temporal lobes, so the CSF can show many erythrocytes as well. MRI of brain may be obtained to evaluate for such hemorrhagic necrosis of the temporal lobes. EEG may show diffuse slowing or periodic lateralized epileptiform discharges.

Cerebral Abscess

Cerebral abscesses typically present with headaches and focal neurological deficits. They do not typically manifest with the common findings of CNS infection such as stiff neck, headache, nausea, vomiting, fever, lethargy, photophobia, or optic disk edema [97, 98]. Many times, cerebral abscesses are discovered in the workup of a patient with a fever of unknown origin or in a stroke workup. The mass effect from the abscess compromises the nearby brain tissue, and therefore symptoms vary based on location. Cerebral abscesses can be a result of either direct spread from the sinuses [99] and also from occasionally dental infections or as a result of hematogenous spread. Hematogenous spread will usually result in multiple abscesses at the gray-white junction, whereas local spread usually results in a single abscess [9]. Hematogenous spread usually takes place in the setting of a compromised immune system. Diagnosis is made using neuroimaging with CT and/or MRI. The abscess is usually hypointense and, if contrast is administered, a rim of peripheral enhancement can be seen. LP is rarely helpful and occasionally can potentiate a herniation syndrome if mass effect is significant. Treatment is with empiric antibiotics and likely neurosurgical drainage of the lesion may be necessary [9].

Intracranial Hypotension

Intracranial hypotension can be either spontaneous or associated with trauma (including fenestration of the dural sac by lumbar puncture) [100]. It is caused by an insufficient hydrostatic pressure to keep the cerebrum, brainstem, and other CNS tissue suspended above the bony calvarium. When this occurs, the base of the brain and brainstem sag down and often rest on the skull base, occasionally causing damage to these structures. These patients almost all universally have headaches, but they can also present with lethargy/stupor, cranial neuropathies, or even as a discrete brainstem syndrome [101]. A frontotemporal dementia-like picture can also be seen in this condition [102]. Due to the compression of the brainstem against the skull base, the ARAS can be compromised, leading to an alteration of mental status. Up to 2/3 of patients have spontaneous intracranial hypotension and have a diagnostic or a physical exam indicative of a connective tissue disorder, leading to the presumption that these disorders have something to do with the pathogenesis [103]. Diagnosis is made by the clinical picture of postural headache worsened by standing or sitting up. The MRI can show diffuse enhancement of the pachymeninges, "slumping" of the midbrain and sometimes subdural hygromas. Treatment with a blood patch is usually attempted first, and if unsuccessful, a surgical repair can be performed.

Epileptiform Activity

Convulsive Status Epilepticus

Convulsive status epilepticus is defined as seizure activity without a recovery of consciousness that lasts longer than 5 min [104]. Convulsive status epilepticus is a life-threatening condition that needs to be identified and treated early to prevent continued neuronal damage to the brain and to other organ systems. This is especially true since the chances that a seizure will resolve spontaneously decrease as the length of time that the seizure lasts increases [105]. Mortality rates are around 20 % according to studies [106]. Aggressive treatment with benzodiazepines and antiepileptic treatment should be initiated. The Veterans Affairs Status Epilepticus Cooperative Study showed us that lorazepam should be considered first-line therapy for patients in status epilepticus [107]. For refractory status, general anesthesia is usually needed in order to suppress epileptic activity. Burst suppression may be needed to break refractory status and to prevent severe neuronal damage from occurring. Different etiologies of status epilepticus include drug toxicity, stroke, alcohol intoxication, chronic epilepsy with subtherapeutic antiepileptic levels, metabolic abnormalities such as hyponatremia or hypocalcemia, CNS infections such as toxoplasmosis, or any space occupying lesions. Patients who end up in status epilepticus due to stroke, anoxic brain injury, and the elderly population have a high incidence of mortality [108].

Nonconvulsive Status Epilepticus (NCSE)

NCSE is a commonly missed diagnosis and is often hard to identify clinically. Morbidity and mortality are difficult to assess in this condition, but an article by Shneker and Fountain indicated that NCSE secondary to a medical condition can have a mortality of 18 % [109], which approaches that of convulsive status epilepticus. They also describe that NCSE can occur without an underlying medical condition and when this occurs it has a much lower mortality rate. EEG is the only way to diagnose this condition, so this test is especially useful in patients with AMS and a known history of seizures who are not having generalized convulsions. Although nonconvulsive status does not seem to be as fatal as convulsive status, it is still important to identify and treat earlier rather than later to prevent neuronal. It should be considered in the setting of AMS when the patient does not have metabolic/toxic/infectious or structural abnormality.

Immune-Mediated Encephalopathies

Recently, immune-mediated encephalopathies have emerged in the literature due to the advent of new assays, increasing recognition, and the concern over missing possible treatable conditions. These encephalopathies can be either idiopathic, autoimmune, or paraneoplastic in nature. As investigation into these entities progresses, the pathogenesis will be elicited and fewer will be classified as idiopathic [110]. Many of these disorders (but not all) are associated with tumors. They all have an immune-mediated pathogenesis and may respond to immune-active therapy as antibody-associated encephalopathies [111].

These disorders have an extremely varied presentation but nearly always have a rapidly progressive encephalopathy with superimposed delirium as a feature. Other manifestations include seizures, movement disorders, psychiatric symptoms (mania, hallucinations, paranoia), and fluctuating symptoms. Many of these disorders have recently had autoantibodies discovered, particularly to neuronal membrane channel proteins. These antibodies can be detected with serological testing. Many of the encephalopathies that affect the limbic system will have MRI T2 signal abnormalities in the mesial temporal lobes. Some of the more common antibodies associated with immune-mediated encephalopathy include voltage-gated potassium channel [112], NMDA receptor [113], amino-3-hydroxy-5-methyl-4-isoxazolepropionic acid (AMPA) receptor [114], and gamma-aminobutyric acid (GABA) B receptor [115]. These antibodies do not necessarily predict clinical course, clinical manifestations, or even whether or not a patient will develop symptoms. The responsiveness to immunosuppressive therapies seems to be greater in patients with subacute onset, fluctuating course, tremor, short delay to treatment, seropositivity for a known antibody, and CSF abnormalities [116].

Another disorder that seems to have immune-mediated pathogenesis is steroid responsive encephalopathy associated with autoimmune thyroiditis (SREAT) [117]. The most common manifestations of this disorder include altered mental status, seizures, stroke-like signs, EEG abnormalities, and increased CSF protein [118]. This disorder is often but not always associated with thyroid function abnormalities and antithyroid peroxidase antibodies.

Evaluation of Brain Death

Brain death evaluation is something often encountered in the ICU. There can be many ethical and cultural dilemmas associated with the notion that a person with devastating neurological disease is brain dead, especially when applying widely accepted criteria [119], while their cardiac and pulmonary functions may be mechanically or chemically supported. It is very important to know the proper clinical criteria to make such a diagnosis and to be aware that these criteria can vary from state to state and from country to country. There have been several published guidelines for determining brain death in adults, and we will focus on those published by the American Academy of Neurology [120, 121]. In Table 23.4, we provide a summary of these guidelines and the ancillary tests that can be performed to aid in the diagnosis of brain death. Once the diagnosis of brain death is made, an organ center should be contacted only if the patient/family has appropriately consented. Once the guidelines discussed next are completed, a checklist should also be completed and signed with the date and time.

Brain death occurs when there is lack of cerebral blood flow to the brain. The respiratory function of the patient is dependent on ventilator support. It is crucial that the cause of coma is established before a diagnosis of brain death is rendered. This is important because if the cause of coma is reversible then the patient will fail to meet criteria for brain death. Many reversible disorders must be ruled out prior to determining that a patient is brain dead. The patient must be

Table 23.4 Summary of guidelines for determining brain death in adults and the ancillary tests that can be performed to aid in the diagnosis of brain death

Requirements for evaluation of brain death	Tests performed
Must rule out causes of reversible coma	Isoelectric EEG indicates cortical damage. However, not necessary for diagnosis
The absence of brainstem reflexes (pupillary reflex, corneal reflex, cold calorics)	Apnea test: CO_2 challenge, $PaCO_2$ above normal level
Complete apnea	TCD
Hypothermic CNS depressant should always be excluded	Cerebral angiography
The absence of respiratory drive after a CO_2 challenge in the setting of normothermia, euvolemia, and absence of hypoxia. Systolic blood pressure should be maintained greater than 100 when evaluating the patient	MRI/MRA brain: documented lack of blood flow in the cavernous portion of the ICA
Absence of confounding factors or reversible causes such as recent administration of neuromuscular blockade or sedatives, severe electrolyte imbalance, hypothermia, hypotension, or substantial acid-base disturbances	
Perform one neurological examination	

Data from The Quality Standards Subcommittee of the American Academy of Neurology [120] and Wijdicks et al. [121]

normothermic and free of any correctible metabolic, endocrine, or acid-base disturbances. The patient must not be receiving a neuromuscular blockade agent and be off of any sedative medications for at least 24 h. The patient must also not be substantially hypotensive (systolic blood pressure of less than 90 mmHg) at the time of declaring brain death, as this could be indicative of a secondary process causing the comatose state. A clinical examination must be performed demonstrating a state of coma and absent brainstem reflexes. This includes failure to respond to painful stimuli, absent corneal reflexes, no pupillary reaction to light, failure of cold calorics to demonstrate a normal response, no gag reflex or cough with suctioning, absent respiratory drive despite hypercapnia (the apnea test is described next), and an absent response of facial muscle movement to external stimuli.

An apnea test must be performed as part of the brain death evaluation. The patient's systolic blood pressure must be greater than or equal to 100 mmHg prior to the test being performed and throughout its duration. This test is performed with preoxygenation with 90 % inspired oxygen for 10 min to a PaO_2 200 mmHg. The patient is then reduced to eucapnia with 10 breaths per minute of the ventilator. Positive end respiratory pressure must be reduced to 5 cmH$_2$O. If pulse oximetry oxygen saturation remains 95 %, then a blood gas is obtained and the clinician may proceed with the test. The patient will then need to be disconnected from the ventilator and oxygenation should be preserved, usually with a catheter inserted into the trachea. Respiratory movements should be observed for at least 10 min, and they are defined as the observation of abdominal or chest excursions [122]. The test should be stopped and deemed inconclusive if the systolic blood pressure decreases to 90 mmHg or below. If no respiratory drive is observed, an arterial blood gas is repeated after 8 min. If the PCO$_2$ has either reached a level of 60 mmHg or greater or 20 mmHg above the pretest measurement, this is considered a positive apnea test and supports the diagnosis of brain death.

While an EEG is often obtained in the ICU setting to aid in the determination of brain death, it is not required to give such a diagnosis. If an EEG is obtained in such a situation, the absence of any electrical potential of more than 2 mV during a 30-min recording, this favors brain death, but it does not always signify brain death. This is termed electrocerebral silence [123]. An EEG can also display a similar pattern in states of severe hypothermia, in intoxications with many sedative drugs, and after hypoxia from cardiac arrest.

Transcranial dopplers (TCDs) may be used to measure cerebral vasospasm. They are particularly useful in the setting of SAH and ischemic stroke. When performing a TCD, the probe should be placed at the temporal bone above the zygomatic arch or the vertebrobasilar arteries through the suboccipital transcranial window. In the setting of brain death, TCD can be useful if there is a lack of diastolic or reverberating flow [121].

Brain death evaluation requires careful examination. The use of ancillary tests can assist in diagnosis. It is important to consider the utility of TCD, EEG, and imaging, but these studies are not mandatory to make this diagnosis. This is a key point to remember, as often clinicians order these tests for confirmation, even if not absolutely necessary.

References

1. Dubin WR, Field HL, Gastfriend DR. Postcardiotomy delirium: a critical review. J Thorac Cardiovasc Surg. 1979;77(4):586–94.
2. Plum F, Posner JB. The diagnosis of stupor and coma. Contemp Neurol Ser. 1972;10:1–286.
3. Tindall SC. Level of consciousness. In: Walker HK, Hall WD, Hurst JW, et al., editors. Clinical methods: the history, physical, and laboratory examinations. 3rd ed. Boston: Butterworths; 1990.
4. Reinoso-Suárez F, de Andrés I, Garzón M. Functional anatomy of the sleep-wakefulness cycle: wakefulness. Adv Anat Embryol Cell Biol. 2011;208:1–128.
5. Fisher CM. Brain herniation: a revision of classical concepts. Can J Neurol Sci. 1995;22(2):83–91.
6. Ropper AH. Lateral displacement of the brain and level of consciousness in patients with an acute hemispheral mass. N Engl J Med. 1986;314(15):953–8.
7. Ropper AH. A preliminary MRI study of the geometry of brain displacement and level of consciousness with acute intracranial masses. Neurology. 1989;39(5):622–7.
8. Young GB. Coma. Ann N Y Acad Sci. 2009;1157(1):32–47.
9. Kaplan PW. The EEG, in metabolic encephalopathy and coma. J Clin Neurophysiol. 2004;21(5):307–18.
10. Fisher CM. The neurological examination of the comatose patient. Acta Neurol Scand. 1969;45 Suppl 36:1–56.
11. Lilly LS. Pathophysiology of heart disease. Philadelphia: Wolters Kluwer/Lippincott Williams & Wilkins; 2007.
12. Pessin M, Panis W, Prager R, Millan V, Scott R. Auscultation of cervical and ocular bruits in extracranial carotid occlusive disease: a clinical and angiographic study. Stroke. 1983;14(2):246–9.
13. Bickley LS, Bates B, Szilagyi PG. Bates' pocket guide to physical examination and history taking. 6th ed. Philadelphia: Wolters Kluwer Health/Lippincott Williams & Wilkins; 2009.
14. Rich MW. Epidemiology, clinical features, and prognosis of acute myocardial infarction in the elderly. Am J Geriatr Cardiol. 2006;15(1):7–11; quiz 12.
15. Garcia AJ, Zanella S, Koch H, Doi A, Ramirez JM. Chapter 3 – networks within networks: the neuronal control of breathing. Prog Brain Res. 2011;188:31–50.
16. Wasserman AM, Sahibzada N, Hernandez YM, Gillis RA. Specific subnuclei of the nucleus tractus solitarius play a role in determining the duration of inspiration in the rat. Brain Res. 2000;880(1–2):118–30.
17. Pauzner R, Mouallem M, Sadeh M, Tadmor R, Farfel Z. High incidence of primary cerebral lymphoma in tumor-induced central neurogenic hyperventilation. Arch Neurol. 1989;46(5):510–2.
18. Mador MJ, Tobin MJ. Apneustic breathing. A characteristic feature of brainstem compression in achondroplasia? Chest. 1990;97(4): 877–83.
19. Wijdicks EF. Biot's breathing. J Neurol Neurosurg Psychiatry. 2007;78(5):512–3.
20. Farney RJ, Walker JM, Boyle KM, Cloward TV, Shilling KC. Adaptive servoventilation (ASV) in patients with sleep disordered breathing associated with chronic opioid medications for nonmalignant pain. J Clin Sleep Med. 2008;4(4):311–9.
21. Levitzky MG, Cairo JM, Hall SM. Introduction to respiratory care. Philadelphia: Saunders; 1990.
22. Rosenthal EN, Riccio CA, Gsanger KM, Jarratt KP. Digit span components as predictors of attention problems and executive functioning in children. Arch Clin Neuropsychol. 2006;21(2):131–9.
23. Pennington LA. The serial sevens test as a psychometric instrument. Am J Orthopsychiatry. 1947;17(3):488–99.
24. Heilman KM, Valenstein E. Mechanisms underlying hemispatial neglect. Ann Neurol. 1979;5(2):166–70.
25. Heilman KM, Watson RT. Mechanisms underlying the unilateral neglect syndrome. Adv Neurol. 1977;18:93–106.
26. Knecht S, Drager B, Deppe M, et al. Handedness and hemispheric language dominance in healthy humans. Brain. 2000;123(Pt 12):2512–8.
27. Huntley A. Documenting level of consciousness. Nursing. 2008;38(8):63–4.
28. Sigg EB, Sigg TD. The modification of the pupillary light reflex by chlorpromazine, diazepam, and pentobarbital. Brain Res. 1973;50(1):77–86.
29. Miller NR, Walsh FB, Hoyt WF. Walsh and Hoyt's clinical neuro-ophthalmology. 6th ed. Philadelphia: Lippincott Williams & Wilkins; 2005.
30. Biller J, Gruener G, Brazis PW, DeMyer W. Technique of the neurologic examination: a programmed text. 6th ed. New York: McGraw-Hill Medical Publishing Division; 2011.
31. Yanovitch T, Buckley E. Diagnosis and management of third nerve palsy. Curr Opin Ophthalmol. 2007;18(5):373–8.
32. Elmalem VI, Hudgins PA, Bruce BB, Newman NJ, Biousse V. Underdiagnosis of posterior communicating artery aneurysm in

noninvasive brain vascular studies. J Neuroophthalmol. 2011;31(2):103–9.

33. Chaudhary N, Davagnanam I, Ansari SA, Pandey A, Thompson BG, Gemmete JJ. Imaging of intracranial aneurysms causing isolated third cranial nerve palsy. J Neuroophthalmol. 2009;29(3): 238–44.

34. Brown SM. The utility of 0.5% apraclonidine in the diagnosis of horner syndrome. Arch Ophthalmol. 2005;123(4):578; author reply 578.

35. Freedman KA, Brown SM. Topical apraclonidine in the diagnosis of suspected Horner syndrome. J Neuroophthalmol. 2005;25(2):83–5.

36. Thompson HS. Diagnosing Horner's syndrome. Trans Sect Ophthalmol Am Acad Ophthalmol Otolaryngol. 1977;83(5):840–2.

37. Goodwill CJ, O'Tuama L. Electromyographic recording of the jaw reflex in multiple sclerosis. J Neurol Neurosurg Psychiatry. 1969;32(1):6–10.

38. Angelaki DE. Eyes on target: what neurons must do for the vestibuloocular reflex during linear motion. J Neurophysiol. 2004;92(1): 20–35.

39. Leigh RJ, Zee DS. The neurology of eye movements. 3rd ed. New York: Oxford University Press; 1999.

40. Roberts TA, Jenkyn LR, Reeves AG. On the notion of doll's eyes. Arch Neurol. 1984;41(12):1242–3.

41. Gonçalves DU, Felipe L, Lima TMA. Interpretação e utilidade da prova calórica. Revista Brasileira de Otorrinolaringologia. 2008; 74:440–6.

42. Davies AE, Kidd D, Stone SP, MacMahon J. Pharyngeal sensation and gag reflex in healthy subjects. Lancet. 1995;345(8948): 487–8.

43. Walker HK. The origins of the history and physical. In: Walker HK, Hall WD, Hurst JW, et al., editors. Clinical methods: the history, physical, and laboratory examinations. 3rd ed. Boston: Butterworths; 1990.

44. Sherrington CS. The integrative action of the nervous system. New York: C. Scribner's Sons; 1906.

45. Brazis PW, Masdeu JC, Biller J. Localization in clinical neurology. 6th ed. Philadelphia: Wolters Kluwer Health/Lippincott Williams & Wilkins; 2011.

46. Floeter MK, Fields HL. Evidence that inhibition of a nociceptive flexion reflex by stimulation in the rostroventromedial medulla in rats occurs at a premotoneuronal level. Brain Res. 1991;538(2): 340–2.

47. Sandrini G, Serrao M, Rossi P, Romaniello A, Cruccu G, Willer JC. The lower limb flexion reflex in humans. Prog Neurobiol. 2005;77(6):353–95.

48. Shah RC, Wilson RS, Tang Y, Dong X, Murray A, Bennett DA. Relation of hemoglobin to level of cognitive function in older persons. Neuroepidemiology. 2009;32(1):40–6.

49. Shah RC, Buchman AS, Wilson RS, Leurgans SE, Bennett DA. Hemoglobin level in older persons and incident Alzheimer disease: prospective cohort analysis. Neurology. 2011;77:219–26.

50. Moschcowitz E. An acute febrile pleiochromic anemia with hyaline thrombosis of the terminal arterioles and capillaries; an undescribed disease. Am J Med. 1952;13(5):567–9.

51. Zaret BS, Beckner RR, Marini AM, Wagle W, Passarelli C. Sodium valproate-induced hyperammonemia without clinical hepatic dysfunction. Neurology. 1982;32(2):206–8.

52. Cook ND. The neuron-level phenomena underlying cognition and consciousness: synaptic activity and the action potential. Neuroscience. 2008;153(3):556–70.

53. Hounsfield GN. Computerized transverse axial scanning (tomography). 1. Description of system. Br J Radiol. 1973;46(552): 1016–22.

54. Ambrose J. Computerized transverse axial scanning of the brain. Proc R Soc Med. 1973;66(8):833–4.

55. Roos KL. Lumbar puncture. Semin Neurol. 2003;23(1):105–14.

56. Husain AM. Electroencephalographic assessment of coma. J Clin Neurophysiol. 2006;23(3):208–20.

57. Bickford RG, Butt HR. Hepatic coma: the electroencephalographic pattern. J Clin Invest. 1955;34(6):790–9.

58. Ch'ien LT, Boehm RM, Robinson H, Liu C, Frenkel LD. Characteristic early electroencephalographic changes in herpes simplex encephalitis. Arch Neurol. 1977;34(6):361–4.

59. Levy SR, Chiappa KH, Burke CJ, Young RR. Early evolution and incidence of electroencephalographic abnormalities in Creutzfeldt-Jakob disease. J Clin Neurophysiol. 1986;3(1):1–21.

60. International Federation of Societies for Electroencephalography and Clinical Neurophysiology. Recommendations for the practice of clinical neurophysiology. Amsterdam/New York: Elsevier; 1983.

61. Wang JT, Young GB, Connolly JF. Prognostic value of evoked responses and event-related brain potentials in coma. Can J Neurol Sci. 2004;31(4):438–50.

62. Dubois MJ, Bergeron N, Dumont M, Dial S, Skrobik Y. Delirium in an intensive care unit: a study of risk factors. Intensive Care Med. 2001;27(8):1297–304.

63. Ely EW, Shintani A, Truman B, et al. Delirium as a predictor of mortality in mechanically ventilated patients in the intensive care unit. JAMA. 2004;291(14):1753–62.

64. Ely EW, Gautam S, Margolin R, et al. The impact of delirium in the intensive care unit on hospital length of stay. Intensive Care Med. 2001;27(12):1892–900.

65. Heymann A, Radtke F, Schiemann A, et al. Delayed treatment of delirium increases mortality rate in intensive care unit patients. J Int Med Res. 2010;38(5):1584–95.

66. American Psychiatric Association. Diagnostic criteria from DSM-IV-TR. Washington DC: American Psychiatric Association; 2000.

67. Campo-Soria C, Chang Y, Weiss DS. Mechanism of action of benzodiazepines on GABAA receptors. Br J Pharmacol. 2006;148(7):984–90.

68. Study RE, Barker JL. Diazepam and (−)-pentobarbital: fluctuation analysis reveals different mechanisms for potentiation of gamma-aminobutyric acid responses in cultured central neurons. Proc Natl Acad Sci U S A. 1981;78(11):7180–4.

69. Benowitz NL. Clinical pharmacology and toxicology of cocaine. Pharmacol Toxicol. 1993;72(1):3–12.

70. Meehan TJ, Bryant SM, Aks SE. Drugs of abuse: the highs and lows of altered mental states in the emergency department. Emerg Med Clin North Am. 2010;28(3):663–82.

71. Williams SR, Turner JP, Crunelli V. Gamma-hydroxybutyrate promotes oscillatory activity of rat and cat thalamocortical neurons by a tonic GABAB, receptor-mediated hyperpolarization. Neuroscience. 1995;66(1):133–41.

72. Mathivet P, Bernasconi R, De Barry J, Marescaux C, Bittiger H. Binding characteristics of gamma-hydroxybutyric acid as a weak but selective GABAB receptor agonist. Eur J Pharmacol. 1997;321(1):67–75.

73. Friedman J, Westlake R, Furman M. "Grievous bodily harm:" gamma hydroxybutyrate abuse leading to a Wernicke-Korsakoff syndrome. Neurology. 1996;46(2):469–71.

74. Okun MS, Boothby LA, Bartfield RB, Doering PL. GHB: an important pharmacologic and clinical update. J Pharm Pharm Sci. 2001;4(2):167–75.

75. Benbadis SR, Sila CA, Cristea RL. Mental status changes and stroke. J Gen Intern Med. 1994;9(9):485–7.

76. Kubik CS, Adams R. Occlusion of the basilar artery; a clinical and pathological study. Brain. 1946;69(2):73–121.

77. Percheron G. The anatomy of the arterial supply of the human thalamus and its use for the interpretation of the thalamic vascular pathology. Z Neurol. 1973;205(1):1–13.

78. Reilly M, Connolly S, Stack J, Martin EA, Hutchinson M. Bilateral paramedian thalamic infarction: a distinct but poorly recognized stroke syndrome. Q J Med. 1992;82(297):63–70.

79. McCormick WF, Rosenfield DB. Massive brain hemorrhage: a review of 144 cases and an examination of their causes. Stroke. 1973;4(6):946–54.

80. Kassell NF, Sasaki T, Colohan AR, Nazar G. Cerebral vasospasm following aneurysmal subarachnoid hemorrhage. Stroke. 1985;16(4):562–72.

81. Byrom FB. The pathogenesis of hypertensive encephalopathy and its relation to the malignant phase of hypertension; experimental evidence from the hypertensive rat. Lancet. 1954;267(6831): 201–11.

82. Bartynski WS. Posterior reversible encephalopathy syndrome, part 1: fundamental imaging and clinical features. AJNR Am J Neuroradiol. 2008;29(6):1036–42.

83. Bartynski WS, Boardman JF, Zeigler ZR, Shadduck RK, Lister J. Posterior reversible encephalopathy syndrome in infection, sepsis, and shock. AJNR Am J Neuroradiol. 2006;27(10): 2179–90.

84. Okun MS, Millar B, Watson R. Early diagnostic magnetic resonance imaging in acute disseminated encephalomyelitis. South Med J. 2000;93(8):793–6.

85. Nishimura A, Fuchigami T, Izumi H, Okubo O, Takahashi S, Harada K. A case of early-onset acute disseminated encephalomyelitis. No To Hattatsu. 1997;29(5):396–400.

86. Stricker RB, Miller RG, Kiprov DD. Role of plasmapheresis in acute disseminated (postinfectious) encephalomyelitis. J Clin Apher. 1992;7(4):173–9.

87. Tan HM, Chan LL, Chuah KL, Goh NS, Tang KK. Monophasic, solitary tumefactive demyelinating lesion: neuroimaging features and neuropathological diagnosis. Br J Radiol. 2004;77(914): 153–6.

88. De Stefano N, Caramanos Z, Preul MC, Francis G, Antel JP, Arnold DL. In vivo differentiation of astrocytic brain tumors and isolated demyelinating lesions of the type seen in multiple sclerosis using 1H magnetic resonance spectroscopic imaging. Ann Neurol. 1998;44(2):273–8.

89. Launay M, Lebrun C, Giordana E, Chanalet S, Thomas P. Clinical, radiographic, prognostic and therapeutic aspects of demelinating disease with tumefactive demyelinating lesions. Rev Neurol (Paris). 2011;167(1):14–22.

90. Zunt JR, Marra CM. Cerebrospinal fluid testing for the diagnosis of central nervous system infection. Neurol Clin. 1999;17(4): 675–89.

91. Arevalo CE, Barnes PF, Duda M, Leedom JM. Cerebrospinal fluid cell counts and chemistries in bacterial meningitis. South Med J. 1989;82(9):1122–7.

92. Chaudhuri A, Martin PM, Kennedy PGE, et al. EFNS guideline on the management of community-acquired bacterial meningitis: report of an EFNS Task Force on acute bacterial meningitis in older children and adults. Eur J Neurol. 2008;15(7):649–59.

93. Tunkel AR, Hartman BJ, Kaplan SL, et al. Practice guidelines for the management of bacterial meningitis. Clin Infect Dis. 2004;39(9):1267–84.

94. Attia J, Hatala R, Cook DJ, Wong JG. Does this adult patient have acute meningitis? JAMA. 1999;282(2):175–81.

95. Whitley RJ. Herpes simplex encephalitis: adolescents and adults. Antiviral Res. 2006;71(2–3):141–8.

96. Whitley RJ, Gnann JW. Viral encephalitis: familiar infections and emerging pathogens. Lancet. 2002;359(9305):507–13.

97. Xiao F, Tseng MY, Teng LJ, Tseng HM, Tsai JC. Brain abscess: clinical experience and analysis of prognostic factors. Surg Neurol. 2005;63(5):442–9; discussion 449–50.

98. Carpenter J, Stapleton S, Holliman R. Retrospective analysis of 49 cases of brain abscess and review of the literature. Eur J Clin Microbiol Infect Dis. 2007;26(1):1–11.

99. Nunez DA, Browning GG. Risks of developing an otogenic intracranial abscess. J Laryngol Otol. 1990;104(6):468–72.

100. Schievink WI, Louy C. Precipitating factors of spontaneous spinal CSF leaks and intracranial hypotension. Neurology. 2007; 69(7):700–2.

101. Fedi M, Cantello R, Shuey NH, et al. Spontaneous intracranial hypotension presenting as a reversible dorsal midbrain syndrome. J Neuroophthalmol. 2008;28(4):289–92.

102. Wicklund MR, Mokri B, Drubach DA, Boeve BF, Parisi JE, Josephs KA. Frontotemporal brain sagging syndrome. Neurology. 2011;76(16):1377–82.

103. Schievink WI, Gordon OK, Tourje J. Connective tissue disorders with spontaneous spinal cerebrospinal fluid leaks and intracranial hypotension: a prospective study. Neurosurgery. 2004;54(1):65–70; discussion 70–1.

104. Lowenstein DH. Status epilepticus: an overview of the clinical problem. Epilepsia. 1999;40 Suppl 1:3–8; discussion S21–2.

105. Garcia Penas JJ, Molins A, Salas Puig J. Status epilepticus: evidence and controversy. Neurologist. 2007;13(6 Suppl 1):62–73.

106. DeLorenzo RJ, Hauser WA, Towne AR, et al. A prospective, population-based epidemiologic study of status epilepticus in Richmond, Virginia. Neurology. 1996;46(4):1029–35.

107. Treiman DM, Meyers PD, Walton NY, et al. A comparison of four treatments for generalized convulsive status epilepticus. Veterans Affairs Status Epilepticus Cooperative Study Group. N Engl J Med. 1998;339(12):792–8.

108. Litt B, Wityk RJ, Hertz SH, et al. Nonconvulsive status epilepticus in the critically ill elderly. Epilepsia. 1998;39(11):1194–202.

109. Shneker BF, Fountain NB. Assessment of acute morbidity and mortality in nonconvulsive status epilepticus. Neurology. 2003;61(8):1066–73.

110. Pruitt AA. Immune-mediated encephalopathies with an emphasis on paraneoplastic encephalopathies. Semin Neurol. 2011;31(02): 158, 168.

111. Tuzun E, Dalmau J. Limbic encephalitis and variants: classification, diagnosis and treatment. Neurologist. 2007;13(5): 261–71.

112. Thieben MJ, Lennon VA, Boeve BF, Aksamit AJ, Keegan M, Vernino S. Potentially reversible autoimmune limbic encephalitis with neuronal potassium channel antibody. Neurology. 2004;62(7):1177–82.

113. Dalmau J, Gleichman AJ, Hughes EG, et al. Anti-NMDA-receptor encephalitis: case series and analysis of the effects of antibodies. Lancet Neurol. 2008;7(12):1091–8.

114. Lai M, Hughes EG, Peng X, et al. AMPA receptor antibodies in limbic encephalitis alter synaptic receptor location. Ann Neurol. 2009;65(4):424–34.

115. Lancaster E, Lai M, Peng X, et al. Antibodies to the GABA(B) receptor in limbic encephalitis with seizures: case series and characterisation of the antigen. Lancet Neurol. 2010;9(1): 67–76.

116. EiP F, McKeon A, Lennon VA, et al. Autoimmune dementia: clinical course and predictors of immunotherapy response. Mayo Clin Proc. 2010;85(10):881–97.

117. Brain L. Hashimoto's disease and encephalopathy. Lancet Neurol. 1966;2(7462):512–4.

118. Chong JY, Rowland LP, Utiger RD. Hashimoto encephalopathy: syndrome or myth? Arch Neurol. 2003;60(2):164–71.

119. Medical Society of the District of Columbia. Natural Death Act of 1981, D.C. Law 4–69: Uniform Determination of Death Act of 1981, D.C. Law 4–68. Washington DC: The Society; 1982.

120. Practice parameters for determining brain death in adults (summary statement). The Quality Standards Subcommittee of the American Academy of Neurology. Neurology. 1995;45(5): 1012–14.

121. Wijdicks EF, Varelas PN, Gronseth GS, Greer DM. Evidence-based guideline update: determining brain death in adults: report

of the Quality Standards Subcommittee of the American Academy of Neurology. Neurology. 2010;74(23):1911–8.

122. Kelly CA, Upex A, Bateman DN. Comparison of consciousness level assessment in the poisoned patient using the alert/verbal/painful/unresponsive scale and the Glasgow Coma Scale. Ann Emerg Med. 2004;44(2):108–13.

123. Ropper AH, Adams RD, Victor M, Samuels MA. Adams and Victor's principles of neurology. 9th ed. New York: McGraw-Hill Medical; 2009.

124. Teasdale G, Jennett B. Assessment of coma and impaired consciousness. A practical scale. Lancet. 1974;2:81–4.

Aneurysmal Subarachnoid Hemorrhage: Evidence-Based Medicine, Diagnosis, Treatment, and Complications

24

Matthew M. Kimball, Gregory J. Velat, J.D. Mocco, and Brian L. Hoh

Contents

M.M. Kimball, MD • B.L. Hoh, MD, FACS, FAHA, FAANS (✉)
Department of Neurological Surgery,
University of Florida College of Medicine,
100265, Gainesville, FL 32610, USA
e-mail: matthew.kimball@neurosurgery.ufl.edu;
brian.hoh@neurosurgery.ufl.edu

G.J. Velat, MD
Department of Neurosurgery,
Lee Memorial Hospital, Fort Myers, FL 33901, USA
e-mail: gvelat@gmail.com

J.D. Mocco, MD, MS, FAANS, FAHA
Department of Neurosurgery,
Vanderbilt University Medical Center,
1161 21st Ave S, RM T4224 MCN, Nashville, TN 37232, USA
e-mail: j.mocco@vanderbilt.edu

Abstract

Aneurysmal subarachnoid hemorrhage is a devastating condition with high mortality and morbidity rates for those that survive the initial hemorrhage. There has been significant research on aneurysmal subarachnoid hemorrhage to better understand how we can diagnose, treat, and manage patients with this disease. Cerebral vasospasm accounts for the majority of morbidity, mortality, and long-term disability in these patients, and a large volume of literature is dedicated to preventing and treating vasospasm. This chapter presents a simplified, evidence-based review of the literature about the modes of diagnosis, medical and surgical management, and treatment options of patients with aneurysmal subarachnoid hemorrhage and cerebral vasospasm.

Keywords

Cerebral aneurysm • Cerebral vasospasm • Evidence-based treatment • Hydrocephalus • Subarachnoid hemorrhage

Introduction

Aneurysmal subarachnoid hemorrhage (SAH) is a devastating condition accounting for about 5 % of all strokes, affecting about 30,000 people in the United States every year [1, 2]. The annual prevalence of aneurysmal SAH is likely higher than 30,000 due to misdiagnosis and those who do not receive medical care. The incidence of aneurysmal SAH varies around the world and has been reported anywhere from 2 to 23 per 100,000 [3, 4]. Mortality rates range from 32 to 67 % [5] with a significant degree of morbidity among those who survive the initial hemorrhage [6, 7]. Recent data have shown that there may be a declining mortality rate after aneurysmal SAH with more recent treatment modalities [8]. However, despite many advancements such as endovascular therapy for the treatment of

A.J. Layon et al. (eds.), *Textbook of Neurointensive Care*,
DOI 10.1007/978-1-4471-5226-2_24, © Springer-Verlag London 2013

aneurysms and the ability to better diagnose and treat cerebral vasospasm, morbidity remains high.

Aneurysmal SAH typically affects adults in the fifth to seventh decades of life and is about 1.6 times more common in females than in males [9, 10]. Some genetic syndromes have a higher risk of aneurysm formation and hemorrhage, such as polycystic kidney disease [11] and Ehlers-Danlos [12] syndrome. Familial intracranial aneurysm syndrome is when two or more first- through third-degree relatives are found to have intracranial aneurysms. Those who have this syndrome are more inclined to harbor multiple intracranial aneurysms and experience aneurysmal SAH at a younger age [13]. Additional risk factors for developing aneurysmal SAH include hypertension, smoking history, and alcohol abuse all of which have been validated on multivariate analyses [14, 15]. Cocaine use and other sympathomimetics have also been shown to increase risk of SAH, particularly in younger patients with SAH [16].

Natural History of Aneurysmal SAH

It is estimated that approximately 15 % of patients die at the time of hemorrhage before receiving medical care. About 30 % of those that survive the initial hemorrhage have moderate to severe disability [5], and about two-thirds who survive to undergo successful aneurysm treatment never regain their baseline quality of life [5]. The overall mortality rate is about 45 %, with most deaths occurring within the first few days following rupture. In one series, the 30-day mortality rate was 46 % [17], and in another study over half of the patients died within 14 days of hemorrhage [18]. For those that survive the initial hemorrhage, approximately 8 % will die from progressive deterioration [19]. Rebleeding before aneurysm treatment remains the major cause of morbidity and mortality following the initial hemorrhage, supporting the need for early treatment (within 72 h) of aneurysm rupture. For those who survive to undergo treatment, cerebral vasospasm accounts for the majority of morbidity and mortality. Angiographic vasospasm occurs in 30–70 % of patients between the fifth and fourteenth days following SAH [20, 21]. Approximately 50 % of patients with angiographic vasospasm will develop delayed ischemic neurologic deficits (DINDS), and 15–20 % of these patients will suffer major stroke or death despite intervention [22, 23].

Bederson and coworkers [24] analyzed patient, aneurysm, and institutional factors on clinical outcomes following aneurysmal SAH. They included patient factors as severity/grade of initial hemorrhage, age, sex, time to treatment, and medical comorbidities including hypertension, atrial fibrillation, congestive heart failure, coronary artery disease, and renal disease. Aneurysm factors included size and location.

Institutional factors included availability of endovascular services, volume of SAH patients treated at a given institution, and the type of facility in which the patient is first evaluated.

Rebleeding after the initial hemorrhage carries a very high mortality rate of approximately 70 % and is highest in the first 24–48 h [25]. The International Cooperative Study on the Timing of Intracranial Aneurysm Surgery [26] found that patients who underwent aneurysm treatment in <72 h had a 5.6 % rebleed rate with 73 % of those occurring in the first 24 h. Overall, they reported a rate of 4.1 % for the first 24 h and 1 % per day for the first two weeks. More recent studies have shown that rebleeding may be more common in the first 2–12 h [27, 28]. Current literature supports early securing of ruptured aneurysms through either microsurgical or endovascular means to prevent rebleeding and improve overall patient outcomes.

Diagnosis and Initial Management

Presentation

The classic presentation of an awake patient with an aneurysmal SAH is the complaint of the worst headache of their life. The headache may also be associated with nausea, vomiting, nuchal rigidity, photophobia, a brief loss of consciousness, cranial neuropathy, or other focal neurologic deficits. Although there has been a drastic improvement in diagnosis by primary care and emergency medical providers, there is still a reported misdiagnosis rate of about 12 %, in which the most common diagnostic error was failure to obtain a noncontrast computed tomographic (CT) scan of the head [24].

Initial Evaluation and Imaging

A noncontrasted head CT is the most important tool for diagnosis of a SAH (Fig. 24.1a). A CT scan is 98–100 % sensitive for the diagnosis of SAH if done within 12 h of hemorrhage. The sensitivity decreases to about 93 % at 24 h and 85 % at 6 days after SAH [29, 30]. In a patient with a known aneurysm and a negative head CT or a patient with a concerning recent history for SAH and a negative head CT, lumbar puncture (LP) can be extremely valuable for diagnosing aneurysmal SAH. It is extremely important that the person performing the lumbar puncture understands how to collect and handle the cerebrospinal fluid (CSF), order the correct labs, and effectively communicate with the laboratory personnel to achieve accurate test results. It is important to know the relationship between the timing of the LP and onset of symptoms, to be able to interpret the results. Lumbar

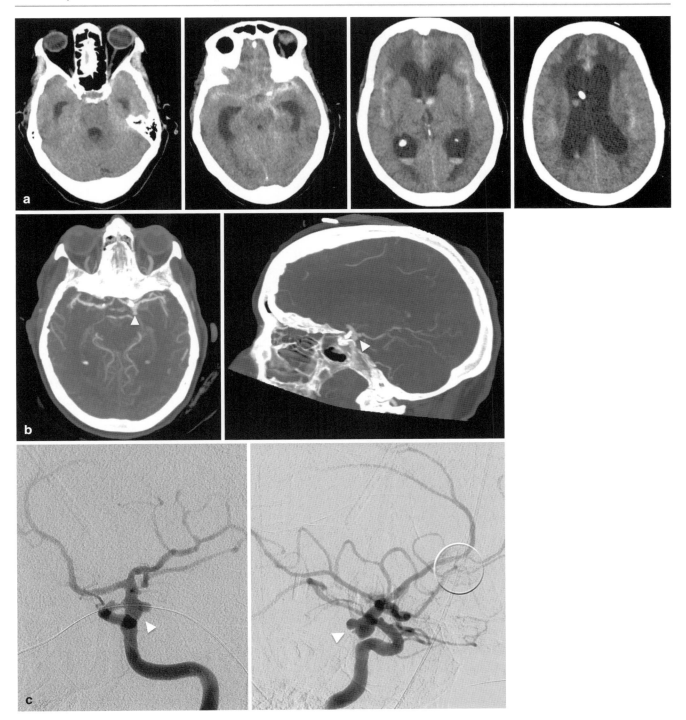

Fig. 24.1 (a–e) Illustrative case. 78-year-old woman with Hunt-Hess grade 3, Fisher score 3 subarachnoid hemorrhage. (a) Noncontrast head computed tomographic (CT) scan demonstrates Fisher score 3 subarachnoid hemorrhage with hydrocephalus. A right frontal ventriculostomy drain catheter has been placed. (b) Maximal intensity projection (MIP) reconstructions of CT angiography (axial on left, sagittal on right) demonstrate a ruptured left posterior communicating artery aneurysm with daughter sac (*arrowheads*). (c) Anteroposterior (AP, *left*) and lateral (*right*) projection cerebral angiography demonstrates a ruptured left posterior communicating artery aneurysm with daughter sac (*arrowheads*). A dime is superimposed on the lateral projection for measurement calibration. (d) Endovascular balloon-assisted coiling of the ruptured left posterior communicating aneurysm is demonstrated on AP (*left*) and lateral (*right*) projection roadmap cerebral angiography (inflated balloon, *arrows*; coiling, *arrowheads*). (e) Completed coil occlusion of the left posterior communicating artery aneurysm is demonstrated on AP (*left*) and lateral (*right*) projection cerebral angiography

Fig. 24.1 (continued)

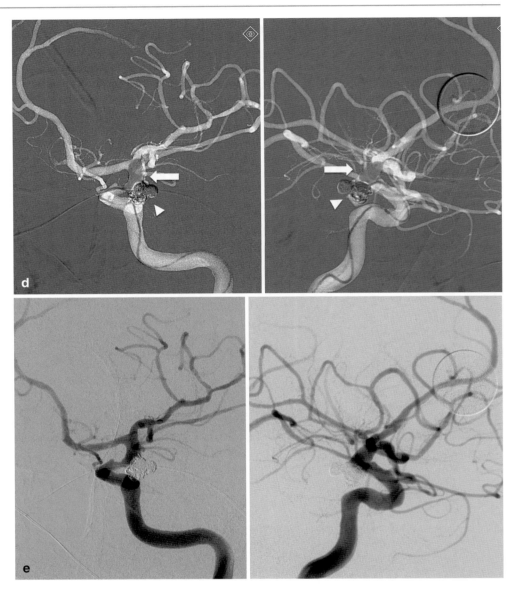

puncture results in SAH have been well studied and are the most sensitive test for SAH [31, 32].

Lumbar puncture should be performed carefully, as some believe that by removing a large volume of CSF, the transmural pressure gradient across the aneurysm dome may increase leading to hemorrhage. Measuring an opening pressure may be helpful, particularly in the setting of hydrocephalus, but is not diagnostic of aneurysmal SAH. Occasionally, patients with a remote history of SAH may present with symptoms of hydrocephalus. It is necessary to be able to differentiate between a traumatic tap and a true SAH [33] (Table 24.1). The most critical data show the comparison of the red blood cell (RBC) count in the first and last tubes, and the presence of xanthochromia in the supernatant fluid. Cerebrospinal fluid in SAH patients is typically bloody or grossly xanthochromic with a yellow or pink color but does not typically clot when collected. Traumatic taps commonly consist of gross blood and clot during collection. The RBC count should remain fairly consistent between the first and last tube, where it will likely decline with a traumatic tap. After the CSF is collected, it is spun down and a supernatant fluid is collected and tested for xanthochromia, which is a discoloration of the CSF due to heme breakdown products from RBCs. This is the most reliable means of differentiating aneurysmal SAH from a traumatic tap. Although gross visual inspection can be helpful, spectrophotometry is much more accurate. Timing of LP and symptoms are very important. Xanthochromia does not appear until 2–4 h after SAH but is present in 100 % of patients at 12 h and remains in the CSF in about 70 % of patients at 3 weeks but drops off significantly between 3 and 4 weeks. If a patient has a normal noncontrasted head CT and CSF profile, aneurysmal SAH is essentially ruled out.

Table 24.1 CSF results in SAH versus traumatic LP

CSF feature	SAH	Traumatic tap
Red blood cell count (RBC)	Usually >100,000 RBC/mm³ (little change between first and last tube)	RBC should decrease between first and last tube
Fluid appearance (gross)	Xanthochromia (yellow/pink)	Bloody
Supernatant appearance (spun)	Xanthochromia	Clear
Clotting	Usually does not clot	Typically clots
WBC/RBC ratio	Slight leukocytosis	Same as peripheral blood
Opening pressure	Commonly elevated	Commonly normal
Protein	Commonly elevated	May be elevated slightly

Magnetic resonance imaging is currently of little diagnostic value for acute aneurysmal SAH due to poor sensitivity to detect methemoglobin molecules in the first 24–48 h following rupture. Patient compliance, duration of time needed to obtain the scan, and increased cost compared to CT scanning have relegated MR imaging in the diagnosis of aneurysmal SAH. Magnetic resonance angiography (MRA) may be used in patients with renal insufficiency, acute renal failure, or pregnant patients to diagnose intracranial aneurysms with reduced sensitivity and specificity compared to CT angiography (CTA). MRA sensitivity ranges from 85 to 100 % for aneurysms >5 mm but drops to approximately 56 % for aneurysms ≤5 mm [34, 35]. MRI and MRA may be helpful when looking for other causes of SAH such as cervical spinal arteriovenous malformations that may be missed by conventional CTA.

The most useful noninvasive imaging modality in acute SAH is CTA (Fig. 24.1b). It can be obtained quickly, provides excellent three-dimensional reconstructions, shows relationship of aneurysms to bony landmarks, may show thrombus or calcification within the aneurysm, is noninvasive, and has a high sensitivity and specificity. Sensitivity of CTA for aneurysms ranges from 95 to 100 % for aneurysms ≥5 mm but drops off to 64–83 % for aneurysms ≤5 mm [36–38]. CTA sensitivity diminishes with small aneurysms, increased blood products, and may vary in accordance with experience of the interpreting neuroradiologist. Potential disadvantages of CTA include the inability to adjust the contrast dose and/or concentration for patients at risk of renal dysfunction, artifact from previous aneurysm clips or embolic material may obstruct aneurysm diagnosis, and small distal vessels may not be well visualized. Currently, CTA is the diagnostic imaging study of choice for initial detection of intracranial aneurysms.

Cerebral angiography, the traditional gold standard diagnostic test for intracranial aneurysms, is typically performed if CT angiography fails to reveal a potential bleeding source. Cerebral angiography holds many advantages over other diagnostic imaging techniques. First, it allows for methodical evaluation of the intracranial vasculature via selective injection of intracranial arteries. PA and lateral projections are obtained simultaneously to better characterize the exact location and morphology of intracranial aneurysms (Fig. 24.1c). Three-dimensional reconstructions can be readily obtained. In addition, cerebral vasculature surrounding an intracranial aneurysm is delineated. Endovascular intervention may be pursued at the time of cerebral angiography, effectively streamlining aneurysm treatment. Contrast load can also be altered, which may benefit patients with renal insufficiency. Despite the improved sensitivity of cerebral angiography for the diagnosis of intracranial aneurysms or other vascular malformation causing SAH, in about 20–25 % a source of hemorrhage will not be found. Many centers repeat a diagnostic cerebral angiogram 1 week after the initial angiogram to evaluate for a small aneurysm that was unable to be visualized on the initial study. In about 1–2 % of patients, an aneurysm is found after repeat angiogram [39]. It is controversial whether the small percentage of aneurysms found on repeat angiography warrants a repeat angiogram on all patients with a single negative diagnostic cerebral angiogram. We feel that the small morbidity of a diagnostic cerebral angiogram of about 1–2 % versus the morbidity and mortality of a re-ruptured undiagnosed aneurysm warrants a repeat angiogram.

Contrast Prophylaxis

The number of diagnostic and therapeutic spinal and cerebral angiograms has gone up exponentially in the last 20 years and therefore the use of iodinated contrast media. Although newer and safer contrast media have been developed and used over recent years, we need to understand the risks of using these agents. The majority of the literature on these agents comes from the cardiology literature where there is a much higher patient population to study. Low-osmolality agents have been in use since the 1980s and have had a direct reduction in the pain associated with administration as well as adverse events. These agents have been proven to be safe but are associated with a small percentage of adverse reactions ranging from rash and flushing to angioedema, vasomotor collapse, and death. The risk for adverse reactions increases with higher osmolarity and ionicity. The risk for all adverse reactions ranges from 4 to 12 % with ionic agents compared to 1–3 % with nonionic agents [40]. The risk for severe reactions such as anaphylaxis and vasomotor collapse was significantly lower for low-osmolality agents 0.03 % compared with 0.16 % for high-osmolality agents [41]. The strongest risk factors for predicting an adverse reaction to contrast are a previous history of contrast reaction and atopic conditions such as asthma. A previous history of a contrast reaction gives a 17–35 % risk of future reaction [42]. Asthma increases the risk of reaction by approximately six times the general population [43]. Other risk factors reported for contrast reactions include underlying heart disease, renal disease, diabetes mellitus, myeloma, sickle cell disease, polycythemia, food or medication allergies, hay fever, non-steroidal anti-inflammatory drug use, beta-blocker use, age greater than 60, and female gender [44]. There has been a long debated argument as to risk of a contrast reaction in a patient with a known shellfish allergy. There has never been a reported case of shellfish allergy where iodine was implicated, and the reaction to radiocontrast media has never been proven to be related in any way to the iodine content in a preparation. Routine premedication for contrast reaction prior to contrast is not supported by the evidence currently available in the literature for those with shellfish allergy. Two major prophylaxis regimens are approved by the American College of Radiology and include:

Pretreatment Protocol 1:

(a) Prednisone 50 mg orally 13, 7, and 1 h prior to procedure

(b) Diphenhydramine 25–50 mg intravenously, intramuscularly, or orally 1 h prior to procedure

(c) Nonionic low-osmolality contrast medium

Pretreatment Protocol 2:

(a) Methylprednisolone 32 mg orally 12 and 2 h prior to procedure

(b) Diphenhydramine 25–50 mg intravenously, intramuscularly, or orally 1 h prior to procedure

(c) Nonionic low-osmolality contrast medium

The use of these preventative protocols has reduced the incidence of severe reactions and should be used in the appropriate populations. In the instance that waiting the 12–13 h is not reasonable for diagnosis or treatment by CTA or cerebral angiogram, a single dose of 100 mg of hydrocortisone sodium succinate can be given intravenously at the time of the procedure.

Initial Stabilization and Management

The patient should be transferred out of the emergency medical setting to a neurosurgical ICU setting as soon as possible. The admission Hunt-Hess grade (Table 24.2), Fisher score (Table 24.3), and World Federation of Neurologic Surgeons (WFNS) grade (Table 24.4) should also be reported, as it

Table 24.2 Hunt-Hess classification

Grade	Description
1	Asymptomatic or minimal headache and slight nuchal rigidity
2	Moderate to severe headache, nuchal rigidity, no neurologic deficit except cranial nerve palsy
3	Drowsy, minimal neurologic deficit
4	Stuporous, moderate to severe hemiparesis, early decerebrate rigidity
5	Deep coma, decerebrate rigidity, moribund

Reproduced with permission from Hunt and Hess [45]

Table 24.3 Fisher score

Fisher grade	Appearance of blood on CT scan
1	No hemorrhage evident
2	Subarachnoid hemorrhage less than 1 mm thick
3	Subarachnoid hemorrhage more than 1 mm thick
4	Subarachnoid hemorrhage of any thickness with intraventricular hemorrhage or intraparenchymal hemorrhage

Modified with permission from Fisher et al. [46]

Table 24.4 World Federation of Neurologic Surgeons (WFNS) grade

WFNS grade	Glasgow coma score	Major focal deficit
0		
1	15	No
2	13–14	No
3	13–14	Yes
4	7–12	Yes or no
5	3–6	Yes or no

Reproduced with permission from Drake [47]

may aid treatment, prognosis, and risk of vasospasm. The Airway management, breathing, and hemodynamic stability are the first priority. All of these should be managed with the understanding that manipulation of the airway may induce gag or cough reflexes, elevations in PCO_2, and intubation may elevate blood pressure, acutely placing the patient at high risk for rebleeding. Preoxygenation should be done prior to intubation. The gag and cough reflex, and reflex cardiac dysrhythmias can be avoided by appropriate pharmacologic agents. Although bed rest and a low-stimulation environment have been accepted as common management for an unsecured aneurysm, there are no data to support that it lowers the risk of early rebleeding; however, it causes no harm to the patient and should probably be followed. There is a large amount of literature in regard to treatment of hypertension in the acute period for an unsecured aneurysm; however, no well-controlled studies have been done to show that strict blood pressure control has any effect on rebleeding rates. A retrospective study has shown that there appears to be a lower risk of rebleeding in those treated with antihypertensive medications, but in this study those treated had higher blood pressures than those not treated, and there did not appear to be a correlation with a lower blood pressure [48]. Another study had stated that rebleeding may be related to greater variations in blood pressure and not an absolute value [49]. A specific goal systolic blood pressure (SBP) remains controversial and variable, but most would agree that a SBP goal <150 mmHg would be safe. When treating elevated SBP, short-acting agents given by continuous infusion are ideal as they can be titrated easily to prevent large fluctuations. Beta-blockers such as labetalol and esmolol and calcium channel blockers such as nicardipine may be used safely with minimal side effects and easy to titrate. Hydralazine can be given intravenously as needed for patients with bradycardia. Sodium nitroprusside should be avoided or used for less than 24 h as it can raise intracranial pressure by direct vasodilation, having greater effect on the arterial than the venous system. It can also cause toxicity by its breakdown products thiocyanate and cyanide. It should be used for acute management until other medications can be titrated to control blood pressure. Blood pressure control should be balanced between preventing rebleeding and hypotensive episodes that reduce cerebral perfusion pressure (CPP) and risk of ischemic events.

Antifibrinolytics

The use of antifibrinolytics for the prevention of early rehemorrhage has been studied since the late 1960s and early 1970s. Early studies showed similar results which included a significant reduction in the incidence of early rebleeding; however, this was offset by an increased risk of cerebral infarction and DINDs. The two major medications used are tranexamic acid and epsilon-aminocaproic acid (EACA). In 1981, Torner [50] reported results from the Cooperative Aneurysm Study in regards to a randomized, double-blinded, placebo-controlled trial using tranexamic acid use for patients after SAH. A slightly greater than 60 % reduction was seen in rebleeding in the treatment group, but there was a significant increased risk of cerebral infarction in the treatment group. In 1984, Kassel [51] gave a report from the Cooperative Aneurysm Study, which showed a 40 % reduction in rebleeding among those patients receiving an antifibrinolytic but a 43 % increase in focal neurologic deficits. Because of the decrease in rebleeding rates but the increase in neurologic deficits, it was believed that, if the antifibrinolytic was used for a short time period until securing of the aneurysm and stopped before the vasospasm period, the increased ischemic complications might decrease.

Since 2002, there have been 3 major studies comparing the use of short-term antifibrinolytics during SAH to prevent rebleeding: 1 randomized controlled trial and 2 retrospective cohort trials. A randomized trial by Hillman [52] included 505 patients of which 254 were treated with tranexamic acid within 48 h of SAH. A significant reduction in rebleeding from 10.8 to 2.4 % was seen among the two groups and a nonsignificant 19 % reduction in poor outcome, and a 4 % increase in good outcome was also noted. A cohort-controlled study by Starke [53] consisted of 72 patients who received EACA on admission that was continued for <72 h, compared to 175 patients that did not receive an antifibrinolytic. A significant reduction in rebleeding was seen in the EACA-treated group 2.7 % versus 11.4 % in the non-treated group. No significant difference was seen between ischemic complications between the two groups; however, an 8-fold increase in deep venous thrombosis (DVT) was found in the EACA-treated group without a difference in pulmonary embolism (PE) incidence. A retrospective review by Harrigan [54] of 356 patients compared to historical controls and determined short-term administration of EACA is associated with rates of rehemorrhage, ischemic stroke, and symptomatic vasospasm that compare favorably with historical controls.

Overall, it appears that there is significant decrease in the incidence of early rehemorrhage with early use of antifibrinolytics which should be discontinued in less than 72 h to decrease the risk of embolic and ischemic complications.

Seizures

There has always been an association between SAH and seizures; however, the true incidence and its effect on clinical outcome are debated. In a study by Lin [55], 217 patients with aneurysmal SAH were reviewed for incidence and timing of seizures and followed for 2 years. Overall, 21 % of all patients experienced one seizure, with 37 % of those being at onset of SAH, 11 % preoperative seizures, and 46 % had at least one seizure after the first week. In total, 6.9 % of the 217 patients developed late epilepsy, but only 3.8 % of patients who had a seizure during the hospitalization developed late epilepsy.

There has been a significant amount of debate in regards to whether seizures associated with SAH have an effect on outcome. Antiepileptic drugs (AEDs) have side effects as well, and some argue that the medications themselves can have an effect on outcome after SAH. A study [56] using the Nationwide Inpatient Sample Database (NISD) reported that generalized convulsive status epilepticus (GCSE) was independently associated with higher in-hospital mortality, longer hospital stays, and higher costs. Literature on nonconvulsive status epilepticus (NCSE) is poor, and the incidence is probably higher than reported. There have been some retrospective studies showing a relationship between phenytoin use in SAH and poor outcome, but because of the retrospective nature and difficulty in interpretation of the data, no recommendations can be made at this time. A study by Chumnanvej [57] reported that 3 days of phenytoin after SAH was adequate for seizure prophylaxis. They compared 79 patients who had previously undergone multi-week phenytoin prophylaxis after SAH versus 370 patients in which only 3 days of phenytoin were given and then discontinued. There was a significant reduction in phenytoin-related complications such as hypersensitivity reactions, but the percentage of patients who had seizures, short or long term, did not change significantly between the two groups. Although this study is not a prospective randomized trial, it may be beneficial to provide a 3-day regimen of phenytoin prophylaxis after SAH to minimize medication side effects such as hypersensitivity reactions, cognitive effects, and interaction with other medications while providing seizure prophylaxis.

Hydrocephalus

Acute hydrocephalus occurs in 15–87 % [58–60] of patients that present with aneurysmal SAH. Of those patients, however, only 8.9–48 % [58–60] develop chronic shunt-dependent hydrocephalus. The management of acute hydrocephalus secondary to aneurysmal SAH is usually managed by external ventricular drainage (EVD) or lumbar drainage (LD). Treatment of acute hydrocephalus with an EVD is associated with neurologic improvement [61–63]. There has been some concern about the risk of rebleeding after placement of an EVD. Three retrospective case series have evaluated this topic. One study found that there was an increased risk of rebleeding with EVD placement [64], and the other two found no increased risk [65, 66]. Lumbar drainage for the treatment of SAH-associated hydrocephalus has only been evaluated in retrospective studies and has been found to be safe and not increase the risk for rebleeding [67–70]. There has been suggestion that lumbar drainage decreases the incidence of vasospasm but has only been studied in retrospective series [68]. Serial lumbar puncture for management of SAH-associated hydrocephalus has also been described as safe and not increasing the risk of rebleeding, but only in small retrospective series [71].

The management of chronic hydrocephalus associated with aneurysmal SAH is usually managed by ventricular shunt placement. External ventricular drainage weaning can be done in a variety of ways. A small single-center prospective randomized control trial studied a method for determining which patients would require permanent ventricular shunt placement [72]. Forty-one patients were randomized to rapid EVD weaning (<24 h), and 40 patients were randomized to gradual EVD weaning (96 h weaning period). There was no difference in rate of shunt placement between the two groups, but the gradual wean group had 2.8 more days in the intensive care unit ($p=0.0002$) and 2.4 more days in the hospital ($p=0.031$).

Several factors have been studied to attempt to identify factors predictive of SAH-associated shunt-dependent hydrocephalus. One factor that has been studied is whether clipping versus coiling affects the incidence of shunting. A meta-analysis [60] of five non-randomized with 1,718 patients (1,336 clipped, 382 coiled) studies showed that the rate of shunt dependency was lower in the clipping group when compared to the coiling group ($p=0.01$); however, only one of the five studies when evaluated independently showed a significant difference [73]. Fenestration of the lamina terminalis has been suggested to reduce the incidence of shunt-dependent hydrocephalus. A meta-analysis of 11 non-randomized studies including 1,973 patients (975 fenestrated, 998 non-fenestrated) found no significant difference in shunt-dependent hydrocephalus between the two groups [74].

Subarachnoid-associated acute hydrocephalus can safely be managed by external ventricular drainage or lumbar drainage. It may potentially improve the neurologic exam and may slightly increase the risk of rebleeding. Although the benefit of neurologic improvement has only been shown in retrospective series, it has been consistently shown in these studies, and the slight risk of rebleeding with placement is not greatly supported in the literature. Chronic hydrocephalus from SAH can be treated with ventricular shunt placement. Determination of shunt dependency by weaning of EVDs within a <24-h period can be done safely without increasing the rate of shunt placement. There is no clear evidence that the modality of aneurysm treatment (clipping versus coiling) is associated with the development of shunt-dependent hydrocephalus. It is unlikely that lamina terminalis fenestration decreases the rate of shunt-dependent hydrocephalus.

Treatment Methods for Ruptured Cerebral Aneurysms

Two basic treatment options exist for ruptured cerebral aneurysms: open surgical clipping or wrapping and endovascular coil embolization. Whether done from inside or outside of the vessel, the goal is to exclude the aneurysm from the cerebral circulation. Ruptured aneurysms should ideally be treated as early as possible, within the first 24 h, to prevent rebleeding.

Surgical Treatment Options

Surgical treatment of aneurysms may involve clipping with titanium clips, wrapping with synthetic substances, or ligation of the feeding vessel. Surgical treatment for ruptured cerebral aneurysms is seated in a long history of courageous and intelligent pioneers developing new ways to treat this deadly pathology. Surgery for ruptured aneurysms first began with what were considered "passive" strategies. Victor Horsley was given credit for successfully treating the first ruptured cerebral aneurysm in 1885 by ligating the ipsilateral cervical carotid artery [75]. In 1931, Dott developed the technique of reinforcing the aneurysm wall by wrapping it with a piece of muscle [76]. Walter Dandy was credited in 1942 with the idea of trapping aneurysms to exclude them from the circulation. All of these methods had high failure rates, morbidity, and mortality. Eventually, a few brilliant and dedicated surgeons came up with the idea that placing a clip at the base of aneurysm while keeping the parent cerebral circulation patent may allow for definitive treatment. On March 23, 1937, Walter Dandy placed a V-shaped silver clip to the neck of an internal carotid artery aneurysm, and since then this has become the gold standard for treatment of ruptured and unruptured aneurysms [77]. Multiple variations and improvements have been made to the clip by many surgeons including Olivecrona, Schwartz, Mayfield, McFadden, Kees, Drake, Heifetz, Sundt, Yasargil, Sugita, Spetzler, and others [78].

Prior to 1970, carotid ligation was a common treatment for ruptured intracranial aneurysms. Studies have shown variable data in regard to rates of rebleeding and treatment morbidity and mortality. In the Cooperative Aneurysm Randomized Treatment Study [79], carotid ligation did not lead to a significant improvement in mortality or rebleeding in the acute period, compared with bed rest in the intent-to-treat analysis. Only 67 % of those patients randomized to carotid ligation actually received that therapy, and in that group there was actually a lower mortality when compared to the bed rest group, and no rebleeding occurred. Long-term follow-up revealed a benefit for carotid ligation in reducing rebleeding at 3 years and mortality at 5 years when compared to bed rest. A large retrospective study by Nishioka [80], however, reported a rebleeding rate of 7.8 % after carotid ligation with other associated complications of treatment. Overall, the treatment of ruptured aneurysms with carotid ligation likely reduces the rate of rebleeding when compared to bed rest alone, but the rate of complications associated with treatment and rebleeding likely exceeds those of surgical clipping.

Surgical clipping and endovascular embolization are preferred over carotid ligation for modern day treatment of ruptured cerebral aneurysms. Aneurysm location, morphology, neck size, patient age, and medical comorbidities are all factors that may make a ruptured aneurysm more likely to be coiled or surgically clipped. There has only been one large trial comparing surgical and endovascular therapy for ruptured cerebral aneurysms. The ISAT [81] trial is a prospective, randomized study that selected 2,143 patients of 9,559 patients with aneurysmal SAH to be randomized to surgical clipping or endovascular treatment, on the assumption that it

was agreed that their aneurysm could be treated by either modality. There was no significant difference in mortality rates at 1 year, 8.1 % in the endovascular group and 10.1 % in the surgical group. Greater disability rates were seen in the surgically treated group 21.6 % versus the endovascularly treated group 15.6 %. This made the overall morbidity and mortality of those treated surgically significantly higher than those treated by endovascular means at 1 year follow-up. The rebleeding rate was reported to be 2.9 % for coil embolization and 0.9 % for clipping, and 139 patients who underwent coiling required further treatment compared to 31 patients that were clipped. The confounding factor in many aneurysmal SAH studies is what makes an aneurysm randomizable? In this study they chose all patients with aneurysms in the anterior circulation, in awake, young patients, which is unclear if that can be extrapolated to other groups.

Surgical clipping of aneurysms has been considered a highly effective method for aneurysm treatment after SAH with its low recanalization and rehemorrhage rates. It has been shown that long-term rebleeding is reduced by either carotid ligation or direct surgical clipping of the aneurysm when compared to hypotension and bed rest [2], but there is a higher rehemorrhage rate and complication rate with carotid ligation when compared to direct surgical clipping. In the Cooperative Study [82], all patients underwent surgical treatment for their ruptured aneurysms. Of the 453 patients, only nine patients (2 %) suffered rehemorrhage, where four of these patients had multiple aneurysms. Sundt [83] also reported a large study of 644 patients who underwent surgical clipping of ruptured aneurysms, with a 1.2 % rate of rehemorrhage after clipping. In a more recent study by David [84] in 1999, 160 aneurysms in 102 patients were treated by surgical clipping and followed for mean of 4.4 years. They reported a complete obliteration rate of 91.8 % on follow-up angiography, with a 0.5 % recurrence rate for completely clipped aneurysms with no rehemorrhages. There was a 1.9 % rehemorrhage rate for incompletely clipped aneurysms with a small "dog-ear" residual. Incompletely clipped aneurysms with a wide residual neck had a 19 % recurrence and 3.8 % rehemorrhage rate. In total, they reported a 2.9 % recurrence rate for all incompletely clipped aneurysms with a total 1.5 % rehemorrhage rate.

Wrapping of aneurysms that are deemed unable to be clipped has been described as a treatment modality with an expected higher rehemorrhage rate than those that are clipped or coiled. Small, older clinical studies have reported a smaller rate of rehemorrhage than conservative management [85, 86]. A more recent long-term study reported an overall risk of rehemorrhage after aneurysm wrapping or coating to be 33 % [87]. A long-term follow-up study of patients who underwent surgical wrapping of ruptured aneurysms showed a rehemorrhage rate of 11.7 % at 6 months and 17.8 % at 6 months to 10 years [88]. The rehemorrhage rate is similar to rates of ruptured aneurysms treated by conservative management. The current data do not support the use of wrapping or coating of ruptured cerebral aneurysms.

Endovascular Treatment

Endovascular management for treatment of cerebral aneurysms is a relatively young field despite the development of cerebral angiography by Egas Moniz in 1927. Guido Guglielmi [89] in 1991 first described the technique of occluding aneurysms by an endovascular approach by using platinum coils called Guglielmi detachable coils that were detachable by applying a small current. The memory of the coils allows them to fill the aneurysm and the coils induce thrombosis. The aneurysm is packed until it is excluded from the normal cerebral circulation. Technology in this field has expanded much faster than our ability to study current modalities. As endovascular methods have become more available, the coil technology, delivery methods, and assistive techniques such as stent-assisted coiling or balloon-assisted coiling (Fig. 24.1d, e) have become more common allowing the morbidity to continue to decrease and ability to coil aneurysms that were initially felt to be uncoilable.

There is great variability in the use of endovascular therapy for ruptured cerebral aneurysms. Some centers use it as a first-line treatment and only clip if coiling cannot be achieved. Other centers use endovascular treatment in critically ill patients or those with significant medical comorbidities that would otherwise be poor surgical candidates. Some centers base their treatment modality on the CTA or angiographic characteristics of the aneurysm. Despite the variability in criteria for use, hospitals where endovascular techniques are available have been linked to improved outcomes [90, 91].

It is difficult to study treatment modalities for SAH, because it is often hard to separate the complications, morbidity, and mortality of the disease from the treatment. When studying aneurysms, the two most important factors when evaluating treatment modalities are the rebleeding rate and recurrence or recanalization rate. Sluzewski [92] reported a rebleeding rate of 1.4 % in 431 patients who underwent endovascular coil embolization of ruptured cerebral aneurysms. Smaller studies have reported between a 0.9 and 2.9 % annual rate of rehemorrhage after endovascular embolization with increasing aneurysm size being an important factor for rehemorrhage [24]. Degree of aneurysm occlusion is also an important factor in risk of rehemorrhage. Murayama [87] reported on their most recent 665 aneurysms in 558 patients treated by endovascular embolization. In small aneurysms (4–10 mm) with small necks (≤4 mm), incomplete coiling occurred in 25.5 % with recurrence in 1.1 % of completely coiled aneurysms and 21 % of incompletely

coiled aneurysms. In small aneurysms with wide necks (>4 mm), incomplete coiling occurred in 59 %, with recurrence in 7.5 % of completely coiled aneurysms and 29.4 % of incompletely coiled aneurysms. In large aneurysms (11–25 mm), incomplete coiling occurred in 56 %, with recurrence in 30 % of completely coiled aneurysms and 44 % of incompletely coiled aneurysms. Giant aneurysms (>25 mm) had incomplete occlusion in 63 %, with recurrence in 42 % of completely coiled aneurysms and 60 % in incompletely coiled aneurysms. Despite the recurrence rates, most patients with incomplete aneurysm obliteration do not rebleed.

Aneurysm recurrence is not uncommon after endovascular embolization, and recanalization can occur even in completely treated aneurysms. Close follow-up of patients treated by endovascular means with formal cerebral angiography, CTA, or MRA is extremely important, as additional embolization can be performed with low morbidity in an elective environment. Timing for follow-up imaging is not defined and can be variable depending upon whether the aneurysm was found after SAH or incidentally, degree of occlusion, size, and location. Derdeyn [88] followed 466 patients with 501 aneurysms for greater than 1 year after coil embolization of cerebral aneurysms. They found recurrence in 33.6 % of patients that occurred at a mean interval of 12.3 months after the initial procedure. Frequent and long-term follow-up of aneurysms treated by endovascular means are recommended to identify recanalization and treat before SAH occurs. Catheter cerebral angiography is the recommended modality of choice for follow-up imaging in previously coiled or clipped aneurysms. Although a small risk of permanent complications exists with diagnostic angiography, felt to be <0.1 % [24], it allows the most precise view of the aneurysm and neck and at the same time allows for retreatment if needed. Coil and clip artifacts are often a problem with using CTA and MRA for follow-up studies, although these are noninvasive modalities.

No matter what treatment modality is chosen for ruptured cerebral aneurysms, treatment should be done early to prevent rebleeding and to have a secured aneurysm prior to the vasospasm window. Surgical clipping and endovascular coiling are both accepted treatment options for ruptured cerebral aneurysms. Surgical wrapping or coating are not supported by the data and may have similar rehemorrhage rates when compared to conservative management, while placing the patient at risk of the morbidity of a craniotomy after SAH. Patient characteristics, medical comorbidities, aneurysm location and morphology, and surgeon experience should all be taken into account when deciding which modality should be chosen. Currently, it is felt that the rate of incomplete obliteration and recurrence is lower with surgical clipping than with endovascular techniques; however, the morbidity of surgical clipping and the long-term disability rates are higher than endovascular treatment.

Cerebral Vasospasm and SAH

After the aneurysm has been secured by surgical or endovascular means, the risk of rebleeding has generally been removed; however, the treatment goals need to now be focused on the prevention and treatment of cerebral vasospasm, delayed cerebral ischemia (DCI), and delayed ischemic neurologic deficits (DINDs). Cerebral vasospasm is a delayed narrowing of the intracranial arteries from vasoconstriction leading to a decrease in cerebral blood flow, which may lead to delayed cerebral ischemia (DCI) or delayed ischemic neurologic deficits (DINDs) and cerebral infarction. There is a significant amount of variation in the literature about how cerebral vasospasm is identified, reported, and defined. Some authors use vasospasm, DINDs, and DCI synonymously, which makes interpretation of the literature and the ability to compare treatment and prevention modalities very difficult. For the purposes if this chapter, vasospasm is defined as the actual narrowing of intracranial arteries diagnosed by cerebral angiography, CTA, or elevated velocities on transcranial dopplers (TCD), with the fact that there is intra-observer error in interpreting these studies. In the setting of SAH, DCI and DINDs are typically secondary to cerebral vasospasm and the reason they get used interchangeably; however, DCI is a clinical change in neurologic status and may occur with or independently of angiographic evidence of vessel narrowing. The opposite may occur as well where angiographic evidence of cerebral vasospasm occurs in the absence of clinical decline. Delayed cerebral ischemia may be reversible or may progress to DIND or cerebral infarction on CT or MRI. The terms delayed cerebral ischemia (DCI) and delayed ischemic neurologic deficit (DIND) are diagnoses of exclusion after all other causes of neurologic decline have been excluded including, seizures, hydrocephalus, hyponatremia, infection, iatrogenic from clipping or coiling, or other metabolic causes. Delayed cerebral ischemia (DCI) and delayed ischemic neurologic deficits (DINDs) will be defined as a neurologic decline that cannot be explained by other means independently of angiographic or TCD evidence of vasospasm. A third outcome measure commonly used in SAH studies is the presence of cerebral infarction on CT or MRI imaging of the brain. Cerebral infarction is the irreversible loss of blood flow, which was presumptively secondary to cerebral vasospasm in the setting of SAH. There has been a push to use cerebral infarct, also known as "hypodensity on CT scan" in the literature, as an independent outcome measure as it has been associated with death or severe disability at 3 months, and is easily measurable in patients in a comatose state where neurologic decline may be difficult to assess [93].

Cerebral vasospasm accounts for the majority of morbidity and mortality for patients who survive to undergo treatment after aneurysmal SAH. Angiographic vasospasm is observed in 30–70 % of patients after SAH and most commonly occurs between day 5 and 14, peaking around day 7 after the hemorrhage [20, 21]. It is estimated that about 50 % of patients with angiographic vasospasm will develop DCI, and about 15–20 % of these patients will develop DINDs, stroke, or death despite aggressive therapy [22, 23]. Many modalities for the prevention and treatment of cerebral vasospasm, DCI and DINDs have been studied over the years with variable results. This will be an evidence-based synopsis for the diagnosis, management, and prevention of cerebral vasospasm.

Modalities for Identifying Cerebral Vasospasm

Clinical evaluation of patients with symptomatic vasospasm and DINDs are easy to identify because a measurable deficit exists; however, a clinical evaluation may not be sensitive enough to detect DCI as some patients may develop asymptomatic cerebral infarctions on CT or MRI. A prospective study by Schmidt [94] studied 580 patients with aneurysmal and non-aneurysmal SAH, where CT scans were done as needed for clinical reasons. Asymptomatic infarcts were noted on CT scans in 26 (4 %) patients and were noted to be more common in patients in comatose states. After data analysis, those with cerebral infarcts were noted to have worse modified Rankin Scores (mRS) at 3 months, which is consistently reported in the literature. Asymptomatic delayed cerebral infarction was also noted on CT scan in 4 % of patients in a retrospective study of 143 aneurysmal SAH patients by Rabinstein [95]. A prospective study by Shimoda [96] followed 125 patients with aneurysmal SAH with MRIs immediately after securing of the aneurysm, 3 days after SAH, 14 days after SAH, and 30 days after SAH. They reported asymptomatic cerebral infarction rates of 23 %. This may be due to the sensitivity of MRI for small ischemic events and may actually represent a higher rate of cerebral infarction than we know, as most studies use CT as the imaging modality of choice. Clinical exam is accurate for identifying patients with symptomatic vasospasm and DINDs when compared to CT findings; however, asymptomatic cerebral infarctions are still missed, especially in comatose patients where the exam is limited. Further imaging modalities such as TCDs, CTA, or angiography may be more beneficial for comatose patients. Digital subtraction angiography (DSA) remains the gold standard for diagnosis of cerebral vasospasm and for which all other modalities are compared.

Transcranial Doppler (TCD)

Transcranial Doppler (TCD) uses ultrasonography to evaluate the major cerebral blood vessels and monitor trends in flow and velocity to diagnose patients at risk for developing and those in cerebral vasospasm. This technique is extremely dependent upon multiple factors including consistency of the individual performing the exam, experience of the individual performing the exam, vascular anatomy, age, intracranial pressure (ICP), hematocrit, mean arterial blood pressure (MAP), and patient anatomical factors allowing for viewing of the temporal window [97]. Transcranial dopplers have been shown to have a high specificity and positive predictive value (PPV) for diagnosing vasospasm in the middle cerebral arteries (MCA). In a meta-analysis by Lysakowski [98], TCD findings were compared with angiographic findings to report sensitivity and specificity of TCDs for diagnosing vasospasm. Those who were assumed to have vasospasm on TCDs of the MCAs were found to have vasospasm on angiography with a sensitivity of 67 % and specificity of 99 % with a PPV of 97 % and negative predictive value (NPV) of 78 %. However, if vasospasm was not predicted on TCDs, it did not exclude vasospasm diagnosed by angiography. They concluded that TCD of the MCA was not likely to show vasospasm if the angiography was negative (high specificity), and that TCDs may be used to identify patients with vasospasm (high PPV). All other vessels studied did not have sufficient data or evidence to support their use in diagnosing vasospasm. Sloan [97] reported that when studying the MCAs with TCD, certain criteria could reliably predict the presence or absence of angiographic vasospasm. MCA flow velocities of >200 cm/s, a rapid rise in flow velocities, and a higher Lindegaard (vMCA/vICA) ratio (6 ± 0.3) were reliably predictive of angiographic vasospasm. An MCA velocity below 120 cm/s also reliably predicted the absence of angiographic vasospasm. Sviri [99] similarly studied the vertebra-basilar system with TCD and comparing them to follow-up angiography. They found that the velocity ratio between the basilar artery (BA) and the vertebral artery (VA) correlated with angiographic vasospasm in the basilar artery. They reported that BA/VA ratio >2 had a 73 % sensitivity and 80 % specificity for basilar artery vasospasm. A ratio higher than 2.5 with BA velocity greater than 85 cm/s was associated with 86 % sensitivity and 97 % specificity for BA narrowing of more than 25 %. A BA/VA ratio higher than 3.0 with BA velocities higher than 85 cm/s was associated with 92 % sensitivity and 97 % specificity for BA narrowing of more than 50 %; however, the NPV and PPV were not reported. The presence of vasospasm based on TCD or angiographic data does not predict DCI or DINDs.

Computed Tomographic Angiogram (CTA)

The use of CTA for the diagnosis of vasospasm is quick, noninvasive, and easily available. CTA is also useful for the quick diagnosis of postoperative bleeding, rehemorrhage, stroke, hydrocephalus, or retraction edema when evaluating for causes of neurologic decline. Almost all studies comparing CTA to DSA for diagnosis of vasospasm are fairly consistent. CTA seems to underestimate the diameter of large cerebral arteries and overestimate the distal smaller cerebral vessels. Surgical clips or coils can lead to artifact and make it difficult to fully evaluate the vessels. CTA has a high accuracy, sensitivity, and specificity for diagnosing severe vasospasm or no vasospasm in larger proximal arteries but loses accuracy in detecting it in distal, smaller vessels when compared to DSA [100, 101]. CTA tended to overestimate the degree of vasospasm when there was a discrepancy. The use of CTA as a screening tool may significantly limit the number of DSA done to diagnose vasospasm; however, CTA is limited in that it lacks the ability to use intra-arterial methods to treat vasospasm.

Vasospasm Prophylaxis and Management

Triple-H Therapy

Triple-H therapy, also known as hypertension, hypervolemia, and hemodilution, has been used since the 1970s in the prophylactic management and treatment of vasospasm following SAH. The idea behind triple-H therapy is to expand the intravascular volume with crystalloid and colloid to increase leptomeningeal collateral perfusion to areas that have been restricted by vasospasm, and improve inflow to counteract vascular resistance, while at the same time diluting the blood viscosity to improve flow rheology to brain tissue. Prophylactic triple-H therapy is that which is done prior to any evidence of vasospasm or clinical decline, whereas therapeutic triple-H therapy is instituted when vasospasm is suspected. The difficulty in studying the literature is that there is no standardization for triple-H therapy for blood pressure parameters or goal hemoglobin levels. Egge [102] randomized 16 patients to prophylactic triple-H therapy and 16 patients to euvolemic therapy. Triple-H therapy was associated with more complications, higher cost, and had no significant difference in vasospasm rates or improvements in TCD velocities when compared to the euvolemic group. Lennihan [103] randomized 82 patients to receive hypervolemia therapy or euvolemic therapy. Cardiac filling pressures were noted to be higher with hypervolemic therapy, but without any evidence of increased cerebral blood flow and significant difference were seen on GOS at 2 weeks, 6 months, or 1 year between the two groups. Complications have been directly attributable to prophylactic triple-H therapy including pulmonary edema and worsening intracranial edema with hemorrhagic transformation [104, 105]. Prophylactic hemodilution has not shown to add any benefit to outcome or vasospasm risk and has the negative effect of decreasing oxygen carrying capacity and cerebral oxygenation. The overall benefit of prophylactic triple-H therapy is not clear and may pose significant physiologic risks including myocardial infarction, pulmonary edema, cerebral edema, renal failure, and even potential rupture of additional intracranial aneurysms. Prophylactic triple-H therapy is not recommended; however, hypotension should be avoided.

Therapeutic induced hypertension and volume expansion have been shown in small studies to improve neurologic deficits if started after the onset of symptoms. Multiple pressors have been studied and many MAP and SBP goals have been suggested. Systolic blood pressures of 160–200 mmHg are commonly quoted for goals, but patient-specific factors need to be taken into account such as baseline cardiac and pulmonary disease. The limited data support that induced hypertension with pressors and volume expansion may improve neurologic deficits but may be at the risk of pulmonary edema, myocardial infarction, and hyponatremia. No randomized trials exist evaluating benefit and risk of induced hypertension in patients that develop a neurologic deficit felt to be secondary to cerebral vasospasm.

Calcium Channel Blockers

Calcium channel blockers act by inhibiting the flow of calcium into arteriolar smooth muscle, causing vascular dilation, and therefore are felt to reduce vasospasm in the cerebral vasculature. Many calcium channel blockers exist; however, the four that have been the most studied for vasospasm prevention are nimodipine, nicardipine, nitroprusside, and verapamil. Nimodipine is the most well-studied drug for vasospasm prophylaxis. It has been shown to have a significant reduction in the incidence of symptomatic vasospasm for patients that received oral nimodipine compared to placebo [106]. The largest randomized clinical trial for nimodipine [107] showed significant reductions in the incidence of cerebral infarction and poor clinical outcome for patients treated with oral nimodipine. Nicardipine has similar pharmacology to nimodipine. It has been studied and used in many forms including intravenous (IV), intra-arterial (IA), intrathecal (IT), and as prolonged-release implants (NPRI). Two randomized controlled trials showed significantly reduced incidence of symptomatic vasospasm when nicardipine was used compared to placebo [108, 109]. Nitroprusside is a medication that is pharmacologically broken down into nitrous oxide which causes relaxation of vascular smooth muscle leading to vasodilation. It is usually used intrathecally due to its short half-life in the blood. One small prospective non-randomized case-control trial showed improved TCD velocities, but large studies are limited on this medication. Verapamil is another calcium channel blocker which specifically blocks the L-type calcium channel. It has been studied in the intra-arterial form in case series with variable results. Among the calcium channel blockers, nimodipine was shown in more randomized controlled trials to significantly reduce symptomatic vasospasm and improve outcomes. A recent meta-analysis on calcium channel blockers showed an overall reduction in poor outcome compared to placebo, with the oral route of nimodipine having the largest reduction in poor clinical outcome [110].

Magnesium Sulfate

Magnesium sulfate directly acts on and antagonizes voltage-dependent calcium channels, which prevents vascular smooth muscle contraction. It has also been shown to have a neuroprotective benefit which is believed to be from blocking N-methyl-D-aspartate (NMDA) receptors and inhibiting the release of glutamate in tissues. Magnesium sulfate is commonly administered by the intravenous route after SAH. Magnesium has been well studied for the prevention of vasospasm. Randomized controlled trials have shown a statistically significant decrease in symptomatic vasospasm when compared to placebo [111], a trend toward reduced MCA TCD velocities and improved clinical outcome [112], a nonsignificant reduction in DCI and poor clinical outcomes at 3 months [113], and a trend toward improved clinical outcomes at 3 months [114]. A meta-analysis [115] done in 2009 reported a statistically significant reduction in poor outcomes including dependency and vegetative state. Known complications of magnesium sulfate infusion include hypocalcemia and hypotension. The evidence shows a significant improvement in outcome possibly from its neuroprotective benefits and a reduction in symptomatic vasospasm in some studies but in others only shows nonsignificant trends toward improved outcome. The evidence is inconclusive at this time and large randomized controlled trials are currently being done for magnesium in SAH.

Statins

Statins, also known as hydroxymethylglutaryl coenzyme-A reductase inhibitors (HMG-CoA reductase inhibitors) are well-known cholesterol-lowering medications that have been shown to decrease inflammation, inhibit thrombogenesis, and induce nitric oxide synthase. Multiple randomized controlled trials (RCT) have been done showing promising results. A meta-analysis of three RCT showed a statistically significant reduction in vasospasm incidence and mortality [116]. Tseng [117] first reported the results of statin use in SAH in 2005. This RCT studied pravastatin versus placebo, which showed a significant reduction in vasospasm incidence, DINDs, and mortality. A RCT by Lynch [118] produced similar results using simvastatin versus placebo where the treatment group showed a significant reduction in vasospasm. Kramer [119] published the most recent meta-analysis of six randomized clinical trials showing a significant reduction in DINDs and a trend toward decreased mortality in those given a statin after aneurysmal SAH. No notable side effects have been reported with statin use after SAH except for the known small risks of elevated liver enzymes and muscle breakdown with general statin use.

Endothelin Receptor Antagonists

Endothelin is a peptide that acts on vascular smooth muscle causing long-acting and severe vascular constriction.

Clazosentan and bosentan are two different endothelin receptor antagonists (ERA) that have been studied in humans. One of the largest and most recent randomized controlled studies [119] assigned 313 patients to receive dose-escalated clazosentan and compared them to 96 placebo patients. A significant reduction in moderate and severe vasospasm was noted in the clazosentan group when given at the high dose compared to placebo, and there was also a reduction in the development of DIND and DCI. Endothelin receptor antagonists are showing promise in the prevention of vasospasm, and further studies are currently being done.

Other Medical Treatments

Many other medical management options for the treatment and prevention of vasospasm and DINDs have been studied. Most of the following have been studied in smaller studies with variable results. Fasudil is a rho-kinase inhibitor administered by the intravenous route that has been studied in Japan. In one RCT [120], it was shown to have a significant reduction in angiographic and symptomatic vasospasm, low-density areas on CT, and improved 1-month Glasgow outcome scores (GOS) when compared to placebo. In a second RCT [121], it was shown to have a nonsignificant reduction in symptomatic vasospasm when compared to nimodipine.

The use of thrombolytics such as urokinase and tissue plasminogen activator (tPA) have been studied for intrathecal use, with the theory that they will break down subarachnoid blood products and decrease the irritation of the blood vessels and prevent vasospasm. Only 2 RCT have been done. One large randomized controlled trial [122] using urokinase showed a significant reduction in symptomatic vasospasm and improved GOS at 6 months compared to placebo when used intrathecally after aneurysm coiling. The second study [123] used intrathecal tPA after aneurysm clipping and was noted to have a trend toward reduced vasospasm severity but was not significant. The data on thrombolytic use are variable and cannot be recommended for use based on current literature.

Papaverine is a well-known cerebral and coronary vasodilator. Its exerts its mechanism of action by inhibiting cyclic adenosine monophosphate (cAMP) and cyclic guanosine 3,5 (cGMP) phosphodiesterase activity. Papaverine has been delivered by many mechanisms including intracisternal use, as a pellet form left at the time of surgery, and intra-arterially by endovascular means. Prophylactic studies using the pellet delivery system and intracisternal use are small; however, they did show some improvement in neurologic outcome and symptomatic vasospasm. No randomized controlled trials have been done to study papaverine in SAH, but non-randomized case-control studies have been reported. Intra-arterial (IA) papaverine given, not prophylactically, but instead for the treatment of vasospasm has been reported to have both improvement in angiographic vasospasm and

clinical symptoms. Kassel [124] was the first to use IA papaverine as a single agent for vasospasm treatment, with two-thirds of patients showing angiographic improvement and one-third showing clinical improvement.

Many other medical therapies have been studied for the prevention and treatment of vasospasm; however, they are small studies. Some of these include antifibrinolytics, thromboxane synthetase inhibitors, low-molecular-weight heparin, and intravenous erythropoietin.

Endovascular Interventions

Medical management of vasospasm consists generally of a combination of medications to prevent vasospasm, as indicated previously. When vasospasm occurs, however, medical options typically only include triple-H therapy, which is associated with many medical complications including heart failure, pulmonary edema, and myocardial infarction. Endovascular interventions include intra-arterial administration of vasodilators (Fig. 24.2a) or transluminal balloon angioplasty (TBA) (Fig. 24.2b).

Transluminal balloon angioplasty is the act of dilating the intracranial arteries with a small balloon. This technique has been used both prophylactically prior to vasospasm and as a therapeutic modality after vasospasm develops. Angioplasty can be used alone or in combination with IA vasodilators such as papaverine and verapamil. Prophylactic TBA was studied in an RCT [125] where 85 patients with SAH underwent TBA of bilateral A1, M1, P1, basilar, and intradural portion of the dominant vertebral artery within 96 h of hemorrhage. Patients who underwent TBA had a trend toward a reduction in DINDs and also had a significant reduction compared to placebo in those requiring therapeutic angioplasty. The risks of TBA include vessel perforation, hemorrhage, and death and are higher if TBA is performed distally in the vessels. During this study, prophylactic angioplasty of the A1 and P1 segments was discontinued due to complications. Prophylactic balloon angioplasty, despite showing a decrease in the need for therapeutic angioplasty, is not recommended due to the risk of vessel perforation and no significant improvement in overall outcome.

Although TBA is not recommended for prophylaxis of vasospasm, it is successful in the treatment of vasospasm when it does develop. Vessels that are treated successfully have been shown to reduce the incidence of DCI [126, 127]. The timing of endovascular intervention after development of cerebral vasospasm has not been well defined. Two studies have reported the timing of endovascular intervention, analyzing early versus delayed intervention after the onset of cerebral vasospasm. Rosenwasser [128] retrospectively reviewed 84 patients that underwent balloon angioplasty with or without IA papaverine. Fifty-five patients were treated within 2 h of neurologic decline, and 33 patients were treated greater than 2 h after neurologic decline. Patients that

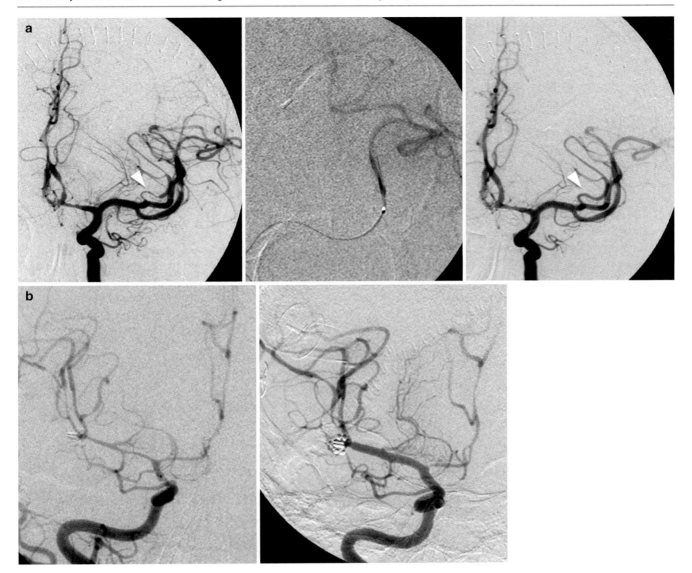

Fig. 24.2 (**a, b**) Cerebral vasospasm. (**a**) Intra-arterial verapamil treatment. *Left panel,* focal vasospasm of M2 branch of the left cerebral artery (*arrowhead*). *Middle panel,* microcatheter injection of verapamil into the affected branch vessel. *Right panel,* immediate improvement in vessel diameter after intra-arterial verapamil treatment (*arrowhead*). (**b**) Transluminal balloon angioplasty. *Left panel,* vasospasm of the right middle cerebral artery after clipping of a ruptured right middle cerebral bifurcation aneurysm. *Right panel,* immediate improvement in vessel diameter after transluminal balloon angioplasty of the right middle cerebral artery

were treated within 2 h had a significantly better neurologic improvement than those that had delayed treatment. Bejjani [129] reported similar findings when they retrospectively studied 21 patients treated within 24 h of neurologic decline and 10 patients treated greater than 24 h after neurologic decline. They reported a more significant improvement in those that underwent early treatment compared to those that had delayed treatment.

The use of intra-arterial agents during endovascular treatment of cerebral vasospasm offers direct delivery of vasodilators to the vessels in vasospasm. Three medications have been well studied for intra-arterial delivery for vasospasm,

papaverine, nicardipine, and verapamil. There have been many case series using IA papaverine showing successful treatment of cerebral vasospasm with both good clinical and angiographic results. Nicardipine in the IA form has been evaluated in retrospective studies to improve angiographic vasospasm and transiently improve neurologic deficits [130]. Verapamil has been shown in retrospective studies to show improvements in arterial diameter without significant side effects [131, 132]. Any agent may be chosen for IA therapy, and dose is limited by systemic hemodynamic response. Further studies need to be done to determine if any agent is more efficacious.

Medical Complications of Subarachnoid Hemorrhage

Medical complications are frequent after SAH and increase the morbidity and mortality; however, they can be managed if recognized early. The Aneurysm Cooperative Study [133] reported the frequency of having at least one life-threatening medical condition after SAH to be 40 %, with a proportion of the deaths from a medical complication to be 23 %. This rate is similar to that quoted to the causes of death from the initial hemorrhage which was 19 %, rehemorrhage which was 22 %, and vasospasm which was 23 %. Pulmonary edema was reported in 23 % of patients, with a 6 % rate of severe pulmonary edema. Renal dysfunction was noted to be 7 % in the whole group, with 15 % of that group that developed severe, life-threatening renal dysfunction. Pulmonary complications were noted to be the most common non-neurologic cause of death. Thrombocytopenia, hepatic dysfunction, and hyponatremia are metabolic disturbances that are also associated with SAH and need to be routinely monitored.

Cardiac and Pulmonary Complications

Cardiac and pulmonary complications have been well documented after aneurysmal SAH. The relationship between SAH and myocardial injury or dysfunction has been hypothesized to be secondary hypothalamic dysfunction or hyperdynamic response to catecholamine release after SAH. Although there has been no specific cause identified, there is clearly an association between the two. It has been shown in clinical studies that there are elevated catecholamine levels early after SAH [134, 135] and that cardiac lesions after SAH when studied pathologically appear very similar to those found in catecholamine-induced myocardial necrosis [136]. It is not felt that cardiac dysfunction is from acute coronary spasm or disease; however, these must be ruled out in patients with cardiovascular risk factors.

Recognizing cardiac and pulmonary complications early better allow the team to maximize medication choices for volume status and induced hypertension if needed. Two of the most commonly studied variables for understanding cardiac dysfunction after SAH are troponin levels and wall motion abnormalities (WMA), also known as regional wall motion abnormalities (RWMA) diagnosed by echocardiography. A large meta-analysis [137] including 2,690 patients from 25 studies, 16/25 studies being prospective, evaluated cardiac complications after SAH and their effect on outcome. Elevation of troponin I was noted in 34 % of patients which was associated with cardiac dysfunction. Poor outcome was associated with elevated troponin levels (RR 2.3) and ST-segment depression (RR 2.4). Factors associated with mortality included wall motion abnormalities (WMA)

(RR 1.9), elevated troponin (RR 2.0) and brain natriuretic peptide (BNP) levels (RR 11.1), tachycardia (RR 3.9), Q waves (RR 2.9), ST-segment depression (RR 2.1), T-wave abnormalities (RR 1.8), and bradycardia (RR 0.6). Occurrence of DCI was associated with WMAs (RR 2.1); elevated troponin (RR 3.2), CK-MB (RR 2.9), and BNP levels (RR 4.5); and ST-segment depression (RR 2.4). There is some variation among these studies of what is considered elevated troponin, which had a range of 0.1–1 ng/ml. Diastolic dysfunction has been reported to occur in 71–89 % [138, 139] of patients after SAH and has been associated with development of pulmonary edema.

Electrocardiogram (ECG) changes are common after SAH and include deep T-wave inversion and QT prolongation. A report by the Cooperative Aneurysm Study [133] reported a frequency of life-threatening cardiac arrhythmias of 5 %, with other cardiac dysrhythmias occurring in about 30 % of patients. Ventricular arrhythmias were more common if troponin I was elevated [140]. No current randomized controlled trials exist evaluating the use of invasive cardiovascular monitoring and its effect on morbidity and mortality after SAH. At this time, the need for invasive cardiovascular monitoring should be evaluated on a patient-by-patient basis. The prophylactic placement of invasive monitoring, excluding arterial lines, is not indicated by the data; however, it may be helpful in preventing cardiopulmonary complications if hyperdynamic or hypertensive therapy is being used. Frequent monitoring of electrolytes and correction of metabolic disturbances such as magnesium and potassium can help prevent arrhythmias.

Wall motion abnormalities (WMA) after SAH are well reported and typically involve left ventricular dysfunction. Kothavale and coworkers [141] prospectively studied 300 patients with aneurysmal SAH with serial echocardiography with a primary outcome of measuring the presence of RWMA. Eight hundred and seventeen echocardiograms were analyzed and RWMA were found in 18 % of patients. Patients with higher admission Hunt-Hess grades had higher rates of RWMA. Patients with Hunt-Hess grades 3–5 had an incidence of 35 %. There was also an association between elevated troponin I and RWMA, where 65 % of patients with troponin I levels greater than 1mcg/L had RWMA. They also reported prior use of cocaine or amphetamine were independent predictors of RWMA. A study by Sugimoto and coworkers [142] studied the prognostic significance of RWMA on outcome. They prospectively enrolled 47 patients after aneurysmal SAH and performed early echocardiography and ECG, within 3 days of SAH. They recorded the incidences of pathologic ECG changes, global hypokinesia defined as a left ventricular ejection fraction (LVEF) <50 %, and RWMA. The incidence of pathologic ECG changes was 62 %, LV ejection fraction <50 % was 11 %, and RWMA was 28 %. Rate-corrected QT interval, LV ejection fraction <50 %, and

RWMA were all significant predictors of death. A specific form of RWMA more commonly being recognized in SAH is what is termed takotsubo cardiomyopathy. This form of cardiomyopathy is defined by left ventricular dysfunction consisting of akinesia of predominantly the apex and mid-ventricle with relative sparing of the basal segment, which gives it a typical appearance on echocardiography. Cardiomyopathy seen in SAH, commonly called neurogenic stress cardiomyopathy (NSC), is defined by hypokinesia of the basal and midventricular portions with relative sparing of the apex. Most cardiomyopathies induced after SAH are believed to be secondary to catecholamine release and not coronary in nature and are felt to be mostly reversible [143]. The original descriptions and studies of takotsubo cardiomyopathy excluded patients with traumatic brain injury and SAH and were not well understood in patients with neurologic diseases. Lee and colleagues [144] reported the largest study of takotsubo cardiomyopathy in SAH patients. They retrospectively reviewed all patients with SAH admitted to the Mayo Clinic Neurological Intensive Care Unit between 1990 and 2005 and found 24 patients that had SAH-induced reversible cardiac dysfunction, and of those, eight met echocardiographic criteria for takotsubo cardiomyopathy. All eight patients were women with a mean age of 55.5. Seven patients presented with Hunt-Hess grade III or IV. Four patients underwent coil embolization and four underwent surgical clipping. The mean initial ejection fraction (EF) was 38 %, and the mean EF at recovery was 55 %. Six of the eight patients developed cerebral vasospasm, but only 3 developed cerebral infarction. Takotsubo cardiomyopathy is a rare form of cardiomyopathy after SAH and is more common in postmenopausal women; is associated with pulmonary edema, prolonged intubation, and vasospasm; but is a reversible form of cardiomyopathy similar to the other neurogenic stress cardiomyopathies.

Pulmonary complications are common after SAH and are the leading non-neurologic cause of morbidity and mortality after aneurysmal SAH. In retrospective trials it is difficult to assess the cause of the pulmonary edema, but it has been documented in the literature to be around 27 %. In one study [145] this was defined by a pulmonary arterial O_2 (PaO_2) to fraction of inspired O_2 (FiO_2) ratio (PaO_2/FiO_2) of <300. A second study [146] used evidence of bilateral pulmonary infiltrates on chest x-ray and found similar incidence of pulmonary edema. Hypervolemia therapy has not shown to have a significant benefit on neurologic outcome and is associated with medical complications including pulmonary edema. Kim and colleagues [147] retrospectively reviewed prospectively collected data on 453 patients after SAH. They were divided into two groups: group 1 were those that were treated with hypervolemic and hypertensive therapy, and group 2 were those that were treated with euvolemic therapy. The rate of pulmonary edema decreased from 14 to 6 % between groups 1 and 2, respectively, and mortality had also decreased from 34 to 29 % between groups 1 and 2, respectively. Patients with pulmonary edema and or cardiac dysfunction may benefit from invasive cardiovascular monitoring to aim for a euvolemic goal to decrease left ventricular dysfunction from volume loading and appropriate balance volume status to improve pulmonary edema.

Anemia and Transfusion

Blood transfusion has always been a controversial topic among physicians treating medical and surgical patients. The risk of blood transfusion includes minor and severe transfusion reactions, and the risk of HIV and hepatitis transmission. Recent data have suggested that patients can tolerate lower hemoglobin levels than we previously thought, and that there may be adverse outcomes associated with blood transfusions. Marik [148] reviewed forty-five studies that reported the independent effect of red blood cell transfusion (RBCT) on patient outcomes. In forty-two of the 45 studies, the risks of RBCT outweighed the benefits, the risk was neutral in two studies, and the benefits outweighed the risks in a subgroup of one study which included elderly patients with acute myocardial infarction and a hematocrit (HCT) less than 30 %. Seventeen of the 18 studies that studied death as a primary outcome showed that BRCT was an independent predictor of death. All twenty-two studies that evaluated the association of RBCT and infection showed that RBCT was an independent predictor of infection. There was also significant association between RBCT and development of multisystem organ failure and acute respiratory distress syndrome (ARDS).

There has also been great debate on what levels of hemoglobin are thresholds for transfusion. The Transfusion Requirements in Critical Care Trial (TRICC) [149] studied two thresholds for transfusion termed "liberal," defined as hemoglobin (Hgb) of 10 g/dl versus "restricted," defined as Hgb of 7 g/dl in 883 ICU patients. The overall 30-day mortality was similar between the two groups, except for those who were younger and less ill where mortality was less in the restrictive RBCT group. Few studies have evaluated RBCT and its effect on patients with brain injury. The best study we have for brain injury patients is a subgroup of the TRICC trial who sustained severe closed traumatic brain injury (TBI) [150]. Twenty-nine patients were randomized to the restrictive (Hgb 7 g/dl) group, and 38 were randomized to the liberal (Hgb 10 g/dl) group. There were no significant differences between the two groups in overall mortality, multisystem organ failure, length of ICU, or length of hospital stay. It is difficult to extrapolate these data to SAH patients who commonly have cardiac dysfunction and may benefit from a liberal Hgb level. The goal in SAH is to maintain normal circulating volume with adequate tissue oxygen delivery. It is a complex relationship between the understanding of adequate tissue oxygenation, volume status, current cardiac and pulmonary dysfunction, and primary medical conditions. Animal studies [151] have shown that a Hgb <10 g/dl is associated with brain hypoxia, and correction with RBCT may improve brain tissue oxygenation, especially in a brain after SAH where normal compensatory cerebrovascular response may be damaged. Preventing hypoxia should be a goal of SAH patient management, as there are limited studies of how RBCT affects patients after SAH. Observational studies show that RBCT can cause medical complications as noted earlier, and there are no consistent data that RBCT improves brain tissue oxygenation. As in many of the RBCT trials, it is often difficult to assess whether RBCT is in fact associated directly with mortality or that those requiring transfusions with persistently low Hgb (7 g/dl) are more critically ill and at baseline have a higher mortality and that transfusion is needed because of that. Anemia is a risk factor for poor outcome after SAH, but it is not clear whether this is an independent risk factor or a measure of the severity of disease. At this time there are no randomized controlled trials or large studies to suggest a threshold hemoglobin level for which SAH patients should be transfused, and each patient should be treated on an individual basis.

Hyponatremia

Hyponatremia is the most common electrolyte abnormality in patients after SAH. It is commonly defined as a serum sodium <135 mmol/l and has been reported to occur in about 30–50 % of aneurysmal SAH patients [152, 153]. Hyponatremia in SAH are often attributed to one of two different mechanisms called cerebral salt wasting (CSW) and syndrome of inappropriate antidiuretic hormone secretion (SIADH). Each of these processes is pathophysiologically different but appears similarly in lab values. Both are associated with low serum sodium and abnormally elevated urine sodium. The mechanism behind CSW is felt to be caused by sympathetic discharge after SAH which stimulates the release of natriuretic peptides causing sodium loss in the urine. This sodium loss causes an osmotic gradient across the tubules, which pulls water with it into the urine, causing an excess of urine output. This excessive urine output causes overall systemic hypovolemic hyponatremia. SIADH is caused by an inappropriate excretion of antidiuretic hormone, causing water reabsorption in the kidney leading to euvolemic or slightly hypervolemic hyponatremia. The ability to measure intravascular volume with central venous lines and strict ins and outs is imperative in diagnosis but also treatment.

Recognition and management of hyponatremia is important because hyponatremia can cause worsening cerebral edema by causing a gradient for water to move into the cerebral space, increasing intracranial pressure and exacerbating neurologic deficits. Hyponatremia by itself is associated with seizures especially at levels <125 mmol/l and in a patient with intracranial pathology places them at increased risk and lowering the threshold for seizures. Hyponatremia has not been associated with worse neurologic outcome.

Treatment strategies aim at raising the sodium slowly, due to the risk of central pontine myelinolysis and aim for normonatremia (135–145 mmol/l). Common treatment options include mineral corticoids and hypertonic saline. Fludrocortisone is a mineralocorticoid often used in the treatment of hyponatremia associated with SAH. Mineralocorticoids act on the renal tubules to form channels that reabsorb sodium from the kidneys, while causing excretion of potassium. Fludrocortisone has the advantage over hydrocortisone of not significantly altering serum glucose levels. There does not appear to be any significant increase in pulmonary edema or congestive heart failure with fludrocortisone use [154]. Hypertonic saline, commonly in the 3 % concentration, is another treatment option for hyponatremia. It can be given as boluses or run as a continuous infusion. Continuous infusions are more commonly given unless seizures occur or acute cerebral edema is present, in which case boluses may be more effective, followed by a continuous infusion to maintain normonatremia. Even though the common treatment for isolated SIADH is volume restriction, in the setting of SAH and vasospasm, this can be dangerous and place the patient at risk for DCI and vasospasm and is not recommended [155]. Sodium should be corrected by the hypertonic saline route, and fludrocortisone may also be used. Only observational studies exist for the use of hypertonic saline and fludrocortisone for hyponatremia in SAH, which both show safety of their use but no definitive dose or duration of treatment can be suggested based on the literature at this time.

Conclusions

Aneurysmal subarachnoid hemorrhage is a multifactorial disease process that requires a treatment team of neurosurgeons and neurointensivists to maximize each patient's outcome. This chapter encompasses the best literature available at the time of publication to manage the intricacies of aneurysmal subarachnoid hemorrhage. There is a vast amount of literature available; however, many uncertainties exist in the literature, and current studies are being done to better optimize our treatment of these patients. At the University of Florida, we have developed treatment practices for the management of aneurysmal SAH patients as outlined in Table 24.5.

Table 24.5 Management practice for aneurysmal SAH patients at the University of Florida

Treatment protocol
Admission to neurosurgical ICU
CT angiogram of head and neck with perfusion
Radial arterial line
Strict systolic BP goals <140 mmHg (until aneurysm secured)
Loaded with fosphenytoin and continued for 3 days unless seizures occur or intraparenchymal hemorrhage
Ventriculostomy placement if hydrocephalus on CT scan or GCS 13 or less
Aminocaproic acid IV infusion for 12–24 h until aneurysm secured[a]
Nimodipine 60 mg PO every 4 h for 14–21 days
Zocor 40 mg PO daily[a]
Magnesium sulfate infusion for 14 days (renally dosed)[a]
Daily transcranial dopplers
Hunt-Hess grades 1–3 undergo coiling or clipping within 24 h
Hunt-Hess grades 4–5 undergo ventriculostomy, if improvement undergoes treatment
Once aneurysm secured, systolic blood pressure range 100–180 mmHg
No prophylactic HHH therapy
If neurologic decline, CT angiogram with perfusion obtained
If vasospasm present on CT angiogram pt taken to angio suite

[a]Optional

References

1. King Jr JT. Epidemiology of aneurysmal subarachnoid hemorrhage. Neuroimaging Clin N Am. 1997;7(4):659–68.
2. Graf CJ, Nibbelink DW. Cooperative study of intracranial aneurysms and subarachnoid hemorrhage: report on a randomized treatment study, 3: intracranial surgery. Stroke. 1974;5:557–601.
3. Inagawa T, Takechi A, Yahara K, et al. Primary intracerebral and aneurysmal subarachnoid hemorrhage in Izumo City, Japan. Part I: incidence and seasonal and diurnal variations. J Neurosurg. 2000;93(6):958–66.
4. Ingall T, Asplund K, Mahonen M, Bonita R. A multinational comparison of subarachnoid hemorrhage epidemiology in the WHO MONICA stroke study. Stroke. 2000;31(5):1054–61.
5. Hop JW, Rinkel GJ, Algra A, van Gijn J. Case-fatality rates and functional outcome after subarachnoid hemorrhage: a systematic review. Stroke. 1997;28(3):660–4.
6. Hijdra A, Braakman R, van Gijn J, Vermeulen M, van Crevel H. Aneurysmal subarachnoid hemorrhage: complications and outcome in a hospital population. Stroke. 1987;18:1061–7.
7. Hop JW, Rinkel GJ, Algra A, van Gijn J. Changes in functional outcome and quality of life in patients and caregivers after aneurysmal subarachnoid hemorrhage. J Neurosurg. 2001;95:957–63.
8. Stegmayr B, Eriksson M, Asplund K. Declining mortality from subarachnoid hemorrhage: changes in incidence and case fatality from 1985 through 2000. Stroke. 2004;35(9):2059–63.
9. Rinkel GJ, Djibuti M, Algra A, van Gijn J. Prevalence and risk of rupture of intracranial aneurysms: a systematic review. Stroke. 1998;29:251–6.
10. van Gijn J, Rinkel GJ. Subarachnoid haemorrhage: diagnosis, causes and management. Brain. 2001;124(pt 2):249–78.
11. Lozano AM, Leblanc R. Cerebral aneurysms and polycystic kidney disease: a critical review. Can J Neurol Sci. 1992;19:222–7.
12. Kato T, Hattori H, Yorifuji T, Tashiro Y, Nakahata T. Intracranial aneurysms in Ehlers-Danlos syndrome type IV in early childhood. Pediatr Neurol. 2001;25:336–9.
13. Wills S, Ronkainen A, van der Voet M, Kuivaniemi H, Helin K, Leinonen E, Frosen J, Niemela M, Jaaskelainen J, Hernesniemi J, Tromp G. Familial intracranial aneurysms: an analysis of 346 multiplex Finnish families. Stroke. 2003;34:1370–4.
14. Qureshi AI, Suri MF, Yahia AM, Suarez JI, Guterman LR, Hopkins LN, Tamargo RJ. Risk factors for subarachnoid hemorrhage. Neurosurgery. 2001;49:607–12.
15. Taylor CL, Yuan Z, Selman WR, Ratcheson RA, Rimm AA. Cerebral arterial aneurysm formation and rupture in 20,767 elderly patients: hypertension and other risk factors. J Neurosurg. 1995;83:812–9.
16. Oyesiku NM, Colohan AR, Barrow DL, Reisner A. Cocaine-induced aneurysmal rupture: an emergent negative factor in the natural history of intracranial aneurysms? Neurosurgery. 1993;32:518–25.
17. Broderick JP, Brott TG, Duldner JE, Tomsick T, Leach A. Initial and recurrent bleeding are the major causes of death following subarachnoid hemorrhage. Stroke. 1994;25:1342–7.
18. Sarti C, Toumilehto J, Salomaa V. Epidemiology of subarachnoid hemorrhage in Finland from 1983-1985. Stroke. 1991;28:848–53.
19. Sahs AL, Nibblelink DW, Torner JC. Aneurysmal subarachnoid hemorrhage: report of the cooperative study. Baltimore-Munich: Urban and Schwarzenberg; 1981. p. 370.
20. Fisher CM, Roberson GH, Ojemann RG. Cerebral vasospasm with ruptured saccular aneurysm – the clinical manifestations. Neurosurgery. 1977;1(3):245–8.
21. Heros RC, Zervas NT, Varsos V. Cerebral vasospasm after subarachnoid hemorrhage: an update. Ann Neurol. 1983;14(6):599–608.
22. Haley Jr EC, Kassell NF, Torner JC. The international cooperative study on the timing of aneurysm surgery. The North American experience. Stroke. 1992;23(2):205–14.
23. Longstreth Jr WT, Nelson LM, Koepsell TD, van Belle G. Clinical course of spontaneous subarachnoid hemorrhage: a population-based study in King County, Washington. Neurology. 1993;43(4):712–8.
24. Bederson JB, Connolly SE, Batjer H, Dacey RG, Dion JE, Diringer MN, Duldner JE, Harbaugh RE, Patel AB, Rosenwasser RH. Guidelines for the management of aneurysmal subarachnoid hemorrhage: a statement for healthcare professionals from a special writing group of the stroke council, American Heart Association. Stroke. 2009;40:994–1025.
25. Kassell NF, Torner JC. Aneurysmal rebleeding: a preliminary report from the cooperative aneurysm study. Neurosurgery. 1983;13:479–81.
26. Kassell NF, Torner JC. The international cooperative study on timing of aneurysm surgery: an update. Stroke. 1984;15:566–70.
27. Ohkuma H, Tsurutani H, Suzuki S. Incidence and significance of early aneurysmal rebleeding before neurosurgical or neurological management. Stroke. 2001;32:1176–80.
28. Laidlaw JD, Siu KH. Poor-grade aneurysmal subarachnoid hemorrhage: outcome after treatment with urgent surgery. Neurosurgery. 2003;53:1275–80.
29. Morgenstern LB, Luna-Gonzales H, Huber Jr JC, Wong SS, Uthman MO, Gurian JH, Castillo PR, Shaw SG, Frankowski RF, Grotta JC. Worst headache and subarachnoid hemorrhage: prospective, modern computed tomography and spinal fluid analysis. Ann Emerg Med. 1998;32(pt 1):297–304.
30. van Gijn J, van Dongen KJ. The time course of aneurysmal haemorrhage on computed tomograms. Neuroradiology. 1982;23:153–6.
31. Edlow JA. Diagnosis of subarachnoid hemorrhage. Neurocrit Care. 2005;2:99–109.

32. Edlow JA. Diagnosis of subarachnoid hemorrhage in the emergency department. Emerg Med Clin North Am. 2003;21:73–87.

33. Shah KH, Edlow JA. Distinguishing traumatic lumbar puncture from true subarachnoid hemorrhage. J Emerg Med. 2002;23:67–74.

34. Horikoshi T, Fukamachi A, Nishi H, Fukasawa I. Detection of intracranial aneurysms by three-dimensional time-of-flight magnetic resonance angiography. Neuroradiology. 1994;36:203–7.

35. Huston 3rd J, Nichols DA, Luetmer PH, Goodwin JT, Meyer FB, Wiebers DO, Weaver AL. Blinded prospective evaluation of sensitivity of MR angiography to known intracranial aneurysms: importance of aneurysm size. AJNR Am J Neuroradiol. 1994;15:1607–14.

36. Hope JK, Wilson JL, Thomson FJ. Three-dimensional CT angiography in the detection and characterization of intracranial berry aneurysms. AJNR Am J Neuroradiol. 1996;17:439–45.

37. Korogi Y, Takahashi M, Katada K, Ogura Y, Hasuo K, Ochi M, Utsunomiya H, Abe T, Imakita S. Intracranial aneurysms: detection with three-dimensional CT angiography with volume rendering: comparison with conventional angiographic and surgical findings. Radiology. 1999;211:497–506.

38. Wilms G, Guffens M, Gryspeerdt S, Bosmans H, Maaly M, Boulanger T, Van Hoe L, Marchal G, Baert A. Spiral CT of intracranial aneurysms: correlation with digital subtraction and magnetic resonance angiography. Neuroradiology. 1996;38 Suppl 1: S20–5.

39. Gilbert JW, Lee C, Young B. Repeat cerebral pan-angiography in subarachnoid hemorrhage of unknown etiology. Surg Neurol. 1990;33:19–21.

40. Canter LM. Anaphylactoid reactions to radiocontrast media. Allergy Asthma Proc. 2005;26:199–203.

41. Caro JJ, Trinidade E, McGregor M. The risk of death and severe nonfatal reactions with high- vs. low-osmolality contrast media: a meta-analysis. AJR Am J Roentgenol. 1990;156:825–32.

42. Bush WH, Swanson DP. Acute reactions to intravascular contrast media: types, risk factors, recognition, and specific treatment. AJR Am J Roentgenol. 1991;157:1153–61.

43. Morcos SK, Thomsen HS. Adverse reactions to iodinated contrast media. Eur Radiol. 2001;11:1267–75.

44. Nayak KR, White AA, Cavendish JJ, Barker CM, Kandzari DE. Anaphylactoid reactions to radiocontrast agents: prevention and treatment in the cardiac catheterization laboratory. J Invasive Cardiol. 2009;21(10):548–51.

45. Hunt WE, Hess RM. Surgical risk as related to time of intervention in the repair of intracranial aneurysms. J Neurosurg. 1968;28:14.

46. Fisher CM, Kistler JP, Davis JM. Relation of cerebral vasospasm to subarachnoid hemorrhage visualized by CT scanning. Neurosurgery. 1980;6:1.

47. Drake CG. Report of World Federation of Neurological Surgeons Committee on a Universal Subarachnoid Hemorrhage Grading Scale. J Neurosurg. 1988;68:985.

48. Wijdicks EF, Vermeulen M, Murray GD, Hijdra A, van Gijn J. The effects of treating hypertension following aneurysmal subarachnoid hemorrhage. Clin Neurol Neurosurg. 1990;92:111–7.

49. Stornelli SA, French JD. Subarachnoid hemorrhage: factors in prognosis and management. J Neurosurg. 1964;21:769–80.

50. Torner JC, Kassell NF, Wallace RB, Adams Jr HP. Preoperative prognostic factors for rebleeding and survival in aneurysm patients receiving antifibrinolytic therapy: report of the Cooperative Aneurysm Study. Neurosurgery. 1981;9:506–13.

51. Kassell NF, Torner JC, Adams Jr HP. Antifibrinolytic therapy in the acute period following aneurysmal subarachnoid hemorrhage: preliminary observations from the cooperative aneurysm study. J Neurosurg. 1984;61:225–30.

52. Hillman J, Fridriksson S, Nilsson O, Yu Z, Saveland H, Jakobsson KE. Immediate administration of tranexamic acid and reduced incidence of early rebleeding after aneurysmal subarachnoid hemorrhage: a prospective randomized study. J Neurosurg. 2002;97(4): 771–8.

53. Starke RM, Kim GH, Fernandez A, Komotar RJ, Hickman ZL, Otten ML, Ducruet AF, Kellner CP, Hahn DK, Chwajol M, Mayer SA, Connolly Jr ES. Impact of a protocol for acute antifibrinolytic therapy on aneurysm rebleeding after subarachnoid hemorrhage. Stroke. 2008;39(9):2617–21.

54. Harrigan MR, Rajneesh KF, Ardelt AA, Fisher 3rd WS. Short-term antifibrinolytic therapy before early aneurysm treatment in subarachnoid hemorrhage: effects on rehemorrhage, cerebral ischemia, and hydrocephalus. Neurosurgery. 2010;67(4):935–9; discussion 939–40.

55. Lin CL, Dumont AS, Lieu AS, Yen CP, Hwang SL, Kwan AL, Kassell NF, Howng SL. Characterization of perioperative seizures and epilepsy following aneurysmal subarachnoid hemorrhage. J Neurosurg. 2003;99(6):978–85.

56. Claassen J, Bateman BT, Willey JZ, Inati S, Hirsch LJ, Mayer SA, Sacco RL, Schumacher HC. Generalized convulsive status epilepticus after nontraumatic subarachnoid hemorrhage: the nationwide inpatient sample. Neurosurgery. 2007;61(1):60–4; discussion 64–5.

57. Chumnanvej S, Dunn IF, Kim DH. Three-day phenytoin prophylaxis is adequate after subarachnoid hemorrhage. Neurosurgery. 2007;60(1):99–102; discussion 102–3.

58. O'Kelly CJ, Kulkarni AV, Austin PC, Urbach D, Wallace MC. Shunt-dependent hydrocephalus after aneurysmal subarachnoid hemorrhage: incidence, predictors, and revision rates. Clinical article. J Neurosurg. 2009;111:1029–35.

59. Little AS, Zabramski J, Peterson M, Goslar PW, Wait SD, Albuquerque FC, McDougall CG, Spetzler RF. Ventriculoperitoneal shunting after aneurysmal subarachnoid hemorrhage: analysis of the indications, complications, and outcome with a focus on patients with borderline ventriculomegaly. Neurosurgery. 2008;62:618–27.

60. de Oliveira JG, Beck J, Setzer M, Gerlach R, Vatter H, Seifert V, Raabe A. Risk of shunt-dependent hydrocephalus after occlusion of ruptured intracranial aneurysms by surgical clipping or endovascular coiling: a single-institution series and meta-analysis. Neurosurgery. 2007;61:924–33.

61. Ransom ER, Mocco J, Komotar RJ, Sahni D, Chang J, Hahn DK, Kim GH, Schmidt JM, Sciacca RR, Mayer SA, Connolly ES. External ventricular drainage response in poor grade aneurysmal subarachnoid hemorrhage: effect on preoperative grading and prognosis. Neurocrit Care. 2007;6:174–80.

62. Rajshekhar V, Harbaugh R. Results of routine ventriculostomy with external ventricular drainage for acute hydrocephalus following subarachnoid haemorrhage. Acta Neurochir (Wien). 1992;115:8–14.

63. Hasan D, Vermeulen M, Wijdicks EF, Hijdra A, van Gijn J. Management problems in acute hydrocephalus after subarachnoid hemorrhage. Stroke. 1989;20:747–53.

64. Paré L, Delfino R, Leblanc R. The relationship of ventricular drainage to aneurysmal rebleeding. J Neurosurg. 1992;76:422–7.

65. Hellingman CA, Van den Bergh WM, Beijer IS, van Dijk GW, Algra A, van Gijn J, Rinkel GJ. Risk of rebleeding after treatment of acute hydrocephalus in patients with aneurysmal subarachnoid hemorrhage. Stroke. 2007;38:96–9.

66. McIver JI, Friedman J, Wijdicks EF, Piepgras DG, Pichelmann MA, Toussaint 3rd LG, McClelland RL, Nichols DA, Atkinson JL. Preoperative ventriculostomy and rebleeding after aneurysmal subarachnoid hemorrhage. J Neurosurg. 2002;97:1042–4.

67. Hoekema D, Schmidt R, Ross I. Lumbar drainage for subarachnoid hemorrhage: technical considerations and safety analysis. Neurocrit Care. 2007;7:3–9.

68. Klimo Jr P, Kestle KJ, MacDonald JD, Schmidt RH. Marked reduction of cerebral vasospasm with lumbar drainage of cerebrospinal

fluid after subarachnoid hemorrhage. J Neurosurg. 2004; 100:215–24.

69. Ochiai H, Yamakawa Y. Continuous lumbar drainage for the pre-operative management of patients with aneurysmal subarachnoid hemorrhage. Neurol Med Chir. 2001;41:576–80.

70. Kwon OY, Kim Y, Kim YJ, Cho CS, Lee SK, Cho MK. The utility and benefits of external lumbar CSF drainage after endovascular coiling on aneurismal subarachnoid hemorrhage. J Korean Neurosurg Soc. 2008;43(6):281–7.

71. Hasan D, Lindsay KW, Vermeulen M. Treatment of acute hydrocephalus after subarachnoid hemorrhage with serial lumbar puncture. Stroke. 1991;22:190–4.

72. Klopfenstein JD, Kim L, Feiz-Erfan I, Hott JS, Goslar P, Zabramski JM, Spetzler RF. Comparison of rapid and gradual weaning from external ventricular drainage in patients with aneurysmal subarachnoid hemorrhage: a prospective randomized trial. J Neurosurg. 2004;100:225–9.

73. Dorai ZHL, Kopitnik TA, Samson D. Factors related to hydrocephalus after aneurysmal subarachnoid hemorrhage. Neurosurgery. 2003;52:763–76.

74. Komotar RJ, Hahn D, Kim GH, Starke RM, Garrett MC, Merkow MB, Otten ML, Sciacca RR, Connolly Jr ES. Efficacy of lamina terminalis fenestration in reducing shunt-dependent hydrocephalus following aneurysmal subarachnoid hemorrhage: a systematic review. Clinical article. J Neurosurg. 2009;111:147–54.

75. Keen WW. Intracranial lesions. Med Newsl. 1890;57:443.

76. Dott NM. Intracranial aneurysms: cerebral arteriography: surgical treatment. Edinburgh Med J. 1933;40:219.

77. Dandy WE. Intracranial aneurysm of internal carotid artery cured by operation. Ann Surg. 1938;107:654.

78. Louw DF, Asfora WT, Sutherland GR. A brief history of aneurysm clips. Neurosurg Focus. 2001;11(2):E4.

79. Sahs AL, Nibbelink DW, Torner JC, editors. Aneurysmal subarachnoid hemorrhage: report of the cooperative study. Baltimore: Urban & Schwarzenberg; 1981.

80. Nishioka H. Results of the treatment of intracranial aneurysms by occlusion of the carotid artery in the neck. J Neurosurg. 1966;25:660–704.

81. Molyneux AJ, Kerr RS, Yu LM, Clarke M, Sneade M, Yarnold JA, Sandercock P, International Subarachnoid Aneurysm Trial (ISAT) Collaborative Group. International Subarachnoid Aneurysm Trial (ISAT) of neurosurgical clipping versus endovascular coiling in 2143 patients with ruptured intracranial aneurysms: a randomised comparison of effects on survival, dependency, seizures, rebleeding, subgroups, and aneurysm occlusion. Lancet. 2005;366:809–17.

82. Sahs AL, Perret GE, Locksley HB, Nishioka H, editors. Intracranial aneurysms and subarachnoid hemorrhage: a cooperative study. Philadelphia: JB Lippincott Co; 1969.

83. Sundt Jr TM, Kobayashi S, Fode NC, Whisnant JP. Results and complications of surgical management of 809 intracranial aneurysms in 722 cases: related and unrelated to grade of patient, type of aneurysm, and timing of surgery. J Neurosurg. 1982;56:753–65.

84. David CA, Vishteh AG, Spetzler RF, Lemole M, Lawton MT, Partovi S. Late angiographic follow-up review of surgically treated aneurysms. J Neurosurg. 1999;91:396–401.

85. Minakawa T, Koike T, Fujii Y, Ishii R, Tanaka R, Arai H. Long term results of ruptured aneurysms treated by coating. Neurosurgery. 1987;21:660–3.

86. Todd NV, Tocher JL, Jones PA, Miller JD. Outcome following aneurysm wrapping: a 10-year follow-up review of clipped and wrapped aneurysms. J Neurosurg. 1989;70:841–6.

87. Murayama Y, Nien YL, Duckwiler G, Gobin YP, Jahan R, Frazee J, Martin N, Vinuela F. Guglielmi detachable coil embolization of cerebral aneurysms: 11 years' experience. J Neurosurg. 2003;98:959–66.

88. Derdeyn CP, Graves VB, Turski PA, Masaryk AM, Strother CM. MR angiography of saccular aneurysms after treatment with Guglielmi detachable coils: preliminary experience. AJNR Am J Neuroradiol. 1997;18:279–86.

89. Guglielmi G, Vinuela F, Dion J, Duckwiler G. Electrothrombosis of saccular aneurysms via endovascular approach, part 2: preliminary clinical experience. J Neurosurg. 1991;75:8–14.

90. Berman MF, Solomon RA, Mayer SA, Johnston SC, Yung PP. Impact of hospital-related factors on outcome after treatment of cerebral aneurysms. Stroke. 2003;34:2200–7.

91. Cross 3rd DT, Tirschwell DL, Clark MA, Tuden D, Derdeyn CP, Moran CJ, Dacey Jr RG. Mortality rates after subarachnoid hemorrhage: variations according to hospital case volume in 18 states. J Neurosurg. 2003;99:810–7.

92. Sluzewski M, van Rooij WJ. Early rebleeding after coiling of ruptured cerebral aneurysms: incidence, morbidity, and risk factors. AJNR Am J Neuroradiol. 2005;26:1739–43.

93. Frontera JA, Fernandez A, Schmidt JM, Claassen J, Wartenberg KE, Badjatia N, Connolly ES, Mayer SA. Defining vasospasm after subarachnoid hemorrhage: what is the most clinically relevant definition? Stroke. 2009;40:1963–8.

94. Schmidt JM, Wartenberg KE, Fernandez A, Claassen J, Rincon F, Ostapkovich ND, Badjatia N, Parra A, Connolly ES, Mayer SA. Frequency and clinical impact of asymptomatic cerebral infarction due to vasospasm after subarachnoid hemorrhage. J Neurosurg. 2008;109(6):1052–9.

95. Rabinstein AA, Weigand S, Atkinson JL, Wijdicks EF. Patterns of cerebral infarction in aneurysmal subarachnoid hemorrhage. Stroke. 2005;36(5):992–7.

96. Shimoda M, Takeuchi M, Tominaga J, Oda S, Kumasaka A, Tsugane R. Asymptomatic versus symptomatic infarcts from vasospasm in patients with subarachnoid hemorrhage: serial magnetic resonance imaging. Neurosurgery. 2001;49(6):1341–8; discussion 1348–50.

97. Sloan MA, Alexandrov AV, Tegeler CH, Spencer MP, Caplan LR, Feldmann E, Wechsler LR, Newell DW, Gomez CR, Babikian VL, Lefkowitz D, Goldman RS, Armon C, Hsu CY, Goodin DS. Assessment: transcranial Doppler ultrasonography: report of the therapeutics and technology assessment subcommittee of the American academy of neurology. Neurology. 2004;62(9):1468–81.

98. Lysakowski C, Walder B, Costanza MC, Tramèr MR. Transcranial Doppler versus angiography in patients with vasospasm due to a ruptured cerebral aneurysm: a systematic review. Stroke. 2001;32(10):2292–8.

99. Sviri GE, Ghodke B, Britz GW, Douville CM, Haynor DR, Mesiwala AH, Lam AM, Newell DW. Transcranial Doppler grading criteria for basilar artery vasospasm. Neurosurgery. 2006;59(2):360–6; discussion 360–6.

100. Anderson GB, Ashforth R, Steinke DE, Findlay JM. CT angiography for the detection of cerebral vasospasm in patients with acute subarachnoid hemorrhage. AJNR Am J Neuroradiol. 2000;21(6):1011–5.

101. Chaudhary SR, Ko N, Dillon WP, Yu MB, Liu S, Criqui GI, Higashida RT, Smith WS, Wintermark M. Prospective evaluation of multidetector-row CT angiography for the diagnosis of vasospasm following subarachnoid hemorrhage: a comparison with digital subtraction angiography. Cerebrovasc Dis. 2008;25(1–2):144–50. Epub 2007 Dec 11.

102. Egge A, Waterloo K, Sjoholm H, Solberg T, Ingebrigtsen T, Romner B. Prophylactic hyperdynamic postoperative fluid therapy after aneurysmal subarachnoid hemorrhage: a clinical, prospective, randomized, controlled study. Neurosurgery. 2001;49(3):593–605; discussion 605–6.

103. Lennihan L, Mayer SA, Fink ME, et al. Effect of hypervolemic therapy on cerebral blood flow after subarachnoid hemorrhage: a randomized controlled trial. Stroke. 2000;31(2):383–91.

104. Medlock MD, Dulebohn SC, Elwood PW. Prophylactic hypervolemia without calcium channel blockers in early aneurysm surgery. Neurosurgery. 1992;30(1):12–6.

105. Shimoda M, Oda S, Tsugane R, Sato O. Intracranial complications of hypervolemic therapy in patients with a delayed ischemic deficit attributed to vasospasm. J Neurosurg. 1993;78(3):423–9.

106. Allen GS, Ahn HS, Preziosi TJ, et al. Cerebral arterial spasm – a controlled trial of nimodipine in patients with subarachnoid hemorrhage. N Engl J Med. 1983;308(11):619–24.

107. Pickard JD, Murray GD, Illingworth R, et al. Effect of oral nimodipine on cerebral infarction and outcome after subarachnoid haemorrhage: British aneurysm nimodipine trial. BMJ. 1989;298(6674):636–42.

108. Barth M, Capelle HH, Weidauer S, et al. Effect of nicardipine prolonged-release implants on cerebral vasospasm and clinical outcome after severe aneurysmal subarachnoid hemorrhage: a prospective, randomized, double-blind phase IIa study. Stroke. 2007;38(2):330–6.

109. Haley Jr EC, Kassell NF, Torner JC. A randomized controlled trial of high-dose intravenous nicardipine in aneurysmal subarachnoid hemorrhage. A report of the cooperative aneurysm study. J Neurosurg. 1993;78(4):537–47.

110. Dorhout Mees SM, Rinkel GJ, Feigin VL, et al. Calcium antagonists for aneurysmal subarachnoid haemorrhage. Cochrane Database Syst Rev. 2007;(3):CD000277.

111. Wong GK, Chan MT, Boet R, Poon WS, Gin T. Intravenous magnesium sulfate after aneurysmal subarachnoid hemorrhage: a prospective randomized pilot study. J Neurosurg Anesthesiol. 2006;18(2):142–8.

112. Veyna RS, Seyfried D, Burke DG, et al. Magnesium sulfate therapy after aneurysmal subarachnoid hemorrhage. J Neurosurg. 2002;96(3):510–4.

113. van den Bergh WM, Algra A, van Kooten F, et al. Magnesium sulfate in aneurysmal subarachnoid hemorrhage: a randomized controlled trial. Stroke. 2005;36(5):1011–5.

114. Muroi C, Terzic A, Fortunati M, Yonekawa Y, Keller E. Magnesium sulfate in the management of patients with aneurysmal subarachnoid hemorrhage: a randomized, placebo-controlled, dose-adapted trial. Surg Neurol. 2008;69(1):33–9; discussion 39.

115. Zhao XD, Zhou YT, Zhang X, Zhuang Z, Shi JX. A meta analysis of treating subarachnoid hemorrhage with magnesium sulfate. J Clin Neurosci. 2009;16(11):1394–7.

116. Sillberg VA, Wells GA, Perry JJ. Do statins improve outcomes and reduce the incidence of vasospasm after aneurysmal subarachnoid hemorrhage: a meta-analysis. Stroke. 2008;39(9):2622–6.

117. Tseng MY, Czosnyka M, Richards H, Pickard JD, Kirkpatrick PJ. Effects of acute treatment with pravastatin on cerebral vasospasm, autoregulation, and delayed ischemic deficits after aneurysmal subarachnoid hemorrhage: a phase II randomized placebo-controlled trial. Stroke. 2005;36(8):1627–32.

118. Lynch JR, Wang H, McGirt MJ, et al. Simvastatin reduces vasospasm after aneurysmal subarachnoid hemorrhage: results of a pilot randomized clinical trial. Stroke. 2005;36(9):2024–6.

119. Macdonald RL, Kassell NF, Mayer S, et al. Clazosentan to overcome neurological ischemia and infarction occurring after subarachnoid hemorrhage (CONSCIOUS-1): randomized, double-blind, placebo-controlled phase 2 dose-finding trial. Stroke. 2008;39(11):3015–21.

120. Shibuya M, Suzuki Y, Sugita K, et al. Effect of AT877 on cerebral vasospasm after aneurysmal subarachnoid hemorrhage. Results of a prospective placebo-controlled double-blind trial. J Neurosurg. 1992;76(4):5.

121. Zhao J, Zhou D, Guo J, et al. Effect of fasudil hydrochloride, a protein kinase inhibitor, on cerebral vasospasm and delayed cerebral ischemic symptoms after aneurysmal subarachnoid hemorrhage. Neurol Med Chir (Tokyo). 2006;46(9):421–8.

122. Hamada J, Kai Y, Morioka M, et al. Effect on cerebral vasospasm of coil embolization followed by microcatheter intrathecal urokinase infusion into the cisterna magna: a prospective randomized study. Stroke. 2003;34(11):2549–54.

123. Findlay JM, Kassell NF, Weir BK, et al. A randomized trial of intraoperative, intracisternal tissue plasminogen activator for the prevention of vasospasm. Neurosurgery. 1995;37(1):168–76; discussion 177–8.

124. Kassell NF, Helm G, Simmons N, Phillips CD, Cail WS. Treatment of cerebral vasospasm with intra-arterial papaverine. J Neurosurg. 1992;77(6):848–52.

125. Zwienenberg-Lee M, Hartman J, Rudisill N, et al. Effect of prophylactic transluminal balloon angioplasty on cerebral vasospasm and outcome in patients with Fisher grade III subarachnoid hemorrhage: results of a phase II multicenter, randomized, clinical trial. Stroke. 2008;39(6):1759–65.

126. Jestaedt L, Pham M, Bartsch AJ, et al. The impact of balloon angioplasty on the evolution of vasospasm-related infarction after aneurysmal subarachnoid hemorrhage. Neurosurgery. 2008; 62(3):610–7; discussion 610–7.

127. Muizelaar JP, Zwienenberg M, Mini NA, Hecht ST. Safety and efficacy of transluminal balloon angioplasty in the prevention of vasospasm in patients with Fisher Grade 3 subarachnoid hemorrhage: a pilot study. Neurosurg Focus. 1998;5(4):5.

128. Rosenwasser RH, Armonda RA, Thomas JE, Benitez RP, Gannon PM, Harrop J. Therapeutic modalities for the management of cerebral vasospasm: timing of endovascular options. Neurosurgery. 1999;44:975–9; discussion 979–80.

129. Bejjani GK, Bank WO, Olan WJ, Sekhar LN. The efficacy and safety of angioplasty for cerebral vasospasm after subarachnoid hemorrhage. Neurosurgery. 1998;42:979–86; discussion 986–7.

130. Linfante I, Delgado-Mederos R, Andreone V, Gounis M, Hendricks L, Wakhloo AK. Angiographic and hemodynamic effect of high concentration of intra-arterial nicardipine in cerebral vasospasm. Neurosurgery. 2008;63:1080–6; discussion 1086–7.

131. Feng L, Fitzsimmons BF, Young WL, Berman MF, Lin E, Aagaard BD, Duong H, Pile-Spellman J. Intraarterially administered verapamil as adjunct therapy for cerebral vasospasm: safety and 2-year experience. AJNR Am J Neuroradiol. 2002;23:1284–90.

132. Keuskamp J, Murali R, Chao KH. High-dose intraarterial verapamil in the treatment of cerebral vasospasm after aneurysmal subarachnoid hemorrhage. J Neurosurg. 2008;108:458–63.

133. Solenski NJ, Haley Jr EC, Kassell NF, Kongable G, Germanson T, Truskowski L, Torner JC. Medical complications of aneurysmal subarachnoid hemorrhage: a report of the multicenter, cooperative aneurysm study. Participants of the multicenter cooperative aneurysm study. Crit Care Med. 1995;23:1007–17.

134. Naredi S, Lambert G, Eden E, Zall S, Runnerstam M, Rydenhag B, Friberg P. Increased sympathetic nervous activity in patients with nontraumatic subarachnoid hemorrhage. Stroke. 2000;31:901–6.

135. Kawahara E, Ikeda S, Miyahara Y, Kohno S. Role of autonomic nervous dysfunction in electrocardio-graphic abnormalities and cardiac injury in patients with acute subarachnoid hemorrhage. Circ J. 2003;67:753–6.

136. Todd GL, Baroldi G, Pieper GM, Clayton FC, Eliot RS. Experimental catecholamine-induced myocardial necrosis. II. Temporal development of isoproterenol-induced contraction band lesions correlated with ECG, hemodynamic and biochemical changes. J Mol Cell Cardiol. 1985;17:647–56.

137. van der Bilt IA, Hasan D, Vandertop WP, Wilde AA, Algra A, Visser FC, Rinkel GJ. Impact of cardiac complications on outcome after aneurysmal subarachnoid hemorrhage: a meta-analysis. Neurology. 2009;72:635–42.

138. Tung PP, Olmsted E, Kopelnik A, Banki NM, Drew BJ, Ko N, Lawton MT, Smith W, Foster E, Young WL, Zaroff JG. Plasma B-type natriuretic peptide levels are associated with early cardiac

dysfunction after subarachnoid hemorrhage. Stroke. 2005;36: 1567–9.

139. Kopelnik A, Fisher L, Miss JC, Banki N, Tung P, Lawton MT, Ko N, Smith WS, Drew B, Foster E, Zaroff J. Prevalence and implications of diastolic dysfunction after subarachnoid hemorrhage. Neurocrit Care. 2005;3:132–8.

140. Frangiskakis JM, Hravnak M, Crago EA, Tanabe M, Kip KE, Gorcsan 3rd J, Horowitz MB, Kassam AB, London B. Ventricular arrhythmia risk after subarachnoid hemorrhage. Neurocrit Care. 2009;10:287–94.

141. Kothavale A, Banki NM, Kopelnik A, Yarlagadda S, Lawton MT, Ko N, Smith WS, Drew B, Foster E, Zaroff JG. Predictors of left ventricular regional wall motion abnormalities after subarachnoid hemorrhage. Neurocrit Care. 2006;4:199–205.

142. Sugimoto K, Watanabe E, Yamada A, Iwase M, Sano H, Hishida H, Ozaki Y. Prognostic implications of left ventricular wall motion abnormalities associated with subarachnoid hemorrhage. Int Heart J. 2008;49:75–85.

143. Bagga S, Sharma YP, Jain M. Cardiac dysfunction after acute subarachnoid hemorrhage: neurogenic stress cardiomyopathy or takotsubo cardiomyopathy. Neurol India. 2011;59(2): 304–6.

144. Lee VH, Connolly HM, Fulgham JR, Manno EM, Brown RD, Wijdicks EF. Tako-tsubo cardiomyopathy in aneurysmal subarachnoid hemorrhage: an underappreciated ventricular dysfunction. J Neurosurg. 2006;105:264–70.

145. Kahn JM, Caldwell EC, Deem S, Newell DW, Heckbert SR, Rubenfeld GD. Acute lung injury in patients with subarachnoid hemorrhage: incidence, risk factors, and outcome. Crit Care Med. 2006;34:196–202.

146. Kramer AH, Bleck TP, Dumont AS, Kassell NF, Olson C, Nathan B. Implications of early versus late bilateral pulmonary infiltrates in patients with aneurysmal subarachnoid hemorrhage. Neurocrit Care. 2009;10:20–7.

147. Kim DH, Haney CL, Van Ginhoven G. Reduction of pulmonary edema after SAH with a pulmonary artery catheter-guided hemodynamic management protocol. Neurocrit Care. 2005;3:11–5.

148. Marik PE, Corwin HL. Efficacy of red blood cell transfusion in the critically ill: a systematic review of the literature. Crit Care Med. 2008;36(9):2667–74.

149. Hebert PC, Wells G, Blajchman MA, Marshall J, Martin C, Pagliarello G, Tweeddale M, Schweitzer I, Yetisir E. A multicenter, randomized, controlled clinical trial of transfusion requirements in critical care. Transfusion requirements in Critical Care Investigators, Canadian Critical Care Trials Group. N Engl J Med. 1999;340(6):409–17. Erratum in: N Engl J Med 1999;340(13):1056.

150. McIntyre LA, Fergusson DA, Hutchison JS, Pagliarello G, Marshall JC, Yetisir E, Hare GM, Hébert PC. Effect of a liberal versus restrictive transfusion strategy on mortality in patients with moderate to severe head injury. Neurocrit Care. 2006;5(1):4–9.

151. Dexter F, Hindman BJ. Effect of haemoglobin concentration on brain oxygenation in focal stroke: a mathematical modelling study. Br J Anaesth. 1997;79:346–51.

152. Qureshi AI, Suri MF, Sung GY, Straw RN, Yahia AM, Saad M, Guterman LR, Hopkins LN. Prognostic significance of hypernatremia and hyponatremia among patients with aneurysmal subarachnoid hemorrhage. Neurosurgery. 2002;50(4):749–55.

153. Audibert G, Steinmann G, de Talancé N, Laurens MH, Dao P, Baumann A, Longrois D, Mertes PM. Endocrine response after severe subarachnoid hemorrhage related to sodium and blood volume regulation. Anesth Analg. 2009;108(6):1922–8.

154. Mori T, Katayama Y, Kawamata T, Hirayama T. Improved efficiency of hypervolemic therapy with inhibition of natriuresis by fludrocortisone in patients with aneurysmal subarachnoid hemorrhage. J Neurosurg. 1999;91(6):947–52.

155. Wijdicks EF, Vermeulen M, Hijdra A, van Gijn J. Hyponatremia and cerebral infarction in patients with ruptured intracranial aneurysms: is fluid restriction harmful? Ann Neurol. 1985;17(2):137–40.

Intracerebral Hemorrhage: Evidence-Based Medicine, Diagnosis, Treatment, and Complications

25

Chad W. Washington, Ahmed N. Hassan, and Gregory J. Zipfel

Contents

C.W. Washington, MS, MPHS, MD
Department of Neurological Surgery,
Washington University in St. Louis,
660 S Euclid, 8057, St. Louis, MO 63110, USA
e-mail: washingtonc@wudosis.wustl.edu

A.N. Hassan, MD
Department of Neurology/Neurocritical Care,
Washington University School of Medicine,
660 S. Euclid Ave, 8111, St. Louis, MI 63110, USA
e-mail: hassana@wustl.edu

G.J. Zipfel, MD (✉)
Department of Neurosurgery,
Barnes-Jewish Hospital, 660 S. Euclid,
8057, St. Louis, MO 63110, USA
e-mail: zipfelg@wustl.edu

Abstract

The treatment of primary intracranial hemorrhage (ICH) is one of the most difficult problems facing neurologists, neurosurgeons, and neurointensivists today, and with an incidence of 10–30 cases per 100,000, it represents a major medical problem. In spite of marked advances in medical technology, the outcomes for patients suffering from a spontaneous ICH remain bleak with mortality rates reaching 62 % within the first year of onset. The difficulty in treating these patients has resulted in substantial research efforts into establishing an appropriate management scheme for ICH.

The purpose of this chapter is to consolidate this information and provide the clinician with evidence-based, up-to-date treatment guidelines for primary ICH. The reader will be led through a discussion of the most current epidemiologic data, use of diagnostic imaging, medical management, and role of surgical intervention. While a significant number of questions exist regarding treatment strategies, following each section is a synopsis of the current literature with treatment recommendations.

Keywords

Primary intracranial hemorrhage • Hemorrhagic stroke • Hypertension • Cerebral amyloid angiopathy • Cerebellar hemorrhage • STICH

Introduction

Intracerebral hemorrhage (ICH) is the end result of a number of pathophysiologic processes where blood is extravasated into the brain parenchyma [1]. These processes are divided

Table 25.1 Causes of spontaneous intracranial hemorrhage

Primary	Hypertension
	Cerebral amyloid angiopathy
Secondary	Aneurysm
	Vascular malformations
	Vasculitis
	Venous thrombosis
	Neoplasm
	Antithrombotics (i.e., warfarin, antiplatelet medication)
	Coagulopathy
	Drugs

into either primary or secondary ICH (Table 25.1). Primary ICH refers to hemorrhage resulting from hypertension or cerebral amyloid angiopathy (CAA) [1]. The focus here will be the diagnosis and management of primary ICH. While many of the principles presented can be applied to the treatment of secondary ICH, we direct the reader to the chapters regarding aneurysmal subarachnoid hemorrhage (Chap. 24), vascular malformations (Chap. 26), and CNS neoplasia (Chap. 34) for details specific to these pathologies.

The treatment of ICH is one of the most difficult problems facing neurologists, neurosurgeons, and neurointensivists today. In spite of marked advances in medical technology, the outcomes for patients suffering from a spontaneous ICH remain bleak with mortality rates reaching 62 % within the first year of onset [2]. The difficulty in treating these patients has resulted in substantial research efforts into establishing an appropriate management scheme for ICH. The purpose of this chapter is to consolidate this information and provide the clinician with evidence-based, up-to-date treatment guidelines for ICH.

Epidemiology

Worldwide, stroke is a major medical problem affecting over 15 million people each year [3] and accounting for 5.5 million deaths annually [1]. In the United States, it is the third leading cause of death [4], and fiscal costs related to stroke are thought to be in excess of $50 billion annually [1].

Incidence

Nontraumatic ICH makes up 10–15 % of reported strokes, with primary ICH making up 78–88 % of these cases [2, 3, 5]. The incidence of ICH varies greatly with regard to the population being studied. There are a number of factors attributable to an increase incidence in ICH (i.e., age, race, genetic predisposition, and hypertension), but in general rates are considered to be in the range of 10–30 cases per 100,000 [6–9]. Interestingly, in spite of significant efforts from the medical community to address known risk factors for ICH, the incidence has not appreciably decreased over the past 30 years [10].

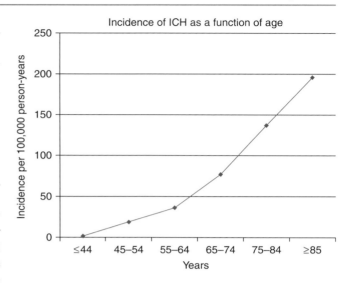

Fig. 25.1 Increasing incidence of ICH is highly correlated with increasing age (Graph extrapolated from data by van Asch et al. [10])

Risk Factors

While the overall incidence of ICH has remained stable over years, many studies show that a number of factors greatly increase an individual's chance of suffering an ICH [2]. Nonmodifiable risk factors include age, ethnicity, genetic factors, and cerebral amyloid angiopathy; major modifiable risk factors include hypertension and excessive alcohol consumption [11].

Age

Perhaps the single most important risk factor related to an increase rate of ICH is advancing age [6, 9, 10]. Sacco and colleagues found the incidence ranged from 1.8 per 100,000 in 0-to-44-year-olds compared to 308.8 per 100,000 in patients over 85 years of age [9]. Similar results were noted by van Asch and colleagues in their meta-analysis demonstrating an exponential progression in ICH incidence related to age (Fig. 25.1) [10]. They found for patients 0–44 years of age, the incidence was 1.9 compared to 196.0 per 100,000 in patients over 85 years of age. Ariesen and colleagues calculated a relative risk with each 10-year increase in age of 1.97 (95 % CI, 1.79–2.16) [11].

Race/Ethnicity

There is a disparate representation of stroke in African-Americans, who are affected at a rate of almost 2–1 compared to Caucasians [7, 8, 12, 13]. The reported incidence for this high-risk population varies from 37 to 50 per 100,000 [7, 8, 12–14]. Much of this burden is carried by middle-aged

(35–54 years old) African-Americans, with relative risks for hemorrhage as high as 9.8 when compared to an aged matched Caucasian population [7]. The etiology of this increased risk has not been fully defined; however, hypertension is likely to play a role, as this condition is an established strong risk factor for ICH and is overrepresented in the African-American community [7]. Underlying genetic factors may also play a role.

Japanese heritage is another patient population that has an increased predilection for ICH [15–17]. Their incidence of ICH is 43–50 per 100,000, which is comparable to the African-American community [15–17].

Hypertension

Hypertension is the single most important modifiable risk factor and the most common cause of primary ICH [18]. Approximately 50 % of ICHs are due to hypertension, and 15 % of patients with chronic hypertension die from ICH [18]. The presence of hypertension leads to a marked increase in ICH risk with an odds ratio (OR) ranging from 2.5 to 5.5 [19–21]. A component of this risk is attributable to the degree of hypertension, as Stage 1 vs. Stage 3 hypertension is associated with relative risks of 1.6 and 7.3, respectively [13]. Importantly, normalization of hypertension with treatment substantially lowers this increased risk of ICH; however, even previously hypertensive patients carry some hemorrhagic risk (OR of 1.4 vs. normotensive patients) [20]. Finally, hypertension has a well-established specificity for ICH type, with the OR for a nonlobar ICH being 4.2 as compared to 1.0 for lobar ICH [21].

The pathophysiology of hypertension-related ICH stems largely from the deleterious effects of persistent elevated blood pressure on penetrating arteries and arterioles [18, 22]. This chronic exposure to elevated pressure causes a progressive hyalinosis and sclerosis of these arteries, resulting in weakening of the vessel walls [22] and in some patients formation of Charcot-Bouchard microaneurysms [18]. The combination of high blood pressure, weakened vessel walls, development of microaneurysms, and low resistance of brain parenchyma leads to a scenario vulnerable to rupture [22].

Cerebral Amyloid Angiopathy

Cerebral amyloid angiopathy (CAA) has been implicated in a number of neurological conditions, especially lobar ICH [23]. It is responsible for 5–10 % of all primary ICHs [23] and is the primary cause of recurrent lobar hemorrhages [24]. CAA is characterized by deposition of amyloid-β peptide (Aβ) into the wall and adventitia of capillaries, arterioles, and small arteries of the cerebral cortex [6]. Advancing age is the strongest risk factor for its development [23], with

approximately 30 % of persons over the age of 60 and more than 50 % of persons over the age of 90 being affected [25, 26]. CAA is also commonly seen in patients with Alzheimer's disease, with at least 80 % of such patients having histologic evidence of CAA [6]. Aβ deposition into cerebral vessels causes severe vascular dysfunction, smooth muscle cell loss, vessel wall weakening, and in many patients blood extravasation into the brain parenchyma [6].

Genetics are also a risk factor for CAA and CAA-related ICH. Specifically, certain apolipoprotein E (APOE) polymorphisms have been linked to the presence and severity of CAA and the incidence of CAA-related ICH. Specifically, carriers of the ε2 and ε4 alleles of APOE have been shown to be at increased risk of lobar ICH, having an OR of 2.30 compared to carriers of the more common ε3 allele [21]. The mechanisms underlying this increased risk, however, differ, as the ε4 allele has been primarily associated with an increased risk of CAA formation [27, 28], while the ε2 allele has been primarily linked to heightened vessel wall fragility [29, 30].

Antithrombotic Medications

ICH related to the use of antithrombotic medications (i.e., warfarin, aspirin, clopidogrel, etc.) is not considered a primary ICH; however, it is a special entity that deserves discussion as ~10 % of patients are receiving warfarin, and ~25 % are receiving aspirin at the time of hemorrhage [31]. Hart and coworkers reviewed the incidences of ICH in elderly patients taking aspirin, aspirin + clopidogrel, warfarin, or warfarin + aspirin. In the patients taking no antithrombotic medications, they noted an ICH incidence of 0.15 % per year. In contrast, patients taking aspirin had a rate of 0.2–0.3 % per year, patients taking aspirin + clopidogrel had a rate of 0.3–0.4 % per year, patients taking warfarin only had a rate of 0.3–1.0 % per year, and patients taking warfarin + aspirin had a rate of 0.5–1.0 % per year [31]. Importantly, the risk related to warfarin therapy is directly related to the degree of anticoagulation, with patients having an INR >4.0 having the greatest risk [31].

Clinical Presentation

Patients presenting with primary ICH have varied neurological symptoms based primarily on the size and location of the hemorrhage. One of the most common symptoms is headache, which occurs in 34–58 % of ICH patients [2, 6]. This symptom is particularly common in patients with hemorrhages occurring in the cerebellum [6]. Seizures are a less frequent symptom, occurring in 10–11 % of ICH patients [6]. This symptom is more common in lobar hemorrhages and generally reflects extension of the ICH into the cerebral cortex. In patients having a large ICH resulting in elevated

Table 25.2 Appearance of ICH on CT and MRI

Stage	CT	T1	T2	T2*
Hyperacute (<12 h)	Hyperdense	Isointense	Hyperintense	Hypointense
Acute (12–48 h)	Hyperdense	Isointense	Hypointense	Hypointense
Early subacute (2–7 days)	Hyperdense	Hyperintense	Hypointense	Hypointense
Late subacute (8–30 days)	Isodense	Hyperintense	Hyperintense	Hypointense
Chronic (>30 days)	Hypodense	Hypointense	Hypointense	Hypointense

intracranial pressure, decreased level of consciousness is very common [2]. This symptom is likely secondary to pressure on the thalamic and brainstem reticular activating systems [32].

Focal neurological deficits are related to the specific location of the ICH, which is typically divided into deep cerebral, lobar, brainstem, and cerebellum. Deep cerebral is the most common location of primary ICH, with incidences ranging from 36 to 69 % [7]. These patients typically present with a combination of symptoms including hemiparesis, hemisensory deficit, gaze paresis, and/or decreased level of consciousness [2, 6]. Lobar is the second most common location of primary ICH, with incidences ranging from 15 to 52 % [7]. These patients present with neurological deficits related to the specific lobe involved and its laterality. Patients with a frontal ICH often present with headache, limb hemiparesis, and gaze deviation [2, 6, 32]. Patients with a dominant temporal ICH usually present with aphasia and/or hemianopsia [2, 6, 32]. Patients with an occipital ICH show evidence of a homonymous visual field deficit [2, 6, 32]. Brainstem and cerebellum are less common locations of primary ICH, with incidences of 4–9 and 7–11 %, respectively [7]. Patients with a brainstem or cerebellar ICH usually present with a combination of neurological deficits including cranial nerve deficits, dysarthria, ataxia, and/or decreased level of consciousness [2, 6, 32].

Morbidity and Mortality

ICH is a devastating and potentially deadly event in the life of a patient. The mortality rate can be as high a 62 % at 1 year [2]. Sacco and coworkers [9] in a prospective analysis of a large cohort of patients with ICH reported 7-day, 30-day, and 1-year mortality rates of 35, 50, and 59 %, respectively. These rates were dependent upon a number of factors including patient age, hemorrhage location, and comorbid conditions [9]. They also reported a 24 % survival rate at 10 years. Other factors associated with prognosis include Glasgow Coma Scale at presentation, ICH volume, and presence of intraventricular hemorrhage [33]. One factor associated with improved mortality rates after ICH is the treatment in a specialized neurologic/neurosurgical intensive care unit [34].

In survivors, ICH is associated with substantial morbidity. For example, in the International Surgical Trial in Intracerebral Haemorrhage (STICH), only 27 % of patients randomized to conservative therapy had favorable functional outcomes in long-term follow-up [35]. In the meta-analysis by van Asch and coworkers [10], only 12–39 % of ICH patients were living independently at last follow-up.

Imaging Diagnostics

One of the hallmark principles in the diagnosis and management of patients with the acute onset of a neurological deficit is neuroimaging [33, 36]. It allows practitioners to rapidly identify patients with ICH vs. subarachnoid hemorrhage vs. ischemic stroke and also permits identification of underlying structural causes of the ICH when they exist. Neuroimaging results are therefore paramount in the initial work-up for all patients suspected of having an ICH.

ICH can be divided into five temporal stages (Table 25.2): hyperacute (<12 h), acute (12–48 h), early subacute (2–7 days), late subacute (8 days to 1 month), and chronic (>1 month) [37, 38]. *Hyperacute hemorrhage* is a liquid composed of oxygenated hemoglobin. As the hemorrhage matures, it converts to a clot form consisting of blood cells, platelets, and serum. Over the course *of acute and early subacute phases* the oxygenated hemoglobin becomes gradually deoxygenated and is eventually converted to methemoglobin. The *late subacute phase* is identified as lysis of red blood cells that releases methemoglobin into the surrounding tissue. The *chronic phase* is the result of macrophages and glial cells migrating into the region of hemorrhage. Methemoglobin is phagocytized and converted into hemosiderin and ferritin [37, 38]. Since these phases are related to the actual physical components of the hemorrhage, there is a correlation to changes found on neuroimaging.

Computed Tomography (CT)

Non-contrast CT is considered the gold standard (sensitivity approaching 100 %) for the detection of intracranial hemorrhage [6, 36]. Because of characteristics such as speed, availability, and relatively low cost, it is often recommended as the first-line imaging study [6, 33, 36].

CT findings in patients with ICH are determined by the density of the hemorrhage that directly affects the attenuation of X-rays [37, 38]. Hence, as a hemorrhage transitions

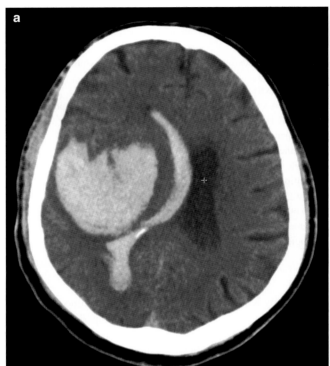 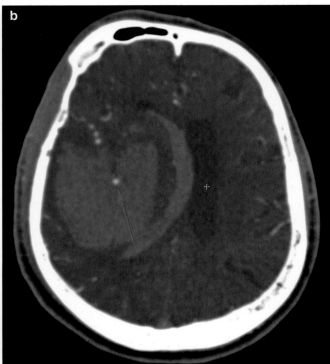

Fig. 25.2 (**a**) Non-contrasted HCT demonstrating a large basal ganglia ICH with intraventricular extension. Size and ventricular involvement are both independent predictors of worsening outcome. (**b**) The "spot sign" (*arrow*), a 1–2 mm focus of enhancement within the hemorrhage volume found on CTA, is associated with hemorrhage enlargement. Abbreviations: *HCT* head computed tomography, *ICH* intracranial hemorrhage, *CTA* computed tomographic angiography

from acute to chronic the relative density compared to brain parenchyma changes from hyperdense to hypodense [37, 38] (Table 25.2). Therefore, CT is able to give an immediate estimate regarding the age of the ICH.

Another important finding assessed by CT is ICH volume, which is a strong predictor of morbidity and mortality in ICH patients. Broderick and colleagues [39] reported that patients with ICH volumes greater than 60 cm³ had a 30 day mortality of 91 % as compared to patients with ICH volumes less than 30 cm³ who had a 30 day mortality of 19 %. A similar association between ICH volume and patient morbidity was found. A clinically useful method for rapidly calculating ICH volume is defined in the following equation: ICH volume $= (A \times B \times C)/2$; where A is the largest cross sectional diameter of the ICH, B is the diameter perpendicular to A, and C equals the number of CT slices showing hemorrhage multiplied by the slice thickness [40, 41].

A factor also found to be related to poor outcomes, which is readily assessed by CT, is hematoma growth. Davis and colleagues [42] in a pooled meta-analysis found that for each 10 % increase in ICH volume the hazard ratio for death increased by 5 %. A similar finding was noted for patient morbidity, as each 10 % increase in ICH volume was associated with a 16 % increase in modified Rankin scale.

Computed Tomographic Angiography (CTA)

Computed tomographic angiography (CTA) is a contrasted CT in which image acquisition is timed to correspond to the late arterial/late venous phase of cerebral perfusion [6, 43]. Similar to non-contrast CT, CTA is rapid, accessible, and relatively inexpensive when compared to magnetic resonance imaging and digital subtraction angiography [6]. CTA provides an assessment of the cerebral vasculature useful in detecting underlying etiologies of ICH such as aneurysms and arteriovenous malformations [6]. A number of studies have shown CTA to be 93–98 % sensitive in detecting cerebral aneurysms [44, 45].

CTA can also be useful in identifying ICH patients that are at high risk for hematoma expansion [43, 46]. Wada and colleagues [43] defined the "spot sign," a finding on CTA which is a 1–2 mm focus of enhancement within the hematoma volume (Fig. 25.2a, b). In their prospective evaluation of 39 patients with spontaneous ICH, they found 33 % demonstrated this so-called spot sign on CTA. This finding was significantly associated with a high likelihood of hematoma progression. Beyond hematoma expansion, the presence of a spot sign has been shown to be an independent predictor of in-hospital mortality (OR of 2.5; 95 % CI 1.3–4.7) and poor outcome (modified Rankin score ≥4) (OR of 2.4; 95 % CI 1.1–4.9) [47].

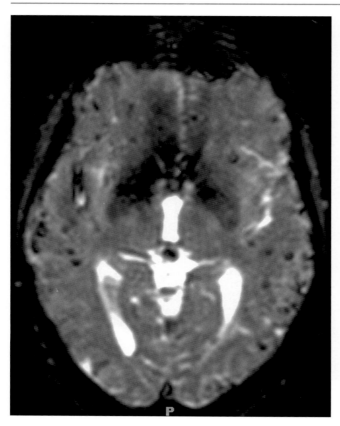

Fig. 25.3 The T2* sequence from the magnetic resonance imaging of a patient with histopathologically proven CAA. Note the multiple areas of hypo-intensity within the bilateral frontal and temporal lobes, which represent multi-focal microhemorrhages

Magnetic Resonance Imaging (MRI)

MRI is considered the most sensitive imaging modality in detecting ICH [37]. In a prospective evaluation of 200 patients comparing CT to MRI, Kidwell and coworkers [48] found these imaging modalities to be equivalent in detecting acute hemorrhage, but that MRI was significantly more sensitive in detecting chronic hemorrhage. In addition to its increased sensitivity for later phases of ICH, MRI provides greater detail as compared to CT in regard to the age of ICH [38]. Specifically, the signal detected by MRI is based on the paramagnetic characteristics of the tissue, the magnetic field strength, and pulse sequence used [6, 37, 38], and therefore, pulse sequence, such as T1, T2, and T2*, and FLAIR all provide unique information about the age of the identified ICH (see Table 25.2 for more details).

An additional MRI finding of particular interest in patients with primary ICH is cerebral microhemorrhage. This finding is defined as a hyperintensity that is most prominent on T2* and gradient-echo MRI sequences (Fig. 25.3) [6]. They have been histopathologically associated with hemosiderin deposition and evidence of angiopathy-related microhemorrhage [49]. This association between primary ICH and microhemorrhages

Table 25.3 Boston criteria for diagnosis of CAA ICH

Definitive CAA: (requires postmortem examination)
Lobar ICH
Histopathologically proven severe, diffuse CAA with vasculopathy
No other ICH etiology
Probable CAA with supporting pathology: (requires pathologic specimen)
Lobar ICH
Histopathologically proven CAA in specimen
No other ICH etiology
Probable CAA:
Multiple lobar ICHs
Age ≥55 years
No other ICH etiology
Possible CAA:
Single lobar ICH
Age ≥55 years

was used by Knudsen and coworkers [50] to define the Boston criteria (Table 25.3). The method was developed to assist clinicians in diagnosing CAA in patients without the necessity of histopathology. For verification, they prospectively followed 39 patients with primary ICH with age ≥55. Of these 13 were categorized as "probable CAA" based on the presence of multiple microhemorrhages on CT and/or MRI. All 13 (100 %) patients were found to have histopathologically proven CAA on biopsy. From the remaining 26 patients with possible CAA, 16 (62 %) were pathologically diagnosed with CAA [50]. These results suggest that CAA may be diagnosed with a degree of certainty based on the combination of clinical details and imaging characteristics.

Digital Subtraction Angiography (DSA)

DSA is considered the gold standard for evaluating the cerebral vasculature [51]. Zhu and coworkers [51] in a prospective evaluation of 206 patients with spontaneous ICH attempted to identify factors indicating which patients should undergo DSA in their work-up for ICH etiology. They found that in young patients (age <45 years) without history of hypertension, the DSA yield was 48 % in basal ganglia and cerebellar ICH and 65 % in lobar ICH. From this they recommend that all patients with spontaneous ICH should be considered for DSA except hypertensive patients who are over 45 years of age and have a prototypic hypertensive ICH on neuroimaging (i.e., ICH based in the basal ganglia, cerebellum, or brainstem).

In attempts to minimize the unnecessary use of DSA, comparisons to CTA and MRI/MRA have been made. In a prospective direct comparison of CTA vs. the gold standard DSA in 109 ICH patients, Wong and coworkers found that CTA had a sensitivity, specificity, positive predictive value, and negative predictive value of 100, 99, 97, and 100 %,

Table 25.4 Issues to address during management of intracerebral hemorrhage

Hematoma expansion/rebleed
Cerebral perfusion/blood pressure
Cerebral edema
Seizures
Indications for surgical intervention

Table 25.5 Stabilizing coagulation status after intracerebral hemorrhage

Discontinue all antiplatelet and anticoagulant medications
Reverse anticoagulation or correct coagulopathy:
Vitamin K 10 mg IV or enterally daily for 3 days
Fresh frozen plasma 15–20 ml/kg
Platelet and coagulation factor replacement as needed for thrombocytopenia and coagulation factor deficiency, respectively
Consider prothrombin complex concentrate or recombinant factor VIIa for coagulopathic patients needing an urgent surgical procedure or those at risk for volume overload
Follow coagulation panel frequently, keep corrected for 24–48 h

respectively. They concluded that CTA compares favorably to DSA in the work-up of ICH patients suspected of having an underlying vascular etiology. In a separate study comparing the utility of MRI/MRA vs. the gold standard DSA in 151 ICH patients, this same group found that MRI/MRA had a sensitivity, specificity, positive predictive value, and negative predictive value of 98, 100, 98, and 100 %, respectively. However, MRI/MRA was found to be more sensitive in detecting angiographically occult lesions such as cavernous malformations, microhemorrhages, and neoplasms. They concluded that MRI/MRA may be a more appropriate screening tool for ICH patients suspected of having an underlying structural etiology.

Recommendations

Initial evaluation of patients with acute neurological deficits should include neuroimaging either via CT or MRI. If an MRI is obtained, blood-sensitive sequences such as T2*, gradient echo, or susceptibility weighted imaging should be included [33, 36]. In cases where the clinical and imaging characteristics are not consistent with a prototypical hypertensive ICH, further analysis with CTA, MRI/MRA, and/or DSA is indicated [33, 36]. CTA is especially useful in identifying patients who are at an increased risk for hemorrhage progression [36]. MRI/MRA is the technique of choice for identifying angiographically occult lesions. DSA is the gold standard for identifying and characterizing underlying vascular etiologies.

Medical Management

Patients with ICH are at high risk for early deterioration and should initially be cared for in an intensive care setting [34, 52] (Table 25.4).

Prevention of Hematoma Expansion and Rebleeding

Even in the absence of coagulopathy, ICH is prone to expand and/or recur, usually in the first 12–24 h. All anticoagulants and antiplatelet agents should be stopped. Normal coagulation should be restored with vitamin K and fresh frozen plasma

[53–55] (Table 25.5). Patients with a severe coagulation factor deficiency or severe thrombocytopenia should receive appropriate factor replacement or platelets. Recombinant factor VIIa or prothrombin complex concentrate may be considered to reverse anticoagulation in those at risk of volume overload or lung injury, but they have not been shown to improve outcomes compared with fresh frozen plasma and may carry a greater risk of thromboembolic events [56, 57].

Maintaining Cerebral Perfusion: Blood Pressure Management

High blood pressure (BP) was thought to contribute to rebleeding; however, there is no convincing evidence that lowering BP improves outcome [58–60]. A higher BP may be necessary to provide adequate blood flow to the brain while ICP is elevated, particularly in chronically hypertensive patients with impaired autoregulation [61]; aggressive BP management may cause hypoperfusion. Even in normotensive patients, ICH may lead to transient hypertension resolving spontaneously over a few days. A modest (~15 %) reduction in BP does not seem to worsen neurological outcome [60]. However, ongoing damage to other organs (heart or kidneys) is a compelling indication to treat elevated BP. If mean arterial pressure is above 130–140 mmHg or end-organ damage is present, short-acting agents are used to gently lower BP. Nitrates are avoided due to the risk of cerebral vasodilatation with worsening edema. Addressing pain may also help control elevated BP (Fig. 25.4).

Treatment of Cerebral Edema

Cerebral edema in ICH can occur as a result of the direct effects of hematoma volume and edema, as well as hydrocephalus due to intraventricular hemorrhage (IVH) or ventricular compression. In patients with a decreased level of consciousness (GCS ≤8), clinical evidence of cerebral herniation, or those with significant IVH or hydrocephalus, ICP monitoring with a ventricular or parenchymal catheter should be considered [62].

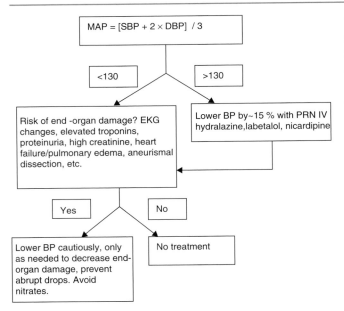

EVD external ventricular drain *ICP* intracranial pressure

Fig. 25.4 Blood pressure management algorithm after intracerebral hemorrhage

Seizures

The primary neuronal damage and blood products increase seizure risk after ICH. Seizures occur in 5–15 % of these patients, usually in the first few days of hospitalization [63]. Prophylactic anticonvulsant therapy is not indicated in ICH [64, 65], but in patients with depressed mental status out of proportion to the degree of brain injury, continuous electroencephalography (EEG) should be considered. Patients with clinical seizures and patients with mental status changes and electrographic seizures should be treated with anticonvulsant therapy.

General Care

Patients with ICH, like all critically ill patients, are at risk for numerous complications including myocardial infarctions, heart failure with pulmonary edema, deep vein thrombosis (DVT), aspiration pneumonia, urinary tract infections, pressure ulcers, and orthopedic complications (contractures, etc.). Sequential compression devices in addition to elastic stockings should be used from admission, and subcutaneous low-molecular-weight heparin or unfractionated heparin for DVT prophylaxis can be started after 48 h if there is no evidence of hematoma expansion [66–68]. Spontaneous lobar ICH in particular carries a relatively high risk of recurrence; thus, avoidance of long-term anticoagulation for nonvalvular atrial fibrillation in these patients is recommended [52]. In the presence of a clear indication for anticoagulation (e.g., mechanical heart

valve) or antiplatelet therapy (e.g., coronary artery stents), it is reasonable to restart anticoagulation in nonlobar ICH in 2–4 weeks and antiplatelet therapy in all ICH 1–2 weeks after documentation of cessation of bleeding.

Surgical Management

With mortality rates for ICH patients being as high as 62 % [3], there has been tremendous effort toward determining whether surgical intervention in this patient population improves outcome. Herein, we present a brief review of the clinical trials that have addressed this question and provide the reader with the most current recommendations provided by the American Heart Association Stroke Council [36] and the European Stroke Initiative [33].

Supratentorial Hemorrhage

One of the first attempts in identifying the role of surgery in primary supratentorial ICH was provided by McKissock and colleagues [69] in their randomized controlled trial comparing surgical intervention via open craniotomy to conservative management in 180 patients with spontaneous ICH. They found no benefit of surgery in regard to mortality or morbidity. They did find increasing age and decreased level of consciousness on admission to be strong predictors of mortality. Of note, ICH diagnosis in this study was based on DSA, as this study was completed in the pre-CT era.

In 1989, Auer and colleagues [70] published their results from a randomized clinical trial evaluating endoscopic surgery (rather than open craniotomy) vs. medical treatment in 100 patients with primary supratentorial ICH. They found that those treated with this minimally invasive surgery had a significant improvement in survival and functional outcome. At 1 week, the mortality was 14 % in the surgical group vs. 28 % in the medical group. At 6 months, the difference in mortality between surgery and medical groups was even greater (42 % vs. 70 %, respectively). They also found that the improved outcome was limited to patients who were less than 60 years of age, who had ICH volumes less than 50 cm³, and who had admission neurologic status of alert or somnolent (vs. comatose). They also found that the improvement related to surgical intervention was only significant in patients with subcortical ICH, while patients with basal ganglia ICH had no apparent benefit related to surgical intervention.

The encouraging findings for surgery in the Auer and colleagues study were soon followed by the discouraging findings of Juvela and colleagues [71] who found no benefit of surgery via open craniotomy in a prospective randomized trial of 52 patients with primary supratentorial ICH. They reported a mortality rate of 46 % for surgery vs. 38 % for conservative therapy. They did find that the length of survival was improved with surgery in the semicomatose or stuporous patients, but found no overall improvement in quality of life. Similar results were reported by Batjer and colleagues [72] in their small prospective randomized trial comparing best medical management vs. best medical management with intracranial pressure monitoring vs. surgery via open craniotomy for patients with primary supratentorial ICH.

In an attempt to build on the favorable results reported by Auer and colleagues [70] who utilized a minimally invasive approach for ICH evacuation, several groups have examined other minimally invasive surgical approaches. Teernstra and colleagues [73] evaluated the utility of stereotactic aspiration + urokinase infusion as a means for treating primary supratentorial ICH. In their randomized clinical trial of 70 patients, they found that surgery resulted in a decrease in ICH volume, but that this hematoma reduction was not associated with a significant improvement in patient outcome. In contrast, Hosseini and coworkers [74] randomized 37 primary supratentorial ICH patients to surgical management via stereotactic aspiration without urokinase infusion vs. conservative therapy and found that surgery led to a significant improvement in mortality (15 % vs. 53 %) and morbidity (Karnofsky's score of 51 vs. 25). Hattori and colleagues [75] also evaluated the potential of minimally invasive surgery for hematoma evacuation. In their trial, 242 patients with primary supratentorial ICH were randomized to stereotactic aspiration without urokinase infusion vs. medical therapy. They reported a nonsignificant trend toward decreased mortality and morbidity in surgical patients.

In an effort to definitively answer the question whether surgical intervention carries clinical benefit in patients with primary supratentorial ICH, Mendelow and colleagues organized STICH – a multicentered randomized controlled trial examining surgical intervention (primarily open craniotomy) vs. best medical therapy [35]. Over an 8-year period, 1,033 patients were randomized to either early surgery vs. initial conservative treatment. They reported unfavorable outcomes in 74 % of surgical patients vs. 76 % of conservatively managed patients. In subgroup analysis, however, an 8 % absolute benefit for surgery in patients with ICH within 1 cm of the cortical surface was found. They also noted that surgery was harmful in patients presenting with Glasgow Coma Scale ≤8, where the relative risk for a poor outcome was raised by 8 %. The main conclusion from this very large, well-conducted randomized controlled trial was that surgery provides no definitive benefit for primary ICH; however, a suggestion that surgical intervention may be beneficial in patients with ICH within <1 cm of the cortical surface was noted.

Recently, Prasad and colleagues [76] published a meta-analysis of ten randomized controlled trials that met pre-defined inclusion and exclusion criteria and addressed the question of surgery vs. medical therapy for patients with supratentorial primary ICH. A total of 2,059 patients were included in their analysis. Their results indicated that surgery provided an overall benefit to this patient population, as the risk of death or dependence was significantly lower in the surgical vs. medical patients (OR of 0.71; 95 % CI 0.58–0.88). Specifically, surgery provided a 26 % relative reduction in being dead and 29 % reduction in being dead or dependent as compared to medical therapy. They also found a suggestion (though this did not reach statistical significance) that minimally invasive surgery (stereotactic or endoscopic techniques) produced better outcomes when compared to open craniotomy (OR of 0.66 vs. 0.82, respectively). Importantly, the authors acknowledged that the benefit of surgery was not consistent across all studies, and, therefore, results from their analysis were not considered robust.

Cerebellar Hemorrhage

There are no randomized controlled trials assessing treatment of spontaneous cerebellar hemorrhage [6]. A number of investigators, however, have proposed a variety of management schemes for patients with cerebellar hemorrhage, primarily based on retrospective data analyses [77–81]. Da Pian and coworkers [77] retrospectively evaluated 205 posterior fossa hemorrhages and found a 38 % mortality in patients with cerebellar hemorrhage, which was primarily determined by hemorrhage size and level of patient consciousness at presentation. They suggested that surgery should be limited to patients with fourth ventricular involvement and hydrocephalus. Koziarski and coworkers [80] retrospectively reviewed 11 cases of cerebellar hemorrhage and found that when hematomas were large (>3 cm), surgical intervention was required. Similar findings were noted by Kobayashi and colleagues [79] who retrospectively reviewed 101 consecutive patients with cerebellar ICH. They proposed a treatment strategy where surgery was performed for patients with hemorrhage size ≥4 cm and/or Glasgow Coma Scale ≤13. In patients who presented in moribund condition, no intensive therapy was recommended. Kirollos and colleagues [78] proposed a management scheme based on a grading scale for fourth ventricular compression along with Glasgow Coma Scale and prospectively applied this protocol to a consecutive series of 50 patients with cerebellar hemorrhage. Three grades of fourth ventricular compression were defined: Grade I, normal size and location; Grade II, partially compressed and shifted; and Grade III, completely obliterated. They recommended the following: expectant management for Grade I and II patients with a Glasgow Come Scale ≥13; CSF diversion for Grade I and II patients with hydrocephalus and a Glasgow Coma Scale <13; surgery for Grade II patients without hydrocephalus and a Glasgow Coma Scale <13; and surgery for all Grade III patients. With this scheme, good outcome (Glasgow Outcome Scale ≥4 at 3 months) for Grade

I, II, and III patients was 100, 58, and 17 %, respectively. Overall mortality was 40 % at 3 months. Interestingly, 60 % of Grade I and II patients had hematomas ≥3 cm and did not require surgical evacuation.

Intraventricular Hemorrhage and Hydrocephalus

Intraventricular hemorrhage (IVH) is a frequent occurrence in spontaneous ICH patients, occurring in approximately 19–45 % of cases [82–84]; and its presence in ICH patients has great impact on patient outcome. Mortality in ICH patients without IVH is 8.5–28.6 % in ICH patients, while mortality in ICH patients with IVH is 29–79 % [82]. Not only is the presence of IVH associated with worse patient outcome, but a dosage effect in which increasing volumes of intraventricular blood are associated with progressively worse patient outcome has also been noted [85]. In addition, the presence of hydrocephalus in ICH patients has been identified as independent risk factor for mortality [86].

The standard treatment for IVH with associated hydrocephalus is placement of an external ventricular drain (EVD); however, whether this treatment leads to improved patient outcomes has not been proven. In a retrospective study of 40 IVH patients with hydrocephalus, Coplin and colleagues [87] noted that the mean initial intracranial pressure was only 16 mmHg and only 15 % of patients had an initial pressure >20 mmHg. Similarly, Ziai and colleagues [88] prospectively followed 11 IVH patients with hydrocephalus who were treated with an EVD and found that only one had increased intracranial pressure. In retrospective studies by Diringer and colleagues [86] and Adams and colleagues [89], placement of an EVD in IVH patients with hydrocephalus was not found to improve overall patient mortality, despite controlling intracranial pressure (<20 mmHg) in 91 % of patients.

In addition to EVD placement, other therapies for IVH have been considered. Use of intraventricular thrombolytics, for example, has been examined as a means for improving patient outcome [83]. The first report presenting a human case where tissue plasminogen activator was injected into the ventricle of a patient with IVH was presented by Findlay and coworkers [90]. They reported a marked decrease in IVH volume and resultant reduction in intracranial pressure. Since this report, a number of small case series have been published suggesting that intraventricular thrombolysis may be a viable treatment strategy [91–93]. There has been one reported prospective, randomized, double-blinded, controlled trial by Naff and colleagues [94]. In their pilot study they presented the results of 12 patients (7 treatment, 5 placebo) who underwent ventriculostomy for IVH and infusion with urokinase vs. placebo. In serial imaging, they found the half-life of the blood products based on imaging was

4.69 days for the urokinase group vs. 8.48 days in the placebo group. The preliminary results from an ongoing study CLEAR-IVH were presented by Morgan and coworkers [84]. For patients receiving intraventricular recombinant tissue plasminogen activator, they found the adverse event profile to be satisfactory for continuation of the study.

In an effort to consolidate the data regarding the treatment of IVH, there have been a number of reviews [91–93]. Nieuwkamp and coworkers [92] in their meta-analysis of 18 publications found the mortality rates for conservative management, EVD, and EVD plus thrombolysis were 78, 58, and 6 % respectively. For these groups the poor outcome rates were 90, 89, and 34 %. From this they felt that EVD plus thrombolysis is a reasonable management strategy but acknowledged that future randomized studies must be initiated. A similar review was attempted by LaPointe and Haines [91]. However, they felt that secondary to flaws in study design and biased control groups, the data were anecdotal and no definitive conclusion could be drawn. Most recently, a review by Staykov and coworkers [93] found mortality rates related to conservative management, EVD, and EVD plus thrombolysis were 71, 53, and 16 %. They also found rates of poor outcomes to be 86, 70, and 45 %. From their findings, they feel that the data supporting the use of EVD plus thrombolysis are increasing, and this will likely be the treatment of choice for a select population of patients with IVH.

Recommendations

The usefulness of surgical intervention for ICH is unclear. It is reasonable to consider hematoma evacuation for those with superficial lobar clots (<1 cm from the cortical surface) and >30 ml in size [33, 36]. Cerebellar hemorrhage showing signs of brainstem compression, hydrocephalus, and/or clinical deterioration should undergo rapid surgical evacuation [36]. Treatment with EVD only is not recommended [36].

Treatment of hydrocephalus with EVD and/or lumbar drain (for nonobstructive hydrocephalus) are considered reasonable [33, 36]. Patients who have a Glasgow Coma Scale of ≤8 and show evidence of herniation may be considered for intracranial pressure monitoring or EVD in setting of hydrocephalus. The use of intraventricular thrombolysis can be considered; however, at this time its use and effectiveness is still considered investigational [33, 36].

References

1. Adams HP. Principles of cerebrovascular disease. New York: McGraw-Hill Medical; 2007.
2. Qureshi AI, Tuhrim S, Broderick JP, Batjer HH, Hondo H, Hanley DF. Spontaneous intracerebral hemorrhage. N Engl J Med. 2001; 344:1450–60.

3. Qureshi AI, Mendelow AD, Hanley DF. Intracerebral haemorrhage. Lancet. 2009;373:1632–44.

4. Lloyd-Jones D, Adams R, Carnethon M, De Simone G, Ferguson TB, Flegal K, et al. Heart disease and stroke statistics – 2009 update: a report from the American Heart Association Statistics Committee and Stroke Statistics Subcommittee. Circulation. 2009;119: 480–6.

5. Fewel ME, Thompson Jr BG, Hoff JT. Spontaneous intracerebral hemorrhage: a review. Neurosurg Focus. 2003;15:E1.

6. Carhuapoma JR, Mayer SA, Hanley DF. Intracerebral hemorrhage. New York: Cambridge University Press; 2010.

7. Flaherty ML, Woo D, Haverbusch M, Sekar P, Khoury J, Sauerbeck L, et al. Racial variations in location and risk of intracerebral hemorrhage. Stroke. 2005;36:934–7.

8. Kleindorfer D, Broderick J, Khoury J, Flaherty M, Woo D, Alwell K, et al. The unchanging incidence and case-fatality of stroke in the 1990s: a population-based study. Stroke. 2006;37:2473–8.

9. Sacco S, Marini C, Toni D, Olivieri L, Carolei A. Incidence and 10-year survival of intracerebral hemorrhage in a population-based registry. Stroke. 2009;40:394–9.

10. van Asch CJ, Luitse MJ, Rinkel GJ, van der Tweel I, Algra A, Klijn CJ. Incidence, case fatality, and functional outcome of intracerebral haemorrhage over time, according to age, sex, and ethnic origin: a systematic review and meta-analysis. Lancet Neurol. 2010;9: 167–76.

11. Ariesen MJ, Claus SP, Rinkel GJ, Algra A. Risk factors for intracerebral hemorrhage in the general population: a systematic review. Stroke. 2003;34:2060–5.

12. Kissela B, Schneider A, Kleindorfer D, Khoury J, Miller R, Alwell K, et al. Stroke in a biracial population: the excess burden of stroke among blacks. Stroke. 2004;35:426–31.

13. Sturgeon JD, Folsom AR, Longstreth Jr WT, Shahar E, Rosamond WD, Cushman M. Risk factors for intracerebral hemorrhage in a pooled prospective study. Stroke. 2007;38:2718–25.

14. Qureshi AI, Giles WH, Croft JB. Racial differences in the incidence of intracerebral hemorrhage: effects of blood pressure and education. Neurology. 1999;52:1617–21.

15. Inagawa T, Ohbayashi N, Takechi A, Shibukawa M, Yahara K. Primary intracerebral hemorrhage in Izumo City, Japan: incidence rates and outcome in relation to the site of hemorrhage. Neurosurgery. 2003;53:1283–97; discussion 1297–8.

16. Suzuki K, Kutsuzawa T, Takita K, Ito M, Sakamoto T, Hirayama A, et al. Clinico-epidemiologic study of stroke in Akita, Japan. Stroke. 1987;18:402–6.

17. Tanaka H, Ueda Y, Date C, Baba T, Yamashita H, Hayashi M, et al. Incidence of stroke in Shibata, Japan: 1976–1978. Stroke. 1981;12: 460–6.

18. Kumar V, Abbas AK, Fausto N, Robbins SL, Cotran RS. Robbins and Cotran pathologic basis of disease. 7th ed. Philadelphia: Elsevier Saunders; 2005.

19. Feldmann E, Broderick JP, Kernan WN, Viscoli CM, Brass LM, Brott T, et al. Major risk factors for intracerebral hemorrhage in the young are modifiable. Stroke. 2005;36:1881–5.

20. Woo D, Haverbusch M, Sekar P, Kissela B, Khoury J, Schneider A, et al. Effect of untreated hypertension on hemorrhagic stroke. Stroke. 2004;35:1703–8.

21. Woo D, Sauerbeck LR, Kissela BM, Khoury JC, Szaflarski JP, Gebel J, et al. Genetic and environmental risk factors for intracerebral hemorrhage: preliminary results of a population-based study. Stroke. 2002;33:1190–5.

22. Plesea IE, Camenita A, Georgescu CC, Enache SD, Zaharia B, Georgescu CV, et al. Study of cerebral vascular structures in hypertensive intracerebral haemorrhage. Rom J Morphol Embryol. 2005; 46:249–56.

23. Vinters HV. Cerebral amyloid angiopathy. A critical review. Stroke. 1987;18:311–24.

24. O'Donnell HC, Rosand J, Knudsen KA, Furie KL, Segal AZ, Chiu RI, et al. Apolipoprotein E genotype and the risk of recurrent lobar intracerebral haemorrhage. N Engl J Med. 2000;342:240–5.

25. McCarron MO, Nicoll JA. Cerebral amyloid angiopathy and thrombolysis-related intracerebral haemorrhage. Lancet Neurol. 2004;3:484–92.

26. Rensink AA, de Waal RM, Kremer B, Verbeek MM. Pathogenesis of cerebral amyloid angiopathy. Brain Res Brain Res Rev. 2003; 43:207–23.

27. Greenberg SM, Rebeck GW, Vonsattel JP, Gomez-Isla T, Hyman BT. Apolipoprotein E epsilon 4 and cerebral hemorrhage associated with amyloid angiopathy. Ann Neurol. 1995;38:254–9.

28. Olichney JM, Hansen LA, Hofstetter CR, Grundman M, Katzman R, Thal LJ. Cerebral infarction in Alzheimer's disease is associated with severe amyloid angiopathy and hypertension. Arch Neurol. 1995;52:702–8.

29. Greenberg SM. Cerebral amyloid angiopathy: prospects for clinical diagnosis and treatment. Neurology. 1998;51:690–4.

30. McCarron MO, Nicoll JA, Stewart J, Ironside JW, Mann DM, Love S, et al. The apolipoprotein E epsilon2 allele and the pathological features in cerebral amyloid angiopathy-related hemorrhage. J Neuropathol Exp Neurol. 1999;58:711–8.

31. Hart RG, Tonarelli SB, Pearce LA. Avoiding central nervous system bleeding during antithrombotic therapy: recent data and ideas. Stroke. 2005;36:1588–93.

32. Andrews BT, Chiles 3rd BW, Olsen WL, Pitts LH. The effect of intracerebral hematoma location on the risk of brain-stem compression and on clinical outcome. J Neurosurg. 1988;69:518–22.

33. European Stroke Initiative Writing C, Writing Committee for the EEC, Steiner T, Kaste M, Forsting M, Mendelow D, et al. Recommendations for the management of intracranial haemorrhage – part I: spontaneous intracerebral haemorrhage. The European Stroke Initiative Writing Committee and the Writing Committee for the EUSI Executive Committee. Cerebrovasc Dis. 2006;22:294–316.

34. Diringer MN, Edwards DF. Admission to a neurologic/neurosurgical intensive care unit is associated with reduced mortality rate after intracerebral hemorrhage. Crit Care Med. 2001;29:635–40.

35. Mendelow AD, Gregson BA, Fernandes HM, Murray GD, Teasdale GM, Hope DT, et al. Early surgery versus initial conservative treatment in patients with spontaneous supratentorial intracerebral haematomas in the International Surgical Trial in Intracerebral Haemorrhage (STICH): a randomised trial. Lancet. 2005;365:387–97.

36. Morgenstern LB, Hemphill 3rd JC, Anderson C, Becker K, Broderick JP, Connolly Jr ES, et al. Guidelines for the management of spontaneous intracerebral hemorrhage: a guideline for healthcare professionals from the American Heart Association/American Stroke Association. Stroke. 2010;41:2108–29.

37. Huisman TA. Intracranial hemorrhage: ultrasound, CT and MRI findings. Eur Radiol. 2005;15:434–40.

38. Kidwell CS, Wintermark M. Imaging of intracranial haemorrhage. Lancet Neurol. 2008;7:256–67.

39. Broderick JP, Brott TG, Duldner JE, Tomsick T, Huster G. Volume of intracerebral hemorrhage. A powerful and easy-to-use predictor of 30-day mortality. Stroke. 1993;24:987–93.

40. Gebel JM, Sila CA, Sloan MA, Granger CB, Weisenberger JP, Green CL, et al. Comparison of the ABC/2 estimation technique to computer-assisted volumetric analysis of intraparenchymal and subdural hematomas complicating the GUSTO-1 trial. Stroke. 1998;29:1799–801.

41. Kothari RU, Brott T, Broderick JP, Barsan WG, Sauerbeck LR, Zuccarello M, et al. The ABCs of measuring intracerebral hemorrhage volumes. Stroke. 1996;27:1304–5.

42. Davis SM, Broderick J, Hennerici M, Brun NC, Diringer MN, Mayer SA, et al. Hematoma growth is a determinant of mortality and poor outcome after intracerebral hemorrhage. Neurology. 2006;66:1175–81.

43. Wada R, Aviv RI, Fox AJ, Sahlas DJ, Gladstone DJ, Tomlinson G, et al. CT angiography "spot sign" predicts hematoma expansion in acute intracerebral hemorrhage. Stroke. 2007;38:1257–62.

44. Chappell ET, Moure FC, Good MC. Comparison of computed tomographic angiography with digital subtraction angiography in the diagnosis of cerebral aneurysms: a meta-analysis. Neurosurgery. 2003;52:624–31; discussion 630–1.

45. Papke K, Kuhl CK, Fruth M, Haupt C, Schlunz-Hendann M, Sauner D, et al. Intracranial aneurysms: role of multidetector CT angiography in diagnosis and endovascular therapy planning. Radiology. 2007;244:532–40.

46. Goldstein JN, Fazen LE, Snider R, Schwab K, Greenberg SM, Smith EE, et al. Contrast extravasation on CT angiography predicts hematoma expansion in intracerebral hemorrhage. Neurology. 2007;68:889–94.

47. Delgado Almandoz JE, Yoo AJ, Stone MJ, Schaefer PW, Oleinik A, Brouwers HB, et al. The spot sign score in primary intracerebral hemorrhage identifies patients at highest risk of in-hospital mortality and poor outcome among survivors. Stroke. 2010;41:54–60.

48. Kidwell CS, Chalela JA, Saver JL, Starkman S, Hill MD, Demchuk AM, et al. Comparison of MRI and CT for detection of acute intracerebral hemorrhage. JAMA. 2004;292:1823–30.

49. Fazekas F, Kleinert R, Roob G, Kleinert G, Kapeller P, Schmidt R, et al. Histopathologic analysis of foci of signal loss on gradient-echo T2*-weighted MR images in patients with spontaneous intracerebral hemorrhage: evidence of microangiopathy-related microbleeds. AJNR Am J Neuroradiol. 1999;20:637–42.

50. Knudsen KA, Rosand J, Karluk D, Greenberg SM. Clinical diagnosis of cerebral amyloid angiopathy: validation of the Boston criteria. Neurology. 2001;56:537–9.

51. Zhu XL, Chan MS, Poon WS. Spontaneous intracranial hemorrhage: which patients need diagnostic cerebral angiography? A prospective study of 206 cases and review of the literature. Stroke. 1997;28:1406–9.

52. American Heart Association Stroke Council and Council on Cardiovascular Nursing. Guidelines for the management of spontaneous intracerebral hemorrhage: a guideline for healthcare professionals from the American Heart Association/American Stroke Association. Stroke. 2010;41:2108–29.

53. Rådberg JA, Olsson JE, Rådberg CT. Prognostic parameters in spontaneous intracerebral hematomas with special reference to anticoagulant treatment. Stroke. 1991;22:571–6.

54. Flaherty ML, Kissela B, Woo D, Kleindorfer D, Alwell K, Sekar P, Moomaw CJ, Haverbusch M, Broderick JP. The increasing incidence of anticoagulant-associated intracerebral hemorrhage. Neurology. 2007;68:116–21.

55. Ansell J, Hirsh J, Hylek E, Jacobson A, Crowther M, Palareti G, American College of Chest Physicians. Pharmacology and management of the vitamin K antagonists: American College of Chest Physicians Evidence-Based Clinical Practice Guidelines (8th edition). Chest. 2008;133(Suppl):160S–98.

56. Mayer SA, Brun NC, Begtrup K, Broderick J, Davis S, Diringer MN, Skolnick BE, Steiner T, Recombinant Activated Factor VII Intracerebral Hemorrhage Trial Investigators. Recombinant activated factor VII for acute intracerebral hemorrhage. N Engl J Med. 2005;352:777–85.

57. Mayer SA, Brun NC, Begtrup K, Broderick J, Davis S, Diringer MN, Skolnick BE, Steiner T, FAST Trial Investigators. Efficacy and safety of recombinant activated factor VII for acute intracerebral hemorrhage. N Engl J Med. 2008;358:2127–37.

58. Willmot M, Leonardi-Bee J, Bath PM. High blood pressure in acute stroke and subsequent outcome: a systematic review. Hypertension. 2004;43:18–24.

59. Leonardi-Bee J, Bath PM, Phillips SJ, Sandercock PA, IST Collaborative Group. Blood pressure and clinical outcomes in the International Stroke Trial. Stroke. 2002;33:1315–20.

60. Anderson CS, Huang Y, Wang JG, Arima H, Neal B, Peng B, Heeley E, Skulina C, Parsons MW, Kim JS, Tao QL, Li YC, Jiang JD, Tai LW, Zhang JL, Xu E, Cheng Y, Heritier S, Morgenstern LB, Chalmers J, INTERACT Investigators. Intensive blood pressure reduction in acute cerebral haemorrhage trial (INTERACT): a randomised pilot trial. Lancet Neurol. 2008;7:391–9.

61. Vemmos KN, Tsivgoulis G, Spengos K, Zakopoulos N, Synetos A, Manios E, Konstantopoulou P, Mavrikakis M. U-shaped relationship between mortality and admission blood pressure in patients with acute stroke. J Intern Med. 2004;255:257–65.

62. Fernandes HM, Siddique S, Banister K, Chambers I, Wooldridge T, Gregson B, Mendelow AD. Continuous monitoring of ICP and CPP following ICH and its relationship to clinical, radiological and surgical parameters. Acta Neurochir Suppl. 2000;76:463–6.

63. Szaflarski JP, Rackley AY, Kleindorfer DO, Khoury J, Woo D, Miller R, Alwell K, Broderick JP, Kissela BM. Incidence of seizures in the acute phase of stroke: a population-based study. Epilepsia. 2008;49:974–81.

64. Messé SR, Sansing LH, Cucchiara BL, Herman ST, Lyden PD, Kasner SE, CHANT Investigators. Prophylactic antiepileptic drug use is associated with poor outcome following ICH. Neurocrit Care. 2009;11:38–44.

65. Naidech AM, Garg RK, Liebling S, Levasseur K, Macken MP, Schuele SU, Batjer HH. Anticonvulsant use and outcomes after intracerebral hemorrhage. Stroke. 2009;40:3810–5.

66. Lacut K, Bressollette L, Le Gal G, Etienne E, De Tinteniac A, Renault A, Rouhart F, Besson G, Garcia JF, Mottier D, Oger E, VICTORIAh (Venous Intermittent Compression and Thrombosis Occurrence Related to Intra-cerebral Acute hemorrhage) Investigators. Prevention of venous thrombosis in patients with acute intracerebral hemorrhage. Neurology. 2005;65:865–9.

67. CLOTS Trials Collaboration, Dennis M, Sandercock PA, Reid J, Graham C, Murray G, Venables G, Rudd A, Bowler G. Effectiveness of thigh-length graduated compression stockings to reduce the risk of deep vein thrombosis after stroke (CLOTS trial 1): a multicentre, randomised controlled trial. Lancet. 2009;373:1958–65.

68. Boeer A, Voth E, Henze T, Prange HW. Early heparin therapy in patients with spontaneous intracerebral haemorrhage. J Neurol Neurosurg Psychiatry. 1991;54:466–7.

69. McKissock W, Richardson A, Taylor J. Primary intracerebral haemorrhage. A controlled trial of surgical and conservative treatment in 180 unselected cases. Lancet. 1961;2:221–6.

70. Auer LM, Deinsberger W, Niederkorn K, Gell G, Kleinert R, Schneider G, et al. Endoscopic surgery versus medical treatment for spontaneous intracerebral hematoma: a randomized study. J Neurosurg. 1989;70:530–5.

71. Juvela S, Heiskanen O, Poranen A, Valtonen S, Kuurne T, Kaste M, et al. The treatment of spontaneous intracerebral hemorrhage. A prospective randomized trial of surgical and conservative treatment. J Neurosurg. 1989;70:755–8.

72. Batjer HH, Reisch JS, Allen BC, Plaizier LJ, Su CJ. Failure of surgery to improve outcome in hypertensive putaminal hemorrhage. A prospective randomized trial. Arch Neurol. 1990;47:1103–6.

73. Teernstra OP, Evers SM, Lodder J, Leffers P, Franke CL, Blaauw G, et al. Stereotactic treatment of intracerebral hematoma by means of a plasminogen activator: a multicenter randomized controlled trial (SICHPA). Stroke. 2003;34:968–74.

74. Hosseini H, Leguerinel C, Hariz M, Medlon E, Palfi S, Deck P, et al. Stereotactic aspiration of deep intracerebral hematomas under computed tomographic control. A multicentric prospective randomised trial. Cerebrovasc Dis. 2003;16:57.

75. Hattori N, Katayama Y, Maya Y, Gatherer A. Impact of stereotactic hematoma evacuation on activities of daily living during the chronic period following spontaneous putaminal hemorrhage: a randomized study. J Neurosurg. 2004;101:417–20.

76. Prasad K, Mendelow AD, Gregson B. Surgery for primary supratentorial intracerebral haemorrhage. Cochrane Database Syst Rev. 2008;(4):CD000200.

77. Da Pian R, Bazzan A, Pasqualin A. Surgical versus medical treatment of spontaneous posterior fossa haematomas: a cooperative study on 205 cases. Neurol Res. 1984;6:145–51.

78. Kirollos RW, Tyagi AK, Ross SA, van Hille PT, Marks PV. Management of spontaneous cerebellar hematomas: a prospective treatment protocol. Neurosurgery. 2001;49:1378–86; discussion 1386–7.

79. Kobayashi S, Sato A, Kageyama Y, Nakamura H, Watanabe Y, Yamaura A. Treatment of hypertensive cerebellar hemorrhage – surgical or conservative management? Neurosurgery. 1994;34:246–50; discussion 250–1.

80. Koziarski A, Frankiewicz E. Medical and surgical treatment of intracerebellar haematomas. Acta Neurochir (Wien). 1991;110:24–8.

81. Mathew P, Teasdale G, Bannan A, Oluoch-Olunya D. Neurosurgical management of cerebellar haematoma and infarct. J Neurol Neurosurg Psychiatry. 1995;59:287–92.

82. Hanley DF. Intraventricular hemorrhage: severity factor and treatment target in spontaneous intracerebral hemorrhage. Stroke. 2009; 40:1533–8.

83. Hinson HE, Hanley DF, Ziai WC. Management of intraventricular hemorrhage. Curr Neurol Neurosci Rep. 2010;10:73–82.

84. Morgan T, Awad I, Keyl P, Lane K, Hanley D. Preliminary report of the clot lysis evaluating accelerated resolution of intraventricular hemorrhage (CLEAR-IVH) clinical trial. Acta Neurochir Suppl. 2008;105:217–20.

85. Tuhrim S, Horowitz DR, Sacher M, Godbold JH. Volume of ventricular blood is an important determinant of outcome in supratentorial intracerebral hemorrhage. Crit Care Med. 1999;27:617–21.

86. Diringer MN, Edwards DF, Zazulia AR. Hydrocephalus: a previously unrecognized predictor of poor outcome from supratentorial intracerebral hemorrhage. Stroke. 1998;29:1352–7.

87. Coplin WM, Vinas FC, Agris JM, Buciuc R, Michael DB, Diaz FG, et al. A cohort study of the safety and feasibility of intraventricular urokinase for nonaneurysmal spontaneous intraventricular hemorrhage. Stroke. 1998;29:1573–9.

88. Ziai WC, Torbey MT, Naff NJ, Williams MA, Bullock R, Marmarou A, et al. Frequency of sustained intracranial pressure elevation during treatment of severe intraventricular hemorrhage. Cerebrovasc Dis. 2009;27:403–10.

89. Adams RE, Diringer MN. Response to external ventricular drainage in spontaneous intracerebral hemorrhage with hydrocephalus. Neurology. 1998;50:519–23.

90. Findlay JM, Weir BK, Stollery DE. Lysis of intraventricular hematoma with tissue plasminogen activator. Case report. J Neurosurg. 1991;74:803–7.

91. Lapointe M, Haines S. Fibrinolytic therapy for intraventricular hemorrhage in adults. Cochrane Database Syst Rev. 2002;(3):CD003692.

92. Nieuwkamp DJ, de Gans K, Rinkel GJ, Algra A. Treatment and outcome of severe intraventricular extension in patients with subarachnoid or intracerebral hemorrhage: a systematic review of the literature. J Neurol. 2000;247:117–21

93. Staykov D, Bardutzky J, Huttner HB, Schwab S. Intraventricular fibrinolysis for intracerebral hemorrhage with severe ventricular involvement. Neurocrit Care. 2011;15(1):194–209.

94. Naff NJ, Hanley DF, Keyl PM, Tuhrim S, Kraut M, Bederson J, et al. Intraventricular thrombolysis speeds blood clot resolution: results of a pilot, prospective, randomized, double-blind, controlled trial. Neurosurgery. 2004;54:577–83; discussion 583–4.

Arteriovenous Malformations: Evidence-Based Medicine, Diagnosis, Treatment, and Complications

26

Muhammad M. Abd-El-Barr, Seth F. Oliveria, Brian L. Hoh, and J.D. Mocco

Contents

Abstract

Cerebral arteriovenous malformations (AVMs) are complex lesions that require specialized, multidisciplinary treatment. Patients may be encountered in the intensive care unit either following intracranial hemorrhage from AVM rupture or following elective surgical resection of an unruptured AVM. This chapter reviews all aspects of clinical management of AVMs including initial assessment and critical care, perioperative considerations, and the available neurosurgical interventions utilized for definitive AVM treatment.

Keywords

Arteriovenous malformation • Radiosurgery • Embolization • Vascular malformation • Spetzler-Martin Grade

Definition

Arteriovenous malformations (AVMs) are a complex tangle of abnormal arteries and veins, with an anatomic absence of the normal capillary bed. This absence of a capillary bed can lead to high-flow shunting through various fistulas [1]. Cerebral AVMs, though relatively rare, are complex entities to diagnose and treat.

Epidemiology and Natural History

It is unclear when the time of onset of cerebral AVMs are, but certain features, such as their presentation in younger patients, including infants, and their abnormal architecture, suggest that at least some are due to a developmental derangement [1, 2]. Other evidence of early incidence is the fact that in the presence of an AVM, there are clear rearrangements of neuronal networks, such as the translocation of eloquent areas, a phenomenon seldom encountered in the face of acute intracranial hemorrhages [3]. This may also

M.M. Abd-El-Barr, MD, PhD
Department of Neurosurgery,
Brigham and Women's Hospital, Harvard Medical School,
75 Francis Street, Boston, MA 02115, USA
e-mail: mabd-el-barr@partners.org

S.F. Oliveria, MD, PhD • B.L. Hoh, MD, FACS, FAHA, FAANS (✉)
Department of Neurological Surgery,
University of Florida College of Medicine,
100265, Gainesville, FL 32610, USA
e-mail: seth.oliveria@neurosurgery.ufl.edu;
brian.hoh@neurosurgery.ufl.edu

J.D. Mocco, MD, MS, FAANS, FAHA
Department of Neurosurgery,
Vanderbilt University Medical Center,
1161 21st Ave S, RM T4224 MCN, Nashville, TN 37232, USA
e-mail: j.mocco@vanderbilt.edu

A.J. Layon et al. (eds.), *Textbook of Neurointensive Care*,
DOI 10.1007/978-1-4471-5226-2_26, © Springer-Verlag London 2013

explain the lower rates of hemorrhages in AVMs compared to other intracranial vascular abnormalities [4]. A point of evidence against an embryonic disturbance is that, whereas there are numerous reports of in utero diagnosis of other vascular abnormalities, the number of AVMs diagnosed in utero are limited to single-digit case reports [5, 6].

Genetic predisposition to cerebral AVMs has been difficult to prove, with only a few candidate genes having been identified to this point [7, 8]. There are a number of germline mutations that have been found to be particularly important in the pathogenesis of AVMs. Some of these candidate proteins include transforming growth factor-beta (TGF-β), vascular endothelial growth factor (VEGF), and the angiopoietin receptor Tie-2 [4, 9–12].

The prevalence of AVMs has been difficult to pinpoint, with ranges from 5 to 600 per 100,000 persons [13, 14]. A retrospective analysis of symptomatic AVMs yielded a rate of 1.1 per 100,000 [15], though this figure may be falsely elevated due to the concurrent existence of other vascular malformations. A prospective, population-based survey yielded an incidence of 1.34 per 100,000 person-years, with approximately one-half presenting with a first-ever hemorrhage (0.51 per 100,000 person-years) [16].

Much of what is known about the natural history of cerebral AVMs is based on a cohort study of 262 symptomatic unoperated patients that presented to a central referral center in Finland [17]. In that study, 40 % of the patients were excluded because they received a treatment upfront, but, for the remaining 160 patients, the incidence of hemorrhage averaged approximately 4 % per year. A recent update to this data set revealed a somewhat similar risk of hemorrhage (2.4 % per year), but this risk was higher in the first 5 years after diagnosis [18]. Multivariate analyses revealed that previous rupture, large AVMs (>50 mm nidus size), and infratentorial and deep locations were independent risk factors to higher hemorrhage rates [18]. Other studies have reported that small AVM size and exclusive deep venous drainage and AVM-related aneurysms are also risk factors associated with higher rates of AMV hemorrhage [19, 20].

Critical Care Management

Acute Evaluation

The most common clinical presentation of cerebral AVMs is hemorrhage (70 %), seizures (25 %), and 5 % of patients will present with headaches and other various vague neurologic complaints [17, 18].

Because hemorrhage is the most common presentation, the hallmark characteristics of hemorrhage must be recognized readily by the medical team. These include the sudden onset of headache, focal neurologic symptoms, and changes in the level of consciousness.

As with all acute presentations, the ABCs of intensive care must be secured. This refers to the airway, breathing or blood pressure, and circulation or coagulation. It is estimated that approximately 30 % of all patients with intracerebral hemorrhage will need to be mechanically ventilated [21]. It has been suggested that any patient with a Glasgow Coma Scale (GCS) of eight or below should be intubated [22].

Importantly, a complete arterial blood gas (ABG) should be drawn, as making sure that the patient is well oxygenated is not enough, since hypercapnia can worsen intracranial hypertension (discussed later in this chapter).

Blood pressure should be controlled to a limited extent, until the etiology of the focal neurological deficit or decrease of consciousness is elucidated. As many of these patients will present with signs and symptoms of a hemorrhagic stroke, recent guidelines suggest that lowering the blood pressure to systolic pressures close to 140 mmHg may be beneficial [23, 24]. As for coagulation, it is important to evaluate if the patient is on anticoagulation medications. It is estimated that approximately 15 % of patients with ICH are on oral anticoagulation (OAC) therapy [25]. If it is found that the patient is on anticoagulation, reversal of this anticoagulation is recommended [26]. The traditional agents for this have been vitamin K and fresh frozen plasma (FFP). Vitamin K, even given intravenously, takes many hours to have an effect [27, 28]. FFP, as a transfused blood product, carries the extra risk of allergic transfusion reactions and requires increased volumes to be effective.

Two classes of drugs that have recently gained some prominence in the treatment of anticoagulation are prothrombin complex concentrates (PCCs) and recombinant factor VIIa (fFVIIa). PCCs are used to treat factor IX deficiency primarily but can also reverse deficiencies of factors II, VII, and X. There is also some interest in using them to counteract warfarin [26]. There is some evidence to suggest that use of these PCCs may decreased the amount of FFP needed to correct abnormal INRs, though clinical outcomes appear to be the same, with perhaps some decrease in adverse effects due to decreased volume overload to patients [26]. rFVIIa, which is licensed to be used by hemophilia patients or those with decreased factor VII or high titers of inhibitors, had originally garnered much attention as a potential potent reversal agent for OAC-associated ICH, but further studies revealed that it does not generate thrombin as effectively as PCCs [29]. A phase 2 trial of rFVIIa showed promising results in terms of limiting hematoma expansion and clinical outcomes, but the phase III failed to reproduce these results and resulted in greater thromboembolic events in the rFVIIa treatment group [30].

Intracranial pressure (ICP) and cerebral perfusion pressures (CPP) are also important parameters that are distinct to this patient population. CPP is defined as the mean arterial pressure minus intracranial pressure (CPP = MAP – ICP). Elevated ICP is usually defined as greater than 20 mmHg for greater than 5 min, and the goal of CPP is to be greater than 60–70 mmHg. To measure intracranial pressure, a fiberoptic ICP wire or an external ventricular drain (EVD) should be placed. Trauma guidelines suggest the insertion of such a device in patients with a GCS of eight or below and abnormal head CT and in the case of a patient with an acute neurological deficit and possible AVM (discussion of radiographic signs follows later in this chapter); this should also be done in the case of a patient without a robust neurological examination that can be followed. An EVD also allows for drainage of cerebrospinal fluid (CSF), which can also be helpful in lowering ICPs.

Lowering intracranial pressure can be accomplished both by decreasing the volume demands of the various intracranial constituents or by sedation, which acts to decrease brain tissue metabolism. The Kellie-Monro hypothesis states that the cranial compartment is incompressible and the volume of the intracranial contents is fixed. Thus, any increase in any of the three main constituents of cranial contents—namely, brain tissue, CSF, and blood—must be accompanied by a decrease in one of the others [31]. It is because of this principle that CSF drainage with the use of an EVD is helpful in the setting of hemorrhage from an AVM. Similarly, brain tissue volume can be decreased by the administration of mannitol or hypertonic saline. Mannitol, which is an osmotic diuretic, works by two mechanisms. The first mechanism is that, when it is given as bolus, it increases oxygen delivery by increasing blood volume. The second mechanism is that, by being an osmotic agent, it draws water out of neurons [32]. In the traumatic brain injury literature, it has been shown to decrease mortality compared to barbiturates [33]. However, mannitol does have some adverse effects, namely nephrotoxicity and causing patients to become hypovolemic [32]. Hypertonic saline, on the other hand, works by the same mechanism of making an osmotic potential across neurons but does not have the same negative effects. A recent meta-analysis comparing the two agents suggested that hypertonic saline does seem to be more efficacious in lowering ICP, though the number of patients (112) was relatively small [34].

Another mechanism used to decrease ICP is causing vasoconstriction through hypocarbia. This can be accomplished by mild hyperventilation with a goal of $PaCO_2$ of 25–30 mmHg. Severe hypocarbia should be avoided as it can cause decreased cerebral blood flow. This therapy is effective when used intermittently, but chronic hyperventilation may cause rebound increased ICP when normocapnea is achieved [35]. Therefore, it is strongly recommended not to pursue prolonged hypocarbia and to use this method of ICP control only for brief periods.

Increased ICP can also be lowered using sedation, which by decreasing agitation, decreases brain tissue metabolic demands. If normal agents (propofol, benzodiazepines such as versed and opioid agonists such as fentanyl) are unable to control ICPs, an induced barbiturate coma with continuous

electroencephalogram (EEG) can be considered. This is usually done until burst suppression is achieved [22]. The last resort for increased ICPs is decompressive craniectomy or craniotomy, discussed elsewhere (Chaps. 27 and 35). Many of the techniques of ICP management are borrowed from the traumatic brain injury (TBI) literature, and, in the author's institute, a detailed algorithm is followed in the cases of severe TBI (GCS ≤8) (Fig. 26.1).

As stated earlier, approximately one-third of patients with cerebral AVMs will present with seizures [36]. A retrospective analysis of 424 patients that presented with cerebral AVMs showed that male sex, age less than 65, AVM size of greater than 3 cm, and location in the temporal lobe were significantly associated with seizures being the presenting symptom [37]. In the acute setting, it is important to initiate antiepileptic prophylaxis in patients presenting with hemorrhage, as this has been shown to increase risk of future seizures [37]. For those patients that present with seizures, antiepileptic therapy is warranted.

Important in the management of patients with AVMs are the systemic complications of neurological insult. Subendocardial ischemia, which has been shown to be in proportion to the neurological insult, may result in a myriad of symptoms from benign elevations in cardiac enzymes to life-threatening arrhythmias and pulmonary edema [38, 39]. It is important to note preexisting cardiac conditions of these ill patients and monitor their progress.

Another organ system at risk in these situations is the pulmonary system. Patients with neurological compromise are at higher risk for atelectasis, aspiration, and pulmonary embolism [22]. Oftentimes, patients with neurological decline with AVMs require pulmonary catheter to keep track of their central venous pressures (CVPs) to avoid pulmonary hypertension, a consequence of hypervolemia for patients undergoing "triple H" therapy for vasospasm, an infrequent but very real potential complication of SAH from an AVM or feeding artery aneurysm associated with an AVM (see Chap. 24 on SAH).

Electrolyte abnormalities must also be monitored in patients with AVMs. The most common abnormality is hyponatremia [40]. There has been a lack of a consensus on the diagnosis and management of hyponatremia in neurosurgical patients. The two most common reasons for hyponatremia, after exclusion of diuretic use, is cerebral salt wasting (CSW) and the syndrome of inappropriate antidiuretic hormone (SIADH). It is important to distinguish between these two etiologies, as the treatment for each is completely different and has significant consequence to the patient. The most important laboratory value to differentiate between the two diagnoses is the patient's volume status. Greatly simplified, patients that are hypovolemic are most likely to have CSW, while those patients with euvolemia or hypervolemia are more likely to harbor SIADH. SIADH is treated with water and volume restriction, while CSW is treated with replacing

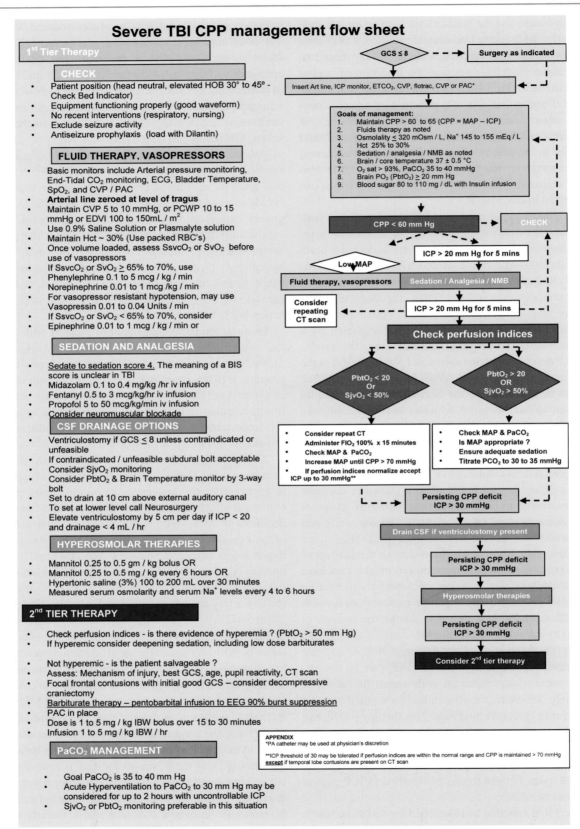

Fig. 26.1 Algorithm for management of patient's decreased Glasgow Coma Scale (GCS ≤8). Although this algorithm is used for patients with traumatic brain injury (TBI), many of the same methods are used in critically ill patients harboring AVMs or other vascular abnormalities

Na and intravenous fluids [40]. Importantly, patients that are vulnerable to cerebral vasospasm due to SAH may suffer irreversible infarcts if heavily volume depleted, so fluid restriction should be avoided in these patients.

Radiographic Assessment

Once the patient has been stabilized, it is important for radiographic imaging to take place. A non-contrast computed tomography (CT) of the brain is the imaging modality of choice when an acute change of consciousness and/or focal neurological symptoms are the presenting signs. This is because a CT will quickly differentiate between an ischemic and hemorrhagic stroke and will also many of times be able to differentiate between a subarachnoid hemorrhage (SAH) and intracerebral hemorrhage (ICH). Due to the vast improvement in imaging technology over the past decade or so, it is not unreasonable to obtain a CT angiogram (CTA) with or without perfusion [41–43]. This does not add much time to the imaging aspect of the initial workup but adds vital information to the possible existence of a cerebral aneurysm or other vascular malformations that may be the etiology behind a hemorrhagic stroke. A recent prospective study comparing 3D-CTA and digital subtraction angiography (DSA), which has long been the gold standard to evaluate AVMs, revealed identical accuracy and slightly decreased sensitivity, though the post processing in the CTAs was more involved than in most centers [44].

For those patients that present with hemorrhage, approximately 60 % will have intraparenchymal hemorrhage (Fig. 26.2), 30 % will have a subarachnoid hemorrhage (SAH) (Fig. 26.3), and 10 % will have intraventricular hemorrhage (IVH) (Fig. 26.4) [45].

Although cerebral aneurysms are the major etiology responsible for SAH, AVMs constitute approximately 10 % of cases of SAH. Importantly, approximately 10 % of AVMs will have an artery feeding the cerebral aneurysm related to the AVM [46]. In these cases, it is more likely that the aneurysm is responsible for the subarachnoid hemorrhage. We will not deal with SAH management in this chapter, but many of the same diagnostic algorithms are similar to aneurysmal SAH. Importantly, the occurrence of cerebral vasospasm, which can be defined by various clinical and radiographic means but usually entails acute neurological decline in the face of focal or global decreases in cerebral vasculature, does not occur frequently with isolated AVMs, though some reports do note its presence [47, 48].

Catheter angiography remains the gold standard for detecting AVMs [44] (Fig. 26.5) and should be instigated once the patient in whom an AVM is suspected is stabilized.

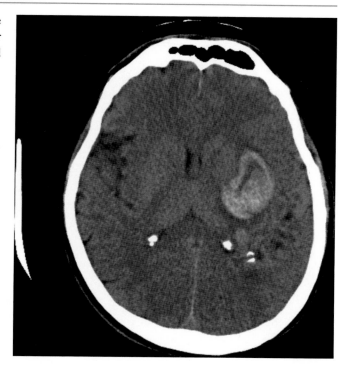

Fig. 26.2 Intracerebral hemorrhage (ICH) from an underlying AVM

Another advantage of catheter angiography is that it allows for evaluation of possible related aneurysm (Fig. 26.6) and instigation of possible endovascular treatment (discussed later in this chapter).

Anesthetic Considerations

Anesthesia plays an important role in all aspects of patient care with AVMs for preoperative investigation, embolization, stereotactic radiosurgery, surgical resection, or long-term ICU care.

Both intravenous and inhaled anesthetics work to decrease the cerebral metabolic rate (CMR). However, most inhaled anesthetics, except N_2O, increase cerebral blood flow (CBF), while intravenous agents cause an increase in cerebral resistance and, hence, a decrease in CBF.

Sedation and monitoring are all that is usually required for CT or CT angiography. A common combination of midazolam and/or fentanyl, with some premedication with glycopyrrolate, usually suffices [49], though care must be taken that there are no increased ICPs.

For diagnostic angiography, either conscious sedation or general anesthesia is used, depending on the neurological status of the patient and his/her ability to cooperate. For embolization, most centers use general anesthesia with

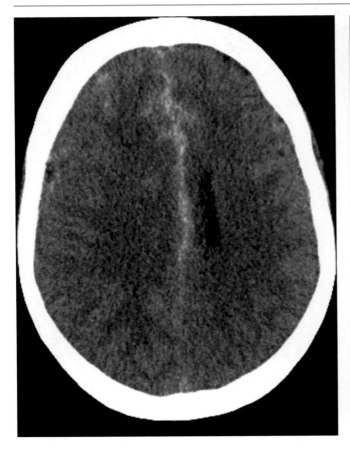

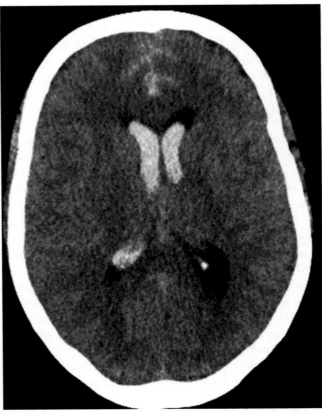

Fig. 26.3 Subarachnoid hemorrhage (SAH) from underlying AVM

Fig. 26.4 The same patient from Fig. 26.3 also had evidence of intraventricular hemorrhage (IVH)

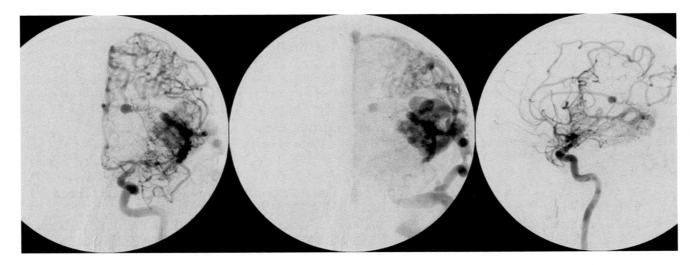

Fig. 26.5 Cerebral angiogram reveals a left frontal AVM with a large nidus and multiple arterial feeders and both superficial and deep venous drainage

endotracheal intubation, though the use of conscious sedation with monitored anesthesia care (MAC) in cooperative patients is also a possibility [50].

Similar to the situation in the preoperative evaluation, blood pressure control is of utmost importance in patients with AVMs, especially those that have hemorrhaged. In certain situations, deliberate hypotension is required, especially in the application of glue for AVM embolization to prevent systemic spread of the glue or onyx [49]. There are also situations where deliberate hypertension may be needed, especially in the case of ischemia. A common drug for this is phenylephrine [49].

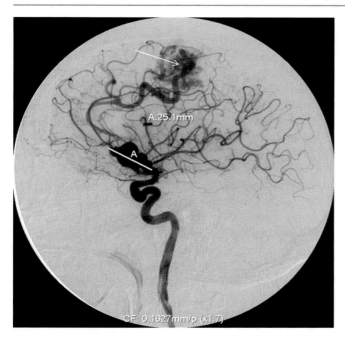

Fig. 26.6 Lateral view of a cerebral angiogram reveals a large (25 mm) feeding artery aneurysm to the AVM, whose nidus is seen (*white arrow*)

Grading and Surgical Management

AVM Grading

The Spetzler-Martin grading system for estimating risk of morbidity or mortality following AVM resection was proposed in 1986 and remains well known and widely referenced [51]. Under this system, lesions are graded based on size, venous drainage pattern, and eloquence of adjacent brain tissue using available imaging modalities including CT, MRI, and cerebral angiography. Lesion grade is calculated by summing a numerical value for each of the three categories described previously as follows: nidus size 1–3 points (small <3 cm, medium 3–6 cm, or large >6 cm, respectively), venous drainage 0–1 point (1 point for drainage into internal cerebral veins, basal veins, or precentral cerebellar vein), and eloquence 0–1 point (1 point for lesions near the sensorimotor, language, and visual cortex, the hypothalamus and thalamus, the internal capsule, the brain stem, the cerebellar peduncles, or the deep cerebellar nuclei). The graded variables of this system address the major issues influencing the overall technical difficulty of AVM resection. Since correlation between AVM grade and incidence of postoperative neurological complications is good, Spetzler-Martin Grade has become a reliable tool for use in preoperative counseling. Both the original manuscript by Spetzler and Martin and subsequent studies [52–57] reveal that resection of Grade I and II lesions was deemed relatively safe with a low incidence of neurologic complications, while Grade IV and V lesions resulted in a significant number of surgically induced neurologic deficits. Indeed, more recently it has been proposed that the Spetzler-Martin grading system be collapsed from a five-tiered (i.e., Grade I–V) to a three-tiered (i.e., Grade A–C) system since the difference in surgical results between Grades I and II and between Grades IV and V are small [58]. Of note, multiple other AVM grading systems have been devised [59–61] that incorporate additional variables—including patient age, diffuseness, nature of feeding artery supply, and clinical status at presentation—to improve surgical risk prediction and patient selection. Nevertheless, the Spetzler-Martin grading remains entrenched as a function of its simplicity and robust applicability.

The primary neurosurgical interventions available for AVM treatment include microsurgical resection, endovascular embolization, and stereotactic radiosurgery. AVM grading prominently influences which of these options are available for any individual patient. In general, low-grade lesions that are small and accessible are often resected directly; small, less accessible lesions are typically treated with radiosurgery; in contrast, high-grade, complex lesions frequently require multidisciplinary management with reductive embolization followed by another definitive treatment modality. These treatment modalities will be considered individually in the following section.

Treatment Modalities for AVM Management

Endovascular Embolization
There are two distinct treatment indications for endovascular AVM embolization. First, for a small number of lesions, AVM nidus embolization may be employed as a definite treatment. While this strategy is desirable because of potential decreased morbidity and mortality relative to open resection, it is essentially limited to small lesions supplied by one or very few feeding arteries. Embolization may fail to completely obliterate an AVM nidus, and it is also subject to late recurrence as a result of either recruitment of additional feeding vessels or true recanalization [62–64]. Partial embolization fails to protect against subsequent hemorrhage [65, 66] and carries the theoretical risk of precipitating hemorrhage via altered flow properties. Therefore, definitive AVM embolization should only be attempted if there is a high likelihood of successful nidus obliteration.

The second indication for endovascular intervention is strategic partial AVM embolization to facilitate subsequent definitive treatment with either open resection or radiosurgery. This adjunctive role for embolization is performed with intent to reduce the size and/or volume of an AVM nidus. When followed by microsurgical resection, AVM embolization creates a more desirable dissection plane by preemptively occluding fragile vessels at the nidus periphery that can complicate microsurgical dissection [67, 68]. By reducing intraoperative blood loss and limiting unintended damage to adjacent tissue, endovascular embolization is generally considered to improve surgical outcomes.

The efficacy and safety of stereotactic radiosurgery decreases as AVM size increases [69–73]. Reductive endovascular embolization can potentially reduce the volume of large AVMs to a size that is amenable to stereotactic radiosurgery, reducing radiation exposure to adjacent normal tissue and potentially reducing the latency period and/or likelihood malformation obliteration [74–76]. However, embolization material can obscure the AVM nidus when imaging is performed for stereotactic radiosurgery treatment planning, and some reports suggest that prior embolization is a significant predictor of radiological failure following SRS treatment of AVMs [77–80]. Therefore, the use of combined endovascular embolization and stereotactic radiosurgery remains somewhat controversial and institution dependent.

Finally, it should be noted that AVM embolization itself poses several risks including embolization of normal vessels and arterial perforation that can cause ischemia and/or hemorrhage, thus compounding the overall risk of patient morbidity or mortality during a staged procedure. For this reason, endovascular embolization may not be indicated prior to definitive treatment of low-grade AVMs.

Stereotactic Radiosurgery

Gamma knife (GK), particle beam (PB), and linear accelerator (LINAC) radiosurgical systems have all successfully been used to treat AVMs in large series, with reported occlusion rates of 60–80 % and complication rates of approximately 2 % [72, 81–84]. Pollock and Flickinger [77] developed the radiosurgery-based arteriovenous malformation (AVM) score (RBAS) from a multivariate analysis of predictive factors of outcome after radiosurgery. The RBAS is calculated as $(0.1 \times \text{volume in cm}^3) + (0.02 \times \text{age in years}) + (0.3 \times \text{location})$, with these location values: frontal/temporal = 0, parietal/occipital/ corpus callosum/cerebellar = 1, and basal ganglia/thalamus/brain stem = 2. This score has been validated using GK, PB, and LINAC systems to accurately predict the likelihood of complete obliteration with no new neurological deficit after single-treatment radiosurgery; patients with an AVM score less than 1.0 are more likely to experience excellent results than those individuals with an AVM score greater than 2.0.

With careful dose planning, stereotactic radiosurgery can avoid injury to critical structures adjacent to an AVM nidus [70, 85]. This treatment modality is therefore potentially ideal for small, deep AVMs that are challenging to resect safely. However, there are several limitations to radiosurgical treatment of AVMs that must be considered: first, there is a well-documented latent period from radiosurgical treatment to complete AVM obliteration of approximately 1–3 years [70, 86, 87]; second, radiosurgery provides no apparent protective effect until complete AVM obliteration is achieved, since the probability of hemorrhage remains similar to the natural history of AVMs, 2–4 % per year, prior to obliteration [88, 89]; finally, the probability of AVM obliteration following radiosurgery declines, and complication risk increases with larger AVM nidus volumes, as predicted by the RBAS equation. Taken together, this suggests that small, surgically inaccessible AVMs should be treated with radiosurgery since the risk of surgical complications outweighs that of hemorrhage during the latent period. In contrast, lesions amenable to resection should often be treated surgically to immediately eliminate the threat of hemorrhage. Again, complex lesions frequently require multimodal therapy as described earlier, though some groups have advocated for staged radiosurgery [84, 90, 91].

Microsurgical Resection

Surgical extirpation remains the gold standard for obliteration of AVMs, because the benefit of surgical therapy is immediate and definitive, and the perioperative risk declines rapidly over the first several postoperative days. The details of AVM resection are largely beyond the scope of this discussion [92, 93], but microsurgical resection generally proceeds as follows: exposure; then subarachnoid, pial, parenchymal, and periventricular dissection; and then finally extirpation. Wide exposure via a relatively large craniotomy and durotomy is preferred to permit close inspection of vessels feeding and draining the AVM nidus. While feeding arteries are meticulously dissected and ligated, great care is taken to preserve venous outflow to avoid intraoperative AVM rupture. This eventually results in gradual AVM involution, until the last venous pedicles can be safely ligated. Prior to closure, the resection bed must be carefully examined for residual AVM and for complete hemostasis. Microsurgery is often performed with the assistance of frameless stereotactic navigation and intraoperative neuromonitoring.

For patients presenting with AVM-associated hemorrhage, surgical intervention may be more clearly indicated than the other treatment modalities described previously. A preexisting neurologic deficit after hemorrhage favors surgical intervention because the risk of surgically induced deficit is lower, while the morbidity and mortality of a nondefinitive approach are higher [68]. Additionally, hemorrhage may facilitate surgery since an intraparenchymal hematoma can create a surgical corridor to better access some lesions by allowing entry into the clot cavity [68, 94, 95]. When the clinical situation permits, subacute microsurgical AVM resection is usually favored to allow time for hematoma organization, relief of brain edema, and resolution of transient neurological deficits [68, 92, 96]. For these reasons and because the risk of nonaneurysmal rebleeding from a ruptured AVM with intact venous drainage is low, the goal of acute surgery for hematoma evacuation when necessary is brain decompression, not AVM resection [93].

Intraoperative and Postoperative Care

The brain parenchyma surrounding AVMs is well known to be subject to hemodynamic perturbations, which may account for both the vascular steal-associated symptoms experienced by some patients with AVMs preoperatively, as well as feared hyperemic complications postoperatively. Chronic arterial hypotension surrounding AVMs has been theorized to induce a loss of cerebrovascular autoregulatory capability, such that perfusion pressure elevation to normal range following AVM shunt obliteration results in reperfusion injury and/or hemorrhage ("normal perfusion pressure breakthrough") [97, 98]. Thus, the cornerstone of perioperative care during and after AVM treatment is strict blood pressure control with absolute prevention of hypertension. Careful administration of anesthesia is paramount, with smooth induction, intubation, and emergence of utmost importance; standard practices of neuroanesthesia otherwise apply, including careful ICP management, though the anesthesiologist should also be prepared for the possibility of sudden, profuse blood loss. Early postoperative complications are often attributed to inadequate blood pressure control [92, 93]. To avoid intra- or postoperative swelling or hemorrhage, systemic hypotension/normotension (mean arterial pressure, 60–70 mmHg) is maintained for 48–72 h postoperatively with sodium nitroprusside and/ or beta-1 blocking agents and then gradually liberalized.

When postoperative bleeding occurs despite adequate blood pressure control, residual malformation should be considered. For this reason, many surgeons perform either intraoperative or postoperative cerebral angiography to document complete resection of the AVM nidus. More rarely, cerebral vasospasm has also been identified as a cause of delayed neurologic decline, perhaps as a result of either subarachnoid hemorrhage or intraoperative vessel manipulation [47]; evaluation with CT or conventional cerebral angiography should therefore be considered for neurologic deterioration once postoperative hemorrhage has been excluded as a cause. In addition to these measures, vigilant postoperative critical care management is necessary, employing the same principles described earlier in the chapter.

Conclusions

Critical care for patients with AVMs is a multidisciplinary challenge, often requiring the close collaboration of neurosurgeons, anesthesiologists, neuroradiologists, and intensivists. It is only with the close collaboration of these different entities that the best care can be administered to these usually critically ill patients.

References

1. Stapf C, Mohr JP, Pile-Spellman J, Solomon RA, Sacco RL, Connolly Jr ES. Epidemiology and natural history of arteriovenous malformations. Neurosurg Focus. 2001;11:e1.
2. Lasjaunias PL. Vascular diseases in neonates, infants, and children: interventional neuroradiology management. New York: Springer; 1996.
3. Lazar RM, Marshall RS, Pile-Spellman J, Hacein-Bey L, Young WL, Mohr JP, Stein BM. Anterior translocation of language in patients with left cerebral arteriovenous malformation. Neurology. 1997;49:802–8.
4. Moftakhar P, Hauptman JS, Malkasian D, Martin NA. Cerebral arteriovenous malformations. Part 1: cellular and molecular biology. Neurosurg Focus. 2009;26:E10.
5. Campi A, Scotti G, Filippi M, Gerevini S, Strigimi F, Lasjaunias P. Antenatal diagnosis of vein of Galen aneurysmal malformation: MR study of fetal brain and postnatal follow-up. Neuroradiology. 1996;38:87–90.
6. DeCesare B, Omojola MF, Fogarty EF, Brown JC, Taylon C. Spontaneous thrombosis of congenital cerebral arteriovenous malformation complicated by subdural collection: in utero detection with disappearance in infancy. Br J Radiol. 2006;79:e140–4.
7. Oikawa M, Kuniba H, Kondoh T, Kinoshita A, Nagayasu T, Niikawa N, Yoshiura K. Familial brain arteriovenous malformation maps to 5p13-q14, 15q11-q13 or 18p11: linkage analysis with clipped fingernail DNA on high-density SNP array. Eur J Med Genet. 2010;53:244–9.
8. Zabel-du Bois A, Wagner-Ecker M, Milker-Zabel S, Schwager C, Wirkner U, Debus J, Abdollahi A, Huber PE. Gene expression signatures in the peripheral blood after radiosurgery of human cerebral arteriovenous malformations. Strahlenther Onkol. 2010;186:91–8.
9. Hatva E, Jaaskelainen J, Hirvonen H, Alitalo K, Haltia M. Tie endothelial cell-specific receptor tyrosine kinase is upregulated in the vasculature of arteriovenous malformations. J Neuropathol Exp Neurol. 1996;55:1124–33.
10. Rothbart D, Awad IA, Lee J, Kim J, Harbaugh R, Criscuolo GR. Expression of angiogenic factors and structural proteins in central nervous system vascular malformations. Neurosurgery. 1996;38:915–24; discussion 924–5.
11. Hashimoto T, Emala CW, Joshi S, Mesa-Tejada R, Quick CM, Feng L, Libow A, Marchuk DA, Young WL. Abnormal pattern of Tie-2 and vascular endothelial growth factor receptor expression in human cerebral arteriovenous malformations. Neurosurgery. 2000;47:910–8; discussion 918–9.
12. Hirschi KK, Rohovsky SA, D'Amore PA. PDGF, TGF-beta, and heterotypic cell-cell interactions mediate endothelial cell-induced recruitment of 10T1/2 cells and their differentiation to a smooth muscle fate. J Cell Biol. 1998;141:805–14.
13. Jellinger K. Vascular malformations of the central nervous system: a morphological overview. Neurosurg Rev. 1986;9:177–216.
14. Sacco RL, Boden-Albala B, Gan R, Chen X, Kargman DE, Shea S, Paik MC, Hauser WA. Stroke incidence among white, black, and Hispanic residents of an urban community: the Northern Manhattan Stroke Study. Am J Epidemiol. 1998;147:259–68.
15. Jessurun GA, Kamphuis DJ, van der Zande FH, Nossent JC. Cerebral arteriovenous malformations in The Netherlands Antilles. High prevalence of hereditary hemorrhagic telangiectasia-related single and multiple cerebral arteriovenous malformations. Clin Neurol Neurosurg. 1993;95:193–8.
16. Stapf C, Labovitz DL, Sciacca RR, Mast H, Mohr JP, Sacco RL. Incidence of adult brain arteriovenous malformation hemorrhage in a prospective population-based stroke survey. Cerebrovasc Dis. 2002;13:43–6.
17. Ondra SL, Troupp H, George ED, Schwab K. The natural history of symptomatic arteriovenous malformations of the brain: a 24-year follow-up assessment. J Neurosurg. 1990;3:387–91.

18. Hernesniemi JA, Dashti R, Juvela S, Vaart K, Niemela M, Laakso A. Natural history of brain arteriovenous malformations: a long-term follow-up study of risk of hemorrhage in 238 patients. Neurosurgery. 2008;63:823–9.

19. Marks MP, Lane B, Steinberg GK, Chang PJ. Hemorrhage in intracerebral arteriovenous malformations: angiographic determinants. Radiology. 1990;176:807–13.

20. Stapf C, Mast H, Sciacca RR, Choi JH, Khaw AV, Connolly ES, Pile-Spellman J, Mohr JP. Predictors of hemorrhage in patients with untreated brain arteriovenous malformation. Neurology. 2006;66:1350–5.

21. Gujjar AR, Deibert E, Manno EM, Duff S, Diringer MN. Mechanical ventilation for ischemic stroke and intracerebral hemorrhage: indications, timing, and outcome. Neurology. 1998;51:447–51.

22. Jabbour PAIHD. Hemorrhagic cerebrovascular disease. In: Layon AGA, Friedman WA, editors. Textbook of neurocritical care. Philadelphia: Saunders; 2004. p. 155–81.

23. Arima H, Anderson CS, Wang JG, Huang Y, Heeley E, Neal B, Woodward M, Skulina C, Parsons MW, Peng B, Tao QL, Li YC, Jiang JD, Tai LW, Zhang JL, Xu E, Cheng Y, Morgenstern LB, Chalmers J. Lower treatment blood pressure is associated with greatest reduction in hematoma growth after acute intracerebral hemorrhage. Hypertension. 2010;56:852–8.

24. Delcourt C, Huang Y, Wang J, Heeley E, Lindley R, Stapf C, Tzourio C, Arima H, Parsons M, Sun J, Neal B, Chalmers J, Anderson C. The second (main) phase of an open, randomised, multicentre study to investigate the effectiveness of an intensive blood pressure reduction in acute cerebral haemorrhage trial (INTERACT2). Int J Stroke. 2010;5:110–6.

25. Nilsson OG, Lindgren A, Stahl N, Brandt L, Saveland H. Incidence of intracerebral and subarachnoid haemorrhage in southern Sweden. J Neurol Neurosurg Psychiatry. 2000;69:601–7.

26. Morgenstern LB, Hemphill 3rd JC, Anderson C, Becker K, Broderick JP, Connolly Jr ES, Greenberg SM, Huang JN, MacDonald RL, Messe SR, Mitchell PH, Selim M, Tamargo RJ. Guidelines for the management of spontaneous intracerebral hemorrhage: a guideline for healthcare professionals from the American Heart Association/American Stroke Association. Stroke. 2010;41:2108–29.

27. Hung A, Singh S, Tait RC. A prospective randomized study to determine the optimal dose of intravenous vitamin K in reversal of over-warfarinization. Br J Haematol. 2000;109:537–9.

28. Watson HG, Baglin T, Laidlaw SL, Makris M, Preston FE. A comparison of the efficacy and rate of response to oral and intravenous vitamin K in reversal of over-anticoagulation with warfarin. Br J Haematol. 2001;115:145–9.

29. Mayer SA, Brun NC, Begtrup K, Broderick J, Davis S, Diringer MN, Skolnick BE, Steiner T. Recombinant activated factor VII for acute intracerebral hemorrhage. N Engl J Med. 2005;352:777–85.

30. Mayer SA, Brun NC, Begtrup K, Broderick J, Davis S, Diringer MN, Skolnick BE, Steiner T. Efficacy and safety of recombinant activated factor VII for acute intracerebral hemorrhage. N Engl J Med. 2008;358:2127–37.

31. Mokri B. The Monro-Kellie hypothesis: applications in CSF volume depletion. Neurology. 2001;56:1746–8.

32. Diringer MN, Zazulia AR. Osmotic therapy: fact and fiction. Neurocrit Care. 2004;1:219–33.

33. Schwartz ML, Tator CH, Rowed DW, Reid SR, Meguro K, Andrews DF. The University of Toronto head injury treatment study: a prospective, randomized comparison of pentobarbital and mannitol. Can J Neurol Sci. 1984;11:434–40.

34. Kamel H, Navi BB, Nakagawa K, Hemphill 3rd JC, Ko NU. Hypertonic saline versus mannitol for the treatment of elevated intracranial pressure: a meta-analysis of randomized clinical trials. Crit Care Med. 2011;39:554–9.

35. Broderick J, Connolly S, Feldmann E, Hanley D, Kase C, Krieger D, Mayberg M, Morgenstern L, Ogilvy CS, Vespa P, Zuccarello M. Guidelines for the management of spontaneous intracerebral hemorrhage in adults: 2007 update: a guideline from the American Heart Association/American Stroke Association Stroke Council, High Blood Pressure Research Council, and the Quality of Care and Outcomes in Research Interdisciplinary Working Group. Circulation. 2007;116:e391–413.

36. Hofmeister C, Stapf C, Hartmann A, Sciacca RR, Mansmann U, terBrugge K, Lasjaunias P, Mohr JP, Mast H, Meisel J. Demographic, morphological, and clinical characteristics of 1289 patients with brain arteriovenous malformation. Stroke. 2000;31:1307–10.

37. Hoh BL, Chapman PH, Loeffler JS, Carter BS, Ogilvy CS. Results of multimodality treatment for 141 patients with brain arteriovenous malformations and seizures: factors associated with seizure incidence and seizure outcomes. Neurosurgery. 2002;51:303–9; discussion 309–11.

38. Lanzino G, Kongable GL, Kassell NF. Electrocardiographic abnormalities after nontraumatic subarachnoid hemorrhage. J Neurosurg Anesthesiol. 1994;6:156–62.

39. Wells C, Cujec B, Johnson D, Goplen G. Reversibility of severe left ventricular dysfunction in patients with subarachnoid hemorrhage. Am Heart J. 1995;129:409–12.

40. Rahman M, Friedman WA. Hyponatremia in neurosurgical patients: clinical guidelines development. Neurosurgery. 2009;65:925–35; discussion 935–6.

41. Kidwell CS, Hsia AW. Imaging of the brain and cerebral vasculature in patients with suspected stroke: advantages and disadvantages of CT and MRI. Curr Neurol Neurosci Rep. 2006;6:9–16.

42. Kidwell CS, Wintermark M. The role of CT and MRI in the emergency evaluation of persons with suspected stroke. Curr Neurol Neurosci Rep. 2010;10:21–8.

43. Delgado Almandoz JE, Romero JM. Advanced CT Imaging in the evaluation of hemorrhagic stroke. Neuroimaging Clin N Am. 2011;21:197–213.

44. Kokkinis C, Vlychou M, Zavras GM, Hadjigeorgiou GM, Papadimitriou A, Fezoulidis IV. The role of 3D-computed tomography angiography (3D-CTA) in investigation of spontaneous subarachnoid haemorrhage: comparison with digital subtraction angiography (DSA) and surgical findings. Br J Neurosurg. 2008;22:71–8.

45. Zhao J, Wang S, Li J, Qi W, Sui D, Zhao Y. Clinical characteristics and surgical results of patients with cerebral arteriovenous malformations. Surg Neurol. 2005;63:156–61; discussion 161.

46. Cunha e Sa MJ, Stein BM, Solomon RA, McCormick PC. The treatment of associated intracranial aneurysms and arteriovenous malformations. J Neurosurg. 1992;77:853–9.

47. Morgan MK, Sekhon LH, Finfer S, Grinnell V. Delayed neurological deterioration following resection of arteriovenous malformations of the brain. J Neurosurg. 1999;90:695–701.

48. Yokobori S, Watanabe A, Nakae R, Onda H, Fuse A, Kushimoto S, Yokota H. Cerebral vasospasms after intraventricular hemorrhage from an arteriovenous malformation: case report. Neurol Med Chir (Tokyo). 2010;50:320–3.

49. Sinha PK, Neema PK, Rathod RC. Anesthesia and intracranial arteriovenous malformation. Neurol India. 2004;52:163–70.

50. Jaeger K, Ruschulte H, Herzog T, Heine J, Leuwer M, Piepenbrock S. Anaesthesiological and criterial care aspects regarding the treatment of patients with arteriovenous malformations in interventional neuroradiology. Minim Invasive Neurosurg. 2000;43:102–5.

51. Spetzler RF, Martin NA. A proposed grading system for arteriovenous malformations. J Neurosurg. 1986;65:476–83.

52. Heros RC, Korosue K, Diebold PM. Surgical excision of cerebral arteriovenous malformations: late results. Neurosurgery. 1990;26:570–7; discussion 577–8.

53. Hamilton MG, Spetzler RF. The prospective application of a grading system for arteriovenous malformations. Neurosurgery. 1994;34:2–6; discussion 6–7.

54. Schaller C, Schramm J, Haun D. Significance of factors contributing to surgical complications and to late outcome after elective surgery of cerebral arteriovenous malformations. J Neurol Neurosurg Psychiatry. 1998;65:547–54.

55. Hartmann A, Stapf C, Hofmeister C, Mohr JP, Sciacca RR, Stein BM, Faulstich A, Mast H. Determinants of neurological outcome after surgery for brain arteriovenous malformation. Stroke. 2000;31:2361–4.

56. Davidson AS, Morgan MK. How safe is arteriovenous malformation surgery? A prospective, observational study of surgery as first-line treatment for brain arteriovenous malformations. Neurosurgery. 2010;66:498–504; discussion 504–5.

57. Lawton MT, Kim H, McCulloch CE, Mikhak B, Young WL. A supplementary grading scale for selecting patients with brain arteriovenous malformations for surgery. Neurosurgery. 2010;66:702–13; discussion 713.

58. Spetzler RF, Ponce FA. A 3-tier classification of cerebral arteriovenous malformations. Clinical article. J Neurosurg. 2011;114:842–9.

59. Tamaki N, Ehara K, Lin TK, Kuwamura K, Obora Y, Kanazawa Y, Yamashita H, Matsumoto S. Cerebral arteriovenous malformations: factors influencing the surgical difficulty and outcome. Neurosurgery. 1991;29:856–61; discussion 861–3.

60. Hollerhage HG. Cerebral arteriovenous malformations: factors influencing surgical difficulty and outcome. Neurosurgery. 1992;31:604–5.

61. Spears J, Terbrugge KG, Moosavian M, Montanera W, Willinsky RA, Wallace MC, Tymianski M. A discriminative prediction model of neurological outcome for patients undergoing surgery of brain arteriovenous malformations. Stroke. 2006;37:1457–64.

62. Goodkin R, McKhann 2nd GM, Haynor DR, Mayberg MR, Eskridge JM, Winn HR. Persistent feeding arteries to angiographically completely embolized arteriovenous malformation demonstrated by intraoperative color-flow Doppler testing: report of two cases. Surg Neurol. 1995;44:326–32; discussion 332–3.

63. Standard SC, Guterman LR, Chavis TD, Hopkins LN. Delayed recanalization of a cerebral arteriovenous malformation following angiographic obliteration with polyvinyl alcohol embolization. Surg Neurol. 1995;44:109–12; discussion 112–3.

64. Gobin YP, Laurent A, Merienne L, Schlienger M, Aymard A, Houdart E, Casasco A, Lefkopoulos D, George B, Merland JJ. Treatment of brain arteriovenous malformations by embolization and radiosurgery. J Neurosurg. 1996;85:19–28.

65. Hurst RW, Berenstein A, Kupersmith MJ, Madrid M, Flamm ES. Deep central arteriovenous malformations of the brain: the role of endovascular treatment. J Neurosurg. 1995;82:190–5.

66. Paulsen RD, Steinberg GK, Norbash AM, Marcellus ML, Lopez JR, Marks MP. Embolization of rolandic cortex arteriovenous malformations. Neurosurgery. 1999;44:479–84; discussion 484–6.

67. Deruty R, Pelissou-Guyotat I, Morel C, Bascoulergue Y, Turjman F. Reflections on the management of cerebral arteriovenous malformations. Surg Neurol. 1998;50:245–55; discussion 255–6.

68. Gross BA, Duckworth EA, Getch CC, Bendok BR, Batjer HH. Challenging traditional beliefs: microsurgery for arteriovenous malformations of the basal ganglia and thalamus. Neurosurgery. 2008;63:393–410; discussion 410–1.

69. Steinberg GK, Fabrikant JI, Marks MP, Levy RP, Frankel KA, Phillips MH, Shuer LM, Silverberg GD. Stereotactic heavy-charged-particle Bragg-peak radiation for intracranial arteriovenous malformations. N Engl J Med. 1990;323:96–101.

70. Lunsford LD, Kondziolka D, Flickinger JC, Bissonette DJ, Jungreis CA, Maitz AH, Horton JA, Coffey RJ. Stereotactic radiosurgery for arteriovenous malformations of the brain. J Neurosurg. 1991;75:512–24.

71. Friedman WA. Radiosurgery for arteriovenous malformations. Clin Neurosurg. 1995;42:328–47.

72. Ellis TL, Friedman WA, Bova FJ, Kubilis PS, Buatti JM. Analysis of treatment failure after radiosurgery for arteriovenous malformations. J Neurosurg. 1998;89:104–10.

73. Chang JH, Chang JW, Park YG, Chung SS. Factors related to complete occlusion of arteriovenous malformations after gamma knife radiosurgery. J Neurosurg. 2000;93 Suppl 3:96–101.

74. Guo WY. Radiological aspects of gamma knife radiosurgery for arteriovenous malformations and other non-tumoural disorders of the brain. Acta Radiol Suppl. 1993;388:1–34.

75. Yoshimoto T, Takahashi A, Kinouchi H, Mizoi K, Jokura H. Role of embolization in the management of arteriovenous malformations. Clin Neurosurg. 1995;42:313–27.

76. Henkes H, Nahser HC, Berg-Dammer E, Weber W, Lange S, Kuhne D. Endovascular therapy of brain AVMs prior to radiosurgery. Neurol Res. 1998;20:479–92.

77. Pollock BE, Flickinger JC, Lunsford LD, Maitz A, Kondziolka D. Factors associated with successful arteriovenous malformation radiosurgery. Neurosurgery. 1998;42:1239–44; discussion 1244–7.

78. Miyawaki L, Dowd C, Wara W, Goldsmith B, Albright N, Gutin P, Halbach V, Hieshima G, Higashida R, Lulu B, Pitts L, Schell M, Smith V, Weaver K, Wilson C, Larson D. Five year results of LINAC radiosurgery for arteriovenous malformations: outcome for large AVMS. Int J Radiat Oncol Biol Phys. 1999;44:1089–106.

79. Schlienger M, Atlan D, Lefkopoulos D, Merienne L, Touboul E, Missir O, Nataf F, Mammar H, Platoni K, Grandjean P, Foulquier JN, Huart J, Oppenheim C, Meder JF, Houdart E, Merland JJ. Linac radiosurgery for cerebral arteriovenous malformations: results in 169 patients. Int J Radiat Oncol Biol Phys. 2000;46:1135–42.

80. Andrade-Souza YM, Ramani M, Scora D, Tsao MN, terBrugge K, Schwartz ML. Embolization before radiosurgery reduces the obliteration rate of arteriovenous malformations. Neurosurgery. 2007;60:443–51; discussion 451–2.

81. Betti OO, Munari C, Rosler R. Stereotactic radiosurgery with the linear accelerator: treatment of arteriovenous malformations. Neurosurgery. 1989;24:311–21.

82. Friedman WA, Bova FJ, Bollampally S, Bradshaw P. Analysis of factors predictive of success or complications in arteriovenous malformation radiosurgery. Neurosurgery. 2003;52:296–307; discussion 307–8.

83. Andrade-Souza YM, Ramani M, Scora D, Tsao MN, TerBrugge K, Schwartz ML. Radiosurgical treatment for rolandic arteriovenous malformations. J Neurosurg. 2006;105:689–97.

84. Liscak R, Vladyka V, Simonova G, Urgosik D, Novotny Jr J, Janouskova L, Vymazal J. Arteriovenous malformations after Leksell gamma knife radiosurgery: rate of obliteration and complications. Neurosurgery. 2007;60:1005–14; discussion 1015–6.

85. Steiner L, Lindquist C, Cail W, Karlsson B, Steiner M. Microsurgery and radiosurgery in brain arteriovenous malformations. J Neurosurg. 1993;79:647–52.

86. Colombo F, Pozza F, Chierego G, Francescon P, Casentini L, De Luca G. Linear accelerator radiosurgery of cerebral arteriovenous malformations: current status. Acta Neurochir Suppl. 1994;62:5–9.

87. Bollet MA, Anxionnat R, Buchheit I, Bey P, Cordebar A, Jay N, Desandes E, Marchal C, Lapeyre M, Aletti P, Picard L. Efficacy and morbidity of arc-therapy radiosurgery for cerebral arteriovenous malformations: a comparison with the natural history. Int J Radiat Oncol Biol Phys. 2004;58:1353–63.

88. Pollock BE, Lunsford LD, Kondziolka D, Maitz A, Flickinger JC. Patient outcomes after stereotactic radiosurgery for "operable" arteriovenous malformations. Neurosurgery. 1994;35:1–7; discussion 7–8.

89. Friedman WA, Blatt DL, Bova FJ, Buatti JM, Mendenhall WM, Kubilis PS. The risk of hemorrhage after radiosurgery for arteriovenous malformations. J Neurosurg. 1996;84:912–9.

90. Firlik AD, Levy EI, Kondziolka D, Yonas H. Staged volume radiosurgery followed by microsurgical resection: a novel treatment for giant cerebral arteriovenous malformations: technical case report. Neurosurgery. 1998;43:1223–8.

91. Pollock BE, Kline RW, Stafford SL, Foote RL, Schomberg PJ. The rationale and technique of staged-volume arteriovenous malformation radiosurgery. Int J Radiat Oncol Biol Phys. 2000;48:817–24.

92. Tew Jr JM, Lewis AI, Reichert KW. Management strategies and surgical techniques for deep-seated supratentorial arteriovenous malformations. Neurosurgery. 1995;36:1065–72.

93. O'Shaughnessy BA, Getch CC, Bendok BR, Batjer HH. Microsurgical resection of infratentorial arteriovenous malformations. Neurosurg Focus. 2005;19:E5.

94. Batjer H, Samson D. Surgical approaches to trigonal arteriovenous malformations. J Neurosurg. 1987;67:511–7.

95. Lee JP. Surgical treatment of thalamic arteriovenous malformations. Neurosurgery. 1993;32:498–503; discussion 503–4.

96. Lewis AI, Tew Jr JM. Management of thalamic-basal ganglia and brain-stem vascular malformations. Clin Neurosurg. 1994;41:83–111.

97. Kader A, Young WL. The effects of intracranial arteriovenous malformations on cerebral hemodynamics. Neurosurg Clin N Am. 1996;7:767–81.

98. Hacein-Bey L, Young WL. Hemodynamic perturbations in cerebral arteriovenous malformations and management implications. Interv Neuroradiol. 1999;5:177–82.

Traumatic Brain Injury: Evidence-Based Medicine, Diagnosis, and Treatment

27

Andres Fernandez, Kristine H. O'Phelan, and M. Ross Bullock

Contents

Abstract

Traumatic brain injury (TBI) is a major cause of death and disability worldwide. The initial trauma triggers a complex cascade of cellular and tissue changes with subsequent secondary injury of the vulnerable brain. Injury can result from derangements of multiple physiological parameters including blood pressure, intracranial pressure, oxygenation, and temperature. The monitoring and treatment of the multiple physiological derangements that can result after TBI are an important aspect of the intensive care management of this patient population, but the specific treatment thresholds for each variable and their relationship to outcome are varied. The focus of this chapter is on severe traumatic brain injury and its treatment with an emphasis on the recommendations from the guidelines of the Brain Trauma Foundation.

Keywords

Trauma • Traumatic brain injury • Intracranial pressure • Brain oxygenation

A. Fernandez, MD
Division of Neurocritical Care, Department of Neurology,
Columbia University, 177 Fort Washington Avenue,
Milstein 8 Center Room 300, New York, NY 10032, USA
e-mail: Af2240@columbia.edu

K.H. O'Phelan, MD
Neurocritical Care Division, Department of Neurology,
University of Miami Miller School of Medicine,
1120 NW 14th Str, Suite 1358, Miami, FL 33136, USA
e-mail: kphelan@med.miami.edu

M.R. Bullock, MD, PhD (✉)
Department of Neurosurgery,
University of Miami/Jackson Memorial Hospital,
1095 NW 14th Terrace, Miami, FL 33136, USA
e-mail: rbullock@med.miami.edu

Epidemiology

Traumatic brain injury (TBI) is the largest cause of death and disability in persons under the age of 45 years, worldwide. According to the latest report on traumatic brain injury in the USA from the Centers for Disease Control and Prevention (CDC), 1.7 million people sustain a TBI annually in the USA [1]. This report identifying TBI cases using the CDC's definition [2] calculates estimates for traumatic brain injuries using emergency department visits, hospitalizations, and deaths based on three national data sources for the years 2002–2006.

TBIs comprised 4.8 and 15.1 % of all injury-related emergency department visits and hospitalizations, respectively.

A.J. Layon et al. (eds.), *Textbook of Neurointensive Care*,
DOI 10.1007/978-1-4471-5226-2_27, © Springer-Verlag London 2013

TBI was a contributing factor in 30.5 % of all injury-related deaths. The CDC report estimated an average age-adjusted annual rate of 468 per 100,000 population TBI-related emergency department visits, 93.6 per 100,000 population TBI-related hospitalizations, and 17.4 per 100,000 population TBI-related deaths [1]. Children, older adolescents, and adults over 65 years old were more likely to sustain a TBI. The highest rates of TBI-related hospitalization and death occurred among adults over 75 years old. Overall, there were approximately 1.4 times as many TBIs in males compared to females [1].

Falls were the leading cause of TBI (35.2 %) and to a greater proportion (60.7 %) in the age group 65 years and older. Falls constituted the greatest number of TBI-related emergency department visits and hospitalizations. Motor vehicle traffic was the second leading cause of TBI (17.3 %) and resulted in the largest percentage of TBI-related deaths (31.8 %), with an average annual rate of 5.6 per 100,000 population compared to 3.3 per 100,000 population TBI-related deaths for the falls category [1].

The incidence of TBI, rate of hospitalization, and subsequent mortality are quite variable across different European countries [3]. The incidence of TBI ranged from 91 to 546 per 100,000 population, and mortality ranged from 5 to 24 per 100,000 population. Of note, out of 13 studies with data on mechanism of injury, most had motor vehicle-related causes as the leading cause of TBI.

Several TBI studies from Asia, Australia, and New Zealand have shown the significant role of motor vehicle and traffic accidents in TBI [4, 5]. In one study of patients with traumatic brain injury in Australia and New Zealand [4], 61 % had TBI due to vehicular trauma. Another study used data on hospitalized patients in South Australia to calculate a statewide incidence of TBI of 322 per 100,000 population, and transport accidents represented 57 % of admissions [5].

In a study of TBI in China, 86 % of the traffic accident TBI patients were motorcyclist, pedestrians, or cyclists, with only 14 % being motor vehicle occupants [6], and there was a nearly twofold increase in TBI caused by traffic accidents compared to a previous survey [7]. Similarly, traffic-related injuries accounted for 45–60 % of brain injury in a review of TBI studies in India [8]. Nakamura and coworkers [9] analyzed national traffic accident data from Japan and reported that even though there was an increase in traffic accidents, there was a decrease in traffic related deaths, with the most significant factor reported to be the reduction of deaths related to head injury. The use of seat belts and helmets and preventive measures for pedestrians and cyclists along with improvement in emergency and neurosurgical care are proposed to have played a role in the decreased mortality from traffic-related head injury [9].

Several limitations and challenges involved in the study of the epidemiology of TBI have been described in the literature [1, 10–12]. These limitations include different study methods, underestimation of TBI due to patients treated in the outpatient setting, exclusion of patients who did not seek medical attention, exclusion of TBI cases from federal, military, or VA hospitals, and limitations relating to coding used to identify the TBI cases [1, 10]. The use of ICD-9 codes to classify subjects in TBI studies also limits the accuracy of the data in TBI studies [11]. Worldwide, TBI incidence is rising, especially in areas with increasing motorization and urbanization, like Asia, South America, and India. In most western countries, TBI due to vehicular accidents is declining, but, sadly, firearm-related TBI continues to increase in the USA.

Pathophysiology

There are cascades of cellular and tissue derangements which are set in motion after an initial traumatic event. Shear forces damage vascular structures and cause direct axonal injury. There is cell membrane depolarization with neurotransmitter release and resulting excitotoxicity [13]. Oxidative stress, inflammation, and calcium-mediated mitochondrial dysfunction also play an important role [14, 15]. Intracellular levels of calcium are elevated in neurons after TBI, leading to the activation of multiple intracellular enzymes which impair mitochondrial function and result in energy failure, apoptosis, and necrotic cell death [16, 17]. Unfortunately, cerebral blood flow is frequently decreased in the first days after TBI. Episodes of ischemia are not uncommon in this population and are a major target for intervention in the critical care of patients with TBI [18]. In addition to decreased cerebral blood flow, brain glucose metabolism may be initially increased and then depressed [19, 20]. This dynamic metabolic impairment serves to heighten brain tissue vulnerability after trauma. These alterations of metabolism and blood flow can be demonstrated at the bedside by low brain tissue oxygen tension and deranged brain chemistry seen with microdialysis monitoring (Chaps. 7 and 8).

This environment of high energy requirements in the setting of impaired substrate delivery caused by systemic hypotension, hypoxia, and local mass effect from elevated intracranial pressure has potentially disastrous consequences. In total, these factors lead to secondary insults that are often fatal to exquisitely vulnerable neural tissue.

Diagnosis

Traumatic brain injury (TBI) has a broad spectrum of severity, pathology, physiology, and sequelae. Because of this, there are numerous ways in which to describe and classify TBI.

Table 27.1 Glasgow Coma Scale

Eye opening	
Spontaneous	4
To sound	3
To pain	2
None	1
Verbal response	
Oriented	5
Confused conversation	4
Inappropriate words	3
Incomprehensible sounds	2
None	1
Motor response	
Obeys commands	6
Localize to pain	5
Flexion (withdrawal)	4
Flexion (abnormal)	3
Extension	2
None	1

Adapted with kind permission of Springer Science + Business Media from Teasdale and Jennett [21]

Primary brain injury is commonly described as those events associated with the acute impact or event. This includes acute depolarization of neuronal membranes and efflux of excitatory neurotransmitters such as glutamate as well as shearing injury to axons and vascular structures.

Secondary injury includes a constellation of hemodynamic, electrical, and metabolic events which can impair the adequate delivery of metabolic substrate and may increase tissue demand. These include hypotension, hypoxia, fever, seizures, elevated intracranial pressure, and anemia.

Mechanistic descriptions of TBI are common: for example, blunt force as opposed to penetrating or blast injury. The terms "mild," "moderate," and "severe" are often used to categorize patients. This is a clinical approach that uses the Glasgow Coma Scale (GCS, Table 27.1) [21] to stratify patients with mild GCS 13–15, moderate GCS 9–12, and severe GCS 3–8.

Categorization of TBI based on the initial CT scan can use an imaging grading system such as the Marshall CT score or the Rotterdam score [22, 23] or describe the structural lesions seen on CT such as subdural, epidural, intraparenchymal hematomas, traumatic subarachnoid hemorrhage, or axonal shearing injury.

In reality, each of these approaches has some strengths and weaknesses, and none are able to completely encompass the heterogeneity of clinical TBI. A combination of a clinical and image-based description is often helpful. For example, a patient has a "severe TBI with an acute subdural and midline shift" would be likely to need urgent surgical therapy.

Patients who sustain a TBI often have associated injuries to the chest, abdomen, or limbs. The Injury Severity Scale (ISS) [24] is often used to document the combined impact of multiple injuries. Patients with TBI and polytrauma are at risk for hypoxic and ischemic complications that may increase their risk of secondary brain injury. Such patients are among the most challenging for the neuro-intensivist to treat, yet their outcome maybe excellent.

Treatment of Severe TBI

The Brain Trauma Foundation (BTF) have five sets of published guidelines on the management of TBI [25]. These include guidelines on medical management, surgical management, field management of combat related injury, prehospital management, and management of pediatric TBI. These form the foundation of evidence-based clinical therapy of patients with acute traumatic brain injuries.

A key aspect in the intensive care management of patients with severe TBI relates to the monitoring, maintenance, and treatment of derangements of multiple physiological parameters that are potential causes for secondary injury in the vulnerable TBI brain. The specific treatment thresholds to target for these variables and the relationship of the different physiological parameters—individually or in combination—to outcome vary depending on the particular variable and at times are not well defined.

Some of the physiological parameters that have been studied in the severe TBI population include blood pressure (BP), intracranial pressure (ICP), cerebral perfusion pressure (CPP), systemic oxygenation, brain oxygen tension (PbtO$_2$), brain chemistry (measured with cerebral microdialysis), and brain temperature (Table 27.2). It is intuitive that derangements in the physiological variables such as hypotension, hypoxia, high ICP, and fever should be avoided, but the range of values in which to maintain the different parameters is not always well defined. Other variables such as CPP, brain oxygen, and brain chemistry also lack consistent treatment threshold values.

Blood pressure, temperature, and oxygenation (PaO$_2$ and SaO$_2$) monitoring should be routinely performed in patients with severe TBI, and ICP monitoring is indicated in most cases. Specifically, patients in coma, with an abnormal CT scan, or those with a nonrevealing CT scan and older age, hypotension, or posturing on exam should receive ICP monitoring. Other variables such as indexes of autoregulation, PbtO$_2$, and measures of brain chemistry by microdialysis may be useful in directing and optimizing the clinical management of these patients. The advent of multimodality monitoring has opened an avenue for exploring the impact of multiple physiological measures on secondary injury and outcome after TBI.

Table 27.2 Key physiological parameters in severe TBI (based on the BTF guidelines)

Blood pressure	Avoid systolic blood pressure <90 mmHg
	Admission hypotension is associated with poor outcome
Oxygenation	Avoid PaO_2 <60 mmHg and SaO_2 <90 %
	Hypoxia on admission is associated with poor outcome
Temperature	Avoid fever (temp >38.3)
Intracranial pressure	Treatment of ICP above 20 mmHg is recommended
Cerebral perfusion pressure (CPP)	A CPP value of approximately 60 mmHg is recommended
	Attempts to keep CPP above 70 mmHg with fluids and pressors are discouraged due to the risk of ARDS
	CPP <50 mmHg should be avoided
Brain oxygen	$PbtO_2$ <15 mmHg and SjO_2 <50 % are recommended as treatment thresholds

Blood Pressure

Hemodynamic monitoring after severe TBI for the avoidance and timely treatment of systemic hypotension (systolic BP <90 mmHg) is a BTF level II recommendation. Several studies show an association between both prehospital and in-hospital hypotension and increased morbidity and mortality [25]. A SBP threshold of 90 mmHg is recommended. Strong data to support maintaining higher SBP are lacking. However, in selected patients, maintaining higher mean arterial pressures may be of value [25]. Additional monitoring modalities, like brain tissue oxygen tension, may help establish appropriate thresholds for a specific patient. The IMPACT (International Mission on Prognosis and Analysis of Clinical Trials) database of TBI [26] compiled data from over 9,000 patients with severe and moderate brain injuries from eight randomized placebo control trials and three observational surveys [26]. This database yielded two observations about blood pressure in patients with acute traumatic brain injuries. There was an 18 % overall prevalence of hypotension on admission, and this was identified as a marker of poor outcome [27]. Furthermore, a U-shaped relationship was found between admission blood pressure and outcome with no obvious threshold effect. The relationship of high blood pressure and outcome was thought to be secondary to increased intracranial pressure as there were higher rates of low motor scores and increased number of mass lesions in patients with SBP >150 mmHg on enrollment. The direct correlation between admission blood pressure and ICP could not be made since ICP was not directly monitored on admission [28].

Systemic Oxygenation

The guidelines offer a level III recommendation supporting the use of oximetry to avoid systemic hypoxia (PaO_2 <60 mmHg or SaO_2 <90 %) [25]. Similar to hypotension, hypoxia is a strong predictor of poor outcome after TBI. McHugh and colleagues analyzed secondary insults (hypotension, hypoxia, and hypothermia) occurring prior to or on admission and their relation to outcome. They reported an overall prevalence of 20 % for hypoxia on admission and identified it as a significant predictor for adverse outcome [27].

Temperature Management

Clinical trials in the area of prophylactic hypothermia in patients with traumatic brain injury have yielded variable results. Overall, there was no clear demonstration of a reduction in all-cause mortality with multiple potential confounders being identified including baseline temperature [25]. The BTF guidelines gave a level III recommendation for prophylactic hypothermia in patients with traumatic brain injury when target temperatures are maintained for more than 48 h based on preliminary findings of reduced mortality [25].

Given the inconsistency of previous trials, the National Acute Brain Injury Study: Hypothermia II (NABIS: HII) trial randomized 232 severe brain injury patients within 2.5 h after injury to hypothermia or normothermia. Ninety-seven patients were included for the primary analysis. No significant difference in outcome was found in the hypothermia group compared to the normothermia group. In subgroup analyses, patients with surgically evacuated hematomas had an improved outcome with hypothermia compared to normothermia. This effect was not seen in the diffuse brain injury group. These authors conclude that further testing of the role of early hypothermia in patients with evacuated hematomas is warranted [29].

Intracranial Pressure (Table 27.3)

Monitoring

The BTF guidelines give a level II recommendation to monitor ICP in salvageable severe TBI patients with abnormal brain CT (a CT scan demonstrating hematomas, contusions, swelling, herniation, or compressed basal cisterns). In patients with a normal brain CT scan, a level III

Table 27.3 ICP management protocol. Targets: Overall aim is to optimize brain perfusion and avoid secondary injury. CPP 60–70 mmHg; ICP <20 mmHg; Temperature <37.5 C; CVP 6–10; maintain CPP with fluids and vasopressors as needed

Stage 1
Head of the bed to 30°
Optimize sedation
Optimize analgesia
Ventilation to normocarbia
Normothermia
Vent ventricular drain for 5 min at a time if ICP >20 mmHg for >5 min
Stage 2
Osmotherapy (see text for discussion)
Stage 3
Mild hyperventilation (use as temporizing measure and avoid in first 24 h after TBI)
Mild hypothermia (34–35 °C using cooling catheter or surface cooling device)
Neuromuscular paralysis
Stage 4
Barbiturates
Decompressive craniectomy for refractory ICP

Adapted from the NSICU University of Miami/Jackson Memorial Hospital protocol
Reproduced with kind permission of Springer Science + Business Media from O'Phelan et al. [56]
*Consider obtaining CT Head at any stage to assess for surgically treatable changes (see discussion on surgical decompression)

recommendation is given for ICP monitoring if two or more of the following features (age >40 years, motor posturing or SBP <90) are present given their risk of high ICP [25]. The guidelines note that ICP is useful for guiding therapy; it can be an early indicator of an evolving mass lesion and is necessary for determination of CPP. ICP lowering treatment without the use of ICP monitoring is not recommended [25].

ICP Treatment

The guidelines give a level II recommendation to treat ICP above 20 mmHg [25]. The management of elevated ICP generally follows a stepwise approach. Initial steps include general measures such as positioning the head of the bed at 30°, providing adequate analgesia and sedation, normalizing pCO_2 and temperature, and CSF drainage. If ICP is not controlled after this initial stage, potential therapies include osmotherapy, hyperventilation, paralysis, hypothermia, and consideration of surgical decompression and barbiturates (discussed later in this chapter).

Osmotherapy

There is a level II recommendation for the use of mannitol to control raised intracranial pressure at doses of 0.25–1 g/kg. There is also a level III recommendation to avoid the use of

mannitol: when ICP monitoring has not been established except in cases of transtentorial herniation or rapidly progressive neurological deterioration not attributable to extracranial causes [25]. There are insufficient data to provide a recommendation regarding the use of continuous vs. intermittent infusions of mannitol. Similarly, there is a lack of evidence to support the recommendations on whether hypertonic saline (HTS) treatment should be used as a bolus or continuous infusion and what the optimal concentration used should be [25]. In general, serum osmolality and sodium should be measured every 4 h to guide osmotic therapy. Mannitol should not be administered if the serum osmolality exceeds 320 mOsm. If hypertonic saline is being administered concomitantly, the osmolar gap can be calculated to monitor renal clearance of mannitol. Mannitol doses should be held if the osmolar gap exceeds 10 mmol/L.

Sorani and colleagues [30] report that mannitol lowers ICP in a dose-dependent fashion with 100 gm doses resulting in a larger and more long lasting reduction in ICP than a 50 gm dose. Interestingly, patients with ICP lower than 20 mmHg at the time of mannitol administration had a lower decrease in ICP, which they conclude argues against prophylactic mannitol administration [30]. Ideally, mannitol dosing should be individualized according to each patient's potential for complications and their need for ICP control. Oddo and coworkers [31] compared hypertonic saline to mannitol for refractory ICP elevation. They found that hypertonic saline reduced ICP as well as improved brain oxygen, CPP, and cardiac output when given as a second tier therapy for refractory ICP in patients with severe TBI. They analyzed 12 patients who had severe TBI, ICP, and $PbtO_2$ monitoring and were treated with mannitol (25 %, 0.75 g/kg) for ICP >20 mmHg or hypertonic saline (7.5 %, 250 ml) if mannitol did not control ICP. Hypertonic saline was associated with an improvement in $PbtO_2$, whereas mannitol was not. They also observed lower ICP and higher CPP and cardiac output with hypertonic saline. The impact of HTS on $PbtO_2$ was thought to be possibly due to its effects on CBF or due to cardiac output augmentation with subsequent increase in oxygen delivery or improvement of flow in the cerebral microcirculation. The authors acknowledge that the question of the superiority of HTS vs. mannitol cannot be drawn from their study given limitations that include small numbers and the treatments not being compared in parallel (HTS was administered after mannitol in all patients); also, there may have been a cumulative effect and the fact that the treatments were not given in equi-osmolar doses [31]. Other studies have also shown the effects of HTS on CPP, brain oxygenation, and ICP. Pascual and coworkers [32] reported a study of 12 hypotensive patients with severe TBI who had CPP and $PbtO_2$ monitoring and received HTS infusions (250 cc of 7.5 % saline over 30 min). HTS administration resulted in ICP reductions by more than 45 % and elevation of CPP and brain oxygen [32]. In another study examining the role of 23.4 % hypertonic saline in patients with severe TBI, Rockswold and colleagues reported 25 patients who received 30 ml of 23.4 % hypertonic saline boluses for ICP >20 mmHg after having failed mild hyperventilation, CSF drainage, and sedation. There was a decrease in ICP with increase in CPP levels and $PbtO_2$ values, with a more significant response in patients with higher baseline ICP and lower CPP [33].

There are currently no definitive data to support the use of one osmotic agent over another (mannitol vs. HTS) for the treatment of elevated ICP. Given the different potential benefits and complication profiles for each therapy, the patient's renal, cardiac, electrolyte, and hemodynamic status may play a role in the determination of which therapy to use in a given patient, e.g., HTS in the setting of hypotension and renal failure vs. mannitol in the setting of hypernatremia or volume overload. Neuro-intensivists should be aware of the potential for cumulative nephrotoxicity in septic patients, those on aminoglycoside antibiotics, the elderly, and those with a history of renal disease, and avoid high osmolarity (>320 mOsm) in those cases in particular.

Hyperventilation

The BTF guidelines give a level II recommendation against the use of prophylactic hyperventilation given the significant risk of cerebral ischemia. A level III recommendation is given for the use of hyperventilation as a temporizing measure for ICP reduction and against its use in the first 24 h after TBI when CBF is often low. Monitoring of oxygen delivery with the use of a brain tissue oxygen monitor or jugular saturation monitor is recommended if hyperventilation is used [25].

Paralysis

In a retrospective review of 514 patients from the traumatic coma data bank, Hsiang and colleagues compared patients that had pharmacological paralysis early in the ICU course and lasting for at least 12 h to patients that did not receive paralytics. They suggested that early routine use of paralytics for ICP management does not improve overall outcome and can lead to greater ICU stay and higher rate of complications such as pneumonia [34]. The use of paralytics in the management of elevated intracranial pressure should be reserved to refractory cases despite the use of first-line therapies.

Hypothermia

The European Society of Intensive Care Medicine is conducting a large multicenter trial (Eurotherm 3235 trial) to study the effects of hypothermia (32–35 °C) on reducing elevated intracranial pressure (>20 mmHg) and on patient outcome. Subjects are randomized to standard of care or standard of care with titrated hypothermia; hypothermia is maintained for at least 48 h and continued as long as necessary to keep ICP <20 mmHg [35].

Surgical Decompression

Some patients will require surgical therapy for their traumatic brain injury. The available literature suggests that the speed and aggressiveness of surgical management will greatly impact patient outcomes [36, 37]. To this end, the Brain Trauma Foundation has developed guidelines for the surgical management of traumatic brain injury based on the available literature published between 1975 and 2001 [38]. We will briefly review the major recommendations and their supporting rationale:

- *Epidural hematoma*: 10 % of patients with severe traumatic brain injury have acute epidural hematomas requiring craniotomy [39, 40]. It is recommended that lesions measuring greater than 30 cc in volume should be surgically evacuated. Nonoperative management is appropriate in awake patients without focal deficits and lesions less than 30 cc, less than 15 mm thickness with less than 5 mm midline shift. The timing of therapy is also important. Comatose patients with pupillary changes should have surgical evacuation as soon as possible. Ipsilateral mydriasis is not associated with adverse outcome if surgical evacuation is performed within 70 min [41]. However, bilateral mydriasis is associated with poor outcomes related to brainstem injury.

- *Acute subdural hematoma*: 15–30 % of severe TBI patients have an acute subdural hematoma on imaging. Surgical evacuation is recommended for lesions that are greater than 10 mm in thickness or associated with a greater than 5 mm midline shift. It is also recommended to perform intracranial pressure monitoring in patients with acute subdural hematomas and a Glasgow Coma Scale score of less than nine. Indications for surgical management of lesions less than 10 mm in thickness or with less than 5 mm shift are recommended if patients deteriorate by two points on the GCS or have an elevated ICP >20.

- *Traumatic parenchymal hemorrhage*: These account for 20 % of operative lesions in patients with severe TBI [42, 43]. Because the mass effect from large parenchymal lesions may cause secondary injury, some patients with this type of injury would likely benefit from surgical therapy. However, the particular characteristics of this group are as yet unclear. The majority of available data are taken from case series and one prospective trial [44]. Thus, the decision to proceed with surgical therapy is often based on a pattern of progressing deficit or uncontrolled ICP. Surgical therapy is recommended for patients with progressive clinical deterioration referable to the lesion, medically refractory elevation in ICP, or evidence of mass effect on CT imaging. Surgical treatment is also recommended for frontotemporal lesions >20 cc in volume associated with midline shift >5 mm or compressed basal cisterns. There is currently insufficient evidence to support a recommendation for decompressive craniectomy vs. craniotomy with lobectomy. Both are treatment options in patients with parenchymal injury and radiographic evidence of impending herniation.

- *Posterior fossa lesions*: Extra-axial lesions in the posterior fossa are relatively rare in severe TBI with the potential to producing rapid clinical deterioration because of the limited size of the posterior fossa and the risk of brainstem compression. Surgical therapy of posterior fossa lesions is recommended if there is evidence of progressive clinical deterioration referable to the lesion or mass effect referable to the lesions such as distortion of the fourth ventricle, compression of the basal cisterns, or obstructive hydrocephalous. Surgical therapy in these patients typically involves evacuation of the hematoma and suboccipital craniectomy.

Steroids

Steroid use is not recommended in TBI [25]. The corticosteroid randomization after significant head injury (CRASH) trial randomized 10,008 head injury patients within 8 h of injury to a 48-h methylprednisolone infusion or placebo. The risk of death and death or severe disability was higher in the steroid group [45].

Barbiturates

Although the existing literature does not support a mortality benefit with the use of barbiturates in patients with traumatic brain injury [46], the BTF guidelines provide a level II recommendation for the use of high-dose barbiturates for control of ICP refractory to maximum medical and surgical treatment. It is noted though that there is no clear benefit on outcome and the potential complications and need for monitoring are stressed as well as the need for hemodynamic stability prior to therapy [25].

CPP/Autoregulation

The BTF guidelines suggest that the CPP value to target lies at the 50–70 mmHg range with a general CPP threshold in the realm of 60 mmHg [25]. They note that the parameters used to calculate CPP (blood pressure and ICP) have been shown to individually correlate to outcome after TBI since both hypotension and elevated ICP have been associated to poor outcome. They also state that there is no defined critical lower threshold of CPP that is associated to cerebral ischemia or poor outcome, but they suggest that a CPP of 50–60 mmHg appears to be a critical lower threshold range for ischemia [25].

The target CPP in a given patient may ultimately vary depending on the individual's autoregulatory status. (For a discussion on the methods and indexes used to measure autoregulation, refer to the neuromonitoring chapters: Chaps. 7

and 8.) A study by Jaeger and colleagues supports the concept of determining individual optimal cerebral perfusion pressure based on measures of cerebrovascular pressure reactivity [47]. Howells and colleagues analyzed a group of patients treated with ICP-oriented vs. CPP-oriented protocols in two different centers. They concluded that the pressure reactivity index can identify the most appropriate treatment strategy in a given patient. They found that in pressure-passive patients, ICP-oriented therapy resulted in better outcomes, and in pressure-active and pressure-stable TBI patients, the CPP-oriented therapy was more beneficial [48]. In a study by Johnson and colleagues, patients with impaired cerebral pressure autoregulation with lower CPP had a more favorable outcome compared to patients with higher CPP. No difference in outcome was seen with different CPP levels in patients with intact autoregulation [49].

Brain Oxygen (PbtO$_2$)

The guidelines give a level III recommendation for the use of jugular venous saturation and brain tissue oxygen monitoring in addition to ICP monitoring in the management of severe TBI. They propose a jugular venous saturation (SjO$_2$) <50 % and brain tissue oxygen tension (PbrO$_2$) <15 mmHg as treatment thresholds [25].

In a study by Bohman and coworkers [50], patients with severe TBI with at least one episode of compromised brain oxygen (defined as PbtO$_2$ <25 mmHg for >10 min) were identified retrospectively. They received medical therapies with goal to maintain PbtO$_2$ >25 mmHg including manipulation of pulmonary function, CPP augmentation, sedation, and elevated ICP control. The response rate to medical treatment of compromised PbtO$_2$ was associated to decreased mortality [50].

Ongoing studies, such as the brain oxygen and outcome in severe traumatic brain injury (BOOST II) phase II trial, are comparing an ICP/CPP-directed therapy to a PbrO$_2$-directed therapy. Patients are randomized within 12 h after TBI to ICP/CPP care or ICP/CPP and brain oxygen care. All patients receive care according to BTF guidelines [51].

Brain Chemistry (Microdialysis)

Assessment of brain chemistry parameters by microdialysis has the potential to aid in the management of severe TBI patients in conjunction with the other physiological variables discussed previously. In one of the largest TBI studies to date on microdialysis monitoring, Timofeev and coworkers studied 223 patients (75 % with severe TBI) and found on multivariate analysis that lactate/pyruvate ratio (>25) had a significant association with increased mortality. Also, higher cerebral glucose was associated with increased mortality, and higher pyruvate was associated with reduced mortality [52]. Definitive data are currently lacking regarding the potential impact that targeting the different derangements in the measured brain chemistry parameters would have on patients with TBI, but ongoing research will likely shed light on the subject; refer to multimodality monitoring chapters—Chaps. 7 and 8—for details.

Seizure Prophylaxis

Seizure prophylaxis is recommended for the first 7 days after severe TBI. In a randomized trial of phenytoin for the prevention of posttraumatic seizures, Temkin and colleagues reported 404 patients with severe head trauma randomized to phenytoin or placebo for 1 year with follow-up continued until 2 years. Seizures occurred significantly more frequently on the first 7 days in the placebo group compared to the phenytoin group (14.2 % vs. 3.6 %, respectively), and the seizure frequency was not significantly different between day 8 and the end of the first year or at the end of year 2 [53]. Newer anticonvulsants such as levetiracetam have also been studied for seizure prophylaxis after severe TBI. Jones and coworkers compared 32 severe TBI cases who received levetiracetam for the first 7 days after injury to 41 historical controls who received phenytoin. Seizure activity was not significantly different between the two groups [54]. Similarly, no difference in seizure occurrence was reported in a prospective, randomized trial of severe TBI and SAH patients randomized to seizure prophylaxis for 7 days with phenytoin or levetiracetam [55].

Conclusion

Overall, outcomes after traumatic brain injury have improved significantly over the past several decades. This is likely due to a combination of improvements in emergency response and prehospital care, early triage, and improved critical care. Because of the brain's exquisite vulnerability to small insults after trauma, excellent critical care is enormously important to mitigate secondary injury and improve long-term outcomes.

References

1. Faul M, Xu L, Wald MM, Coronado VG. Traumatic brain injury in the United States: emergency department visits, hospitalizations and deaths 2002–2006. Atlanta: Centers for Disease Control and Prevention, National Center for Injury Prevention and Control; 2010.
2. Marr A, Coronado V, editors. Central nervous system injury surveillance data submission standards—2002. Atlanta: Centers for Disease Control and Prevention, National Center for Injury Prevention and Control; 2004.
3. Tagliaferri F, Compagnone C, Korsic M, Servadei F, Kraus J. A systematic review of brain injury epidemiology in Europe. Acta Neurochir (Wien). 2006;148(3):255–68.
4. Myburgh JA, Cooper DJ, Finfer SR, Venkatesh B, Jones D, Higgins A, Bishop N, Higlett T. Epidemiology and 12-month outcomes from traumatic brain injury in Australia and New Zealand. Australasian Traumatic Brain Injury Study (ATBIS) Investigators for the Australian; New Zealand Intensive Care Society Clinical Trials Group. J Trauma. 2008;64(4):854–62.
5. Hillier SL, Hiller JE, Metzer J. Epidemiology of traumatic brain injury in South Australia. Brain Inj. 1997;11(9):649–59.
6. Wu X, Hu J, Zhuo L, Fu C, Hui G, Wang Y, Yang W, Teng L, Lu S, Xu G. Epidemiology of traumatic brain injury in eastern China, 2004: a prospective large case study. J Trauma. 2008 ;64(5):1313–9.
7. Wang CC, Schoenberg BS, Li SC, Yang YC, Cheng XM, Bolis CL. Brain injury due to head trauma. Epidemiology in urban areas of the People's Republic of China. Arch Neurol. 1986;43:570–2.
8. Gururaj G. Epidemiology of traumatic brain injury: Indian scenario. Neurol Res. 2002;24(1):24–8.
9. Nakamura N, Yamaura A, Shigemori M, Ono J, Kawamata T, Sakamoto T. Epidemiology, prevention and countermeasures against severe traumatic brain injury in Japan and abroad. Japanese Data Bank Committee for traumatic brain injury. Neurol Res. 2002;24(1):45–53.
10. Langlois JA, Rutland-Brown W, Wald MM. The epidemiology and impact of traumatic brain injury: a brief overview. J Head Trauma Rehabil. 2006;21(5):375–8.
11. Jennett B. Epidemiology of head injury. J Neurol Neurosurg Psychiatry. 1996;60(4):362–9.
12. Bruns Jr J, Hauser WA. The epidemiology of traumatic brain injury: a review. Epilepsia. 2003;44 Suppl 10:2–10.
13. Zauner A, Bullock R. The role of excitatory amino acids in severe brain trauma: opportunities for therapy: a review. J Neurotrauma. 1995;12:547–54.
14. Bullock R, Zauner A, Woodward JJ, Myseros J, Choi SC, Ward JD, Marmarou A, Young HF. Factors affecting excitatory amino acid release following severe human head injury. J Neurosurg. 1998;89:507–18.
15. Reinert MM, Bullock R. Clinical trials in head injury. Neurol Research. 1999;21:330–8.
16. Clausen T, Bullock R. Medical treatment and neuroprotection in traumatic brain injury. Curr Pharm Des. 2001;7:1517–32.
17. Fiskum G. Mechanisms of neuronal death and neuroprotection. J Neurosurg Anesthesiol. 2004;16:108–10.
18. Robertson CS, Valadka AB, Hannay HJ, Contant CF, Gopinath SP, Cormio M, Uzura M, Grossman RG. Prevention of secondary ischemic insults after severe head injury. Crit Care Med. 1999;27:2086–95.
19. Bergsneider M, Hovda DA, Shalmon E, Kelly DF, Vespa PM, Martin NA, Phelps ME, McArthur DL, Caron MJ, Kraus JF, Becker DP. Cerebral hyperglycolysis following severe traumatic brain injury in humans: a positron emission tomography study. J Neurosurg. 1997;86(2):241–51.
20. Giza CC, Hovda DA. The neurometabolic cascade of concussion. J Athl Train. 2001;36(3):228–35.
21. Teasdale G, Jennett B. Assessment and prognosis of coma after head injury. Acta Neurochir (Wien). 1976;34(1–4):45–55.
22. Marshall LF, Marshall SB, Klauber MR, Clark MB, Eisenberg HM, Jane JA, Luerssen TG, Marmarou A, Foulkes MA. A new classification of head injury based on computerized tomography. J Neurosurg. 1991;75:S14–20.
23. Maas AI, Hukkelhoven CW, Marshall LF, Steyerberg EW. Prediction of outcome in traumatic brain injury with computed tomographic characteristics: a comparison between the computed tomographic classification and combinations of computed tomographic predictors. Neurosurgery. 2005;57(6):1173–82.
24. Baker SP, O'Neill B, Haddon Jr W, Long WB. The injury severity score: a method for describing patients with multiple injuries and evaluating emergency care. J Trauma. 1974;14:187–96.
25. Brain Trauma Foundation; American Association of Neurological Surgeons; Congress of Neurological Surgeons; Joint Section on Neurotrauma and Critical Care, AANS/CNS. Guidelines for the

management of severe traumatic brain injury 3rd edition. J Neurotrauma. 2007;24 Suppl 1:S1–106.

26. Marmarou A, Lu J, Butcher I, McHugh GS, Mushkudiani NA, Murray GD, Steyerberg EW, Maas AI. IMPACT database of traumatic brain injury: design and description. J Neurotrauma. 2007;24(2):239–50.

27. McHugh GS, Engel DC, Butcher I, Steyerberg EW, Lu J, Mushkudiani N, Hernández AV, Marmarou A, Maas AI, Murray GD. Prognostic value of secondary insults in traumatic brain injury: results from the IMPACT study. J Neurotrauma. 2007;24(2):287–93.

28. Butcher I, Maas AI, Lu J, Marmarou A, Murray GD, Mushkudiani NA, McHugh GS, Steyerberg EW. Prognostic value of admission blood pressure in traumatic brain injury: results from the IMPACT study. J Neurotrauma. 2007;24(2):294–302.

29. Clifton GL, Valadka A, Zygun D, Coffey CS, Drever P, Fourwinds S, Janis LS, Wilde E, Taylor P, Harshman K, Conley A, Puccio A, Levin HS, McCauley SR, Bucholz RD, Smith KR, Schmidt JH, Scott JN, Yonas H, Okonkwo DO. Very early hypothermia induction in patients with severe brain injury (the National Acute Brain Injury Study: Hypothermia II): a randomised trial. Lancet Neurol. 2011;10(2):131–9.

30. Sorani MD, Morabito D, Rosenthal G, Giacomini KM, Manley GT. Characterizing the dose-response relationship between mannitol and intracranial pressure in traumatic brain injury patients using a high-frequency physiological data collection system. J Neurotrauma. 2008;25(4):291–8.

31. Oddo M, Levine JM, Frangos S, Carrera E, Maloney-Wilensky E, Pascual JL, Kofke WA, Mayer SA, LeRoux PD. Effect of mannitol and hypertonic saline on cerebral oxygenation in patients with severe traumatic brain injury and refractory intracranial hypertension. J Neurol Neurosurg Psychiatry. 2009;80(8):916–20.

32. Pascual JL, Maloney-Wilensky E, Reilly PM, Sicoutris C, Keutmann MK, Stein SC, LeRoux PD, Gracias VH. Resuscitation of hypotensive head-injured patients: is hypertonic saline the answer? Am Surg. 2008;74(3):253–9.

33. Rockswold GL, Solid CA, Paredes-Andrade E, Rockswold SB, Jancik JT, Quickel RR. Hypertonic saline and its effect on intracranial pressure, cerebral perfusion pressure, and brain tissue oxygen. Neurosurgery. 2009;65(6):1035–41; discussion 1041–2.

34. Hsiang JK, Chesnut R, et al. Early, routine paralysis for intracranial pressure control in severe head injury: is it necessary? Crit Care Med. 1994;22:1471–6.

35. Andrews PJ, Sinclair HL, Battison CG, Polderman KH, Citerio G, Mascia L, Harris BA, Murray GD, Stocchetti N, Menon DK, Shakur H, De Backer D; Eurotherm3235Trial collaborators. European society of intensive care medicine study of therapeutic hypothermia (32–35°C) for intracranial pressure reduction after traumatic brain injury (the Eurotherm3235Trial). Trials. 2011;12:8.

36. Concensus conference: rehabilitation of persons with traumatic brain injury. NIH Consensus Development Panel on Rehabilitation of Persons with Traumatic Brain Injury. JAMA. 1999;282:974–83.

37. Picard J, Bailey S, Sanderson H, Reese M, Garfeld JS. Steps towards cost benefits analysis of regional neurosurgical care. BMJ. 1990;301:629–35.

38. Bullock MR, Chesnut R, Ghajar J, Gordon D, Hartl R, Newell DW, Servadei F, Walters BC, Wilberger J. Guidelines for the surgical management of traumatic brain injury. Neurosurgery. 2006; 58 Suppl 3:S21–62.

39. Gennarelli T, Spielman G, Langfitt T, Gildenberg P, Harrington T, Jane J, Marshall L, Miller J, Pitts L. Influence of the type of intracranial lesion on outcome from severe head injury. J Neurosurg. 1982;56:26–32.

40. Seelig J, Marshall L, Toutant S, Toole B, Klauber M, Bowers S, Varnell J. Traumatic acute epidural hematoma: unrecognized high lethality in comatose patients. Neurosurgery. 1984;15:167–620.

41. Cohen J, Montero A, Israel Z. Prognosis and clinical revelance of anisocoriacraniotomy lantency for epidural hematoma in comatose patients. J Trauma. 1996;41:120–2.

42. Miller JD, Butterworth JF, Gudeman SK, Faulkner JE, Choi SC, Selhorst JB, Harbison JW, Lutz HA, Young HF, Becker DP. Further experience in the management of severe head injury. J Neurosurg. 1981;54:289–99.

43. Wu J, Hsu C, Liao S, Wong Y. Surgical outcome of traumatic intracranial hematoma at a regional hospital in Taiwan. J Trauma. 1999;47:39–43.

44. Taylor A, Butt W, Rosenfeld J, Shann F, Ditchfield M, Lewis E, Klug G, Wallace D, Henning R, Tibballs J. A randomized trial of very early decompressive craniectomy in children with traumatic brain injury and sustained intracranial hypertension. Childs Nerv Syst. 2001;17:154–62.

45. Edwards P, Arango M, Balica L, Cottingham R, El-Sayed H, Farrell B, Fernandes J, Gogichaisvili T, Golden N, Hartzenberg B, Husain M, Ulloa MI, Jerbi Z, Khamis H, Komolafe E, Laloë V, Lomas G, Ludwig S, Mazairac G, Muñoz SanchézMde L, Nasi L, Olldashi F, Plunkett P, Roberts I, Sandercock P, Shakur H, Soler C, Stocker R, Svoboda P, Trenkler S, Venkataramana NK, Wasserberg J, Yates D, Yutthakasemsunt S, CRASH trial collaborators. Final results of MRC CRASH, a randomised placebo-controlled trial of intravenous corticosteroid in adults with head injury-outcomes at 6 months. Lancet. 2005;365(9475):1957–9.

46. Roberts I, Sydenham E. Barbiturates for acute traumatic brain injury. Cochrane Database Syst Rev. 1999;(3):CD000033. doi:10.1002/14651858.CD000033.

47. Jaeger M, Dengl M, Meixensberger J, Schuhmann MU. Effects of cerebrovascular pressure reactivity-guided optimization of cerebral perfusion pressure on brain tissue oxygenation after traumatic brain injury. Crit Care Med. 2010;38(5):1343–7.

48. Howells T, Elf K, Jones PA, Ronne-Engström E, Piper I, Nilsson P, Andrews P, Enblad P. Pressure reactivity as a guide in the treatment of cerebral perfusion pressure in patients with brain trauma. J Neurosurg. 2005;102(2):311–7.

49. Johnson U, Nilsson P, Ronne-Engström E, Howells T, Enblad P. Favorable outcome in traumatic brain injury patients with impaired cerebral pressure autoregulation when treated at low cerebral perfusion pressure levels. Neurosurgery. 2011;68(3):714–21; discussion 721–2.

50. Bohman LE, Heuer GG, Macyszyn L, Maloney-Wilensky E, Frangos S, Le Roux PD, Kofke A, Levine JM, Stiefel MF. Medical management of compromised brain oxygen in patients with severe traumatic brain injury. Neurocrit Care. 2011;14(3):361–9.

51. http://neurocriticalcare.org/sites/default/files/pdfs/1015LeRoux.pdf. Accessed 25 July 2011.

52. Timofeev I, Carpenter KL, Nortje J, Al-Rawi PG, O'Connell MT, Czosnyka M, Smielewski P, Pickard JD, Menon DK, Kirkpatrick PJ, Gupta AK, Hutchinson PJ. Cerebral extracellular chemistry and outcome following traumatic brain injury: a microdialysis study of 223 patients. Brain. 2011;134(Pt 2):484–94.

53. Temkin NR, Dikmen SS, Wilensky AJ, Keihm J, Chabal S, Winn HR. A randomized, double-blind study of phenytoin for the prevention of post-traumatic seizures. N Engl J Med. 1990;323(8): 497–502.

54. Jones KE, Puccio AM, Harshman KJ, Falcione B, Benedict N, Jankowitz BT, Stippler M, Fischer M, Sauber-Schatz EK, Fabio A, Darby JM, Okonkwo DO. Levetiracetam versus phenytoin for seizure prophylaxis in severe traumatic brain injury. Neurosurg Focus. 2008;25(4):E3.

55. Szaflarski JP, Sangha KS, Lindsell CJ, Shutter LA. Prospective, randomized, single-blinded comparative trial of intravenous levetiracetam versus phenytoin for seizure prophylaxis. Neurocrit Care. 2010;12(2):165–72.

56. O'Phelan KH, Mangat HS, Olvey SE, Bullock MR. Multimodal monitoring in acute brain injury. In: Bhardwaj A, Mirski MA, editors. Handbook of neurocritical care. 2nd ed. New York: Springer Science+Business Media; 2011.

Pediatric Traumatic Brain Injury: Evidence-Based Medicine, Diagnosis, Treatment, and Complications

28

Kyle M. Fargen and David W. Pincus

Contents

Abstract

Traumatic brain injury (TBI) is the most common cause of long-term morbidity and mortality in pediatric trauma. It is estimated that over 400,000 children in the United States are evaluated in emergency departments after sustaining a TBI annually, resulting in over 3,000 deaths and ten times as many hospitalizations. This chapter reviews the epidemiology, pathophysiology, clinical presentation, and imaging findings associated with TBI in children. A diagnostic and management algorithm is then reviewed. Finally, the representative evidence and risks/benefits of intracranial pressure monitoring, hyperosmolar therapy, barbiturate coma, decompressive craniectomy, and other therapeutic modalities are explained in detail.

Keywords

Decompressive craniectomy • Hyperosmolar therapy • Hypothermia • Intracranial pressure monitoring • Pediatric Traumatic brain injury

K.M. Fargen, MD, MPH • D.W. Pincus, MD, PhD (✉)
Department of Neurological Surgery,
University of Florida College of Medicine,
100265, Gainesville, FL 32610, USA
e-mail: kyle.fargen@neurosurgery.ulf.edu;
pincus@neurosurgery.ufl.edu

Introduction

Traumatic brain injury (TBI) is the most common cause of long-term morbidity and mortality in pediatric trauma [1]. Brain injury in this population remains a significant public health concern both in the United States and abroad, despite efforts to reduce such injuries. It is estimated that over 400,000 children in the United States are evaluated in emergency departments after sustaining a TBI annually, resulting

A.J. Layon et al. (eds.), *Textbook of Neurointensive Care*,
DOI 10.1007/978-1-4471-5226-2_28, © Springer-Verlag London 2013

in over 3,000 deaths and ten times as many hospitalizations [2]. Although the vast majority of head injuries in children are classified as mild injuries, moderate to severe brain injuries result in a substantial burden to families both emotionally and financially [3]. Deficits sustained in childhood from TBI incur tremendous weight upon family members and may necessitate long-term medical and nursing care. Successful recognition of potential brain injury, accurate diagnosis, and expedient initiation of therapy is essential in minimizing secondary injury, providing the best possible chance for good outcome.

Complicating the management of pediatric TBI is the relative paucity of scientific evidence for commonly accepted practices. The majority of therapies used today in pediatric intensive care units around the world rely on evidence of treatment effect in adults; many are supported by little or no evidence in children. As most neurotrauma experts would attest, children are not simply "little adults." The pediatric brain has a higher water content than the adult brain, imparting less compliance and skewing the traditional understanding of intracranial pressure (ICP) and volume. In infants and toddlers, open fontanelles and sutures provide less protection to acutely injured brain. Furthermore, children demonstrate a higher rate of apoptosis, portending a potentially exaggerated sensitivity to secondary injury. Children respond differently to medications than adults, particularly in regards to sedatives, and many of these medications have not been evaluated effectively in the pediatric population. In addition, children demonstrate a lower cerebral blood flow per gram of tissue than adults. Using traditional, adult blood pressure or cerebral perfusion pressure (CPP) goals does not consider differences in metabolic demands or the integrity of the blood-brain barrier of children and may lead to unintended exacerbations of cerebral edema. These reasons are thought to contribute to the increased TBI-associated mortality seen in children, particularly given that the adult therapies used in pediatric TBI management may not be fully applicable [4, 5]. In 2003, experts in the field of pediatric neurotrauma convened and attempted to develop guidelines for management of brain injury in children based upon the Brain Trauma Foundation's adult treatment guidelines [6]. Unfortunately, due to the paucity of class one or two evidence, the report merely provided treatment options for pediatric patients, with most treatment options originating from evidence gained from adult studies. Since 2003, little ground has been gained in this regard.

This chapter will discuss current practices in diagnosis and management of pediatric TBI. When applicable, differences in adult and pediatric therapies will be mentioned. Evidence-based recommendations will be provided. Common practices with little evidence supporting their use in the pediatric population will be highlighted.

Epidemiology

The Center for Disease Control and Prevention reports approximately 1.7 million people suffer a TBI annually, of which over 50,000 die. Overall, TBI is a contributing factor to 30 % of all deaths in the United States related to injury [7]. It is estimated that the health-care burden of TBI in the United States is approximately 60 billion dollars annually. Of the 1.7 million sustaining TBI, it is estimated that over 400,000 children in the United States are evaluated in emergency departments after sustaining a TBI annually, resulting in over 3,000 deaths and ten times as many hospitalizations. While motor vehicle collisions represent the most common cause of fatal TBI in all age groups, alternative sources of injury, such as domestic violence and all-terrain vehicle use, are especially common in pediatric patients. In children 0–14 years of age, falls account for 50 % of TBI emergency room visits, followed by injuries from being struck by or against an object (25 %), unknown or other causes (15 %), motor vehicle traffic (7 %), and assault (3 %) [7]. Of note, all-terrain vehicle-related TBI continues to be on the rise and represents a growing public health concern, accounting for approximately 4,000 pediatric hospitalizations in 2006 [8]. Falls and assault share a disproportionately high incidence in children 4 years of age or less. Risk factors for child abuse-related TBI include children less than 2 years of age, male gender, young age of mother, substance abuse, multiple siblings, and living with unrelated adults [9–11].

Children are thought to be more susceptible to TBI due to multiple factors. First, children have a larger head-to-body size ratio, resulting in a larger angular rotational force which may increase risk for axonal shearing injuries and explain the higher rate of diffuse injuries seen. In addition, children have thinner skull bones with open fontanelles and sutures in infants, providing less protection to the underlying intracranial contents. Poorly myelinated neural tissue seen in young children may also play a pivotal role in the increased vulnerability to trauma [12].

Given the mechanical forces associated with TBI, such injuries are frequently associated with calvarial fractures, extremity fractures, and solid organ injuries. However, TBI remains the most common cause of mortality in pediatric trauma [1]. Life-threatening intracranial abnormalities may consist of cerebral contusions, subdural hematomas, epidural hematomas, subarachnoid hemorrhage, diffuse axonal injury (DAI), or a combination of these. Diffuse TBI, ranging from concussion to DAI, is thought to represent the most common form of pediatric TBI and is a result of shearing of axons from linear and angular forces. Due to the range of injuries sustained in such patients, care of pediatric trauma patients usually involves the coordinated action of multiple specialists including intensivists, neurosurgeons, neurologists, orthopedic surgeons, and general surgeons. In addition, social service workers play an integral role in providing financial, emotional, and spiritual assistance to families during this difficult time period. Furthermore, there is evidence supporting better outcomes of patients with severe TBI treated at high-volume, level-1 pediatric trauma centers [13, 14], as these centers usually have the means and specialists necessary to recognize and manage all potential complications. Unfortunately, however, one recent population-based study suggested that up to one-third of children with TBI failed to receive care in higher-level trauma centers [15].

Pathogenesis

Primary injury refers to the damage accumulated by neural tissue upon the transfer of energy during the acute traumatic event. Brain contusions or lacerations, shearing of axons, or disruption and subsequent hemorrhage of bridging veins or cortical arteries are all examples of primary injuries. Primary brain injuries may be fatal if severe in nature; furthermore, such injuries may require urgent or emergent operative intervention if mass effect is present to decompress critical neural structures. In many patients with contusions or hematomas, primary injuries may be dynamic; for instance, contusions may blossom over days and epidural hematomas may increase in size over minutes to hours. In patients with survivable primary injuries, prevention of secondary injury remains paramount. Secondary injury refers to the evolution of neuronal cell death due to delayed injury to neurons which have been made more vulnerable due to the previously sustained primary injury. Prevention of secondary injury is the major focus of pediatric TBI management and, as such, will be a recurring focus of this chapter.

Secondary brain injury is a direct result of the metabolic failure of neurons after primary injury. Most commonly, secondary injury is a result of hypoxia or hypotension, both of which result in failure of oxidative phosphorylation and cause collapse of the metabolic machinery necessary to keep vulnerable neurons alive. Such neurons may undergo necrosis or proceed toward cell death through apoptosis. Hypotension and hypoxia may have numerous causes in the trauma patient, including significant blood loss, circulatory compromise, respiratory failure, decreased vasomotor tone, or sepsis. Furthermore, diffuse cerebral edema after primary injury due to blood-brain barrier disruption is a common, and potentially avoidable, cause of secondary injury. Control of ICP and maintenance of adequate CPP following TBI are of utmost importance as dysregulation of either of these parameters may result in metabolic failure and secondary injury. Therapies have been developed with the aim of ameliorating secondary injury by reducing the cerebral metabolic rate of oxygen, such as hypothermia and barbiturate coma.

Neuroprotective therapies, which aim to maintain adequate oxygen delivery to vulnerable brain, will be discussed in detail in the sections that follow.

Diagnosis

Initial Evaluation

Pediatric patients presenting to the trauma bay after acute trauma should undergo immediate evaluation by Advanced Trauma Life Support protocol. These measures ensure adequate oxygen exchange and cardiovascular tone such that a thorough evaluation of injuries can be performed. Patients with Glasgow Coma Scale (GCS) less than or equal to eight should undergo endotracheal intubation for establishment of a secure and definitive airway. Prior to administration of sedation or neuromuscular blockade, it is important that a thorough neurologic examination is recorded as these medications will prevent further evaluation. Fluid resuscitation in the setting of hypotension or significant blood loss is a priority. Hypotension, defined as a systolic blood pressure less than the fifth percentile for age, present in the field or in the emergency department, is a strong predictor of poor outcome after pediatric TBI [16]. In the setting of pediatric TBI and volume depletion, hypertonic saline has demonstrated superiority over lactated Ringer's in a randomized trial; patients resuscitated with saline demonstrated lower ICP, higher CPP, and shorter intensive care unit (ICU) stays [17]. Furthermore, resuscitation with saline is associated with lower mortality than resuscitation with albumin in children with TBI [18]. In many trauma patients, routine laboratory analysis including arterial blood gas, coagulation panel, and complete blood count is indicated to ensure adequate resuscitation and detect potential coagulopathy. After the initial primary evaluation, a secondary survey should be performed to identify associated injuries, such as long bone fractures.

Grading Scales

Evaluating the severity of a TBI in a validated and consistent manner is essential in appropriately directing treatment. The modified Glasgow Coma Scale (GCS) remains the most widely used method for characterizing the extent of neurologic injury and has three elements: eye opening, verbal response, and motor response. GCS scoring differs based upon age, as infants and toddlers cannot be expected to perform the same verbal or motor responses on command as can older children. The most widely used scales are presented in Table 28.1. GCS has been extensively studied with satisfactory inter-rater reliability and validity [19]. Patients presenting with a GCS of 8 or less are considered comatose and

Table 28.1 Modified Glasgow Coma Scale. The best scores from each category are added for a total score of 3–15

Child or adult	Score	Infant or toddler
Eye opening		Eye opening
Spontaneous	4	Spontaneous
To speech	3	To speech
To pain	2	To pain
None	1	None
Eyes swollen shut	1c	Eyes swollen shut
Verbal response		Verbal response
Oriented	5	Coos, babbles, age appropriate
Confused	4	Irritable, cries
Inappropriate words	3	Cries to pain
Incomprehensible sounds	2	Moans to pain
None	1	None
Intubated patient	1T	Intubated patient
Motor response		Motor response
Follows commands	6	Spontaneous movement
Localizes to pain	5	Withdraws to touch
Withdraws to pain	4	Withdraws to pain
Abnormal flexion	3	Abnormal flexion
Extensor response	2	Extensor response
None	1	None

Data from Teasdale and Jennett [129], Davis et al. [130], James et al. [131], and Morray et al. [132]

Table 28.2 The Pediatric Trauma Score. Scores range from −6 to +12

Score	+2	+1	−1
Weight (kg)	>20	10–20	<10
Airway	Patent	Maintainable	Unmaintainable
Systolic blood pressure (mmHg)	>90	50–90	<50
Level of consciousness	Awake	Loss of consciousness	Comatose
Fractures	None	Closed or suspected	Multiple
Wounds	None	Minor	Major, penetrating, burns

Data from Tepas et al. [24]

require endotracheal intubation. In most clinical settings, GCS of 13–15 is considered "mild" TBI, while GCS of 9–12 is considered "moderate" and 8 or less is "severe." In one study of over 300 children presenting with TBI, GCS was found to be the most important predictor of survival when compared to alternative factors such as imaging findings or other organ injuries [20]. Interestingly, poor outcome in adults is traditionally associated with a GCS of 8 or less; however, in this study and in a second pediatric series, the threshold for poor outcome was a GCS of 5 or less [20, 21]. Although GCS is composed of three separate entities, most clinicians consider the motor response the most critical, as patients who have facial trauma with swelling may have an underestimated score (and therefore overestimated brain injury). Similarly, ventilated patients at time of arrival frequently have mistakenly overestimated brain injuries [22]. In an attempt to overcome some of these challenges, alternate scales have been developed, such as the FOUR score, which evaluates level of consciousness based upon 4-point eye, motor, brainstem, and respiration scales [23].

Other grading scales designed to take into account systemic factors have been developed to further direct care of the acute pediatric trauma patient and predict prognosis. The Pediatric Trauma Score (PTS) assesses six factors and the summated score has a linear association with mortality. PTS totals range from −6 to +12 (Table 28.2). Mortality is approximately 9 % with a PTS greater than 8 and 100 % with a PTS less than or equal to zero [24, 25]. Perhaps the most encompassing scale is the Pediatric Risk of Mortality score (PRISM; most recent of which is the PRISM III scale) that assesses 17 different physiologic variables to predict mortality risk [26].

Imaging

After initial patient assessment, clinicians must assess the need for brain imaging based upon examination findings. Computed tomography (CT) remains the mainstay imaging modality to evaluate for brain, spine, thoracic, and abdominal injuries in the acute setting. CT imaging is widely available

Table 28.3 Three management protocols used to assess the need for CT imaging in the acute pediatric trauma patient

NICE [30]	Beaudin and colleagues [31]	Willis and colleagues [32]
1. GCS <13 at any time since injury	1. GCS 14 or less	1. GCS <13 on initial assessment
2. GCS 13 or 14 at 2 h after injury	2. Seizures at any time after injury	2. GCS 13 or 14 at 2 h after adequate resuscitation
3. Two or more episodes of emesis	3. Linear skull fracture over 4 mm or depressed or open skull fractures	3. Four or more episodes of emesis or vomiting 2 h after injury

Indications for CT are listed herewith. These include the UK National Institute of Health and Clinical Excellence (NICE) guidelines [30] and those provided by Beaudin et al. [31] and Willis et al. [32]

and is highly sensitive in identifying mass lesions requiring emergent surgical intervention; for these reasons, it remains the ideal imaging technique for pediatric patients presenting with acute TBI [27]. Given the rapid advancements in CT technology over the last 10 years and the limited time needed to acquire high-resolution imaging on most modern CT scanners, the use of CT in evaluation of TBI continues to rise in the United States [28]. The downside to routine CT imaging in all trauma patients is the potentially unnecessary exposure to radiation. Such doses were initially thought to be trivial; however, recent evidence suggests that the radiation burden of even a single head CT in a young child may impart a future risk of cancer as high as 0.07 % [29]. Therefore, CT imaging guidelines weighing both the risks and benefits of CT scanning in the pediatric population are needed. Although no current consensus exists, several groups have attempted to provide recommendations for CT imaging after trauma. Three different proposed management protocols are presented in Table 28.3.

CT imaging is very useful in the acute setting for multiple reasons. First, CT imaging of the head, cervical spine, chest, abdomen, and pelvis can be performed in several minutes or less on the acute pediatric trauma patient and is highly sensitive in demonstrating acute injuries to bony structures as well as soft tissue and internal organs. Furthermore, CT imaging is highly sensitive for acute intracranial hemorrhage and therefore is useful in recognizing patients in need of immediate operative intervention. Subdural hematomas, epidural hematomas, depressed skull fractures, cerebral contusions, DAI, intraventricular hemorrhage, and acute hydrocephalus are readily apparent on CT imaging (Figs. 28.1, 28.2, 28.3, and 28.4). Furthermore, CT findings may assist in differentiating non-accidental (inflicted) from accidental trauma in children. Non-accidental injuries are frequently associated with combinations of both acute and chronic injuries such as subdural or multifocal extra-axial hematomas of varying ages, hygromas, atrophy, and ventricular dilatation from ex vacuo; accidental injuries more frequently involve skull fractures, epidural hematomas, or intraparenchymal hemorrhages [33, 34].

CT remains the most common imaging modality performed beyond the initial trauma evaluation. However, indications for repeat imaging are not clearly defined in children with TBI. One retrospective review of pediatric TBI identified epidural hematomas, subdural hematomas, cerebral

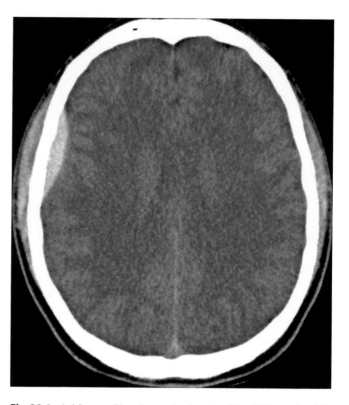

Fig. 28.1 A 16-year-old male sustained a closed head injury after falling into a brick wall and was GCS 15 on presentation. Non-contrast CT imaging demonstrated a right-sided convex hyperdensity posterior to the coronal suture consistent with an acute epidural hematoma. The patient remained neurologically intact and did not require operative intervention

edema, and intraparenchymal hemorrhages as "high-risk" lesions that were more likely to progress on repeat CT and more likely to require operative intervention. "Low-risk" lesions, such as subarachnoid hemorrhage, intraventricular hemorrhage, and DAI, demonstrated no increased risk of progression [35]. A second large retrospective study revealed only 30 % of pediatric TBI patients had worsening of CT scan findings on repeat imaging. Only 20 % of patients with mild TBI had worsening of imaging findings, while nearly 50 % of those with moderate to severe TBI demonstrated progression on repeat CT. Interestingly, progression on CT rarely required operative intervention (1 % in mild TBI, 6 % in moderate and severe) [36]. These findings suggest that repeat CT imaging should be performed in patients with

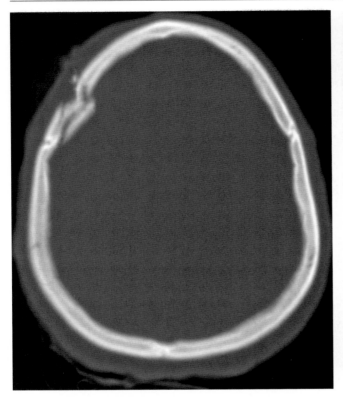

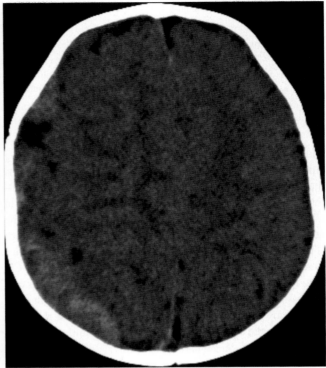

Fig. 28.2 A 16-year-old male was thrown from an all-terrain vehicle and was GCS 15 on presentation. Non-contrast CT imaging demonstrated a depressed skull fracture underlying a large scalp laceration. The patient was taken to the operating room for debridement and repair of the cosmetic defect

Fig. 28.3 A 4-month-old female was dropped from standing height by her father onto concrete. On presentation she was GCS 13 but she quickly deteriorated. A CT of the head revealed a large right acute subdural hematoma (note the midline shift with bowing of the falx cerebri from right to left). She was taken emergently to the operating room and underwent hematoma evacuation with decompressive craniectomy

higher risk lesions, such as space-occupying hematomas, and those with more severe brain injuries based on GCS.

The use of magnetic resonance imaging (MRI) in pediatric TBI has been on the rise in the last decade given its high sensitivity to detect DAI; MRI provides highly detailed brain imaging without the associated radiation exposure. Due to long acquisition times and the need for patient immobility, complete MRI remains a poor initial imaging study in the acute setting. Rapid MRI sequences that take less than 1 min and allow for patient movement (Half-fourier Acquisition Single shot Turbo spin-Echo or HASTE) may provide useful information but is probably not as useful as CT due to the inability to visualize fractures. However, there is increasing evidence that MRI findings may have utility in predicting prognosis after TBI, and, for this reason, MRI use after pediatric brain injury has become more commonplace. Furthermore, susceptibility weighted imaging, a relatively new MRI sequence, may be the most sensitive of all imaging modalities for detecting brain hemorrhages after pediatric TBI [37]. Areas of ischemia and hemorrhage are also detected with high sensitivity on diffusion-weighted imaging. Several

studies have identified that location and volume of lesions on MRI may be correlated to neuropsychological outcomes. Deeper and more centrally located lesions are associated with poorer global functioning [38, 39]. An increasing lesion burden, both in number and volume, outside of the frontal or temporal lobes is associated with diminished executive, memory, and attention function at delayed follow-up [40, 41]. Finally, diffusion tensor tractography, which allows for visualization of individual fiber tracts based on the three-dimensional diffusion of water, may provide enhanced prognostic data by revealing damage to individual, critical white matter tracts.

Transcranial Doppler ultrasonography (TCD) is also being more commonly employed due to its sensitivity for detecting vasospasm and in quantifying arterial velocities after neurologic injury in a noninvasive manner. Recent evidence suggests that TCD may help predict which children are at risk for elevated ICP and low CPP after trauma and guide early management. One such trial reported a sensitivity of 94 % in detecting intracranial hypertension and 80 % in detecting low CPP [42].

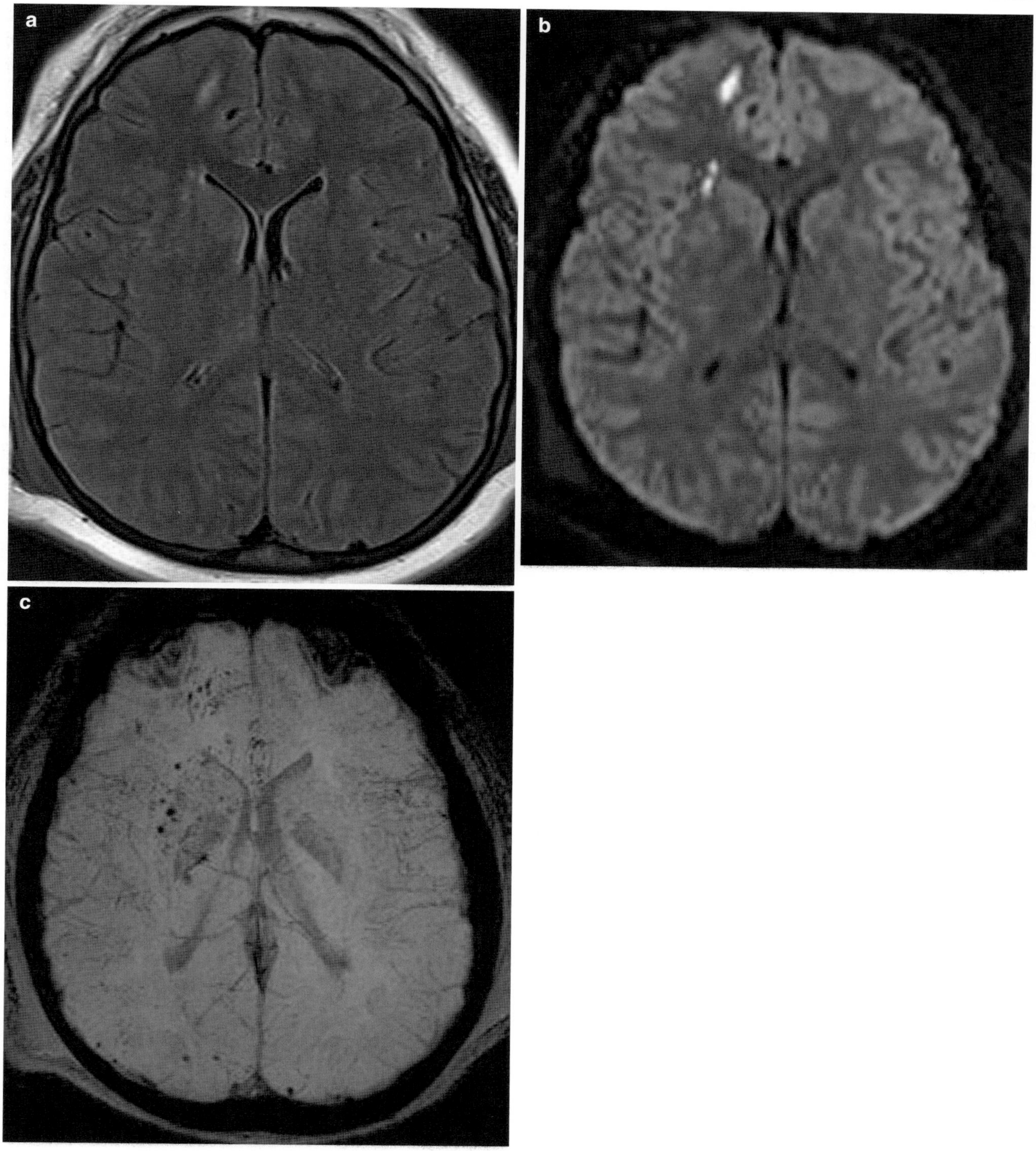

Fig. 28.4 A 13-year-old male was involved in a motor vehicle collision and presented with a GCS of 7. Head CT demonstrated no abnormalities. MRI was consistent with DAI. Flair imaging revealed multiple small areas of signal abnormality (**a**), confirmed by DWI (**b**). Susceptibility imaging (**c**) revealed numerous small areas of subcortical hypointensity in the right hemisphere consistent with microhemorrhages

The Role of Biomarkers in Diagnosis

The measurement of serum biomarkers and their relation to the diagnosis of acute injury and prognosis after TBI has been the subject of considerable investigatory efforts over the last decade. Interestingly, analysis of select biomarkers may assist clinicians in differentiating between accidental trauma and inflicted injuries. Berger and colleagues studied three serum biomarkers of brain injury (neuron-specific enolase, myelin basic protein, and S100B) in 127 infants after accidental trauma, inflicted injury, or hypoxic-ischemic insults. Peak levels of neuron-specific enolase were reached quickly after accidental trauma but were delayed after inflicted injury, suggesting that this biomarker may be useful in differentiating the two etiologies [43]. Furthermore, elevation of serum biomarkers in well-appearing infants with non-specific symptoms may help identify occult inflicted trauma [44]. Biomarker analysis may also predict prognosis after TBI. Higher initial serum concentrations of these three biomarkers appear to be predictive of more severe injuries and are associated with worse outcomes [45]. Increased levels of CSF endothelin-1, a vasoactive peptide that is upregulated after injury, have also shown to be predictive of poor outcome in children sustaining brain injuries [46].

Management Algorithm

Strict adherence to protocol in the trauma bay is necessary to ensure adequate cardiopulmonary resuscitation. Furthermore, a streamlined hospital-based protocol for the acute management of multi-trauma patients is essential in expediting care in those with life-threatening injuries. However, given the multitude of potential intracranial and extracranial injuries, varying ages and sizes of patients, and other individual factors, defining a universal management algorithm for pediatric TBI once the patient reaches the intensive care unit is extraordinarily difficult. Regardless, utilizing treatment principles generated from predominantly adult evidence-based literature, a generalized algorithm for pediatric TBI management can be provided (Fig. 28.5). General recommendations for the management of individual parameters are listed in Table 28.4. It is important to understand, however, that individual patient factors must be considered on a case-by-case basis. For instance, a child with an abnormal CT of the brain, a good neurologic exam, and a serious abdominal organ injury may require placement of intracranial monitoring devices such that ICP may be monitored while the patient is in the operating room receiving treatment for his/her other injuries and unable to be examined, regardless of a GCS higher than 8 prior to undergoing anesthesia.

The management algorithm begins in the trauma bay with the primary assessment. A child with suspected TBI undergoes primary assessment on arrival in which an adequate airway is obtained, hemodynamic resuscitation is performed, and the neurologic exam is assessed. Those presenting with GCS less than or equal to 8 should undergo endotracheal intubation. Following these measures, the child should undergo CT imaging of the brain and, based upon suspected additional injuries, imaging of the spine, chest, abdomen, pelvis, or extremities. Those with mass lesions (such as epidural or subdural hematoma) require an emergent neurosurgical consultation to assess the need for surgical decompression. Those without space-occupying lesions should be admitted to the pediatric ICU for further management.

Patients presenting with a GCS of 9 or more should undergo serial neurologic examinations and/or imaging examinations to detect potential worsening. Children presenting with a GCS less than 9 and no intracranial mass lesion should undergo placement of intracranial monitoring devices, such as an external ventricular drain, intracranial pressure transducing device, and/or brain oxygen tension monitor. ICP can be monitored and, when elevated, therapeutic measures may be undertaken. These include optimizing sodium, draining cerebrospinal fluid (CSF), intravenous sedation, hyperosmotic therapies, neuromuscular blockade, barbiturate coma, and decompressive craniectomy, among others.

Neuromonitoring

It is standard practice at most centers to place intracranial monitoring devices in children presenting with GCS of 8 or less. This is based on the general, yet unproven, consensus that children with severe brain injuries will benefit from continuous monitoring of ICP and manipulation of either ICP or CPP should ICP be elevated [47]. No class 1 evidence exists in the pediatric literature to suggest that the adult TBI management strategy of neuromonitoring in those with a GCS of 8 or less is beneficial. However, most authorities recognize that accurate measurement of the ICP and subsequent monitoring and manipulation of CPP provides children with the best chance for good outcome.

Neuromonitoring devices available for use include ventriculostomy catheters, intraparenchymal fiber-optic or strain gauge pressure transducers, and cerebral oxygen tension monitors. In most instances, one or more devices may be placed through the same burr hole when monitoring is deemed necessary. Placement of these devices is performed at the bedside under sterile conditions. Ventricular catheters are considered the most accurate means of measuring ICP as the pressure waves are obtained directly from a continuous column of CSF. However, catheter occlusion or obstruction may result in incorrect values and pressures cannot be

Fig. 28.5 Management algorithm for children presenting with TBI

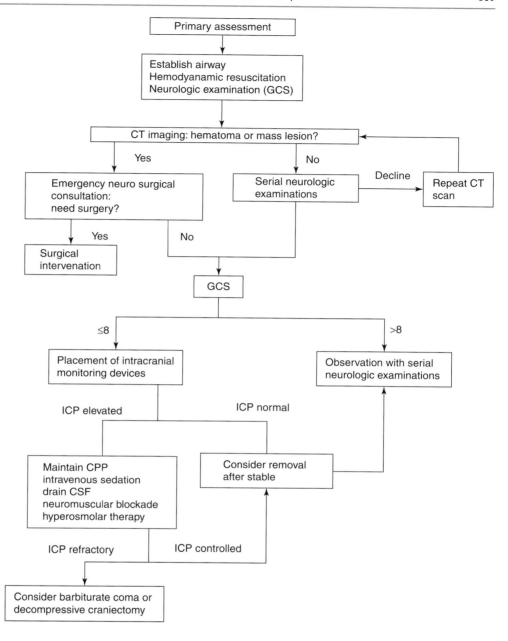

Table 28.4 General recommendations for individual physiologic parameters in pediatric TBI

Factor	Recommendation
ICP	Neuromonitoring if GCS less than 9, maintain ICP less than 15–20 mmHg (based on patient age)
CPP	Keep CPP>45–63 mmHg (based on patient age)
Blood pressure	Correct hypovolemia and hypotension
PaCO₂	Avoid hyperventilation (PaCO₂ less than 35) unless herniation exists
Temperature	Avoid hyperthermia, goal temperature 36–37 °C

transduced while CSF is actively being drained. For this reason, placement of a ventriculostomy catheter with intermittent ICP measurements only may fail to detect elevations in ICP while the catheter is open to drain; placement of an additional pressure transducer may reduce such detection errors [48]. Fiber-optic or strain gauge pressure transducers are usually inserted into the brain parenchyma and supply continuous ICP measurements. However, drifting of the zero point over time may result in falsely elevated, or underestimated, ICP readings. Even with advancements in these technologies, drifting of the zero point remains a concern in modern pressure transducers [49, 50]. Brain tissue oxygen tension ($PbtO_2$) monitors reflect the balance between cerebral oxygen supply and demand and are useful in determining brain hypoxia. However, such devices measure local brain oxygen tension at the site where the device is deployed, and therefore, the reading obtained may not necessarily be a global measurement of brain ischemia. Furthermore, the technology is not fully understood at this point, and a consensus regarding $PbtO_2$ protocols in TBI is lacking [51].

Although complications associated with intracranial monitoring are well described in the adult literature, data are considerably more scarce in the pediatric population. One small retrospective review of 80 children undergoing placement of one or more monitoring devices revealed hemorrhagic complications in 16 patients (24 %), with a fourfold increased risk in those receiving ventriculostomy catheters compared to fiber-optic monitors [52].

Intracranial Hypertension

A normal ICP in adults or older children is 5–15 mmHg compared with 2–4 mmHg in infants or younger children. ICP elevation is common after moderate to severe TBI due to blood-brain barrier disruption, cerebral edema, mass lesions, and hydrocephalus. It is universally understood that marked elevations in ICP are associated with poor outcome due to the resultant cerebral herniation and restricted blood flow that occurs in accordance with the Monro-Kellie doctrine. An ICP greater than 20 mmHg has become the universally accepted threshold for adult patients at which aggressive therapies are implemented; target ICP in most settings is less than 20. There are no universally accepted ICP thresholds in infants and children, although some experts advocate initiating treatment for pressures 15 mmHg or greater in infants, 18 mmHg or greater in children less than 8 years of age, and 20 or greater in children 8 years or older [53]. Monitoring of ICP in children with severe brain injury provides integral information to the clinician and is essential in guiding management and detecting the patient's response to therapies. Initial ICP measurements upon placement of neuromonitoring may be important in predicting prognosis. In a recent study, 80 % of children presenting with an initial ICP of less than 20 mmHg had a good outcome, while only 50 % of those with initial ICP greater than 20 mmHg had good outcomes after TBI [54]. In addition, monitoring ICP allows for calculation of CPP, defined as mean arterial pressure minus ICP. As will be discussed in the next section, monitoring CPP is important in ensuring adequate cerebral oxygen delivery after TBI. The continuous monitoring of ICP is useful in determining the child's response to hyperosmolar agents, intravenous sedation, or other therapies aimed at lowering ICP. Spikes in ICP may be treated aggressively, while persistently normal ICP may indicate the acute injury has been successfully weathered. Markedly elevated ICP that is refractory to all therapeutic interventions frequently signifies a fatal injury. Given the importance of ICP in clinical decision making in pediatric TBI, ICP represents the most widely used clinical guide for treatment after severe injury. However, there is considerable disagreement among practicing clinicians regarding optimal ICP thresholds based on age, use of hyperventilation, serum osmolality thresholds for hyperosmolar therapy, and other practices, underscoring the need for randomized clinical trials in pediatric TBI [55].

Interventions to lower ICP are performed in a stepwise fashion with those having the highest benefit-to-risk ratio employed first. Such "first-tier" therapies are useful in controlling ICP in severe brain injuries but are frequently insufficient in those with significant intracranial pathology. More aggressive therapies that impart a higher degree of risk ("second-tier" therapies) are undertaken only if first-tier measures fail. Table 28.5 lists first- and second-tier therapies used for controlling ICP. Of note, prophylactic hyperventilation is no longer recommended in the treatment of TBI as its benefit is short-lived and it may lead to vasoconstriction and reduced cerebral blood flow and therefore increased secondary injury from ischemia. Maintaining the $PaCO_2$ between 35 and 40 is recommended, although transient hyperventilation in the setting of acute herniation may be beneficial in quickly reducing ICP until other measures can be initiated. There is no role for prophylactic steroid administration after pediatric TBI as steroids appear to increase infection rates without providing benefits in reducing edema or controlling ICP [56].

Table 28.5 Interventions for lowering ICP after TBI

First-tier therapies	Second-tier therapies
Elevation of head	Barbiturate coma
Maintaining head straight and cervical collar loose	Decompressive craniectomy
Analgesia	Hypothermia (questionable benefit)
Intravenous sedation	
Neuromuscular blockade	
Hyperosmolar therapy	
CSF drainage	

First-tier therapies have a high benefit-to-risk ratio and therefore are utilized first. Second-tier therapies are utilized when ICP is refractory to first-tier measures

Initial therapies for ICP control include adequate patient positioning. Elevating the head of the bed reduces ICP in a linear fashion in children by promoting venous return, yet does not have a detrimental effect on CPP [57]. Similarly, maintaining the patient's head in a neutral position and ensuring the cervical collar is loose allow for optimization of jugular and cerebral venous drainage. Intravenous analgesia and sedation in mechanically ventilated patients are useful measures for lowering ICP and may offer neuroprotection by reducing ischemia secondary to excitotoxicity. Ketamine, previously thought to be detrimental in pediatric TBI, has recently been shown to decrease ICP without causing hypotension or lowering CPP after pediatric TBI [58]. Propofol is an additional agent that may lower ICP and has a short half-life allowing for serial neurologic examinations; however, propofol may lower blood pressure and therefore have a detrimental effect on CPP. Prolonged administration of propofol may result in the propofol infusion syndrome, a fatty acid-based mitochondrial dysfunction that may result in rhabdomyolysis, cardiac failure, electrolyte abnormalities, and death. Propofol infusion syndrome is more common in children, and therefore, propofol is usually used for short periods only after TBI in children. Neuromuscular blockade may lower ICP by several mechanisms including reducing venous pressure by eliminating muscle contraction and shivering and may facilitate ventilation and PCO_2 control. Patients under neuromuscular blockade are at increased risk for pressure sores and may be at higher risk for ventilator-associated pneumonias. Hyperosmolar therapy, CSF drainage, and second-tier therapies will be discussed in detail later in this chapter.

Cerebral Perfusion Pressure

Cerebral perfusion pressure has become an important measurement of brain perfusion and oxygenation in adult and pediatric TBI. CPP is calculated by subtracting ICP from mean arterial pressure and represents the net blood pressure supplied to the brain in the setting of increased resistance to perfusion due to elevated ICP. When the autoregulatory capabilities of the cerebral vasculature are impaired, or when mean arterial pressure is below the lower limit of autoregulation, brain perfusion is entirely dependent on CPP. Poor CPP is therefore indicative of poor cerebral perfusion and is thought to correlate with increased secondary injury. Therefore, clinicians must take into account the effect on CPP when administering any ICP-lowering therapies. Therapies directed primarily at increasing CPP while having negligible effects on ICP, such as intravenous vasopressor support, may be required. Furthermore, avoidance of hypotension is critical in this patient population due to its deleterious effect on CPP.

Identifying target CPP for children of various ages has been a focus of pediatric TBI research during the last several decades. Research from the 1980s and 1990s had suggested that CPP targets between 40 and 65 mmHg were associated with favorable outcomes after TBI [59–62]. More recent studies have attempted to establish specific age-appropriate CPP targets in children. Chambers and colleagues, in a study of 235 children with TBI, divided patients into three age groups including 2–6, 7–10, and 11–16 years and analyzed CPP in regards to outcome. Target CPPs of 53, 63, and 66 mmHg were identified as being threshold values for good outcome in the three age groups, respectively [63]. In addition, a recent analysis of outcomes in 22 children less than 2 years of age has identified a CPP threshold value of 45 mmHg as being an important determinant of good outcome [64].

Brain Oxygen Tension

The principle of maintaining adequate $PbtO_2$ after TBI is based on evidence in the adult literature of an association between low $PbtO_2$ and poor outcome [65–68]. Although the technology is still poorly understood, lower measured brain oxygen tension is thought to be an indicator of generalized cerebral ischemia, hypoxia, and poor oxidative metabolism, and therefore, a lower measured $PbtO_2$ may be a marker of increased secondary injury. However, the relationship between aggressive measures to improve $PbtO_2$ and better outcomes is less clear. In the adult literature, several studies have indicated that therapies directed primarily at maintaining $PbtO_2$ may be superior to traditional ICP-directed therapies [67, 68], although limited evidence does exist to the contrary [69].

Studies evaluating the relationship between $PbtO_2$ and outcome in children appear to demonstrate similar results. In a prospective pediatric study of 52 TBI patients undergoing both brain oxygen tension and ICP monitoring, low $PbtO_2$ was an independent risk factor for poor outcome and had the strongest independent association with poor outcome compared to other factors [70]. Interestingly, one study revealed that up to one-third of pediatric patients with severe TBI may have periods of low-oxygen tension ($PbtO_2$ less than 10 mmHg) despite strict adherence to standard treatment goals for ICP, CPP, and even blood oxygen tension [71]. Furthermore, children who displayed periods of low $PbtO_2$ in the study of 52 TBI patients were poorly predicted by other measures of TBI severity [72]. Although it is apparent that maintaining adequate $PbtO_2$ may be important in optimizing outcomes in pediatric TBI by reducing secondary injury, the role of oxygen tension-directed therapies in children remains poorly understood and, for the most part, experimental at this time.

Hyperosmolar Therapy

The two most common hyperosmolar agents used in TBI are mannitol and hypertonic saline, both of which have demonstrated efficacy in reducing ICP when given intravenously [73–75]. These agents are effective in reducing ICP due to two distinct effects: first, plasma expansion with a resultant decrease in hematocrit and cerebral blood volume and second, by the creation of an osmotic gradient that results in shifting of fluid from the cerebral to the intravascular compartment. Mannitol is administered in doses of 0.25–1 g/kg while keeping measured serum osmolarity less than 320 mOsm/L to prevent mannitol-induced acute renal insufficiency. Hypertonic saline is usually administered either as a 3 % continuous infusion of 0.1–1 mL/kg/h or in 23.4 % bolus injections while keeping osmolarity below 360 mOsm/L. Recent evidence in both adult and pediatric patients may indicate superiority of hypertonic saline over mannitol in controlling ICP [73, 76]. In one trial, children with elevated ICP randomized to hypertonic saline had significantly shorter coma lengths than those receiving mannitol [76]. At this time, both agents remain effective measures for reducing ICP in pediatric TBI.

Induced Hypothermia

In 1997, a landmark article was published by Marion and colleagues that showed improved neurologic recovery in adults randomized to moderate hypothermia compared to those randomized to normothermia after severe TBI. In this trial, 40 adults were randomized to the cooling group which entailed cooling to a mean of 33 °C, maintained at 32–33 °C for 24 h, then slowly rewarmed at a rate not exceeding 1 °C/h. Those randomized to hypothermia had significantly improved outcomes at 3 and 6 months compared to controls, but no difference was noted at 12 months [77]. Unfortunately, a large multicenter trial that followed failed to reproduce these results, showing no difference among adults randomized to hypothermia versus controls [78].

Hypothermia has shown efficacy in reducing mortality and neurological impairment in newborns with perinatal hypoxic-ischemic encephalopathy [79, 80]. Furthermore, the results from Marion and colleagues indicated that younger adults may have improved outcomes compared to older adults [77], suggesting that the benefits of hypothermia may be age dependent. To test the safety of induced hypothermia in children after TBI, a phase II trial was performed involving 48 children randomized to moderate hypothermia or normothermia within 6 h of injury. Although definitive conclusions could not be drawn regarding its effective on outcomes, hypothermia was associated with a trend of improved neurologic outcome [81]. In 2008, the results of a large multicenter trial were published in which 225 children were randomized to hypothermia versus normothermia. Hypothermia was associated with a trend of increased mortality and poor neurologic outcome compared to those kept normothermic; in addition, hypotension and need for pressor support were significantly increased in the group that was cooled [82]. Although these results have seriously questioned the role of induced hypothermia after pediatric TBI, many authorities believe hypothermia still holds promise given its purported neuroprotective effects. Further large-scale studies evaluating different hypothermia protocols are necessary. Until that time, induced hypothermia after pediatric TBI remains experimental.

Cerebrospinal Fluid Drainage

Placement of an external ventricular drain allows for both measurement of ICP as well as drainage of CSF to help control elevated ICP. Strategies for CSF drainage include both intermittent drainage, such as draining CSF only when ICP is elevated, and continuous drainage, where the ventricular catheter is left open and allowed to drain by gravity with the system fixed to a target height above the tragus. There are little data comparing these two strategies although one small study of 19 pediatric TBI patients revealed that continuous drainage resulted in lower mean ICP, increased CSF drained, and lower CSF biomarkers of neuronal injury [83]. Interestingly, in one small study, the use of lumbar drainage of CSF in pediatric patients who failed to show ICP improvement after ventricular drainage and had patent cisterns without a mass lesion resulted in persistently lowered ICP and obviated the need for other ICP-lowering therapies [84]. While ventricular drainage remains standard practice, lumbar drainage is controversial and is not used at most centers.

Decompressive Craniectomy

Decompressive craniectomy after TBI is employed in two settings: first, in the presence of a mass lesion necessitating surgery where the craniotomy bone flap is left off to reduce ICP from expected postsurgical swelling, and, second, to treat medically refractory ICP in the absence of a mass lesion. Surgical decompression as a treatment for refractory intracranial hypertension alone after brain trauma continues to be a topic of considerable debate. Currently, there is no class 1 evidence to support or refute the use of routine decompression in adults with severe brain injuries and elevated ICP. There is a single randomized study in the pediatric literature in which 27 patients were randomized to either early craniectomy and medical therapy or maximal medical therapy alone; 14 % of those receiving medical therapy only had no or mild disability at 6 months, while 54 % of those undergoing craniectomy had good outcomes [85]. Furthermore, several retrospective reviews of severe pediatric TBI have indicated that craniectomy may be a successful salvage therapy in those with refractory ICP [86–88] and may be useful if performed in the first few hours after the injury in those where further ICP elevations are expected [89]. The benefits of decompression appear to be a result of immediate (and frequently persistent) reduction in ICP and the associated improvements in cerebral oxygenation and perfusion pressures [90]. In patients who survive, the skull defect is usually replaced several months after the injury with the original craniectomy flap or with a synthetic cranioplasty. Complications associated with decompressive craniectomy include posttraumatic hydrocephalus and epilepsy, which were reported in 40 and 20 % of children in one series, respectively [91].

Barbiturate Coma

Hemodynamically stable patients with ICP refractory to first-tier therapies may be candidates for continuous infusion of barbiturates, which slows cerebral metabolism and reduces cerebral oxygen consumption. This treatment may reduce secondary injury after TBI by temporarily decreasing cerebral oxygen demand. When initiated on barbiturate therapy, patients are monitored for adequate suppression of brain activity (referred to as "burst suppression") by electroencephalography. The effectiveness of barbiturate coma for refractory intracranial hypertension has come into question recently, particularly given its systemic effects such as myocardial depression and hypotension [92], although there is some evidence of benefit [93]. There is, however, little evidence suggesting the benefits outweigh the risks in the pediatric population. In a review of children receiving barbiturates for elevated ICP, 90 % required the use of vasopressors or intravascular volume resuscitation due to barbiturate-induced hypotension [94]. In addition, barbiturate therapy may potentially have lasting developmental consequences on the developing nervous system due to its effects on synaptic activity. For these reason, barbiturate coma remains a controversial treatment option for children with severe brain injuries.

Cardiopulmonary Considerations

Cardiac arrhythmias are common after severe traumatic brain injury in children and are likely reflective of increased serum catecholamine concentrations [95, 96]. In addition, elevated ICP or low CPP after TBI is associated with marked autonomic dysfunction and heart rate variability in children that is proportional to the severity of the injury [97]. Ventilator management and the optimization of cardiac function are important in the management of the pediatric TBI patient. However, these principles are not unique to TBI and are beyond the scope of this chapter. These topics are covered in detail in other chapters in this text.

Seizure Prophylaxis

Early posttraumatic seizures (EPTS) may cause increased metabolic demand after TBI and are speculated to promote secondary injury by exacerbating brain hypoxia, hypercarbia, and ICP. Therefore, identifying and treating patients considered high risk for seizures after TBI has the theoretical benefit of reducing secondary injury burden. In children with accidental or non-accidental brain injuries, EPTS are associated with worse outcomes [98–100]. Younger age (less than 2 years), more severe injury, non-accidental trauma, and SDH are established risk factors for EPTS after TBI [11, 98, 101–103]. However, data regarding the prophylactic use of antiepileptic drugs (AED) in this setting are mixed. The 2003 guidelines for severe TBI management recommended consideration of prophylactic AED in patients who are expected to be high risk for EPTS based on adult and limited pediatric evidence of benefit after TBI [6]. A trial of 102 children after moderate to severe blunt head injury randomized to either phenytoin or placebo revealed no significant difference between EPTS and outcome at 30 days [104]. Seizures only occurred in 6 patients (3 in each group), questioning the utility for AED after trauma. A more recent retrospective analysis of 275 children with moderate or severe TBI, of which nearly half were administered an AED as prophylaxis, demonstrated a 12 % rate of EPTS. Antiepileptic prophylaxis significantly reduced the odds of EPTS in this analysis by a factor of five [105]. In summary, the theoretical benefits of seizure suppression by AED administration have not consistently been demonstrated after pediatric TBI, with a randomized trial failing to demonstrate benefit. Administration of such agents to patients deemed high risk for EPTS based on clinical factors likely represents the best management approach at this time.

Glycemic Control

Several retrospective reviews evaluating glucose levels during the hospitalization for children with TBI have indicated an association between hyperglycemia and poor outcome [106–108]. In these reviews, admission hyperglycemia in particular appeared to be the strongest glycemic predictor of poor outcome. These findings suggest that marked hyperglycemia on admission may be an indicator of more severe brain injury and larger stress response, although the pathophysiology of this relationship is poorly understood. Unfortunately, there are currently little data to support the use of tight glycemic control after head injury in children, but the absence of evidence does not imply absence of benefit. Tight glycemic control while in the pediatric ICU has reduced morbidity and mortality associated with other disease processes, particularly in severely burned children [109, 110], and will likely play an important role in pediatric TBI management in the future.

Venous Thromboembolism Prophylaxis

In stark contrast to adult critical care literature, the risk of venous thromboembolism (VTE) in critically ill children is exceedingly low, estimated at approximately 6 VTE per 1,000 discharges [111]. The presence of a central venous line, more than any other factor, appears to impart the greatest risk of VTE in children after trauma [111–113]. Overall, venous thromboembolism is exceedingly rare in those less than 17 years of age, and, therefore, prophylaxis is not recommended in this age group [114].

Nutrition

Adequate nutritional support during the acute phase after TBI in infants and children has theoretical benefits of optimizing nutritional status and providing the necessary energy substrates for recovery after injury. Based on the 2003 brain injury recommendations, initiation of nutrition should be performed within 72 h of injury [6]. However, nutritional support in the pediatric ICU has not been well investigated, and there are no clear guidelines for timing or type (parenteral versus enteral) of nutrition in the critically ill child [115].

Coagulopathy

The development of coagulopathy is common after adult multi-trauma and represents an independent predictor of mortality [116]. Traumatic brain injury-associated coagulopathy, defined as a platelet count less than 100,000 and/or elevated international normalized ratio and/or activated partial thromboplastin time in the setting of TBI, occurred in approximately one-third of adult patients after severe brain injury in a prospective trial of over 400 patients by Talving and colleagues. Risk factors for the development of coagulopathy were penetrating injury, GCS less than 9, hypotension, and CT findings of cerebral edema, midline shift, or subarachnoid hemorrhage. The authors concluded that the development of coagulopathy in the adult population increased the risk of death tenfold and resulted in longer ICU stays [117]. Although few studies have evaluated coagulopathy in pediatric TBI, risk of coagulopathy

appears to be directly related to injury severity and therefore inversely related to GCS in children [118–120]. In the largest retrospective analysis of pediatric TBI, coagulopathy developed in 40 % of patients but was not independently associated with increased mortality. Risk factors for coagulopathy included increasing injury severity, increasing age, and the presence of intraparenchymal lesions on CT [119].

Adrenal Insufficiency

It is estimated that acute adrenal insufficiency (AI) occurs in approximately one-quarter of adult patients after TBI [121]. In a study of 28 children with TBI in which serial cortisol and adrenocorticotropin levels were obtained while hospitalized, 36 % demonstrated laboratory evidence of AI. Adrenal insufficiency was more common in patients with elevated ICP, and those with AI required significantly longer periods of mechanical ventilation than those without AI [122]. Chronic endocrinopathies are common after pediatric TBI and are easily treatable when detected. Laboratory work-up for AI is important while in the acute phase; however, children should be monitored closely in the years that follow for the development of chronic AI or delayed growth that may be secondary to TBI-related pituitary dysfunction [123].

Future Therapies

A pilot study evaluating the safety of intravenous, autologous bone marrow-derived mononuclear cells, thought to be neuroprotective based on preclinical evidence, after severe TBI in ten pediatric patients revealed no delayed changes in MRI findings, with 7 of the 10 displaying good outcomes at 6 months [124]. The authors concluded that autologous mononuclear cell administration is safe and feasible for larger clinical trials.

Outcome

Of the approximately 400,000 brain injuries sustained annually by children, approximately 3,000 are fatal injuries and 29,000 require hospitalization. CDC data from 1997 regarding the risk of mortality in children from TBI by age group indicated an increasing risk with increasing age, with those 15–19 years having the highest mortality rate (17 %). Using an algorithm to predict disability based on injury severity, disposition, and type of injury based on acute care hospital discharges for pediatric TBI data from one US state from 1996 to 1999, the CDC predicted that approximately 8 % of all discharged patients would "probably" have disabilities,

47 % would "possibly" have disabilities, and 45 % were "unlikely" to have disabilities [125]. Although these data appear crude, it underscores the sheer number of newly disabled children due to TBI.

Physical, cognitive, and emotional deficits are common in children who survive after TBI. In the first year after severe TBI, executive dysfunction is common and affects approximately 20–40 % of children [126]. Children with more severe injuries demonstrate slower recovery and poorer cognitive outcomes up to 5 years after the insult, although most children stabilize after approximately 30 months and begin to make appropriate gains in the realms of verbal and nonverbal skills, attention, and other measures of intellectual function [127]. In one study of 49 patients 10 years after TBI, those with severe injuries displayed persistent reductions in gray and white matter volume, while patients with any degree of TBI (mild through severe) demonstrated smaller hippocampi and larger CSF spaces compared to age-matched controls [128]. These studies indicate that any degree of TBI may have lasting effects on cognitive, emotional, and physical development of children well beyond the time of injury and even into adulthood.

Conclusions

Traumatic brain injury remains the most common cause of mortality and is a leading cause of persistent disability in children. The primary goals of pediatric TBI ICU therapies revolve around reducing secondary injury to neurons by optimizing CPP and oxygen delivery to the brain while controlling elevations in ICP. Upon initial evaluation of a child who sustained a TBI, a primary assessment should be performed in which an adequate airway is obtained, hemodynamic stabilization is performed, and a neurologic exam is recorded. Patients should then undergo brain and associated imaging by CT scan to detect intracranial mass lesions or solid organ injuries necessitating emergency operative intervention. Those with GCS of 8 or less should undergo placement of intracranial monitoring for measurement of ICP, CPP, and PbtO$_2$, while those with GCS of 9 or more should be followed with serial neurologic examinations. In patients with elevated ICP, high benefit-to-risk (first-tier) therapies are initiated in a stepwise fashion. These include optimizing patient positioning, sedation, neuromuscular blockade, hyperosmolar therapies, and CSF drainage. Patients with ICP refractory to first-tier measures may benefit from second-tier interventions, such as decompressive craniectomy. The most important predictor of outcome is GCS. Although patients with severe injuries have the highest risk of persistent cognitive and emotional dysfunction, even children with mild TBI may have lasting disabilities secondary to their injuries. This fact underscores the importance of preventative measures in reducing TBI incidence.

References

1. Langlois JA, Rutland-Brown W, Wald MM. The epidemiology and impact of traumatic brain injury: a brief overview. J Head Trauma Rehabil. 2006;21:375–8.
2. Bishop NB. Traumatic brain injury: a primer for primary care physicians. Curr Probl Pediatr Adolesc Health Care. 2006;36:318–31.
3. Tilford JM, Aitken ME, Anand KJ, et al. Hospitalizations for critically ill children with traumatic brain injuries: a longitudinal analysis. Crit Care Med. 2005;33:2074–81.
4. Giza CC, Mink RB, Madikians A. Pediatric traumatic brain injury: not just little adults. Curr Opin Crit Care. 2007;13:143–52.
5. Morrow SE, Pearson M. Management strategies for severe closed head injuries in children. Semin Pediatr Surg. 2010;19:279–85.
6. Adelson PD, Bratton SL, Carney NA, et al. Guidelines for the acute medical management of severe traumatic brain injury in infants, children, and adolescents. Chapter 1: Introduction. Pediatr Crit Care Med. 2003;4:S2–4.
7. Faul M, Xu L, Wald MM, Coronado VG. Traumatic brain injury in the United States: emergency department visits, hospitalizations and deaths 2002–2006. Centers for Disease Control and Prevention, National Center for Injury Prevention and Control; 2010.
8. Bowman SM, Aitken ME. Still unsafe, still in use: ongoing epidemic of all-terrain vehicle injury hospitalizations among children. J Trauma. 2010;69:1344–9.
9. Walsh C, MacMillan HL, Jamieson E. The relationship between parental substance abuse and child maltreatment: findings from the Ontario Health Supplement. Child Abuse Negl. 2003;27:1409–25.
10. Schnitzer PG, Ewigman BG. Child deaths resulting from inflicted injuries: household risk factors and perpetrator characteristics. Pediatrics. 2005;116:e687–93.
11. Keenan HT, Runyan DK, Marshall SW, Nocera MA, Merten DF, Sinal SH. A population-based study of inflicted traumatic brain injury in young children. JAMA. 2003;290:621–6.
12. Sookplung P, Vavilala MS. What is new in pediatric traumatic brain injury? Curr Opin Anaesthesiol. 2009;22:572–8.
13. Potoka DA, Schall LC, Ford HR. Improved functional outcome for severely injured children treated at pediatric trauma centers. J Trauma. 2001;51:824–32; discussion 32–4.
14. Hall JR, Reyes HM, Meller JL, Loeff DS, Dembek R. The outcome for children with blunt trauma is best at a pediatric trauma center. J Pediatr Surg. 1996;31:72–6; discussion 6–7.
15. Hartman M, Watson RS, Linde-Zwirble W, et al. Pediatric traumatic brain injury is inconsistently regionalized in the United States. Pediatrics. 2008;122:e172–80.
16. Coates BM, Vavilala MS, Mack CD, et al. Influence of definition and location of hypotension on outcome following severe pediatric traumatic brain injury. Crit Care Med. 2005;33:2645–50.
17. Simma B, Burger R, Falk M, Sacher P, Fanconi S. A prospective, randomized, and controlled study of fluid management in children with severe head injury: lactated Ringer's solution versus hypertonic saline. Crit Care Med. 1998;26:1265–70.
18. Myburgh J, Cooper DJ, Finfer S, et al. Saline or albumin for fluid resuscitation in patients with traumatic brain injury. N Engl J Med. 2007;357:874–84.
19. Prasad K. The Glasgow Coma Scale: a critical appraisal of its clinimetric properties. J Clin Epidemiol. 1996;49:755–63.
20. Chung CY, Chen CL, Cheng PT, See LC, Tang SF, Wong AM. Critical score of Glasgow Coma Scale for pediatric traumatic brain injury. Pediatr Neurol. 2006;34:379–87.
21. Grinkeviciute DE, Kevalas R, Saferis V, Matukevicius A, Ragaisis V, Tamasauskas A. Predictive value of scoring system in severe pediatric head injury. Medicina (Kaunas). 2007;43:861–9.
22. Stocchetti N, Pagan F, Calappi E, et al. Inaccurate early assessment of neurological severity in head injury. J Neurotrauma. 2004;21:1131–40.

23. Wijdicks EF, Bamlet WR, Maramattom BV, Manno EM, McClelland RL. Validation of a new coma scale: the FOUR score. Ann Neurol. 2005;58:585–93.

24. Tepas 3rd JJ, Mollitt DL, Talbert JL, Bryant M. The pediatric trauma score as a predictor of injury severity in the injured child. J Pediatr Surg. 1987;22:14–8.

25. Ramenofsky ML, Ramenofsky MB, Jurkovich GJ, Threadgill D, Dierking BH, Powell RW. The predictive validity of the pediatric trauma score. J Trauma. 1988;28:1038–42.

26. Pollack MM, Patel KM, Ruttimann UE. PRISM III: an updated pediatric risk of mortality score. Crit Care Med. 1996;24:743–52.

27. Suskauer SJ, Huisman TA. Neuroimaging in pediatric traumatic brain injury: current and future predictors of functional outcome. Dev Disabil Res Rev. 2009;15:117–23.

28. Blackwell CD, Gorelick M, Holmes JF, Bandyopadhyay S, Kuppermann N. Pediatric head trauma: changes in use of computed tomography in emergency departments in the United States over time. Ann Emerg Med. 2007;49:320–4.

29. Brenner DJ, Hall EJ. Computed tomography – an increasing source of radiation exposure. N Engl J Med. 2007;357:2277–84.

30. Smits M, Dippel DW, de Haan GG, et al. Minor head injury: guidelines for the use of CT – a multicenter validation study. Radiology. 2007;245:831–8.

31. Beaudin M, Saint-Vil D, Ouimet A, Mercier C, Crevier L. Clinical algorithm and resource use in the management of children with minor head trauma. J Pediatr Surg. 2007;42:849–52.

32. Willis AP, Latif SA, Chandratre S, Stanhope B, Johnson K. Not a NICE CT protocol for the acutely head injured child. Clin Radiol. 2008;63:165–9.

33. Ewing-Cobbs L, Prasad M, Kramer L, et al. Acute neuroradiologic findings in young children with inflicted or noninflicted traumatic brain injury. Childs Nerv Syst. 2000;16:25–33; discussion 4.

34. Keenan HT, Runyan DK, Marshall SW, Nocera MA, Merten DF. A population-based comparison of clinical and outcome characteristics of young children with serious inflicted and noninflicted traumatic brain injury. Pediatrics. 2004;114:633–9.

35. Durham SR, Liu KC, Selden NR. Utility of serial computed tomography imaging in pediatric patients with head trauma. J Neurosurg. 2006;105:365–9.

36. Hollingworth W, Vavilala MS, Jarvik JG, et al. The use of repeated head computed tomography in pediatric blunt head trauma: factors predicting new and worsening brain injury. Pediatr Crit Care Med. 2007;8:348–56; CEU quiz 57.

37. Beauchamp MH, Ditchfield M, Babl F, et al. Detecting traumatic brain lesions in children: CT vs conventional MRI vs susceptibility weighted imaging (SWI). J Neurotrauma. 2011;28(6):915–27.

38. Levin HS, Mendelsohn D, Lilly MA, et al. Magnetic resonance imaging in relation to functional outcome of pediatric closed head injury: a test of the Ommaya-Gennarelli model. Neurosurgery. 1997;40:432–40; discussion 40–1.

39. Grados MA, Slomine BS, Gerring JP, Vasa R, Bryan N, Denckla MB. Depth of lesion model in children and adolescents with moderate to severe traumatic brain injury: use of SPGR MRI to predict severity and outcome. J Neurol Neurosurg Psychiatry. 2001;70:350–8.

40. Power T, Catroppa C, Coleman L, Ditchfield M, Anderson V. Do lesion site and severity predict deficits in attentional control after preschool traumatic brain injury (TBI)? Brain Inj. 2007;21:279–92.

41. Slomine BS, Gerring JP, Grados MA, et al. Performance on measures of executive function following pediatric traumatic brain injury. Brain Inj. 2002;16:759–72.

42. Melo JR, Di Rocco F, Blanot S, et al. Transcranial Doppler can predict intracranial hypertension in children with severe traumatic brain injuries. Childs Nerv Syst. 2011;27:979–84.

43. Berger RP, Adelson PD, Richichi R, Kochanek PM. Serum biomarkers after traumatic and hypoxemic brain injuries: insight into the biochemical response of the pediatric brain to inflicted brain injury. Dev Neurosci. 2006;28:327–35.

44. Berger RP, Dulani T, Adelson PD, Leventhal JM, Richichi R, Kochanek PM. Identification of inflicted traumatic brain injury in well-appearing infants using serum and cerebrospinal markers: a possible screening tool. Pediatrics. 2006;117:325–32.

45. Berger RP, Beers SR, Richichi R, Wiesman D, Adelson PD. Serum biomarker concentrations and outcome after pediatric traumatic brain injury. J Neurotrauma. 2007;24:1793–801.

46. Salonia R, Empey PE, Poloyac SM, et al. Endothelin-1 is increased in cerebrospinal fluid and associated with unfavorable outcomes in children after severe traumatic brain injury. J Neurotrauma. 2010;27:1819–25.

47. Adelson PD, Bratton SL, Carney NA, et al. Guidelines for the acute medical management of severe traumatic brain injury in infants, children, and adolescents. Chapter 5. Indications for intracranial pressure monitoring in pediatric patients with severe traumatic brain injury. Pediatr Crit Care Med. 2003;4:S19–24.

48. Exo J, Kochanek PM, Adelson PD, et al. Intracranial pressure-monitoring systems in children with traumatic brain injury: combining therapeutic and diagnostic tools. Pediatr Crit Care Med. 2011;12(5):560–5.

49. Al-Tamimi YZ, Helmy A, Bavetta S, Price SJ. Assessment of zero drift in the Codman intracranial pressure monitor: a study from 2 neurointensive care units. Neurosurgery. 2009;64:94–8; discussion 8–9.

50. Gelabert-Gonzalez M, Ginesta-Galan V, Sernamito-Garcia R, Allut AG, Bandin-Dieguez J, Rumbo RM. The Camino intracranial pressure device in clinical practice. Assessment in a 1000 cases. Acta Neurochir (Wien). 2006;148:435–41.

51. Rohlwink UK, Figaji AA. Methods of monitoring brain oxygenation. Childs Nerv Syst. 2010;26:453–64.

52. Anderson RC, Kan P, Klimo P, Brockmeyer DL, Walker ML, Kestle JR. Complications of intracranial pressure monitoring in children with head trauma. J Neurosurg. 2004;101:53–8.

53. Mazzola CA, Adelson PD. Critical care management of head trauma in children. Crit Care Med. 2002;30:S393–401.

54. Catala-Temprano A, Claret Teruel G, Cambra Lasaosa FJ, Pons Odena M, Noguera Julian A, Palomeque Rico A. Intracranial pressure and cerebral perfusion pressure as risk factors in children with traumatic brain injuries. J Neurosurg. 2007;106:463–6.

55. Dean NP, Boslaugh S, Adelson PD, Pineda JA, Leonard JR. Physician agreement with evidence-based recommendations for the treatment of severe traumatic brain injury in children. J Neurosurg. 2007;107:387–91.

56. Fanconi S, Kloti J, Meuli M, Zaugg H, Zachmann M. Dexamethasone therapy and endogenous cortisol production in severe pediatric head injury. Intensive Care Med. 1988;14:163–6.

57. Agbeko RS, Pearson S, Peters MJ, McNames J, Goldstein B. Intracranial pressure and cerebral perfusion pressure responses to head elevation changes in pediatric traumatic brain injury. Pediatr Crit Care Med. 2012;13(1):e39–47.

58. Bar-Joseph G, Guilburd Y, Tamir A, Guilburd JN. Effectiveness of ketamine in decreasing intracranial pressure in children with intracranial hypertension. J Neurosurg Pediatr. 2009;4:40–6.

59. Kaiser G, Pfenninger J. Effect of neurointensive care upon outcome following severe head injuries in childhood – a preliminary report. Neuropediatrics. 1984;15:68–75.

60. Barzilay Z, Augarten A, Sagy M, Shahar E, Yahav Y, Boichis H. Variables affecting outcome from severe brain injury in children. Intensive Care Med. 1988;14:417–21.

61. Elias-Jones AC, Punt JA, Turnbull AE, Jaspan T. Management and outcome of severe head injuries in the Trent region 1985–90. Arch Dis Child. 1992;67:1430–5.

62. Downard C, Hulka F, Mullins RJ, et al. Relationship of cerebral perfusion pressure and survival in pediatric brain-injured patients. J Trauma. 2000;49:654–8; discussion 8–9.

63. Chambers IR, Stobbart L, Jones PA, et al. Age-related differences in intracranial pressure and cerebral perfusion pressure in the first 6 hours of monitoring after children's head injury: association with outcome. Childs Nerv Syst. 2005;21:195–9.

64. Mehta A, Kochanek PM, Tyler-Kabara E, et al. Relationship of intracranial pressure and cerebral perfusion pressure with outcome in young children after severe traumatic brain injury. Dev Neurosci. 2010;32:413–9.

65. Valadka AB, Gopinath SP, Contant CF, Uzura M, Robertson CS. Relationship of brain tissue PO2 to outcome after severe head injury. Crit Care Med. 1998;26:1576–81.

66. van den Brink WA, van Santbrink H, Steyerberg EW, et al. Brain oxygen tension in severe head injury. Neurosurgery. 2000;46:868–76; discussion 76–8.

67. Stiefel MF, Spiotta A, Gracias VH, et al. Reduced mortality rate in patients with severe traumatic brain injury treated with brain tissue oxygen monitoring. J Neurosurg. 2005;103:805–11.

68. Narotam PK, Morrison JF, Nathoo N. Brain tissue oxygen monitoring in traumatic brain injury and major trauma: outcome analysis of a brain tissue oxygen-directed therapy. J Neurosurg. 2009;111:672–82.

69. Martini RP, Deem S, Yanez ND, et al. Management guided by brain tissue oxygen monitoring and outcome following severe traumatic brain injury. J Neurosurg. 2009;111:644–9.

70. Figaji AA, Zwane E, Thompson C, et al. Brain tissue oxygen tension monitoring in pediatric severe traumatic brain injury. Part 1: relationship with outcome. Childs Nerv Syst. 2009;25:1325–33.

71. Figaji AA, Fieggen AG, Argent AC, Leroux PD, Peter JC. Does adherence to treatment targets in children with severe traumatic brain injury avoid brain hypoxia? A brain tissue oxygenation study. Neurosurgery. 2008;63:83–91; discussion –2.

72. Figaji AA, Zwane E, Thompson C, et al. Brain tissue oxygen tension monitoring in pediatric severe traumatic brain injury. Part 2: relationship with clinical, physiological, and treatment factors. Childs Nerv Syst. 2009;25:1335–43.

73. Kamel H, Navi BB, Nakagawa K, Hemphill 3rd JC, Ko NU. Hypertonic saline versus mannitol for the treatment of elevated intracranial pressure: a meta-analysis of randomized clinical trials. Crit Care Med. 2011;39:554–9.

74. Sakellaridis N, Pavlou E, Karatzas S, et al. Comparison of mannitol and hypertonic saline in the treatment of severe brain injuries. J Neurosurg. 2011;114:545–8.

75. Wakai A, Roberts I, Schierhout G. Mannitol for acute traumatic brain injury. Cochrane Database Syst Rev. 2007:CD001049.

76. Upadhyay P, Tripathi VN, Singh RP, Sachan D. Role of hypertonic saline and mannitol in the management of raised intracranial pressure in children: a randomized comparative study. J Pediatr Neurosci. 2010;5:18–21.

77. Marion DW, Penrod LE, Kelsey SF, et al. Treatment of traumatic brain injury with moderate hypothermia. N Engl J Med. 1997;336:540–6.

78. Clifton GL, Miller ER, Choi SC, et al. Lack of effect of induction of hypothermia after acute brain injury. N Engl J Med. 2001;344:556–63.

79. Edwards AD, Brocklehurst P, Gunn AJ, et al. Neurological outcomes at 18 months of age after moderate hypothermia for perinatal hypoxic ischaemic encephalopathy: synthesis and meta-analysis of trial data. BMJ. 2010;340:c363.

80. Jacobs S, Hunt R, Tarnow-Mordi W, Inder T, Davis P. Cooling for newborns with hypoxic ischaemic encephalopathy. Cochrane Database Syst Rev. 2007:CD003311.

81. Adelson PD, Ragheb J, Kanev P, et al. Phase II clinical trial of moderate hypothermia after severe traumatic brain injury in children. Neurosurgery. 2005;56:740–54; discussion –54.

82. Hutchison JS, Ward RE, Lacroix J, et al. Hypothermia therapy after traumatic brain injury in children. N Engl J Med. 2008;358:2447–56.

83. Shore PM, Thomas NJ, Clark RS, et al. Continuous versus intermittent cerebrospinal fluid drainage after severe traumatic brain injury in children: effect on biochemical markers. J Neurotrauma. 2004;21:1113–22.

84. Levy DI, Rekate HL, Cherny WB, Manwaring K, Moss SD, Baldwin HZ. Controlled lumbar drainage in pediatric head injury. J Neurosurg. 1995;83:453–60.

85. Taylor A, Butt W, Rosenfeld J, et al. A randomized trial of very early decompressive craniectomy in children with traumatic brain injury and sustained intracranial hypertension. Childs Nerv Syst. 2001;17:154–62.

86. Jagannathan J, Okonkwo DO, Dumont AS, et al. Outcome following decompressive craniectomy in children with severe traumatic brain injury: a 10-year single-center experience with long-term follow up. J Neurosurg. 2007;106:268–75.

87. Rutigliano D, Egnor MR, Priebe CJ, et al. Decompressive craniectomy in pediatric patients with traumatic brain injury with intractable elevated intracranial pressure. J Pediatr Surg. 2006;41:83–7; discussion –7.

88. Thomale UW, Graetz D, Vajkoczy P, Sarrafzadeh AS. Severe traumatic brain injury in children – a single center experience regarding therapy and long-term outcome. Childs Nerv Syst. 2010;26:1563–73.

89. Josan VA, Sgouros S. Early decompressive craniectomy may be effective in the treatment of refractory intracranial hypertension after traumatic brain injury. Childs Nerv Syst. 2006;22:1268–74.

90. Figaji AA, Fieggen AG, Argent AC, Le Roux PD, Peter JC. Intracranial pressure and cerebral oxygenation changes after decompressive craniectomy in children with severe traumatic brain injury. Acta Neurochir Suppl. 2008;102:77–80.

91. Kan P, Amini A, Hansen K, et al. Outcomes after decompressive craniectomy for severe traumatic brain injury in children. J Neurosurg. 2006;105:337–42.

92. Roberts I. Barbiturates for acute traumatic brain injury. Cochrane Database Syst Rev. 2000:CD000033.

93. Marshall GT, James RF, Landman MP, et al. Pentobarbital coma for refractory intra-cranial hypertension after severe traumatic brain injury: mortality predictions and one-year outcomes in 55 patients. J Trauma. 2010;69:275–83.

94. Kasoff SS, Lansen TA, Holder D, Filippo JS. Aggressive physiologic monitoring of pediatric head trauma patients with elevated intracranial pressure. Pediatr Neurosci. 1988;14:241–9.

95. Goldstein B, Kempski MH, DeKing D, et al. Autonomic control of heart rate after brain injury in children. Crit Care Med. 1996;24:234–40.

96. Bourdages M, Bigras JL, Farrell CA, Hutchison JS, Lacroix J. Cardiac arrhythmias associated with severe traumatic brain injury and hypothermia therapy. Pediatr Crit Care Med. 2010;11:408–14.

97. Biswas AK, Scott WA, Sommerauer JF, Luckett PM. Heart rate variability after acute traumatic brain injury in children. Crit Care Med. 2000;28:3907–12.

98. Ong LC, Dhillon MK, Selladurai BM, Maimunah A, Lye MS. Early post-traumatic seizures in children: clinical and radiological aspects of injury. J Paediatr Child Health. 1996;32:173–6.

99. Chiaretti A, De Benedictis R, Polidori G, Piastra M, Iannelli A, Di Rocco C. Early post-traumatic seizures in children with head injury. Childs Nerv Syst. 2000;16:862–6.

100. Keenan HT, Hooper SR, Wetherington CE, Nocera M, Runyan DK. Neurodevelopmental consequences of early traumatic brain injury in 3-year-old children. Pediatrics. 2007;119:e616–23.

101. Ratan SK, Kulshreshtha R, Pandey RM. Predictors of posttraumatic convulsions in head-injured children. Pediatr Neurosurg. 1999;30:127–31.

102. Barlow KM, Spowart JJ, Minns RA. Early posttraumatic seizures in non-accidental head injury: relation to outcome. Dev Med Child Neurol. 2000;42:591–4.

103. Hahn YS, Fuchs S, Flannery AM, Barthel MJ, McLone DG. Factors influencing posttraumatic seizures in children. Neurosurgery. 1988;22:864–7.

104. Young KD, Okada PJ, Sokolove PE, et al. A randomized, double-blinded, placebo-controlled trial of phenytoin for the prevention of early posttraumatic seizures in children with moderate to severe blunt head injury. Ann Emerg Med. 2004;43:435–46.

105. Liesemer K, Bratton SL, Zebrack CM, Brockmeyer D, Statler KD. Early post-traumatic seizures in moderate to severe pediatric traumatic brain injury: rates, risk factors, and clinical features. J Neurotrauma. 2011;28:755–62.

106. Smith RL, Lin JC, Adelson PD, et al. Relationship between hyperglycemia and outcome in children with severe traumatic brain injury. Pediatr Crit Care Med. 2012;13(1):85–91.

107. Asilioglu N, Turna F, Paksu MS. Admission hyperglycemia is a reliable outcome predictor in children with severe traumatic brain injury. J Pediatr (Rio J). 2011;87:325–8.

108. Cochran A, Scaife ER, Hansen KW, Downey EC. Hyperglycemia and outcomes from pediatric traumatic brain injury. J Trauma. 2003;55:1035–8.

109. Jeschke MG, Kulp GA, Kraft R, et al. Intensive insulin therapy in severely burned pediatric patients: a prospective randomized trial. Am J Respir Crit Care Med. 2010;182:351–9.

110. Pham TN, Warren AJ, Phan HH, Molitor F, Greenhalgh DG, Palmieri TL. Impact of tight glycemic control in severely burned children. J Trauma. 2005;59:1148–54.

111. O'Brien SH, Candrilli SD. In the absence of a central venous catheter, risk of venous thromboembolism is low in critically injured children, adolescents, and young adults: evidence from the National Trauma Data Bank. Pediatr Crit Care Med. 2011;12(3):251–6.

112. Hanson SJ, Punzalan RC, Greenup RA, Liu H, Sato TT, Havens PL. Incidence and risk factors for venous thromboembolism in critically ill children after trauma. J Trauma. 2010;68:52–6.

113. Vavilala MS, Nathens AB, Jurkovich GJ, Mackenzie E, Rivara FP. Risk factors for venous thromboembolism in pediatric trauma. J Trauma. 2002;52:922–7.

114. Azu MC, McCormack JE, Scriven RJ, Brebbia JS, Shapiro MJ, Lee TK. Venous thromboembolic events in pediatric trauma patients: is prophylaxis necessary? J Trauma. 2005;59:1345–9.

115. Joffe A, Anton N, Lequier L, et al. Nutritional support for critically ill children. Cochrane Database Syst Rev. 2009:CD005144.

116. MacLeod JB, Lynn M, McKenney MG, Cohn SM, Murtha M. Early coagulopathy predicts mortality in trauma. J Trauma. 2003;55:39–44.

117. Talving P, Benfield R, Hadjizacharia P, Inaba K, Chan LS, Demetriades D. Coagulopathy in severe traumatic brain injury: a prospective study. J Trauma. 2009;66:55–61; discussion −2.

118. Keller MS, Fendya DG, Weber TR. Glasgow Coma Scale predicts coagulopathy in pediatric trauma patients. Semin Pediatr Surg. 2001;10:12–6.

119. Talving P, Lustenberger T, Lam L, et al. Coagulopathy after isolated severe traumatic brain injury in children. J Trauma. 2011;71(5):1205–10.

120. Becker S, Schneider W, Kreuz W, Jacobi G, Scharrer I, Nowak-Gottl U. Post-trauma coagulation and fibrinolysis in children suffering from severe cerebro-cranial trauma. Eur J Pediatr. 1999;158 Suppl 3:S197–202.

121. Powner DJ, Boccalandro C. Adrenal insufficiency following traumatic brain injury in adults. Curr Opin Crit Care. 2008;14:163–6.

122. Dupuis C, Thomas S, Faure P, et al. Secondary adrenal insufficiency in the acute phase of pediatric traumatic brain injury. Intensive Care Med. 2010;36:1906–13.

123. Einaudi S, Bondone C. The effects of head trauma on hypothalamic-pituitary function in children and adolescents. Curr Opin Pediatr. 2007;19:465–70.

124. Cox Jr CS, Baumgartner JE, Harting MT, et al. Autologous bone marrow mononuclear cell therapy for severe traumatic brain injury in children. Neurosurgery. 2011;68:588–600.

125. Langlois JA. Summary and recommendations from the Expert Working Group. Traumatic brain injury in the United States: assessing outcomes in children. Centers for Disease Control and Prevention; 2000.

126. Sesma HW, Slomine BS, Ding R, McCarthy ML. Executive functioning in the first year after pediatric traumatic brain injury. Pediatrics. 2008;121:e1686–95.

127. Anderson V, Catroppa C, Morse S, Haritou F, Rosenfeld JV. Intellectual outcome from preschool traumatic brain injury: a 5-year prospective, longitudinal study. Pediatrics. 2009;124:e1064–71.

128. Beauchamp MH, Ditchfield M, Maller JJ, et al. Hippocampus, amygdala and global brain changes 10 years after childhood traumatic brain injury. Int J Dev Neurosci. 2011;29:137–43.

129. Teasdale G, Jennett B. Assessment of coma and impaired consciousness. A practical scale. Lancet. 1974;2:81–4.

130. Davis RJ, et al. Head and spinal cord injury. In: Rogers MC, editor. Textbook of pediatric intensive care. Baltimore: Williams & Wilkins; 1987.

131. James H, Anas N, Perkin RM. Brain insults in infants and children. New York: Grune & Stratton; 1985.

132. Morray JP, Tyler DC, Jones TK, Stuntz JT, Lemire R. Coma scale for use in brain-injured children. Crit Care Med. 1984;12:1018.

Spinal Cord Injury: Evidence-Based Medicine, Diagnosis, Treatment, and Complications

29

Alexander Taghva and Daniel J. Hoh

Contents

Abstract

Traumatic spinal cord injury can result in devastating motor and sensory deficits with resulting significant morbidity. Sequelae of spinal cord injury can include not only loss of upper and lower extremity function but potentially respiratory, urinary, and autonomic dysfunction with both acute and chronic complications. Currently, there is no available effective treatment for reversing neurologic deficits after traumatic spinal cord injury. Minimizing primary injury and preventing secondary injury depend on appropriate multidisciplinary management by first responders, trauma and spinal surgeons, and neurocritical care physicians. In this chapter, key clinical and neurologic assessment modalities, injury classification schemes, and critical care and surgical treatment strategies are outlined.

Keywords

Spinal cord injury • Spine trauma • Spine surgery • Neuroprotection • Paraplegia • Quadriplegia

Epidemiology

Traumatic spinal cord injury (SCI) remains a significant public health issue worldwide. The incidence of SCI is estimated to be between 10.4 and 83 per million [1], with approximately 15,000 new cases of SCI per year in the United States and Canada [2, 3]. The Centers for Disease Control estimates that nearly 9.7 billion dollars are spent annually in the United States for SCI alone, creating a huge socioeconomic burden [4].

There are an estimated 200,000 individuals in the United States currently living with SCI [5]. Quadriplegia occurs in 54.1 % of cases, with complete SCI occurring in 55.6 % [6]. The most common etiology of SCI is motor vehicle collisions, followed by falls, gunshot wounds, and diving

A. Taghva, MD
Department of Neurological Surgery,
Ohio State University,
410 W 10 Avenue, N1047 Doan Hall,
Columbus, OH 43210, USA
e-mail: alextaghva@gmail.com

D.J. Hoh, MD (✉)
Department of Neurological Surgery,
University of Florida College of Medicine,
BDF 100265, Gainesville, FL 32610, USA
e-mail: daniel.hoh@neurosurgery.ufl.edu

A.J. Layon et al. (eds.), *Textbook of Neurointensive Care*,
DOI 10.1007/978-1-4471-5226-2_29, © Springer-Verlag London 2013

accidents [6, 7]. Males are four times more likely to suffer from SCI than females; however, there has been a rising incidence among women recently [6]. Further, over half of individuals affected by traumatic SCI are between age 16 and 30 years old, but there has been an increasing population of SCI patients older than 60 years of age since 1990 (4.5 % in 1970 vs. 11.5 %) [6–8]. Despite this concerning data, significant advances in the diagnosis, medical, and surgical management of traumatic spinal cord and spinal column injury have led to fewer severe cord injuries seen in spinal cord rehabilitation centers and improved overall clinical outcomes for survival and recovery [2].

Initial Management and Evaluation

The initial management and resuscitation of trauma patients including those with suspected SCI is dictated by the Advanced Trauma Life Support (ATLS) protocols as outlined by the American College of Surgeons (ACS). Evaluation by first responders consists of the standard "ABCs" of airway, breathing, and circulation. First, establishment of a competent and protected airway is of critical importance. An awake, talking patient is likely to have an adequate airway; however, frequently SCI occurs in the setting of head injury or polytrauma, and, therefore, priority must be made for establishing an airway in unconscious patients or those with compromised mental status. Emergent intubation may be necessary, particularly for those individuals presenting with a Glasgow Coma Scale score less than or equal to 8. In the case of a mechanically obstructed airway, such as by a foreign body, the blockage must be cleared immediately from the oropharynx. Common maneuvers to establish an airway, including the jaw thrust, may be attempted; however, any attempts to establish an airway, including intubation, should be performed using manual in-line traction if a cervical spine injury is suspected.

A critical aspect of the ATLS protocol for airway management is protection and maintenance of cervical spine alignment until proper cervical spine clearance can be demonstrated. Rigid external cervical spine immobilization is an essential first step in potentially preventing devastating neurologic deterioration in the setting of a suspected cervical spine injury [2, 3, 9, 10]. The significant overall decrease in complete SCI in the past 30 years is likely attributable to this simple yet critical practice by trauma first responders [11, 12], with an estimated 1/4 of all spinal cord injuries suspected to occur after the initial trauma [3, 13–15] secondary to excessive movement of an unstable spine causing further mechanical injury to the spinal cord. ACS guidelines recommend the use of a cervical collar, a backboard, and a lateral support device upon initial assessment and for transport, with the goal of cervical spine immobilization being to maintain anatomic, neutral position, keeping the neck free from flexion, extension, or rotation.

After establishment of an adequate, protected airway, the second important step is to assess for sufficient breathing and ventilation. Inspection, palpation, percussion, and auscultation of the chest are means for determining if the patient is able to independently ventilate appropriately. Mid- to upper cervical SCI can significantly compromise spontaneous ventilatory function (C5 and rostral), with injuries at these levels resulting in apnea potentially requiring assisted ventilatory support. It is important to note that even lower cervical and/or thoracic SCI can compromise ventilatory function via dysfunction of the intercostal muscles. Even with intact phrenic nerve and diaphragmatic function, intercostal muscle and chest wall impairment can reduce forced vital capacity (FVC) and maximum negative inspiratory force (NIF) by roughly two-thirds of normal [16, 17]. One-third of patients with cervical spine injuries will require intubation, most of these in the first 24 h [18]; therefore, hospital admission to an intensive care unit setting for respiratory monitoring is essential in any patient with a suspected upper cervical spinal cord injury. As with other critically ill patients, decreasing vital capacity and increasing respiratory rate or PCO_2 are all indications for possible emergent or urgent intubation, with manual in-line traction by experienced practitioners [19, 20].

Adequate cardiovascular support and systemic circulation for sufficient tissue perfusion is the third critical component of the initial assessment. Aggressive resuscitation and/or intervention in the setting of any shock syndrome or ongoing hemorrhage is essential. SCI patients may present initially in neurogenic shock with autonomic dysfunction and loss of sympathetic tone, leading to decreased chronotropic input to the heart and peripheral vasculature. The hallmark of neurogenic shock unlike other shock syndromes is the presence of bradycardia in the setting of hypotension, hemodynamic instability, and acute SCI. Therefore, volume resuscitation alone is inadequate in treating neurogenic shock even in polytrauma patients with concomitant hypovolemic shock. Resuscitation with intravenous pharmacologic alpha and beta adrenergic pressors is necessary, the most common being dopamine and norepinephrine [21]. Persistent bradycardia may require atropine to prevent further cardiovascular collapse [22].

Maintaining normotension may be essential to reduce secondary ischemic neural tissue injury, leading to worsening neurologic function. Studies have demonstrated that optimizing hemodynamic support improves neurologic outcome [23–25]. Vale and colleagues prospectively analyzed 77 patients presenting with acute spinal cord injury utilizing Swan-Ganz catheter monitoring, aggressive volume resuscitation, and vasopressor support to maintain a goal mean arterial pressure of 85 mmHg [22]. They found that 60 % of cervical complete SCI and 33 % of thoracic complete SCI patients on admission improved one or more Frankel or ASIA grades. Furthermore, 92 % of cervical incomplete SCI and 99 % of thoracic incomplete SCI patients on admission regained ambulatory function [26].

Neurologic Examination

A directed history and physical and neurologic examination are important aspects of the initial evaluation of suspected spinal cord injury. A focused history includes the mechanism of injury and importantly the presence of motor or sensory deficits either immediately following trauma or in a delayed fashion. Palpation of the entire spine is essential for assessing for step-offs, malalignment, widening of the interspinous distances, bruising, swelling, hematoma, or tenderness. "Logrolling" of the patient is performed to maintain alignment throughout the examination; however, it is important to note that even despite careful, meticulous maintenance of spinal precautions, abnormal motion through the spine can still occur [27].

Standard classification of neurologic function is by the American Spinal Injury Association (ASIA) grade and motor score and includes the level of neurologic injury (Table 29.1) [28]. The level of neurologic injury is the most caudal spinal cord level with normal neurologic function. The ASIA grade is a five-letter classification system, graded by increasing loss of spinal cord function. ASIA grade A indicates a complete SCI, as defined by loss of all motor or sensory function in the sacral segments S4–5. ASIA grades B–D are incomplete spinal cord injuries. ASIA grade B is consistent with preserved sensory but not motor function below the neurologic level of injury including the sacral segments. ASIA grade C indicates presence of motor function below the neurologic level of injury; however, it is less than antigravity strength in over half of these muscle groups. ASIA grade D indicates the presence of preserved motor function below the neurologic level and with at least half of the key muscle groups below the neurologic level of injury having greater

than antigravity strength. ASIA grade E is consistent with a normal motor and sensory exam throughout.

The ASIA Standard of Neurological Classification is a composite motor score and sensory score, evaluating key muscle groups and sensory dermatomes (Fig. 29.1). The motor score is determined by evaluation of five separate muscle groups in each of the upper and lower extremities, both left and right sides, and including the anal sphincter. The motor score is graded on a six-point scale: 5 represents full strength, 4 represents movement against resistance, 3 is movement against gravity alone, 2 is equal to movement across a joint without resistance from gravity, 1 is palpable or visible movement or muscle activity, and 0 is complete absence of any movement or muscle activity. The deltoids and biceps (C5) participate in shoulder abduction and elbow flexion. Wrist extensors (C6) are checked by having the patient cock his/her wrists. Triceps (C7) extend the elbow. Flexor digitorum profundus (C8) can be checked by having the patient squeeze his/her hand, and hand intrinsics (T1) are commonly evaluated by having the patient abduct his/her small finger. In the lower extremities, iliopsoas (L2) governs hip flexion, quadriceps (L3) performs knee extension, and tibialis anterior (L4) and extensor hallucis longus (L5) perform dorsiflexion of the foot and big toe, respectively. Gastrocnemius (S1) is evaluated by foot plantar flexion.

The sensory score is based on a three-point scale to light touch and pinprick, evaluating 28 separate dermatomes. Normal sensation is graded 2, impaired sensation is equal to a score of 1, and complete absence of sensation is graded 0. Retained perianal sensory or motor function is the key motor and sensory finding that differentiates an incomplete SCI from a complete injury. Spinal cord reflexes such as deep tendon reflexes and bulbocavernosus reflex are critical aspects of the evaluation. Particularly, presence or absence of a bulbocavernosus reflex is necessary before classifying any SCI as complete or incomplete. The absence of a bulbocavernosus reflex despite the presentation of complete motor and sensory loss throughout may represent temporary spinal shock, with potential for reversible partial recovery of motor and/or sensory function once spinal shock resolves. The presence or return of a bulbocavernosus reflex, however, indicates the absence of spinal shock, and therefore, the motor and sensory exam and neurologic level at that time represents an accurate assessment of true neurologic function. Priapism indicates loss of sympathetic tone and poor prognosis for recovery. Urinary retention is often present in severe SCI, and consideration should be made for placement of a Foley catheter.

There are other commonly encountered spinal cord injury syndromes with unique presentation of motor and sensory findings. Central cord syndrome is characterized by more prominent weakness of the upper extremities compared to the lower extremities, with varying degree of sensory

Table 29.1 ASIA grade for spinal cord injury

Grade	ASIA
A	No sensory or motor function preserved in sacral segments
B	Sensory but not motor function is preserved below injury level, extends through sacral segments
C	Motor function preserved below the injury level, most key muscles with unable to resist gravity
D	Motor function preserved below the injury level, most key muscles able to resist gravity
E	Normal motor and sensory exam

Data from Ditunno et al. [28]

Patient Name _____

Examiner Name _____   Date/Time of Exam_____

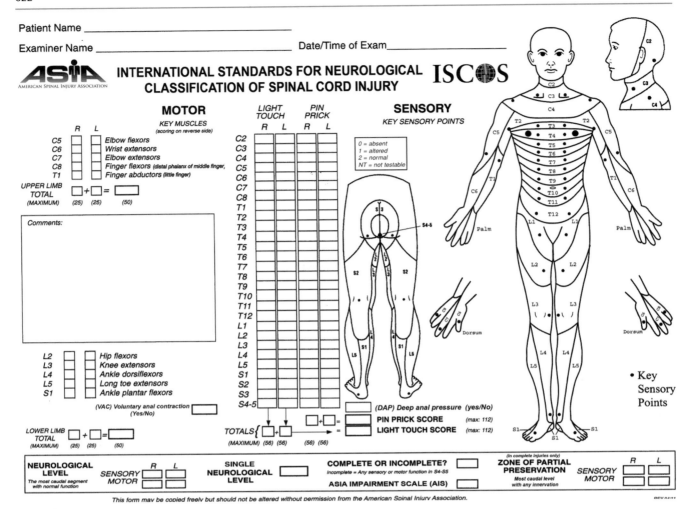

Fig. 29.1 Diagram of the ASIA Standard Neurological Classification of Spinal Cord Injury: motor and sensory exam (From American Spinal Injury Association: International Standards for Neurological Classification of Spinal Cord Injury, revised 2011; Atlanta, GA. Reprinted 2011. Used with permission)

disturbance, most commonly hyperalgesia. Myelopathic findings such as hyperreflexia and urinary retention are frequently present [29, 30]. Central cord syndrome is often secondary to a hyperextension injury in the setting of preexisting cervical stenosis. It is not uncommon for patients to have even dramatic improvement initially with conservative therapy which eventually reaches a plateau, followed by late deterioration [31]. Timing and indications for surgery in central cord syndrome remain controversial; however, early surgical decompression is recommended in cases with ongoing compression from a fracture or acutely herniated disc [32].

Less commonly encountered patterns of incomplete SCI include anterior cord syndrome, Brown-Séquard syndrome, and posterior cord syndrome. Anterior cord syndrome presents with paraplegia and dissociated sensory loss below the lesion (intact posterior column function) [33] and carries the worst prognosis of incomplete injuries with only 10–20 % recovery of motor function. Brown-Séquard (or spinal cord

hemisection) carries the best prognosis (90 % eventually ambulatory with bowel and bladder control) and presents with contralateral pain and temperature loss with ipsilateral motor and posterior column loss [34]. Posterior cord syndrome is rare and presents with pain and paresthesias of the neck, arms, and torso along with mild paresis of the upper extremities.

Imaging

Advances in radiology and imaging modalities have significantly improved timely and accurate diagnosis of spinal cord and spinal column injury, particularly in patients who are unconscious and a thorough neurologic examination is not possible. In the initial evaluation of a suspected spine injury, plain radiographs are the most expeditious first imaging modality. Anterior-posterior, lateral, and open-mouth views of the cervical spine are necessary radiographs in any patient with a suspected neck injury or significant head trauma. For adequate visualization of the cervicothoracic junction, a swimmer's view x-ray with the patient's arm raised over the head allows better evaluation through the bulk of the shoulder girdle. For complete radiographic assessment of the cervical spine, one must be able to clearly visualize the C7–T1 junction. Assessment of spinal alignment, interspinous distance, and presence of soft tissue swelling is included in the evaluation. In addition to relatively low cost and generally immediate availability of these studies, complete plain film radiography demonstrates a high sensitivity (96 %) and specificity (94 %) for identifying clinically significant cervical spine injuries [35, 36].

Helical computed tomography (CT) is increasingly becoming the imaging modality of choice for evaluating cervical, thoracic, lumbar, and sacral spinal column injuries. Helical CT provides a high degree of bony detail and is invaluable for detecting even subtle fractures. Current CT imaging processing software has the capability to reconstruct sagittal, coronal, and even three-dimensional views for better evaluation of spinal alignment in multiple planes. Several studies have indicated nearly 100 % sensitivity in detecting clinically significant fractures as well as greater than 90 % sensitivity in detecting cervical instability [37–42]. CT may also be more accurate than plain films alone in detecting clinically significant injuries in the thoracolumbar spine which may affect management [43], as approximately 25 % of burst fractures may be misclassified as stable compression fractures on plain films [44].

CT imaging, however, is limited in the ability to assess soft tissue structures, such as ligamentous integrity, as well as the spinal cord and nerve roots. Magnetic resonance imaging (MRI) is the modality of choice for evaluation of ligamentous and nervous tissue [45–50]. Conversely, MRI is poorly capable of assessing fractures and demonstrates a low sensitivity for fracture detection [51, 52], with low specificity in the upper cervical spine and low sensitivity in the posterior cervical spine for clinically significant injuries. Furthermore, longer duration to acquire MR studies, cost, and limited availability compared with CT imaging make the routine use of MRI a cost-ineffective measure for screening trauma patients, particularly those without neurologic deficit [53].

The major value of MRI, however, is the superior imaging detail of neural structures that MRI provides, making it the gold standard measure for radiologic evaluation of patients with neurologic deficit of unknown etiology or for further anatomic assessment in the setting of a known injury. Furthermore, MRI may provide important prognostic information in the setting of SCI. The degree of spinal canal compromise, spinal cord compression, hemorrhage, or edema is a poor prognosticator for recovery of neurologic function [54]. Increasing size of hemorrhage is also a predictor of degree of injury, with hemorrhages smaller than 4 mm in length being associated with better outcomes [55].

Perhaps the most significant value of radiologic imaging modalities is assessing for spinal instability in a trauma patient presenting with known significant head, neck, or trunk injuries. Given ATLS standards, all patients with a potential spinal column injury are transported to the hospital setting with external cervical immobilization and on a flat board, maintained in spinal precautions. For patients with true spinal instability, these measures are appropriate and critically necessary. However, it is important to note that only a small percentage of patients who are evaluated in a hospital emergency department with external cervical immobilization have clinically significant spinal cord or column injuries. Delayed clearance of the cervical spine with prolonged external cervical immobilization, particularly in obtunded patients, is associated with significant morbidity [56–59]. Hard cervical orthoses are associated with increased risk of pressure sores and ulcerations, elevated intracranial pressure from compression of jugular venous outflow, poor line care, and increasing nursing demands [56, 57].

Numerous studies have evaluated criteria for radiographic assessment of suspected cervical spine injuries for presence of instability. The National Emergency X-Radiography Utilization Study Group (NEXUS) Low-Risk Criteria and Canadian C-Spine Rule (CCR) are two well-accepted clinical protocols used to evaluate for cervical spine injuries. The NEXUS Low-Risk Criteria for evaluating cervical spine injuries are the absence of midline cervical tenderness, focal neurologic deficit, intoxication, and painful or distracting injury in a patient with otherwise normal alertness. Patients that meet these criteria do not require any cervical spine imaging, whereas patients with either midline cervical tenderness, neurologic deficit, presence of intoxication or a painful or distracting injury, or altered mental status require imaging. Of 34,069 patients and 818 cervical spine injuries, these criteria demonstrated 99.0 % sensitivity and 12.9 % specificity for significant cervical spine injuries [60, 61].

The Canadian C-Spine Rule (CCR) was devised as a decision tool for determining the necessity for obtaining cervical spine imaging. Patients with any one of three high-risk clinical factors (age >65 years, dangerous mechanism, paresthesias in the extremities) were mandated to obtain imaging. Patients with any one of five low-risk clinical factors (simple rear-end motor vehicle collision, sitting position in emergency department, ambulatory at any time after accident, delayed onset of neck pain, or absence of midline cervical spine tenderness) were then assessed for neck range of motion. Individuals unable to axially rotate their head 45° in either direction also required further imaging. Patients with any low-risk clinical factor and who were able to axially rotate their head 45° in both directions did not require imaging [62]. Using these criteria for obtaining cervical spine imaging, the study found a 100 % sensitivity and 42.5 % specificity for identifying clinically significant cervical spine injuries. A follow-up Canadian study found the CCR more sensitive and specific for cervical spine injuries with fewer radiographic studies mandated compared to NEXUS Low-Risk Criteria [63]. Despite these two studies, there remains significant variability in protocols for cervical spine clearance at different institutions [64, 65].

Controversy exists regarding the utility of dynamic flexion-extension radiography in the setting of trauma to evaluate cervical instability in symptomatic or obtunded patients. Some studies suggest a low false-negative rate of flexion-extension x-rays [66, 67]. However, approximately one-third of these studies are inadequate secondary to poor visualization or degree of flexion [68, 69], and there is a documented risk of neurologic injury in passive fluoroscopic flexion-extension imaging in obtunded patients [70]. A recent study suggests low utility in obtaining MRI or flexion-extension imaging in the setting of trauma in obtunded patients, with one missed injury (found on MRI and managed nonoperatively) in 367 comatose patients with negative CT [71]. In another study of 366 patients, multi-detector row CT had negative predictive values of 98.9 % for ligamentous injury and 100 % for unstable cervical spine injury [72]. The proper standard evaluation of cervical instability in obtunded and comatose patients remains unresolved, and better data are needed before suggesting universal guidelines.

Classifications of Spinal Column Injuries

Traumatic spinal cord injury most commonly occurs in the setting of spinal column injury, whether fracture, dislocation, or ligamentous disruption. Often, appropriate timely management of acute spinal cord injury requires expeditious identification of the underlying spinal column injury with immediate reduction and stabilization as necessary. Various classification systems have existed for identifying and characterizing traumatic spinal column injuries. Improved imaging modalities have provided better bony detail and resolution to better categorize fractures and ligamentous injuries, as well as mechanisms of injury and instability. A comprehensive review of all traumatic spinal column injuries is beyond the scope of this chapter; however, a general overview of region specific injuries is included.

Injuries to the Craniocervical Junction

Occipital condyle fractures are poorly visualized on plain films and frequently necessitate fine-cut CT imaging through the craniocervical junction with multiplanar reconstructions for adequate detection [73]. Patients with occipital condyle fractures may present with neurologic deficits ranging from lower cranial nerve deficits to quadriparesis or may be completely neurologically intact. Generally, MR imaging is recommended to evaluate the integrity of ligaments about the occiput and atlantoaxial complex, and, for most fractures, treatment consists of external immobilization in a halo vest or cervical collar for 6–8 weeks [74]. Those failing external mobilization with pain, neurologic deficit, or instability may require posterior occipitocervical fusion.

Atlanto-occipital dislocation is a potentially catastrophic injury and is estimated to account for 5–8 % of fatal traffic injuries and 8–5 % of all fatal cervical spine injuries [75, 76] (Fig. 29.2a, b). Atlanto-occipital dislocation occurs more commonly in children than in adults and is generally secondary to extension and rotational forces. Mortality generally results from upper cervical cord injury with loss of spontaneous respiratory function. Survivors may present with either minimal deficits or bulbar-cervical dislocation. Twenty percent or greater of individuals 20 % of individuals present with a normal neurologic exam [77]. In general, cervical traction is to be avoided as it is associated with a 10 % risk of neurologic deterioration [78] and should be completely avoided in longitudinal dislocations. In the case of lateral or anteroposterior dislocations, light traction of 5 lb may be applied for reduction; however, it must be performed in conscious patients in which continuous awake, neurologic assessment can be made. Initial management should include placement in a halo vest, with most patients eventually going on to posterior occipitocervical fusion [79, 80].

Jefferson fracture is a burst fracture of the ring of C1 occurring under axial loading of the head and neck (Fig. 29.3). Most patients are neurologically intact at presentation secondary to the generous canal diameter for the spinal cord at this level; however, Jefferson fractures frequently occur in conjunction with an associated C2 fracture [81]. Therefore, radiographic assessment of a suspected C1 fracture also includes thin-cut evaluation of C2 for any concomitant fractures. An open-mouth odontoid plain film x-ray for the evaluation of Jefferson fractures is essential for indirect assessment of the integrity of the transverse ligament. In an axial loading injury, burst fracture of the ring of C1, the comminuted fracture fragments displace radially outward. Therefore, on a two-dimensional open-mouth cervical x-ray, the sum total of the overhang of the C1 lateral masses on C2 indicates whether the transverse ligament has been disrupted. A total overhang of 7 mm or greater indicates that the transverse ligament has been compromised and indicates an unstable atlantoaxial complex [82, 83]. MR imaging with focused images through the transverse ligament may also detect ligamentous disruption of an avulsion injury. Because the

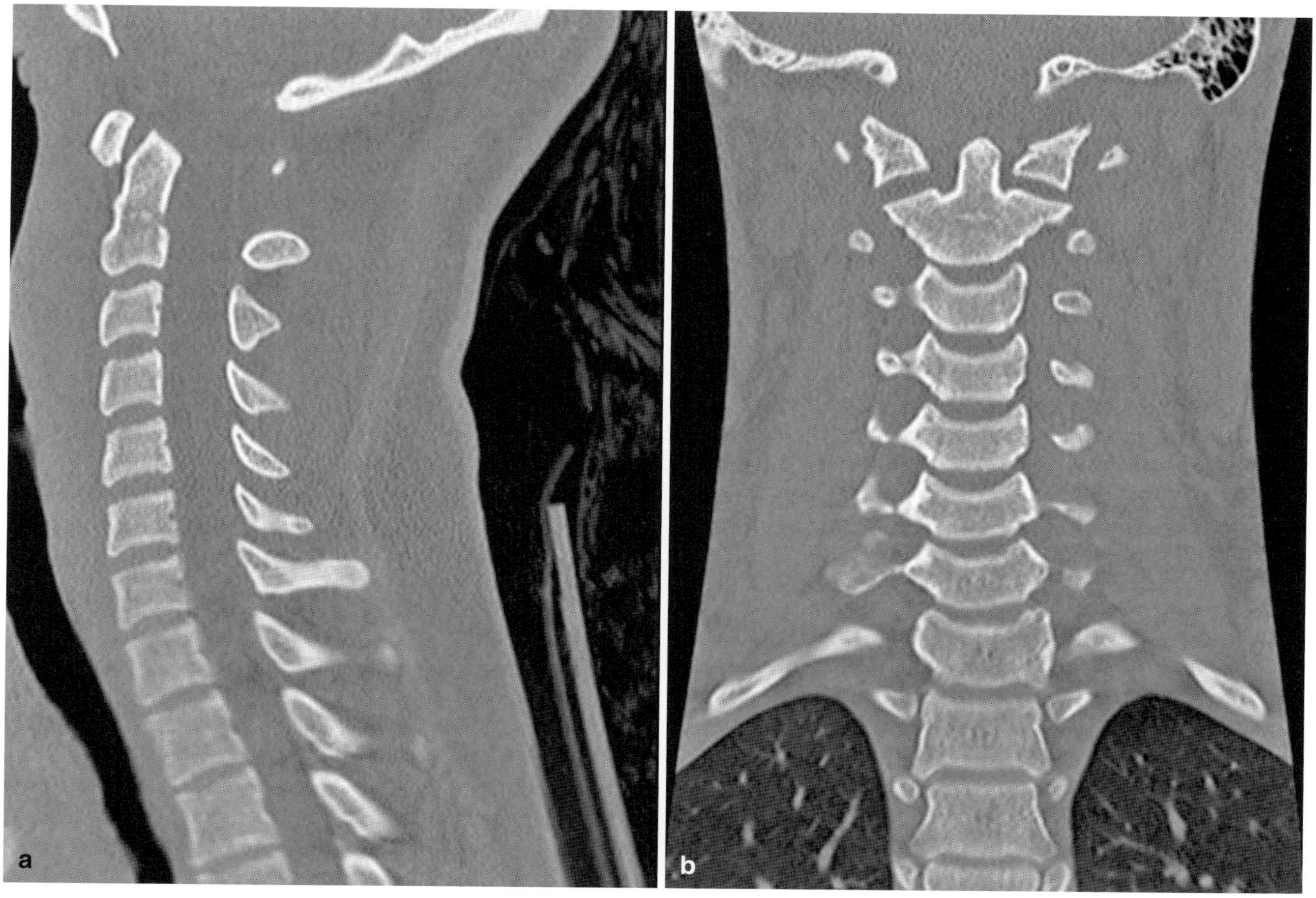

Fig. 29.2 (**a**) Sagittal reconstructed CT image demonstrating atlanto-occipital dislocation with increased distance between the skull base and the dens. (**b**) Coronal reconstructed CT image of the same patient demonstrating widening of the space between the skull base and C1

transverse ligament is responsible for maintaining C1–C2 alignment particularly in flexion-extension and for resisting translation, an atlanto-dental interval greater than 3.5 mm is suggestive of an incompetent transverse ligament. Fractures with intact transverse ligaments can be treated in cervical collar or halo vest; however, if a transverse ligament disruption has occurred, then surgical fusion of C1–C2 is required [84–90].

Atlantoaxial rotatory subluxation is most commonly seen in children, can occur spontaneously, and is frequently associated with Down's syndrome, rheumatoid arthritis, congenital dens abnormalities, major or minor trauma, or Grisel's syndrome [91–93]. Rotatory subluxation is often initially suspected by the classic clinical sign of a "cock robin" head appearance, such that the head is tilted toward and rotated away from the side of the dislocation. Subluxation can often be managed with traction starting at 7 lb in children and increasing to 15 lb or in adults, starting at 15 lb and increasing to 20 lb. If the rotatory subluxation is able to be close reduced, halo immobilization for 3 months can be an effective treatment option [91]. Open reduction and fixation of C1–C2 is recommended in cases that fail to reduce with closed traction [91, 93].

Odontoid fractures comprise approximately 7–15 % of all cervical spine fractures [94, 95] (Fig. 29.4a, b). It is estimated that odontoid fractures may be fatal at the time of the accident in 25–40 % of patients [96]. Individuals with an odontoid fracture may present neurologically intact or may have significant neurologic deficits [97, 98]. Most odontoid fractures may be successfully treated with external immobilization; however, risk factors for fracture non-healing with conservative measures include older age and significant fracture displacement or angulation. Fracture nonunion is treated with surgical fusion.

Traumatic fracture of the pars or pedicles of the axis, or a hangman's fracture [99], was classically described as hyperextension and distraction injuries obtained during judicial hangings [100] but presently is more commonly associated with flexion-distraction forces or combination hyperflexion, extension, and distraction. Minimally displaced fractures can be successfully treated with immobilization [101, 102], with open surgical reduction and fusion reserved for patients with severe angulation or displacement [103].

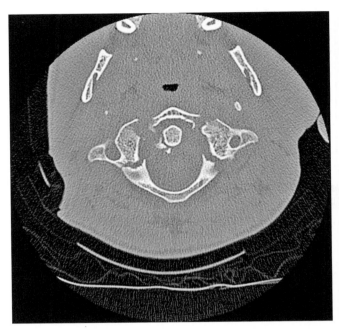

Fig. 29.3 Axial CT image demonstrating a burst fracture (Jefferson fracture) of C1

Subaxial Cervical Spine Injuries

Subaxial cervical spine injuries account for 65 % of all spine fractures and greater than 75 % of all spinal dislocations [104]. Several classification schemes exist for subaxial injuries [105, 106]; however, more recently Vaccaro and colleagues and the Spine Trauma Study Group proposed the Subaxial Cervical Spine Injury Classification System (SLIC) that includes morphology based on mechanism, along with evaluation of disco-ligamentous disruption and neurologic status in an effort to develop a treatment algorithm for these fractures [107].

Compression fractures involve loss of height of the anterior portion of the vertebral body with a resulting kyphosis of varying degrees, with preservation of the posterior vertebral body wall. On imaging, compression fractures demonstrate a wedge appearance of the vertebral body. Burst fractures are similar to compression fractures except the posterior aspect of the vertebral body is also involved. The posterior vertebral body wall is violated with retropulsion of bony fragments into the spinal canal and a resultant loss of vertebral body height.

Flexion teardrop fractures were originally described by Schneider and colleagues [108] and generally result from a flexion-axial loading force [108–110] (Fig. 29.5a, b). The injury is identified classically by the presence of a small chip of

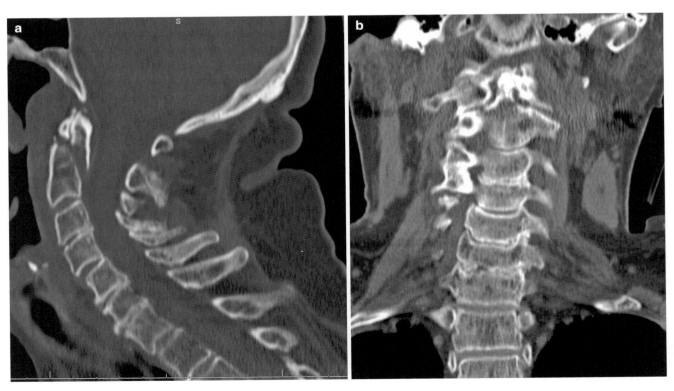

Fig. 29.4 (a) Sagittal reconstructed CT demonstrating a fracture through the base of the odontoid process. (b) Coronal reconstructed CT image of the same patient showing fracture through the base of the odontoid process

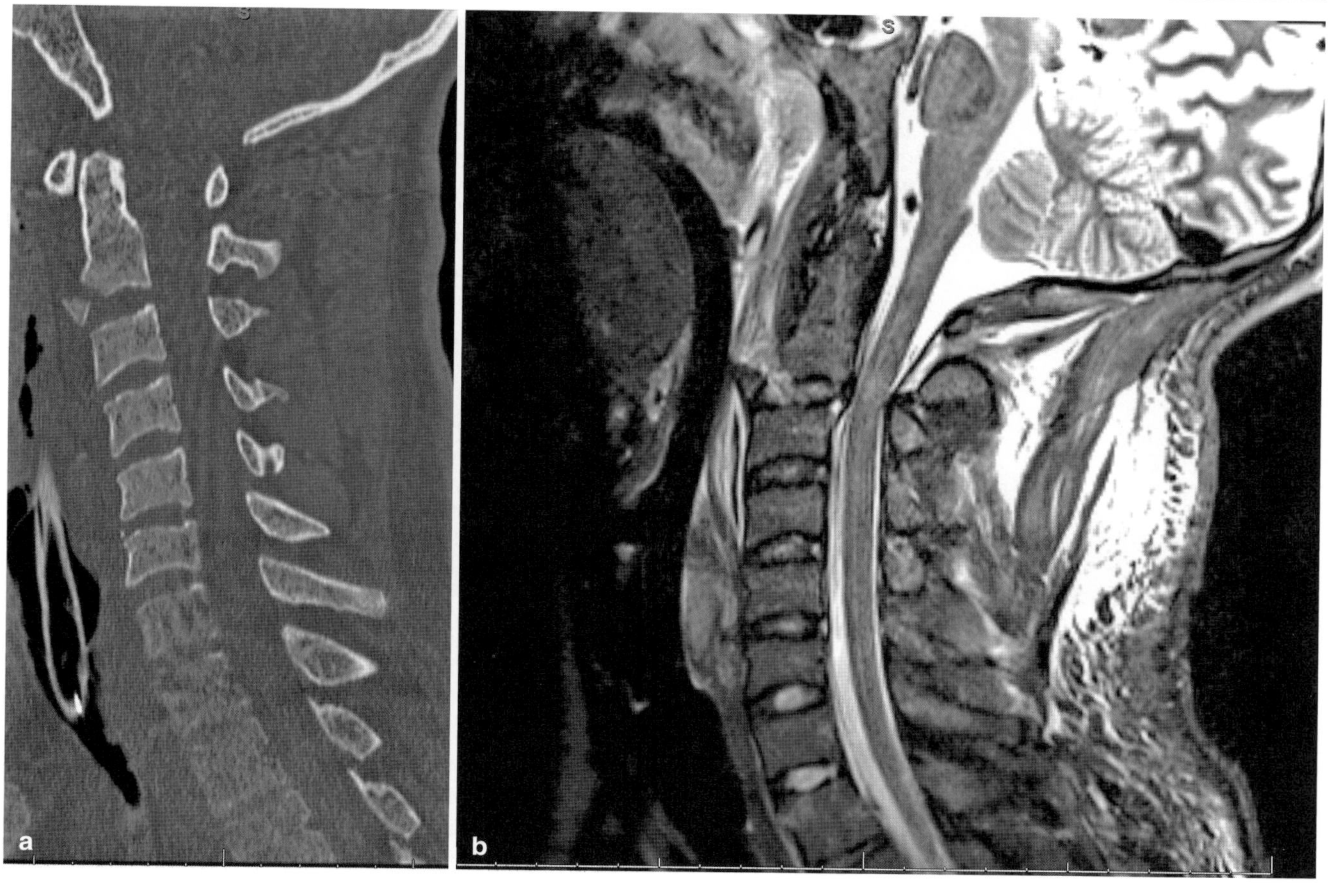

Fig. 29.5 (a) Sagittal reconstructed CT image demonstrating a "teardrop fracture" of C2. (b) Sagittal T2-weighted MRI of the same patient demonstrating instability at C2 with T2 signal abnormality within the spinal cord at the corresponding level

bone ("teardrop") beyond the anterior inferior edge of the vertebral body. As injury severity increases, retrolisthesis with canal compromise, sagittal fracture, and bilaminar fractures of the vertebra may be present [105, 109, 111]. Flexion teardrop fractures are associated with a significant risk of spinal cord injury (more severe with increasing retrolisthesis) [105, 108], and half of patients present with quadriplegia [111].

Severe flexion injuries can lead to facet dislocations, known as perched, jumped, or locked facets (Fig. 29.6a–c). In these cases, the cervical facet capsule is disrupted, and the inferior articulating process is dislocated ventral to its companion superior articulating process (Fig. 29.3). These injuries can be either unilateral or bilateral; 25 % of patients with unilateral locked facets are neurologically intact, 37 % have root injuries, 22 % have incomplete cord injuries, and 15 % have complete cord injuries [112]. Approximately 70–90 % of patients with bilateral jumped facets have complete SCI, 10–30 % are incomplete, and less than 10 % present neurologically intact [105, 113].

Criteria suggestive of instability include angulation of greater than or equal to 11° or 3.5 mm of translation

[114, 115]. Pre-MRI closed reduction should be considered in cases of cervical spine subluxation, and particularly, urgent reduction is recommended in individuals presenting with facet dislocation and incomplete SCI.

Thoracolumbar Injuries

Various classification schemes exist for characterizing thoracolumbar injuries; however, the Denis classification system has gained widespread acceptance for its ease of application [116]. The Denis system is based on a three-column model of spinal instability in which the anterior column consists of the anterior half of the disc and vertebral body, including the anterior longitudinal ligament and annulus fibrosis. The middle column consists of the posterior half of the vertebral body and disc, including the posterior longitudinal ligament. The posterior column consists of the bony neural arch, facet joints, the interspinous and supraspinous ligaments, and the ligamentum flavum. Minor spinal injuries in this classification include isolated transverse process fractures, spinous

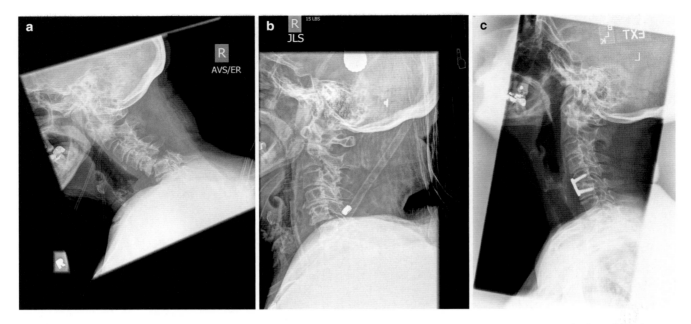

Fig. 29.6 (**a**) Lateral x-ray demonstrating bilateral jumped facets at C5–C6. (**b**) Lateral x-ray after halo closed reduction in the same patient. (**c**) Lateral x-ray after anterior cervical stabilization and fusion demonstrating stable, maintained alignment

process fractures, and pars and isolated facet fractures. The remaining fractures are divided into compression fractures, burst fractures, fracture-dislocations, and "seat-belt"-type injuries. Instability is defined as failure of two or more columns.

Compression fractures are the result of a flexion injury with failure of the anterior column and generally preservation of the middle and posterior columns (Fig. 29.7a, b). Compression fractures are generally successfully managed nonoperatively with a TLSO or Jewett extension brace with early ambulation [105, 117]. Surgical intervention may be indicated in cases of greater than 20°–30° of kyphosis or more than 50 % loss of height [118], with percutaneous cement augmentation being a potentially less invasive option for management of compression fractures.

Burst fractures indicate failure of both anterior and middle columns primarily under axial loading (Fig. 29.8a–e). Unstable fractures are considered in patients with progressive neurologic deterioration, greater than 50 % loss of anterior vertebral body height, or a kyphotic deformity of greater than 20° [119]. Stable fractures are managed nonoperatively with a thoracolumbar orthosis [120], whereas highly unstable fractures may require surgical stabilization with decompression (Fig. 29.4a, b).

"Chance" fractures are transverse fractures through the vertebral body and posterior elements; soft tissue injuries through the disc space, facet joint, and ligaments; or a combination of both bony and soft tissue disruptions [121].

Chance fractures are failure of the anterior column in flexion with posterior column disruption under simultaneous distraction [116]. Bony injuries alone can be treated with external immobilization; however, complex injuries or soft tissue injuries require surgical stabilization.

Fracture-dislocation is a failure of all three columns and is a highly unstable injury (Fig. 29.9a, b). Fracture-dislocation can occur due to flexion-rotation, shear, or flexion distraction [116]. All fracture-dislocation types are associated with a high rate of neurologic deficit, and often individuals present with complete SCI [116]. Operative intervention may consist of a posterior only, anterior only, or combined anterior-posterior approach for open reduction, decompression, and surgical stabilization [122].

Gunshot wounds and other types of penetrating trauma while associated with significant neurologic impairment generally do not compromise spinal column stability. Management is typically nonoperative, and corticosteroids have not been shown to improve neurologic outcome [123]. Relative indications for surgery in penetrating spinal column injuries include cauda equina injuries [124, 125], copper jacketed bullets causing severe inflammatory reactions [126], or lead poisoning (when the bullet is in the joint or disc space) [127]. A study of 90 patients with gunshot wounds to the spine demonstrated modest motor improvement with removal of retained fragments when the bullet was lodged between T12 and L4; however, no significant improvement from bullet or bone fragment removal at more rostral levels was demonstrated [128].

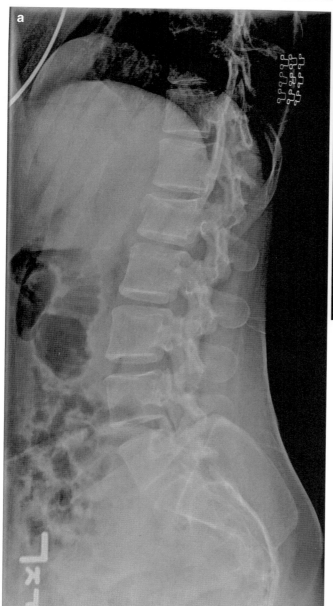

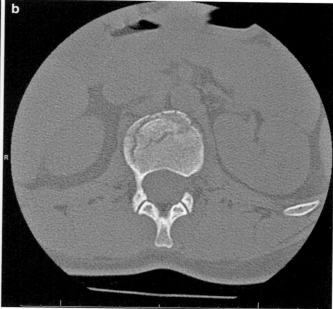

Fig. 29.7 (**a**) Lateral x-ray demonstrating an L1 compression fracture with minimal loss of anterior vertebral body height. (**b**) Axial CT image of the same patient demonstrating fracture of only the anterior portion of L1 with preservation of the dorsal vertebral body wall and posterior elements

Medical Management of SCI

The medical management of SCI patients is complex, owing to the multisystem implications of the disorder. Many advances have been made in diagnosis and treatment of the medical aspects of SCI that influence current clinical practice. These measures are aimed at managing the comorbidities of SCI as well as mitigating injury to the spinal cord itself.

Respiratory complications rank among the most common causes of early and late morbidity and mortality after SCI [8], with pneumonia accounting for the majority of respiratory-related deaths [129, 130]. Risk of pneumonia is directly correlated with the level of injury, with a greater than 60 % incidence in patients with SCI at C4 or above [129]. Vigilant attention to pulmonary management and respiratory therapy is paramount in reducing ventilator-associated pneumonia (VAP) and for optimizing treatment with its occurrence. A recent meta-analysis reports that the presence of a new radiographic infiltrate with at least 2 of fever, leukocytosis, or purulent sputum increases the likelihood of VAP [130]. Treatment of suspected VAP without a clearly identified organism is empiric coverage of suspected pathogens, *Streptococcus pneumoniae* or *Hemophilus influenza*, in the first 4 days following intubation and *Staphylococcus aureus* or gram-negative bacilli, especially *Pseudomonas aeruginosa*, thereafter [21]. In addition, the NASCENT randomized trial published in 2008 suggests that the incidence of VAP may be significantly reduced by the use of silver-coated endotracheal tubes [131].

The number of ventilator days is also significantly correlated to the level of injury and thereby related to risk of respiratory complications with patients with C1–C4 levels of injury having an average 65 days of ventilator dependence, 22 days for patients with C5–C8 levels, and 12 days for patients with thoracic injuries [129]. Common ventilator weaning strategies include pressure support ventilation with progressively decreasing amounts of support, on/off ventilator cycling, T-piece trials, and obtaining weaning parameters such as negative inspiratory force and spontaneous tidal volumes.

Tracheostomy should be considered in patients when prolonged intubation is anticipated. Complications of prolonged endotracheal intubation include vocal cord ulceration, subglottic inflammation, and tracheal stenosis. In addition, tracheostomy tends to be more comfortable for patients and results in less dead space ventilation than endotracheal intubation [21]. Some data suggest that early tracheostomy is associated with lower rates of pneumonia [132] and shorter periods of mechanical ventilation in trauma patients [133]. Other benefits of tracheostomy include low surgical and airway risk; however, patients also undergoing anterior cervical spine surgery should allow generally 2 weeks for appropriate wound healing prior to tracheostomy.

Recently, there has been interest in the surgical placement of diaphragm pacing stimulators to replace or delay the need for long-term positive pressure mechanical ventilation in patients with upper cervical spinal cord injuries. Diaphragm stimulator placement is performed laparoscopically, in which mapping of the motor point of the diaphragm where the greatest muscle contraction occurs first occurs. Then, permanent electrodes are implanted both at the motor point as well as at additional supplementary points, which are subsequently connected to a stimulator programmed to provide a stimulus that provides a tidal volume of 15 % over basal needs. In a study of 50 patients with spinal cord injury and diaphragm pacing stimulation, 98 % of patients were able to produce tidal volumes of 15 % over their basal requirements [134]. Ninety-six percent of patients presently use the diaphragm pacing stimulation for greater than 4 continuous hours, with over 50 % utilizing stimulation for over 24 continuous hours.

Patients with severe SCI are at risk for developing neurogenic shock. Neurogenic shock, which is the loss of sympathetic tone, is to be differentiated from spinal shock, which is characterized by hypotonia and areflexia. Neurogenic shock results in decreased systemic vascular resistance due to generalized vasodilatation with a concomitant inability to generate tachycardia. Care must be made in treating patients in neurogenic shock with aggressive fluid resuscitation since with the exception of significant hemorrhage from polytrauma, most patients are relatively euvolemic. The

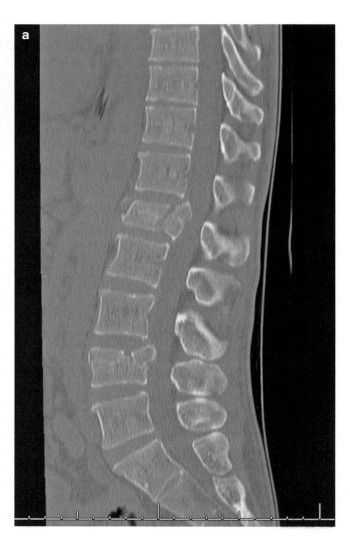

Fig. 29.8 (**a**) Sagittal reconstructed CT image demonstrating simultaneous burst fractures at L1 and L4. (**b**) Axial CT image of the same patient at L1 demonstrating fracture of both the anterior and posterior aspects of the vertebral body with significant retropulsion of bone fragments into the spinal canal. (**c**) Axial CT image of the same patient at L4 demonstrating a similar fracture pattern with retropulsed bone fragments. (**d**) Axial CT image 6 months after injury and surgical stabilization at L1 demonstrating healing of the fracture and resorption of the retropulsed bone fragments. (**e**) Axial CT image at 6 months of the same patient at L4 demonstrating a healed L4 fracture with resorption of bone fragments and restoration of the spinal canal

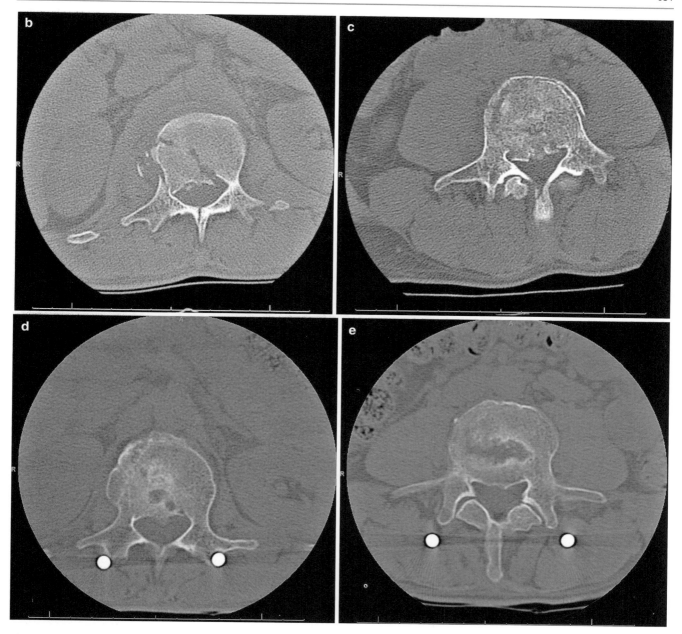

Fig. 29.8 (continued)

consequence of excessive fluid administration is to induce congestive heart failure with pulmonary edema.

Alternatively, appropriate management of neurogenic shock involves the judicious use of vasopressors to counteract the loss of systemic vasoconstriction. Norepinephrine is an ideal agent for treatment of neurogenic shock as it combines alpha vasoconstrictive properties with beta chronotropic and inotropic effects. Dopamine is also effective and likely works through primarily norepinephrine pathways, as dopamine is a norepinephrine precursor. Phenylephrine is a pure alpha agent that is also useful at increasing vascular resistance; however, it may also induce a rebound bradycardia

that in some instances can lead to asystole. Bradyarrhythmia secondary to loss of sympathetic tone can be managed either by anticholinergics such as atropine or with chronotropic agents such as norepinephrine or dopamine. In severe cases, a pacemaker may be necessary.

Loss of sympathetic tone may also lead to gastrointestinal dysfunction secondary to absent autonomic innervation to the bowel. Complications that may result include impaired gastric emptying and the development of a paralytic ileus with gastric dilatation. Abdominal distension is further aggravated by swallowing large volumes of air or premature feeding in the acute phase after injury. Severe abdominal

Fig. 29.9 (a) Sagittal reconstructed CT image demonstrating fracture-dislocation at T11–T12. (b) Lateral x-ray after surgical reduction of the dislocation and instrumented stabilization and fusion

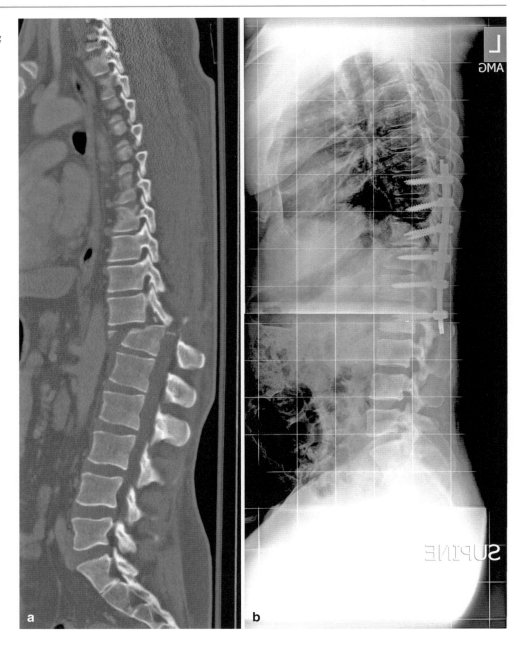

distention can compound respiratory dysfunction by compressing the diaphragm and reducing total lung volume. Management primarily consists of withholding enteral feeding until spontaneous bowel activity has occurred and routine use of suppositories, enemas, and stimulants. Additional gastrointestinal complication to consider is the risk for gastrointestinal bleeding secondary to stress-induced ulcers. Careful attention to hematocrit and routine prophylactic use of H_2 blockers is recommended.

Venous thromboembolic disease also represents a major source of morbidity in SCI. Spinal cord injury patients demonstrate the highest risk of venous thromboembolism compared to all other non-SCI hospitalized patients [135].

Reports suggest that the incidence of deep venous thrombosis (DVT) is exceedingly high in patients with spinal cord injury, ranging from 50 to 100 % of all patients undergoing routine screening [135–137]. Approximately 10 % of mortality following SCI is attributable to pulmonary embolism [138–141]. Several advances have improved DVT prevention including use of low-molecular-weight heparin (LMWH), intermittent pneumatic compression (IPCs), low-dose unfractionated heparin (LDH), and inferior vena cava (IVC) filters.

Choosing appropriate DVT prophylaxis involves selecting an optimal method, dose, and time of intervention. Most class I evidence suggests the use of LMWH for routine prophylaxis of DVT following SCI. A multicenter, randomized trial published in 2003 compared 107 patients randomized to receive either low-dose heparin (5,000 units every 8 h) and IPCs or enoxaparin 30 mg every 12 h [137]. The trial found similar rates of DVTs in both groups (63.3 % with LDH-IPC vs. 65.5 % with enoxaparin, $p=0.81$) but lower incidence of pulmonary embolism in the enoxaparin group (18.4 % with LDH-IPC vs. 5.2 % with enoxaparin, $p=0.03$). There was also a trend toward fewer major bleeding complications in the enoxaparin group (5.3 % with LDH-IPC versus 2.6 % with enoxaparin, $p=0.14$). Regarding dosing, evidence suggests that enoxaparin 40 mg subcutaneously once daily is similar in efficacy and safety to twice daily dosing [142]. Early initiation of pharmacologic prophylaxis for DVT following spinal trauma carries risk of bleeding complications including epidural hematoma. In concurrence, evidence suggests that the risk of thromboembolism is actually low in the first 72 h following SCI [143]. Therefore, use of mechanical prophylaxis immediately following injury with initiation of pharmacologic prophylaxis 72 h after injury may prove to be an optimal balance between decreasing risk of thromboembolism acutely and not increasing risk for bleeding complications [21]. Inferior vena cava filters are an alternative measure for decreasing risk of pulmonary embolus, but not, however, deep venous thrombosis [144]. The use of inferior vena cava filters is not recommended for routine use in all SCI patients; however, they may be an effective option for patients in whom pharmacologic management is contraindicated or who have failed drug therapy [145].

Genitourinary complications are another source of significant morbidity and mortality after SCI. Loss of innervation to the bladder and the external urethral sphincter results in urinary retention often requiring bladder catheterization. In the acute phase, continuous Foley catheterization is ideal as it allows for closer monitoring of overall fluid status, particularly in polytrauma patients. However, continuous bladder catheterization poses increased risk of urinary tract infections, renal and bladder calculi, and chronic bladder hyperreflexia [146]. Ultimately, transitioning to clean intermittent catheterization or suprapubic cystostomy is likely to reduce the risk of developing urinary tract infections and other renal complications.

Patients with severe SCI are at high risk for developing pressure ulcers. Inadequate tissue perfusion, prolonged maintenance on a spine backboard, immobilization with inadequate logrolling, and the patient's impaired sensation for tissue injury contribute to increased risk for skin ulceration. Standard care should include manual logrolling, use of oscillating beds, and, most importantly, meticulous care toward frequent inspection and hygiene.

Last, particular sensitivity to the patient and family's emotional reaction to what is a significant life-altering event is essential. As with any grieving process, patients progress through the typical stages of grief including denial, anger, depression, and finally acceptance. The role of critical care providers in caring for these patients must include an awareness of these stages of grief and fostering of completion of the grieving process leading to ultimate resolution. While there is no clear ideal method for helping patients through this extraordinary time, in general, compassion and honesty in discussing care, prognosis, education, and counseling are advocated.

Phamacologic Adjuncts in SCI: NASCIS and Sygen® (Fidia Pharmaceuticals Corporation, Parsippany, NJ) Studies

The role of pharmacologic agents designed for treating SCI and improving neurologic recovery is limited and controversial (Table 29.2). Administration of intravenous high-dose methylprednisolone (MP) for the treatment of acute SCI has been the subject of considerable scrutiny and debate. The first randomized trial of MP in the setting of acute spinal cord injury was reported by Bracken and colleagues in 1984 [147]. In this double-blinded trial, 330 patients were randomized to either high-dose (1,000 mg intravenously for 10 days) or standard-dose MP (100 mg intravenously for 10 days). The investigators found no difference in motor or sensory recovery between the two groups at 6 weeks or 6 months. Furthermore, the high-dose MP group had higher early mortality rates and wound infection rates than the lower dose group.

Following this trial, an experimental model of spinal cord injury in cats demonstrated functional improvement using a higher dose of MP than that used in the clinical trial [148]. In addition, animal studies suggest that the opioid antagonist naloxone may demonstrate therapeutic benefit for spinal cord injury [149–151]. The Second National Acute Spinal Cord Injury Study (NASCIS II) was designed to address the concern for MP under-dosing and also incorporate an investigation of naloxone [152]. In this double-blinded, randomized study, 162 patients were given MP as a 30 mg/kg bolus followed by 5.4 mg/kg/h for 23 h. Naloxone was given to 154 patients as a bolus of 5.4 mg/kg, followed by infusion at 4.0 mg/kg/h for 23 h. Placebo treatment was administered to 171 patients by bolus and infusion. Motor scores were calculated by evaluation of 14 muscle groups on a 0–5 scale, and sensation to pinprick and touch was calculated based on a 3-point scale (absent, decreased, normal) at 29 segments. The results of the trial demonstrated a significant difference in sensation to pinprick and touch in the MP group, without accompanying motor improvement. However, a subgroup analysis of those patients treated within 8 h of injury demonstrated a modest but statistically significant (10.6 vs. 7.2

Table 29.2 A summary of the study design, enrollment, intervention, and results of the NASCIS I, II, III and Sygen® (Fidia Pharmaceuticals Corporation, Parsippany, NJ) clinical trials

Study	Study design and enrollment	Intervention	Results
NASCIS I	330 patients. Motor and sensory scores based on ASIA disability score measured at 6 weeks and 6 months	High-dose MP (1,000 mg IV × 10 days) vs. standard-dose (100 mg IV × 10 days)	No difference in motor sensory scores at 6 weeks or 6 months.
NASCIS II	162 patients receiving MP, 154 receiving naloxone, 171 receiving placebo. ASIA disability score as NASCIS I	MP: 30 mg/kg bolus then 5.4 mg/kg/h for 23 h. Naloxone 5.4 mg/kg, then 4.0 mg/kg/h for 23 h	Statistically significant sensory improvement in MP group. Statistically significant motor (16.0 vs. 11.2 motor points at 6 months) and sensory improvement in MP group for subgroup receiving treatment within 8 h
NASCIS III	499 patients comparing 24 h MP, 48 h MP, and 48 h tirilazad regimens. Outcome measures include FIM	All patients receive 30 mg/kg MP bolus then: 24 h MP, 48 h MP, or 48 h tirilazad	Statistically significant difference in motor improvement for 48 h MP group in patients treated between 3 and 8 h after injury. No difference between 24 h MP and tirilazad
Sygen®	760 patients comparing low-dose and high dose GM1 ganglioside, and placebo. ASIA or Modified Benzel grade as primary outcome measure	All patients receive 30 mg/kg MP bolus then either low-dose GM1 ganglioside (300 mg loading dose and 100 mg daily for 56 days), high-dose (600 mg then 200 mg daily), or placebo	Trend toward quicker recovery in GM1 ganglioside group, but no difference in eventual recovery

motor score, $p = 0.048$ at 6 weeks; 16.0 vs. 11.2 motor score, $p = 0.033$ at 6 months) improvement in motor function in the MP group compared to placebo. Wound infection and gastrointestinal bleeding were more common in the MP group, but this did not reach statistical significance. No significant improvement was observed in patients treated with naloxone. The proposed mechanism of MP was suppression of the breakdown of cell membranes via inhibition of lipid peroxidation and neurofilament degradation, a process which peaks at 8 h following injury [148, 153, 154]. In addition, a secondary proposed mechanism was increased spinal cord perfusion due to reduction of vasoreactive by-products from arachidonic acid metabolism [155].

Critics have targeted primarily the methodology and data analysis of the NASCIS II trial including outcome measures and statistical methods used [156]. Using a post hoc subgroup analysis of patients receiving steroids within 8 h of injury when other analyses demonstrated no statistical significance has raised questions regarding the validity of the results. Also, use of raw motor scores versus functional outcome as the primary end point raises issues of the clinical significance of the results.

NASCIS III was a randomized, controlled, double-blinded trial of 499 patients comparing 24 h methylprednisolone, 48 h methylprednisolone, and 48 h tirilazad regimens [157]. In this study, it should be noted that all patients received a 30 mg/kg bolus of methylprednisolone prior to randomization. The primary outcome measures of NASCIS III were similar to NASCIS II but also included Functional Independence Measure (FIM) assessment. Again, a subgroup analysis demonstrated a statistically significant difference in motor improvement for patients receiving 48 h versus

24 h of methylprednisolone in patients treated between 3 and 8 h after injury. There was a trend toward better improvement in FIM in this group as well. Of note, motor improvement comparisons between the 24-h methylprednisolone and tirilazad groups were not significantly different. In addition, patients receiving 48 h methylprednisolone had a higher incidence of severe sepsis and pneumonia than other groups. Other studies indicate that complications of high-dose methylprednisolone therapy include increased risk of infection and pulmonary issues [158]. In light of these issues, recent guidelines indicate that use of high-dose methylprednisolone is considered optional in the setting of spinal cord injury without any strong recommendation for either its use or lack thereof.

The Sygen® Multicenter Acute Spinal Cord Injury Study investigated GM1 ganglioside as a potential medical therapy in the setting of acute spinal cord injury [159]. A prior single-center trial of 28 patients demonstrated a statistically significant improvement in patients receiving GM1 ganglioside versus placebo [160]. Seven hundred and sixty patients were randomized to receive placebo, low-dose GM1 (300 mg loading dose, then 100 mg daily for 56 days) or high-dose GM1 (600 mg loading dose, then 200 mg daily). All patients also received the methylprednisolone protocol per NASCIS II. Neurologic assessment was performed based on the ASIA Impairment Scale and the Modified Benzel Scale, and the primary outcome measure was the proportion of patients improved at 26 weeks. Secondary outcome measures were time course of recovery, motor and sensory score improvement, and bowel and bladder improvement. Primary outcome measures did not demonstrate a benefit to use of GM1 ganglioside. The results appeared to trend toward quicker recovery in the treatment group versus placebo group with both groups eventually reaching the same level of recovery. The use of GM1 ganglioside is therefore only considered an optional adjunct in the management of SCI.

Surgical Management of Spinal Cord and Spinal Column Injuries

While most patients who suffer from traumatic spine injuries are primarily managed medically, a significant number of patients ultimately require some form of surgical intervention. Surgical management of spine injuries can involve decompression of the neural elements, namely, the spinal cord and nerves, as well as stabilization of the unstable spinal column and its supporting structures. Surgery directed toward neural decompression is focused primarily on reducing risk of further neurologic deterioration post injury and optimizing potential for neurologic recovery. Surgical treatment of the spinal column functions to restore spinal alignment and stabilize unstable injuries, both acutely and long term.

The last several decades have witnessed a paradigm shift in the surgical management of patients with traumatic spinal cord and spinal column injuries. Traditionally, patients with spine injuries were treated conservatively with bed rest and external immobilization. Spinal decompression was performed in a delayed fashion to avoid higher risk of surgical complications in acutely injured patients. Improved modern surgical and anesthetic techniques, however, have allowed for earlier operative intervention with minimized patient morbidity. Additionally, development of improved technology for spinal fixation has resulted in better reduction and stabilization of fractures compared to more conservative modalities. As a result, earlier operative spinal stabilization is being performed to aggressively treat unstable injuries and promote patient mobilization and rehabilitation.

Surgical Treatment of Spinal Cord Injuries

There are currently no available effective surgical means for directly repairing the injured spinal cord. Surgical treatment of spinal cord injuries is primarily focused toward reducing risk of further neurologic deterioration and optimizing potential for neurologic recovery via decompression of bony or soft tissue compression or hematoma. Neurologic deficit secondary to traumatic compressive spinal cord lesions may be potentially reversible with emergent decompression. Causes of traumatic spinal cord compression include fractured bony elements in the spinal canal, acute disc herniation, epidural or subdural hematoma, or compromised space available for the cord due to subluxation, dislocation, or other malalignment.

Prior studies initially suggested that early surgical decompression in the setting of acute spinal cord injury led to increased patient morbidity. As a result, most advocated that decompression when indicated be performed in a delayed fashion. Marshall and colleagues found that patients treated with early surgical intervention demonstrated a higher risk of medical complications [161]. Larson and coworkers recommended delaying surgical decompression until >1 week post injury [162]. Concern for increased complications with early intervention arose from performing surgery in medically compromised patients and for risk of causing further tissue damage in the setting of an acutely injured edematous spinal cord.

Recently, however, there has been renewed enthusiasm for considering early decompression in spinal cord injury. The results of the NASCIS II and III clinical trials demonstrating a modest yet significant benefit for medical therapy when administered within 8 h post injury suggest a potential role for earlier intervention. Furthermore, animal models of acute spinal cord compression demonstrate that earlier removal of compression results in better neurologic recovery.

Despite scientific rationale to suggest that early decompression may improve neurologic recovery, the timing of surgical intervention in the setting of acute spinal cord injury remains unresolved. Largely, debate regarding this issue stems from the lack of any large-scale class I evidence demonstrating the benefit of either early or delayed surgery for acute spinal cord injury. Difficulty in performing a prospective randomized clinical trial investigating timing of surgery in SCI is due to multiple issues. Determining the appropriate therapeutic window in which decompression must be performed to mitigate secondary injury is unclear. Recruiting patients with an appropriate diagnosis and surgically intervening within a narrow time period is challenging and may be feasible in only a limited number of institutions. Finally, ethical issues arise in randomization of patients with incomplete injuries to delayed or nonsurgical intervention when there exists the potential for reversal of a significant neurologic deficit.

To address these issues, a prospective pilot study was performed to assess the feasibility and safety of performing acute decompressive procedures within 8 h of cervical spinal cord injury [163]. Eight different institutions within North America that treat patients with cervical spinal cord injury secondary to trauma participated. The protocol for the study included immediate imaging with MRI or CT for diagnosis of patients arriving within 8 h post injury and emergent decompression via either traction with closed reduction, traction plus surgery, or surgery alone. The study was prospective and nonrandomized with the objective of determining whether emergent decompression can be performed in a high proportion of patients with acceptable outcomes.

In a 4 month period, only 26 patients among the 8 institutions met criteria for enrollment within the study, which was estimated to represent less than 10 % of the patients admitted to these centers for cervical SCI. Low enrollment was attributed to delay in patient transport to the institution and difficulty obtaining immediate imaging studies. Among the 26 patients, 5 patients underwent traction alone, 17 patients underwent traction plus surgery, and 5 patients had surgery alone. Among the 22 patients that had surgery with or without traction, an average of 38 ± 9.6 h transpired between injury and surgical intervention. Only 2 patients had surgical decompression within 8 h of injury. Only 6 patients achieved decompression via traction within 8 h. Therefore, only 8 of 26 patients with SCI had spinal cord decompression within 8 h of injury. The investigators concluded that it is not feasible to acquire the appropriate diagnostic studies and perform emergent decompression within 8 h post injury under the system of care at the study centers. To proceed with a large-scale clinical trial for emergent decompression within 8 h post injury would require an improvement in factors resulting in delay of patient admission to the treating centers and in attaining diagnostic imaging.

Papadopoulos and coworkers prospectively studied 66 patients arriving within 9 h of spinal cord injury and who underwent emergency decompression via either closed traction or operative decompression [164]. The mean time to closed reduction was 3.7 h and the average time until surgical decompression was 9.6 h. Forty-eight percent of patients underwent traction as the primary means of decompression, whereas 52 % had primarily surgical decompression. These study patients were compared to 25 control patients who were managed outside of this treatment protocol due to either contraindication to MRI, need for other more emergent surgical procedures, or the admitting surgeon's preference. Fifty percent of patients that underwent emergent decompression improved in Frankel grade compared to only 24 % of control patients. Patients treated with emergent decompression also demonstrated less ICU days and shorter total hospitalization. This study, however, provides only class II evidence regarding the benefit of emergent decompression due to the lack of randomization.

Vaccaro and colleagues performed a prospective randomized investigation of patients undergoing early decompression within 72 h of injury compared to delayed decompression (after 5 days) [165]. Sixty-four patients were admitted within 48 h of spinal cord injury. The investigators found that patients undergoing early surgical decompression within 72 h did not demonstrate any significant difference in neurologic outcome, length of acute postoperative ICU stay, or length of rehabilitation compared to patients treated with delayed surgery. While the authors concluded that surgery within 72 h did not confer any benefit with regard to outcome, an earlier time period for intervention may be necessary to positively impact neurologic recovery.

In a large-scale retrospective study, McKinley reviewed 779 patients with spinal cord injury treated at 1 of 18 model spinal cord injury centers [166]. Patient outcomes were analyzed based on nonsurgical treatment, surgery within 3 days of injury, or delayed surgery. Upon review of the data, the investigators observed that patients in the nonsurgical group were more likely to demonstrate improvements in ASIA motor index; however, these were also more likely to include patients with incomplete cord injuries, whereas surgical patients were more likely to have more severe injuries. They also found that patients undergoing early surgery had shorter acute care and total length of hospital stay than patients with late surgery. More medical complications were noted in patients treated with late surgery compared to early surgery. Otherwise, no significant difference in functional outcome as assessed by functional independence measurement was observed between patients undergoing early surgery, late surgery, or nonsurgical management.

An evidence-based review of the literature, unfortunately, fails to recommend any current standards regarding the timing of surgical decompression for acute spinal cord injury [167]. This stems from a lack of class I evidence demonstrating that early decompression results in better outcome than delayed surgery. Few limited studies suggest that early decompressive surgery or closed reduction can be performed in the setting of acute SCI safely and effectively and provide class II evidence that early intervention leads to better neurologic recovery and shorter hospitalization. Therefore, early decompression is generally recommended in patients with incomplete SCI or neurologic deterioration with ongoing compression and who are medically stable to undergo surgery. Ultimately, however, the determination of the optimal timing for surgical decompression remains to be demonstrated by a large prospective randomized clinical trial.

Surgical Treatment of Spinal Column Injuries

While many traumatic spinal column injuries can be successfully managed conservatively, improved surgical techniques and fixation devices have made operative treatment for unstable spinal fractures a more common practice. Currently, open reduction and stabilization of spinal fractures are performed with better clinical outcomes, decreased morbidity, and improved long-term function. The primary objective of surgical treatment for spinal column injuries is to protect the neural elements in the setting of spinal instability and to potentially recover neurologic function by correcting spinal malalignment causing spinal cord compression. Additional objectives include restoration of normal spinal mechanics and prevention of chronic instability which may lead to segmental collapse, deformity, pain, and disability. Operative intervention also functions to promote early mobilization and rehabilitation in patients with spinal instability.

Surgical treatment of unstable spinal column injuries has several advantages compared to nonsurgical management. Operative fixation provides immediate stabilization, thereby avoiding prolonged bed rest or external immobilization. With early operative stabilization, patients may initiate prompt mobilization, rehabilitation, and an earlier return to function. In doing so, potential reduction in complications associated with prolonged bed rest and immobilization, as well as a more rapid return to a satisfactory quality of life, may be attained. Particularly in medically compromised polytrauma patients, prolonged recumbency poses risk of potentially severe complications such as deep venous thrombosis, infection, impaired pulmonary function, decubitus ulcers, and muscle atrophy. Immediate surgical stabilization may allow multiply injured patients to undergo other necessary surgeries or procedures. Surgical stabilization also is better equipped than external immobilization to restore natural spinal alignment and facilitate fracture healing. Inadequately treated fractures may lead to chronic nonunion resulting in chronic pain, deformity progression, neurologic deterioration, and impaired function. Finally, rapid surgical reduction and stabilization of spinal column injuries in conjunction with spinal cord decompression may serve to better preserve neurologic function.

Surgical techniques and instrumentation are constantly evolving to provide better spinal column stabilization, reconstruction, and restoration of normal alignment. Fixation devices are available for stabilization of the full neuraxis ranging from the occiput to the sacrum and pelvis. Implants are designed to be used in a variety of surgical approaches including anterior, posterior, and lateral exposures depending on the primary location of injury, instability, or mechanical failure. Further discussion of complex spine surgical techniques and instrumentation for the treatment of spinal column injuries is presented in separate chapters (Chaps. 30 and 31).

Conclusion

Major progress in our understanding of the pathophysiology of spinal cord injury coupled with improved diagnostic and therapeutic modalities have significantly advanced our management of patients with acute SCI. Improvement in overall care begins with better awareness of initial responders appropriately immobilizing and expediting transport of SCI patients to the hospital. Advanced intensive care and medical management of critically ill patients have resulted in better survival with reduction of complications. Surgical interventions for spinal cord decompression and stabilization of spinal column injuries are being performed with improved clinical outcomes and decreased morbidity. Better awareness, prevention, and management of late complications associated with SCI are improving rehabilitation, with greater functional independence, and longer satisfactory quality of life. Ultimately, however, effective therapies capable of altering the pathogenic mechanisms of spinal cord injury and reversing neurologic deficit are unavailable and remain the targets for future investigation.

References

1. Wyndaele M, Wyndaele JJ. Incidence, prevalence and epidemiology of spinal cord injury: what learns a worldwide literature survey? Spinal Cord. 2006;44:523–9.
2. Waters RL, Meyer Jr PR, Adkins RH, Felton D. Emergency, acute, and surgical management of spine trauma. Arch Phys Med Rehabil. 1999;80:1383–90.
3. Toscano J. Prevention of neurological deterioration before admission to a spinal cord injury unit. Paraplegia. 1988;26:143–50.
4. Centers for Disease Control: National Center for Injury Prevention and Control. Spinal cord injury: fact sheet, 2011. Accessed at: http://www.cdc.gov/ncipc/factsheets/scifacts.htm.
5. Berkowitz M, O' Leary P, Kruse D, Harvey C. Spinal cord injury: an analysis of medical and social costs. New York: Demos Medical Publishing; 1998.
6. Jackson AB, Dijkers M, Devivo MJ, Poczatek RB. A demographic profile of new traumatic spinal cord injuries: change and stability over 30 years. Arch Phys Med Rehabil. 2004;85:1740–8.
7. Nobunaga AI, Go BK, Karunas RB. Recent demographic and injury trends in people served by the Model Spinal Cord Injury Care Systems. Arch Phys Med Rehabil. 1999;80:1372–82.
8. Banovac K, Sherman A. Spinal cord injury rehabilitation. In: Herkowitz HN, Garfin SR, Eismont FJ, Bell GR, Balderston RA, editors. Rothman-Simeone: the spine. 5th ed. Philadelphia: Saunders Elsevier; 2006. p. 1220–31.
9. Dyson-Hhudson TA, Stein AB. Acute management of traumatic cervical spinal cord injuries. Mt Sinai J Med. 1999;66:170–8.
10. Horn EM, Forage J, Sonntag VK. Acute treatment of patients with spinal cord injury. In: Herkowitz HN, Garfin SR, Eismont FJ, Bell GR, Balderston RA, editors. Rothman-Simeone: the spine. Philadelphia: Saunders-Elsevier; 2006. p. 1185–96.
11. Green BA, Eismont FJ, O'Heir JT. Spinal cord injury – a systems approach: prevention, emergency medical services, and emergency room management. Crit Care Clin. 1987;3:471–93.
12. Garfin SR, Shackford SR, Marshall LF, Drummond JC. Care of the multiply injured patient with cervical spine injury. Clin Orthop Relat Res. 1989;239:19–29.
13. Brunette DD, Rockswold GL. Neurologic recovery following rapid spinal realignment for complete cervical spinal cord injury. J Trauma. 1987;27:445–7.
14. Prasad VS, Schwartz A, Bhutani R, Sharkey PW, Schwartz ML. Characteristics of injuries to the cervical spine and spinal cord in polytrauma patient population: experience from a regional trauma unit. Spinal Cord. 1999;37:560–8.
15. Podolsky S, Baraff LJ, Simon RR, Hoffman JR, Larmon B, Ablon W. Efficacy of cervical spine immobilization methods. J Trauma. 1983;23:461–5.
16. Ledsome JR, Sharp JM. Pulmonary function in acute cervical cord injury. Am Rev Respir Dis. 1981;124:41–4.
17. McMichan JC, Michel L, Westbrook PR. Pulmonary dysfunction following traumatic quadriplegia. Recognition, prevention, and treatment. JAMA. 1980;243:528–31.
18. Gardner BP, Watt JW, Krishnan KR. The artificial ventilation of acute spinal cord damaged patients: a retrospective study of forty-four patients. Paraplegia. 1986;24:208–20.

19. Grande CM, Barton CR, Stene JK. Appropriate techniques for airway management of emergency patients with suspected spinal cord injury. Anesth Analg. 1988;67:714–5.

20. Shatney CH, Brunner RD, Nguyen TQ. The safety of orotracheal intubation in patients with unstable cervical spine fracture or high spinal cord injury. Am J Surg. 1995;170:676–9; discussion 9–80.

21. Ball PA. Critical care of spinal cord injury. Spine. 2001;26: S27–30.

22. Vale FL, Burns J, Jackson AB, Hadley MN. Combined medical and surgical treatment after acute spinal cord injury: results of a prospective pilot study to assess the merits of aggressive medical resuscitation and blood pressure management. J Neurosurg. 1997;87:239–46.

23. Zach GA, Seiler W, Dollfus P. Treatment results of spinal cord injuries in the Swiss Paraplegic Centre of Basle. Paraplegia. 1976;14:58–65.

24. Levi L, Wolf A, Belzberg H. Hemodynamic parameters in patients with acute cervical cord trauma: description, intervention, and prediction of outcome. Neurosurgery. 1993;33:1007–16; discussion 16–7.

25. Tator CH, Rowed DW, Schwartz ML, et al. Management of acute spinal cord injuries. Can J Surg. 1984;27:289–93, 96.

26. Blood pressure management after acute spinal cord injury. Neurosurgery. 2002;50:S58–62.

27. Conrad BP, Horodyski M, Wright J, Ruetz P, Rechtine 2nd GR. Log-rolling technique producing unacceptable motion during body position changes in patients with traumatic spinal cord injury. J Neurosurg Spine. 2007;6:540–3.

28. Ditunno Jr JF, Young W, Donovan WH, Creasey G. The international standards booklet for neurological and functional classification of spinal cord injury. American Spinal Injury Association. Paraplegia. 1994;32:70–80.

29. Schneider RC, Cherry G, Pantek H. The syndrome of acute central cervical spinal cord injury; with special reference to the mechanisms involved in hyperextension injuries of cervical spine. J Neurosurg. 1954;11:546–77.

30. Merriam WF, Taylor TK, Ruff SJ, McPhail MJ. A reappraisal of acute traumatic central cord syndrome. J Bone Joint Surg Br. 1986;68:708–13.

31. Levi L, Wolf A, Mirvis S, Rigamonti D, Fianfaca MS, Monasky M. The significance of dorsal migration of the cord after extensive cervical laminectomy for patients with traumatic central cord syndrome. J Spinal Disord. 1995;8:289–95.

32. Guest J, Eleraky MA, Apostolides PJ, Dickman CA, Sonntag VK. Traumatic central cord syndrome: results of surgical management. J Neurosurg. 2002;97:25–32.

33. Schneider RC. The syndrome of acute anterior spinal cord injury. J Neurosurg. 1955;12:95–122.

34. Roth EJ, Park T, Pang T, Yarkony GM, Lee MY. Traumatic cervical Brown-Sequard and Brown-Sequard-plus syndromes: the spectrum of presentations and outcomes. Paraplegia. 1991;29: 582–9.

35. Woodring JH, Lee C. Limitations of cervical radiography in the evaluation of acute cervical trauma. J Trauma. 1993;34:32–9.

36. Blackmore CC, Deyo RA. Specificity of cervical spine radiography: importance of clinical scenario. Emerg Radiol. 1997;4:283–6.

37. Mace SE. Emergency evaluation of cervical spine injuries: CT versus plain radiographs. Ann Emerg Med. 1985;14:973–5.

38. Mann FA, Cohen WA, Linnau KF, Hallam DK, Blackmore CC. Evidence-based approach to using CT in spinal trauma. Eur J Radiol. 2003;48:39–48.

39. Berne JD, Velmahos GC, El-Tawil Q, et al. Value of complete cervical helical computed tomographic scanning in identifying cervical spine injury in the unevaluable blunt trauma patient with multiple injuries: a prospective study. J Trauma. 1999;47: 896–902; discussion –3.

40. Blackmore CC, Mann FA, Wilson AJ. Helical CT in the primary trauma evaluation of the cervical spine: an evidence-based approach. Skeletal Radiol. 2000;29:632–9.

41. Blackmore CC, Ramsey SD, Mann FA, Deyo RA. Cervical spine screening with CT in trauma patients: a cost-effectiveness analysis. Radiology. 1999;212:117–25.

42. Demetriades D, Charalambides K, Chahwan S, et al. Nonskeletal cervical spine injuries: epidemiology and diagnostic pitfalls. J Trauma. 2000;48:724–7.

43. Dai LY, Chen WH, Jiang LS. Anterior instrumentation for the treatment of pyogenic vertebral osteomyelitis of thoracic and lumbar spine. Eur Spine J. 2008;17:1027–34.

44. Flanders AE. Thoracolumbar trauma imaging overview. Instr Course Lect. 1999;48:429–31.

45. Flanders AE, Schaefer DM, Doan HT, Mishkin MM, Gonzalez CF, Northrup BE. Acute cervical spine trauma: correlation of MR imaging findings with degree of neurologic deficit. Radiology. 1990;177:25–33.

46. Schaefer DM, Flanders AE, Osterholm JL, Northrup BE. Prognostic significance of magnetic resonance imaging in the acute phase of cervical spine injury. J Neurosurg. 1992;76:218–23.

47. Tien RD. Fat-suppression MR, imaging in neuroradiology: techniques and clinical application. AJR Am J Roentgenol. 1992;158:369–79.

48. Hall AJ, Wagle VG, Raycroft J, Goldman RL, Butler AR. Magnetic resonance imaging in cervical spine trauma. J Trauma. 1993;34:21–6.

49. Benzel EC, Hart BL, Ball PA, Baldwin NG, Orrison WW, Espinosa MC. Magnetic resonance imaging for the evaluation of patients with occult cervical spine injury. J Neurosurg. 1996;85:824–9.

50. D'Alise MD, Benzel EC, Hart BL. Magnetic resonance imaging evaluation of the cervical spine in the comatose or obtunded trauma patient. J Neurosurg. 1999;91:54–9.

51. Klein GR, Vaccaro AR, Albert TJ, et al. Efficacy of magnetic resonance imaging in the evaluation of posterior cervical spine fractures. Spine. 1999;24:771–4.

52. Katzberg RW, Benedetti PF, Drake CM, et al. Acute cervical spine injuries: prospective MR imaging assessment at a level 1 trauma center. Radiology. 1999;213:203–12.

53. Vaccaro AR, Kreidl KO, Pan W, Cotler JM, Schweitzer ME. Usefulness of MRI in isolated upper cervical spine fractures in adults. J Spinal Disord. 1998;11:289–93; discussion 94.

54. Miyanji F, Furlan JC, Aarabi B, Arnold PM, Fehlings MG. Acute cervical traumatic spinal cord injury: MR imaging findings correlated with neurologic outcome – prospective study with 100 consecutive patients. Radiology. 2007;243:820–7.

55. Boldin C, Raith J, Fankhauser F, Haunschmid C, Schwantzer G, Schweighofer F. Predicting neurologic recovery in cervical spinal cord injury with postoperative MR imaging. Spine. 2006;31: 554–9.

56. Richards PJ. Cervical spine clearance: a review. Injury. 2005;36:248–69; discussion 70.

57. Morris CG, McCoy EP, Lavery GG. Spinal immobilisation for unconscious patients with multiple injuries. BMJ. 2004;329:495–9.

58. Ackland HM, Cooper DJ, Malham GM, Kossmann T. Factors predicting cervical collar-related decubitus ulceration in major trauma patients. Spine. 2007;32:423–8.

59. Morris CG, McCoy E. Clearing the cervical spine in unconscious polytrauma victims, balancing risks and effective screening. Anaesthesia. 2004;59:464–82.

60. Hoffman JR, Mower WR, Wolfson AB, Todd KH, Zucker MI. Validity of a set of clinical criteria to rule out injury to the cervical spine in patients with blunt trauma. National Emergency X-Radiography Utilization Study Group. N Engl J Med. 2000;343: 94–9.

61. Hoffman JR, Schriger DL, Mower W, Luo JS, Zucker M. Low-risk criteria for cervical-spine radiography in blunt trauma: a prospective study. Ann Emerg Med. 1992;21:1454–60.

62. Stiell IG, Wells GA, Vandemheen KL, et al. The Canadian C-spine rule for radiography in alert and stable trauma patients. JAMA. 2001;286:1841–8.

63. Stiell IG, Clement CM, McKnight RD, et al. The Canadian C-spine rule versus the NEXUS low-risk criteria in patients with trauma. N Engl J Med. 2003;349:2510–8.

64. Bandiera G, Stiell IG, Wells GA, et al. The Canadian C-spine rule performs better than unstructured physician judgment. Ann Emerg Med. 2003;42:395–402.

65. Stiell IG, Wells GA, Vandemheen K, et al. Variation in emergency department use of cervical spine radiography for alert, stable trauma patients. CMAJ. 1997;156:1537–44.

66. Lewis LM, Docherty M, Ruoff BE, Fortney JP, Keltner Jr RA, Britton P. Flexion-extension views in the evaluation of cervical-spine injuries. Ann Emerg Med. 1991;20:117–21.

67. Insko EK, Gracias VH, Gupta R, Goettler CE, Gaieski DF, Dalinka MK. Utility of flexion and extension radiographs of the cervical spine in the acute evaluation of blunt trauma. J Trauma. 2002;53:426–9.

68. Anglen J, Metzler M, Bunn P, Griffiths H. Flexion and extension views are not cost-effective in a cervical spine clearance protocol for obtunded trauma patients. J Trauma. 2002;52:54–9.

69. Sees DW, Rodriguez Cruz LR, Flaherty SF, Ciceri DP. The use of bedside fluoroscopy to evaluate the cervical spine in obtunded trauma patients. J Trauma. 1998;45:768–71.

70. Davis JW, Parks SN, Detlefs CL, Williams GG, Williams JL, Smith RW. Clearing the cervical spine in obtunded patients: the use of dynamic fluoroscopy. J Trauma. 1995;39:435–8.

71. Harris TJ, Blackmore CC, Mirza SK, Jurkovich GJ. Clearing the cervical spine in obtunded patients. Spine. 2008;33:1547–53.

72. Hogan GJ, Mirvis SE, Shanmuganathan K, Scalea TM. Exclusion of unstable cervical spine injury in obtunded patients with blunt trauma: is MR imaging needed when multi-detector row CT findings are normal? Radiology. 2005;237:106–13.

73. Bloom AI, Neeman Z, Slasky BS, et al. Fracture of the occipital condyles and associated craniocervical ligament injury: incidence, CT imaging and implications. Clin Radiol. 1997;52:198–202.

74. Occipital condyle fractures. Neurosurgery. 2002;50:S114–9.

75. Bucholz RW, Burkhead WZ, Graham W, Petty C. Occult cervical spine injuries in fatal traffic accidents. J Trauma. 1979;19:768–71.

76. Alker Jr GJ, Oh YS, Leslie EV. High cervical spine and craniocervical junction injuries in fatal traffic accidents: a radiological study. Orthop Clin North Am. 1978;9:1003–10.

77. Management of pediatric cervical spine and spinal cord injuries. Neurosurgery. 2002;50:S85–99.

78. Diagnosis and management of traumatic atlanto-occipital dislocation injuries. Neurosurgery 2002;50:S105–13.

79. Eismont FJ, Bohlman HH. Posterior atlanto-occipital dislocation with fractures of the atlas and odontoid process. J Bone Joint Surg Am. 1978;60:397–9.

80. Montane I, Eismont FJ, Green BA. Traumatic occipitoatlantal dislocation. Spine. 1991;16:112–6.

81. Levine AM, Edwards CC. Fractures of the atlas. J Bone Joint Surg Am. 1991;73:680–91.

82. Spence Jr KF, Decker S, Sell KW. Bursting atlantal fracture associated with rupture of the transverse ligament. J Bone Joint Surg Am. 1970;52:543–9.

83. Fielding JW, Cochran GB, Lawsing 3rd JF, Hohl M. Tears of the transverse ligament of the atlas. A clinical and biomechanical study. J Bone Joint Surg Am. 1974;56:1683–91.

84. Hadley MN, Dickman CA, Browner CM, Sonntag VK. Acute traumatic atlas fractures: management and long term outcome. Neurosurgery. 1988;23:31–5.

85. Sonntag VK, Hadley MN, Dickman CA, Browner CM. Atlas fractures: treatment and long-term results. Acta Neurochir Suppl (Wien). 1988;43:63–8.

86. Isolated fractures of the atlas in adults. Neurosurgery. 2002;50:S120–4.

87. Lee TT, Green BA, Petrin DR. Treatment of stable burst fracture of the atlas (Jefferson fracture) with rigid cervical collar. Spine. 1998;23:1963–7.

88. Levine AM, Edwards CC. Treatment of injuries in the C1-C2 complex. Orthop Clin North Am. 1986;17:31–44.

89. Fowler JL, Sandhu A, Fraser RD. A review of fractures of the atlas vertebra. J Spinal Disord. 1990;3:19–24.

90. McGuire Jr RA, Harkey HL. Primary treatment of unstable Jefferson's fractures. J Spinal Disord. 1995;8:233–6.

91. Fielding JW, Hawkins RJ. Atlanto-axial rotatory fixation. (Fixed rotatory subluxation of the atlanto-axial joint). J Bone Joint Surg Am. 1977;59:37–44.

92. Lourie H, Stewart WA. Spontaneous atlantoaxial dislocation. A complication of rheumatoid disease. N Engl J Med. 1961;265:677–81.

93. Phillips WA, Hensinger RN. The management of rotatory atlanto-axial subluxation in children. J Bone Joint Surg Am. 1989;71:664–8.

94. Husby J, Sorensen KH. Fracture of the odontoid process of the axis. Acta Orthop Scand. 1974;45:182–92.

95. Amyes EW, Anderson FM. Fracture of the odontoid process; report of sixty-three cases. AMA Arch Surg. 1956;72:377–93.

96. Crockard HA, Heilman AE, Stevens JM. Progressive myelopathy secondary to odontoid fractures: clinical, radiological, and surgical features. J Neurosurg. 1993;78:579–86.

97. Przybylski GJ. Management of odontoid fractures. Contemp Neurosurg. 1998;20:1–6.

98. Clark CR, White 3rd AA. Fractures of the dens. A multicenter study. J Bone Joint Surg Am. 1985;67:1340–8.

99. Schneider RC, Livingston KE, Cave AJ, Hamilton G. "Hangman's fracture" of the cervical spine. J Neurosurg. 1965;22:141–54.

100. Wood-Jones F. The ideal lesion produced by judicial hanging. Lancet. 1913;1:53.

101. Levine AM, Edwards CC. The management of traumatic spondylolisthesis of the axis. J Bone Joint Surg Am. 1985;67:217–26.

102. Francis WR, Fielding JW, Hawkins RJ, Pepin J, Hensinger R. Traumatic spondylolisthesis of the axis. J Bone Joint Surg Br. 1981;63-B:313–8.

103. Tay BK-B, Eismont FJ. Injuries of the upper cervical spine. In: Herkowitz HN, Garfin SR, Eismont FJ, Bell GR, Balderston RA, editors. Rothman-Simeone: the spine. 5th ed. Philadelphia: Saunders-Elsevier; 2006. p. 1073–99.

104. Watson-Jones R. The results of postural reduction of fractures of the spine. J Bone Joint Surg Am. 1938;20:567–86.

105. Allen Jr BL, Ferguson RL, Lehmann TR, O'Brien RP. A mechanistic classification of closed, indirect fractures and dislocations of the lower cervical spine. Spine. 1982;7:1–27.

106. Harris Jr JH, Edeiken-Monroe B, Kopaniky DR. A practical classification of acute cervical spine injuries. Orthop Clin North Am. 1986;17:15–30.

107. Dvorak MF, Fisher CG, Fehlings MG, et al. The surgical approach to subaxial cervical spine injuries: an evidence-based algorithm based on the SLIC classification system. Spine. 2007;32:2620–9.

108. Kahn EA, Schneider RC. Chronic neurological sequelae of acute trauma to the spine and spinal cord. I. The significance of the acute-flexion or tear-drop fracture-dislocation of the cervical spine. J Bone Joint Surg Am. 1956;38-A:985–97.

109. Torg JS, Pavlov H, O'Neill MJ, Nichols Jr CE, Sennett B. The axial load teardrop fracture. A biomechanical, clinical and roentgenographic analysis. Am J Sports Med. 1991;19:355–64.

110. Korres DS, Stamos K, Andreakos A, Spyridonos S, Kavadias K. The anterior inferior angle fracture of a lower cervical vertebra. Eur Spine J. 1994;3:202–5.

111. Lee C, Kim KS, Rogers LF. Triangular cervical vertebral body fractures: diagnostic significance. AJR Am J Roentgenol. 1982;138:1123–32.

112. Andreshak JL, Dekutoski MB. Management of unilateral facet dislocations: a review of the literature. Orthopedics. 1997;20:917–26.

113. Payer M, Schmidt MH. Management of traumatic bilateral locked facets of the subaxial cervical spine. Contemp Neurosurg. 2005;27:1–4.

114. White AA 3rd, Johnson RM, Panjabi MM, Southwick WO. Biomechanical analysis of clinical stability in the cervical spine. Clin Orthop Relat Res. 1975;109:85–96.

115. White AA, Southwick WO, Panjabi MM. Clinical instability in the lower cervical spine – a review of past and current concepts. Spine. 1976;1:15–27.

116. Denis F. The three column spine and its significance in the classification of acute thoracolumbar spinal injuries. Spine. 1983;8:817–31.

117. Ferguson RL, Allen Jr BL. A mechanistic classification of thoracolumbar spine fractures. Clin Orthop Relat Res. 1984;189:77–88.

118. Singh K, Kim D, Vaccaro AR. Thoracic and lumbar spinal injuries. In: Herkowitz HN, Garfin SR, Eismont FJ, Bell GR, Balderston RA, editors. Rothman-Simeone: the spine. Philadelphia: Saunders-Elsevier; 2006. p. 1132–56.

119. McAfee PC, Yuan HA, Fredrickson BE, Lubicky JP. The value of computed tomography in thoracolumbar fractures. An analysis of one hundred consecutive cases and a new classification. J Bone Joint Surg Am. 1983;65:461–73.

120. Cantor JB, Lebwohl NH, Garvey T, Eismont FJ. Nonoperative management of stable thoracolumbar burst fractures with early ambulation and bracing. Spine. 1993;18:971–6.

121. Chance C. Note on a type of flexion fracture of the spine. Br J Radiol. 1948;21:452.

122. Denis F, Burkus JK. Shear fracture-dislocations of the thoracic and lumbar spine associated with forceful hyperextension (lumberjack paraplegia). Spine. 1992;17:156–61.

123. Heary RF, Vaccaro AR, Mesa JJ, et al. Steroids and gunshot wounds to the spine. Neurosurgery. 1997;41:576–83; discussion 83–4.

124. Robertson DP, Simpson RK. Penetrating injuries restricted to the cauda equina: a retrospective review. Neurosurgery. 1992;31:265–9; discussion 9–70.

125. Benzel EC, Hadden TA, Coleman JE. Civilian gunshot wounds to the spinal cord and cauda equina. Neurosurgery. 1987;20:281–5.

126. Messer HD, Cerza PF. Copper jacketed bullets in the central nervous system. Neuroradiology. 1976;12:121–9.

127. Linden MA, Manton WI, Stewart RM, Thal ER, Feit H. Lead poisoning from retained bullets. Pathogenesis, diagnosis, and management. Ann Surg. 1982;195:305–13.

128. Waters RL, Adkins RH. The effects of removal of bullet fragments retained in the spinal canal. A collaborative study by the National Spinal Cord Injury Model Systems. Spine. 1991;16:934–9.

129. Jackson AB, Groomes TE. Incidence of respiratory complications following spinal cord injury. Arch Phys Med Rehabil. 1994;75:270–5.

130. Klompas M. Does this patient have ventilator-associated pneumonia? JAMA. 2007;297:1583–93.

131. Kollef MH, Afessa B, Anzueto A, et al. Silver-coated endotracheal tubes and incidence of ventilator-associated pneumonia: the NASCENT randomized trial. JAMA. 2008;300:805–13.

132. Rodriguez JL, Steinberg SM, Luchetti FA, Gibbons KJ, Taheri PA, Flint LM. Early tracheostomy for primary airway management in the surgical critical care setting. Surgery. 1990;108:655–9.

133. Arabi Y, Haddad S, Shirawi N, Al Shimemeri A. Early tracheostomy in intensive care trauma patients improves resource utilization: a cohort study and literature review. Crit Care. 2004;8:R347–52.

134. Onders RP, Elmo M, Khansarinia S, et al. Complete worldwide operative experience in laparoscopic diaphragm pacing: results

and differences in spinal cord injured patients and amyotrophic lateral sclerosis patients. Surg Endosc. 2009;23:1433–40.

135. Geerts WH, Pineo GF, Heit JA, et al. Prevention of venous thromboembolism: the Seventh ACCP Conference on Antithrombotic and Thrombolytic Therapy. Chest. 2004;126:338S–400.

136. Prevention of thromboembolism in spinal cord injury. Consortium for Spinal Cord Medicine. J Spinal Cord Med. 1997;20:259–83.

137. Spinal Cord Injury Thromboprophylaxis Investigators. Prevention of venous thromboembolism in the acute treatment phase after spinal cord injury: a randomized, multicenter trial comparing low-dose heparin plus intermittent pneumatic compression with enoxaparin. J Trauma. 2003;54:1116–24; discussion 25–6.

138. Deep venous thrombosis and thromboembolism in patients with cervical spinal cord injuries. Neurosurgery. 2002;50:S73–80.

139. Attia J, Ray JG, Cook DJ, Douketis J, Ginsberg JS, Geerts WH. Deep vein thrombosis and its prevention in critically ill adults. Arch Intern Med. 2001;161:1268–79.

140. Wade WE, Chisholm MA. Venous thrombosis after acute spinal cord injury: cost analysis of prophylaxis guidelines. Am J Phys Med Rehabil. 2000;79:504–8.

141. DeVivo MJ, Krause JS, Lammertse DP. Recent trends in mortality and causes of death among persons with spinal cord injury. Arch Phys Med Rehabil. 1999;80:1411–9.

142. Hebbeler SL, Marciniak CM, Crandall S, Chen D, Nussbaum S, Mendelewski S. Daily vs twice daily enoxaparin in the prevention of venous thromboembolic disorders during rehabilitation following acute spinal cord injury. J Spinal Cord Med. 2004;27:236–40.

143. Green D, Rossi EC, Yao JS, Flinn WR, Spies SM. Deep vein thrombosis in spinal cord injury: effect of prophylaxis with calf compression, aspirin, and dipyridamole. Paraplegia. 1982;20:227–34.

144. Shackford SR, Cook A, Rogers FB, Littenberg B, Osler T. The increasing use of vena cava filters in adult trauma victims: data from the American College of Surgeons National Trauma Data Bank. J Trauma. 2007;63:764–9.

145. Maxwell RA, Chavarria-Aguilar M, Cockerham WT, et al. Routine prophylactic vena cava filtration is not indicated after acute spinal cord injury. J Trauma. 2002;52:902–6.

146. Lloyd LK, Kuhlemeier KV, Fine PR, Stover SL. Initial bladder management in spinal cord injury: does it make a difference? J Urol. 1986;135:523–7.

147. Bracken MB, Collins WF, Freeman DF, et al. Efficacy of methylprednisolone in acute spinal cord injury. JAMA. 1984;251:45–52.

148. Braughler JM, Hall ED, Means ED, Waters TR, Anderson DK. Evaluation of an intensive methylprednisolone sodium succinate dosing regimen in experimental spinal cord injury. J Neurosurg. 1987;67:102–5.

149. Faden AI, Jacobs TP, Holaday JW. Opiate antagonist improves neurologic recovery after spinal injury. Science. 1981;211:493–4.

150. Faden AI, Jacobs TP, Mougey E, Holaday JW. Endorphins in experimental spinal injury: therapeutic effect of naloxone. Ann Neurol. 1981;10:326–32.

151. Young W, Flamm ES, Demopoulos HB, Tomasula JJ, DeCrescito V. Effect of naloxone on posttraumatic ischemia in experimental spinal contusion. J Neurosurg. 1981;55:209–19.

152. Bracken MB, Shepard MJ, Collins WF, et al. A randomized, controlled trial of methylprednisolone or naloxone in the treatment of acute spinal-cord injury. Results of the Second National Acute Spinal Cord Injury Study. N Engl J Med. 1990;322:1405–11.

153. Braughler JM, Hall ED. Correlation of methylprednisolone levels in cat spinal cord with its effects on (Na+ + K+)-ATPase, lipid peroxidation, and alpha motor neuron function. J Neurosurg. 1982;56:838–44.

154. Braughler JM, Hall ED. Effects of multi-dose methylprednisolone sodium succinate administration on injured cat spinal cord neurofilament degradation and energy metabolism. J Neurosurg. 1984;61:290–5.

155. Young W. Blood flow, metabolic and neurophysiological mechanisms in spinal cord injury. In: Becker D, Povlishock J, editors. Central nervous system trauma status report. Rockville: National Institutes of Health; 1985.

156. Hurlbert RJ. Methylprednisolone for acute spinal cord injury: an inappropriate standard of care. J Neurosurg. 2000;93:1–7.

157. Bracken MB, Shepard MJ, Holford TR, et al. Administration of methylprednisolone for 24 or 48 hours or tirilazad mesylate for 48 hours in the treatment of acute spinal cord injury. Results of the Third National Acute Spinal Cord Injury Randomized Controlled Trial. National Acute Spinal Cord Injury Study. JAMA. 1997;277:1597–604.

158. Matsumoto T, Tamaki T, Kawakami M, Yoshida M, Ando M, Yamada H. Early complications of high-dose methylprednisolone sodium succinate treatment in the follow-up of acute cervical spinal cord injury. Spine. 2001;26:426–30.

159. Geisler FH, Coleman WP, Grieco G, Poonian D. The Sygen multicenter acute spinal cord injury study. Spine. 2001;26:S87–98.

160. Geisler FH, Dorsey FC, Coleman WP. Recovery of motor function after spinal-cord injury – a randomized, placebo-controlled trial with GM-1 ganglioside. N Engl J Med. 1991;324:1829–38.

161. Marshall LF, Knowlton S, Garfin SR, et al. Deterioration following spinal cord injury. A multicenter study. J Neurosurg. 1987;66:400–4.

162. Larson SJ, Holst RA, Hemmy DC, Sances AJ. Lateral extracavitary approach to traumatic lesions of the thoracic and lumbar spine. J Neurosurg. 1976;45:628–37.

163. Ng WP, Fehlings MG, Cuddy B, et al. Surgical treatment for acute spinal cord injury study pilot study #2: evaluation of protocol for decompressive surgery within 8 hours of injury. Neurosurg Focus. 1999;6:e3.

164. Papadopoulos SM, Selden NR, Quint DJ, Patel N, Gillespie B, Grube S. Immediate spinal cord decompression for cervical spinal cord injury: feasibility and outcome. J Trauma. 2002;52:323–32.

165. Vaccaro AR, Daugherty RJ, Sheehan TP, et al. Neurologic outcome of early versus late surgery for cervical spinal cord injury. Spine. 1997;22:2609–13.

166. McKinley W, Meade MA, Kirshblum S, Barnard B. Outcomes of early surgical management versus late or no surgical intervention after acute spinal cord injury. Arch Phys Med Rehabil. 2004;85:1818–25.

167. Fehlings MG, Perrin RG. The timing of surgical intervention in the treatment of spinal cord injury: a systematic review of recent clinical evidence. Spine. 2006;31:S28–35; discussion S6.

Complex Spine Surgery

30

Daniel J. Hoh and R. Patrick Jacob

Contents

Abstract

Recent developments in surgical technique and technology have advanced the capabilities for surgical treatment of complex spinal pathology. Various surgical approaches allow for anterior, lateral, posterior, and circumferential exposure of the vertebral column, spinal cord, and nerves from the skull base to the pelvis. Contemporary spinal instrumentation provides optimal three-dimensional spinal fixation with improved biomechanical advantage for correction of spinal malalignment and long-term stabilization. The combination of these advances has resulted in broadened capabilities for treating traumatic, infectious, oncologic, and spinal deformity conditions in patients with complicated underlying primary disease as well as comorbidities. Optimal care includes a collaborative multidisciplinary effort including spine surgeons, neuro-anesthesiologists, and advanced neuro-critical care physicians. In this chapter, surgical approaches, techniques, and instrumentation are outlined with focus on specific anatomic and clinical considerations as well as potential complications.

Keywords

Spine surgery • Spinal instrumentation • Spinal deformity • Scoliosis • Spine tumor • Spine trauma

Introduction

The surgical management of spinal conditions has significantly evolved over the last several decades. Specifically, *complex spine surgery* has emerged as a growing area of subspecialty practice within both neurosurgery and orthopedics, as advanced surgical techniques and instrumentation facilitate the treatment of complicated spinal pathologies. Previously, traditional spine surgery primarily consisted of posterior midline approaches to

D.J. Hoh, MD (✉) • R.P. Jacob, MD
Department of Neurological Surgery,
University of Florida College of Medicine,
BDF 100265, Gainesville, FL 32610, USA
e-mail: daniel.hoh@neurosurgery.ufl.edu;
jacob@neurosurgery.ufl.edu

A.J. Layon et al. (eds.), *Textbook of Neurointensive Care*,
DOI 10.1007/978-1-4471-5226-2_30, © Springer-Verlag London 2013

decompress the neural elements via laminectomy for degenerative stenosis, herniated discs, infection, tumors, or traumatic hematoma. In cases of segmental spinal instability, immobilization either via bed rest or external orthosis was required until either the underlying pathology such as a fracture spontaneously healed or a surgical onlay fusion was achieved. Techniques for correction of spinal deformity were relegated to prolonged, sequential traction or manipulation with external casting and subsequent fusion.

While there have been many important developments in spine surgery, two major paradigm shifts ushered in the modern era of complex spine surgery. With these advancements, spine surgeons became significantly better equipped to manage complicated spinal disorders including traumatic spinal instability, spinal column tumors, infection, and spinal deformity. First, expansion of surgical exposures and approaches beyond conventional posterior midline surgery allowed for better access to ventral-based pathology, particularly in the thoracic and lumbar spine. Second, the development of instrumentation for internal spinal fixation provided the opportunity for immediate spinal stabilization, correction and maintenance of spinal alignment, and the capability for spinal reconstruction for conditions in which the normal weight-bearing architecture of the spine has been compromised.

The advent of complex spine surgery has also seen a nascent collaboration between spine surgeons and neuro-critical care providers to improve the management of these complicated patients. Complex spine surgical patients frequently suffer from significant medical conditions, whether they be related to the underlying primary pathology or to other comorbidities that can compromise outcome. Furthermore, the nature of these surgical procedures with prolonged operative time, increased blood loss, prone positioning, and elevated risk of injury to critical neurologic, vascular, or other visceral organs can significantly impact immediate and long-term clinical and functional status. Therefore, as complex spine surgery grows as a subspecialty, the role of neuro-critical care in the management of complex spine patients similarly increases. While a detailed description of the treatment of all complex spine pathologies is beyond the scope of this chapter, the following provides an introduction to clinical indications, surgical approaches, instrumentation techniques, and potential complications of complex spine surgery.

Complex Thoracic and Lumbar Surgical Approaches

Traditional spine surgery consists of conventional posterior midline approaches for laminectomy to expose the thecal sac and its contents for decompression. A direct posterior approach allows adequate access for most dorsal-based

intradural and extradural pathology throughout the cervical, thoracic, and lumbar spine. For ventral extradural compression, a posterior laminectomy can achieve an indirect decompression at the cervical and lumbar spine if there is sufficient lordosis to allow the neural elements to migrate posteriorly away from the ventral pathology.

Posterior midline exposures, however, have significant limitations. A posterior approach does not allow direct resection of a ventral-based lesion such as a tumor or abscess, particularly in the cervical or thoracic spine, as the spinal cord is susceptible to injury with even minimal manipulation or retraction. A laminectomy approach also does not create access to the vertebral body for reconstruction and stabilization for conditions in which the load-bearing capacity of the spinal column has been compromised. And, because the thoracic spine is naturally kyphotic, laminectomy for thoracic ventral-based pathology does not only affect an indirect decompression but can increase risk for neurologic injury.

Various complex surgical approaches have been developed to circumnavigate these issues, particularly for the treatment of thoracic and lumbar pathology. In the cervical spine, anterior neck exposures to the ventral spine have been readily appropriated by spinal surgeons given the natural cleavage planes between the strap muscles, carotid sheath, and the trachea and esophagus. As a result, anterior cervical spine surgery has become a standard approach in the armamentarium of most spine surgeons for routine degenerative, as well as traumatic, oncologic, infectious, and deformity-related conditions. Gaining surgical access to the ventral thoracic and lumbar spine, however, requires more advanced surgical techniques, as organ structures adjacent to the spine in these regions pose potential risk for significant morbidity if injured. Cardiopulmonary structures in the thorax and gastrointestinal, urologic, and vascular structures in the abdomen present particularly unique obstacles for exposing the thoracic and lumbar spine, respectively. These complex surgical approaches, however, have gained increasing acceptance for their exceptional exposure of the ventral thoracic and lumbar spine for decompression, stabilization, and reconstruction.

Anterior Approaches to the Thoracic Spine

The most direct corridor of access to the ventral thoracic spine is via an anterior or anterolateral approach. Unlike a posterior midline approach in which surgical dissection disrupts only the posterior paraspinal musculature, anterior and anterolateral thoracic surgery must navigate significant cardiovascular and pulmonary structures that occupy the chest and lower neck, with unique anatomic considerations and limitations at various rostral–caudal segments within the thoracic spine.

Access to upper thoracic levels (T1–T3) is limited by the thoracic inlet and accompanying structures, including the esophagus, trachea, vagus and recurrent laryngeal nerves, and the aortic arch. A standard thoracotomy is unfeasible in this region due to obstruction by the scapula. A standard anterior neck exposure to the rostral thoracic levels is impeded by the manubrium. Therefore, the trans-manubrial, trans-clavicular approach was developed to provide direct surgical exposure of T1–T3.

This surgical approach is commonly performed in conjunction with either a cardiothoracic or thoracic surgeon. General anesthesia with single-lumen endotracheal intubation is generally sufficient. Surgical exposure involves a T-shaped incision made on the anterior upper neck and chest, with dissection of the overlying muscles to expose the left 2/3 of the manubrium and the medial 1/3 of the clavicle. A drill or oscillating saw is used to remove a portion of the lateral aspect of the manubrium, thereby providing exposure to the ventral aspect of T1, T2, and the uppermost portion of T3. Critical at-risk structures encountered in this exposure include the contents of the carotid sheath, esophagus, trachea, recurrent laryngeal nerve, thoracic duct, and the aortic arch at the level of T3.

A conventional thoracotomy provides the best anterior exposure of the mid-thoracic spine (T4–T11) for the treatment of thoracic disc herniation, traumatic fracture, vertebral body tumor, and osteomyelitis. Excellent visualization of the ventral and ipsilateral thecal sac is achieved for decompression as well as single or multiple vertebrae for vertebrectomy, reconstruction, and stabilization. The only limitation of this approach is exposure of the contralateral pedicle and the posterior spinal elements.

The thoracotomy approach to the thoracic spine is generally performed in collaboration with a cardiothoracic, thoracic, or vascular surgeon. Generally, a right-sided approach is taken for upper thoracic lesions (T2–T6) to avoid the heart and great vessels. Mid- and lower thoracic levels, however, are most commonly accessed via a left thoracotomy as the aorta is easier to mobilize than the vena cava and is more amenable to surgical repair in the event of inadvertent perforation. Double-lumen endotracheal intubation is necessary to allow for unilateral lung deflation. A flank type incision is made corresponding to the level of interest with exposure of the overlying rib. After disarticulation of the rib, further surgical exposure can be performed either retropleural or intrapleural. Retropleural exposure is achieved by dissecting between the endothoracic fascia of the thoracic wall and the parietal pleura, avoiding entering into the pleural cavity and thereby obviating the need for a postoperative chest tube. For an intrapleural approach, the parietal pleura is opened and the chest cavity is entered. The ipsilateral lung is deflated and retracted to gain access to the anterolateral spine. A pleural flap overlying the spine is elevated and the segmental

vessels are ligated at the midpoint of the vertebral body to preserve anastomotic feeders entering into the foramen. Whether a retropleural or intrapleural exposure is made, at this point the vertebra and disc spaces are accessible for decompression, resection, or stabilization as indicated. Postoperatively, a chest tube is placed to prevent pneumothorax after an intrapleural approach or if the pleura is accidentally violated during retropleural exposure.

Thoracotomy at the thoracolumbar junction must also include exposure and detachment of the diaphragm from its periphery to allow access to the lower thoracic and upper lumbar levels. After entering the chest cavity, a circumferential incision is made in the medial portion of the diaphragm along its peripheral attachment to the rib to enter into the upper portion of the abdomen. A retroperitoneal dissection is performed to sweep the contents of the upper abdomen including the stomach, spleen, and kidney away from the rostral lumbar segments. The crus of the diaphragm is also cut at its attachment to the anterior longitudinal ligament, with later re-approximation of the diaphragm both medially and peripherally upon closure of the wound.

Trans-manubrial, trans-clavicular, and thoracotomy approaches are generally well tolerated by most patients; however, significant complications can occur. The most common complications after thoracotomy are pulmonary related and include atelectasis, pneumonia, pleural effusion, and bronchopulmonary fistula. Aggressive chest physical therapy as well as rapid mobilization in the early postoperative period is critical to avoid or minimize pulmonary complications, and decrease risk of venous thromboembolic events. In the upper thoracic spine, there is risk of injury to the esophagus, trachea, and carotid artery as they enter the neck from the thoracic inlet. Transection or retraction injury to the recurrent laryngeal nerve may impair airway protection against aspiration. Horner's syndrome may result from injury to the sympathetic chain. Violation of the thoracic duct can result in a persistent leak and chylothorax. Vascular injuries in the thoracic spine to either the aorta or vena cava can result in catastrophic sequelae. Sacrifice of segmental vessels is generally well tolerated; however, unexpected postoperative paraplegia after exposure of T10–L2 should raise concern for possible compromise of the artery of Adamkiewicz and spinal cord infarction.

Anterior Approaches to the Lumbar Spine

Exposure of the ventral lumbar spine can be performed via either a retroperitoneal or transperitoneal approach; however, the retroperitoneal approach is generally preferred to minimize morbidity related to bowel exposure. Special care must be made during the retroperitoneal approach to avoid gastrointestinal, urologic, and major vascular structures as they lie in close proximity to the lumbar spine. Anterior approaches to the lumbar spine are commonly performed in conjunction with a vascular or general surgeon, although, many experienced spine surgeons provide their own exposure. Access to the rostral lumbar spine (L1–L2) is achieved via a thoracotomy approach with splitting of the diaphragm as described previously. Exposure of L2–L4 is achieved via a flank incision, whereas, L4–S1 is obtained with an anterior abdominal incision. After dissection of the abdominal musculature, blunt dissection is carried out to separate the peritoneal sac from the retroperitoneal space, exposing the psoas muscle overlying the anterolateral aspect of the vertebra and disc space. For exposure of L5, a direct anterior approach is performed with mobilization of the iliac arteries. Major anatomic structures encountered during these approaches include the iliac arteries, veins, ureters, and potentially bowel in the event of inadvertent violation of the peritoneal sac.

Anterior exposure of the lumbar spine is generally better tolerated than anterior thoracic surgery. Potential complications include wound dehiscence, abdominal hernia, retroperitoneal hematoma, paralytic ileus, and ureteral, bowel, or vascular injury. Direct major arterial or venous injuries are rare; however, they can be catastrophic and are at most risk during placement of instrumentation or retractor positioning. The left iliolumbar vein is particularly susceptible to avulsion during exposure of the L4–L5 disc space. Elderly patients with significant atherosclerosis can develop plaque rupture and thrombosis with excessive traction of diseased arteries resulting in ischemia to the leg. Damage to the superior hypogastric plexus can cause retrograde ejaculation in males and is an important risk to be discussed preoperatively in those patients who may have future plans to procreate.

Posterior Approaches to the Ventral Thoracic and Thoracolumbar Spine

Anterior approaches provide the most direct access to the ventral thoracic and thoracolumbar spine; however, they have several limitations. First, anterior approaches do not provide access to the dorsal or contralateral thecal sac or the posterior spinal elements. Therefore, pathology that is both anterior and posterior to the spinal cord cannot be treated via a single-stage anterior approach. Second, spinal instability across multiple vertebral segments or secondary to compromise of the posterior osseous, ligamentous, or facet joint complex often cannot be adequately treated with anterior stabilization alone and subsequently requires a posterior approach for spinal fixation. Third, certain patients may not be able to tolerate a thoracotomy approach secondary to underlying medical comorbidities or prior thoracic surgery.

As a result, single-stage posterior approaches to gain simultaneous access to the ventral and dorsal spine have been developed. The goal of these approaches is to achieve adequate exposure of the thecal sac for circumferential decompression and the anterior and posterior spinal column for discectomy or vertebrectomy and anterior and/or posterior instrumented stabilization. These posterior approaches represent a significant advance over a conventional midline approach for laminectomy, which is limited in providing only exposure to the dorsal thecal sac. Compared to a midline laminectomy, these complex posterior surgical approaches are optimally designed for pathologies such as traumatic fracture dislocations, vertebral column tumors, and spinal deformity in which there is a need for 360° access to the spinal cord and spinal column for decompression and instrumented stabilization.

The transpedicular approach was developed primarily as a technique for excision of paramedian or lateral soft thoracic disc herniations. The transpedicular approach makes use of removal of a portion or all of the pedicle and superior articular process of the level caudal to the involved disc space. Through this small aperture, the intervertebral disc can be entered and herniated fragments removed. Bilateral transpedicular approaches allow for more extensive discectomy; however, disruption of bilateral facet joints creates iatrogenic instability at the involved motion segment, and therefore surgical fusion is required to prevent progressive deformity. Limited vertebrectomy can be performed through a unilateral or bilateral transpedicular approach for tumor resection, osteomyelitis debridement, or fracture reduction; however, the exposure is too restricted to allow for anterior stabilization or reconstruction.

The costotransversectomy approach provides considerably better and more expansive exposure of the ventrolateral spine by extending the posterior muscle dissection out laterally beyond the tips of the transverse processes onto the rib. The rib corresponding to the involved level is transected and disarticulated, allowing retropleural dissection to expose the lateral pedicle and vertebral body. The costotransversectomy approach can be performed over multiple levels to allow access to one or more disc spaces or vertebra for discectomy or vertebrectomy. Because this approach exposes both the posterior and anterolateral spine, ventral and dorsal spinal cord decompression can be performed as well as anterior spinal column reconstruction with posterior spinal fixation. A bilateral costotransversectomy provides complete circumferential exposure to the vertebral column for decompression and instrumented fusion. Therefore, costotransversectomy approaches are ideal for anterior–posterior disease such as complex traumatic fractures or tumors that involve both the vertebral body and the posterior elements. An advanced refinement of this technique is the total en bloc vertebrectomy, in which an entire vertebra is removed in two pieces (anterior and posterior to the spinal cord) through a bilateral costotransversectomy. With this approach, both pedicles are transected allowing removal of the complete posterior neural arch as one piece. Subsequent blunt dissection to free the vertebral body anteriorly from the surrounding soft tissues allows delivery of the remaining portion of the vertebra for en bloc removal. This technique has been advocated for wide margin resection of primary bony tumors in which en bloc removal has been associated with better outcomes than intralesional tumor resection [1].

Unlike anterior approaches which are partially limited at the thoracic inlet or by the diaphragm, the costotransversectomy approach can be performed throughout the full extent of the thoracic and thoracolumbar spine. The costotransversectomy approach also minimizes risks associated with entering the pleural cavity such as pneumothorax, pulmonary contusion, vascular injury, and intercostal neuralgia. The primary drawback of the costotransversectomy approach is that direct visualization of the ventral midline dura is inadequate, and therefore resection of central ventral pathology may pose significant risk of dural violation or potential spinal cord injury with overly aggressive surgical maneuvers.

The lateral extracavitary approach is a modification of the costotransversectomy approach in which a hockey-stick incision is made such that, instead of a conventional midline opening in the paraspinal musculature, a paramedian tissue plane is developed between fascial layers. This creates a myocutaneous flap which can be mobilized medially to provide a much more lateralized trajectory to the anterolateral vertebral column. After ventral decompression and/or anterior column reconstruction, the myocutaneous flap can then be directed laterally to gain access to the posterior midline spine for dorsal decompression and/or instrumentation.

Spinal Instrumentation

Perhaps the principal common element of nearly all complex spine surgery is the use of spinal instrumentation. The advent of modern spinal instrumentation increased the capability to treat complicated spinal pathology, as internal spinal fixation afforded the opportunity for immediate spinal stabilization as well as optimal biomechanical forces of implants applied directly to the spine for spinal reconstruction and deformity correction. Improved technology and surgical technique for spinal stabilization allows treatment of pathology causing critical instability that, if left otherwise untreated, could lead to either dynamic compressive injury to the spinal cord or progressive deformity with resulting pain and loss of function. The superior biomechanical advantage of internal spinal fixation provides the opportunity to reconstruct the spinal column after vertebrectomy for tumor resection, traumatic fracture, or osteomyelitis and to apply various implant forces to facilitate correction of subluxation or spinal deformity.

Posterior Instrumentation

Early spinal instrumentation consisted of posteriorly placed hooks and Harrington distraction rods for the treatment of spinal deformity in patients with poliomyelitis. The initial constructs were a hook–rod system, in which incremental compression and/or distraction was performed to achieve fixation. Particularly for treating deformity, the ability to apply compressive or distractive forces directly to the spine offered improved capability for curve correction than with external orthoses. Because of initial success with these constructs for deformity surgery, Harrington distraction rod instrumentation was readily applied as a means for stabilizing traumatic fractures, spinal reconstruction after tumor resection, and to facilitate bony fusion for the treatment of degenerative lumbar disease. With widespread use of Harrington rod instrumentation, however, clear recognition of its limitations surfaced. The use of primarily nonsegmental hook fixation of only the posterior elements necessitated excessively long fusion constructs to accommodate for the limited points of implant – bone contact – and the inadequate capability for load sharing of axially compressive forces. Furthermore, the method of posterior-based distraction to achieve spinal fixation and correction of coronal curves also resulted in a concomitant shift in sagittal alignment into overall kyphosis.

As a result, Eduardo Luque pioneered segmental spinal fixation to partially address these issues [2]. In contrast to Harrington nonsegmental fixation (in which hooks were only applied at the terminal ends of the construct), Luque instrumentation consisted of multilevel sublaminar wires or hooks which, when connected to rods, provided polysegmental fixation not only at the ends of the construct but also at multiple intermediate points. Segmental fixation offered the advantage of improved corrective and stabilization forces while decreasing overall stress upon each individual fixation point, by increasing the number of fixators across multiple vertebral levels. Furthermore, Luque instrumentation allowed for simultaneous compression and distraction over different levels spanning the instrumented spine to create relative lordosis or kyphosis as appropriate.

The advent of pedicle screws by Roy-Camille in 1963, however, ushered in the modern era of spinal instrumentation [3]. Pedicle screws were originally designed for the treatment of thoracic and lumbar fractures and to provide stabilization after tumor resection. Because of the unique biomechanical advantages of pedicle screws compared to hooks or wires, pedicle screws were quickly appropriated for the treatment of various conditions requiring spinal stabilization. Unlike hooks or wires which fixate only the dorsal osseous elements (e.g., lamina, transverse process), pedicle screws are placed down the shaft of the pedicle and into the vertebral body. As a result, pedicle screws simultaneously fixate both the anterior (vertebral body) and the posterior (pedicle) aspects of the spinal column. Therefore, a multi-level construct consisting of bilateral pedicle screws with a connecting rod and transverse rod connector is optimally designed to resist motion in all six planes, as well as exert three-dimensional control of the spine for corrective maneuvers. Furthermore, an appropriately sized pedicle screw engages both the cancellous bone at the core of the pedicle and a portion of the cortical rim, offering the strongest point of fixation at the implant–bone interface, compared to wires or hooks which merely make surface-surface contact with bony structures.

The integration of pedicle screws in complex spine surgery allowed for aggressive surgical treatment of complex pathologies that were once considered either untreatable or were relegated to poor outcomes related to suboptimal treatment, chronic instability, or deformity progression. Pedicle screws, however, have several disadvantages. Principal among these is the steep learning curve required for safe implantation. The intimate proximity of the pedicle to the thecal sac and exiting nerve roots poses risk of potential neurologic injury with an improperly placed pedicle screw that breaches either the spinal canal or the neural foramen. Excessively long pedicle screws that perforate the ventral cortex of the vertebral body can result in direct arterial injury, as the aorta and iliac arteries course along the ventral or ventrolateral aspect of the thoracic and lumbar spine. Unlike hooks, pedicle screws achieve their fixation by purchasing the cancellous portion of the pedicle and vertebral body. Conditions that decrease bone mineral density or compromise cancellous bone, such as osteoporosis, tumor, or infection, can impair the integrity of the screw–bone interface and weaken construct stability. Lastly, as with any device or implant, pedicle screws are subject to hardware fracture or loosening with excessive or repetitive biomechanical loading and can subsequently result in worsening spinal instability, threatening associated neural or vascular structures.

Anterior Instrumentation

Various techniques for anterior fixation of the cervical, thoracic, and lumbar spine exist. Anterior cervical instrumentation has enjoyed widespread popularity and acceptance. The primary advantage of anterior cervical instrumentation is the relative ease by which the ventral aspect of the cervical spine can be accessed with minimal disruption to overlying soft tissues structures. Unlike posterior approaches which require extensive dissection of paraspinal musculature, anterior cervical surgery is performed by developing natural cleavage planes between the strap muscles, trachea, esophagus, and carotid sheath. Considerable exposure across multiple segments can be achieved through a single transverse or longitudinal neck incision. As a result, anterior cervical surgery is ideal for resection of ventral compressive spinal cord lesions such as herniated discs, osteophytes, ossification of the posterior longitudinal ligament, tumor, or infection. Via the same anterior exposure, reconstruction, stabilization, and fusion of the anterior vertebral column can be performed after single or multilevel discectomy and vertebrectomy or to treat cervical fractures, dislocation, or deformity.

Anterior cervical instrumentation serves to stabilize the spine, to provide rigid immobilization to facilitate fusion, and to prevent intervertebral graft extrusion, collapse, or subsidence. Current anterior instrumentation employs a low-profile plate design with vertebral body screws that either lock to the plate or are semi-constrained to allow for minor compressive loading onto the intervertebral graft or cage. Use of current anterior cervical plate fixation has been shown to improve fusion rates and clinical outcomes compared to uninstrumented anterior cervical decompression and fusion [4]. Another important advantage of anterior plating, particularly with respect to complex vertebral column reconstruction, is to prevent graft extrusion or collapse with multilevel vertebrectomy [5]. The ventral plate serves as a buttress to physically block graft migration as well as load share to prevent excessive subsidence. However, it should be noted that ventral plating alone may be inadequate to prevent deformity progression after multilevel vertebrectomy without supplemental posterior spinal fixation, particularly in the setting of combined anterior and posterior spinal instability.

Anterior thoracic instrumentation is designed as a means for anterior spinal column reconstruction and stabilization when an anterior approach to the spine is performed. The initial anterior thoracic instrumentation was developed to treat scoliosis and consisted of a vertebral body screw connected to a tension cable, such that spinal correction was achieved by applying compressive forces through the cable along the convexity of the curve. Excessive force applied to the anterior spine, however, results in an undesirable degree of concomitant thoracic kyphosis or loss of lumbar lordosis. The initial screw-tension cable design eventually evolved into various screw–rod and screw–plate systems which provide increased construct rigidity and stability. Current systems have an improved low-profile design with the added ability to apply distraction or compressive forces at the screw–plate or screw–rod junction. The primary advantage of anterior spinal fixation is that it allows for a single-stage approach for spinal stabilization when an anterior approach is best indicated for treatment of the underlying pathology. Anterior instrumentation, however, is limited in addressing posterior osseous or ligamentous instability and therefore may be inadequate when the posterior elements are compromised or when more than one vertebral segment is involved.

Intervertebral cages have become an integral component of anterior column reconstruction. The vertebral body provides approximately 80 % of the load-bearing function of the spinal column. Pathology that compromises the vertebral body such as traumatic fracture, tumor, or infection significantly reduces the capacity of the vertebral column to support axial loading forces, maintain alignment, and ultimately protect the neural elements. Posterior-based instrumentation is not optimally designed to support excessive or cyclical axial loading and is prone to failure when used alone to stabilize significant anterior column defects. As a result, intervertebral cages designed from either titanium, carbon fiber, or polyetheretherketone were introduced. Cages are inserted to span a vertebral defect created by either a destructive pathologic process or after resection of a vertebral body tumor, osteomyelitis, or collapsed fracture, thereby reconstructing the anterior vertebral column, generally in combination with anterior and/or posterior spinal fixation. With intervertebral cage reconstruction after discectomy or vertebrectomy, the native axial loading characteristics of the spine are restored to provide optimal biomechanical stability. Disadvantages of intervertebral cages include the surgical approach morbidity frequently necessary to place an adequately sized cage to accommodate the vertebral defect, risk of cage collapse into the adjacent vertebral body resulting in kyphotic deformity, and cage extrusion either dorsally into the spinal canal or into the surrounding viscera creating neurologic or other organ system injury.

Sacro-Pelvic Instrumentation

Long-segment fusion extending into the lumbosacral region requires adequate fixation at the caudal most extent of the construct. Particularly when performing multilevel lumbar and thoracolumbar fusion for deformity, tumor, or trauma surgery, the caudal fixation points serve as the anchor for the entire construct. With long instrumented fusion, the sacral fixation point is generally subjected to large cantilever forces that may lead to screw pullout. Traditional sacral fixation consists of screws placed transpedicularly at S1. The S1 pedicle, however, is predominantly a broad cancellous channel and therefore provides less biomechanical fixation compared to thoracic or lumbar pedicle screws and is particularly susceptible to failure. While S1 pedicle screws may be adequate for shorter segment lumbar fusion, high rates of screw failure with longer segment fusion to S1 demonstrated a need to identify alternate means for caudal fixation.

Various techniques exist for fortifying caudal fixation to the sacrum. Recently, the addition of pelvic fixation with iliac screws has provided a means for improving stability at the lumbosacral junction. Placement of bilateral long variable angle iliac screws obliquely through the iliac crest, joined by a transverse connector, creates a tripod effect for load sharing and increased resistance to cantilever forces and

screw pullout. Furthermore, an L5–S1 discectomy with intervertebral cage placement provides additional load sharing to reduce stress on the sacro-pelvic fixation and may serve as a crucial additional degree of stability in patients with osteoporosis and high risk for implant failure.

The advent of segmental iliac screw fixation that can be joined to lumbosacral pedicle screws provides a biomechanically advantageous method for the treatment of sacral fractures. The sacrum is an integral part of the spinal column and its attachment to the pelvic ring. Besides protecting the sacral nerve roots, the sacrum maintains pelvic and spinal column alignment. Injuries to the sacrum can result in deformity, chronic pain, and loss of bowel, bladder or sexual function. Lumbo-pelvic fixation provides the best biomechanical fixation for stabilizing complex sacral fractures, or other pathologies that compromise the stability of the sacrum. By anchoring bilateral iliac crest screws in combination with rostrally placed segmental lumbar pedicle fixation, the construct spans the sacrum and mimics the normal load transfer from the lumbar spine to the pelvis. With adequate lumbo-pelvic fixation, the strength of the construct permits immediate weight-bearing without the need for external bracing in the setting of unstable sacral fractures.

Clinical Applications of Complex Spine Surgery

A comprehensive overview of clinical applications of complex spine surgery is beyond the scope of this chapter. However, the development of complex surgical approaches and the use of instrumentation for spinal stabilization and reconstruction have had a significant impact on the management of various traumatic, neoplastic, infectious, and deformity-related conditions.

Spinal Trauma

The advent of spinal instrumentation has significantly changed the management and prognosis for patients with spinal column injuries. Spinal instrumentation allows for immediate stabilization of unstable fractures and ligamentous injuries to protect the neural elements and preserve neurologic function. Furthermore, the biomechanical advantage of implants applied directly to the spine allows for improved capability for reduction of subluxation, dislocation, or rotational injuries, particularly with pedicle screw fixation which provides three-dimensional control of the spine. Perhaps, the most critical benefit of spinal instrumentation in the treatment of spinal column injuries is that, with immediate spinal stabilization, patients can be mobilized earlier and initiate rehabilitation. With earlier mobilization, one can potentially

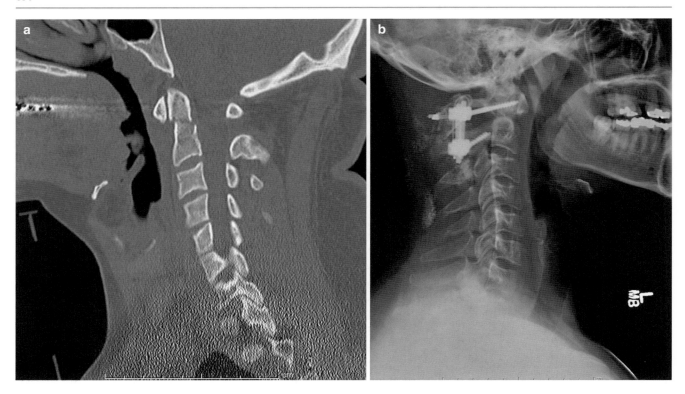

Fig. 30.1 (**a**) Sagittal CT scan demonstrating a linear horizontal fracture through the base of the odontoid process. (**b**) Postoperative lateral x-ray demonstrating posterior C1–C2 fixation with C1 lateral mass screw, C2 pars screw–rod construct in combination with posterior graft–wiring

reduce risk of pulmonary complications, skin breakdown, venous thromboembolic events, and muscle atrophy. Furthermore, aggressive surgical treatment of unstable spine injuries may allow for earlier transitioning from the acute inpatient hospital setting to rehabilitation, improving long-term functional outcomes.

Atlantoaxial Fractures

The atlantoaxial complex constitutes an important motion segment, with distinct anatomy compared to the subaxial spine, thereby accounting for its unique range of mobility. Specifically, the axially oriented facet joints, absence of an intervertebral disc between C1 and C2, and their complex ligamentous attachments allow for significant rotation about C1–C2 without translation or flexion–extension. Because of these features, however, traumatic injury to these ligaments, their attachments, or to the interposed odontoid process is grossly unstable in flexion or translation. High risk of devastating neurologic injury can occur with atlantoaxial instability and generally requires operative spinal stabilization.

Early methods for achieving internal fixation at C1–C2 involved various wiring or graft–wiring techniques; however, these proved unsuccessful in providing adequate immobilization of C1–C2 and demonstrated unacceptable fusion rates [6]. Furthermore, these constructs frequently degraded with cyclical, repetitive loading and therefore generally

required supplemental halo immobilization. Transarticular screw placement was introduced in the mid-1980s as an improved technique for spinal fixation of C1–C2. This posterior technique involved directing a screw from C2 across the facet joint into C1 and, when used in combination with a graft–wiring construct, provided better rigid biomechanical fixation and a superior fusion rate compared to prior techniques [7, 8]. As a result, this procedure gained widespread popularity for a number of indications which result in C1–C2 instability including odontoid process fracture, traumatic disruption of the transverse ligament, or rheumatologic conditions with increased ligamentous laxity at C1–C2.

Transarticular screw fixation, however, is a technically demanding procedure with potential risk of vertebral artery perforation as it courses within the C2 lateral mass. Patients with a high-riding, torturous, or hyperplastic vertebral artery are at significant risk for vertebral artery injury which could lead to a potentially devastating brainstem stroke [9, 10]. As a result, various alternative techniques for posterior C1–C2 fixation have been developed which avoid screw placement in such close proximity to the vertebral artery, such as screw–rod constructs employing a C1 lateral mass screw in combination with a C2 pars or intralaminar screw (Fig. 30.1a, b) [11, 12].

Ventral techniques at the atlantoaxial complex involve primarily screw fixation across a fractured odontoid process. Odontoid process fractures, particularly at the base of the dens, are associated with a high nonhealing rate with conservative management or external immobilization [13]. Direct ventral odontoid screw fixation was first described in 1980 and has gained significant popularity with the advent of specially designed retractors systems that allow ventral access to the vertebral body of C2, as well as the introduction of intraoperative spinal navigation systems which provide virtual three-dimensional imaging during screw placement [14]. Compared to posterior C1–C2 fixation such as with transarticular screws, anterior odontoid screw fixation offers the primary advantage of maintaining normal anatomic rotation at the C1–C2 joint and avoiding risk of vertebral artery violation. Clinical indications for odontoid screw placement, however, are limited primarily to acute odontoid fractures with an intact transverse ligament and minimal displacement. Contraindications include chronic nonhealing fractures of >6 months duration, comminuted or severely displaced fractures, pathologic fractures, or injuries occurring in individuals with severe osteoporosis.

Subaxial Cervical Facet Dislocation

The subaxial cervical spine is the most common site of traumatic spinal column injury and is particularly vulnerable to mechanical disruption of disco-ligamentous and/or bony structures. Particularly, hyperflexion–distraction injuries can disrupt the capsular facet complex as well as the interspinous ligaments, with failure of the dorsal tension band, predisposing the spinal column to translational forces, dislocation, and subsequent neurologic injury. The primary goals of management of any unstable cervical spine injury are immediate reduction of dislocation when present and spinal stabilization to protect neurologic function and potentially recover compromised, salvageable neural tissue. A posterior approach is often ideal for open reduction of dislocated facets via osteotomy through the dislocated facet joint and then spinal fixation across the unstable segment.

Cervical lateral mass screw fixation is a popular technique for surgical treatment of traumatic cervical facet dislocation. The initial techniques for posterior internal fixation of the subaxial cervical spine consisted of spinous process wiring. However, since then various instrumentation techniques and designs have developed. Lateral mass screw and rod fixation involves placement of screws in the cervical lateral mass via a posterior approach and has gained widespread acceptance due to the relative ease and safety of implantation, capability for spanning the cervicothoracic junction, and the ability to place instrumentation in the absence of an intact lamina or spinous processes (as with wiring or hooks). In experienced hands, cervical lateral mass screw fixation can be performed across multiple segments with significantly less operative time than segmental wiring or hooks and obviates the need for placement of instrumentation within the spinal canal. Unlike pedicle screws, however, lateral mass screw fixation

only obtains purchase within the lateral mass and therefore is susceptible to lower pullout forces and lacks the same capacity for axial load sharing as pedicle screws.

Thoracic and Lumbar Fractures

There are various approaches for the treatment of unstable thoracic and lumbar fractures. Determining the optimal treatment strategy is dependent on a number of factors including the degree of instability, number of involved segments, presence of neural compression, and the integrity of the load-bearing capacity of the spine. Numerous classification schemes for thoracic and lumbar fractures exist to facilitate treatment decision-making. The Denis classification is widely used secondary to its ease of applicability and communicability [15]. The Denis system divides the spine into anterior, middle, and posterior columns. The anterior column consists of the ventral 2/3 of the vertebral body, the middle column consists of the dorsal 1/3 of the vertebral body, and the posterior column consists of the osseous and ligamentous structures dorsal to the vertebral body (i.e., pedicles, facet joints, lamina, spinous processes, interspinous ligaments). The anterior and middle columns provide the primary load-bearing function of the spine under axial compression, whereas the posterior column is responsible for resisting flexion, extension, translation, and distraction.

These biomechanical characteristics are relevant in understanding mechanisms of failure during traumatic injury. Denis described four basic thoracolumbar injury types. Compression fractures are a flexion injury in which compression occurs at the anterior column while the middle and posterior columns remain intact. Burst fractures are a pure axial loading injury with failure of the anterior and middle columns, with an intact posterior column. Flexion–distraction injuries are those in which the ventral ligamentous complex acts as a hinge such that hyperflexion and compression occur in the anterior column in combination with excessive distraction disrupting the posterior column. Fracture–dislocation injury is perhaps the most severe injury mechanism in which all three columns are disrupted through bony and/or ligamentous structures via either severe flexion–distraction or translational or rotational forces.

Indications for surgical treatment are to rigidly fixate spinal instability, maintain or correct alignment, protect the neural elements, and prevent deformity progression. Using the Denis system, unstable thoracolumbar injuries are those in which two or more columns are disrupted. Therefore, compression fractures with intact middle and posterior columns are generally considered stable. Burst fractures, however, in which both the anterior and middle columns have failed under axial compressive loads can be highly unstable with risk of neurologic deterioration or deformity progression.

Because burst fractures represent primarily anterior and middle column axial loading failure, surgical intervention designed to treat these fractures is best approached by restoring the overall load-bearing function of the spine. This is optimally achieved by resection of the comminuted fracture fragments, reconstruction of the anterior and middle columns with a load-sharing intervertebral cage, and placement of anterior instrumentation for supplemental stabilization. Conversely, posterior-based hook–rod constructs are poorly equipped to stabilize burst fractures as these implants only fixate the posterior elements and therefore are incapable of compensating for a deficient anterior and middle column. Pedicle screw–rod constructs fixate the anterior and middle columns as pedicle screws traverse the posterior elements as well as the vertebral body and can be effective for treating burst fractures [16, 17]. However, it should be noted that without an intervertebral cage to axially load share, a pedicle screw–rod construct alone is subject to potential failure with repetitive, cyclical loading. Therefore, posterior pedicle screw–rod stabilization for burst fractures frequently requires longer instrumented fusions involving more motion segments in order to adequately distribute load sharing across multiple points of fixation.

Pedicle screw instrumentation, however, is particularly effective for the treatment of flexion–distraction injuries [18]. Flexion–distraction injuries result in compression of the anterior column with distraction through the posterior osseous and/or ligamentous elements. Because pedicle screws traverse all three columns, they provide ideal spinal fixation for restoring proper alignment and spinal stabilization and are optimal in resisting torsional, translational, and flexion–distraction forces (Fig. 30.2a–d). Frequently, with flexion–distraction injuries, a portion of the anterior and/or middle columns remain intact to provide primary load bearing, and therefore an anterior approach is not necessary to reconstruct the anterior column. Further, an anterior-only approach for stabilization may prove to be inadequate with these types of injuries as anterior constructs do not adequately address the disrupted posterior column.

Spinal Infections

Management of spinal infections has significantly evolved over the last several decades. Advances in imaging allow for prompt diagnosis with initiation of appropriate antimicrobial pharmacotherapy, often early in the clinical course. Most patients with vertebral osteomyelitis respond successfully to nonsurgical treatment [19]. However, some patients fail medical therapy either through continued infection or sepsis despite treatment, progressive neurologic deficit, or development of deformity leading to pain and disability. Complex spine surgical treatment has become a viable option for the treatment of spinal infections in many of these situations. Improved surgical technique combined with advances in

spinal instrumentation has resulted in decreased surgical morbidity and better long-term clinical outcomes.

Several important issues require consideration once it is determined that a patient necessitates surgical intervention. First, one must determine the appropriate surgical approach and technique for stabilization and fusion when indicated. Anterior approaches include anterior debridement and fusion with or without instrumentation. Posterior approaches involve a posterior decompression, debridement, and instrumented fusion. Circumferential approaches include anterior debridement with strut grafting and instrumentation with posterior supplemental fixation in a single-stage or two-stage fashion. Ultimately, surgical decision-making is dependent upon whether the primary pathology is ventral, dorsal, or circumferential and whether the infected tissue requires complete or partial debridement. Additional factors include the degree of preexisting deformity, determining the optimal technique for restoring spinal alignment, and whether spinal reconstruction and stabilization are necessary. Lastly, given the propensity for significant medical comorbidities in this patient population, serious consideration must be given towards selecting a surgical approach that the patient can tolerate with minimized morbidity.

Timing of surgical intervention is also a critical factor. Patients with acute neurologic deficits secondary to spinal cord compression require emergent decompression to prevent irreversible injury. Persistent sepsis despite medical therapy with significant abscesses and infected or necrotic tissue may necessitate urgent drainage or debridement to decrease the overall infectious burden and facilitate antimicrobial penetration. Acute instability that threatens neurologic structures demands immediate immobilization and may require urgent operative stabilization. Delayed surgical intervention is indicated for patients that are stable neurologically and clinically; however, have disabling pain or evidence of chronic progressive deformity. Generally, in these instances, surgical instrumented stabilization and arthrodesis are performed after the acute infection is cleared.

Posterior Approach

Posterior decompression for spinal infection is primarily reserved for evacuation of isolated epidural abscesses without involvement of the bony anterior spinal column or intervertebral discs. Epidural abscesses, particularly in the thoracic and lumbar spine, preferentially occur dorsal to the thecal sac and therefore are amenable to laminectomy for decompression and drainage. The extent of the laminectomy ideally does not involve the facet joints to prevent iatrogenic destabilization. Posterior decompression alone, however, is not recommended in the setting of osteomyelitis, discitis, or osteo-discitis. Laminectomy with removal of the posterior tension band further destabilizes the spine in patients with already impaired anterior column support, with demonstrated

Fig. 30.2 (**a**) Sagittal CT scan demonstrating multilevel thoracic vertical split fracture with mild transverse displacement. (**b**) Coronal CT scan of the same patient demonstrating moderate vertebral column collapse. (**c**) Postoperative lateral x-ray demonstrating restoration of alignment and reduction of vertebral collapse with posterior pedicle screw instrumentation. (**d**) Anteroposterior x-ray of the same patient demonstrating reconstruction of anterior vertebral height

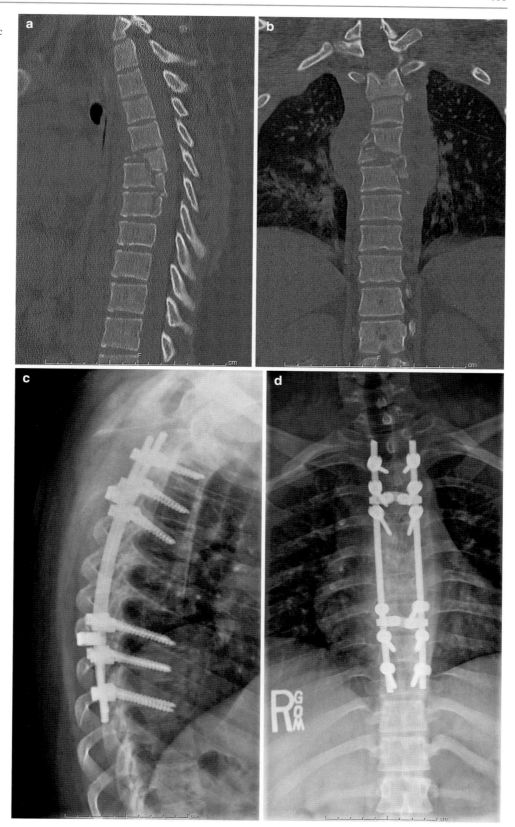

unfavorable outcomes related to deformity progression, increased instability, and neurologic deterioration.

With the advent of pedicle screw–rod fixation, a single-stage posterior approach for decompression, debridement, and instrumented stabilization may be an appropriate alternative surgical modality [20]. Various posterior approaches for accessing anterior thoracic and lumbar pathology are available. Costotransversectomy, lateral extracavitary, and transpedicular techniques allow access to the anterior spinal column via a posteriorly based approach (Fig. 30.3a–h). With these techniques, debridement of varying degrees of the anterior column may be performed, although complete vertebrectomy via solely a posterior approach is technically challenging given limited visualization of the anterior aspect of the thecal sac.

After debridement of infected, necrotic tissue, anterior column reconstruction may be achieved using either stackable or expandable intervertebral cages that are designed to be inserted from a posterior approach. Particularly in the thoracic spine, a unilateral single nerve root may be ligated to facilitate insertion of an interbody cage. Again, limited exposure via a posterior approach, however, may restrict the size of the intervertebral cage that can be inserted, thereby presenting potential risk for graft subsidence, kyphosis, or nonunion. Supplemental posterior fixation with a pedicle screw–rod construct provides instrumented stabilization and thereby prevents progressive sagittal deformity as well as facilitates arthrodesis. A single-stage posterior approach for debridement, decompression, and stabilization may be particularly suited for medically compromised patients with osteomyelitis who may not tolerate a thoracotomy for anterior exposure.

Anterior Approach

Anterior procedures to surgically treat osteomyelitis have become increasingly popular since Hodgson first reported anterior debridement and fusion for spinal tuberculosis in 1960 and has since become the standard treatment for bacterial osteomyelitis. Because the pathology is generally ventral, an anterior approach allows for thorough debridement of infected and necrotic tissue, with simultaneous drainage of psoas or paravertebral abscesses [21]. With an anterior approach, it is possible to completely remove all necrotic tissue until bleeding, well-vascularized bone is encountered and to decompress the ventral thecal sac. Anterior spinal column reconstruction with an intervertebral graft for arthrodesis, anterior column support, and restoration of sagittal alignment is also best attained from an anterior approach. Spinal fixation for stabilization can also be performed from an anterior approach during the same procedure.

Initially, anterior procedures incorporated autologous strut grafting without instrumented stabilization because of concern of placing a foreign body in a contaminated wound. As a result, patients were immobilized and maintained on prolonged bed rest postoperatively. While initial reports demonstrated successful clinical outcomes, subsequent studies have observed loss of correction, progressive deformity, and pseudarthrosis without the use of instrumentation. Recently, numerous studies have described successful use of titanium-based implants in the setting of spinal infection without evidence of persistent infection or relapse (Fig. 30.4a–c) [22]. The use of anterior spinal fixation in combination with anterior debridement and grafting allows for early patient mobilization thereby reducing the risk of complications associated with prolonged recumbency such as pneumonia, pulmonary embolism, decubitus ulcer, and muscle atrophy.

The anterior-only approach provides the benefit of thorough debridement, reconstruction, fusion, and stabilization in a single-stage, single approach. With a single surgical procedure, there is less morbidity associated with prolonged anesthesia, lengthy operative time, blood loss, and potential tissue injury in patients who are generally medically compromised and may be predisposed to poor wound healing.

Single-Stage Anterior and Posterior Procedure

A combined anterior and posterior procedure to treat vertebral osteomyelitis provides several benefits over a single anterior approach. Circumferential access to the spinal canal allows for complete neural decompression in patients who may have both ventral compression from retropulsed bone fragments as well as dorsal compression from epidural abscess or posterior spinal arch involvement.

Combined anterior and posterior instrumentation provides an optimal biomechanical construct to treat advanced bony destruction, spinal instability, and deformity secondary to vertebral osteomyelitis [23]. Anterior removal of necrotic tissue with anterior column reconstruction provides ideal load sharing and restoration of sagittal

Fig. 30.3 (a) Sagittal MR imaging of a patient presenting with thoracic osteo-discitis, epidural abscess, pathologic fracture, and spinal cord compression. (b) Axial MR imaging of the same patient revealing severe spinal cord compression as well as presence of paravertebral abscesses. (c) Sagittal CT image demonstrating significant vertebral endplate and bony erosion. (d) Axial CT image showing retropulsion of pathologic fracture fragments into the spinal canal. (e) Intraoperative photograph demonstrating a left posterior thoracic costotransversectomy approach after two-level vertebral corpectomy. Pedicle screw instrumentation is placed on both sides with a connecting rod locked into the contralateral side, prior to final placement of the ipsilateral connecting rod. Black sutures are used to ligate and transect two thoracic nerve roots. (f) Intraoperative photograph after anterior column reconstruction with an intervertebral titanium cage. (g) Intraoperative lateral x-ray demonstrating complete spinal reconstruction with an anterior intervertebral cage and posterior pedicle screw stabilization. (h) Intraoperative anteroposterior x-ray demonstrating the same spinal reconstruction construct

supplemental fixation results in poor sagittal correction and long-term increase in kyphosis [21]. An anterior fusion alone may be appropriate for a single-level corpectomy with an intact posterior tension band. However, patients with multi-level involvement, significant bony endplate destruction, or disease that crosses the thoracolumbar junction may be

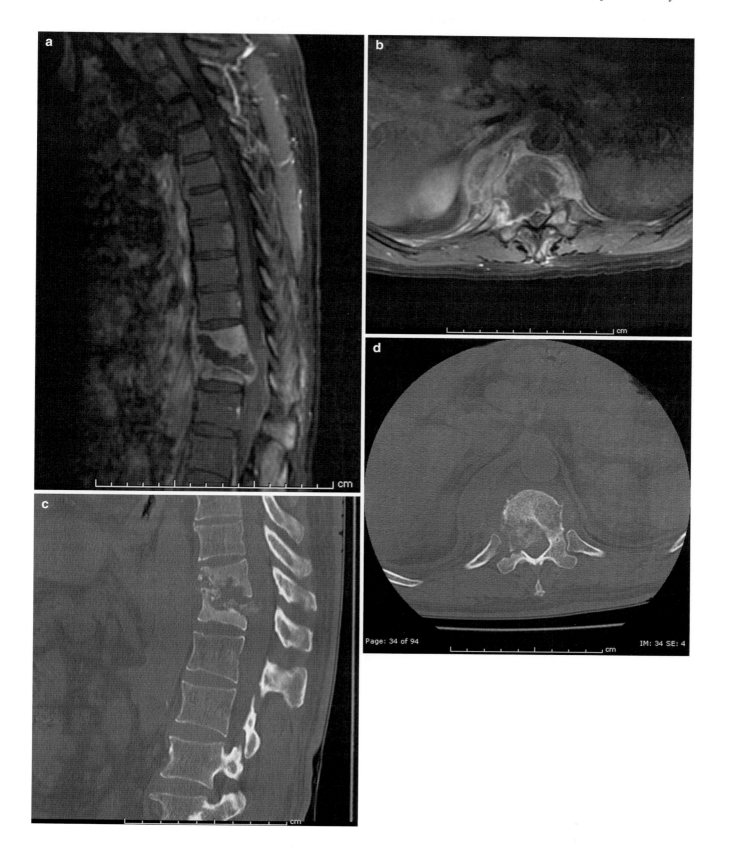

Page: 34 of 94

IM: 34 SE: 4

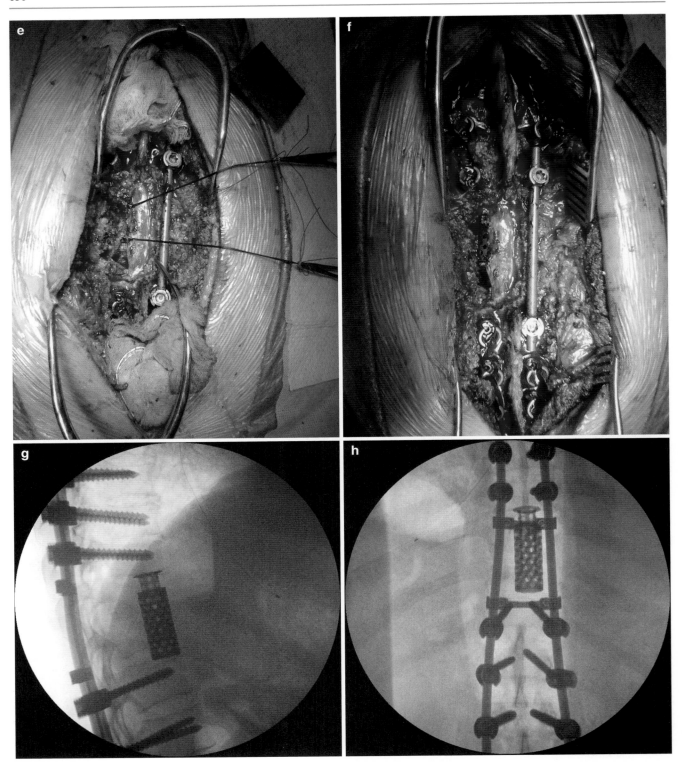

Fig. 30.3 (continued)

alignment in cases of vertebral height loss. Posterior supplemental fixation recreates the posterior tension band to restrict potential for long-term loss of sagittal plane correction [24].

The primary advantage of a combined anterior–posterior approach for stabilization arises from concern regarding long-term stability with an anterior-only procedure. Some have observed that an anterior procedure without posterior

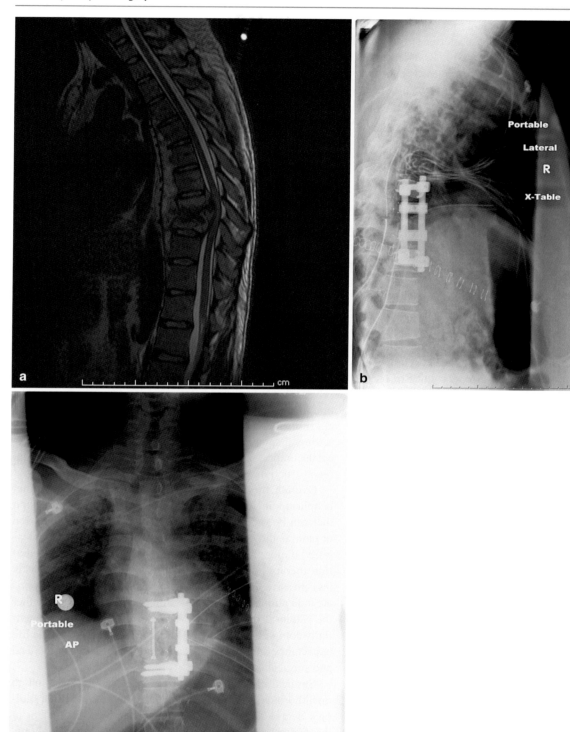

Fig. 30.4 (**a**) Sagittal MR image demonstrating a mid-thoracic osteo-discitis with pathologic fracture and retropulsion of bony fragments into the canal. (**b**) Postoperative lateral x-ray of the same patient show-ing single-stage anterior debridement, corpectomy, anterior column reconstruction, and anterior instrumented stabilization. (**c**) Anteroposterior x-ray demonstrating the final anterior reconstruction and stabilization construct

predisposed to failure with an anterior-only construct. Particularly, patients with loss of the posterior tension band either through extensive posterior spinal arch involvement, such as in spinal tuberculosis, or from iatrogenic destabilization via laminectomy may also require supplemental posterior instrumentation. Excellent restoration of sagittal alignment with long-term maintenance of correction has been demonstrated with a combined anterior–posterior procedure.

Two-Stage Anterior–Posterior Procedure

Circumferential treatment of vertebral osteomyelitis can be performed as a single-stage procedure or in a two-stage fashion, with initial anterior debridement and then delayed posterior fixation [25]. Staged spinal surgery has gained popularity for the treatment of various other complex spinal disorders such as deformity, trauma, oncologic, and rheumatologic conditions. The benefit of staged surgery is shorter operative time and less blood loss for each individual procedure, which may be particularly relevant for patients with worse overall general health. A two-stage surgery allows for a convalescent period to bridge between the two procedures in which the patients may have an opportunity to recover clinically and neurologically. Also, performing supplemental posterior instrumentation in a delayed manner allows for a longer course of antimicrobial therapy to further reduce the infected environment prior to implantation of hardware. Disadvantages of a two-stage procedure is an overall increased length of hospitalization, delay in transition to rehabilitation, and concerns regarding prolonged recumbency and impaired mobilization and nutrition status in the intermediary period between stages.

Spinal Neoplasms

Treatment strategies for spinal neoplasms are continually evolving. Recent improvement in both short- and long-term outcomes for patients with spine tumors is largely due in part to advances in early diagnosis, staging, chemotherapy, and various radiation treatment modalities. An essential component of successful multimodal treatment of spinal tumors, however, is the integration of complex surgical therapies for tumor resection, neural decompression, and spine stabilization. As with all oncologic management, the primary goal of surgical treatment is to obtain a tissue diagnosis, tumor cure or control, preservation of neurologic function, maintenance of spinal stability, and to minimize pain and disability.

Spine tumors may originate from local lesions within the spine, tissue adjacent to the spinal column, or metastatic spread from distant malignancies. Local lesions consist of primary bony or soft tissue tumors or tumors arising from the spinal cord or its covering. Metastatic spinal column tumors account for the majority of spinal neoplasms seen and arise from paraspinal or distant sites with lung, breast, prostate, kidney, and gastrointestinal cancer being the most prevalent.

Appropriate treatment of metastatic spinal column tumors is dependent on several important factors. Harrington devised a classification scheme based on an assessment of spinal stability and neurologic status [26]. Class I patients have no significant neurologic involvement. Class II patients have bone involvement with tumor but no collapse or instability. Class III patients have major neurologic impairment without significant bone involvement. Class IV patients have vertebral collapse or instability causing pain but without significant neurologic compromise. Class V patients have vertebral collapse or instability with significant neurologic impairment.

Pain in the absence of spinal instability or neurologic impairment is generally managed medically with chemotherapy, bisphosphonates, and radiation therapy. Spinal instability frequently necessitates surgical intervention which can range from less-invasive percutaneous cement augmentation to open multilevel instrumented spinal fixation and stabilization. Neurologic compromise particularly with acute deterioration should be treated urgently to potentially recover salvageable neurologic function with either emergent radiation therapy for radiosensitive lesions or otherwise immediate surgical decompression. Spinal cord compression in the setting of spinal instability may require both emergent surgical decompression with instrumented stabilization and spinal reconstruction as indicated.

Overall, the indications for surgical treatment in spinal neoplasms include an isolated primary or metastatic lesion that can be radioresistant, causing spinal cord compression or pain; pathologic fracture, deformity, or acute spinal instability; tumor progression despite chemotherapy and/or radiation therapy; and inability to obtain a tissue diagnosis by less-invasive measures. While these may represent appropriate indications for surgery, one must always consider whether the patient is reasonably medically sound to undergo potentially complex spine surgery and can expect a reasonable life expectancy and functional capacity with aggressive medical and surgical therapy.

Surgical treatment requires an organized approach based on a thorough preoperative understanding of the tumor biology, degree of neurologic compromise, anatomic extent of the lesion, and structural integrity of the spinal column. A crucial initial determination is deciding the most appropriate single or combined approach that will provide adequate access for tumor resection, neural decompression, and stabilization as necessary. An inappropriate surgical approach may result in an inability to completely resect the tumor or adequately decompress the spinal cord.

Once the approach is identified, the extent of tumor resection is largely determined by the underlying tumor biology and systemic disease burden. Obtaining a wide or marginal resection for primary and some metastatic spinal tumors has been demonstrated to improve survival and decrease local recurrence compared to a subtotal or intralesional resection [1]. En bloc tumor resection including wide margins is important for locally aggressive or radioresistant lesions and particularly beneficial for malignant primary bony tumors, as this minimizes the risk of tumor "spill" into surrounding tissues during resection.

Surgical decompression is essential for patients with progressive neurologic deficit in the setting of epidural spinal cord compression. Epidural spinal cord compression is reported to occur in 5–20 % of patients with metastatic cancer [27, 28]. Spinal cord compression can occur due to either direct compression from an epidural mass, mechanical compression from pathologic fracture and retropulsion of bony fragments into the canal, vertebral collapse resulting in severe kyphosis, and intradural disease. Aggressive early treatment is recommended as presurgical neurologic status is strongly correlated with postsurgical outcome. Therefore, the prognosis for significant functional recovery, extent of recovery, maintenance or regaining ambulation, and bowel and bladder function are largely determined by the neurologic status on presentation. A recent prospective randomized clinical trial demonstrated that the combination of surgical decompression with radiation therapy for patients with metastatic epidural spinal cord compression significantly improved neurologic outcomes compared to radiation therapy alone [29].

Specific surgical approach and technique is largely determined by the anatomic extent of the lesion. Metastatic tumors commonly arise from the vertebral body and therefore lie ventral to the spinal cord. Ventral compression particularly in the thoracic spine is poorly treated by laminectomy alone, and prior studies demonstrate suboptimal neurologic outcomes after laminectomy, often due to postoperative instability [26]. Various complex surgical approaches including thoracotomy, transpedicular, costotransversectomy, and lateral extracavitary were designed to circumnavigate this issue and provide improved access for tumor resection and spinal cord decompression. Decision-making with regard to which surgical approach is ideal also depends on the rostral–caudal level of involvement, as anterior versus posterior approaches can be limited at various spinal levels, as well as on consideration of the patient's overall medical status for tolerating potentially morbid approaches such as a thoracotomy.

Surgical management must also account for the structural integrity of the diseased spinal column. Instability may be due in part to an osteolytic underlying tumor process, as well as iatrogenic destabilization from either the surgical approach or tumor resection. Metastatic tumors most commonly involve the vertebral body, and, therefore, significant instability with axial loading can occur due to a deficient anterior and middle column from either pathologic vertebral collapse or partial or complete vertebrectomy for tumor resection.

Spinal reconstruction is recommended when the anterior weight-bearing column of the spine has been impaired. Vertebrectomy generally necessitates anterior spinal reconstruction to prevent vertebral collapse and focal angular kyphosis [30]. Instrumented posterior stabilization is necessary to restore the posterior tension band after extensive laminectomy or when the facet joints have been compromised by either tumor or surgically. Combined anterior reconstruction with posterior spinal fixation is indicated for cases with both anterior and posterior disease, significant deformity, or in which total spondylectomy or multilevel vertebrectomy is required (Fig. 30.5a–d) [31]. The last component of surgical decision-making is anticipation of disease progression and potential for spinal instability at adjacent levels. Future problems may be avoided by including more levels in the instrumentation construct above and below the tumor, combining anterior and posterior instrumentation, and maximizing multiple points of fixation.

Spinal Deformity

A growing area in complex spine surgery is the treatment of adult spinal deformity. Adult spinal deformity is defined as an abnormal spinal curvature that presents or undergoes treatment after skeletal maturity. This includes deformity that developed during childhood that is subsequently treated as an adult, or deformity that developed de novo after skeletal maturity secondary to degenerative processes or osteoporosis. Adult spinal deformity can also occur iatrogenically after prior spinal decompression or fusion surgery. Rising incidences of spine surgery in the United States in combination with a growing elderly population likely explain an increased awareness of patients presenting with adult deformity. Furthermore, recently there is growing consciousness of the significant potential morbidity related to adult spinal deformity. A study in 2003 in which patients with adult deformity were assessed using the Medical Outcomes Survey Short-Form 36 found that patients with adult deformity averaged much lower scores for the US population, including comparison with patients with comorbid conditions such as back pain [10].

Unlike the pediatric deformity population, adult patients present most commonly with pain. Back pain is frequently seen in the area of the spinal curvature and may be related to asymmetric disc collapse, degeneration, subluxation, and lateral listhesis. Generalized low back pain is further compounded by progressive muscle fatigue as paraspinal core muscles strain to maintain proper head and truncal posture in the face of gross spinal imbalance. Neurogenic claudication

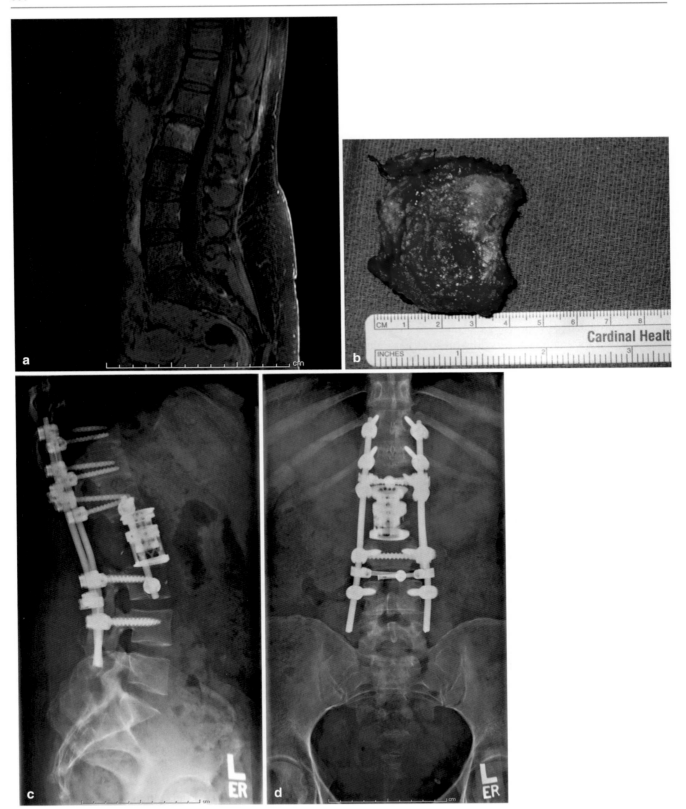

Fig. 30.5 (a) Sagittal MR image of a patient with an L2 Ewing sarcoma. (b) Intraoperative photograph of the vertebral body specimen after en bloc resection of an L2 Ewing sarcoma. (c) Postoperative lateral x-ray demonstrating anterior and posterior spinal reconstruction after en bloc resection of an L2 Ewing sarcoma. (d) Postoperative anteroposterior x-ray of the same patient showing the final spinal reconstruction construct

and leg pain may be due to nerve root compression secondary to ligamentum flavum hypertrophy, disc protrusions, or decreased foraminal height, most commonly on the concavity of the curve or at the level of a subluxation or lateral listhesis. Radiographic evidence of curve progression has been well documented in the adult population [32, 33], with significant increase in pain correlated with more severe curves [34].

Conservative treatment is generally the first-line therapy for patients with adult scoliosis, consisting of physical therapy, NSAIDs, and nonsurgical pain management modalities. However, for patients with progressive deformity, disabling pain, and loss of function refractory to medical therapy, advances in complex surgical techniques and instrumentation for deformity correction offer potential for clinical benefit and improvement in quality of life. Several factors must be considered prior to pursuing surgical treatment for adult spinal deformity. The individual's overall medical and health status is critical as frequently these patients suffer from significant medical comorbidities that may result in an unacceptable level of surgical risk. Among these comorbidities, osteopenia or osteoporosis is a specific major concern in the elderly population as low bone mineral density will compromise the ability for achieving and maintaining spinal correction with instrumentation. Before pursuing any surgical treatment for adult deformity, an in-depth preoperative discussion with the patient must be had with regard to potential risks and foreseeable benefits, as well as the expected lengthy recovery time, in order to align patient and physician expectations for a reasonable expected clinical outcome.

Various surgical modalities for the treatment of adult idiopathic deformity exist and are dictated by the location of the primary structural curve and the presence of additional structural or compensatory curves. A primary thoracic curve with a flexible compensatory lumbar curve can frequently be treated with a posterior instrumented fusion. Patients with a thoracolumbar or lumbar curve are often ideal candidates for anterior correction and instrumented fusion. An anterior approach in these situations provides several advantages, including the need to fuse fewer motions segments, superior spinal correction, and better fusion rates. However, in the setting of concomitant lumbar stenosis, a posterior or combined approach may be preferable to allow for both curve correction and neural decompression. Individuals with both structural thoracic and lumbar curves are more challenging. The primary objective in adult deformity, unlike pediatric patients, is to achieve an overall well-balance spine such that the head is centered over the pelvis [35, 36]. Therefore, despite significant thoracic and lumbar curves, frequently a posterior instrumented fusion directed towards stabilizing and maintaining overall balance may be adequate for achieving long-term symptomatic benefit and halting deformity progression. Patients with severe multi-planar curves and profound overall imbalance may require a combined anterior

and posterior approach. An anterior approach for multilevel discectomy and placement of large intervertebral grafts restores lumbar lordosis while releasing the spine for further correction. A subsequent posterior approach allows for decompression as needed, with final curve correction and instrumented stabilization and fusion to maintain long-term alignment.

Unlike idiopathic spinal deformity, degenerative spinal deformity poses altogether unique challenges. Patients with degenerative spinal deformity commonly present for revision surgery after having prior decompression or fusion procedures with significant scar formation, preexisting instrumentation, and relatively fixed deformities. Patients with degenerative spinal deformity may present with symptomatic adjacent segment degeneration with stenosis and progressive deformity, failed prior fusion with painful pseudarthrosis and instrumentation failure, or progressive sagittal imbalance from prior lumbar fusion with relative loss of lordosis ("flat-back" syndrome). The combination of these factors increases the potential morbidity of surgical treatment, as well as the complexity of surgical decision-making and approach. Overall, however, the primary goals of surgical treatment are to decompress the neural elements, achieve a balanced, stable spine, and obtain solid fusion.

Revision or salvage spine surgical techniques are employed for the management of symptomatic adjacent segment stenosis with progressive deformity and for painful pseudarthrosis with instrumentation failure. Generally, a posterior approach is indicated in the lumbar spine to decompress adjacent segment stenosis. At the level of the thoracic and thoracolumbar spine, an anterior approach or transpedicular or costotransversectomy approach may be necessary to treat ventral-based compression. Once neural decompression is achieved, the presence of junctional kyphosis or angular deformity is addressed as necessary either though the incorporation of intervertebral grafts to restore lordosis or a variety of osteotomy techniques to recreate lordosis. Extension of the instrumentation and fusion to incorporate the revision levels is necessary to maintain alignment and prevent restenosis or progressive deformity.

Management of painful pseudarthrosis with instrumentation failure requires careful preoperative assessment of CT and MR imaging to assess for nonunion levels, careful inspection of fractured or loosened hardware, and identification of areas of residual or new neural compression. During surgery, meticulous exploration of the prior fusion mass is performed. Frequently, pseudarthrosis occurs in the setting of a failed posterolateral fusion or fusion ending or extending across a junction. In these situations, consideration for interbody fusion with the use of intervertebral grafts is ideal as the loading of the graft in compression increases likelihood of successful fusion. Decompression as necessary is performed in the same setting and may be achieved from a posterior, anterior, or combined approach as dictated by the level and location of pathology. Generally, in the setting of symptomatic pseudarthrosis, the preexisting hardware is explanted, and new instrumentation is reinserted. If the prior hardware has fractured and is retained or if there has been significant loosening of previous hardware, then the revision fusion may need to be extended across additional levels in order to achieve adequate fixation for stabilization.

Fixed sagittal imbalance or "flat-back" syndrome is a particularly challenging spinal deformity. In general, lumbar lordosis progressively decreases with age, secondary to age-related loss of intervertebral disc height. Prior lumbar fusion with Harrington distraction rods or surgical fusion performed with the patient in a lumbar flexed or relatively flat alignment can further contribute to overall sagittal imbalance. Flat-back syndrome leads to a crouched stance or walking position in which worsening back pain occurs secondary to progressive fatigue of paraspinal and thigh muscles, straining to maintain upright head and truncal posture. Frequently, multilevel spinal stenosis occurs in the setting of sagittal imbalance, particularly adjacent to previously fused segments, resulting in neurogenic claudication and leg pain.

Surgical treatment of sagittal imbalance is primarily directed towards obtaining a well-balance spine such that the head is positioned squarely over the pelvis. Largely, correction of sagittal imbalance is best achieved by restoring or increasing lumbar lordosis. Various complex osteotomy techniques have been developed to recreate lumbar lordosis in the setting of a fixed or fused spinal deformity. The original Smith–Petersen osteotomy technique for the correction of fixed spinal deformity was described in 1945 for patients with ankylosing spondylitis. The surgical technique involves removal of the posterior elements, undercutting of the adjacent spinous processes, and then closing the posterior osteotomy, thus creating an opening-wedge osteotomy through the anterior aspect of the disc space. This extension-type osteotomy creates lumbar hyperextension, thereby exaggerating lordosis at that segment via a closure of the posterior elements and an opening of the anterior elements.

Although this extension osteotomy technique can achieve dramatic deformity correction, the true Smith–Petersen osteotomy carries significant morbidity. By lengthening the anterior column with disruption of the anterior longitudinal ligament to create the opening-wedge osteotomy, there is risk of injury to adjacent anterior vascular structures. In an early review in 1959 of 80 patients treated with this procedure, 10 % of patients died secondary to surgery-related complications. Neurologic complications were reported in up to 30 % of patients [37]. Forceful hyperextension of the spine may cause rupture of the aorta or inferior vena cava, which are frequently calcified in the elderly patients and particularly in those with ankylosing spondylitis for whom the original technique was described.

Since then, a variation of this technique known as the polysegmental osteotomy has been described in which a similar surgical removal of the posterior elements and facet joints is performed at multiple levels [38]. Subsequent compression of the remaining posterior elements creates a minor degree of extension at each level without disruption or significant lengthening of the anterior column. The correction is obtained through deformation of the disc spaces without rupture of the anterior longitudinal ligament as with the Smith–Petersen osteotomy. As a result, less degrees of correction are achieved with each level of osteotomy; however, the sum result across multiple levels may be sufficient to achieve adequate deformity correction.

The primary benefit of the polysegmental osteotomy is that it is not associated with the same degree of surgical complications as with the Smith–Petersen technique. In a review of 177 patients with ankylosing spondylitis undergoing polysegmental osteotomies for deformity correction, the mortality rate was only 2.3 % with a 2.3 % incidence of nonreversible neurologic complications, which compares favorably to much higher complication rates with the Smith–Petersen osteotomy [39]. However, there are several limitations with this technique; first and foremost is the substantially decreased overall correction obtained from a single segment osteotomy. The average correction achieved at each level of a polysegmental osteotomy is about 10° compared to nearly 30° with the original description of the Smith–Petersen osteotomy for ankylosing spondylitis. Therefore, multiple levels (i.e., "polysegmental" osteotomy) are necessary to achieve any significant degree of spinal correction. Further, the polysegmental osteotomy achieves correction through deformation of the anterior disc space and therefore is dependent on disc spaces that are not fused or significantly collapsed secondary to degenerative disease.

An alternative more advanced surgical technique for achieving spinal correction is the pedicle subtraction osteotomy (or "closing-wedge" osteotomy) [40]. Similar to the Smith–Petersen osteotomy, the posterior elements are removed as well as a portion of the adjacent segments rostral and caudal to the index level. However, in addition, complete removal of both pedicles as well as a wedge of bone from the vertebral body is taken with the base of the wedge at the dorsal vertebral body wall and the apex at the ventral vertebral body. This aggressive technique with removal of a significant wedge of bone can result in a sagittal plane correction of up to 40° (Fig. 30.6a–d). By performing asymmetric removal of the posterior elements, correction of both sagittal and coronal plane deformities can be performed simultaneously.

The advantage of this technique is that unlike the Smith–Petersen osteotomy, the osteotomy is primarily a closing wedge, and overall spinal-shortening procedure, thereby obviating the risks associated with lengthening the spinal column and potential injury to neurologic or vascular

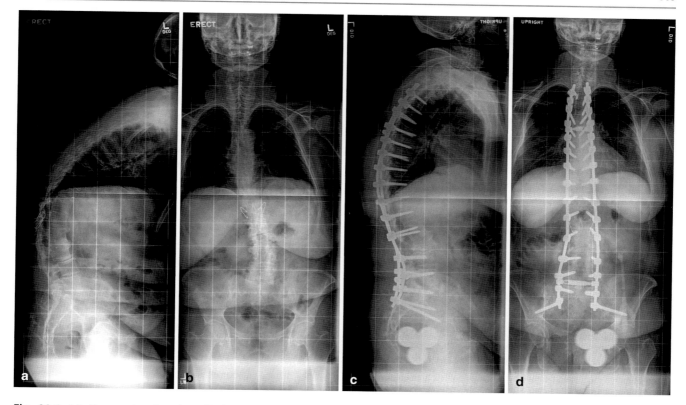

Fig. 30.6 (**a**) Preoperative lateral scoliosis x-ray demonstrating marked positive sagittal imbalance. (**b**) Preoperative anteroposterior scoliosis x-ray of the same patient demonstrating rightward truncal shift. (**c**) Postoperative lateral scoliosis x-ray after pedicle subtraction osteotomy and T4–pelvic posterior fixation demonstrating spinal deformity correction with appropriate sagittal balance. (**d**) Postoperative anteroposterior x-ray of the same patient demonstrating correction of rightward truncal shift

structures. Furthermore, a dramatic degree of correction can be achieved at a single segment, therefore not requiring multiple levels of osteotomy as with the polysegmental osteotomy approach. The pedicle subtraction osteotomy, however, is a technically demanding procedure and associated with risk of substantial intraoperative blood loss related to the epidural venous plexus surrounding the dorsal vertebral body as well as the exposed cancellous bone surfaces after wedge removal. Furthermore, with the closing-wedge procedure, care must be made to ensure that nerve roots do not become pinched as the thecal sac buckles during the closure.

Complications

Complication avoidance is particularly relevant in adult deformity surgery as many patients are generally of advanced age and suffer from significant medical comorbidities. With improving complex surgical techniques, instrumentation, and neuro-anesthesia, the incidence of spinal deformity complications have decreased. However, complications are still a significant concern as reported rates of total minor and major complications after adult spinal deformity surgery range from 22 to 58.2 % [41–44]. Significant neurologic injury after deformity surgery is rare and occurs in less than 1–5 % of cases [45]. Significant risk factors for neurologic injury,

however, include hyper-kyphosis and combined anterior and posterior surgery. Neurologic deficits do not always appear immediately after surgery, as delayed paraplegia is a devastating complication that can occur several hours after deformity correction surgery. Postoperative hypovolemia and mechanical tension on spinal vessels along the concavity of the corrected curve have been implicated as causing delayed spinal cord ischemia and postoperative neurologic deficit. Postoperative visual loss is a rare but serious neurologic complication after adult deformity surgery with the risk estimated to be 0.05–1 % after major spinal surgery [46]. Risk factors associated with postoperative visual loss include hypotension, low hematocrit, prone positioning, use of a ProneView head positioning device (as opposed to a skull clamp), and coexisting disease.

Significant bleeding with resulting hypovolemia and anemia can occur at the time of surgery or in the early postoperative period. The primary causative factor is bleeding from the surgical site which may present as a low hematocrit during or immediately after surgery or a gradual decrease in hematocrit over a number of days secondary to persistent blood loss via subfascial drains or chest tube (in cases of thoracotomy). Other causative factors to consider for anemia after surgery include platelet washout, acute thrombocytopenia, platelet dysfunction, heparin administration, disseminated intravascular coagulation, impaired coagulation, decreased hepatic function, undiagnosed hereditary coagulation disorder, or laboratory error.

Deep venous thrombosis and pulmonary embolism are significant potential complications after spine surgery. While the incidence of deep venous thromboembolism after spine surgery is unknown, it is estimated to range from 0.47 to 12.4 % depending on the condition [47]. Prophylaxis for thromboembolism should be strongly considered after major spine surgery with heparin and sequential compression devices and stockings.

Impaired nutritional status is a significant concern after major spinal surgery. The daily caloric requirement has been shown to markedly increase after spinal fusion surgery, upwards of 9 % above the average baseline determination, with increased caloric needs remaining elevated until 6 weeks after surgery [48]. Optimization of nutrition, in certain cases requiring hyperalimentation, is critical as poor nutrition status is correlated with wound complications, increased infection, and prolonged recovery from surgery. Impairment of nutrition is further confounded by the potential for postoperative paralytic ileus, of which the incidence is 5–12 % of spine patients [49]. Postoperative paralytic ileus is the temporary loss of gastrointestinal motility after surgery. Vomiting and abdominal distention and discomfort are the primary symptoms, with abdominal radiographs demonstrating distended loops of bowel. Treatment consists of restricting gastric intake and placement of a nasogastric tube to decompress the gastrointestinal tract.

Spine surgical infection rates depend on the approach and the age of the patient, but in the adult population, these rates are estimated at 3–5 % [45]. A deep surgical site infection can have significant sequelae including the need for multiple reoperations to treat the infection, as well as the potential need to explant instrumentation and bone graft for persistent infection. Wound infection should be suspected if persistent fever occurs over several days postoperatively, with presence of erythema, swelling, tenderness, and drainage from the incision.

Other wound-related complications include wound dehiscence and the development of pressure ulcers. Elderly patients have normal age-related changes to epidermal turnover as well as progressive decreased collagen synthesis which impairs wound healing and increases risk of wound complications. Patients with spinal cord injury, compromised neurologic status, or other factors resulting in impaired mobility are at highest risk for wound breakdown or pressure ulcer formation. Malnutrition reduces overall tissue tolerance and vitality. Body weight is a considerable factor with regards to wound healing and risk for pressure ulcers. Emaciated patients have little padding over bony prominences and therefore are at greater risk for pressure injury.

Obese patients have poor tissue perfusion and are frequently less mobile and therefore are at increased risk for wound and skin complications. Patients that are less than 90 % or greater than 120 % of their ideal body weight are at greatest risk of pressure ulcers [50].

The most common significant complication relates to failed fusion and implant failure. Particularly in the elderly population in whom osteopenia, inadequate nutrition, vasculopathy, and other metabolic disorders impair bone healing, pseudarthrosis can lead to increasing pain and disability, hardware failure, loss of correction, and deformity progression.

Conclusion

Complex spine surgery encompasses a broad spectrum of advanced surgical and spinal instrumentation techniques to improve the treatment of complicated spinal pathology. Major advancements in these arenas have occurred in the last few decades which have allowed for better management of conditions that compromise the spinal cord and nerve roots and spinal column stability. In addition to the complex surgical management of these patients, successful clinical outcome is dependent on an interdisciplinary approach with proper collaboration with approach surgeons, anesthesiologists, and neuro-critical care physicians. With better understanding of these pathologies and the surgical techniques available to treat them, we can expect improved patient outcomes with reduced morbidity.

References

1. Boriani S, Bandiera S, Biagini R, et al. Chordoma of the mobile spine: fifty years of experience. Spine (Phila Pa 1976). 2006;31:493–503.
2. Luque ER. Segmental spinal instrumentation of the lumbar spine. Clin Orthop Relat Res. 1986;203:126–34.
3. Roy-Camille R, Saillant G, Mazel C. Plating of thoracic, thoracolumbar, and lumbar injuries with pedicle screw plates. Orthop Clin North Am. 1986;17:147–59.
4. Connolly PJ, Esses SI, Kostuik JP. Anterior cervical fusion: outcome analysis of patients fused with and without anterior cervical plates. J Spinal Disord. 1996;9:202–6.
5. Wang JC, Hart RA, Emery SE, Bohlman HH. Graft migration or displacement after multilevel cervical corpectomy and strut grafting. Spine (Phila Pa 1976). 2003;28:1016–21; discussion 21–2.
6. Coyne TJ, Fehlings MG, Wallace MC, Bernstein M, Tator CH. C1-C2 posterior cervical fusion: long-term evaluation of results and efficacy. Neurosurgery. 1995;37:688–92; discussion 92–3.
7. Melcher RP, Puttlitz CM, Kleinstueck FS, Lotz JC, Harms J, Bradford DS. Biomechanical testing of posterior atlantoaxial fixation techniques. Spine (Phila Pa 1976). 2002;27:2435–40.
8. Gluf WM, Brockmeyer DL. Atlantoaxial transarticular screw fixation: a review of surgical indications, fusion rate, complications, and lessons learned in 67 pediatric patients. J Neurosurg Spine. 2005;2:164–9.

9. Yoshida M, Neo M, Fujibayashi S, Nakamura T. Comparison of the anatomical risk for vertebral artery injury associated with the C2-pedicle screw and atlantoaxial transarticular screw. Spine (Phila Pa 1976). 2006;31:E513–7.

10. Wright NM, Lauryssen C. Vertebral artery injury in C1-2 transarticular screw fixation: results of a survey of the AANS/CNS section on disorders of the spine and peripheral nerves. American Association of Neurological Surgeons/Congress of Neurological Surgeons. J Neurosurg. 1998;88:634–40.

11. Harms J, Melcher RP. Posterior C1-C2 fusion with polyaxial screw and rod fixation. Spine (Phila Pa 1976). 2001;26:2467–71.

12. Menendez JA, Wright NM. Techniques of posterior C1-C2 stabilization. Neurosurgery. 2007;60:S103–11.

13. Koivikko MP, Kiuru MJ, Koskinen SK, Myllynen P, Santavirta S, Kivisaari L. Factors associated with nonunion in conservatively-treated type-II fractures of the odontoid process. J Bone Joint Surg Br. 2004;86:1146–51.

14. Apfelbaum RI, Lonser RR, Veres R, Casey A. Direct anterior screw fixation for recent and remote odontoid fractures. J Neurosurg. 2000;93:227–36.

15. Denis F. The three column spine and its significance in the classification of acute thoracolumbar spinal injuries. Spine (Phila Pa 1976). 1983;8:817–31.

16. Guven O, Kocaoglu B, Bezer M, Aydin N, Nalbantoglu U. The use of screw at the fracture level in the treatment of thoracolumbar burst fractures. J Spinal Disord Tech. 2009;22:417–21.

17. McLain RF, Burkus JK, Benson DR. Segmental instrumentation for thoracic and thoracolumbar fractures: prospective analysis of construct survival and five-year follow-up. Spine J. 2001;1:310–23.

18. McLain RF. The biomechanics of long versus short fixation for thoracolumbar spine fractures. Spine (Phila Pa 1976). 2006;31:S70–9; discussion S104.

19. Euba G, Narvaez JA, Nolla JM, et al. Long-term clinical and radiological magnetic resonance imaging outcome of abscess-associated spontaneous pyogenic vertebral osteomyelitis under conservative management. Semin Arthritis Rheum. 2008;38:28–40.

20. Gonzalvo A, Abdulla I, Riazi A, De La Harpe D. Single-level/single-stage debridement and posterior instrumented fusion in the treatment of spontaneous pyogenic osteomyelitis/discitis: long-term functional outcome and health-related quality of life. J Spinal Disord Tech. 2011;24:110–5.

21. Kuklo TR, Potter BK, Bell RS, Moquin RR, Rosner MK. Single-stage treatment of pyogenic spinal infection with titanium mesh cages. J Spinal Disord Tech. 2006;19:376–82.

22. Dai LY, Chen WH, Jiang LS. Anterior instrumentation for the treatment of pyogenic vertebral osteomyelitis of thoracic and lumbar spine. Eur Spine J. 2008;17:1027–34.

23. Sundararaj GD, Babu N, Amritanand R, et al. Treatment of haematogenous pyogenic vertebral osteomyelitis by single-stage anterior debridement, grafting of the defect and posterior instrumentation. J Bone Joint Surg Br. 2007;89:1201–5.

24. Korovessis P, Repantis T, Iliopoulos P, Hadjipavlou A. Beneficial influence of titanium mesh cage on infection healing and spinal reconstruction in hematogenous septic spondylitis: a retrospective analysis of surgical outcome of twenty-five consecutive cases and review of literature. Spine. 2008;33:E759–67.

25. Dimar JR, Carreon LY, Glassman SD, Campbell MJ, Hartman MJ, Johnson JR. Treatment of pyogenic vertebral osteomyelitis with anterior debridement and fusion followed by delayed posterior spinal fusion. Spine. 2004;29:326–32; discussion 32.

26. Harrington KD. Metastatic disease of the spine. J Bone Joint Surg Am. 1986;68:1110–5.

27. Wong DA, Fornasier VL, MacNab I. Spinal metastases: the obvious, the occult, and the impostors. Spine (Phila Pa 1976). 1990;15:1–4.

28. Constans JP, de Divitiis E, Donzelli R, Spaziante R, Meder JF, Haye C. Spinal metastases with neurological manifestations. Review of 600 cases. J Neurosurg. 1983;59:111–8.

29. Patchell RA, Tibbs PA, Regine WF, et al. Direct decompressive surgical resection in the treatment of spinal cord compression caused by metastatic cancer: a randomised trial. Lancet. 2005;366:643–8.

30. Dvorak MF, Kwon BK, Fisher CG, Eiserloh 3rd HL, Boyd M, Wing PC. Effectiveness of titanium mesh cylindrical cages in anterior column reconstruction after thoracic and lumbar vertebral body resection. Spine (Phila Pa 1976). 2003;28:902–8.

31. Hu Y, Xia Q, Ji J, Miao J. One-stage combined posterior and anterior approaches for excising thoracolumbar and lumbar tumors: surgical and oncological outcomes. Spine (Phila Pa 1976). 2010;35:590–5.

32. Weinstein SL, Ponseti IV. Curve progression in idiopathic scoliosis. J Bone Joint Surg Am. 1983;65:447–55.

33. Weis JC, Betz RR, Clements 3rd DH, Balsara RK. Prevalence of perioperative complications after anterior spinal fusion for patients with idiopathic scoliosis. J Spinal Disord. 1997;10:371–5.

34. Kostuik JP, Bentivoglio J. The incidence of low back pain in adult scoliosis. Acta Orthop Belg. 1981;47:548–59.

35. Kim YJ, Bridwell KH, Lenke LG, Cheh G, Baldus C. Results of lumbar pedicle subtraction osteotomies for fixed sagittal imbalance: a minimum 5-year follow-up study. Spine (Phila Pa 1976). 2007;32:2189–97.

36. Yagi M, Akilah KB, Boachie-Adjei O. Incidence, risk factors and classification of proximal junctional kyphosis: surgical outcomes review of adult idiopathic scoliosis. Spine (Phila Pa 1976). 2011;36:E60–8.

37. McMaster MJ. A technique for lumbar spinal osteotomy in ankylosing spondylitis. J Bone Joint Surg Br. 1985;67:204–10.

38. Geck MJ, Macagno A, Ponte A, Shufflebarger HL. The Ponte procedure: posterior only treatment of Scheuermann's kyphosis using segmental posterior shortening and pedicle screw instrumentation. J Spinal Disord Tech. 2007;20:586–93.

39. Hehne HJ, Zielke K, Bohm H. Polysegmental lumbar osteotomies and transpedicled fixation for correction of long-curved kyphotic deformities in ankylosing spondylitis. Report on 177 cases. Clin Orthop Relat Res. 1990;258:49–55.

40. Bridwell KH, Lewis SJ, Edwards C, et al. Complications and outcomes of pedicle subtraction osteotomies for fixed sagittal imbalance. Spine (Phila Pa 1976). 2003;28:2093–101.

41. Lapp MA, Bridwell KH, Lenke LG, et al. Long-term complications in adult spinal deformity patients having combined surgery a comparison of primary to revision patients. Spine (Phila Pa 1976). 2001;26:973–83.

42. Cho SK, Bridwell KH, Lenke LG, et al. Major complications in revision adult deformity surgery: risk factors and clinical outcomes with two- to seven-year follow-up. Spine (Phila Pa 1976). 2012;37(6):489–500.

43. Cho SK, Bridwell KH, Lenke LG, et al. Comparative analysis of clinical outcome and complications in primary vs. revision adult scoliosis surgery. Spine (Phila Pa 1976). 2012;37(5):393–401.

44. Glassman SD, Hamill CL, Bridwell KH, Schwab FJ, Dimar JR, Lowe TG. The impact of perioperative complications on clinical outcome in adult deformity surgery. Spine (Phila Pa 1976). 2007;32:2764–70.

45. Smith JS, Sansur CA, Donaldson 3rd WF, et al. Short-term morbidity and mortality associated with correction of thoracolumbar fixed sagittal plane deformity: a report from the scoliosis research society morbidity and mortality committee. Spine (Phila Pa 1976). 2011;36:958–64.

46. Patil CG, Lad EM, Lad SP, Ho C, Boakye M. Visual loss after spine surgery: a population-based study. Spine (Phila Pa 1976). 2008;33:1491–6.

47. Smith JS, Fu KM, Polly Jr DW, et al. Complication rates of three common spine procedures and rates of thromboembolism following

spine surgery based on 108,419 procedures: a report from the Scoliosis Research Society Morbidity and Mortality Committee. Spine (Phila Pa 1976). 2010;35:2140–9.

48. McMulkin ML, Ferguson RL. Resting energy expenditure and respiratory quotient in adolescents following spinal fusion surgery. Spine (Phila Pa 1976). 2004;29:1831–5.

49. Kang BU, Choi WC, Lee SH, et al. An analysis of general surgery-related complications in a series of 412 minilaparotomic anterior lumbosacral procedures. J Neurosurg Spine. 2009;10:60–5.

50. Scott SM, Mayhew PA, Harris EA. Pressure ulcer development in the operating room. Nursing implications. AORN J. 1992;56: 242–50.

Spinal Cord Injury Rehabilitation and the ICU

31

Janice M. Cohen and Alan K. Novick

Contents

Abstract

Spinal cord injury, previously regarded as a fatal illness, now affects approximately 265,000 survivors today in the United States. Due to improved medical technology and trauma response systems, the spinal cord-injured patient has a longer life expectancy than previously observed. The rehabilitation of a patient with an acute spinal cord injury (SCI) begins in the intensive care unit. A comprehensive neurological exam is performed early during the hospitalization of the SCI patient. The American Spinal Injury Association's Impairment Scale is widely used for classification of severity of injury for tetraplegia and paraplegia. This tool can also be used as an aid for prognostication of neurological and functional recovery, as well as for patient and caregiver education. Rehabilitation efforts require a team approach led by a rehabilitation specialist. Early rehabilitation goals include prevention of complications of immobility. Such complications include contracture, pressure ulcer formation, orthostatic hypotension, and respiratory complications. Physical and occupational therapists work closely with the SCI patient in the ICU setting. Common medical issues in the SCI patient are also addressed in the rehabilitation plan of care. Issues such as autonomic dysreflexia, neurogenic bowel and bladder, spasticity, pain, heterotopic ossification, and psychological adjustment are treated by the rehabilitation team. Each SCI patient requires an individualized plan of care based on his or her physical, psychological, and social needs. Early rehabilitation is vital to achieving long-term functional goals.

J.M. Cohen, MD • A.K. Novick, MD (✉)
Department of Neuroscience/Physical Medicine and Rehabilitation,
Memorial Regional Hospital South/Memorial Healthcare System,
1150 N 35th Avenue, Suite 390, Hollywood, FL 33021, USA
e-mail: jmcohen07@gmail.com; novicka@bellsouth.net

Keywords

Spinal cord • Spinal cord injury • Rehabilitation • Tetraplegia • Paraplegia • Physical therapy • Occupational therapy • Neurogenic bladder • Neurogenic bowel • Spasticity • Pressure ulcer

A.J. Layon et al. (eds.), *Textbook of Neurointensive Care*,
DOI 10.1007/978-1-4471-5226-2_31, © Springer-Verlag London 2013

Introduction

Rarely does the thought of a patient's rehabilitation and recovery drive the initial care of a critically ill trauma patient. For these patients, the medical team's focus is resuscitation: securing an airway, ventilation and perfusion of the lungs, and providing hemodynamic stability. For the traumatic spine and spinal cord-injured patient, further efforts are aimed at immobilization, decompression, and stabilization of the spine. However, once stabilized, attention should be given to the recovery of a patient with acute spinal cord injury (SCI). Early consideration of rehabilitation needs benefits not only the patient and caregivers but also impacts the burden of care and cost on the medical system as a whole.

For a relatively rare condition, the economic impact of caring for a spinal cord injury survivor is large. For a 25-year-old with tetraplegia resulting from cervical spinal cord injury, the lifetime cost directly attributable to SCI has been estimated as high as $4,373,912, not including the cost of indirect losses such as wages and productivity [1]. Previously regarded as a fatal illness, SCI is a medical condition that, at present, affects approximately 265,000 survivors in the United States. A 20-year-old survivor of a high-level SCI resulting in tetraplegia has a life expectancy of an additional 35.7 years [1]. The increased survival rate and prevalence may be attributed to many factors. The efforts by first responders to improve immobilization of trauma patients, the use of life-saving technology not previously available, and the designation of trauma treatment centers have all contributed to the SCI patient's survival and extended life expectancy.

In the care of an SCI patient, the involvement of a physiatrist is ideally initiated once the patient is stabilized. Physiatrists are physicians trained in the practice of physical medicine and rehabilitation, having completed a 4-year residency program approved, in the United States, by the Accreditation Council of Graduate Medical Education. Upon completion of the training program, the physiatrist is proficient in management of the rehabilitation of patients with spinal cord injury. Further expertise may also be obtained through fellowship training and examination in the subspecialty of spinal cord injury medicine [2]. A physiatrist coordinates efforts aimed at mobilizing the patient and preventing secondary complications. The ultimate goal of rehabilitation is restoring function to the injured patient and improving quality of life.

Classification of Injury

Once an SCI has been recognized, the neurological level of injury should be identified. The American Spinal Injury Association's (ASIA) Impairment Scale (AIS), published in the International Standards for Neurological and Functional Classification of Spinal Cord Injury, is a widely accepted method of classifying patients with traumatic spinal cord injury [3]. Though limitations of the AIS exist, routine use of this scale provides a common, standardized language that serves as a tool for prognostication and family and patient education. Based on the classification of injury, the team can focus on appropriate rehabilitation goals. For instance, a patient with a high-level, complete cervical injury may steer the rehabilitation team's short-term goals toward sitting tolerance and balance and family or caregiver training for longer-term goals. In contrast, rehabilitation goals for a patient with an incomplete lower lumbar injury may involve transferring from a bed to wheelchair and eventual ambulation.

The AIS exam is ideally performed once the patient has been stabilized. In addition, an exam performed at 72 h may be more reliable than one performed within 24 h of injury; present recommendations are to perform the examination between 3 and 7 days after injury [4–6]. However, many factors may delay the formal AIS exam. For example, concomitant injuries requiring further surgical interventions may limit the initial exam, while the presence of induced sedation or acquired brain injury prevents adequate patient interaction that is required to perform an accurate AIS evaluation. In addition, the presence of spinal shock – a clinical syndrome often seen in patients with severe spinal cord injury, in which the triad of motor loss, sensory loss, and sympathetic autonomic dysfunction are observed – may confound the initial neurological exam. The resolution of spinal shock was previously indicated by presence or return of the bulbocavernosus reflex. However, recent research suggests a multiphasic model of spinal shock spanning from the onset of injury to 6 months [7, 8]. The implication is that neurological examination for the sake of prognostication should take into account the evolution of spinal shock and timing of the exam should be optimized to provide the most reliable information.

The purpose of the AIS exam is to establish a neurological level of injury and determine the severity of the injury. By testing bilateral individual dermatome and myotome segments, one can discern the levels of motor and sensory preservation. The lowest segment maintaining normal sensory and motor levels bilaterally becomes the neurological level of injury. The impairment of function in the cervical segments is referred to as tetraplegia. The impairment of function in the thoracic, lumbar, or sacral segments is referred to as paraplegia. To determine the severity of the SCI, a rectal exam is performed. Presence of anal sensation or voluntary external anal sphincter contraction means the injury is incomplete. Depending on the presence of motor preservation based on the manual muscle test scoring system, an incomplete injury can be classified as ASIA B, C, or D. If neither motor nor sensory function is preserved in the sacral segments of S4–S5 and deep anal sensation is absent, then

Patient Name_____

Examiner Name_____ Date/Time of Exam_____

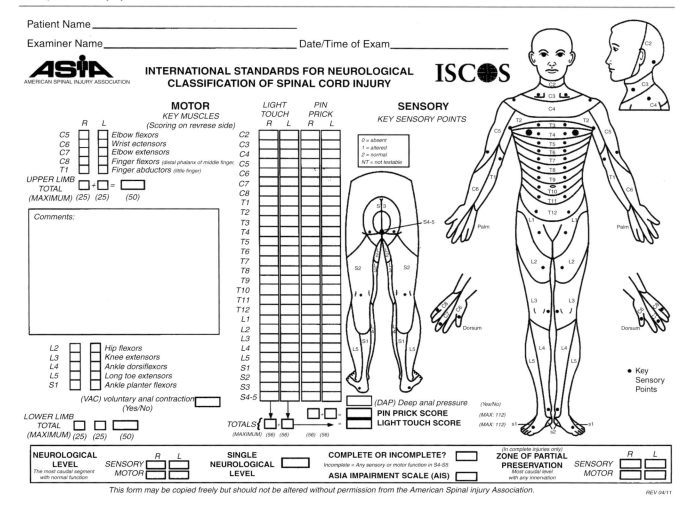

Fig. 31.1 International Standard for Neurological Classification of Spinal Cord Injury (From American Spinal Injury Association: International Standards for Neurological Classification of Spinal Cord Injury, revised 2011; Atlanta, GA, Reprinted 2011. With permission)

the injury is considered complete, or ASIA A classification. In addition to the neurological level of injury, one may also denote the sensory level and motor level for each side. The advantage of specifically notating each side is a decreased propensity to be deceived of preserved function, which may otherwise be overlooked by relying solely on the neurological level (Fig. 31.1).

According to the National Spinal Cord Injury Statistical Center, the most frequent neurological injury is incomplete tetraplegia (39.5 %) followed by complete paraplegia (22.1 %), incomplete paraplegia (21.7 %), and complete tetraplegia (16.3 %) [1]. In addition to tetraplegia and paraplegia, other clinical syndromes may be identified. Central cord syndrome is an incomplete injury distinguished by arm weakness greater than leg weakness, commonly seen in hyperextension injuries of the cervical spine with existing spondylosis. Brown-Sequard syndrome describes ipsilateral muscle weakness and loss of proprioception with contralateral loss of pinprick and thermal sensation due to

cord hemisection. Injury to the anterior two-thirds of the spinal cord, either from trauma or anterior spinal artery injury, results in pain and motor deficits but spares proprioception and light touch. Whereas the aforementioned syndromes are mainly upper motor neuron injuries, the presentation in conus medullaris syndrome and cauda equina syndrome may be a mixed picture of both upper and lower motor neuron syndromes. Injury in conus medullaris syndrome produces saddle anesthesia, flaccid anal sphincter tone, and areflexic bowel and bladder function. Injury in cauda equina syndrome produces asymmetric areflexic paralysis and sphincter dysfunction.

Functional Independence Outcomes

Determination of the level and severity of SCI can be used as a tool to prognosticate functional recovery, providing a basis for a plan of care for the rehabilitation team, including short-term and long-term goals. For the purpose of this text, short-term goals will be discussed, but it is important to remember that achieving short-term goals is imperative to achieving long-term independence both functionally and psychosocially.

In general, 70–90 % of patients with complete injuries, or ASIA A classification, will not progress to an incomplete injury status. Marino [9] found that 22 % of subjects classified as AISA A converted to AISA B or better by rehabilitation discharge; 30 % converted by 1 year. Only 3–6 % of those with ASIA A injuries will achieve ambulation [10–12]. About 50 % of those classified as ASIA B, or more specifically sensory incomplete and motor complete, become ambulatory. Three-quarters or more of those with ASIA C or ASIA D injuries will ambulate. Additionally, those who recover the ability to ambulate may need assistance of bracing or assistive devices.

Further prediction of functional capabilities can be made based on muscle strength testing alone and has been studied [9, 13, 14]. Several studies have examined neurological prognosis in patients with complete and incomplete tetraplegia. By determining the motor score at particular motor levels in these patients, functional outcomes could be predicted at 1 month post-injury and even possibly as early as 1 week [13]. In one study, motor level was unchanged or ascended in 35 % and improved one level in 42 %, two levels in 14 %, and more than two levels in 9 %. However, motor recovery has been noted to decline at a rapid rate in the first 6 months [9, 14–16].

A widely accepted measurement tool for documenting and describing functional status is the Functional Independence Measure (FIM). The FIM instrument consists of an ordinal scale of levels of independence assigned to each of 18 items. The levels are scored as 1 (the subject only contributes less than 25 % effort to complete a task) to 7 (the subject performs the task safely and independently, without the assistance of a person or device). The 18 measured tasks are eating, grooming, bathing, upper body dressing, lower body dressing, toileting, bladder management, bowel management, bed, chair and wheelchair transfers, toilet transfers, tub and shower transfers, ambulation or wheelchair mobility, stair mobility, comprehension, expression, social interaction, problem solving, and memory [17, 18].

Translating the motor level of injury into a functional prognosis requires knowledge of basic functional anatomy and familiarity with the key muscles tested in the AIS exam. For instance, in a patient determined to have a C7 ASIA B injury, the elbow extensors (C7 muscle group) will remain intact, as will those involved in elbow flexion (C5 muscle group) and wrist extension (C6 muscle group). One can predict that this patient will be able to bear weight on extended arms in a seated position, thus allowing for independent bed mobility and transfers from a bed to a chair. In contrast, a patient with a high-level injury, C5 perhaps, would not be expected to perform independent transfers due to the lack of

elbow extension. Of course, there are other factors influencing the level of independence obtained by a person with spinal cord injury. These factors include, but are not limited to, concomitant injury, premorbid health status, age, psychological factors, and social factors. Therefore, it is imperative that the patient be involved in a comprehensive rehabilitation process addressing the patient in a holistic manner to achieve the best possible outcome.

Rehabilitation of the Patient with Acute Spinal Cord Injury

Rehabilitation of a spinal cord-injured patient is complex and requires a team approach. The physiatrist assumes the role of leader of the rehabilitation team, which consists of the nursing staff, physical therapist, occupational therapist, speech language pathologist, registered dietician, respiratory therapist, recreational therapist, psychologist, orthotist, pharmacist, and the patient and family. The team works closely with physicians in the acute setting, including trauma surgeons, intensivists, neurosurgeons, and orthopedic surgeons, given that many of these patients require adherence to postoperative or post-injury range of motion, bracing, weight-bearing, and limb dangle precautions in addition to having concomitant internal injuries.

One distinctive feature of the rehabilitation team is individualizing the plan of care based on the patient's specific medical, functional, psychological, and social needs. The plan should be goal oriented and realistic. The inclusion of patients and family in list of team members is not superfluous. It is imperative that the patient and family are involved in the initial goal setting and ongoing education and training by all members of the team. This ensures that expectations are clear and, in addition, may provide added psychological benefit to the patient as well, who may feel he or she has some control in an otherwise seemingly dire situation that is out of their control.

Early rehabilitation efforts in the intensive care setting are aimed at prevention of complications of immobility. Common complications in the SCI patient population in the acute and subacute setting include joint contractures, pressure ulcers, edema, orthostatic hypotension, and respiratory problems. Deep vein thrombosis is a complication that is discussed in detail elsewhere in this textbook (Chap. 17) but is important to recognize in this population and is briefly reviewed here.

Contraction and Edema

Contracture is a limitation of joint range of motion (ROM) and can be due to changes in the bone, surrounding soft tissues of the joint, muscle, or tendon [19]. The physiologic changes can begin as early as 1 week from the start of immobilization [20].

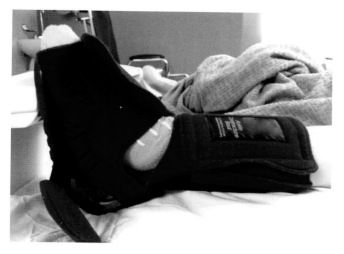

Fig. 31.2 Anti-contracture orthosis

Immobilized patients with tetraplegia are at particular risk of developing contractures of shoulder internal rotation and adduction, elbow flexion, wrist flexion, and finger flexion. Both tetraplegics and paraplegics are prone to contractures of hip and knee flexion and ankle plantar flexion. Loss of ROM leads to movement abnormalities and joint deformities that in turn cause loss of functional activity.

Proper positioning of the patient is vital to prevention of contractures. Recall that a patient with a C7 ASIA B injury maintains the ability to extend the elbows, which in turn allows the patient to support his or her body weight on the arms and subsequently perform transfers. If such a patient were to develop elbow flexion contractures in the ICU, the preserved strength in the elbow extensor muscles would be rendered useless. Use of support cushions or pillows should not promote the limb positions that lead to contracture. Support cushions are helpful, however, in managing dependent limb edema. The therapy staff is involved in educating the patient and caregivers in this practice.

ROM exercise should begin as soon as possible, provided there are no contraindications. ROM may be classified as passive ROM or active ROM. Passive ROM is the motion observed at a particular joint that is at rest, with the observer moving the joint instead of the patient. Active ROM requires voluntary movement of a joint without assistance from another person. ROM is often passive in this setting due to induced sedation or concomitant brain injury and performed with the patient supine in the bed. ROM may be carried out by the physical therapist or occupational therapist and should be performed daily at the minimum. Due to time and resource constraints in high-volume trauma centers, twice daily therapy sessions may not be feasible. In such cases, the family may be trained by the therapy staff to perform passive ROM exercises for the patient. Patients who develop spasticity of the limbs should have a higher frequency of ROM exercise.

Orthoses can also be used for added joint protection in the acute setting. A resting hand splint or wrist-hand orthosis prevents hand and wrist contractures, particularly of concern in patients with high-level tetraplegia. The resting hand splint keeps the hand in a more functional position, with the fingers extended and the thumb abducted. Similarly, an ankle-foot orthosis or anti-contracture boot (Fig. 31.2) is applied to the lower extremities to prevent plantar flexion contracture by positioning the ankle in dorsiflexion. By preserving ROM and preventing joint contracture in the acute setting, the patient may maximize his or her potential for functional recovery in the subacute rehabilitation phase.

Orthostatic Hypotension and Respiratory Complications

Once the situation allows, the physical therapist and occupational therapist will advance from ROM exercises to strengthening exercise and sitting tolerance. Initiation of sitting allows for the patient to increase endurance and work on controlling and strengthening the trunk muscles. The therapists from each discipline may work together during these initial efforts of mobility and transferring to a bedside chair, often a specialized positioning chair.

The benefits of early mobilization in the ICU appear to outweigh the risks in a patient who has been properly screened for initiation of mobilization [21, 22]. Furthermore, it is known that immobilization has a negative effect on the cardiovascular and respiratory systems. In fact, the leading cause of death in patients with SCI is respiratory complication [1]. Assisting the patient to develop tolerance for upright positioning may in turn alleviate factors such as reduced clearance of secretions and atelectasis. Immobilized patients develop a restriction of intercostal muscle motion that leads to impaired breathing. When coupled with paralysis, these patients are at high risk for mucous plugging, pneumonia, and hypoxemia [23]. Patients with tetraplegia are at a disadvantage due to paralysis of the abdominal muscles (innervated by T7 through T12), diaphragm (innervated by C3 through C5), intercostals, and accessory muscles of breathing, including the sternohyoid, mylohyoid, platysma, and sternocleidomastoid (innervated by the mid-thoracic levels and above). Employing the manually assisted cough, or "quad cough," may circumvent lack of adequate cough, provided there are no contraindications such as recent thoracic spine or abdominal surgery. This is a maneuver in which the staff member places the hands over the patient's abdomen and applies pressure timed with the cough efforts of the patient to increase expiratory force. Another treatment for insufficient cough is the mechanical insufflator-exsufflator, which is an electrical device that simulates a cough via noninvasive positive and negative pressures. Besides being noninvasive, an advantage of the mechanical insufflator-exsufflator is its ability to produce effective expiratory flow rates that can be administered orally or via a tracheostomy tube [24]. Respiratory therapists are vital in maintaining pulmonary toilet and assisting in re-expansion of lung tissue affected by atelectasis or pneumonia. Other interventions by respiratory therapists and physical therapists are incentive spirometry, suctioning, chest percussion, and postural drainage. Speech therapists can assist with breathing techniques such as glossopharyngeal breathing, also known as "frog breathing," and breath stacking. Frog breathing is a technique in which the trachea and pharyngeal muscles force air into the trachea. Breath stacking is a technique in which consecutive breaths are taken and held to increase the lung volume [25].

In contrast to non-SCI patients, patients with tetraplegia may have a mechanical advantage when in the supine position, in that the diaphragm has a greater excursion allowing for greater vital capacity. The contrast between non-SCI and SCI patients is again seen in the upright position. The weakened diaphragm in the SCI patient, with lack of abdominal support and at the mercy of gravity, is now at a mechanical disadvantage with regard to diaphragm excursion, with low vital capacity resulting. This may be combated with the use of an abdominal binder while in the upright position, which theoretically splints the abdominal contents by simulating the supine position.

It should be noted that pulmonary management of the acute SCI patient is complex and that the techniques discussed here may be of more relevance in patients not dependent on mechanical ventilation. The reader is referred to previous chapters for detailed discussion on airway management (Chap. 10) and noninvasive and invasive mechanical ventilation (Chap. 11), which should be strongly considered for patients in whom the vital capacity has fallen below 10–15 mL/kg of ideal body weight [25, 26]. Likewise, pharmacologic intervention is discussed in detail elsewhere. However, it is important to note that venous thromboembolism and subsequent pulmonary embolism are common complications in this population. The Consortium for Spinal Cord Medicine Clinical Practice Guidelines suggest prophylaxis with unfractionated heparin or low molecular weight heparin should be initiated within 72 h of injury, provided that hemostasis has been achieved. The recommended treatment duration is at least 8 weeks for uncomplicated complete motor lesions and 12 weeks or until discharge in those with complicated complete motor lesions. Patients with ASIA C and ASIA D injury are recommended for anticoagulation prophylaxis for the duration of hospitalization [25, 27]. Traditionally, bed rest has been prescribed after diagnosis of acute venous thromboembolism or pulmonary embolism. However, a recent review of literature found that early ambulation, compared with bed rest, was not associated with a higher risk of progression of venous thromboembolism, new pulmonary embolism, or mortality [28, 29].

Orthostatic hypotension is ubiquitous in this patient population; an incidence of up to 74 % has been reported [30]. Some patients are asymptomatic, but others experience lightheadedness, dizziness, or nausea [31]. An acutely injured patient with tetraplegia in spinal shock may even experience loss of consciousness. The positional drop in blood pressure and elevation of heart rate is a result of many physiologic changes in the SCI patient but likely mostly due to venous stasis as well as sympathetic nervous system disruption. Venous stasis has been anecdotally combated by the use of compression stockings to the lower extremities and an abdominal binder, in effect restricting venous pooling. Some patients may require these interventions just to sit up in bed, as may be seen in cervical or high thoracic injuries. Pharmacologic treatments are available if needed and include salt tablets, midodrine, and fludrocortisone. Salt tablets and fludrocortisone, a systemic corticosteroid, act to increase plasma volume. Midodrine is an α (alpha)-1 adrenergic agonist that causes peripheral vasoconstriction. Other modalities, such as tilt table and functional electrical stimulation (FES), have been shown to modulate the effects of orthostatic hypotension but are more likely to be employed in the post-acute rehabilitation setting [32].

Pressure Ulcers

Members of the acute care staff and rehabilitation staff should be vigilant about skin protection and wound prevention. Wound formation in the spinal cord-injured patient is a serious, costly, and preventable complication that, if left untreated, may delay rehabilitation efforts and even lead to mortality. These patients are at high risk of pressure ulcer formation due to insensate skin and prolonged immobilization. Linares and colleagues [33, 34] found patients who developed a pressure ulcer were more likely to have had a prolonged immobilization at the onset of the injury. Pressure ulcers occur more frequently in patients with more complete SCI. Areas of particular risk are bony prominences such as the occiput, sacrum, and heels. The patient should be turned from side to side every 2 h to offload these areas. Applying heel suspension ankle-foot orthoses may provide additional offloading of the heels. Instead of a regular mattress, a low air loss mattress or overlay should be used in patients with SCI. Mechanical forces contributing to pressure wounds also include shear forces, such as the friction that may be encountered during transfers and repositioning of the patient. Other contributing factors include moisture and poor nutrition; therefore, bowel and bladder incontinence, as well as nutritional status, should be addressed routinely. Many centers have wound prevention protocols in place and use risk assessment tools such as the Braden scale, a widely accepted scale used to identify patients at high risk for pressure ulcer formation [16, 34].

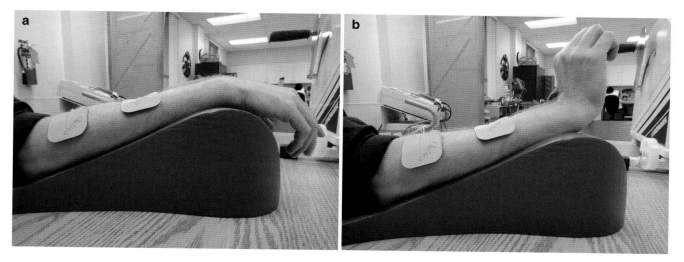

Fig. 31.3 Electrical stimulation has multiple uses in neurological diseases, including facilitation of motor recovery and prevention of disuse atrophy. Electrodes are placed on the skin surface at rest (**a**) and cause contraction of the wrist extensors during stimulation (**b**)

Wound prevention is a lifelong practice, and education for the patient and family begins in the ICU and continues in the rehabilitation setting to include techniques such as pressure relief in the seated position (by use of arm extension in paraplegics and reclining power wheelchair in tetraplegics), use of low air loss seating cushions on wheelchairs, and routine skin inspections. Patients may be issued a skin mirror for self-assessment of skin.

Promoting Functional Mobility and Recovery

For rapidly recovering patients with incomplete tetraplegia and paraplegia, the therapist may initiate transfer training and initial gait training with assistive devices such as a rolling walker. A rolling walker increases the area of support while facilitating movement.

There are a myriad of orthoses and assistive and adaptive devices to increase functional independence in SCI patients. These devices are introduced in the post-acute setting such as a rehabilitation facility. In addition, wheelchair prescription for positioning and mobility takes place in the post-acute rehabilitation setting. The rehabilitation team, under the care of a SCI specialist or physiatrist, continues to work with the patient and caregivers in the post-ICU period to ensure continued recovery and reintegration into the community (Fig. 31.3a, b).

Common Medical Issues in Rehabilitation

Autonomic Dysreflexia

SCI may result in dysregulation of the autonomic nervous system. One potentially life-threatening condition that

results is called autonomic dysreflexia, reported to occur in up to 85 % of those at risk and requiring treatment as soon as recognized [35]. The hallmark of the syndrome is markedly elevated blood pressure. Those at risk have complete or incomplete injuries at the T6 level or higher, though autonomic dysreflexia has been reported with levels as low as T8 and even T10 [16, 36, 37]. Recall that the splanchnic sympathetic outflow is located at T6 through L2 and remains functional despite SCI. Noxious afferent signals are transmitted via intact sensory nerves below the level of injury and ascend to stimulate sympathetic neurons. Normal inhibitory impulses above the injury level are blocked at the injury site as they descend. Consequentially, there is unopposed sympathetic outflow from the sympathetic chain. The result is vasoconstriction below the lesion causing the severe hypertension and reflex vasodilatation above the lesion. Relative bradycardia results from intact vagus nerve innervation to the heart but is not adequate to offset the severe vasoconstriction. Other clinical signs include headache, nasal congestion, and flushing and sweating of the skin above the lesion. It is important to note that the resting blood pressure in patients with SCI will generally be lower. When monitoring blood pressure for signs of autonomic dysreflexia, one should use the SCI patient's post-morbid blood pressure as the new baseline. A typical blood pressure reading may appear normal, when in fact it may be a sign of autonomic dysreflexia, especially if it is 20–40 mmHg above the new baseline.

Once identified, the treatment is aimed at lowering the blood pressure and eliminating the cause. The most common causes of autonomic dysreflexia are bladder distension (from kinked catheter, stone, or sphincter obstruction) or bowel dysfunction (distension or impaction). Other common causes include urinary tract infection, cholelithiasis, pressure ulcer, appendicitis, and menstruation. Even seemingly benign

Table 31.1 Common causes of autonomic dysreflexia

Genitourinary
  Overdistended bladder
  Bladder catheterization
  Kinked Foley catheter
  Tight Foley catheter leg bag strap
  Detrusor-sphincter dyssynergia
  Kidney stone
  Bladder stone
  Urinary tract infection
Gastrointestinal
  Fecal impaction
  Gastroesophageal reflux
  Hemorrhoids
  Biliary disease
Integumentary
  Infection
  Ingrown toenail
  Pressure ulcer
Gynecological
  Menstrual cramps
Musculoskeletal
  Heterotopic ossification
  Fracture
Cardiovascular
  Deep vein thrombosis
Pharmacologic
  Local anesthesia

Data from Gala et al. [7], Frost [16], Kirschblum et al. [64]

causes may be the cause of autonomic dysreflexia, including an ingrown toenail and constrictive clothing or braces (Table 31.1).

The first action to correct the high blood pressure is to immediately put the patient into a sitting from a supine position, in effect causing orthostasis. Any tight clothing or devices, such as indwelling catheter leg bags, abdominal binders, or belts, should be loosened or removed. The blood pressure and pulse should be monitored every 2–5 min until the patient is stabilized. A cursory exam should focus first on the urinary tract. As the most common cause of autonomic dysreflexia is bladder distention, efforts are aimed at emptying the bladder via catheterization with use of lidocaine jelly at the urethral meatus. If a catheter is already in place, identify and correct any kinks or obstruction to the catheter and collection system. The second most common cause of autonomic dysreflexia is fecal impaction. If initial efforts fail to reduce blood pressure, then the focus moves from the urinary system to the gastrointestinal system and manual disimpaction.

Systolic blood pressure that is at or above 150 mmHg during an episode of autonomic dysreflexia warrants pharmacologic treatment with rapid-onset, short-duration antihypertensive medications. Oral treatment options include immediate-release nifedipine and hydralazine [38]. Nitroglycerin 2 % ointment, 1 in., may be applied above the level of the SCI. The patient's medication profile should be noted to identify any drug-drug interactions. The patient's blood pressure should be monitored for at least 2 h after resolution of the episode. Left untreated, the patient may develop complications from the severe hypertension, including stroke, intracranial hemorrhage, seizure, cardiac arrhythmia, and/or death.

Neurogenic Bladder

Although respiratory complications are the current leading cause of mortality in SCI patients, urologic complications once took the blame. Urologic complications still contribute to considerable morbidity in this patient population, however, more so from urinary tract infection than the previously ubiquitous renal failure. Many SCI patients develop some degree of neurogenic bladder, which is a term generally used to describe bladder dysfunction caused by a neurological condition [39]. It is imperative to recognize and treat neurogenic bladder not only to prevent urologic complications but also for promoting continence, social reintegration, and overall psychosocial well-being.

Knowledge of normal anatomy and physiology of the urinary tract is necessary to determine the best management option for SCI patients with neurogenic bladder. In a normally functioning urinary system, the kidneys act to form urine and excrete it into the collecting system. The urine flows from the kidney collecting system to the bladder via the ureters. The area where the ureters connect to the bladder is called the ureterovesical junction. The ureterovesical junction acts as a valve to prevent retrograde flow from the bladder to the ureter. The bladder itself is smooth muscle called the detrusor and innervated by S2, S3, and S4 parasympathetic fibers via the pelvic nerve and T10–L2 sympathetic fibers via the hypogastric nerve. Normal parasympathetic stimulation of the detrusor results in acetylcholine release and binding to muscarinic receptors with subsequent contraction or emptying of the bladder. The bladder neck is predominantly innervated by T10–L2 sympathetic fibers via the hypogastric nerve. Normal sympathetic stimulation of the detrusor results in norepinephrine release and binding to β (beta)-adrenergic receptors with subsequent relaxation, or storing, of urine in the bladder. Normal sympathetic stimulation of the bladder neck and urethra results in norepinephrine release and binding to α (alpha)-adrenergic receptors with subsequent contraction, or storing, of urine in the bladder. The external sphincter is made up of the pelvic floor striated muscles and is innervated by S2–S4 somatic fibers via the pudendal nerve. Normal somatic stimulation of the external sphincter results in subsequent contraction, or storing, of the urine in the bladder. Continence is maintained by supraspinal control in the cerebral cortex and the pons, in turn controlling the local sacral reflex arc involving the systems mentioned previously, to promote bladder storage by inhibiting detrusor contraction. Voluntary voiding is initiated by relaxation of the external sphincter and release of inhibition of detrusor contraction, thus promoting bladder emptying [40]. Patients with SCI will usually exhibit neurogenic bladder due to either suprasacral injury (resulting in spastic or "upper motor" bladder) or sacral injury (resulting in areflexic or "lower motor" bladder). However, suprapontine injury should not be overlooked, as some SCI patients also have concomitant traumatic brain injury, though they clinically appear similar to suprasacral injuries. During initial injury, there is no bladder contraction. Contraction appears to reappear with resolution of spinal shock [41]. In patients with suprasacral injury, the inhibitory control of the sacral reflex arc is lost and detrusor-sphincter dyssynergia commonly results. Coordination is lost in detrusor-sphincter dyssynergia, and the external sphincter fails to relax during detrusor contraction. Sacral cord injury may result in detrusor areflexia and loss of reflex voiding, eventually leading to loss of bladder compliance and overdistention.

Acute management of neurogenic bladder in the SCI patient involves the placement of an indwelling urethral catheter to accurately monitor urine output and to avoid complications of urinary retention. Urethral catheterization should be avoided in patients with suspected urethral injury, such as those with hematuria, pelvic fracture, or other penetrating trauma, and a urologist should be consulted [6].

The SCI patient should be placed on a bladder program once strict monitoring of urine output, and the need for an indwelling catheter, is no longer needed. The main purpose of a bladder program is to avoid further damage to the urinary system and to maintain continence by establishing regular patterns of voiding. An intermittent catheterization program should be started in SCI patients who maintain hand dexterity or who have a caregiver who will continue the process after discharge from the rehabilitation program. The nursing staff (or the patient or caregiver, once comprehension is demonstrated) empties the bladder at frequent intervals (commonly every 4–6 h) to maintain bladder volumes less than 500 mL [41]. This intermittent catheterization is accomplished by inserting a catheter only to drain the bladder then removing it immediately afterward.

Intermittent catheterization is one of the most common methods of neurogenic bladder management in the acute and subacute period. There are a host of other methods, especially for complicated patients or those with chronic SCI. The choices range from timed voiding, indwelling catheters, or surgical augmentation of the urinary system to adjunctive oral medication or botulinum toxin injections into the sphincter.

The reader is referred to literature specific to chronic spinal cord injury management or chronic neurogenic bladder management for further discussion.

Neurogenic Bowel

Neurogenic bowel is prevalent in this patient population. One study found 39.4 % of SCI patients with severe dysfunction, which had a positive correlation with high level of cord lesion and completeness and chronicity of injury [42]. As is the case with neurogenic bladder, neurogenic bowel is a condition of bowel dysfunction resulting from spinal cord injury and denervation of the bowels and may have serious medical and psychosocial consequences. However, these complications can be prevented or alleviated with development and adherence to a bowel management program which includes both bowel function and defecation. In addition to the common encounter with bowel incontinence or constipation, other manifestations of neurogenic bowel include nausea, bloating, gastric ulcers, ileus, impaction, diverticulosis, hemorrhoids, and autonomic dysreflexia [43–45]. In the acute setting, complications of ileus, peptic ulcer, and pancreatitis were noted within the first month post-injury. The main purpose of a bowel program is to establish timely, predictable bowel evacuations and prevent complications and incontinence.

Fecal formation, movement, and continence are maintained via a network of autonomic and somatic control of several anatomic components of the bowel. The colon has both intrinsic reflex activity provided by the Auerbach's plexus and Meissner's plexus in the gut wall and extrinsic innervation by the parasympathetic (vagus and pelvic nerves), sympathetic (hypogastric and mesenteric nerves), and somatic (pudendal nerve) systems. In a normal functioning bowel, the intrinsic reflexes provided by the Auerbach's plexus and Meissner's plexus sense stool content and cause muscle wall coordination to form stool and propel contents toward the anus. This reflex activity is rarely affected directly by SCI. Normal parasympathetic vagus nerve stimulation promotes movement of contents of small intestine through the ascending and transverse colon. Normal parasympathetic stimulation of the remaining distal gut to the rectum is provided by S2–S4 via the pelvic nerve and further acts to promote bowel emptying. The rectocolic reflex is modulated by the pelvic nerve and promotes colon motility with rectal stimulation. In a normal resting state, sympathetic stimulation to the internal anal sphincter (via L1–2) and somatic stimulation to the puborectalis (via S1–5) and external anal sphincter by the pudendal nerve (via S2–4) are contracted to maintain continence [44, 46, 47]. Normal defecation occurs when stool in the rectum causes rectal stretch, inducing relaxation of the puborectalis and external anal sphincter muscles coupled with increased intra-abdominal pressure [48].

SCI patients usually exhibit either upper motor neuron neurogenic bowel or lower motor neuron neurogenic bowel. The upper motor neuron, or reflexic bowel, is caused by lesions above the conus medullaris and is characterized by increased anal tone with loss of voluntary external anal sphincter control. This in turn causes fecal retention and constipation. Lower motor neuron, or flaccid bowel, is caused by lesions at the conus or cauda equina and is characterized by slowed colonic transit time and low anal sphincter tone which in turn causes constipation with fecal incontinence. One must note, however, the possibility of loss of all autonomic reflex in the acute period of spinal shock.

Physical exam at the onset of injury should include a rectal exam to assess for presence of reflexic or flaccid neurogenic bowel. Resting anal tone may be high in reflexic bowel or hypotonic in flaccid bowel. The bulbocavernosus reflex is present in reflexic bowel and returns with the resolution of spinal shock. Testing of the bulbocavernosus reflex involves applying pressure to the dorsal glans penis in males or clitoris in females during the rectal exam, eliciting external anal sphincter contraction. Alternatively, one may gently tug on an indwelling Foley catheter, if present, to elicit the bulbocavernosus reflex during rectal examination. The patient will also be tested for voluntary contraction of the external anal sphincter and puborectalis as well as for deep sensation.

A bowel program is initiated in the acute setting. A consistent time of the day should be set for the bowel program in an attempt to develop predictable defecation. The patient and all caregivers should be part of the process. The reiteration of the goals of the bowel program is often necessary, as patients may become discouraged due to the weeks or months that may be required to establish an adequate bowel program. Furthermore, due to fluctuations in fluid intake, diet, and activity in the intensive care unit, frequent adjustments to the bowel program may be needed initially to avoid impaction and obstruction.

Patients with acute reflexic neurogenic bowel are usually managed with a rectal suppository, such as bisacodyl or glycerin, followed by digital stimulation provided by the caregiver while the patient is in a side-lying position. These patients may need stool softeners to maintain soft-formed stool that is easily eliminated with rectal stimulation. For those with flaccid neurogenic bowel and those in spinal shock, the method of choice is manual evacuation [49]. In contrast to those with reflexic neurogenic bowel, these patients may need bulk-forming supplements or medications to produce firm stool to maintain continence between bowel evacuations. Once the patient enters the rehabilitation phase, medications will be adjusted for optimal bowel program effectiveness. Equipment to improve the individual's independence with the bowel program will be prescribed, or, alternately, the caregivers will be trained in proper bowel program technique.

Spasticity

Patients with SCI often develop spasticity, defined as abnormal, velocity-dependent increase in stretch reflex [50, 51]. Spasticity manifests as an excessive muscle contraction in response to passive stretch of the peripheral joints. The cause of spasticity is alpha-motor neuron hyperexcitability within the spinal cord due to loss of inhibition from descending neural pathways as a result of the spinal cord injury. Spasticity is a component of the upper motor neuron syndrome, which also includes abnormalities such as primitive reflexes, loss of precise autonomic control, rigidity, relaxed cutaneous reflexes, paresis, and fatigability, to name a few. Spasticity follows the period of flaccidity initially seen in the acute spinal cord injury and may occur after several weeks. Often times, patients and families will mistake involuntary muscle contractions for return of voluntary control of the muscle.

A widely accepted tool used to assess spasticity is the Modified Ashworth Scale (MAS). The MAS scale ranks the level of spasticity of a joint on a scale of 0–4, with 0 meaning no increase in tone is noted and 4 indicating the joint is in rigid flexion or extension (Table 31.2). Treatment of spasticity is individualized to each patient. At times, patients with SCI may find the increase in muscle tone from the spasticity assists with functional activities such as transferring or ambulating. In such cases, aggressive treatment of spasticity would serve no advantage. However, spasticity must be treated if it interferes with positioning and hygiene care or causes pain. Initial treatment includes intermittent stretching by passive range of motion or tonic stretching by serial casting. Oral pharmacologic treatment may be used in the acute and subacute period and includes oral baclofen, tizanidine, diazepam, and dantrolene sodium (Table 31.3). Other treatment options that may be considered in subacute or chronic patients include phenol or botulinum toxin injection, intrathecal baclofen, and neurosurgical procedures.

Pain

Pain after SCI has a reported prevalence of 77–81 %. There are a multitude of types of pain in this population but mostly falling under the categories of neuropathic/neurological or musculoskeletal/nociceptive [52]. Musculoskeletal pain appeared more common, whereas neuropathic pain appeared more severe. Some of these pains develop over time and are briefly mentioned here, while others can be frequently encountered in the acute period.

Pain that originates from damaged bone or tissue falls under the category of musculoskeletal pain, seen commonly in the acute trauma injury phase. Chronic musculoskeletal conditions include overuse injuries (commonly to the shoulders), muscle spasm, degenerative joint disease, and spasticity-related pain.

Table 31.2 Modified Ashworth Scale

0	No increase in tone
1	Slight increase in muscle tone, manifested by a catch and release or by minimal resistance at the end of the range of motion when the affected part(s) is moved in flexion or extension
1+	Slight increase in muscle tone, manifested by a catch, followed by minimal resistance throughout the remainder (less than half) of the range of motion
2	More marked increase in muscle tone through most of the range of motion but affected part(s) easily moved
3	Considerable increase in muscle tone, passive movement difficult
4	Affected part(s) rigid in flexion or extension

Data from Bohannon and Smith [65]

Table 31.3 Oral pharmacologic management of spastic hypertonia in SCI

Oral medication	Mechanism of action	Dose	Cautions
Baclofen	Spinal GABA-B receptor agonist; presynaptic inhibition of alpha-motor neuron excitation	5–80 mg/day, in three or four divided doses	Avoid sudden withdrawal Caution use in concomitant TBI/stroke patients due to potential negative supraspinal effects
Clonidine	Alpha-2 adrenergic agonist	Maximum 0.4 mg/day	Hypotension
Diazepam	Facilitates spinal postsynaptic effects of GABA	2–10 mg three to four times per day	Caution use in concomitant TBI/stroke patients
Tizanidine	Alpha-2 adrenergic agonist	Maximum dose 8 mg three times per day	Monitor liver function test Hypotension

Neuropathic pain is associated with injury to nerve roots, spinal cord, or cauda equina. In chronic SCI, compression mononeuropathies may also be seen, such as median mononeuropathy. Acute neuropathic pain may be described as radicular when originating from nerve root damage. Transition zone or segmental pain describes hyperalgesia or hypersensitivity in the adjacent dermatomes to the level of the spinal cord lesion [16, 52]. In patients with thoracic level injury, transition zone or segmental pain is often described as a "band" sensation around the trunk. In patients with incomplete tetraplegia, segmental pain may be described as "burning hands."

A commonly utilized tool to measure pain is the Numerical Rating Scale (NRS), which ranks pain intensity on a scale of 0 (no pain) to 10 (severe pain). Once pain is identified and characterized, a treatment plan should be initiated. Musculoskeletal pain due to acute spine instability is addressed with spine immobilization surgery and postsurgical pain treated with physical modalities, nonnarcotic medication, and/or opioid medication. Neuropathic pain is initially treated with anticonvulsant medication such as gabapentin, pregabalin, or carbamazepine. Alternative or adjunctive medication includes the tricyclic antidepressant class, including amitriptyline or nortriptyline. Opioids have been used for management of neuropathic pain, though are not first-line treatment [53, 54]. Physical modalities or transcutaneous electrical stimulation (TENS) may be helpful in managing neuropathic pain. Psychological treatment approaches and interdisciplinary methods show promise in the management of SCI pain as well.

Heterotopic Ossification

Heterotopic ossification (HO) is a condition resulting from abnormal lamellar ossification within para-articular soft tissue planes in persons with neurological injury. The tissues below the level of injury may be affected in 16–53 % of SCI patients, but only 10–20 % result in clinically significant complications. It is more common in complete injuries in which spasticity is also seen. HO has been reported as early as 20 days post-injury, though generally the onset is within 6 months of the injury.

The most common site of HO in SCI patients is in the hips, followed by the knees, shoulders, and elbows. Initial clinical presentation may be a painful, warm, erythematous, and swollen extremity; therefore, deep vein thrombosis, septic arthritis, and cellulitis should be ruled out. The clinician may also notice a restriction of range of motion and pain with range of motion. One should also be aware that the presence of HO may trigger autonomic dysreflexia.

The gold standard for confirmation of HO is the three-phase bone scan, which can provide early detection but is limited by its lack of specificity [55]. For this test, the patient receives intravenous technetium Tc 99m-labeled diphosphonate which records accumulation of the substance at areas of active bone growth. During the procedure, blood flow and uptake is recorded at three different intervals: dynamic flow immediately after injection, static pooling after injection, and repeated static scan after several hours. Plain radiograph may also be used to detect HO but has a lag time of 4–6 weeks after bone scan detection. Serum alkaline phosphatase may be elevated in HO, but its use in initial diagnosis is limited by lack of specificity.

Range of motion therapy is an important preventive measure and treatment for HO. Recent literature reviews found that management with NSAIDs was the most efficacious for prevention of HO when compared to other pharmacologic treatments. There was also strong support for bisphosphonates as a treatment for HO when compared with other pharmacologic and non-pharmacologic treatment strategies [56, 57]. Surgical resection is indicated in severe cases of HO that result in nerve impingement, joint ankylosis, or pressure ulcers. However, surgical intervention should be delayed until the bone has reached full maturity, often 1 year.

Psychological Adjustment

Sustaining a traumatic SCI can be a devastating event in a person's life. Recent surveys have shown the presence of probable major depression in 21 % of SCI survivors at 1 year post-injury and as high as 23 % in patients with SCI living in the community [58, 59]. Premorbid issues with substance abuse and psychological or behavioral disorders have an effect on long-term outcome, and psychosocial issues may play a larger role in functional outcome than even the neurological level of injury [60, 61]. Poor health and decreased satisfaction with life have been associated with depression [62]. While addressing acute physical and medical needs, the treatment team must not overlook the need for psychosocial support. Psychologists play an important role in the rehabilitation team effort toward the ultimate goal of improved quality of life for SCI patients. The psychologist may directly assist the patient and family with acceptance of the new impairments and disability as well as guide the rehabilitation team in providing the type of support that most benefits the patient. A positive screening for depression may be answered with cognitive-behavioral intervention or pharmaceutical intervention. When conducted in the inpatient rehabilitation phase, cognitive-behavioral therapy resulted in fewer hospital admissions, less medication use, and improved mood 2 years after injury [63].

Summary

The acute stabilization of a traumatic SCI patient is just the beginning of the road to recovery. Early involvement of the rehabilitation team may decrease secondary complications and provide a smooth transition from the acute setting to the rehabilitation phase. To date, there is no single treatment to reverse the devastating impairments and disability caused by SCI. Regenerative medicine as a potential treatment modality continues to advance in the research field, but human studies are lacking. The combination of surgical, pharmacologic, and rehabilitation methods remains the standard intervention. Individualized therapy and discharge planning with return to the community underscores the need for early involvement of the rehabilitation team, with the ultimate goal of improving the SCI patient's quality of life.

References

1. Spinal cord injury facts and figures at a glance. https://www.nscisc.uab.edu/public_content/pdf/Facts%202011%20Feb%20Final.pdf. Accessed 12 Oct 2011.
2. American Board of Medical Specialties: specialties and subspecialties. http://www.abms.org/who_we_help/physicians/specialties.aspx. Accessed 12 Oct 2011.
3. American Spinal Injury Association. International standards for neurological and functional classification of spinal cord injury. Spinal Cord. 1997;35(5):266–74.
4. Brown PH, Marino RJ, Herbison GL, et al. The 72 hour examination s a predictor of recovery in motor complete quadriplegia. Arch Phys Med Rehabil. 1991;72:546–50.
5. Herbison GJ, Zerby SA, Cohen ME, Marino RJ, Ditunno Jr JF. Motor power differences within the first two weeks post-SCI in cervical spinal cord-injured quadriplegic subjects. J Neurotrauma. 1992;9(4):373–80.
6. Consortium for Spinal Cord Medicine. Early acute management in adults with spinal cord injury: a clinical practice guideline for health-care providers. Washington DC: Paralyzed Veterans of America; 2008.
7. Gala VC, Voyadzis JM, Kim DH, Asir A, Fessler RG. Trauma of the nervous system: spinal cord trauma. In: Bradley WG, Daroff RB, Fenichel GM, Jankovic J, editors. Neurology in clinical practice. 5th ed. Philadelphia: Butterworth Heinemann Elsevier; 2008. p. 1121.
8. Ditunno JF, Little JW, Tessler A, Burns AS. Spinal shock revisited: a four-phase model. Spinal Cord. 2004;42(7):383–95.
9. Marino RJ, Burns S, Graves DE, Leiby BE, Kirshblum S, Lammertse DP. Upper- and lower-extremity motor recovery after traumatic cervical spinal cord injury: an update from the national spinal cord injury database. Arch Phys Med Rehabil. 2011;92(3):369–75.
10. Consortium for Spinal Cord Medicine. Outcomes following traumatic spinal cord injury: clinical practice guidelines for health – care professionals. Washington DC: Paralyzed Veterans of America; 1999.
11. Maynard FM, Reynolds GG, Fountain S, et al. Neurological prognosis after traumatic quadriplegia: three-year experience of California regional spinal cord injury care system. J Neurosurg. 1979;50:611–6.
12. Ditunno JF, Cohen ME, Formal C. Functional outcomes. In: Stover SL, Whiteneck GG, DeLisa JA, editors. Spinal cord injury: clinical outcomes from the model systems. Gaithersburg: Aspen; 1995. p. 170–84.
13. Ditunno Jr JF, Cohen ME, Hauck W, Jackeon AB, Sipski ML. Recovery of upper-extremity strength in complete and incomplete tetraplegia: a multicenter study. Arch Phys Med Rehabil. 2000;81:389–93.
14. Waters RL, Adkins RH, Yakura JS, et al. Motor and sensory recovery following complete tetraplegia. Arch Phys Med Rehabil. 1993;74:242–7.
15. Ditunno Jr JF, Stover SL, Freed MM, et al. Motor recovery of the upper extremities in traumatic quadriplegia: a multicenter study. Arch Phys Med Rehabil. 1992;73:431–6.
16. Frost FS. Spinal cord injury medicine. In: Braddom RL, editor. Physical medicine & rehabilitation. 2nd ed. Philadelphia: Saunders; 2000. p. 1230–82.

17. Guide for the uniform data set for medical rehabilitation, version 5.1. Buffalo: State University of New York at Buffalo; 1997.

18. Granger CV, Kelly-Hayes M, Johnston M, Deutsch A, Braun S, Fiedler RC. Quality and outcome measures for medical rehabilitation. In: Braddom RL, editor. Physical medicine & rehabilitation. 2nd ed. Philadelphia: Saunders; 2000. p. 151–64.

19. Dudek N, Trudel G. Joint contractures. In: Frontera WR, Silver JK, Rizzo Jr TD, editors. Frontera: essentials of physical medicine and rehabilitation. 2nd ed. Philadelphia: Saunders Elsevier; 2008. p. 651–5.

20. Kottke FJ, Pauley DL, Ptak RA. The rationale for prolonged stretching for correction of shortening of connective tissue. Arch Phys Med Rehabil. 1966;47:345–52.

21. Wang D, Teddy PJ, Henderson NJ, Shine BS, Gardner BP. Mobilization of patients after spinal surgery for acute spinal cord injury. Spine. 2001;26(20):2278–82.

22. Stiller K. Safety issues that should be considered when mobilizing critically ill patients. Crit Care Clin. 2007;23(1):35–53.

23. Buschbacher RM, Porter CD. Deconditioning, conditioning, and the benefits of exercise. In: Braddom RL, editor. Physical medicine & rehabilitation. 2nd ed. Philadelphia: Saunders; 2000. p. 702–26.

24. Benditt JO, McCool FD. The respiratory system and neuromuscular disease. In: Mason RJ, Broaddus VC, Martin TR, King Jr TE, Schraufnagel DE, Murray JF, Nadel JA, Mason RJ, editors. Murray and Nadel's textbook of respiratory medicine. 5th ed. Philadelphia: Saunders Elsevier; 2010. p. 2047–66.

25. Consortium for Spinal Cord Medicine. Respiratory management following spinal cord injury: a clinical practice guideline for health-care professionals. Washington DC: Paralyzed Veterans of America; 2005.

26. Bott J, Blumenthal S, Buxton M. Guidelines for the physiotherapy management of the adult, medical, spontaneously breathing patient. Thorax. 2009;64 Suppl 1:i1–51.

27. Consortium for Spinal Cord Medicine. Prevention of thromboembolism in spinal cord injury. 2nd ed. Washington DC: Paralyzed Veterans of America; 1999.

28. Aissaoui N, Martins E, Mouly S, Weber S, Meune C. A meta-analysis of bed rest versus early ambulation in the management of pulmonary embolism, deep vein thrombosis, or both. Int J Cardiol. 2009;137(1):37–41.

29. Blumenstein MS. Early ambulation after acute deep vein thrombosis: is it safe? J Pediatr Oncol Nurs. 2007;24(6):309–13.

30. Illman A, Stiller K, Williams M. The prevalence of orthostatic hypotension during physiotherapy treatment in patients with an acute spinal cord injury. Spinal Cord. 2000;38(12):741–7.

31. Claydon VE, Steeves JD, Krassioukov A. Orthostatic hypotension and spinal cord injury: understanding clinical pathophysiology. Spinal Cord. 2006;44:341–51.

32. Krassioukov A, Eng JJ, Warburton DE, Teasell R. A systematic review of the management of orthostatic hypotension after spinal cord injury. Arch Phys Med Rehabil. 2009;90(5):876–85.

33. Linares HA, Mawson AR, Suarez E, et al. Association between pressure sores and immobilization in the immediate postinjury period. Orthopedics. 1987;10:571–3.

34. Consortium for Spinal Cord Medicine. Pressure ulcer prevention and treatment following spinal cord injury: a clinical practice guideline for health-care professionals. Washington DC: Paralyzed Veterans of America; 2000.

35. Colachis 3rd SC. Autonomic hyperreflexia with spinal cord injury. J Am Paraplegia Soc. 1992;15(3):171–86.

36. Consortium for Spinal Cord Medicine. Acute management of autonomic dysreflexia: individuals with spinal cord injury presenting to health-care facilities. Washington DC: Paralyzed Veterans of America; 2001.

37. Gimovsky ML, Ojeda A, Ozaki R, et al. Management of autonomic hyperreflexia associated with a low thoracic spinal cord lesion. Obstet Gynecol. 1985;153:223–4.

38. Braddom RL, Rocco JF. Autonomic dysreflexia: a survey of current treatment. Am J Phys Med Rehabil. 1991;70:234.

39. Stoffel JT, McGuire EJ. Treating the adult neurogenic bladder. Preface. Urol Clin North Am. 2010;37(4):xi–xii.

40. Cardenas DD, Mayo ME. Management of bladder dysfunction. In: Braddom RL, editor. Physical medicine & rehabilitation. 2nd ed. Philadelphia: Saunders; 2000. p. 561–78.

41. Consortium for Spinal Cord Medicine. Bladder management for adults with spinal cord injury: a clinical practice guideline for health-care providers. Washington DC: Paralyzed Veterans of America; 2006.

42. Liu CW, Huang CC, Chen CH, Yang YH, Chen TW, Huang 3rd MH. Prediction of severe neurogenic bowel dysfunction in persons with spinal cord injury. Spinal Cord. 2010;48(7):554–9.

43. Branco F, Cardenas DD, Svircev JN. Spinal cord injury: a comprehensive review. Phys Med Rehabil Clin N Am. 2007;18(4): 651–79.

44. Consortium for Spinal Cord Medicine. Neurogenic bowel management in adults with spinal cord injury. Washington DC: Paralyzed Veterans of America; 1998.

45. Kirk PM, King RB, Temple R, Bourjaily J, Thomas P. Long-term follow-up of bowel management after spinal cord injury. SCI Nurs. 1997;14(2):56–63.

46. Pedersen E. Regulation of bladder and colon–rectum in patients with spinal lesions. J Auton Nerv Syst. 1983;7(3–4):329–38.

47. King JC, Stiens SA. Neurogenic bowel: dysfunction and management. In: Braddom RL, editor. Physical medicine & rehabilitation. 2nd ed. Philadelphia: Saunders; 2000. p. 579–91.

48. Stiens SA, Bergman SB, Goetz LL. Neurogenic bowel dysfunction after spinal cord injury: clinical evaluation and rehabilitative management. Arch Phys Med Rehabil. 1997;78(3 Suppl):S86–102.

49. Halm MA. Elimination concerns with acute spinal cord trauma. Assessment and nursing interventions. Crit Care Nurs Clin North Am. 1990;2(3):385–98.

50. Lance JW. Symposium synopsis. In: Feldman RG, Young RR, Koella WP, editors. Spasticity: disordered motor control. Chicago: Yearbook Medical; 1980. p. 485–94.

51. Gracies JM, Simpson DM. Spastic dystonia. In: Brin MF, Comella C, Jankovic J, editors. Dystonia: etiology, clinical features and treatment. Philadelphia: Lippincott Williams & Wilkins; 2004. p. 195–211.

52. Ullrich PM. Pain following spinal cord injury. Phys Med Rehabil Clin N Am. 2007;18(2):217–33, vi.

53. Levendoglu F, Ogun CO, Ozerbil O, et al. Gabapentin is a first line drug for the treatment of neuropathic pain in spinal cord injury. Spine. 2004;29:743–51.

54. Siddall PJ, Cousins MD, Otte A, et al. Pregabalin in central neuropathic pain associated with spinal cord injury: a placebo-controlled trial. Neurology. 2006;67:1792–800.

55. Harrington AL, Blount PJ, Bockenek WL. Heterotopic ossification. In: Frontera WR, Silver JK, Rizzo Jr TD, editors. Essentials of physical medicine and rehabilitation. 2nd ed. Philadelphia: Saunders Elsevier; 2008. p. 691–5.

56. Teasell RW, Mehta S, Aubut JL, Ashe MC, Sequeira K, Macaluso S, Tu L. A systematic review of the therapeutic interventions for heterotopic ossification after spinal cord injury. Spinal Cord. 2010;48(7):512–21.

57. Aubut JA, Mehta S, Cullen N, Teasell RW. A comparison of heterotopic ossification treatment within the traumatic brain and spinal cord injured population: an evidence based systematic review. NeuroRehabilitation. 2011;28(2):151–60.

58. Hoffman JM, Bombardier CH, Graves DE, Kalpakjian CZ, Krause JS. A longitudinal study of depression from 1 to 5 years after spinal cord injury. Arch Phys Med Rehabil. 2011;92(3):411–8.

59. Fann JR, Bombardier CH, Richards JS, Tate DG, Wilson CS, Temkin N. Depression after spinal cord injury: comorbidities, mental health service use, and adequacy of treatment. Arch Phys Med Rehabil. 2011;92(3):352–60.

60. Scelza WM, Kirshblum SC, Wuermser LA, Ho CH, Priebe MM, Chiodo AE. Spinal cord injury medicine. 4. Community reintegration after spinal cord injury. Arch Phys Med Rehabil. 2007; 8(3 Suppl 1):S71–5.
61. Holicky R, Charlifue S. Aging with spinal cord injury: the impact of spousal support. Disabil Rehabil. 1999;21:250–7.
62. Bombardier CH, Richards JS, Krause JS, Tulsky D, Tate DG. Symptoms of major depression in people with spinal cord injury: implications for screening. Arch Phys Med Rehabil. 2004;85:1749–56.
63. Craig A, Hancock K, Dickson H. Improving the long-term adjustment of spinal cord injured persons. Spinal Cord. 1999;37: 345–50.
64. Kirschblum SC, Priebe MM, Ho CH, Scelza WM, Chiodo AE, Wuermser LA. Spinal cord injury medicine. 3. Rehabilitation phase after acute spinal cord injury. Arch Phys Med Rehabil. 2007;88(3 Suppl 1):S62–70.
65. Bohannon RW, Smith MB. Interrater reliability of a modified Ashworth scale of muscle spasticity. Phys Ther. 1986;67:206–7.

Special Issues in Pediatric Neurocritical Care After Neurosurgery

32

Robert C. Tasker

Contents

R.C. Tasker, MA, MBBS, MD
Division of Critical Care Medicine, Department of Anesthesiology,
Perioperative and Pain Medicine, Boston Children's Hospital,
300 Longwood Avenue, Bader 627,
Boston, MA 02115, USA

Department of Neurology, Boston Children's Hospital,
300 Longwood Avenue, Bader 627,
Boston, MA 02115, USA
e-mail: robert.tasker@childrens.harvard.edu

Abstract

The postoperative management of pediatric neurosurgical patients presents many challenges to neurointensivists. Many conditions and complications are unique to small children. A basic understanding of age-related physiology and pharmacology is essential in minimizing perioperative morbidity.

Keywords

Child • Neurosurgery • Intensive care • Neurocritical care

Introduction

Neurocritical care in children represents a "special issue" [1]. Specific clinical programs have started in a number of centers with the purpose of improving outcome in critically ill children with acute brain disorders. Although the exact model that develops may be dependent on the needs of individual institutions [2], the next 10 years will determine whether there is a case for special expertise in pediatric neurocritical care that is independent of pediatric critical care, as well as pediatric neurology and neurosurgery. In centers where programs are developing, the typical sequence for organization follows the adult neurocritical care model and includes seven key steps [3]: (1) training clinical staff, (2) building and equipping the facility, (3) developing special standards and protocols for monitoring and other support techniques, (4) training of allied health professionals, (5) provision of continuing education, (6) full-time coverage by specialists, and (7) developing a research program.

To set pediatric neurocritical care in context, it should be appreciated that, in general, the practice covers 17 % of all critical care in children [4, 5]. Four separate categories of patients are incorporated, including neurosurgery, spine surgery, neurotrauma, and neurovascular (7 % of the entire population); general critical care for children with chronic encephalopathy or neurogenetic, neurologic, or peripheral

A.J. Layon et al. (eds.), *Textbook of Neurointensive Care*,
DOI 10.1007/978-1-4471-5226-2_32, © Springer-Verlag London 2013

Table 32.1 Three categories of specific *neurocritical care* in columns with conditions in each category grouped by cell

Neurosurgery and vascular	Chronic encephalopathy or neurogenetic, neurologic, or peripheral nervous system disease	Acute neurology of illness
Neurosurgery	*General surgery*	*Seizure or status epilepticus*
Hydrocephalus	Gastrointestinal	Fever associated
Tumors	Orthopedics	Complicated/complex febrile convulsion
Special surgery	Airway	Part of encephalopathy in medical condition (hematology/oncology, gastrointestinal, sepsis, endocrine)
	Bladder	
Spinal surgery	*Acute medical disease*	*Coma or cerebral edema*
	Acute kidney injury and failure	Encephalopathy
	Stevens-Johnson syndrome	Post-cardiac arrest and hypoxia-ischemia
	Liver and gastrointestinal	Inborn error of metabolism
		Metabolic disease
		Intoxication
		Diabetic ketoacidosis
Neurovascular	*Thoracic pump disorder*	*CNS infection*
Extradural	Demyelinating condition	Meningitis
Subdural	Spinal muscular atrophy	Encephalitis
Intracranial hemorrhage	Guillain-Barre syndrome	Cerebral abscess
Acute ischemic stroke	Neuromuscular junction diseases	
Venous thrombosis	Muscle disease	
Vascular malformation		
Neurotrauma	*Sepsis, septicemia, and septic shock*	
	Mechanical ventilation (MV) alone	
	MV and inotropes	
	Seizures or status epilepticus	

nervous system disease (3 % of population); acute neurology of critical illness (4 % of population); and seizures or status epilepticus (3 % of population). Table 32.1 summarizes this range of conditions, and in many respects, our management follows principles and practices developed from neurocritical care in adults, pediatric Reye syndrome, and neonatal hypoxic-ischemic encephalopathy. Most of the topics and conditions mentioned in Table 32.1 are covered elsewhere in this book, and there is little to distinguish children except for special attention to etiology and certain aspects of developmental physiology, pharmacology, and fluid therapy. Therefore, the main focus of this chapter will be the general principles of pediatric neurosurgical and neurocritical care practice that differ from practice in adults. Issues in which pediatric traumatic brain injury differs from adult injury as well as emergency care, including pediatric airway management and mechanical ventilation, hemodynamic support, and intracranial pressure management, are addressed elsewhere (Chap. 28).

Developmental Considerations

The "pediatric" age range starts with newborns and runs through to adults; thought of in another way, this is 1–100 kg – a change in mass of two orders of magnitude.

If we just consider the changing brain, we are treating an organ that has a sixfold increase in weight from birth to maturity, with most of the change in weight occurring by the age of 2 years.

Hemodynamic Physiology

Normal values of intracranial pressure (ICP) are less in newborns (2–6 mmHg) and children (less than 15 mmHg) than in adults [6]. So, too, are normal values for blood pressure (BP), which means that a calculation of cerebral perfusion pressure (CPP = MAP [mean arterial pressure] – ICP$_{mean}$) will be very different to the values found in adults (Fig. 32.1). The impact of the cranial vault on intracranial hydrodynamics is also different in children. The infant's cranium has the potential for growth, with open fontanels and sutures, so that there is greater total compliance of the system. For example, a slow growing tumor will not have an acute mass effect, as the increase in intracranial volume occurring with tumor expansion results in the widening of sutures and fontanels in a compensatory manner. As a result, infants and young children may have advanced intracranial pathology at the time of presentation, with little remaining reserve.

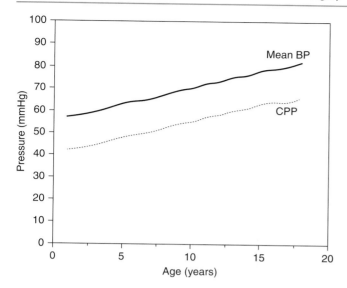

Fig. 32.1 Mean blood pressure (mean BP, mean arterial pressure [MAP]) and cerebral perfusion pressure (*CPP*) by age using normative date for BP and upper limit of normal for ICP of 15 mmHg

Cerebral Blood Flow

Cerebral blood flow (CBF) is coupled to metabolic demand (or rate) for oxygen ($CMRO_2$), and both increase proportionately after birth. Whole-brain CBF peaks between the ages of 5–8 years (~70 mL/100 g/min) and then declines to the adult level (~50 mL/100 g/min) in early teenage [7]. Despite these changes, oxygen extraction fraction (OEF) is constant even in early childhood [8]. CBF responsiveness or reactivity to changes in carbon dioxide (CO_2), O_2, and perfusion pressure clearly occurs in the developing brain. Critical questions such as "how low can perfusion pressure go" [9] are very difficult to address. The answer is different for adults, but when should we be concerned? Figure 32.1 summarizes normal MAP in infants and children, and this, at least, is a starting point for tight BP control. In the perioperative patient, we need noninvasive monitoring that would enable valid assessment of adequacy of cerebral perfusion.

Postoperative Neurocritical Care

One should not – indeed cannot – manage a child in the postoperative period without knowing what has gone on before. Considering the pathway from preoperative treatments to induction of anesthesia and the surgical procedure, to recovery room care, and then to admission to the intensive care unit (ICU) as a continuum is absolutely essential. Postoperative neurosurgical children will have been exposed to a number of therapies before and during surgery. At the time of "hand-off," a formal assessment should be made of pre-, intra-, and postoperative issues; an essential component of the "hand-off" assessment is medicines and anesthetics.

For example, the patient may have been hyperhydrated in preparation for a cerebrovascular procedure (see discussion later in this chapter). They will have received anesthetics that have been specifically used because they depress cerebral metabolism. However, it is the other unwanted cerebrovascular effects that may be of concern postoperatively.

Intraoperative Anesthetic Drugs and Agents

The volatile anesthetics act as potent vasodilators in the cerebral circulation. They are capable of uncoupling the usual relationship between CBF and $CMRO_2$. Such uncoupling increases cerebral blood volume (CBV) and, in consequence, elevated ICP with worsening of intracranial hypertension [10]. Desflurane and isoflurane increase transcranial Doppler (TCD)-measured CBF velocity, as well as blunt the autoregulatory response that maintains CBF with changes in perfusion pressure; both isoflurane and sevoflurane decrease $CMRO_2$, but flow-metabolism coupling is maintained; nitrous oxide has vasodilatory effects [11, 12].

Intravenous anesthetics, sedative/hypnotic drugs, and opioids also have cerebral metabolic effects, but they do not cause cerebrovascular vasodilatation. For example, barbiturates and propofol maintain autoregulation and flow-metabolism coupling while reducing CBF, CBV, and $CMRO_2$. Propofol maintains cerebrovascular reactivity to CO_2 when the latter is above 30 mmHg [13]. However, propofol at high doses lowers MAP and TCD-measured CBF velocity [14]. The maintenance of anesthesia during neurosurgery with an opioid (i.e., fentanyl or other related synthetic opioids such as sufentanil or remifentanil) along with nitrous oxide (70 %) and low-dose (0.2–0.5 %) isoflurane is a frequently used technique [15, 16], and when it comes to postoperative considerations, those caring for such patients should be aware of cumulative dosing and timings. For example, nitrous oxide may contribute to postoperative nausea and vomiting and dose-dependent increase in CBF [16]. Clearly, we do not want a postoperative infant following a procedure on an arteriovenous malformation to be vomiting such that there are episodic rises in intrathoracic pressure transmitted to intracranial vessels.

Perioperative Intravenous Fluids

The prescription of intravenous (IV) maintenance fluids for children unable to tolerate oral therapy is fundamental in pediatric critical care, and, in recent years, it has proved to be a topic of much debate. What we want to know is: How much and what type of fluid should we give postoperatively? The main aims of fluid therapy are as follows: first, to have a hemodynamically stable patient; second, to avoid electrolyte abnormalities; and third, to ensure adequate glucose control.

The first aim requires careful maintenance of intravascular volume. Preoperative fluid restriction and the use of mannitol, hypertonic saline, or diuretics may lead to blood pressure instability and even cardiovascular collapse intraoperatively, with problems carrying over into the postoperative phase. It is therefore important to know what has happened intraoperatively, the estimated blood loss as a proportion of blood volume, as well as fluid inputs and outputs before intensive care unit admission.

Normal Saline

Normal saline is the preferred IV fluid during and after neurosurgery since its osmolality (308 mOsm/L) should minimize the risk of hyponatremia (serum sodium less than 135 mMol/L) and cerebral edema. It is conventional in pediatric practice to calculate the rate of maintenance fluid administration scaled to weight of the patient using the classic Holliday and Segar [17] formula for daily fluids: 100 mL/kg for the first 10 kg in body weight, plus 50 mL/kg for the next 10 kg in body weight (i.e., weight 10–20 kg), plus 20 mL/kg for weight above 20 kg (Table 32.2).

These rates are based on normal conditions in health, and they may not reflect what is needed in the operating room. Issues that may need consideration are: How long was the procedure? How much maintenance fluid has been given? It is not unusual for long procedures to necessitate maintenance fluid up to 10 mL/kg/h. Were boluses of saline needed to stabilize BP? When more than 60 mL/kg has been used, there is the risk of hyperchloremic metabolic acidosis, which may not be appreciated unless serum chloride was measured [18]. Lastly, was there any evidence of diabetes insipidus (DI)?

Postoperatively, there is a significant risk of hospital-acquired hyponatremia, which approaches 30 % [19]. In this setting, postoperative pain, stress, nausea, vomiting, narcotics, and volume depletion all have the potential to stimulate vasopressin production and induce a state of euvolemic hyponatremia not dissimilar to the syndrome of inappropriate antidiuretic hormone release (SIADH); in fact, ADH secretion may well be an *appropriate* survival response. To date, there have been three prospective trials of intravenous fluids in postoperative patients (not specifically neurosurgical patients): two studies in the pediatric ICU [20, 21] and one study in the postoperative ward [22]. Unfortunately, the end points in these studies differed in respect to what and when either an absolute change in serum sodium [20] or proportion of cases with hyponatremia defined as below 135 mMol/L [20] or below 130 mMol/L [22] and measurements at 8, 12, or 24 h [20–22]. The general message from these studies is that isotonic fluids prevent postoperative falls in serum sodium concentration and hypotonic fluids result in decreased sodium concentration. In none of these three

Table 32.2 Example of calculated fluid maintenance volume in a 23 kg child

24-h total:	0–10 kg	First 10 kg = (10 × 100) mL
	10–20 kg	Second 10 kg = (10 × 50) mL
	20–23 kg	Final 3 kg = (3 × 20) mL
		Total = 1,560 mL
Rate per hour = 65 mL/h or 2.8 mL/kg/h		

studies was fluid overload or significant hypernatremia a complication. We do not know the epidemiology of perioperative pediatric neurosurgical intravenous fluid management, but a recent survey of practice in general pediatric surgeons and anesthesiologists using infant and child clinical scenarios showed that significant numbers of clinicians were using hypotonic fluids or fluid restriction [23].

Modeling the Effect "Too Much Water or Too Much Salt"

The debate about volume and type of intravenous fluids arises because the maintenance requirements for the postoperative child are not clear. We have all seen the edematous child who has received too much free water or who has received too much salt. Which is worse?

Figures 32.2 and 32.3 illustrate the arguments for and against volume and concentration by modeling salt and water handling [24, 25]. Figure 32.2 shows responses in extracellular (V_e) and intracellular (V_i) volumes in a closed system with two compartments separated by a membrane that permits the movement of water but is impermeable to sodium (Na^+) and potassium (K^+), which are, respectively, the sole V_e and V_i cations. If the V_i component of the model functions as a perfect osmometer, then the sloping lines represent isopleths, lines of constant overall volume ($V_e + V_i$). The numbers have been normalized to body water, with loss or gain in percent for each compartment, relative to the origin (point O), which is steady-state euvolemia. The two vectors represent an accumulated positive balance in the system, either 20 mL/kg of water (vector OW) or 20 mL/kg of normal saline (vector OS). In this model, which is applicable between 10 and 30 kg body weight, the effect of gaining 20 mL/kg of saline is an 8 % increase in V_e, without any change in V_i or serum osmolality. The effect of gaining 20 mL/kg of water is an expansion in both V_e and V_i, each by over 3 % with an associated fall in serum osmolality. (The vector SW represents a desalination of 1.5 mMol/kg, and any movement along this same axis above horizontal can be considered as net loss of salt from a particular initial condition.)

The homeostatic challenges are different for the two conditions OW and OS. In the case of gain in saline, the theoretical system must deal with the acute salt load, the change in interstitial compliance as V_e increases, and resulting edema. These issues are not trivial. For example, in healthy adults, in

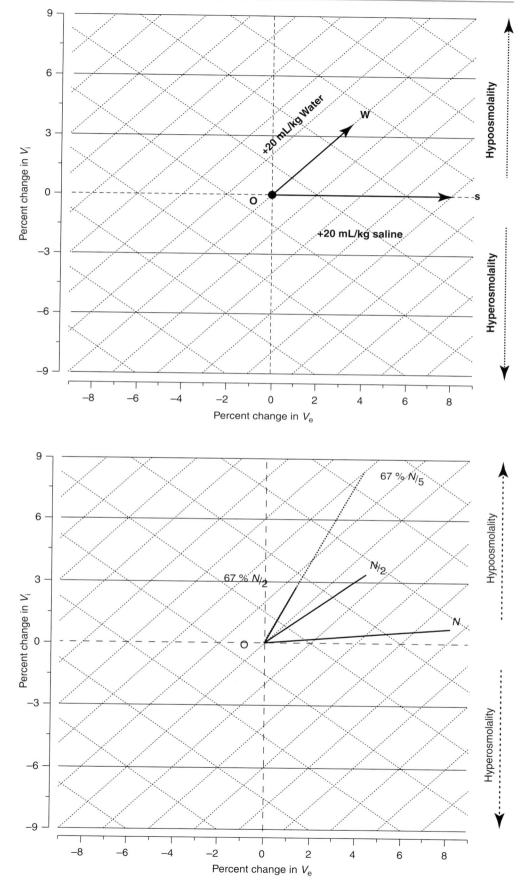

Fig. 32.2 Model of fluid shifts due to addition of 20 mL/kg intravenous water or normal saline

Fig. 32.3 Model of fluid shifts due to different tonicities of saline

the supine position, it takes 2 days to regulate the amount of salt and water provided by an acute saline infusion [26, 27]. Experimentally, generalized edema will accelerate after ~15 % expansion in V_e, although this response will be different in different tissues as well as being influenced by plasma colloid osmotic pressure [28–30]. In the case of gain in water, the main difference to saline is that the system must defend changes in V_i induced by the hypoosmolality. Is this threat real for the range of values typically seen in postoperative neurosurgical children on maintenance intravenous fluids? In other words, which tissues function as perfect osmometers, like the model?

Experimental studies show that skeletal muscle, containing the bulk of an organism's water and K^+, is important as a buffer during acute hyponatremia since it serves as a near-perfect osmometer [31, 32]. In contrast, within the brain, increases in water content are less than expected, but there are regional differences [33, 34]. For example, during acute hyponatremia (in which the Na^+ is reduced from 138 ± 1 to 123 ± 2 mMol/L), the water content of the whole brain and white matter increases but it is less than expected for perfect osmotic behavior, whereas in the thalamus, water content increases as expected for a perfect osmometer [32]. These data provide the experimental context for interpreting the significance of change in electrolytes and osmolality summarized in the previous section. It is true that symptomatic hyponatremia with encephalopathy in previously well children has the potential for high neurologic morbidity [34, 35]. How likely is this complication in the first 24 h after an operation and admission to the intensive care unit?

Figure 32.3 uses similar principles to Fig. 32.2, but in addition, the model takes account of mass balance for Na^+ and K^+, where the input comes from IV fluid and the output in water and electrolytes is considered as solely via urine [36]. The three prospective studies of postoperative and intensive care children provide information about urine tonicity and volume [20–22]. Maintenance fluids were calculated using the Holliday and Segar equation [17] in all three studies. Urine tonicity across the studies is almost fixed: in those receiving normal saline (N) at full maintenance, urine tonicity is about 200 mOsm/L; in those receiving any other prescription, urine tonicity is lower, about 160 mOsm/L. Only one study reports urine output [22], and it appears that, irrespective of fluid prescribed, mean output over 12–24 h was about 1.2 mL/kg/h. These data have been used to generate the four vectors for the 12-h cumulative fluid and tonicity balance in Fig. 32.3. Starting from the origin (point O), the greatest increase in V_e is seen with full maintenance N. The likelihood of increased V_i and hypoosmolality is in the following increasing order: N, two-thirds restricted half-normal saline (67 % $N/2$), full maintenance $N/2$, and two-thirds one-fifth-normal saline (67 % $N/5$). The severe derangement occurring with 67 % $N/5$ is nearly three times the theoretical

expansion of V_e and hypoosmolality occurring during the other prescriptions. The problem of hypernatremia is not seen in the model, but more complexity in the volume relationships can be added with other variables common in postoperative neurosurgical children, e.g., the sequestration of extracellular water within injured tissues necessitating saline replacement, neuroendocrine stress physiology, and consideration of gains, losses, and urinary desalination [37–40].

Postoperative Renal Salt and Water Handling

Disorders of salt and water homeostasis are common in postoperative neurosurgical patients. The three main renal salt and water handling problems that occur in these children are euvolemic states of ADH excess (i.e., SIADH), cerebral salt wasting (CSW), and DI. Therefore, regular monitoring of intravascular volume, urine output and tonicity, and serum electrolytes are needed during the postoperative period and while administering IV fluids. It is also advisable that children with significant cerebrospinal fluid (CSF) drainage have adequate replacement of this source of sodium loss as well. The overall calculation will depend on the size of the child and usual maintenance level of sodium replacement. An example for a 25 kg child is as follows:

$$Usual\ Na^+\ maintenance = 2 - 4mMol/kg/day$$
$$\cong 50 - 100mMol\ Na^+/day;$$

$$CSF\ drainage\ up\ to\ 0.35mL/min = 500\ mL\ CSF/day$$
$$\cong 75\ mMol\ Na^+/day.$$

In this instance, the child could require up to 175 mMol Na^+/day (7 mMol/kg/day), and we have not even addressed urinary losses. Therefore, making an assumption that subsequent hyponatremia is due to SIADH, volume restricting the child, without first checking that adequate sodium replacement has occurred, is the wrong course of action. Another, often unappreciated, cause of hyponatremia is pseudohyponatremia due to the use of perioperative radiologic nonionic hyperosmolar contrast medium [41].

Syndrome of Inappropriate Antidiuretic Hormone (SIADH) Secretion

The risk of postoperative hyponatremia is a major concern, as it may go unrecognized until the onset of a seizure [42]; this is one of the reasons for frequent post-procedure Na^+ checks. If the cause of the hyponatremia is perioperative SIADH, and not inadequate sodium prescription (see previous discussion), it has occurred because of free water retention that follows natriuresis so that fluid balance is maintained at the expense of serum osmolality. Because of this risk, many clinicians avoid hypotonic solutions altogether in the perioperative period. It should be noted that Ringer's lactate sodium (136 mMol/L) might result in a fall in serum sodium. This fluid is often used intraoperatively as it is a balanced solution with a physiologic amount of base, calcium, and K^+ and will limit the hyperchloremic acidosis that occurs with large volumes of normal saline.

The usual treatment of SIADH is to reduce free water excess by fluid restriction and diuretics. If a hyponatremic seizure occurs, then hypertonic (3 %) saline solution should be used to correct serum sodium; the level to be targeted is that at which the seizure comes under control, often about 130 mMol/L. Taking 0.6 L/kg body weight as the apparent volume of distribution for sodium, one should anticipate an immediate increase of 3–5 mMol/L in serum sodium concentration with a rapid IV bolus of 4–6 mL/kg body weight of 3 % saline [43]; the utilization of continuous infusion 3 % saline solution is an alternative to the usual treatment of SIADH with fluid restriction/diuresis.

Cerebral Salt Wasting (CSW)

The diagnosis of CSW is one of exclusion, based upon clinical criteria. It appears to be common in children after all types of neurosurgical procedures [44–46], and it results from excessively high atrial (ANP) or brain natriuretic peptide (BNP) levels [47]. The essential features are renal sodium and chloride wasting in a patient with a *contracted effective arterial blood volume*, where other causes of excess sodium excretion have been excluded. Volume contraction is likely to be present when there is a deficit of sodium that exceeds 2 mMol/kg [48]; hyponatremia is a nonspecific clue. Table 32.3 lists some of the diagnoses that should be excluded before concluding that the patient has CSW. It is worth noting that ANP level is high in the patient who has been managed with hypervolemic fluid management. Hence, in this instance, natriuresis as a response to volume control is part of homeostasis, and not CSW.

As CSW has become more generally recognized as a condition, the syndrome has been diagnosed with increasing frequency. The incidence is apparently on the order of 1–5 % of neurosurgical procedures, and it has been reported in association with calvarial remodeling, tumor resection and hydrocephalus [44–46]. Recently, Hardesty and colleagues [46] reported a 5-year review of postoperative pediatric brain tumor patients they managed. CSW was defined retrospectively as one laboratory measurement of hyponatremia (less than 135 mMol/L) with brisk diuresis (more than 3 mL/kg/h) and elevated urine sodium (greater than 120 mMol/L), when

Table 32.3 Diagnosis of cerebral salt wasting in a patient who has a cerebral lesion is one of exclusion. There must be excretion of Na^+ and Cl^- without an obvious cause

1. Rule out:

A physiologic cause for the excretion of Na^+ and Cl^- (e.g., an expanded extracellular fluid (ECF) volume from hyperhydration)

A non-cerebral cause for natriuresis:

Diuretics

States with low aldosterone

Bartter syndrome

Ligands for the calcium receptor in the loop of Henle (e.g., hypercalcemia, gentamicin)

Obligatory excretion of Na^+ by the excretion of anions other than Cl^-

High-output renal failure

Sodium wasting from cerebrospinal fluid drainage

2. Possible explanations for salt wasting:

Natriuretic agents of cerebral origin

Downregulation of renal Na^+ transport by chronic ECF volume expansion

Pressure natriuresis from adrenergic agents

Suppression of the release of aldosterone

available, or elevated urinary osmolarity (greater than 300 mOsm/kg water). The authors did not have any assessment of volume status (see earlier discussion), but all patients in their institution were treated with normal saline intra- and postoperatively. However, they found that 5 % of all pediatric tumor patients undergoing craniotomy in their center developed CSW, which was more frequently observed than SIADH (3 %). The median onset of CSW was on postoperative day 3, lasting a median of 2.5 days. Patients with CSW were more likely to have suffered postoperative stroke, have chiasmatic or hypothalamic tumors, and be younger than patients with normal postoperative sodium concentration. Almost half of the patients with CSW had postoperative hyponatremic seizures (serum sodium range 118–128 mMol/L). The treatment of CSW involves sodium administration to match urinary losses and correction of intravascular volume contraction. In some instances, more rapid resolution of hyponatremia after volume expansion has been achieved with fludrocortisone [49].

Diabetes Insipidus

DI results from a deficiency of vasopressin and is an expected complication of surgical procedures near the pituitary or hypothalamus. It is most frequently seen in association with craniopharyngioma, where it can be a presenting symptom in 40 % of cases [50]. In most patients, DI is transient, but in approximately 6 %, it is permanent [51, 52]. The diagnosis should be suspected when serum sodium rises above 145 mMol/L in association with urine output above

2.5 mL/g/h for three consecutive hours or more than 4 mL/kg/h in any 1 h. The urine osmolality should be hypotonic (less than 300 mOsm/L) in the face of increased plasma osmolality (greater than 300 mOsm/L) and in the absence of glycosuria, mannitol use, and renal failure. An important consequence of this condition is severe dehydration and hypovolemia since urine output is driven by lack of vasopressin.

Knowledge of the several patterns of DI that can occur following surgery in the hypothalamic-pituitary area is important. The most common is that associated with local edema as a result of traction or manipulation of the pituitary stalk. This lesion usually results in transient polyuria that begins 2–6 h after surgery and resolves as edema diminishes in 1–7 days [53, 54].

A "triphasic pattern" has also been described [51]. The initial phase is associated with polyuria in the first postoperative days [55, 56]. The second phase is the resumption of normal urinary output or SIADH, probably resulting from the release of previously stored ADH from damaged neurons. Ultimately, transection of the pituitary stalk or destruction of the hypothalamic median eminence will result in permanent DI [56, 57]. Frequently, permanent DI, either partial or complete, develops without interphase changes [53, 55].

There are a variety of successful approaches to treating DI. It is useful to have a neuroendocrine assessment preoperatively, with a perioperative care plan, since deficiencies of thyroid and/or adrenocortical hormones can coexist. In the child with known DI, preoperatively, some endocrinologists prefer not to replace vasopressin and to restrict total fluid intake to approximately twice-normal maintenance (scaling to body surface area rather than weight, i.e., 3 L/m²/day), recognizing that this can result in mild hypernatremia and thirst but minimizing the more dangerous risk of water intoxication with vasopressin administration. Others prefer to withhold long-acting DDAVP in the perioperative period and instead manage DI with intermittent injections of intramuscular vasopressin. The administration of excessive fluids in this setting, as with the perioperative maintenance of DDAVP, can result in hyponatremic seizures [46, 58, 59].

Typically, postoperative DI develops 2–12 h after surgery (average, 6 h following completion of surgery). When DI is recognized, the strategy discussed next should lead to serum sodium concentrations between 130 and 150 mMol/L. In such patients, new-onset postoperative DI responds to an infusion of aqueous vasopressin (20 units/500 mL). Aqueous vasopressin is used because of its rapid onset of action and brief duration of effect [60]. However, its potential vascular effects (i.e., hypertension) means that close observation in a monitored setting is required. The infusion is started at 0.5 mUnits/kg/h and titrated upward in 0.5 mUnits/kg/h increments every 5–10 min until urine output decreases to

less than 2 mL/kg/h. It is rare to require more than 10 mUnits/kg/h [61]. Once a urine output of less than 2 mL/kg/h is achieved, the vasopressin infusion is not adjusted downward. Neither is fluid administration adjusted according to urine output. Antidiuresis with vasopressin is essentially an "all-or-none" phenomenon, and the aqueous infusion is being used to produce a "functional SIADH" state [54]. This strategy recognizes that renal blood flow remains normal in the normovolemic, but maximally antidiuresed, child. Because urine output is minimal (0.5 mL/kg/h), other clinical markers of volume status must be followed closely. For example, anuria together with increased heart rate or decreased BP may be evidence of hypovolemia. Vasopressin infusion does not induce acute tubular necrosis, and severe oliguria or anuria is an indication for additional fluid and not for decreasing or discontinuing the infusion. A major caveat when using vasopressin infusion is that management necessitates careful fluid restriction. In the presence of full antidiuresis, excessive fluids (oral or intravenous) can lead to intravascular volume overload. In addition, administration of hypotonic fluids (oral or intravenous) can result in dangerous hyponatremia. This complication can be prevented by fluid restriction limited to replacing insensible losses, which is generally considered to be about two-thirds of the usual maintenance rates [62].

In children at risk of developing permanent DI, in whom adequate oral intake has been established, IV fluids and the vasopressin infusion can be discontinued while permitting free oral intake. Subsequent treatment of DI is withheld until the child demonstrates polyuria. At this time, treatment with DDAVP rather than restarting a vasopressin infusion is recommended. DDAVP is a synthetic vasopressin with duration of action of 12–24 h. It is usually administered intranasally at a dose of 5–10 μg. Oral DDAVP can be used at 10–20 times the nasal dose. Antidiuresis generally begins within 1 h. In children with nasal packing (e.g., transsphenoidal surgery), oral DDAVP is used. In children with known DI, DDAVP treatment can be resumed once an intact thirst mechanism has returned and oral intake without vomiting.

Glucose or No Glucose in Perioperative Intravenous Fluids

Pediatric patients, particularly infants, are at particular risk for perioperative hypoglycemia. Infants, with limited reserves of glycogen and limited gluconeogenesis, require continuous infusions of glucose at 5–6 mg/kg/min in order to maintain serum levels. At the same time, the stress of critical illness and resulting insulin resistance can produce hyperglycemia that, in turn, has been associated with neurologic injury and poor outcomes in adult studies. Hyperglycemia has been linked to poor outcome and it may worsen ischemia, but it remains unclear that the opposite – tight glycemic control – offers significant benefits to children [63]. There is also evidence that tight control carries a 20 % risk of hypoglycemia [64, 65]. It is prudent to follow a conservative approach that maintains random serum glucose level in the normal (140–150 mg/dL) range and certainly below 180 mg/dL. Intraoperatively, the stress response is generally able to maintain normal serum glucose levels without exogenous glucose administration [66]. However, in postoperative infants and small children, particularly if there has been an effective fast of 6–12 h, it is advisable to use glucose-containing fluids to meet baseline demands. Normal saline in 2.5–5 % dextrose should suffice. In general, older children and adolescents can tolerate 18–24 h of fasting.

Postoperative Sedation and Pain Management

Pain control and sedation present unique challenges in pediatric neurocritical care. Ideally, postoperative neurosurgical patients are comfortable, awake, and sufficiently cooperative so as to complete serial neurological examinations. In pediatrics, these goals can be difficult to maintain due to differences in development and cognitive ability of the child. Frequently, a low level of sedation is needed, and in the first two postoperative days, attention to post-craniotomy pain is also required [67]. These targets are achieved using a combination of opioid and benzodiazepine via continuous infusion [68, 69]. Ideal sedation includes short-acting or reversible agents that can be withdrawn intermittently to permit assessment. Some agents suitable for adults are unsuitable in children, and some agents used widely in pediatrics are less useful in adults. In the mechanically ventilated child, the most commonly used sedative agent is midazolam. Titration to a validated sedation score is recommended as is a regular "drug holiday" to help prevent excessive sedation and tolerance [70, 71]. Infants and children receiving sedative infusion for more than 5 days are at risk of withdrawal when infusions are discontinued abruptly. In regard to analgesia, opioids such as morphine and fentanyl should be carefully titrated so as to minimize post-craniotomy pain yet maintain consciousness; in this context, patient-controlled analgesia with a programmable infusion pump may be helpful [72].

Propofol, a potent, ultrashort-acting, sedative/hypnotic agent, is extremely useful in adult neurocritical care but has only limited utility in pediatrics. This is because of its association with the propofol infusion syndrome, a potentially fatal syndrome of bradycardia, rhabdomyolysis, metabolic acidosis, and multiple organ failure when the agent is used over extended periods [73]. While the mechanism of the syndrome remains unclear, it appears related to both the duration of therapy and the cumulative dose; these difficulties are much less common in adults. Some centers have advocated its use in children only under strict controls, but propofol is generally limited to operative anesthesia, procedural sedation, and continuous infusions of limited duration (less than 24 h) [74].

Dexmedetomidine, an IV central alpha-2 agonist, is a newer ultrashort-acting single-agent sedative sometimes used in the postoperative period. Studies involving children are primarily in centers reporting case series. The drug appears to be effective when used for periods of 24 h or less [75, 76]. Opioid cross-tolerance makes it a useful agent for treatment of fentanyl or morphine withdrawal [77]. Transient increases in blood pressure can be seen with boluses followed by hypotension and bradycardia as sedation deepens. Further experience and safety studies are needed before this agent is used in routine perioperative care of pediatric neurosurgical patients.

Blood Loss

Some degree of blood loss during and after brain tumor resection is to be expected and should be replaced [78]. There is a high prevalence of massive blood loss in young infants undergoing intracranial tumor surgery who, invariably, have a significantly longer stay on the intensive care unit [79]. When blood loss (intra- and postoperative) reaches 50–75 % of the preoperative blood volume (or 40–60 mL/kg), some derangement in coagulation is likely. At this level, serum prothrombin (PT) and partial thromboplastin times (aPTT) should be obtained and fresh frozen plasma given if necessary [80]. The derangements in the balance between coagulation and anticoagulation may follow one of the three patterns or any combination, for example, some degree of *hypercoagulability* [81, 82], which may be related to hemodilution [83, 84]. However, the issue of antithrombotic therapy for hypercoagulability is debated. Alternatively, as hemorrhage approaches 100 % of blood volume, coagulopathy is due to factor depletion [85].

Seizures and Status Epilepticus

Postoperative seizures are uncommon but potentially devastating. In known epileptics, there should be a postoperative plan for seizure control. Phenytoin is commonly used for prophylaxis, but maintaining therapeutic serum levels can be a challenge. Levetiracetam is being used more frequently, possibly because of the ease of use. Both drugs can be given intravenously, but unlike phenytoin, the administration of levetiracetam does not require electrocardiographic and hemodynamic monitoring. Again, unlike phenytoin, serum drug level monitoring to avoid toxicity is not required with levetiracetam. The other antiepileptic drugs frequently used in pediatrics include phenobarbital, carbamazepine, and valproic acid.

Status epilepticus can be treated with lorazepam (0.1 mg/kg) as an IV push over 2 min. Lorazepam may be repeated after 10 min and accompanied by IV fosphenytoin (20 mg/kg) if the initial doses are ineffective. Phenobarbital (20 mg/ kg) is also an effective first-line antiepileptic drug [86].

Brain Death

The determination of brain death in infants and children is a clinical diagnosis based on the absence of neurologic function with a known reversible cause of coma. In the United States, the *American Academy of Pediatrics* has recently updated the *1987 Task Force Recommendation* for *Guidelines for the Determination of Brain Death in Infants and Children* [87]. In this latest document, after establishing a known mechanism and cause of coma, the diagnosis requires normothermia, normotension, normal system oxygenation, and the absence of confounding toxins or medications. The examination seeks to establish the complete absence of cortical and brainstem function. An apnea test, documenting the absence of respiratory effort despite $PaCO_2$ greater than or equal to 60 mmHg, from a baseline of 40 mmHg, is conducted last. In order to establish irreversibility, age-related observation periods are necessary. An observation period of 24 h for infants up to 30 days of age and 12 h for infants and children older than 30 days and younger than 18 years. The first examination determines the child has met the accepted neurologic examination criteria for brain death. In the new pediatric guidelines [87], the second examination confirms brain death based on an unchanged and irreversible condition. This guideline is certainly different to the 2010 American Academy of Neurology evidence-based guideline update on determining brain death in adults [88], which changed the 1995 two-examination recommendation [89] to a single examination. It should be noted that all current and previous pediatric recommendations from North America have been consistent in recommending two examinations [90, 91]. It is also recommended that assessment of neurologic function after cardiopulmonary arrest or other severe acute brain injuries should be deferred for 24 h or longer if there are concerns or inconsistency in the examination.

Ancillary studies such as electroencephalography and radionuclide cerebral blood flow studies are not required to establish the diagnosis of brain death, nor are they a substitute for the clinical examination. These studies are used when components of the clinical examination or apnea testing cannot be completed safely because of the patient's medical instability, or if there is uncertainty about the results of the neurologic examination, or if a medication or metabolic effect is present.

References

1. Tasker RC. Pediatric neurocritical care: is it time to come of age? Curr Opin Pediatr. 2009;21:724–30.
2. Bell MJ, Carpenter J, Au KK, et al. Development of a pediatric neurocritical care service. Neurocrit Care. 2009;10:4–10.
3. Safar P, Grenvik A. Critical care medicine. Organizing and staffing intensive care units. Chest. 1971;59:535–47.
4. Tasker RC, Fleming TJ, Young AE, et al. Severe head injury in children: intensive care unit activity and mortality in England and Wales. Br J Neurosurg. 2011;25:68–77.
5. Paediatric Intensive Care Audit Network. PICANet 2011 summary report. http://www.picanet.org.uk.
6. Avery RA, Shah SS, Licht DJ, et al. Reference range for cerebrospinal fluid opening pressure in children. N Engl J Med. 2010;363: 891–3.
7. Chiron C, Raynaud C, Maziere B, et al. Changes in regional cerebral blood flow during maturation in children and adolescents. J Nucl Med. 1992;33:696–703.
8. Takahashi T, Shirane R, Sato S, Yoshimoto T. Developmental changes of cerebral blood flow and oxygen metabolism in children. AJNR Am J Neuroradiol. 1999;20:917–22.
9. Hayward R, Gonsalez S. How low can you go? Intracranial pressure, cerebral perfusion pressure, and respiratory obstruction in children with complex craniosynostosis. J Neurosurg. 2005;102 (1 Suppl):16–22.
10. Hansen TD, Warner DS, Todd MM, Vust LJ. The role of cerebral metabolism in determining the local cerebral blood flow effects of volatile anesthetics: evidence for persistent flow-metabolism coupling. J Cereb Blood Flow Metab. 1989;9:323–8.
11. Fairgrieve R, Rowney DA, Karsli C, Bissonnette B. The effect of sevoflurane on cerebral blood flow velocity in children. Acta Anaesthesiol Scand. 2003;47:1226–30.
12. Wong GT, Luginbuehl I, Karsli C, Bissonnette B. The effect of sevoflurane on cerebral autoregulation in young children as assessed by the transient hyperemic response. Anesth Analg. 2006;102:1051–5.
13. Karsli C, Luginbuehl I, Bissonnette B. Cerebrovascular response to hypocapnia in children receiving propofol. Anesth Analg. 2004; 99: 1049–52.
14. Karsli C, Luginbuehl I, Farrar M, Bissonnette B. Propofol decreases cerebral blood flow velocity in anesthetized children. Can J Anaesth. 2002;49:830–4.
15. Todd MM, Warner DS, Sokoll MD, et al. A prospective, comparative trial of three anesthetics for elective supratentorial craniotomy. Anesthesiology. 1993;78:1005–20.
16. McGregor DG, Lanier WL, Pasternak JJ, et al. Effect of nitrous oxide on neurologic and neuropsychological function after intracranial aneurysm surgery. Anesthesiology. 2008;108:568–79.
17. Holliday MA, Segar WE. The maintenance need for water in parenteral fluid therapy. Pediatrics. 1957;19:823–32.
18. Stephens R, Mythen M. Optimizing intraoperative fluid therapy. Curr Opin Anaesthesiol. 2003;16:385–92.
19. Moritz ML, Ayus JC. Water water everywhere: standardizing postoperative fluid therapy with 0.9% normal saline. Anesth Analg. 2010;110:293–5.
20. Yung M, Keeley S. Randomised controlled trial of intravenous maintenance fluids. J Paediatr Child Health. 2009;45:9–14.
21. Montanana PA, Alapont V, Ocon AP, et al. The use of isotonic fluid as maintenance therapy prevents iatrogenic hyponatremia in

pediatrics: a randomised, controlled open study. Pediatr Crit Care Med. 2008;9:589–97.

22. Neville KA, Sandeman DJ, Rubinstein A, et al. Prevention of hyponatremia during maintenance intravenous fluid administration: a prospective randomized study of fluid type versus fluid rate. J Pediatr. 2010;156:313–9.

23. Way C, Dhamrait R, Wade A, Walker I. Perioperative fluid therapy in children: a survey of current prescribing practice. Br J Anaesth. 2006;97:371–9.

24. Darrow DC, Yannet H. The changes in the distribution of body water accompanying increase and decrease in extracellular electrolyte. J Clin Invest. 1935;14:266–75.

25. Carpenter RHS. Beyond the Darrow-Jannet diagram: an enhanced plot for body fluid spaces and osmolality. Lancet. 1993;342: 968–70.

26. Crawford B, Ludemann H. The renal response to intravenous injection of sodium chloride solutions in man. J Clin Invest. 1951;30: 1456–62.

27. Drummer C, Gerzer R, Heer M, et al. Effects of an acute saline infusion on fluid and electrolyte metabolism in humans. Am J Physiol. 1992;262:F744–54.

28. Guyton AC. Interstitial fluid pressure: II. Pressure-volume curves of interstitial space. Circ Res. 1965;16:452–60.

29. Meyer BJ, Meyer A, Guyton AC. Interstitial fluid pressure: V. Negative pressure in the lungs. Circ Res. 1968;22:263–71.

30. Guyton AC, Granger HJ, Taylor AE. Interstitial fluid pressure. Physiol Rev. 1971;51:527–63.

31. Usher-Smith JA, Huang CL, Fraser JA. Control of cell volume in skeletal muscle. Biol Rev. 2009;84:143–59.

32. Overgaard-Steensen C, Stodkilde-Jorgensen H, Larsson A. Regional differences in osmotic behavior in brain during acute hyponatremia: an in vivo MRI-study of brain and skeletal muscle in pigs. Am J Physiol Regul Integr Comp Physiol. 2010;299: R521–32.

33. Holliday MA, Kalayci MN, Harrah J. Factors that limit brain volume changes in response to acute and sustained hyper- and hyponatremia. J Clin Invest. 1968;47:1916–28.

34. Arieff AI, Ayus JC, Fraser CL. Hyponatremia and death or permanent brain damage in healthy children. Br Med J. 1992;304:1218–22.

35. Moritz ML, Ayus JC. New aspects in the pathogenesis, prevention, and treatment of hyponatremic encephalopathy in children. Pediatr Nephrol. 2010;25:1225–38.

36. Carlotti AP, Bohn D, Mallie J-P, Halperin ML. Tonicity balance, and not electrolyte-free water calculations, more accurately guides therapy for acute changes in natremia. Intensive Care Med. 2001; 27:921–4.

37. Le Quesne LP, Lewis AAG. Postoperative water and sodium retention. Lancet. 1953;i:153–8.

38. Shafiee MAS, Bohn D, Hoorn EJ, Halperin ML. How to select optimal maintenance intravenous fluid therapy. Q J Med. 2003;96: 601–10.

39. Bailey AG, McNaull PP, Jooste E, Tuchman JB. Perioperative crystalloid and colloid fluid management in children: where are we and how did we get here? Anesth Analg. 2010;110:375–90.

40. Steele A, Gowrishankar M, Abrahamson S, et al. Postoperative hyponatremia despite near-isotonic saline infusion: a phenomenon of desalination. Ann Intern Med. 1997;126:20–5.

41. Dennhardt N, Schoof S, Osthaus WA, et al. Alterations of acid-base balance, electrolyte concentrations, and osmolality caused by nonionic hyperosmolar contrast medium during pediatric cardiac catheterization. Paediatr Anaesth. 2011;21:1119–23.

42. Hardesty DA, Sanborn MR, Parker WE, Storm PB. Perioperative seizure incidence and risk factors in 223 pediatric brain tumor patients without prior seizures. J Neurosurg Pediatr. 2011;7:609–15.

43. Sarnaik A, Meert K, Hackbarth R, Fleischmann L. Management of hyponatremic seizures in children with hypertonic saline: a safe and effective strategy. Crit Care Med. 1991;19:758–62.

44. Levine JP, Stelnicki E, Weiner HL, et al. Hyponatremia in the postoperative craniofacial pediatric patient population: a connection to cerebral salt wasting syndrome and management of the disorder. Plast Reconstr Surg. 2001;108:1501–8.

45. Jimenez R, Casado-Flores J, Nieto M, Garcia-Teresa MA. Cerebral salt wasting syndrome in children with acute central nervous system injury. Pediatr Neurol. 2006;35:261–3.

46. Hardesty DA, Kilbaugh TJ, Storm PB. Cerebral salt wasting syndrome in post-operative brain tumor patients. Neurocrit Care. 2011. doi:10.1007/s12028-011-9618-4.

47. Singh S, Bohn D, Carlotti AP, et al. Cerebral salt wasting: truths, fallacies, theories, and challenges. Crit Care Med. 2002;30:2575–9.

48. Hollenberg NK. Set point for sodium homeostasis: surfeit, deficit, and their implications. Kidney Int. 1980;17:423–9.

49. Papadimitriou DT, Spiteri A, Pagnier A, et al. Mineralocorticoid deficiency in post-operative cerebral salt wasting. J Pediatr Endocrinol Metab. 2007;20:1145–50.

50. Di RC, Caldarelli M, Tamburrini G, Massimi L. Surgical management of craniopharyngiomas – experience with a pediatric series. J Pediatr Endocrinol Metab. 2006;19 Suppl 1:355–66.

51. Lindsay RC, Seckl JR, Padfield PL. The triple-phase response – problems of water balance after pituitary surgery. Postgrad Med J. 1995;837:439–41.

52. Hopper N, Albanese A, Ghirardello S, Maghnie M. The preoperative assessment of craniopharyngiomas. J Pediatr Endocrinol Metab. 2006;19(Suppl):325–7.

53. Paja M, Lucas T, Garcia-Uria J, et al. Hypothalamic-pituitary dysfunction in children with craniopharyngioma. Clin Endocrinol. 1995;42:467–73.

54. Hensen J, Henig A, Fahlbusch R, et al. Prevalence, predictors and patterns of postoperative polyuria and hyponatremia in the immediate course after transsphenoidal surgery for pituitary adenomas. Clin Endocrinol. 1999;50:431–9.

55. Thomas Jr WC. Diabetes insipidus. J Clin Endocrinol. 1957;17: 565–8.

56. Poon WS, Lolin TF, Yeung CP, et al. Water and sodium disorders following surgical excision of pituitary region tumors. Acta Neurochir. 1996;138:921–7.

57. Davis BB, Bloom ME, Field JB, et al. Hyponatremia in pituitary insufficiency. Metabolism. 1969;18:821–32.

58. Robson WL, Leung AK. Hyponatremia in children treated with desmopressin. Arch Pediatr Adolesc Med. 1998;152:930–1.

59. Bhalla P, Eaton FE, Coulter JB, et al. Lesson of the week: hyponatremic seizures and excessive intake of hypotonic fluids in young children. Br Med J. 1999;11:1554–7.

60. Balestrieri FJ, Chernow B, Rainey TG. Postcraniotomy diabetes insipidus, who's at risk? Crit Care Med. 1982;10:108–10.

61. Chanson P, Jedynak CP, Dabrowski G, et al. Ultra-low doses of vasopressin in the management of DI. Crit Care Med. 1987;15: 44–6.

62. Wise-Faberowski L, Soriano SG, Ferrari L, et al. Perioperative management of diabetes insipidus in children. J Neurosurg Anesthesiol. 2004;16:220–5.

63. Vlasselaers D. Blood glucose control in the intensive care unit: discrepancy between belief and practice. Crit Care. 2010;14:145.

64. Vlasselaers D, Milants I, Desmet L, et al. Intensive insulin therapy for patients in paediatric intensive care: a prospective, randomized controlled study. Lancet. 2009;373:547–56.

65. Branco RG, Xavier L, Garcia PC, et al. Prospective operationalization and feasibility of a glycemic control protocol in critically ill children. Pediatr Crit Care Med. 2011;12:265–70.

66. Sandstrom K, Nilsson K, Andreasson S, et al. Metabolic consequences of different perioperative fluid therapies in the neonatal period. Acta Anaesthesiol Scand. 1993;37:170–5.

67. Gottschalk A, Berkow LC, Stevens RD, et al. Prospective evaluation of pain and analgesic use following major elective intracranial surgery. J Neurosurg. 2007;106:210–6.

68. Chiaretti A, Viola L, Pietrini D, et al. Preemptive analgesia with tramadol and fentanyl in pediatric neurosurgery. Childs Nerv Syst. 2000;16:93–100.

69. Sudheer PS, Logan SW, Terblanche C, et al. Comparison of the analgesic efficacy and respiratory effects of morphine, tramadol and codeine after craniotomy. Anaesthesia. 2007;62:555–60.

70. Marx CM, Smith PG, Lowrie LH, et al. Optimal sedation of mechanically ventilated pediatric critical care patients. Crit Care Med. 1994;22:163–70.

71. Ista E, van Dijk M, Tibboel D, de Hoog M. Assessment of sedation levels in pediatric intensive care patients can be improved by using the COMFORT "behavior" scale. Pediatr Crit Care Med. 2005;6:58–63.

72. Chiaretti A, Genovese O, Antonelli A, et al. Patient-controlled analgesia with fentanyl and midazolam in children with postoperative neurosurgical pain. Childs Nerv Syst. 2008;24:119–24.

73. Hutchens MP, Memtsoudis S, Sadovnikoff N. Propofol for sedation in neuro-intensive care. Neurocrit Care. 2006;4:54–62.

74. Wheeler DS, Vaux KK, Ponaman ML, Poss BW. The safe and effective use of propofol sedation in children undergoing diagnostic and therapeutic procedures: experience in a pediatric ICU and a review of the literature. Pediatr Emerg Care. 2003;19:385–92.

75. Diaz SM, Rodarte A, Foley J, Capparelli EV. Pharmacokinetics of dexmedetomidine in postsurgical pediatric intensive care unit patients: preliminary study. Pediatr Crit Care Med. 2007;8:419–24.

76. Olutoye OA, Glover CD, Diefenderfer JW, et al. The effect of intraoperative dexmedetomidine on postoperative analgesia and sedation in pediatric patients undergoing tonsillectomy and adenoidectomy. Anesth Analg. 2010;111:490–5.

77. Tobias JD. Dexmedetomidine to treat opioid withdrawal in infants following prolonged sedation in the pediatric ICU. J Opioid Manag. 2006;2:201–5.

78. Spentzas T, Escue JE, Patters AB, Varelas PN. Brain tumor resection in children: neurointensive care unit course and resource utilization. Pediatr Crit Care Med. 2010;11:718–22.

79. Piastra M, Di Rocco C, Caresta E, et al. Blood loss and short-term outcome of infants undergoing brain tumour removal. J Neurooncol. 2008;90:191–200.

80. O'Shaughnessy DF, Atterbury C, Bolton MP, et al. Guidelines for the use of fresh-frozen plasma, cryoprecipitate and cryosupernatant. Br J Haematol. 2004;126:11–28.

81. Iberti TJ, Miller M, Abalos A, et al. Abnormal coagulation profile in brain tumor patients during surgery. Neurosurgery. 1994;34:389–94.

82. Goobie SM, Soriano SG, Zurakowski D, et al. Hemostatic changes in pediatric neurosurgical patients as evaluated by thromboelastograph. Anesth Analg. 2001;93:887–92.

83. Ruttmann TG. Hemodilution enhances coagulation. Br J Anaesth. 2002;88:470–2.

84. Hsieh V, Molnar I, Ramadan A, et al. Hypercoagulability syndrome associated with cerebral lesions. Prospective study of coagulation during surgery of primary brain tumors (17 cases). Neurochirurgie. 1986;32:404–9.

85. Williams GD, Ellenbogen RG, Gruss JS. Abnormal coagulation during pediatric craniofacial surgery. Pediatr Neurosurg. 2001;35:5–12.

86. Tasker RC. Emergency treatment of acute seizures and status epilepticus. Arch Dis Child. 1998;79:78–83.

87. Nakagawa TA, Ashwal S, Mathur M, et al. Clinical report – guidelines for the determination of brain death in infants and children: an update of the 1987 task force recommendations. Pediatrics. 2011;128:e720–40.

88. Wijdicks EFM, Varelas PN, Gronseth GS, Greer DM. Evidence-based guideline update: determining brain death in adults. Report of the Quality Standards Subcommittee of the American Academy of Neurology. Neurology. 2010;74:1911–8.

89. The Quality Standards Subcommittee of the American Academy of Neurology. Practice parameters for determining brain death in adults (summary statement). Neurology. 1995;45:1012–4.

90. Report of special task force. Guidelines for the determination of brain death in children. American Academy of Pediatrics Task Force on Brain Death in Children. Pediatrics. 1987;80:298–300.

91. Canadian Neurocritical Care Group. Guidelines for the diagnosis of brain death. Can J Neurol Sci. 1999;26:64–6.

Acute Ischemic Stroke: Therapy and Guidelines

33

Vishnumurthy Shushrutha Hedna, Brian L. Hoh, and Michael F. Waters

Contents

V.S. Hedna, MD
Department of Neurology, University of Florida College of
Medicine, 1600 SW Archer Road, Gainesville, FL 32611, USA
e-mail: v.hedna@neurology.ufl.edu

B.L. Hoh, MD, FACS, FAHA, FAANS
Department of Neurological Surgery,
University of Florida College of Medicine,
100265, Gainesville, FL 32610, USA
e-mail: brian.hoh@neurosurgery.ufl.edu

M.F. Waters, MD, PhD (✉)
Department of Neurology, McKnight Brain Institute,
University of Florida College of Medicine, 100236,
Gainesville, FL 32610, USA
e-mail: mwaters@neurology.ufl.edu

Abstract

The focus of this chapter is ischemic stroke necessitating intensive care unit (ICU) level of care, including discussions of pathophysiology and stroke subtypes, relative outcomes, and potential treatment modalities. Consideration is given to current therapies and guidelines in the management of all types of ischemic stroke including intravenous and intra-arterial thrombolysis, blood pressure management, and supportive care.

Keywords

Stroke • Thrombotic stroke • Hemorrhagic stroke • Neurological outcome • Stroke therapy, mechanical • Stroke therapy, pharmacological

Introduction

The focus of this chapter will be ischemic stroke necessitating intensive care unit (ICU) level of care and will include discussions of pathophysiology and stroke subtypes, relative outcomes, and potential treatment modalities. Consideration will be given to current therapies and guidelines in the management of all types of ischemic stroke including intravenous and intra-arterial thrombolysis, blood pressure management, and supportive care.

Ischemic Stroke Pathophysiology

Ischemic strokes are divided into five main categories as per TOAST criterion [1–3] (Table 33.1 and Fig. 33.1): lacunar strokes, large vessel atherosclerosis, cardio-embolism, cryptogenic, and strokes of undetermined causes.

Small vessel (lacunes) infarctions are due to fibrinoid necrosis and or progressive lipohyalinosis leading to symptoms

A.J. Layon et al. (eds.), *Textbook of Neurointensive Care*,
DOI 10.1007/978-1-4471-5226-2_33, © Springer-Verlag London 2013

Table 33.1 Classification of ischemic stroke (TOAST criteria)

1. Small vessel (lacunar) stroke

2. Large vessel atherosclerotic stroke (includes both extra and intracranial disease)

3. Cardio-embolic stroke

4. Cryptogenic stroke

5. Stroke of undetermined causes (which includes dissection, vasculitis and others)

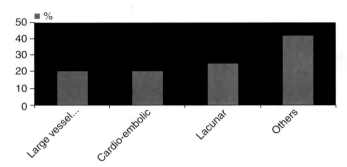

Fig. 33.1 Distribution of ischemic stroke as per etiology

arising from a single perforating artery distribution. The infarcts by imaging definition are usually less than 15 mm in diameter. Classic lacunar syndromes are mainly due to hypertension, diabetes, dyslipidemia, smoking, and metabolic syndromes and less commonly related to genetic causes, age, and substance abuse. Classic lacunar syndromes reported include pure motor hemiparesis (internal capsule or pons), pure sensory symptoms (thalamus), sensorimotor, clumsy-hand dysarthria with facial weakness (pons, internal capsule cerebral peduncle), and ataxic hemiparesis (internal capsule, pons, thalamo-capsular, corona radiata, ACA, red nucleus).

Brain stem small vessel ischemic strokes include:

- *Midbrain syndromes*: Weber's (third nerve palsy with contralateral hemiparesis), Claude's (third cranial nerve palsy with contralateral ataxia), and Benedict's (third cranial nerve palsy with contralateral tremor)
- *Pontine syndromes*: Millard-Gubler (sixth and seventh cranial nerve palsy with contralateral hemiparesis) and Foville's syndrome
- *Medullary syndromes*: Medial medullary (tongue weakness with contralateral ataxia and hemiparesis) and lateral medullary syndrome (ipsilateral ataxia, loss of pain and temperature in face) and Horner's syndrome with contralateral loss of pain and temperature in arm and leg

Large vessel ischemic stroke events are comprised of *atherosclerotic and cardio-embolic events* which constitute almost 40 % of all ischemic strokes [4]. Large vessel ischemic stroke events are mainly due to atherosclerosis in the major extra- or intracranial artery. Atherosclerosis can lead to either plaque ulceration with thrombosis (and subsequent local occlusion) or distal embolization from plaque rupture (leading to artery to artery embolism). When young patients

with no risk factors present with larger vessel occlusion, dissection of the large vessel is an important consideration. When dissection is the etiology, the presentation is dramatic with neck pain and eye pain with or without associated Horner syndrome and may coincide with traumatic neck manipulation or underlying fibromuscular dysplasia (FMD) (Fig. 33.2). There is also a subset of *ischemic strokes due to cerebral hypoperfusion blood pressure drops* in the setting of hemodynamically significant narrowing of the intra- or extracranial blood vessels. This will cause watershed injury which can be readily identified by advanced brain imaging. The most common sites of extracranial atherosclerosis are the origin of internal carotid artery (ICA) and vertebral artery (VA). In the intracranial circulation, the most common sites for atherosclerosis are supraclinoid ICA, carotid siphon, proximal MCA at the origin (M1 segment), distal vertebral artery, and proximal to mid-basilar artery.

Cerebral embolism is the next large category responsible for ischemic strokes. Even though emboli may originate from multiple sources including atrial fibrillation, artificial valve, endocarditis, intracardiac thrombus, or right-to-left shunt, a large number of embolic cerebral infarcts may remain *cryptogenic*.

Clinical Syndromes Associated with Large Vessel Occlusion (Fig. 33.3)

MCA Stroke

The clinical syndromes of M1 segment occlusion are altered sensorium, neglect (nondominant lobe), aphasia (dominant lobe), gaze deviation towards the lesion, homonymous hemianopia, and face/arm/leg weakness and numbness. M2 segment occlusion (superior division) presents with Broca's aphasia and gaze deviation towards the lesion associated with face/arm/leg weakness and numbness. M2 segment occlusion (inferior division) presents with Wernicke's aphasia and homonymous hemianopia with or without neglect.

ACA Stroke

ACA stroke presents with psychomotor slowing, abulia, mono-paresis of the contralateral leg and, rarely, paraplegia (if both ACAs are arising from a single origin in the ICA).

Dominant parietal lobe strokes can cause Gerstmann syndrome (finger anomia, right-left confusion, acalculia, and agraphia) and apraxia (e.g., ideomotor, limb kinetic, or ideational apraxia). Nondominant parietal lobe strokes can cause delirium, dressing apraxia, and constructional apraxia. Bilateral parietal-occipital stroke can cause Balint's syndrome (visual apraxia, optic ataxia, simultanagnosia).

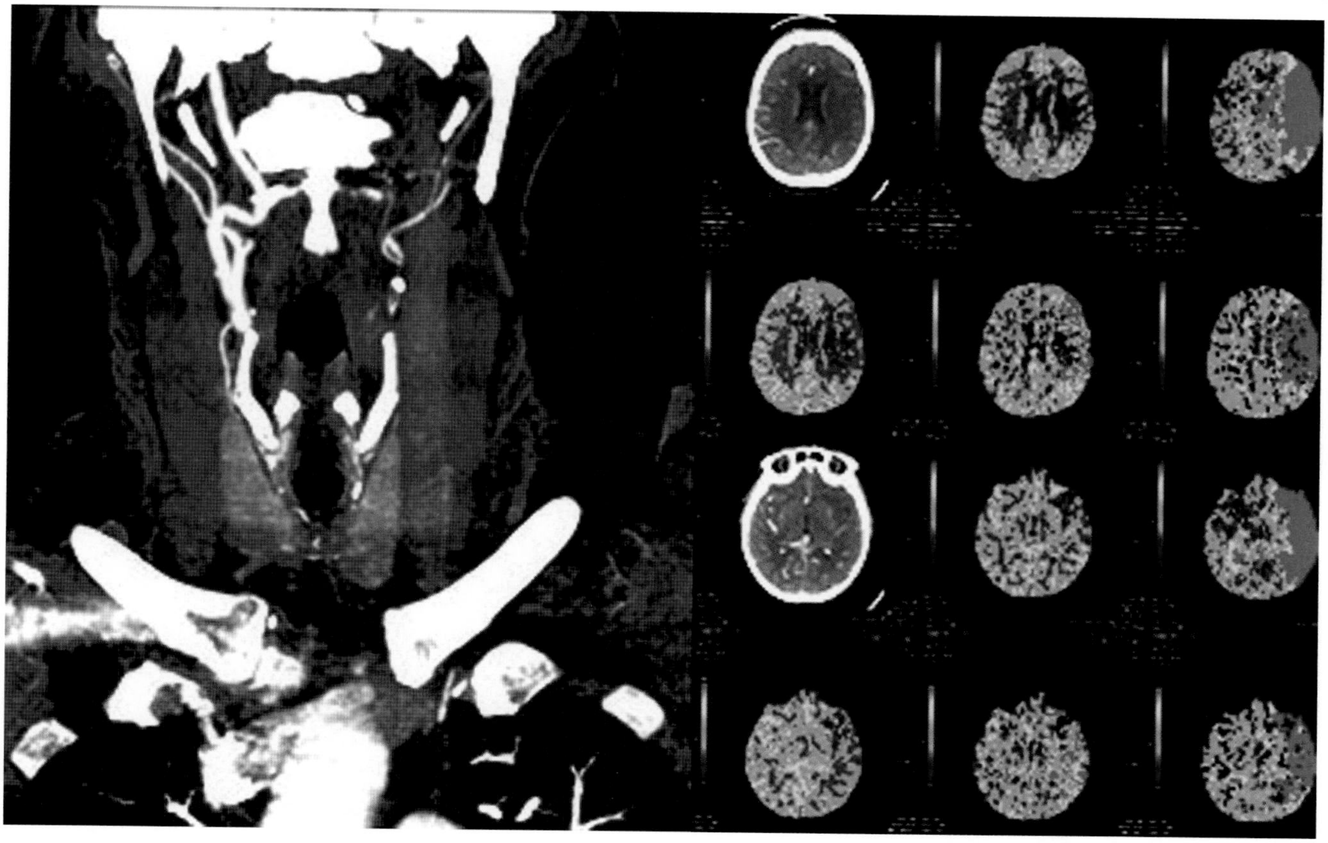

Fig. 33.2 Cervical artery dissection is more commonly seen in young patients. The neck CT angiogram in a 28-year-old male who experienced sudden onset of severe left neck pain after bouts of cough due to chest infection shows occluded left internal carotid artery (*left panel*).

Examination revealed left Horner's syndrome, global aphasia, and right hemiplegia. CT perfusion of the brain (*right panel*) shows elevated time to peak (TTP), reduced cerebral blood flow (CBF), and reduced cerebral blood volume (CBV) in the entire left MCA territory

PCA Stroke Involvement of the Occipital Lobe

PCA stroke involvement of the occipital lobe will present with homonymous hemianopia with or without contralateral weakness/numbness, Anton's syndrome (denial of blindness), Charles Bonnet syndrome (visual hallucinations), and alexia without agraphia (occipital lobe and splenium of the corpus callosum involvement). PCA stroke involvements of the occipital-temporal lobe (nondominant lobe) can cause prosopagnosia which is inability to recognize a face.

Other Important Causes of Ischemic Stroke

Other important causes of ischemic stroke include primary or secondary vasculitis, substance abuse, hypercoagulable states including malignancy, genetic disorders, and prothrombotic conditions. The prothrombotic conditions which can be associated with ischemic strokes are antiphospholipid syndrome, prothrombin gene mutation, lupus anticoagulant, anticardiolipin antibodies, activated protein C resistance, factor V mutation, MTHFR gene mutation, protein C, protein S, and antithrombin III. Gene disorders primarily causing strokes

are CADASIL, CARASIL, COL4A1, and cystatin C mutation. Other conditions include Fabry's disease, Marfan's syndrome, sickle cell disease, moyamoya syndrome, and chromosome 9P21 disorders, among others [5].

Stroke Mimics

Consideration should be given to stroke mimics which – constituting up to 15 % of stroke admissions – may present with acute focal neurological deficit. Common conditions mimicking stroke are seizures, migraines, AV malformations, brain tumors, posterior reversible encephalopathy syndrome (PRES), infective emboli, hypoglycemia, hyperglycemia, meningoencephalitis, and psychogenic etiology.

Evaluation

The initial basic diagnostic studies in all acute ischemic stroke patients include blood studies (blood glucose, basic metabolic panel, complete blood count, cardiac enzymes, coagulation labs), oxygen saturation, EKG, and non-contrast

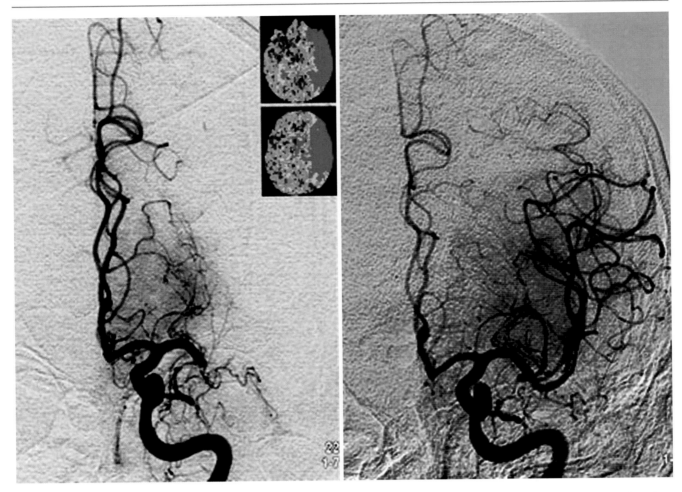

Fig. 33.3 Left middle cerebral artery (M1 segment) occlusion. The cerebral angiogram (*left*) shows occluded left MCA M1 segment (cutoff) in a 68-year-old male who presented with aphasia, left gaze deviation, and right hemiparesis. The CT perfusion (*inset*) shows elevated time to peak (TTP) in entire left MCA distribution. Patient had mechanical thrombectomy with complete recanalization of left M1 segment (*right*)

brain CT or brain MRI. In some patient populations, evaluation includes liver function tests, urine toxicology, a pregnancy test, arterial blood gas, chest x-ray, advanced coagulation labs, EEG, and lumbar puncture. The guidelines published by the American Heart Association/American Stroke Association (AHA/ASA) in 2013 suggest that although it is desirable to know the results of these tests before giving intravenous thrombolytics, therapy should not be delayed until results are available unless the patient is on anticoagulation, there is a suspicion of a bleeding disorder, or the patient has recently received heparin [6].

The clinical evaluation of acute stroke usually begins in the emergency department. The dedicated stroke centers have protocols to reduce the door-to-therapy time. The abbreviated neurological assessment, such as the National Institutes of Health Stroke Scale (NIHSS), is one of the easily administered standard neurological scoring systems employed in many institutions (Table 33.2).

The most important consideration in patients presenting with focal neurological deficit is to determine whether they qualify for thrombolytic therapy. Hence, the crucial step is to exclude intracerebral hemorrhage and stroke mimics. The first-line investigation will be brain computed tomography (CT) without contrast, which is a quick and readily available modality of imaging. In some institutions, CT perfusion or magnetic resonance (MR) perfusion along with angiogram has become part of the initial stroke evaluation. CT perfusion and MR diffusion-perfusion-weighted (Fig. 33.4) imaging play an important role to detect the volume of salvageable brain tissue, the "penumbra." This information becomes important especially when endovascular intervention is considered. In the perfusion studies, time to peak (TTP), cerebral blood volume (CBV), cerebral blood flow (CBF), and mean transit time (MTT) will give vital information about the infarct zone and penumbra.

Table 33.2 Adapted National Institute of Heath Stroke Scale (NIHSS)

Six tests for higher cognitive functions						*Total score=*	
Level of consciousness	Alert-0	Drowsy-1	Stupor-2	Corno-3			
Orientation (month, age)	Both correct-0	One correct-1	Both incorrect-2				
Obey commands (open and close eyes) (make first and let go)	Both correct-0	One correct-1	Both incorrect-2				
Dysarthria	Normal-0	Mild/moderate-1	Incomprehensible-2	Intubated-UT			
Aphasia	Normal-0	Mild/moderate-1	Severe-2	Mute-3			
Neglect – double simultaneous stimulation	Normal-0	Partial-I	Complete-2				
Three tests for cranial nerve functions							
Gaze deviation	Normal-0	Partial-1	Complete-2				
Visual field deficit (Hemianopia)	Normal-0	Partial-1	Complete-2	Bilateral-3			
Facial palsy	Normal-0	Minor-1	Partial-2	Complete-3			
One test for motor function							
Drift testing in right UE (10 s)	Normal-0	Drift-1	Some effort against gravity-1	No effort against gravity-2	No movements-4	Amputation-UT	
Drift testing in left UE (10 s)	Normal-0	Drift-1	Some effort against gravity-1	No effort against gravity-2	No movements-4	Amputation-UT	
Drift testing in right LE (5 s)	Normal-0	Drift-1	Some effort against gravity -1	No effort against gravity-2	No movement-4	Amputation-UT	
Drift testing in left LE (5 s)	Normal-0	Drift-1	Some effort against gravity-1	No effort against gravity-2	No movement-4	Amputation-UT	
One test for sensory function							
Pain sensation	Normal-0	Partial loss-1	Severe loss-2				
One test for cerebellar function							
Limb Ataxia	Absent-0	Present one limb-1	Present both limbs-2				

Data from Ref. [7]

Since the perfusion studies involve contrast administration, caution must be exercised regarding potential renal toxicity. Magnetic resonance imaging (MRI) helps in acute stroke imaging not only by confirming the stroke but also in delineating the exact stroke size and location, both of which bear on prognosis. Other modalities, including CT angiogram (CTA) and MR angiogram (MRA), are used to delineate the vessels more clearly. Noninvasive investigations employed in stroke evaluation are transcranial Doppler (TCD) and duplex carotid ultrasound. TCD is used mainly for noninvasive evaluation of the intracranial vessels but can also be used in conjunction with intravenous thrombolytics to facilitate thrombolysis (Fig. 33.5). In the setting of ischemic strokes, the diseased extracranial vessel has to be identified in order to pursue further therapeutic options including carotid endarterectomy or stenting. Carotid duplex ultrasound is one of the most commonly used investigations to identify the hemodynamically significant stenosis in the extracranial circulation. Conventional cerebral angiogram can be used in acute stroke scenarios for both therapeutic and diagnostic reasons. The catheter access in this procedure can be used for intra-arterial thrombolysis, for mechanical thrombectomy, or, when there is a diagnostic dilemma, to diagnose vasculitis, moyamoya syndrome, or vessel dissection. Recently, MRI of the head and neck with T1 fat suppression imaging modality has become an important test to rule out vessel dissection. Routine stroke laboratory tests, comprised of complete blood count (CBC), complete metabolic panel (CMP), fasting lipid panel, thyroid function, hemoglobin A1c, vitamin B12, and folate levels, should be obtained. In special circumstances, drug screen, ESR, CRP, blood cultures, ANA, syphilis test, antiphospholipid panel, lupus panel, vasculitis panel, and thrombophilia screening are used to rule out underlying systemic conditions. Baseline EKG, telemetry, transthoracic echocardiogram, swallow assessment by speech and language therapist, and physical therapy and occupational therapy assessment constitute the standard workup in any stroke patient, in general.

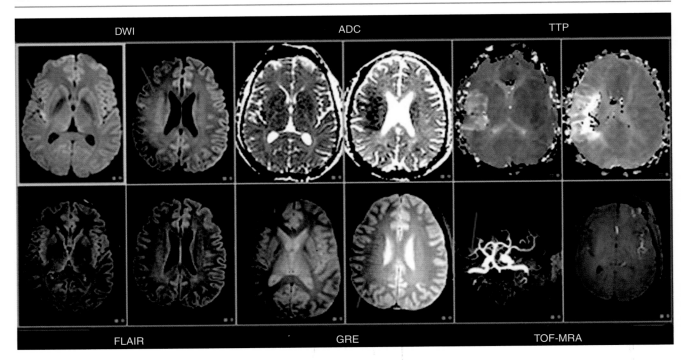

Fig. 33.4 Multimodal brain MRI will help to differentiate infarct from penumbra. A 54-year-old man presented with acute onset of left-sided weakness, facial droop, and slurred speech with NIHSS of seven. On diffusion-weighted imaging (*DWI*), there is a subtle hyperintense signal in the right insular cortex and subcortical white matter. On apparent diffusion coefficient (*ADC*), the hypointense lesion appears more prominently in the corresponding DWI region, suggesting it is cytotoxic edema seen in acute ischemic stroke. The time to peak scan shows a delay for the contrast to arrive in the right MCA territory. There is a diffusion/perfusion mismatch indicating that there is a zone of ischemic penumbra which can be salvaged if intervened and blood flow is restored. There are no early FLAIR changes. Sometimes there are hyperintense vessels in the distal branches which indicate sluggish flow likely due to collaterals. Gradient echo (*GRE*) is good to evaluate for micro bleeds, hemorrhage, and blood clot. In acute stroke, dilated veins appear as several hypointense transverse lines as seen here as in the right MCA territory. It probably indicates that the vessels are dilated with increase in blood volume in early stages of ischemia. The brain tries to extract more oxygen from the available circulation to meet the metabolic demands. On time of flight (*TOF*) MRA, there is a cutoff in the M2 segment of the right MCA, and fewer blood vessels are seen on the right compared to the left

Management (Fig. 33.6)

Intravenous Thrombolysis

The main therapy in acute ischemic stroke is intravenous (IV) tissue plasminogen activator (t-PA). The goal is to complete a quick evaluation and to begin IV thrombolysis therapy within 1 h of the patient's arrival. It is crucial to rapidly evaluate the patient using the NIH stroke scale, and, once it is determined that there is no intracerebral hemorrhage on brain imaging, a quick decision has to be made to administer the thrombolytics using the inclusion and exclusion criteria published by the NINDS trial [6, 7]. This trial, in the past, has helped us to establish the strict inclusion criteria for the administration of t-PA in acute stroke patients. IV t-PA received FDA approval in 1996 for acute ischemic stroke after NINDS trial showed an increase in the odds of a favorable outcome (OR, 1.9; 95 % CI, 1.2–2.9). While IV t-PA has a higher risk of intracerebral hemorrhage when compared to placebo (6 % vs. 0.6 %), its benefit by far outweighs the risk. IV t-PA, when compared to placebo, showed a better chance of recovery and functional measures in global disability (40 % vs. 28 %), global outcome (43 % vs. 32 %), activities of daily living (53 % vs. 38 %), and neurological deficits (34 % vs. 20 %), when measured 90 days after its administration. The benefit was sustained even 1 year after stroke [6]. IV t-PA in a dose of 0.9 mg/kg (maximum dose is 90 mg) is recommended for patients who may be treated within 3 h of onset of ischemic stroke, once the patient is selected according to the inclusion and exclusion criteria. Ten percent of the total dose is given as bolus and the rest as infusion over 1 h. Ideally, the door-to-needle time should be within 60 min from arrival.

Recently the inclusion and exclusion criteria have been updated by the AHA/ASA [6]. These criteria are (1) symptoms consistent with acute brain infarction, with a clearly defined onset of within 3 h (if the onset was not witnessed the ictus is measured from the time the patient was last seen to be at baseline); (2) a significant neurological deficit expected to result in a long-term disability; and (3) age greater than 18 years.

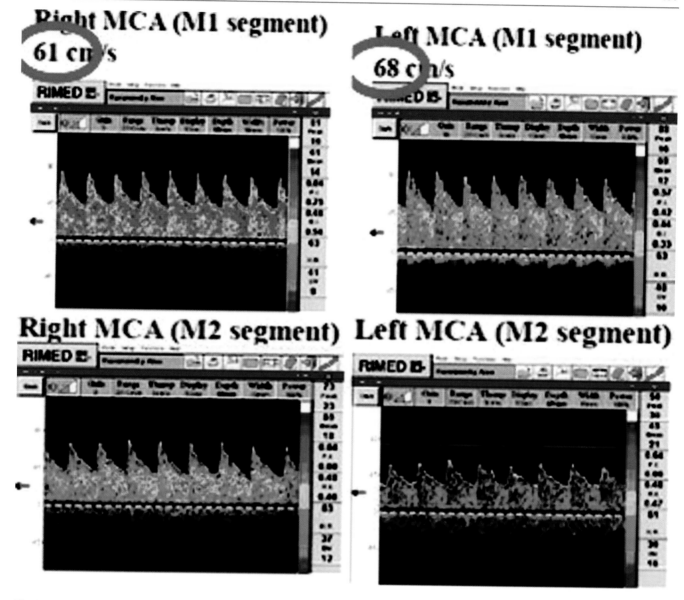

Fig. 33.5 Transcranial Doppler (TCD) study in a normal patient. This study demonstrates normal flow velocity in the right and left MCA distribution. In patients with significant intracranial vessel stenosis, TCD will demonstrate higher velocities (>200 cm/s)

The exclusion criteria can be divided into absolute and relative contraindications. The absolute contraindications are:

- Frank hemorrhage on brain imaging
- Frank hypo-density in more than one-third of the middle cerebral artery (MCA) territory
- Presence of structural lesions in the brain which contraindicates thrombolysis (including brain tumor, abscess, aneurysm, and vascular malformation)
- Heparin use within 48 h resulting in abnormally elevated activated partial thromboplastin time (aPTT) greater than the upper limit of normal
- A history of intracranial bleed or symptoms suggestive of subarachnoid hemorrhage
- Recent intracranial or intraspinal surgery
- Significant head trauma within 3 months
- Known bleeding diathesis including renal or hepatic insufficiency
- Current use of anticoagulation with international normalized ratio (INR) more than 1.7 or partial thromboplastin time (PT) more than 15 s
- Current use of direct thrombin inhibitors or direct factor Xa inhibitors with elevated sensitive laboratory tests such as aPTT, INR, platelet count, and ecarin clotting time (ECT); thrombin time (TT); or appropriate factor Xa activity assays
- Platelet count less than 100,000 cells/μL

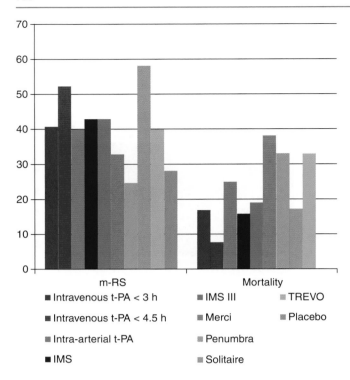

Fig. 33.6 Comparison of outcomes from different recanalization techniques in acute ischemic stroke. Functional outcome, mortality, and morbidity vary from intervention to intervention in acute stroke management. Favorable modified Rankin scale (m-RS) and survival rate is seen with Solitaire device

- Glucose concentration less than 50 mg/dL
- Systolic blood pressure greater than 185 mmHg or diastolic blood pressure greater than 110 mmHg
- Arterial puncture at the noncompressible site within 7 days
- Stroke within 3 months.
  The relative contraindications are:
- Rapidly improving symptoms
- Pregnancy
- Seizure at onset
- Major surgery or trauma within 14 days
- Recent myocardial infarction within 3 months
- Internal bleed (including gastrointestinal, urologic, respiratory) within 21 days

The patient should be admitted to the intensive care or stroke unit for monitoring. During the IV t-PA administration, if the patient has worsening neurological examination or develops severe headache, acute hypertension, nausea, or vomiting, the infusion should be discontinued and a stat CT scan obtained to rule out intracranial bleed. If there is development of angioedema (incidence is 1.3–5.1 %), the drug should be stopped and standard allergic reaction therapy initiated. For the first 24 h post-infusion, avoid any invasive procedures such as nasogastric tubes, indwelling bladder catheters, or central/arterial/PICC lines, if patient safety is

not compromised by doing so. Obtain a follow-up brain CT or MRI scan at 24 h after IV t-PA before starting anticoagulants or antiplatelet agents.

Blood Pressure Management During and After Thrombolysis

Treatment of elevated blood pressure in thrombolytic eligible acute stroke patients is very important to prevent hemorrhagic conversion of the infract zone and to improve outcome. At the time of t-PA administration, if the BP is greater than 185/110 mmHg, IV labetalol (10–20 mg over 1–2 min, may repeat once) or nicardipine infusion (5 mg/h IV, titrate up by 2.5 mg/h every 5–15 min, to a maximum of 15 mg/h) is usually recommended. If there are contraindications for these drugs, other IV agents such as hydralazine or enalaprilat may be considered. If BP is not maintained at or below 185/110 mmHg, do not administer t-PA. Measure blood pressure and perform neurological assessments every 15 min during and after t-PA infusion for 2 h, then every 30 min for 6 h, and then hourly until 24 h after t-PA therapy [6].

When the desired BP is reached, adjust the medications to maintain it in less than 180/105 mmHg range for the entirety of the first 24 h. If the systolic blood pressure increases to greater than 180 mmHg or if diastolic blood pressure increases to greater than 105 mmHg, an increase in the frequency of blood pressure measurements is advocated, and a continuous infusion with either labetalol at 2–8 mg/min or nicardipine 5 mg/h (titrate to desired effect by 2.5 mg/h every 5–15 min, maximum 15 mg/h) can be used. If BP not controlled with measures just discussed or if diastolic BP is greater than 140 mmHg, IV sodium nitroprusside infusion is recommended [6].

The usefulness of other intravenous thrombolytics, fibrinolytics, and defibrinogenetic agents like urokinase, tenecteplase, reteplase, desmoteplase, streptokinase, and ancrod is still under investigation and currently not recommended in acute ischemic stroke [6].

Current AHA/ASA recommendations for t-PA administration in ischemic stroke of onset between 3 and 4.5 h as studies show favorable results. The ECASS (I, II, III), ATLANTIS A, and ATLANTIS B have shown the benefit of t-PA for patients in the 3–4.5 h window with better outcomes (adjusted OR, 1.40; 95 % CI, 1.05–1.85) in relation to post-stroke disability with no increase in mortality (13 % vs. 12 %) but with higher rates of ICH (5.9 % vs. 1.7 %) when compared to placebo [8]. But the FDA has not approved the extended window for IV t-PA. IV t-PA (0.9 mg/kg, maximum dose 90 mg) can be recommended in patients presenting between 3 and 4.5 h after stroke onset if they qualify using the inclusion and exclusion criteria just discussed. However, the extended window will not apply in the following patient category: (1) those greater than 80 years, (2) those on oral anticoagulants regardless of their INR, (3) NIHSS score greater than 25, (4) imaging evidence of ischemic injury involving more than 1/3 of the MCA territory, and (5) history of stroke associated with diabetes mellitus.

Some trials, such as the international stroke trial (IST-III), have addressed the safety of extending the time window of t-PA up to 6 h, but results were disappointing as they tend to show increase in the ICH rates (7 % vs. 1 %) with no significant difference in outcome and mortality [9]. Current guidelines do not recommend IV t-PA beyond 4.5 h.

Thrombolysis in the Setting of Oral Anticoagulation

When patients on traditional or newer oral anticoagulants (OA) present with ischemic stroke and t-PA is under consideration, the issue of safety arises. Recently, newer oral anticoagulants like dabigatran (direct thrombin inhibitor), rivaroxaban, and apixaban (factor Xa inhibitors) have been approved by FDA for primary and secondary stroke prophylaxis in patients with atrial fibrillation. The current guidelines for t-PA administration in Coumadin-consuming patients are well established. However, for newer anticoagulants, traditional coagulation tests are not reliable for measuring the anticoagulant effect. In patients using dabigatran, the suggestion is to use sensitive tests like TT and ECT, which show a good linear correlation with dabigatran plasma concentration. If normal, t-PA might be considered. A major limitation is the time duration for the results to become available in the ED. With the direct factor Xa inhibitors (rivaroxaban and apixaban), direct factor Xa activity assays may be used; as these tests are not routinely performed, results may take hours before becoming available. Until more data looking at the safety of these newer OA agents become available, the current AHA/ASA recommendations are that the use of IV t-PA in patients taking newer OA is not recommended unless [1] tests such as ECT, TT, APTT, INR, platelet count, and direct factor Xa activity assays are normal or [2] the patient has not received these agents for at least 2 days (assuming normal renal function). The same rules apply to patients who are on OA, in whom intra-arterial t-PA is being considered [6].

Intra-arterial and Mechanical Endovascular Therapy in Acute Stroke

The overall recanalization rate with IV thrombolytics is only 46.2 %. IV thrombolysis has a variable effect on large vessel occlusive thrombus and shows high failure rates [10]. The recanalization rate depends on various factors, including the

Table 33.3 Variation in recanalization rate in different vasculature. ICA recanalization varies from 14 to 30 %. Vertebral-basilar circulation has better recanalization chances

%	IV t-PA	IA	Combined (IV+IA)	Mechanical
MCA/ACA	55	66	66	78
Vertebral/basilar artery	80	63	66	100
ICA	14	49	60	77

vessel involved, duration, and modality used for recanalization; for example, the recanalization rate for the extracranial ICA from intravenous thrombolysis is only 30 % [11] (Table 33.3). The recanalization rate is slightly better for middle cerebral artery (MCA) and highest for posterior circulation. This led to the development of alternative recanalization techniques including endovascular approach mainly in patients failing intravenous thrombolysis or in patients who do not qualify for intravenous thrombolysis.

Intra-arterial Thrombolysis

Intra-arterial thrombolysis has shown some promise in acute ischemic stroke. There are a few advantages: (1) the thrombolytic dose is about one-third that of the IV dose, so it can be used in cases where there are contraindications for IV thrombolysis; (2) it can be used in patients who have failed to recanalize with IV thrombolysis; (3) there is direct visualization and confirmation of thrombolysis; (4) if intra-arterial thrombolysis fails, mechanical thrombectomy can be achieved using the same access.

Results from two major studies – The Prolyse in Acute Cerebral Thromboembolism (PROACT) II [12] and the Middle Cerebral Artery Embolism Local Fibrinolytic Intervention Trial (MELT) [13] – support the use of intra-arterial approach. The PROACT II enrolled 180 patients with acute middle cerebral artery occlusion into two randomized groups. One group received 9 mg of intra-arterial recombinant pro-urokinase (pro-UK) and heparin, the other group heparin alone within 6 h of symptom onset. Patients receiving pro-UK were more likely to have recanalization (66 % vs. 18 %) and higher functional independence at 90 days (40 % vs. 25 %); there was not much difference in the mortality between the two groups [12].

The MELT trial randomized patients to receive either local intra-arterial pro-UK (infusion of 12,000 U per 5 min to achieve complete recanalization or until a total dose of 60,000 U had been given) or no intervention. IV infusion of thrombolytic agents was prohibited in the both groups [13]. The primary end point was the proportion of patients with favorable outcomes (m-RS scores of 0–2) at 90 days; secondary end points were symptomatic intracranial hemorrhage within 24 h, mortality, recanalization rate of the MCA, and other functional outcomes including the Barthel index. The independent monitoring committee recommended stopping the trial after approval of IV infusion of r-tPA in Japan.

The primary end point did not reach statistical significance (OR 1.54; 95 % CI, 0.73–3.23; $p = 0.345$). However, the secondary end points showed excellent outcome in the pro-UK treated group, highlighting the beneficial role of intra-arterial fibrinolysis acute ischemic stroke therapy. Currently, the FDA has not approved intra-arterial pro-UK or t-PA in acute ischemic stroke thrombolysis. The optimal dose of intra-arterial t-PA is not well established, and tertiary centers use variable doses of t-PA during intra-arterial approach of thrombolysis.

Use of Transcranial Ultrasound in Augmenting Thrombolysis

The favorable biologic effect of ultrasound when combined with thrombolytic agents has been employed to enhance thrombolysis in patients with acute stroke treated with IV t-PA. The recanalization rate is higher in cases in which t-PA is combined with TCD in comparison to t-PA alone (37 % vs. 17 %). The CLOTBUST trial enrolled 126 acute middle cerebral artery stroke patients and randomly assigned them to receive t-PA combined with continuous 2 MHz TCD ultrasound or t-PA with placebo [14]. The rate of sustained complete recanalization at 2 h was significantly higher for the treatment group compared with placebo (38 % vs. 13 %) and showed a higher trend towards good clinical outcome at 3 months. Ultrasound-enhanced thrombolysis definitely shows some promise, and studies are underway in this direction.

Mechanical Thrombectomy

Mechanical thrombectomy or clot retrieval can be combined with either IV thrombolysis, the intra-arterial approach, or used alone. In order to identify the appropriate patient, there is a need for advanced imaging in the form of CT or MR angiogram with or without perfusion/diffusion studies. In the last decade, there has been a huge interest in establishing the safety of various devices for mechanical thrombectomy; the data in this regard are quite conflicting and controversial.

Studies have shown the safety of various devices for the purpose of mechanical thrombectomy in acute ischemic stroke. In the Multi MERCI® (Concentric Medical, Mountain View, CA) trial, 164 patients within 8 h of symptom onset who had large vessel occlusion were treated with newer-generation retriever MERCI devices. Patients with persistent vessel occlusion after t-PA were included in the study. Treatment with the new-generation L5 MERCI retriever resulted in successful recanalization in 57 % of treated vessels. When this therapy was combined with other adjunctive therapy including intra-arterial thrombolysis the recanalization, rate was higher at 70 % [15].

The Penumbra® (Penumbra Inc, Alameda, CA) trial enrolled 125 patients who presented within 8 h of symptom onset with NIHSS scores greater than or equal to 8 and were treated with the Penumbra System. Partial or complete recanalization rate was 82 %, and favorable clinical outcomes with an m-RS score of less than or equal to 2 were seen in 25 % of the patients [16].

In the SWIFT study, the non-inferiority of Solitaire device was compared to traditional MERCI devices. In this study, 113 subjects were randomized for mechanical thrombectomy using either Solitaire™ (ev3, Irvine, CA) or MERCI Retrieval System within 8 h of symptom onset. The recanalization rate was 61 % in Solitaire arm and 24 % in the MERCI arm ($p < 0.001$). The m-RS scale less than or equal to 2 at 90 days was 58 % (Solitaire device) versus 33 % (MERCI device), which was statistically significant [17].

In another non-inferiority trial, which recruited 178 patients, Trevo® Retriever (Stryker, Kalamazoo, MI) was compared with the traditional MERCI device. There was statistically significant higher recanalization rate (86 %) in the Trevo device arm when compared to in the MERCI arm [18] (60 %).

Currently, FDA has approved devices like MERCI (2004), Penumbra (2007), Solitaire (2012), and Trevo (2012) for mechanical clot disruption and extraction.

Recent NIH-/NINDS-funded studies such as IMS III and MR Rescue and Italian Medicines Agency-funded SYNTHESIS study failed to demonstrate superiority of endovascular therapy when compared to IV thrombolysis. In the SYNTHESIS trial, 362 patients with acute ischemic stroke within four and a half hours of symptom onset were randomly assigned to receive any of the following therapies: IV t-PA, or intra-arterial thrombolysis in conjunction to t-PA, or mechanical clot retrieval, or a combination of these approaches. Treatments were started as soon as possible after randomization. The primary outcome was modified Rankin score less than or equal to 1 at 90 days. At 90 days, after adjusting for age, sex, and stroke severity, 55 patients in the endovascular-therapy group (30.4 %) and 63 in the IV t-PA group (34.8 %) were alive without disability (OD 0.71; 95 % CI, 0.44–1.14; $p = 0.16$). There were no significant differences between the two groups in relation to mortality or fatal symptomatic intracranial hemorrhage rate. This study concluded that endovascular therapy was not superior to standard treatment with IV t-PA [19]. In the IMS III trial, 656 patients who had received IV t-PA within 3 h of symptom onset were randomly assigned to receive additional endovascular therapy or IV t-PA alone in a 2:1 ratio. The primary outcome measure was an m-RS score of less than or equal to 2 at 90 days. The study was prematurely halted because of futility. The primary end point did not differ significantly between the two groups (40.8 % for endovascular therapy versus 38.7 % for IV t-PA with 95 % CI 6.1–9.1). This trial concluded that there were similar safety outcomes and no significant difference in functional independence when combined therapy (endovascular therapy with t-PA) was compared with IV t-PA alone [20].

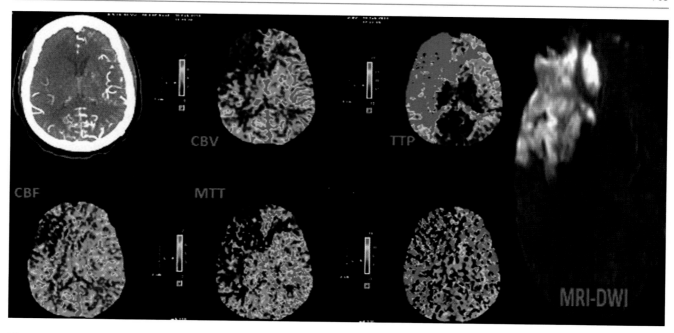

Fig. 33.7 Predictors of malignant MCA stroke. The CT angiogram with perfusion (*left*) demonstrates the entire right MCA territory ischemic involvement, putting this patient at high risk for brain edema and subsequent brain herniation. In addition there is involvement of ACA territory which has poor prognostic implication. The DWI (*right*) images show cytotoxic edema in the affected territory. Mortality can be up to 80 % from this condition

Current guidelines mandate that when patients present with acute ischemic stroke to a tertiary center with endovascular intervention capability, this should not preclude patients from receiving IV t-PA, which is the first-line therapy. Intra-arterial t-PA can be considered in carefully selected patients who have relative contraindications for IV thrombolysis and present less than 6 h after symptom onset. In cases in which endovascular mechanical thrombectomy is considered, the devices of choice should be Solitaire and Trevo [6]. However, any of these devices can be used to depending upon the expertise of the performer in carefully selected patients. In carefully selected patients, mechanical thrombectomy can be used alone or in combination with IV t-PA especially in large vessel occlusions resistant to IV t-PA alone.

Acute Neurological Complications in Intensive Care Unit

Up to 25 % of ischemic stroke patients have neurological or systemic deterioration. The usual causes are recurrent stroke, hemorrhagic transformation, cerebral edema and subsequent herniation, seizures, infection, metabolic disturbance, deep venous thrombosis (DVT), myocardial infarction, arrhythmia, heart failure, pulmonary edema, and encephalopathy due to various etiologies.

Cerebral Edema and Subsequent Herniation

Ischemic strokes involving the entire middle cerebral artery territory and large cerebellar territory are notorious for causing elevated intracranial pressure and brain herniation. The complete infarction of the middle cerebral artery territory leading to mass effect and herniation is termed a malignant MCA stroke. It is important to recognize this condition which has an incidence of 10 %, with a mortality rate of 80 % [21]. It is usually seen within 5 days of the initial event; however, development of brain edema even after 1 week has been reported. Experts suggest several patient characteristics predicting malignant transformation of MCA stroke; these are high NIH stroke scale (greater than 15), depressed level of consciousness, early nausea and vomiting, unequal pupils, history of hypertension, and heart failure. The radiological predictors (Fig. 33.7) are involvement of both ACA and PCA territories along with entire MCA territory stroke, more than 82 mL stroke lesion volume (specificity of 98 % and sensitivity of 52 %) and greater than 145 mL stroke volume (specificity of 94 % and sensitivity of 100 %) [22–25].

Conservative management of elevated ICP to minimize the edema development are head of bed elevation to 20–30°, avoiding dextrose-containing fluids, correction of hypoxia and hypercarbia, avoiding cerebral vasodilators, temporary hyperventilation, hypertonic saline, mannitol, and CSF drainage using invasive catheters. In actual practice, these

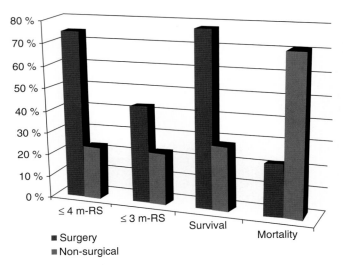

Fig. 33.8 Comparison of decompressive hemicraniectomy with conservative management using the pooled analysis of the results from three studies (DECIMAL, DESTINY, and HAMLET). The diagram demonstrates statistical significance in mortality and functional outcome in the pooled analysis from the major decompressive hemicraniectomy trials

conservative strategies are temporary and have not shown to alter the outcome. Hence, they are used in conjunction with more definitive therapy such as a decompressive hemicraniectomy, which has shown some promise. Several studies, including DECIMAL, HAMLET, and DESTINY, have shown that decompressive hemicraniectomy can be beneficial and lifesaving in malignant MCA strokes. The pooled analysis (Fig. 33.8) from these hemicraniectomy trials showed an increased chance of survival (78 % vs. 29 %) and better functional outcome in the surgical arm when compared to conservative nonsurgical therapy [24].

Factors to be considered strictly before deciding on hemicraniectomy are stroke onset less than 48 h, age between 18 and 80 years, NIH stroke scale greater than 15, decreased level of consciousness, infarct affecting at least 50 % of MCA territory with or without involvement of ACA or PCA territory on CT scan, and infarct volume more than 145 mL on MRI-DWI images. Although the surgery may improve survival and help in functional outcome, the patient's family should be made aware of the realistic potential outcomes including severe disability in patients surviving decompressive hemicraniectomy [22–25].

In cases of cerebellar stroke showing mass effect and tonsillar herniation, urgent neurosurgical evaluation for a suboccipital craniectomy or external ventricular drainage placement is considered. Current guidelines from American Heart and Stroke Associations recommend decompressive surgical evacuation of a space-occupying cerebellar infarction to treat brainstem herniation and compression from a cerebellar infarction.

Hemorrhagic Transformation

Both cerebral and cerebellar ischemic stroke can have hemorrhagic transformation. IV t-PA has a risk of hemorrhagic transformation of up to 6 %. This is usually seen within 24 h of t-PA administration. The management of t-PA-induced bleeding is not well established. Some experts suggest using cryoprecipitate to correct fibrinogen levels if it is below 100 mg/dL. If bleeding is refractory or life-threatening, aminocaproic acid can be considered. Some have used tranexamic acid when blood product use is contraindicated [6]; hematologic consultation may be helpful.

If the hemorrhagic transformation is small, or a non-t-PA patient has a hemorrhagic transformation, the management will be same as in spontaneous intracerebral hemorrhage cases. The conservative approach of avoiding anticoagulants, blood pressure control, and very careful monitoring is appropriate.

Seizures

Poststroke seizures are commonly encountered in cases of hemorrhagic stroke, hemorrhagic conversion of ischemic stroke, large ischemic strokes, or in strokes due to a cardioembolic etiology. The incidence is up to 15 % and depends on the etiology, location, and extent of the brain injury. Prophylactic seizure medications are not recommended. Patients with recurrent seizures are treated in the same manner as epilepsy patients. The choice of the antiepileptic drug (AED) depends on the patient characteristics including age and underlying comorbidities.

Supportive Care

In patients receiving t-PA, aspirin or other anticoagulants, including prophylactic heparin, should be withheld for at least 24 h. If the patient did not receive t-PA, aspirin and statin therapy are initiated within 24 h. DVT and gastrointestinal prophylaxis is administered as for any ICU patient. Stroke patients who have decreased level of consciousness and/or bulbar weakness would need urgent evaluation for airway support and potential ventilator assistance. Supplemental oxygen should be provided to maintain oxygen saturation greater than 94 % to preserve cerebral oxygenation. In the neurocritical care setting, cardiac monitoring is recommended to detect any serious cardiac dysrhythmias for at least first 24 h. Hypovolemia, hypoglycemia, hyperglycemia, and dysrhythmias should be corrected aggressively as they are associated with poor outcomes in the setting of acute ischemic stroke. Hyperthermia needs be aggressively investigated for an infectious cause and treated if one is found; hyperthermia can lead to poor outcome after strokes [6].

Patients who have systolic blood pressure more than 185 mmHg and are eligible for treatment with IV thrombolytic should have their blood pressure carefully lowered so that systolic blood pressure is less than 185 mmHg and diastolic blood pressure less than 110 mmHg before thrombolysis is initiated. It is imperative that the systolic blood pressure be maintained below 180/105 mmHg for at least the first 24 h after IV thrombolysis. In patients who do not receive thrombolytics and have markedly elevated systolic (greater than 220 mmHg) or diastolic blood pressure (greater than 120 mmHg), a reasonable goal is to lower blood pressure by 15 % during the first 24 h after onset of stroke. In known hypertensive patients, it is recommended to start their routine antihypertensive medications after the first 24 h, once they are neurologically stable, if there are no specific contraindication [6].

Palliative Care

Some patients have early clinical deterioration from a large ischemic stroke. In cases of advanced brain damage, a realistic discussion with the family, explaining the prognosis and disability, will give the family an opportunity to respect the patient wishes and consider a DO NOT RESUSCITATE order or palliative care. Even though stroke is the fourth leading cause of death in United States, there are no large studies in which these issues have been addressed, especially in stroke scenario.

References

1. Arsava EM, Ballabio E, Benner T, Cole JW, Delgado-Martinez MP, Dichgans M, Fazekas F, Furie KL, Illoh K, Jood K, Kittner S, Lindgren AG, Majersik JJ, Macleod MJ, Meurer WJ, Montaner J, Olugbodi AA, Pasdar A, Redfors P, Schmidt R, Sharma P, Singhal AB, Sorensen AG, Sudlow C, Thijs V, Worrall BB, Rosand J, Ay H. The causative classification of stroke system: an international reliability and optimization study. Neurology. 2010;75:1277–84.
2. Ay H, Benner T, Arsava EM, Furie KL, Singhal AB, Jensen MB, Ayata C, Towfighi A, Smith EE, Chong JY, Koroshetz WJ, Sorensen AG. A computerized algorithm for etiologic classification of ischemic stroke: the causative classification of stroke system. Stroke. 2007;38:2979–84.
3. Ay H, Furie KL, Singhal A, Smith WS, Sorensen AG, Koroshetz WJ. An evidence-based causative classification system for acute ischemic stroke. Ann Neurol. 2005;58:688–97.
4. Singer DE, Albers GW, Dalen JE, Go AS, Halperin JL, Manning WJ. Antithrombotic therapy in atrial fibrillation: the seventh ACCP conference on antithrombotic and thrombolytic therapy. Chest. 2004;126:429S–56.
5. Elkind MS. Epidemiology and risk factors. Continuum (Minneap Minn). 2011;17:1213–32.
6. Jauch EC, Saver JL, Adams Jr HP, Bruno A, Connors JJ, Demaerschalk BM, Khatri P, McMullan Jr PW, Qureshi AI, Rosenfield K, Scott PA, Summers DR, Wang DZ, Wintermark M,

Yonas H. Guidelines for the early management of patients with acute ischemic stroke: a guideline for healthcare professionals from the American Heart Association/American Stroke Association. Stroke. 2013;44:870–947.
7. The National Institute of Neurological Disorders and Stroke rt-PA Stroke Study Group. Tissue plasminogen activator for acute ischemic stroke. N Engl J Med. 1995;333:1581–7
8. Lees KR, Bluhmki E, von Kummer R, Brott TG, Toni D, Grotta JC, Albers GW, Kaste M, Marler JR, Hamilton SA, Tilley BC, Davis SM, Donnan GA, Hacke W, Allen K, Mau J, Meier D, del Zoppo G, De Silva DA, Butcher KS, Parsons MW, Barber PA, Levi C, Bladin C, Byrnes G. Time to treatment with intravenous alteplase and outcome in stroke: an updated pooled analysis of ECASS, ATLANTIS, NINDS, and EPITHET trials. Lancet. 2010;375:1695–703.
9. Sandercock P, Wardlaw JM, Lindley RI, Dennis M, Cohen G, Murray G, Innes K, Venables G, Czlonkowska A, Kobayashi A, Ricci S, Murray V, Berge E, Slot KB, Hankey GJ, Correia M, Peeters A, Matz K, Lyrer P, Gubitz G, Phillips SJ, Arauz A. The benefits and harms of intravenous thrombolysis with recombinant tissue plasminogen activator within 6 h of acute ischaemic stroke (the third international stroke trial [IST-3]): a randomised controlled trial. Lancet. 2012;379:2352–63.
10. Rha JH, Saver JL. The impact of recanalization on ischemic stroke outcome: a meta-analysis. Stroke. 2007;38:967–73.
11. Pechlaner R, Knoflach M, Matosevic B, Ruecker M, Schmidauer C, Kiechl S, Willeit J. Recanalization of extracranial internal carotid artery occlusion after i.V. Thrombolysis for acute ischemic stroke. PLoS One. 2013;8:e55318.
12. Furlan A, Higashida R, Wechsler L, Gent M, Rowley H, Kase C, Pessin M, Ahuja A, Callahan F, Clark WM, Silver F, Rivera F. Intra-arterial prourokinase for acute ischemic stroke. The PROACT II study: a randomized controlled trial. Prolyse in acute cerebral thromboembolism. JAMA. 1999;282:2003–11.
13. Ogawa A, Mori E, Minematsu K, Taki W, Takahashi A, Nemoto S, Miyamoto S, Sasaki M, Inoue T. Randomized trial of intraarterial infusion of urokinase within 6 hours of middle cerebral artery stroke: the middle cerebral artery embolism local fibrinolytic intervention trial (MELT) Japan. Stroke. 2007;38:2633–9.
14. Alexandrov AV. Ultrasound identification and lysis of clots. Stroke. 2004;35:2722–5.
15. Smith WS, Sung G, Saver J, Budzik R, Duckwiler G, Liebeskind DS, Lutsep HL, Rymer MM, Higashida RT, Starkman S, Gobin YP, Frei D, Grobelny T, Hellinger F, Huddle D, Kidwell C, Koroshetz W, Marks M, Nesbit G, Silverman IE. Mechanical thrombectomy for acute ischemic stroke: final results of the multi merci trial. Stroke. 2008;39:1205–12.
16. Penumbra Pivotal Stroke Trial Investigators. The penumbra pivotal stroke trial: safety and effectiveness of a new generation of mechanical devices for clot removal in intracranial large vessel occlusive disease. Stroke. 2009;40:2761–8.
17. Saver JL, Jahan R, Levy EI, Jovin TG, Baxter B, Nogueira RG, Clark W, Budzik R, Zaidat OO. Solitaire flow restoration device versus the merci retriever in patients with acute ischaemic stroke (SWIFT): a randomised, parallel-group, non-inferiority trial. Lancet. 2012;380:1241–9.
18. Nogueira RG, Lutsep HL, Gupta R, Jovin TG, Albers GW, Walker GA, Liebeskind DS, Smith WS. Trevo versus merci retrievers for thrombectomy revascularisation of large vessel occlusions in acute ischaemic stroke (TREVO 2): a randomised trial. Lancet. 2012;380:1231–40.
19. Ciccone A, Valvassori L, Nichelatti M, Sgoifo A, Ponzio M, Sterzi R, Boccardi E. Endovascular treatment for acute ischemic stroke. N Engl J Med. 2013;368:904–13.
20. Broderick JP, Palesch YY, Demchuk AM, Yeatts SD, Khatri P, Hill MD, Jauch EC, Jovin TG, Yan B, Silver FL, von Kummer R, Molina CA, Demaerschalk BM, Budzik R, Clark WM, Zaidat OO,

Malisch TW, Goyal M, Schonewille WJ, Mazighi M, Engelter ST, Anderson C, Spilker J, Carrozzella J, TR R, Ryckborst KJ, Janis LS, Martin RH, Foster LD, Tomsick TA. Endovascular therapy after intravenous t-PA versus t-PA alone for stroke. N Engl J Med. 2013;368:893–903.

21. Hacke W, Schwab S, Horn M, Spranger M, De Georgia M, von Kummer R. 'Malignant' middle cerebral artery territory infarction: clinical course and prognostic signs. Arch Neurol. 1996;53: 309–15.

22. Treadwell SD, Thanvi B. Malignant middle cerebral artery (MCA) infarction: pathophysiology, diagnosis and management. Postgrad Med J. 2010;86:235–42.

23. Simard JM, Sahuquillo J, Sheth KN, Kahle KT, Walcott BP. Managing malignant cerebral infarction. Curr Treat Options Neurol. 2011;13:217–29.

24. Vahedi K, Hofmeijer J, Juettler E, Vicaut E, George B, Algra A, Amelink GJ, Schmiedeck P, Schwab S, Rothwell PM, Bousser MG, van der Worp HB, Hacke W. Early decompressive surgery in malignant infarction of the middle cerebral artery: a pooled analysis of three randomised controlled trials. Lancet Neurol. 2007;6:215–22.

25. National Collaborating Centre for Chronic Conditions (UK). Stroke: national clinical guideline for diagnosis and initial management of acute stroke and transient ischaemic attack (TIA). London: Royal College of Physicians (UK); 2008.

Central Nervous System Neoplasia: Evidence-Based Medicine, Diagnosis, Treatment, and Complications

34

Erin M. Dunbar

Contents

E.M. Dunbar, MD
Department of Neurological Surgery,
University of Florida College of Medicine,
100 South Newell Drive, Bldg 59,
Gainesville, FL 32610, USA
e-mail: edunbar@neurosurgery.ufl.edu

Abstract

This chapter is a practical summary of the best available evidence for the comprehensive management of CNS tumors. In the USA, an estimated 40,000 new cases of primary CNS tumors, both benign and malignant, are diagnosed in adults annually. Overarching goals of treatment include the minimization of the known risks and symptoms of tumor with simultaneous minimization of the potential risks and symptoms of treatment. Determination of treatment remains highly individualized, influenced by evolving radiographic and clinical response criteria, challenges to the comparison of treatments, as well as patient-, provider-, and tumor-specific factors. Interdisciplinary teams are best suited to balance these influences and provide optimal care. This chapter is a practical summary of the best available evidence for the comprehensive management of CNS tumors.

Keywords

Brain (CNS) tumor • Meningioma • Glioma • Pituitary tumor • Radiation • Surgery

Introduction

Overarching goals include the minimization of the known risks and symptoms of tumor with simultaneous minimization of the potential risks and symptoms of treatment. Determination of treatment remains highly individualized, influenced by evolving radiographic and clinical response criteria, challenges to the comparison of treatments, as well as patient-, provider-, and tumor-specific factors. Interdisciplinary teams are best suited to balance these influences and provide optimal care.

A.J. Layon et al. (eds.), *Textbook of Neurointensive Care*,
DOI 10.1007/978-1-4471-5226-2_34, © Springer-Verlag London 2013

Epidemiology

In the USA, an estimated 40,000 new cases of primary brain tumors, both benign and malignant, are diagnosed in adults annually. Although primary brain tumors represent only ~2 % of adult malignancies, they incur disproportionate morbidity and mortality. In adults, 70 % of primary brain tumors are supratentorial and, proportional to the size of the lobes, most commonly occur in the frontal lobes. Several adult primary tumors have varying gender predisposition, including a slight predisposition for gliomas in males, a slight predisposition for schwannomas in females, and a significant predisposition for meningiomas in females (both brain and spine). Race is not a significant factor [1]. By comparison, in the USA, an estimated 150,000 new cases of secondary brain tumors (a.k.a. brain metastases (BMs)) are diagnosed in adults annually. This represents a ten-time higher incidence than primary brain tumors. This translates to a 25 % chance of US adults diagnosed with systemic cancers developing symptomatic BMs during their lifetime and a 20 % chance that BMs will be the first diagnosed site of their systemic malignancy [2]. Thirty-three percent of BMs present as solitary, oligometastatic (2–3 lesions), or polymetastatic (>4) lesions, respectively. Race is not a significant factor. The incidence of BMs is increasing due to the aging population, the increased detection by advanced imaging, the blood–brain barrier's (BBB) sanctuary site for tumors and

against most systemic agents, the select improved control of certain systemic cancers, and the select improved control of BMs [3, 4].

In contrast, CNS tumors affect children very differently. In the USA, CNS tumors are the second most common primary tumor site. Race and gender are not factors. Risk factors include RT and a few genetic syndromes, including neurofibromatosis types 1 and 2, tuberous sclerosis, Li-Fraumeni syndrome, and Gorlin syndrome. Although many systemic malignancies present diffusely, traditional metastatic disease to the CNS is rare in children.

Classification of Common CNS Tumors

Tables 34.1 and 34.2 list common CNS tumors in adults and children, respectively [5, 6].

Gliomas

Eighty percent of adult primary brain tumors are gliomas. The only definitive risk factors include RT and rare genetic syndromes. Based on criteria detailed next, the World Health Organization (WHO) divides gliomas into grade I–IV. The median onset of I and II gliomas (collectively referred to as low-grade gliomas (LGGs)) is the third and fourth decade,

Table 34.1 The percent incidence of adult CNS tumors

Origin	Percent incidence (%)
Neuroepithelial	34.4
Glioma	50
Astrocytoma (WHO I–IV)	75
Ependymoma	6
Medulloblastoma	6
Oligodendroglioma	5
Choroid plexus papilloma	2
Colloid cysts	1
Other neuroepithelial, neuronal/glial	1
Tumors of cranial and spinal nerves (malignant and nonmalignant)	8.7
Tumors of the meninges	35.1
Meningioma	34
Other mesenchymal, including hemangioblastoma	1.1
Lymphomas and hematopoietic neoplasms	2.4
Germ cell tumors	0.4
Sella tumors	13.5
Pituitary	12.7
Craniopharyngioma	0.7
Local extension from regional tumors including chordoma and chondrosarcomas	0.1
Unclassified, including hemangiomas and other	5.5
Total	100

Data from States CBTRotU [5]

Table 34.2 The percent incidence of adult CNS tumors

Astrocytomas (I–IV)	43 %
Supratentorial	22 %
Infratentorial	13 %
Brainstem gliomas	8 %
Oligodendrogliomas	2 %
Medulloblastomas	20 %
Ependymomas	8 %
Supratentorial	3 %
Infratentorial	5 %
Craniopharyngioma	7 %
Pineal region and germ cell tumors (GCTs)	4 %
Choroid plexus	2 %
Gangliogliomas	2 %
Meningiomas	2 %
Primitive embryonal tumors and others	2 %
Total	100 %

Data from DeAngelis [6]

respectively. The median onset of WHO III–IV gliomas (a.k.a. high-grade gliomas (HGGs)) is the sixth decade, respectively [1]. HGGs make up 75 % of gliomas, occur more often in older adults, and constitute 40 % of the ~18,000 new cases of malignant CNS tumors in the USA annually. Median survival of adults with treated HGGs is 3–5 years for WHO III HGGs (5-year survival less 20 %), 16–18 months for WHO IV HGGs (5-year survival less than 5 %), and even longer in younger ages if a significant oligodendrial component is present. LGGs make up 25 % of gliomas and occur more often in younger adults. Median survival of adults with treated LGGs is 5–7 years and also longer in younger ages and when an oligodendroglial component is present. Many LGGs in children are curable, including completely resected WHO I juvenile pilocytic astrocytomas.

Gliomas represent a heterogeneous group of tumors that originate from one or more cell types making up the normal brain (e.g., astrocytes, oligodendrocytes, and ependymal cells). Accordingly, histologic subtypes of gliomas include astrocytoma, oligodendroglioma, ependymoma, and mixed glioma. Histologic grading of astrocytic gliomas incorporates the degree of cellularity, atypia, mitoses, endothelial proliferation, and necrosis (mitoses, nuclear pleomorphism, pseudopalisading necrosis, and endothelial proliferation) into a WHO grade between I and IV. Numerous retrospective and prospective studies correlate WHO grade with biologic aggressiveness [7]. HGGs originate either as HGGs or having malignantly transformed from LGGs. This distinction has increasing relevance as recent evidence suggests that WHO IV gliomas (glioblastomas (GBs)) originating from transformed LGGs (secondary GBs) have distinct molecular-genetic profiles, prognosis, and possibly response to treatment. This is exemplified by a recent publication by Yan and

colleagues that identifies somatic mutations of the NADP(+)-dependent isocitrate dehydrogenase 1 gene (IDH1), most frequently found in secondary GBs, and correlates them to improved outcomes [8].

The heterogeneity in gliomas extends far beyond histology and grade. Diverse molecular, genetic, and signal transduction aberrations are differential factors in the genesis, maintenance, resistance, and survival of gliomas [9]. This is exemplified by the recent publication by The Cancer Genome Atlas (TCGA) that describes pathways altered GB genesis, correlates O_6-methylguanine-DNA methyltransferase (MGMT) promoter methylation in treated GB with improved outcome and response to treatment, and details the incidence of certain gene expressions and mutations, including epidermal growth factor receptor type 2 (ERBB2), neurofibromatosis gene type 1 (NF1), and tumor promoter 53 (TP53) [10]. Lastly, heterogeneous functions of stem cells and the microenvironment in and around gliomas are differential factors in migration, resistance, vascularity, invasion, and repair.

Brain Metastases

By default, they are classified as stage IV systemic disease. BMs most commonly originate from lung, breast, and kidney, and the median onset is 60 years old. BMs most commonly to have microscopic or macroscopic hemorrhage include renal cell carcinoma, embryonal, and melanoma. Several recent studies have shown that the profile of tumor markers identified in BMs, such as progesterone, estrogen, and Her-2/Neu, can be significantly different than the profile identified in the original systemic malignancy ~1/3 of the time. Given the profound impact that tumor marker status has in treatment and prognosis, retesting tumor markers in BMs is ever-important [11]. Risk factors include poor systemic disease control, presentation of BMs late in the disease course of the systemic disease, and neurotropism of certain histologies, such as melanoma, small cell lung cancer, and possibly her-2/neu breast adenocarcinoma.

The classifications of other common CNS tumors are detailed in the treatment section in this chapter.

Presentation of Common CNS Tumors

CNS tumors present with symptoms and signs attributable to one or more phenomena, including focal destruction, focal irritation, and, unique to the CNS, elevated intracranial pressure (ICP) [12]. Elevated ICP originates from local or general mass effect (including from the tumor, hemorrhage, or surrounding edema), which may involve hydrocephalus (including communicating and obstructive). Symptoms of progressively elevated ICP include headache, nausea, vomiting, changes in cognition and level of consciousness, papilledema, and cranial nerve palsy. Treatments, depending on the urgency, involve dexamethasone, ventriculostomy or ventriculoperitoneal shunt, and/or resection. Focal destruction originates from invasion of tumor and associated inflammatory cells into surrounding brain. Symptoms include deficits correlated to the affected anatomy, whether sensory, motor, vision, endocrine, cognitive, language, or vascular. Symptoms usually present gradually enough that they can be distinguished from acute cerebrovascular accidents; however, notable exceptions include intratumoral hemorrhage (apoplexy) or seizure. Treatments, depending on the pattern and severity, involve dexamethasone, other supportive care, or less commonly procedural and resection. Focal irritation originates from abnormal functioning of normal brain as a result of the tumor. Symptoms most commonly include deficits emanating from some type of seizure (a.k.a. convulsion or epilepsy), whether dysfunctions of motor, sensory (including auras), or emotion or alterations of level of consciousness or bowel/bladder control. Treatments include an ever-increasing number of antiepileptic drugs (AEDs) described in Chap. 39 on Seizures.

Radiographic Evaluation

While a careful history and physical remains essential, diagnostic imaging is increasingly important to the formulation of the differential diagnosis and treatment plan. Although CT scans are frequently the first noninvasive imaging modality obtained, secondary to availability, relative inexpensiveness, and ability to detect acute intracranial bleeding or trauma, MRI using gadolinium-contrast MRI is far superior. Location, number, and pattern of lesions; involvement of the dura or ventricles, edema, necrosis, or hemorrhage; and appearance on MRI (T1-weighted (w), T2-w, FLAIR, other sequences) are important considerations. Although neuroimaging is detailed in Chap. 40, a few generalities are presented here.

LGGs are commonly supratentorial, infiltrative, with little mass effect, non-enhancing on T1-w, best seen on T2-w, and commonly include calcifications, especially if there is an oligodendroglioma component (Fig. 34.1a–c). HGGs are commonly enhancing on T1-w and commonly include surrounding vasogenic edema, mass effect, central necrosis, and hemorrhage (Fig. 34.2a, b). Radiographic evaluation of other common CNS tumors is detailed in the treatment section in this chapter.

Preoperative imaging narrows the differential diagnosis, predicts postoperative deficits, maximizes safe resection, and minimizes injury to eloquent brain [13, 14]. This is often accomplished by "frameless" stereotaxis, a computer system that continually integrates preoperative MRI and/or CT images [15–18]. Intraoperative imaging, when available, allows assessment of tumor volume and eloquent brain in its real-time anatomic location [19]. Postoperative MRI (within 48 h) confirms extent of resection, absence of hemorrhage, ischemia, and other factors impacting future treatment.

Diagnosis

The determination of whether the initial diagnostic procedure is a stereotactic biopsy, open biopsy, or more extensive resection depends on the clinical presentation, diagnostic imaging, and available medical expertise. Frozen section, when available, assists "real-time" decision-making regarding extent of resection and intraoperative staging. Although histopathologic diagnosis is detailed in Chap. 6 on neuropathology, clinically relevant issues are discussed here.

Glial fibrillary acidic protein (GFAP) via immunohistochemistry identifies astrocytic gliomas, and its WHO grade is defined, as noted earlier. Mitotic rate and Ki-67 (MIB-1) nuclear labeling index and TP53 mutation rate correlate with grade and proliferative capacity and inversely correlate with survival. Predictive, prognostic, confirmatory information (particularly with stereotactic biopsies) is available through the judicious use of ancillary testing. Chromosomal deletion of 1p and/or 19q identifies a glioma with an oligodendroglioma component, correlates to improved prognosis, and predicts response to treatment [20, 21]. Methylated MGMT (O_6-methylguanine-DNA methyltransferase) identifies a glioma with an astrocytic component; correlates to improved prognosis, via "silencing" of enzymatic DNA repair; and

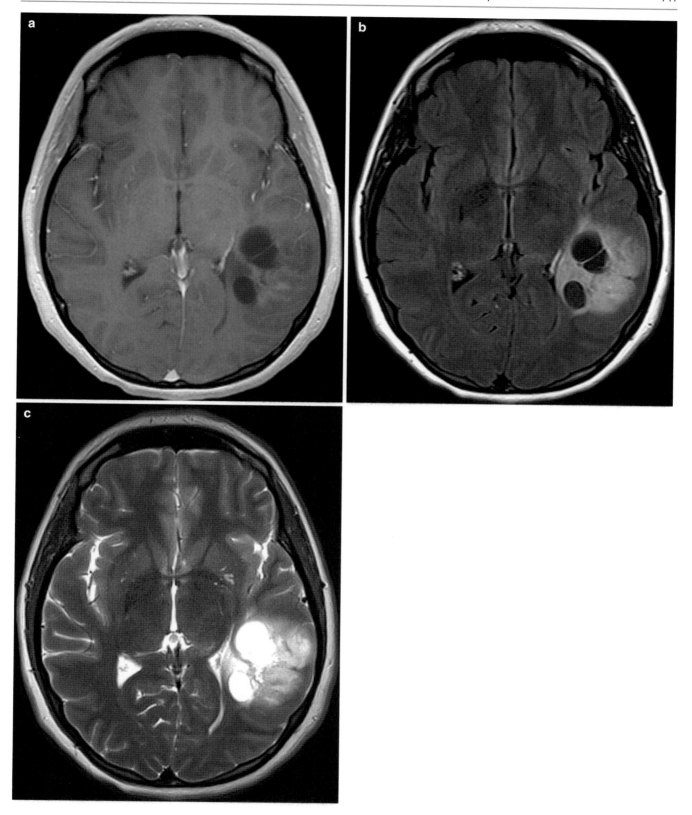

Fig. 34.1 (**a–c**) T1-w, FLAIR, and T2-w images of a WHO II oligodendroglioma in the left temporal lobe, with cystic and solid components and slight contrast enhancement. It demonstrates moderate vasogenic edema and local mass effect on the occipital horn of the lateral ventricle

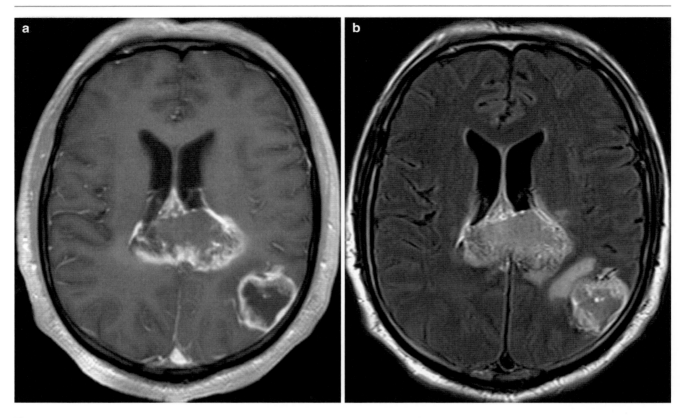

Fig. 34.2 (**a, b**) T1-w and FLAIR images of a WHO IV glioblastoma involving the left parietal lobe and splenium of the corpus callosum. It demonstrates ring enhancement, central necrosis, and early subependymal spread along the lateral ventricle

predicts response to treatment [22, 23]. This is exemplified by temozolomide, first-line chemotherapy in malignant gliomas, which terminally damages DNA by adding methyl groups to the O_6 position of guanine. This effect can be reversed by the endogenous DNA repair enzyme MGMT, thus providing a mechanism of relative chemoresistance to alkylating agent chemotherapies. MGMT methylation also correlates with increased posttreatment effect (a.k.a. pseudoprogression) seen in 40–50 % of patients within several weeks of chemoradiation and may correlate to a "hypermutated tumor" that is resistant to subsequent treatments. Unfortunately, widespread utilization of MGMT methylation status is limited by inconsistency in availability and results between academic centers, within a given patient's tumor, and throughout a patient's lifetime. The co-occurrence of epidermal growth factor receptor (EGFR) mutant variant III (EGFRvIII) and wild-type phosphatase and tensin homolog (PTEN) appears to correlate to sensitivity with anti-EGFR agents. Mutation of the NADP+ -dependant isocitrate dehydrogenase-1 (IDH1) gene, hypothesized to be an early event in GB tumorigenesis, occurring in 50–80 % of GBs transformed from LGGs but only 1–2 % of primary GBs, appears to correlate to improved survival [8]. Such complimentary tests highlight the importance of individualizing treatment, including clinical trial design, stratification, and analysis.

Treatment

Optimal treatment requires the careful integration of *cancer-specific factors*, including the size, location, and pathologic profile of the cancer; *patient-specific factors*, including age, comorbidities, and performance status; as well as *provider-specific factors*, including training, biases, and resources. These factors are incorporated into the simultaneous goals of maximizing cancer control while also minimizing the morbidity of both cancer and its treatment. Prognostic factors, including age, WHO grade, extent of resection (EOR), Karnofsky Performance Status (KPS), and sometimes tumor location [24–26], form the basis of common treatment planning tools. Two such planning tools include the prospectively validated prognostic recursive partitioning analysis (RPA) nomograms for gliomas and BMs [27, 28].

Response criteria, both radiographic and clinical, are essential to optimal treatment, including its selection, assessment, and discontinuation. Since the 1990s, the modified Macdonald criteria have served as the traditional radiographic response criteria for gliomas but are commonly extrapolated to other primary/secondary CNS tumors. The modified Macdonald criteria incorporate steroid dose, neurologic findings, and 2-dimensional T1-w post-gadolinium MRI measurements to determine complete response (CR), partial response (PR), stable disease (SD), or progressive disease (PD) [29]. More recently, the Response Assessment in Neuro-Oncology (RANO) radiographic response criteria have received attention for incorporation of T2-w and FLAIR sequences, the temporal relationship of serial MRIs to the completion of RT (less than or greater to 12 weeks), and use of agents that alter the contrast enhancements of scans (including steroids and antiangiogenic agents) [30]. Although exciting, RANO requires prospective validation. RANO helps to distinguish pseudo-progression and pseudo-response, both a result of the indiscriminant leak of contrast through a blood–brain barrier broken by one or more situations not related to tumor progression, including radiation necrosis, infection, and inflammation. Pseudo-progression is defined as the development of MRI features consistent with progression that occur within 4–6 weeks of completing a given regimen's RT and the absence of further progression on that regimen during the subsequent 6 months. It occurs as high as 40–60 % in GB patients whose treatments include chemo-RT. Pseudo-response is usually defined as the resolution of imaging features discordant to the clinical situation or biologic principles of cancer and is commonly seen in the use of antiangiogenic agents [30]. Given the inability of imaging to definitively differentiate true from pseudo-progression, it remains the domain of the individual patient and physician to determine the best course of action. Irrespective of specific criteria, radiographic response assessment in LGGs is inherently difficult since LGGs are typically non-enhancing and infiltrative. For example, a meaningful clinical response may occur in the absence of radiographic response [31, 32]. This dichotomy is also seen with several agents discussed later in this chapter.

Clinical response criteria represent a qualitative summary of subjective and objective findings, including the patient's symptoms, the provider's exam findings, and the performance status. Recent advances in the ability to differentiate effects from the tumor from effects of the treatment, as well as improvements in supportive treatments, are increasing the importance of clinical response as an independent endpoint of treatment. As a result, the need for adequate and universally used response criteria is ever-important [33].

Surgery

Factors involved in the decision between a stereotactic biopsy, for diagnosis, and a craniotomy, for more extensive resection and palliation, include the *patient's* performance status, general health, and preferences; the *tumor's* presentation, location, and size; and the *provider's* expertise, biases, and resources [34]. The optimally recommended extent of resection is often referred to as maximal safe resection in an attempt to acknowledge the goals of maximal cytologic reduction without significant neurologic sequela. In benign tumors, this "complete resection" usually results in a cure. Although stereotactic and functional neurosurgery (as appropriate in various chapters) and intraoperative care (Chap. 41) are detailed elsewhere, pertinent concepts are summarized here.

A stereotactic biopsy involves the placement of a stereotactic head ring under local anesthetic, followed by imaging in a CT scanner. A stereotactic computer system creates 3D coordinates of the brain and head ring using the CT images, and often using a non-stereotactic MRI recently obtained, to plan the target and trajectory. The target point is set up on a device called a phantom. The stereotactic frame is then connected to the phantom to accurately determine coordinates. The involved skin is shaved and prepped and the stereotactic frame is attached to the head ring. Following administration of local anesthetic, a burr hole is placed, the dura is opened and coagulated, the biopsy needle is advanced to the target, and several biopsies are performed. After the retrieval of diagnostic tissue is confirmed, the needle is removed, the site is closed, and the stereotactic frame is removed. Complications occur in less than 2 % of cases and include failure to obtain diagnostic tissue, seizures, other focal deficits, and arterial hemorrhage. The latter, usually occurring in surgery, may require conversion to an open craniotomy.

A craniotomy and resection involves the induction of general anesthesia, positioning to optimize the technical aspects of the surgery and protect the patient, opening the skin sufficiently to access to the brain while preserving adequate blood supply, removing the skull flap (sometimes requiring synthetic creation), opening and retracting the dura, excising the tumor using various techniques and instruments (including the microscope and neurologic monitoring), and closing [35]. Complications are relatively rare and include seizures, unanticipated neurologic deficits, cerebral edema, cerebrovascular ischemia, meningitis (infectious and noninfectious), endocrine sequela (such as hyponatremia), hemorrhage, and hydrocephalus. These may be immediate or delayed and require a high index of suspicion, and the latter two may require an immediate non-contrast CT if suspected [36].

Radiation Therapy

Once histologic diagnosis is established, external beam RT serves an integral role in many CNS tumors and involves the delivery of high-energy photon beams to both visible (macroscopic) tumor and a select area surrounding the visible tumor representing a high probability of microscopic tumor cells. The dose and fractionation are selected to optimize the cell death of cancer cells (via DNA damage) while preventing treatment-related side effects (a.k.a. complications). Complications increase with increased dose and volume treated, decreased fractionation, extremes of age, and concurrent use of chemotherapy [37, 38]. When RT is delivered in one fraction, it is referred to as stereotactic radiosurgery (SRS). When it is delivered in more than one fraction, it is referred to as fractionated RT.

SRS involves the use of special devices to precisely deliver one large fraction of RT to a specific target while sparing surrounding tissue. Special devices include *Gamma knife*, which uses 201 fixed cobalt sources, and *LINAC*, which uses a linear accelerator. For example, one of the most commonly used devices for producing and focusing radiation beams is the linear accelerator (LINAC), which accelerates electrons near the speed of light and then collides them with heavy metals to produce braking radiation, whereby high-energy photons (called x-rays) result and are focused by a series of shaping collimators onto the tumor. SRS is commonly used, often in combination with other treatments, in BMs, acoustic schwannomas, meningiomas, pituitary microadenomas, and occasionally others. Complications are very rare and most commonly include radiation necrosis (RN), typically occurring 3–18 months post-SRS.

FRT involves computer assistance to precisely deliver RT in a 3D conformal and/or intensity-modulated (IMRT) technique. FRT is commonly used, often in combination with other treatments, with technique, dose, and fractionation algorithms tailored to specific CNS tumors. Complications, although relatively common, are rarely severe. Acute complications (less than 2 months) include dermatitis, hair loss, nausea, vomiting, fatigue/malaise, exacerbation of neurologic issues, and rarely encephalopathy. Delayed complications (2–3 months) include somnolence, cognitive sequela (usually memory), transient worsening of specific neurologic symptoms, pseudo-progression, and, less commonly, RN. Late complications (more than 3 months) include leukoencephalopathy syndrome (lethargy, dysarthria, seizures, ataxia, memory loss, and possibly dementia) [39].

Chemotherapy and Other Systemic Therapies

Chemotherapy and other systemic agents involve various mechanisms that either kill the tumor cell or modify the behavior of the tumor cell or its microenvironment. Examples include traditional cytotoxic agents (damage to single- or double-stranded DNA and ultimately leading to cell death), antiangiogenic agents, small molecular inhibitors, and immunomodulators. They are selected for their CNS penetration, efficacy, and tolerability. At diagnosis, they are most commonly used in combination with other treatments, often as part of a curative-intent strategy. At recurrence/progression, they are commonly used alone and are almost always palliative intent. Common agents used in CNS tumors are detailed in Table 34.3 [40]. Complications are agent-specific and increase with extremes of age, concurrent RT, and increased dose or duration of treatment [41–43]. However, it is important to note that the distinct/unique complications to antiangiogenic agents (Table 34.3) historically excluded their use in primary/secondary CNS tumors. However, recent evidence suggests that they may not only be safe but also efficacious. For example, Rohr and coworkers reported on a

Table 34.3 Chemotherapy and systemic agents commonly used in CNS tumors

Agent[a]	Name	Uses	Complications
Cytotoxic agents			
Alkylators			
	BCNU[b] (IV) (carmustine) or wafer (Gliadel) or CCNU[c] (lomustine) (PO)	Gliomas, BMs, medulloblastomas, others	Myelosuppression (occasionally secondary MDS/AML), nausea/vomiting, transaminitis, optic neuroretinitis, nephritis, and idiopathic pulmonary fibrosis (usually with BNCU, can be severe)
	Platinum agents (IV) (carboplatin (Paraplatin)) or (cisplatin (Platinol))	Gliomas, skull-based tumors, BMs	Myelosuppression, nausea/vomiting, alopecia, renal toxicity, neurotoxicity, mainly (sensorineural hearing loss and sensory peripheral neuropathy, occasionally vision)
	Procarbazine (Matulane) (PO) CYP450 metabolism[d]	Gliomas, medulloblastomas, others	Myelosuppression, nausea/vomiting, mucositis (stomatitis, diarrhea, ulcerative colitis), monoamine oxidase reaction (including with sympathomimetics, anesthetics, tricyclic antidepressants, tyramine-rich foods), disulfiram-like reaction with alcohol, various neurologic (can be severe: emotional, psychiatric, neuropathies, coma, tremor, HA, insomnia), and various pulmonary and constitutional symptoms
	Temozolomide (TMZ) (MTIC[e]) (PO, IV)	Gliomas, BMs, PCNSL, others	Headache, constipation, nausea/vomiting, myelosuppression (including secondary MDS), thrombocytopenia (nadir ~26 days) > neutropenia (nadir ~28 days)

Table 34.3 (continued)

Agent[a]	Name	Uses	Complications
DNA topoisomerase II inhibitors	VP-16 (etoposide) (Vepesid) (PO, IV)	Gliomas, BMs, medulloblastomas and other PNET, BMS, others	Myelosuppression (including secondary MDS), nausea/vomiting, alopecia, mucositis, Stevens-Johnson syndrome, IV infusion-related reactions (including hypotension, dyspnea, angioedema syndrome)
Antimetabolites (folate antagonists)	Methotrexate (IV, PO, IT)	Gliomas, PCNSL, BMs, others	Myelosuppression, mucositis, transaminitis, renal impairment, ileus, 3rd spacing, various neurologic (severity and acuity depends on the route (headache, nausea, limb spasticity, sensory peripheral neuropathy, dementia, coma, nuchal rigidity, chemical arachnoiditis))
DNA topoisomerase I inhibitors	Irinotecan (CPT-11) (Camptosar) (IV) CYP450 metabolism[d]	Gliomas, CNSL, others	Hyperbilirubinemia, diarrhea (acute and chronic), thrombocytopenia > neutropenia (nadir ~ 15 days), nausea/vomiting, alopecia, mucositis
Monoclonal antibodies (MA)			
Immunomodulators	Ipilimumab (Yervoy) MA against CTLA-4 a negative regulator of T-cell activation (thereby increasing T-cell activation and proliferation)	Metastatic melanoma	Life-threatening immune reactions, transaminitis, hyperbilirubinemia, various neuropathies (Guillain-Barre syndrome, myasthenia gravis, peripheral motor neuropathy), endocrinopathy, fatigue, diarrhea/colitis, pruritus/rash
	Rituximab (Rituxan) MA against CD-20+ B-cells	PCNSL, metastatic systemic lymphoma	Infusion reactions (fevers, chills, rarely severe hyposensitivity reactions), atypical infections, and rarely mucocutaneous reactions (can be severe/life-threatening)
Antiangiogenic agents	Bevacizumab (Avastin) (IV) MA against VEGFR	Gliomas, BMs, RN	Pseudo-response, bleeding, poor wound healing (varies in severity and depends on tumor type; half-life is 20 days; no reversal agent), venous and arterial thromboembolism, exacerbation of vascular disease (such as proteinuria and hypertension (most common), CVA, CAD, CHF), fatigue, and rarely, reversible posterior leukoencephalopathy syndrome
Small-molecule inhibitors	Erlotinib (Tarceva) TKI against EGFR/Her-1 (PO) CYP450 metabolism[d]	Gliomas with EGFRvIII mutation, BMs with EGFR	Cutaneous acneiform rash (can be severe), diarrhea, nausea/vomiting, mucositis, pruritus, fatigue, hand-foot syndrome (palmar-plantar erythrodysesthesia (painful tingling, erythema, and edema of palms and/or soles))
	Imatinib (Gleevec) TKI against PDGFR, c-kit, stem cell factor, bcr-abl fusion protein, etc. (PO) CYP450 metabolism[d]	Gliomas, BMs with EGFR, chordomas	Fluid retention (peripheral, third spacing), myelosuppression, hepatotoxicity, cardiotoxicity (mostly exacerbation of known CHF)
Supportive agents	Rasburicase (Elitek) (IV) urate oxidase inhibitor (allopurinol is a xanthine oxidase inhibitor)	Prevention and treatment of tumor lysis syndrome (used with other TLS care)	Severe hypersensitivity reaction, including anaphylaxis, hemolysis (G6PD-deficient patients)
	Zoledronic acid (Zometa) bisphosphonate (IV)	Prevention of BMs and bone-related events related to BMs (fracture, pain), malignancy-related hypercalcemia	Osteonecrosis (usually the mandible), nephrotoxicity, electrolyte abnormalities
Investigational agents	Various		Refer to trial sponsor or search agent via www.fda.gov, www.clinicaltrial.gov

Key:
[a]All are considered teratogenic, carcinogenic, and causing infertility, unless proven otherwise. IV (intravenous), PO (oral), IT (intrathecal), PCNSL (primary CNS lymphoma)
[b]1, 3-bis(2-chloroethyl)-1-nitrosurea (BCNU)
[c]*N*-(2-chloroethyl)-*N'*-cyclohexyl-*N*-nitrosourea (CCNU (lomustine))
[d]Watch drug-drug/herb/diet interactions: other CYP450 metabolizing chemotherapies, dexamethasone, cimetidine, fluoxetine, St John's wart, "azoles," rifampin, antiretrovirals, EIAEDs (phenytoin, fosphenytoin, carbamazepine), grapefruit, erythromycin, clarithromycin, diltiazem, amiodarone, verapamil, barbiturates
[e]5-(3-methyltriazen-1-yl)imidazole-4-carboxamide

retrospective analysis evaluating >13,000 patients randomized to 1 of 17 systemic tumor trials involving bevacizumab and who were subsequently diagnosed with BMs. It showed that the collective incidence of cerebral hemorrhage was less than 1–3 % compared to the historical incidence of 3.5–29 % and there was no difference in all-cause mortality [42]. Many others have reported similar results in various primary/secondary CNS tumors, including safety with concurrent use of antiangiogenic agents and anticoagulation.

Treatment of Common CNS Tumors

Gliomas

Treatment of HGGs and LGGs is very different and, thus, detailed separately.

HGGs

Refer to Fig. 34.2a, b for typical MRI characteristics. Acknowledging a lack of prospective randomized trials, existing evidence suggests that an initial approach to treatment involving maximal safe resection improves postoperative neurologic function, performance status, and survival, especially as compared to biopsy alone [44, 45]. With the exception of Gliadel, techniques designed to improve the efficacy of resection including brachytherapy, convection-enhanced delivery, and SRS have not improved outcome.

RT is most commonly used as part of initial therapy and may be used at progression. The most common initial regimen includes a total dose of 60 Gy delivered at 1.8–2 Gy per 30 fraction [46–48]. This is exemplified by the 2005 landmark paper by Stupp and colleagues [49]. For HGG patients not well represented in the literature, such as the elderly and frail (>70 years old and <70 KPS), existing evidence suggests that RT, often delivered at a lowered dose and in a shortened course, improves symptoms and may nominally improve survival [50].

Chemotherapy is commonly used as part of initial treatment, almost always with RT, and with the goals of enhancing the local effect of radiation while preventing or delaying distant recurrence. This is exemplified by the landmark 2005 publication by Stupp and colleagues on behalf of the European Organization for the Research and Treatment of Cancer (EORTC) and National Cancer Institute of Canada (NCIC), who reported a phase III trial of newly diagnosed GB patients treated with either biopsy or resection, then randomized to either traditional RT alone or RT plus concurrent daily temozolomide (TMZ) followed by adjuvant TMZ for up to 6 months (RT/TMZ → TMZ). In long-term follow-up (>5 years), those who received TMZ showed improved overall survival (from 12.1 to 14.6 months), progression-free survival (from 5.0 to 6.9 months), and 2-year survival (from 10.4 to 26.5 %)

and declined in neither neurologic function nor health-related quality of life [41, 51]. Benefit was most pronounced in patients with MGMT methylation [52]. In another example, the addition of the surgically placed BCNU impregnated biodegradable polymer (Gliadel) to maximal safe resection, and RT demonstrated improved survival over RT alone (13.9 vs. 11.6 months) yet remains minimally used secondary to potentially life-threatening symptoms (cerebral edema and infection), poor reimbursement, and the frequent exclusion of such patients from subsequent enrollment into clinical trials [53, 54]. Similar improvements in progression-free survival and overall survival in HGGs are seen with systemic BCNU, CCNU, and PCV [55]. For HGG patients not well represented in the literature (>70 years old or KPS < 70), many reports suggest a non-inferior or improved outcome with chemotherapy, either with RT or alone, over supportive care [56].

Other systemic agents are most commonly used at progression or experimentally with initial therapy. The former is exemplified by the prospective report by Vredenburg and colleagues showing improved progression-free survival and neurologic function, but not overall survival, with bevacizumab [43]. The latter is exemplified by the ongoing RTOG 0825 trial exploring the addition of concurrent and adjuvant bevacizumab to RT/TMZ → TMZ [57]. However, it is important to realize the limits to assessing the impact of antiangiogenic and other systemic agents for HGGs. For example, as a class, antiangiogenic agents often produce a clinical response by minimizing cerebral edema and mass effect in a fashion similar to steroids. However, they also often produce a radiographic response (reduction of T1-w enhancement), which may not correlate to tumor reduction, and thus, "pseudoresponse" [58]. In another example, and in contrast, as a class, small-molecule inhibitors often produce radiographically stable disease, which may not translate to traditional response criteria nor reflect clinical benefit and outcome [59].

There is significantly less consensus on treatment at progression, partially resulting from the diversity in patient presentation, the increased number of agents and strategies under evaluation, and the inherent difficulties in getting prospectively, randomized comparisons. One increasingly used, yet woefully incompletely understood, agent commonly used at progression deserves mention. The antiangiogenic agent bevacizumab was FDA approved in 2009 for progressive GB after demonstrating durable radiographic responses and, in many cases, maintained or improved symptoms. However, such responses may only represent pseudoresponse, as evidenced by mounting literature consistently failing to show a survival advantage.

LGGs

Refer to Fig. 34.1a–c for typical MRI characteristics. Acknowledging that the varied presentations of LGGs and biases (patient and provider) preclude a uniform treatment strategy, existing evidence suggests that an initial approach to treatment involving maximal safe resection of ≥90 % of visible LGG improves survival and minimizes morbidity [60, 61]. In children, LGGs are commonly curable, both because they tend to occur in locations where complete resection is achievable (such as the cerebellum) and because many are WHO I juvenile pilocytic astrocytomas. In adults, LGGs are less commonly curable, even when aggressive resection is achievable, partly because most are grade II and infiltrative.

RT is commonly used for LGGs having (1) undergone only a biopsy or subtotal resection, (2) high-risk features, or (3) undergone progression. The former is exemplified by the prospective EORTC trial 22845 that randomized patients who had undergone either a biopsy or subtotal resection to either RT (54 Gy in 6 weeks) or reservation of RT until progression. Long-term follow-up revealed statistically improved seizure control, prolongation of progression-free survival (5.4 vs. 3.7 years), but no improved survival for those undergoing initial RT [62]. High-risk features commonly used by international researchers include age >40 years old, astrocytic dominant histology, size >6 cm, location crossing the corpus callosum or involving more than one lobe, neurologic symptoms, and Ki-67 >3 % [47, 60]. Several ongoing trials, including RTOG 0424, are evaluating whether initial RT, regardless of extent of resection, will improve outcome.

Chemotherapy is commonly used for LGGs having undergone progression and, occasionally, when treatment is desired but resection and/or RT is undesirable or unachievable. The former is exemplified by numerous studies failing to prolong survival, including RTOG 9802 that showed that adding PCV (procarbazine, CCNU, vincristine) chemotherapy to initial RT in subtotally resected LGGs only slightly improved progression-free survival and at the expense of moderate toxicity [63].

Oligodendrogliomas are a possible exception, and studies are ongoing [32, 64]. Interpreting the benefit of chemotherapy has been limited by the following: (1) difficulty assessing radiographic response in a tumor that is inherently diffuse and non-contrast enhancing, (2) difficulty assessing the results of trials that combine numerous treatments and LGG histologies, and (3) difficulty assessing the results of a tumor with an expected prolonged course. Treatment at progression is similar to HGGs.

Brain Metastases

Clinical presentation, classification, and risk factors are detailed previously. Typical MRI characteristics include well-circumscribed T-1w contrast-enhancing lesion(s), often at the gray-white junction, with significant surrounding vasogenic edema (Fig. 34.3a, b). Treatment centers around simultaneous control of the existing BMs (local brain control), prevention of future BMs (distant brain control), and control of the systemic cancer (systemic control). A prognostic nomogram aiding treatment planning includes RTOG's RPA. RPA class I (16–20 % of BMs) includes patients with KPS > 70, age < 65, controlled primary tumor, and no extracranial metastases (median survival 7.7 months). RPA class III (10–15 %) represents KPS < 70 (median survival 2.3 months). RPA class II (60–65 %) represents the rest (median survival 4.5 months) [28]. RPA is limited by nonrigorous estimation of systemic tumor control and total BMs, two factors known to influence survival. These are incorporated into the more recent Graded Prognostic Assessment (GPA). The GPA uses four factors (age, KPS, number of metastasis, and the presence or absence of extra-neural disease) to partition patients into one of four categories with median overall survival from 2.6 to 11 months [65]. To date, no nomogram incorporates other known prognostic factors (histology, size, or location) nor has been validated using modern treatment. Ultimately, control of the systemic cancer remains the dominant factor impacting overall survival.

In general, patients considered to have a poor prognosis are more likely to receive symptom management alone or a monotherapy, usually WBRT. In contrast, patients considered to have a good prognosis are more likely to receive multimodality therapy, usually a combination of therapies. In general, median survivals for patients who receive steroids alone, WBRT alone, or combination therapy are 1–2, 3–4, and 6+ months, respectively.

Acknowledging that the varied presentations of BMs and biases (patient and provider) precludes a uniform treatment strategy, existing evidence demonstrates that an initial treatment involving maximal safe resection of symptomatic BMs improves survival and minimizes morbidity [66]. Complications are similar to other indications for resection. After resection, or if resection is unachievable or undesirable, available treatments include SRS, WBRT, chemotherapy, and other systemic agents. Individualizing multimodality therapy remains highly evolving and somewhat controversial.

RT is commonly used. Historically, patients received WBRT, either alone or with local treatments (surgery or SRS), and patients receiving both predominantly have improved brain control and time to neurologic decline, and minimal impact on overall survival [67, 68]. However, growing concern over the treatment effects of WBRT, coupled with the improvements in local control, and in select patients, survival, with the combination with local treatment, resulted in a reconsideration regarding the role of WBRT. This is exemplified by Swinson and colleagues, who reported on 619 patients who underwent SRS (N = 1,569) as part of their BM treatment and showed comparable outcomes to series including WBRT. Overall local control rate was 84.3 % and

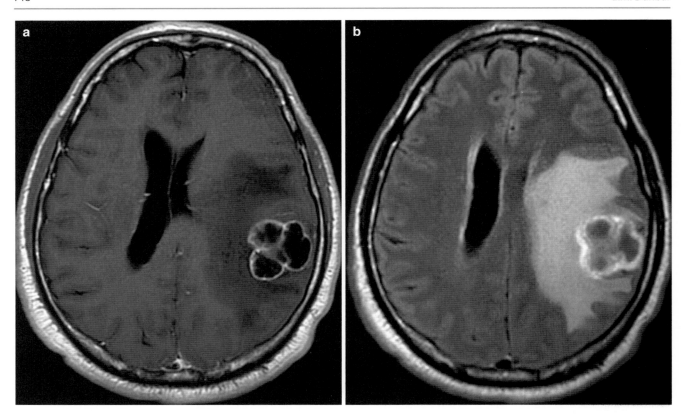

Fig. 34.3 (**a**, **b**) Brain metastasis. T1-w and FLAIR images of a multilobulated brain metastasis within the left parietal lobe, originating from non-small cell lung carcinoma. It demonstrates central necrosis, peripheral enhancement, marked local vasogenic edema, and local mass effect

1- and 2-year actuarial local control probabilities were 0.82 and 0.72, respectively. Median actuarial survival was 7.9 months and 1- and 2-year actuarial survival probabilities were 0.36 and 0.14, respectively. The prognostic value of age, KPS, systemic disease status, and RTOG RPA class was confirmed. In addition, female gender, nonmelanoma BMs, asynchronous presentation of BM, fewer and smaller BMs, resection prior to SRS, and >1 SRS treatment correlated to survival. Lastly, WBRT prior to SRS correlated to improved regional control [69]. Complications are detailed earlier.

Chemotherapy and systemic agents are increasingly being used, especially if there is a need to impact both systemic and CNS disease, but remain mostly palliative. They are used alone or with RT and are chosen either for their efficacy crossing the BBB or for their efficacy with specific histologies [70]. Quantifying their impact in isolation remains challenging because most studies include patients with various histologies, uncontrolled systemic disease, unreported numbers of prior recurrences or treatments, and subjective response criteria. Thus, when generalizing across dissimilar studies, response range between 10 and 30 %, stable disease range between 20 and 30 %, and outcomes in palliation and survival range widely. This is exemplified by a randomized phase III trial by Cameron and coworkers, who reported the oral combination of Xeloda and lapatinib in 399 refractory

metastatic HER2-positive beast showed improved time to progression (HR of 0.57), trended toward improved overall survival (HR of 0.78), and showed fewer cases with CNS involvement at first progression (4 vs. 13, $P = 0.045$) [71]. Complications are detailed in Table 34.3.

Ependymoma

Ependymomas are rare gliomas that originate within or around the ependymal lining of the ventricular system. They represent <10 % of all CNS tumors, 25 % of those occurring in the spine, and most commonly occur in children <20 years old (median age 5 years old) [6]. No gender, race, or other risk factors are known. Prognostic factors include age, histologic grade, extent of resection (determined by postoperative MRI within 48 h), and possibly infratentorial location and KPS. WHO subtypes include myxopapillary ependymoma (WHO grade I), subependymoma (WHO grade I), ependymoma (WHO grade II), and anaplastic ependymoma (WHO grade III), with the latter considered highly malignant. Infratentorial tumors most commonly present with symptoms related to obstructive hydrocephalus. Typical MRI characteristics include homogeneous T1-w hypointensity, T2-w hyperintensity, and possibly cysts or calcifications (Fig. 34.4a–c).

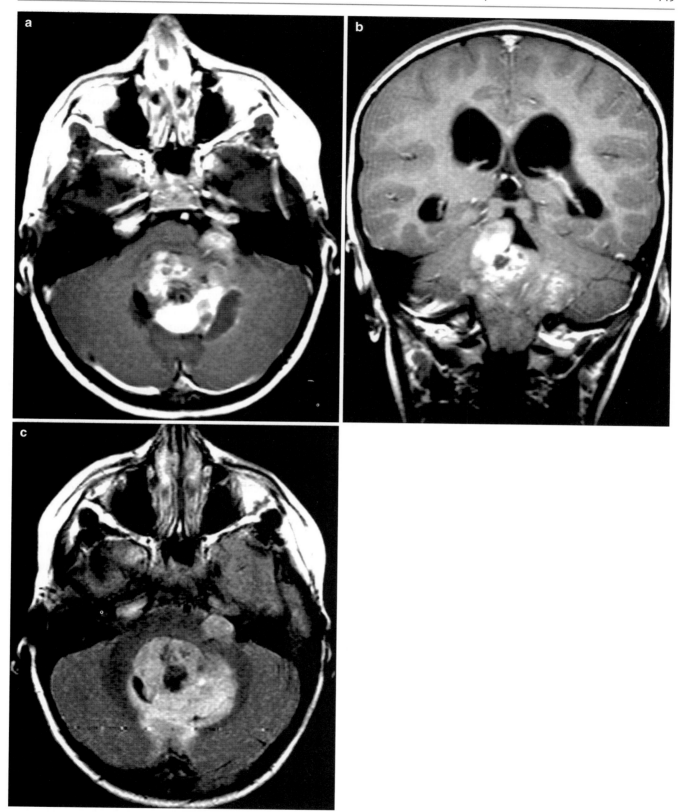

Fig. 34.4 (a–c) T1-w axial/coronal FLAIR images of a WHO II ependymoma arising around the posterior fossa. It demonstrates cystic components and causes hydrocephalus

Staging commonly involves surgical staging, spinal imaging, and CSF. Pathologic characteristics include perivascular pseudorosettes and tapering GFAP-immunoreactive processes. Treatment begins with maximal safe resection, including correcting obstructive hydrocephalus, if present. Given the absence of randomized trials, adjuvant therapy with RT ± chemo (etoposide and platinums) is common, depending on age (usually after 3 years old) and especially when GRT is not achievable or gross metastatic disease is present. Care within academic centers and/or trials are encouraged. Treatment at recurrence is palliative, ideal treatment is undefined, and prognosis is poor.

Medulloblastoma/PNET

Medulloblastomas are CNS primitive neuroectodermal tumors (PNETs) that arise from embryonal cells within the posterior fossa, most commonly around the fourth ventricle, where they present with obstructive hydrocephalus. In children, they are the most common malignant CNS tumor, representing ~33 % of all CNS tumors, and predominantly occur by age 20 years old (>70 %) and rarely after 40 years old. In adults, CNS PNETs are more commonly supratentorial, have a worse prognosis, and receive care similarly to children. No gender or race risk factors are known. Prognostic factors include age, extent of resection, and histopathology (positive if desmoplasia/nodularity is present). Typical MRI characteristics include a heterogeneous T-1w enhancing midline tumor with fourth ventricle compression, cysts, necrosis, hemorrhage, and, one-third of the time, metastasis throughout the neuroaxis (Fig. 34.5a–c). Thus, staging must involve surgical staging, MRI of the brain and spine, and CSF (Table 34.4) [72]. Treatment begins with maximal safe resection (documented by post-op MRI within 48 h), including correcting obstructive hydrocephalus, if present. Adjuvant therapy with RT to the tumor bed (~5,000 cGy) and the entire neuroaxis (~3,000 cGy, usually after 3 years old), as well as chemotherapy (platinums, cyclophosphamide, CCNU, vincristine), are most common and yield 5-years survival rate of 50–70 %. Long-term survivors often have profound treatment-related complications, including neuron-cognitive, hearing, endocrine, and secondary cancers. Treatment at recurrence, which may include systemic disease, is varied and prognosis is poor. Care within academic centers and trials are encouraged.

Intracranial Germ Cell Tumors

Intracranial germ cell tumors (GCTs) are rare tumors that arise within the pineal and suprasellar regions and commonly present with symptoms related to obstructive hydrocephalus

and possibly endocrinopathies (Fig. 34.6a–d). No gender, race, or other risk factors are known. Staging involves MRI (brain and spine), CSF (cytology and tumor markers), blood (tumor markers (alpha-fetoprotein, beta-human chorionic gonadotropin), and systemic imaging. Determination of germinomas and non-germinomatous subtypes is essential because the latter require more intensive treatment, usually RT (both tumor (~45 Gy) and neuroaxis (~21 Gy)) and chemotherapy. Pure germinomas commonly receive whole ventricle RT with boost to the tumor. Chemotherapy in pure germinoma is most commonly used for metastases or recurrence. Especially for non-germinomatous GSTs, trials are encouraged.

Meningioma

Meningiomas represent up to one-third of all CNS tumors, originating from meningothelial cells throughout the dura, most commonly at sites of dural reflection (falx cerebri, tentorium cerebelli, venous sinuses). They are twice as common in females (especially spine). Risk factors include prior RT. Presentation is variable and largely depends on location. Typical MRI characteristics include strong homogeneous T1-w enhancement, iso- to hyperintense T2-w, and, classically, a dural "tail." Most are WHO I (slow growing, benign) (Fig. 34.7a, b), but occasionally WHO II (atypical) and WHO III (fast growing, malignant) occur (Fig. 34.8a, b). In any one individual, they can grow unpredictably. Prognostic factors include age, histologic grade, and extent of resection (most commonly denoted by Simpson grade [73], as detailed in Table 34.5).

Historically, treatment had centered around maximal safe resection, which is commonly curative, especially in WHO I–II lesions and locations ideal for surgery (high-convexity, parasagittal, lateral sphenoid wing). Complications are uncommon and relate to general surgical risks or location. Historically, FRT has been used upfront for unresectable and grade III lesions, or at recurrence. This is exemplified by Condra and colleagues, who reported 15-years local control rates of 30 % (incomplete resection), 76 % (complete resection), and 87 % (incomplete resection + FRT), with survival rates 51, 88, and 86 %, respectively [74]. However, more recently, SRS is being increasingly used for <3 cm or unresectable lesions (such as cavernous sinus). Advantages to SRS include a minimally invasive, single-session, outpatient procedure with long-term control rates >90 %. This is exemplified by Friedman and coworkers, retrospectively reporting on 210 patients undergoing SRS using LINAC and with a minimum of 2-year follow-up. Actuarial local control rates for WHO I lesions were 100 % at both 1 and 2 years and 96 % at 5 years. Actuarial local control rate for WHO II lesions were 100 % at 1 year, 92 % at 2 years, and 77 % at

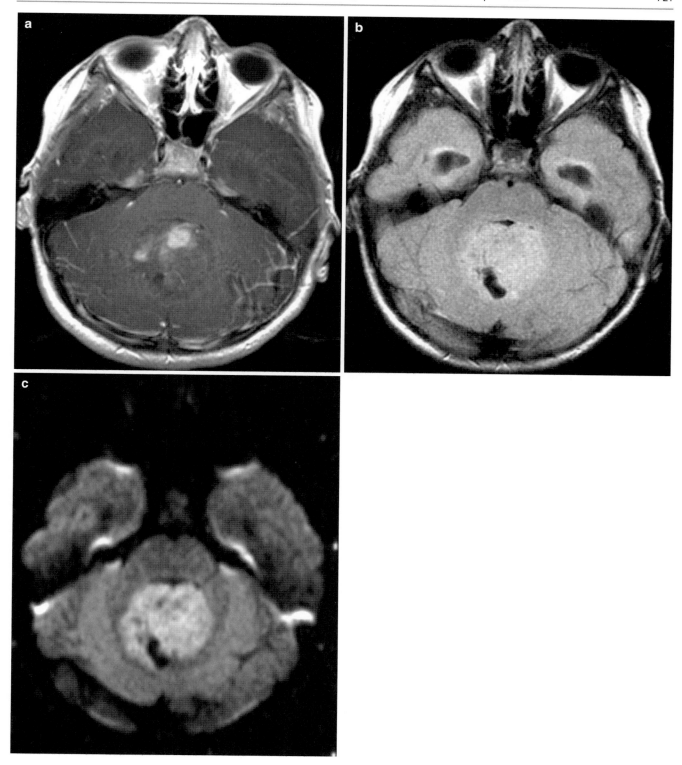

Fig. 34.5 (a–c) T1-w axial, FLAIR, diffusion axial images of a medulloblastoma (PNET) within the posterior fossa. It demonstrates a heterogeneous mass with cystic components and local mass effect

5 years. Actuarial control rates for WHO III lesions were 100 % at both 1 and 2 years and only 19 % at 5 years [75]. Complications to various treatments are uncommon and equivalent to similar CNS tumors. Chemo is uncommonly used at progression/recurrence and is considered investigational and palliative.

Table 34.4 Modified Chang criteria for medulloblastoma

Extent of tumor	No consideration is given to the presence of hydrocephalus or the number of structures invaded
T1	Tumor less than 3 cm in diameter
T2	Tumor greater than 3 cm in diameter
T3a	Tumor greater than 3 cm in diameter and with disease extending into the aqueduct of Sylvius and/or the foramen of Luschka
T3b	Tumor greater than 3 cm in diameter and with gross extension into the brain. This includes surgical staging, regardless of imaging
T4	Tumor greater than 3 cm in diameter and with disease extending past the aqueduct of Sylvius and/or past the foramen magnum
Extent of metastasis	
M0	None, including surgical staging and evaluation of CSF, blood, marrow, and viscera
M1	Only positive CSF cytology (obtained pre- or post-op)
M2	Gross metastasis within the cerebellar/cerebral subarachnoid space or in the third or lateral ventricles
M3	Gross metastasis within the spinal subarachnoid space
M4	Gross metastasis outside the CNS (blood, marrow, viscera)

Data from Chang et al. [72]

Vestibular Schwannoma

Vestibular schwannomas (a.k.a. acoustic neuromas) represent 10 % of primary CNS tumors, yet >80 % of tumors at the cerebellopontine angle, and originate from Schwann cells arising from the myelin sheath of the vestibular branch of the CNVIII. In adults, they have a median onset of 50 years old, slight female predominance, and are unilateral >90 % (without sidedness), unless as part of autosomal dominant neurofibromatosis, type II. In children, they are rare, unless as part of neurofibromatosis. Presentation reflects cranial nerve involvement or compression, including sensorineural hearing loss, tinnitus, ataxia, and facial paresis, paresthesia, hypesthesia, or pain. Race is not a factor, and risk factors include neurofibromatosis, prior RT, and possibly vestibular injury (including occupational). Evaluation includes physical exam, audiometry, vestibular testing, and imaging. Typical MRI characteristics, using millimeter sections through the auditory meatus, include homogeneously T1-w enhancing lesions in the region of the internal auditory canal with variable extension into the cerebellopontine angle (Fig. 34.9a, b). Treatment is individualized to incorporate the variable natural history between patients (averaging 2 mm/year), lesion characteristics, symptoms, presence of genetic syndrome, and preferences (patient and provider). Historically, initial treatment has centered around resection as the primary recommended modality, as exemplified by numerous large series. Although local control rates averaged >90 %, hearing rarely improved after surgery, and long-term follow-up is lacking [76]. Complications increase with lesion size and decrease with increased surgical volume and experience and (despite microscopic techniques and intraoperative neurophysiologic monitoring) include hearing loss, facial paresis/paresthesias, and vestibular disturbances. However, more recently, SRS is increasingly used for lesions, preferentially for <3 cm and after hearing loss, and provides an outpatient, single-session, cost-effective alternative with improved long-term results. This is exemplified by Friedman and coworkers, who report on over 450 patients, receiving SRS using LINAC, and showed a local control rate of 90 % (5-year actuarial control data) and resulting in 99 % of patients requiring no further treatment. With modern dosing (12.5 Gy), complications of facial and trigeminal neuropathies are reported less than 1 % [77]. FRT is less commonly used. Observation is reasonable for the aged and medically ill. Antiangiogenic agents are under investigation, predominantly for their ability to delay time to hearing loss and other palliation [78].

Pituitary Adenomas

Pituitary macroadenomas represent 15 % of primary CNS tumors and present with symptoms of local mass effect (bitemporal hemianopsia and extraocular muscle dysfunction) and/or endocrine dysfunction. Additionally, intratumoral hemorrhage (a.k.a., pituitary apoplexy) can cause sudden visual loss and endocrine failure (Addisonian crisis). Hypo-functioning (nonsecreting) lesions are most common and result in low levels of follicle-stimulating hormone and luteinizing hormone (amenorrhea and impotence) and sometimes low TSH. Hyper-functioning (hypersecreting) lesions result in elevated levels of adrenocorticotropin hormone (Cushing's disease), prolactin (amenorrhea and galactorrhea),

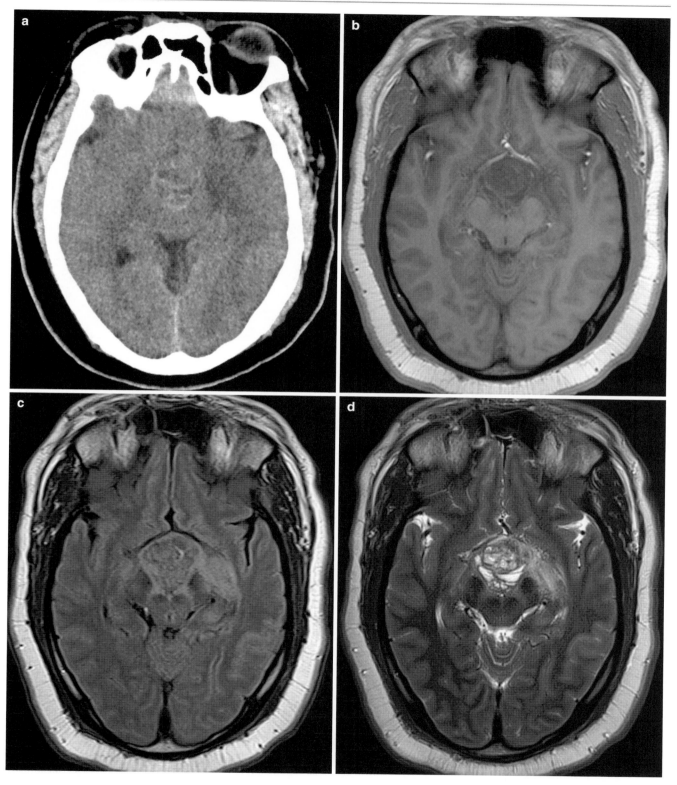

Fig. 34.6 (**a–d**) T and T1-w MRI images, performed without contrast secondary to acute renal failure, of a large suprasellar intracranial germ cell tumor. It demonstrates cystic components, peripheral density representing calcifications, and an absence of infiltrative features

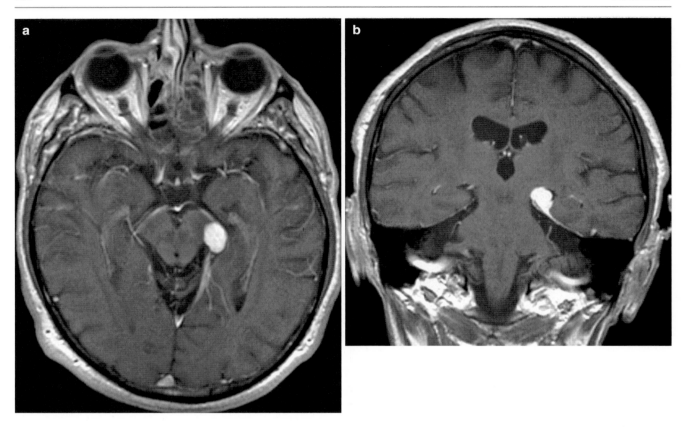

Fig. 34.7 (**a, b**) T1-w, T2-w, and FLAIR images of a WHO grade I meningioma. It demonstrates a densely contrasting enhancing mass and classic "dural tail"

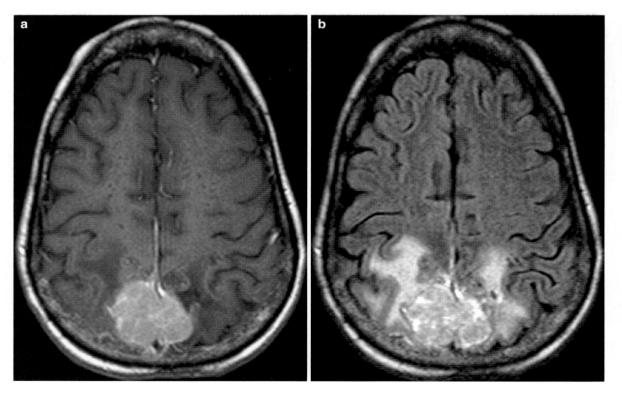

Fig. 34.8 (**a, b**) 1-w and FLAIR images of a parafalcine bilobed WHO grade II atypical meningioma of the parietal cortex. It demonstrates local venous collateralization and encephalomalacia in the mesial brain the parenchyma in the left parietal-occipital area from prior treatment

Table 34.5 Simpson grade resection criteria for meningiomas

Grade	Description	10-years recurrence rates*
I	Complete resection, including dural attachment and abnormal bone	9 %
II	Complete resection with coagulation of dura	19 %
III	Complete resection without dural resection or coagulation	29 %
IV	Incomplete resection	40 %
V	Decompression only	Not reported
		*Similar rates reported in subsequent series

Data from Simpson [73]

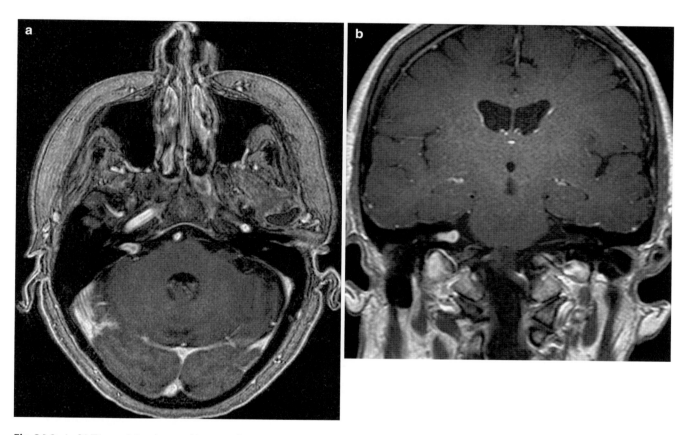

Fig. 34.9 (a, b) T1-w axial and coronal images of a uniformly contrast-enhancing vestibular schwannoma arising from the right cranial nerve VIII

and growth hormone (acromegaly). Typical MRI characteristics include a relatively homogeneously T1-w enhancing lesion within the pituitary fossa (Fig. 34.10a, b). Treatment begins with the knowing secretory status, which impacts the selection of initial treatment and perioperative safety. Historically, complete surgical resection was most commonly used and usually curative (10-years tumor control rate ~90 % in across modern series) for most secretory microadenomas and many of the macroadenomas. Complications are rare and include CSF leak, visual and pituitary deficits, and very rarely, vascular complications. FRT is used upfront for unresectable lesions, unusually aggressive rare histologies (such as Crooke's hyaline change) or at recurrence/progression. However, more recently, SRS is increasingly used for microadenomas, with benefits and results equivalent to similar CNS tumors. Chemotherapy is investigational and palliative.

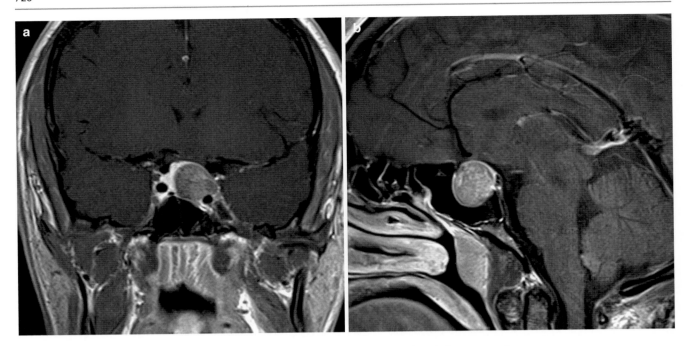

Fig. 34.10 (a, b) T1-w axial and sagittal images of a homogeneously contrast-enhancing pituitary macroadenoma

Summary and Conclusion

Secondary (metastatic) CNS tumors are ten times as common as primary CNS tumors. Symptoms and signs from CNS tumors originate from any combination of the following: elevated intracranial pressure, local destruction, and local irritation. Once treatment begins, signs and symptoms may also originate from the treatment (such as radiation necrosis or myelosuppression) or factors associated with malignancy (such as immunocompromise or venous thromboembolism) and are important to differentiate and treat separately.

Although CT is often the first best imaging technique performed on patients presenting with CNS tumors, MRI is far superior to formulating the differential diagnosis and planning treatment.

Most patients with secondary (metastatic) CNS tumors die from causes unrelated to the CNS, whereas most patients with malignant primary CNS tumors die from CNS causes.

Supportive treatment is distinct from tumor treatment. It is important to simultaneously consider both throughout the disease continuum, spanning diagnosis, curative-intent treatment and palliative/end-of-life.

The development of individualized treatment plans for CNS tumors at progression can be aided by the involvement of tumor boards, academic centers, and enrollment in clinical trials. Mining and contributing to tissue repositories that also prospectively collect clinical information are ever-important.

References

1. Wen PY, Kesari S. Malignant gliomas in adults. N Engl J Med. 2008;359(5):492–507.
2. Norden AD, Wen PY, Kesari S. Brain metastases. Curr Opin Neurol. 2005;18(6):654–61.
3. Brem SN. Central nervous system cancers. NCCN guidelines. J Natl Compr Canc Netw. 2011;9:352–400.
4. Gori S, Rimondini S, De Angelis V, et al. Central nervous system metastases in HER-2 positive metastatic breast cancer patients treated with trastuzumab: incidence, survival, and risk factors. Oncologist. 2007;12(7):766–73.
5. States CBTRotU. CBTRUS statistical report, central brain tumor registry of the United States 2004: primary brain tumors in the United States, 1997–2001. http://www.cbtrus.org/reports/reports.html. Accessed 1 Sept 2009.
6. DeAngelis LM. Brain tumors. N Engl J Med. 2001;344(2):114–23.
7. Louis D, Ohgaki H, Wiestler OD, Cavenee WK. WHO classification of tumours of the nervous system. Lyon: IARC Press; 2007.
8. Yan H, Parsons DW, Jin G, et al. IDH1 and IDH2 mutations in gliomas. N Engl J Med. 2009;360(8):765–73.
9. Furnari FB, Fenton T, Bachoo RM, et al. Malignant astrocytic glioma: genetics, biology, and paths to treatment. Genes Dev. 2007;21(21):2683–710.
10. Cancer Genome Atlas Research Network. Comprehensive genomic characterization defines human glioblastoma genes and core pathways. Nature. 2008;455(7216):1061–8.
11. Wilking U, Karlsson E, Skoog L, et al. HER2 status in a population-derived breast cancer cohort: discordances during tumor progression. Breast Cancer Res Treat. 2011;125(2):553–61.
12. Sawaya R. Considerations in the diagnosis and management of brain metastases. Oncology (Williston Park). 2001;15(9):1144–54, 1157–8; discussion 1158, 1163–5.
13. Ganslandt O, Buchfelder M, Hastreiter P, Grummich P, Fahlbusch R, Nimsky C. Magnetic source imaging supports clinical decision

making in glioma patients. Clin Neurol Neurosurg. 2004;107(1): 20–6.

14. Pirotte B, Goldman S, Dewitte O, et al. Integrated positron emission tomography and magnetic resonance imaging-guided resection of brain tumors: a report of 103 consecutive procedures. J Neurosurg. 2006;104(2):238–53.

15. Patel N, Sandeman D. A simple trajectory guidance device that assists freehand and interactive image guided biopsy of small deep intracranial targets. Comput Aided Surg. 1997;2(3–4):186–92.

16. Young GS. Advanced MRI of adult brain tumors. Neurol Clin. 2007;25(4):947–73, viii.

17. Pirotte BJ, Levivier M, Goldman S, et al. Positron emission tomography-guided volumetric resection of supratentorial high-grade gliomas: a survival analysis in 66 consecutive patients. Neurosurgery. 2009;64(3):471–81; discussion 481.

18. Hermann EJ, Hattingen E, Krauss JK, et al. Stereotactic biopsy in gliomas guided by 3-tesla 1H-chemical-shift imaging of choline. Stereotact Funct Neurosurg. 2008;86(5):300–7.

19. Asthagiri AR, Pouratian N, Sherman J, Ahmed G, Shaffrey ME. Advances in brain tumor surgery. Neurol Clin. 2007;25(4):975–1003, viii–ix.

20. Cairncross G, Berkey B, Shaw E, et al. Phase III trial of chemotherapy plus radiotherapy compared with radiotherapy alone for pure and mixed anaplastic oligodendroglioma: Intergroup Radiation Therapy Oncology Group Trial 9402. J Clin Oncol. 2006;24(18): 2707–14.

21. van den Bent MJ, Carpentier AF, Brandes AA, et al. Adjuvant procarbazine, lomustine, and vincristine improves progression-free survival but not overall survival in newly diagnosed anaplastic oligodendrogliomas and oligoastrocytomas: a randomized European Organisation for Research and Treatment of Cancer phase III trial. J Clin Oncol. 2006;24(18):2715–22.

22. Dunn J, Baborie A, Alam F, et al. Extent of MGMT promoter methylation correlates with outcome in glioblastomas given temozolomide and radiotherapy. Br J Cancer. 2009;101(1):124–31.

23. Brandes AA, Tosoni A, Franceschi E, et al. Recurrence pattern after temozolomide concomitant with and adjuvant to radiotherapy in newly diagnosed patients with glioblastoma: correlation with MGMT promoter methylation status. J Clin Oncol. 2009;27(8): 1275–9.

24. Laws ER, Parney IF, Huang W, et al. Survival following surgery and prognostic factors for recently diagnosed malignant glioma: data from the Glioma Outcomes Project. J Neurosurg. 2003;99(3): 467–73.

25. Lamborn KR, Chang SM, Prados MD. Prognostic factors for survival of patients with glioblastoma: recursive partitioning analysis. Neuro Oncol. 2004;6(3):227–35.

26. Gorlia T, van den Bent MJ, Hegi ME, et al. Nomograms for predicting survival of patients with newly diagnosed glioblastoma: prognostic factor analysis of EORTC and NCIC trial 26981-22981/ CE.3. Lancet Oncol. 2008;9(1):29–38.

27. Curran Jr WJ, Scott CB, Horton J, et al. Recursive partitioning analysis of prognostic factors in three Radiation Therapy Oncology Group malignant glioma trials. J Natl Cancer Inst. 1993;85(9): 704–10.

28. Gaspar L, Scott C, Rotman M, et al. Recursive partitioning analysis (RPA) of prognostic factors in three Radiation Therapy Oncology Group (RTOG) brain metastases trials. Int J Radiat Oncol Biol Phys. 1997;37(4):745–51.

29. Macdonald DR, Cascino TL, Schold Jr SC, Cairncross JG. Response criteria for phase II studies of supratentorial malignant glioma. J Clin Oncol. 1990;8(7):1277–80.

30. van den Bent MJ, Vogelbaum MA, Wen PY, Macdonald DR, Chang SM. End point assessment in gliomas: novel treatments limit usefulness of classical Macdonald's criteria. J Clin Oncol. 2009;27(18): 2905–8.

31. Liu R, Solheim K, Polley MY, et al. Quality of life in low-grade glioma patients receiving temozolomide. Neuro Oncol. 2009;11(1):59–68.

32. Kesari S, Schiff D, Drappatz J, et al. Phase II study of protracted daily temozolomide for low-grade gliomas in adults. Clin Cancer Res. 2009;15(1):330–7.

33. Grossman SA, Ye X, Piantadosi S, Desideri S, Nabors, LB, Rosenfeld M, Fisher J, NABTT CNS Consortium. Current survival statistics for patients with newly diagnosed glioblastoma treated with radiation and temozolomide on research studies in the United States. Paper presented at: ASCO annual meeting, Orlando; June 2009.

34. Olson JD, Riedel E, DeAngelis LM. Long-term outcome of low-grade oligodendroglioma and mixed glioma. Neurology. 2000;54(7):1442–8.

35. Meyer FB, Bates LM, Goerss SJ, et al. Awake craniotomy for aggressive resection of primary gliomas located in eloquent brain. Mayo Clin Proc. 2001;76(7):677–87.

36. Sawaya R, Hammoud M, Schoppa D, et al. Neurosurgical outcomes in a modern series of 400 craniotomies for treatment of parenchymal tumors. Neurosurgery. 1998;42(5):1044–55; discussion 1055–6.

37. Merchant TE, Conklin HM, Wu S, Lustig RH, Xiong X. Late effects of conformal radiation therapy for pediatric patients with low-grade glioma: prospective evaluation of cognitive, endocrine, and hearing deficits. J Clin Oncol. 2009;27(22):3691–7.

38. Ruben JD, Dally M, Bailey M, Smith R, McLean CA, Fedele P. Cerebral radiation necrosis: incidence, outcomes, and risk factors with emphasis on radiation parameters and chemotherapy. Int J Radiat Oncol Biol Phys. 2006;65(2):499–508.

39. Ricard D, Taillia H, Renard JL. Brain damage from anticancer treatments in adults. Curr Opin Oncol. 2009;21(6):559–65.

40. George TJ, Leather H, et al. "University of Florida hematology-oncology handbook", 2009. http://www.medicine.ufl.edu/hemonc/ fellowship/Handbook/HOH-TOC.htm. Accessed 30 May 2011.

41. Stupp R, Hegi ME, Mason WP, et al. Effects of radiotherapy with concomitant and adjuvant temozolomide versus radiotherapy alone on survival in glioblastoma in a randomised phase III study: 5-year analysis of the EORTC-NCIC trial. Lancet Oncol. 2009;10(5): 459–66.

42. Rohr U, Augustus S, Lasserre SF, et al. Safety of bevacizumab in patients with metastases to the central nervous system (abstract). J Clin Oncol. 2009;27:88s. Abstract available on line at: http:// www.abstract.asco.org.lp.hscl.ufl.edu/. Accessed on 5 June 2009.

43. Vredenburgh JJ, Desjardins A, Herndon 2nd JE, et al. Bevacizumab plus irinotecan in recurrent glioblastoma multiforme. J Clin Oncol. 2007;25(30):4722–9.

44. Bucci MK, Maity A, Janss AJ, et al. Near complete surgical resection predicts a favorable outcome in pediatric patients with non-brainstem, malignant gliomas: results from a single center in the magnetic resonance imaging era. Cancer. 2004;101(4):817–24.

45. Lacroix M, Abi-Said D, Fourney DR, et al. A multivariate analysis of 416 patients with glioblastoma multiforme: prognosis, extent of resection, and survival. J Neurosurg. 2001;95(2):190–8.

46. Coughlin C, Scott C, Langer C, Coia L, Curran W, Rubin P. RP Phase, II two-arm RTOG trial (94–11) of bischloroethyl-nitrosourea plus accelerated hyperfractionated radiotherapy (64.0 or 70.4 Gy) based on tumor volume (>20 or < or = 20 cm(2), respectively) in the treatment of newly-diagnosed radiosurgery-ineligible glioblastoma multiforme patients. Int J Radiat Oncol Biol Phys. 2000;48(5): 1351–8.

47. Shaw E, Arusell R, Scheithauer B, et al. Prospective randomized trial of low- versus high-dose radiation therapy in adults with supratentorial low-grade glioma: initial report of a North Central Cancer Treatment Group/Radiation Therapy Oncology Group/Eastern Cooperative Oncology Group study. J Clin Oncol. 2002;20(9): 2267–76.

48. Karim AB, Maat B, Hatlevoll R, et al. A randomized trial on dose–response in radiation therapy of low-grade cerebral glioma: European Organization for Research and Treatment of Cancer (EORTC) Study 22844. Int J Radiat Oncol Biol Phys. 1996;36(3):549–56.

49. Stupp R, Mason WP, van den Bent MJ, et al. Radiotherapy plus concomitant and adjuvant temozolomide for glioblastoma. N Engl J Med. 2005;352(10):987–96.

50. Keime-Guibert F, Chinot O, Taillandier L, et al. Radiotherapy for glioblastoma in the elderly. N Engl J Med. 2007;356(15):1527–35.

51. Taphoorn MJ, Stupp R, Coens C, et al. Health-related quality of life in patients with glioblastoma: a randomised controlled trial. Lancet Oncol. 2005;6(12):937–44.

52. Mirimanoff RO, Gorlia T, Mason W, et al. Radiotherapy and temozolomide for newly diagnosed glioblastoma: recursive partitioning analysis of the EORTC 26981/22981-NCIC CE3 phase III randomized trial. J Clin Oncol. 2006;24(16):2563–9.

53. Westphal M, Hilt DC, Bortey E, et al. A phase 3 trial of local chemotherapy with biodegradable carmustine (BCNU) wafers (Gliadel wafers) in patients with primary malignant glioma. Neuro Oncol. 2003;5(2):79–88.

54. Weber EL, Goebel EA. Cerebral edema associated with Gliadel wafers: two case studies. Neuro Oncol. 2005;7(1):84–9.

55. Stewart LA. Chemotherapy in adult high-grade glioma: a systematic review and meta-analysis of individual patient data from 12 randomised trials. Lancet. 2002;359(9311):1011–8.

56. Brandes AA, Vastola F, Basso U, et al. A prospective study on glioblastoma in the elderly. Cancer. 2003;97(3):657–62.

57. Gilbert M. RTOG 0825: temozolomide and radiation therapy with or without bevacizumab in treating patients with newly diagnosed glioblastoma or gliosarcoma. http://clinicaltrials.gov/ct2/show/NCT00884741?term=0825&rank=3. Accessed 1 Sept 2009.

58. Wen PY, Macdonald DR, Reardon DA, et al. Updated response assessment criteria for high-grade gliomas: response assessment in neuro-oncology working group. J Clin Oncol. 2010;28(11):1963–72.

59. van den Bent MJ, Brandes AA, Rampling R, et al. Randomized phase II trial of erlotinib versus temozolomide or carmustine in recurrent glioblastoma: EORTC brain tumor group study 26034. J Clin Oncol. 2009;27(8):1268–74.

60. Pignatti F, van den Bent M, Curran D, et al. Prognostic factors for survival in adult patients with cerebral low-grade glioma. J Clin Oncol. 2002;20(8):2076–84.

61. Keles GE, Lamborn KR, Berger MS. Low-grade hemispheric gliomas in adults: a critical review of extent of resection as a factor influencing outcome. J Neurosurg. 2001;95(5):735–45.

62. van den Bent MJ, Afra D, de Witte O, et al. Long-term efficacy of early versus delayed radiotherapy for low-grade astrocytoma and oligodendroglioma in adults: the EORTC 22845 randomised trial. Lancet. 2005;366(9490):985–90.

63. Shaw EG, Berkey B, Coons SW, Brachman D, Buckner JC, Stelzer KJ, Barger GR, Brown RD, Gilbert MR, Mehta M. Initial report of Radiation Therapy Oncology Group (RTOG) 9802: prospective studies in adult low-grade glioma (LGG). Paper presented at: ASCO, Journal of Clinical Oncology; June 2006.

64. Mohile NA, Forsyth P, Stewart D, et al. A phase II study of intensified chemotherapy alone as initial treatment for newly diagnosed anaplastic oligodendroglioma: an interim analysis. J Neurooncol. 2008;89(2):187–93.

65. Sperduto PW, Berkey B, Gaspar LE, Mehta M, Curran W. A new prognostic index and comparison to three other indices for patients with brain metastases: an analysis of 1,960 patients in the RTOG database. Int J Radiat Oncol Biol Phys. 2008;70(2):510–4.

66. Patchell RA, Tibbs PA, Walsh JW, et al. A randomized trial of surgery in the treatment of single metastases to the brain. N Engl J Med. 1990;322(8):494–500.

67. Andrews DW, Scott CB, Sperduto PW, et al. Whole brain radiation therapy with or without stereotactic radiosurgery boost for patients with one to three brain metastases: phase III results of the RTOG 9508 randomised trial. Lancet. 2004;363(9422):1665–72.

68. Patchell RA, Tibbs PA, Regine WF, et al. Postoperative radiotherapy in the treatment of single metastases to the brain: a randomized trial. JAMA. 1998;280(17):1485–9.

69. Swinson BM, Friedman WA. Linear accelerator stereotactic radiosurgery for metastatic brain tumors: 17 years of experience at the University of Florida. Neurosurgery. 2008;62(5):1018–31; discussion 1031–2.

70. Gerstner ER, Fine RL. Increased permeability of the blood–brain barrier to chemotherapy in metastatic brain tumors: establishing a treatment paradigm. J Clin Oncol. 2007;25(16):2306–12.

71. Cameron D, Casey M, Press M, et al. A phase III randomized comparison of lapatinib plus capecitabine versus capecitabine alone in women with advanced breast cancer that has progressed on trastuzumab: updated efficacy and biomarker analyses. Breast Cancer Res Treat. 2008;112(3):533–43.

72. Chang C, Housepain EM, Herbert Jr C. An operative staging system and a megavoltage radiotherapeutic technic for cerebellar medulloblastomas. Radiology. 1969;93:1351–9.

73. Simpson D. The recurrence of intracranial meningiomas after surgical treatment. J Neurol Neurosurg Psychiatry. 1957;20(1):22–39.

74. Condra KS, Buatti JM, Mendenhall WM, Friedman WA, Marcus Jr RB, Rhoton AL. Benign meningiomas: primary treatment selection affects survival. Int J Radiat Oncol Biol Phys. 1997;39(2):427–36.

75. Friedman WA, Murad GJ, Bradshaw P, et al. Linear accelerator surgery for meningiomas. J Neurosurg. 2005;103(2):206–9.

76. Samii M, Matthies C. Management of 1000 vestibular schwannomas (acoustic neuromas): surgical management and results with an emphasis on complications and how to avoid them. Neurosurgery. 1997;40(1):11–21; discussion 21–3.

77. Friedman WA. Linear accelerator radiosurgery for vestibular schwannomas. In: Régis J, Roche P-H, editors. Modern management of acoustic neuroma. Prog Neurol Surg, vol. 21. Basel: Karger; 2008. p. 228–37, 78.

78. Plotkin SR, Stemmer-Rachamimov AO, Barker 2nd FG, et al. Hearing improvement after bevacizumab in patients with neurofibromatosis type 2. N Engl J Med. 2009;361(4):358–67.

Elevated Intracranial Pressure

35

Shelly D. Timmons

Contents

S.D. Timmons, MD, PhD, FACS, FAANS
Department of Neurological Surgery, Geisinger Health System,
100 North Academy Ave, Danville, PA 17822, USA
e-mail: stimmons@mac.com

Abstract

Understanding the physiology underlying intracranial pressure is critical to developing sound management plans for central nervous system pathology. Principles of treatment are based upon a variety of complex interactions between cerebral blood supply and drainage, tissue oxygenation and ischemia, brain tissue edema, and a variety of other pathophysiological mechanisms. Molecular, cellular, tissue, and organ pathologies vary according to the primary insult, but management of ICP elevation is crucial for the reduction of further injury, debility, and death.

Keywords

Intracranial pressure • Monro-Kellie doctrine • Blood–brain barrier • Cerebral edema • Cerebral compliance • Autoregulation • Cerebral herniation • Neuromonitoring

Introduction

Intracranial pressure is the pressure inside the skull, typically measured in mmHg or cmH_2O. Any discussion of intracranial pressure (ICP) must begin with the Monro-Kellie doctrine, the principles of which were first described by Monro in 1783 [1] and expounded upon by Kellie in 1824 [2]. The intracranial compartment can be conceptualized as a closed container with three primary tissues comprising the intracranial contents: the brain, cerebrospinal fluid (CSF), and blood. If one of the components within the cranium increases in volume, one of the others must decrease, or else the intracranial pressure will increase. This relationship is characterized by the pressure-volume curve (Fig. 35.1). If the volume of the brain expands due to cerebral edema, the pressure will eventually increase, unless the volume of either the circulating blood or CSF is decreased. An increase in intracranial pressure can likewise decrease the circulating blood volume, leading to a cascade of ischemia, cellular dysfunction,

A.J. Layon et al. (eds.), *Textbook of Neurointensive Care*,
DOI 10.1007/978-1-4471-5226-2_35, © Springer-Verlag London 2013

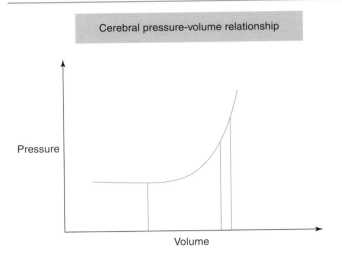

Fig. 35.1 Pressure-volume relationship to intracranial pressure. Monro-Kellie doctrine

worsening edema, and cellular and tissue death. Development of mass lesions such as tumors or hemorrhages can contribute slowly or rapidly to the intracranial volume. Depending on the patient's age and degree of cerebral atrophy, additional volumes of 100–150 mL can be accommodated, especially if the increase is slowly developing, but beyond this, elevated ICP is seen.

In order to properly understand the development of elevated ICP or intracranial hypertension, its evolution if left unchecked, and the various mechanisms of preventing and treating it, there are several key concepts of brain physiology that need to be understood.

The Blood–Brain Barrier

The blood–brain barrier (BBB) is constituted by tight junctions between endothelial cells lining the intracranial vasculature [3]. (Likewise, a "blood-CSF" barrier exists due to similar junctions between choroid plexus epithelial cells.) This barrier prevents the entry of pathogens and other molecules to the extracellular space of the brain parenchyma from the bloodstream, thereby providing a relatively protected environment for the brain. This barrier is actually a dynamic interface responding to a variety of states, and can be altered by drugs, such as methamphetamine and other drugs of abuse [4], and in a variety of pathological states, including ischemic stroke, trauma, subarachnoid hemorrhage, CNS infection, hepatic encephalopathy, hyperammonemia, multiple sclerosis, AIDS encephalopathy, and Alzheimer's disease. Disruption of the blood–brain barrier contributes to vasogenic cerebral edema through the entry of water into the interstitium of the brain.

Cerebrospinal Fluid

In adults, CSF is constantly produced at a rate of 0.4 mL/min (approximately 450 mL/day), while the normal total CSF volume in an adult is approximately 150 mL, with approximately half within the cranial vault and the remainder in the spine. Normal flow after production, which is primarily by intraventricular choroid plexus at the trigones of the lateral ventricles and fourth ventricle, is through the ventricular system out the foramina of Magendie and Luschka over the surfaces of the brain and spinal cord, and absorption via arachnoid granulations. Increased secretion or decreased absorption of CSF can result in excess CSF volume and therefore an increase in ICP. In the setting of aneurysmal or traumatic subarachnoid hemorrhage, the passive absorption of CSF by the arachnoid granulations may be impaired, resulting in over-accumulation of CSF, increased ICP, or hydrocephalus. Tumors or intraventricular hemorrhages may likewise obstruct the flow of CSF, especially if the fourth ventricle is compressed or directly compromised by the mass lesion.

Displacement of CSF out of the cranial vault and into the subarachnoid space of the spinal cord is a compensatory mechanism to eliminate significant elevations in intracranial pressure if the volume of brain is increased by small amounts of edema. As cerebral edema worsens to a point beyond which no CSF can be displaced, cerebral blood volume (CBV) and cerebral blood flow (CBF) decrease, ultimately resulting in cerebral ischemia, brain herniation, and death if left unchecked.

Cerebral Edema

Vasogenic Edema

Vasogenic edema results from opening of tight endothelial junctions between the cells forming the blood–brain barrier. This may be caused by mechanical forces such as trauma or pressure-induced transudation of fluid as seen in arterial hypertension. It can also be caused by chemical or cellular interactions, such as the release of compounds that attack the endothelium, as by some types of brain tumors. Finally, ischemia-induced endothelial damage, as seen in high-altitude sickness or trauma, can produce breakdown of the BBB. In addition to allowing plasma components into the tissues, molecules normally excluded from brain tissue by this endothelial layer and kept confined to the intravascular space can enter the extracellular space of the brain parenchyma forming an osmotic gradient that pulls additional water into the extracellular environment.

Cytotoxic (Cellular) Edema

Cytotoxic edema is a result of alterations in cellular metabolism that impair the ion pumps of glial cells, resulting in accumulation of intracellular sodium and water. This can be seen in a variety of clinical scenarios, including toxin or drug ingestion, ischemia, encephalopathy, or even hypothermia.

Osmotic Edema

Failure to maintain normal osmolality in blood can result in development of osmotic edema. When plasma becomes dilute, as in hyponatremia or hemodialysis, an osmotic gradient is set up promoting flow of water down the osmotic gradient from the serum to the brain tissue, resulting in brain edema.

Interstitial Edema

Obstructive hydrocephalus can produce direct pressure on the ependyma of the ventricles, pushing fluid from the CSF spaces into the extracellular spaces of the periventricular areas. This can be seen as transependymal flow on T2-weighted MRI scans.

Coma and Herniation Syndromes

The end result of unchecked intracranial hypertension is herniation and ultimately death. Cushing's triad consisting of hypertension, bradycardia, and respiratory dysfunction may be seen with cerebral herniation. Since the intracranial compartment is divided into supratentorial and infratentorial compartments by the tentorium cerebelli, depending on the location of the intracranial process producing high ICP, herniation may occur downward (from the supratentorial to the infratentorial compartment and ultimately through the foramen magnum) or, much less commonly, upward in select circumstances. Mass lesions producing compression on the supratentorial hemisphere can result in uncal herniation.

Central Herniation

This form of herniation may also be described as downward herniation, transtentorial herniation, or tentorial herniation. The diencephalic stage [5] is characterized by an early change in alertness followed by agitation or drowsiness, stupor, and coma. Respiratory patterns of sighs, yawns, and pauses with progression to Cheyne-Stokes respirations are

typical. Pupils are small and reactive. Intact oculocephalic and oculovestibular responses are present early and later become easier to elicit (without nystagmus). Appropriate motor responses to noxious stimuli, but sometimes accompanied by Babinski responses and increased tone, may be seen early with progression to motionlessness and decorticate posturing.

The midbrain-upper pons stage is typified by hyperventilation; mid-position, irregular, fixed pupils; impaired oculocephalic and oculovestibular reflexes; and lack of motor response or decerebrate posturing [5].

Finally, the lower pons-upper medullary stage follows, as exemplified by shallow rapid breathing at normal rates or ataxic breathing, fixed mid-position pupils, absent oculocephalic and oculovestibular reflexes, and flaccidity or isolated lower extremity flexion or Babinski [5].

Uncal Herniation

Uncal herniation is most often the result of a rapidly expanding unilateral hematoma, usually from trauma. This form of herniation is characterized by the early third nerve stage, the late third nerve stage, and the midbrain-upper pons stage, followed by central herniation [5]. The process is begun by compression of the temporal lobe typically from a middle fossa or hemispheric lesion, displacing the medial uncus and hippocampal gyrus over the tentorial edge, compressing or entrapping the third nerve which runs along the tentorial edge, and ultimately compressing the midbrain. The posterior cerebral artery (PCA) may also be compressed or occluded.

The early third nerve stage is identified by a unilateral, usually ipsilateral, dilating pupil that may also become sluggishly reactive. While patients may retain consciousness at this point, there is typically some alteration in the neurological status, such as agitation or confusion. A contralateral Babinski may be seen early on in this stage.

The late third nerve stage consists of a fully dilated unreactive pupil, ptosis – often obscured by unconsciousness – external oculomotor ophthalmoplegia, progression to stupor and coma, hyperventilation (if not mechanically ventilated), and contralateral weakness. (The Kernohan's notch phenomenon may be seen in which the false-localizing sign of ipsilateral hemiplegia occurs from compression of the contralateral cerebral peduncle against the opposite tentorial edge.) Bilateral decerebration follows, with or without preceding decorticate posturing, but most often without.

The midbrain-upper pons stage consists of the contralateral pupil becoming unreactive, followed by return of both pupils to a mid-position (5–6 mm) and fixed state. Oculomotor function becomes decreased or absent; sustained hyperpnea and bilateral decerebrate rigidity ensue. Following this, progression to central herniation occurs.

Upward Herniation

Upward herniation can occur in the setting of posterior fossa mass lesions or cerebellar edema [5]. This can be aggravated by ventricular drainage; however, compression of the aqueduct of Sylvius and basilar cisterns may result in acute hydrocephalus requiring CSF drainage. As the cerebellar tissues ascend through and above the tentorium, direct compression of the midbrain and superior cerebellar arteries or deep central draining veins can occur, producing worsening ischemia and edema.

ICP Waveforms

Normal ICP waveforms consist of several peaks produced by pulsations transmitted from the systemic blood pressure to the intracranial contents superimposed on slower peaks from respirations. The blood pressure pulsations can be subdivided into three main peaks, the so-called A, B, and C waves. The "A wave" corresponds to the arterial systolic pressure and has a 1–2 mmHg variability and a dicrotic notch. The "B wave" follows the A wave and consists of smaller less distinctive peaks. The "C wave" corresponds to the central venous "A" wave from the right atrium. The spectral properties of ICP vary with different intracranial states, such as alterations in brain compliance, autoregulation, cerebral perfusion pressure, site of measurement, and time differences in vascular inflow and outflow.

Compliance

Cerebral compliance is defined as the "stiffness" of the brain and can be described by the relationship between the ICP and brain volume as follows, where Δv = change in volume and Δp = change in pressure:

$$C = \frac{\Delta v}{\Delta p}$$

Elasticity or elastance is the reverse:

$$E = \frac{\Delta p}{\Delta v}$$

The reason that the pressure/volume curve is not linear is that brain compliance decreases as ICP increases. The pressure-volume index is defined as the volume required to increase the ICP tenfold and is the slope of the volume

plotted logarithmically against the ICP [6]. The degree of compliance can be estimated in the intensive care unit (ICU) by evaluation of the ICP waveforms. The noncompliant brain will be demonstrated by higher peaks and wider pulse pressures on the ICP waveform; these patients will benefit the most from small volume reduction, such as removal of even small volumes of CSF, in terms of ICP control, but may also suffer from acute elevations with minor increases in blood volume, such as can be seen with obstructed venous outflow from raided intrathoracic or intra-abdominal pressure or direct compression from head turning.

Autoregulation and Cerebral Energy Requirements

Cerebral metabolism relies upon a constant supply of CBF. CBF is defined by the following equation, where CPP is cerebral perfusion pressure, MAP is mean arterial pressure, and CVR is cerebrovascular resistance:

$$CBF = \frac{CPP}{CVR} = \frac{MAP - ICP}{CVR}$$

Low CBF may result from elevated ICP, low MAP, or increased cerebrovascular resistance, e.g., from diffuse cerebral edema. In normal physiologic states, CBF is directly related to CBV, but this relationship may be altered in pathological states such as trauma, ischemic stroke, or aneurysmal subarachnoid hemorrhage.

The energy requirements for the brain are provided by aerobic metabolism, i.e., from the oxidation of glucose in the presence of oxygen. The cerebral metabolic rate for oxygen consumption ($CMRO_2$) ranges from 3.1 to 3.7 mL/100 g of brain tissue per minute and comprises 20 % of the oxygen consumption of the body. $CMRO_2$ is estimated by the following equation:

$$CMRO_2 = CBF \times AVjDO_2$$

where $AVDO_2$ is the arterial-jugular venous oxygen difference. $AVjDO_2$ is kept at a relatively constant 6.5 mL of O_2 per 100 mL of blood; so to meet alternating demands of $CMRO_2$, CBF must change.

Autoregulation normally occurs to maintain blood flow to the brain in the face of varying conditions. This occurs via arterial constriction and dilation for baroregulation (response to changes in BP) and chemoregulation (response to changes in pCO_2 and pH). In pathological states, autoregulation may be impaired regionally or globally within the brain. Complete loss of autoregulation results in a linear relationship between MAP and ICP (Fig. 35.2).

Normally, autoregulation of the cerebral vasculature maintains adequate perfusion at mean arterial blood pressures ranging from 50 to 150 mmHg. In the classic work of

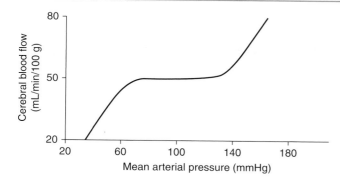

Fig. 35.2 Autoregulation between MAP and ICP

Kety and Schmidt, normal CBF was defined at approximately 50 mL/100 g/min (46–63 at normal $PaCO_2$ levels). Regional alterations in CBF are known to occur. When an area of the brain performs "work," its metabolic needs (and therefore regional CBF) may increase. The ability to measure regional cerebral blood flow (rCBF) has aided in the definition of thresholds for cerebral dysfunction. For example, Morawetz and colleagues, using an awake *Macaca irus* monkey model of reversible ischemia via middle cerebral artery occlusion, showed that at 20 mL/100 g/min, EEG and evoked potential abnormalities were seen, and paralysis was noted; at 15 mL/100 g/min, EEG and evoked potentials were lost. CBF at ~12 mL/100 g/min for >120 min resulted in cerebral infarction; at 6 mL/100 g/min, cell membrane integrity was lost.

CBF alterations have been extensively studied in the setting of severe TBI. Severe TBI results in immediate decreases in CBF [7–11], and reduction in CBF can result in either regional or global cerebral ischemia. Regional reductions in CBF in pericontusional areas and under SDH have also been demonstrated [12, 13]. TBI-associated vasospasm increases intravascular resistance and thereby decreases CBF [14–16]. Cerebral metabolism also initially decreases, resulting in decreased CBF after TBI [11]. Decreased CBF is associated with increases in mediators of secondary brain injury, such as production of extracellular oxygen radicals, lactate, glutamate, and intracellular ionized calcium [17] as well as altered cerebral metabolism as demonstrated by glucose metabolism variability near hematomas seen on positron emission tomography (PET) [18].

In clinical practice, CBF is not easily measured at the bedside; therefore, it is more commonly estimated using measurements of cerebral perfusion pressure (CPP). Patients with conditions resulting in elevated ICP may require maintenance of a higher CPP to maintain adequate CBF.

Again, studies from the TBI arena have greatly informed our understanding of the clinical use of CPP. The most recent evidence-based guidelines for management of severe TBI indicated that a range of 50–70 mmHg is likely optimal for adults [19]. This represented a change from the first guidelines published in 1996 which recommended maintenance of CPP greater than 70 mmHg [20] and the 2000 second edition that had recommended maintenance of CPP greater than 60 mmHg [21].

Early studies from animal models of TBI demonstrated that elevation and maintenance of MAP aborted ICP plateau waves and rapid rises in ICP [22]. Human studies showed improvement in outcomes of TBI patients whose CPP was kept above 70 mmHg when compared to a historical control group using Traumatic Coma Data Bank (TCDB) data, while sometimes allowing ICP to range from 20 to 25 mmHg [23]. Others have variably demonstrated effects of different CPP thresholds on outcome. One study demonstrated that the percentage of time the CPP was less than 70 mmHg was associated with poor outcome [24], while CPP less than 50 mmHg correlated with poor outcome but not values less than 60 or 70 mmHg [25]. Still other studies showed that CPP less than 60 mmHg correlated with poor outcomes [26–30], with one of these using decision tree analysis to identify the two most important variables among eight, which were hypotension and CPP less than 60 mmHg (even more important than ICP in that series). However, two of these series showed no improvement in outcome when CPP was kept above 60 mmHg, suggesting potential confounders [28, 29]. Furthermore, subsequent evaluation of CPP-driven therapy using vasopressors and fluids to keep CPP above a minimum of 70 mmHg showed that the therapy was associated with significant pulmonary morbidity from a fivefold increase in adult respiratory distress syndrome [31].

Pericontusional increases in extracellular lactate and increased lactate/pyruvate ratios indicating ischemia have been shown when CPP is less than 50 mmHg [32]. These changes were not seen in normal-appearing brain or when CPP was maintained greater than 50 mmHg. Others have shown that a reduction of mean CPP from 73 to 62 mmHg resulted in reductions in extracellular lactate and glutamate and lactate/pyruvate ratios or "normalization" of cerebral metabolism [33]. This is in keeping with the "Lund concept" of brain trauma management, the goals of which are to prevent elevated ICP and to improve perfusion and oxygenation around contusions [34]. Measurements of arterial-jugular venous oxygen content difference ($AVDO_2$) or saturation ($S_{jv}O_2$) have also been used to further define optimal CPP. When CPP was kept above 50 mmHg, no $S_{jv}O_2$ drops below 50 % were seen [35]. When kept above 60 mmHg, increases in $S_{jv}O_2$ were seen along with decreases in $AVDO_2$ [36] without further benefit noted when CPP was pushed to more than 70 mmHg. Finally, when clinical effects of CPP thresholds on partial pressure of brain tissue oxygen ($P_{bt}O_2$) were studied, increases in $P_{bt}O_2$ were seen up to 67 mmHg but beyond that were not improved [37]. Logistic regression analysis done for that study identified CPP greater than 60 mmHg as the most important determinant of sufficient $P_{bt}O_2$, even more important than mannitol, hyperventilation, elevation of HOB, and decompressive craniectomy as other therapeutic measures employed to reduce ICP and improve CPP in TBI patients. Another trial determined that the incidence of $P_{bt}O_2$ less than 20 mmHg (a critical threshold for ischemia) was no different for CPP measurements ranging from 48 to 70 mmHg than for measurements greater than 70 mmHg [38].

In the absence of intact autoregulation, the concern is that increasing the MAP and CPP will increase ICP. When the absence of autoregulation was defined by a greater than 30 % increase in CBF, an increase in MAP from 92 to 123 mmHg showed no significant increases in ICP [39]. In more recent research, various methods of imputing the optimal CPP have been used [40, 41]. In one such examination, when autoregulation was considered to be defective by increases in ICP of greater than or equal to 2 mmHg associated with increases in MAP greater than or equal to 15 mmHg, better outcomes were seen when CPP was 50–60 mmHg and ICP was kept below 20 mmHg. Those patients who had intact autoregulation did better with higher MAP/CPP levels. Such use of the ICP/MAP relationship proves to be the most straightforward means of estimating whether autoregulation is intact or not in the ICU, as xenon CT to measure CBF is not widely available and bedside CBF measurements are not yet widely employed.

It is also important to remember that even brain-injured patients who undergo aggressive therapy to maintain ICP and CPP at normal levels may still experience periods of severe brain hypoxia [42]. Likewise, interventions previously thought to improve tissue oxygenation may improve ICP and CPP but actually decrease $P_{bt}O_2$ [43]. Therefore, more advanced neuromonitoring techniques may be justified in many of these patients.

Optimizing CPP in the setting of aneurysmal subarachnoid hemorrhage has been associated with improved outcomes as well [44]. Other pathological states may impact on autoregulatory management in the ICU. For example, the cerebral autoregulatory curve is shifted to the right in patients with chronic arterial hypertension, so that a higher pressure is required to maintain adequate perfusion of the brain parenchyma. The implication is that in chronically hypertensive individuals, the lower limit of autoregulation may be as high as 110–130 mmHg [45] rather than 60 mmHg in non-hypertensives.

Impact on Prognosis

In the setting of TBI, elevated ICP is associated with poor outcome, as shown in numerous clinical studies. Marmarou and colleagues demonstrated that the proportion of ICP

measurements greater than 20 mmHg was highly significant in explaining worse outcomes in severely brain-injured patients [46, 47]. Others have demonstrated similar findings with aggressive treatment of TBI including ICP monitoring and targeted therapy going back several decades [48–53]. Similar results have been shown in other pathogenic states such as stroke [54] and spontaneous intracranial hemorrhage [55].

Indications for Monitoring Intracranial Pressure

Traumatic Brain Injury

Evidence-based guidelines [19] recommend ICP monitoring for all salvageable patients with severe TBI (post-resuscitation GCS 3–8) and an abnormal computed tomography (CT) scan as a Level II recommendation. Abnormal CT is defined as demonstrating hematoma, contusion, swelling, herniation, or compressed basal cisterns. Level III recommendations are also included for monitoring severe TBI patients with a normal head CT and two of more criteria as follows: age greater than 40 years, motor posturing (unilateral or bilateral), or any SBP measurement less than 90 mmHg.

Other Conditions

Conditions such as ischemic infarction, aneurysmal subarachnoid hemorrhage (aSAH), hepatic encephalopathy, infectious conditions, or any other condition resulting in significant cerebral edema may prompt measurement of ICP. In the setting of aSAH, the use of external ventricular drainage is often employed for both the measurement of ICP and drainage of CSF, the circulation of which can be obstructed by the presence of the aSAH, resulting in interstitial edema superimposed on other potential types of edema caused by ischemia from vasospasm, for example.

Techniques for Monitoring Intracranial Pressure

Fluid-Coupled Monitoring/Ventriculostomy

The gold standard for monitoring of ICP is a fluid-coupled mechanism using external ventricular drainage (EVD) via a ventricular catheter. This remains a relatively low-cost means of measuring ICP. In addition to the diagnostic benefit of measuring ICP, there is also the potential for therapeutic benefit, via the drainage of CSF thereby reducing volume of CSF and lowering ICP. As previously noted, on the higher portion of the pressure-volume curve where compliance is poor, the removal of very small volumes of CSF can have profoundly advantageous impact on the ICP. Other advantages include ability to recalibrate the catheter in situ.

A right (non-dominant) frontal approach is typically used, but the left side may be required in some instances, such as the presence of significant right IVH. Prophylactic antibiotics are not indicated [19], except perhaps for the utilization of a single pre-procedural dose, as skin contamination at insertion has been shown to be the most common risk factor for infection. Colonization of the device is more often seen than significant infection [56]. Risk factors [57–66] for infection include intraventricular hemorrhage, subarachnoid hemorrhage, open skull fracture, basilar skull fracture with CSF leak, elevated ICP, duration of monitoring, previous neurosurgical operation, irrigation of the closed EVD system, leakage around the catheter, and presence of other infections. Not associated with infection are location of insertion, previous EVD, CSF drainage, or use of steroids.

Surveillance cultures and CSF profiles for cell count with differential, protein, and glucose measurements are sometimes performed. These are performed more frequently in the setting of fever, and less frequently without fever. Arguing for routine use of surveillance cultures is early detection and therefore potential for treatment, of CSF infection. However, obtaining specimens for study requires opening the closed CSF drainage system and therefore increasing the potential for contamination. Treatment with appropriate antibiotics when infections are identified is indicated. Routine catheter exchanges are not recommended [19, 60].

Other disadvantages of this ICP monitoring technique include difficulty in placement in the setting of small or slit ventricles as in severe cerebral edema, difficulty maintaining patency in the presence of intraventricular hemorrhage or hemorrhage on the tip of the catheter, and relatively more complex and intricate maintenance and troubleshooting needs.

Parenchymal Monitoring

Monitoring of ICP with fiber-optic techniques is also a commonly employed technique. While this technique has been found to be reliable, it is also prone to minor inaccuracies which have resulted in it not being considered as the gold standard. However, it is simpler technically to place these monitors, and they have been shown to be associated with fewer complications, including very low hemorrhage rates and nearly negligible infection rates.

Other Forms of ICP Monitoring

Developed in the early days of ICP monitoring, other forms have largely been abandoned. These include subarachnoid, subdural, and epidural monitors.

Other Forms of Advanced Neuromonitoring

Brain Tissue Oxygenation
Parenchymal catheters are now available for the routine monitoring of continuous brain tissue oxygenation ($P_{bt}O_2$). $P_{bt}O_2$ measurements with currently available commercial technology require simultaneous measurement of brain temperature, which can be done with either the same catheter or a separate one. Double-lumen or triple-lumen bolts are available to accommodate simultaneous placement of an intraparenchymal ICP catheter.

Cerebral Blood Flow
Bedside CBF monitoring employing thermal diffusion probe technology has been described in neurosurgical intraoperative and critical care settings, often for aneurysmal subarachnoid hemorrhage [67, 68]. This technique most accurately can be described as measuring regional CBF.

Electroencephalography (EEG)
Many ICUs are employing utilization of continuous video EEG monitoring for broader and broader indications. Given emerging literature to suggest frequent incidence of nonconvulsive seizures (with potential implications for ICP control) in comatose patients [69], utilization of this modality may become even more widespread.

Hemodynamic Monitoring
For critically ill patients undergoing ICP or other neuromonitoring, use of arterial line continuous blood pressure measurements is vital for the simultaneous measurement of CPP. Central venous catheters or pulmonary artery (PA) catheters are also commonly employed for measurement of central venous pressure or pulmonary artery pressure to aid in management. Understanding of systemic volume status is key to the management of the patient with intracranial hypertension. Core body temperature is measured with bladder probes or PA catheter probes.

Techniques for Treatment of Elevated Intracranial Pressure

Resuscitation

Maintenance of airway, breathing, and circulation are critical to limiting the degree of ischemia and resultant brain edema.

Maintenance of cerebral blood volume is important for maintaining perfusion of the brain for adequate oxygenation, as previously elucidated.

Techniques to Reduce CSF Volume and CBV

Cerebrospinal Fluid Drainage

External ventricular drainage is a mainstay of treatment for elevated ICP due to hydrocephalus or diffuse cerebral edema related to traumatic brain injury. Fluid-coupled transducers or fiber-optic catheters can be incorporated into the drain for continuous or intermittent measurement of ICP.

Hyperventilation

Hyperventilation results in vasoconstriction and a concomitant decrease in blood volume. Rebound vasodilation with rapidly rising pCO_2 can result in abrupt worsening of edema and ICP elevation. In the setting of severe TBI, chronic prolonged or prophylactic hyperventilation to pCO_2 less than or equal to 25 mmHg is to be avoided as a Level II recommendation [19, 70] hyperventilation within the first 24 h may compromise perfusion at a time when CBF is already low. Hyperventilation *is* recommended as a temporizing measure (Level III evidence) to reduce ICP, as in patients with measured ICP or signs of impending cerebral herniation, such as unilateral or bilateral posturing, unilateral or bilateral fixed dilated pupils, or unilateral hemiparesis. Measurements of $S_{jv}O_2$ or $P_{bt}O_2$ are recommended to approximate oxygen delivery to the brain. Hyperventilation has historically been used to control ICP in the setting of brain tumors as well. Pericontusional [12] ischemic penumbra and peritumoral tissue may be at particular risk with the use of hyperventilation, due to loss of chemoregulation of the cerebral vasculature in those areas.

Positioning

The head of bed is elevated to 30° to enhance the venous outflow by the aid of gravity and to maximize the cerebral perfusion by limiting the amount of elevation. The use of neuromonitoring to guide the positioning of the patient for optimization of both ICP and CPP is recommended.

The presence of an external cervical orthosis may inhibit cerebral venous outflow, thereby increasing intracranial pressure. Likewise, the postural weakness conferred by the neurological insult may result in the head turning to the side if no collar is in place, thereby kinking the jugular veins and obstructing venous outflow.

Initial efforts at controlling ICP elevations should always first include the simple maneuvers of making sure that the HOB is elevated, that the neck is in the neutral position, and that there is no compression of the neck vessels by orthoses or other medical equipment or positioning.

Techniques to Reduce Cerebral Edema

Osmotic Agents

Historically, the osmotic diuretic urea was used to reduce ICP. Mannitol has enjoyed a longer life in the treatment armamentarium due to fewer side effects. Administration of mannitol in bolus doses of 0.25 g/kg to 1 g/kg body weight is effective for control of elevated ICP [19]. Care should be taken to avoid hypovolemia and associated hypotension (SBP less than 90 mmHg). Use in TBI patients prior to initiation of ICP monitoring is restricted to those with signs of transtentorial herniation or to those with progressive neurological deterioration not attributable to systemic or hemodynamic causes.

The mechanisms of action of mannitol are thought to be twofold [71–73]. First, there is an immediate rheological effect from reductions in hematocrit and blood viscosity resulting from plasma expansion. This eventuates in increased CBF, microvascular circulation of erythrocytes, and O_2 delivery, and reduction of ICP ensues within minutes. The next phase is characterized by the osmotic effect brought about by increased serum tonicity drawing cerebral edema fluid down the osmotic gradient into the intravascular space. This occurs only after osmotic gradients are established, which takes 15–30 min after administration and may last up to 1.5–6 h.

Bolus administration is preferred over continuous infusion due to the fact that mannitol opens the BBB and itself may cross the BBB and draw fluid into the interstitial space of the brain [74]. If used regularly, tapering doses off will aid in prevention of rebound ICP elevations.

Loop diuretics (furosemide 10–40 mg IV in multiple doses) are sometimes employed alone or in combination with mannitol to increase the serum osmolarity. Although serum osmolarity greater than 320 mOsm/L may be safe in some circumstances, osmotic and loop diuretics, as well as hypertonic solutions, are typically only used when the intravascular volume is adequate and the serum osmolarity is less than 320 mOsm/L. Acute renal failure can occur with repeated doses of these agents (acute tubular necrosis). Extra caution should be employed in patients with hypovolemia, use of other drugs that are potentially nephrotoxic, septic patients, and those with preexisting renal disease.

Evidence is emerging regarding the use of hypertonic saline as both an osmotic treatment of ICP and a small volume resuscitation fluid that can increase the intravascular volume through osmotic gradients [75]. While there is lack of consensus on the exact dose and timing of delivery, studies support the use of bolus therapies over continuous infusions for TBI. In addition to being more efficacious, bolus administration may help prevent sudden significant hypernatremia and hyperosmolarity that may be seen with large fluid shifts in polytrauma patients. Continuous drips are used in other circumstances, but in the face of hyponatremia upon presentation, it must be used with extreme caution in order to avoid central pontine myelinolysis.

The use of HTS may help avoid hypotension, one of the two cardinal insults after TBI, the other being hypoxia. There has been repeated documentation of the efficacy of HTS in improving and maintaining MAP in animal models of resuscitation through volume expansion, reduction in peripheral and pulmonary vascular resistance, and centrally mediated effects on cardiac output, effects that have been borne out in human studies [75, 76]. Improvements in ICP, CPP, and CBF in brain-injured humans have also been demonstrated [77–80]. Like mannitol, HTS has osmotic effects that enhance CBF by reduction of blood viscosity, but without the disadvantage of accumulating in cerebral tissue [74]. Although HTS has been extensively studied in human resuscitation and trauma (reviewed in [75]), the most recent edition of the TBI treatment guidelines [19] lists HTS only as an option to treat elevated ICP based upon Level III evidence consisting of just two studies which met inclusion criteria at that time [81, 82]. Limited conclusions for clinical management can be drawn from these studies. Certainly the preponderance of evidence indicates that HTS is safe in humans with severe TBI and may mitigate several pathophysiological processes contributing to secondary injury. If used, close monitoring of serum sodium and osmolarity, volume status and fluid balance, ICP, and CPP should be performed, and the patient's clinical examination and imaging should guide therapeutic use.

Steroids

Steroids may be employed to treat edema caused by brain tumors or patients undergoing cerebral radiation. Based upon the early work of French and Galicich [83], once the appropriateness of steroid use has been determined, a loading dose of dexamethasone 10 mg IV is typically given, followed by initial treatment of 4 mg IV every 6 h followed by a taper, the rapidity of which is dictated by the clinical circumstance and imaging. Dexamethasone is the preferred agent due to minimal mineralocorticoid effects.

The single guideline for treatment of traumatic brain injury that is supported by Level I evidence is the *avoidance* of corticosteroid therapy, as demonstrated in multiple trials, but most definitively in the Corticosteroid Randomization After Significant Head Injury (CRASH) trial [84]. Studies of the 21-aminosteroid non-glucocorticoid analog of methylprednisolone, tirilazad mesylate showed no improvement in TBI patients in a randomized prospective trial [84], although several important observations were made from this trial regarding the role of hypotension and hypoxia and lessons learned in the conduct of large-scale multicenter trials for TBI.

Techniques to Reduce Cerebral Metabolism

Barbiturates

Barbiturate therapy decreases the metabolic expenditures of the brain via a variety of putative mechanisms [85]. Only one study has shown efficacy of pentobarbital in improving outcomes *if* the drug was effective at treating elevated ICP [84], and this study concluded that the indications applied only to a small subset of patients with severe TBI. Not all patients respond to barbiturates. Patients receiving barbiturates who are also hypovolemic actually fare worse. The main drawback to the use of barbiturates in patients with brain insults is the propensity to cause hypotension via decreased sympathetic tone and suppression of myocardial contractility with reduction in cardiac output, thereby negatively affecting brain perfusion. Therefore, if employed, invasive hemodynamic monitoring and maintenance of adequate intravascular volume are required. Pentobarbital coma also requires continuous EEG monitoring to guide appropriate dosing to achieve burst suppression. This is typically achieved with administering a loading dose 10 mg/kg IV over 30 min followed by 5 mg/kg every hour for three additional doses. This is followed by a continuous infusion of 1 mg/kg/h. For those unfortunate patients who progress to brain death, the determination of brain death may be delayed until serum pentobarbital levels drop to a negligible level, which may take several days. Likewise, an accurate neurological examination is not achievable during this period for those who may improve. Finally, higher rates of infection may also be seen with prolonged use.

Hypothermia

Hypothermia also decreases cerebral metabolic demands. Normothermia is defined as 36.5–38.5 °C. Mild hypothermia is generally accepted to range from 34 to 36 °C and moderate hypothermia from 32 to 33 °C, with deep or severe hypothermia being less than 32 °C. Several clinical trials have demonstrated efficacy in reduction of ICP with hypothermia after TBI, but no large-scale trials have demonstrated definitive improvements in outcome. Due to the propensity for negative side effects, recommendations are currently to use in research settings only for TBI [75]. No Phase III randomized trials have yet been conducted in ischemic stroke, although a European study is planned to begin in late 2012 [86].

Seizure Treatment and Prophylaxis

Seizures have been shown to increase intracranial pressure. Conversely, elevated ICP has been shown to induce seizures. For critical care patients with neurological impairment who may be subject to seizure activity, consideration should be given to seizure prophylaxis, especially those in coma or under sedation who may experience subclinical seizure activity.

For patients with traumatic brain injury, Level II evidence for seizure prophylaxis in the first week is indicated for those with post-resuscitation Glasgow Coma Scale scores less than 10, seizure within 24 h of injury, subdural hematoma, epidural hematoma, cortical contusion, intracerebral hematoma, depressed skull fractures, or penetrating brain trauma [84]. Phenytoin and valproate have been shown to be effective at preventing early (less than 7 days post-injury) post-traumatic seizures, with valproate being associated with a trend toward higher mortality [84]. Use of novel agents such as levetiracetam has started to be evaluated in the setting of TBI in recent years, with somewhat mixed results thus far. In one study, patients with TBI were studied with EEG monitoring and given phenytoin or levetiracetam, and those given levetiracetam had more abnormal EEG findings and electroencephalographic seizure tendency. No differences were seen in outright seizure activity or Glasgow Outcome Scores, although not originally statistically powered for outcomes differences [84]. However, another randomized clinical trial examining levetiracetam versus phenytoin in patients with severe TBI and aneurysmal SAH showed improvement in later Disability Rating Scales and Glasgow Outcome Scores in the levetiracetam group, although no differences were seen in side effects, mortality, or seizure rates on continuous EEG in the first 72 h [84]. The same group concluded that, while generalized slowing on early EEG in TBI and SAH patients was associated with worse long-term outcomes, EEG findings of focal slowing, epileptiform discharges, and seizures were not linked to long-term outcome [84].

In the setting of aSAH, some endovascular treatments have been shown to induce seizure activity (intra-arterial verapamil [84], intra-arterial fasudil [84], but not coil embolization [84]). Prophylactic use after aSAH has remained somewhat controversial. Seizures often occur only at the time of initial hemorrhage or rehemorrhage but may occur in up to 2 % of patients after invasive treatment [87]. Furthermore, nonconvulsive seizures may occur in comatose patients. Short-term prophylaxis for 3 days has therefore been advocated by some.

Patients with CNS tumors who will be undergoing chemotherapy or radiation therapy may require different agents that are not hepatically metabolized [88], such as gabapentin or levetiracetam. Agents inducing the hepatic cytochrome p450 system may result in increased clearance and decreased efficacy of corticosteroids and chemotherapeutic agents. Furthermore, anticonvulsants with propensity for cutaneous reactions may be associated with increased complications of irradiation therapy to the cranium and scalp.

In summary, anticonvulsant therapy in the critical care setting is an important adjunct for treatment, but has not been shown to be effective at preventing long-term seizures in post-traumatic or post-aSAH settings or for prevention of first seizures in the setting of cerebral neoplasm.

Mixed Mechanisms of Action

Minimization of Stimulation

Many procedures and care activities in the ICU can increase ICP. Fiber-optic bronchoscopy [84] has been shown to increase ICP, for example, albeit without concomitant reductions in CPP (due to increase in MAP). This study showed that neither pretreatment with topical 4 % lidocaine to the trachea nor sedation or paralysis prevented this effect, but no patients exhibited neurological deterioration. Another study corroborated the findings of increased ICP and CPP with endotracheal suctioning and further showed that estimations of cerebral oxygenation (using $S_{jv}O_2$) were unchanged [84]. For those patients with particularly reactive ICP or reduced compliance, minimization of stimulation can sometimes aid in ICP control.

Sedation/Neuromuscular Blockade

Analgesia for pain control can aid in ICP control and should be a first-line of treatment for postoperative patients or those with painful traumatic injuries. Use of intravenous morphine or fentanyl may aid in the smooth treatment of pain, but care must be taken to monitor and respond to potential decreases in CPP. Furthermore, narcotics may lower the seizure threshold. Patients with dysautonomia, on the other hand, may benefit from the use of narcotics, which dissipate the effects of "storming." Another advantage is reversibility. Care must be taken when using these agents and weaning from mechanical ventilation, as respiratory suppression may occur.

Sedation and neuromuscular blockade can be used if patients are agitated, but their use outside this scenario is unproven in terms of improving outcome after TBI and other neurocritical care illnesses. Patients who are agitated, posturing, or shivering may experience elevations in ICP that are responsive to sedative and/or paralytic agents. Propofol is an excellent choice for most neurocritical care patients due to its short duration of effect and the ability to titrate patients to a sedated yet responsive state. Since its introduction, use of neuromuscular blockade has significantly diminished for use in control of ICP in the ICU. Sedation with or without paralytics may be needed for those patients in whom mechanical ventilation induces coughing, bucking, or "fighting the ventilator."

Benzodiazepines are less desirable due to less predictability of effect on the neurological examination, particularly with the elderly and obese, and with prolonged use. If needed, shorter-acting drugs such as midazolam should be considered.

Dexmedetomidine, a centrally acting α_2-receptor agonist, has been emerging as a sedative agent in critical care in recent years; however, its use in neurocritical care patients, especially those with TBI, has not yet been studied extensively. Specifically, its use has not yet been proven safe in patients with neurological disorders in whom it is critical to maintain normal CBF [89]. The FDA has approved its use with a loading dose of 0.1 mcg/kg infused over 10 min followed by 0.2–0.7 mcg/kg/h continuous infusion for less than or equal to 24 h [84].

Agents such as antipsychotics commonly used in the setting of ICU delirium should be avoided due to their potentially prolonged effects on the neurological examination and, with some drugs, harmful effects on outcome [90].

Glucose Control

Both hypoglycemia and hyperglycemia can exacerbate secondary neuronal injury. Hypoglycemia (serum glucose <50 mg/dL in adults and <30 mg/dL in neonates) can result in direct neuronal injury [91], as cerebral aerobic metabolism relies on continuous delivery of glucose. However, in hypoxic states, hyperglycemia (serum glucose greater than 150 mg/dL) may also be deleterious, by causing a shift to anaerobic metabolism resulting in intracellular acidosis and magnification of the secondary injury cascade. Clinical studies have demonstrated better results in patients with controlled serum glucose in the face of acute brain injury, e.g., stroke or TBI [92]. Hyperglycemia may be induced by corticosteroid therapy employed in the treatment of brain tumors and should be controlled, as elevated glucose can exacerbate cerebral edema.

Temperature Control

Avoidance of hyperthermia is desirable with most brain pathology that results in edema, ischemia, and elevated ICP. The deleterious effects of fever on cell survival [75] compound other cytotoxic effects of elevated ICP.

Surgical Techniques to Expand the Cranial Vault

Evacuation of Mass Lesions

Removal of mass lesions such as hematomas and tumors is important to reduce the intracranial volume occupied by these lesions and to accommodate the surrounding edematous brain. Removal of tumors will often result in rapid reduction of edema from the surrounding brain tissue over the ensuing several days, in addition to the volume occupied by the tumor. Removal of sizeable hematomas will result in immediate reduction in ICP. For traumatic hematoma, guidelines for removal exist based upon volume and degree of midline shift associated with the lesion.

Removal of deep cerebral hematomas, while associated with reduction in ICP and direct mass effect, may not impact eventual outcome [84] due to the destruction of vital paramedian tissues such as the basal ganglia that are often associated. Likewise surgical evacuation of very large spontaneous cerebral hematomas (more than 85 mL in volume) may not confer improvement in outcome [93].

Evidence-based surgical guidelines for evacuation of traumatic mass lesions were published in 2006. While evidence bases relied upon Level III evidence, due to the nature of the ethics of research in this area, several recommendations were made based upon volume and mass effect of mass lesions, while taking into account the clinical examination and circumstances.

Epidural hematomas [94] greater than 30 mL should generally be evacuated regardless of the GCS. An EDH less than this volume *and* less than 15 mm thick *and* less than 5 mm midline shift *and* GCS greater than 8 *without* focal deficit can sometimes be managed non-operatively with serial CT and close neurological observation in a neurosurgical center.

Regardless of GCS, subdural hematomas with thickness greater than 10 mm *or* midline shift more than 5 mm should be evacuated [95]. Patients with SDH and GCS less than 9, i.e., in coma, should generally undergo ICP monitoring. Finally, a comatose patient not meeting the above surgical evacuation size criteria may still require surgery if GCS decreased between time of injury and admission by 2 or more points *and/or* if initial examination reveals asymmetrical or fixed and dilated pupils *and/or* the ICP is greater than 20 mmHg.

For those patients with traumatic intraparenchymal hematomas and contusions, signs of neurological deterioration referable to the lesion, ICP refractory to medical treatments, or signs of significant mass effect on CT should be considered for surgical evacuation [96]. Patients with GCS 6–8 and frontal or temporal contusions more than 20 mL and midline shift of 5 mm or more *and/or* cisternal compression on CT *or* those with lesion volume more than 50 mL should be considered for surgery. For those patients without neurological compromise, no elevated ICP, and no significant mass effect, non-operative management with intensive care neuromonitoring and serial imaging can be done. In addition to surgical evacuation of the mass lesion, other surgical techniques that may be employed in these scenarios include bifrontal decompressive craniectomy and decompressive hemicraniectomy. In either case, subtemporal decompression is critical. Temporal lobectomy may sometimes be employed. These techniques bear consideration especially in the setting of clinical or radiographic impending transtentorial herniation.

Posterior fossa hematomas should be evacuated in those patients with mass effect on imaging or neurological dysfunction or deterioration referable to the lesion [97]. Compression of the basilar cisterns, shift or compression of the fourth ventricle, and obstructive hydrocephalus are signs of mass effect in the posterior fossa.

Decompressive Hemicraniectomy and Duraplasty

Decompressive hemicraniectomy (DHC) has been shown to help control ICP in numerous studies [75]. Its use has become more and more widespread in the last decade in cases of medically refractory ICP in the face of TBI, stroke, and other pathologies. Keys to success of this procedure are patient selection, timing, adequate bone removal, and opening of the dura. Unsalvageable patients due to prolonged herniation and those who are late in the course of refractory ICP are not likely to do well after DHC [75]. The bony removal must be large enough and incorporate adequate temporal bone removal down to the floor of the middle fossa floor to prevent herniation of already vulnerable brain tissue over the bone edges compressing venous outflow and arterial blood supply or causing direct tissue damage. For patients with malignant middle cerebral artery stroke-related edema, outcome is typically more favorable in younger patients with better GCS scores done as early intervention prior to herniation [84] and in non-dominant hemispheric lesions [84].

Bifrontal Craniectomy

Bifrontal craniectomy is typically used in a subset of patients in whom there is diffuse cerebral edema with cisternal effacement and lack of lateralizing findings on CT. The same principles of management apply as with DHC.

Summary

A variety of mechanisms for treating intracranial hypertension exist, based upon principles of CSF drainage, reduction in cerebral blood volume, reduction in tissue edema, removal of mass lesions, and expansion of the cranial vault. Contemporaneous utilization of a variety of techniques is often required in the critical care unit, and meticulous attention to detail is a must. Modification of treatments based upon response may be required several times during the course of an episode of care. Thorough understanding of the physiology coupled with a constant awareness of potentially conflicting treatment strategies and possible side effects will enhance the care of the patient with neuropathological illness resulting in intracranial hypertension.

Acknowledgments Thank you to A. Joseph Layon and Andrea Gabrielli for provision of the chapter on Elevated Intracranial Pressure from the first edition of this title as guidance.

References

1. Monro A. Observations on the structure and function of the nervous system. Edinburgh: Creech & Johnson; 1783.
2. Kellie G. An account of the appearances observed in the dissection of two of the three individuals presumed to have perished in the storm of the 3rd, and whose bodies were discovered in the vicinity of Leith on the morning of the 4th November 1821 with some reflections on the pathology of the brain. Trans Medico-Chirurgical Soc Edinburgh. 1824;1:84–169.
3. Naik P, Cucullo L. In vitro blood–brain barrier models: current and perspective technologies. J Pharm Sci. 2012;101(4):1337–54.
4. Kousik SM, Napier TC, Carvey PM. The effects of psychostimulant drugs on blood brain barrier function and neuroinflammation. Front Pharmacol. 2012;3:121.
5. Plum FP, Posner JB. The diagnosis of stupor and coma. 3rd ed. Philadelphia: FA Davis; 1982.
6. Marmarou A, Shulman K, Rosende RM. A nonlinear analysis of the cerebrospinal fluid system and intracranial pressure dynamics. J Neurosurg. 1978;48(3):332–44.
7. Marion DW, Bouma GJ. The use of stable xenon-enhanced computed tomographic studies of cerebral blood flow to define changes in cerebral carbon dioxide vasoresponsivity caused by a severe head injury. Neurosurgery. 1991;29(6):869–73.
8. Bouma GJ, Muizelaar JP, Choi SC, Newlon PG, Young HF. Cerebral circulation and metabolism after severe traumatic brain injury: the elusive role of ischemia. J Neurosurg. 1991;75(5):685–93.
9. Bouma GJ, Muizelaar JP, Bandoh K, Marmarou A. Blood pressure and intracranial pressure-volume dynamics in severe head injury: relationship with cerebral blood flow. J Neurosurg. 1992;77(1):15–9.
10. Bouma GJ, Muizelaar JP. Cerebral blood flow, cerebral blood volume, and cerebrovascular reactivity after severe head injury. J Neurotrauma. 1992;9 Suppl 1:S333–48.
11. Obrist WD, Langfitt TW, Jaggi JL, Cruz J, Gennarelli TA. Cerebral blood flow and metabolism in comatose patients with acute head injury. Relationship to intracranial hypertension. J Neurosurg. 1984;61(2):241–53.
12. McLaughlin MR, Marion DW. Cerebral blood flow and vasoresponsivity within and around cerebral contusions. J Neurosurg. 1996;85(5):871–6.
13. Salvant Jr JB, Muizelaar JP. Changes in cerebral blood flow and metabolism related to the presence of subdural hematoma. Neurosurgery. 1993;33(3):387–93; discussion 393.
14. Martin NA, Doberstein C, Alexander M, et al. Posttraumatic cerebral arterial spasm. J Neurotrauma. 1995;12(5):897–901.
15. Servadei F, Murray GD, Teasdale GM, et al. Traumatic subarachnoid hemorrhage: demographic and clinical study of 750 patients from the European brain injury consortium survey of head injuries. Neurosurgery. 2002;50(2):261–7; discussion 267–9.
16. Taneda M, Kataoka K, Akai F, Asai T, Sakata I. Traumatic subarachnoid hemorrhage as a predictable indicator of delayed ischemic symptoms. J Neurosurg. 1996;84(5):762–8.
17. McIntosh TK. Neurochemical sequelae of traumatic brain injury: therapeutic implications. Cerebrovasc Brain Metab Rev. 1994 Summer;6(2):109–62.
18. Bergsneider M, Hovda DA, Lee SM, et al. Dissociation of cerebral glucose metabolism and level of consciousness during the period of metabolic depression following human traumatic brain injury. J Neurotrauma. 2000;17(5):389–401.
19. Bratton SL, Chestnut RM, Ghajar J, et al. Guidelines for the management of severe traumatic brain injury. J Neurotrauma. 2007;24 Suppl 1:S37–44.
20. Bullock R, Chesnut R, Clifton G, et al. Guidelines for the management of severe head injury. Brain Trauma Foundation, American Association of Neurological Surgeons, Joint Section on Neurotrauma and Critical Care. J Neurotrauma. 1996;13(11):641–734.
21. Bullock M, Chesnut R, Clifton G, et al. Guidelines for the management of severe traumatic brain injury. J Neurotrauma. 2000;17(6–7):457–627.
22. Rosner MJ, Becker DP. Origin and evolution of plateau waves. Experimental observations and a theoretical model. J Neurosurg. 1984;60(2):312–24.
23. Rosner MJ, Rosner SD, Johnson AH. Cerebral perfusion pressure: management protocol and clinical results. J Neurosurg. 1995;83(6):949–62.

24. Dunham CM, Ransom KJ, Flowers LL, Siegal JD, Kohli CM. Cerebral hypoxia in severely brain-injured patients is associated with admission Glasgow Coma Scale score, computed tomographic severity, cerebral perfusion pressure, and survival. J Trauma. 2004;56(3):482–9; discussion 489–91.

25. Vath A, Meixensberger J, Dings J, Roosen K. Advanced neuromonitoring including cerebral tissue oxygenation and outcome after traumatic brain injury. Neurol Res. 2001;23(4):315–20.

26. Andrews PJ, Sleeman DH, Statham PF, et al. Predicting recovery in patients suffering from traumatic brain injury by using admission variables and physiological data: a comparison between decision tree analysis and logistic regression. J Neurosurg. 2002;97(2):326–36.

27. Changaris DG, McGraw CP, Richardson JD, Garretson HD, Arpin EJ, Shields CB. Correlation of cerebral perfusion pressure and Glasgow Coma Scale to outcome. J Trauma. 1987;27(9):1007–13.

28. Clifton GL, Miller ER, Choi SC, Levin HS. Fluid thresholds and outcome from severe brain injury. Crit Care Med. 2002;30(4):739–45.

29. Juul N, Morris GF, Marshall SB, Marshall LF. Intracranial hypertension and cerebral perfusion pressure: influence on neurological deterioration and outcome in severe head injury. The Executive Committee of the International Selfotel Trial. J Neurosurg. 2000;92(1):1–6.

30. Tan H, Feng H, Gao L, Huang G, Liao X. Outcome prediction in severe traumatic brain injury with transcranial Doppler ultrasonography. Chin J Traumatol. 2001;4(3):156–60.

31. Robertson CS, Valadka AB, Hannay HJ, et al. Prevention of secondary ischemic insults after severe head injury. Crit Care Med. 1999;27(10):2086–95.

32. Nordstrom CH, Reinstrup P, Xu W, Gardenfors A, Ungerstedt U. Assessment of the lower limit for cerebral perfusion pressure in severe head injuries by bedside monitoring of regional energy metabolism. Anesthesiology. 2003;98(4):809–14.

33. Stahl N, Ungerstedt U, Nordstrom CH. Brain energy metabolism during controlled reduction of cerebral perfusion pressure in severe head injuries. Intensive Care Med. 2001;27(7):1215–23.

34. Grande PO. The "Lund Concept" for the treatment of severe head trauma – physiological principles and clinical application. Intensive Care Med. 2006;32(10):1475–84.

35. Vigue B, Ract C, Benayed M, et al. Early SjvO$_2$ monitoring in patients with severe brain trauma. Intensive Care Med. 1999;25(5):445–51.

36. Chan KH, Dearden NM, Miller JD, Andrews PJ, Midgley S. Multimodality monitoring as a guide to treatment of intracranial hypertension after severe brain injury. Neurosurgery. 1993;32(4):547–52; discussion 552–3.

37. Kiening KL, Hartl R, Unterberg AW, Schneider GH, Bardt T, Lanksch WR. Brain tissue pO$_2$-monitoring in comatose patients: implications for therapy. Neurol Res. 1997;19(3):233–40.

38. Sahuquillo J, Amoros S, Santos A, et al. Does an increase in cerebral perfusion pressure always mean a better oxygenated brain? A study in head-injured patients. Acta Neurochir Suppl. 2000;76:457–62.

39. Bouma GJ, Muizelaar JP. Relationship between cardiac output and cerebral blood flow in patients with intact and with impaired autoregulation. J Neurosurg. 1990;73(3):368–74.

40. Steiner LA, Czosnyka M. Assessing drug effects on cerebral autoregulation using the static rate of autoregulation. Anesth Analg. 2002;95(5):1463; author reply 1463–4.

41. Howells T, Elf K, Jones PA, et al. Pressure reactivity as a guide in the treatment of cerebral perfusion pressure in patients with brain trauma. J Neurosurg. 2005;102(2):311–7.

42. Bardt TF, Unterberg AW, Hartl R, Kiening KL, Schneider GH, Lanksch WR. Monitoring of brain tissue PO$_2$ in traumatic brain injury: effect of cerebral hypoxia on outcome. Acta Neurochir Suppl. 1998;71:153–6.

43. Zauner A, Doppenberg E, Soukup J, Menzel M, Young HF, Bullock R. Extended neuromonitoring: new therapeutic opportunities? Neurol Res. 1998;20 Suppl 1:S85–90.

44. Rasulo FA, Girardini A, Lavinio A, et al. Are optimal cerebral perfusion pressure and cerebrovascular autoregulation related to long-term outcome in patients with aneurysmal subarachnoid hemorrhage? J Neurosurg Anesthesiol. 2012;24(1):3–8.

45. Lassen NA. Control of cerebral circulation in health and disease. Circ Res. 1974;34(6):749–60.

46. Marmarou AA, Anderson RL, Ward JD, et al. Impact of ICP instability and hypotension on outcome in patients with severe head injury. J Neurosurg. 1991;75:S59.

47. Marmarou A. Increased intracranial pressure in head injury and influence of blood volume. J Neurotrauma. 1992;9 Suppl 1: S327–32.

48. Marshall LF, Smith RW, Shapiro HM. The outcome with aggressive treatment in severe head injuries. Part I: the significance of intracranial pressure monitoring. J Neurosurg. 1979;50(1):20–5.

49. Miller JD, Butterworth JF, Gudeman SK, et al. Further experience in the management of severe head injury. J Neurosurg. 1981;54(3):289–99.

50. Saul TG, Ducker TB. Intracranial pressure monitoring in patients with severe head injury. Am Surg. 1982;48(9):477–80.

51. Jennett B, Teasdale G, Galbraith S, et al. Severe head injuries in three countries. J Neurol Neurosurg Psychiatry. 1977;40(3):291–8.

52. Becker DP, Miller JD, Ward JD, Greenberg RP, Young HF, Sakalas R. The outcome from severe head injury with early diagnosis and intensive management. J Neurosurg. 1977;47(4):491–502.

53. Lu J, Marmarou A, Choi S, Maas A, Murray G, Steyerberg EW. Mortality from traumatic brain injury. Acta Neurochir Suppl. 2005;95:281–5.

54. Koennecke HC, Belz W, Berfelde D, et al. Factors influencing in-hospital mortality and morbidity in patients treated on a stroke unit. Neurology. 2011;77(10):965–72.

55. Nikaina I, Paterakis K, Paraforos G, et al. Cerebral perfusion pressure, microdialysis biochemistry, and clinical outcome in patients with spontaneous intracerebral hematomas. J Crit Care. 2012;27(1):83–8.

56. Sundbarg G, Nordstrom CH, Soderstrom S. Complications due to prolonged ventricular fluid pressure recording. Br J Neurosurg. 1988;2(4):485–95.

57. Mayhall CG, Archer NH, Lamb VA, et al. Ventriculostomy-related infections. A prospective epidemiologic study. N Engl J Med. 1984;310(9):553–9.

58. Aucoin PJ, Kotilainen HR, Gantz NM, Davidson R, Kellogg P, Stone B. Intracranial pressure monitors. Epidemiologic study of risk factors and infections. Am J Med. 1986;80(3):369–76.

59. Blomstedt GC. Results of trimethoprim-sulfamethoxazole prophylaxis in ventriculostomy and shunting procedures. A double-blind randomized trial. J Neurosurg. 1985;62(5):694–7.

60. Holloway KL, Barnes T, Choi S, et al. Ventriculostomy infections: the effect of monitoring duration and catheter exchange in 584 patients. J Neurosurg. 1996;85(3):419–24.

61. Lozier AP, Sciacca RR, Romagnoli MF, Connolly Jr ES. Ventriculostomy-related infections: a critical review of the literature. Neurosurgery. 2002;51(1):170–81; discussion 181–2.

62. Lyke KE, Obasanjo OO, Williams MA, O'Brien M, Chotani R, Perl TM. Ventriculitis complicating use of intraventricular catheters in adult neurosurgical patients. Clin Infect Dis. 2001;33(12):2028–33.

63. Poon WS, Ng S, Wai S. CSF antibiotic prophylaxis for neurosurgical patients with ventriculostomy: a randomised study. Acta Neurochir Suppl. 1998;71:146–8.

64. Stenager E, Gerner-Smidt P, Kock-Jensen C. Ventriculostomy-related infections – an epidemiological study. Acta Neurochir. 1986;83(1–2):20–3.

65. Winfield JA, Rosenthal P, Kanter RK, Casella G. Duration of intracranial pressure monitoring does not predict daily risk of infectious complications. Neurosurgery. 1993;33(3):424–30; discussion 430–1.

66. Zabramski JM, Whiting D, Darouiche RO, et al. Efficacy of antimicrobial-impregnated external ventricular drain catheters: a prospective, randomized, controlled trial. J Neurosurg. 2003;98(4): 725–30.

67. Thome C, Vajkoczy P, Horn P, Bauhuf C, Hubner U, Schmiedek P. Continuous monitoring of regional cerebral blood flow during temporary arterial occlusion in aneurysm surgery. J Neurosurg. 2001;95(3):402–11.

68. Vajkoczy P, Roth H, Horn P, et al. Continuous monitoring of regional cerebral blood flow: experimental and clinical validation of a novel thermal diffusion microprobe. J Neurosurg. 2000;93(2): 265–74.

69. Vespa PM, Nuwer MR, Nenov V, et al. Increased incidence and impact of nonconvulsive and convulsive seizures after traumatic brain injury as detected by continuous electroencephalographic monitoring. J Neurosurg. 1999;91(5):750–60.

70. Muizelaar JP, Marmarou A, Ward JD, et al. Adverse effects of prolonged hyperventilation in patients with severe head injury: a randomized clinical trial. J Neurosurg. 1991;75(5):731–9.

71. McGraw CP, Howard G. Effect of mannitol on increased intracranial pressure. Neurosurgery. 1983;13(3):269–71.

72. Barry KG, Berman AR. Mannitol infusion. III. The acute effect of the intravenous infusion of mannitol on blood and plasma volumes. N Engl J Med. 1961;264:1085–8.

73. James HE. Methodology for the control of intracranial pressure with hypertonic mannitol. Acta Neurochir. 1980;51(3–4):161–72.

74. Kaufmann AM, Cardoso ER. Aggravation of vasogenic cerebral edema by multiple-dose mannitol. J Neurosurg. 1992;77(4):584–9.

75. Timmons SD. Current trends in neurotrauma care. Crit Care Med. 2010;38(9 Suppl):S431–44.

76. Ramires JA, Serrano Junior CV, Cesar LA, Velasco IT, Velasco IT, Rocha e Silva Jr M, Pileggi F. Acute hemodynamic effects of hypertonic (7.5%) saline infusion in patients with cardiogenic shock due to right ventricular infarction. Circ Shock. 1992;37(3): 220–5.

77. Prough DS, Johnson JC, Poole Jr GV, Stullken EH, Johnston Jr WE, Royster R. Effects on intracranial pressure of resuscitation from hemorrhagic shock with hypertonic saline versus lactated Ringer's solution. Crit Care Med. 1985;13(5):407–11.

78. Einhaus SL, Croce MA, Watridge CB, Lowery R, Fabian TC. The use of hypertonic saline for the treatment of increased intracranial pressure. J Tenn Med Assoc. 1996;89(3):81–2.

79. Shackford SR. Effect of small-volume resuscitation on intracranial pressure and related cerebral variables. J Trauma. 1997;42(5 Suppl):S48–53.

80. Simma B, Burger R, Falk M, Sacher P, Fanconi S. A prospective, randomized, and controlled study of fluid management in children with severe head injury: lactated Ringer's solution versus hypertonic saline. Crit Care Med. 1998;26(7):1265–70.

81. Shackford SR, Bourguignon PR, Wald SL, Rogers FB, Osler TM, Clark DE. Hypertonic saline resuscitation of patients with head injury: a prospective, randomized clinical trial. J Trauma. 1998; 44(1):50–8.

82. Qureshi AI, Suarez JI, Castro A, Bhardwaj A. Use of hypertonic saline/acetate infusion in treatment of cerebral edema in patients with head trauma: experience at a single center. J Trauma. 1999; 47(4):659–65.

83. French LA, Galicich JH. The use of steroids for control of cerebral edema. Clin Neurosurg. 1964;10:212–23.

84. Roberts I, Yates D, Sandercock P, et al. Effect of intravenous corticosteroids on death within 14 days in 10,008 adults with clinically significant head injury (MRC CRASH trial): randomized placebo controlled trial. Lancet. 2004;364:1321–8.

85. Lyons MKM, Mayer FB. Cerebrospinal fluid physiology and the management of increased intracranial pressure. Mayo Clin Proc. 1990;65:684–707.

86. Watson R. European research is launched into hypothermia stroke treatment. BMJ. 2012;344:e2215.

87. Lanzino G, D'Urso PI, Suarez J. Seizures and anticonvulsants after aneurysmal subarachnoid hemorrhage. Neurocrit Care. 2011;15(2): 247–56.

88. Michelucci R. Optimizing therapy of seizures in neurosurgery. Neurology. 2006;67(12 Suppl 4):S14–8.

89. Farag E. Dexmedetomidine in the neurointensive care unit. Discov Med. 2010;9(44):42–5.

90. Timmons SD, Toms SA. Comparative effectiveness research in neurotrauma. Neurosurg Focus. 2012;33(1):E3.

91. Sieber FE, Traystman RJ. Special issues: glucose and the brain. Crit Care Med. 1992;20(1):104–14.

92. Fukuda S, Warner DS. Cerebral protection. Br J Anaesth. 2007;99(1):10–7.

93. Volpin L, Cervellini P, Colombo F, Zanusso M, Benedetti A. Spontaneous intracerebral hematomas: a new proposal about the usefulness and limits of surgical treatment. Neurosurgery. 1984;15(5):663–6.

94. Bullock MR, Chesnut R, Ghajar J, et al. Surgical management of acute epidural hematomas. Neurosurgery. 2006;58(3 Suppl):S7–15; discussion Si–iv.

95. Bullock MR, Chesnut R, Ghajar J, et al. Surgical management of acute subdural hematomas. Neurosurgery. 2006;58(3 Suppl):S16–24; discussion Si–iv.

96. Bullock MR, Chesnut R, Ghajar J, et al. Surgical management of traumatic parenchymal lesions. Neurosurgery. 2006;58(3 Suppl):S25–46; discussion Si–iv.

97. Bullock MR, Chesnut R, Ghajar J, et al. Surgical management of posterior fossa mass lesions. Neurosurgery. 2006;58(3 Suppl):S47–55; discussion Si–iv.

Therapeutic Hypothermia in Neurocritical Care

36

Adam Schiavi and Romergryko G. Geocadin

Contents

A. Schiavi, PhD, MD
Division of Neuroanesthesia and Neurosciences
Critical Care, Anesthesiology and Critical Care Medicine,
Johns Hopkins University and Hospital,
Baltimore, MD 21287, USA

ACCM-Neurology, Johns Hopkins University and Hospital,
600 N. Wolfe Street, Meyer 8-140,
Baltimore, MD 21287, USA
e-mail: aschiav1@jhmi.edu

R.G. Geocadin, MD (✉)
ACCM-Neurology, Johns Hopkins University and Hospital,
600 N. Wolfe Street, Meyer 8-140,
Baltimore, MD 21287, USA
e-mail: rgeocad1@jhmi.edu

Abstract

Therapeutic hypothermia (TH) is the intentional cooling of a patient by artificial means for a specific therapeutic purpose. Cooling of patients has been used to treat a large number of diseases over the years. Only recently, however, has its use been subject to scientific scrutiny. Patients who have suffered cardiac arrest and are comatose in the post-resuscitation phase have been shown to benefit from the use of TH. This chapter discusses the use of TH in patients who have not suffered cardiac arrest but are in the neurocritical care unit for other diseases such as ischemic stroke, subarachnoid hemorrhage, intracerebral hemorrhage, seizures, spinal cord injury, acute liver failure, and traumatic brain injury. While this is an intriguing therapy with enormous potential for both treating patients and for research, there is scant evidence to support its routine use clinically. Basic definitions and methods for cooling are described, timing of cooling and rewarming is given, and side effects of the use of TH are also presented. In summary, this chapter will assist anyone considering the use of TH in neurologically injured patients by providing a review of the current literature and integrating it in to the risk/benefit analysis applied daily to their patients.

Keywords

Therapeutic hypothermia • Targeted temperature management • Neurological disease • Neurocritical care

Introduction

Therapeutic hypothermia (TH) is the intentional cooling of a patient by artificial means for a specific therapeutic purpose. It is also referred to as targeted temperature management (TTM), whereby a specific temperature is set and the patient is maintained there for a period of time. The intentional cooling of patients for neurologic protection from a wide variety of insults has a long history. Induced hypothermia as

A.J. Layon et al. (eds.), *Textbook of Neurointensive Care*,
DOI 10.1007/978-1-4471-5226-2_36, © Springer-Verlag London 2013

a treatment for acute brain injury was described as early as the 1940s by Fay [1]. Bigelow described the use of deep hypothermia during cardiac surgery in the 1950s [2], Benson described its use in cardiac arrest patients in 1959 [3], and in the 1960s Rosomoff extensively studied the use of hypothermia [4, 5]. While these early studies provided a basic understanding of the physiology of hypothermia, it was not until the 1980s that researchers in Pittsburgh [6–9] and Miami [10, 11], working mainly with animal models, performed a more systematic investigation of the use of hypothermia. Two early reviews on the topic of brain preservation, or "cerebral resuscitation," by Safar [9] and Ginsberg [11] argue that preservation of cerebral function post injury is of paramount importance and describe hypothermia as a mechanism to accomplish this goal.

While there has been active interest in the concept of preservation of brain function for many years, it is not until relatively recently that investigators have attempted to determine whether the use of TH as a therapeutic modality actually improves outcomes. In 2002, two randomized clinical trials using mild hypothermia following resuscitation from cardiac arrest showed a significant positive impact on patient survival and functional outcomes [12, 13]. Consequently, in 2003, the early success of these two studies led the Task Force of the International Liaison Committee on Resuscitation (ILCOR) to recommend the use of TH as a modality in caring for patients in the post-cardiac arrest recovery [14]. This recommendation is summarized by the committees' consensus statement: "Unconscious adult patients with spontaneous circulation after out-of-hospital cardiac arrest should be cooled to 32 C–34 C for 12–24 h when the initial rhythm is ventricular fibrillation (VF). Such cooling may also be beneficial for other rhythms or in-hospital cardiac arrest." With additional evidence demonstrating the beneficial effects of TH post-cardiac arrest, the American Heart Association (AHA) has endorsed this recommendation in the Post-Cardiac Arrest Care Section of the 2010 Guideline for Cardiopulmonary Resuscitation and Emergency Cardiovascular Care [15].

The use of TH has been described in the literature for over 60 years. While much of the early work was anecdotal and did not meet current, more rigorous standards of scientific investigation, there has been consistent interest in TH as a therapeutic modality. Despite all of this early work, a study from 2006 looking the clinical usage of TH in the emergency department (ED) and in the intensive care unit (ICU) demonstrated that in most cases it was simply not used. Seventy-four percent of clinicians in these areas did not use TH for *any reason* [16]. Additionally, despite the fact that ILCOR had publicized their recommendation several years earlier, over 40 % of clinicians reported that TH was not supported by the advanced cardiac life support (ACLS) guidelines. Reasons cited for not using TH were lack of awareness of TH as a therapeutic option, difficulty in implementing a hypothermia protocol, and lack of sufficient convincing evidence for its clinical usefulness.

The therapeutic value of TH in cardiac arrest survivors has led to a reevaluation of its use in other acute neurological injuries as well as non-neurological injuries. It is essential for those with an interest in TH to understand its application in cardiac arrest patients where it has been proven definitively to be beneficial. The use of TH after cardiac arrest is considered elsewhere in this text and will only be discussed here at a cursory level for the purpose of illustrating physiology, theory, or techniques. This chapter will focus on the use of TH for noncardiac arrest, neurologically injured patients in the ICU, an emerging area of interest and research.

Mechanism of Action

Although acute neuronal injury may be a consequence of a number of distinct etiologies, a common process is shared, namely, primary injury followed by secondary injury. In the neurocritical care unit, most primary neuronal injury is a result of ischemia, trauma, or a combination of the two. Primary injury incites subsequent secondary injury at the site of the initial insult or in adjacent areas. Secondary injury is a result of a cascade of destructive physiology frequently called reperfusion injury, post-resuscitative disease, or simply secondary brain injury. It is believed that hypothermia acts to inhibit or at least diminish the progression of this cascade at multiple levels.

Secondary neuronal injury, regardless of antecedent cause, has a tendency to follow a similar progression and similar mechanisms underlie the pathology. These complex cellular pathological mechanisms are only beginning to be elucidated. The majority of scientifically sound research on these pathological mechanisms and the use of TH to ameliorate this process has been done in post-cardiac arrest patients, a population where the greatest therapeutic benefit of TH thus far has been realized. Therefore, a brief review of the mechanisms of neuronal injury after cardiac arrest that appear to be the targets for TH will be discussed. For a more detailed account of the complex pathophysiology, please refer to the following sources in the reference list: [16–21].

In global cerebral ischemia from cardiac arrest, the injury cascade starts with cerebral hypoxia which results in a loss of ATP production and dysfunction of the ATP-dependent Na-K pumps in the cell membrane. Subsequent loss of cellular integrity triggers the release of glutamate, which causes excitotoxic injury [22] mediated largely through *N-methyl-D*-aspartate (NMDA) receptors [23]. Inhibitory neurotransmitters, such as glycine and gamma-aminobutyric acid (GABA), which act to dampen this excitotoxic effect, are decreased following the initiation of this cascade further exacerbating injury [24]. Activation of NMDA receptors leads to an elevation of intracellular calcium [25] that in turn

Table 36.1 Summary of the key mechanisms believed to contribute to the neuroprotective effects of hypothermia

Proposed mechanisms	Explanation	Time frame
Prevention of apoptosis	Ischemia can induce apoptosis and calpain-mediated proteolysis. Hypothermia can prevent or reduce this process	Hours to weeks
Reduced mitochondrial dysfunction	Mitochondrial dysfunction is a frequent occurrence after an episode of ischemia. Hypothermia reduces metabolic demands	Hours to days
Reduction of excessive free radical production	Production of free radicals such as superoxide, peroxynitrite, hydrogen peroxide, and hydroxyl radicals is typical in ischemia	Hours to days
Mitigation of reperfusion injury	Cascade of reactions following reperfusion, partly mediated by free radicals but with distinctive and a range of features	Hours to days
Reduced permeability of the blood–brain barrier and the vascular wall; reduced edema formation	Blood–brain barrier disruptions induced by trauma or ischemia are moderated by hypothermia. The same effect occurs with vascular permeability and capillary leakage	Hours to days
Reduced permeability of cellular membranes/cell nucleus membrane	Decreased leakage of cellular membranes, with associated improvements in cell function and cellular homoeostasis, including decrease of intracellular acidosis and mitigation of DNA injury	Hours to days
Improved ion homoeostasis	Ischemia induces accumulation of excitatory neurotransmitters such as glutamate and prolonged excessive influx of Ca_2^+ into the cell. This activates numerous enzyme systems (kinases) and induces a state of permanent hyperexcitability (excitotoxic cascade), which can be moderated by hypothermia	Minutes to 72 h
Reduction of metabolism	Cellular oxygen and glucose requirements decrease by an average of 5–8 % per degree Celsius decrease in temperature	Hours to days
Depression of the immune response and potentially harmful proinflammatory reactions	Sustained destructive inflammatory reactions and secretion of proinflammatory cytokines after ischemia can be blocked or mitigated by hypothermia	Hours to days
Reduction in cerebral thermopooling	Some areas in the brain have significantly higher temperatures than the surrounding areas and measured core temperature. These differences can increase dramatically during injury, with up to 2–3 °C higher temperatures in injured areas of the brain. Hyperthermia can increase the damage to injured brain cells	Minutes to days
Anticoagulant effects	Microthrombus formation might add to brain injury after CPR. Anticoagulant effects of hypothermia might protect against thrombus formation. Thrombolytic therapy has been shown to improve outcome after CPR	Minutes to days
Suppression of epileptic activity and seizures	Many patients experience seizures after ischemic episodes or trauma, or both, which might add to injury. Hypothermia has been shown to mitigate epileptic activity	Hours to days

Adapted with permission of Elsevier from Polderman [29]

contributes to an increase in oxygen free radicals [25, 26]. In the setting of mitochondrial dysfunction, reperfusion of an ischemic area results in the creation of free radicals [27]. These reactive oxygen species cause damage through lipid peroxidation, protein oxidation, and DNA fragmentation, which leads to more extensive secondary injury and cell death [28].

This core cascade of pathological processes also occurs in focal insults such as ischemic strokes and acute spinal cord injury. The same pathology is present in traumatic brain injury and intracerebral hemorrhage, but patients suffer additional direct injury to the brain from mass effect (TBI and ICH) and diffuse axonal injury in TBI. In status epilepticus, the excitotoxic process shares many common elements of the injury process in global ischemia. These similarities have led investigators to study the effect of TH in these conditions.

While the precise mechanism underlying the neuroprotective effect of TH is not fully understood, numerous hypotheses have been suggested [11]. The effect of TH does not appear to be limited to a single physiologic mechanism. Rather, observations that hypothermia impacts multiple points along the injury cascade point to the pleiotropic nature of TH as a therapeutic intervention. This multifactorial effect is believed to be the reason for its success as a neuroprotective agent. Table 36.1 provides a summary of the key mechanisms believed to contribute to the neuroprotective effects of hypothermia [29].

Technologies for Cooling

The body naturally cools itself via the mechanisms of radiation, evaporation, conduction, and convection. The technologies used to augment cooling utilize one of these natural mechanisms. There are many methods available to cool patients, but it is important to note that currently there is no FDA-approved device or technology for the induction of hypothermia. Rather, most devices are approved for fever prevention and temperature control, and their use for the induction of therapeutic hypothermia is considered off-label.

Table 36.2 Methods and devices for inducing and maintaining hypothermia

Surface cooling (air)	Surface cooling (liquid)	Core cooling
Exposure of skin	Ice packs	Intravascular catheter
Skin exposure + water/alcohol	Water immersion	Peritoneal lavage
Fans	Circulating cold water to skin	Intravenous infusion (iced saline)
Air-circulating blankets	Pre-refrigerated cooling pads	ECMO
Special beds	Water-circulating cooling blankets	Drugs
	Water-circulating cooling pads/garment	
	Hydrogel-coated water-circulating pads	

Table 36.3 Therapeutic temperature definitions

Hypothermia	Core temperature <36.0 °C regardless of the cause
Induced hypothermia	An intentional reduction of core temperature <36.0 °C
Therapeutic hypothermia	Controlled induced hypothermia
Controlled normothermia/therapeutic normothermia	Maintaining temperature within a range of 36.0–37.5 °C
Temperature range definitions	
Mild therapeutic hypothermia	An intentional and controlled reduction of core temperature to 34.0–35.9 °C
Moderate therapeutic hypothermia	An intentional and controlled reduction of core temperature to 32.0–33.9 °C
Moderate/deep therapeutic hypothermia	An intentional and controlled reduction of temperature to 30.0–31.9 °C
Deep therapeutic hypothermia	An intentional and controlled reduction of temperature to <30.0 °C
Mild hyperthermia	Core temperature 37.5–38.0 °C
Moderate hyperthermia	Core temperature 38.1–38.5 °C
Moderate/severe hyperthermia	Core temperature 38.6–38.9 °C
Severe hyperthermia	Core temperature >39.0 °C

Reprinted with permission from Polderman and Herold [74]

Table 36.2 lists several common methods and devices used for inducing and maintaining hypothermia, although none has been established as clearly superior. The treatment team must consider several factors when choosing a method and device for cooling. These include the (1) venue where hypothermia is initiated (i.e., in the field, emergency department, or intensive care unit (ICU)), (2) capacity of first responders to initiate hypothermia, (3) rapidity of induction and stability of temperature during treatment, (4) ability to control rewarming, (5) portability of the device used for cooling, (6) management of specific adverse effects, (7) likelihood that the method used will hamper the provision of care in the critical care environment, and (8) cost [30]. Table 36.3 defines the common terms used in the clinical implementation of TH. The therapeutic range of 32.0–33.9 C has been shown to be the most clinically effective [21, 30].

Specific Disease States

Traumatic Brain Injury

In a review of traumatic brain injury (TBI) literature, Polderman [29] describes at least 29 clinical studies that have assessed the efficacy of hypothermia. Twenty-seven of these studies were in adults and 18 used controlled designs. Eighteen studies, all performed in specialized neurotrauma centers, used hypothermia to treat patients with high intracranial pressure (ICP) that was refractory to conventional treatments such as sedation and osmotic therapy. All of the patients in these studies had decreased ICP while being cooled. Of these 18 studies, four reported a positive trend and 13 reported significant improvements in outcome associated with hypothermia treatment. While these results seem to be promising, the study protocols vary considerably and the actual randomization of patients was questioned in many of the studies.

There is one large prospective randomized multicenter trial that was conducted in 2001 [31]. Surface cooling was used to maintain a temperature of 33°C for 48 h in 392 patients with severe TBI, but failed to show any benefit in mortality or functional outcome. Several explanations have been put forth to explain these results, most notably variability by the participating centers in the treatment protocols, delays in the institution of hypothermia induction, and mandatory rewarming at 48 h independent of ICP at that time. Post hoc subgroup analysis, however, showed potential benefit in the patients who were hypothermic at presentation [31].

Based on the level of evidence available, the 2007 Guidelines of Severe Traumatic Brain Injury give a level III recommendation (therapeutic "option") for the use of TH in TBI. There are insufficient data to support a level I ("standard") or level II ("guideline") recommendation for TH in

TBI. The authors argue that, while TH was not associated with decreased mortality compared to normothermic controls, preliminary findings suggest that a greater decrease in mortality is observed when target temperature is maintained for greater than 48 h [32].

A systematic review by Sydenham and colleagues for the Cochrane group in 2009 [33] found 23 trials with a total of 1,614 randomized patients where therapeutic hypothermia (<35 °C) was utilized for at least 12 h. Twenty-one trials, involving 1,587 patients, reported data on mortality rates and unfavorable outcomes (death, vegetative state, or severe disability). There were fewer deaths in patients treated with hypothermia than in control groups (OR 0.84, 95 % CI 0.67–1.05). Similarly, patients treated with hypothermia were less likely to have an unfavorable outcome than those in the control group (OR 0.76, 95 % CI 0.61–0.93). However, nine trials that were selected for good allocation concealment showed no decrease in the likelihood of death compared with the control group, a result that was not statistically significant (OR 1.08, 95 % CI 0.79–1.47). Patients treated with hypothermia showed a trend toward decreased likelihood to have an unfavorable outcome than those in the control group, but the reduction was small and nonsignificant (OR 0.91, 95 % CI 0.69–1.20). Hypothermia may be effective in reducing death and unfavorable outcomes for traumatic head-injured patients, but significant benefit was only found in low-quality trials [33]. Thus, the authors of this analysis concluded that there is no evidence that hypothermia is beneficial in the treatment of head injury.

The use of therapeutic hypothermia should be used with caution in patients with traumatic brain injury. Evidence suggesting a benefit to TH is equivocal. Given that there are side effects and complications to the use of TH, such as coagulopathy, it seems reasonable to conclude that only mild hypothermia should be used in order to minimize these adverse effects in trauma patients. It also seems reasonable to cool patients in an effort to avoid hyperthermia in trauma patients, but until further consistent evidence shows benefit to trauma patients as a whole, each patient should be evaluated individually with consideration for the other medical and surgical issues inherent to trauma patients.

Ischemia and Stroke

The use of therapeutic hypothermia in the treatment of acute ischemic stroke has been investigated in several studies. A recent review by Linares and Mayer provides a more in-depth discussion [34]. Some of the key studies are discussed next.

Krieger and colleagues examined the potential for additional benefit from hypothermia when added to thrombolysis (intra-arterial or intravenous) in patients with acute MCA ischemic stroke in Cooling for Acute Ischemic Brain Damage

1 study [35]. Eligible patients were randomized to the hypothermia or control group. Moderate hypothermia was induced for at least 12 h and up to 72 h, with initiation of rewarming 12 h after the establishment of MCA patency by sonographic or angiographic evidence. In this study, mortality was 30 % in the hypothermia (3 of 10) group versus 22.2 % in the control group (2 of 9) and the modified Rankin Scale score was ~3 in the hypothermia group versus ~4 in the control group at 3 months. De Georgia and coworkers [36] proceeded with the Cooling for Acute Ischemic Brain Damage 2 study, enrolling 40 ischemic stroke patients who presented within 12 h of symptom onset. An endovascular cooling device cooled patients to 33 °C for 24 h. Eighteen patients were randomized to hypothermia and 22 to receive standard medical management. Mean diffusion-weighted imaging lesion growth in the hypothermia group compared with control group was not statistically significant.

The impact of hypothermia on postischemic edema was studied by Guluma and colleagues [37]. The investigators cooled 18 patients with acute ischemic stroke to 33 °C for 12 or 24 h using an endovascular system, followed by 12 h of controlled rewarming. At 48 h, total cerebrospinal fluid volume was significantly lower in the normothermia group compared with the hypothermia group ($p < 0.05$), but no significant differences in the mean volume of ischemia assessed by morphometric analysis of CT scans were identified. At 30 days, the difference in cerebrospinal fluid volumes had resolved, and infarct volumes and functional outcomes were comparable [37].

Another trial in 2001 enrolled 50 patients with hemispheric infarction [38]. Cooling was started on average 22 h after stroke onset. ICP values were reduced from 20 ± 14 mmHg before the beginning of hypothermia to 12 ± 5 mmHg when a steady state of hypothermia was reached. Faster rewarming was associated with larger rebound increases in ICP, and most deaths occurred during the rewarming period; overall mortality was 38 % [38].

Recently, a feasibility and safety trial combining intravascular cooling after thrombolysis was undertaken in 2010. The Intravenous Thrombolysis Plus Hypothermia for Acute Treatment of Ischemic Stroke (ICTuS-L) trial examined the impact of hypothermia and intravenous tissue plasminogen activator on patients treated within 6 h after presentation of ischemic stroke [39]. Patients were stratified into two groups based on how long after symptom onset they received initial treatment. Those presenting within 3 h of symptom onset received standard dose intravenous alteplase and were randomized to undergo 24 h of endovascular cooling to 33 °C followed by 12 h of controlled rewarming versus normothermia treatment. Those presenting between 3 and 6 h were randomized twice: to receive tissue plasminogen activator or not and to receive hypothermia versus normothermia. The trial had 28 patients randomized to receive hypothermia and 30 received normothermia. Cooling was achieved in all patients except two in whom there were technical difficulties. The median time to target temperature after catheter placement was 67 min. At 3 months, there was no difference in outcome; 18 % of patients treated with hypothermia had a modified Rankin Scale score of 0 or 1 versus 24 % in the normothermia groups (NS). Six patients in the hypothermia and five in the normothermia groups died within 90 days (NS). The incidence of pneumonia was noted to be higher in the hypothermia group. Although none of the outcomes achieved statistical significance, nonetheless, this study demonstrated the feasibility and preliminary safety of combining therapeutic hypothermia after stroke with intravenous thrombolysis [39]. A definitive efficacy trial is needed at this stage.

The combined effect of hypothermia plus hemicraniectomy was studied in a prospective randomized study by Els and coworkers [40]. Twenty-five consecutive patients with an ischemic infarction of more than two thirds of one hemisphere were enrolled and randomized to either hemicraniectomy alone or in combination with hypothermia. Overall mortality was 12 % (2/13 vs. 1/12), but none of the three deaths were due to treatment-related complications. No severe side effects of hypothermia were identified. There was a trend toward improved outcome in the hemicraniectomy plus moderate hypothermia group after 6 months, but these findings did not reach statistical significance.

A 2009 systematic review by the Cochrane group looked at the effects of pharmacological and physical strategies to reduce body or brain temperature in patients with acute stroke [41]. This included five pharmacological temperature reduction trials and three physical cooling trials involving a total of 423 participants. None of the pharmacological or physical temperature-lowering therapies resulted in statistically significant reductions in the risk of death or dependency (odds ratio (OR) 0.9, 95 % confidence interval (CI) 0.6–1.4) or death (OR 0.9, 95 % CI 0.5–1.5). The authors concluded that evidence from randomized trials did not support routine use of physical or pharmacological strategies to reduce temperature in patients with acute stroke [41].

The American Heart Association 2007 Guidelines for the Early Management of Adults with Acute Ischemic Stroke, in reference to the use of hypothermia in ischemic strokes, states: "At present, no intervention with putative neuroprotective actions has been established as effective in improving outcomes after stroke, and therefore none currently can be recommended (Class III, Level of Evidence A)" [42].

Ischemic stroke is one of the greatest causes of disability among adults and has a devastating effect on the lives of the patients and society. Once the acute phase is resolved, ischemic damage remains, and little can be done to recover the injured brain tissue. It is clear that the sooner a patient is treated with acute interventions to minimize ischemia, the better the outcome. Hypothermia has the potential to help

patients with ischemic stroke if implemented early, but it is difficult to employ TH in the field and to maintain consistent hypothermia. Inadvertent premature or rapid rewarming may be more harmful than no therapy at all. Additionally, TH may interfere with those early interventions known to be beneficial and delay evidence-based care. The data on TH in stroke do not indicate a clear benefit with the possible exception of use when brain edema is so severe that hemicraniectomy is indicated. TH should not be used as a routine intervention in the treatment of ischemic stroke until higher quality evidence can demonstrate how and when to utilize it effectively.

Intracerebral Hemorrhage

At present, there is little evidence to support the use of TH in spontaneous intracerebral hemorrhage (ICH). The 2010 American Heart Association Guidelines for the Management of Spontaneous Intracerebral Hemorrhage has officially stated that therapeutic cooling has not been systematically investigated in ICH [43]. Acute ICH accounts for 10–15 % of new strokes and is associated with a 30-day mortality rate of up to 52 % [44, 45]. There are a number of factors that contribute to this unfavorable outcome, namely, size of the hematoma [46], rebleeding or expansion of hematoma [47], and intraventricular extension [48]. When the acute phase of an ICH is resolved, the most common cause of mortality is the development of peri-hemorrhage edema that causes increased ICP [49]. It appears that relative peri-hematomal edema volume can predict outcomes within the first 24 h independent of other indicators such as hematoma volume, hydrocephalus, and GCS score [50]. In ICH, the extent of secondary damage to otherwise healthy tissue contributes to significant morbidity and mortality. TH may not be able to effect change in tissue that is primarily damaged by the hemorrhage, but, by modifying the amount of edema and subsequent secondary damage from the ensuing cascade of pathological processes, TH may be very important to improving outcomes.

A 2010 study by Kollmar and coworkers looked at a group of 37 patients with ICH, 12 of which were treated with mild hypothermia (35 °C) and 25 did not have an intervention. They found that in the hypothermia group, edema volume remained stable during the first 14 days, compared to the control group who had on average a 100 % increase in relative edema [51]. The side effects of therapeutic hypothermia, including ventilator-associated pneumonia and shivering, were relatively minor and amenable to treatment. There was no coagulopathy noted, and the volume of the hemorrhage in the hypothermia versus the control group was not significantly different. These data appear promising that mild TH can help to reduce mortality in ICH by controlling one of the main causes of mortality, namely, relative peri-hematomal edema. In this study, there does not appear to be an increased risk of continued hemorrhage expansion with the use of mild hypothermia. More studies are clearly warranted to elucidate this promising area.

In ICH, a hemorrhage volume of about 30 ml can be considered the cutoff value for high morbidity and mortality [46]. As with any intervention, the use of TH must only be considered for use in those patients who may receive benefit. Based on this reasoning, those with small ICH volumes generally have favorable outcomes and may not necessarily receive any additional benefit from TH; thus, its use is not recommended. Conversely, for those with very large catastrophic hemorrhage, the potential harm from TH such as coagulopathy and cardiac arrhythmias in patients who may be hemodynamically unstable constitutes high risk while offering little benefit. Brokerick [46] demonstrated that hemorrhages larger than 60 ml are associated with 91 % mortality. While there is not an established upper limit to define when the burden of bleed is too great for survival, it is difficult to decide when interventions should not be offered and should be evaluated on a case-by-case basis and in accordance with patient and family wishes.

Aneurysmal Subarachnoid Hemorrhage

Several studies examining therapeutic hypothermia in small groups of patients with poor-grade subarachnoid hemorrhage (SAH) and refractory vasospasm have shown promising results [52]. A study by Gasser and colleagues [53] evaluated the feasibility and safety of long-term hypothermia (greater than 72 h) in the treatment of severe brain edema after poor-grade (Hunt and Hess grade 4–5) SAH. This study demonstrated that functional independence at 3 months (defined by the Glasgow Outcome Scale (GOS) score of 4 or 5) did not differ significantly between patients who were treated with TH for >72 h versus <72 h.

The utility of hypothermia as a neuroprotective agent during intracranial aneurysm surgery has been studied in a large prospective multicenter trial of intraoperative hypothermia in patients with good-grade (World Federation of Neurological Surgeons (WFNS) score I, II, III) SAH. The study did not show any treatment benefit with the use of intraoperative hypothermia (target temperature 33 °C) versus normothermia (36.5 °C) [54]. The 2009 Guidelines for the Management of Aneurysmal Subarachnoid Hemorrhage states that induced hypothermia during aneurysm surgery may be a reasonable option in some cases but is not routinely recommended (Class III, Level of Evidence B) [55]. These guidelines do not provide a statement on the use of therapeutic hypothermia outside of surgery for SAH.

There are insufficient data at this time to determine whether TH should be used in SAH at all. In patients with good-grade SAH in which there are no significant neurological deficits, or where there is no severe vasospasm, TH may provide little benefit. It is less clear, however, in poor-grade SAH where there is severe neurological deficit, brain swelling, or severe vasospasm leading to hypoperfusion as to whether TH could be of benefit. Hypothermia may not currently be indicated for use in SAH, but, as in other neurological injuries, strict temperature control with a goal of normothermia should be implemented in the continuing supportive role during the acute phase of SAH [29].

Seizures

Seizures are a common complication of acute brain injury. Following cardiac arrest, the presence of myoclonic status epilepticus is known to be associated with poor outcome [56]. A causal relationship has not been established, however, and it is not known if seizures and myoclonus are a cause of a poor outcome or, rather, a marker of more severe injury that is refractory to recovery. Similarly, status epilepticus (SE) has a high mortality and frequently fails to respond to conventional treatments. In refractory SE, one of the therapeutic goals is to suppress all seizure and epileptiform activity on the EEG. This is typically accomplished with pharmacologic intervention with agents such as pentobarbital. This therapy can progress to general anesthesia in an effort to produce burst suppression and sometimes electrical silence. Because hypothermia can also lead to electrical silence on EEG, there has been a growing interest in the use of TH in the treatment of refractory status epilepticus, as described in a few small case series. In a recent study, 4 cases of refractory SE were treated concurrently with TH and midazolam or pentobarbital [57]. These patients were cooled to 31–35 °C, and when EEG evidence of seizure control was achieved, the medications were tapered off. After 24 h of seizure-free EEG, the patients were rewarmed with successful resolution of SE in all 4 cases. However, complications include shivering, coagulopathy, and venous thromboembolism; of the 4 patients, there were 2 deaths, 1 due to sepsis. In another small case series of three pediatric patients with refractory SE, hypothermia with a temperature of 30–31 °C was combined with barbiturate coma to achieve successful control of seizure activity [58].

The temperatures needed to achieve burst suppression with TH vary from patient to patient but fall outside of the definition of mild hypothermia, the category that is associated with the least amount of risk. If a patient cannot tolerate induction of burst suppression with pentobarbital or all other treatments have failed, the use of TH can be considered as a way to control brain activity. However, the use of TH must be tempered with the caveat that the deeper to the patient is cooled in TH, the greater the potential for side effects. This risk/benefit ratio must be carefully considered for each patient in association with goals of care. Refractory SE is associated with high mortality, and TH appears to be effective in controlling seizures but is not without the potential for significant harm. Additional research in this area is necessary to elucidate which patients will benefit the most from the use of TH [59].

Spinal Cord Injury

There is currently only anecdotal evidence that the use of TH in spinal cord injury (SCI) is beneficial and available literature on the topic is scarce. There are experimental animal models that show that early cooling strategies using systemically administered mild hypothermia at 33 °C improved locomotive function as well as forelimb gripping strength and coordination in both thoracic and cervical contusive spinal cord injury. These animal studies have been thoroughly reviewed by Deitrich [60], and promising animal studies have sparked interest in clinical research. Levi and coworkers studied the clinical use of TH in cervical spine injury and concluded that the use of moderate hypothermia (33 °C) using an intravascular catheter was safe, with only minor complications all of which were easily treatable. Hypothermia did not increase in severe side effects such as DVT coagulopathy or pulmonary embolism. Additionally, there was modest improvement in the patients treated with TH compared to the control group [61, 62]. These encouraging results with the use of moderate TH have prompted that group to initiate a large-scale, randomized, multicenter clinical trial.

The use of TH in SCI is currently a promising therapy and is being aggressively pursued based on a large body of laboratory data and encouraging preliminary clinical data. Given the large burden of injury associated with SCI and the fact that there are virtually no treatments other than supportive care and rehabilitation, TH should be used conservatively and only in appropriate patients, where any potential side effects do not prohibit ongoing care. The American Association of Neurological Surgeons/Neurological and Spinal Surgery Joint Sections of the Disorders of the Spine and Joint Section of Trauma currently state that there is not enough evidence available to recommend for or against the practice of TH as a treatment for SCI [63]. This is an active area of research, and with the current clinical trials underway, a clear direction should emerge.

Acute Liver Failure

There is a subset of patients with acute liver failure complicated by hepatic encephalopathy who are admitted to the neurointensive care unit while awaiting liver transplant for management of ICP. Intracranial pressure can become so great that these patients are at risk of a herniation syndrome and death before transplant can occur. Conventional ICP management, such as mannitol and ultrafiltration, may be inadequate, and more aggressive measures can be lifesaving. There are a few small studies that describe the use of TH in the management of these patients. One case series suggests that, in patients who are candidates for orthotopic liver transplant, TH can be used as a bridge to transplant to decrease ICP and preserve neurologic function until suitable organs are available [64]. Of the seven acute liver failure patients who were cooled, four were transplant candidates and survived to receive a liver transplant. The three patients who were not candidates and were rewarmed to normothermia all experienced increases in ICP and died [65]. There is also an encouraging case series where patients with acute liver failure and increased ICP were treated with TH to 32–33 °C. Thirteen of 14 patients survived to transplant with complete neurologic recovery and no significant complications related to cooling [66]. These studies are indeed encouraging, and it seems that the use of TH can be beneficial for acute liver failure patients with severe neurologic compromise for the temporary control of ICP while awaiting transplant. Larger controlled studies may further elucidate the utility of TH in this growing population.

Risks and Side Effects

Mild hypothermia (34–35.9 °C) is relatively well tolerated. It can be a challenge to distinguish complications resulting from the disease indicating the use of TH versus those from TH itself. In a study by Bernard and coworkers that looked at hypothermia (33 °C) after out-of-hospital cardiac arrest, the hypothermia group had a trend toward lower cardiac index, higher systemic vascular resistance, and more hyperglycemia than the control group, but no difference in the frequency of adverse events. The proportion of patients with any complication, however, was high in both the TH (73 %) and the normothermic groups (70 %) [12]. Most investigations on the physiologic effects of hypothermia in isolation are animal studies. Human clinical trials have investigated TH in patients with severe physiologic perturbations from their underlying disease process. Studies by Levi and coworkers [61, 62] have demonstrated that the use of moderate hypothermia (33 °C) in patients with spinal cord injury is safe in the phase 1 safety and efficacy trial. Complications of hypothermia were minor and easily treatable. Deep hypothermia (below 32 °C) appears to be associated with more deleterious side effects that are directly attributable to the intervention itself. Careful consideration and monitoring for side effects of TH are essential. These physiologic changes are routinely closely monitored in the intensive care unit, and any patient for whom TH is being considered should be admitted to an ICU.

The side effects of TH can be categorized broadly as cardiac, hematologic, immunologic, and metabolic. Problems with hypotension, increased systemic vascular resistance, and decreased cardiac output are possible, but the greatest risk is cardiac arrhythmia as colder temperatures are used. These complications should be treated with supportive care. Coagulation deficits including platelet dysfunction and coagulation enzyme dysfunction should be monitored. Immunosuppression can increase the risk of infection in cooled patients. Cooling a patient suppresses the normal adaptive fever response to stress, infection, and inflammation, so a high degree of suspicion for occult infection and other tissue damage is warranted. Metabolic effects such as hypokalemia and metabolic acidosis are possible perturbations [67]. Calcium, magnesium, and glucose levels may also be altered. Careful surveillance of blood chemistry values and correction where appropriate are important, with the understanding that glucose and electrolytes tend to return to baseline during the rewarming phase as physiologic parameters normalize.

From a neurologic perspective, seizures have been noted to occur in both normothermic patients and those treated with hypothermia. This phenomenon is likely secondary to the global ischemic injury sustained during and reperfusion in cardiac arrest [68, 69] and in other forms of acute brain injury. It is advisable to have a low threshold for using electroencephalogram (EEG) monitoring in patients who are suspected to have seizure activity, especially in those patients who are paralyzed or heavily sedated because these pharmacologic interventions can mask any clinical manifestations of seizures.

Shivering in response to hypothermia can generate heat leading to an increase in core temperature and increased oxygen consumption, thus significantly impeding the goal of intentional therapeutic cooling [14, 70]. European and American studies have both addressed shivering with paralytic agents and midazolam for sedation [12, 13]. Shivering is most prominent during the induction of TH; therefore, more attention needs to be given to the use of sedatives and paralytics during this period. Pharmacologic paralysis requires full ventilator support; however, these patients are typically comatose and likely require this level of ventilator assistance in any case. Surface counter-warming of thermoreceptors in the face and hands can suppress shivering while permitting core temperatures to be within the target range chosen during the maintenance phase of cooling. Other agents that are useful in the suppression of shivering include meperidine, buspirone, magnesium sulfate [71], opiates, and alpha-2 agonist agents, namely, clonidine or dexmedetomidine. A detailed neurologic evaluation is essential prior to initiation of paralysis and sedation and should be repeated once the drugs have been discontinued, with the caution that patients may metabolize these agents more slowly as a result of hypothermia.

Rewarming

The process of cooling a patient is an active one, requiring energy to continuously remove heat that is generated from metabolism. Once the maintenance phase of TH is completed, the rewarming phase begins by the removal of active cooling.

There are no clear data about how quickly a person with neurologic injury should be warmed, but it seems that a slower process is better. A study of cardiopulmonary bypass patients indicated that, although rapid rewarming helps postoperative coagulopathy, it also leads to increases in cognitive deficits after bypass surgery. Cognitive outcomes are improved with slow rewarming [72]. In patients with traumatic brain injury treated by TH, rapid rewarming increases the risk for a rapid rise in intracranial pressure [31]. There are a few clinical trials that indicate that slow rewarming, at a rate ranging from 0.25 to 0.5 °C, is superior [12, 13, 31]. It can be difficult to warm a patient this slowly. Metabolic processes warm different patients at different rates as the body is allowed to return to a non-hypothermic state. If a fever has been suppressed during TH, the temperature may rise quickly once active cooling is removed. Additionally, if medications were used to suppress shivering, discontinuation of these medications can permit residual shivering and increased metabolic rates before normothermia is achieved. The cooling device should be kept in place during the rewarming phase to control the rate of warming and to prevent the overshoot of temperature into the hyperthermic range which can be deleterious to neurologically injured patients.

The reversal of TH also reverses the physiologic changes that occurred as a result of cooling. The same considerations for physiologic monitoring in the intensive care unit for the induction and maintenance of TH should be considered for the rewarming phase. Just as in the induction and maintenance of TH, electrolyte levels will change in rewarming as well. Potassium and magnesium levels may rise during rewarming and should be closely monitored. In addition, the vasculature may dilate in response to warming, and the patients may have relative hypovolemia requiring the administration of intravenous fluid.

Seizures are of particular concern during the rewarming phase because the seizure threshold may be lowered for many reasons. A recent study in pediatric patients for whom TH was used after cardiac arrest demonstrated that a significant increase in seizures was seen during the rewarming phase compared to both the normothermic and hypothermic phases on continuous EEG monitoring [73]. It is unclear if this is a phenomenon that is unique to the global ischemia of cardiac arrest or to pediatric patients. In either case, the increased metabolic demand of seizing is detrimental to the damaged brain in the warming phase. Cooling reduces brain metabolism and as a result increases the seizure threshold. If a patient has been sedated with agents that act as anticonvulsants, removal of these agents coupled with the decrease in the seizure threshold as the brain is rewarmed confers additional risk during this phase. It is reasonable to consider monitoring patients who are at risk for seizures with continuous EEG. If not available, monitoring for motor activity from seizures or transient vital sign variations followed by spot EEG is indicated.

Conclusions

Therapeutic hypothermia is a medical intervention with tremendous potential to treat a wide variety of medical and surgical conditions. Its use has been described in the literature for many years, and anecdotal evidence of its miraculous properties may tempt one to think of it as a "silver bullet." However, the clinical use of TH must be approached with caution. In most cases, the gold standard of what is considered to be acceptable therapy, namely, the randomized, controlled clinical trial, has not been applied to the use of TH. The clear exception to this is the recovery or post-resuscitation phase after a cardiac arrest, where the evidence supports its efficacy in comatose survivors. There are extensive laboratory and animal data that describe how TH affects or mitigates pathological processes, but little, if any, exist for humans. It is tempting to try to generalize these laboratory studies for use in the clinical arena, but these results are not necessarily transferrable, and caution is warranted. TH affects a wide array of physiology and appears to have multiple mechanisms of action. This is a double-edged sword because while it has the potential to treat a wide variety of pathologic conditions, each of those states will have to be studied in isolation. Different pathologic conditions may respond to different timing of induction and maintenance of TH, to a varying degree of temperatures, and to different rewarming strategies. Various mechanisms of cooling (i.e., surface cooling vs. intravascular catheters) may also prove to have differing degrees of efficacy, as in the case of spinal cord injury.

Varying degrees of hypothermia may be required to achieve the desired goal (i.e., stop seizure activity, reduce brain edema, reduce ICP) for any particular pathologic state. The deeper the degree of cooling needed, the greater the potential for adverse effects. This necessitates a careful risk–benefit balance not only for each patient depending on the severity of their disease state but also for each

type of pathology. For instance, with liver transplant patients, coagulopathy and immunosuppression may be of greater concern than for other types of patients. Similarly, SAH might have greater risk of cardiac arrhythmias. The complications from the disease state itself combined with the depth and time of hypothermia needed to be beneficial, and thus the risk of further derangement in those areas will also affect the decision to implement TH. Most guidelines at this time cannot provide recommendation for the use of TH. For the general population of patients, this may be true at this time given the lack of compelling evidence of the effectiveness of TH in most conditions. However, there will always be cases in which no other therapeutic option exists and the determination to attempt TH in the treatment of these patients is made. These considerations may help determine what the greatest threat to life is and when the use of TH might be appropriate despite high stakes.

As a pleiotropic intervention, TH has a strong potential to provide beneficial effects for acute neurologic injuries in the neurocritical care unit. However, at this time, its role for routine use outside of the immediate post-cardiac arrest setting is not well defined and therefore not recommended. Well-designed clinical trials are needed to define its role in other acute neurologic injuries, and this area of research provides fertile ground for investigation on how to use this intervention to its greatest potential.

References

1. Fay T. Observations on generalized refrigeration in cases of severe cerebral trauma. Assoc Res Nerv Ment Dis Proc. 1943;24:611–9.
2. Bigelow WG, Lindsay WK, Greenwood WF. Hypothermia; its possible role in cardiac surgery: an investigation of factors governing survival in dogs at low body temperatures. Ann Surg. 1950;132:849–66.
3. Benson DW, Williams Jr GR, Spencer FC, Yates AJ. The use of hypothermia after cardiac arrest. Anesth Analg. 1959;38:423–8.
4. Rosomoff HL. Protective effects of hypothermia against pathological processes of the nervous system. Ann N Y Acad Sci. 1959;80:475–86.
5. Rosomoff HL, Shulman K, Raynor R, Grainger W. Experimental brain injury and delayed hypothermia. Surg Gynecol Obstet. 1960;110:27–32.
6. Bleyaert AL, Nemoto EM, Safar P, Stezoski SM, Mickell JJ, Moossy J, Rao GR. Thiopental amelioration of brain damage after global ischemia in monkeys. Anesthesiology. 1978;49:390–8.
7. Abramson NS, Safar P, Detre K, Kelsey S, Reinmuth O, Snyder J. An international collaborative clinical study mechanism for resuscitation research. Resuscitation. 1982;10:141–7.
8. Vaagenes P, Cantadore R, Safar P, Mossy J, Rao G, Diven W, Alexander H, Stezoski W. Amelioration of brain damage by lidoflazine after prolonged ventricular fibrillation after cardiac arrests in dogs. Crit Care Med. 1984;12:846–55.
9. Safar P. Cerebral resuscitation after cardiac arrest: a review. Circulation. 1986;74:IV138–53.

10. Ginsberg MD, Sternau LL, Globus MY, Dietrich WD, Busto R. Therapeutic modulation of brain temperature: relevance to ischemic brain injury. Cerebrovasc Brain Metab Rev. 1992;4: 189–225.

11. Ginsberg M, Belayev L. The effects of hypothermia and hyperthermia in global cerebral ischemia. In: Maier C, Steinberg G, editors. Hypothermia and cerebral ischemia. Totowa: Humana Press; 2004.

12. Bernard SA, Gray TW, Buist MD, Jones BM, Silvester W, Gutteridge G, Smith K. Treatment of comatose survivors of out-of-hospital cardiac arrest with induced hypothermia. N Engl J Med. 2002;346:557–63.

13. The Hypothermia after Cardiac Arrest Study Group. Mild therapeutic hypothermia to improve the neurologic outcome after cardiac arrest. N Engl J Med. 2002;346:549–56.

14. Nolan JP, Morley PT, Vanden Hoek TL, Hickey RW, Kloeck WG, Billi J, Bottiger BW, Okada K, Reyes C, Shuster M, Steen PA, Weil MH, Wenzel V, Carli P, Atkins D. Therapeutic hypothermia after cardiac arrest: an advisory statement by the advanced life support task force of the International Liaison Committee on Resuscitation. Circulation. 2003;108:118–21.

15. Peberdy MA, Callaway CW, Neumar RW, Geocadin RG, Zimmerman JL, Donnino M, Gabrielli A, Silvers SM, Zaritsky AL, Merchant R, Vanden Hoek TL, Kronick SL. Part 9: post-cardiac arrest care: 2010 American Heart Association Guidelines for Cardiopulmonary Resuscitation and Emergency Cardiovascular Care. Circulation. 2010;122:S768–86.

16. Merchant RM, Soar J, Skrifvars MB, Silfvast T, Edelson DP, Ahmad F, Huang KN, Khan M, Vanden Hoek TL, Becker LB, Abella BS. Therapeutic hypothermia utilization among physicians after resuscitation from cardiac arrest. Crit Care Med. 2006;34: 1935–40.

17. Froehler MT, Geocadin RG. Hypothermia for neuroprotection after cardiac arrest: mechanisms, clinical trials and patient care. J Neurol Sci. 2007;261:118–26.

18. Greer DM. Mechanisms of injury in hypoxic-ischemic encephalopathy: implications to therapy. Semin Neurol. 2006;26:373–9.

19. Harukuni I, Bhardwaj A. Mechanisms of brain injury after global cerebral ischemia. Neurol Clin. 2006;24:1–21.

20. Hoesch RE, Koenig MA, Geocadin RG. Coma after global ischemic brain injury: pathophysiology and emerging therapies. Crit Care Clin. 2008;24:25–44, vii–viii.

21. Polderman KH. Mechanisms of action, physiological effects, and complications of hypothermia. Crit Care Med. 2009;37:S186–202.

22. Vaagenes P, Ginsberg M, Ebmeyer U, et al. Cerebral resuscitation from cardiac arrest: pathophysiologic mechanisms. Crit Care Med. 1996;24:S57–68.

23. Lipton SA, Rosenberg PA. Excitatory amino acids as a final common pathway for neurologic disorders. N Engl J Med. 1994;330: 613–22.

24. Globus MY, Ginsberg MD, Busto R. Excitotoxic index – a biochemical marker of selective vulnerability. Neurosci Lett. 1991;127: 39–42.

25. Choi DW. Excitotoxic cell death. J Neurobiol. 1992;23:1261–76.

26. Traystman RJ, Kirsch JR, Koehler RC. Oxygen radical mechanisms of brain injury following ischemia and reperfusion. J Appl Physiol. 1991;71:1185–95.

27. Chan PH. Role of oxidants in ischemic brain damage. Stroke. 1996;27:1124–9.

28. Chan PH. Reactive oxygen radicals in signaling and damage in the ischemic brain. J Cereb Blood Flow Metab. 2001;21:2–14.

29. Polderman KH. Induced hypothermia and fever control for prevention and treatment of neurological injuries. Lancet. 2008;371: 1955–69.

30. Geocadin RG, Koenig MA, Jia X, Stevens RD, Peberdy MA. Management of brain injury after resuscitation from cardiac arrest. Neurol Clin. 2008;26:487–506, ix.

31. Clifton GL, Miller ER, Choi SC, Levin HS, McCauley S, Smith Jr KR, Muizelaar JP, Wagner Jr FC, Marion DW, Luerssen TG, Chesnut RM, Schwartz M. Lack of effect of induction of hypothermia after acute brain injury. N Engl J Med. 2001;344:556–63.

32. Bratton SL, Chestnut RM, Ghajar J, McConnell Hammond FF, Harris OA, Hartl R, Manley GT, Nemecek A, Newell DW, Rosenthal G, Schouten J, Shutter L, Timmons SD, Ullman JS, Videtta W, Wilberger JE, Wright DW. Guidelines for the management of severe traumatic brain injury. III. Prophylactic hypothermia. J Neurotrauma. 2007;24 Suppl 1:S21–5.

33. Sydenham E, Roberts I, Alderson P. Hypothermia for traumatic head injury. Cochrane Database Syst Rev. 2009;(1):CD001048.

34. Linares G, Mayer SA. Hypothermia for the treatment of ischemic and hemorrhagic stroke. Crit Care Med. 2009;37:S243–9.

35. Krieger DW, De Georgia MA, Abou-Chebl A, Andrefsky JC, Sila CA, Katzan IL, Mayberg MR, Furlan AJ. Cooling for acute ischemic brain damage (cool aid): an open pilot study of induced hypothermia in acute ischemic stroke. Stroke. 2001;32:1847–54.

36. De Georgia MA, Krieger DW, Abou-Chebl A, Devlin TG, Jauss M, Davis SM, Koroshetz WJ, Rordorf G, Warach S. Cooling for Acute Ischemic Brain Damage (COOL AID): a feasibility trial of endovascular cooling. Neurology. 2004;63:312–7.

37. Guluma KZ, Oh H, Yu SW, Meyer BC, Rapp K, Lyden PD. Effect of endovascular hypothermia on acute ischemic edema: morphometric analysis of the ICTuS trial. Neurocrit Care. 2008;8:42–7.

38. Schwab S, Georgiadis D, Berrouschot J, Schellinger PD, Graffagnino C, Mayer SA. Feasibility and safety of moderate hypothermia after massive hemispheric infarction. Stroke. 2001;32: 2033–5.

39. Hemmen TM, Raman R, Guluma KZ, Meyer BC, Gomes JA, Cruz-Flores S, Wijman CA, Rapp KS, Grotta JC, Lyden PD, ICTuS-L Investigators. Intravenous thrombolysis plus hypothermia for acute treatment of ischemic stroke (ICTuS-L): final results. Stroke. 2010; 41(10):2265–70.

40. Els T, Oehm E, Voigt S, Klisch J, Hetzel A, Kassubek J. Safety and therapeutical benefit of hemicraniectomy combined with mild hypothermia in comparison with hemicraniectomy alone in patients with malignant ischemic stroke. Cerebrovasc Dis. 2006;21:79–85.

41. Den Hertog HM, van der Worp HB, Tseng MC, Dippel DW. Cooling therapy for acute stroke. Cochrane Database Syst Rev. 2009;(1):CD001247.

42. Adams Jr HP, del Zoppo G, Alberts MJ, Bhatt DL, Brass L, Furlan A, Grubb RL, Higashida RT, Jauch EC, Kidwell C, Lyden PD, Morgenstern LB, Qureshi AI, Rosenwasser RH, Scott PA, Wijdicks EF. Guidelines for the early management of adults with ischemic stroke: a guideline from the American Heart Association/American Stroke Association Stroke Council, Clinical Cardiology Council, Cardiovascular Radiology and Intervention Council, and the Atherosclerotic Peripheral Vascular Disease and Quality of Care Outcomes in Research Interdisciplinary Working Groups: the American Academy of Neurology affirms the value of this guideline as an educational tool for neurologists. Stroke. 2007;38:1655–711.

43. Morgenstern LB, Hemphill 3rd JC, Anderson C, Becker K, Broderick JP, Connolly Jr ES, Greenberg SM, Huang JN, MacDonald RL, Messe SR, Mitchell PH, Selim M, Tamargo RJ. Guidelines for the management of spontaneous intracerebral hemorrhage: a guideline for healthcare professionals from the American Heart Association/American Stroke Association. Stroke. 2010;41:2108–29.

44. Broderick JP, Brott T, Tomsick T, Miller R, Huster G. Intracerebral hemorrhage more than twice as common as subarachnoid hemorrhage. J Neurosurg. 1993;78:188–91.

45. Broderick J, Connolly S, Feldmann E, Hanley D, Kase C, Krieger D, Mayberg M, Morgenstern L, Ogilvy CS, Vespa P, Zuccarello M, American Heart Association; American Stroke Association Stroke

Council; High Blood Pressure Research Council, Quality of Care and Outcomes in Research Interdisciplinary Working Group. Guidelines for the management of spontaneous intracerebral hemorrhage in adults: 2007 update: a guideline from the American Heart Association/American Stroke Association Stroke Council, High Blood Pressure Research Council, and the Quality of Care and Outcomes in Research Interdisciplinary Working Group. Stroke. 2007;38:2001–23.

46. Broderick JP, Brott TG, Duldner JE, Tomsick T, Huster G. Volume of intracerebral hemorrhage: a powerful and easy-to-use predictor of 30-day mortality. Stroke. 1993;24:987–93.

47. Brott T, Broderick J, Kothari R, Barsan W, Tomsick T, Sauerbeck L, Spilker J, Duldner J, Khoury J. Early hemorrhage growth in patients with intracerebral hemorrhage. Stroke. 1997;28:1–5.

48. Daverat P, Castel JP, Dartigues JF, Orgogozo JM. Death and functional outcome after spontaneous intracerebral hemorrhage: a prospective study of 166 cases using multivariate analysis. Stroke. 1991;22:1–6.

49. Fernandes HM, Siddique S, Banister K, Chambers I, Wooldridge T, Gregson B, Mendelow AD. Continuous monitoring of ICP and CPP following ICH and its relationship to clinical, radiological and surgical parameters. Acta Neurochir Suppl. 2000;76:463–6.

50. Gebel Jr JM, Jauch EC, Brott TG, Khoury J, Sauerbeck L, Salisbury S, Spilker J, Tomsick TA, Duldner J, Broderick JP. Relative edema volume is a predictor of outcome in patients with hyperacute spontaneous intracerebral hemorrhage. Stroke. 2002;33:2636–41.

51. Kollmar R, Staykov D, Do''rfler A, Schellinger PD, Schwab S, Bardutzky J. Hypothermia reduces perihemorrhagic edema after intracerebral hemorrhage. Stroke. 2010;41:1684–9.

52. Axelrod YK, Diringer MN. Temperature management in acute neurologic disorders. Neurol Clin. 2008;26:585–603, xi.

53. Gasser S, Khan N, Yonekawa Y, Imhof HG, Keller E. Long-term hypothermia in patients with severe brain edema after poor-grade subarachnoid hemorrhage: feasibility and intensive care complications. J Neurosurg Anesthesiol. 2003;15:240–8.

54. Todd MM, Hindman BJ, Clarke WR, Torner JC. Mild intraoperative hypothermia during surgery for intracranial aneurysm. N Engl J Med. 2005;352:135–45.

55. Bederson JB, Connolly Jr ES, Batjer HH, Dacey RG, Dion JE, Diringer MN, Duldner Jr JE, Harbaugh RE, Patel AB, Rosenwasser RH. Guidelines for the management of aneurysmal subarachnoid hemorrhage: a statement for healthcare professionals from a special writing group of the Stroke Council, American Heart Association. Stroke. 2009;40:994–1025.

56. Young GB, Doig G, Ragazzoni A. Anoxic ischemic encephalopathy: clinical and electrophysiological associations with outcome. Neurocrit Care. 2005;2:159–64.

57. Corry J, Dhar R, Murphy T, Diringer M. Hypothermia for refractory status epilepticus. Neurocrit Care. 2008;9:189–97.

58. Orlowski JP, Erenberg G, Lueders H, Cruse RP. Hypothermia and barbiturate coma for refractory status epilepticus. Crit Care Med. 1984;12:367–72.

59. Robakis TK, Hirsch LJ. Literature review, case report, and expert discussion of prolonged refractory status epilepticus. Neurocrit Care. 2006;4:35–46.

60. Dietrich 3rd WD. Therapeutic hypothermia for spinal cord injury. Crit Care Med. 2009;37:S238–42.

61. Levi AD, Casella G, Green BA, Dietrich WD, Vanni S, Jagid J, Wang MY. Clinical outcomes using modest intravascular hypothermia after acute cervical spinal cord injury. Neurosurgery. 2010; 66:670–7.

62. Levi AD, Green BA, Wang MY, Dietrich D, Brindle T, Vanni S, Casella G, Elhammady G, Jagid J. Clinical application of modest hypothermia after spinal cord injury. J Neurotrauma. 2009;26: 407–15.

63. Kwon BK, Mann C, Sohn HM, Hilibrand AS, Phillips FM, Wang JC, Fehlings MG. Hypothermia for spinal cord injury. Spine J. 2008;8:859–74.

64. Jalan R, Damink SWMO, Deutz NEP, Lee A. Moderate hypothermia for uncontrolled intracranial hypertension in acute liver failure. Lancet. 1999;354:1164–8.

65. Jalan R, Damink SWMO, Deutz NEP, Davies NA, Garden OJ, Madhavan KK, Hayes PC, Lee A. Moderate hypothermia prevents cerebral hyperemia and increase in intracranial pressure in patients undergoing liver transplantation for acute liver failure. Transplantation. 2003;75:2034–9.

66. Jalan R, Damink SWMO, Deuts NEP, Hayes PC, Lee A. Moderate hypothermia in patients with acute liver failure and uncontrolled intracranial hypertension. Gastroenterology. 2004;127:1338–46.

67. Boelhouwer RU, Bruining HA, Ong GL. Correlations of serum potassium fluctuations with body temperature after major surgery. Crit Care Med. 1987;15:310–2.

68. Krumholz A, Stern BJ, Weiss HD. Outcome from coma after cardiopulmonary resuscitation: relation to seizures and myoclonus. Neurology. 1988;38:401–5.

69. Sunde K, Dunlop O, Rostrup M, Sandberg M, Sjoholm H, Jacobsen D. Determination of prognosis after cardiac arrest may be more difficult after introduction of therapeutic hypothermia. Resuscitation. 2006;69:29–32.

70. Nolan JP, Morley PT, Hoek TL, Hickey RW. Therapeutic hypothermia after cardiac arrest. An advisory statement by the advancement life support task force of the international liaison committee on resuscitation. Resuscitation. 2003;57:231–5.

71. Neumar RW, Nolan JP, Adrie C, Aibiki M, Berg RA, Bottiger BW, Callaway C, Clark RS, Geocadin RG, Jauch EC, Kern KB, Laurent I, Longstreth Jr WT, Merchant RM, Morley P, Morrison LJ, Nadkarni V, Peberdy MA, Rivers EP, Rodriguez-Nunez A, Sellke FW, Spaulding C, Sunde K, Vanden HT. Post-cardiac arrest syndrome: epidemiology, pathophysiology, treatment, and prognostication. A consensus statement from the International Liaison Committee on Resuscitation (American Heart Association, Australian and New Zealand Council on Resuscitation, European Resuscitation Council, Heart and Stroke Foundation of Canada, InterAmerican Heart Foundation, Resuscitation Council of Asia, and the Resuscitation Council of Southern Africa); the American Heart Association Emergency Cardiovascular Care Committee; the Council on Cardiovascular Surgery and Anesthesia; the Council on Cardiopulmonary, Perioperative, and Critical Care; the Council on Clinical Cardiology; and the Stroke Council. Circulation. 2008; 118:2452–83.

72. Grigore AM, Grocott HP, Mathew JP, et al. Neurologic Outcome Research Group of the Duke Heart Center. The rewarming rate and increased peak temperature alter neurocognitive outcome after cardiac surgery. Anesth Analg. 2002;94:4–10.

73. Abend NS, Topjian A, Ichord R, Herman ST, Helfaer M, Donnelly M, Nadkarni V, Dlugos DJ, Clancy RR. Electroencephalographic monitoring during hypothermia after pediatric cardiac arrest. Neurology. 2009;72:1931–40.

74. Polderman K, Herold I. Therapeutic hypothermia and controlled normothermia in the intensive care unit: practical considerations, side effects, and cooling methods. Crit Care Med. 2009;37: 1101–20.

Cerebral Resuscitation from Cardiac Arrest

37

Clifton W. Callaway

Contents

Abstract

Brain injury is the principal barrier to good survival after cardiac arrest. Assessment of brain injury should include clinical imaging and neurophysiological measurements. Intensive care management focuses on optimizing cerebral blood flow through blood pressure and ventilator management. Targeted temperature management or mild hypothermia also improves outcomes. Current research seeks to determine optimal goals and monitors with which to titrate care.

Keywords

Hypothermia • Nonconvulsive status epilepticus • Cardiac arrest • Brain death • Persistent vegetative state • Cerebral blood flow • Evoked potentials

Introduction

Brain injury is the principal barrier to good survival after cardiac arrest. Improvements in cardiopulmonary resuscitation (CPR) have increased the rate of return of pulses to as much as 50 % [1], and mechanical rescue strategies can restore circulation when hearts do not respond to CPR [2]. Many organ systems have transient dysfunction after restoration of circulation, but modern intensive care can support patients through

C.W. Callaway, MD, PhD
Department of Emergency Medicine, University of Pittsburgh,
400A Iroquois, 3600 Forbes Avenue, Pittsburgh, PA 15260, USA
e-mail: callawaycw@upmc.edu

A.J. Layon et al. (eds.), *Textbook of Neurointensive Care*,
DOI 10.1007/978-1-4471-5226-2_37, © Springer-Verlag London 2013

this time period. However, brain injury begins after only a few minutes without circulation and increases over time. Severe brain injury can prompt withdrawal of life-sustaining treatments [3], and intermediate brain injury can severely compromise the quality of survival [4, 5].

The past decade has provided much new information about the basic physiology of post-cardiac arrest brain injury, as well as new clinical experience with the application of neurointensive care to this population. Intense interest surrounds therapeutic hypothermia or targeted temperature management to improve cerebral recovery after cardiac arrest [6, 7]. Because this targeted temperature management requires a bundle of associated care to implement, new clinical observations have multiplied. In general, studies of implementation of bundles of neurointensive care, including temperature management, report improved quality of survival after cardiac arrest [8, 9].

Heterogeneity of Functional Outcomes

Among patients with restoration of pulses after cardiac arrest, neurological and functional outcomes vary widely [10]. Severe brain injury and cerebral edema can progress to brain death. Intermediate injury leads to coma, which may resolve over time. However, coma does not resolve in a subset of patients who are left in a persistent vegetative state (PVS). Many families and most physicians who perceive that a patient is on trajectory for a PVS elect to withdraw life-sustaining treatment [11]. Thus, PVS is not a common outcome in North America and Europe at the present time. When coma does resolve to wakefulness, patients may exhibit reduced function and quality of life [4, 5, 12]. These may be evident on superficial examination or require more detailed testing to detect. Common deficits in awake survivors of cardiac arrest include depressed mood, impaired memory, and impaired executive function. Patients continue to improve for several months after cardiac arrest.

Anatomical Pattern of Brain Injury

Imaging studies provide some information about the areas of the brain that are most affected after cardiac arrest (Fig. 37.1a–f). These studies must be interpreted with some caution because patients with the most severe injury may not survive long enough to be imaged. Acknowledging this potential bias, cortical and basal ganglia gray matter are most frequently abnormal in imaging studies.

CT Scans

An initial non-contrast CT scan of the brain provides important information about etiology of cardiac arrest and degree of cerebral edema. CT scan does not have the sensitivity to detect subtle changes that might be associated with functional impairments. Over weeks to months, atrophic areas appear in patients with PVS or severe brain injury [13]. Therefore, little specific anatomical information about post-cardiac arrest brain injury is provided acutely by CT scan. Nevertheless, this test can provide important information about structural lesions precipitating arrest. In one series, 4 % of cardiac arrest patients were discovered to have unexpected intracerebral hemorrhage on initial CT scan [14]. A separate series identified a 9.8 % incidence of intracranial hemorrhage [15]. These hemorrhages are distinct from the pseudosubarachnoid hemorrhage observed with pial venous congestion in the setting of severe cerebral edema [16]. It is important to detect intracranial hemorrhage in order to modify estimates of prognosis and to safely plan or discontinue anticoagulation for other indications.

Cerebral edema appears on CT scan as a loss of contrast between gray matter and white matter, primarily because of decreased attenuation in edematous gray matter. Decreased ratios of gray matter attenuation to white matter attenuation (gray-white ratio, GWR) have been reported in patients with poor outcomes [17, 18]. Specific locations to measure GWR have been proposed in studies: basal ganglia to deep white matter (putamen, caudate to internal capsule, and corpus callosum) and superior cortex (mesial cortex to centrum semiovale) [17]. All of these regions and the thalamus display bilateral edema, with changes in cortex slightly more common than basal ganglia [14, 17]. When GWR was quantified in patients after cardiac arrest, patients with an average GWR less than 1.20 rarely awakened from coma [14, 17, 19].

The fact that cerebral edema is apparent on CT scan at very short times after restoration of pulses suggests a vasogenic rather than a cytotoxic cause of edema [20]. It is conceivable that rapid blood pressure changes, capillary leak, and loss of cerebral autoregulation converge to produce a pattern of edema similar to a hypertensive emergency. In severe cases, this edema may progress to herniation. It is unclear whether any of these events are preventable. Furthermore, there are no data about the efficacy of treating CT-recognized edema with hypertonic agents or other interventions. Regardless, it seems prudent to gather this information to help set expectations for progression and to inform specific therapeutic choices.

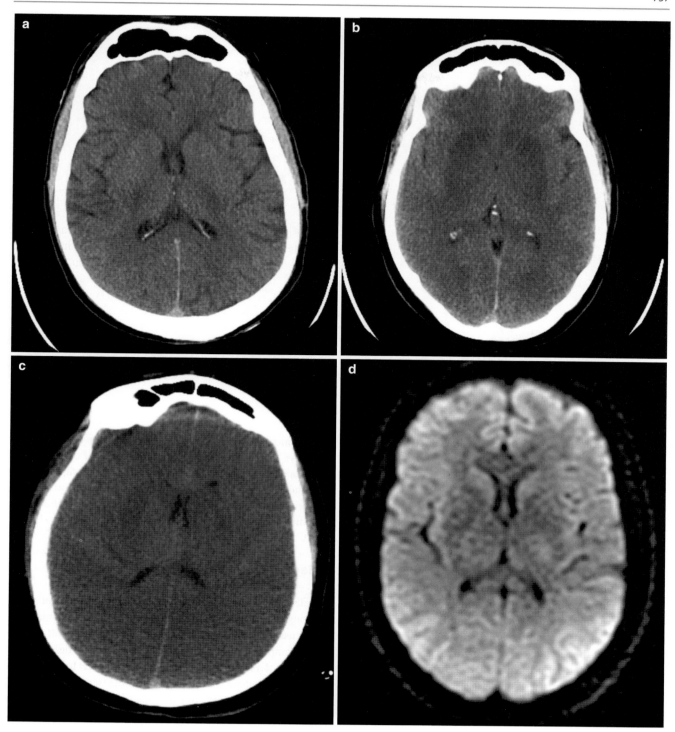

Fig. 37.1 (**a**–**f**) Non-contrast CT scan of the brain within a few hours after cardiac arrest can indicate the degree of cerebral edema. Edema can be none or minimal (**a**); moderate, in this case particularly severe in basal ganglia (**b**); or severe and diffuse, in this case with complete effacement of sulci and loss of gray-white differentiation (**c**). Diffusion-weighted images (DWI) on MRI obtained in comatose patients 3–7 days after cardiac arrest can reveal areas of damage. Increased DWI signal can be absent (normal, **d**) or appear in any focal area. Increased DWI signal can appear in isolated cortical regions (**e**) or basal ganglia (**f**). Increased signal in any combination of sites, or diffuse signal affecting the entire brain, is possible

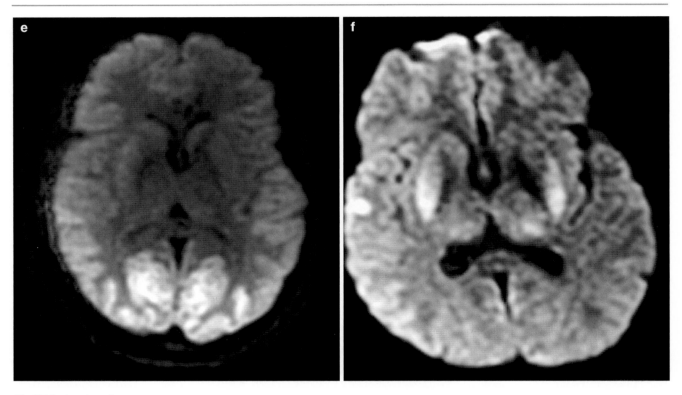

Fig. 37.1 (continued)

Magnetic Resonance Imaging (MRI) Studies

Magnetic resonance imaging (MRI) performed within 1–2 weeks after cardiac arrest can delineate the anatomical extent of cerebral injury, as an increase on diffusion-weighted images (DWI) and decrease of apparent diffusion coefficient (ADC) [21, 22]. While these techniques are sensitive indicators of cerebral edema, not tissue damage or cell death, MRI abnormalities do correlate with areas of damage identified on autopsy [23]. MRI studies definitely can distinguish patients with undetectable or focal abnormalities from patients with diffuse cerebral edema. Other MRI techniques include magnetic resonance spectroscopy (MRS). MRS provides information about the relative concentrations of energy substrates and metabolites in brain regions. However, systematic data from cardiac arrest patients beyond case reports are lacking.

Decreased ADC in cortex and basal ganglia are common [24]. Patients with poor outcome frequently have decreased ADC in putamen, occipital cortex, and temporal cortex and, in this series, always had at least one abnormal area. The peak MRI abnormalities are evident 3–5 days after cardiac arrest [22, 24]. Occipital, parietal, and putamen abnormalities were noted in other series, where total brain ADC or DWI were associated with survival [21, 22]. Other studies are limited by small sample sizes but support the finding that worse outcomes are associated with more extensive MRI abnormalities [25–27].

Taken together, MRI studies suggest that cortex is very sensitive to the ischemia-reperfusion injury of cardiac arrest and that the extent of cortical involvement contributes to the likelihood of functional recovery. However, all other brain regions and white matter can also be affected in individual patients [16].

Selective Neuronal Injury

Preclinical studies have noted that some brain cells and regions are more vulnerable to global ischemia and reperfusion than others. Specifically, CA1 region of the hippocampus has been extensively studied in rodent models of cardiac arrest and cerebral ischemia [28–31]. Neurons in the CA1 region are selectively vulnerable to ischemia, in that CA1 neurons will die after periods of ischemia that do not affect neighboring brain regions and that are not lethal to the animal [28, 29]. These facts have made CA1 cell loss a popular histological outcome measure for cerebral ischemia studies. Loss of hippocampal function from any cause is associated with specific memory deficits [32]. Loss of hippocampal volume also occurs after hypoxia in humans and is associated with post-hypoxia memory deficits [33]. Other brain regions that are notably affected by global ischemia include the reticular nuclei of the thalamus, dorsal striatum (caudate-putamen), and specific layers of the cortex [29–31].

Moreover, certain glia, particularly oligodendrocytes, may be as sensitive as neurons to ischemia [34].

Despite years of study, there is no unifying hypothesis to explain the selective vulnerability of specific neurons. Proposed mechanisms include increased susceptibility to oxidative stress, increased basal metabolic rate, increased exposure to excitotoxic neurotransmitters, and increased activity of cell pathways that mediate programmed cell death. While selective neuronal vulnerability is interesting from a mechanistic standpoint and attractive from a laboratory standpoint, the neurological morbidity after cardiac arrest involves less selective injury such as cerebral edema and global cortical injury as described by the CT and MRI studies. Clinically relevant interventions, such as targeted temperature management, do improve survival of selectively vulnerable neurons. For example, CA1 neurons are spared in rats subjected to cardiac arrest and resuscitation followed by hypothermia at 33–35 °C for 12–48 h [35–37]. Therefore, the animal models that focus on selectively vulnerable neurons may be most relevant for understanding how interventions will reduce the subtle neurological deficits such as memory loss among patients who awaken from coma. These animal models may be less relevant for understanding how to improve the rate of awakening from coma.

Cerebral Blood Flow

Cardiac arrest disrupts cerebral blood flow (CBF) autoregulation, but responsivity to hypercapnia and hypocapnia is preserved (Fig. 37.2a–c). These alterations in the usual effects of ventilation and blood pressure manipulation on cerebral blood flow may modify the management of the patient in the intensive care unit. Unfortunately, there are no clinical trials demonstrating improvements in outcome with any particular strategy, despite relatively detailed knowledge about the physiology of cerebral blood flow.

Cerebral Perfusion Pressure

Global cerebral ischemia disrupts autoregulation of cerebral blood flow across different arterial blood pressures. Prior to ischemia, cerebral blood flow remains constant across a wide range of arterial blood pressures and increases or decreases in proportion to cerebral metabolic rate. Immediately after reperfusion from cardiac arrest, cerebral vascular resistance increases [38] and cerebral autoregulation is either absent or right shifted [39, 40]. Using transcranial Doppler and jugular bulb oxygen saturation measurements, studies indicate that brain perfusion declines when mean arterial pressure decreases below 80–120 mmHg. These data suggest that a higher blood pressure would benefit the post-cardiac arrest

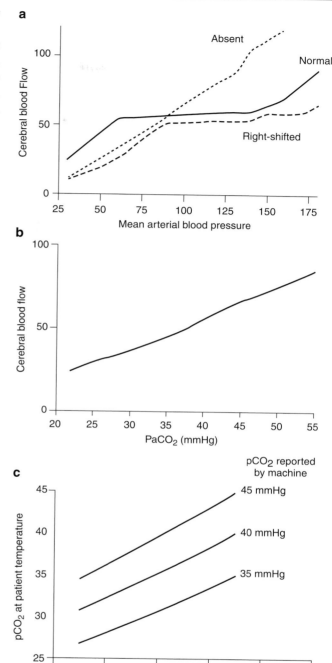

Fig. 37.2 (a–c) Changes in cerebral blood flow (*CBF*) with blood pressure, $PaCO_2$, and temperature. (**a**) In normal physiology, CBF is constant across a range of blood pressures. After cardiac arrest, autoregulation is absent or right shifted, suggesting that higher blood pressures may be required to maintain normal CBF. (**b**) Both in normal physiology and after cardiac arrest, CBF declines significantly with hypocapnia. Hyperventilation that lowers $PaCO_2$ may be poorly tolerated especially when blood pressure is low. (**c**) When using induced hypothermia, it is important to consider that $PaCO_2$ in the patient will be lower than $PaCO_2$ reported in the machine. Differences of 6–8 mmHg may occur between 37 and 32–34 °C, increasing the risk of accidental hypocapnia

brain. In fact, patients admitted to the hospital with mean arterial pressures >78 mmHg during the first 2 h after cardiac arrest had better neurological recovery in one series [41].

Combined with impaired autoregulation of cerebral blood flow, intracranial pressure may be elevated as a result of cerebral edema [14]. Increased intracranial pressure would also favor maintaining higher than normal mean arterial pressures to maintain cerebral perfusion. However, as noted previously, the early appearance of edema on CT scans suggests some vasogenic contribution to the cerebral edema, and increased blood pressures may result in deleterious hyperemia [42]. Therefore, the optimal blood pressure management strategy for an individual patient is unclear. To date, no study has examined a strategy of individualized cerebral perfusion optimization after cardiac arrest. Likewise, acute treatment of cerebral edema or intracranial hypertension in this setting is unproved.

The cerebral blood flow data do suggest general approaches for managing patients after cardiac arrest. Hypotension should be avoided, and mean arterial pressure maintained at least normal (>65 mmHg) and perhaps higher (80–100 mmHg) if tolerated. Routine maneuvers to avoid exacerbating raised intracranial pressure from cerebral edema also should be considered: elevation of the head, avoidance of hypotonic fluids, and minimal rotation of the neck.

CO$_2$ Reactivity of Cerebral Blood Flow

Reactivity of cerebral blood flow to changes in CO$_2$ is preserved after cardiac arrest in contrast to cerebral autoregulation which is impaired (Fig. 37.2a–c). Even at short times after cardiac arrest, hyperventilation with hypocapnia can decrease global cerebral blood flow [43–45]. Thus, strategies for management of ventilation after cardiac arrest are similar to that in other neurological conditions. Routine hyperventilation with hypocapnia should be avoided to prevent global decreases in cerebral blood flow.

Clinically important effects of PaCO$_2$ on cerebral blood flow are still present when patients are treated with mild hypothermia. For example, in eight subjects at 33 °C after ventricular fibrillation cardiac arrest, decreasing ventilation from normocapnia (5.0 kPa, 38 mmHg) to hypercapnia (6.0 kPa, 45 mmHg) increased jugular bulb O$_2$ saturation by 23 %, decreased transcranial Doppler-measured median flow velocity in the middle cerebral artery, and increased microdialysis-measured lactate/pyruvate ratios in the frontal cortex [43]. Conversely, transition from normocapnia to hypocapnia (4.3 kPa, 32 mmHg) reduced jugular bulb O$_2$ saturation by 26 %. With hypocapnia, cerebral venous oxygen saturation in most patients fell below the ischemic threshold of 55 %. A similar study in comatose patients after

out-of-hospital cardiac arrest estimated a ~4 % decline in cerebral blood flow per 1 mmHg decrease in PaCO$_2$ [44]. These studies emphasize that even mild hyperventilation with hypocapnia can compromise cerebral perfusion sufficiently to cause signs of ischemia.

Heterogeneity of Microvascular Blood Flow

The global changes in cerebral blood flow in response to ventilation and blood pressure may not correlate with local or microvascular changes. In some animal models, regional hypoperfusion and microvascular collapse occur despite normal blood pressure and normal global perfusion. Preclinical studies describe a phenomenon of patchy no-reflow after global cerebral ischemia [46]. With increasing durations of ischemia, reperfusion may be inadequate in patchy areas, largely because of edema and swelling of perivascular cells. These areas may experience additional ischemia and damage despite restoration of circulation. When studied with xenon-CT scan in dogs, these patchy areas of low flow appeared 1–4 h after return of pulses [47]. Increased blood pressure immediately (within minutes) after reperfusion improves cerebral blood flow and reduces the heterogeneity of reflow [48]. Promotion of cerebral blood flow with hypertension (MAP 110–140) and hemodilution reduced the heterogeneity of cerebral reflow, with more areas approaching normal blood flow [49]. However, caution is warranted when promoting cerebral blood flow with vasopressor drugs. In swine after cardiac arrest, epinephrine infusions reduce blood flow in small brain capillaries imaged using orthogonal polarization microscopy despite increased blood pressure [50]. This effect is attributable to the alpha-1 agonist effects of epinephrine.

While clinical data with patient-oriented outcomes are lacking, it appears reasonable to avoid hyperventilation (hypocapnia) when cerebral blood flow is compromised. Likewise, episodes of hypotension may add to prior brain ischemia, and global cerebral blood flow declines during the hours after reperfusion. Support of blood pressure during this sensitive phase seems warranted. An optimal vasopressor that does not produce adverse effects on cerebral vessels remains to be determined.

Seizures

Clinical seizures have been reported in 8–18 % of patients after cardiac arrest [6, 51], but the definitions and neurophysiological evaluation of these seizures vary widely between studies. Studies agree that patients who seize have worse outcomes than those who do not [52, 53]. However, no studies have tested if treating seizures will improve outcome or alternatively if seizures represent a sign of irreversible and

Table 37.1 Taxonomy for continuous EEG findings in 101 comatose patients after cardiac arrest

EEG finding	Definition	Incidence (%)	Survivors (%)
Electrographic seizure	Repetitive, generalized, or focal spikes, sharp waves, spike-and-wave or sharp-slow wave complexes at ≥3 Hz, or sequential rhythmic, periodic, or quasi-periodic waves at ≥1 Hz with unequivocal evolution in frequency, morphology, or location, lasting ≥10 s	6	17
Nonconvulsive status epilepticus (NCSE)	Continuous single electrographic seizure lasting 30 min or greater or recurrent electrographic seizures lasting for over 30 min	12	8
	GPEDs lasting at least 30 min at a rate >2.5 Hz		
	GPEDs lasting at least 30 min at a rate >1 Hz with unequivocal evolution in frequency, morphology, or location over time		
Myoclonic status epilepticus (MSE)	More than 30 min period of myoclonic jerks or subtle facial movements locked in with bursts in a burst-suppression pattern or associated GPEDs	21	0
Epileptiform discharges	Spikes, polyspikes, sharp waves, spike-and-wave, or sharp-slow waves occurring independently, periodically (GPEDs), or during burst suppression	20	10

Data from Rittenberger et al. [56]

severe brain damage. In the latter case, treating seizures may be futile.

Implementation of continuous EEG monitoring in the population of comatose intensive care patients, including post-cardiac arrest patients, has provided much more precise characterization of occult seizures and epileptiform discharges [54–56]. Several types of electrographic and convulsive syndromes can be distinguished after cardiac arrest (Table 37.1). It is important to recognize that post-cardiac arrest epileptiform activity is not epilepsy, causing some incongruencies when using standard EEG nomenclature. Most significantly, post-cardiac arrest EEG is dynamic, and multiple phenomena can appear in a single patient within a few hours. One recent paper recommended some definitions of findings in this setting and reported the relative incidence of epileptiform discharges in a series of 101 cases [56].

Epileptiform Discharges

Epileptiform discharges are often detected and can include spikes, sharp waves, and triphasic waves. When these epileptiform discharges are recorded bilaterally and repeatedly across the whole cortex, they are referred to as generalized periodic epileptiform discharges (GPEDs). While localized epileptiform occurs in epilepsy or focal brain injury, GPEDs are more common after cardiac arrest. GPEDs may be detected at a low frequency (<3 Hz) and are worrisome because they may progress to seizure or NCSE. GPEDs may be suppressed with anticonvulsant drugs. However, the effect of this treatment on patient outcome is unknown.

Nonconvulsive Status Epilepticus (NCSE)

Nonconvulsive status epilepticus (NCSE) is characterized by epileptiform discharges exceeding a defined frequency

(e.g., GPEDs at >2.5–3 Hz) without clinical convulsions and lasting for an extended period of time (e.g., >30 min). NCSE has been recognized as a potential cause of coma in many ICU patients [54]. A series of post-cardiac arrest patients report that NCSE occurs in 12–32 % of adults [52, 56] or 32 % of children [55]. Survival with good neurological outcome has been reported after NCSE [57], suggesting that this syndrome is not simply an epiphenomenon of bad brain and deserves aggressive treatment. The optimal anticonvulsant regimen for post-cardiac arrest NCSE is unknown. In addition, there are some patients with refractory NCSE that cannot be suppressed despite multiple anticonvulsants over days. Refractory status probably represents one end point of neurological resuscitation.

Myoclonic Status Epilepticus (MSE)

Myoclonic status epilepticus (MSE) is the most ominous and least survivable finding. Clinically, MSE is characterized by repetitive myoclonic jerks that most often involve the face but can extend to all of the extremities. These myoclonic jerks can appear very shortly after restoration of circulation but are most common 12–48 h after cardiac arrest [58]. The frequency of jerks can vary from once every 1–2 min to almost continuously every 1–2 s. Electrographically, myoclonic jerks are associated with bursts of electrical activity. The most common pattern is a burst followed by nearly complete suppression of the EEG (burst suppression). The burst may or may not contain spikes or sharp waves.

Association of the burst-suppression pattern on EEG with clinical myoclonic jerks, typically for 30 min or longer, is required for the diagnosis of MSE. This combined electrographic and clinical definition is important, because some patients who have burst-suppression pattern on EEG, but not MSE, may recover [56]. In addition, sedatives such as propofol can cause burst-suppression patterns independently of ischemic injury. Finally, clinical signs of tonic-clonic sei-zures, which also might be treatable, may be confused with myoclonic jerks if EEG is not examined. When MSE is accu-rately diagnosed, the probability of awakening using current therapy is vanishingly small. Many series report that all sub-jects who survive MSE develop a persistent vegetative state. Other series suggest that a small percentage of patients who exhibit myoclonus may recover [57]. However, the literature is confused by many reports without clear correlation between clinical and EEG features.

Taken together, these data support frequent or continuous monitoring of EEG in comatose patients after cardiac arrest. Potentially treatable epileptiform discharges or NCSE may be detected in over 30 % of patients. Furthermore, proper diagnosis of MSE may temper family and caregiver expecta-tions for recovery and alter decisions about other aspects of care.

Targeted Temperature Management

The landscape for the critical care of patients resuscitated from cardiac arrest changed dramatically over the past decade because of the clinical trials demonstrating improved outcome when temperature was maintained at 32–34 °C for 12–24 h after restoration of pulses [6, 7]. These papers prompted widespread application of therapeutic hypother-mia or targeted temperature management protocols. Although the published trials were conducted in a narrowly defined population (out-of-hospital cardiac arrest with ventricular fibrillation or ventricular tachycardia as the initial rhythm), many hospitals offered these protocols to all patients with coma after cardiac arrest. This practice seems biologically plausible and is endorsed by organizations that write treat-ment guidelines [59–61]. Registry data, although nonran-domized and prone to reporting bias, suggested that survival for post-cardiac arrest patients improved as targeted temper-ature management was adopted [62, 63].

A direct consequence of the adoption of hypothermia protocols has been the regimentation of post-cardiac arrest care. Each hospital that created a clinical pathway for tar-geted temperature management had to address blood pres-sure goals, choice of sedation, ventilation goals, and other physiological variables that were associated with cooling and rewarming. As a consequence, this past decade has wit-nessed the development of a "multidisciplinary" and "mul-tiorgan" approach to post-cardiac arrest care. Almost without exception, investigators report implementation of these protocols is associated with improved survival and neurological recovery [8, 9]. It is impossible from these various before-and-after reports to determine whether ben-efits derive from temperature management or from increas-ingly protocolized care.

Therapeutic Window for Targeted Temperature Management

Animal and clinical data suggest that it is necessary to initi-ate hypothermia less than 6–8 h after return of pulses. It is unknown whether there is incremental benefit from even faster cooling within this 6-h time window. Animal data sup-port durations of temperature management for at least 5 h and preferably for 72 h after reperfusion. Clinical data sup-port durations of 12 or 24 h of hypothermia, but have not compared durations. Most animal data and all clinical stud-ies have employed target temperatures of 32–34 °C. This temperature range was selected for its lack of adverse effects on cardiovascular performance and its demonstrated neuro-logical benefit.

Animal studies suggest that there are two phases during which induced hypothermia affects recovery from cardiac arrest. First, brief (<1 h) episodes of mild (32–34 °C) hypo-thermia induced prior to reperfusion improve survival in multiple species when achieved during ischemia prior to reperfusion [64, 65]. This benefit is lost when hypothermia starts more than 20 min into the attempted resuscitation [66] or more than 15 min after reperfusion [65]. Second, more prolonged (>5 h) hypothermia improves outcomes in multi-ple animal models of cardiac arrest even when initiation is delayed for 4–6 h after reperfusion [67, 68]. Benefit declines with delays beyond 6 h. A duration of at least 5 h of hypo-thermia is required for this effect [69], and the best improve-ment in outcome after global cerebral ischemia results from 72 h of temperature control [37, 67].

Timing of Initiation of Hypothermia

The optimal time to initiate hypothermia after cardiac arrest is debated. In the clinical trials that demonstrated efficacy of induced hypothermia after cardiac arrest, tem-peratures <34 °C were achieved within 2 h or at a median of 8 h (IQR 4–16) [6] after return of pulses. A registry-based case series ($n = 465$) of comatose post-cardiac arrest patients with varying times to initiate cooling (IQR 1–1.8 h) and varying times to reach target temperature (IQR 3–6.7 h) found no association between timing of initiation or time to reach target temperature and neurological outcome [62]. A case series ($n = 49$) of comatose post-cardiac arrest patients reaching target temperature at median of 6.8 h (IQR 4.5–9.2 h) after return of pulses found no association of time to initiate cooling or time to reach target temperature with neurological outcome [70]. However, shorter times to cold-est temperature were associated with better outcome. These data support the conclusion that hypothermia should be achieved in less than 6–8 h, similar to the results of animal studies.

Clinical trials find no benefit from extremely early initiation of hypothermia. For example, outcomes were similar between cardiac arrest patients treated with 4 °C intravenous fluid in the ambulance ($n=63$) or standard care in the hospital ($n=62$) [71]. Likewise, there was no difference in outcome between adults resuscitated from out-of-hospital VF who received 2 L of intravenous, ice-cold Hartmann's solution in the ambulance ($n=118$) versus standard hypothermia in the emergency department ($n=116$) [72]. These studies suggest that ambulance versus emergency department initiation of hypothermia does not produce any large clinical effects. While it seems unwise to intentionally delay initiation of hypothermia, these data suggest that start of temperature management can be prioritized along with other aspects of stabilization and care.

Duration of Hypothermia Treatment

Most data in adults have been obtained with protocols using 12 or 24 h of hypothermia. In clinical practice, 24 h of hypothermia is the most common protocol [73]. Effects of different durations of hypothermia have not been studied in humans. However, up to 72 h of hypothermia has been used safely in newborns [74]. Longer durations of hypothermia up to 72 h are used successfully in Japanese practice for adult patients with clinical features suggesting worse injury (e.g., longer total no-flow and low-flow time) [2].

Rewarming after induced hypothermia must proceed slowly. For example, rewarming from hypothermia used to treat traumatic brain injury can lead to hyperemia-induced cerebral edema [75], and similar hyperemia occurs 12–24 h after cardiac arrest without temperature manipulation [42]. Rates of <0.5 °C/h (typically targeting 0.25 °C/h) have been used in most studies [6, 51].

Techniques for Targeted Temperature Management

There are multiple methods to control temperature for therapeutic benefit. There are no data to suggest that one method is more beneficial to the patient than another [51, 76]. However, the side-effect profile and resource requirements do differ. Therefore, clinicians should choose temperature management methods that are familiar and that minimize procedural risk and chances of complication for the individual patient.

The first priority in targeted temperature management is accurate measurement of patient temperature. Central venous monitors are the gold standard for core temperature, but may not be available in every patient. Because the esophageal lumen is separated from the great vessels by only a thin layer of muscle, esophageal temperature most accurately estimates core temperature during temperature manipulation [77, 78]. An esophageal probe should be placed with its tip in the middle of the mediastinum on chest x-ray. Bladder temperature is also accurate when urine output exceeds 0.5 ml/kg/h. Accurate rectal temperature measurements require that the probe be passed 15–20 cm past the anus. Because of decreased blood flow in this region and because of the thermal mass of colonic contents, rectal temperature may lag behind the core temperature by up to 1.5 °C during active temperature manipulation [77]. Axillary and tympanic measurements are not well related to core temperature during hypothermia induction because of technical limitations and influence of peripheral blood flow. Proper tympanic measurements require the probe to be in contact with the tympanic membrane, which is unlikely in clinical practice. These sites should never be used to guide active temperature control.

Options to lower the temperature to 32–34 °C after cardiac arrest include infusions of cold intravenous fluids, endovascular cooling catheters, and surface cooling. As a result of mixing cool peripheral blood with core blood compartments during circulatory collapse and CPR, the initial temperature for patients after cardiac arrest averages 35–35.5 °C [6, 7, 71, 79]. Therefore, induction of hypothermia to the target range (32–34 °C) requires only a 1–1.5 °C additional change. Regardless of the method used to accomplish this final temperature change, measures to prevent shivering and rewarming should be in place within the first hour [71].

Cold intravenous fluids are the simplest and fastest method to lower temperature. Rapid infusion of 30–40 ml/kg of cold (4 °C) intravenous fluid is well tolerated after cardiac arrest [80] and can reduce core body temperature by 1–1.5 °C within 20 min [71, 72, 81–83]. The large temperature change observed with this small volume of fluids results from the fact that the fluids are delivered quickly into the thermal mass of the core blood compartment (e.g., 20–30 kg) and not the entire body (e.g., >80 kg). To achieve this compartment-specific effect, the infusion of fluids must be rapid (e.g., 1 l/20 min or faster using pressure bags) into the torso (e.g., large antecubital vein or central line). This technique is limited by the ability of the patient to tolerate the volume load. For example, this method will be unusable in patients with severe pulmonary edema. In addition, the effect of cold intravenous fluids is transient and must be followed by a maintenance cooling methods and shivering suppression [71].

Endovascular cooling devices can reduce core temperature by up to 1.0 °C/h [62, 84]. These devices are inserted as central venous catheters and require proprietary consoles to function. Complications do not differ from other central venous catheters. In general, the precision of temperature control achieved with endovascular devices is excellent. Disadvantages include the time required for placement and limited availability in some locations. For example, a standard central venous catheter might be placed emergently during resuscitation, and the intensivist must subsequently decide whether to replace this line with an endovascular cooling catheter or to place a second line strictly for temperature management. Because of these logistical and procedural delays, times to initiate cooling and to reach goal temperatures are actually longer in patients cooled with endovascular devices compared to surface devices [62].

Surface cooling devices can reduce core temperature by 0.5 °C/h [6, 7, 51]. The simplest surface cooling is to place ice bags or cold blankets on the patient. Thermostatically controlled, water-filled blankets are available in most hospitals and departments. Maintenance of hypothermia can be accomplished with any of these devices, although the temperature controller and wattage of some devices may improve the precision of temperature control [51]. One reported disadvantage of surface cooling is that core temperature is being manipulated via physical manipulation of the peripheral compartment, creating a time lag between adjustments and responses. Consequently, temperature overshoot (<32 °C) and temperature out of range are more common with surface cooling techniques [85].

Induction of hypothermia requires adequate sedation and muscle relaxation to control shivering and prevent rewarming. Without adequate sedation, core temperature rapidly rebounds [71]. Many protocols for induced hypothermia include neuromuscular blocking agents routinely or as needed to facilitate cooling [8]. Continued neuromuscular blockade during hypothermia maintenance may not be necessary. If neuromuscular blockade is used, adequate monitoring should be in place to detect and treat seizures or other acute changes.

Complications of Targeted Temperature Management

Induced hypothermia produces predictable changes in cardiovascular parameters, blood coagulation, immune function, blood volume, and electrolytes [86]. Most of these changes require little alteration of therapy. However, increased monitoring of certain parameters (e.g., serum potassium) during cooling and rewarming is prudent. Overall, studies suggest the risk-benefit profile favors induced hypothermia during the first hospital day after cardiac arrest for non-bleeding patients.

Cooling from 37 °C to about 32 °C produces a negative chronotropic effect but a positive inotropic effect on the heart. Heart rate may slow to 40 beats per minute or even lower when patients are cooled to 33 °C (Fig. 37.3a–c). However, blood pressure and cardiac output are preserved because of increased stroke volume and contractility [87]. Repolarization may be altered, with prolongation of QT

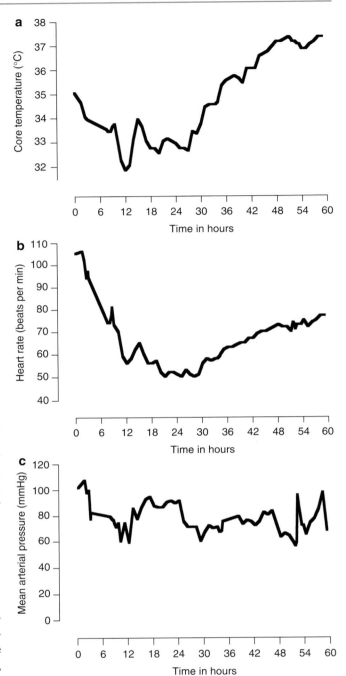

Fig. 37.3 (**a–c**) Example of temperature measurements (**a**), heart rate (**b**), and mean arterial pressure (**c**) in a patient undergoing induced hypothermia after cardiac arrest. As temperature declines to 32–33 °C, heart rate can also decline to the low 40s or high 30s without any compromise in blood pressure. Rewarming should be slow, over 8–12 h, during which time heart rate will also rise

intervals [88]. The decreased heart rate reduces some of the risk for R-on-T events, but caution is advised when hypothermic patients are also given QT-prolonging drugs such as amiodarone. Despite this effect on repolarization, the reported incidence of ventricular dysrhythmias is reported to be lower in hypothermia-treated patients. Finally, there is no decrease and perhaps even an increase in defibrillation shock efficacy with hypothermia in the 32–37 °C range [89].

Blood coagulation requires multiple enzymatic steps. With decreasing temperature, particularly below 35 °C, the kinetics of these steps are slowed. Likewise, activation of platelets requires active steps that may be slowed at lower temperatures. Consequently, thrombogenesis and actual bleeding time may be prolonged in the hypothermic patient despite normal levels of coagulation factors and platelets [86]. Vigilance for noncompressible bleeding is warranted during induced hypothermia, and any occurrence of bleeding should prompt reconsideration of the risk-benefit profile for hypothermia. One response to new onset of bleeding in a hypothermic patient is to warm above 35 °C while trying to achieve hemostasis. If bleeding is controlled, very mild hypothermia of 35 °C may be continued for the remainder of the prescribed time period. Hypothermia of 35 °C was equivalent in neurological benefit to 33 °C in rat studies [36].

Like coagulation, leucocyte function declines with hypothermia. As a consequence, the incidence of infections increases with prolonged hypothermia. In the randomized trial of hypothermia after cardiac arrest, hypothermia increased the incidence of sepsis from 29 to 37 % and the incidence of pneumonia from 7 to 13 % [6]. Although not statistically significant, these effects were probably real. Pneumonia rates as high as 65 % have been reported when induced hypothermia is used [90]. In other patient populations, pneumonia and other infections are definitely increased when hypothermia is maintained for periods longer than 24 h.

Initial cooling results in diuresis, loss of electrolytes in the urine, and shifting of potassium into cells. After cardiac arrest, decreased serum levels of potassium, magnesium, and phosphorus occur [91]. The diuresis with cooling may cause patients to be relatively hypovolemic when rewarmed, an effect that was thought to be important for morbidity in some patients during clinical trials of hypothermia for traumatic brain injury [92]. These changes should prompt clinicians to monitor electrolytes, particularly potassium, more frequently during cooling and rewarming. There are no data to suggest changes in replacement doses or target goals for these electrolytes. Likewise, volume status can be monitored with central venous pressures and urine output during the temperature management.

Blood Gas Interpretation and Hypothermia

Temperature affects the solubility of gases and also shifts the oxygen-hemoglobin dissociation curve (Fig. 37.2a–c). Blood gases are measured in machines where the electrodes are usually held at 37 °C. When the patient temperature differs from 37 °C, some correction is required to estimate the true partial pressures of gases in the body [93]. During induced hypothermia, the physiological pCO_2 is lower than the reported pCO_2 (about 7–8 mmHg lower at 32–33 °C). Likewise, pO_2 may be 20 % lower in the body at 32–33 °C than what is reported by the blood gas machine. Consequently, it is reasonable to avoid hyperventilation that might lead to severe hypocapnia during hypothermia (e.g., keep pCO_2 ~40–45 mmHg) and to maintain an adequate margin to avoid hypoxemia (e.g., keep pO_2 ~100–130 mmHg).

There is no consensus about whether ventilator management during mild induced hypothermia should target temperature-corrected or uncorrected blood gas values. A strategy in which the clinician titrates ventilation to "normalize" the uncorrected pCO_2 values (perhaps resulting in respiratory alkalosis) is termed "alpha-stat," and a strategy in which the clinician normalizes the corrected pCO_2 values (more normal pH) is termed "pH-stat." While compared extensively in cardiopulmonary bypass, anesthesia, and other settings, there are no data comparing patient outcomes with alpha-stat and pH-stat strategies during induced hypothermia for cardiac arrest. Available data recommend only that the clinician have awareness of the issue and take caution to avoid inadvertent hyperventilation.

Neurological Monitoring After Cardiac Arrest

Ideally, monitors are placed in order to allow titration of care and early detection of correctable problems. After cardiac arrest, the evolution of brain injury may involve changes in CBF, seizures, cellular homeostasis, intracellular signaling pathways, and a variety of other physiological changes that will affect neurological recovery. Unfortunately, the utility of only a few monitors has been examined in this population.

Arterial Blood Pressure

Arterial catheters are not a specific neurological monitor but must be emphasized as a critical component of the monitoring of post-cardiac arrest patients. There is a high incidence of hemodynamic instability. After initial resuscitation, blood pressure may fall over minutes to hours as catecholamines are metabolized or receptors become desensitized. At the same time, myocardial stunning is common over the first 24 h after cardiac arrest. Continuous arterial blood pressure monitoring is essential for rapid titration of vasoactive medicines and inotropic medicines in order to avoid hypotensive episodes or rearrest. In addition, the important interaction between ventilation and CBF will require frequent blood gas sampling, which also will be expedited with arterial catheters.

Electroencephalography (EEG)

EEG has been studied primarily as an aid in determining prognosis after cardiac arrest, but the high incidence (8–18 %) of seizures after cardiac arrest suggests EEG should be used as a continuous monitor to detect treatable, nonconvulsive epileptiform activity. Diagnostic EEG patterns obtained on intermitted EEGs that are associated with poor neurological recovery include generalized suppression (<20 μV), burst-suppression pattern associated with generalized epileptic activity, or diffuse periodic complexes on a flat background [94]. NCSE and other epileptiform activity are increasingly recognized as a feature of the comatose ICU patient [54]. Current research will need to determine if treating these EEG findings can alter the natural history of coma from many causes including cardiac arrest.

Continuous EEG monitoring reveals that the brain electrical activity is very dynamic and evolving during the first few days after cardiac arrest. Frequent, but not continuous, NCSE or other epileptiform activity has been reported in children [55] and adults [56] after cardiac arrest. Therefore, spot EEG may miss potentially treatable pathology. In one series, transient hemodynamic instability in post-arrest patients was discovered to be the only manifestation of nonconvulsive seizures when continuous EEG was applied [56]. This finding dramatically altered patient management.

Amplitude-integrated EEG (aEEG) was developed for monitoring of infants with hypoxic-ischemic encephalopathy. Using a reduced electrode set, this machine collects continuous EEG data and displays them as the integrated amplitude with some automated reading. Using this instrument, one series noted that evolution to a continuous EEG pattern was associated with awakening and that nonconvulsive epileptiform activity could be identified in 27 % of patients [95]. Studies have not compared the clinical utility of aEEG to full-montage EEG after adult cardiac arrest.

Bispectral EEG (BIS) is a tool developed for anesthesia to measure depth of sedation. Using four electrodes, this device collects continuous EEG from the two frontal hemispheres. The cross-correlation of the power spectrum of each side of the brain is displayed as number from 0 to 100. Lower numbers reflect greater desynchrony of the cortices, corresponding to greater sedation with many anesthetics. In two studies of post-cardiac arrest patients, BIS values of zero at any time during the ICU care were associated with poor outcome (death or PVS) [96, 97]. Rising BIS values over time are associated with better outcome. However, there are too few observations to consider BIS reliable for excluding awakening.

Somatosensory Evoked Potentials (SSEP)

SSEPs are primarily used as a test to determine prognosis. Advantages include the fact that this test can be performed at the bedside and is robust to a variety of temperature and sedative regimens. Absence of the N20 cortical response after median nerve stimulation is very specific for poor neurological outcome [53, 94]. In over 250 reported cases in the literature who were not treated with hypothermia, no patient with N20 absent more than 24 h after cardiac arrest awakened. However, a recent case series reported two patients treated with hypothermia with absent N20 responses 3 days or more after cardiac arrest, who later recovered cognition [98]. Based on this latter report, repeat examination to confirm a persistently absent N20 might be a reasonable practice. SSEP responses vary with the elapsed time since resuscitation [99]. While not specific, recovery of longer latency event-related potentials in the cortex may precede awakening [99–101].

Jugular Bulb Oximetry

Several studies have reported jugular bulb oxygen saturation ($SjbO_2$) or jugular bulb lactate as quantitative way to follow global brain oxygen extraction. $SjbO_2$ values below 55 % suggest ischemia and should prompt maneuvers to increase cerebral oxygen delivery [102]. A significant limitation of $SjbO_2$ monitoring is that it is a global measure and will be insensitive to focal or patchy areas of ischemia. Nevertheless, cerebral oxygen extraction increases more than systemic oxygen extraction in dogs during the first day after cardiac arrest [103], corresponding to the time that global and focal cerebral blood flow may be impaired. Clinical studies in post-cardiac arrest patients confirm that hyperventilation with hypocapnia [43–45] as well as decreases in blood pressure [39] can increase cerebral oxygen extraction (decrease $SjbO_2$). These studies confirm that $SjbO_2$ assesses the balance between global cerebral oxygen delivery and demand after cardiac arrest.

Clinical studies of $SjbO_2$ after cardiac arrest reveal a dynamic pattern of $SjbO_2$ after cardiac arrest. In the first few hours after cardiac arrest, $SjbO_2$ tends to be lower than mixed-venous oxygen saturation [104] and may fall more quickly than mixed-venous saturations with cardiogenic shock [105]. These studies did not find any early distinction between patients with good or poor outcomes. In some patients with poor outcome, $SjbO_2$ increases (cerebral oxygen extraction decreases) over the next day or days [105–108]. This declining oxygen extraction by injured brains may represent global metabolic failure or even progression to brain death. No studies exist about titration of care based on $SjbO_2$ after cardiac arrest. In summary, jugular bulb monitoring is one technique to assess the balance of cerebral oxygen delivery and extraction, but it is not yet established whether any subgroup of patients benefits from care titrated to this monitor.

Near-Infrared Spectroscopy (NIRS)

Near-infrared spectroscopy (NIRS) can measure cerebral hemoglobin and cytochrome oxygenation after cardiac arrest [109]. Because infrared light can penetrate some distance into the tissue, NIRS probes placed on the forehead may detect some signal from the underlying cortex (regional cerebral oxygenation). However, it is unclear in actual practice to what extent the scalp and superficial tissues dominate this signal. Advantages of NIRS include the fact that it is noninvasive and provides continuous data. In cardiac arrest patients, NIRS signals can detect the presence or absence of cerebral perfusion [110]. However, once circulation is restored, manipulating arterial CO_2 concentrations sufficiently to alter jugular bulb oxygen saturation does not reliably alter NIRS readings [111]. Similar lack of sensitivity has been reported after traumatic brain injury [112]. These data suggest that NIRS lacks the sensitivity to fine-tune care but may have a role as warning monitor that can detect severe disruptions of perfusion.

Transcranial Doppler (TCD)

The effect of interventions on cerebral blood flow can be estimated by looking at changes in transcranial Doppler (TCD) signals from the middle cerebral artery. TCD has the advantage of being noninvasive, repeatable, and portable. However, TCD is limited by the need for an experienced operator, limited ultrasonographic windows for some individuals, and the difficulty of interpreting the absolute values for any TCD finding. TCD is sensitive to changes in blood flow in post-cardiac arrest patients. For example, decreased arterial CO_2 concentrations are associated with reduced mean flow velocity in the middle cerebral artery [43–45]. Conversely, hypertension can increase flow [40]. In general, changes in the flow velocity and pulsatility index measured by TCD are highly correlated with changes measured by jugular bulb oximetry [43, 44, 108]. There are no studies reporting on modification of treatment regimens based on real-time TCD monitoring.

Intracranial Monitoring

Data from intracranial probes have been reported for select patients after cardiac arrest. Common disadvantages include the invasive nature of these probes and the fact that the probe

only samples a small region of the brain (usually nondominant frontal lobe). Patients on anticoagulation will incur risk of intracranial bleeding. All patients will incur risk of intracerebral infection. Only case reports are available about intracranial tissue oxygen sensors [113]. This report confirmed that the probe is sensitive to the expected changes during cardiac arrest. More reports are available for microdialysis probes which can continuously sample extracellular fluid and have the ability to measure multiple metabolites. For example, increases in cerebral lactate and lactate/pyruvate ratios closely parallel declines in $SjbO_2$ in patients after cardiac arrest [43]. Dynamic and multiphasic increases in the excitatory amino acid glutamate and lipid breakdown product glycerol also occur [114]. While these data are very useful for research studies, it is unclear how to titrate care with these monitors.

Pharmacological Considerations

The entire range of drugs used in any intensive care patient may be necessary for post-cardiac arrest patients. Several physiological changes after cardiac arrest may modify the usual doses or timing for drugs. Specifically, cardiac arrest may impair enteral absorption, as well as renal and hepatic elimination, because of ischemia-reperfusion injury to the gut, kidney, and liver. The absolute incidence of renal and hepatic impairment after cardiac arrest is unknown, but transient elevations of creatinine and transaminases are common. Special caution is required when using drugs that may exacerbate the original cause of cardiac arrest.

Induced hypothermia can impair drug transport and elimination. Gut motility is decreased during hypothermia, and enteral drug administration is unreliable and should be avoided until after rewarming. Induced hypothermia reduces active renal excretion of drugs [115]. Hypothermia reduces hepatic metabolism of drugs by several cytochrome P450 (CYP) isoforms [116]. For example, a study in normal volunteers found that clearance of the CYP3A substrate midazolam decreases 11 % per °C decrease below 36.5 °C [117]. There is a similar 11 % per °C reduction in vecuronium clearance with hypothermia [118]. Reduced clearance can result in clinically important doubling or tripling of the duration of drug effects at 33–34 °C.

It is impossible to list all drugs that might increase the risk of recurrent cardiac arrest, and the risk for any given drug will differ from patient to patient. For example, many antipsychotic drugs that would be used to control agitation also can prolong cardiac QT intervals. This effect is worrisome for patients who suffered primary ventricular dysrhythmias resulting from repolarization abnormalities but is probably inconsequential for patients who suffered cardiorespiratory arrest from impaired oxygenation. Similarly, propofol as a sedative may cause more myocardial depression than midazolam, but this effect is offset by the short half-life and ease of titration of propofol. In general, clinicians should consider the prodysrhythmic and cardiodepressant effects of all routinely administered drugs in patients who are recovering from cardiac arrest.

Non-neurological Organ Support

Cardiac arrest is a situation that is followed by a syndrome of global ischemia-reperfusion. This syndrome can affect every organ system in the body [119], although individual patients can display changes in none, some, or all of these systems.

Nevertheless, data are available to recommend several specific approaches for the post-cardiac arrest patients. Specifically, the intensivist should consider specific parameters for treatment of acute coronary syndromes, ventilator management, and other organ system support.

Acute Cardiovascular Interventions and Hemodynamic Support

Acute coronary syndromes are common among patients who are resuscitated from cardiac arrest outside the hospital [120–123]. As many as 70 % of patients admitted to the hospital after cardiac arrest have an acute coronary occlusion [121]. Interventions to accomplish reperfusion are associated with improved outcomes [8, 122, 123]. Combination of percutaneous coronary intervention and induced hypothermia has been demonstrated to be safe and feasible [124, 125].

Consequently, all patients resuscitated from cardiac arrest should be evaluated for acute ST-elevation myocardial infarction (STEMI). Even in the absence of STEMI, evaluation of coronary anatomy may be considered if there are suggestive historical features, rising troponin levels, or hemodynamic instability attributable to cardiogenic shock. Echocardiogram may also detect focal wall motion abnormalities that would prompt examination for coronary occlusion. Placement of circulatory support devices such as intra-aortic balloon pumps often accompanies coronary interventions, but definitive data are lacking about whether these devices independently improve outcomes after cardiac arrest [122]. In the setting of cardiogenic shock, these devices may reduce the need for vasoconstricting drugs to support blood pressure, with consequent improvement in microcirculation.

Ventilator Strategies

In addition to avoiding hypocapnia that might reduce cerebral blood flow, there are some data specifically addressing ventilator strategies after cardiac arrest. Fortunately, lung injury and difficulty oxygenating are very rare causes of death in this population. Available data suggest the same attention to and strategies for ventilator management in post-cardiac arrest patients that are required for other respiratory failure. Specifically, avoiding high airway pressures, hypoxemic episodes, and excessive hyperoxia is important.

In one large ($n = 6{,}326$) database, excessive oxygenation ($PaO_2 > 300$ mmHg) was associated with higher in-hospital mortality (63, 95 % CI 60–66 %) compared to patients with normal PaO_2 (45, 95 % CI 43–48 %) [82]. Mortality was also higher (57, 95 % CI 56–59 %) in patients with hypoxemia ($PaO_2 < 60$ mmHg). This observation was biologically plausible given the vulnerability of brain and other organs to oxygen-derived free radicals after ischemia-reperfusion and to secondary insult from hypoxemia. However, another large ($n = 12{,}108$) series did not confirm this association [126]. A prospective study comparing FiO_2 of 1.0 ($n = 14$) to FiO_2 of 0.3 ($n = 14$) for the first 60 min after resuscitation found no large difference in survival or outcome but did note lower serum levels of neuron-specific enolase in the low oxygen group [127]. Taken together, these data suggest that patients should receive adequate oxygenation (PaO_2 60–300 mmHg) with the lowest feasible FiO_2, but that aggressive attempts to rapidly lower FiO_2 deserve more study.

Bundles of care designed to reduce aspiration, barotrauma, and other complications will benefit post-cardiac arrest patients in the same manner as all ICU patients. Avoiding excessive plateau pressures (<35 mmHg) and peak pressures (<50 mmHg) is associated with improved outcomes in cohorts that included post-cardiac arrest patients [128]. Lower tidal volumes (6–8 ml/kg) have been adopted over time in many ICUs over the past two decades. This strategy has resulted in no significant change in post-cardiac arrest outcomes or pulmonary complications [129]. However, lower tidal volumes do result in a greater incidence of atelectasis. Thus, choices of ventilator volumes and pressures need little modification specifically for cardiac arrest patients.

Glycemic Control

Many studies examined the effects of intensive glycemic control in ICU patients, and the ischemic brain is well known to be sensitive to glucose levels in the laboratory. However, relative to a strategy of conventional glucose control (<10 mmol/l, <180 mg/dl), targeting low target glucose ranges 4.5–6 mmol/l (81–108 mg/dl) is associated with increased risk of hypoglycemic episodes and higher mortality [130]. One trial specifically in post-cardiac arrest patients compared glycemic control strategies aimed at 4–6 mmol/l (72–108 mg/dl) or 6–8 mmol/l (108–144 mg/dl) [131]. Again, the lower target range resulted in more hypoglycemic episodes without any measurable improvement in outcome.

Therefore, it is reasonable to treat hyperglycemia, but available data indicate no incremental benefit from trying to lower glucose levels below 8 or 10 mmol/l (144 or 180 mg/dl).

Inflammatory and Hematological Changes

Several hematological disturbances have been noted after cardiac arrest, but the clinical significance of these findings is uncertain. For example, inflammatory cytokines and endotoxin increase in serum during the first day after cardiac arrest [132]. Tumor necrosis factor-α (alpha) is the most prominent cytokine in most studies. Similarly, there is a prothrombotic state, with evidence of increased intravascular thrombosis [133]. These biochemical changes prompted the hypothesis that the ischemia-reperfusion after cardiac arrest is a "sepsis-like" state with diffuse activation of or injury to endothelium. This sepsis-like state might respond to volume resuscitation and hemodynamic optimization similar to protocols used for sepsis. However, this hypothesis leads to little change in clinical care, because all patients undergoing active resuscitation should have hemodynamic optimization and titration of volume. Moreover, cardiac arrest patients are prone to all of the infections of other ICU patients. Pneumonitis, albeit without microbiological confirmation of pneumonia, occurs in 33–41 % of patients after cardiac arrest [6, 134]. Therefore, clinicians must consider that the post-cardiac arrest patient may have actual sepsis rather than "sepsis-like" physiology. As in other ICU patients, appropriate evaluation for a source of infection should precede empiric antibiotics.

Nutritional Support and Electrolyte Management

There are no data about specific feeding regimens after cardiac arrest. However, the application of induced hypothermia has specific effects. First, intestinal motility is decreased during hypothermia. Bowel sounds are often absent and gastric residuals are large. For this reason, enteral feeding and enteral drug administration should be deferred until after rewarming.

Second, the process of inducing hypothermia causes predictable changes in potassium and other electrolytes. Cooling can cause diuresis as well as shifting of potassium from the extracellular space to the intracellular space [91, 92, 135]. Consequently, potassium levels will decrease by 0.5–1.0 mEq/l during induction of hypothermia. Similar decreases in serum magnesium and phosphorus levels also occur [91, 135]. With rewarming, potassium levels will rise again. There are no data to suggest that electrolytes should be managed any differently at higher and lower temperatures.

However, it is important that clinicians anticipate these electrolyte shifts: more frequent monitoring should be routinely employed when manipulating temperature.

Neurological Prognostication

A large proportion of care for the comatose patient after cardiac arrest involves determining the likelihood of meaningful neurological recovery. Meaningful recovery is generally defined to be awakening, although it is critical to educate families that the patient may have residual functional deficits even if they awaken. Understanding the prior wishes of the patient about ongoing life-sustaining treatment in any of the several possible outcomes is critical to providing proper advice and care. A regimented evaluation and initial treatment for the patient will help provide early and quantitative information to assist families with decision-making. Concurrent with this initial evaluation, the intensivist can educate the family and assess whether the patient's wishes are accurately represented. Based on these discussions, reduced intensity of evaluation or deviation from the general approach to care might occur at any time after the cardiac arrest.

The simplest outcome to recognize is brain death. All of the usual criteria for this determination apply to the post-cardiac arrest patient. However, the diagnosis of brain death usually must be delayed for 24 h or more in order to correct all of the potential confounders that are common after cardiac arrest: metabolic derangement, shock, and drugs. Because induced hypothermia also may be instituted during this time period using drugs which may have prolonged elimination, it is even more difficult to obtain an untainted examination during the first 24–36 h of support. Therefore, clinical practice usually does not allow proper brain death examination until the second or third ICU day after cardiac arrest [136]. Exceptions might include patients with radiographic evidence of herniation or patients with documented absence of cerebral blood flow.

No single finding can completely exclude awakening (Table 37.2). Because an advanced directive or a family may ask to withdraw life-sustaining treatment for a patient with no chance of awakening, near-perfect certainty is required. Different decision-makers will tolerate different false-positive rates (FPR) (rate of awakening when a clinical test predicts no awakening) when making these decisions. Certainly, results from EEG, SSEP, MRI, and clinical examination can revise the estimates about the odds of awakening, even when the FPR >0 %. Improving the statistical precision of these estimates and determining the prognostic value of combinations of findings is a critical need in the literature.

One approach to systematically approach prognosis after cardiac arrest is depicted in the figure (Fig. 37.4). Evaluations

Table 37.2 Examples of clinical findings that predict prognosis

Clinical finding	N	Good outcome in cohort	Yield of test (number with finding/number tested)	Good outcome with finding	Good outcome without finding	Odds ratio for good outcome (95 % CI)	False-positive rate (95 % CI), percent with finding, and good outcome
Cerebral edema (ratio of attenuation in gray matter to white matter <1.20) (some treated with hypothermia) [14]	240	87/240 (36 %)	58/240 (24 %)	2/58 (3 %)	85/182 (47 %)	0.04 (0.01–0.17)	3 % (1–9 %)
Somatosensory evoked potential with absent N20 cortical response (no hypothermia) [94]	687	141/687 (21 %)	249/687 (36 %)	0/249 (0 %)	141/438 (32 %)	Perfect prediction	0 % (0–1.5 %)
Somatosensory evoked potential with absent N20 cortical response (some treated with hypothermia) [98]	112	47/112 (42 %)	36/112 (32 %)	1/36 (3 %)	46/75 (61 %)	0.02 (0.00–0.14)	3 % (1–10 %)
Myoclonic status epilepticus on continuous EEG (all treated with hypothermia) [56]	101	30/101 (30 %)	21/101 (21 %)	0/20 (0 %)	30/80 (38 %)	Perfect prediction	0 % (0–14 %)
Epileptiform discharges on EEG (all treated with hypothermia) [56]	101	30/101 (30 %)	20/101 (20 %)	2/21 (10 %)	28/81 (35 %)	0.20 (0.04–0.92)	10 % (1–24 %)
MRI showing diffuse injury (whole-brain ADC<665 μm²/s) (some treated with hypothermia) [21]	80	14/80 (18 %)	27/80 (34 %)	0/27 (0 %)	14/53 (26 %)	Perfect prediction	0 % (0–10 %)

Good outcome is variously defined in different studies as survival, survival with awakening, or survival with good functional status. Good outcome varies between cohorts because of different clinical criteria and different times for ordering any given test. When considering limitation of life-sustaining treatment, decision-makers should pay particular attention to uncertainty described by the false-positive rate

can be divided into three stages based on time after cardiac arrest: immediate data (0–6 h after arrest), first day in the ICU (24–48 h), and first week in the ICU (3–7 days). Serial neurological examination of the patient provides information about the trajectory of recovery. As long as there is improvement over time, it is reasonable to continue support. However, when the examination has plateaued, some ancillary tests may help revise the probability of recovery. The most desirable outcome is immediate or rapid resolution of coma into awakening.

For patients who are indeterminate in their outcome after 7 days or so, the intensivist and family must agree whether or not to embark on long-term support (tracheostomy, feeding tubes, etc.). In North America during the past two decades, few families opt for long-term support if risk of PVS is high, but that pathway is chosen more often in Asian cultures. A small percentage of patients awaken and recover after weeks of support, but the majority of patients who awaken do so in the first week or two. Therefore, decisions must be individualized for the local culture, family preferences, and clinical scenario.

Rehabilitation

At the end of acute hospitalization, three distinct categories are noted among cardiac arrest patients (Fig. 37.5). First, some patients die or do not awaken in the hospital (modified Rankin score, MRS, 5–6). Second, some patients are minimally injured after their cardiac arrest, perhaps receiving only a single rescue shock or brief CPR. These patients awaken quickly and have excellent functional outcome by the time of hospital discharge (MRS 0–1). Third, some patients with post-cardiac arrest brain injury recover to wakefulness after a prolonged period of coma. These patients may recover in the hospital to intermediate functional status (MRS of 3–4). Their ultimate disposition is to be discharged to subacute hospitals, skilled nursing facilities, or even home with the hope of continuing recovery. The third group, and to a lesser extent the second group, has significant potential benefit from rehabilitation therapies.

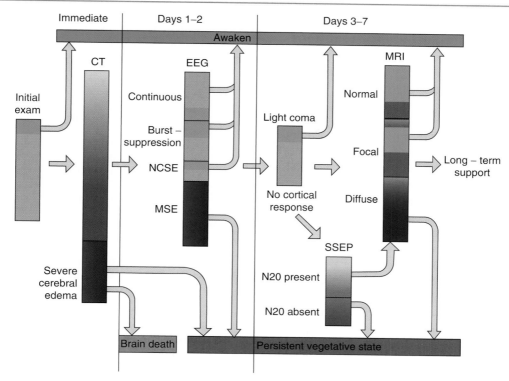

Fig. 37.4 One approach to estimate probability of awakening versus persistent vegetative state in patients who are comatose after cardiac arrest. Each evaluation alters the estimated probability of good or poor outcome, and no evaluation provides 100 % certainty. Immediate evaluation includes assessment of depth of coma as well as cranial CT scan. During the first 1–2 days in the ICU, additional data can be obtained by EEG and serial examination. For patients after hypothermia and rewarming, further refinement of prognosis can be obtained over the days 3–7 with SSEP for patients without clinical signs of cortical function and MRI with DWI for patients with persistent coma. Brain death usually requires 1–2 days to determine because of the need to correct metabolic or toxicological confounders, unless there is obvious herniation or absence of cerebral blood flow

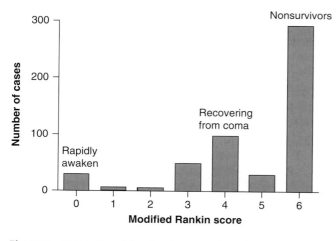

Fig. 37.5 Distribution of functional status at time of hospital discharge after cardiac arrest. Many patients die (MRS 6). Patients with coma recover over days to weeks. Once they achieve moderate function (MRS 3–5), they will be discharged from the acute care hospital for longer-term rehabilitation. However, recovery may continue for 6–12 months. Other patients awaken quickly and recover to near-normal functional status while in the hospital (MRS 0–2) (Data from Rittenberger et al. [140])

Even after hospital care is complete, it is important to recognize the dynamic state of neurological recovery. In one cohort of patients from a clinical trial, 23 % of subjects had mild improvement on neuropsychiatric tests between the 3 and 12 months after cardiac arrest [137]. These and similar observations illustrate that patients continue to improve over at least the first 3–12 months after cardiac arrest and deserve ongoing therapy during this time frame.

Early physical and occupational therapy can stimulate neurological recovery. In a general ICU population, starting these interventions within 72 h can reduce delirium, increase ventilator-free days, and decrease disability at hospital discharge [138]. In addition, early therapy begins the process of evaluation for rehabilitation after the acute hospitalization. Thus, the intensivist has opportunity to impact the path of recovery far beyond the ICU. Recent studies of post-cardiac arrest patients indicate that many patients who might benefit from rehabilitation therapies do not receive this care [56].

Organ Donation After Brain Death or Withdrawal of Life-Sustaining Treatment

Failure to survive after cardiac arrest can result from several clinical situations. After admission to the intensive care unit, intractable shock or multiple organ failure may prompt withdrawal of care. Secondly, the most devastated subjects may progress to brain death. Finally, a poor neurological trajectory in which the treating team and family anticipate that the patient will reach a PVS can prompt withdrawal of life-sustaining treatment. In the latter two instances, there is potential for the patient to be considered as an organ donor. Transplanted organs derived from donor who reached brain death after a cardiac arrest are reported to be as successful as organs from other types of donors [136]. In contrast, a smaller proportion of non-brain-dead cardiac arrest patients for whom ICU care was futile or discontinued were suitable donors in another series [139]. These experiences do suggest that the potential for organ donation should be considered for individual patients who are approaching end of life after cardiac arrest.

Conclusion

Resuscitation from cardiac arrest creates a clinical scenario that is often dominated by brain injury. Modern ICU care has optimized acute cardiovascular interventions and treatment of shock and its sequelae. Only a few modifications of the usual care for non-neurological organ systems are required for the cardiac arrest patients. However, attention to optimization of cerebral perfusion, avoidance of cerebral edema, vigilance of the common epileptiform activity, and application of targeted temperature management impart a distinct flavor to post-cardiac arrest ICU care. The intensivist will also need to help the family assess the likelihood of meaningful neurological recovery while providing ongoing care. Awareness of the uncertainty in prognostication along with the available quantitative data is essential. The past decade has identified multiple specific clinical questions about management that were previously unrecognized (optimal anticonvulsant, optimal sedative regimen, optimal blood pressure goal, optimal choice of imaging, etc.). Future clinical trials may fill in these knowledge gaps.

References

1. Hostler D, Everson-Stewart S, Rea TD, Stiell IG, Callaway CW, Kudenchuk PJ, Sears GK, Emerson SS, Nichol G, Resuscitation Outcomes Consortium Investigators. Effect of real-time feedback during cardiopulmonary resuscitation outside hospital: prospective, cluster-randomised trial. BMJ. 2011;342:d512.

2. Nagao K, Kikushima K, Watanabe K, Tachibana E, Tominaga Y, Tada K, Ishii M, Chiba N, Kasai A, Soga T, Matsuzaki M, Nishikawa K, Tateda Y, Ikeda H, Yagi T. Early induction of hypothermia during cardiac arrest improves neurological outcomes in patients with out-of-hospital cardiac arrest who undergo emergency cardiopulmonary bypass and percutaneous coronary intervention. Circ J. 2010;74(1):77–85.

3. Laver S, Farrow C, Turner D, Nolan J. Mode of death after admission to an intensive care unit following cardiac arrest. Intensive Care Med. 2004;30(11):2126–8.

4. Raina KD, Callaway C, Rittenberger JC, Holm MB. Neurological and functional status following cardiac arrest: method and tool utility. Resuscitation. 2008;79(2):249–56.

5. Tiainen M, Poutiainen E, Kovala T, Takkunen O, Häppölä O, Roine RO. Cognitive and neurophysiological outcome of cardiac arrest survivors treated with therapeutic hypothermia. Stroke. 2007;38(8):2303–8.

6. Hypothermia after Cardiac Arrest Study Group. Mild therapeutic hypothermia to improve the neurologic outcome after cardiac arrest. N Engl J Med. 2002;346:549.

7. Bernard SA, Gray TW, Buist MD, et al. Treatment of comatose survivors of out-of-hospital cardiac arrest with induced hypothermia. N Engl J Med. 2002;346:557.

8. Sunde K, Pytte M, Jacobsen D, et al. Implementation of a standardised treatment protocol for post resuscitation care after out-of-hospital cardiac arrest. Resuscitation. 2007;73:29.

9. Rittenberger JC, Guyette FX, Tisherman SA, et al. Outcomes of a hospital-wide plan to improve care of comatose survivors of cardiac arrest. Resuscitation. 2008;79:198.

10. Khot S, Tirschwell DL. Long-term neurological complications after hypoxic-ischemic encephalopathy. Semin Neurol. 2006;26(4):422–31.

11. Marik PE, Varon J, Lisbon A, Reich HS. Physicians' own preferences to the limitation and withdrawal of life-sustaining therapy. Resuscitation. 1999;42(3):197–201.

12. Nichol G, Stiell IG, Hebert P, Wells GA, Vandemheen K, Laupacis A. What is the quality of life for survivors of cardiac arrest? A prospective study. Acad Emerg Med. 1999;6(2):95–102.

13. Manish M, Veenu S. Persistent vegetative state. Neurology. 2007;68(19):1635.

14. Metter RB, Rittenberger JC, Guyette FX, Callaway CW. Association between a quantitative CT scan measure of brain edema and outcome after cardiac arrest. Resuscitation. 2011;82(9):1180–5.

15. Cocchi MN, Lucas JM, Salciccioli J, Carney E, Herman S, Zimetbaum P, Donnino MW. The role of cranial computed tomography in the immediate post-cardiac arrest period. Intern Emerg Med. 2010;5(6):533–8.

16. Gutierrez LG, Rovira A, Portela LA, Leite Cda C, Lucato LT. CT and MR in non-neonatal hypoxic-ischemic encephalopathy: radiological findings with pathophysiological correlations. Neuroradiology. 2010;52(11):949–76.

17. Torbey MT, Selim M, Knorr J, Bigelow C, Recht L. Quantitative analysis of the loss of distinction between gray and white matter in comatose patients after cardiac arrest. Stroke. 2000;31(9):2163–7.

18. Wu O, Batista LM, Lima FO, Vangel MG, Furie KL, Greer DM. Predicting clinical outcome in comatose cardiac arrest patients using early noncontrast computed tomography. Stroke. 2011;42(4):985–92.

19. Choi SP, Park HK, Park KN, Kim YM, Ahn KJ, Choi KH, Lee WJ, Jeong SK. The density ratio of grey to white matter on computed tomography as an early predictor of vegetative state or death after cardiac arrest. Emerg Med J. 2008;25(10):666–9.

20. Geocadin RG, Kowalski RG. Imaging brain injury after cardiac arrest resuscitation when it really matters. Resuscitation. 2011;82(9):1124–5.

21. Wu O, Sorensen AG, Benner T, Singhal AB, Furie KL, Greer DM. Comatose patients with cardiac arrest: predicting clinical outcome with diffusion-weighted MR imaging. Radiology. 2009;252(1): 173–81.

22. Wijman CA, Mlynash M, Caulfield AF, Hsia AW, Eyngorn I, Bammer R, Fischbein N, Albers GW, Moseley M. Prognostic value of brain diffusion-weighted imaging after cardiac arrest. Ann Neurol. 2009;65(4):394–402.

23. Järnum H, Knutsson L, Rundgren M, Siemund R, Englund E, Friberg H, Larsson EM. Diffusion and perfusion MRI of the brain in comatose patients treated with mild hypothermia after cardiac arrest: a prospective observational study. Resuscitation. 2009;80(4):425–30.

24. Mlynash M, Campbell DM, Leproust EM, Fischbein NJ, Bammer R, Eyngorn I, Hsia AW, Moseley M, Wijman CA. Temporal and spatial profile of brain diffusion-weighted MRI after cardiac arrest. Stroke. 2010;41(8):1665–72.

25. Wijdicks EF, Campeau NG, Miller GM. MR imaging in comatose survivors of cardiac resuscitation. AJNR Am J Neuroradiol. 2001;22(8):1561–5.

26. Arbelaez A, Castillo M, Mukherji SK. Diffusion-weighted MR imaging of global cerebral anoxia. AJNR Am J Neuroradiol. 1999;20(6):999–1007.

27. Topcuoglu MA, Oguz KK, Buyukserbetci G, Bulut E. Prognostic value of magnetic resonance imaging in post-resuscitation encephalopathy. Intern Med. 2009;48(18):1635–45.

28. Pulsinelli WA, Brierley JB. A new model of bilateral hemispheric ischemia in the unanesthetized rat. Stroke. 1979;10(3):267–72.

29. Smith ML, Auer RN, Siesjö BK. The density and distribution of ischemic brain injury in the rat following 2–10 min of forebrain ischemia. Acta Neuropathol. 1984;64(4):319–32.

30. Radovsky A, Katz L, Ebmeyer U, Safar P. Ischemic neurons in rat brains after 6, 8, or 10 minutes of transient hypoxic ischemia. Toxicol Pathol. 1997;25(5):500–5.

31. Bottiger BW, Schmitz B, Wiessner C, Vogel P, Hossman KA. Neuronal stress response and neuronal cell damage after cardiocirculatory arrest in rats. J Cereb Blood Flow Metab. 1998;18(10): 1077–87.

32. Yonelinas AP, Kroll NE, Quamme JR, Lazzara MM, Sauve MJ, Widaman KF, Knight RT. Effects of extensive temporal lobe damage or mild hypoxia on recollection and familiarity. Nat Neurosci. 2002;5:1236–41.

33. Di Paola M, Caltagirone C, Fadda L, Sabatini U, Serra L, Carlesimo GA. Hippocampal atrophy is the critical brain change in patients with hypoxic amnesia. Hippocampus. 2008;18(7): 719–28.

34. Petito CK, Olarte JP, Roberts B, Nowak Jr TS, Pulsinelli WA. Selective glial vulnerability following transient global ischemia in rat brain. J Neuropathol Exp Neurol. 1998;57(3):231–8.

35. Hicks SD, DeFranco DB, Callaway CW. Hypothermia during reperfusion after asphyxial cardiac arrest improves functional recovery and selectively alters stress-induced protein expression. J Cereb Blood Flow Metab. 2000;20(3):520–30.

36. Logue ES, McMichael MJ, Callaway CW. Comparison of the effects of hypothermia at 33 degrees C or 35 degrees C after cardiac arrest in rats. Acad Emerg Med. 2007;14(4):293–300.

37. Che D, Li L, Kopil CM, Liu Z, Guo W, Neumar RW. Impact of therapeutic hypothermia onset and duration on survival, neurologic function, and neurodegeneration after cardiac arrest. Crit Care Med. 2011;39(6):1423–30.

38. Buunk G, van der Hoeven JG, Frolich M, Meinders AE. Cerebral vasoconstriction in comatose patients resuscitated from a cardiac arrest. Intensive Care Med. 1996;22:1191–6.

39. Nishizawa H, Kudoh I. Cerebral autoregulation is impaired in patients resuscitated after cardiac arrest. Acta Anaesthesiol Scand. 1996;40(9):1149–53.

40. Sundgreen C, Larsen FS, Herzog TM, Knudsen GM, Boesgaard S, Aldershvile J. Autoregulation of cerebral blood flow in patients resuscitated from cardiac arrest. Stroke. 2001;32(1):128–32.

41. Mullner M, Sterz F, Binder M, Hellwanger K, Meron G, Herkner H, Laggner AN. Arterial blood pressure after human cardiac arrest and neurologic recovery. Stroke. 1996;27:59–62.

42. Iida K, Satoh H, Arita K, Nakahara T, Kurisu K, Ohtani M. Delayed hyperemia causing intracranial hypertension after cardiopulmonary resuscitation. Crit Care Med. 1997;25(6):971–6.

43. Pynnönen L, Falkenbach P, Kämäräinen A, Lönnrot K, Yli-Hankala A, Tenhunen J. Therapeutic hypothermia after cardiac arrest – cerebral perfusion and metabolism during upper and lower threshold normocapnia. Resuscitation. 2011;82(9):1174–9.

44. Bisschops LL, Hoedemaekers CW, Simons KS, van der Hoeven JG. Preserved metabolic coupling and cerebrovascular reactivity during mild hypothermia after cardiac arrest. Crit Care Med. 2010;38(7):1542–7.

45. Buunk G, van der Hoeven JG, Meinders AE. Cerebrovascular reactivity in comatose patients resuscitated from a cardiac arrest. Stroke. 1997;28(8):1569–73.

46. Ames 3rd A, Wright RL, Kowada M, Thurston JM, Majno G. Cerebral ischemia. II. The no-reflow phenomenon. Am J Pathol. 1968;52(2):437–53.

47. Wolfson Jr SK, Safar P, Reich H, Clark JM, Gur D, Stezoski W, Cook EE, Krupper MA. Dynamic heterogeneity of cerebral hypoperfusion after prolonged cardiac arrest in dogs measured by the stable xenon/CT technique: a preliminary study. Resuscitation. 1992;23(1):1–20.

48. Fischer EG, Ames 3rd A, Lorenzo AV. Cerebral blood flow immediately following brief circulatory stasis. Stroke. 1979;10:423–7.

49. Leonov Y, Sterz F, Safar P, Johnson DW, Tisherman SA, Oku K. Hypertension with hemodilution prevents multifocal cerebral hypoperfusion after cardiac arrest in dogs. Stroke. 1992;23(1): 45–53.

50. Ristagno G, Tang W, Huang L, Fymat A, Chang YT, Sun S, Castillo C, Weil MH. Epinephrine reduces cerebral perfusion during cardiopulmonary resuscitation. Crit Care Med. 2009;37(4): 1408–15.

51. Heard KJ, Peberdy MA, Sayre MR, Sanders A, Geocadin RG, Dixon SR, Larabee TM, Hiller K, Fiorello A, Paradis NA, O'Neil BJ. A randomized controlled trial comparing the Arctic Sun to standard cooling for induction of hypothermia after cardiac arrest. Resuscitation. 2010;81(1):9–14.

52. Rossetti AO, Logroscino G, Liaudet L, Ruffieux C, Ribordy V, Schaller MD, Despland PA, Oddo M. Status epilepticus: an independent outcome predictor after cerebral anoxia. Neurology. 2007;69(3):255–60.

53. Wijdicks EF, Hijdra A, Young GB, et al. Practice parameter: prediction of outcome in comatose survivors after cardiopulmonary resuscitation (an evidence-based review): report of the Quality Standards Subcommittee of the American Academy of Neurology. Neurology. 2006;67:203.

54. Oddo M, Carrera E, Claassen J, Mayer SA, Hirsch LJ. Continuous electroencephalography in the medical intensive care unit. Crit Care Med. 2009;37(6):2051–6.

55. Abend NS, Topjian A, Ichord R, Herman ST, Helfaer M, Donnelly M, Nadkarni V, Dlugos DJ, Clancy RR. Electroencephalographic monitoring during hypothermia after pediatric cardiac arrest. Neurology. 2009;72(22):1931–40.

56. Rittenberger JC, Popescu A, Brenner RP, Guyette FX, Callaway CW. Frequency and timing of nonconvulsive status epilepticus in comatose post-cardiac arrest subjects treated with hypothermia. Neurocrit Care. 2012;16(1):114–22.

57. Rossetti AO, Oddo M, Logroscino G, Kaplan PW. Prognostication after cardiac arrest and hypothermia: a prospective study. Ann Neurol. 2010;67(3):301–7.

58. Wijdicks EF, Parisi JE, Sharbrough FW. Prognostic value of myoclonus status in comatose survivors of cardiac arrest. Ann Neurol. 1994;35(2):239–43.

59. Nolan JP, Morley PT, Vanden Hoek TL, Hickey RW, Kloeck WG, Billi J, Böttiger BW, Morley PT, Nolan JP, Okada K, Reyes C, Shuster M, Steen PA, Weil MH, Wenzel V, Hickey RW, Carli P, Vanden Hoek TL, Atkins D, International Liaison Committee on Resuscitation. Therapeutic hypothermia after cardiac arrest: an advisory statement by the advanced life support task force of the International Liaison Committee on Resuscitation. Circulation. 2003;108(1):118–21.

60. Morrison LJ, Deakin CD, Morley PT, Callaway CW, Kerber RE, Kronick SL, Lavonas EJ, Link MS, Neumar RW, Otto CW, Parr M, Shuster M, Sunde K, Peberdy MA, Tang W, Hoek TL, Böttiger BW, Drajer S, Lim SH, Nolan JP, Advanced Life Support Chapter Collaborators. Part 8: advanced life support: 2010 International Consensus on Cardiopulmonary Resuscitation and Emergency Cardiovascular Care Science With Treatment Recommendations. Circulation. 2010;122(16 Suppl 2):S345–421.

61. Peberdy MA, Callaway CW, Neumar RW, Geocadin RG, Zimmerman JL, Donnino M, Gabrielli A, Silvers SM, Zaritsky AL, Merchant R, Vanden Hoek TL, Kronick SL. Part 9: post-cardiac arrest care: 2010 American Heart Association Guidelines for Cardiopulmonary Resuscitation and Emergency Cardiovascular Care. Circulation. 2010;122(18 Suppl 3):S768–86.

62. Arrich J, European Resuscitation Council Hypothermia After Cardiac Arrest Registry Study Group. Clinical application of mild therapeutic hypothermia after cardiac arrest. Crit Care Med. 2007;35(4):1041–7.

63. Nielsen N, Friberg H, Gluud C, Herlitz J, Wetterslev J. Hypothermia after cardiac arrest should be further evaluated-a systematic review of randomized trials with meta-analysis and trial sequential analysis. Int J Cardiol. 2011;151(3):333–41.

64. Zhao D, Abella BS, Beiser DG, Alvarado JP, Wang H, Hamann KJ, Hoek TL, Becker LB. Intra-arrest cooling with delayed reperfusion yields higher survival than earlier normothermic resuscitation in a mouse model of cardiac arrest. Resuscitation. 2008;77(2):242–9.

65. Kuboyama K, Safar P, Radovsky A, Tisherman SA, Stezoski SW, Alexander H. Delay in cooling negates the beneficial effect of mild resuscitative cerebral hypothermia after cardiac arrest in dogs: a prospective, randomized study. Crit Care Med. 1993;21(9):1348–58.

66. Nozari A, Safar P, Stezoski SW, Wu X, Kostelnik S, Radovsky A, Tisherman S, Kochanek PM. Critical time window for intra-arrest cooling with cold saline flush in a dog model of cardiopulmonary resuscitation. Circulation. 2006;113(23):2690–6.

67. Colbourne F, Corbett D. Delayed postischemic hypothermia: a six month survival study using behavioral and histological assessments of neuroprotection. J Neurosci. 1995;15(11):7250–60.

68. Colbourne F, Corbett D. Delayed and prolonged post-ischemic hypothermia is neuroprotective in the gerbil. Brain Res. 1994;654(2):265–72.

69. Coimbra C, Wieloch T. Hypothermia ameliorates neuronal survival when induced 2 hours after ischaemia in the rat. Acta Physiol Scand. 1992;146(4):543–4.

70. Wolff B, Machill K, Schumacher D, Schulzki I, Werner D. Early achievement of mild therapeutic hypothermia and the neurologic outcome after cardiac arrest. Int J Cardiol. 2009;133(2):223–8.

71. Kim F, Olsufka M, Longstreth Jr WT, Maynard C, Carlbom D, Deem S, Kudenchuk P, Copass MK, Cobb LA. Pilot randomized clinical trial of prehospital induction of mild hypothermia in out-of-hospital cardiac arrest patients with a rapid infusion of 4 degrees C normal saline. Circulation. 2007;115(24):3064–70.

72. Bernard SA, Smith K, Cameron P, Masci K, Taylor DM, Cooper DJ, Kelly AM, Silvester W, Rapid Infusion of Cold Hartmanns

73. (RICH) Investigators. Induction of therapeutic hypothermia by paramedics after resuscitation from out-of-hospital ventricular fibrillation cardiac arrest: a randomized controlled trial. Circulation. 2010;122(7):737–42.

73. Binks AC, Murphy RE, Prout RE, Bhayani S, Griffiths CA, Mitchell T, Padkin A, Nolan JP. Therapeutic hypothermia after cardiac arrest - implementation in UK intensive care units. Anaesthesia. 2010;65(3):260–5.

74. Shankaran S, Laptook AR, Ehrenkranz RA, Tyson JE, McDonald SA, Donovan EF, Fanaroff AA, Poole WK, Wright LL, Higgins RD, Finer NN, Carlo WA, Duara S, Oh W, Cotten CM, Stevenson DK, Stoll BJ, Lemons JA, Guillet R, Jobe AH, National Institute of Child Health and Human Development Neonatal Research Network. Whole-body hypothermia for neonates with hypoxic-ischemic encephalopathy. N Engl J Med. 2005;353(15):1574–84.

75. Iida K, Kurisu K, Arita K, Ohtani M. Hyperemia prior to acute brain swelling during rewarming of patients who have been treated with moderate hypothermia for severe head injuries. J Neurosurg. 2003;98(4):793–9.

76. Tømte Ø, Drægni T, Mangschau A, Jacobsen D, Auestad B, Sunde K. A comparison of intravascular and surface cooling techniques in comatose cardiac arrest survivors. Crit Care Med. 2011;39(3):443–9.

77. Robinson J, Charlton J, Seal R, et al. Oesophageal, rectal, axillary, tympanic and pulmonary artery temperatures during cardiac surgery. Can J Anaesth. 1998;45:317.

78. Erickson RS, Kirklin SK. Comparison of ear-based, bladder, oral, and axillary methods for core temperature measurement. Crit Care Med. 1993;21:1528.

79. Callaway CW, Tadler SC, Katz LM, Lipinski CL, Brader E. Feasibility of external cranial cooling during out-of-hospital cardiac arrest. Resuscitation. 2002;52(2):159–65.

80. Kim F, Olsufka M, Carlbom D, Deem S, Longstreth Jr WT, Hanrahan M, Maynard C, Copass MK, Cobb LA. Pilot study of rapid infusion of 2 L of 4 degrees C normal saline for induction of mild hypothermia in hospitalized, comatose survivors of out-of-hospital cardiac arrest. Circulation. 2005;112(5):715–9.

81. Bernard S, Buist M, Monteiro O, Smith K. Induced hypothermia using large volume, ice-cold intravenous fluid in comatose survivors of out-of-hospital cardiac arrest: a preliminary report. Resuscitation. 2003;56(1):9–13.

82. Kilgannon JH, Jones AE, Shapiro NI, Angelos MG, Milcarek B, Hunter K, Parrillo JE, Trzeciak S, Emergency Medicine Shock Research Network (EMShockNet) Investigators. Association between arterial hyperoxia following resuscitation from cardiac arrest and in-hospital mortality. JAMA. 2010;303(21):2165–71.

83. Kliegel A, Losert H, Sterz F, Kliegel M, Holzer M, Uray T, Domanovits H. Cold simple intravenous infusions preceding special endovascular cooling for faster induction of mild hypothermia after cardiac arrest–a feasibility study. Resuscitation. 2005;64(3):347–51.

84. Al-Senani FM, Graffagnino C, Grotta JC, Saiki R, Wood D, Chung W, Palmer G, Collins KA. A prospective, multicenter pilot study to evaluate the feasibility and safety of using the CoolGard System and Icy catheter following cardiac arrest. Resuscitation. 2004;62(2):143–50.

85. Merchant RM, Abella BS, Peberdy MA, Soar J, Ong ME, Schmidt GA, Becker LB, Vanden Hoek TL. Therapeutic hypothermia after cardiac arrest: unintentional overcooling is common using ice packs and conventional cooling blankets. Crit Care Med. 2006;34(12 Suppl):S490–4.

86. Nielsen N, Sunde K, Hovdenes J, Riker RR, Rubertsson S, Stammet P, Nilsson F, Friberg H, Hypothermia Network. Adverse events and their relation to mortality in out-of-hospital cardiac arrest patients treated with therapeutic hypothermia. Crit Care Med. 2011;39(1):57–64.

87. Dae MW, Gao DW, Sessler DI, Chair K, Stillson CA. Effect of endovascular cooling on myocardial temperature, infarct size, and cardiac output in human-sized pigs. Am J Physiol Heart Circ Physiol. 2002;282(5):H1584–91.

88. Storm C, Hasper D, Nee J, Joerres A, Schefold JC, Kaufmann J, Roser M. Severe QTc prolongation under mild hypothermia treatment and incidence of arrhythmias after cardiac arrest–a prospective study in 34 survivors with continuous Holter ECG. Resuscitation. 2011;82(7):859–62.

89. Boddicker KA, Zhang Y, Zimmerman MB, Davies LR, Kerber RE. Hypothermia improves defibrillation success and resuscitation outcomes from ventricular fibrillation. Circulation. 2005;111(24):3195–201.

90. Perbet S, Mongardon N, Dumas F, Bruel C, Lemiale V, Mourvillier B, Carli P, Varenne O, Mira JP, Wolff M, Cariou A. Early onset pneumonia after cardiac arrest: characteristics, risk factors and influence on prognosis. Am J Respir Crit Care Med. 2011;184(9):1048–54.

91. Polderman KH, Peerdeman SM, Girbes AR. Hypophosphatemia and hypomagnesemia induced by cooling in patients with severe head injury. J Neurosurg. 2001;94:697–705.

92. Clifton GL, Miller ER, Choi SC, Levin HS. Fluid thresholds and outcome from severe brain injury. Crit Care Med. 2002;30:739–45.

93. Gabel RA. Algorithms for calculating and correcting blood-gas and acid–base variables. Respir Physiol. 1980;42:211–32.

94. Zandbergen EG, de Haan RJ, Stoutenbeek CP, Koelman JH, Hijdra A. Systematic review of early prediction of poor outcome in anoxic-ischaemic coma. Lancet. 1998;352(9143):1808–12.

95. Rundgren M, Westhall E, Cronberg T, Rosén I, Friberg H. Continuous amplitude-integrated electroencephalogram predicts outcome in hypothermia-treated cardiac arrest patients. Crit Care Med. 2010;38(9):1838–44.

96. Stammet P, Werer C, Mertens L, Lorang C, Hemmer M. Bispectral index (BIS) helps predicting bad neurological outcome in comatose survivors after cardiac arrest and induced therapeutic hypothermia. Resuscitation. 2009;80(4):437–42.

97. Leary M, Fried DA, Gaieski DF, Merchant RM, Fuchs BD, Kolansky DM, Edelson DP, Abella BS. Neurologic prognostication and bispectral index monitoring after resuscitation from cardiac arrest. Resuscitation. 2010;81(9):1133–7.

98. Leithner C, Ploner CJ, Hasper D, Storm C. Does hypothermia influence the predictive value of bilateral absent N20 after cardiac arrest? Neurology. 2010;74:965.

99. Gendo A, Kramer L, Häfner M, Funk GC, Zauner C, Sterz F, Holzer M, Bauer E, Madl C. Time-dependency of sensory evoked potentials in comatose cardiac arrest survivors. Intensive Care Med. 2001;27(8):1305–11.

100. Madl C, Kramer L, Domanovits H, Woolard RH, Gervais H, Gendo A, Eisenhuber E, Grimm G, Sterz F. Improved outcome prediction in unconscious cardiac arrest survivors with sensory evoked potentials compared with clinical assessment. Crit Care Med. 2000;28(3):721–6.

101. Zingler VC, Krumm B, Bertsch T, Fassbender K, Pohlmann-Eden B. Early prediction of neurological outcome after cardiopulmonary resuscitation: a multimodal approach combining neurobiochemical and electrophysiological investigations may provide high prognostic certainty in patients after cardiac arrest. Eur Neurol. 2003;49(2):79–84.

102. MacMillan CSA, Andrews PJD. Cerebrovenous oxygen saturation monitoring: practical considerations and clinical relevance. Intensive Care Med. 2000;26:1028–36.

103. Oku K, Kuboyama K, Safar P, Obrist W, Sterz F, Leonov Y, Tisherman SA. Cerebral and systemic arteriovenous oxygen monitoring after cardiac arrest. Inadequate cerebral oxygen delivery. Resuscitation. 1994;27(2):141–52.

104. van der Hoeven JG, de Koning J, Compier EA, Meinders AE. Early jugular bulb oxygenation monitoring in comatose patients after an out-of-hospital cardiac arrest. Intensive Care Med. 1995;21(7):567–72.

105. Takasu A, Yagi K, Ishihara S, Okada Y. Combined continuous monitoring of systemic and cerebral oxygen metabolism after cardiac arrest. Resuscitation. 1995;29(3):189–94.

106. Buunk G, van der Hoeven JG, Meinders AE. Prognostic significance of the difference between mixed venous and jugular bulb oxygen saturation in comatose patients resuscitated from a cardiac arrest. Resuscitation. 1999;41(3):257–62.

107. Zarzuelo R, Castañeda J. Differences in oxygen content between mixed venous blood and cerebral venous blood for outcome prediction after cardiac arrest. Intensive Care Med. 1995;21(1):71–5.

108. Lemiale V, Huet O, Vigué B, Mathonnet A, Spaulding C, Mira JP, Carli P, Duranteau J, Cariou A. Changes in cerebral blood flow and oxygen extraction during post-resuscitation syndrome. Resuscitation. 2008;76(1):17–24.

109. Xiao F, Rodriguez J, Arnold TC, Zhang S, Ferrara D, Ewing J, Alexander JS, Carden DL, Conrad SA. Near-infrared spectroscopy: a tool to monitor cerebral hemodynamic and metabolic changes after cardiac arrest in rats. Resuscitation. 2004;63(2):213–20.

110. Newman DH, Callaway CW, Greenwald IB, Freed J. Cerebral oximetry in out-of-hospital cardiac arrest: standard CPR rarely provides detectable hemoglobin-oxygen saturation to the frontal cortex. Resuscitation. 2004;63(2):189–94.

111. Buunk G, van der Hoeven JG, Meinders AE. A comparison of near-infrared spectroscopy and jugular bulb oximetry in comatose patients resuscitated from a cardiac arrest. Anaesthesia. 1998;53(1):13–9.

112. Lewis SB, Myburgh JA, Thornton EL, Reilly PL. Cerebral oxygenation monitoring by near-infrared spectroscopy is not clinically useful in patients with severe closed-head injury: a comparison with jugular venous bulb oximetry. Crit Care Med. 1996;24(8):1334–8.

113. Imberti R, Bellinzona G, Riccardi F, Pagani M, Langer M. Cerebral perfusion pressure and cerebral tissue oxygen tension in a patient during cardiopulmonary resuscitation. Intensive Care Med. 2003;29(6):1016–9.

114. Nordmark J, Rubertsson S, Mörtberg E, Nilsson P, Enblad P. Intracerebral monitoring in comatose patients treated with hypothermia after a cardiac arrest. Acta Anaesthesiol Scand. 2009;53(3):289–98.

115. Zhou J, Poloyac SM. The effect of therapeutic hypothermia on drug metabolism and response: cellular mechanisms to organ function. Expert Opin Drug Metab Toxicol. 2011;7(7):803–16.

116. Tortorici MA, Kochanek PM, Poloyac SM. Effects of hypothermia on drug disposition, metabolism, and response: a focus of hypothermia-mediated alterations on the cytochrome P450 enzyme system. Crit Care Med. 2007;35(9):2196–204.

117. Hostler D, Zhou J, Bies R, Tortorici MA, Rittenberger JC, Callaway CW, Poloyac SM. Mild hypothermia decreases the metabolism of midazolam in normal healthy subjects. Drug Metab Dispos. 2010;28(5):781–8.

118. Caldwell JE, Heier T, Wright PM, Lin S, McCarthy G, Szenohradszky J, Sharma ML, Hing JP, Schroeder M, Sessler DI. Temperature-dependent pharmacokinetics and pharmacodynamics of vecuronium. Anesthesiology. 2000;92(1):84–93.

119. Neumar RW, Nolan JP, Adrie C, Aibiki M, Berg RA, Böttiger BW, Callaway C, Clark RS, Geocadin RG, Jauch EC, Kern KB, Laurent I, Longstreth Jr WT, Merchant RM, Morley P, Morrison LJ, Nadkarni V, Peberdy MA, Rivers EP, Rodriguez-Nunez A, Sellke FW, Spaulding C, Sunde K, Vanden HT. Post-cardiac arrest syndrome: epidemiology, pathophysiology, treatment, and prognostication. A consensus statement from the International Liaison

Committee on Resuscitation (American Heart Association, Australian and New Zealand Council on Resuscitation, European Resuscitation Council, Heart and Stroke Foundation of Canada, InterAmerican Heart Foundation, Resuscitation Council of Asia, and the Resuscitation Council of Southern Africa); the American Heart Association Emergency Cardiovascular Care Committee; the Council on Cardiovascular Surgery and Anesthesia; the Council on Cardiopulmonary, Perioperative, and Critical Care; the Council on Clinical Cardiology; and the Stroke Council. Circulation. 2008;118(23):2452–83.

120. Spaulding CM, Joly LM, Rosenberg A, Monchi M, Weber SN, Dhainaut JF, Carli P. Immediate coronary angiography in survivors of out-of-hospital cardiac arrest. N Engl J Med. 1997;336(23):1629–33.

121. Dumas F, Cariou A, Manzo-Silberman S, Grimaldi D, Vivien B, Rosencher J, Empana JP, Carli P, Mira JP, Jouven X, Spaulding C. Immediate percutaneous coronary intervention is associated with better survival after out-of-hospital cardiac arrest: insights from the PROCAT (Parisian Region Out of hospital Cardiac Arrest) registry. Circ Cardiovasc Interv. 2010;3(3):200–7.

122. Reynolds JC, Callaway CW, El Khoudary SR, Moore CG, Alvarez RJ, Rittenberger JC. Coronary angiography predicts improved outcome following cardiac arrest: propensity-adjusted analysis. J Intensive Care Med. 2009;24(3):179–86.

123. Anyfantakis ZA, Baron G, Aubry P, Himbert D, Feldman LJ, Juliard JM, Ricard-Hibon A, Burnod A, Cokkinos DV, Cokkinos DV, Steg PG. Acute coronary angiographic findings in survivors of out-of-hospital cardiac arrest. Am Heart J. 2009;157(2):312–8.

124. Wolfrum S, Pierau C, Radke PW, Schunkert H, Kurowski V. Mild therapeutic hypothermia in patients after out-of-hospital cardiac arrest due to acute ST-segment elevation myocardial infarction undergoing immediate percutaneous coronary intervention. Crit Care Med. 2008;36(6):1780–6.

125. Batista LM, Lima FO, Januzzi Jr JL, Donahue V, Snydeman C, Greer DM. Feasibility and safety of combined percutaneous coronary intervention and therapeutic hypothermia following cardiac arrest. Resuscitation. 2010;81(4):398–403.

126. Bellomo R, Bailey M, Eastwood GM, Nichol A, Pilcher D, Hart GK, Reade MC, Egi M, Cooper DJ, The Study of Oxygen in Critical Care (SOCC) Group. Arterial hyperoxia and in-hospital mortality after resuscitation from cardiac arrest. Crit Care. 2011;15(2):R90.

127. Kuisma M, Boyd J, Voipio V, Alaspää A, Roine RO, Rosenberg P. Comparison of 30 and the 100% inspired oxygen concentrations during early post-resuscitation period: a randomised controlled pilot study. Resuscitation. 2006;69(2):199–206.

128. Esteban A, Anzueto A, Frutos F, Alía I, Brochard L, Stewart TE, Benito S, Epstein SK, Apezteguía C, Nightingale P, Arroliga AC, Tobin MJ, Mechanical Ventilation International Study Group. Characteristics and outcomes in adult patients receiving mechanical ventilation: a 28-day international study. JAMA. 2002;287(3):345–55.

129. Wongsurakiat P, Pierson DJ, Rubenfeld GD. Changing pattern of ventilator settings in patients without acute lung injury: changes over 11 years in a single institution. Chest. 2004;126:1281–91.

130. NICE-SUGAR Study Investigators, Finfer S, Chittock DR, Su SY, Blair D, Foster D, Dhingra V, Bellomo R, Cook D, Dodek P, Henderson WR, Hébert PC, Heritier S, Heyland DK, McArthur C, McDonald E, Mitchell I, Myburgh JA, Norton R, Potter J, Robinson BG, Ronco JJ. Intensive versus conventional glucose control in critically ill patients. N Engl J Med. 2009;360(13):1283–97.

131. Oksanen T, Skrifvars MB, Varpula T, Kuitunen A, Pettilä V, Nurmi J, Castrén M. Strict versus moderate glucose control after resuscitation from ventricular fibrillation. Intensive Care Med. 2007;33(12):2093–100.

132. Adrie C, Adib-Conquy M, Laurent I, Monchi M, Vinsonneau C, Fitting C, Fraisse F, Dinh-Xuan AT, Carli P, Spaulding C, Dhainaut JF, Cavaillon JM. Successful cardiopulmonary resuscitation after cardiac arrest as a "sepsis-like" syndrome. Circulation. 2002;106(5):562–8.

133. Böttiger BW, Motsch J, Böhrer H, et al. Activation of blood coagulation after cardiac arrest is not balanced adequately by activation of endogenous fibrinolysis. Circulation. 1995;92:2572–8.

134. Nielsen N, Hovdenes J, Nilsson F, Rubertsson S, Stammet P, Sunde K, Valsson F, Wanscher M, Friberg H, Hypothermia Network. Outcome, timing and adverse events in therapeutic hypothermia after out-of-hospital cardiac arrest. Acta Anaesthesiol Scand. 2009;53(7):926–34.

135. Abiki M, Kawaguchi S, Maekawa N. Reversible hypophosphatemia during moderate hypothermia therapy for brain-injured patients. Crit Care Med. 2001;29:1726–30.

136. Adrie C, Haouache H, Saleh M, Memain N, Laurent I, Thuong M, Darques L, Guerrini P, Monchi M. An underrecognized source of organ donors: patients with brain death after successfully resuscitated cardiac arrest. Intensive Care Med. 2008;34(1):132–7.

137. Roine RO, Kajaste S, Kaste M. Neuropsychological sequelae of cardiac arrest. JAMA. 1993;269(2):237–42.

138. Schweickert WD, Pohlman MC, Pohlman AS, Nigos C, Pawlik AJ, Esbrook CL, Spears L, Miller M, Franczyk M, Deprizio D, Schmidt GA, Bowman A, Barr R, McCallister KE, Hall JB, Kress JP. Early physical and occupational therapy in mechanically ventilated, critically ill patients: a randomised controlled trial. Lancet. 2009;373(9678):1874–82.

139. Gratrix AP, Pittard AJ, Bodenham AR. Outcome after admission to ITU following out-of-hospital cardiac arrest: are non-survivors suitable for non-heart-beating organ donation? Anaesthesia. 2007;62(5):434–7.

140. Rittenberger JC, Raina K, Holm MB, Kim YJ, Callaway CW. Association between cerebral performance category, Modified Rankin Scale, and discharge disposition after cardiac arrest. Resuscitation. 2011;82(8):1036–40.

Neuromuscular Disorders in the ICU

38

Arash Salardini and William J. Triggs

Contents

Abstract

Neuromuscular diseases are conditions of the motor unit affecting the nervous system, inclusively between the anterior horn cells and the muscle. The occurrence of some of these conditions can lead to admission to the intensive care unit (ICU): weakness can impair breathing and disrupt airway protection. Many neuromuscular diseases are also associated with autonomic instability. Furthermore, critically ill patients may develop neuromuscular involvement as a consequence of long ICU stays. In this chapter, we describe a general approach to the problems of the neuromuscular disease in the neurological ICU.

Keywords

Neuromuscular disorders • Hypercapnic respiratory failure • Guillain-Barre • Myasthenia gravis • Critical illness neuromyopathy

Introduction

Neuromuscular disorders (NMDs) refer to a subset of neurological conditions that affect the motor unit. The motor unit is a lower motor neuron, with its axon and branches, the muscle fibers it supplies, and the related neuromuscular junctions. NMDs are thus a heterogeneous group of diseases that may affect any part of this chain from the anterior horn of the spinal cord or cranial nerve motor nuclei to the muscle fiber itself. Some neuromuscular disorders result in pervasive weakness, which can become critical if they affect the ventilatory machinery or the reflexes which subserve airway protection. Some neuromuscular conditions are also associated with autonomic and circulatory instability. Whenever the airway, breathing, or circulation of an NMD sufferer is compromised, the appropriate venue of care is the neurological intensive care unit (NICU).

A. Salardini, BSc, MBBS
Department of Radiology, University of Florida College
of Medicine, 1600 SW Archer Road,
Gainesville, FL 32601, USA
e-mail: arash.salardini@neurology.ufl.edu

W.J. Triggs, MD (✉)
Department of Neurology, University of Florida College
of Medicine, 100 S. Newell Drive L3-100,
Gainesville, FL 32611, USA
e-mail: triggswj@neurology.ufl.edu

A.J. Layon et al. (eds.), *Textbook of Neurointensive Care*,
DOI 10.1007/978-1-4471-5226-2_38, © Springer-Verlag London 2013

In this chapter, we will outline a general approach to neuromuscular diseases in the critically ill patient, explore conditions that require ICU admission, and discuss the implications of NMDs associated with ICU hospitalization. As weakness is the main reason for admission to the ICU, we will concentrate on the motor aspects of NMDs. We will begin with the assessment and management of NMD patients possibly requiring admission to the NICU and end the chapter with a discussion of the signs, symptoms, and tests commonly encountered in critical illness NMD. But first, a summary working knowledge of pathophysiology of weakness may be a good place to start.

Pathophysiology

Between the brain's motor centers and the effectors of movement in the periphery, i.e., the muscles, there are two orders of neurons: the upper motor neuron and the lower motor neuron. Weakness occurs with the dysfunction of the upper motor neuron, the lower motor neuron, or the muscle.

The upper motor neuron may be interrupted anywhere in the motor pathway: in the cortex of the precentral gyrus and along the course of its descending axon in the subcortical cerebrum, the brainstem, or the spinal cord. The upper motor neuron and its descending fibers have a moderating role on spinal reflexes. With the interruption of descending tracts, the motor response to stretch and somatosensation is exaggerated and some primitive reflexes are unmasked. The increased stretch reflex leads to enhanced deep tendon reflexes, which are elicited by rapid stretch of muscles achieved by percussing their tendons, and spasticity, a velocity-dependent resistance to muscle stretch [1]. Triple flexion reflex, another classic sign of upper motor neuron dysfunction, is essentially an exaggerated withdrawal reflex, where stroking the plantar surface of the foot leads to dorsiflexion of the ankle, with the flexion of knee and hip on the same leg. This is seen mostly in myelopathies [2]. Finally, most famously, Babinski response is elicited by stroking the lateral aspect of the bottom of the foot. The normal response is flexion of all toes. In the case of an upper motor lesion, the big toe dorsiflexes and the other toes fan out [3]. These signs are important in the diagnosis of certain motor neuron diseases and more importantly in ruling out myelopathy or cerebrovascular accident in the event of critical weakness.

The lower motor neurons reside in the anterior horn of the spinal cord as well as the cranial nerve nuclei in the brainstem. Nerve fibers and their presynaptic terminals are physiologically and anatomically continuous with the somata of neurons. As such, damage to any part of this apparatus will affect the other parts. However, conceptually, neurologists tend to divide lower motor neuron diseases into anatomical categories of motor neuron disease, neuropathy, neuromuscular junction, and muscle diseases. This provides a framework for discussion of diseases of the peripheral nervous system [4].

Neuropathies can be caused by damage to the axolemma or its myelin sheath. Some of the etiologies of damage are more prosaic such as compression and trauma, due to either direct mechanical damage or neural sheath thickening secondary to connective tissue diseases or chronic meningoencephalitides. Arteriopathy of vasa nervorum can also cause neuropathy. This is thought to be the mechanism of many vasculitic neuropathies causing mononeuritis multiplex. Pathology may affect the myelin sheath, the axolemma, and the axoplasmic transport or disrupt the nodes of Ranvier. The latter is a specialized part of the axon membrane that intervenes between two Schwann cells and contains ion channels necessary for saltatory conduction. Damage to the axolemma and the axoplasmic transport, as seen in metabolic disorders, tends to initially affect nerve fibers of greatest length and smallest caliber. The longest nerves in the body may be found, in order of length, in the lower limbs, upper limbs, and midline axial, lateral axial, and paraspinal areas. This is often the order in which the derangement of function occurs. As smaller-caliber fibers are preferentially affected, small fiber-mediated sensation such as pain and temperature is affected first in a glove and stocking distribution. "Gain of function" abnormalities such as dysesthesias and allodynias are also more common in this subgroup. In contrast, large nerve fibers are affected more by demyelinating conditions which affect proximal and distal muscles and tend to affect motor function and proprioception. Simplistically, most peripheral neuropathies fall into these two categories of demyelinating and axonal neuropathies with characteristic electromyographic findings for each. Small fiber neuropathies may have normal nerve conduction responses [5, 6].

The pathologic response of the axon to damage is threefold: segmental demyelination, Wallerian degeneration, and axonal degeneration. Segmental demyelination is caused by damage to Schwann cells and denuding an interval of the axon of its covering. In contrast to the other two pathological responses, demyelination is not associated with muscle atrophy. Wallerian degeneration is commonly seen with mechanical damage to the axon where the distal part of the axon degenerates but a connective tissue framework remains in place. Axonal degeneration occurs proximally and distal to the lesion and is associated with the loss of the myelin sheath. Both these two latter entities are associated with muscle wasting [7].

Muscle diseases may be congenital or acquired. Acquired conditions of the muscle may affect the muscle itself or the neuromuscular junction. They can cause acute reversible weakness leading to respiratory compromise. Inflammatory myopathies can either be secondary to systemic autoimmune diseases, primary myositis (polymyositis, dermatomyositis, and inclusion body myositis), infection, and toxins or due to endocrinopathies. Neuromuscular junction disease could be due to interference with release of acetylcholine into the synapse (tick paralysis, Lambert-Eaton myasthenic syndrome, and botulism) or due to scarcity of postsynaptic acetylcholine receptors (myasthenia gravis) [8].

Inherited myopathies come to the attention of the intensivist when there is concomitant pulmonary disease leading to disproportionate distress and respiratory failure. Inherited myopathies may be due to deficient structural gene products (muscular dystrophies), defective gene transcription mechanisms (myotonic dystrophies), channelopathies (myotonias and periodic paralyses), aberrant contractile mechanism (some congenital myopathies), and metabolic enzymopathies (metabolic and mitochondrial myopathies). These are mostly slowly progressive diseases of varying severity that can lead to worsening swallow and respiratory function. Some are associated with potentially fatal arrhythmias. These patients find their way into the ICU when they are being supported during a respiratory perturbation, commonly an infection, or as a temporizing measure when they are being transitioned to tracheostomy and home ventilation or pacemaker. Among the inherited myopathies, channelopathies can present with acute episodes of weakness which are largely reversible [9–11].

Diseases of the anterior horn of the spinal cord do not neatly fit into either upper or lower motor neuron disease categories. Some affect the inhibitory interneurons by autoimmune (stiff person syndrome) or infectious (tetanus) mechanisms. Both can be associated with significant respiratory and airway complications. Motor neurons are affected in a variety of conditions: some have predominantly lower motor neuron presentation (spinal muscular atrophy and primary muscular atrophy), others have mostly upper motor neuron features (hereditary spastic paraparesis and primary lateral sclerosis), while the most common phenotype is a mixture of the two (amyotrophic lateral sclerosis). Like inherited myopathies, these conditions come to the attention of the intensivist mainly during reversible respiratory conditions or transitional periods [12, 13].

Finally, a mention of the disease that started the discipline of intensive care, during the Copenhagen polio epidemic of 1952–1953, an anesthetist, Bjorn Ibsen, pioneered the use of invasive ventilation, in response to shortage of "iron lung" devices for the critically ill patients. Thus, the first intensive care unit was born. Poliomyelitis is an infection of the motor neurons which classically occurs with the poliovirus, but can occur with other viridae, namely, West Nile and Coxsackie viridae. The deterioration in muscle and respiratory function is often rapid but there is variable degree of recovery [14].

General Approach to Patients with Weakness in the ICU

History

A detailed history and examination are particularly important in the management of neuromuscular disease in the ICU. A focused and competent clinical history and examination in

cerebrovascular disease, for example, may be sufficient where testing is likely to locate the pathology and perhaps even the etiology. In the neuromuscular field, testing is essentially meaningless unless it is interpreted in the context of the clinical information and extensive knowledge of disease processes (with the exception of some compressive neuropathies and a few others). Further, if the patient requires intubation, the opportunity to obtain a detailed history will be rapidly lost.

The clinical interview aims to answer the following questions:

- What is the time course of the disease (antecedents, age of onset, acuity, progression, and fluctuation or recurrence)?
- What is the distribution and characteristics of the weakness (anatomical distribution, symmetry, and fluctuations in weakness)?
- What are the associated symptoms accompanying the weakness (positive and negative sensory changes, presence of pain, autonomic and behavioral symptoms)?
- Is there respiratory distress, signs of bulbar weakness, or signs of circulatory changes (dyspnea, aspiration, presyncope, or palpitations)?
- Is the respiratory distress, when present, due to acute onset of severe weakness or respiratory decompensation in the presence of static or slowly progressive weakness?
- Is there anything in the background history of the patient that may narrow the differential diagnosis (primary muscle disease, systemic diseases including endocrinopathies, hematopathologies, and autoimmune diseases, as well as list of medications)?

Physical Examination

By the end of the general examination, the clinician should have answered the following questions:

- Are there any underlying systemic diseases that may explain the neuromuscular disease (e.g., thyroid disease, vasculitis, or malignancy)?
- Are there any findings consistent with a neuromuscular syndrome (e.g., characteristic facies of myasthenia and myotonia)?
- What is the general state of patient's health in particular in reference to the cardiorespiratory function (airway function, breathing, circulation)?
- What is the likely diagnosis?

The components of the examination may include the following:

- ABCs and vitals:
  - *Airway protection*: This may be gauged by examining the strength of the cough and a bedside swallow test if the patient is alert.
  - *Breathing*: One should assess pump function as well as the presence of fibrosis due to previous aspiration and

systemic inflammatory states. The use of accessory muscles of respiration, visible distress, and the ability to speak in full sentences should be noted. The patient can be asked to count numbers on a single breath. The respiratory digit span can then be compared when the patient is supine versus erect, and if there are serious discrepancies, then diaphragmatic paralysis is suspected. In some cases neck flexion strength may be used as a surrogate for diaphragmatic function. This is because many neuromuscular disorders seem to affect regions of the peripheral nervous system differentially and the innervations of the diaphragm and neck flexor muscles overlap [15, 16].

– *Circulation*: Circulatory stability, postural symptoms, and the heart rhythm and pump function are assessed early in the assessment of the patient.

• General physical examination:

– *General appearance*: A general inspection of the skin and the habitus should be performed from the foot of the bed. Attention should be paid to the presence of rashes and trophic changes.

– *HEENT*: This should include ophthalmoscopy and the inspection of the eye, mouth, and the nose (for dryness and ulcers).

– *Neck*: Look for goiter, venous and arterial pulsations, as well as use of accessory muscles of respiration.

– *Abdominal examination*: One looks for the presence of masses and organomegaly.

• Neurological examination:

– *Higher mental state examination*: In our experience, this is somewhat low yield in the acute setting. The presence of altered mental state in a weak patient should lead to brain imaging, but beyond this, a detailed mental state examination is not required.

– *Cranial nerve testing*: With the exception of cranial nerve I (and sometimes VIII), all other cranial nerves are examined in this patient population. The cranial nerves are part of the peripheral nervous system, and their involvement or otherwise assists in diagnosis:

• CN II: Acuity and fields.

• CNs III, IV, and VI: Pupillary reflexes and eye movement.

• CN V: Facial sensation, masticatory strength, and jaw jerk.

• CN VII: Facial strength and symmetry.

• CN VIII: A crude hearing test and head impulse test may suffice.

• CNs IX, X, and XI: Palatal rise, swallowing a cup of liquid, and phonation.

• CN XII: Tongue strength, atrophy, and fasciculations.

– *Sensory testing*: The object of the sensory testing is to document the distribution of sensory changes. Fine touch, pin prick, temperature, position sense, and vibration are typically tested.

– *Cerebellar testing*: This can be brief and include rapid alternating movement and the point-to-point tests.

– *Motor testing*:

• *Observation*: Look for involuntary movements including fasciculations, myokymia, neuromyotonia, myotonia, and pseudoathetosis. Look for muscle atrophy.

• *Muscle tone*: Ask the patient to relax, then move the joints passively: first slowly, then more rapidly. Take note of flaccidity versus rigidity or spasticity.

• *Muscle strength*: The Medical Research Council grading system remains the most popular strength grading system. It scores muscle strength by asking the patient to move voluntarily against the examiner's resistance:

– *0/5*: No movement whatsoever

– *1/5*: Muscle contraction but no discernible movement

– *2/5*: Movement at the joint but not against gravity

– *3/5*: Movement against gravity with no added resistance

– *4/5*: Movement against added resistance but not normal

– *5/5*: Normal [17]

Pronator drift is often examined with strength testing.

– *Reflexes*: Tendon reflexes are attempted at the biceps, triceps, brachioradialis, patella, and the Achilles tendons. Often forgotten is the all-important abdominal reflex that gives some indication of reflex function between the two limb girdles. The abdomen is divided into four quadrants and scratched obliquely, and the resultant movement of the umbilicus is observed. For the rest, a simple grading system is most commonly used:

• *0*: Absent

• *1+*: Less active than average

• *2+*: Average reflex activity

• *3+*: More brisk than average without clonus

• 4+: Brisk with clonus [2]

Plantar reflexes are examined by stroking the lateral part of the foot.

• *Gait and balance*: The weak patient coming to the attention of the ICU is commonly unable to ambulate.

Testing

This is guided by the findings on history and examination and should not be ordered in a blanket manner. More commonly ordered tests are in bold lettering:

• Laboratory testing:

– *CK*

– *Routine testing*: CMP, **CBC with diff.**, B12, folate, HbA1c, RPR, and TSH

Fig. 38.1 A general approach to acute weakness in the ICU

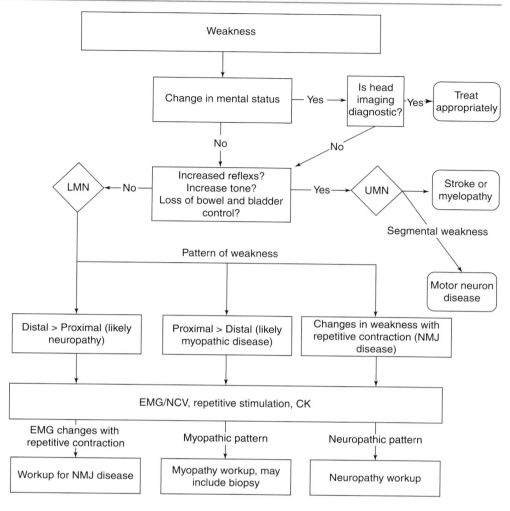

- *Autoimmune testing*: UPEP, SPEP, IFE, ESR, CRP, RF, ANA, SSA, SSB, and ANCA
- *CSF testing*: Protein, glucose, cell count, oligoclonal band, and serology based on clinical suspicion
- *Demyelination-related testing*: anti-GM1, anti-GD1, MAG, and anti-GQ1b
- *Neuromuscular junction-related testing*: anti-AChR, anti-MuSK, and anti-P/Q calcium channel
- Respiratory testing :
  - *Lung function test*
  - *Blood gases*
  - *Sniff test*: Is rarely required except in the case of suspected diaphragmatic paresis
- Imaging, when indicated:
  - *Imaging of the head and the spinal cord*: commonly an MRI
  - *Imaging of plexuses*: MRI
  - *Imaging of muscle*: MRI or ultrasound
- Neurophysiology:
  - *Nerve conduction test*
  - *Electromyography*
  - *Repetitive nerve stimulation*

- Tissue testing:
  - *Nerve biopsy*: The sural nerve is most commonly biopsied in selected patients.
  - *Muscle biopsy*
  - *Other tissue biopsy*: For example, lymph nodes in the case of lymphoma or sarcoidosis.
- Genetic testing: When appropriate for hereditary causes of motor weakness

Management

Synthesis

Figure 38.1 summarizes our approach to neuromuscular disorders. By this stage, the clinician will be able to decide on the appropriate management of weakness. This is driven by two variables. The first is the extent of the weakness, which regardless of cause will require support of respiratory function, airway protection, and prophylaxis of complications following a reduction in mobility. We will address these under the heading of general management. The second consideration is the diagnosis, which will drive the specific treatment geared towards the pathology. We will address these under the heading of specific treatment and again when discussing the individual conditions.

General Management

General critical care management of neuromuscular disorders consists of three main components: protection of airway, ensuring adequate ventilation, and anticipating and managing complication.

Assessment of Ventilator Need

Lung Function Testing

In our practice, we use the 20-30-40 rule: this is a crude rule of thumb for the timing of elective intubation. If the forced vital capacity (FVC) is less than 20 ml/kg, maximum inspiratory pressure (MIP) less than 30, or maximum expiratory pressure (MEP) less than 40 cmH_2O, we are prompted to consider ventilation support, invasive or noninvasive based on the presumptive diagnosis and prognosis. The MIP and FVC are better predictors of the need for mechanical ventilation and the MEP for intubation for airway protection purposes [18, 19].

Blood Gases

Commonly, patients with ventilatory failure do not exhibit hypoxia until quite late in the course of their decline. Increased pCO_2 is a much more sensitive sign of reduction in minute ventilation. The interpretation of the pCO_2 is more complex in the NMD population. Many patients with chronic respiratory disease may at baseline have higher CO_2. pH and the degree of metabolic compensation may be used as an adjunct to assess the degree of decompensation [20].

Clinical Judgment

Finally, there is no lab substitute for clinical judgment; a patient may have above-threshold values for pulmonary volumes or blood gases but look exhausted and unwell, and the clinician might anticipate rapid deterioration of the respiratory function and go ahead and intubate the patient.

Management of Ventilation and Airway Protection

When it comes to ventilation, the choices are noninvasive ventilation and invasive ventilation. Although noninvasive ventilation provides several theoretical benefits compared to invasive ventilation, in practice we find that there are several important practical limitations to its use.

Noninvasive Ventilation

NIPPV may be used as a temporizing measure to avoid intubation. It is also used intermittently while the patient may have borderline weakness, as a way of transitioning the patient to the ward [21]. In our practice its wider use is limited by:

- *Complications of prolonged use*: NIPPV cannot be used for long periods of time as use of the mask can lead to the formation of pressure sores.
- *It does not provide airway protection*: The patient needs to be able to protect her airway in order for mask ventilation to be clinically safe. In practice, loss of cough reflex, which is a consequence of expiratory weakness, often accompanies ventilatory failure [21].

Invasive Mechanical Ventilation

The need for intubation should be anticipated in advance as special measures are taken in the endotracheal intubation of neuromuscular patients. The use of succinylcholine should be avoided in this patient population as it may lead to severe electrolyte disturbance. Topical anesthetics may be used instead of systemic anesthetic where possible. This approach provides better airway protection.

Another advantage of early intubation in patients with acute weakness is a reduction in the risk of aspiration pneumonia as it improves airway protection. Airway protection strategy should include aggressive secretion clearance: these can include the use of chest vibration and physiotherapy, bronchodilators and nebulized saline combined with suction, and intermittent positive pressure breathing. Cough assistance including mechanical insufflation-exsufflation and hyperinflation maneuvers should be instituted in all patients with NMD [19].

Extubation

Extubation of patients with neuromuscular disease follows the same standard criteria as other ICU patients. Some differences are worth noting:

- *Airway protection and management of secretions*: The risk of reintubation is related not only to ventilatory recovery but also control of secretion – more so that of the general ICU patient. The vast majority of our NMD patients have prolonged stays in the ICU and thus have tracheostomies which may facilitate management of airway secretions.
- *Rate of recovery*: The second important difference is that the rate of recovery is likely to be comparatively slower; thus, the weaning process is likely to be lengthier. We use the 4-5-6 rule of thumb: patients with improvement in FVC of more than 4 ml/kg compared to the pre-intubation status, MIP of more than $-50\ cmH_2O$, and MEP >60 cmH_2O should be considered for extubation [22, 23].

Circulation

The management of circulation in NMD is mostly the same as the general ICU patient. When our patients are more resistant to pressors, there are a number of factors we routinely investigate:

- *Adrenal insufficiency*: Many NMD patients are on fluctuating doses of steroids and thus might suffer from iatrogenic addisonism. We may start with a morning cortisol and look at the electrolytes, but to diagnose adrenal insufficiency definitively, we perform the cosyntropin test.
- *Infections*: Many of the patients with NMD are immunosuppressed, so there should be a high index of suspicion for sepsis even without the classic signs of fever and increased white blood cell count.
- *Acid–base abnormalities (–osis)*: For example, inotropes may not work properly in the presence of severe respiratory.
- *Autonomic dysfunction*: In the face of continuing orthostasis and autonomic instability, the use of fludrocortisone and midodrine might help weaning off the vasopressors.

Prophylaxis and Maintenance
Nutrition and Electrolytes
Nutritional approach in a patient with NMD should take into account several considerations:

- *Electrolyte management*: A weak patient is more vulnerable to fluctuations in electrolyte, and thus close monitoring and replacement of abnormalities including phosphate and especially potassium should be routine. Special care should be taken during refeeding when these electrolyte serum levels may plummet.
- *Adequate protein and calories*: Care should also be taken to provide adequate supply of calories and protein to reduce the rate of utilization of muscle proteins for metabolic purposes. Overfeeding should also be avoided as it leads to excess carbon dioxide production and risks hypercarbia [24].
- *Need for enteric feeding*: We recommend some measure of enteric feeding to maintain the integrity of the blood/gut lumen barrier. This in our view reduces the risk of ICU-associated infections [25].
- *Prophylactic measures*: There is no excuse for not having ICU patients on deep venous thrombosis prophylaxis; in our institution, we combine subcutaneous heparins with sequential compression devices [26]. We have our patients at 30° head up to reduce the risk of aspiration. Stress ulcer prophylaxis is especially important in this patient population.

Symptomatic Care
Pain
The use of opiates and benzodiazepine is deferred until other classes of medications have been tried. NSAIDs including intravenous and rectal formulations are used as first line. For nerve pain, antiepileptics including Depakote and tricyclics can be useful. However, ultimately our priority is to insure that the patient is not in pain even if it means prolongation of ICU stay.

Table 38.1 A representative list of conditions that can lead to ICU admission, by anatomical localization

Anatomical substrate	Clinical condition
Anterior horn cells	Acute poliomyelitis
Motor neuropathy	Guillain-Barre syndrome
	Acute porphyria
Neuromuscular junction	Myasthenia gravis
	Lambert-Eaton
	Botulism
	Tetanus
	Diphtheria
	Tick paralysis
	Puffer fish poisoning
Muscle	Hypokalemic periodic paralyses
	Myositis

Medication Use
Clinical pharmacists have a relatively larger role in helping choose the medication to use in NMD patients. Many pharmaceuticals, especially antibiotics, have actions at the neuromuscular junction or may cause a myopathy.

Other Autonomic Treatment
The presence of gastroparesis and constipation is common in our patient population, and bowel movements and feeding tube residuals should be recorded and monitored. Gastroparesis may become apparent if there are large amount of post-feed residuals. The treatment with metoclopramide and erythromycin can be effective. The main precaution when instituting the latter is to make sure that magnesium levels are high normal and to monitor the QT interval. Bulking agents and laxatives are used for constipation. Urinary catheterization mitigates the complications of bladder dysfunction [27].

Psychiatric Consideration
Some NMD is associated with severe depression including GBS. Early recognition improves compliance during follow-up [28].

Specific Treatments
There are three groups of NMDs that come to the attention of the intensivists:

1. Acute onset weakness requiring ICU care
2. Chronic weakness with acute respiratory decompensation
3. ICU-acquired weakness

Table 38.1 lists some of the common causes of acute reversible weakness requiring ICU care. These conditions usually have specific treatments which are outlined in the sections that follow. Chronic causes of weakness with respiratory decompensation often do not have specific therapies. Exceptions include the short-term use of steroids in muscular dystrophy for improved strength, and the use of acetazolamide may be used in myotonic dystrophy. These interventions make marginal contributions, and, given the long list of chronic neuromuscular diseases, it is not practical to include them all in the following section. Our own practice is to stay "on board" as neurologists when patients with chronic neuromuscular disease are admitted for any reason to any inpatient unit. Finally, ICU-acquired weakness is a topic of great import, and we have included a separate section.

Acute Poliomyelitis

This disease is of mostly historical interest to first world intensivists. Poliomyelitis was the most common neuromuscular cause of respiratory failure before vaccination became widespread. The choice of ventilation for polio patients at that stage was to mimic the physiology of breathing with the use of negative ventilation mechanisms called iron lungs. During the 1952–1953 polio epidemic in Denmark, the widespread use of invasive positive pressure ventilation was pioneered (mostly due to a shortage of iron lungs), and thus critical care medicine was born. Today, polio is seen rarely but several polio-like syndromes are described with Coxsackie and West Nile viruses [29, 30].

Poliovirus enters the blood via the oral or respiratory mucosa, causing a viremia. This first phase causes a prodrome of 1–4 days which is associated with flu-like and gastrointestinal symptoms. The viridae then are picked by nerve endings in the periphery and are transported antidromically to the spinal cord leading to degeneration of motor neurons. This can lead to asymmetrical weakness of axial and bulbar muscles. Recovery is often slow. Pain is a common feature of poliomyelitis [31]. Treatment is mostly supportive.

Guillain-Barre Syndrome (GBS)

Guillain-Barre is now the main reason for critical weakness leading to ICU hospitalization. GBS has a mortality of roughly 5 % in the ICU environment. The basic mechanism is thought to be immune destruction of the peripheral nerves, perhaps instigated by an antecedent infection classically with *Campylobacter jejuni* but also Epstein-Barr virus, cytomegalovirus, and *Mycoplasma pneumoniae*. The antigens from these infectious agents cause an early humoral (ant-GM1 for *C. jejuni* and anti-GM2 for CMV) and a later cell-mediated attack on myelin, where a lymphocytic infiltrate accompanies a macrophage-mediated stripping of the myelin sheath and appearance of a conduction block. Inflammation can also cause axonal damage, an important determinate of prognosis, though it remains unclear whether this axonal damage is a primary or secondary process. Other less common precipitants of GBS include human immunodeficiency virus. "Postsurgical GBS" might mostly be due to critical illness polyneuropathy [32].

Clinical Features

In almost all patients weakness starts in the proximal lower limb and ascends to the arms. Facial and bulbar weakness happens in about half the patients. The duration of the weakness usually reaches its peak in up to 3 weeks. Areflexia is often the sign that alerts the clinician to the presence of GBS. It is found in the paretic limb. Sensory symptoms are somewhat more variable with a glove and stocking loss of large fiber modalities and delayed sacral paresthesia being the most common. Occasionally, a sciatica-like syndrome may intervene which complicates early diagnosis. Early diagnosis is critical in cases where respiratory failure occurs within hours to days. These patients, in our experience, have a more severe and prolonged course of disease. Some degree of dysautonomia is common in GBS.

There are a number of clinical variants, the most dramatic of which is the Miller-Fischer variant which presents with areflexia, ophthalmoparesis, and ataxia. There are patients in whom the weakness is descending and affects the bulbar muscles and may be mistaken for myasthenia or botulism. There are cases where there is a preponderance of sensory, motor, cerebellar, and autonomic symptoms. But these are the exceptions rather than the rule [33].

Diagnosis

The diagnosis is made clinically and supported by electrophysiological and laboratory testing. The EMG is often normal very early in the disease, but later the patient may develop motor blocks and delay of late responses. The former is noted when there is significant amplitude attenuation when the nerve is stimulated proximal to the block. F-waves, which are due to the retrograde transmission of a supramaximal stimulus, may be delayed. It is important to note that even though electrodiagnosis is helpful, it lags behind clinical changes and in our experience has little utility for monitoring improvements. Other supportive laboratory testing includes raised CSF protein and the absence of CSF findings consistent with other diagnosis. Of academic interest may be mild hepatic enzyme changes (usually following EBV and CMV infections), campylobacter cultures of the stool, and raised anti-GM1 circulating antibodies [34].

There are several GBS patterns commonly described by EMG/NCV criteria:
1. Acute inflammatory demyelinating polyneuropathy
2. Acute motor sensory axonal neuropathy
3. Acute motor axonal neuropathy [35]

We feel that this classification may in fact be confusing. There are no characteristic electromyographic features of an axonal Guillain-Barre syndrome. Axonal GBS, as defined by immune destruction of axons in the absence of an inflammatory demyelinating process, is likely to be exceedingly rare. Conduction block can be seen in acute inflammatory demyelinating polyneuropathy giving low amplitude but normal conduction velocities. There is also axonal degeneration and muscle denervation in severe inflammatory demyelinating disease. Why this matters is that "an axonal pattern" on the EMG/NCV does not necessarily portend a dire outcome. Unexcitable nerves in the first 2 weeks of disease, unresponsive to supramaximal stimulation, are likely to have heterogeneous pathologies. We think better prognostication may be achieved with repeat EMG/NCV after 2 weeks and the following risk stratification, dividing our patients into three types:

- Type 1: These show conduction block in the first 2 weeks but only mild evidence of denervation on needle electromyography. These will likely have transient motor weakness.
- Type 2: These show an axonal pattern of conduction and early denervation. These may include both severe distal inflammatory degeneration but also the more pure acute motor axon neuropathy. The prognosis in these cases is usually but not uniformly poor.
- Type 3: Shows delayed muscle denervation but prolonged abnormalities indicating a persistent inflammatory pathology. These have the worst prognosis of the three groups [36, 37].

Management

Like all neuromuscular diseases in the ICU, the main morbidities are loss of airway protection and ventilatory failure. These have been addressed elsewhere in the chapter. Dysautonomia is a more pronounced feature of the GBS compared to the other entities discussed here. In its pure form, the patient is said to have panautonomia. The most common manifestation is a "fixed" sinus tachycardia (fixed because sinus arrhythmia is attenuated). Malignant arrhythmias are uncommon. When present, they can include ventricular tachyarrhythmias, heart block, and asystole. Occasionally, nonspecific T and ST changes are seen which may be confused clinically with coronary artery events.

Blood pressure abnormalities including orthostasis, hypertension (fixed or labile), and hypotension can be seen in this condition. Hypertension can be episodic and extreme and, when alternating with low blood pressure, may be a therapeutic challenge. Sweating anomalies as well as bowel and urinary issues including ileus, incontinence, urinary retention, and diarrhea are not uncommon. Gastroparesis and ileus, though uncommon, can complicate tube feeding [27].

Immunotherapy
Plasmapheresis
The standard treatment since the late 1970s has been plasmapheresis, which seems to reduce the time to recovery by about a half. There is no standard regimen, but we use approximately 200 ml/kg spread over about five sessions. In preparation for plasmapheresis, a large-bore apheresis catheter is placed. We measure ionized calcium and fibrinogen before every session and supplement them with calcium gluconate and FFP if they are less than 5 and 100 mg/dl, respectively. The main complications are increased risk of infections, coagulopathy, and fluid overload. These are usually not of great consequence when managed well.

Intravenous Immunoglobulin (IVIg)
Due to the ease of use, our preferred mode of treatment is the use of intravenous gamma globulins at 0.4 g/kg given over 3–5 days. Renal failure, fluid overload, and allergic reaction, most ominously anaphylaxis, are the main potential complications. We typically test renal function and when clinically relevant cardiac function. Headache with IVIg due to aseptic meningitis is usually not trivial and requires a change in management.

Some cases of GBS that appear unresponsive to immunotherapy are likely associated with extensive axonal injury and may require prolonged periods of supportive therapy [38–40].

Acute Porphyria
This is a treatable albeit rare mimic of GBS. Porphyrias are a group of genetic diseases in which there are deficiencies in the production of the porphyrin ring, a major constituent of heme. There are several different kinds of acute porphyrias with different biochemistries and semiologies, but their neurological symptoms are relatively uniform.

Semiology
An acute episode is precipitated by hormonal and diet changes or by medications, typically the ones that interfere with the P450 system. The patient often complains of abdominal and limb pain followed by delirium which can lead to frank psychosis and seizures. Within 2–3 days, the patient develops weakness and autonomic instability which may need ICU care. The pattern of weakness and its progression resembles that of GBS. Autonomic instability is usually in the form of sympathetic overdrive.

Diagnosis
The diagnosis is made by measuring, in the urine and feces, certain metabolites which are intermediaries in the metabolism of porphyrins including delta-aminolevulinic acid, porphobilinogen, uroporphobilinogen, coproporphyrinogen, and protoporphyrinogen. The most common acute porphyria, acute intermittent porphyria, has a routine genetic test which may be performed for confirmation.

Treatment
Management of acute porphyria should be done under close supervision of a hematologist. Typically glucose

(at 10–20 g/h) and hematin (1–5 mg/kg/day) are given for days to weeks until the symptoms improve. Education and avoidance of triggers are important parts of prevention of further episodes. Supportive respiratory therapy and autonomic monitoring are instituted for as long as required as discussed under the general management section [41, 42].

Myasthenia Gravis

Acquired myasthenia gravis is an autoimmune disease against the postsynaptic cholinergic receptors in muscles. There is an association with thymic growths and autoimmune conditions including autoimmune thyroid disease, connective tissue disease, and arthritis. The disease has a bimodal distribution: young women in their teens to thirties (associated with autoimmune diseases) and older men in their sixth to eighth decades (greater coincidence with thymic hyperplasia).

Clinical Features

The hallmark of myasthenia gravis is fatigability of muscle strength which is a diminution of strength with repeated contractions. The most commonly affected muscles are ocular muscles and bulbofacial muscles. Acute exacerbations of weakness are termed crises. There are two kinds of crises in myasthenic and cholinergic. The former is a worsening of weakness that occurs as a result of worsening of generalized weakness. Most of these patients have a known history of MG and are often in the early stages of disease; a minority have unmasked their latent disease with the use of neuromuscular blockade or certain antibiotics, for example, around the time of surgery. Cholinergic crisis, the minority of cases encountered in the ICU, is due to weakness caused by depolarization block due to excessive cholinesterase inhibitor usage [43].

Diagnosis

The diagnosis of myasthenia gravis is a clinical one and is supported by electrophysiological and laboratory testing. A decremental response to a train of stimuli or increased jitter is diagnostic of myasthenia gravis. Serological evidence of myasthenia in majority of cases includes the presence of antibodies against cholinergic receptors. In our practice, we do not use Tensilon test in the ICU diagnosis of myasthenia gravis. A trial of cholinesterase inhibitors such as intramuscular neostigmine is rarely used except to rule out cholinergic crisis and gauge therapeutic response.

Pulmonary Treatment

Respiratory management of myasthenic patients follows the same general principles outlined in the general management of neuromuscular disease. The physiology of myasthenia should be taken into consideration when managing airway in these patients. Firstly, given that the patients are commonly

on cholinesterase inhibitors, the amount of airway secretion is increased significantly. Secondly, the use of depolarizing neuromuscular blockers should be avoided as much as possible due to prolonged action and unpredictable dosing [44].

Pharmacological Treatment
Cholinesterase Inhibitors

The continuation or cessation of cholinesterase inhibitors is an individualized clinical choice. Pyridostigmine can be given via a Dobhoff tube to a maximum of 120 mg q8h or as an infusion starting at 2 mg/h and titrated to response. Cholinesterase medications have marginal roles in the management of critically weak individuals and may be omitted if their side effects such as diarrhea or excessive airway secretions become problematic.

Steroids

The mainstay treatment of myasthenia is the use of steroids for long-term immunosuppression at the rate of 1 mg/kg initially then 2 mg/kg every second day for the maintenance of pituitary-adrenal axis. The dose may be weaned after discharge over weeks to months, and if resistant to weaning, then azathioprine can be used for steroid sparing. Although lacking supporting evidence, it is our practice to give pulses of methylprednisone in the first 3 days.

Immunotherapy

The main problem with the use of steroids in myasthenia is that it exacerbates weakness, often in the second week of treatment. For this reason, we supplement steroid therapy with plasmapheresis or IVIg. We use 0.4 g/kg for IVIg over 4 or 5 days. Plasmapheresis can be used until respiratory function improves to a level of 80 % predicted. Typically, we do not go much beyond 5 l of exchange. Other immunosuppressive drugs are also used, but they need to be prescribed by a neurologist familiar with them or in consultation with a clinical immunologist [45].

Surgical Considerations

Thymectomy is recommended in myasthenia. This is usually delayed until the patient has recovered, the exception being in patients who continue to remain ventilator dependent in spite of other therapy. Plasma exchange may be used preoperatively on patients with MG whose FVC is below 80 % of predicted for age, gender, and height [46].

Lambert-Eaton Myasthenic Syndrome (LEMS)

This is another autoimmune neuromuscular disease that physiologically resembles myasthenia gravis. The majority of cases are paraneoplastic, often related to small cell carcinoma of the lung, where the anti-VGCC antibody interferes with the presynaptic P/Q type of calcium channel, thus reducing vesicular fusion and synaptic acetylcholine.

Clinically, however, LEMS differs markedly from MG, in that bulbar and ocular symptoms are relatively mild and there is dysautonomia and proximal weakness, which, in our experience, is generally fixed. The diagnosis is made clinically and is confirmed by repetitive nerve stimulation studies and presence of anti-VGCC antibodies. Other paraneoplastic antibodies can coexist, most notably anti-Hu and anti N-type calcium channel [47].

The main fact to remember about LEMS is that the majority of the cases are paraneoplastic, where the life expectancy is determined more by the malignancy than the LEMS. A concerted effort should be made to ascertain the existence of a malignancy in any patient presenting with LEMS. The non-paraneoplastic autoimmune variety often responds well to immunosuppressive medications. The protocols used for steroid, azathioprine, plasma exchange, and IVIg are similar to the ones used for MG. Mestinon (pyridostigmine) might have a minor role in the treatment of LEMS. 3,4-Diaminopyridine (3,4-DAP) has been used for prolongation of potassium current which improves strength. Our own experience with 3,4-DAP has been limited [48].

Botulism

This is a classic but uncommon disease caused by the neurotoxin produced by *C. botulinum*, an anaerobic gram-positive organism which produces neurotoxins. The mechanism of action of botulinum toxins, which are seven in number, is by inhibiting the mechanisms required for the docking and release of acetylcholine from the presynaptic receptors [49].

Several clinical forms of botulism are recognized:

- *Foodborne*: Classically, as the name suggests, botulism occurred in consumers of improperly preserved and stored meats where the clostridia would proliferate and produce its toxin. When ingested, this would cause botulism. With improved food safety standards, this form of botulism is exceedingly rare.
- *Intestinal*: In infants (and exceedingly rarely in adults), the intestines are colonized with the organism which can cause botulism.
- *Wound botulism*: The most common form of adult botulism involves wound infection. A note of caution regarding wound botulism: the patients are typically drug users, with difficult histories and personalities who present with slurred speech and blurring of sight and are thus dismissed as being intoxicated and not credible. If any doubt, such patient should have two hourly neurological checks for at least 12 h looking for the onset of descending flaccid paralysis.
- *Iatrogenic*: There are rare reports of iatrogenic botulism thought to be due to aerosolization of the Botox.
- *Weaponized*: There are also fears that governments and terrorist groups may have weaponized botulinum toxin and may use it in the future against civilian targets.

Presentation

Botulism presents with cranial nerve abnormalities as facial weakness, drooling, loss of swallowing reflexes, and blurring of vision and proceeds to cause a descending paralysis often affecting the digits last. There are no sensory symptoms. There is often a variable incubation period related to the dose of the toxin.

Diagnosis and Treatment

The only specific treatment for botulism is antitoxin which neutralizes the unbound toxin and should be given early in the course of the disease. The testing though often lags clinical urgency, and thus the decision to give the antitoxin is on the clinical index of suspicion. Gastric lavage or cleaning a putatively contaminated wound may also be useful. During the admission to the ICU, apart from the routine tests ordered, samples of feces, NG aspirate, saliva, and serum should be sent for testing for *C. botulinum*.

Our most important advice is to contact the Center for Disease Control and Prevention and speak to their botulism experts. They will patiently gather information from history taken by the intensivist and offer advice on testing and treatment. Typically they will be interested in the clinical presentation, neurological examination, food history for the last week, and history of drug abuse. Outbreaks of botulism are public health emergencies and should be reported as soon as possible to health authorities [50].

Tick Paralysis

This is a flaccid paralysis caused by the toxin of gravid ticks belonging to a heterogeneous group of ticks. The Australian *Ixodes holocyclus* (a dog tick) produces the most severe syndrome, often in afflicted children. The treatment is extremely simple: support the patient in the ICU and remove the tick organism as a whole. There may be a brief exacerbation of weakness initially, but typically the symptoms are self-limited after the removal of the causative organism. The challenge of tick paralysis is its diagnosis; inspection for ticks is not a common part of neurological examination, and the symptoms resemble more common conditions such as botulism, diphtheria, or Guillain-Barre. The tick is commonly found fortuitously. Once found, other tick-borne diseases such as Lyme disease should be considered and ruled out [51].

Neurotoxic Fish Poisoning

Various edible marine animals consume dinoflagellates and concentrate sodium channel poisons produced by these tiny creatures. The classic ones, which played an important role in the elucidation of the mechanism of action potentials, included tetrodotoxin, ciguatoxin, saxitoxin, and brevetoxin. Puffer fish, an accumulator of tetrodotoxin, is a delicacy in Japanese cuisine because of the numbness it causes around the mouth after it is prepared in a particular way to minimize the toxin. In larger doses, all these toxins cause severe gastrointestinal and neurological symptoms. The gastrointestinal symptoms include nausea, vomiting, pain, and diarrhea. The neurological symptoms include paresthesia around the mouth and in the digits, allodynia where temperature is perceived as pain and weakness, and in severe cases respiratory failure. The history of consumption of puffer fish, snails, and shellfish in endemic areas is sufficient for the diagnosis. The treatment is supportive. Mannitol diuresis is said to hasten recovery [52].

Diphtheria

Diphtheria is commonly not a diagnostic dilemma for the neurologist, as the preponderance of systemic symptoms often leads to diagnosis earlier than neurological symptoms appear. The condition is caused by *Corynebacterium diphtheriae*, infecting the upper respiratory tract leading to sore throat, nasal discharge, hoarseness, and fever. It is spread by respiratory secretions. A gray pharyngeal pseudomembrane is pathognomic but culture is diagnostics. The neurological symptoms of diphtheria are due to a neurotoxin produced by the organism. This causes a neuropathy with a propensity for cranial nerves and occasionally respiratory muscles. The treatment is supportive, including circulation when there is concomitant myocarditis. Specific therapy includes antitoxin and antibiotics (penicillin or erythromycin if allergic). The doses should be determined in consultation with infectious disease physicians [53].

Tetanus

Among the neuromuscular disorders requiring ICU hospitalization, tetanus stands apart. Whereas most of the other conditions discussed require ventilator support due to weakness, tetanus is associated with severe spasms that require iatrogenic muscle paralysis and ventilation. Tetanus toxin is produced by *Clostridium tetani*, a gram-positive anaerobic organism commonly found in the soil. Tetanus toxin interferes with inhibitory transmission of the spinal cord and causes hyperreflexia, tetanic contractions, trismus, and dysphagia. Tonic spastic responses are elicited by minimal sensory stimulation. When spasms affect the larynx or the respiratory musculature, asphyxiation may result. The patient is paralyzed and ventilated. If a wound is the source of the infection, it will be debrided and cleaned. The patient should be immunized passively and actively and started on intravenous penicillin chemotherapy [54].

Hypokalemic Periodic Paralysis

This is the most common of the channelopathies which cause weakness, in particular acute weakness. The problem is the lack of sensitivity of the voltage-gated calcium or sodium channels (to voltage changes) which makes the muscle more sensitive to low potassium (increase potassium gradient leads to more rapid repolarization with non-sustained Na or Ca current). Thus, the triggers for hypokalemic paralysis are anything that might reduce extracellular potassium concentration, and these include exercise, high adrenergic state, and carbohydrate-rich meals. The treatment is correction of hypokalemia while supporting the ABCs. Long-term management includes the use of acetazolamide, potassium supplementation, and potassium-sparing diuretics [55, 56].

Polymyositis/Dermatomyositis (PM/DM)

Inflammatory myopathies are by far the most common causes of acute myopathy. Three general entities are recognized: polymyositis, dermatomyositis, and inclusion body myositis. The latter is a chronic milder form and will not be discussed here. Both PM and DM are inflammatory, likely autoimmune, conditions that cause acute proximal symmetrical weakness and can affect bulbar and respiratory muscles. The former is a result of T-cell-mediated cytotoxicity, rarely as a stand-alone entity but mostly secondary to systemic autoimmune or connective tissue diseases and certain viral infections and as a paraneoplastic phenomenon. DM is an immune complex muscle and skin vasculitis. Dermatomyositis presents similarly to PM but has characteristic skin findings such as Gottron's papules and heliotropic rash (Fig. 38.2a, b). It is more commonly idiopathic but can be paraneoplastic for up to 15 % of cases. Diagnosis is made with EMG, creatine phosphokinase (CPK) (raised in PM), and muscle biopsy showing perivascular (DM) or intrafascicular inflammatory infiltrates. Autoantibodies anti-Jo1 and anti-Mi2 may be raised in these conditions. The treatment has three parts: (1) supportive measures as in all NMD with special attention to arrhythmias which are more common in myositides; (2) looking for neoplasms in dermatomyositis, we usually perform a surveillance CT of chest, abdomen, and pelvis, with fecal occult blood test and mammogram where indicated; and (3) we start the patient on prednisone and seek the assistance of a rheumatologist for long-term management of the immunosuppressive drugs [57–59].

Discharge Planning

Neuromuscular patients present a special set of challenges on discharge, and planning should occur early in the course of hospitalization. We encourage social work intervention in all such patients because the length of disease, the level of care, and the slow rate of recovery put inordinate financial, psychological, and relationship pressures on the sufferer and family. Most patients will require a period of rehabilitation. This is not only to provide a step-down environment for the patient to regain her confidence, but also to strengthen muscles as much as possible and improve quality of life. Vaccination should also be updated before the day of the discharge if no contraindications. There are several

Fig. 38.2 (**a**, **b**) Gottron's papules and heliotropic rash seen in dermatomyositis (Used with permission under the Creative Commons Attribution-Share Alike Unported License/ Wikipedia Common GNU License. From http:// dermatology.cdlib.org/1502/ reviews/photoessay)

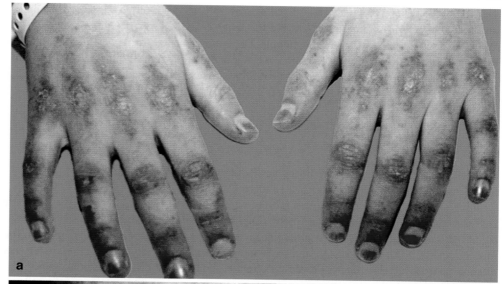

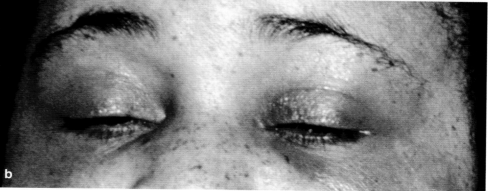

commonly encountered scenarios that require careful planning:

- *Chronic weakness with acute deterioration*: Apart from rehabilitation, several other issues should be taken into account. An estimate of the rate of recovery might encourage the placement of a permanent tracheostomy for control of secretion in anticipation of prolonged or permanent weakness of cough. Many patients with neuromuscular disease are also transitioned to nocturnal BiPAP, through a mask or tracheostomy, to mitigate nighttime hypoventilation. This may be discussed with the patient and the family, and follow-up arrangements made. An inpatient pulmonary consult is a good way to start. Finally, some patient will require transitional or permanent skilled nursing facility; this is decided after a period of rehabilitation [60]

- *Acute weakness with slow recovery*: GBS with denervation is the prototype of acute and severe weakness with slow recovery. The period of weakness often exceeds months. The use of step-down facilities that accept ventilated patients facilitates patient flow but often requires minimal ventilator settings and lower percentage of inspired oxygen. It is a good practice to be aware of the parameters acceptable to such facilities within the area.

- *Transition to permanent ventilation*: Invasive and noninvasive ventilator options are available. In chronic weakness which has progressed to a point where the conditions for discharge from ICU may not be reached, intermittent or chronic noninvasive ventilation may be an option, especially if the weakness is borderline. If weakness is profound, then ventilation through tracheostomy is an unsatisfactory alternative to end-of-life plans [61].

ICU-Acquired Weakness

It has long been noted that patients with multiorgan failure, sepsis, and prolonged ventilation develop neuromuscular dysfunction. The presence of changes to nerve and muscle function is almost universal in this patient population, but the data on incidence are variable and depend on the diagnostic threshold of severity and methods of diagnosis. Using the paradigm of polyneuropathy versus myopathy, we believe, is less useful in this condition. All relevant patients have degrees of concurrent myopathy and distal axonal polyneuropathy. The former is more pervasive but the latter is less reversible and determines long-term outcome. Depending on what element predominates, ICU-acquired weakness may be called critical illness polyneuropathy, critical illness myopathy, or critical illness polyneuromyopathy (CIPM).

Clinical Presentation

Patients with ICU-acquired neuromuscular disease come to the attention of the clinician usually when there is difficulty weaning off ventilation. Rarely, it may present with generalized weakness or quadriparesis in a conscious, often intubated, patient. Weakness is more pronounced in the lower limb compared to the upper limb and axial muscles and is often last to recover. Examination reveals a symmetrical flaccid quadriparesis. If the patient is sedated, then strength testing is likely to be difficult. Serial testing of representative groups of muscle may provide a good clinical correlate of pathology.

Electrophysiology

In the face of often unreliable neurological examination, electrophysiology plays an important role in the diagnosis of critical illness polyneuromyopathy. The nerve conduction study shows distal sensorimotor axonopathy with reduced compound muscle action potential and sensory action potential. The patient may have no evidence of demyelination. Evidence of denervation forebodes severe and refractory weakness. The pattern of muscle electrophysiology is a myopathic one with short low-amplitude polyphasic motor unit discharges. There is also early recruitment when the patient is awake enough for voluntary action [62, 63].

Diagnosis

The diagnosis of critical illness polyneuromyopathy is one of the exclusions as the clinical and electrophysiological features are not unique to this condition. In the case of failure to wean, the diagnosis is entertained as a differential. It is safe to say in all such cases CIPM is a contributing factor. In the case of the quadriparetic patient, other more ominous and potentially reversible causes need to be ruled out before a diagnosis of this entity is made. These investigations should include the central nervous system causes of quadriparesis. Muscle biopsy can be confirmatory and may show a predominantly type II muscle fiber pattern of atrophy, loss of thick filaments, loss of ATP staining, and in severe cases necrosis. Loss of myosin fibers is relatively specific to CIPM. Given the high morbidity of muscle biopsy, core biopsy may be used in conjunction with electrophoresis to ascertain the ratio of the thick to thin filaments. Some effort should be made on the part of neurophysiologist to distinguish the relative contributions of muscle and nerve to the weakness. This is of some practical value given that axonal neuropathy recovers poorly and slowly. The details of these techniques are outside the scope of this chapter.

Risk Factors

Several classic risk factors are identified for ICU-acquired weakness:
- Mechanical ventilation for more than 7 days
- Systemic inflammatory response syndromes, in particular when related to sepsis
- Multiorgan system failure [64]

Management

The approach to CIPM should take into account that there is no specific therapy for this condition. There are preventative measures which need to be taken, but these interventions occur prior to the making of diagnosis. The only real benefit in making a specific diagnosis is prognostication. This only becomes important in cases where this potentially reversible condition can prevent overly dire predictions for survival:
- Preventative measures: The only evidence-based intervention is intensive insulin therapy [65].
- Careful use of medication: The use of corticosteroids and neuromuscular blocking agents is associated with an increased risk of CIPM [66].
- Homeostatic measures: Careful correction of electrolytes especially magnesium, phosphate, and potassium. Adequate nutrition with adequate calories and protein intake.
- Other measures: Reduced sedation and early mobilization.
  In our ICU, we use standardized electrolyte and insulin protocols and emphasize early physiotherapy and nutrition. In high-risk patients, we avoid higher doses of steroids, neuromuscular blockers where possible, and begin weaning sedation as soon as clinically possible. We reserve the use of electrodiagnostics to patients with severe weakness.

Interpretation of Symptoms, Signs, and Testing

Symptoms
The main purpose of an NMD history is the establishment of the temporal evolution of symptoms and the order and location in which they first appeared. These symptoms include

weakness and sensory changes but also autonomic and behavioral changes.

Weakness

Weakness can present proximally or distally, locally or generally, and subacutely or chronically:

- Temporal characteristics:
  - *Age of onset*: Congenital and genetic disorders are more common in childhood and adolescence, paraneoplastic and ischemic events in old age, and autoimmune diseases in between (especially in women).
  - *Acuity*: Most neuromuscular diseases have a chronic or subacute mode of onset; an acute onset should alert one to the possibilities of an upper motor neuron disease such as a vascular event in the brain or the spinal cord. The exception is periodic paralysis which may start abruptly. Among the neuromuscular diseases, inflammatory and toxic causes typically present more rapidly than other etiologies.
  - *Time course*: The time from the onset to the nadir of strength might also help the neurologist decide between diagnoses. The time from the onset to the nadir of strength may distinguish between diagnoses (e.g., Guillain-Barre syndrome [GBS] versus chronic inflammatory demyelinating polyneuropathy [CIDP]).
  - *Recurrence and fluctuations*: Recurrent episodes of weakness can point to one of the periodic paralyses or – when associated with abdominal symptoms, seizures, and behavioral problems – to acute porphyrias. Myasthenia (gravis and congenital forms) and CIDP can also present with severe fluctuation which may mimic discrete recurrent episodes.
  - *Antecedents*: The use of medications that block neuromuscular junction, classically aminoglycosides, can worsen myasthenia. Guillain-Barre is commonly preceded by respiratory or GI symptoms. Mosquito bites and fevers can be features of West Nile virus infection. Tick bites can lead to Lyme disease or tick paralysis. Other infectious diseases have characteristic presentations also; for example, diphtheria is preceded by upper respiratory tract symptoms, whereas patients with tetanus have a history of exposure to anaerobic environments such as soil and rusty implements.
- Patterns of weakness:
  - Distribution:
  - *Neuropathic patterns of weakness*: Although motor or sensory patterns may predominate, they are often characterized by mixed deficits. In some acute neuropathies such as AIDP and porphyrias, the sensory symptoms may be subtle. Neuropathies commonly present in a single nerve, symmetrically or asymmetrically:
    - *Single nerve*: The affliction of a single nerve is unlikely to come to the attention of an intensivist,

the exception being phrenic neuropathy which commonly presents with orthopnea.
    - *Asymmetrical weakness*: This is seen in mononeuritis multiplex. The associated conditions are due to nerve damage secondary to a systemic disease such as metabolic or hemato-oncological disorders. Most of these etiologies are treatable. Plexopathies can also be asymmetrical but rarely present to the ICU. They can be seen in postoperative patients due to stretch on the plexuses in particular brachial plexus during, for example, thoracotomy.
    - *Symmetrical weakness*: Typically axonal neuropathies present in a length- and fiber size-dependent manner, i.e., they tend to affect smaller nerves at a distance from the spinal cord, so that they tend to affect the legs and small fibers first [6].
  - *Myopathic patterns of weakness*: Myopathic weakness is often symmetrical and proximal. It is not associated with sensory symptoms. The exceptions are myopathies affecting distal muscle or having predilection for particular muscle group. Also, some processes may cause neuropathy and myopathy together. Proximal weakness manifests itself with the patient having problems climbing stairs or getting out of a chair [67, 68].
- Fluctuations:
  - Relation to Exercise:
    - Fatigability: This is a characteristic of neuromuscular junction disease in particular myasthenia. Using muscles during the day causes worsening of weakness. This contrasts with chronic fatigue and functional causes where the weakness is often felt, not during the exertion, but the next few hours, where the patient seems to "pay a price" with fatigue.
    - Dynamic weakness: This is seen in some inherited metabolic myopathies where exercise can lead to myoglobulinuria and lactic acidosis.
    - Periodic paralysis: Some muscle channelopathies can have severe exacerbation of symptoms with exercise [67, 68].

Sensory Changes

Somatosensation in neuropathy:

- Positive symptoms: These mostly represent small fiber modalities: the feelings of pins and needles (dysesthesia), decreased pain threshold (hypoesthesia), and soreness to touch (allodynia) can be symptoms of small fiber neuropathies.
- Negative symptoms: The loss of pain and temperature and fine touch can be perceived as numbness. The loss of proprioception can be associated with loss of gait balance often preceding the presentation to the hospital.

Pain in myopathy:

- Other sensory changes are rare in myopathies.
- Muscle pain can distinguish between different kinds of myopathies: Infectious and ischemic myopathies are painful. Metabolic myopathies can present with exercise-induced discomfort.
- Back pain is seen in myelopathic and compressive radiculopathies. These are not detailed in this chapter but are important differential diagnoses for neuromuscular disease. However, the presence of pain does not rule out the presence of NMD, as back pain can be a feature of Guillain-Barre syndrome and some kinds of diabetic neuropathy.
- Certain neuropathies are more prone to be associated with pain. These are most common in systemic and metabolic diseases such as connective tissue diseases, diabetes, hemato-oncological disorders, renal failure, nutritional deficiencies, and toxic neuropathy.

Autonomic and Other Symptoms

The presence of autonomic symptoms may be subtle and include excessive sweating, diarrhea, impotence, pupillary abnormalities, and urinary retention. From the point of view of the neurointensivist, the most important symptoms are those that are associated with cardiovascular instability. Syncope and presyncope are ominous symptoms as are palpitations and episodes of high or low pulse rate.

Some motor neuron disease is associated with behavioral and cognitive changes. Frontotemporal dementia is associated with amyotrophic lateral sclerosis (ALS). Acute porphyria is also associated with bizarre behaviors. Most importantly, the presence of confusion and acute onset of weakness should encourage brain imaging.

Cardiorespiratory Considerations

Ultimately, the neurointensivist is interested in the stability of respiration, circulation, and airway protection. The interviewer should direct part of the interview to the functional aspect of the disease, i.e., having established the impairment, one should ascertain the handicap in terms of mobility but most importantly shortness of breath, episodes of presyncope, and coughing while swallowing.

Other History

Past medical history and review of systems should be reviewed in detail with regard to:

- *Primary neuromuscular diseases*: The patients presenting with acute respiratory disease superimposed on chronic weakness are likely to have previous testing and even a diagnosis. When not available from patient and family, outside medical records must be sought to ascertain testing already done by outside institutions.

- *Secondary neuromuscular diseases*: Effort should be made to detail previous medical history especially history of endocrinopathies especially diabetes and thyroid disease, autoimmune disease and vasculitis, chronic infections such as hepatitis C, and hematological disorders in particular porphyria. Review of systems should include inquiries regarding dryness of mouth and rashes, photosensitivity, and rashes.

It is imperative to review all medication in the patient's history with regard to:

- *Medications that cause myopathy*: The prototypic medications causing myopathy are statins and steroids. These are usually not a cause of de novo respiratory failure but can compound weakness or delay weaning. Medications used in rheumatological conditions can rarely cause myopathies: antimalarials, colchicine, and penicillamine can cause myositis and other myopathies. Antivirals including HAART drugs and interferon therapy can cause myotoxicity [6].
- *Medications that cause neuromuscular junction blockade*: Many drugs should be used with caution in patient with neuromuscular junction disease. Classically class 1 antiarrhythmics, aminoglycosides, and lincosamide antibiotics (e.g., gentamicin, amikacin, tobramycin, clindamycin, and lincomycin) and botulinum toxin are contraindicated. The use of neuromuscular blocking medications should be done with extreme cautiousness in the critically weak patient [69, 70].
- *Medications that cause neuropathy*: Medications such as chemotherapeutics (platinum drugs and taxoids), amiodarone, and HIV medications can cause neuropathies, but these are typically small fiber in presentation and do not cause critical weakness [69, 70].

Social history is another aspect that is essential to a thorough review with regard to:

- *Occupational and exposure history*: Heavy metals often as environmental contaminants cause chronic neuropathies. Thallium used in hair removal products and rat poison can produce an acute syndrome with weakness and encephalopathy. Critical weakness can also be cause by acetylcholinesterase inhibitors found in pesticides.
- *Social habits*: Alcohol can cause an acute as well as chronic myopathy. Cocaine can cause muscle necrosis via a vasospastic ischemic mechanism. Nutritional history can also be valuable as an exacerbating factor in severe neuromuscular disease.

Signs
Vital Signs and Cardiorespiratory Examination
Airway

An intricate balance separates the sterile lower respiratory tract and the bacteriologically rich alimentary tract. Bulbar muscles, those arising from the pharyngeal arches, may be affected by NMD. This manifests as tongue weakness, dysphagia, dysarthria, retained secretion, masticatory weakness, facial paresis, and nasal voice. Additionally alertness is required for normal swallowing function, and the important protective mechanism of cough relies on expiratory strength.

Breathing

The main function of respiration is to oxygenate the blood and maintain normal physiological pH. It achieves this by matching two separate but complementary processes: ventilation and perfusion. The latter is the distribution of blood to capillary beds to allow the greatest area of exchange possible. Ventilation is the process of moving air into and out of the lungs to optimize the pickup of oxygen and expulsion of carbon dioxide. For this to occur, volumes of air are cycled through the lung, driven by respiratory muscles. There are three sets of respiratory muscles in humans:

- Inspiratory muscles: These are muscles which are the main drivers of respiration as expiration in most circumstances represents a passive process employing the recoil of the lung and thoracic wall. The most important of these muscles is the diaphragm, which is responsible for the bulk of inspiratory effort, with contributions from intercostals, parasternal muscles, and accessory muscles mainly trapezius and sternocleidomastoid. Weakness of inspiratory muscles causes a reduction in vital capacity and total lung capacity. One way to assess the total inspiratory function is to measure maximal negative inspiratory pressure at the mouth. Another way is to measure nasal pressure during a sniff test [15].
- Expiratory muscles: Abdominal muscles with help from intercostal muscles aid the expulsion of air during expiration. During normal respiration, expiration is achieved passively through the recoil of the elastic tissues in the lungs and the chest wall. Expiratory muscles are used during hyperventilation and to achieve high enough expiratory pressures for coughing. The latter is an essential mechanism for airway protection. Weakness of these muscles leads to increased residual volume and reduced expiratory pressure [19].
- Bulbar muscles: Both the respiratory and alimentary tracts embryologically arise from foregut and as such share many anatomical structures. In order to keep the sterile lungs safe from the microbiologically rich gastrointestinal tract, elaborate bulbar mechanisms are required for airway protection. Weakness of bulbar muscles can lead to aspiration both during deglutition but also with reflux and normal physiological salivation. Recurrent aspiration can lead to fibrosis and changes in lung compliance in chronic NMDs.

Circulation

Autonomic instability may be suspected in the presence of a percussible bladder, abnormal sweating, presence of postural symptoms, and blood pressure and pulse rate variability. These change periodically but the beat-to-beat variation is in fact reduced. In the presence of respiratory distress, there is an exaggeration of the physiological beat-to-beat R-R interval, the so-called sinus arrhythmia. In the presence of autonomic dysfunction, this response is blunted, and the experienced clinician may discern this from an EKG tracing or by examination of the pulse [71].

Neurological Signs

Cranial Nerve Examination

Several infectious causes of weakness may be associated with cranial nerve signs, in particular Lyme disease, diphtheria, and tetanus. They are also seen in botulism, hypothyroidism, certain paraneoplastic conditions, and botulism. Occasionally, AIDP can present with cranial nerve symptoms. Optic neuropathies are seen in hereditary and toxic causes of weakness including arsenic, lead, and lysosomal storage diseases. Thallium toxicity can affect all cranial nerves.

Sensory Examination

The main aim of the sensory examination is to determine the following:

- *Distribution*: Proximal versus distal as well as symmetrical versus asymmetrical. The significance of these is explained under symptoms.
- *Modality*: Pinprick and temperature are small fiber modalities, whereas position sense and vibration are mediated by large neural fibers.
- *Sensory level*: The presence of a sensory level should alert one of a spinal process rather than a neuromuscular condition.

Motor and Reflex Examination

The motor examination is directed towards three aims:

- *Distribution of weakness and atrophy*: Proximal versus distal as well as symmetrical versus asymmetrical. The significance of these is explained under symptoms.
- *Upper motor neuron* versus *lower motor neuron lesions*: The difference between the upper motor neuron disease and lower motor neuron disease is important in determining localization and etiology:
  - Upper motor neuron (UMN) disease is characterized by the presence of increased tone and brisk reflexes. Hypertonus may be spastic or rigid. Spasticity is a velocity-dependent resistance to passive movement and marks an increase in the myotatic reflex. It is often associated with brisk reflexes and is due to loss of descending upper motor neuron influences. This is also the mechanism underlying increased reflexes and clonus. Spasticity is associated with the clasp-knife phenomenon when the tone gives way at the end of the

range of movement due to the activation of Golgi organ. The differentials are rigidity – a velocity-independent increase in tone with or without supervening cog wheeling seen in extrapyramidal conditions – and paratonia where involuntary variable resistance is supplied by a patient who commonly suffers from a dementing process. Babinski response accompanies UMN lesions.

- Lower motor neuron (LMN) disease is characterized by a decrease in tone and less brisk reflexes. Flaccid paresis results from the disruption of either the afferent or efferent limb of the myotatic reflex. The differentials include mitgehen (and mitmachen) that is the involuntary facilitation of movement of joint performed by the examiner. It is also seen mostly in demented patients.

- Mixed signs: The presence of both upper and lower motor signs can be seen in multifocal nervous system conditions, myelopathies, and motor neuron diseases. Spinal cord syndromes have characteristic findings which distinguish them from the motor neuron diseases.

Presence of Abnormal Movements

Muscle twitches come in many flavors in neuromuscular disease. Fasciculations are the result of denervation of muscles and are asynchronous muscle twitches, which commonly do not result in movement at the joint. They are seen physiologically after exercise, for example, but also in motoneuron disease and some neuropathies. Myokymia shows a greater degree of organization than fasciculation and resembles "a bag of worms" under the skin. It is seen with CNS disease and in response to radiation injury. It is also seen in conditions associated with neuromyotonia which results in stiffness and apparent myotonia. It can occur in toxic and autoimmune diseases. Myotonia is the muscle's inability to relax after voluntary contraction. Percussion myotonia, commonly elicited in the tongue and thenar eminence, is a transient increase in muscle tone in response to percussion. Pseudoathetosis and "moving toes" can occur in response to loss of position sense. Neuropathic tremor can resemble orthostatic tremor. Muscle cramps are painful muscle contractions which are seen in motor neuron disease and myopathies [6, 67].

Test Results
Laboratory Testing
CPK

Creatine phosphokinase is an enzyme which converts creatine to phosphocreatine. The latter is a ready and rapid source of energy in tissues that consume ATP rapidly. CK has the highest concentration in the muscle, and a raised CK is a sign of muscle damage, be it in the heart or the musculoskeletal system. Many myopathies are associated with increased CK levels while others are not. CK in conjunction with EMG provides important diagnostic information to a trained neuromuscular neurologist. CK can also be used as a marker of ongoing muscle damage in myopathic processes.

Routine Testing (CMP, CBC with Differential, B12, Folate, HbA1c, RPR, and TSH)

Several of the muscle channelopathies present with paroxysmal weakness. Out of all such genetic myopathies, only periodic hypokalemic paralysis is likely to be severe enough to require ICU attention. In such patients, during the attack, the potassium level is low. Rhabdomyolysis can cause kidney failure. A raised creatinine may complicate the interpretation of CPK results. Changes in potassium, phosphate, and calcium can also cause weakness. Baseline cell counts are important because many of the specific treatments used in neuromuscular diseases affect the bone marrow. Concomitant vitamin deficiencies and tertiary syphilis can complicate the clinical picture. Thyrotoxicosis could be the cause of profound weakness in hyperthyroid periodic paralysis and less plausibly in hyperthyroid myopathy.

Autoimmune and Hematological Testing (UPEP, SPEP, IFE, ESR, CRP, RF, ANA, and ANCA)

Plasma dyscrasias can lead to severe and progressive weakness, sometimes leading to death. The presence of plasma dyscrasias may be subtle and absent from the plasma electrophoresis. Small-chain gammopathies present in the urine as they are easily excreted and do not accumulate in the urine. Immunoelectrophoresis is used either when the suspicion is very high or there is a positive finding on the UPEP and SPEP. Rarely even the IFE is negative in a case of gammopathy and a lambda/kappa ratio may be needed. POEMS is rare enough for us to stop at IFE if SPEP and UPEP are negative. General inflammatory workup, as well as ANA and RF, are nonspecific but may point to a connective tissue or vasculitis process requiring further testing. ANA is raised in more than half of patients with myositis. ANCA is raised in vasculitis: in Churg-Strauss, for example, mononeuritis multiplex may progress to polyneuropathy. The presence of concomitant respiratory difficulties may erroneously lead the clinician to diagnose respiratory muscle weakness. A positive ANCA is often followed by more specific testing such as evaluating the presence of antibodies raised against PR3 or MPO [72, 73].

CSF Testing (Protein, Glucose, Cell Count, Oligoclonal Band, Serology Based on Clinical Suspicion)

A clear CSF is reassuring to a neurologist, but specifically the presence of oligoclonal bands can confirm GBS. We also rule out infections, in particular tertiary syphilis in our patients by performing VDRL on the CSF. Given the difficulty with which CSF samples are obtained, when compared to serum, for example, we recommend sending for other routine tests including cultures and HSV PCR. In suspected cases of polio, serology for HTLV-1 and poliovirus should be done. It is prudent to take out additional CSF and freeze it, in case other tests may be required in the future.

Demyelination-Related Testing

The antiganglioside antibodies are more of a scientific curiosity than useful clinical tools. Anti-GM1 and GD1 are more common in the "axonal" forms of GBS. The only situations in which we have used them in the past have been in cases of early GBS presenting with predominantly bulbar symptoms. Anti-GQ1b is seen in Miller-Fischer syndrome and in GBS affecting the eye muscles. Serological testing for HIV, CMV, HSV, mycoplasma pneumonia, and campylobacter (also fecal cultures) is also of academic interest, but, in our experience, adds little to the management of GBS and related disorders [72, 73].

Neuromuscular Junction-Related Testing
(Anti-AChR, Anti-MuSK, Anti-P/Q Calcium Channel)

Serology and repetitive muscle stimulation studies are key to the diagnosis of autoimmune neuromuscular diseases. Antibodies against the acetylcholine receptor are a sensitive test for the diagnosis of myasthenia gravis. Most of the "seronegative" MG cases are anti-MuSK positive but usually have more limited anatomical distribution and are less likely to cause generalized weakness. Antibodies against voltage-gated calcium channels are used as confirmatory tests in cases of Lambert-Eaton myasthenic syndrome [72, 73].

Respiratory Testing

Lung Function Test

The first step in providing proficient care is to assess the degree of decompensation caused by neuromuscular disease. Like all muscle testing, the strength of respiratory musculature is tested by probing its function. Pulmonary function testing is a dynamic study of lung volumes and flows. As a general rule of thumb, ventilatory failure is reflected in inspiratory weakness and a pattern of pulmonary restriction; and loss of adequate cough reflex is indicated by poor maximal expiratory force. In a restrictive pattern of weakness, both forced expiratory volume in one second (FEV_1) and forced vital capacity (FVC) are reduced, though the ratio often remains the same or may be increased. FVC measured in the supine position should be no more than 10 % reduced compared to erect readings. Greater reductions are seen in diaphragmatic dysfunction. Maximal voluntary ventilation, maximal inspiratory pressure, and maximal expiratory pressures are all reduced. The first of these measurements correlates with the degree of respiratory failure; MIP reflects diaphragmatic weakness and MEP correlates with expiratory force and the strength of a patient's cough. Diffusing capacity

for carbon monoxide (DLCO) is normal in acute neuromuscular function, but with chronic muscle weakness and coexistent recurrent aspiration, the DLCO may be increased. In the presence of significant bulbar dysfunction, limitations of respiratory testing are related to the ability of the patient to form an adequate seal around the mouthpiece. In this patient population, sniff nasal inspiratory pressure offers a good alternative.

Blood Gases

Blood gases divide respiratory failure into two types:

- *Hypoxemic respiratory failure* ($PaO_2 < 60$ mmHg), which is caused by shunting and V/Q mismatch; the etiologies include alveolar failure due to edema, infection, interstitial disease, or pulmonary disease. These can be seen as complication of NMD.
- Hypercarbic respiratory failure ($PaCO_2 > 45$ mmHg), which is caused by ventilator failure including in NMD. There are various ways to ascertain the chronicity of the perturbation which are beyond the scope of this chapter.

Sniff Test

The sniff test is rarely required except in the case of suspected diaphragmatic paresis.

Imaging

Imaging is commonly performed on patients who present with weakness often inappropriately. In the presence of stroke-like symptoms such as hemiparesis, neglect, or language deficits, brain imaging will be required. If there is a sensory level or loss of bowel and bladder function, then spinal imaging is indicated. Imaging of muscle is not usually indicated in acute weakness but may be useful in chronic weakness.

Neurophysiology

Understanding the rudiments of clinical neurophysiology will not enable the nonspecialist to interpret the test, but it may be useful in having a better understanding of an EMG/NCV report. Given the limitations of space here, we are offering the most superficial glance at neurophysiological testing in the following section.

EMG

Needle electromyography records the electrical activity of muscle at rest and during contraction. This activity is both displayed visually and transduced into sound. The muscle is probed initially in the resting state. Except at the neuromuscular junction, a resting muscle should be electrically silent. Spontaneous activity in a resting muscle is a sign of pathology. When it pertains to muscle fibers, as in fibrillation, for example, it points to denervation (although not acutely) or an inflammatory myopathy. In the case of fasciculation where the motor units fire spontaneously, suspicion for motor neuron disease is raised. A particular pattern of spontaneous firing, the sound of which has been compared to the sound of a vintage dive bomber, is seen in myotonic disorders and rarely polymyositis. The electromyography typically shows progressive recruitment. Physiologically smaller motor units are recruited first, and as effort is increased, larger units are activated. At maximal effort, these potentials are summated into an interference pattern, where individual motor unit potentials can no longer be distinguished. In myopathies, the individual motor unit potentials are smaller and more units are recruited for a given degree of effort. In contrast in neuropathic conditions, the degree of recruitment is decreased with denervation. With reinnervation, a single nerve may subserve a larger number of muscle fibers than initially, so that the motor unit potentially may become larger. Certain conditions have characteristic patterns on testing including myokymia seen in plexus injury, for example. Myokymia clinically looks like a bag of worms under the skin and on the speaker sounds like soldiers marching in unison.

Nerve Conduction Studies

Conduction velocity of nerves can be measured by looking at nerve response at several points along its length, after stimulating its motor component. The compound muscle action potential is recorded and compared to normalized values. Sensory recordings are of more limited in utility and are best utilized in localizing the neuropathic lesion proximal or distal to the dorsal root ganglion. Nerve conduction studies are used for localization and for determining the extent of deficit. They can also suggest underlying pathology. In acquired demyelinating disease, there is a dispersion (spreading out) of the CMAP and a delay. There can be conduction blocks. In axonal neuropathies, the amplitude of the CMAP is decreased without any slowing or dispersion.

H-Reflex and F-Wave Studies

H-reflex is the electrophysiological correlate of the ankle reflex. The tibial nerve is stimulated, and the response in the soleus muscle is recorded. F-waves are obtained by antidromically stimulating motor nerves to activate the anterior horn. The cells in the anterior horn then fire off an orthodromic signal which is then recoded. This test is often used to confirm Guillain-Barre where the F-wave is slowed or absent.

Muscle Response to Repetitive Nerve Stimulation and Single-Fiber Electromyography

Repetitive muscle stimulation is used to probe the function of the neuromuscular junction. In normal muscle, repetitive supramaximal electrical stimulation after half a minute of sustained contraction elicits the same magnitude of response. In myasthenia gravis when the muscle is stimulated at

2–5 Hz, there is a decremental response to repeat stimulus. In presynaptic pathologies notably Eaton-Lambert myasthenic syndrome and botulism, repeated stimulation at 10 Hz leads to increments in the muscle activity. Single-fiber electromyography is a more sensitive test of myasthenia gravis. The time delay between the discharges of two muscle fibers within a motor unit is averaged. This quantity, termed neuromuscular jitter, is increased in neuromuscular disorders [74].

Tissue Testing

Nerve Biopsy

The sural nerve is biopsied in the investigation of neuropathies. This is rarely needed in acute weakness.

Muscle Biopsy

Muscle biopsy, along with CPK and EMG, provides the third important pillar of muscle diagnostics. In acute weakness, given that the differential is more limited, the incidence of biopsy may be less than is the case in the clinic. Several conditions, notably the myositides, are best diagnosed histopathologically.

Other Tissue Biopsy

Examples of other tissue testing would be, for example, lymph nodes in the case of lymphoma or sarcoidosis.

Genetic Testing

Genetic testing may be appropriate for diagnosis of hereditary causes of motor weakness, but the results will rarely be available or useful in the cases of acute weakness.

References

1. Logan LR. Rehabilitation techniques to maximize spasticity management. Top Stroke Rehabil. 2011;18(3):203–11.
2. Campbell WW. DeJong's the neurologic examination. Philadelphia: Lippincott Williams & Wilkins; 2005.
3. Walker HK. The plantar reflex. In: Walker HK, Hall WD, Hurst JW, editors. Clinical methods: the history, physical, and laboratory examinations. 3rd ed. Boston: Butterworths; 1990, Chapter 73.
4. Barohn RJ. Approach to peripheral neuropathy and neuronopathy. Semin Neurol. 1998;18(1):7–18.
5. England JD, Asbury AK. Peripheral neuropathy. Lancet. 2004;363:2151.
6. Ropper AH, Samuels MA. Chapter 46. Diseases of the peripheral nerves. In: Ropper AH, Samuels MA, editors. Adams and Victor's principles of neurology, 9e. 2009. http://www.accessmedicine.com/content.aspx?aID=3641268.
7. Amato AA, Russell JA. Neuromuscular disorders. New York: McGraw-Hill; 2008.
8. Engel AG, Franzini-Armstrong C, editors. Myology. 3rd ed. New York: McGraw-Hill; 2004.
9. Smith EC, El-Gharbawy A, Koeberl DD. Metabolic myopathies: clinical features and diagnostic approach. Rheum Dis Clin North Am. 2011;37(2):201–17, vi.

10. Amato AA, Griggs RC. Overview of the muscular dystrophies. Handb Clin Neurol. 2011;101:1–9.

11. Ashizawa T, Sarkar PS. Myotonic dystrophy types 1 and 2. Handb Clin Neurol. 2011;101:193–237.

12. Meininger V. ALS, what new 144 years after Charcot? Arch Ital Biol. 2011;149(1):29–37.

13. Alexopoulos H, Dalakas MC. A critical update on the immunopathogenesis of Stiff Person Syndrome. Eur J Clin Invest. 2010;40(11):1018–25.

14. Reisner-Sénélar L. The birth of intensive care medicine: Björn Ibsen's records. Intensive Care Med. 2011;37(7):1084–6.

15. Wilcox PG, Pardy RL. Diaphragmatic weakness and paralysis. Lung. 1989;167(6):323–41. Review.

16. Ali SS, O'Connell C, Kass L, Graff G. Single-breath counting: a pilot study of a novel technique for measuring pulmonary function in children. Am J Emerg Med. 2011;29(1):33–6.

17. Guarantors of Brain. Aids to the examination of the peripheral nervous system. 2nd ed. London: Baillière-Tindall; 1986.

18. Sharshar T, Chevret S, Bourdain F, et al. Early predictors of mechanical ventilation in Guillain-Barré syndrome. Crit Care Med. 2003;31:278.

19. Mehta S. Neuromuscular disease causing acute respiratory failure. Respir Care. 2006;51:1016.

20. Severinghaus JW, Astrup P, Murray JF. Blood gas analysis and critical care medicine. Am J Respir Crit Care Med. 1998;157 (4 Pt 2):S114–22.

21. Vianello A, Bevilacqua M, Arcaro G, et al. Non-invasive ventilatory approach to treatment of acute respiratory failure in neuromuscular disorders. A comparison with endotracheal intubation. Intensive Care Med. 2000;26:384.

22. Nguyen TN, Badjatia N, Malhotra A, et al. Factors predicting extubation success in patients with Guillain-Barré syndrome. Neurocrit Care. 2006;5:230.

23. Rabinstein AA, Mueller-Kronast N. Risk of extubation failure in patients with myasthenic crisis. Neurocrit Care. 2005;3:213.

24. Reid C. Frequency of under- and overfeeding in mechanically ventilated ICU patients: causes and possible consequences. J Hum Nutr Diet. 2006;19(1):13–22.

25. Marik PE, Zaloga GP. Early enteral nutrition in acutely ill patients: a systematic review. Crit Care Med. 2002;29(12):2264–70. Review. Erratum in: Crit Care Med. 2002;30(3):725.

26. Sud S, Mittmann N, Cook DJ, Geerts W, Chan B, Dodek P, Gould MK, Guyatt G, Arabi Y, Fowler RA, E-PROTECT Investigators and the Canadian Critical Care Trials Group. Screening and prevention of venous thromboembolism in critically ill patients: a decision analysis and economic evaluation. Am J Respir Crit Care Med. 2011;184(11):1289–98.

27. Zochodne DW. Autonomic involvement in Guillain-Barré syndrome: a review. Muscle Nerve. 1994;17:1145–55.

28. Neroutsos E, et al. Guillain-Barre syndrome and mood disorders. Ann Gen Psychiatry. 2010;9 Suppl 1:S204.

29. Sejvar JJ. West Nile virus and "poliomyelitis". Neurology. 2004;63(2):206–7.

30. Gorson KC, Ropper AH. Nonpoliovirus poliomyelitis simulating Guillain-Barré syndrome. Arch Neurol. 2001;58(9):1460–4.

31. Corrales-Medina VF, Shandera WX. Chapter 32. Viral and Rickettsial infections. In: McPhee SJ, Papadakis MA, editors. Current medical diagnosis and treatment. 2011. http://www.accessmedicine.com/content.aspx?aID=17051.

32. Winer JB. Guillain Barré syndrome. Mol Pathol. 2001;54(6):381–5.

33. Ropper AH, Wijdicks EFM, Truax BT. Guillain-Barré syndrome. Philadelphia: Davis; 1991.

34. Ropper AH. Intensive care of acute Guillain-Barré syndrome. Can J Neurol Sci. 1994;21:S23.

35. Hadden RD, Cornblath DR, Hughes RA, Zielasek J, Hartung HP, Toyka KV, et al. Electrophysiological classification of Guillain-Barré syndrome: clinical associations and outcome. Plasma Exchange/Sandoglobulin Guillain-Barré Syndrome Trial Group. Ann Neurol. 1998;44(5):780–8.

36. Triggs WJ, Cros D, Gominak SC, Zuniga G, Beric A, Shahani BT, Ropper AH, Roongta SM. Motor nerve inexcitability in Guillain-Barré syndrome. The spectrum of distal conduction block and axonal degeneration. Brain. 1992;115:11–302.

37. Cros D, Triggs WJ. There are no neurophysiologic features characteristic of "axonal" Guillain-Barré syndrome. Muscle Nerve. 1994;17(6):675–7.

38. Guillain-Barré Syndrome Study Group. Plasmapheresis and acute Guillain-Barré syndrome. Neurology. 1985;35:1096–104.

39. Plasma Exchange/Sandoglobulin Guillain-Barré Syndrome Trial Group. Randomised trial of plasma exchange, intravenous immunoglobulin, and combined treatments in Guillain-Barré syndrome. Lancet. 1997;349(9047):225–30.

40. van der Meché FG, Schmitz PI. A randomized trial comparing intravenous immune globulin and plasma exchange in Guillain-Barré syndrome. Dutch Guillain-Barré Study Group. N Engl J Med. 1992;326(17):1123–9.

41. Meyer UA, Schuurmans MM, Lindberg RL. Acute porphyrias: pathogenesis of neurological manifestations. Semin Liver Dis. 1998;18(1):43–52.

42. Kauppinen R. Porphyrias. Lancet. 2005;365(9455):241–52.

43. Engel AG. Acquired autoimmune myasthenia gravis. In: Engel AG, Franzini-Armstrong C, editors. Myology: basic and clinical. 2nd ed. New York: McGraw-Hill; 1994. p. 1769–97.

44. Thomas CS, Mayer SA, Gungor Y, et al. Myasthenic crisis: clinical features, mortality, complications and risk factors for prolonged mechanical ventilation. Neurology. 1997;48:1253–60.

45. Lisak RP. Myasthenia gravis. Curr Treat Options Neurol. 1999;1(3):239–50.

46. Takanami I, Abiko T, Koizumi S. Therapeutic outcomes in thymectomied patients with myasthenia gravis. Ann Thorac Cardiovasc Surg. 2009;15(6):373–7.

47. Wirtz PW, Sotodeh M, Nijnuis M, Van Doorn PA, Van Engelen BG, Hintzen RQ, et al. Difference in distribution of muscle weakness between myasthenia gravis and the Lambert-Eaton myasthenic syndrome. J Neurol Neurosurg Psychiatry. 2002;73(6):766–8.

48. Keogh M, Sedehizadeh S, Maddison P. Treatment for Lambert-Eaton myasthenic syndrome. Cochrane Database Syst Rev. 2011;(2):CD003279.

49. Shapiro RL, Hatheway C, Swerdlow DL. Botulism in the United States: a clinical and epidemiologic review. Ann Intern Med. 1998;129(3):221–8.

50. Cherington M. Botulism: update and review. Semin Neurol. 2004;24(2):155–63.

51. Diaz JH. A 60-year meta-analysis of tick paralysis in the United States: a predictable, preventable, and often misdiagnosed poisoning. J Med Toxicol. 2010;6(1):15–21.

52. Isbister GK, Kiernan MC. Neurotoxic marine poisoning. Lancet Neurol. 2005;4(4):219–28.

53. Bishai WR, Murphy JR. Chapter 138. Diphtheria and other infections caused by corynebacteria and related species. In: Fauci AS, Braunwald E, Kasper DL, Hauser SL, Longo DL, Jameson JL, Loscalzo J, editors. Harrison's principles of internal medicine, 18e. 2011. http://www.accessmedicine.com/content.aspx?aID=9120730.

54. Bleck TP. Clostridium tetani. In: Mandell GL, Bennett JE, Dolin R, editors. Bennett's principles and practice of infectious diseases. Philadelphia: Churchill Livingstone; 1995. p. 2373–8.

55. Venance SL, Cannon SC, Fialho D, et al. The primary periodic paralyses: diagnosis, pathogenesis and treatment. Brain. 2006;129(Pt 1):8–17.

56. Levitt JO. Practical aspects in the management of hypokalemic periodic paralysis. J Transl Med. 2008;6:18.

57. Amato AA, Barohn RJ. Evaluation and treatment of inflammatory myopathies. J Neurol Neurosurg Psychiatry. 2009;80(10):1060–8.

58. Hengstman GJ, van den Hoogen FH, van Engelen BG. Treatment of the inflammatory myopathies: update and practical recommendations. Expert Opin Pharmacother. 2009;10(7):1183–90.

59. Marinelli WA, Leatherman JW. Neuromuscular disorders in the intensive care unit. Crit Care Clin. 2002;18(4):915–29.

60. Annane D, Chevrolet JC, Chevret S, Raphael JC. Nocturnal mechanical ventilation for chronic hypoventilation in patients with neuromuscular and chest wall disorders. Cochrane Database Syst Rev. 2007;(4):CD001941. PubMed: 10796839.

61. Bourke SC, Tomlinson M, Williams TL, et al. Effects of non-invasive ventilation on survival and quality of life in patients with amyotrophic lateral sclerosis: a randomised controlled trial. Lancet Neurol. 2006;5:140.

62. Lacomis D, Zochodne DW, Bird SJ. Critical illness myopathy. Muscle Nerve. 2000;23:1785–8.

63. Latronico N, Peli E, Botteri M. Critical illness myopathy and neuropathy. Curr Opin Crit Care. 2005;11:126–32.

64. de Letter MA, Schmitz PI, Visser LH, et al. Risk factors for the development of polyneuropathy and myopathy in critically ill patients. Crit Care Med. 2001;29:2281–6.

65. Van den Berghe G, Wilmer A, Hermans G, et al. Intensive insulin therapy in the medical ICU. N Engl J Med. 2006;354:449–61.

66. Rouleau G, Karpati G, Carpenter S, et al. Glucocorticoid excess induces preferential depletion of myosin in denervated skeletal muscle fibers. Muscle Nerve. 1987;10:428–38.

67. Ropper AH, Samuels MA. Chapter 48. Principles of clinical myology: diagnosis and classification of diseases of muscle and neuromuscular junction. In: Ropper AH, Samuels MA, editors. Adams and Victor's principles of neurology, 9e. 2009. http://www.accessmedicine.com/content.aspx?aID=3642131.

68. DiMauro S, Tonin P, Servidei S. Metabolic myopathies. In: Vinken PJ, Bruyn GW, editors. Handbook of clinical neurology, vol. 18. Amsterdam: North Holland; 1992. p. 479–526.

69. Ahmed A, Simmons A. Drugs which may exacerbate or induce myasthenia gravis: a clinician's guide. Int J Neurol. 2009; 10(2):11.

70. Olesen LL, Jensen TS. Prevention and management of drug-induced peripheral neuropathy. Drug Saf. 1991;6(4):302–14. PubMed: 1653573.

71. Goldberger JJ, Challapalli S, Tung R, Parker MA, Kadish AH. Relationship of heart rate variability to parasympathetic effect. Circulation. 2001;103(15):1977–83.

72. Czaplinski A, Steck AJ. Antibody testing in peripheral neuropathies: a critical approach. Schweizer Archiv für Neurologie und Psychiatrie. 1985 (A. 2002);153(7):301–7.

73. Agius MA, Richman DP, Vincent A. Myasthenia gravis and related disorders. In: Autoantibody testing in the diagnosis and management of autoimmune disorders of neuromuscular transmission and related diseases. Davis: Humana Press; 2009. p. 143–56.

74. Ropper AH, Samuels MA. Chapter 45. Electrophysiologic and laboratory aids in the diagnosis of neuromuscular disease. In: Ropper AH, Samuels MA, editors. Adams and Victor's principles of neurology, 9e. 2009. http://www.accessmedicine.com/content.aspx?aID=3641085.

Seizures

39

Robin L. Gilmore, Jean E. Cibula, Stephan Eisenschenk, and Steven N. Roper

Contents

R.L. Gilmore, MD
Department of Neurology, Maury Regional Medical Center,
927 N. James Campbell Blvd,
Columbia, TN 38401, USA
e-mail: gilmore2003@bellsouth.net

J.E. Cibula, MD
Department of Neurology, University of Florida College of Medicine,
Gainesville, FL 32611, USA
e-mail: jean.cibula@neurology.ufl.edu

S. Eisenschenk, MD (✉)
Department of Neurology, University of Florida College of Medicine,
1149 Newell Drive, Gainesville, FL 32611, USA
e-mail: stephan.eisenschenk@neurology.ufl.edu

S.N. Roper, MD
Department of Neurological Surgery,
University of Florida College of Medicine,
100 South Newell Drive, Gainesville, FL 32610, USA
e-mail: roper@neurosurgery.ufl.edu

Abstract

Prompt recognition of seizures and status epilepticus depends on maintaining a high degree of suspicion; early treatment is important. Seizures are a frequent occurrence in the neuro-ICU and may be reactive or secondary to another condition. We review the basic recognition and treatment of seizures and their differential diagnosis. Nonconvulsive status epilepticus should be suspected in patients with unexplained alteration of consciousness or coma. Consultation with a neurologist or epileptologist is recommended.

Keywords

Nonconvulsive status epilepticus • Status epilepticus • Seizures • Epilepsy • Alteration of consciousness • Coma • EEG/electroencephalography • Anticonvulsant medication

Introduction

Because seizures are a symptom of central nervous system dysfunction, seizures are frequently encountered in the critically ill patient in the neuro-ICU. Yet seizures may be so subtle as to be unrecognized or so dramatic as to shake the patient's bed and instrumentation. The first difficulty, then, is the identification of seizures. When a patient has an unexpected or unexplained change in level of consciousness, always consider the possibilities of brief sporadic seizures or

A.J. Layon et al. (eds.), *Textbook of Neurointensive Care*,
DOI 10.1007/978-1-4471-5226-2_39, © Springer-Verlag London 2013

nonconvulsive status epilepticus. Since seizures are a symptom of central nervous system dysfunction, the possibility of seizure should always be considered even when other conditions such as masses, bleeds, and vasospasm are "ruled in." In the neurologic intensive care unit, up to 34 % of patients undergoing EEG monitoring have nonconvulsive seizures, and 76 % of these cases are nonconvulsive status epilepticus [1]. In addition 8 % of comatose patients have nonconvulsive seizures [2].

How to Suspect Seizures

One must have a high index of suspicion in order to identify seizures in the ICU. For patients with persistent mental status changes, there may be no or minimal examination findings to identify underlying seizures. This is even more difficult when the patient is sedated or paralyzed. When a patient has an unexpected or unexplained change in level of consciousness or ability to interact with nursing and medical personnel, always consider the possibility of sporadic, brief seizures with a prolonged postictal or interictal state, or nonconvulsive status epilepticus. Seizures may reflect a change in the underlying central nervous system condition such as bleeds or vasospasm and be symptomatic of others, including metabolic, neoplastic, hypoxic/ischemic, and traumatic [3]. An electroencephalogram (EEG) is an extremely useful diagnostic tool and should be immediately available for clinicians caring for the critically ill, neurologically impaired patient. After experienced clinical personnel, the EEG is the best diagnostic tool for the diagnosis of seizures in the critically ill patient.

The EEG: When to Get It and What to Do with It

While intensive care units are hostile recording environments, the experienced EEG technologist will almost always be able to record a clinically useful study. The technologist is able to record the relevant activity occurring at the patient's bedside and note those activities which produce artifacts that might interfere with the accurate interpretation of the study. The technologist is the "eyes, ears, and hands" of the interpreting physician and makes observations relevant to record interpretation, which cannot be done by the physician since he or she is not continuously at the bedside. Current digital EEG equipment will commonly have the capacity for video recording, and video recording should be performed if possible to assist the interpreting physician in identifying patient behaviors and events of interest.

When the EEG technologist cannot record an interpretable record due to patient movement, spasms, agitation, or other artifact-inducing activity at the patient's bedside, the technologist will troubleshoot, attempt to identify the sources of artifact, and minimize their effect on the recording. This may even include asking the patient's nurse or physician to consider obtaining an order to use neuromuscular blockade to paralyze the patient if he or she is already on a ventilator. Movement or electromyographic artifact can produce a waveform resembling epileptiform activity. If not identified, a false-positive interpretation of such an EEG could result in unnecessary treatment of seizures. The well-trained technologist will call the interpreting physician when there is a question of ongoing electrographic seizure activity so that the electroencephalographer can diagnose the issue and work with the treating team to immediately address it. Once an interpretable record is obtained, the technologist alerts the physician that the emergent or urgent EEG is available for interpretation so that the treating team receives the result and necessary treatments can be undertaken promptly.

Nonconvulsive status epilepticus (NCSE) occurs when seizures with minimal or no clinical manifestation last continuously or nearly continuously for at least 30-min duration [1, 4, 5]. Some patients may have subtle signs associated with nonconvulsive seizures including myoclonus, nystagmus, eye deviation, papillary abnormalities, and autonomic instability [5].

A single EEG may not provide sufficient information for patients having waxing and waning mental status changes. Extending the duration of recording the EEG may enhance detection of subclinical seizures. A standard, 30-min EEG may detect subclinical seizures in 15 % of cases, while extending the EEG to 60 min may detect seizures in approximately 50 % of patients having seizures. The indications for continuous EEG monitoring include (1) detection of nonconvulsive seizures and assessment of patients with altered mental status, (2) monitoring ongoing therapy such as anticonvulsant therapy or intracranial pressure management with pentobarbital coma, and (3) prognostication following acute brain injury or cardiac arrest. To achieve the 95th percentile for subclinical seizure detection, patients who are not comatose require a minimum 24 h of continuous EEG monitoring and 48 h if the patient is comatose [3]. For technical details regarding monitoring in the ICU, please see Chaps. 7 and 8 which cover neurologic monitoring in the ICU.

EEG Patterns

Interpretation of EEG takes a great deal of practice and skill and is beyond the intended scope of this chapter. However, the report may also require some explanations. The first part is typically a summary of the clinical presentation, including medications, with the second part describing the technical aspects of the test administered. Then, the EEG patterns are

Fig. 39.1 This is the EEG of a patient in nonconvulsive status epilepticus (NCSE); he has a history of medically refractory epilepsy due to Lennox-Gastaut syndrome and presented in convulsive status epilepticus. The precipitant was thought to be VNS generator battery end-of-life. After initial treatment, he reverted to nonconvulsive status

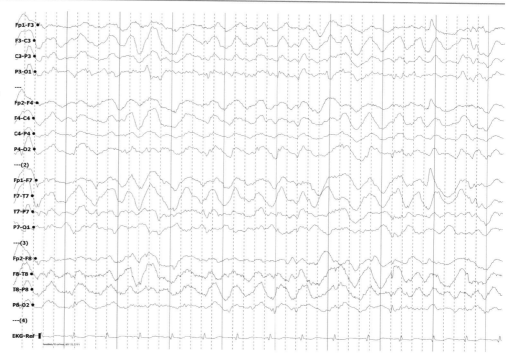

described, and the interpretation summary, usually with a clinical correlation or differential diagnosis, follows. A normal EEG is rarely seen in the neuro-ICU. The EEG with focal or lateralized slowing (theta frequency is 4–8 Hz and delta <4 Hz) implies a destructive process ipsilateral to the slowing. The greater the slowing, the more severely abnormal the EEG. A destructive process may be structural or functional. Cerebral contusion, hemorrhage, and tumor are examples of structural destructive processes. Functional destructive processes include the postictal state and regional ischemia as in vasospasm. Epileptiform transients or paroxysmal activity include spikes, sharp waves, and repetitive, rhythmic, or periodic activity. "Epileptiform" generally means that the waveform is consistent with what may be seen before, during, or after a seizure. Spikes are discharges lasting less than 80 ms; sharp waves last less than 200 ms. Epileptiform periodic activity usually has a frequency of 1–2 Hz or faster and may last <5 s. Epileptiform activity may be focal, lateralized, or generalized. When it occurs between seizures, it is called interictal activity and suggests a predilection for seizures.

There is often confusion about the difference between seizures and epilepsy. "Epilepsy" is defined as recurrent seizures and is synonymous with the term "seizure disorder." When repetitive epileptiform activity is present continuously for more than 5 s at a frequency of more than 1.5–2 Hz, a seizure is occurring and the EEG is referred to as ictal. The ictal EEG may or may not be associated with clinical manifestations. When no *simultaneous clinical* behavior is recognized during the ictal EEG, the seizure is referred to as a subclinical seizure, or an electrographic seizure. The significance of subclinical seizures is varied and depends on both the underlying condition and the period of time the patient has been having the seizures.

Subclinical seizures may contribute to the patient's altered mental status [6]. Appropriate treatment may lead to prompt and significant improvement in the patient's neurological status, but not always, particularly if the condition has been ongoing or the underlying central nervous system disease is severe. When the electrographic seizures become continuous (at some arbitrary time limit – usually several minutes), nonconvulsive status epilepticus is said to exist (Fig. 39.1). The clinical significance and management of NCSE is a controversial issue [2, 6–9]. Some authorities regard this condition as almost equivalent to convulsive status epilepticus in severity and significance and advocate its emergent treatment, while others are less aggressive, considering NCSE an epiphenomenon of irreversibly injured brain which does not warrant aggressive treatment. The answer is likely in between and likely highly individualized depending upon the underlying etiologies of the NCSE.

Convulsive status epilepticus is a life-threatening neurological emergency and can be a challenge to treat. It is defined as a seizure or series of seizures lasting at least 30 min without a return to baseline cognitive function. Functionally, however, epileptologists treat a patient as having status if their seizures are more prolonged than usual or begin clustering without remission before the 30-min mark. The sooner the treatment begins, the easier the seizures should be to stop. A large randomized controlled trial conducted through the VA medical centers concluded that the best first-line therapy for status epilepticus out of four options in common use at the time was lorazepam; however, the short-time line used for outcome measures may have affected this as well [10].

What to Consider

Seizures should be regarded as a symptom of central nervous system (CNS) dysfunction. The urgency to determine the cause is based on the patient's vital signs, level of consciousness, focality on examination, and other clinical findings. The health-care provider should also remember that there are certain drug-related syndromes that produce seizures or paroxysmal events that resemble seizures. They may be provoked by the addition or withdrawal of certain drugs or substances and are summarized in Table 39.1. The need for emergent neuroimaging studies and lumbar puncture will depend on the likelihood of the diagnosis of a new or expanding intracranial lesion, infection (CNS or systemic), and metabolic state. Factors predisposing patients to seizures include (1) changes in blood-brain barrier permeability due to infection, hypoxia, dysautoregulation of cerebral blood flow, or microdeposition of hemorrhage or edema secondary to vascular endothelial damage; (2) alteration of neuronal excitability by exogenous or endogenous substances including excitatory and inhibitory neurotransmitters; (3) inability of glial cells to regulate the neuronal extracellular environment; (4) electrolyte imbalances; (5) and hypoxia-ischemia. Some patients without a history of epilepsy may be genetically prone to have seizures triggered by systemic factors.

Post-traumatic Seizures

Post-traumatic seizures (PTS) can be a serious complication of head injury, causing secondary brain damage through increased metabolic requirements, raised intracranial pressure, cerebral hypoxia, and/or excessive release of neurotransmitters. The occurrence of an immediate seizure and post-traumatic status epilepticus may thus complicate the patient's management [11]. Damage to the hippocampus, especially the CA1 region, occurs in a high proportion of fatal head injuries [12–14] and may be important to the development of epilepsy in survivors.

Fluctuating changes in the patient's level of consciousness, intermittent changes in behavior, and changes in staffing may lead to diagnostic problems, especially in the first 1–2 weeks after injury. Determining which changes are really related to the patient, which are related to post-traumatic syndrome, and which may be caused by seizure activity may be difficult but are very important for management. Careful hand-off communication as caregivers change is important to

Table 39.1 Syndromes producing seizures or seizure-like events

| Syndromes | Clinical findings | |
	CNS effects	Peripheral effects
Central anticholiergicn	Hallucinations, confusion, sedation, seizures, mydriasis, hyperthermia	Decreased gut motility, dry skin and oral mucosa, tachycardia, urinary retention
Cholinergic	Confusion, lethargy, seizures	Salivation, lacrimation, urination, diarrhea, increased gut motility, emesis, bradycardia, bronchorrhea, bronchospasm
Sympathomimetics	Agitation, seizures	Diaphoresis, hypertension, hyperthermia, tachycardia, cardiac dysrhythmias
Serotonin	Confusion, agitation, myoclonus, hypomania, dysarthria, orobuccal dyskinesias, tremor, rigidity with cogwheeling, hyperreflexia, incoordination	Dysautonomia, hyperthermia, diaphoresis, diarrhea, mydriasis, tachycardia
Malignant hyperthermia	Marked rigidity, consciousness disturbance	Hyperthermia, dysautonomia, rhabdomyolysis

Reproduced with permission from Gilmore [104]

establishing a baseline and identifying changes in clinical status quickly. Video-EEG monitoring may be necessary for definitive diagnosis in some cases [14]. These patients are often unstable and particularly vulnerable to the consequences of seizures. Phenytoin and its prodrug fosphenytoin are the drugs of choice for preventing and treating early seizures because of demonstrated efficacy and the availability of a formulation for intravenous administration. Recommended concentration of the unbound or free phenytoin is 1–2.0 μg/ml. Phenytoin has been the most consistently studied and utilized antiepileptic drugs for post-traumatic prophylaxis, but other IV agents including levetiracetam and valproic acid may be utilized depending on the clinical presentation and concurrent medical conditions.

Seizures and Vascular Lesions

Subarachnoid Hemorrhage

Subarachnoid hemorrhage is a common condition in the neuro-ICU and may be seen following trauma or in association with aneurysmal or AVM rupture. Convulsive seizures may occur in 10–25 % of aneurysms that rupture or rebleed

[15, 16]. In approximately one-third of patients with AVMs, the presenting and only manifestation may be a seizure. Cavernous malformations or cavernous angiomas may also present with seizures; the incidence of this presentation is not known. Seizures that present at onset are an independent risk factor for later seizures and a predictor of poor outcome [16].

Natriuresis is a common systemic manifestation of aneurysmal subarachnoid hemorrhage (SAH). Natriuresis and its accompanying hypovolemia may be a major contributing factor in the pathophysiology of symptomatic cerebral vasospasm. This may also contribute to seizures. Management of seizures related to hyponatremia is discussed later in this chapter.

Stroke

Both hemorrhagic and ischemic stroke may produce acute mental status changes and may also produce seizures acutely. The incidence is far more common with hemorrhagic insults (28 %) than with ischemic stroke (6 %) [17]. Clinical manifestations assist in assessment. With stroke, patients will typically have "negative" symptoms with loss of function associated with the cortical injury. With seizures, patients typically will have "positive" symptoms generated by activation of the cortical area (e.g., clonic movements). For example, the eyes may be tonically deviated towards the side of the insult with stroke, whereas there may be subtle eye movements away from the side of the focus with seizures.

Vasculitis

Seizure as a manifestation of vasculitis may occur as a feature of encephalopathy or as a focal neurologic deficit. The incidence of seizures increases with duration and severity of the underlying vasculitis [18], ranging from 24 to 45 %. The relationship of the seizure disorder to the underlying disease may not always be clear, however. A confounding feature of anticonvulsant drug treatment is the occurrence of drug-induced systemic lupus erythematosus [19]. Antiphospholipid antibody syndrome is also associated with seizures; most are associated with focal brain infarction [20]. Systemic necrotizing vasculitis and granulomatous vasculitis rarely present with seizures. Among patients with giant-cell arteritis with non-ocular signs, seizures occur in 1.5 % [21]. Behcet's disease has neurological involvement in 10–25 % of patients. The onset is more often acute and is occasionally associated with seizures [22].

Malignancy

Mechanisms for seizures in cancer patients include direct invasion of cortex or leptomeninges, metabolic derangements, opportunistic infection, and chemotherapeutic agents [23]. Seizures may be an early symptom of CNS malignancy or may appear after surgical procedures for diagnosis or treatment. Following biopsy for diagnosis or resection, single seizures may occur, or a first seizure of an epileptic disorder may occur.

In approximately 50 % of patients with low-grade astrocytomas, a focal or generalized seizure is the first symptom. More than one-half of patients with oligodendrogliomas present with partial or generalized seizures; seizures may persist for years before other symptoms or signs develop. Other tumor types are associated with seizures as well. Glioblastomas, ependymomas, and meningiomas are all well represented among patients with tumors and seizures. Metastatic carcinoma frequently presents with seizures. Over the course of the illness, 60–75 % of all patients with tumors will experience seizures.

Seizures associated with remote effects of malignancy or paraneoplastic syndromes are much less common than direct effects of malignancy, but do occur. Limbic encephalitis is a paraneoplastic syndrome seen in patients with small cell carcinoma or, less commonly, Hodgkin's disease. Patients usually present with amnestic dementia, affective disturbance, and sometimes a personality change. During the course of the illness, both complex partial and generalized seizures may occur. Paraneoplastic limbic encephalitis associated with anti-Hu antibodies may present with seizures and precede the diagnosis of cancer [24].

Opsoclonus myoclonus occurs most frequently in young children (mean age, 18 months). Approximately half of the cases have been diagnosed with neuroblastoma, but only about 3 % of all the cases of neuroblastoma have this complication. Opsoclonus myoclonus may occur in adults as well, having been reported with carcinoma, but also occurring on an idiopathic basis. Since the idiopathic and paraneoplastic syndromes are indistinguishable clinically, the appearance of opsoclonus myoclonus should always lead to a search for neuroblastoma or other occult neoplasm. In the adult, these neoplasms are most commonly small cell lung cancer or breast cancer. Symptoms are responsive to steroids or corticotropin [25]. Intravenous immunoglobulin has also been used [26].

Other Causes of Seizures and Altered Mental States

Hyperbaric oxygenation precipitates seizures, possibly as a toxic effect of oxygen itself. Some antineoplastic drugs such as chlorambucil and methotrexate precipitate seizures. Other drugs reported to precipitate seizures are seen in Table 39.2.

Obstructive sleep apnea is also common in the general population and medically refractory epilepsy patients [27]. It may also be seen in patients with malformations and trauma of anterior cranial structures [28]. While doing a full

Table 39.2 Medications that may cause seizures

Analgesics	Fantasy, meperidine, mefenamic acid, pentazocine, propoxyphene, tramadol
Antibiotics	β (beta)-lactam (penicillin, ampicillin, etc.) cephalosporins, carbapenems (imipenem, etc.), isoniazid, lindane, metronidazole, nalidixic acid, pyrimethamine
Antidepressants	Amitriptyline, bupropion, citalopram, doxepin, fluoxetine, maprotiline, mianserine, nomifensine, nortriptyline, paroxetine, sertraline
Antineoplastic drugs	BCNU, busulfan, chlorambucil, cytosine arabinoside, methotrexate, vincristine
Antipsychotics	Chlorpromazine, haloperidol, olanzapine, perphenazine, prochlorperazine, thioridazine, trifluoperazine, ziprasidone
Bronchial agents	Aminophylline, theophylline
General anesthetics	Enflurane, ketamine
Local anesthetics	Bupivacaine, lidocaine, procaine
Sympathomimetics	Ephedrine, phenylpropanolamine, terbutaline
Others	Alcohol, amphetamines, anticholinergics, antihistamine, atenolol, baclofen, cyclosporin A, domperidone, ergonovine, FK506 flumazenil, folic acid, foscarnet, hyperbaric oxygen, insulin, aqueous iodinated contrast, lithium, methylphenidate, methylxanthines, oxytocin, phencyclidine

Modified with permission from Gilmore [104]

sleep study in the ICU setting is not practical, consider the possibility of CO_2 retention in patients with high BMI. Sleep apnea may cause fragmentation of sleep, just as the often overly stimulating atmosphere of the ICU may contribute to ICU psychosis [29]. Sleep deprivation exacerbates seizures and is often used as a provocative measure in the epilepsy monitoring unit where seizures are intentionally recorded for localization and classification with the purpose of tailoring the medical and surgical treatment of refractory epilepsy.

Gastrointestinal disease is occasionally associated with seizures. Approximately 7–10 % of patients with nontropical sprue have seizure disorders [30]. Deficiencies of calcium, magnesium, and vitamins, genetic factors [31], and isolated CNS vasculitis [32] are potential mechanisms. Inflammatory bowel disease (ulcerative colitis and Crohn's disease) is associated with a low incidence of focal or generalized seizures. Whipple's disease is a multisystem granulomatous disease caused by *Tropheryma whippelii* [33]. About 10 % of patients with Whipple's disease have neurologic involvement; as many as 25 % of these patients have seizures [34].

Sawka and colleagues [35] described four patients with tension pneumocranium who presented with seizures or impaired mental status after transsphenoidal pituitary surgery.

Heavy metal intoxication, especially with lead and mercury, is a well-known seizure precipitant. Ingestion of lead from paint and inhalation of lead oxide are especially hazardous for young children.

Transplantation and Seizures

Organ transplantation has led to newly recognized CNS disorders and new manifestations of old disorders. Seizures in patients awaiting or having undergone transplantation may be difficult to manage for several reasons: (1) these patients are frequently metabolically stressed; (2) preexisting diseases and preceding therapies may have affected the CNS (e.g., bone marrow transplant patients may have received L-asparaginase, which is associated with acute intracerebral hemorrhage and infarction, and ischemic seizures); and (3) immunosuppressive drugs, especially cyclosporine and *tacrolimus* (*FK506*), may provoke seizures.

Certain populations of transplant patients appear to have higher risks for seizures.

Liver

In one large series Wijdicks and colleagues [36] concluded that the majority of new-onset seizures in liver transplant patients were secondary to immunosuppressant neurotoxicity (cyclosporine and FK506). They also concluded that new-onset seizures were not indicative of poor outcome.

Lung

Vaughn and coworkers [37] found that of 85 lung transplant cases, 22 patients had seizures (including 15 of 18 patients with cystic fibrosis) and patients less than 25 years old, particularly those on intravenous methylprednisolone for rejection, may be at increased risk for seizures.

Bone Marrow

Among patients undergoing bone marrow transplantation, it has recently been shown that the risk of seizures from cyclosporine neurotoxicity increases in patients with HLA-mismatched and unrelated donor transplant [38]. Foscarnet, used to treat cytomegalovirus hepatitis following bone marrow transplantation [39], may also precipitate seizures [40]. Patients requiring antibiotics may be commonly given carbapenems, which have seizure-inducing potential likely due to the β (beta)-lactam ring structure and their binding to gamma-aminobutyric acid (GABA) receptors. In particular, imipenem-cilastatin has reported seizure rates of 3–33 % [41].

For acute management of prolonged seizures, benzodiazepines are least likely to induce the enzyme system responsible for metabolizing immunosuppressant drugs [42]. Long-term management is determined after the etiology has been ascertained. Because allograft survival is decreased in patients treated with phenytoin or phenobarbital and steroids, the use of these older antiepileptic drugs has been discouraged [43]. The half-lives of prednisolone [44] and probably cyclosporine [42] are decreased when phenobarbital, phenytoin, and carbamazepine are used for treatment of seizures. Levetiracetam has become the agent of choice in transplantation since it has broad efficacy and no drug interactions. Lacosamide does not have any drug interactions with the immunosuppressants but has potentially more side effects, with dizziness being prominent; gabapentin has no drug interactions with low side effects but may have lower efficacy and is excreted renally. In patients other than those having undergone hepatic transplantation and bone marrow transplantation during engraftment, valproic acid may also be a reasonable antiepileptic choice. Levetiracetam, lacosamide, and valproic acid are all available as IV formulations as well as oral formulations; gabapentin is only available in oral formulations.

Levetiracetam and gabapentin may be useful for hepatic transplantation and bone marrow transplantation patients. These drugs are eliminated from systemic circulation by renal excretion as unchanged drug. Very little gabapentin (<3 %) and levetiracetam (<10 %) are protein bound. Obviously, use of these agents in patients with renal disease must be modified. Phenytoin might be considered for partial seizures, except during bone marrow engraftment, when carbamazepine is also relatively contraindicated. Both of these drugs may have toxic hematologic side effects. During the 2- to 6-week period of engraftment, phenobarbital is acceptable. When anticonvulsant drugs other than valproic acid, gabapentin, or levetiracetam are used, the doses of immunosuppressive drugs should be increased to ensure therapeutic immunosuppression. Cyclosporine levels should be periodically assessed. Experience with other anticonvulsant drugs such as lamotrigine and topiramate in these setting is limited.

Management of Seizures

Patients in the neuro-ICU may have coexisting conditions which make the management of anticonvulsant drug regimens challenging. For instance, a CNS trauma patient may also have liver lacerations and/or contusions with consequent acute hepatic failure. Understanding the interaction of other organ systems is therefore necessary for appropriate management of seizures. Hepatic and renal dysfunction will induce changes in pharmacokinetics which then necessitate

adjustment of the anticonvulsant regimen. In cases of hepatic dysfunction, plasma drug concentrations must be correlated with serum albumin and protein levels, and free (unbound) drug levels measured if possible. Patients with hepatic and renal failure may have normal serum and albumin levels but altered protein binding that results in elevated free drug concentrations [45]. Changes in temperature also may be associated with increased protein binding by phenytoin [46].

Metabolic Disorders

Metabolic disorders are considered in this chapter because the management of seizures is intricately related to the patient's metabolic state.

Hyponatremia

In the hospital setting, disorders of electrolytes and fluid balance are some of the more common metabolic disorders noted. Hyponatremia is defined as serum sodium level less than 115 mEq/l, and is one of the most frequent metabolic abnormalities, occurring in 2.5 % of hospitalized patients [47]. Acute hyponatremia is a frequent event in neurosurgery practice and is usually associated with subarachnoid hemorrhage, head trauma, infections, and neoplasms [48]. The two common clinical manifestations are the syndrome of inappropriate antidiuretic hormone (SIADH) secretion and the cerebral salt wasting syndrome (CSWS), which have previously been attributed to each other due to identical clinical presentation. Neurologic symptoms, including seizures, are seen more frequently in acute rather than chronic hyponatremia [49–51]. The critical difference between SIADH and CSWS is that CSWS involves renal salt loss leading to hyponatremia and volume loss, whereas SIADH is a euvolemic/hypervolemic condition [52]. Attention to volume status in patients with hyponatremia is essential. The primary treatment for CSWS is water and salt replacement. Urgent, but not immediate, correction to serum sodium levels greater than 120 mEq/l is essential when hypovolemia is absent. When hypovolemia is present, more rapid correction is necessary.

The critical difference between SIADH and CSWS is that CSWS involves renal salt loss leading to hyponatremia and volume loss, whereas SIADH is a euvolemic/hypervolemic condition.

Serum sodium is commonly reduced as a result of sodium depletion [53] resulting in hypo-osmolar hyponatremia. Hyponatremia with normal osmolality is rare but may be seen in patients with hyperlipidemia or hyperproteinemia. Hyperosmolar hyponatremia occurs in hyperosmolar states such as hyperglycemia. Hypo-osmolar hyponatremia may be associated with normal extracellular fluid volume, hypovolemia, or hypervolemia [54]. Hypo-osmolar hyponatremia with hypovolemia may be seen from renal (diuretic use, Addison's disease) or extrarenal loss (vomiting, diarrhea, or "third spacing") and CSWS. SIADH, hypothyroidism, and certain drugs including the antiepileptic drugs carbamazepine and oxcarbazepine and psychotropic agents may cause hypo-osmolar hyponatremia with normal volume. Hypo-osmolar hyponatremia associated with hypervolemia, frequently manifested by a patient's clinical edema, occurs in cardiac failure, nephrotic syndrome, and acute or chronic renal failure. The therapeutic implications of these conditions are significant since appropriate therapy for normovolemic or hypervolemic hyperosmolar hyponatremia is water restriction. Hypovolemic hyponatremia is managed by replacement of water and sodium [54]. Because these disturbances are usually secondary processes, management of associated seizures requires identification and treatment of the primary disorder in conjunction with correction of the fluid and/or electrolyte disturbance. When hypovolemia is absent, rapid correction of hyponatremia has been associated with central pontine myelinolysis (CPM), manifested clinically by pseudobulbar palsy and spastic quadriparesis. Norenberg and colleagues [55] noted that, in each of 12 patients with CPM, there had been a recent rapid rise in serum sodium. Thus, caution and careful monitoring of serum sodium are advised.

Disturbances of Glucose Metabolism

Hypoglycemia and nonketotic hyperglycemia may be associated with focal seizures, but these do not occur with ketotic hyperglycemia [56], possibly due to the anticonvulsant action of ketosis. Ketosis also involves intracellular acidosis with augmented activity of glutamic acid decarboxylase which increases gamma-aminobutyric acid (GABA) levels, thereby increasing seizure threshold.

Nonketotic hyperglycemia with or without hyperosmolarity may be associated with seizures. Hyperglycemia increases the frequency of seizures through brain dehydration in animal models with cortical lesions [57]. Focal motor seizures and *epilepsia partialis continua* are well-known complications of nonketotic hyperglycemia, occurring in approximately 20 % of cases [58].

Hypocalcemia

Seizures due to severe hypocalcemia (<6 mg/dl) are relatively infrequent, but do occur. Severe acute hypocalcemia most frequently follows thyroid or parathyroid surgery. Although not well understood, late-onset hypocalcemia with seizures rarely may develop years after extensive thyroid surgery [59]. Hypocalcemia frequently complicates renal failure and acute pancreatitis [53]. Tetany is the most frequent neuromuscular symptom in patients with hypocalcemia [60] and can be mistaken for seizure activity. Tetany is the clinical manifestation of spontaneous, irregular, repetitive action

potentials originating in peripheral nerves. Latent tetany may be unmasked by hyperventilation or regional ischemia (Trousseau test). In the average adult, a slow intravenous (IV) bolus of 15 ml of 10 % calcium gluconate solution (9 mg calcium/ml) with careful cardiac monitoring followed by slow infusion of the equivalent of 10 ml/h of 10 % calcium gluconate solution should alleviate seizures [61].

Hypomagnesemia

Hypomagnesemia is associated with seizures most often when serum levels are less than 0.8 mEq/l. Because secondary hypocalcemia may be produced by a decrease in circulating levels of or end-organ resistance to parathyroid hormone, magnesium levels should be measured in the hypocalcemic patient who does not respond to calcium supplementation. Treatment requires administration of intramuscular 50 % magnesium sulfate every 6 h or intravenous infusion. Because respiratory muscle paralysis may be precipitated by transient hypermagnesemia [62], intravenous calcium gluconate should be administered concurrently.

Hypophosphatemia

Profound hypophosphatemia may accompany alcohol withdrawal, diabetic ketoacidosis, chronic intake of phosphate binding antacids, recovery from extensive burns, hyperalimentation, and severe respiratory alkalosis. A sequence of symptoms consistent with metabolic encephalopathy occurs, involving irritability, apprehension, muscle weakness, numbness, paresthesias, dysarthria, confusion, obtundation, convulsive seizures, and coma [63]. Generalized tonic-clonic seizures may occur with levels less than 1.0 mg/dl and may not be controlled by anticonvulsant drugs [64].

Hypoparathyroidism

Thirty to 70 % of patients with hypoparathyroidism experience seizures, usually in association with tetany and hypocalcemia. These seizures may be generalized tonic-clonic, focal motor, and, less frequently, atypical absence and akinetic attacks. Restoration of normal calcium levels is necessary for control. Because anticonvulsant drugs may partially suppress seizures as well as tetany and Trousseau's sign, hypocalcemia must be considered.

Uremia

Mental status changes are the hallmark of uremic encephalopathy involving simultaneous neural depression (obtundation) and neural excitation (twitching, myoclonus, generalized seizures). Phenytoin is a typical anticonvulsant drug utilized to treat seizures in non-transplanted uremic patients. However, the physician should remember that critical changes in anticonvulsant drug pharmacokinetics occur, including (1) increased volume of distribution producing lowered plasma drug levels, (2) decreased protein binding creating higher free drug levels, and (3) increased hepatic enzyme oxidation yielding increased plasma elimination [45]. Because uremic patients have plasma protein-binding abnormalities and because phenytoin is highly plasma bound, administration is different than in non-uremic patients. In non-uremic patients, up to 10 % of phenytoin is not protein bound. In uremic patients, as much as 75 % may not be protein bound, and therefore it is necessary to use free phenytoin levels (between 1 and 2 μg/ml) instead of total phenytoin levels to assess therapeutic efficacy [65]. Since fosphenytoin is preferred over phenytoin for parenteral administration, the neuro-ICU physician should be familiar with its use as well. For drugs such as gabapentin [66], pregabalin, levetiracetam, topiramate, and zonisamide that are eliminated largely via renal excretion, the usual total dose should be reduced equivalently to the reduction in creatinine clearance.

Hepatic Encephalopathy

Hepatic encephalopathy is classified into four stages: stage III is associated with focal or generalized seizures; stage IV is marked by coma and decerebrate posturing. The incidence of seizures varies widely, from 2 to 33 % [67, 68]. Hypoglycemia, complicating liver failure, may be responsible for some seizures. Therapy should be directed at the underlying etiology of the hepatic failure with intervention focused on reduction of gastrointestinal protein and administration of lactulose. Anticonvulsant drug treatment of hepatic encephalopathy does not usually require chronic therapy unless there is a known predisposition to seizures (e.g., previous cerebral injury). Little experience with the use of anticonvulsant drugs has been reported. Anticonvulsant drugs with sedative effects may precipitate coma [68] and are generally contraindicated. Anticonvulsant drugs not metabolized by the liver such as gabapentin, pregabalin, lacosamide, or levetiracetam should be considered first, although gabapentin and pregabalin are not available parenterally. Fosphenytoin or phenytoin is less sedating than phenobarbital. Oral or parenteral valproate derivatives should be avoided.

Intoxication

This section is not to be used as a guide to the management of drug intoxication but rather to deal with specific instances of intoxication that may arise in the neurointensive care setting.

Recreational Drug-Induced Seizures

Alcohol and recreational drugs are often factors in cerebral trauma. For this reason, it is important for the clinician to recognize the occurrence of drug- and substance-induced and substance withdrawal-induced seizures. Alldredge and colleagues [69] retrospectively identified 49 cases of recreational drug-induced seizures in 47 patients. Most patients experienced a single generalized tonic-clonic seizure associated with acute drug intoxication, but seven patients had multiple seizures and two patients developed status epilepticus. The recreational drugs implicated were cocaine (32 cases), amphetamine [10], heroin [7], phencyclidine, and combinations of substances. Marijuana is unlikely to alter seizure threshold [70]. However, seizures occurring in patients with toxicology screens positive for marijuana should be tested for additional illicit drug use and alcohol.

Cocaine, a biologic compound, is one of the most abused recreational drugs in the United States. Common neurological complications include tremors, stroke, and generalized seizures [71]. Cocaine can provoke seizures, exacerbate a preexisting seizure disorder, or cause an ischemic or hemorrhagic stroke that leads to seizures [72].

Seizures can occur immediately after drug administration without other signs of toxicity. Convulsions and death may occur within minutes of overdose. The majority of seizures are single and generalized, induced by intravenous or "crack" cocaine, and not associated with any lasting neurological deficits. Most focal or repetitive events are associated with an acute intracerebral complication or concurrent use of other drugs [73]. The treatment of choice is diazepam or lorazepam. Bicarbonate for acidosis, artificial ventilation, and cardiac monitoring are also useful, depending upon the duration of the seizures. Urinary acidification accelerates excretion of the drug. Chlorpromazine use has also been recommended since it raised rather than lowered the seizure threshold in cocaine-intoxicated primates [74]. Tricyclic antidepressants may also be useful by decreasing vasoconstrictor and cardiac action [75].

Methamphetamine is a synthetic drug similar to cocaine with toxic effects, including seizures, similar to those of amphetamine and cocaine [76]. The amphetamine derivative 3,4-methylenedioxymethamphetamine is known as MDMA. Also known as "ecstasy," it has become a frequently abused substance in the United States, especially popular at "raves." It may cause seizures with rhabdomyolysis and hepatic dysfunction [77]. Treatment of methamphetamine-induced seizures is similar to cocaine-induced seizures. Hyperthermia is a life-threatening complication of MDMA use [78]. While protracted seizure activity may be associated with hyperthermia, the degree of hyperthermia is lower than that associated with MDMA use. Very high temperatures (>104 °F) should raise the suspicion of MDMA intoxication.

Nonrecreational Drug-Induced Seizures

Many medications have been associated with provocation of seizures in both epileptic and nonepileptic patients (Table 39.2). Predisposing factors include family history of seizures, concurrent illness, and high-dose intrathecal and intravenous administration. More commonly, these are generalized convulsions with or without focal features, and status epilepticus may occur. Because multiple medical conditions are associated with polypharmacy, drug-induced seizures may be even more common in the elderly patient [79]. The prescribing information should be consulted to determine the seizure potential of drugs for specific conditions.

Serotonin Syndrome

This syndrome is increasingly recognized. The "serotonin syndrome" consists of delirium, tremors, and occasionally seizures [80]. In part, it is occurring more frequently due to the increasing use of SSRI antidepressant agents. The syndrome is characterized by confusion, agitation, diaphoresis, tachycardia, myoclonus, and hyperreflexia. Sometimes the myoclonus may be confused with seizures. Seizures are less frequent with this condition than previously reported. The EEGs recorded from patients with this syndrome may be quite disorganized with slowing of the background both generalized and lateralized. The increased use of serotonergic agents (alone and in combination) across multiple medical disciplines presents the possibility that the prevalence and clinical significance of this condition will increase in the future. The syndrome of inappropriate antidiuretic hormone (SIADH) has been reported with most antidepressant drugs but appears to be more common with serotonergic agents and in elderly patients. Thus, while the nature of the patient's surgery may suggest SIADH as a reasonable complication, be sure to check the patient's medication list (before and after admission) for possible contributing factors.

Central Anticholinergic Syndrome

Many drugs used in anesthesia and the intensive care unit can precipitate seizures. Although listing of each drug is not possible, we will review the central anticholinergic syndrome [81], a common disorder associated with blockade of central cholinergic neurotransmission. Acetylcholine modulates many interactions among most other central transmitters. The clinical picture of central cholinergic blockade is identical with the central symptoms of atropine intoxication, including seizures, agitation, hallucinations, disorientation, stupor, coma, and respiratory depression. Such disturbances may be induced by opiates, ketamine, etomidate, propofol, nitrous oxide, and halogenated inhalation anesthetics as well as by H_2-blocking agents such as cimetidine. While there is an individual predisposition for central anticholinergic syndrome, it is unpredictable from laboratory findings or other signs. The postanesthetic syndrome can be prevented by administration of physostigmine during anesthesia.

Analgesics

Meperidine, pentazocine, and propoxyphene, among other analgesic drugs, infrequently cause seizures [82]. Nonetheless, caution should be utilized in critically ill and postsurgical patients. Tramadol is a centrally acting synthetic analgesic whose mechanism is unknown. It has been associated with seizures even when taken within the recommended dosage range. Seizure risk is increased with doses above the recommended range. Simultaneous use with certain drugs also increases the risk of seizures. These drugs include the SSRI antidepressants and anorectics, tricyclic antidepressants, and opioids. Other drugs that may increase the seizure risk include the MAO inhibitors and neuroleptics.

Antidepressants

Intoxication from tricyclic antidepressants has caused generalized tonic-clonic seizures. In fact, seizures may occur at therapeutic levels in about 1 % of patients [83]. Because desipramine is believed to have a lower risk of precipitating seizures than other drugs of this class, it is preferred in patients with known seizure disorders [84] when this class of antidepressant is needed. Since amitriptyline and imipramine depress the level of consciousness, utilization of barbiturates is relatively contraindicated to treat seizures, and diazepam or paraldehyde is recommended. Physostigmine may reverse the neurologic manifestations of tricyclic antidepressant toxicity; however, because it may also cause asystole, hypotension, hypersalivation, and convulsions, it should not be used to treat tricyclic-induced seizures.

Fluoxetine and sertraline are selective serotonin reuptake inhibitors (*SSRIs*). These drugs may have an associated seizure risk of approximately 0.2 %. The SSRIs may have an antiepileptic effect at therapeutic doses [85]. However, when combined with other serotonergic agents or MAO inhibitors, the "serotonin syndrome" may occur; see discussion on this topic earlier in this chapter.

Antipsychotics

Antipsychotic drugs have long been known to precipitate seizures [86, 87]. Both phenothiazines and haloperidol have been implicated, but the potential is greater with phenothiazines and seizures occur more frequently with increasing dosage. Clozapine is an atypical antipsychotic drug (dibenzodiazepine class) for treatment in patients with intractable schizophrenia. Like other antipsychotic agents, the incidence of seizures increases with increasing dosage [88]. Seizures rarely occur with newer antipsychotic agents such as ziprasidone and olanzapine.

Methylxanthines

Theophylline and other methylxanthines may lead to generalized tonic-clonic seizures. In rare patients, theophylline at nontoxic concentration may provoke seizures. When seizures are a result of overdosage, they are best treated acutely with intravenous diazepam. Massive overdosage may produce hypocalcemia and other electrolyte abnormalities [89].

Anesthetics

Lidocaine may precipitate seizures, usually in the setting of congestive heart failure, shock, or hepatic insufficiency. General anesthetics such as ketamine and enflurane are also implicated in precipitating seizures [90]. (See also section on "Central Anticholinergic Syndrome".)

Antibiotics

Many antiparasitic drugs and antimicrobials, particularly penicillins and cephalosporins in high concentrations, precipitate seizures. Lindane, an antiparasitic shampoo against head lice (pediculosis capitis), has a rare association with self-limited, generalized seizures. However, it is best to use another agent should reinfestation occur. Seizures have not been reported with permethrin, another anti-pediculosis agent.

Isoniazid (INH)

Isoniazid combines with pyridoxine inhibiting pyridoxine kinase that forms the active cofactor for the enzyme glutamic acid decarboxylase that forms GABA. Therefore, INH depletes GABA altering seizure threshold [91]. Severe INH intoxication involves coma and severe, intractable seizures and metabolic acidosis. Ingestion of more than 80 mg/kg bodyweight produces severe CNS symptoms that are rapidly reversed with intravenous administration of pyridoxine [92] at 1 mg for every 1 mg of isoniazid. Conventional doses of short-acting barbiturates, phenytoin, or diazepam are also recommended to potentiate the effect of pyridoxine [93].

Treatment: How to Use the AEDs, Old and New

If patients are actively seizing, parenteral formulations should always be utilized since gastrointestinal absorption and metabolism may vary considerably in patients in the neurological intensive care unit.

Benzodiazepines

Benzodiazepines remain the antiepileptic drug (AED) of choice in the initial treatment of acute seizures or status epilepticus [10]. Either lorazepam or diazepam may be used, although lorazepam is preferred since it produces a longer antiepileptic effect. The dose for lorazepam is 0.1–0.2 mg/kg over 2–4 min. Maximum dose is 8 mg. For diazepam, the dose is 0.1–0.3 mg/kg over 2–4 min. Maximum dose is

20 mg. Rectal diazepam gel is a formulation that can be used when IV access is delayed or difficult and is unlikely to be used in the ICU setting. Lorazepam and diazepam are available for oral administration but are not commonly used for maintenance antiepileptic treatment. When oral benzodiazepines are used in chronic seizure disorders for maintenance, a more useful frequently used drug is clonazepam, which has a longer half-life of 20–50 h. Dosage ranges from 0.25–5 mg/day in the drug non-naive patient.

Phenytoin and Fosphenytoin

Although several newer antiepileptic drugs have been released in the last 5 years, there are still only a few AEDs for acute and chronic seizure treatment that are available for parenteral use. Phenytoin is still used extensively in ICUs. Fosphenytoin is the phosphate ester prodrug of phenytoin. It has several advantages over phenytoin that are detailed in the discussion to come.

Phenytoin is soluble in saline and only at high pH. It is quite toxic to tissue when inadvertently extravasated. For acute seizure management, it should only be administered intravenously and should *never* be administered via the intramuscular route. Fosphenytoin can be safely administered intramuscularly. Phenytoin is administered parenterally at a maximum rate of 50 mg/min. Typical loading dose for the treatment of status epilepticus is 18–20 mg/kg. Fosphenytoin can be administered intravenously at a higher maximum rate than phenytoin (150 PE/min) [94]. All fosphenytoin doses are expressed as the amount of phenytoin equivalents (PE) delivered. When administering phenytoin or fosphenytoin using the intravenous route, cardiac and blood pressure monitoring are necessary. Never use phenytoin IM. You *can* use fosphenytoin IM. However, when treating status epilepticus, *always* use the IV route.

For chronic phenytoin use, the typical dose is 300–400 mg/day. Obviously, levels should be followed; discussion regarding serum free and bound phenytoin levels covered previously in this chapter.

Coma in the Treatment of Refractory Status Epilepticus

When status epilepticus fails to respond to one or two parenteral anticonvulsants, the ICU physician may opt to induce coma and burst suppression in order to control the seizures. Phenobarbital is used in the treatment of status epilepticus and acute seizures and for chronic seizure management. For treatment of status, the loading dose is 20 mg/kg over 10 min. Thereafter, it is delivered at 0.75 mg/min. It is typically used after benzodiazepines and phenytoin (or fosphenytoin) have been used without adequate seizure response. Because of the risk of respiratory compromise, it is essential to be prepared for endotracheal intubation of the patient. When treating refractory status epilepticus, continuous EEG monitoring is recommended to verify that the seizures are stopping and not converting to subclinical status epilepticus or intermittent subclinical seizures [95]. If using coma induction with barbiturates or other sedatives, titrate the drug to burst suppression on the EEG. Some clinicians prefer pentobarbital when it appears that the patient may be entering refractory status epilepticus. From the standpoint of sedation, respiratory compromise, and duration of sedating effects, there is little difference. However, it is believed that for long-term use pentobarbital has fewer adverse effects on myocardial contractility. Nonetheless, hypotension is an adverse effect with both drugs. When using pentobarbital in the treatment of refractory status epilepticus, the dosage is 5–15 mg/kg followed by a continuous infusion of 1–3 mg/kg/h titrating to burst suppression on the EEG. When managing chronic seizures with phenobarbital, the usual dose is 100–240 mg/day.

Other drugs are being studied for the treatment of refractory status epilepticus [96]. Midazolam is loaded IV in a 0.15–0.3 mg/kg bolus and followed with a continuous infusion of 2–6 μg/kg/min. Propofol is also being used for managing refractory status epilepticus. The loading dose is 1–2 mg/kg bolus followed with a continuous infusion of 3–10 mg/kg/h.

Other Drugs in the Treatment of Status Epilepticus

Although The Veterans Cooperative Study 265 was the largest multicenter study of status epilepticus to date, other studies have looked at the use of some of the newer parenteral anticonvulsants in status epilepticus. Recently, investigators at the University of Lausanne compared phenytoin, valproic acid, and levetiracetam after benzodiazepines in the treatment of status epilepticus and found that valproic acid seemed to control status epilepticus more efficiently than levetiracetam. However, this was a retrospective unblinded study, and although postanoxic seizures were excluded, the etiologies of the seizures were not necessarily similar across groups [97].

Valproic Acid/Depacon® (Abbott Laboratories, Abbott Park, IL)

The parenteral formulation of valproic acid has been used at doses of 15–44 mg/kg using infusion rates of 0.25–0.73 mg/kg/min with serum concentrations ranging from 71 to 277 μg/min [98]. Although studies of its use in status epilepticus are generally not large scale, it may well be useful in that setting [97, 99].

Levetiracetam

Levetiracetam is a very good anticonvulsant drug with few adverse effects. It is available in parenteral form and is rapidly and almost completely absorbed after oral administration. It is not protein bound (<10 %), and the major metabolic pathway is hydrolysis of the acetamide group to the inactive carboxylic derivative. Since urinary excretion of the unchanged drug accounts for approximately 50 % of the administered dose, dosage adjustment may be necessary in patients with moderate and severe renal impairment. Its metabolism is independent of the hepatic cytochrome P450 system. There is little potential for pharmacokinetic interactions with other drugs, including oral contraceptives [100]. Usual daily dosing is 1,000–3,000 mg in 2–3 divided doses.

Lacosamide

Although no definitive loading dose is known for lacosamide IV, it has also been a useful AED for seizures in the neuro-ICU. Its mechanism of action is inactivation of low voltage-sensitive sodium channels. It is metabolized by the cytochrome P450 system with the 2C19 substrate and inhibition. It is excreted in the urine (40 % unchanged). Adult dosages may start at 50 mg twice daily and increase to 200 mg twice daily. Case reports regarding use of lacosamide in status epilepticus have reported variable results, but in two recent larger case series, results have been encouraging [101, 102].

Gabapentin

Despite its structural similarity to GABA, gabapentin does not bind to GABA receptors in the CNS. Gabapentin is not metabolized and not plasma protein bound. It neither induces nor inhibits hepatic metabolism. It is eliminated by the kidney. Thus, drug-drug interactions are not an issue with gabapentin. The gabapentin $T_{1/2}$ in otherwise healthy patients is 4–9 h and is dosed three to four times per day. The usual daily dose as an antiepileptic is 3,600 mg. Patients with renal insufficiency need lower dosages and less frequent dosing. Adverse effects are usually mild and transient [103].

Epilepsy Surgery

Over recent years, the surgical treatment of intractable epilepsy has evolved from a rare therapy practiced in only a handful of centers in the USA to a much more common practice. Today, most major academic centers have an epilepsy surgery program. For this reason, it is important to understand some special considerations when managing these patients in the neuro-ICU. The diagnostic evaluation of potential epilepsy surgery patients can be divided into three phases. Phase I is the noninvasive portion and includes initial outpatient evaluation, imaging (MRI, PET, SPECT, magnetoencephalography), and inpatient video-EEG monitoring. Since long-term video-EEG usually occurs in specialized epilepsy monitoring units (EMUs), it will not be addressed here.

Phase II consists of invasive recording of electrocorticography (ECoG) through surgically implanted electrodes. At many centers, these patients may spend their first few postoperative days in the neuro-ICU. Invasive electrodes can be roughly divided into subdural electrodes (grids and strips) and depth electrodes. Subdural electrodes are usually placed via craniotomy and brain coverage may be extensive. These patients may show evidence of mass effect from their electrodes, associated brain swelling, and/or slowly accumulating subdural hematomas. They must be followed closely for declining neurological status that may indicate that they are not tolerating their invasive electrodes. Depth electrodes are thin tubular structures that are placed stereotactically into the brain parenchyma, often the hippocampi, through burr holes. In general, mass effect from the electrodes themselves is not an issue; although intracerebral hemorrhage can complicate these procedures in rare instances.

In addition to concerns for mass effect, these patients will almost certainly be experiencing seizures. In fact, that is the main goal of the phase II evaluation. In order to encourage seizures in a timely fashion, AEDs are often withdrawn. This raises the possibility of having too many seizures or frank status epilepticus. To counterbalance these concerns, we usually order PRN lorazepam (1–2 mg, IV) to be given for two partial complex or one generalized seizures per 8-h shift. This event also requires evaluation by the epilepsy team.

Phase III consists of the therapeutic surgery. These range from small lesionectomies through larger anterior temporal lobectomies to even larger extratemporal resections and hemispherectomies. Once again, postoperative seizures may be seen due to inflammation and brain irritation from surgery. Most postoperative seizures require evaluation by the epilepsy team. Otherwise, they are treated similarly to seizures during Phase II, i.e., observation of small, sporadic seizures and benzodiazepines for more prolonged seizures. Adequate AED levels, when appropriate, should also be confirmed. As with seizures in the general neuro-ICU population, it can sometimes be difficult to differentiate postictal confusion or a Todd's paralysis from a new deficit related to a postoperative hematoma or stroke. The epilepsy team should be involved in all such situations to help avoid both under- and overdiagnosis of other postoperative problems (e.g., multiple emergency CT scan per day).

Summary

Seizures are symptomatic of underlying central nervous system disease; frequent, uncontrollable seizures are a neurological emergency not uncommon in the neuro-ICU setting, but they may go unrecognized. Close collaboration with neurological colleagues will be necessary to optimally manage these patients, particularly given the constant evolution of medical therapy. Early prolonged EEG monitoring may be particularly helpful in the early recognition and treatment of seizures in the critically ill patient.

Some points to remember are as follows:

- Seizures may be so subtle as to be unrecognized or so dramatic as to shake the patient's bed and instrumentation.
- When a patient has an unexpected or unexplained change in level of consciousness or ability to interact with nursing and medical personnel, one should always consider the possibilities of sporadic, brief seizures with a prolonged postictal or interictal state, or nonconvulsive status epilepticus.
- After experienced clinical personnel, the EEG is the best diagnostic tool for the diagnosis of seizures in the critically ill patient.
- Natriuresis is a common systemic manifestation of aneurysmal subarachnoid hemorrhage (SAH). Natriuresis and its accompanying hypovolemia may be a major contributing factor in the pathophysiology of symptomatic cerebral vasospasm. This may also contribute to seizures.
- Seizures may be an early symptom of CNS malignancy or may appear after surgical procedures for diagnosis or treatment.
- Since the idiopathic and paraneoplastic syndromes are indistinguishable clinically, the appearance of opsoclonus myoclonus should always lead to a search for neuroblastoma or other occult neoplasm.
- Obstructive sleep apnea is also common in medically refractory epilepsy patients.
- For *acute* management of prolonged seizures, benzodiazepines are least likely to induce the enzyme system responsible for metabolizing immunosuppressant drugs.
- In cases of hepatic dysfunction, plasma concentrations must be correlated with serum albumin and protein levels, and free (unbound) levels measured if possible.
- Rapid correction of hyponatremia has been associated with central pontine myelinolysis (CPM), manifested clinically by pseudobulbar palsy and spastic quadriparesis.

References

1. Jordan KG. Nonconvulsive seizures (NCS) and nonconvulsive status epilepticus (NCSE) detected by continuous EEG monitoring in the neuro ICU. Neurology. 1992;42:180. Abstract.
2. Towne AR, Waterhouse EJ, Boggs JG, et al. Prevalence of nonconvulsive status epilepticus in comatose patients. Neurology. 2000;54: 340–5.
3. Claassen J, Mayer SA, Kowalski RG, Emerson RG, Hirsch LJ. Detection of electrographic seizures with continuous EEG monitoring in critically ill patients. Neurology. 2004;62(10): 1743–8.

4. Young GB, Jordan KG, Doig GS. An assessment of nonconvulsive seizures in the intensive care unit using continuous EEG monitoring: an investigation of variables associated with mortality. Neurology. 1996;47:83–9.

5. Jirsch J, Hirsch LJ. Nonconvulsive seizures: developing a rational approach to the diagnosis and management in the critically ill population. Clin Neurophysiol. 2007;118:1660–70.

6. Privitera M, Hoffman M, Moore JL, Jester D. EEG detection of nontonic-clonic status epilepticus in patients with altered consciousness. Epilepsy Res. 1994;18:155–66.

7. Drislane FW, Schomer DL. Clinical implications of generalized electrographic status epilepticus. Epilepsy Res. 1994;19:111–21.

8. Vespa PM, Nuwer MR, Nenov V, et al. Increased incidence and impact of nonconvulsive seizures after traumatic brain injury as detected by continuous electroencephalographic monitoring. J Neurosurg. 1999;91:750–60.

9. Treiman DM. Therapy of status epilepticus in adults and children. Curr Opin Neurol. 2001;14:203–10.

10. Treiman DM, Meyers PD, Walton NY, Collins JF, Colling C, Rowan AJ, Handforth A, Faught E, Calabrese VP, Uthman BM, Ramsay RE, Mamdani MB. A comparison of four treatments for generalized convulsive status epilepticus. Veterans Affairs Status Epilepticus Cooperative Study Group. N Engl J Med. 1998;339(12):792–8.

11. Willmore LJ. Prophylactic treatment. In: Engel J, Pedley TA, et al., editors. Epilepsy: a comprehensive textbook. Philadelphia: Lippincott-Raven Publishers; 2008. p. 1333.

12. Kotapka MJ, Graham DI, Adams JH, Doyle D, Gennarelli TA. Hippocampal damage in fatal paediatric head injury. Neuropathol Appl Neurobiol. 1993;19:128–33.

13. Kotapka MJ, Graham DI, Adams JH, Doyle D, Gennarelli TA. Hippocampal pathology in fatal human head injury without high intracranial pressure. J Neurotrauma. 1994;11:317–24.

14. Langendorf F, Pedley TA, Langendorf F, Pedley TA, et al., editors. Epilepsy: a comprehensive textbook. Philadelphia: Lippincott-Raven Publishers; 2008. p. 2469.

15. Hart RG, Byer JA, Slaughter JR, et al. Occurrence and implication of seizures in subarachnoid hemorrhage due to ruptured intracranial aneurysms. Neurosurgery. 1981;8:417.

16. Butzkueven H, Evans AH, Pitman A, Leopold C, Jolley D, Kaye AH, Kilpatrick CJ, Davis SM. Onset seizures independently predict poor outcome after subarachnoid hemorrhage. Neurology. 2000;55:1315–20.

17. Vespa PM, O'Phelan K, Shah M, et al. Acute seizures after intracerebral hemorrhage: a factor in progressive midline shift and outcome. Neurology. 2003;60:1441–6.

18. Adelman DC, Saltiel E, Klinenberg JR. The neuropsychiatric manifestations of systemic lupus erythematosus: an overview. Semin Arthritis Rheum. 1986;15:185–99.

19. Alarcon-Segovia D, Palacios R. Differences in immunoregulatory T cell circuits between diphenylhydantoin-related and spontaneously occurring systemic lupus erythematosus. Arthritis Rheum. 1981;24:1086–92.

20. Levine SR, Brey RL. Neurological aspects of antiphospholipid antibody syndrome. Lupus. 1996;5:347–53.

21. Nadeau S, Watson RT. Neurologic manifestations of vasculitis and collagen vascular syndromes. In: Joynt R, editor. Clinical neurology. Philadelphia: Harper and Row; 1996. p. 1–166.

22. Schotland DL, Wolf SM, White HH, Dubin HV. Neurologic aspects of Behcet's disease. Am J Med. 1963;34:544–53.

23. Stein DA, Chamberlain MC. Evaluation and management of seizures in the patient with cancer. Oncology. 1991;5:33–9.

24. Dalmau J, Graus F, Rosenblum MK, Posner JB. Anti-Hu associated paraneoplastic encephalitis/sensory neuropathy: a clinical study of 71 patients. Medicine. 1992;71:59–72.

25. Lott I, Kinsbourne M. Myoclonic encephalopathy of infants. In: Fahn S, Marsden CD, Van Woert MH, et al., editors. Myoclonus, vol. 43. New York: Raven Press; 1986; 43:127–46. Advances in Neurology.

26. Bataller L, Graus F, Saiz A, Vilchez JJ. Clinical outcome in adult onset idiopathic or paraneoplastic opsoclonus-myoclonus. Brain. 2001;124:437–43.

27. Malow BA, Levy K, Maturen K, Bowes R. Obstructive sleep apnea is common in medically refractory epilepsy patients. Neurology. 2000;55:1002.

28. Gilmore RL, Falace P, Kanga J, Baumann R. Sleep disordered breathing in Mobius syndrome. J Child Neurol. 1991;6:73–7.

29. Gelling L. Causes of ICU psychosis: the environmental factors. Nurs Crit Care. 1999;4:22–6.

30. Finelli PF, McEntee WJ, Ambler M, Restenbaum D. Adult celiac disease presenting as cerebellar syndrome. Neurology. 1980;30:245–9.

31. Albers JW, Nostrant TT, Riggs JE. Neurologic manifestations of gastrointestinal disease. Neurol Clin. 1989;7:525–48.

32. Rush PJ, Inman R, Berstein M, Carlen P, et al. Isolated vasculitis of the central nervous system in a patient with celiac disease. Am J Med. 1986;81:1092–4.

33. Relman DA, Schmidt TM, MacDermott RP, Falkow S. Identification of the uncultured bacillus of Whipple's disease. N Engl J Med. 1992;327:293–301.

34. Louis ED, Lynch T, Kaufmann P, Fahn S, Odel J. Diagnostic guidelines in central nervous system Whipple's disease. Ann Neurol. 1996;40:561–8.

35. Sawka AM, Aniszewski JP, Young WF, et al. Tension pneumocranium, a rare complication of transsphenoidal pituitary surgery: mayo clinic experience 1976-1998. J Clin Endocrinol Metab. 1999;84:4731.

36. Wijdicks EMF, Plevak DJ, Wiesner RH, Steers JL. Causes and outcome of seizures in liver transplant recipients. Neurology. 1996;47:1523–5.

37. Vaughn BV, Olivier KN, Lackner RP, Robertson KR, Messenheimer JA, Paradowski LJ, Egan TM. Seizures in lung transplant recipients. Epilepsia. 1996;37:1175–9.

38. Zimmer WE, Hourihane JM, Wang HZ, Schriber JR. The effect of human leukocyte antigen disparity on cyclosporine neurotoxicity after allogeneic bone marrow transplantation. AJNR Am J Neuroradiol. 1998;19:601–8.

39. Zomas A, Mehta J, Powels R, Treleaven J, et al. Unusual infections following allogeneic bone marrow transplantation for chronic lymphocytic leukemia. Bone Marrow Transplant. 1994;14:799–803.

40. Lor E, Liu YQ. Neurologic sequelae associated with foscarnet therapy. Ann Pharmacother. 1994;28:1035–7.

41. Miller AD, Ball AM, Bookstaver PB, Dornblaser EK, Bennett CL. Epileptogenic potential of carbapenem agents: mechanism of action, seizure rates, and clinical considerations. Pharmacotherapy. 2011;31(4):408–23.

42. Gilmore R. Seizures and antiepileptic drug use in transplant patients. Neurol Clin. 1988;6:279–96.

43. Wassner SJ, Malekzadeh MH, Pennisi AJ, et al. Allograft survival in patient receiving anticonvulsant medications. Clin Nephrol. 1977;8:293–7.

44. Gambertoglio JG, Holford NHG, Kapusnik JE, Nishikawa R, et al. Disposition of total and unbound prednisolone in renal transplant patients receiving anticonvulsant. Kidney Int. 1984;25:119–23.

45. Boggs JG. Seizures in medically complex patients. Epilepsia. 1997;38 Suppl 4:S55–9.

46. Anderson GD, Pak C, Doane KW, Griffy KG, Temkin NR, Wilensky AJ, Winn HR. Revised Winter-Tozer equation for normalized phenytoin concentrations in trauma and elderly patients with hypoalbuminemia. Ann Pharmacother. 1997;31:279.

47. Anderson RJ, Chung HM, Kluge R, Shrier RW. Hyponatremia: a prospective analysis of its epidemiology and the pathogenetic role of vasopressin. Ann Intern Med. 1985;102:164–8.

48. Oruckaptan HH, Ozisik P, Akalan N. Prolonged cerebral salt wasting syndrome associated with the intraventricular dissemination of brain tumors. Report of two cases and review of the literature. Pediatr Neurosurg. 2000;33:16.

49. Arieff AI, Guisardo R. Effects on the central nervous system of hypernatremic and hyponatremic states. Kidney Int. 1976;10: 104–16.

50. Daggett P, Deanfield J, Moss F. Neurological aspects of hyponatremia. Postgrad Med J. 1982;58:737–40.

51. Epstein FH. Signs and symptoms of electrolyte disorders. In: Maxwell MJ, Kleemand CR, editors. Clinical disorders of fluid and electrolyte metabolism. 3rd ed. New York: McGraw-Hill Book Co; 1979. p. 499–530.

52. Harrigan MR. Cerebral salt wasting syndrome. Crit Care Clin. 2001;17:125–38.

53. Riggs JE. Neurologic manifestations of fluid and electrolyte disturbances. Neurol Clin. 1989;7:509–23.

54. Rossi NF, Schrier RW. Hyponatremic states. In: Maxwell MH, Cleeman CR, Narins RG, Maxwell MH, Cleeman CR, Narins RG, et al., editors. Clinical disorders of fluid and electrolyte metabolism. 5th ed. New York: McGraw-Hill Book Co; 1987. p. 461–70.

55. Norenberg MD, Leslie KO, Robertson AS. Association between rise in sodium and central pontine myelinolysis. Ann Neurol. 1982;11:128–35.

56. Singh BM, Strobos R. Epilepsia partialis continua associated with nonketotic hyperglycemia: clinical and biochemical profile of 21 patients. Ann Neurol. 1980;8:155–60.

57. Vastola EF, Maccario M, Homan RO. Activation of epileptogenic foci by hyperosmolality. Neurology. 1967;17:520–6.

58. Singh BM, Gupta DR, Strobos RJ. Nonketotic hyperglycemia and epilepsia partialis continua. Arch Neurol. 1973;29:189–90.

59. Halperin I, Nubiola A, Vendrell J, Vilardell E. Late-onset hypocalcemia appearing years after thyroid surgery. J Endocrinol Invest. 1989;12(6):419–22.

60. Layzer RB. Neuromuscular manifestations of systemic disease. Philadelphia: FA Davis Co; 1985. p. 58–62.

61. Reber PM, Heath H. Hypocalcemic emergencies. Med Clin North Am. 1995;79:93–106.

62. Whang R. Clinical disorders of magnesium metabolism. Compr Ther. 1997;23(3):168–73.

63. Silvis SE, Paragas PD, Silvis SE, Paragas PD. Paresthesias, weakness, seizures, and hypophosphatemia in patients receiving hyperalimentation. Gastroenterology. 1972;62:513–20.

64. Knochel JP. The pathophysiology and clinical characteristics of severe hypophosphatemia. Arch Intern Med. 1977;137: 203–20.

65. Lockwood AH. Neurologic complications of renal disease. Neurol Clin. 1989;7(3):617–27.

66. Beydoun VA, Uthman BM, Sackellares JC. Gabapentin: pharmacokinetics, efficacy, and safety. Clin Neuropharmacol. 1995;18(6): 469–81.

67. Adams RD, Foley JM. The neurological disorder associated with liver disease. In: Metabolic and toxic diseases of the nervous system. New York, Baltimore: Williams & Wilkins; 1953. p. 198–231.

68. Plum F, Posner JB. Diagnosis of stupor and coma. Philadelphia: FA Davis Co; 1984. p. 222–5.

69. Alldredge BK, Lowenstein DH, Simon RP. Seizures associated with recreational drug abuse. Neurology. 1989;39(8):1037–9.

70. Brust JCM, Ng SKC, Hauser AW, Susser M. Marijuana use and the risk of new onset seizures. Trans Am Clin Climatol Assoc. 1992;103:176–81.

71. Jeri FR, Sanchez CC, Del Pozo T, Fernandez M, Carbajal C. Further experience with the syndromes produced by coco paste smoking. Bull Narc. 1978;30:1–7.

72. Koppel BS, Samkoff L, Daras M. Relation of cocaine use to seizures and epilepsy. Epilepsia. 1996;37:875.

73. Pascual- Leone A, Dhuna A, Altafullah I, Anderson DC. Cocaine - induced seizures. Neurology. 1990;40(3, Part 1):404–7.

74. Johnson S, O'Meara M, Young JB. Acute cocaine poisoning. Importance of treating seizures and acidosis. Am J Med. 1983; 75:1061–4.

75. Antelman SM, Kocan D, Rowland N, de Giovanni L, Chiodo LA. Amitriptyline provides long-lasting immunization against sudden cardiac death from cocaine. Eur J Pharmacol. 1981;69: 119–20.

76. Jaffe JH. Drug addiction and drug abuse. In: Gilman AG, Goodman LS, Rall TW, Murrad F, editors. Goodman and Gilman's the pharmacologic basis of therapeutics. New York: Macmillan; 1985. p. 550–4.

77. Henry JA, Jeffreys KJ, Dawling S. Toxicity and death from 3,4-methylenedioxymethamphetamine ("ecstasy"). Lancet. 1992; 340:384–7.

78. Burgess C, O'Donohoe A, Gill M. Agony and ecstasy: a review of MDMA effects and toxicity. Eur Psychiatry. 2000;15:287.

79. Eisenschenk S, Gilmore RL. Strategies for successful management of older patients with seizures. Geriatrics. 1999;54:31, 34, 39–40.

80. Bodner RA, Lynch T, Lewis L, Kahn D. Serotonin syndrome. Neurology. 1995;45:219–23.

81. Schneck HJ, Rupreht J. Central anticholinergic syndrome (CAS) in anesthesia and intensive care. Acta Anaesthesiol Belg. 1989; 40(3):219–28.

82. Blain PG, Stewart-Wynne E. Neurologic disorders. In: Davies DM et al., editors. Textbook of adverse drug reactions. 3rd ed. New York: Oxford University Press; 1985. p. 494.

83. Lowry MR, Dunner FJ. Seizures during tricyclic therapy. Am J Psychiatry. 1980;137:1461–2.

84. Richardson III JW, Richelson R. Antidepressants: clinical update for medical practitioners. Mayo Clin Proc. 1984;59:330–7.

85. Favale E, Rubino V, Mainardi P, Lunardi G, Albano C. Anticonvulsant effect of fluoxetine in humans. Neurology. 1995; 45:1926–7.

86. Messing RO, Simon RP. Seizures as a manifestation of systemic disease. Neurol Clin. 1986;4:563–84.

87. Logothetis J. Spontaneous epileptic seizures and electroencephalographic changes in the course of phenothiazine therapy. Neurology. 1967;17:869–77.

88. Devinsky O, Honigfeld G, Patin J. Clozapine-related seizures. Neurology. 1991;41:369–71.

89. Eshleman SH, Shaw LM. Massive theophylline overdose with atypical metabolic abnormalities. Clin Chem. 1990;36:398–9.

90. Steen PA, Michelfelder JD. Neurotoxicity of anesthetics. Anesthesiology. 1979;50:437–53.

91. Wood JD, Peesker SJ. The effect of GABA metabolism in brain of isonicotinic acid hydrazide and pyridoxine as a function of time after administration. J Neurochem. 1972;19:1527–37.

92. Watkins RC, Hambrick EL, Benjamin G, Chavda SN. Isoniazid toxicity presenting as seizures and metabolic acidosis. J Natl Med Assoc. 1990;2(1):57–64.

93. Chin L, Sievers ML, Herrier RN, Pichionni AL. Potentiation of pyridoxine by depressants and anticonvulsants in the treatment of acute isoniazid intoxication in dogs. Toxicol Appl Pharmacol. 1981;58:504–9.

94. Fierro LS, Savulich DH, Benerza DA. Safety of fosphenytoin sodium. Am J Health Syst Pharm. 1996;53:2707–12.

95. DeLorenzo RJ, Waterhouse EJ, Towne AR, Boggs JG, Ko D, DeLorenzo GA, Brown A, Garnett L. Persistent nonconvulsive

status epilepticus after the control of convulsive status epilepticus. Epilepsia. 1998;39(8):833–40.

96. Prasad A, Worrall BB, Bertram EH, Bleck TP. Propofol and midazolam in the treatment of refractory status epilepticus. Epilepsia. 2001;42:380–6.

97. Alvarez V, Januel JM, Burnand B, Rosetti AO. Second-line status epilepticus treatment: comparison of phenytoin, valproate, and levetiracetam. Epilepsia. 2011;52:1292–6.

98. Wheless JW, Venkataraman V. Safety of high dose intravenous valproate loading doses in epilepsy patients. J Epilepsy. 1998;11:319–24.

99. Hovinga CA, Chicella MF, Rose DF, Eades SK, Eades SK, Dalton JT, Phelps SJ. Use of intravenous valproate in three pediatric patients with nonconvulsive or convulsive status epilepticus. Ann Pharmacother. 1999;33:579–84.

100. Nicolas JM, Collart P, Gerin B, et al. In vitro evaluation of potential drug interactions with levetiracetam, a new antiepileptic agent. Drug Metab Dispos. 1999;27:250–4.

101. Kellinghaus C, Berning S, Immisch I, Larch J, Rosenow F, Rossetti AO, Tilz C, Trinka E. Intravenous lacosamide for treatment of status epilepticus. Acta Neurol Scand. 2011;123(2):137–41.

102. Koubeissi MZ, Mayor CL, Estephan B, Rashid S, Azar NJ. Efficacy and safety of intravenous lacosamide in refractory nonconvulsive status epilepticus. Acta Neurol Scand. 2011;123(2):142–6.

103. Morris GL. Efficacy and tolerability of gabapentin in clinical practice. Clin Ther. 1995;17:891.

104. Gilmore RL. Seizures. In: Layon AJ, Gabrielli A, Friedman WA, et al., editors. Textbook of neurointensive care. Philadelphia: WB Saunders; 2004.

Part VI

Situations of Special Interest

Neuroradiological Imaging

40

Jeffrey A. Bennett and Sandip Patel

Contents

J.A. Bennett, MD (✉) • S. Patel, MD
Department of Radiology,
University of Florida College of Medicine,
Gainesville, FL 32610, USA
e-mail: bennja@radiology.ufl.edu; patsan@radiology.ufl.edu

Abstract

The role of radiology in the setting of neurocritical care is discussed in detail. The author initially outlines the various modalities along with their specific indications that are utilized when imaging patients in the neuro ICU. These include CT and MRI as well as CT and MRI angiography of the head and neck. In addition, the significance of key imaging sequences in both CT and MRI and their associated findings are also described. In the second part of this chapter, the author continues to illustrate common radiologic findings that are encountered with patients in the neuro ICU that range from intracranial hemorrhage to herniation syndromes and hydrocephalus.

Keywords

MRI • CT • CT angiography • Herniation • Hemorrhage • Hydrocephalus • Stroke • Perfusion

Introduction

Neuroradiology is an essential tool in critical care medicine. The goals of this chapter are to help the reader understand how images are created using the modalities of magnetic resonance imaging (MRI) and computed tomography (CT). This understanding will then be elaborated upon to inform the reader in interpretation of images. Pattern recognition essential for recognizing brain herniation syndromes is addressed, as are common findings seen in acute cerebral infarction, hemorrhage, and hydrocephalus. Although the initial sections on understanding MRI and CT are somewhat technical, it is worth making the effort to understand the material and to better speak the language of the radiologist. This will aid knowing which study to order and will help clear communication in critical care situations.

A.J. Layon et al. (eds.), *Textbook of Neurointensive Care*,
DOI 10.1007/978-1-4471-5226-2_40, © Springer-Verlag London 2013

Understanding Magnetic Resonance Imaging (MRI)

To understand the modality of MRI, it is necessary to delve into some of the physics that goes into the creation of the images. This is important in order to differentiate tissue types on T1-weighted and T2-weighted images and to recognize artifacts which could potentially be confused with pathology. This section will accomplish this with a minimum of mathematical formulae by building on some basic physical principles of electromagnetism. The understanding of where signal and contrast comes from in MRI will help the neurointensivist to speak the language of the radiologist and will help when ordering studies to know whether special sequences or intravenous contrast are necessary. The spin echo sequence and the gradient-recalled echo sequence will be discussed first as these are the only two methods available to create signal. All other pulse sequences, some of which will be discussed subsequently, are variations of these two fundamental procedures.

The Main Magnetic Field

In 1831, Michael Faraday discovered that if he moved a magnet through a coil of wire, an electric current was produced in the wire. Faraday's law of electromagnetic induction is critical to the workings of MR units. The main magnetic field of an MR machine, termed B_0, is produced by an electric current flowing through a coil of wire. The magnetic field induced by this current is perpendicular to the coil. In order to induce the very strong magnetic fields used in clinical scanners, typically 1.5 T or 3 T, a very large current is necessary. To avoid the generation of heat from this current, the wire is immersed in liquid helium at a very low temperature to allow superconduction. A great deal of work is spent by vendors to create very strong main magnetic fields that are uniform within the bore of the magnet. Differences in the magnetic field at different locations, termed magnetic field inhomogeneities, degrade the quality of images, as will be shown later.

Protons, Resonance, and the Radiofrequency (RF) Pulse

Clinical MRI uses hydrogen protons to obtain signal because of their abundance in the body in the form of water, fat, and other organic compounds. Other charged particles, such as sodium, can also be imaged, and this is being developed on a research basis using high-field magnets, for cerebral infarction and other indications. This chapter will only discuss proton MRI. A hydrogen proton is positively charged and spins about its axis, making it act like a tiny bar magnet.

When protons are put into a strong magnetic field, some align in the direction of the main magnetic field (the longitudinal or z direction), and others align in the opposite direction. Those aligned opposite to the field are at a higher energy state. It turns out that slightly more protons are aligned with the magnetic field than against it, and it is this difference, termed the net magnetization, that is acted upon to become the source of signal for MRI.

The spinning protons in the main magnetic field wobble, or precess, about their axis at a specific frequency which is dependent on the strength of the magnetic field. Precession is similar to the motion of a spinning top being acted upon by gravity. The frequency of precession is determined by the Larmor equation:

$$F = \gamma B_0$$

where F is the frequency of precession, γ is the gyromagnetic ratio (a constant characteristic of each type of nucleus), and B_0 is the strength of the magnetic field. At 1.5 T this frequency is about 64 MHz for hydrogen protons, in the radiofrequency range of energy. This is the resonant frequency of protons in the magnetic field, and, thus, if energy is delivered to the protons at this radiofrequency, there will be efficient transfer of energy to the protons. This is why the term resonance is used in MRI.

A radiofrequency energy pulse is produced by way of rapidly alternating currents in loops of wire called an RF transmit coil. This magnetic field energy is transferred to the spinning protons and causes their net magnetization to rotate or flip away from the longitudinal axis of the main magnet to the transverse plane. The amount of rotation is called the flip angle and depends on the strength and duration of the RF pulse. An RF pulse designed to change net magnetization to the transverse plane is called a 90° RF pulse. A 180° RF pulse flips net magnetization to the $-z$ axis.

T1 Relaxation and T1-Weighted Contrast

After a 90° RF pulse, protons absorb energy which results in their net magnetization being at a higher energy level in the transverse plane. The net longitudinal magnetization is zero. When the RF pulse is turned off, the protons give up their energy to the environment, termed the lattice, and realign back to the longitudinal axis. This process of regaining longitudinal magnetization is termed T1 relaxation or recovery. This change in the direction of net magnetization can be detected by a receiver coil (often the same coil as the transmit coil) where the changing magnetic field induces a current which can be measured and turned into an image.

The rate at which protons relax is different for protons in different tissue. White matter has a very short T1 relaxation time. Gray matter has an intermediate T1 relaxation time. CSF has a very long T1 relaxation time. If an image is created

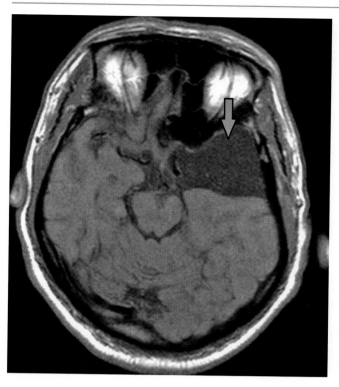

Fig. 40.1 Axial T1-weighted MR image showing a left middle cranial fossa arachnoid cyst (*orange arrow*). Note that the fluid within the cyst follows CSF signal intensity, which is dark on T1-weighted images. Differentiation of this lesion from an epidermoid cyst would require comparison with T2-weighted images, FLAIR images, and diffusion-weighted images. An arachnoid cyst would follow CSF signal intensity on all these sequences

at a time when these tissues are at different stages of relaxation, we can see T1-weighted contrast. On a T1-weighted image, CSF is assigned to dark pixels, gray matter is intermediate gray, and white matter is assigned to lighter shaded pixels (Fig. 40.1).

Even without understanding the physics of image creation, it is useful to know what is high signal, or bright, on T1-weighted images. The protons in fat actually recover their longitudinal magnetization the fastest, and so fat is bright on T1-weighted images; also bright are forms of intracellular calcium, methemoglobin blood breakdown products, melanin, and high proteinaceous material. Contrast material, such as gadolinium, also shortens the relaxation of protons in structures that take up the contrast, resulting in high signal (Fig. 40.2a, b).

T2 Relaxation and T2-Weighted Contrast

The protons in the magnetic field all precess at the Larmor frequency, but are not in phase. The RF pulse gives energy to the protons and causes them to precess in phase. When the RF pulse is turned off, the protons lose this energy by dephasing. This is secondary to several mechanisms, including spin-spin interactions, magnetic field inhomogeneities, magnetic susceptibility, and chemical shift. Immediately after a 90° RF pulse, magnetization in the transverse plane is at its maximum. Transverse magnetization decreases over time, and the rate of dephasing or loss of transverse magnetization is called T2 relaxation. Like T1, T2 is tissue specific. If we measure the amount of transverse magnetization with a receiver coil at a time when different tissues are at different stages of T2 relaxation, we can create a T2-weighted image. CSF has a very long T2 and is assigned to white pixels; white matter has a short T2 and is gray on T2-weighted images. Gray matter has an intermediate T2 value and so is a lighter gray than white matter on T2-weighted images. Tissue that is bright or high signal on T2-weighted images is high free water tissue such as CSF, proteinaceous material, and certain blood products (oxyhemoglobin, extracellular methemoglobin) (Fig. 40.3). T1 relaxation and T2 relaxation happen simultaneously, so all images have some factor of T1 and some factor of T2 in them. Pulse sequence timing is designed to weight images toward T1 or T2 contrast, hence the terms T1-weighted or T2-weighted images.

Remember that protons are being imaged, and so material with a low density of protons will be dark on both T1- and T2-weighted images. For example, air has no protons and appears black. Mineral-rich tissue such as cortical bone and dystrophic calcifications also appears dark on MRI (Fig. 40.4a–c).

Spin Echo

After a 90° RF pulse, longitudinal magnetization increases and transverse magnetization decreases. What is measured as signal on MRI is transverse magnetization, and so it can be seen that the maximum signal is present immediately after the RF pulse. The signal then drops in a manner called free induction decay. The spin echo pulse sequence is designed to recover signal and measure it later. This is achieved with a 180° refocusing RF pulse given after the 90° RF pulse. This reverses the axis of the precessing protons which then recover their phase, and therefore signal, at time TE (the echo time).

TR

TR (repetition time) is the time it takes to run through a pulse sequence one time. This generates one row of data in k-space, where MR raw data are stored. If we want to make an image with a 256 pixel × 256 pixel matrix, we have to repeat the pulse sequence 256 times to fill k-space. This takes time (256 × TR). It is important to realize that each row of data in

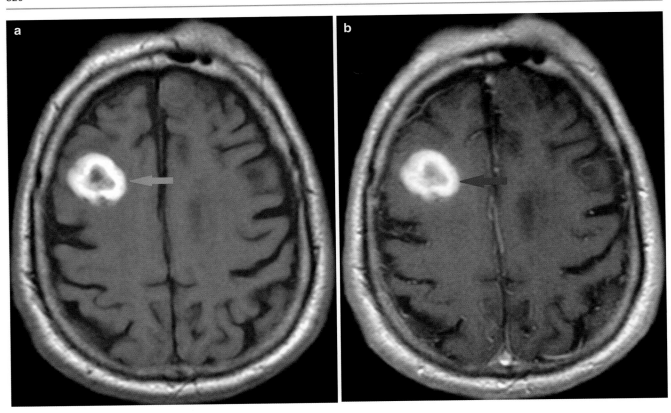

Fig. 40.2 Axial noncontrast (**a**) and post-contrast (**b**) T1-weighted MR images of a right frontal melanoma metastasis. Notice that the mass is spontaneously high signal on the noncontrast T1-weighted image (*orange arrow*, **a**) and shows some minimal enhancement (*blue arrow*, **b**). The high T1 signal may be from melanin in the tumor or from methemoglobin if the lesion is hemorrhagic. Additional sequences such as GRE or SWI could be performed to determine the presence of blood products within the lesion

k-space contains data about the entire image to be created. This idea will be discussed more in the section on artifacts, where it will be seen how motion affects the image.

Spatial Localization

Gradient pulses must be turned on in three orthogonal directions to localize the signal in three dimensions and thus create images in different slices. Embedded in the pulse sequence are the slice select gradient, the phase-encoding gradient, and the frequency-encoding (or read-out) gradient. These gradients make linear changes to the magnetic field in different directions to allow localization of signal in space.

Contrast on Spin Echo Sequences

The timing of TE and TR can be changed by the operator to make images with T1-weighting, T2-weighting, or proton density-weighting. A short TE minimizes T2-weighting. A long TE maximizes T2-weighting. An intermediate TR maximizes T1-weighting. A long TR minimizes T1-weighting. If both T1 and T2 effects are minimized (short TE and long TR), a proton density-weighted image results. Typical values at 1.5 T for T1-weighting are TE = 20 ms and TR = 500 ms. Typical values at 1.5 T for T2-weighting are TE = 80 ms and TR = 2,000 ms.

Fast Spin Echo Techniques

Fast spin echo or turbo spin echo is a variation of the conventional spin echo pulse sequence where additional 180° refocusing pulses are given to produce multiple echos (when signal can be detected) in one TR. This results in faster filling of k-space and thus decreased overall imaging time.

Inversion Recovery

The inversion recovery sequence is a frequently used imaging technique and is a variation of the conventional spin echo technique. The difference is that a 180° RF pulse is

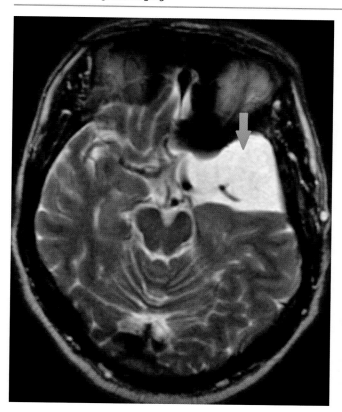

Fig. 40.3 Axial T2-weighted MR image of the same left middle cranial fossa arachnoid cyst shown in Fig. 40.1. On the T2-weighted sequence fluid including CSF is high signal (*orange arrow*). Notice the dark signal within the cyst representing a flow void in the left middle cerebral artery

Gradient-Recalled Echo (GRE) Sequence

The gradient-recalled echo sequence is a different technique compared to spin echo sequences for obtaining signal from tissue. The RF pulse that is given is less than 90°, say 20° or 30°, and there is no 180° refocusing pulse. Gradient pulses are used to dephase and rephase net transverse magnetization, which is less than the net transverse magnetization in the spin echo sequence. The advantage of a smaller flip angle is that it takes less time for recovery of longitudinal magnetization and therefore a shorter TR can be used. This allows overall decreased imaging time but less signal to noise than a spin echo sequence. GRE sequences can be T1 weighted or T2 weighted.

The spin echo sequence has an advantage of refocusing dephased protons regardless of slight irregularities in the magnetic field. The GRE sequence does not do this, and therefore signal can be lost if there is not a truly uniform magnetic field. Technically, GRE sequences with long TEs are not T2 weighted, but are T2* weighted, because of the magnetic field inhomogeneities and magnetic susceptibility which increase the rate of dephasing. This can be used to advantage to identify hemosiderin, which alters the local magnetic field and causes signal loss within the affected voxels (Fig. 40.7a, b).

A recently developed pulse sequence is susceptibility-weighted imaging (SWI). This is a long TE flow-compensated GRE sequence which is designed to detect small differences in magnetic susceptibility and lose signal in the voxels affected. The sequence is very sensitive to high iron content in the basal ganglia; hemosiderin, for example, from amyloid angiopathy or hypertensive microhemorrhages; and deoxy-hemoglobin in venous structures (Fig. 40.8).

Gradient-recalled echo sequences also have a role in volumetric acquisitions. The increased speed of the GRE sequence can be used to advantage to collect very thin, 1 mm, contiguous section images. These images can be reformatted in multiple planes and used with image guidance systems in surgery or radiation therapy. T1-weighted imaging with intravenous contrast administration is often used to optimally display tumor prior to image-guided biopsy (Fig. 40.9).

The Effect of Intravenous Contrast Material

Gadolinium is a heavy metal which increases the rate of T1 relaxivity in tissues that retain it during image acquisition. This is the cause of high signal on T1-weighted images in tissues that enhance. The basis of abnormal contrast enhancement is similar for both CT (using iodinated contrast material) and MR and is the result of an expanded intravascular pool or to breakdown of the blood-brain barrier allowing diffusion of contrast into the brain parenchyma. An expanded intravascular

delivered first, flipping net magnetization into the −z axis. The different tissues then recover their longitudinal magnetization at different rates. The 90° RF pulse can be timed to be given when the net magnetization of a certain tissue in the longitudinal plane is zero. If it is timed for fluid, it is called FLAIR (fluid attenuated inversion recovery). If it is timed for fat, it is called STIR (short tau inversion recovery). The advantage is that if fluid or fat is excited by a 90° RF pulse when it has zero longitudinal magnetization, it will have zero transverse magnetization and thus will give no signal. STIR is a very effective fat suppression technique when the magnetic field in the main magnet is homogenous. FLAIR images are extremely useful in evaluating brain pathology as most pathological conditions have high signal on T2-weighted images (Fig. 40.5). If the fluid is suppressed, the contrast of the pathology is enhanced. This is especially true for white matter disease. FLAIR images are also very good for detecting blood or pus in the subarachnoid space. The blood or pus is high signal on T2-weighted images and is obscured on routine T2-weighted images. The suppression of CSF allows visualization of the pathology (Fig. 40.6).

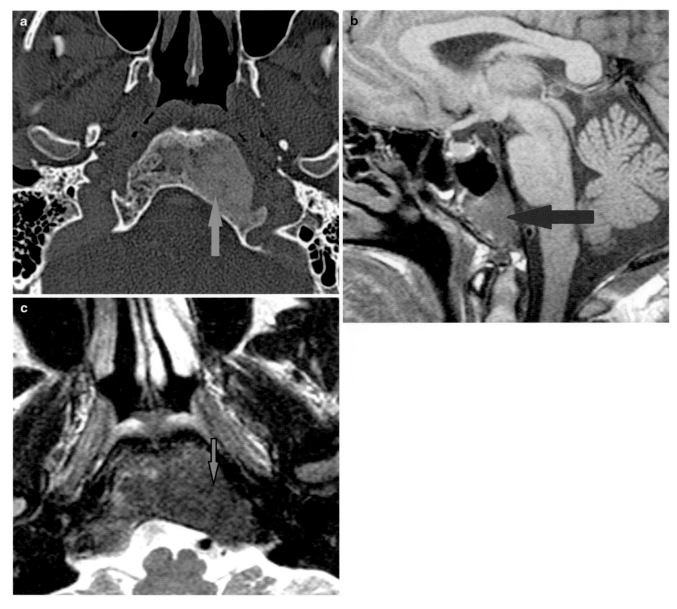

Fig. 40.4 Axial CT scan (**a**), noncontrast sagittal T1-weighted MR image (**b**), and axial T2-weighted MR image (**c**) of a fibro-osseous lesion of the clivus. CT shows a ground glass mineralized lesion (*orange arrow*, **a**). The T1-weighted (*blue arrow*, **b**) and T2-weighted (*orange arrow*, **c**) images both show relatively dark signal within the lesion. Most pathology is bright on T2-weighted images unless the lesion is mineralized or fibrous, as in this case, or is hemorrhagic

pool occurs in tissue that has impaired autoregulation and thus an increased capacity of regional capillary volume. This can be seen following a seizure, stroke, or following head trauma. An expanded vascular pool can also be present in vascular malformations. Finally, neoplasms with angiogenesis may have an expanded vascular pool from increased number and size of vessels and so can enhance.

Leaky blood vessels from a lack of endothelial tight junctions or from pathological processes will also result in contrast enhancement. This occurs from extravasation of contrast out of the blood vessels and into the interstitium. This occurs

normally in the pituitary gland and stalk, the choroid plexus, and dural structures. Abnormal contrast enhancement secondary to breakdown of the blood-brain barrier can take various forms including nodular (or mass-like), gyriform, or nonspecific (Fig. 40.10a, b).

Echo-Planar Imaging

An echo-planar sequence is one form of fast MR imaging. In this type of sequence, which can be either spin echo or GRE,

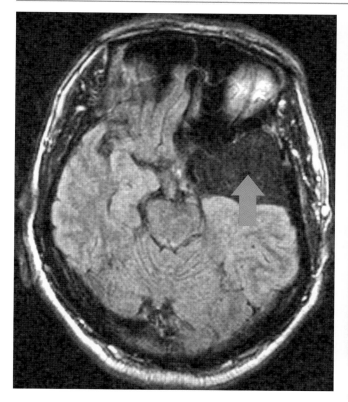

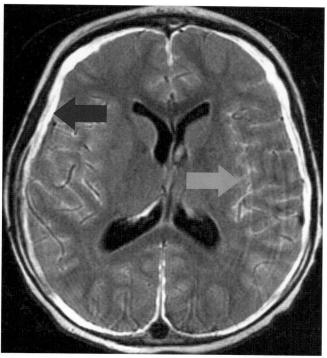

Fig. 40.5 Axial FLAIR MR image of the same left middle cranial fossa arachnoid cyst (*orange arrow*) shown in Fig. 40.1. On the FLAIR sequence, fluid including CSF is suppressed and appears as dark signal

Fig. 40.6 Axial FLAIR MR image of a patient with bacterial meningitis shows thickened high signal dura (*blue arrow*) and high signal in the sulci (*orange arrow*) from pus. Normally the CSF in the sulci should be low signal on FLAIR images

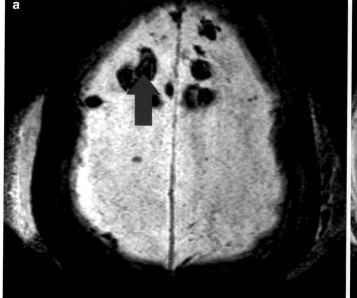

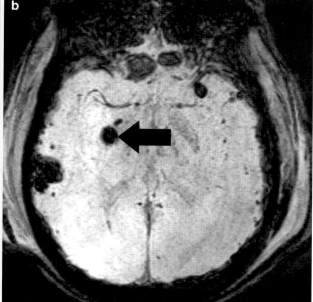

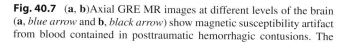

Fig. 40.7 (**a, b**)Axial GRE MR images at different levels of the brain (**a**, *blue arrow* and **b**, *black arrow*) show magnetic susceptibility artifact from blood contained in posttraumatic hemorrhagic contusions. The inhomogeneity of the magnetic field from the blood products causes signal loss and a "blooming" artifact of very dark signal in the contusions

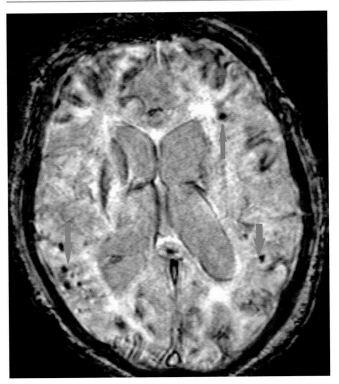

Fig. 40.8 Axial susceptibility-weighted MR image shows multiple foci of signal loss (*orange arrows*) at the gray-white junction in this elderly patient with amyloid angiopathy. The signal loss is from magnetic susceptibility artifact from the blood products

a long echo train is used to fill all lines of k-space in one TR. To achieve this, the phase-encoding gradient and the frequency-encoding gradient must be turned on and off very rapidly, resulting in a very loud sequence for the patient; it is the method of choice for diffusion-weighted imaging.

Diffusion-Weighted Imaging (DWI)

This is a form of physiological imaging that utilizes two equal strength opposing gradients to sensitize the protons for rapid motion by diffusion. If there is no motion of the water, the first gradient dephases the spins of the protons, and the second gradient refocuses them, resulting in high signal intensity. However, if there is motion of the protons in the time between the two gradients, they may not be refocused, and so there will be signal loss. The amount of diffusion weighting is often described by a "b value." The b value is defined as the product of the square of the diffusion gradient strength and the time between the two gradient pulses. A b value of 1,000 is typically used in the clinical setting. A $b=0$ image is one taken without the diffusion gradients being turned on. This is essentially just a low resolution T2-weighted image. The $b=0$ and $b=1,000$ images can be used to calculate an apparent diffusion coefficient (ADC) map, which effectively takes the

T2-weighting out of the image. The ADC values are scaled to the negative logarithm of the signal intensity ratio between the $b=0$ and the $b=1,000$ images. Therefore, areas of restricted diffusion are dark on ADC maps, whereas they are bright on diffusion-weighted images.

The main clinical application of DWI is acute stroke. After an acute cerebral infarction, the dead cells swell, and there is restricted motion of water in both the intracellular and extracellular space, resulting in high signal intensity on the diffusion-weighted image and low signal on the ADC map. Similar restricted diffusion is seen in bacterial abscesses and some tumors such as lymphoma. Often tumors with a high nuclear to cytoplasm ratio will also have restricted diffusion, but typically the DWI images are not as bright as is seen with infarction (Fig. 40.11a, b).

Diffusion-weighted imaging can also be performed with multiple direction gradients, six directions or more, to create diffusion tensor imaging (DTI). This technique allows the direction of fiber tracts to be determined. Currently there is little utility of DTI in the acute clinical setting, but much research is being done in the fields of traumatic brain injury, seizures, dementias, and others which are revealing that this technique may be sensitive to brain injury.

MR Perfusion

Another physiological imaging technique is perfusion. There are various techniques available for perfusion imaging. Probably the most commonly used method is dynamic susceptibility contrast-enhanced perfusion. This technique uses rapid T2*-weighted imaging of the brain as contrast flows in and out. There is signal loss on the images as a result of the magnetic susceptibility artifact of the gadolinium as it flows through tissue. The different intensity of pixels over time can be used to calculate relative perfusion maps of mean transit time (MTT), cerebral blood volume (CBV), and cerebral blood flow (CBF). These maps show relative values over the brain but are not quantitatively accurate. The images are useful in acute stroke and also for differentiating recurrent brain tumor from radiation necrosis. Radiation necrosis will often enhance and be difficult to distinguish from tumor on anatomic imaging but will have decreased blood flow and volume on perfusion imaging. Recurrent tumor, such as glioblastoma multiforme (GBM), will have increased perfusion (Fig. 40.12a, b).

A more recent technique for acquiring MR perfusion imaging is arterial spin labeling (ASL). This is a noninvasive technique as no intravenous contrast is required. Inflowing blood is magnetically tagged and can then be imaged to create similar perfusion maps. This technique can be used to tag individual vessels, for example, the left internal carotid artery, and show the territory of the brain perfused by this vessel.

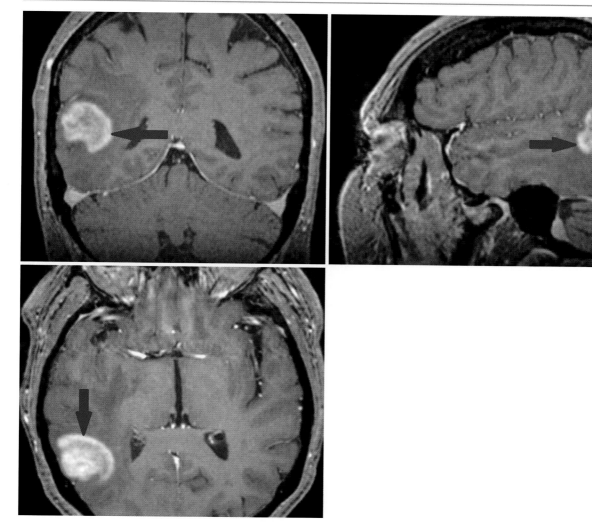

Fig. 40.9 A thin section axial T1-weighted GRE MR volumetric acquisition has been reformatted in sagittal and coronal planes using post-processing software. This type of volumetric GRE sequence can be used with intraoperative software for the purpose of image guidance. *Blue arrows* points out the enhancing tumor

MR Angiography (MRA) and MR Venography (MRV)

There are various methods available to obtain MR angiographic images, including time-of-flight (TOF) imaging, phase – contrast imaging, and contrast-enhanced angiography. In TOF imaging, stationary tissue is suppressed by multiple RF pulses with short TRs to saturate the proton spins. Inflowing protons in blood are not suppressed and therefore generate signal. TOF images can be 2D, with different slice acquisition, or 3D, where a volumetric acquisition is performed. The images can be sensitized for inflowing blood (MRA) or outflowing blood (MRV) (Fig. 40.13). Phase-contrast imaging uses two acquisitions sensitized to flow in opposite directions, which are subtracted to reveal signal only from flowing blood. This technique in used in CSF flow studies where pulsatile motion of CSF is sensitized to generate signal.

Contrast-enhanced MR angiography is typically used for imaging the neck vessels as this technique has the advantage of greater coverage, allowing visualization of the carotid and vertebral vessels from their origins to the skull base. T1-weighted images are obtained as gadolinium flows through the vessels. The contrast shortens the T1 relaxation time and therefore is seen as high signal intensity in the vessels. This technique requires accurate timing of acquisition so that data are acquired while the gadolinium is in the cervical vessels (Fig. 40.14).

Restrictions to the Use of MR

In critical care patients it may be difficult to perform the routine screening of patients to determine safety prior to entering the magnet. Patients may have implanted metallic devices

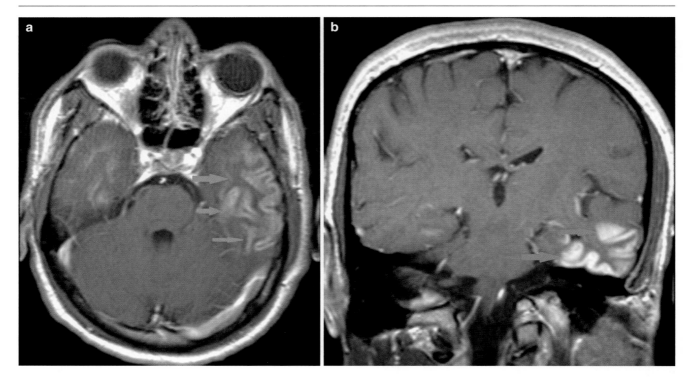

Fig. 40.10 Axial (**a**) and coronal (**b**) post-contrast T1-weighted MR images of a subacute infarct show gyriform cortical enhancement (*orange arrows*). The enhancement results from reperfusion of infarcted tissue with leakage of contrast into the parenchyma from damage of the blood-brain barrier

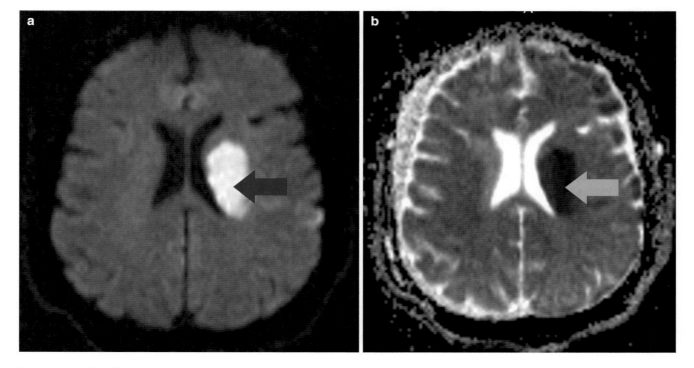

Fig. 40.11 Axial diffusion-weighted MR image with $b = 1,000$ (**a**) and corresponding ADC map (**b**) shows an acute periventricular infarction demonstrating high signal on the DWI image (*blue arrow*) and low signal on the ADC map (*orange arrow*)

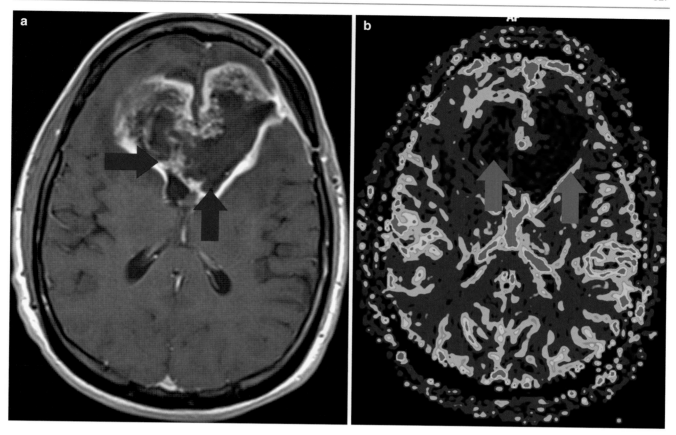

Fig. 40.12 Axial post-contrast T1-weighted MR image (**a**) has the appearance of a glioblastoma multiforme crossing the genu of the corpus callosum (*blue arrows*). The corresponding MR perfusion image (**b**) shows low blood flow (*red arrows*) suggesting that this is not tumor, but is radiation necrosis

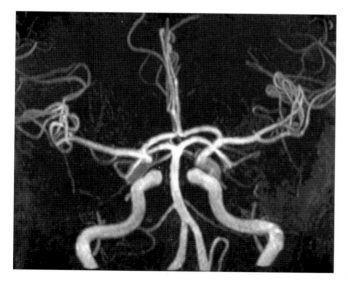

Fig. 40.13 3D reformation of a 2D time-of-flight noncontrast MRA of the intracranial vessels. This is a noninvasive technique requiring no contrast to obtain images of the vessels

or pacemakers which may be incompatible with strong magnetic fields. The reader is referred to www.mrisafety.com, which discusses the safety of many implants. Often it is necessary to check with the implant manufacturer to determine safety. Issues include implant heating, malfunction, and torqueing, all of which can cause patient injury.

The presence of metallic foreign bodies in a patient can be a contraindication to MRI. Plain films of the orbit are often performed in metal workers to determine whether there are foreign bodies in the orbits that could potentially be dislodged by the magnetic field causing blindness. Patients that have been shot create another dilemma as it is usually unknown what metals are present in the bullet fragments. Often metal will cause severe magnetic susceptibility artifact, making the images uninterpretable. This can be a problem with spine imaging with implanted metallic rods and screws, or in the head in a patient with metallic dental hardware (Fig. 40.15).

Another problem with MR is the claustrophobic or uncooperative patient. Motion degrades the images and creates

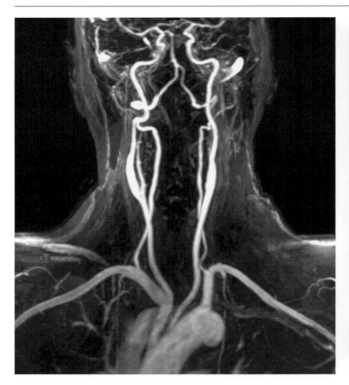

Fig. 40.14 3D reformatted image of a contrast-enhanced MRA of the cervical vessels. This method uses contrast bolus tracking to create an image that covers the entire extent of the cervical vessels

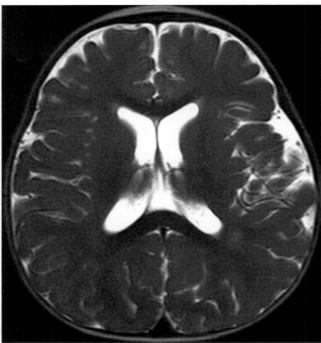

Fig. 40.16 Axial T2-HASTE image is a useful fast imaging technique in the uncooperative patient and in pediatric patients requiring frequent imaging to follow ventriculoperitoneal shunt function. The images of the whole brain are acquired in approximately 60 s

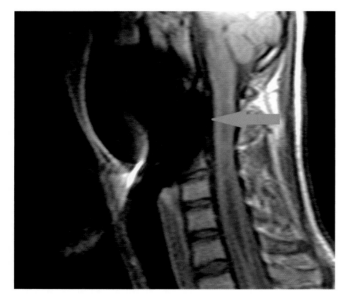

Fig. 40.15 Sagittal T1-weighted MR image of the upper cervical spine shows extensive signal loss (*orange arrow*) from metal artifact in this patient wearing braces

significant artifact, especially in the phase-encoding direction, as phase information takes much longer to acquire than frequency information. MR sequences take much longer to perform than CT acquisitions and so suffer from motion

artifact. Sedation of the patients or anesthesia may be required. Faster imaging techniques are being developed to help reduce motion-related image degradation. These techniques use clever techniques to fill portions of k-space and calculate values to fill k-space and thus allow image formation. These techniques have been used to great advantage in pediatric patients to look for hydrocephalus using fast imaging without sedation, such as a T2-HASTE sequence. This can acquire axial images of the entire brain in about 60 s and has the advantage of not exposing the child to the ionizing radiation of computed tomography (Fig. 40.16).

Restrictions to the Use of Intravenous Gadolinium Contrast Agents

Renal function needs to be determined prior to administering gadolinium because of the rare but serious condition of nephrogenic systemic fibrosis (NSF). In our institution we do not give gadolinium to patients with a glomerular filtration rate (GFR) of less than 30 mL/min, and we get informed consent from patients with a GFR of 30–60 mL/min.

Pregnant women should also not receive gadolinium contrast agents. The contrast crosses the placenta and is circulated through the fetus and excreted by the fetal kidneys. It then is excreted into the amniotic fluid where it is swallowed and absorbed, repeating the process. It is unknown whether this has any deleterious effects on the fetus, but contrast manufacturers do not support the use of contrast agents in pregnant women.

Understanding Computed Tomography (CT)

CT has undergone rapid technological advancements to increase acquisition speed, provide physiological data, and decrease radiation dose. CT images are obtained by passing a highly collimated rapidly rotating x-ray beam through a patient and detecting the photons transmitted through the patient on the opposite side of the gantry. Similar to conventional x-ray plain films, different tissue types absorb or scatter the photons to different degrees. The result is that the number of photons detected depends on the electron density of tissue through which they pass. The signal detected is translated into shades of gray. Structures which absorb more photons such as cortical bone appear white, and structures that do not absorb many photons, such as the lungs, appear dark.

The gray scale used for displaying images ranges from +1,000 to −1,000 Hounsfield units (HU), named after Sir Godfrey Hounsfield who developed CT for clinical use in 1972–1973. Water is designated zero HU. Bone is generally close to 1,000 HU and air is −1,000 HU. Gray matter is about 30–40 HU and white matter is about 20–30 HU. Calcium is 150 HU or greater. Acute hemorrhage is 50–80 HU, whereas fat is about −40 to −100 HU. The differential x-ray attenuation of these tissues accounts for the contrast. The images can be windowed and leveled using post-processing software to change the range of the scale presented to accentuate different contrasting tissues.

The spatial resolution, or ability to distinguish small adjacent structures, is dependent on the quality of the x-ray beam collimation; the number, size, and quality of the detectors; and the slice thickness. *The thinner the slice, the greater the detail and ability to spatially resolve different structures.* The downside is an increased radiation dose. A greater number of detectors are being built into the newer generation of CT scanners, with 64 detector row scanners being common on the market. A 320-detector row scanner is also available which allows a 16 cm field of view. This allows volumetric imaging of the brain in a single rotation of the gantry. The speed advantage of CT over MRI can thus be clearly seen.

CT Contrast Agents

The intravenous contrast agents used for CT are iodine-containing compounds that increase the attenuation of the x-ray beam, and thus contrast-enhancing structures appear higher density on the images. Older ionic forms of contrast medium have largely been replaced by nonionic forms which have a lower osmolality and fewer idiosyncratic reactions. Reactions vary from urticarial, mild bronchospasm, and wheezing to airway edema and serious anaphylaxis. A mild contrast reaction can be a harbinger of a more severe reaction, and so patients with a prior mild reaction are premedicated prior to receiving an additional dose of intravenous contrast. The current most widely used pretreatment algorithm is prednisone 50 mg orally given at 13, 7, and 1 h prior to the procedure and diphenhydramine 50 mg orally given 1 h prior to contrast injection.

CT contrast agents are excreted by the kidneys and can have renal toxicity. The status of renal function should be determined prior to giving the contrast agent because kidney function could be worsened.

CT Angiography and CT Perfusion

Thin section CT scanning can be performed during the administration of IV contrast to produce high-quality CT angiographic images. These can be post-processed by various software packages to produce multiplanar reformations and 3D reformations of the cervical and intracranial vasculature. This technique has almost replaced conventional catheter angiography for the detection of aneurysms, vascular malformations, vascular stenosis, dissections, or occlusions. This anatomic data can be combined with physiological data obtained by CT perfusion to obtain more diagnostic information about the effects of vascular stenosis or occlusions (Fig. 40.17).

CT perfusion is obtained by imaging the brain sequentially over time as intravenous contrast is injected. As the contrast enters and leaves the brain, the density of each pixel increases and then decreases. This data can be manipulated to create maps of time to peak (TTP), mean transit time (MTT), cerebral blood flow (CBF), and cerebral blood volume (CBV). These maps are extremely useful in the evaluation of acute cerebral infarction to determine the size of the infarct core and the presence of a penumbra of oligemic tissue. A simple way to analyze the data in the setting of acute stroke is to look at the TTP and MTT maps first. If these are symmetric and normal, there are no infarctions or no tissue is at risk. If there is a vascular territory that has delayed TTP or prolonged MTT, the other maps should be analyzed. If there is an area of significantly decreased CBV, this corresponds to dead tissue in the infarcted core. If there is decreased CBF but preserved CBV, this tissue is oligemic and at risk for infarction but is potentially salvageable. The CTA data together with CT perfusion data can be used to guide therapy in the setting of acute cerebral infarction, in terms of when it may be appropriate to perform clot lysis (Fig. 40.18).

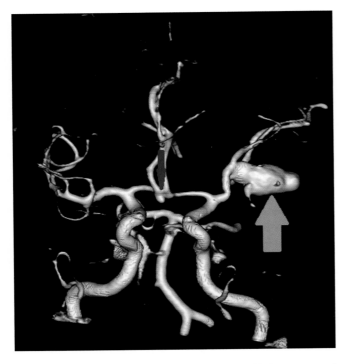

Fig. 40.17 3D reformation of a CT angiogram with bone removed shows exquisite detail of the intracranial vasculature. A large MCA bifurcation aneurysm (*orange arrow*) can be seen as well as a very small anterior communicating artery aneurysm (*blue arrow*)

A disadvantage of CT perfusion over MR perfusion is that on many CT scanners, only selected slices can be used to obtain perfusion data, dependent on the detector row size: 32-detector row scanners can generate two 1 cm slices of perfusion data; a 64-detector row scanner can give four slices. The newer 320-detector row scanners can perform whole brain perfusion as the detector thickness is 16 cm (Fig. 40.19).

Neuroradiological Clinical Issues

Brain Herniation

One of the primary reasons for obtaining noncontrast CT scans of the brain from the emergency department or from the inpatient service is to evaluate for altered mental status. Often, there is a significant clinical history associated with the patient that would aid the referring clinicians to give an etiology for the sudden change in mental status such as elevated white count, drop in hemoglobin, or other imaging studies which demonstrate widespread metastatic disease. However, there are many instances when no obvious cause is present clinically, and further investigation with interventional procedures such as lumbar puncture may be

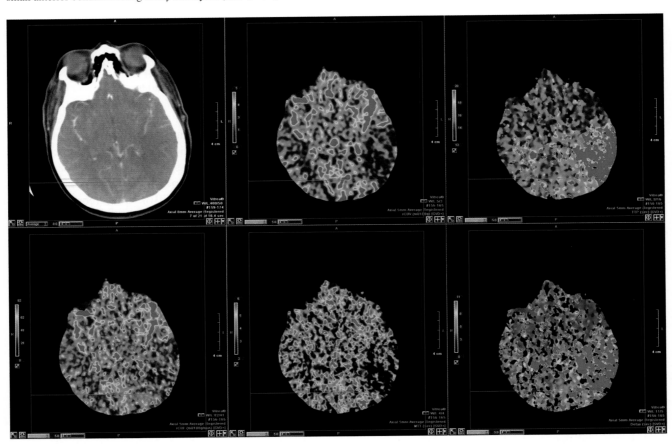

Fig. 40.18 Axial slice from a CT perfusion study demonstrates an area of increased time to peak (TTP) in *red* in the *top right image* and decreased cerebral blood volume (CBV) in *dark blue* in the *top middle image* indicating a completed infarct

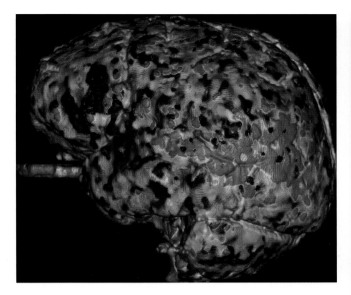

Fig. 40.19 3D reformation of a time to peak (TTP) map from a whole brain CT perfusion study. The image shows increased TTP in the posterior temporal lobe and occipital lobe. This surface-rendered image can be compared to other maps such as CBV to determine the volume of tissue at risk during an episode of acute cerebral ischemia

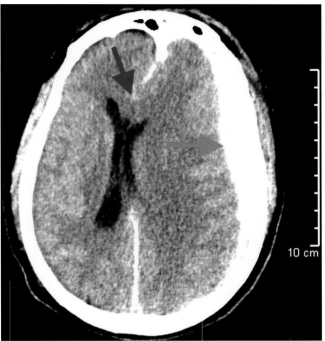

Fig. 40.20 Axial CT scan shows a left subdural hematoma (*orange arrow*) with resultant left-to-right subfalcine herniation (*blue arrow*). The left lateral ventricle has been compressed

necessary to evaluate for etiologies that may not always be present on radiographic images such as meningitis. However, prior to proceeding with such procedures, findings of brain herniation syndrome must be excluded before it is safe to "tap" the patient.

Brain herniation is the displacement of brain from one cranial compartment to another by a space-occupying lesion. The effects of brain herniation are most severe in children and young adults due to the lack of space within the calvarium and a non-atrophic brain. Older patients have more CSF within the ventricular system and in the extra-axial space allowing for less compression of the brain tissue by mass effect. For significant mass effect to occur, the size of the mass must be large enough to displace vital anatomic structures into adjacent cranial compartments. The mass itself will exert a pressure in the form of a vector that will be directional and thus determine the type of herniation that will occur.

Herniation syndromes include subfalcine herniation (produced by a mesial mid-convexity vector), downward transtentorial uncal herniation (produced by a mesial, low convexity, midtemporal vector), downward transtentorial parahippocampal herniation (produced by a mesial, low convexity, posterior temporal vector), upward herniation (produced by a cerebellar region vector), and downward cerebellar tonsillar herniation (produced by a mid to inferior, cerebellar region vector).

Subfalcine Herniation

Subfalcine herniation is also called midline shift and occurs when the mid-convexity brain structures such as the corpus callosum and cingulate gyrus shift beneath the falx cerebri

and are compressed against the free margin of the falx. Subfalcine herniation is usually secondary to space-occupying lesions occurring in the frontoparietal region, basal ganglia, and perisylvian region. Extra-axial fluid collections such as subdural hematomas and empyemas in the frontoparietal regions can also produce similar findings. Even a minimal midline shift is significant as the falx is composed of tough fibrous tissue and subsequently is relatively resilient to compression by adjacent structures. In addition, careful attention should also be made to vascular structures that course through the midline such as branches of the anterior cerebral artery and venous drainage pathways especially posteriorly (Fig. 40.20).

Downward Transtentorial Herniation

Transtentorial herniation can be further subdivided into descending, ascending, and uncal. This occurs when there is mass effect that causes shift of normal brain structures into the tentorial notch, which contains the brainstem and traversing vessels.

In descending herniation, there is medial and then downward displacement of the temporal lobe, particularly the parahippocampal gyrus. The center of the lesion is usually in the posterior temporal lobe which exerts a vector that points medially and inferiorly. The parahippocampal gyrus then herniates compressing the brainstem resulting in inferior displacement of the midbrain and pons. The initial sign of impending herniation is effacement of the ambient cistern on the ipsilateral side. Due to stretching of the brainstem, there

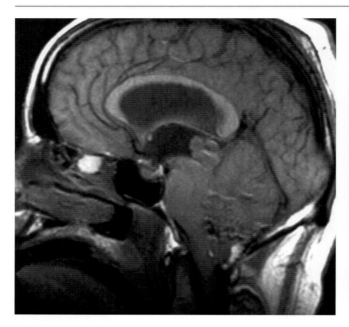

Fig. 40.21 Midline sagittal T1-weighted MR image shows downward transtentorial herniation with resultant crowding of the posterior fossa structures and fourth ventricular obstruction resulting in hydrocephalus

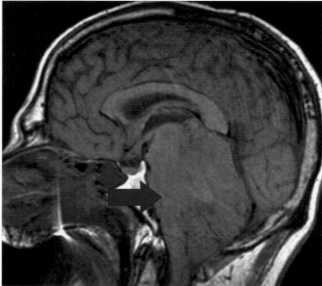

Fig. 40.22 Midline sagittal T1-weighted MR image shows upward transtentorial herniation. Brainstem structures are seen ascending across the plane of the incisura (*blue arrow*)

may be a resultant Duret hemorrhage which is secondary to stretching and eventually rupture of the perforating vessels supplying the brainstem. Another important consequence is compromise of flow into the parietal occipital branch of the posterior cerebral artery (Fig. 40.21).

Ascending Transtentorial Herniation

Ascending herniation occurs when the center of the mass is in the posterior fossa, and it exerts mass affect and superior displacement of the cerebellar vermis into the tentorial notch, displacing the brainstem toward the clivus. There is secondary obliteration of the quadrigeminal plate cistern as well as the prepontine cistern and interpeduncular fossa. Obliteration of the cerebral aqueduct may also occur resulting in obstructive hydrocephalus. Vascular complications resulting from this type of herniation are compression of the venous structures in the supratentorial brain such as the vein of Galen and basal vein of Rosenthal (Fig. 40.22).

Uncal Herniation

Descending uncal herniation occurs when the uncus is displaced inferiorly secondary to mass lesion of the midtemporal region. The uncus is displaced medially first into the suprasellar cistern and then inferiorly into the crural cistern. This results in obliteration of the circumesencephalic cistern. Uncal herniation results in mass effect on the cerebral peduncles as well as the oculomotor nerve which can result in clinical findings of a "blown" pupil and contralateral hemiparesis. The key to diagnosis is effacement of the suprasellar cistern (Fig. 40.23).

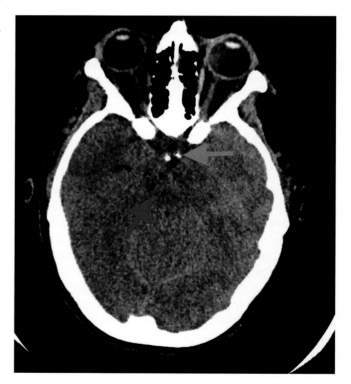

Fig. 40.23 Axial CT scan shows downward transtentorial and uncal herniation. Notice obliteration of the paramesencephalic cisterns (*blue arrow*) from the downward transtentorial herniation and compression of the suprasellar cistern (*orange arrow*) from uncal herniation

Tonsillar Herniation

Tonsillar herniation occurs when there is downward displacement of the cerebellar tonsils inferiorly into the cisterna magna. The center of the lesion is in the posterior fossa and depending on its location medially or laterally, the tonsils may or may not be splayed. Downward displacement of the cerebellar tonsils is an imaging finding that is often present; however, not all of them demonstrate impending doom.

Tonsillar ectopia is a common imaging finding that is found incidentally on both CT and MRI and may have no clinical significance to the patient. Misdiagnosing tonsillar ectopia for tonsillar herniation may result in inappropriate management. Other entities that are often misdiagnosed are Chiari 1 malformation and intracranial hypotension, which can often be mistaken for tonsillar herniation, but understanding the mechanism and key anatomic structures involved in these diagnoses may lead the radiologist and clinician down the appropriate path (Figs. 40.24, 40.25, and 40.26).

To differentiate these entities, one must understand that in order to diagnose tonsillar herniation, the relationship of the vallecula and circummedullary cistern to the tonsils should be established. Herniation can be diagnosed if either of these two cisterns is obliterated. If the cisterns are not obliterated,

then other etiologies such as Chiari, tonsillar ectopia, and intracranial hypotension should be entertained, and relationship of other structures such as the obex, which is the opening for CSF into the central canal, and the plane of the incisura should be established to help further narrow the differential diagnosis.

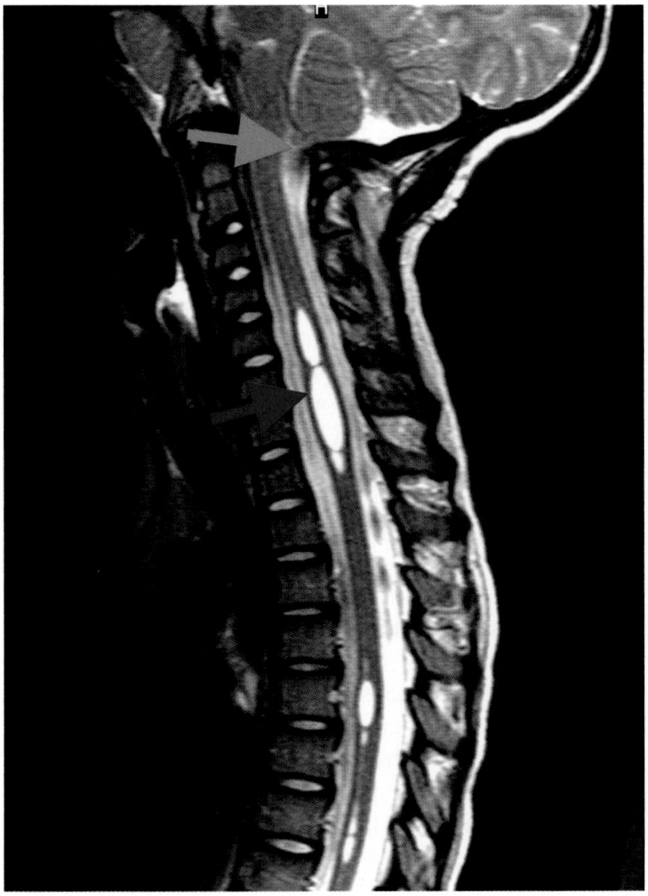

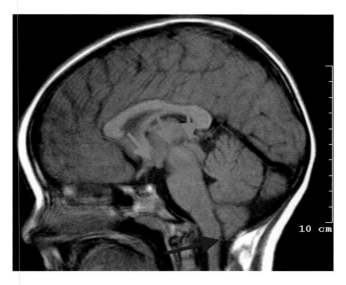

Fig. 40.25 Midline sagittal T1-weighted MR image demonstrates a low position of the cerebellar tonsils below the plane of the foramen magnum (*blue arrow*). The relationship of structures at the plane of the incisura (*orange arrows*) is normal

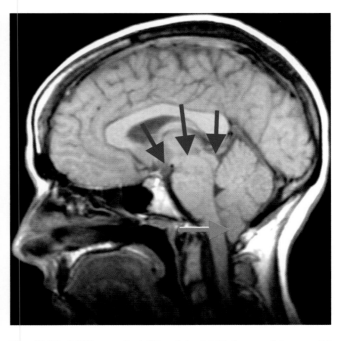

Fig. 40.26 Midline sagittal T1-weighted MR image of intracranial hypotension. In this case there is sagging of the brainstem and cerebellar tonsillar ectopia (*orange arrow*). The position of structures relative to the plane of the incisura (*blue arrows*) is abnormal

Fig. 40.24 Sagittal T2-weighted MR image of the cervical spine demonstrates a Chiari 1 malformation with low-lying cerebellar tonsils (*orange arrow*) and a syrinx (*blue arrow*)

Evaluation of Oligemia, Stroke, and Dural Sinus Thrombosis

Brain perfusion is an important parameter that can be analyzed using CT or MRI. Adequate blood flow in the major feeding arteries of the brain is crucial to maintaining cerebral function. There is extensive autoregulation that occurs within the brain to help maintain adequate blood flow to the brain. Any disruption in autoregulation, whether increased and resulting in hyperemia, or decreased and resulting in oligemia, can result in neurologic symptoms and possibly death. The recent advances in both CT perfusion and MR perfusion have allowed radiologists to play an active role in decreasing the gap between onset of clinical symptoms and diagnosis. Ischemia to the brain is being detected much earlier in onset and thus increased the chance of successful treatment.

Oligemia is a result of decreased flow to the brain that may be secondary to proximal obstruction or stenosis from atherosclerotic disease, dissection, mass effect, etc. Decreased cerebral blood flow results in ischemia to the corresponding vascular territory affected with eventual shift from ischemia to infarction. Once infarcted, brain tissue previously at risk from ischemia is dead, and revascularization with interventional methods may be futile. The goal of early diagnosis is to determine the "tissue at risk," or penumbra, based on the CT or MR imaging findings. The amount of penumbra that is present is based on a variety of factors, most importantly whether or not there has been development of collateral vessels.

At our institution, the algorithm for acute stroke is initial CT scanning comprised of a noncontrast CT of the brain, CTA of the brain, CTA of the neck, and perfusion imaging. The goal of imaging is to exclude hemorrhage, to differentiate between irreversibly compromised brain tissue and reversibly impaired tissue, and to identify stenosis or occlusion of major extra- and intracranial arteries. CT has the advantage of being available 24 h a day and is extremely sensitive to evaluate for a bleed.

The initial noncontrast CT allows for diagnosis of acute bleeds, extent of edema if visible, along with other etiologies that may cause neurologic decline, such as a subdural hematoma. Early signs of ischemia on CT are hypoattenuating brain tissue corresponding to edema, obscuration of the lentiform nucleus, dense MCA sign, insular ribbon sign, and loss of sulcal effacement. Hypoattenuation is a result of cytotoxic edema within the brain from the failure of ion pumps which results in water entry. If edema is present within the first 6 h, this finding is highly specific for irreversible brain damage. Both obscuration of the lentiform nucleus and insular ribbon sign are very subtle early CT findings of infarction in the middle cerebral artery territory. This region is very sensitive to ischemia due to the lack of collateral flow. The findings of dense intracranial vasculature should be correlated with clinical findings as, often, vessels which appear dense on noncontrast CT – when there is no focal neurologic deficit – are likely due to an underlying volume status abnormality, making blood more dense than normal, or anemia (Fig. 40.27a, b).

The second component of a stroke workup includes evaluation of the cervical and intracranial arterial supply, which is performed with CT or MR angiography. Images are obtained of the aortic arch, and vessels are traced superiorly into the third or fourth order branches within the brain to evaluate for aneurysms, stenosis, and dissections. If further confirmation or evaluation is needed, the diagnostic 4-vessel angiography is recommended. To further evaluate for dissections, MR is the preferred study of choice, as it allows for better visualization of the lumen and wall of the vessel and also may be used to visualize an intramural hematoma. The main role of imaging is to clarify the status of the cervical and intracranial arteries and thereby help define the occlusion site (if present), grade collateral flow, and evaluate for extent of atherosclerotic disease. This information will provide guidance for the interventional radiologist prior to intraarterial thrombolysis.

The third component is the perfusion study. This is performed in CT by monitoring the first pass of the iodinated contrast agent bolus through the cerebral circulation. It involves continuous cine imaging over the same piece of brain tissue to help produce a perfusion curve. Based on this information, color-coded maps are produced which include cerebral blood volume, cerebral blood flow, and mean transit time. When evaluating these components of the perfusion study, it is important to not only analyze each component but to analyze them as a whole to help get an overall picture of the brain's perfusion status. In at risk ischemic tissue, there is elevated mean transit time with slightly decreased blood flow and slightly decreased or normal blood volume. This means that blood takes a longer amount of time to get to that specific portion of the brain, but blood volume to that region is maintained. In contrast, infarcted tissue has elevated mean transit time, with decreased blood flow and volume, indicating that there is essentially no blood flow to this region.

Venous Obstruction

Cerebral venous thrombosis is an important cause of stroke especially in children and young adults. It is more common than previously thought and frequently missed on initial imaging. It is a difficult diagnosis because of its nonspecific clinical presentation and subtle findings on imaging. The clue to diagnosing venous infarcts is that when there is hemorrhage in an atypical location, not conforming to a vascular territory, venous stenosis/occlusion should be excluded. Typical locations are in the high frontal/parietal convexity

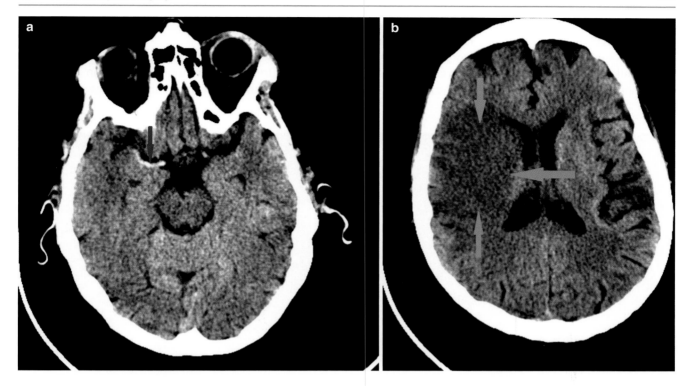

Fig. 40.27 Axial CT scan images show a hyperdense right MCA sign (*blue arrow*) (**a** and **b**) edema in the right MCA territory (*orange arrow*) with loss of gray-white differentiation and loss of high density in the caudate nucleus and putamen on the right from cytotoxic edema

due to thrombosis of the draining cortical veins or superior sagittal sinus. This results in increased back pressure which causes capillary rupture; cerebral edema is often present. Both CT and MR venographies are the diagnostic tests of choice with the former being a better tool for evaluating venous thrombosis. The imaging features include evidence of clot within the lumen on nonenhanced scan and abnormal enhancement of the wall of the dural sinus (Fig. 40.28).

Evaluation of Hypoxia and Metabolic Insufficiency

Regardless of cause, the common underlying process that occurs in hypoxia is decreased cerebral blood flow and decreased blood oxygenation to the brain. This can be focal or global, depending on the type of injury and the affected vasculature – anterior circulation, posterior circulation, or both. When there is a combination of decreased flow and decreased blood oxygenation, the ability to the make ATP for the brain is inhibited, and cell function/integrity cannot be maintained.

The areas in the brain that require the most energy are more prone to injury and thus are seen earlier as abnormalities on MRI. The globus pallidus, periaqueductal gray matter, dorsal pons, dentate cerebellar nuclei, hippocampus, cerebral

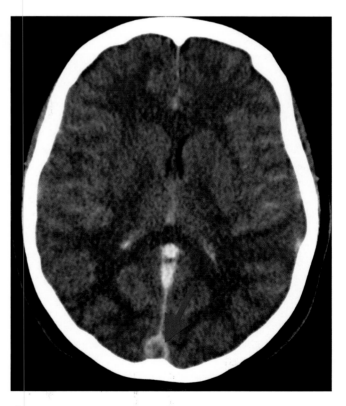

Fig. 40.28 Axial post-contrast CT scan shows an empty delta sign where there is thrombosis of the superior sagittal sinus (*blue arrow*)

cortex, and cerebellar cortex are the structures which require the highest ATP per gram of tissue. However, note should be made that other etiologies such as hypoglycemia can also cause similar findings, and correlation with clinical and laboratory values is recommended (Fig. 40.29a–c).

Seizure Disorder

The role of an imaging study in evaluating seizure disorder is to provide information that can help guide patient treatment. There are numerous causes of seizure

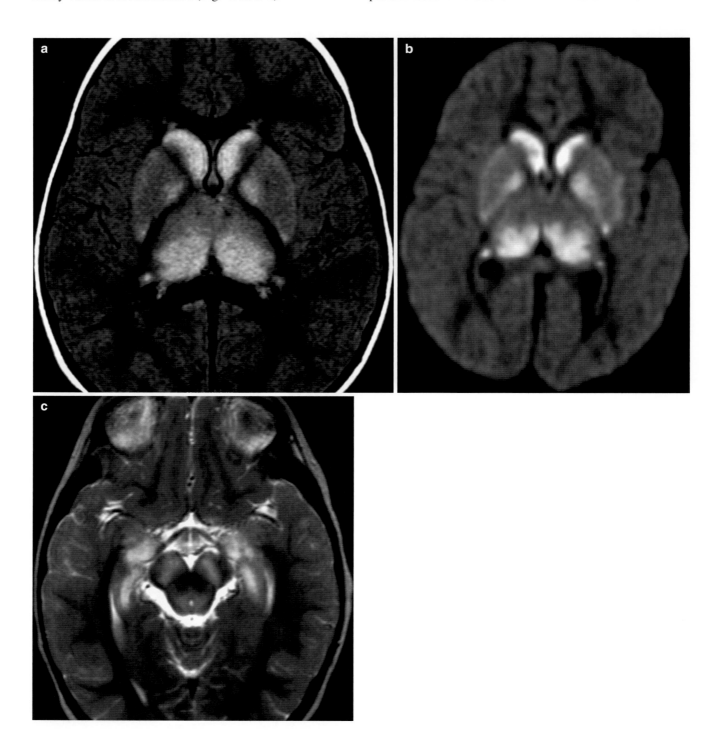

Fig. 40.29 Axial T1-weighted MR images (**a**) and axial diffusion-weighted image with $b=1,000$ (**b**) show high signal in the high ATP demand zones of the basal ganglia and thalami as a result of acute hypoxic injury. Axial T2-weighted MR image (**c**) at a lower level shows high signal from edema in the parahippocampal gyrus and periaqueductal gray matter which are also high ATP demand zones

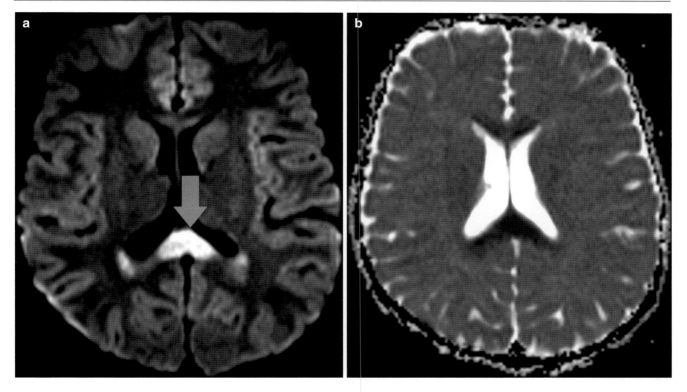

Fig. 40.30 Axial diffusion-weighted image with $b = 1,000$ (**a**) and axial ADC map (**b**) show acute restricted diffusion in the splenium of the corpus callosum (*orange arrow*, **a**). This is a fairly common finding following secondary generalization of a seizure

disorder that range from pharmacologic imbalance to structural causes within the brain. When seizures occur, the appropriate initial study to obtain is a noncontrast CT of the brain to evaluate for space-occupying lesions such as masses, hemorrhages, or edema that will result in the patient's clinical symptoms. If the CT is inconclusive, then an MRI contrasted with gadolinium is the next study of choice.

The degree of abnormal signal intensity on MRI will depend upon whether the patient is scanned in the ictal or interictal phase. In the interictal phase, one can expect to find signal changes on T2 sequences in addition to diffusion restriction involving the splenium of the corpus callosum, hippocampus, and parahippocampal gyrus. A CT perfusion study, often ordered if the patient develops weakness following a stroke, can also demonstrate increased blood flow and volume with decreased mean transit time in the affected region (Fig. 40.30a, b).

Patients with a history of epilepsy can be evaluated with a noncontrasted MRI if a structural cause for convulsions has been excluded in the past. The role of imaging for patients with epilepsy is to better characterize the gray matter and the hippocampus and to determine a seizure focus with additional correlation to the EEG findings.

Evaluation of Ventricular Size

Changes in ventricular size are an important prognostic indicator. Baseline ventricular size should be established and note should be made that this varies physiologically based upon age. Once baseline ventricular size is determined, comparison should be made to demonstrate whether there has been an acute change in the size of the ventricles. The most important radiographic clue that helps determine an acute change in CSF pressure is transependymal migration of CSF which is exemplified by hypoattenuation within the periventricular white matter and suggests an acute hydrocephalus (Fig. 40.31).

In the emergency setting, any change in size of the ventricles – whether increased or decreased – should be examined. If ventricular size has increased, then etiologies such as shunt malfunction or obstructing lesion should be excluded. If ventricular size has decreased, then correlation for overshunting is recommended.

Evaluation of Intracranial Hemorrhage

Understanding the MR characteristics of blood has allowed radiologists the ability to render rather sophisticated diagnostic opinions and help referring physicians with establishing the appropriate time frame when brain events have occurred. MR signal changes are based mainly on the state of hemoglobin within the red blood cells. Stages of

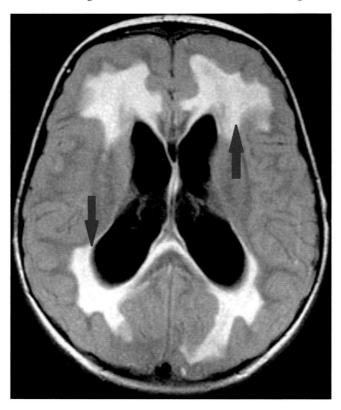

Fig. 40.31 Axial FLAIR MR image in a patient with acute hydrocephalus showing ventriculomegaly and high signal in the periventricular region representing transependymal fluid migration (*blue arrow*)

hemorrhage can be differentiated into hyperacute, acute, early subacute and late subacute, and finally chronic, all of which have different signal intensities on T1- and T2-weighted sequences.

Hyperacute hemorrhage occurs within the first 3–6 h and is rarely seen on imaging due to the time frame of onset. In the first 3–6 h, the intact red cells still contain mostly oxyhemoglobin. The T2WI image is hyperintense with peripheral hypointensity and the T1WI is hypointense.

Acute hemorrhage (Fig. 40.32a, b) lasts about a week and occurs after the initial accumulation of oxyhemoglobin and secondary clot formation with retraction and reabsorption of serum. There is increase in lactic acid and carbon dioxide within the hematoma which results in less hemoglobin saturation and more deoxyhemoglobin. The high protein content of clot which is evident on CT where it is hyperdense causes T1 shortening which results in isointense to hypointense signal on T1-weighted MR imaging. In addition, there is marked susceptibility which is secondary to local field inhomogeneity produced by the paramagnetic deoxyhemoglobin within the RBC which all results in a hypointense signal on T2-weighted imaging also.

The next stage of hematoma evolution is the subacute phase. The subacute phase may be subdivided into early and late stages, based on whether hemoglobin molecules are intra- or extracellular. The overall change that occurs from the acute to subacute phase is the conversion of deoxyhemoglobin to methemoglobin. The early subacute phase occurs within 3–7 days, and signal changes are a result of the ability of water molecules to approach the paramagnetic heme of methemoglobin. This results in increased T1 signal with decreased T2 signal. The late subacute phase

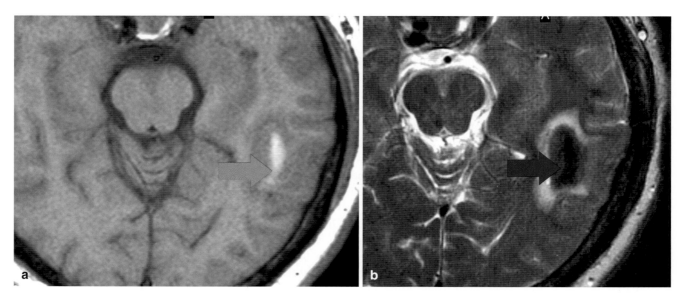

Fig. 40.32 Axial noncontrast T1-weighted MR image (**a**) shows high signal from intracellular methemoglobin (*orange arrow*). Axial T2-weighted image (**b**) shows low signal from methemoglobin (*blue arrow*) with surrounding edema in this patient with an acute hemorrhage

occurs when there is lysis of the methemoglobin molecule, formed from the conversion from deoxyhemoglobin to methemoglobin.

The chronic phase occurs months later when there is complete breakdown and resorption of the fluid and protein within the clot which results in susceptibility effects resulting in hypointense signal on T1- and T2-weighted sequences.

Subarachnoid Hemorrhage

Patients presenting with subarachnoid hemorrhage typically have a severe acute onset headache and may have nausea or vomiting or an altered mental status. The acute hemorrhage is best detected on noncontrast CT, where it is seen as high attenuation in the subarachnoid space. It can be posttraumatic in which case the blood is often detected over the convexities. Most commonly the cause is a ruptured cerebral aneurysm. The blood is then often seen centered at the site of the aneurysm. For example, a ruptured anterior communicating artery aneurysm will often present with symmetric midline hemorrhage centered in the cistern of the lamina terminalis and usually extending into the suprasellar cistern and sylvian fissures. A middle cerebral artery aneurysm on the other hand typically presents with blood in the ipsilateral sylvian fissure.

Following a noncontrast CT scan showing subarachnoid hemorrhage, a CT angiogram is usually performed to look for a cause of the bleed, such as a ruptured aneurysm, AVM, or rarely benign perimesencephalic subarachnoid hemorrhage

from a venous bleed. The Fisher grading scale is used to classify the appearance of the hemorrhage on CT scan. Grade 1 is no hemorrhage evident, grade 2 is less than 1 mm thick, grade 3 is more than 1 mm thick, and grade 4 is any thickness with intraventricular or parenchymal extension. Multiplanar and 3D reformations of the CT angiogram are very helpful to identify an aneurysm or AVM. If the CT angiogram does not show the cause of the bleed and there is no other plausible explanation such as trauma, a catheter arteriogram is indicated. If this is also negative, repeat catheter arteriogram in 2 weeks can sometimes reveal an abnormality which was thrombosed on the initial imaging (Fig. 40.33a, b).

Brain Tumors

When evaluating patients with altered mental status, referring clinicians often ask radiologists to exclude underlying mass lesions. The first test often ordered is a noncontrast CT. The initial step is to determine if the study is normal or not. If the study is normal, then the likelihood that underlying mass lesion is present is low. However, without the addition of contrast, these scans are limited, and complete exclusion of an underlying mass lesion cannot always be confirmed. If post-contrast images demonstrate a mass lesion, it is important to assist the referring physician in the development of an appropriate differential diagnosis to help with biopsy and eventually treatment.

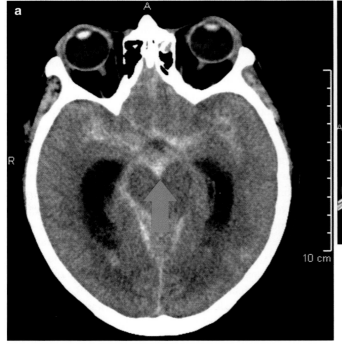
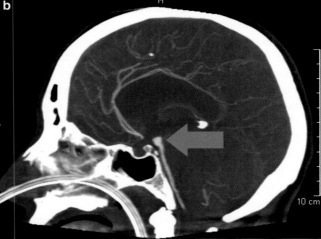

Fig. 40.33 Axial noncontrast CT scan of the head (**a**) demonstrates diffuse subarachnoid hemorrhage within the basilar cisterns (*orange arrow*, **a**) with extension into the ventricular system making this a

Fisher Grade 4 hemorrhage. Sagittal reformation of the CT angiogram (**b**) demonstrates a basilar tip aneurysm (*blue arrow*)

When attempting to create a differential diagnosis for brain lesions, it is important to first group lesions as being either intra-axial or extra-axial. If lesions are extra-axial in location, they are separate from the brain parenchyma and can be localized to the subarachnoid/subdural space, dural lining, or calvarium. Often T2-weighted MR sequences can help in localizing lesions to the extra-axial space if there is mass effect and buckling of the adjacent gray matter. The differential diagnosis for extra-axial masses is quite wide, but common entities in this location are meningiomas, dural-based metastases, lymphoma, or calvarial metastatic disease.

If the lesion is intra-axial in location, the differential transforms to tumors that occur in the brain parenchyma. First, the age of the patient must be established, as adults and children are predisposed to a variety of different tumors. Second, the location of the lesion – whether it is infratentorial or supratentorial in location – will also help tailor the differential diagnosis. Finally, if a supratentorial lesion is in question, then it is important to determine whether the mass is localized to the gray matter, white matter, or a combination of both.

Most brain tumors are centered in the white matter and grow along the white matter tracts. These tumors are primarily astrocytomas of varying grades. Tumors at the gray-white junction are often metastatic foci due to increased flow in this region. Tumors involving predominately the gray matter are often histologically oligodendrogliomas. It is important to note that enhancement does not always signify underlying tumor, and other sequences and tests should be correlated to properly conclude that the mass that is present on the scan is actually a neoplasm and not a tumefactive demyelinating plaque, abscess, or stroke, all of which can enhance. In addition, the advances in MR spectroscopy and MR perfusion have improved the ability to accurately diagnose a mass as a tumor. Low-grade neoplasms often occur in children and adolescents, rather than in infants. Low-grade tumors that are often present in children are gangliomas, dysembryoplastic neuroepithelial tumors (DNET), pleomorphic xanthoastrocytoma, and pilocytic astrocytoma. The low-grade nature of these tumors means that they have low biological activity and are less aggressive then high-grade neoplasms. They demonstrate a slow growth pattern which is exhibited over serial imaging studies which show stable size of these lesions.

High-grade neoplasms, on the other hand, have high biological activity and exhibit more aggressive growth patterns. These tumors often occur later in life, mostly affecting older adults, especially in cases of metastatic disease. These tumors demonstrate an infiltrative growth pattern that is rapid and can be seen on serial imaging studies. In addition, these tumors often outgrow their normal blood supply eventually undergoing central necrosis. There is edema, which is often out of proportion to the size of the lesion, in conjunction with increasing venous drainage secondary to angiogenesis which is often referred to as AV shunting. Common high-grade tumors include glioblastoma multiforme, metastatic disease, and lymphoma among other etiologies.

Posttreatment imaging is critical to determine the extent of treatment changes and follow-up residual tumor if present. Imaging with MRI plays a key role in establishing whether the current treatment regimen is appropriate or not. Thus, it is imperative to have serial scans following therapy to reliably illustrate whether there is an appropriate response to the therapy. Immediate scans following surgery are also important to determine a baseline study to help compare future follow-ups.

Following the operative state, a variety of changes are common. Changes range from obvious encephalomalacic defect to hematomas within the surgical site. Enhancement is a common finding in the postoperative state and often represents either reactive changes or hematoma. Enhancement is often not a good indicator of whether there is recurrence or progression of disease, as postradiation changes can look similar and be misleading. When evaluating for residual/recurrent disease, an appropriate search pattern is important to establish. Initially, T1-weighted MR sequences determine whether brain tissue changes are secondary to radiation changes (hyperintense T1 signal) or persistent tumor (hypointense T1 signal). Subsequently, T2-weighted sequences should be analyzed as persistent solid tumor in the resection cavity appears isointense to gray matter on T2-weighted sequences, and infiltrating disease is often mildly hyperintense on T-weighted sequences but not as hyperintense as edema. Finally, correlation with susceptibility-weighted images can help determine whether the signal abnormality on T1 and T2 sequences is due to hemorrhage or not.

Radiation therapy is often used in conjunction with surgical therapy to treat brain tumors. The imaging characteristics of radiation changes vary and can occur anywhere from 1 month after initiation to 10 years. The most common findings associated with radiation therapy are mucositis in the ipsilateral mastoid air cells, along with fatty replacement of the bone marrow, especially in the clivus and skull. However, in the brain parenchyma, evidence of radiation changes is noted by a hyperintense T1 signal surrounding the resection cavity and in the field of prior therapy. In addition, common places such as the basal ganglia often demonstrate signal changes. Within and surrounding the resection cavity, radiation changes appear as soft hyperintense signal which appears more distinct than residual tumor. MR perfusion is often used to help decipher whether the changes evident on MRI represent residual/recurrent tumor or sequela of prior RT therapy. However, relying primarily on perfusion imaging can be misleading due to leaky capillaries and increased flow that may result in increased blood flow on perfusion studies resembling tumor. Correlation with other sequences is important when determining whether changes present are due to RT or tumor. Radiation dosage that exceeds neuronal tolerance can produce radiation necrosis, progressive necrotizing leukoencephalopathy, and radiation-induced second primary tumor formation, usually a sarcoma. Progressive necrotizing leukoencephalopathy is characterized by multiple ill-defined areas of contrast enhancement primarily involving the cerebral white matter particularly in the periventricular distribution.

Acknowledgement Thank you to the authors of the first edition of this chapter, Drs. Ronald G. Quisling and Dr. Lorna Sohn-Williams, for inspiring in part the organization for this totally rewritten chapter for this second edition.

Bibliography

Atlas S. Magnetic resonance imaging of the brain and spine. 4th ed. Philadelphia: Lippincott Williams & Wilkins; 2008.

Bitar L, Leung G, Perng R, et al. MR pulse sequences: what every radiologist wants to know but is afraid to ask. Radiographics. 2006; 26:513–37.

Cobourn M, Rodriquez F. Cerebral herniations. Appl Radiol. 1998;25(5):10–6.

de Lucas EM, Sánchez E, Gutiérrez A, et al. CT protocol for acute stroke: tips and tricks for general radiologists. Radiographics. 2008;28:1673–87.

Fisher C, Kistler J, Davis J. Relation of cerebral vasospasm to subarachnoid hemorrhage visualized by computerized tomographic scanning. Neurosurgery. 1980;6:1–9.

Grossman R, Yousem D. Neuroradiology: the requisites. 2nd ed. Philadelphia: Mosby; 2003.

Hagmann P, Jonasson L, Maeder P, et al. Understanding diffusion MR imaging techniques: from scalar diffusion-weighted imaging to diffusion tensor imaging and beyond. Radiographics. 2006; 26:S205–23.

Hendriske J, van Raamt AF, van der Graaf Y, et al. Distribution of cerebral blood flow in the circle of willis. Radiology. 2005;235:184–9.

Huang B, Castillo M. Hypoxic ischemic brain injury: imaging findings from child to adulthood. Radiographics. 2008;28:417–39.

Jacobs MA, Ibrahim TS, Ouwerkerk R. AAPM/RSNA physics tutorial for residents. MR imaging: brief overview and emerging applications. Radiographics. 2007;27:1213–29.

Konstas AA, Goldmakher GV, Lee TY, Lev MH. Theoretic basis and technical implementations of CT perfusion in acute ischemic stroke. Part 1: theoretic basis. AJNR Am J Neuroradiol. 2009;30:662–8.

Lee SH, Rao K, Zimmerman R. Cranial MRI and CT. 4th ed. New York: McGraw-Hill; 1999.

Morelli JN, Runge VM, Ai F, et al. An image-based approach to understanding the physics of MR artifacts. Radiographics. 2011; 31:849–66.

Osborn A. Diagnostic neuroradiology. Philadelphia: Mosby; 1994.

Pooley R. AAPM/RSNA physics tutorial for residents. Fundamental physics of MR imaging. Radiographics. 2005;25:1087–99.

Wintermark M, Sesay M, Barbier E, et al. Comparative overview of brain perfusion imaging techniques. J Neuroradiol. 2005;32:294–314.

Zhuo J, Gullapalli RP. AAPM/RSNA physics tutorial for residents. MR artifacts, safety, and quality control. Radiographics. 2006; 26:275–97.

Intraoperative Neuroanesthesia

41

Elizabeth Brady Mahanna, Dietrich Gravenstein,
Nikolaus Gravenstein, and Steven A. Robicsek

Contents

E.B. Mahanna, MD
Division of Critical Care Medicine,
Department of Anesthesiology,
University of Florida College of Medicine,
1600 SW Archer Road, 100254,
Gainesville, FL 32610, USA
e-mail: emahanna@anest.ufl.edu

D. Gravenstein, MD • S.A. Robicsek, MD, PhD (✉)
Department of Anesthesiology,
University of Florida College of Medicine,
1600 SW Archer Road, 100254,
Gainesville, FL 32610, USA
e-mail: dgravenstein@anest.ufl.edu; robicsek@ufl.edu

N. Gravenstein, MD
Departments of Anesthesiology and Neurological Surgery,
University of Florida College of Medicine,
1600 SW Archer Road, 100254,
Gainesville, FL 32610, USA

Department of Periodontology,
University of Florida College of Dentistry,
Gainesville, FL, USA
e-mail: ngravenstein@anest.ufl.edu

Abstract

This chapter broadly describes considerations and objectives that are included in the formulation of a neuroanesthetic management plan. There are unique intraoperative issues confronting the anesthesiologist for all neurosurgical procedures as anesthetic agents and technique may significantly affect cerebral oxygen consumption ($CMRO_2$), cerebral oxygen delivery (CDO_2), cerebral blood flow (CBF), intracranial tissue volume, intracranial pressure (ICP), arterial oxygen content (CaO_2), and the autoregulation of CBF. Recognition and treatment of concurrent comorbidities, optimization of the surgical exposure, and avoidance and management of surgery-related events in the operating room and during the perioperative period broadly define secondary objectives of the anesthetic intervention.

A.J. Layon et al. (eds.), *Textbook of Neurointensive Care*,
DOI 10.1007/978-1-4471-5226-2_41, © Springer-Verlag London 2013

A selection of representative clinical scenarios including surgeries for mass lesions, lesions in the posterior fossa, transphenoidal hypophysectomies, open and endovascular surgeries for aneurysms and other vascular malformations, surgical treatment of stroke, spine surgeries, and functional operations are presented. Unique considerations and complications such as positioning, postoperative visual loss, venous air embolism, neuroprotection, and neuromonitoring are reviewed in detail.

Keywords

Neural autoregulation • Postoperative visual loss • Venous air embolism • Trigeminal-cardiac reflex • Neuroprotection • Neuromonitoring • Cerebral aneurysmal clipping • Carotid endarterectomy • Functional surgeries • Pituitary adenoma • Posterior fossa

Introduction

Surgical intervention on the central nervous system (CNS) requires an in-depth appreciation of intracranial and spinal cord physiology and pathophysiology. The dynamic course of a surgical intervention can be quite challenging and requires an actively involved and informed anesthesiologist to assure the most favorable outcome.

This chapter will broadly describe considerations and objectives that are included in the formulation of a neuroanesthetic management plan. We will discuss the intraoperative issues confronting the anesthesiologist for a selection of representative clinical scenarios. Upon completion of surgery, the outcome of the intraoperative anesthetic and surgical management often does not become fully manifest until the patient is in the intensive or postanesthesia care unit. Familiarity with both the anesthetic and surgical characters of postoperative recovery can help one distinguish findings that are related to the anesthetic and are ephemeral from more ominous ones that may require aggressive intervention.

Anesthesia and Basic Neuropathophysiology

The balance of cerebral and spinal cord oxygen delivery with its consequences (e.g., induced systemic hypertension, lactate acidosis, free radical formation, vasodilation) is the foundation of every neuroanesthetic plan. These tasks are interrelated because agents used to accomplish surgical anesthesia also influence cerebral and spinal cord hemodynamics. Anesthetic agents and technique may significantly affect cerebral oxygen consumption ($CMRO_2$), cerebral oxygen delivery (CDO_2), cerebral blood flow (CBF), intracranial tissue volume, intracranial pressure (ICP), arterial oxygen content (CaO_2), and the autoregulation of CBF. Recognition and treatment of concurrent comorbidities, optimization of the surgical exposure, and avoidance and management of surgery-related events in the operating room and during the perioperative period broadly define secondary objectives of the anesthetic intervention.

Cerebral Oxygen Consumption

Approximately 40 % of oxygen consumed by the brain is used to maintain the cellular integrity of its neural tissue. The remaining 60 % of oxygen is consumed accomplishing cellular electrophysiologic functions [1]. Inhalational agents (IA), narcotics, and commonly used hypnotic agents all lower cellular metabolism (i.e., $CMRO_2$) by decreasing cortical neuron electrical activity. Isoflurane is perhaps the most studied IA for neurosurgical procedures. In addition to decreasing $CMRO_2$, isoflurane uniquely and substantially lowers the critical CBF at which the EEG begins to demonstrate cerebral ischemia from a baseline lower CBF flow threshold of 20 ml/100 g brain tissue/min to nearer 10 ml/100 g brain tissue/min [2, 3]. For example, the incidence of ischemia suggested by electroencephalography (EEG) during carotid endarterectomy (CEA) is lower with isoflurane than with the other IAs [4]. These observations have led to a body of work generally supportive of the use of isoflurane as a neuroprotective agent in low cerebral blood flow states. However, it is not clear if these effects are temporary or permanent [4]. Sodium thiopental and propofol, along with all other intravenous hypnotic agents (except ketamine), reduce $CMRO_2$ along with CBF and will in sufficient dose produce an isoelectric EEG pattern.

Cerebral oxygen consumption increases with cortical seizure activity and during hyperthermia. Conversely, cooling a patient slows all enzymatic and chemical reactions and lowers $CMRO_2$ by slowing processes responsible for maintaining cellular integrity and those responsible for electrical function [5]. Hence, cooling is one modality used to protect the brain from transient ischemic events. When autoregulation is intact, cooling the brain produces an approximate 5–7 % decrease in $CMRO_2$ per degree Celsius cooled [6]. Any decrease in CBF reduces cerebral blood volume (CBV) and decreases intracranial pressure (ICP). Induced hypothermia is not completely benign as it has associated risks of impaired coagulation, cardiac arrhythmias, leftward shift of the oxygen-hemoglobin dissociation curve, increased infection, and slowed metabolism of many medications.

While the effectiveness of hypothermia for neuroprotection in "global" ischemia continues to accumulate, evidence suggests that there may be a difference for "focal" ischemia [7–13]. In 2002, two studies showed improved neurological outcomes and mortality for patients who had medically induced mild hypothermia after cardiac arrest [8, 9]. Since then, therapeutic mild hypothermia has been incorporated into the American Heart Association cardiac arrest guidelines [10]. For patients with traumatic brain injury, there are conflicting results regarding whether induced hypothermia is effective for neuroprotection [11, 12]. Studies are underway to further investigate the effectiveness of hypothermia in stroke patients [13].

For the management of temporary ischemia during aneurysm clipping, the Intraoperative Hypothermia for Aneurysm Surgery Trial (IHAST) published in 2005 did not find any outcome differences from mild hypothermia (33.5 °C) in this setting [7]. The majority of patients enrolled into the study had low-grade aneurysms, World Federation of Neurological Surgeons score of I, II, or III, where little difference in neurological outcome between any treatment groups would be expected. Many neuroanesthesiologists would employ normothermia in patients with these lower-grade diseases to avoid the associated risks (arrhythmias, prolonged intubation, increased infection, increased coagulation), while others maintain the potential benefit of decreased CMRO$_2$ outweigh these risks.

Intracranial Pressure

The intracranial space is a fixed volume with three major components: brain tissue (80–85 %), cerebrospinal fluid (7–10 %), and blood (5–8 %). In 1783, Alexander Monro described the cranium as a "rigid box" filled where the total volume tends to remain constant and that any increase in the volume of the cranial contents (e.g., brain, blood, or cerebrospinal fluid) will elevate intracranial pressure. Additionally, if any of the three volumes increase, it must occur at the expense of volume of the other two elements. George Kellie confirmed and published these observations in the early nineteenth century [14]. Now known as the Monro-Kellie doctrine, it describes a hyperbolic compliance curve relating ICP changes to intracranial volume. Normal ICP is approximately 10 mmHg. If the volume of one component increases, the volume of another must decrease or else the ICP rises. Brain tissue volume comprises both neural cells and extracellular fluid which can expand by tumor growth, intracranial bleed, and/or edema. There are two types of edema: vasogenic and cytotoxic. Vasogenic edema occurs in brain tissue surrounding tumors and is a consequence of the breakdown of the blood–brain barrier. This type of edema is amenable to steroid therapy. Cytotoxic edema, on the other hand, is a result of tissue ischemia and trauma and does not respond to steroid therapy. It will, however, respond to some degree to osmotic agents, although not to the same degree as normal brain tissue. Hydrocephalus occurs when there is excess cerebral spinal fluid (CSF). This can be due to impaired CSF

absorption and is also referred to as communicating hydrocephalus, or impaired CSF circulation also referred to as obstructive hydrocephalus. Finally, cerebral blood volume can expand by either vasodilation with increased cerebral blood flow or obstruction to cerebral venous drainage.

Cerebral Blood Flow and Its Influences

Cerebral blood flow (CBF) is normally under autoregulatory control and dependent on cerebral oxygen demand (CMRO$_2$), cerebral perfusion pressure (CPP), arterial CO$_2$ (PaCO$_2$), and arterial O$_2$ (PaO$_2$). CBF in adults is normally approximately 50 ml/100 g/min. Gray matter has blood flow of approximately 75 ml/100 g/min and white matter 25 ml/100 g/min. The higher blood flow to gray matter is mostly secondary to the higher gray matter metabolic rate and related oxygen consumption. CMRO$_2$ is a major determinate of CBF. The exact mechanism of this regulation is not precisely known. Temperature, as previously mentioned, also has a great effect on CMRO$_2$, with a 5–7 % decrease per degree Celsius cooling (in the temperature range from 27 to 37 °C), and therefore also cerebral blood flow [6].

Changes in mean arterial pressure (MAP) and therefore cerebral perfusion pressure (CPP) normally cause changes in cerebral blood flow only when outside the limits of autoregulation which have been conventionally characterized between mean arterial pressure of 50 and 150 mmHg in normotensive patients and higher in chronically hypertensive patients (Fig. 41.1). When the MAP falls below the lower autoregulation limit, the brain is considered at risk for hypoperfusion and ischemia, and when the MAP is above the upper autoregulatory limit, hyperperfusion, hyperemia, and cerebral edema become risks. Cerebral blood flow autoregulatory response may not function properly at MAPs below 60–70 mmHg in

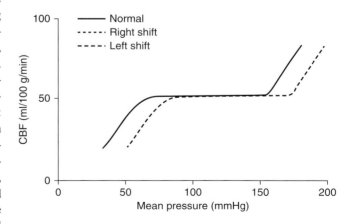

Fig. 41.1 Normal autoregulatory curve with right shift and left shift depicted (Reproduced with permission from Gravenstein and Gravenstein [75])

normotensive adults or at even higher levels in the uncontrolled chronically hypertensive patient and is slower in adolescents [15–17]. When autoregulation of regional CBF is compromised by acute injury, tumor-associated factors, vascular malformation, ischemia, or deeper planes of general anesthesia, CBF becomes increasingly pressure dependent. Proper intra- and perioperative blood pressure management are thus even more critical in these cases.

The effect of MAP on CBF, cerebral blood volume, and ICP is dependent on the volume of brain tissue under autoregulatory control. In situations where ICP is elevated but a substantial part of the brain remains under normal autoregulatory control, elevation of blood pressure will augment CPP by both increasing mean arterial pressure and through autoregulatory arteriolar constriction causing a slightly lowered CBV in the autoregulated part of the brain that exceeds the CBV increase experienced in the poorly autoregulated part of the brain. The combined effect causes a decrease of CBV followed by decreased ICP. In the scenario where a more extensive cerebral insult has occurred and autoregulation is fully compromised, ICP changes will follow MAP and CBV changes in the same direction. Because similar treatment can produce very different effects on patients with variable level of cerebral blood flow autoregulation, multimodality monitoring (jugular venous bulb oximetry [S_jvO_2], transcranial Doppler, cerebral oximetry, EEG, tissue pO_2, and invasive ICP monitoring) has all been used to guide therapy in selective cases [16, 18].

The primary influence of tissue pH on CBF is via the arterial partial pressure of CO_2 (PaCO$_2$). As PaCO$_2$ decreases, CBF is reduced and consequently CBV and ICP are also lowered. For PaCO$_2$ levels between 20 and 70 mmHg for each 1 mmHg change, there is an approximately 4 % change in cerebral blood flow (increase for CBF for increased PaCO$_2$ and decreased CBF for decreased PaCO$_2$). Outside of these levels, there is a plateau and no further cerebral vascular tone effects are seen. Aggressive hyperventilation poses the risk of inducing cerebral ischemia through the powerful vasoconstrictive effect of hypocapnia [19]. Deep hyperventilation therapy to control ICP has been associated with less favorable outcomes compared to normocapneic management. Intraoperatively, a mild hypocapneic state (PaCO$_2$, 35–40 mmHg) is the currently preferred goal.

Oxygenation (PaO$_2$) also exerts an effect on CBF. When administered in sufficient quantity to elevate the PaO$_2$ above 300 mmHg, it produces a mild (10 %) reduction of CBF [20]. Profound hypoxemia (PaO$_2$ < 50 mmHg) causes cerebral vasodilation and an exponential rise in cerebral blood flow, blood volume, and ICP. This is thought to be due to a decrease in pH secondary to lactic acidosis.

Ventilation parameters affect PaCO$_2$ and PaO$_2$. Anesthetic agents simultaneously influence CMRO$_2$, CPP [CPP=MAP – (the greater of CVP or ICP)], as well as diminishing in

a dose-dependent fashion the CBF autoregulatory response [21]. All IAs (halothane, enflurane, isoflurane, sevoflurane, desflurane) attenuate cerebral autoregulation. Additionally, CMRO$_2$ is disproportionately decreased (uncoupled) compared to its effect on cerebrovascular resistance (CVR) and CBF. Halothane, the most potent cerebral vasodilator among the IAs, was therefore seldom used during neurosurgery because of this attribute. When IAs are used as part of a balanced neuroanesthetic, they are limited to being used in low concentrations and in conjunction with mild hypocapnia when there is concern about limited intracranial or intraspinal elastance (such as with elevated ICP or spinal cord injury).

Both general anesthesia and surgery have effects on cerebral physiology which may continue into the postoperative period. Cerebral hyperemia may persist for up to 30 min following extubation from an anesthetic combination of isoflurane /N$_2$O/O$_2$/fentanyl/atracurium or propofol/O$_2$/air/fentanyl/atracurium [22]. Whether these more prolonged effects result from trace anesthetic-induced impairment of autoregulation, hemodilution, recovery from prolonged hyperventilation, or a nonspecific response to stress is not known [23]. The intraoperative and postoperative management of blood pressure is also potentially related to the incidence of postoperative intracranial hemorrhage (ICH). When intraoperative or postoperative blood pressure (within the first 12 h of operation) remained above 160/90 mmHg for two or more consecutive measurements made 5 min apart, the incidence of postoperative ICH after craniotomy was higher in one study [24]. At the time of this writing, it is still not clear whether blood pressure control can prevent hyperemia.

The brain can recover from brief episodes of ischemia but has little chance of return to normal following traumatic herniation. Therefore, when the potential for mechanical brain injury via herniation exists, aggressive acute hyperventilation (PaCO$_2$, 20–25 mmHg) can in conjunction with other measures decrease cerebral volume even though it may risk cerebral ischemia. A PaCO$_2$ as low as 20 mmHg will decrease CBF to near 10 ml/100 g/min. Although this blood flow normally produces profound cerebral ischemia, in the presence of isoflurane anesthesia, it represents, at least in normal brain, the lowered threshold of where the EEG first demonstrates a pattern of ischemia [2, 3].

The anesthesiologist can perform several clinically simple maneuvers that can further improve CPP in the perioperative period. A non-neutral head position, a tight tracheostomy tie, or ECG lead stretched tightly across the neck can all cause obstruction to jugular venous drainage [25, 26]. Placing the patient into a head-elevated position to augment venous drainage, short-term judicious hyperventilation to produce mild hypocapnia with decreased CBV and lowered ICP, hyperosmolar or hypertonic therapy based on intravascular volume, ventriculostomy drainage, infusion of a vasopressor to maintain cerebral inflow, and institution of muscle relaxation to increase chest wall compliance (and decrease intrathoracic and consequently CVP) can all improve CPP.

The reference (zero) all blood pressure transducers to the brain is by convention to the ear tragus at the Willis circle level.

Arterial Oxygen Content

Principal determinants of CDO_2 include hemoglobin concentration, oxygen saturation, and cardiac output. The Fick equation describes that oxygen delivery is equal to $1.36 \times CO \times SaO_2 + 0.003 \times PaO_2$. Coexisting disease states, such as pulmonary or cardiac contusion, heart failure, and aspiration, may substantially influence transfusion, ventilation, and cardiovascular support limits. The need for and benefit of transfusion is based on an estimate of probable cardiovascular reserve that is balanced against the current hemoglobin concentration, pulmonary function, and an estimate of the risk and severity of any additional bleeding. Currently, the optimum hemoglobin level for neurocritically ill patients is unknown. Very few studies have looked at the specific population of patients with neurological disease and optimum transfusion goals [27].

Fluid and Electrolyte Management

Fluid replacement during neurosurgical procedures differs from that used during non-CNS surgery. The tight-intercellular junctions found in the CNS and collectively referred to as the blood–brain barrier, with an effective pore size of only 8 Å, are essentially impermeable to sodium, other ions, or proteins. They are, however, freely permeable to water [28]. Hence, to avoid cerebral or spinal cord edema, intravenous solutions that are at least isotonic, i.e., 285 mOsm/kg, should be used. Thus, normal saline, i.e., 0.9 % NaCl, or hypertonic saline (without glucose) is preferred over solutions like lactated Ringer's (LR) that are relatively hypotonic. Clinicians will observe that 0.9 % NaCl solution has a calculated osmolality of 308 mOsm/kg water, suggesting that it is hypertonic, while LR solution has a calculated osmolality of 273 mOsm/kg water. These calculations that are printed on the solution bags represent the simple summation of the component electrolytes. These solutions are actually isotonic and hypotonic, respectively, because the *calculated* osmolalities do not account for solute ion interactions that are responsible for a *measured* osmolality that is actually considerably (approximately 20 mOsm/kg/water) less than the calculated value (Table 41.1). The labeling on the solution bags is always of the calculated and never the measured osmolality.

Solutions with glucose are generally avoided in neurosurgical patients for two reasons. First, although the

Table 41.1 Calculated osmolarity and osmolality of common intravenous fluids

Fluid	Osmolarity	Osmolality
Water	0	0
D5W	252	259
D5 .2NS	325	321
NS	308	282
LR	273	250
D5LR	525	524
3 % saline	1,027	921
6 % hetastarch	310	307
20 % mannitol	1,098	1,280
Plasma protein fraction	–	261

Reproduced with permission from Gravenstein and Gravenstein [75]
Abbreviations: D5W 5 % dextrose in water, D5 .2NS 5 % dextrose in 0.2 normal saline, D5NS 5 % dextrose in normal saline, D5LR 5 % dextrose in lactated Ringer's solution

glucose-containing solution may be iso- or hypertonic (Table 41.1), the glucose is rapidly metabolized. Thus its osmotic contribution of 252 mOsm/kg water is lost and a net free water gain results. This resulting free water will aggravate edema. Secondly, uncontrolled hyperglycemia has been associated with worsened neurologic outcome in patients with focal ischemic injuries. One theory for the mechanism of injury suggests that the presence of glucose increases neuronal metabolism and thereby decreases cellular viability during ischemia. Infants below 5 kg are at some risk for intraoperative hypoglycemia as they have very limited glycogen stores and in anticipation of potential hypoglycemia may therefore receive slightly hypertonic (from the transient glucose contribution intravenous maintenance therapy with D2.5 % normal saline) at our institution. This regimen addresses neuronal dependence on glucose as a metabolic substrate, the limitations of gluconeogenesis, and the high metabolic rate observed in this population. It also yields an isotonic fluid after the glucose is consumed. However, when fluid boluses are needed, 0.9 % NaCl solution, rather than the D2.5 % maintenance normal saline, is used. While the relative risk of hyper- vs hypoglycemia has been well addressed in ICU patient, clear guidelines on blood sugar control in the perioperative period are still unclear but in general maintained below 150 mg/ml in patients with poor glucose tolerance.

Intravascular volume replacement therapy does not differ between neurosurgical and non-CNS procedures. Suggested replacement of blood loss is a 3:1 (isotonic crystalloid to blood loss) volume ratio for 0.9 % saline solutions and 1:1 for colloid, 3 % NaCl, and blood products. Deficits calculated from fasting, insensible losses, urine output, and third-space losses are replaced 1:1. When blood or crystalloid replacement therapy exceeds a few liters (caused by hemorrhage, diabetes insipidus, or a pharmacologically induced diuresis), electrolytes, especially calcium, potassium, and sodium, are followed serially and corrected.

Blood transfusion during neurosurgical procedures may be viewed as somewhat more aggressive compared to other surgery, but the management objective remains to keep the hematocrit in the 24–30 % range. Anemia provokes increased cardiac output and cerebral vasodilatation.

Getting Started

Surgical intervention dictates that the anesthesiologist prepares an anesthetic management plan. This requires that pathophysiology be involved and implications of the surgical approach or procedure be considered.

Stable, controlled cerebral and cardiovascular hemodynamics are the goals prior to surgery. Induction of general anesthesia, laryngoscopy, intubation, positioning, application of the head pinioning apparatus, and eventually skin incision are all profound yet transient insults that make attainment of this goal challenging.

Careful timing and communication to allow coordination of drug effects with stimulation are essential to smoothly navigate the assorted surgical stimuli. Laryngeal or intravenous administration of lidocaine (1–1.5 mg/kg) prior to intubation attenuates endotracheal stimulation. Pinioning of the head may be accomplished in most adults with only a 5–10 % variation of the vital signs. One approach is just prior to pinion placement administer 1–1.5 mg/kg esmolol and 0.5 mg/kg propofol. Thiopental, widely used in the past, is currently not available in the US market.

If the heart rate is lower than preoperative values, the dose of esmolol is reduced. Similarly, if the blood pressure has not recovered from induction, the propofol or STP dose is reduced. Once the drugs have been administered, allowing sufficient time for the heart rate or the blood pressure shows a drug effect before proceeding to pinion the head is recommended. This coordination accomplishes matching the peak surgical stimulus with the peak drug effect, regardless of circulation time. Other regimens, including preemptive local anesthetic infiltration of the pinion sites and a titrated remifentanil infusion, have also been advocated for pinioning [29].

Positioning

Following induction, the task of positioning is undertaken. Both the presence of anesthesia and muscle relaxation during patient transfer and positioning present conditions where the patient is unable to protect himself and is more susceptible to nerve and spinal injury with the removal of muscular tone.

The different positions into which a patient may be placed for surgery are associated with various known risks [30]. The supine position places pressure on the heels and occiput, reduces lumbar lordosis, and may cause flexion of the neck or pressure on peripheral nerves. The ulnar nerve at the elbow is the most frequent place for position-related nerve injury. Injury of the brachial plexus can be caused by aggressive abduction and in the lateral position by a chest roll that slips into the axilla from its intended upper thoracic location. The lateral position further risks lateral flexion of the cervical spine, pressure from the surgical table on the "down arm" and the fibula, threatening the brachial plexus and superficial peroneal nerve. Regardless of body position, one must be cautious with rotation or extension of the head as it may cause venous congestion and is associated with elevated ICP [26, 27]. The prone position requires the abdomen to be properly suspended and knees, testicles, and breasts to be free from pressure.

Special Perioperative Clinical Considerations

Postoperative Visual Loss

Postoperative blindness is a catastrophic complication, the etiology of which is not fully understood. In the prone position the risk of ischemic optic neuropathy (ION) and central retinal artery occlusion (CRAO) is increased. It has been described both when the head has been rested on a foam cushion with a cutout for the eyes, nose, and lips and when the head has been suspended by a pinioning system. Young and old patients are at risk as are patients of any physical status. Pediatric patients (<18 years of age) and the elderly (>84 years) may be more susceptible to visual loss following spine surgery [31]. Speculation is that the pathogenesis involves length of surgery, low arterial perfusion pressure, elevated episcleral venous and intraocular pressures, anemia, embolic events, Wilson frame, and the use of pressor agents [32, 33]. According to the ASA's 2012 Practice Advisory for Perioperative Visual Loss Associated with Spine Surgery, the length of the procedure is also an important risk factor with the vast majority (94 %) of ION occurring in cases lasting longer than 6 h [34]. Therefore patients considered at high risk are ones undergoing prolonged procedures (greater than 6.5 h), in the prone position, with substantial blood loss. Staging procedures is an option to consider but must be balanced against the risks of a staged procedure: possible increase in infection rates, neurological injury, thromboembolism, and cost [34]. Deliberate hypotension has not been shown to definitely increase risk but is not commonly employed anymore. Central (or peripheral) [35] venous pressure monitoring may be considered in high-risk patients and colloid plus crystalloid can be employed to help minimize periorbital edema. There is no set low level of hemoglobin, but commonly a level of 9 is used as a trigger for transfusion [34]. In January 2012, risk factors for ION were assessed in a large, multicenter, case-controlled study [36]. Eighty patients were from the American Society of Anesthesiologist Postoperative Visual Loss Registry with ION and 315 control subjects without ION after prone spinal surgery [36]. Using multivariate analysis, risk factors found for ION after spinal fusion surgery were male sex (OR 2.53), obesity (OR 2.83), Wilson frame use (OR 4.3), anesthesia duration (OR per 1 h = 1.39), estimated blood loss (OR per 1 l = 1.34), and colloid as percent of non-blood replacement (OR per 5 % = 0.67) [36]. Direct pressure on the eye obviously places patients at increased risk for CRAO (not ION) and should be avoided. In the postoperative period a visual exam should be performed as soon as possible. If any visual disturbance is identified, an ophthalmology consult should be placed and consideration given to optimization of the patient's hemoglobin and hematocrit [35].

Venous Air Embolism

Venous air embolism (VAE) is best known as a danger associated with the sitting position but also is well described in association with the lateral, prone, and supine positions [37, 38]. The incidence of air detectable in neurosurgical cases (craniotomy, cervical laminectomy) using the sitting position is near 45 % but can exceed 70 % [38, 39]. About 20 % of VAE cases in adults produce clinically significant effects, while in children the significant effects are twice that of adults [39]. Because the morbidity of VAE is significant, prevention and monitoring that allow early detection of intravascular gas are key elements of a successful management plan.

Continuous positive end-expiratory pressure (PEEP) in the airway and adequate intravascular volume help to reduce VAE occurrence. Early detection is readily accomplished with continuous precordial Doppler monitoring. Transesophageal echocardiography (TEE) is more sensitive and specific but is used less frequently due to the patient's position and the need for direct observation to make the diagnosis of VAE. Additionally, if fluoroscopy is being used, the probe is not radiolucent. The observance of acute changes, during an otherwise stable anesthetic, of decreased exhaled CO_2, increased central venous, pulmonary artery or decreased systemic blood pressure, or SpO_2 are also suggestive of VAE. Successful management of VAE includes several maneuvers. For a head-elevated operation, the surgeon is notified of the suspicion of a VAE, the wound is flooded with irrigating fluid if possible, the surgical site is lowered to a dependent position relative to the heart, and light manual jugular venous pressure is applied to arrest further entrainment of air and increase cerebral venous pressure. The elevated cerebral venous pressure from manual external jugular compression will in many cases demonstrate a new site of bleeding, i.e., the site of air ingress prior to the arti-

factual elevation of venous pressure. All myocardial depressants (e.g., any potent IA) are discontinued and ventilation switched to 100 % oxygen. Nitrous oxide poses a special risk because it has low blood solubility and can aggravate a serious condition through its rapid diffusion into an intravascular gas collection, doubling its size in less than 15 min. The effectiveness of repositioning the patient head down with left side down to sequester gas away from the right ventricular outflow track has been challenged and may interfere with other resuscitation maneuvers [40]. In the face of an air-filled right ventricle, pulmonary hypertension, and diminishing systemic pressure, aggressive administration of volume to support preload and intravenous inotropic support and CPR are begun. Aspiration of air or foam from a multi-orifice central venous catheter if present may also be attempted but is unlikely to be therapeutic. As many interventions may be necessary, early calls for assistance are advised.

The addition of positive end-expiratory pressure (PEEP) is not recommended for treatment of VAE even though it may lessen the volume of additional air entrained. Application of PEEP after hemodynamic consequences are observed will increase intrathoracic pressure when air is already in the right heart and pulmonary circulation. Consequently, addition of PEEP will further compromise right ventricular preload just when it is most needed. Furthermore, with an approximately 25 % incidence of patent foramen ovale in adults and a 35 % incidence in children and adolescents, PEEP may increase the likelihood of causing a paradoxical (left heart) air embolus, particularly upon release when right atrial pressure is transiently higher than the left atrial pressure [40–44]. Air traversing from the right atrium across a patent foramen ovale into the left atrium bypasses the lung that normally filters out most air bubbles. Once in the left heart circulation, these air bubbles can travel to the brain or heart, causing acute cerebral or myocardial ischemia, respectively. Clinicians must remain vigilant to this devastating complication, especially if an intraoperative VAE occurred and PEEP was being used. Hemodynamically significant air embolism after intracranial or spinal surgery may also occur upon moving the patient to a supine position [43]. Air sequestered in the originally nondependent vertebral or splanchnic veins gains access to the heart when the patient is returned to a supine position or upon release of PEEP. Spine, paraspinal, and splanchnic venous air simply floats up to the heart level in the supine position.

Mass Lesions

Tumors present unique risks to patients in the perioperative period because of features related to size, vascularity, endocrine activity, and location. Rapidly growing tumors and those causing obstructive hydrocephalus can be associated with diminished intracranial elastance and elevated ICP. When ICP concerns exist, mild hyperventilation, reverse Trendelenburg position, hyperosmolar therapy, and decompression with CSF diversion are all ICP decreasing options to consider. CPP and oxygenation are defended throughout induction and until the dura has been opened. Once resection of the tumor is underway, bleeding becomes a primary focus of concern. The anesthesiologist will have secured intravenous access proportionate to the presumed risk of bleeding. When the arterial supply and venous drainage of a tumor are known to be high-flow vessels, analogous to those in an arteriovenous malformation, the CPP will be adjusted downward as the tumor is excised. Failure to moderate CPP once the high flow, low resistance diversion is removed risks bleeding from the tumor bed and significant postoperative cerebral hyperemia and edema. The CPP may gradually be returned to normal over 24–72 h as the cerebral vessels' muscularis layer recovers its ability to modulate the vessels' tone, i.e., local cerebral vascular autoregulation normalizes.

Posterior Fossa Surgery

Surgery in the posterior fossa, especially when near the vestibulocochlear nerves, has a greater than 50 % incidence of postoperative nausea associated with it. The nausea alone has been attributed to increasing the length of stay for some patients. Intraoperative anesthetic management can influence the incidence and the severity of postoperative nausea. We use a multifaceted pharmacological approach to reduce postoperative nausea. In addition to administration of intravenous ondansetron (4 mg) 30 min prior to the end of surgery, we typically administer dexamethasone (4 mg) and promethazine (6.25 mg) at the start of the procedure and run an infusion of propofol at 25–50 mcg/kg/min throughout the case. Anecdotally, this technique slightly slows the emergence from anesthesia, but dramatically decreases the incidence and severity of postoperative nausea. Other techniques, such as simply using higher infusion doses of propofol, may also be effective nausea prophylaxis.

Brainstem

Resection of tumors in the brainstem can result in dramatic intraoperative and postoperative findings. When the tumor is located on the floor of the fourth ventricle and areas near the ventral medulla (vasomotor center) are manipulated, hypotension or profound hypertension and bradycardia or even asystole may occur. Surgery in this vicinity may stimulate the dorsal motor nucleus of the vagus or the nucleus ambiguous, reducing cardiac contractility and blocking conduction through the atrioventricular node. To address this possibility,

a transthoracic pacer or pacing pulmonary artery catheter (PAC) may be employed in stand-by mode. A transesophageal pacer would not be effective as it paces the atrium and the A-V node will not transmit atrial impulses in this scenario. In the absence of a PAC with pacing capability or transthoracic pacer, pharmacological treatment with anticholinergic medications will also terminate episodes of bradycardia, but this approach eliminates the valuable surgical feedback that the episodes of bradycardia provide.

Finally, this surgery may impair swallowing reflexes by damage of the cranial nerves VIII, IX, and X, a consideration that may affect the decision to extubate the patient early (in the OR) or late (in the ICU).

Transphenoidal Hypophysectomy

Pituitary tumors are often small tumors, microadenomas that are discovered by their unique presenting signs and symptoms. Enlargement of the sella turcica can cause visual disturbances by pressure on the optic chiasm causing bitemporal hemianopsia or extraocular muscle palsies by pressure on cranial nerves III, IV, and VI. Presenting symptoms may also be related to hypersecretion of any one of the pituitary hormones. The anterior pituitary secretes adrenocorticotropic hormone (ACTH), growth hormone (GH), prolactin (PRL), thyroid-stimulating hormone (TSH), luteinizing hormone (LH), follicle-stimulating hormone (FSH), and melanocyte-stimulating hormone (MSH). Prolactin-secreting tumors are the most common secreting tumors but usually do not pose special anesthetic risks to the patient. Patients with long-term GH-secreting tumors may present with acromegaly, placing them at risk for having a difficult airway and postoperative respiratory complications. These patients can have large, immobile mandibles and narrowing of the mandible and the airway below the level of the vocal cords. They also frequently have obstructive sleep apnea. ACTH-secreting tumors cause Cushing disease which again could cause the patient to have a difficult airway and the possibility of hyperglycemia. TSH-secreting tumors can cause hyperthyroidism that should be medically treated and stabilized with antithyroid medication and beta-adrenergic blockade prior to coming to the operating room. Patients may also present with panhypopituitarism, requiring replacement of these hormones. The posterior pituitary secretes antidiuretic hormone (ADH) and deficiency of this is manifested as diabetes insipidus (DI). Intraoperative occurrence of DI must be continually monitored for by the anesthesiologist. Suspicion of this acute syndrome should occur if urine output suddenly greatly increases disproportionately to the intravenous fluids infused and investigated with intraoperative analysis of urine specific gravity, urine osmolality, and serial plasma Na levels. A low urine osmolality (less than 200 mOsm/kg), urine specific gravity of less than 1.005, and urine Na less than 25 are diagnostic. Unique features of this procedure are predominately in the emergence phase where hypertension and valsalva must be avoided due to the consequences of a hematoma in this region. If a transnasal surgical approach is utilized, rescue mask ventilation should include an oral airway to try to avoid pneumocephalus. A nasal airway should not be placed and nasal CPAP should not be applied postoperatively.

Vascular Neurosurgery

Cerebral Aneurysms

Cerebral aneurysms are abnormal outpouching of cerebral arteries due to weakness of the vessel wall either from congenital causes or secondary to environmental stress and exposures, i.e., hypertension, cigarette smoke, and cocaine. The majority of cerebral aneurysms are found along the circle of Willis at arterial bifurcations. About 90 % are in the anterior circulation and 10 % in the posterior circulations with these mostly occurring at the basilar tip. The rate of rupture is 0.05–6 % per year with resultant subarachnoid hemorrhage. Subarachnoid hemorrhage (SAH) is traditionally graded by multiple systems: the World Federation of Neurological Surgeons Grading System (WFNS), Hunt Hess, and Fisher Grade and modified Fisher Grade scale [45–47]. The WFNS scale (Table 41.2) and the Hunt Hess grading scale (Table 41.3) are clinical scores that assess prognosis. The WFNS is based on the Glasgow coma scale and the score is inversely related to the prognosis. Hunt Hess (HH) 0 is an unruptured aneurysm. HH-1 is asymptomatic or minor headache with no neurological deficits and carries a 2 % mortality. HH-2 is described by headache that can be severe, nuchal rigidity, and possibly a cranial nerve palsy as its only deficit. HH-2 carries a 5 % mortality. HH-3 is described by altered mental status, lethargy, and minor neurological deficits and carries a 15–20 % mortality. HH-4 entails stupor and hemiparesis with a 30–40 % mortality. HH-5 includes patients in deep coma with a motor exam no better than decerebrate and carries a 50–80 % mortality.

Following subarachnoid hemorrhage, vasospasm is a significant risk (20–40 %). The Fisher Grade scale is

Table 41.2 The World Federation of Neurological Surgeons (WFNS) scale

Grade	GCS	Motor deficit
I	15	Absent
II	13–14	Absent
III	13–14	Present
IV	7–12	Absent/present
V	3–6	Absent/present

Data from Anonymous [45]

Table 41.3 Hunt Hess score

Scale	Symptoms
0	Unruptured aneurysm
1	Asymptomatic or minor headache with no neurological deficits
2	Headache that can be severe, nuchal rigidity, and possibly a cranial nerve palsy
3	Altered mental status, lethargy, and minor neurological deficits
4	Stupor and hemiparesis
5	Deep coma with a motor exam no better than decerebrate

Data from Hunt and Hess [46]

Table 41.4 Fisher and modified Fisher Grade scale

Grade	Radiologic findings	Vasospasm risk (%)
Fisher scale		
1	No SAH or focal thin SAH	21
2	Diffuse thin SAH (<1 mm)	25
3	Thick SAH (>1 mm)	37
4	IVH	31
Modified Fisher		
0	No SAH or IVH	
1	Thin SAH (<1 mm) and no IVH	24
2	Thin SAH (<1 mm) and IVH	33
3	Thick SAH (>1 mm) and no IVH	33
4	Thick SAH (>1 mm) with IVH	40

Data from Frontera et al. [47]

a radiological grading system to help predict the rate of symptomatic vasospasm. The modified Fisher scale was developed to better correlate with symptomatic vasospasm (Table 41.4). Grade 0 has no SAH or IVH. Grade 1 has thin SAH (less than 1 mm) and no IVH and carries a 24 % risk of vasospasm. Grade 2 has thin SAH with IVH and carries a 33 % risk. Grade 3 has thick SAH without IVH and has a 33 % risk. Grade 4 has thick SAH with IVH and has a 40 % risk of symptomatic vasospasm [47]. Vasospasm most frequently occurs in the first 14 days post bleed with the highest incidence between days 3 and 7. Management strategies have included nimodipine, statins, and magnesium sulfate infusions [48–51]. However, recently the MASH-2 trial demonstrated a lack of efficacy in magnesium infusion to prevent vasospasm [51].

Rebleeding is a feared complication that has a significant mortality associated with it. Early surgical or endovascular securing of the aneurysm within 24–48 h has improved outcome and is the only definitive way to prevent rebleeding. The International Subarachnoid Aneurysm Trial (ISAT) compared neurosurgical clipping or endovascular coiling in 2,143 patients and found low rates of rebleeding in both groups at a mean of 9 years in the long-term follow-up [52]. Before the aneurysm is secured, steps must be taken to prevent rebleeding by maintaining stable transmural vessel pressure. Prior to the operating room, this is accomplished by controlling the systemic arterial blood pressure with a goal of the systolic blood pressure less than 140 mmHg via short-acting antihypertensives, controlling pain and anxiety, and preventing seizures.

In the operating room, induction of anesthesia must be a slow, controlled event with the goal to limit sympathetic response to laryngoscopy. The rate of rupture on induction is 0.5–2 % and carries a 75 % mortality. Ventilation parameters are initially maintained near normal to prevent altering CBF or ICP and maintaining a stable transmural pressure. For procedures requiring a craniotomy, it is common to gradually induce mild hypocapnia to decrease brain size after craniotomy, but prior to opening of the dura and also to facilitate a better surgical exposure. When the dura is taut, additional hyperosmolar or diuretic (mannitol, furosemide) may be considered, with transitory hyperventilation, and the patient may be placed into a reverse Trendelenburg position. When additional steps are taken, plasma electrolytes, arterial CO_2 end-tidal CO_2 gradient, and urine output are followed closely. Electrolytes lost with diuresis are replaced in the operating room and immediate postoperative phase. If the diuresis is brisk and sustained, and the urine dilute, the possibility of induced diabetes insipidus should be explored by checking the urine specific gravity or urine osmolality and following serial serum sodium.

Blood pressure and heart rate are kept stable during clipping of simple aneurysms that present with a favorable orientation. Not infrequently, however, clipping an aneurysm will first require placement of temporary clips to completely occlude the arterial cerebral circulation upstream of the aneurysm. In anticipation of this possibility and the implications for the regional cerebral ischemic insult, patients have been traditionally cooled via conduction and a water blanket to approximately 34.5 °C. Intraoperative prophylactic cooling, although traditionally employed, has been called into question by the Intraoperative Hypothermia for Aneurysm Surgery Trial (IHAST) [7]. IHAST did not demonstrate any improvement in 3-month neurologic outcome with the use of short-duration intraoperative hypothermia during craniotomy for good-grade patients, WFNS grades I to III, with aneurysmal SAH [7]. Preoperative discussion with the neurosurgeon on temperature management is appropriate in light of these conflicting data. Temperature can be measured from esophageal, rectal, or bladder probes, although the brain is likely to be cooler than measured core temperature because the surgical site is exposed to ambient room temperature. Blood pressure is maintained by a vasopressor (commonly phenylephrine because of its preference for peripheral over intracranial vasoconstriction), while either barbiturate or propofol is administered to near 90 % burst suppression monitored by EEG. No compelling clinical data currently support the use of propofol for neuroprotection. One study which compared the use of propofol and isoflurane in 20 patients during coronary artery bypass grafting showed no difference in neuropsychological outcomes between the two groups [53]. The hypnotic infusions are titrated to an EEG pattern showing at least 90 % burst suppression. A deeper

coma with barbiturates, i.e., isoelectric EEG (100 % burst suppression), has not been demonstrated to convey any additional cerebral protection and may result in diminished hemodynamic stability, a slowed emergence and extended respiratory support. The limit to which perfusion pressure during temporary clip times can be augmented is determined by the cardiovascular reserve (i.e., onset of myocardial ischemia). Usually, a 20 % increase above baseline blood pressure is sufficient additional pressure support to protect normal cerebral function. However, if myocardial ischemia develops, efforts must be made to improve myocardial oxygen delivery/consumption balance. When a temporary or permanent clip application produces an alteration in a monitored evoked potential, the mean arterial pressure is augmented further, usually with an alpha agonist intravenous infusion. When placement of the clip occludes one or more lenticulostriate perforating vessels, the mean arterial pressure necessary to perfuse ischemic and vasodilated tissues through collateral vessels is augmented to 10–30 % above baseline [54]. Once the perfusion pressure has been adjusted, a gradual recovery of evoked potential waves is often observed (Fig. 41.2).

Vessel rupture and hemorrhage are major complications of neurovascular surgery. Ideally, the patient is rapidly cooled to a mild hypothermia goal (35 °C), and a hypnotic agent (in general propofol if hemodynamically tolerated) is administered before a temporary clip is applied and the bleeding halted. When the aneurysm rupture occurs without a temporary clip in place, acute and profound hypotension is induced in the attempt to decrease bleeding rate. Placement of the temporary clip defines the start of a regional ischemic event. The temperature of the brain and the total ischemic time will predict the likelihood of cerebral infarction. The longest ischemic time usually tolerated by the brain (approximately 60 min) is achieved in controlled situations when the patient is cooled to 18 °C and while on low-flow cardiopulmonary bypass or induced total circulatory arrest. Severe hypothermia is predictably associated with a coagulopathy and should be reversed before emerging from anesthesia.

Arteriovenous Malformations

Arteriovenous malformations (AVM) are abnormal collection of arteries and veins that lack the capillary system and therefore have shunting between the arterial and venous system. This resulting high-pressure flow to the venous system becomes at risk for rupture secondary to fibromuscular thickening and weakened elastic lamina [55]. Hemorrhage is the most common presenting symptom of AVMs. There are multiple options for treating AVMs. The Spetzler-Martin scale is used to guide therapy and scores the AVMs on the basis of surgical outcome. It looks at three characteristics: the maximum diameter, its location either within or outside of eloquent

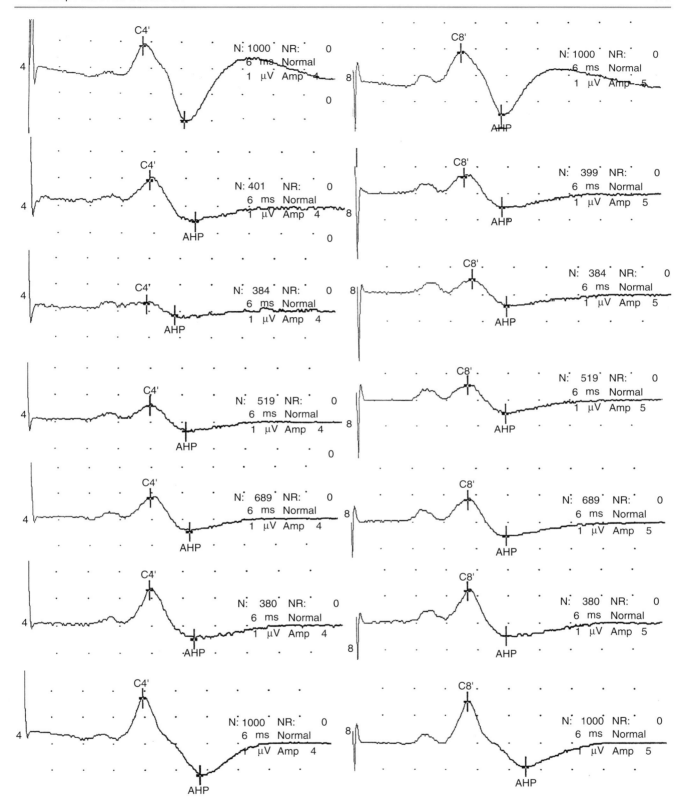

Fig. 41.2 Once the perfusion pressure has been adjusted, a gradual recovery of evoked potential waves is observed. Leads 4 and 8 follow progression of C4' and C8' (Reproduced with permission from Gravenstein and Gravenstein [75])

cortex, and the presence or absence of deep venous drainage. According to the 2001 American Stroke Association guidelines, grades 1 and 2 should be considered for surgical resection, grade 3 for endovascular treatment, and grades 4 and 5 for conservative management [56].

Anesthetic management of the excision or embolization of AVMs is similar to that of a vascular tumor. The need for intravenous access will be substantial secondary to the risk of significant bleeding during the surgical resection. Pharmacological coma to EEG burst suppression is not induced in this disease because bleeding is not typically amenable to temporary clip placement. Patients are kept normothermic to avoid impairment of coagulation or risks of hypothermia (arrhythmias, shivering, slowed drug metabolism, left-shifted oxygen-hemoglobin dissociation curve). As the AVM is successfully removed, local CBF is expected to increase due to cerebral vasodilatation in areas that were previously chronically hypoperfused [57]. The increase in CBF can cause cerebral edema and hemorrhage. Hence, CPP will be lowered to guard against hyperemia and cerebral edema. Strict avoidance of hypertension is a continued goal for at least 24 h postoperatively. Staged procedures are another option to attempt to reduce incidence of post AVM resolution hyperemic hemorrhage from cerebral hyperperfusion.

Carotid Endarterectomy

Carotid endarterectomy (CAE) differs from intracranial vascular surgery in its association with coronary and peripheral vascular disease and proximity to the carotid sinus. If no temporary arterial shunt is applied by the surgeon, the mean arterial pressure is augmented during the time of carotid artery occlusion, just as it is for temporary clip application during cerebral aneurysm surgery. Blood pressure and heart rate can be erratic when the carotid sinus is surgically manipulated. This intraoperative and postoperative hemodynamic lability may not be improved with the use of local anesthetic field blocks of the carotid sinus [58, 59]. When the surgical procedure during carotid endarterectomy causes denervation of the carotid body, an altered chemoreceptor function and a diminished hypoxic response may result [60]. The loss of the hypoxic response is a particularly relevant postoperative consideration in the patient with a prior CEA who may now have bilateral carotid body chemoreceptor dysfunction and postoperative respiratory status should be closely monitored in the recovery room or intensive care unit before discharge to the neurosurgical ward.

Blood pressure and blood flow are reduced prior to removal of the carotid artery clamps to minimize hyperemia and the risk of postsurgical bleeding. Arterial hemorrhage into the surgical site can be provoked or worsened during emergence by perioperative coughing, bucking, and uncontrolled hypertension. Hence, the target blood pressure in this phase of the anesthetic is at the lower end of the patient's normal range. Emergence from anesthesia often utilizes narcotics for their combined analgesic, sedative, and cough suppressant effects. Intravenous lidocaine to reduce tracheal reactivity to the endotracheal tube during extubation may reduce bucking and coughing.

Neuromonitoring during neurovascular surgery aids in detection of ischemic strokes. Strokes may originate from embolic sources, as from plaque loosened during carotid endarterectomy or shunt placement and during the time of temporary clip placement or by misapplication or rotation of permanent clips during surgery for intracranial aneurysm. In recognition of these risks, CNS monitoring to alert the surgeon and anesthesia provider of such events is a priority. The mental status of awake patients who are operated for carotid endarterectomy with field block anesthesia serves as neuromonitors for cerebral ischemia. Patients are asked to verbally respond to questions or complete simple tasks such as squeezing a rubber toy, so their compliance with the request is unmistakable. When patients are under general anesthesia, CNS monitoring is accomplished with the use of electroencephalography (EEG) and/or continuous somatosensory evoked potential (SSEP) monitoring. Transcranial electrical motor- and visual evoked potential (TceMEP and VEP, respectively) and facial nerve monitoring are other modalities that have been utilized intraoperatively and described in detail elsewhere in the book. TceMEP and VEP are difficult to obtain as they are exquisitely sensitive to conventional anesthetics and can limit the surgical field because of the physical setup. When any of these monitoring modalities are used, the anesthetic technique is biased towards using reduced concentration of volatile agents and increased narcotic infusions, preferably shorter acting agents.

Endovascular

Endovascular treatment of cerebral vascular disease is minimally invasive and entails the interventional radiological access to the vessel of interest via intra-arterial catheters. This is usually accomplished by accessing the femoral artery and then the carotid or vertebral arteries, depending on the target vessel of interest. The anesthetic considerations specific to the disease state are the same for endovascular treatment as for open craniotomy. Anesthesia can be accomplished either through intravenous sedation with continual mental status monitoring or through general anesthesia. Endovascular treatment of aneurysms entails deploying of coils into the aneurysm to occlude flow. Depending on the shape of the aneurysm, additional therapeutic maneuvers such as placement of stents or temporary balloon angioplasty may be required. The manipulation of these vessels poses the possible risk of rupture of the aneurysm or stroke from embolic or occlusive complications. The anesthesiologist must be prepared for these events and have a ready armamentarium to rapidly manipulate cerebral blood flow and perfusion. Patients with subarachnoid hemorrhage may also present for angioplasty for vasospasm. If the aneurysm is already secured, hypertensive therapy will most likely be employed and should be continued throughout the angioplasty procedure.

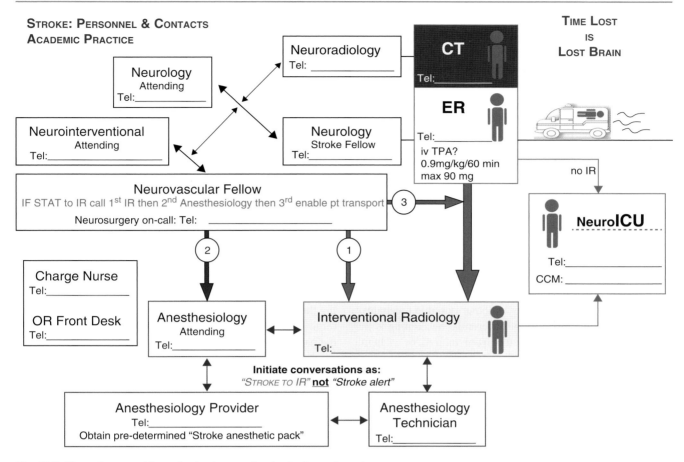

Fig. 41.3 Example protocol for activating interventional suite for stroke patient

Alleviation of the vasospasm can be attempted through balloon angioplasty or through direct intra-arterial injection of vasodilators, usually calcium channel blockers such as verapamil and nicardipine. Systemic circulation of these medications can occur with resultant profound hypotension.

Stroke

Patients suffering acute stroke are now undergoing more and more interventional procedures in attempts to reestablish cerebral blood flow. Stroke affects more than 795,000 people annually in the USA with 85 % of these being ischemic in origin and 15 % hemorrhagic. Over the past decade, there have been vast improvements in treatment of acute stroke. In 1995, IV tissue plasminogen activator (tPA) was first shown to improve outcomes if given within 3 h of symptom onset [61]. In 1999, the PROACT II study showed that intra-arterial administration of pro-urokinase within 6 h of onset improved clinical outcomes at 90 days but with an increased risk of intracranial hemorrhage (10 % vs. 2 %) [62]. In 2005, the use of the MERCI device, a clot retrieval catheter to allow recanalization of the cerebral arterial vessels, was approved for up to 8 h post onset of stroke symptoms [63]. In 2007, the Interventional Management of Stroke (IMS) II study showed

decreased mortality at 3 months with a combined intravenous and intra-arterial tPA approach [64]. In 2008, Hacke and colleagues reported that alteplase could be used from 3 to 4.5 h with improved clinical outcomes at 90 days and no increase in mortality [65]. At the time of this writing, ongoing trials are looking at the safety and efficacy of new and improved devices to mechanically disrupt and remove the clot.

Currently, the use of intravenous tPA may be considered within 4.5 h from the onset of symptoms of an ischemic stroke. At our institution, an intravascular recanalization approach is performed if the patient does not improve clinically with intravenous tPA but shows a CT angiography and perfusion scans with less than one third of the vessel's territory compromised. In this case, the presence of a large amount of salvageable brain tissue penumbra, a brain territory that is ischemic but not yet infarcted, is assumed. When cerebral blood flow falls below 20 ml/100 g/min, neuronal function declines. CBF from 15–20 ml/100 g/min causes decreased synaptic activity but can still be salvaged. When CBF falls below 15 ml/100 g/min, irreversible ischemic injury occurs and below 6 ml/100 g/min neuronal cell membrane failure occurs. Because "Time is Brain," well-organized protocols need to be in place at each institution to activate all the necessary personnel if a patient is to go to the interventional suite (example protocol in Fig. 41.3).

Anesthetic management of the acute stroke patient requires fast preparation. If the patient has received IV tPA, strict blood pressure control (systolic pressures less than 185 mmHg and diastolic pressure less than 110 mmHg) needs to occur. Permissive hypertension to this point is allowed in order to improve perfusion through collaterals.

Anesthetizing a patient who has recovered function from a prior stroke either partially or wholly is accompanied by the risk of the patient and surgeon potentially experiencing the phenomenon of the patient awakening from anesthesia with some or all of the deficits that occurred at the time of the original CVA. This recapitulation phenomenon has been termed "differential awakening" of the brain and related to patients as a "reliving" of their stroke [66]. It is postulated that the patient with a remote stroke has regained function by learning to utilize new pathways that require vastly more synapses than the original pathway. The normal brain recovers function with a certain low partial pressure of anesthetic agent along neurons and at receptors. Another possible mechanism explaining the phenomenon of differential awakening is that anesthetic agents are eliminated from injured or ischemic brain more slowly than normal brain, perhaps because of differential blood flow. Finally, it has been suggested that the cumulative amounts of the same low partial pressure anesthetic along the much longer neuronal pathways and vastly larger number of receptors used to overcome the CVA deficit are sufficient to keep those pathways nonfunctional. In general these residual anesthetic effects dissipate within hours of discontinuation of anesthesia as the partial pressures and concentrations of the agents used continue to diminish. However, if memory within the pathways has also been disturbed, full recovery to preoperative baseline may require days, weeks, and possibly an even longer period of rehabilitation, but full recovery is eventually expected.

The patient with preoperative paralysis of more than several days, whether from central or peripheral neural injury, poses other anesthetic and postoperative concerns. The paralyzed patient may have up-regulated neuromuscular junctions to a degree that administration of a depolarizing muscle relaxant, i.e., succinylcholine can precipitate an acute hyperkalemic event. Monitoring of neuromuscular blockade is also complicated when attempted on an affected limb of a patient with a prior CVA. Electrically stimulating the ulnar or posterior tibial nerve in an affected limb, where there is an increased neuromuscular junction density, produces exaggerated responses compared with the normal limb. Thus, well-intentioned titration of neuromuscular blocking agent to monitored twitches on a paretic or plegic limb can lead to significant overdosage of neuromuscular blocker and subsequently an inability to reverse the patient for extubation. Simply monitoring on a non-affected side or following the activity of the levator palpebrae muscle with facial nerve stimulation or performance of a head lift for greater than 5 s will confirm suitable strength is recovered for extubation.

Spine Surgery

Spinal cord dynamics are similar to those of the brain. The cord responds to anesthetic agents, ventilation parameters, temperature, perfusion pressure, and ischemia in essentially the same fashion as the brain. Perioperative edema of the spinal cord presents with similar concerns of ischemia and infarction. The decompression, instrumentation, distraction, and fusion of vertebral elements are unique to surgery of the spine. Bleeding or the entrainment of air results most commonly from violation of the epidural veins. Intraoperative neurological injury, unless catastrophic, is not hemodynamically apparent but can usually be detected with ideally continuous neurological monitoring (e.g., SEP or MEP) or less sensitively with an intraoperative wake-up test. In at-risk patients, these monitoring and exam modalities do not, unfortunately, guarantee functional outcomes. They demonstrate pathway integrity only of the monitored tracts and only during the period they are interrogated. The monitors are usually removed at the conclusion of the case, often prior to turning the patient from a prone position to a supine position or upon emergence from anesthesia. During these events and this unmonitored time, hardware or fusion grafts can dislocate and ischemia or edema of the spinal cord may still develop.

Prolonged surgery in the prone position may produce generalized edema of the face and neck. This edema will be increased by large volume fluid administration, trauma (from a difficult intubation), and the head-down position as might be used for cervical spine surgery or as a result of positioning on a Wilson frame. Patients demonstrating significant facial and airway swelling must be carefully evaluated to establish their appropriateness for extubation, and a combined plan with the neurointensivist should be formulated if necessary. Generally, once the patient is supine and the head elevated, edema will resolve gradually over the same time course as it developed. Therefore, patients might require a planned period of postoperative mechanical ventilation.

In addition to operative management of acute spinal cord injury, medical management with methylprednisolone has been a common but controversial occurrence. This is based off of the National Acute Spinal Cord Injury Studies: NASCIS-2 and NASCIS-3, which recommended giving methylprednisolone 30 mg/kg bolus followed by an infusion of 5.4 mg/kg/h for 24 h if initial bolus was given within 3 h or for 48 h if initial bolus was given between 3 and 8 h post injury [67, 68]. While these studies showed an improvement in motor function at 6 weeks and 6 months, they lost statistical significance at 1 year and a higher trend to postoperative complication rates in the methylprednisolone arm. Specifically in the NASCIS-3 trial, the 48 h methylprednisolone group had statistically significant greater incidence of severe sepsis and severe pneumonia [68]. Evidence for complications, pneumonia, urinary tract infections, wound infections, and GI bleeding from the steroids has been more consistently shown [69, 70]. These trials have been greatly criticized since their publications and their results have not been duplicated. Currently, methylprednisolone therapy is not recommended for routine use in acute spinal cord injury, and its use for reasons different than spinal cord ischemia should be weighed against the possibilities of complications [70].

A significant complication after spine surgery is a surgical site infection. In addition to complying with SCIP measures of antibiotic timing and normothermia, there is compelling evidence that using an FIO_2 of at least 50 % during surgery reduces the likelihood of postoperative infection in spine surgery patients [71].

Functional Operations

Functional or awake craniotomies are undertaken when the area being operated on is in the vicinity of eloquent cerebral cortex such as language, motor, sensory, and vision. It was first used for surgical resection of epileptic foci then extended to the placement of deep brain stimulators.

Awake procedures require special planning and vigilance on the part of the anesthesiologist to ensure patient safety and comfort. Preoperative evaluation and discussion with the patient is key. The patient's airway should be assessed with consideration that a patient with a difficult airway, obstructive sleep apnea, or features that put him at risk for acute obstruction under sedation can be considered relative contraindications. However, the only true contraindication is an uncooperative patient. This means that all patients need to be preemptively assessed for their level of maturity and ability to handle stressful situations. Extensive counseling and explanation of the operation is necessary to help preparing the patient. Positioning of the patient is also very important. The surgeon, anesthesiologist, and neurologist must all be able to have access to full verbal and visual communication with the patient. The patient is placed in pinions and his face visible and free of drapes not only for his comfort, to assess the level of consciousness and for neurologic and speech evaluation [72]. The patient's head should be straight with minimization of jugular compression that could raise the venous pressure. Reverse Trendelenburg positioning may also be necessary to aid in venous drainage. Airway equipment should be immediately available for possible need of emergent intubation if the patient becomes uncooperative and unresponsive and has intractable seizures or other reasons resulting in loss of airway protection. Intraoperative airway complications have been documented to occur in 1.6–2.2 % of patients [72]. An asleep-awake-asleep technique has also been described during which the patient is fully anesthetized for initial skin incision and craniotomy and is allowed to awaken and then anesthetized for closure [73]. Other potential complications or problems also may occur that need to have advanced preparation. Seizure is an obvious possible occurrence with an incidence of 0.8–4.5 % [72]. This may be due to the patient's underlying epilepsy or more commonly cortical stimulation. In the patient in pinions, seizure could pose a serious threat of facial injury. In general the seizure will terminate when the neurosurgeon stops manipulation of the field [73]. If it does not, propofol can be used in small increasing increments. Nausea is common and can be reduced with dexamethasone 4–8 mg iv, ondansetron, and low-dose propofol.

Sedation prior to mapping can be accomplished by small increments of fentanyl 25–100 µg, propofol, or remifentanil infusions. Boluses of propofol and esmolol are commonly given during pinion placement. After cortical mapping has taken place, dexmedetomidine infusion can also be used along with a remifentanil infusion [73].

Extubation Logistics in the OR

A clinical assessment of the airway and patient, taken in the context of the course of surgery, the anesthetic agents used, re-dosing intervals for drugs, and reversal or antagonizing agents given, allows for a determination of the patient's suitability for extubation. When a patient is left intubated, it is either at the surgeon's request or in situations where the clinical assessment suggests extubation would be unsafe to allow adequate airway protection. The determination for leaving a patient intubated will also be influenced by a number of intraoperative scenarios and should be communicated from the operating room to the neurointensivist for a combined plan.

Several neurosurgical procedures need special consideration on extubation of the trachea. It may be difficult to predictably emerge from anesthesia a patient following resection of tumor using a surgical approach necessitating prolonged frontal lobe retraction. These patients remain intubated until they are able to follow commands or demonstrate the ability to protect their own airway with a cough, swallow, or gag reflex. Postoperatively, patients with surgical injury or edema to structures within the brainstem may also fail to "emerge from anesthesia" and not regain consciousness. When the reticular activating system, which resides in the upper pons and mesencephalon, has been disrupted, consciousness can be affected. Similarly, spontaneous breathing can be impaired with injury to respiration-related cells located low in the medulla, parabrachial nucleus injury in the mid to caudal pons, as well as injury to suprapontine anatomy, most notably the limbic structures. Surgery in the posterior fossa may lead to dysfunction of cranial nerves VII, IX, and X. Impaired function of these cranial nerves can lead to difficulty swallowing, loss of a gag reflex, airway obstruction from vocal cord paresis, and increased risk of aspiration. When no evidence of a gag, coughing, or swallowing can be elicited by manipulation of the endotracheal tube or with oropharyngeal suctioning, the patient will be transported to the ICU intubated.

Conclusion of any operation on the cervical spine or surgery requiring a prone position always includes a reassessment of the airway for a determination of the suitability for extubation. Oropharyngeal or laryngeal edema and macroglossia are recognized complications [74]. Prolonged or vigorous lateral retraction of the trachea as can accompany anterior cervical spine approaches can provoke edema that may compromise the airway. The decision to extubate in the presence of upper airway edema, whether from local retractor-associated trauma, neck flexion during posterior cervical approach, or massive volume resuscitation, is aided by performing a few tests: the patient should be strong—with objectively verified recovery of neuromuscular function—and warm and follow commands appropriately so that the only variable is the adequacy of the airway itself. In this situation, a positive pressure leak test will give a gauge of the airway edema present. It is performed by deflating the endotracheal tube cuff and then slowly increasing the airway pressure until gas leaking around the cuff is heard at the mouth. When the threshold leak pressure is under $20 \, cmH_2O$, the airway can typically be safely extubated and maintained by the patient. If one is contemplating extubation of a patient with difficulty placing the endotracheal tube, a more cautious approach is taken by also after oropharyngeal suctioning performing a negative pressure leak test. This test is performed by deflating the endotracheal tube cuff, disconnecting the breathing circuit from the endotracheal tube, and instructing the patient (after an exhalation) to breathe in while one occludes the endotracheal tube. With a stethoscope placed over the trachea, it is readily determined if the patient is successfully ventilating around the occluded endotracheal tube. If air movement is auscultated, this demonstrates that the patient is able to stent open his airway despite the negative pressure in the oropharynx and the space occupying endotracheal tube present. Because posttraumatic swelling may continue to increase for several hours after surgery and the level of stimulation will decrease following removal of the tracheal tube and the addition of any analgesics or sedatives, we will on occasion extubate these patients over an exchange catheter. The tube changer is taped in place just like an endotracheal tube and is generally well tolerated and can be removed several hours later or, if necessary, used to jet ventilate or re-intubate in the event worsening edema leads to evidence of obstruction.

Summary

Anesthetic agents and technique may significantly affect cerebral oxygen consumption ($CMRO_2$), cerebral oxygen delivery (CDO_2), cerebral blood flow (CBF), intracranial tissue volume, intracranial pressure (ICP), arterial oxygen content (CaO_2), and the autoregulation of CBF.

Potent inhalational agents (PIAs), narcotics, and commonly used hypnotic agents all lower cellular metabolism (i.e., $CMRO_2$) by decreasing cortical neuron electrical activity. All PIAs attenuate cerebral autoregulation and uncouple $CMRO_2$ from cerebrovascular resistance (CVR) and CBF.

Cooling the brain or spinal cord reduces $CMRO_2$ by 5–7 % per degree Celsius decrease.

While the effectiveness of hypothermia for neuroprotection in "global" ischemia continues to accumulate, evidence suggests that there may be a difference for "focal" ischemia. The longest "safe" ischemic time (approximately 60 min) is achieved in controlled situations when the patient is slowly cooled to 18 °C and placed on low-flow cardiopulmonary bypass or circulatory arrest.

The ICP follows the net decrease of CBV downward. In the scenario where a more extensive cerebral insult has occurred and autoregulation is compromised, ICP changes will follow MAP and CBV changes.

As $PaCO_2$ decreases, CBF is reduced and consequently CBV and ICP are also lowered. For $PaCO_2$ levels between 20 and 70 mmHg for each 1 mmHg change, there is an approximately 4 % change in cerebral blood flow. Profound hypoxemia ($PaO_2 < 50$ mmHg) causes cerebral vasodilation and an exponential rise in cerebral blood flow, blood volume, and ICP. This is thought to be due to a decrease in pH secondary to lactic acidosis. Cerebral hyperemia may persist for up to 30 min following extubation.

The brain can recover from brief episodes of ischemia but has little chance of return to normal following traumatic herniation. Therefore, when the potential for mechanical brain injury via herniation exists, aggressive acute hyperventilation ($PaCO_2$: 20–25 mmHg) can in conjunction with other measures decrease cerebral volume even though it may risk cerebral ischemia.

The tight-intercellular junctions found in the CNS and collectively referred to as the blood–brain barrier, with an effective pore size of only 8 Å, are essentially impermeable to sodium, other ions, or proteins. They are however freely permeable to water. To avoid cerebral or spinal cord edema, solutions that are isotonic, i.e., 285 mOsm/kg should be used.

Suggested replacement of blood loss is a 3:1 (isotonic crystalloid to blood loss) volume ratio for 0.9 % saline solutions and 1:1 for colloid, 3 % NaCl, and blood products. Deficits calculated from fasting, insensible losses, urine output, and third-space losses are replaced 1:1.

Careful timing and communication to allow coordination of drug effects with stimulation are essential to smoothly navigate the assorted surgical stimuli.

Pediatric patients (<18 years of age) and the elderly (>84 years) may be more susceptible to visual loss following spine surgery. Speculation is that the pathogenesis involves length of surgery, low arterial perfusion pressure, elevated episcleral venous and intraocular pressures, anemia, embolic events, Wilson frame, and the use of pressor agents.

The incidence of air detectable in neurosurgical cases (craniotomy, cervical laminectomy) using the sitting position is near 45 % but can exceed 70 %.

When ICP concerns exist, mild hyperventilation, reverse Trendelenburg position, diuretics, and decompression with CSF diversion are all ICP decreasing options to consider.

Surgery in the posterior fossa, especially when near the vestibulocochlear nerves, has a greater than 50 % incidence of postoperative nausea. When the tumor is located on the floor of the fourth ventricle and areas near the ventral medulla (vasomotor center) are manipulated, hypotension or profound hypertension and bradycardia or even asystole may occur. Patients with GH-secreting tumors will eventually develop acromegaly, placing them at risk for having a difficult airway and postoperative respiratory complications.

Before the aneurysm is secured, steps must be taken to prevent rebleeding by maintaining stable transmural vessel pressure. Prior to the operating room, this is accomplished by controlling the systemic arterial blood pressure with a goal of the systolic blood pressure less than 140 mmHg via short-acting antihypertensives, controlling pain and anxiety, and preventing seizures.

Hypothermia has been called into question by the Intraoperative Hypothermia for Aneurysm Surgery Trial (IHAST).

"Time is Brain" protocols at each institution need to be in place to activate all the necessary personnel if a patient is to go to the interventional suite.

Spinal cord dynamics are similar to those of the brain. The cord responds to anesthetic agents, ventilation parameters, temperature, perfusion pressure, and ischemia in essentially the same fashion as the brain.

Methylprednisolone therapy is now not recommended for routine use in acute spinal cord injury and its use should be weighed against the possibilities of complications.

Awake procedures require special planning and vigilance on the part of the anesthesiologist to ensure patient safety and comfort.

Conclusion

A careful review and understanding of the intraoperative anesthetic management and surgical events will assist in forming a perioperative plan and differential diagnoses for clinical findings observed in the intensive care unit. Communication among neurosurgeon, anesthesiologist, and neurointensivist is essential to better guide patients' postoperative care and the recovery expectations of family and healthcare staff, to everyone's benefit.

References

1. Michenfelder JD. The interdependency of cerebral functional and metabolic effects following massive doses of thiopental in the dog. Anesthesiology. 1974;41:231–6.
2. Jones TH, Morawetz RB, Crowell RM, Marcoux FW, FitzGibbon SJ, DeGirolami U, Ojemann RG. Thresholds of focal cerebral ischemia in awake monkeys. J Neurosurg. 1981;54:773–82.
3. Messick Jr JM, Casement B, Sharbrough FW. Correlation of regional cerebral blood flow (rCBF) with EEG changes during isoflurane anesthesia for carotid endarterectomy: critical rCBF. Anesthesiology. 1987;66:344–9.
4. Kitano H, Kirsch J, Hurn P, Murphy S. Inhalational anesthetics as neuroprotectants or chemical preconditioning agents in ischemic brain. J Cereb Blood Flow Metab. 2007;27(6):1108–28.
5. Verhaegen M, Iaizzo PA, Todd MM. A comparison of the effects of hypothermia, pentobarbital, and isoflurane on cerebral energy stores at the time of ischemic depolarization. Anesthesiology. 1995;82:1209–15.
6. Hagerdal M, et al. Protective effects of combinations of hypothermia and barbiturates in cerebral hypoxia in the rat. Anesthesiology. 1978;49(3):165–9.
7. Todd MM, Hindman BJ, Clarke WR, et al. Mild intraoperative hypothermia during surgery for intracranial aneurysm. N Engl J Med. 2005;352:135–45.
8. Bernard SA, Gray TW, Buist MD, et al. Treatment of comatose survivors of out-of-hospital cardiac arrest with induced hypothermia. N Engl J Med. 2002;346:557–63.
9. The Hypothermia after Cardiac Arrest Study Group. Mild therapeutic hypothermia to improve the neurologic outcome after cardiac arrest. N Engl J Med. 2002;346:549–56.
10. Nolan M, Morley PT, et al. ILCOR advisory statement. Therapeutic hypothermia after cardiac arrest: an advisory statement by the advance life support task force of the international liaison committee on resuscitation. Circulation. 2003;108:118–21.
11. Clifton GL, Miller ER, et al. Hypothermia on admission in patients with severe brain injury. J Neurotrauma. 2002;19(3):293–301.
12. Clifton GL, Valadka A, et al. Very early hypothermia induction in the patients with severe brain injury (the National Acute Brain Injury Study: Hypothermia II): a randomized trial. Lancet Neurol. 2011;10(2):131–9.
13. The Internet Stroke Center. The intravascular cooling in the treatment of stroke 2/3 trial "ICTuS2/3" *clinical trials registry*. 2013. Available at: www.strokecenter.org. Accessed 04 June 2013.
14. Kellie G. An account of the appearances observed in the dissection of two of the three individuals presumed to have perished in the storm of the 3rd, and whose bodies were discovered in the vicinity of Leith on the morning of the 4th November 1821 with some reflections on the pathology of the brain. Trans Medico-Chir Soc Edinb. 1824;1:84–169.
15. Olsen KS, Svendsen LB, Larsen FS. Validation of transcranial near-infrared spectroscopy for evaluation of cerebral blood flow autoregulation. J Neurosurg Anesthesiol. 1996;8(4):280–5.
16. Unterberg AW, Kiening KL, Hartl R, et al. Multimodal monitoring in patients with head injury: evaluation of the effects of treatment on cerebral oxygenation. J Trauma. 1997;42(5 Suppl):S32–7.
17. Vavilala MS, Newell DW, Junger E, et al. Dynamic cerebral autoregulation in healthy adolescents. Acta Anaesthesiol Scand. 2002;46(4):393–7.
18. Meixensberger J, Jager A, Dings J, et al. Multimodal hemodynamic neuromonitoring – quality and consequences for therapy of severely head injured patients. Acta Neurochir Suppl. 1998;71:260–2.
19. Laffey JG, Kavanagh BP. Hypocapnia. N Engl J Med. 2002;347(1):43–53.
20. Rossi S, Stocchetti N, Longhi L, et al. Brain oxygen tension, oxygen supply, and oxygen consumption during arterial hyperoxia in a model of progressive ischemia. J Neurotrauma. 2001;18:163–74.

21. Strebel S, Lam A, Matta B, et al. Dynamic and static cerebral autoregulation during isoflurane, desflurane, and propofol anesthesia. Anesthesiology. 1995;83:66–76.

22. Bruder N, Pellissier D, Grillot P, et al. Cerebral hyperemia during recovery from general anesthesia in neurosurgical patients. Anesth Analg. 2002;94:650–4.

23. Shubert A. Cerebral hyperemia, systemic hypertension, and perioperative intracranial morbidity: is there a smoking gun? Anesth Analg. 2002;94:485.

24. Basali A, Mascha E, Kalfas I, et al. Relation between perioperative hypertension and intracranial hemorrhage after craniotomy. Anesthesiology. 2000;93:48–54.

25. Mavrocordatos P, Bissonnette B, Ravussin P. Effects of neck position and head elevation on intracranial pressure in anesthetized neurosurgery patients. J Neurosurg Anesthesiol. 2000;12(1):10–4.

26. Seoane E, Rhoton AL. Compression of the internal jugular vein by the transverse process of the atlas as the cause of cerebral hemorrhage after supratentorial craniotomy. Surg Neurol. 1999;51: 500–5.

27. Desjardins P, et al. Hemoglobin levels and transfusion in neurocritically ill patients: a systemic review of comparative studies. Crit Care. 2012;16(2):R54.

28. Fenstermacher JD, Johnson JA. Filtration and reflection coefficients of the rabbit blood–brain barrier. Am J Physiol. 1966;211(2): 341–6.

29. Agarwal A, Sinha PK, Pandey CM, et al. Effect of a subanesthetic dose of intravenous ketamine and/or local anesthetic infiltration on hemodynamic responses to skull-pin placement. J Neurosurg Anesthesiol. 2001;13(3):189–94.

30. Rozit I, Vavilala MS. Rozit risks and benefits of patient positioning during neurosurgical care. Anesthesiol Clin. 2007;25(3):631–53.

31. Patil CG, Lad EM, Lad SP, Ho C, Boakye M. Visual loss after spine surgery. A population based study. Spine. 2008;33(13):1491–6.

32. Nuttall GA, Garrity JA, Dearani JA, et al. Risk factors for ischemic optic neuropathy after cardiopulmonary bypass: a matched case/control study. Anesth Analg. 2001;93(6):1410–6.

33. Lee LA. ASA postoperative visual loss (POVL) registry. APSF Newsletter Winter. 2001–2002;16(4):56.

34. American Society of Anesthesiologists Task Force on Perioperative Visual Loss. Practice advisory for perioperative visual loss associated with spine surgery. Anesthesiology. 2012;116:274–85.

35. Tobias JD. Measurement of central venous pressure from a peripheral intravenous catheter in the prone position during spinal surgery. South Med J. 2009;102(3):256–9.

36. The Post Operative Visual Loss Study Group. Risk factors associated with ischemic optic neuropathy after spinal fusion surgery. Anesthesiology. 2012;116:15–24.

37. Albin MS, Carroll RG, Maroon JC. Clinical considerations concerning detection of venous air embolism. Neurosurgery. 1978;3:380–4.

38. Black S, Ockert DB, Oliver Jr WC, et al. Outcome following posterior fossa craniectomy in patients in the sitting or horizontal positions. Anesthesiology. 1988;69:49–56.

39. Papadopoulos G, Kuhly P, Brock M, et al. Venous and paradoxical air embolism in the sitting position: a prospective study with transesophageal echocardiography. Acta Neurochir (Wien). 1994;126(2–4):140–3.

40. Schmitt HJ, Hemmerling TM. Venous air emboli occur during release of positive end-expiratory pressure and repositioning after sitting position surgery. Anesth Analg. 2002;94:400–3.

41. Losasso TJ, Muzzi DA, Dietz NM, et al. Fifty percent nitrous oxide does not increase the risk of venous air embolism in neurosurgical patients operated upon in the sitting position. Anesthesiology. 1992;77:21–30.

42. Fuchs G, Schwartz G, Stein J, et al. Doppler color-flow imaging: screening of a patent foramen ovale in children scheduled for neurosurgery in the sitting position. J Neurosurg Anesthesiol. 1998;10:5.

43. Geissler HJ, Allen SJ, Mehlhorn U, et al. Effect of body repositioning after venous air embolism: an echocardiographic study. Anesthesiology. 1997;86:710–7.

44. Hagen PT, Scholz DG, Edwards WD. Incidence and size of patent foramen ovale during the first 10 decades of life: an autopsy study of 965 normal hearts. Mayo Clin Proc. 1984;59:17–20.

45. Anonymous. Report of World Federation of Neurological Surgeons committee on a universal subarachnoid hemorrhage grading scale. J Neurosurg. 1988; 68:985–6.

46. Hunt WE, Hess RM. Surgical risk as related to time of intervention in the repair of intracranial aneurysms. J Neurosurg. 1968;28:14–20.

47. Frontera JA, Claassen J, et al. Prediction of symptomatic vasospasm after subarachnoid hemorrhage: the modified fisher scale. Neurosurgery. 2006;59(1):21–7.

48. Dorhout Mees S, Rinkel G, Feigin V, et al. Calcium antagonists for aneurysmal subarachnoid haemorrhage. Cochrane Database Syst Rev. 2007;(3):CD000277.

49. Tseng MY, Participants in the International Multidisciplinary Consensus Conference on the Critical Care Management of Subarachnoid Hemorrhage. Summary of evidence of immediate statins therapy following aneurysmal subarachnoid hemorrhage. Neurocrit Care. 2011;15(2):298–301. Review.

50. Sugawara T, Ayer R, Zhang JH. Role of statins in cerebral vasospasm. Acta Neurochir Suppl. 2008;104:287–90.

51. Mees SM, Algra A, Vandertop WP, et al. Magnesium for aneurysmal subarachnoid haemorrhage (MASH-2): a randomized placebo-controlled trial. Lancet. 2012;380(9836):44–9.

52. Molyneux AJ, Kerr RS, et al. Risk of recurrent subarachnoid haemorrhage, death or dependence and standardized mortality ratios after clipping or coiling of an intracranial aneurysm in the International Subarachnoid Aneurysm Trial (ISAT): long-term follow-up. Lancet Neurol. 2009;8(5):427–33.

53. Kanbrak M, Saricaoglu F, Avci A, et al. Propofol offers no advantage over isoflurane anesthesia for cerebral protection during cardiopulmonary bypass: a preliminary study of S-100beta protein levels. Can J Anaesth. 2004;51:712–7.

54. Taylor CL, Selman WR, Kiefer SP, et al. Temporary vessel occlusion during intracranial aneurysm repair. Neurosurgery. 1996;39: 893–905.

55. Friedlander R. Arteriovenous malformations of the brain. N Engl J Med. 2007;356:2704–12.

56. Ogilvy CS, Stieg PE, Awad I, et al. AHA Scientific Statement: recommendations for the management of intracranial arteriovenous malformations: a statement for healthcare professionals from a special writing group of the Stroke Council, American Stroke Association. Stroke. 2001;32:1458–71.

57. Hashimoto T, Young WL, Prohovnik I, et al. Increased cerebral blood flow after brain arteriovenous malformation resection is substantially independent of changes in cardiac output. J Neurosurg Anesthesiol. 2002;14:204–8.

58. Fardo DJ, Hankins WT, Houskamp W, et al. The hemodynamic effects of local anesthetic injection into the carotid body during carotid endarterectomy. Am Surg. 1999;65:648–51; discussion 651–2.

59. Maher CO, Wetjen NM, Friedman JA, et al. Intraoperative lidocaine injection into the carotid sinus during endarterectomy. J Neurosurg. 2002;97:80–3.

60. Vanmaele RG, De Backer WA, Willemen MJ, et al. Hypoxic ventilatory response and carotid endarterectomy. Eur J Vasc Surg. 1992;6:241–4.

61. The National Institute of Neurological Disorders and Stroke rt-PA Stroke Study Group. Tissue plasminogen activator for acute ischemic stroke. N Engl J Med. 1995;333:1581–8.

62. Furlan A, et al. PRO-ACT II: prospective randomized controlled trial of IV heparin vs. IV heparin + IA pro-urokinase. JAMA. 1999;282(21):2003–11.

63. Smith WS, et al. Safety and efficacy of mechanical embolectomy in acute ischemic stroke results of the MERCI trial. Stroke. 2005;36:1432–40.

64. IMS II Trial Investigators. The interventional management of stroke (IMS) II study. Stroke. 2007;38:2127–35.

65. Smith WS, et al. Mechanical thrombectomy for acute ischemic stroke final results of the multi MERCI trial. Stroke. 2008;39:1205–12.

66. Cucchiara RF. Differential awakening (letter). Anesth Analg. 1992;75:467.

67. Bracken MB, et al. Administration of methylprednisolone for 24 or 48 hours or tirilazad mesylate for 48 hours in the treatment of acute spinal cord injury. Results of the Third National Acute Spinal Cord Injury Randomized Controlled Trial. National Acute Spinal Cord Injury Study. JAMA. 1997;277(20):1597–604.

68. Bracken MB, et al. A randomized, controlled trial of methylprednisolone or naloxone in the treatment of acute spinal-cord injury. Results of the Second National Acute Spinal Cord Injury Study. N Engl J Med. 1990;322(20):1405–11.

69. Ito Y, et al. Does high dose methylprednisolone sodium succinate really improve neurological status in patient with acute cervical cord injury?: A prospective study about neurological recovery and early complications. Spine (Phila Pa 1976). 2009;34(20):2121–4.

70. AANS/CNS Guidelines. Pharmacological therapy after acute cervical spinal cord injury. Neurosurgery. 2002;50(3 Suppl):S663–72.

71. Maragakis LL, Crosgrove SE. Intraoperative fraction of inspired oxygen is a modifiable risk factor for surgical site infection after spinal surgery. Anesthesiology. 2009;110:556–62.

72. Venkatraghavan L, Luciano M, Manninen P. Anesthetic management of patients undergoing deep brain stimulator insertion. Anesth Analg. 2010;110(4):1138–45.

73. Erikson K, Cole D. Anesthetic considerations for awake craniotomy for epilepsy. Anesthesiol Clin. 2007;25:535–55.

74. Sinha A, Agarwal A, Gaur A, et al. Pharyngeal swelling and macroglossia after cervical spine surgery in the prone position. J Neurosurg Anesthesiol. 2001;13:237–9.

75. Gravenstein D, Gravenstein N. Intraoperative and immediate postoperative neuroanesthesia. In: Layon AJ, Gabrielli A, Friedman WA, editors. Textbook of neurointensive care. Philadelphia: WB Saunders; 2004.

Postoperative Neurosurgical Care: Recovery Room Misadventures and Immediate Concerns

42

Mary A. Herman, Nikolaus Gravenstein, and Dietrich Gravenstein

Contents

M.A. Herman, MD, PhD • D. Gravenstein, MD (✉)
Department of Anesthesiology,
University of Florida College of Medicine,
1600 SW Archer Road, 100254, Gainesville, FL 32610, USA
e-mail: mherman@anest.ufl.edu; dgravenstein@anest.ufl.edu

N. Gravenstein, MD
Departments of Anesthesiology and Neurological Surgery,
University of Florida College of Medicine,
1600 SW Archer Road, 100254, Gainesville, FL 32610, USA

Department of Periodontology, University of Florida College
of Dentistry, Gainesville, FL, USA
e-mail: ngravenstein@anest.ufl.edu

Abstract

This chapter presents numerous cases in which patients demonstrated postoperative complications. These presentations segue into broader discussions of problems that may be encountered by patients following assorted neurosurgical interventions and various anesthetic techniques.

Keywords

Postoperative • Complication • Localized • Systemic
Case review

Introduction

The typical neurosurgical intervention addresses a specific problem of concern following which the patient transitions through a postanesthesia care unit (PACU) for up to a few hours before being discharged to home or, more likely, to a ward; alternatively, the patient may be sent directly from the operating room (OR) to the intensive care unit (ICU). This transition period, during which time the patient continues to emerge from anesthesia and regains full consciousness and strength, represents a period of dynamic physiological changes that are fraught with a variety of potential complications and misadventures that need to be anticipated and planned for.

The outcome and any complications of the intraoperative anesthetic and surgical management often do not become fully manifest until the patient has arrived in the PACU or ICU. Because patients presenting with new clinical findings in the PACU can present a diagnostic challenge to the clinician at bedside, familiarity with the anesthetic (and surgical procedure) impact on the character of postoperative recovery can help the clinician distinguish findings that are related to the anesthetic and are thus expected to be ephemeral from more ominous ones that require intervention. While patients undergoing neurosurgical interventions may be expected to have neurological complications, many of the complications are, in fact, common to most surgeries.

A.J. Layon et al. (eds.), *Textbook of Neurointensive Care*,
DOI 10.1007/978-1-4471-5226-2_42, © Springer-Verlag London 2013

Herein we will discuss clinical situations similar to ones actually encountered by the authors (with a liberal use of literary license) in the PACU following neurological surgeries. The cases, ranging from relatively minor to critical, will be followed by a general discussion of the etiology and treatment of the complications.

Postoperative Nausea and Vomiting (PONV)

A 37-year-old woman is admitted to the PACU following microvascular decompression of the trigeminal nerve. Her intraoperative course was unremarkable; she had been induced with propofol, fentanyl, and rocuronium; intubated; placed into a 3/4 prone position; and her head pinioned. She was maintained on remifentanil, isoflurane, and an oxygen-air mixture achieving an FiO$_2$ of 0.5. During dissection of the vessel away from the nerve, she experienced a brief episode of hypertension and bradycardia responding to a small remifentanil bolus. At the conclusion of the operation, she received full reversal of her neuromuscular blockade with neostigmine and glycopyrrolate, PONV prophylaxis with ondansetron 4 mg to augment the Decadron 4 mg that she received at the start of the case, and was extubated and awake before transfer to the PACU.

After 3 h of recovery, the PACU nurse calls for assistance with this patient, who is bradycardic with a heart rate of 32 beats per minute (bpm) and mildly hypotensive with a blood pressure of 86/45 mmHg. Upon arrival, we find her sitting, with her head leaning forward over an emesis basin. She is pale and complains of severe vertigo. The nurse reports she had been re-treated with ondansetron in PACU 30 min earlier and was given isopropyl alcohol swabs to sniff without improvement. The symptoms are diagnosed as likely caused by a vagal response to surgery in the posterior fossa. The patient is given small intravenous (IV) doses of glycopyrrolate (0.2 mg) to support the heart rate and promethazine (Phenergan, 6.25 mg) for the nausea. The heart rate stabilized above 40 bpm but the nausea remained. Because droperidol had been removed from formulary, propofol 10 mg IV was given by the anesthesiologist achieving nearly immediate symptomatic relief. Improvement persisted for approximately 15 min before the vertigo recurred. Another propofol bolus is administered with resolution of the dizziness and bradycardia. An antiemetic propofol infusion of 10 mcg/kg/min was begun in the PACU with excellent result. After 6 h, the propofol was discontinued, and the patient was transferred to the ward.

The two most common complications encountered in the PACU are PONV and pain. PONV is often dismissed as a minor postoperative complication; however, the significant vascular stresses that result from the forceful Valsalva and retching that precede vomiting risk provoking rebleeding into a closed spine, head, or neck. Therefore, prevention and expeditious treatment of this common problem takes on additional significance. At its core, PONV is a complex neurological complication with many aggravating factors and chemical triggers.

The vomiting center and chemoreceptor trigger zone (CTZ), located in the highly vascularized area postrema within the medulla oblongata, receive stimuli from the oropharynx, peritoneum, and genitalia via the vagus nerve. Additional inputs arise from the labyrinth of the inner ear, limbic area, and the cerebral cortex. Without an effective blood-brain barrier, the CTZ can be activated by exogenous irritants like mustard gas, cisplatin, digoxin, and anesthetic agents, to name but a few. Medical management, however, is directed at blocking receptors for the common stimulants: histamine, serotonin, dopamine, opiates, and muscarinic receptor agonists.

Surgery in the posterior fossa, especially when near the vestibular-cochlear nerves, has a greater than 50 % incidence of troublesome postoperative nausea associated with it; the nausea alone has been attributed to increasing the length of stay for some patients. Intraoperative anesthetic management can influence the incidence and the severity of postoperative nausea. We use a multifaceted pharmacological approach to reduce postoperative nausea in patients at high risk for PONV, which are aligned with recent recommendations on the treatment of PONV [1]. The first choice for antiemetic prophylaxis or treatment would be a serotonin antagonist, unless the patient had prolonged QT syndrome. If this therapy is not effective for at least 6 h, a second agent with a different site of action is introduced; thereafter, additional agents are added until symptoms are improved. A therapy that successfully improves nausea for 6 or more hours is simply repeated, with the exception of steroids.

In addition to administration of IV ondansetron (4 mg) 30 min prior to the end of surgery, we also give dexamethasone (4 mg) and promethazine (6.25 mg) at the start of the procedure and run an infusion of propofol at 25–50 mcg/kg/min throughout the case. Addition of a small amount of diphenhydramine (10 mg) helps block H1 receptors without causing increased drowsiness. We generally avoid use of scopolamine in our elderly patients out of concern that central effects may cloud the neurological exam. We inform the neurosurgeons when a transdermal scopolamine patch is applied to the patient because of the resulting mydriasis.

Anecdotally, this multimodal technique slightly slows the emergence from anesthesia but, in our experience, dramatically decreases the incidence and severity of postoperative nausea. Other techniques, such as simply using higher doses of propofol, may demonstrate the same or better nausea prophylaxis.

Postoperative Obtundation Without Localizing Findings

Case 1

A 55-year-old athletic 55 kg woman with mild hypertension, controlled with hydrochlorothiazide therapy and who is otherwise healthy, undergoes a one-level anterior cervical discectomy and fusion (ACDF) for neck and shoulder pain. The procedure begins in the late afternoon. She receives a balanced anesthetic with fentanyl, isoflurane, nitrous oxide, oxygen, and a nondepolarizing muscle relaxant. Her intraoperative course lasts 135 min and is uneventful. The neuromuscular blockade is reversed; she is extubated and taken to the PACU. After 40 min in PACU, she complains of a pain in her neck and is administered hydromorphone 2 mg IV. This drug-naïve patient falls asleep and is allowed to rest for 50 min. When the bedside RN tries to reassess her, she is unresponsive, although her vital signs remain stable. The nurse calls and requests naloxone. On exam, the patient is very lethargic and has unintelligible verbal responses to questions. Her pupils are symmetric and responsive to light. Her reflexes are normal. A bedside glucose test reports her serum glucose to be 42 mg/dL. She awakens after dextrose 50 mg is administered intravenously.

Solutions with glucose are generally avoided in neurosurgical patients and may place patients at increased risk for hypoglycemia postoperatively. One rationale for use of glucose-free solutions is that although glucose-containing solutions may be iso- or hypertonic (Table 42.1), the glucose is rapidly metabolized. Thus, its osmotic contribution of 252 mOsm/kg water is lost, and a net free water gain results; this free water will aggravate CNS edema. Additionally, elevated serum glucose has been associated with worsened neurologic outcome.

One theory for the mechanism of injury suggests that the presence of glucose increases neuronal metabolism

Table 42.1 Calculated osmolarity and osmolality of common intravenous fluids

Fluid	Osmolarity calculated	Osmolality physiological	Osmolarity* no dextrose
Water	0	0	0
D5W	252	259	0
D5 0.2NS	325	321	73
NS	308	282	282
LR	273	250	273
D5LR	525	524	273
3 % saline	1,027	921	1,027
6 % hetastarch	310	307	310
20 % mannitol	1,098	1,280	1,098
Plasma protein fraction	–	261	–

Modified with permission from Gravenstein and Gravenstein [25]
Abbreviations: *D5W* 5 % dextrose in water, *D5 0.2NS* 5 % dextrose in 0.2 normal saline, *D5NS* 5 % dextrose in normal saline, *D5LR* 5 % dextrose in lactated Ringer's solution, * denotes calculated osmolarity of solution after dextrose has been metabolized

and thereby decreases cellular viability during ischemia. Finally, the stress response to surgery will typically produce and maintain a more than sufficient elevation of the serum glucose. Infants below 5 kg are at some risk for intraoperative hypoglycemia and may therefore at our institution receive intravenous maintenance therapy with 2.5 % dextrose solution in 0.9 % saline. This regimen addresses the central nervous system's (CNS's) dependence on glucose as a metabolic substrate, the limitations of gluconeogenesis, and the high metabolic rate observed in this young population. It also yields an isotonic fluid after the glucose is consumed. However, when fluid boluses are needed, 0.9 % NaCl solution, rather than the dextrose containing solution, is used.

Case 2

A 74-year-old man with a history of spinal stenosis, mild hypertension, and chronic pain from a "failed back" syndrome underwent an anterior-posterior revision of broken T11–L3 hardware. His intraoperative course was typical for this procedure, lasting 7 h and requiring transfusion of 4 units of PRBC. At the end of the case, electrolyte and blood count laboratory studies were normal. The patient was given morphine 10 mg and extubated after meeting

extubation criteria. He was delivered comfortable, responsive, and moving all extremities to the PACU. Over the next 3 h, he would intermittently attempt to move and complain of pain. He would report a "12-out-of-10" pain and beg, "Please help me!" Small additional doses of IV morphine (2–4 mg) to a total of 30 mg were administered to provide comfort. A patient controlled analgesia pump (PCA) was programmed to deliver a basal infusion of 1 mg/h morphine. Oxygen via nasal cannula was applied, first at 2 L/min and then increased stepwise to 8 L/min until the pulse oximeter saturations stabilized above 97 %. Due to the level of oxygen support he required, the patient was held in the PACU until an ICU bed became available. Now late into the evening, he was allowed to sleep and appeared to be resting comfortably with stable vital signs. During early morning rounds, the neurosurgeons attempt to examine the patient, and he is unresponsive. Blood pressure is 92/50 mmHg, heart rate is 102 bpm, temperature is 36.5 °C, SpO_2 is 100 %, and respirations are 6 breaths per minute and shallow. A blood gas drawn immediately after (re)intubation reveals a pH of 7.15, PaO_2 45 of mmHg, HCO_3 of 19 mEq/L, $PaCO_2$ of 105 mmHg, and a mild anemia with Hgb of 9 g/dL but otherwise normal electrolytes and blood work. The patient "awakens" approximately 35 min after institution of mechanical ventilation and a slow back-titration of the narcotics with 160 mcg naloxone IV over 15 min.

This case represents a common complication occurring in the PACU. Treatment of pain, a priority for patients and PACU staff (trying to transition patients home, the ward, or the ICU), is most commonly accomplished as it

was here, by titration of opiate analgesic medications. Often, aggressive medication leads to progressive hypoventilation and desaturation which, with the best of intentions, is then treated by the addition of supplemental oxygen. This narcotic and then oxygen are incrementally ratcheted up every time the patient complains of pain. Even as the patient becomes severely hypercarbic, the bedside nurse only sees a comfortably sleeping patient with reassuring pulse oximeter readings near 100 % and a mildly tachycardic heart rate, consistent with a postoperative state. The clinician evaluating the patient at beside, however, is aware of the alveolar gas equation which, in simplified form, is

$$P_A O_2 = [(P_{atm} - P_{H_2O})FiO_2 - (P_A CO_2 / R)]$$

and understands that supplemental oxygen with FiO_2 of only 0.5 will allow an SpO_2 of 100 % even with a $PaCO_2$ of 150 mmHg. Hypercarbia, in addition to being sympathomimetic, becomes an anesthetic in excess of 80 mmHg and may further diminish ventilation until respiratory arrest ensues.

Case 3

A 66-year-old active man with prior medical history of migraine headaches treated conservatively with extra strength Tylenol and ibuprofen at onset of symptoms undergoes release of a Dupuytren's contracture at the scheduled midmorning time. He is given midazolam 2 mg to address significant anxiety. This patient, who has never had surgery, requests a general anesthetic. The surgery is performed with Fentanyl 100 mcg, a propofol infusion, and a laryngeal mask airway. The patient breathes spontaneously throughout, maintaining $ETCO_2$ always less than 65 mmHg. At the conclusion of the procedure, the propofol infusion is discontinued, the LMA removed, and the

patient is brought to recovery, sleeping, breathing spontaneously, and with stable vital signs. After 2 h, the patient has not awakened further. Eye findings are normal, vital signs are unchanged, and he localizes and withdraws from painful stimuli. Neither reversal of the benzodiazepine nor the narcotic improved the neurological exam. His wife is advised of the concerning findings. She conveys that he always has difficulty awakening until he has had his morning coffee. Seeking clarification, we learn that he is a farmer and typically drinks 4 pots of coffee per day, starting at 0430 h; one pot brews 16 cups of coffee. Intravenous caffeine 800 mg is administered, and the patient awakens.

Case 4

A 60-year-old woman with history of hypertension suffered a small subarachnoid hemorrhage and had just undergone clipping of a 13 mm middle cerebral artery (MCA) aneurysm. She had been on beta-blocker for blood

pressure control and a magnesium infusion since admission the prior day for vasospasm prophylaxis. Her anaphylactic allergy to penicillin led to her receiving vancomycin 1 g prior to surgical incision. The intraoperative course was uneventful, although a temporary clip was applied for

6 min while the aneurysm was definitively clipped. Intraoperative exam with indocyanine green and also conventional angiograms using contrast confirm the aneurysm is excluded from the cerebral circulation. There were no changes observed on the intraoperative neurological monitoring of median nerve somatosensory evoked potentials (SSEPs). The patient did not require burst suppression, and she was intentionally kept warm with a bladder temperature reading 36.6 °C at the end of the case. She was extubated after awakening, had moved all extremities, and followed simple commands. Because the neurointensive care unit accepted an emergent admission into her open room, the patient was to be boarded in the PACU until an ICU bed became available. The patient was moved to the PACU with the same catheters and infusions with which she had come to the OR. Upon arrival in the PACU, the woman became progressively somnolent, her SpO₂ decreased, her breathing became shallower, and she then became unresponsive. She remained hemodynamically stable and with no localizing findings. Her ventilation was assisted, and she was emergently reintubated. While examining the patient, the pump alarm sounded indicating the magnesium infusion had finished. It was discovered that the magnesium infusion bag had been moved to a new pump prior to transporting the patient from the OR to the PACU, and a programming error resulted in administering 8 g of magnesium sulfate over 20 min. The patient received 10 % calcium gluconate 1 g IV at the bedside. She was placed on mechanical ventilation and, after she returned to spontaneous breathing, was extubated 5 h later. She was discharged home after approximately 1 week without new deficits.

Magnesium sulfate is given to reduce vasospasm and control hypertension following aneurysm rupture [2, 3]. At low concentrations, magnesium ions facilitate calcium entry through voltage-dependent calcium channels. However, at high concentrations, magnesium competes with calcium entry, thereby partially blocking these channels. Magnesium also competes for the low-affinity calcium-binding site on the outside of the sarcoplasmic reticulum and prevents increases in intracellular free calcium necessary for myosin light-chain kinase activity necessary for muscle contraction. Furthermore, magnesium antagonizes the effect of alpha-1 and alpha-2 adrenergic agonists and angiotensin II on cerebral vasculature, inhibits calcium-facilitated presynaptic release of neurotransmitters, attenuates the release of acetylcholine at the neuromuscular junction, enhances sensitivity to all nondepolarizing and depolarizing neuromuscular relaxant drugs, inhibits catecholamine release, and provides seizure prophylaxis.

The observed effects of magnesium correspond with the magnesium level in the blood. Patients lose deep tendon reflexes at 8–10 mg/dL of magnesium. Respiratory depression occurs at 10–15 mg/dL of magnesium. Cardiac conduction defects (widened QRS complex, increased PR interval) and cardiac arrest can occur at magnesium levels greater than 15 mg/dL. Administering intravenous calcium reverses these effects.

Case 5

An 18-year-old 45 kg boy with cerebral palsy and severe spasticity is non-communicative but alert, slightly agitated, and still able to sit in a wheelchair. His past medical history is remarkable for four prior ventricular peritoneal shunt (VPS) placements/revisions and a baclofen pump insertion at age 14, which has now malfunctioned. He presents to PACU following an uneventful replacement of his baclofen pump under general anesthesia. He arrives in PACU extubated, breathing spontaneously, eyes open, and in no apparent discomfort. Forty-five minutes after transferring care, a code is called for a new onset seizure and apparent ventilatory arrest. At bedside are the nurse, colleagues from the ICU and anesthesia, as well as the ARNP who manages all of the neurosurgical pumps and stimulators. His seizure was treated with lorazepam 1 mg IV and resolved. He was reintubated, placed on mechanical ventilation with pressure support, and was extubated at close to his baseline status 3.5 h later and eventually discharged home.

After review of events in temporal association with the seizure, it was determined to have most likely been caused by a re-initiation of the baclofen pump at bedside, although initially disputed by the experienced ARNP. Only later was it realized that the baclofen pump had been set to prime the line extending from the pump into the intrathecal space before starting its chronic infusion. However, the line had not been replaced and was therefore already primed. As a consequence, the patient was administered 0.25 mL of baclofen 2,000 mcg/mL during the priming sequence.

Case 6

A 46-year-old man, who had been previously healthy, presents with a 6-week history of inappropriate behaviors, progressively severe headaches, double vision, and new onset nausea and incontinence. He undergoes a bifrontal craniotomy for resection under general anesthesia of a large superior convexity frontal lobe glioma that extends to the optic chiasm. The maintenance anesthetic is remifentanil, sevoflurane, and propofol infusion at 25 mcg/kg/min that is stopped 30 min before applying the dressing. The intraoperative course is uncomplicated although only a subtotal resection was ultimately possible. The surgeon requests that the patient recover in the PACU and return to the floor. The patient remains nonresponsive 15 min after completion of the case during which time all infusions were stopped and no measurable anesthetic agent was in the exhaled gases. He was then taken intubated to the PACU. After an additional 30 min in PACU, the patient continues to sleep but will withdraw from painful stimuli and does localize. The surgeon asks if the patient's condition is a result of the anesthetic or whether a radiological study is necessary. He is reassured that without localized findings and stable vital signs, this most likely represents the variable emergence that can occur following significant frontal lobe retraction. The patient gradually awakens over the next 30 min.

Patients will occasionally "fail to awaken" immediately upon conclusion of surgery. Delayed emergence is a recognized complication of prolonged frontal lobe retraction. However, residual anesthetic drugs, whether given during surgery or taken prior to surgery, are surely the most common culprits. Long-acting benzodiazepines, narcotics, barbiturates, and residual muscle relaxants can prevent a patient from demonstrating wakefulness. Even caffeine withdrawal by heavy coffee or soda drinkers can manifest as an unarousable patient following surgery. It is crucial to maintain a broad differential diagnosis. In the context of the patient's coexisting medical conditions, the surgical intervention, and intraoperative and postoperative management, less common etiologies of delayed emergence may be more plausible. For example, in the diabetic patient requiring intraoperative insulin and glucose management, one must consider hypoglycemia, along with other systemic metabolic derangements such as hypoxia, hypercapnia, and hyponatremia.

When patients do not recover consciousness as expected, they are likely to be taken to a PACU and remain intubated until they are able to follow commands or demonstrate an ability to protect their own airway by swallowing, coughing, or gagging on the endotracheal tube. When no evidence of these reflexes can be elicited, by manipulation of the endotracheal tube or with oropharyngeal suctioning, the patient will generally remain intubated.

Patients with surgical injury or edema to structures within the brainstem may also fail to "emerge from anesthesia" and not regain consciousness. When the reticular activating system, which resides in the upper pons and mesencephalon, has been disrupted, consciousness can be affected. Similarly, spontaneous breathing can be impaired with injury to respiration-related cells located low in the medulla, parabrachial nucleus injury in the mid to caudal pons, as well as injury to suprapontine anatomy, most notably the limbic structures. Surgery in the posterior fossa may lead to dysfunction of cranial nerves IX, X, and XII. Impaired function of these cranial nerves can lead to difficulty swallowing, loss of a gag reflex, airway obstruction from vocal cord paresis, and increased risk of aspiration.

Following surgery for brain injury, aneurysm (without barbiturates), or a difficult tumor resection, an intracranial event such as intracerebral hemorrhage or ischemia from a slipped clip are but two examples where one might anticipate delayed awakening [4]. However, even uncomplicated neuroendoscopies performed with endoscope pressures that exceeded 30 mmHg have been associated with delayed emergence [4]. Although beyond the scope of this chapter's objectives, a well-performed neurological examination to establish presence or absence of new localized or global findings is fundamental to addressing the question of whether an anesthetic or metabolic derangement (global events) or surgical event is the more probable culprit in delayed awakening.

Case 7

A 42-year-old man, previously healthy, develops worsening headaches and occasional odd behavior. Brain imaging reveals a 14 mm lesion in the parietal lobe. There is no significant mass effect. The patient undergoes a general anesthetic for craniotomy and tumor excision using standard monitors, a radial arterial, and urinary bladder catheters. The intraoperative course is unremarkable; estimated blood loss is under 75 mL. The anesthetic is discontinued and his neuromuscular blockade is reversed. He emerges from anesthesia uneventfully, is awake and extubated, then moves himself to the transport gurney, and is taken to PACU for recovery. Forty minutes after arrival, the patient is found unresponsive but breathing and with otherwise normal vital signs. No drugs had been administered recently, and no eye or other localizing findings are present. Serum electrolytes and osmolality as well as a CT are ordered when it is realized the patient had a bowel movement in the bed. The suspicion is high that the patient had an unwitnessed seizure and was now in a postictal state. He had not been on seizure prophylaxis. Lorazepam and fosphenytoin are ordered along with a neurology consult. In hindsight, it was believed that increasing pain led to mild hyperventilation and a lowered seizure threshold which was superimposed on the new surgical wound seizure nidus.

Patients undergoing any type of surgery where the brain cortex can be irritated are at risk of experiencing a perioperative seizure. If a seizure is witnessed, a postictal state can be expected. However, in the event of a subclinical seizure, diagnosing a postictal state will depend on maintaining a high level of clinical suspicion.

Postoperative seizures can occur in the PACU following high doses of intraoperative ketamine or as a consequence of acute narcotic or alcohol withdrawal, or electrolyte disturbance such as severe hyponatremia caused by diabetes insipidus. Intraoperative hypoxemia with injury may also provoke postoperative seizures. Recent research suggests a linkage between propofol and seizures in neonatal animals. A possible linkage between sevoflurane and seizures in neonates is also under investigation. While some have speculated on how well the animal models may apply to humans and how well the neonatal outcomes may be extrapolated to adults, there currently are no guidelines, cautions, or black box warnings for the use of either of these agents in adults.

Seizure-like myoclonic jerking is known to occur with injection of propofol and etomidate and during recovery from high doses of etomidate. Additionally, drugs that block dopamine receptors, a common feature of many antiemetic drugs such as droperidol, metoclopramide, and promethazine, chlorpromazine, or other phenothiazines, may provoke similar repetitive movements, especially in patients with Parkinson disease or other repetitive movement disorders, such as those who undergo deep brain stimulator placements.

Violent whole-body rigors as a response to cooling can also mimic seizures. Patient cooling occurs through the radiation, conduction, evaporation, and convection of heat. Patients may passively cool or be actively cooled in the operating room and require ongoing rewarming in the PACU. Triggering and modulation mechanisms of shivering are complex and poorly understood [5].

Hypothermia almost immediately provokes vasoconstriction and release of norepinephrine. It can induce shivering with a lowering of core temperature by only 1.5 °C [6]. If shaking rigors develop, oxygen consumption can increase 400 % or more [7]. Hypothermia also causes a leftward shift in the oxygen-hemoglobin dissociation curve and is associated with cardiac dysrhythmias, ranging from bradycardia, atrial fibrillation, and ventricular tachycardia to ventricular fibrillation and asystole (temp 28, 25, 22, and 18 °C, respectively). These factors, coupled with the presence of platelet-activating factors in the postsurgical patient with postoperative pain, are speculated to contribute to a 2.2 relative risk of experiencing cardiac morbidity (unstable angina/ischemia, cardiac arrest, or myocardial infarction) in the hypothermic patient compared with the normothermic patient [8].

Anesthetic agents are themselves associated with producing a shivering response, the so-called halothane shakes which may be vigorous enough to be confused with seizure activity, during emergence. This has been attributed to the loss of spinal cord inhibition from cortical inputs that remain under the influence of anesthesia. Patients will not report being cold. Hypothermia and anesthetic-induced shivering do not impair communication, cause loss of bowel or bladder control, are generally of brief duration, and have no postictal period. They are responsive to rewarming and small doses of IV meperidine (12.5–25 mg) or clonidine (25–50 mcg). When the patient remains intubated and mechanically ventilated, it is tempting to use neuromuscular blockade to eliminate shivering; however, that will also mask the motor signs of a seizure.

The patient being warmed in PACU must be watched for "recurarization," i.e., the reappearance of neuromuscular blockade after demonstrating strength. This may occur because hypothermia decreases the sensitivity of neuromuscular junctions to the effects of nondepolarizing neuromuscular blocking (NMB) agents. Hence, a patient who is cold but strong may become warm and weak, especially if no reversal agents were given, as the warmed neuromuscular junctions become increasingly sensitive to residual NMB.

New Localized Neurological Deficit

Case 1

An 84-year-old man with history of colon cancer undergoes diagnostic resection of one of three small temporoparietal brain lesions believed to represent metastatic disease. His past medical history is significant for CAD, HTN controlled on meds, partial colectomy for colon cancer 2 prior to this admission (PTA), and left carotid endarterectomy 5 years PTA which was complicated by an embolic stroke that caused significant right-sided arm and leg weakness. After 6 months in a rehabilitation center, and an additional year of physical therapy, he had only very subtle residual weakness but required a walker for stability. After an uneventful general anesthetic using a short-acting narcotic, one-half MAC of inhalational agent, and nondepolarizing muscle relaxants that were reversed, the patient awakens. He opens his eyes and mouth to command, has a cough, and good strength as assessed by the 5-s sustained tetany elicited from the twitch monitor. He is extubated, although still sleepy he maintains his airway, and is taken to the PACU. Exam in the PACU reveals that he will follow commands on his left side but will not move his dominant right side. As arrangements for an emergent CT are made, the patient begins to show weak movement of the affected side. The CT shows postsurgical changes and a small operative-side pneumocephalus, but no hemorrhage. His strength continues to improve, recovering nearly to his baseline exam by the time of his discharge home 2 days later.

The patient who has recovered function from a prior stroke either partially or wholly is at risk of awakening from anesthesia with some or all of the deficits that occurred at the time of the original CVA. This recapitulation phenomenon has been termed "differential awakening" of the brain and related to patients as a "reliving" of their stroke [9]. It is postulated that the patient with a remote stroke has regained function by learning to utilize new pathways that require vastly more synapses than the original pathway and is thus more vulnerable to the anesthetic effects, while the normal brain recovers function with a low partial pressure of anesthetic agent still present. One possible mechanism explaining the phenomenon of differential awakening is that anesthetic agents are eliminated from injured or ischemic brain more slowly than normal brain, perhaps because of differential blood flow. Another suggests that the cumulative amounts of the same low partial pressure anesthetic along the much longer neuronal pathways and vastly larger number of receptors used to overcome the CVA deficit are sufficient to keep those pathways quiescent. These anesthetic effects should dissipate within hours of discontinuation of anesthesia as the partial pressures and concentrations of drug continue to diminish. But if memory within the pathways has also been disturbed, full recovery to preoperative baseline may require days, weeks, and possibly even as long as the original rehabilitation—but full recovery is expected.

The patient with preoperative paralysis of more than several days, whether from central or the more worrisome peripheral neural injury, warrants additional postoperative consideration when testing muscle twitches to assess recovery from residual neuromuscular blocking agents or selecting a neuromuscular blocking agent to give prior to an (re)intubation.

The patient paralyzed from a lower motor neuron injury in the spinal cord may have upregulated the population of neuromuscular junctions to a degree that administration of a depolarizing muscle relaxant can precipitate an acute hyperkalemic event. Monitoring of neuromuscular blockade is also complicated when attempted on an affected limb of a patient with a prior CVA. Electrically stimulating the ulnar or posterior tibial nerve in an affected limb—where there is an increased neuromuscular junction density—produces exaggerated responses compared with the normal limb. Thus, well-intentioned assessment for the recovery of strength by evaluating twitches on a paretic or plegic limb can lead to an incorrect determination that the patient has recovered sufficient strength to tolerate extubation. Almost invariably, this error will necessitate providing some form of ventilator support and possibly reintubation.

Simply monitoring twitches on a non-affected side or following the activity of the levator palpebrae muscle with facial nerve stimulation or performance of a head lift for greater than 5 s will confirm suitable strength is recovered for extubation.

Case 2

A 22-year-old man diagnosed with acromegaly is scheduled for transsphenoidal resection of the pituitary tumor via a transnasal approach. The intraoperative course is reported to be uncomplicated, without difficulties ventilating or intubating at the onset. Anesthesia is maintained with muscle relaxant, fentanyl 350 mcg, isoflurane, air, and oxygen. The resection is completed in less than 1 h.

The anesthetic is discontinued and the muscle relaxant reversed. The patient swallows, breathes spontaneously, follows simple commands, and is successfully extubated and transported to the PACU. On admission to the PACU, the patient has blood pressure, heart rate, saturation, and temperature at his baseline but is lethargic and bradypneic, and a new "blown" pupil is discovered on the side of the operative nares. Closer examination shows the pupil to be unresponsive to light, while the contralateral pupil is constricted and produces a pupillary light reflex. The eye

is not a prosthetic glass eye. Before a CT exam is ordered, the operative record is reviewed and reveals that the nares were treated with pledgets soaked with the vasoconstrictor oxymetazoline (Afrin). Oxymetazoline (and phenylephrine) can reach the eye if the nasolacrimal duct is patent. Topical application of these vasoconstrictors on the eye will cause mydriasis that can take several hours to resolve. Administration of several small (40 mcg) boluses of naloxone awakened the patient from his over-narcotized state.

Case 3

A 12-year-old boy with attention deficit/hyperactivity disorder (ADHD) and hydrocephalus undergoes his third ventriculoperitoneal shunt (VPS) revision. The intraoperative course is unremarkable. General anesthesia is conducted without difficulty. The surgical team tests the proximal (cranial) and distal portions of the shunt and elects to replace the entire shunt but to convert to a programmable valve. Following successful surgery, the patient is awakened, extubated, and taken to the PACU where he tells the nurse he is hungry. One hour later, he has maintained normal vital signs, tolerated some juice, and is sitting without complaints on his gurney. He is discharged from the PACU. While hugging his nurse "goodbye," he suddenly states not feeling well and becomes unresponsive. Examination shows a flaccid paralysis, apnea, a fixed 5 mm right pupil, and absent brainstem reflexes. Systolic blood pressures (SBPs) are in the 80s mmHg with heart rates (HRs) of 160–180 bpm and SpO_2 in the low 80 %. Mask ventilation is initiated and phenylephrine and naloxone (400 mcg in divided doses) are administered without improvement. Shortly thereafter, pink, frothy sputum begins bubbling from the boy's mouth.

The patient is emergently intubated and ventilated with PEEP. Within minutes, a bedside transthoracic echo shows a dilated heart, with global severe biventricular hypokinesis and an ejection fraction of 15–20 %; he is taken emergently to the CT scanner. Upon arrival in the scanner, the transport monitor is unable to measure a blood pressure, the pulse oximeter fails to display a plethysmogram, and only intermittently can femoral pulses be palpated. Capnometry is not available at this time, but chest rise and breath sounds are appreciated bilaterally. Epinephrine 50 mcg is administered, which makes pulses globally palpable and produces a systolic BP in the 80s mmHg. The CT scan demonstrates an acute intraventricular hemorrhage. The patient is rushed to the operating room where an arterial catheter is placed and additional intravenous access established. A ventriculostomy is

performed and an epinephrine infusion started to maintain cerebral perfusion pressure. His postoperative course is notable for epinephrine and milrinone infusion requirements until the second postoperative day (POD #2). He is extubated on POD #3. Cardiac enzymes are elevated. In the absence of any other identifiable cause for myocardial dysfunction, this appears to be a case of neurogenic myocardial stunning (Takotsubo cardiomyopathy). At a clinic visit 4 weeks later, the patient had returned nearly to preoperative function and was without obvious new neurological deficit.

A patient will be influenced by the general anesthesia and surgery for some time into the postanesthetic period. Cerebral hyperemia persisted for at least 30 min following extubation from an isoflurane/N_2O/O_2/fentanyl/atracurium- or propofol/O_2/air/fentanyl/atracurium-based anesthetic [10]. Whether these prolonged effects result from trace anesthetic-induced impairment of autoregulation, hemodilution, recovery from prolonged hyperventilation, or a nonspecific response to stress is not known [11]. The intraoperative and postoperative management of blood pressure is further related to the incidence of postoperative intracranial hemorrhage (ICH) [12]. When intraoperative or postoperative blood pressure (within the first 12 h of operation) remained above 160/90 mmHg for two or more consecutive measurements made 5 min apart, the incidence of postoperative ICH after craniotomy was significantly higher (62 and 62 %, respectively) than compared with non-hypertensive controls (34 and 25 %, respectively) [13].

The phenomenon of myocardial injury following cerebral hemorrhage, specifically aneurysmal subarachnoid hemorrhage (SAH), is well known in the literature and has been reported after many different procedures presumed to otherwise be a low risk for this complication [14]. It consists of impairment of left ventricular (LV) function, including structural cardiac damage, and ECG changes (ST segment, T wave, QT interval). The mechanism is believed to be an excessive release of catecholamines modulated by cardiac adrenoceptors [15]. Cardiac decompensation results from failure to meet inotropic demands. A contraction band necrosis has been found in cardiac pathologies of fatal SAH. Postmenopausal women may be at higher risk of being affected by LV dysfunction although this may represent observational bias since aneurysmal SAH is a disease of middle-aged to older women [14].

This experience is a reminder that critical events can occur in new patient populations even when associated with "routine" cases. Acute intracerebral hemorrhage has been described following ventriculoscopy, ventriculostomy, temporal grid placement, and deep brain stimulator placement. Rapid diagnosis is essential to securing the best outcomes but requires a high level of suspicion, even after low-risk surgery.

Case 4

A 56-year-old pediatric nurse has reported right-sided weakness, lethargy, confusion, and is reported by family to have altered personality. Work-up reveals a large right frontotemporal tumor with extension into the optic chiasm, brainstem, and cavernous sinus with encasement of the carotid artery. She undergoes an uneventful intraoperative course, with a stable induction, head pinioning, and insertion of arterial catheter. No urinary bladder catheter is placed because this procedure expected to take less than 2 h. The procedure is completed within 10 min after the biopsy specimen is submitted. The patient is reversed and extubated once eye opening, gag, and cough are observed (it is not believed she will be able to understand or follow simple commands). She is taken to PACU to recover and await the pathological diagnosis and treatment plan options. Within 15 min of arriving, she becomes hypertensive, then almost immediately unresponsive, with a blown pupil on the right side. Mask ventilation is begun but is difficult. Because she has had a transsphenoidal resection through her nose, instead of inserting a nasal trumpet, an oral airway is used. Once the emergent airway equipment is brought to the bedside, she is intubated and hyperventilated, with mannitol 1 g/kg ordered, and taken emergently to the CT scanner. It reveals a massive right-sided hemorrhage, but no blood near the surgical site, with 8 mm right-to-left midline shift, slit-like ventricles, and severe, non-survivable uncal herniation through the foramen magnum. A CT angiogram does not show an aneurysm or arteriovenous malformation as the cause for bleeding. Autopsy finds the tumor had extended to the right MCA, from where the bleeding had originated. It was believed that the manipulation of the "tough" tumor during biopsy transmitted shear forces to where the MCA failed.

Transsphenoidal resection of pituitary tumors (TSRPT) and other procedures done through the nose are often relegated to the category of "less risky" surgeries; however, they too can be prone to misadventures because once the nasal drip dressing is removed, it is not apparent that any surgery has been done, let alone which surgery. The patient having had a craniopharyngioma resected looks just like a patient might who had a pituitary tumor resected, or one who had undergone a lumbar microdiscectomy. When intracranial surgery has been performed through the nose—or there has been a recent history of basilar skull fracture—it is imperative that the nose not be instrumented, likely for several months, with a nasal trumpet or nasogastric tube out of concern the appliance will find a path into the brain [16, 17].

Case 5

A thin 73-year-old woman with progressive cervical stenosis, rheumatoid arthritis, and limited mobility underwent a C4–T1 posterior cervical decompression with instrumentation. She had prior anesthetics for cholecystectomy and hysterectomy in the past without difficulties. She underwent a smooth induction and was intubated using a fiber-optic bronchoscope. The tube was secured and her eyes taped with preformed adhesive plastic ovals because the lids did not remain closed over the eyes. The head was pinioned and she was flipped prone onto the operating table. Due to a fixed kyphotic spinal deformity, she was placed in a significantly head-elevated position. The surgery and anesthetic were uneventful. Physiological data showed a stable 4 h intraoperative course. She is returned to her bed, and after reversal of neuromuscular blockade, she demonstrated eye opening and strong hand squeezing bilaterally before successful extubation. She was pleasant and conversant but remarks she cannot see well. Her visual fields are tested, and she is able to distinguish light from dark, and she is able to discriminate between one finger and two. She is reassured that her vision should return to normal and was wheeled to the PACU. After 45 min in the PACU, she continues to report severely blurred vision. She cannot read large font type. On exam, cranial nerves I, II, III, and VI are intact, and her visual testing remains grossly blurred; ophthalmology is consulted. The exam with a Woods lamp shows a desiccated cornea, presumably from her eyelids retracting under the nonocclusive adhesive, exposing the cornea to dry room air. With patching and saline eye drops, her vision fully recovers over 3 days.

Postoperatively, when evaluating patients in the PACU for postoperative visual loss (POVL), one assumes that the intraoperative management properly addressed the concerns associated with patients in the prone position. It requires the abdomen to be properly suspended and knees, testicles, and breasts to be free from pressure. Unfortunately, even when positioning has been done with meticulous care, the risk of central retinal artery thrombosis, cortical blindness, and ischemic optic neuropathy remains [18]. This catastrophic outcome of POVL has been described when a headrest foam cushion with a cut-out for the eyes, nose, and lips was used and even when the head has been fixed by a pinioning system. POVL has also been reported in patients who remained supine throughout their procedure, although the risk is about 2/3

of that in the prone position and about 1/7th of that associated with a combined anterior-posterior operation (Fig. 42.1) [19]. Young and old patients are at highest risk, but patients of any physical status can suffer this catastrophe [18]. Speculation is that the pathogenesis involves low arterial perfusion pressure, elevated episcleral venous and intraocular pressures, anemia, embolic events, the use of pressor agents, and an exposure time for these conditions [20, 21]. Periorbital edema is likely an important variable in the etiology. Postoperatively, efforts are made empirically to defend perfusion and oxygen delivery while limiting venous pressure to the eyes by positioning the patient with periorbital edema with the head elevated and avoiding conditions promoting coagulation, such as vascular volume contraction. See Tables 42.2 and 42.3.

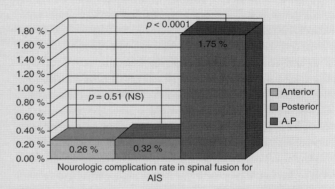

Fig. 42.1 Neurologic complications in spinal fusion for AIS. *A/P* indicates anterior-posterior, *NS* not significant, *AIS* adolescent idiopathic scoliosis (Reproduced with permission from Jeffrey et al. [19])

Table 42.2 Frequency of specific types of perioperative visual loss (POVL) by surgical procedure for years 1996–2005

Procedure	All POVL	Ischemic optic neuropathy	Cortical blindness	Retinal vascular occlusion	Total discharges
Hip/femur treatment	226	43	68	113	1,207,542
Knee replacement	84	>10[a]	<10	65	771,528
Cholecystectomy	51	<10	<10	34	796,284
Cardiac surgery[b]	704	114	53	541	815,856
Appendectomy	<10	<10	<10	<10	550,945
Colorectal resection	69	>10[a]	<10	43	543,201
Laminectomy without fusion	45	<10	<10	32	528,721
Spinal fusion	140	39	68	32	465,345
Total	1,326	245	215	864	5,679,422

Reproduced with permission from Shen et al. [18]

The numerical result when less than ten may not be reported according to Nationwide Inpatient Sample (NIS) regulations

[a]Count is reported as >10 to avoid indirectly revealing value of count <10 for cortical blindness

[b]Cardiac surgery includes valve and coronary artery bypass grafting surgery

Table 42.3 Perioperative visual loss (POVL) by patient demographic, clinical, and surgical characteristics—incidence and univariate associates

Covariates	Covariate levels	Subgroup percent	POVL cases	Incidence per 10,000		Univariate logistic regression		
				Estimate	95 % CI	Odds ratio	95 % CI	P
Age group	<18	434	107	4.37	2.95–6.46	4.75	3.14–7.18	
	18–49	25.10	128	0.92	0.74–1.14	Referent		<0.0001
	50–64	23.17	323	2.46	2.17–2.79	2.68	2.13–3.37	
	≥65	47.39	768	2.87	2.62–3.14	3.12	2.50–3.89	

Reproduced with permission from Shen et al. [18]

The numerical result when less than ten may not be reported according to Nationwide Inpatient Sample (NS) regulations

Case 6

A 19-year-old, 76 in. 130 kg man, who is an active and healthy sport archer, suffers progressive lower extremity weakness and undergoes a posterior T6–T9 thoracic laminectomy for removal of an extra-axial spinal cord tumor. After induction of anesthesia, additional access is placed including arterial and intravenous catheters. He is positioned, pinned, and carefully flipped. His arms are brought forward into a so-called "surrender" position, where they rest on arm board memory foam cushions. The operation is successfully completed in 6 h; the patient is extubated, awake, and able to move his legs. He is taken to PACU on a gurney with side rails up. Over the 90 min there his pain is managed with additional opiate analgesics, and he rests comfortably. On the Aldrete survey done prior to discharge from PACU, it is discovered that he has lost feeling and strength in his nondominant hand.

The ulnar nerve at the elbow is the most frequent place for position-related nerve injury in anesthesia and is often not recognized until the patient is near full recovery from anesthesia. This injury may have occurred in the OR as a result of a combination of ulnar nerve compression and stretch. These risks are manifest when the elbow is flexed and the hand pronated on the arm board, exposing the nerve in the cubital tunnel to the risk of compression by either the top cushion or its edge, if the arms do not fit well on the cushions. Stretch at the elbow and brachial plexus compression as it tracks through the thoracic outlet may also contribute. Although nerve injury is also possible with attempts at ulnar arterial catheter placement, this was not the case here. The actual mechanism of injury is often only speculative as it is also possible the injury occurred postoperatively when the patient rested his elbows on the gurney rails while he slept, and positioning was not a primary concern.

Injury of the brachial plexus is also a mechanism through which an ulnar neuropathy may occur, caused by the head and neck being fixed while unsupported shoulders sag, pulling at the brachial plexus and nerve roots. Procedures utilizing aggressive arm abduction or a shoulder harness or a lateral position with a chest roll that slips into the axilla from its intended upper thorax location are other mechanisms for upper-extremity nerve injury.

The lateral position further risks lateral flexion of the cervical spine, pressure from the surgical table on the "down arm" and the fibula, threatening the brachial plexus and superficial peroneal nerve, respectively. The supine position places pressure on the heels and occiput. Neurology consultation is indicated and reassurance that recovery is expected within days to months, depending on the location and severity of nerve injury

Case 7

A 70-year-old woman with history of transient ischemic attacks is found to have a high-grade 85 % left carotid artery stenosis. She is morbidly obese with a BMI of 52, has hypertension that is controlled on lisinopril, and obstructive sleep apnea, but is not compliant with her CPAP at night. She has a Mallampati Class 3 airway exam.

She undergoes what is reported to be an uncomplicated endarterectomy under general anesthesia. Induction of anesthesia occurs after a radial arterial catheter is placed and is smooth, utilizes a videolaryngoscope to intubate, but is unable to administer tracheal lidocaine. A superficial cervical block is placed by the anesthesiologist, and the surgeon elects to utilize a shunt. The 4-channel EEG and compressed spectral array are monitored throughout the case and show only changes consistent with depth of anesthesia and no unilateral changes. Total cross-clamp time is 54 min. The procedure ends; the patient awakens and meets extubation criteria but is extubated over an endotracheal tube exchange catheter (EEC) out of caution. The patient is transferred to the PACU in stable condition and the EEC removed 30 min later. The patient experiences some pain and hypertension that are successfully treated with morphine. She becomes nauseated and after some retching vomits. Her nausea resolves and she is treated with ondansetron prophylactically. Twenty-five minutes later she complains of difficulty breathing. Although her obesity obscures physical exam findings, close examination reveals her left neck to have a "fullness" that is absent on the right side. Over the next 10 min, her breathing becomes labored, and she appears to be in distress.

Carotid endarterectomy (CAE) differs from intracranial vascular surgery in its association with coronary and peripheral vascular disease and proximity to the carotid sinus. Blood pressure can be erratic after work near the carotid sinus. Postoperative labile hemodynamics may not be improved with the intraoperative use of local anesthetic field blocks of the sinus [22, 23]. When exposure for carotid endarterectomy injures or denervates the carotid body, an altered chemoreceptor function and a diminished hypoxic response may also result [24]. The loss of the hypoxic response is a particularly relevant postoperative consideration in the patient with a prior CEA who has just begun to recover from a CEA on the contralateral side.

Arterial hemorrhage into the surgical site can be provoked or worsened during the perioperative period by coughing, bucking, and elevated blood pressures. Hence, the target blood pressure is at the lower end of the patient's normal range. Emergence and recovery from anesthesia often utilizes narcotics for their combined analgesic, sedative, and cough suppressant effects.

Perioperative hemorrhage following CAE represents a significant complication and usually first manifests as swelling in the neck. When the source is venous, the swelling typically is limited and takes some time before it is obvious. An arterial bleeding source may continue to expand a hematoma to the point where the trachea is deviated and progress to airway obstruction. This process may take several hours to become apparent and can be diagnosed in the recovery room, ICU, or ward. In addition to the observation of neck fullness or swelling, which may obscure the lateral shift of airway structures, the patient with incipient airway obstruction will become progressively short of breath, tachypneic, hoarse, and either agitated or obtunded as he becomes more hypoxic and hypercarbic. Early detection requires a vigilant clinician. Aggressive management of pain with narcotics will blunt ventilatory drive. Addition of supplemental oxygen, as many do routinely, may delay arterial desaturation even as the patient becomes severely hypercarbic (e.g., $PaCO_2$ greater than 80 mmHg) and acidotic (pH less than 7.2). Treatment prior to respiratory compromise involves emergent return to surgery and intubation, followed with a decompression and re-exploration of the wound. If the airway has become compromised prior to arrival in the operating room, emergent airway management is facilitated by first effecting a surgical decompression at the bedside, that is, emergent removal of sutures/staples to decompress the wound.

Another concern in the CEA patients is coronary artery disease and the associated increased risk of a perioperative myocardial infarction. It makes sense to monitor precordial V_5 lead in the PACU. This is possible even if only a three-lead ECG system is used. In such a case, placing the left arm's lead—which is (+)—in the V_5 position (anterior axillary line fifth intercostal space) and monitoring lead I is essentially equivalent in sensitivity to a true V_5 lead.

Case 8

A 63-year-old 95 kg woman with worsening vision and headaches is found to have a craniopharyngioma extending from her sella turcica to her optic chiasm. Her pituitary function is intact. She is admitted for an endoscopic resection. Her anesthetic induction for surgery occurs without difficulty; additional vascular access, an arterial catheter, and an orogastric tube are placed. She is given antibiotics (cefazolin and gentamicin) as prophylaxis for the transnasal surgery before incision with a plan to intraoperatively re-dose every 3 and 6 h, respectively. Her head is pinioned for surgery, and muscle relaxation is maintained throughout the duration of the procedure. Phenylephrine-soaked pledgets are placed into the nose in preparation for incision. The surgical resection, done in conjunction with otolaryngology, is uneventful and completed in 7 h. At the conclusion of the case, she has a single twitch and is given a full reversal dose of glycopyrrolate and neostigmine.

The stomach and hypopharynx are suctioned to eliminate blood and secretions and she is extubated. She is awake and extubated and taken to the PACU where report is given. Within 15 min of arrival, it is clear she is short of breath and is having difficulty breathing. A resident physician assessing the patient determines she is obstructing, likely due to residual weakness, and administers a second full reversal dose of glycopyrrolate and neostigmine. Rather than improve, she requires increasing levels of oxygen support and a jaw thrust to maintain the airway. An arterial blood sample result reveals inadequate ventilation with a $PaCO_2$ of 78 mmHg. After reviewing these results it is clear that ventilator assistance is required. Although discussed, a nasal trumpet was not placed for fear it could be advanced into the brain through the hidden cranial defect left by the surgery. Similarly, when a bag valve mask is requested, the risk of producing a pneumocephalus drives the management towards early reintubation. The patient is successfully reintubated and recovers full strength by twitch monitor and clinical assessments after an additional 5 h in the PACU.

Postoperative weakness may not be immediately apparent upon extubation in the OR and may lead to patients developing respiratory distress some time later in the PACU. Often, prior to extubation, patients are given 100 % oxygen as they emerge from anesthesia. A slightly weak but present exam may be assessed as being within expected during the emergence period. Unrecognized myasthenia gravis, Eaton-Lambert, muscular dystrophy, and glycogen storage or pulmonary diseases would be in the differential as a cause for postoperative respiratory failure, but these would present differently in the operating room. Likewise, prolonged weakness following succinylcholine administration would portend a pseudocholinesterase deficiency. This patient may have had weakness from two less well-appreciated causes: gentamicin, neostigmine, or both. Gentamicin and other aminoglycoside drugs have been associated with prolonging muscle weakness. Further, neostigmine in excess effectively inhibits all acetylcholinesterase activity, allowing acetylcholine released into the neuromuscular junction to keep the cell membrane depolarized.

Summary

The possibility of incomplete rewarming precipitating a shaking rigor and increased oxygen consumption would place the patient at considerable risk for perioperative cardiac ischemia, arrhythmia, and infarction. In addition to the observation of neck fullness or swelling, which may obscure the lateral shift of airway structures, the patient with incipient airway obstruction will become progressively short of breath, tachypneic, hoarse, and either agitated or obtunded and desaturate as he becomes more hypoxic and hypercarbic. Spinal cord dynamics are similar to those of the brain. The cord responds to anesthetic agents, ventilation parameters, temperature, perfusion pressure, and ischemia in essentially the same fashion as the brain. The patient who has recovered function from a prior stroke either partially or wholly is at risk of awakening from anesthesia with some or all of the deficits that occurred at the time of the original CVA. This recapitulation phenomenon has been termed "differential awakening" of the brain and related to patients as a "reliving" of their stroke.

Conclusion

In conclusion, a careful review and understanding of the intraoperative anesthetic management and surgical events will assist in forming differential diagnoses for clinical findings observed in the PACU. As surveyed in this chapter, the differential for altered emergence is broad (Table 42.4). Determination of likely etiologies quickly is valuable for directing care with the proper urgency.

Table 42.4 Causes of prolonged postoperative "wake-up"

Drugs	Narcotics
	Residual anesthetic agent
	Nondepolarizing neuromuscular relaxants
	Neostigmine
	Gentamicin
	Baclofen
	Magnesium
	Drug dependence
	Alcohol withdrawal
	Medication error (dose or substitution)
Disease	Eaton-Lambert syndrome
	Multiple sclerosis
	Muscular dystrophy
	Myasthenia gravis
	Glycogen storage disease
	Pseudocholinesterase deficiency
	Developmental delay
	Alzheimer disease
	Cerebral palsy
Neurological	Stroke
	Hypoperfusion
	Relative hypotension
	Seizure/postictal
	"Differential awakening" from previous stroke
	Retraction of frontal lobe/frontal lobe pressure
	Elevated ICP
	Pneumocephalus
	Cerebral edema

Table 42.4 (continued)

Metabolic	Hypoglycemia
	Hyponatremia
	Liver failure
	Renal failure
	Acidosis
CV	Hypotension
	Thrombus
	Severe anemia
Other	Hypothermia
	Elderly
	Acute alcohol intoxication
	Baclofen or narcotic pump malfunction
Pulmonary	Hypoxia
	Hypercarbia
	Carbon monoxide poisoning

References

1. Gan TJ, Meyer TA, Apfel CC. Society for ambulatory anesthesia guidelines for the management of postoperative nausea and vomiting. Anesth Analg. 2007;105:1615–28.
2. Wong GK, Chan MT, Poon WS, et al. Magnesium therapy within 48 hours of an aneurysmal subarachnoid hemorrhage: neuropanacea. Neurol Res. 2006;28:431–5.
3. Westermaier T, Stetter C, Vince GH. Prophylactic intravenous magnesium sulfate for the treatment of aneurysmal subarachnoid hemorrhage: a randomized, placebo-controlled clinical study. Crit Care Med. 2010;38:1284–90.
4. Black S, Enneking FK, Cucchiara RF. Failure to awaken after general anesthesia due to cerebrovascular events. J Neurosurg Anesthesiol. 1998;10:10–5.
5. De Witte J, Sessler DI. Perioperative shivering: physiology and pharmacology. Anesthesiology. 2002;96:467–84.
6. Xiong J, Kurz A, Sessler DI, et al. Isoflurane produces marked and nonlinear decreases in the vasoconstriction and shivering thresholds. Anesthesiology. 1996;85:240–5.
7. MacIntyre PE, Pavlin EG, Dwersteg JF. Effect of meperidine on oxygen consumption, carbon dioxide production, and respiratory gas exchange in post anesthesia shivering. Anesth Analg. 1987;66:751–5.
8. Frank SM, Fleisher LA, Breslow MJ, et al. Perioperative maintenance of normothermia reduces the incidence of morbid cardiac events: a randomized clinical trial. JAMA. 1997;277:1127–34.
9. Cucchiara RF. Differential awakening. Anesth Analg (Letter). 1992;75:467.
10. Strebel S, Lam A, Matta B, et al. Dynamic and static cerebral autoregulation during isoflurane, desflurane, and propofol anesthesia. Anesthesiology. 1995;83:66–76.
11. Bruder N, Pellissier D, Grillot P, et al. Cerebral hyperemia during recovery from general anesthesia in neurosurgical patients. Anesth Analg. 2002;94:650–4.
12. Shubert A. Cerebral hyperemia, systemic hypertension, and perioperative intracranial morbidity: is there a smoking gun? Anesth Analg. 2002;94:485.
13. Basali A, Mascha E, Kalfas I, et al. Relation between perioperative hypertension and intracranial hemorrhage after craniotomy. Anesthesiology. 2000;93:48–54.
14. Lee VH, Connolly HM, Fulgham JR, Manno EM, Brown RD, Wijdicks EFM. Tako-tsubo cardiomyopathy in aneurysmal subarachnoid hemorrhage: an underappreciated ventricular dysfunction. J Neurosurg. 2006;105:264–70.
15. Balkin DM, Cohen LS. Takotsubo syndrome. Coron Artery Dis. 2011;22:206–14.
16. Hanna AS, Grindle CR, Patel AA, Rosen MR, Evans JJ. Inadvertent insertion of nasogastric tube into the brain stem and spinal cord after endoscopic skull base surgery. Am J Otolaryngol. 2012;33:178–80.
17. Schade K, Borzotta A, Michaels A. Intracranial malposition of nasopharyngeal airway. J Trauma. 2000;49:967–8.
18. Shen Y, Drum M, Roth S. The prevalence of perioperative visual loss in the United States: a 10-year study from 1996 to 2005 of spinal, orthopedic, cardiac, and general surgery. Anesth Analg. 2009;109:1534–45.
19. Jeffrey D, Coe JD, Arlet V, et al. Complications in spinal fusion for adolescent idiopathic scoliosis in the new millennium. A Report of the Scoliosis Research Society Morbidity and Mortality Committee. Spine. 2006;31:345–9.
20. Agarwal A, Sinha PK, Pandey CM, et al. Effect of a subanesthetic dose of intravenous ketamine and/or local anesthetic infiltration on hemodynamic responses to skull-pin placement. J Neurosurg Anesthesiol. 2001;13:189–94.
21. Nuttall GA, Garrity JA, Dearani JA, et al. Risk factors for ischemic optic neuropathy after cardiopulmonary bypass: a matched case/control study. Anesth Analg. 2001;93:1410–6.
22. Hashimoto T, Young WL, Prohovnik I, et al. Increased cerebral blood flow after brain arteriovenous malformation resection is substantially independent of changes in cardiac output. J Neurosurg Anesthesiol. 2002;14:204–8.
23. Fardo DJ, Hankins WT, Houskamp W, et al. The hemodynamic effects of local anesthetic injection into the carotid body during carotid endarterectomy. Am Surg. 1999;65:648–51; discussion 651–2.
24. Maher CO, Wetjen NM, Friedman JA, et al. Intraoperative lidocaine injection into the carotid sinus during endarterectomy. J Neurosurg. 2002;97:80–3.
25. Gravenstein D, Gravenstein N. Intraoperative and immediate postoperative neuroanesthesia. In: Layon AJ, Gabrielli A, Friedman WA, editors. Textbook of neurointensive care. Philadelphia: WB Saunders; 2004.

Neurorehabilitation

43

Rita Formisano, Eva Azicnuda, Umberto Bivona,
Maria Paola Ciurli, Andrea Gabrielli, and Sheila Catani

Contents

R. Formisano, MD, PhD (✉) • E. Azicnuda, PsyD
U. Bivona, PhD • M.P. Ciurli, PsyD • S. Catani, MD
IRCCS Santa Lucia Foundation, Rome, Italy
e-mail: r.formisano@hsantalucia.it; e.azicnuda@hsantalucia.it;
u.bivona@hsantalucia.it; p.ciurli@hsantalucia.it;
s.catani@hsantalucia.it

A. Gabrielli, MD, FCCM
Departments of Anesthesiology and Surgery,
University of Florida College of Medicine, Gainesville, FL, USA
e-mail: agabrielli@anest.ufl.edu

Neurorehabilitation and Disorders of Consciousness

The logistics of neurorehabilitation of this group of patients differ based on their unique clinical status. Disorders of consciousness (DOC) after severe acquired brain injury (ABI) include coma, vegetative state (VS), and minimally conscious state (MCS). Coma is primarily assessed via the Glasgow Coma Scale (GCS) [1] in the acute phase, whereas the Disability Rating Scale (DRS) [2], Levels of Cognitive Function (LCF) [3], Glasgow Outcome Scale (GOS), and Glasgow Outcome Scale-Extended (GOS-E) [4, 5] are the most commonly used scales in the post-acute phase.

Coma

The definition of coma includes the clinical triad of "closed eyes, not obeying simple commands, no comprehensible verbal utterances" [6]. Coma has also been defined as a complete failure of the arousal system, with no spontaneous eye opening in patients who are unable to be awakened by application of vigorous sensory stimulation [7].

The rehabilitation process of a comatose patient is complex and requires an accurate and articulate plan. Specific protocols concerning adequate positioning to contrasting pathological postures are based on maintaining a passive range of motion, daily nursing activity, and promoting emotional stimulation by significant others. The presence of muscular hypertonia, vegetative dysautonomia (defined as paroxysmal sympathetic hyperactivity) [8], and/or psychomotor agitation often antagonizes this plan, and, consequently, these conditions have to be generally addressed with sedation, which may, in turn, compromise the goal of early rehabilitation.

Vegetative State

The vegetative state (VS) is a condition that follows coma when the patient recovers vigilance or alertness (eyes

A.J. Layon et al. (eds.), *Textbook of Neurointensive Care*,
DOI 10.1007/978-1-4471-5226-2_43, © Springer-Verlag London 2013

opening), but not awareness—the latter defined as the ability to obey simple commands. The patient is unable to interact with the surroundings in spite of the eyes opening and partial recovery of the sleep-wake circadian cycle. The term "persistent" has been used in the past to indicate a potentially reversible process, whereas the term "permanent" indicated an irreversible condition. The time interval for the recovery potential is presently 1 year for trauma cases and 3–6 months for all other etiologies. Vegetative state remains a commonly used term, but qualifying the VS with "persistent" or "permanent" has been recently challenged [9] considering the increasing number of late recoveries reported with this diagnosis [10–13]. A number of complex neurological syndromes may affect the likelihood of appropriate rehabilitation at this stage. Undiagnosed epileptic activity, as nonconvulsive seizures, has been detected in 6.3 % of the cases [14]. Parkinsonism is also common [15, 16], especially as an evolution of diffuse axonal injury (DAI) [17–20] generally consisting of akinesia, rigidity, hypomimia, and hypersalivation.

The Multi-Society Task Force for the Study of Vegetative State has recommended the utilization of a common terminology for this condition, suggesting that any other term describing this state of DOC, such as "coma vigile" (French literature) and "apallic syndrome" (Austrian and German literature), should be abandoned [21]. The term "akinetic mutism" remains an exception to the rule and is characterized as a condition with severe quadriparesis, mutism, akinesia, visual fixation, and pursuit [22]. More recently, a European task force has introduced the definition of unresponsive wakefulness syndrome (UWS) [23] to replace the term vegetative state, although it has not been universally accepted [24].

Minimally Conscious State (MCS)

The MCS may follow either coma or VS as a transition or a permanent condition [25], usually between the VS and "severe disability" categories of the GOS [4, 5]. However, the evaluation of the consciousness level may be affected by recurrent infections; convulsive and nonconvulsive seizures [14]; psychomotor agitation, restlessness, aggressiveness, and erratic behaviors [26]; normotensive or hypertensive hydrocephalus [27]; and sedative, antiepileptic, and muscle-relaxant drugs.

Many MCS patients may be able to exhibit visual fixation and eye pursuing and tracking, in addition to being mute and akinetic; therefore, akinetic mutism should be considered a subcategory of MCS. Psychomotor agitation and aggressiveness are frequent behaviors in individuals with severe ABI who may be unable to follow simple commands. Agitated patients often display intentional aggressive behaviors against themselves or others, and only rarely can they obey simple commands [26]. Aggressiveness may be the manifestation of physical or emotional discomfort or mental confusion that the patient is not able to express otherwise. For these reasons, agitated patients should be also diagnosed with a MCS instead of VS, even if not able to follow commands [28, 29].

Neurological Evaluation of Patients with Disorders of Consciousness

Rare blinking and absent threat reflex, consisting of the lack of blinking at the rapid approach of the hand to the eye, is a common feature demonstrating the lack of responsivity in VS patients and may be generally interpreted as confirmation of unconsciousness, although blindness due to bilateral lesion of the optic nerve can also be the cause of the absence of blinking in response to visual stimuli.

In the acute and post-acute phase, endocrine disorders—hypopituitarism being the most common—should be investigated [30, 31]. Vigilance disorders, electrolyte imbalance, immunological deficits, dysautonomic symptoms, and cognitive and behavioral disturbances also may be secondary to dysfunction of the hypothalamic-pituitary axis [32–42]. Prediction of recovery of consciousness in patients with prolonged DOC is more difficult, since the severity and duration of coma are similar in all subjects with severe ABI, i.e., $GCS \leq 8$ and duration of unconsciousness of at least 1 month in the VS.

The Medical Disability Society [43] defines severe ABI as all states of coma lasting at least 6 h. The definition of "prolonged coma" has also been suggested as an indicator of "very severe brain injury" for patients with unconsciousness lasting at least 15 days [29, 44, 45]. In patients with prolonged DOC, the time interval from coma to the achievement of some rehabilitation goals [45] seems to be predictive of the final outcome at 1-year follow-up according to the GOS [4] and Barthel Index (BI) [46]. The most significant predictive clinical features are the presence of spontaneous motor activity and the time interval to the recovery of sustained visual fixation, eye tracking, and safe oral feeding, the latter tending to be correlated with neuropsychological recovery [45]. Psychomotor agitation and bulimia during recovery from DOC may be considered favorable prognostic indicators of the final prognosis. In fact, the diagnosis of a confused-agitated state upon admission to the rehabilitation ward, evaluated by means of the LCF scale [3], predicted a statistically significant better outcome at discharge compared to patients without any agitation [26].

Posttraumatic psychomotor agitation (PPA) represents, according to some authors [47–49], a positive indicator of consciousness recovery, especially if it occurs in the early stages of coma [26]. Nevertheless, aggressiveness may be considered a predictive indicator of an unfavorable neuro-psychological prognosis when persisting for several months. Posttraumatic psychomotor agitation has been classified as a subtype of delirium, with onset during the period of posttraumatic amnesia (PTA). It is characterized by extreme behaviors, including aggressiveness, akathisia, disinhibition, and emotional lability [50], and occurs during the period after the onset of coma when the patient is not able to recall everyday events of the last 24 h [51]. Some recovery phases from DOC may be characterized not only by psychomotor agitation but also by the Klüver-Bucy syndrome, defined as a transient phase with behavioral disinhibition, as well as increased primitive oral automatisms and hypersexuality, described as a possible recovery phase of prolonged DOC [52, 53]. Undergoing the Klüver-Bucy syndrome after DOC has been previously reported as a favorable predictive indicator of the final prognosis [54]. During this remission phase, patients may have extreme attention lability (hypermetamorphosis) and restlessness, and therefore, they are only rarely able to follow commands. This condition, generally transient, should be diagnosed as MCS and, in some cases, may evolve to bulimia lasting also several months.

Pathological postures in decortication (flexion and intrarotation of the upper limbs along with intrarotation and hyperextension of the lower limbs) and decerebration (intrarotation and hyperextension of the upper and lower limbs) are rarely described in the literature in DOC patients [15, 55]. In general, they represent a negative indicator of long-term functional outcome in comparison with patients without these postures and earlier recovery of spontaneous motility of the upper and/or lower limbs [55]. Pathological postures are also frequently associated with severe spasticity, akinesia, rigidity, parkinsonian posture, and dysautonomic symptoms. Baguley et al. [56] found dysautonomic syndrome in about 30 % of individuals in the VS, with a simultaneous and paroxysmal increase in at least five of the following seven autonomic parameters: heart rate (tachycardia), respiratory rate (tachypnea), muscle tone (increased), posture (decerebrate or decorticate), blood pressure (arterial hypertension), sweating (profuse), and temperature (increased or decreased). Dysautonomia or paroxysmal sympathetic hyperactivity has been reported as a negative prognostic indicator of the final outcome of severe ABI patients [8, 55, 57]. Passive range of motion may be also limited by muscle contractures and ankylosis at the level of the major joints, frequently due to periarticular ossification (PAO) and tendon retractions or shortenings [58–61].

Sensorial deficits of central or peripheral origin, such as blindness or deafness, may be due to cerebral lesions or cranial nerve paralysis and may often cause diagnostic errors when evaluating the consciousness disorder. Similarly, patients with language disorders (aphasia) or gesture execution deficit (apraxia) may be not able to obey simple commands because of comprehension deficits or difficulty in executing gestures, respectively. A right hemiparesis or quadriparesis with right prevalence may be factors for aphasia and apraxia, while a left hemiplegia or quadriparesis with left prevalence may be associated with neglect or hemi-inattention.

In individuals with VS, the presence of primitive oral automatisms, such as chewing, sucking, and yawning, may also predict a worse prognosis in patients with DOC [55]. Focal deficits after severe head injury were commonly found in a group of 150 survivors from severe head injury [5]: hemiparesis was present in 49 %, dysphagia in 29 %, deficit in one or more cranial nerves in 32 %, posttraumatic epilepsy (PTE) in 15 %, ataxia in 9 %, and homonymous hemianopia in 5 % of the cases. Among cranial nerve deficits, the optic nerve was the most commonly involved, followed by involvement of one of the ocular muscle nerves. Deficits of the oculomotor, trochlear, or abducens nerves may be responsible of monolateral or bilateral ptosis, strabismus, and diplopia, all of which can complicate the evaluation of visual fixation and eye tracking movements. In some cases, after eye opening, the patients may voluntary close one eye during visual fixation or pursuing, most likely due to diplopia. Monolateral or bilateral blepharospasm may also impair the patient's attempts at communication via eyelid closure. Additionally, approximately 5 % of all patients with head trauma manifest some visual loss following TBI [62].

Motor recovery generally starts with distal to proximal limb motility, likely due to the relative sparing of the cerebral cortex, where the cortical representation of the hand and foot is more extended, and there is more involvement of the muscles of the major joints, especially shoulder and hip contractures. Asymmetric motor recovery between the upper and lower limbs is a possible clinical indicator of either spinal cord injury, critical illness polyneuropathy (CIP) or critical illness mio-neuropathy (CRIMINE), or hydrocephalus. The most significant clinical features of hydrocephalus are regression or arrest of previous consciousness improvement, fever, epileptic seizures, and cognitive and behavioral disorders poorly responsive to pharmacologic and rehabilitative treatment [27]. Diffuse muscle atrophy, recurrent sepsis, and PAO, especially at the level of the hips, elbows, and knees, should suggest the diagnosis of CIP [63] or compressive neuropathies, often secondary to entrapment by PAO, fibrous retractions by muscle hemorrhagic contusions, or prolonged pathological postures.

Parkinsonian [64] and cerebellar symptoms [65] may be both associated with pyramidal paralysis, with mixed features and frequent lateralization (pyramidal-cerebellar syndrome). Occasionally, the improvement of rigidity or spasticity, or of mixed features of rigidity and spasticity, may exacerbate the intentional cerebellar tremor because of the reduction in muscular tone. The main parkinsonian symptoms are rigidity, akinesia, trunk flexion, and hypomimia, whereas tremor is only rarely present. Hypersalivation (sialorrhea), rare blinking, and seborrhea of the face are common adjunctive extrapyramidal symptoms.

A transient period of posttraumatic mutism (PTM) is commonly associated with parkinsonian symptoms. These patients may recover alternative forms of communication through gestures or sometimes by writing, but they do not demonstrate any verbal communication or the intention to vocalize. This condition may last several weeks and sometimes a few months but only rarely persists as permanent unless associated with verbal inertia or severe dysarthria. Posttraumatic mutism has been reported with a frequency of 3 % in individuals with severe TBI [66], but in our database, its incidence in survivors with DOC seems much higher, up to 30 % of the cases, especially when associated with severe frontal damage to brainstem lesions or disconnection syndrome. Recovery of verbal communication during the period of PTM has been widely described in the literature [67].

Trismus secondary to bilateral masseter contraction or focal dystonia should be dealt with early because of the high risk of muscle contracture and temporomandibular ankylosis, especially after maxillary and jaw fractures. Myoclonic jerks may be secondary to cortical or brainstem lesions or cerebral hypoxic damage; they are, in general, early predictive indicators of poor prognosis for long-lasting disability [55].

Neurophysiological Investigations in Neurorehabilitation

Electroencephalogram

The electroencephalogram (EEG) is a physiologic measure of cerebral function that has been used to assess coma and prognosticate survival and global outcomes after TBI. A single EEG can help with broad diagnostic categorization, whereas continuous and serial EEGs provide monitoring for unstable and potentially treatable conditions and for monitoring the effects of therapy. The EEG plays a supplemental role in establishing the prognosis for severe ABI. The prognostic value of electrophysiological monitoring thus far has been consolidated by several studies in the literature [68–70]. In order to determine the predictive value of the EEG, several authors have tried to characterize EEG patterns that could be related to the following possibilities of recovery of the patient. Bricolo [68] studied EEG patterns in patients with head trauma and established a classification that correlated various EEG patterns with the outcome. Subsequently, Synek [69], Rae-Grant [71], and Gutling [72] developed further classifications of the EEG patterns in such patients

using a series of hierarchical levels based on the progressive reduction of EEG frequency (from alpha to delta) and of amplitude (from normal until plate) and noticed particular patterns, such as the delta and theta coma. Kane et al. [73] found that the measures most significantly correlating with outcome were over the left hemisphere, with beta activity power in the frontocentral and centrotemporal regions and alpha activity power in the centrotemporal region. The EEG patterns that have a defined prognostic value are the alpha coma, the theta coma, the triphasic waves, and the spontaneous burst suppression. These are considered signs of unfavorable outcome in terms of both survival and quality of life. A particular kind of reactivity with unfavorable prognostic value is the manifestation of a focal burst suppression pattern after a bolus of thiopental in patients already under sedation [74].

The presence of exclusively rudimentary forms of oscillation has also been described in association with poor prognosis [75]. Sleep patterns have been shown to continue to improve during rehabilitation, and REM sleep percentage increases with the recovery of cognitive functions [76, 77]. In a series of ten patients with posttraumatic VS, the absence of a defined sleep pattern was observed in the only patient who never recovered from the VS but died before the sixth month of follow-up [78]. More recently, the sleep-wake organization pattern based on 24-h polysomnographic recordings in the subacute stage of posttraumatic coma has been demonstrated to be a very reliable prognostic marker for both survival and functional recovery. In particular, the presence of organized sleep patterns is highly predictive of a better outcome [79].

Somatosensory Evoked Potentials

Evoked potentials (EP) are generated from a very defined system and are not significantly influenced by sedation therapy. Their prognostic efficacy varies based on the sensory modality explored and the type of results obtained; this approach seems to provide further prognostic information when multimodal EPs are performed and repeated during the evolution of the clinical picture [80]. Short-latency somatosensory EP (SL-SEP) abnormalities provide significant prognostic value [81]. For example, the overwhelming majority of patients (90 % to nearly 100 %) with a bilateral absence of N20 associated with bilateral cerebral lesions either does not survive or develops VS; in the rare case of recovery of awareness, severe neurological disabilities are present. On the contrary, the bilateral absence of N20 due to primary damage of the brainstem is associated with a more variable outcome depending on the extent and severity of the lesion but still with the possibility of a good recovery in a discrete amount of cases. However, it has also been emphasized that a bilateral N20 within normal limits does not guarantee a favorable prognosis.

Somatosensory EPs have been commonly used as an objective and reproducible electrophysiological means of evaluating the integrity of sensory pathways in neurologically impaired patients, including head trauma. In acute TBI, somatosensory EP (SEP) abnormalities often correlate with the severity of the trauma and are helpful in predicting the extent of the patient's recovery. There is a general consensus that the presence or absence of SEPs over one or both hemispheres represents an excellent predicting parameter for discriminating between a globally good or bad outcome. Somatosensory EPs have been used in determining the diagnosis, prognosis, presence of secondary lesions, and follow-up treatment methods for brain injury patients. Greenberg et al. [82] grouped patients according to the quality of their short-latency SEPs, and compared these SEP values with GOS scores, computed tomography (CT) findings, and other clinical parameters. They found that SEPs had a reliability of 91 % for determining prognosis. Visual evoked potential (VEPs) are somewhat less useful than SEPs in predicting the prognosis of comatose patients. Further, the variability of this category of potentials in normal subjects is the greatest deterrent for their use as predictors of outcome.

Motor evoked potentials (MEPs) may have also a prognostic value; however, they do not add further information with respect to clinical indicators, such as GCS [83]. Alterations of SEPs, acoustic evoked potentials (AEPs), and visual evoked potentials (VEPs) have a wide predictive value when considered together, both for outcome in the acute phase of coma and, subsequently, after the first years after head trauma [72]. Prediction of outcome approximates 100 % of accuracy when EPs are combined with EEG.

Mismatch Negativity and P300

The recent opportunity to evaluate EEG event-related potential components, such as mismatch negativity (MMN) and P300, has allowed a redefinition of some prognostic criteria. The patterns of EEG responses evoked by auditory paradigms eliciting classical P300 waveform and its subcomponents, and the more recent auditory paradigms based on the patient's own name, have shown to be significant predictors of recovery from DOC or signs of islands of consciousness [84].

Mismatch negativity is typically seen as a frontocentral negativity of approximately 0.5–5 lV in amplitude, occurring in the latency range of 100–250 ms. The peak latency, thus, occurs well after the sensory N100 component. The capacity of MMN to predict awakening from coma has been investigated in five cohort studies in which MMN and N100 have reliably reflected the functional status of comatose patients [85]. Mismatch negativity can be useful in the efforts to ascertain the perceptual capabilities of the comatose patient as well as the likelihood of awakening from coma. The presence of MMN recorded during the comatose state is the best

predictor of awakening within a 12-month period [86]. A positive predictive value for awakening has been reported in 100 % of cases in one study [87], whereas the absence of MMN was predictive of nonawakening in 84 % of cases. In predicting awakening, MMN was superior to auditory N100, early SEPs, N20 and P40, middle latency auditory event-related potentials (ERPs), auditory brainstem potentials, and pupillary light reflex [88].

Neuroimaging

In the acute setting, neuroimaging techniques can determine the presence and extent of injury and can be used to guide surgical planning and minimally invasive interventions. Neuroimaging can also be important in the chronic treatment of TBI and severe ABI, as well as identifying chronic sequelae, determining the prognosis, and supporting the rehabilitation plan.

Computed Tomography

Computed tomography is considered the imaging modality of choice in the management of acute brain injury. The Marshall classification [89] is widely utilized in the acute phase and is especially indicated for assessment of cerebral edema, discrimination of focal or diffuse damage, and severity of DAI. The functional outcome ultimately depends on how many neurons are preserved after injury. The sites of damage and the ability of existing neurons to reorganize their connections to recover functions are also critical. Neuronal injury is caused by direct injury, compression, ischemia, DAI, and secondary damage. The number of lesions correlates with a poorer prognosis, and lesions present in the supratentorial white matter, corpus callosum, and corona radiata correlate with a greater likelihood that the patient will remain in a VS [90].

Magnetic Resonance Imaging

Magnetic resonance imaging is generally more sensitive than CT for detecting neuronal damage. Patients with widespread MRI abnormalities or brainstem injuries usually show poor neurological recovery, even when their CT scans are normal [91]. However, aside from the obvious cases of devastating injury, a consistent relationship between MRI lesions and clinical or neuropsychological outcomes has not been demonstrated [92]. More recent MRI technologies, such as diffusion tensor imaging (DTI) techniques [93–100], perfusion MRI [101], Turbo-PEPSI [102], and voxel-based morphometry may provide, respectively, better information for prognosis, rehabilitation guidance, shorter time of acquisition, and final prognosis [17, 103]. Recent studies have indicated the relevance of advanced neurophysiological and neuroimaging techniques in the evaluation of DOC [104–107].

Owen et al. [104] first described the case of "hidden islands of consciousness" in a young woman who sustained a severe head injury in a traffic accident and afterward was diagnosed with a VS. Although the patient was still unresponsive and unable to communicate 5 months after the accident, a functional MRI (fMRI) showed that she retained some ability to process language and produce some visual imagery on request similar to healthy subjects [104]. Monti et al. showed that a small proportion of patients with a VS or MCS have brain activation reflecting some awareness and cognition when fMRI was used to assess the patient's ability to generate willful, neuroanatomically specific, blood oxygenation level-dependent responses during established mental-imagery tasks. This technique, as well as using EEG for the same tasks [108], may be useful in establishing basic communication with patients who appear to be unresponsive [109]. More recently these individuals have been defined as with functional locked-in syndrome [110, 111].

Single Photon Emission Computed Tomography

Single photon emission computed tomography (SPECT) appears to be better than CT or MRI in determining long-term prognosis. A negative initial SPECT scan after trauma seems to strongly predict a favorable clinical outcome [112], and an abnormal SPECT can be predictive of neuropsychological deficits [113]. Some studies found that decreased blood flow to various parts of the brain correlates with different types of behaviors: frontal lobes (disinhibitive behavior), left cerebral hemisphere (increased social isolation), and right hemispheric areas (increased aggressive behavior) [114]. However, no consistent correlation between SPECT abnormalities and neuropsychological tests scores has been established. Single photon emission computed tomography studies have demonstrated that changes in regional cerebral blood flow (CBF) induced by auditory stimulation consisted of stronger functional connectivity between the secondary auditory cortex and temporal and prefrontal cortices in MCS patients compared to those with VS [115].

Positron Emission Tomography

Positron emission tomography can be used to measure the cerebral metabolism of various substrates, most commonly by utilizing the fluorodeoxyglucose (FDG) method, which involves the measurement of glucose metabolism that should correspond to neuronal changes. This imaging technique can be also used to diagnose patients with DAI to determine the

extent of cerebral damage and possibly the prognosis. The metabolic effects of cortical contusions, intracranial hematoma, and resultant encephalomalacia are primarily confined to the site of the injury; subdural and epidural hematomas are often widespread and may even affect the contralateral hemisphere [90], whereas DAI results in diffuse hypometabolism. Alavi [116] found that a CGS score of ≤13 was associated with whole-brain hypometabolism of FDG. However, studies have shown that PET can uncover areas of cerebral hypometabolism not detected by CT, MRI, or EEG that are associated with neurological and behavioral dysfunction [117].

Transcranial Doppler

Alteration in cerebral circulation has been shown in head-injured patients by various studies and include impaired autoregulation, altered CO_2 reactivity, hyperemia (increased CBF), oligemia (decreased CBF), and vasospasm [118, 119]. Transcranial Doppler (TCD) does not yield absolute CBF values; however, linear correlation has been established between the changes in flow velocities of basal cerebral arteries and changes in CBF [120]. An understanding of the timing and evolution of trauma-induced circulatory changes is critically important in order to provide new insights on the pathophysiology and possible therapeutic strategies for cerebrovascular disturbances after brain injury at the appropriate time.

Neurorehabilitation Protocols

Physical and rehabilitation medicine (PRM) guidelines have been developed as a biopsychosocial approach to rehabilitation in cooperation with the World Health Organization (WHO) International Classification of Functioning Disability and Health (ICF), which was approved by the World Health Assembly in May 2001 [121] (see Fig. 43.1). Physical and rehabilitation medicine is an independent medical specialty

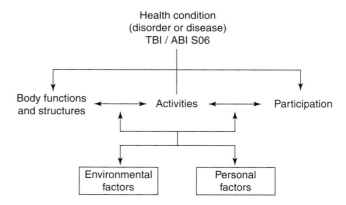

Fig. 43.1 PM&R Guideline Approach. Adapted from the current framework of functioning and disability – the WHO International Classification of Functioning and Health (ICF) [20]

concerned with the promotion of physical and cognitive functioning, activities (including behavior), participation (including quality of life), and the modification of personal and environmental factors. Accordingly, it is responsible for the prevention, diagnosis, treatment, and rehabilitation management of people with disabling medical conditions and comorbidity across all ages [122].

Rehabilitation has been shown to be effective not only in enhancing individual functioning and independent living, but in reducing the costs of dependency [123]. Acute rehabilitation affects respiratory dynamics, blood pressure, the perception of body and space, arousal, circadian rhythms, and deconditioning and muscle tone disorders, as well as playing a role in preventing joint deformity, excessive bed rest, and reducing the incidence of gastroesophageal reflux and aspiration.

Prone positioning improves the functional residual respiratory capacity, gas exchange, and ventilation/perfusion, thereby enhancing and prolonging the effect of oxygenation maneuvers [124] in line with what has been observed in acute respiratory failure patients in the ICU [125]. For these reasons, the use of a tilt table to aid patients in recovering the standing position is widespread among physical therapists [126].

Frequent postural mobilization induces a positive effect in terms of an inflammatory response; indeed, in the ICU, it was observed that only 15 min of postural mobilization in bed significantly reduces circulating levels of proinflammatory cytokines in critically ill patients [127]. The duration of bed rest is the main factor responsible for the reduction of muscle function: 5 weeks produces muscle strength reduction of 26 % in the ankle plantiflexor muscle [128], while 12–16 weeks leads to a reduction of 30 % of muscle strength over the same muscles [129] and a negative nitrogen balance [130]. Acquired brain injury may cause two distinct functional impairments of muscle and tendons [131, 132]: paresis from immobilization in pathological postures, with secondary plasticity reorganization of muscles and tendons leading towards muscle contracture, and central spasticity such as muscle hyperactivity, contractions, and dystonia. After 8 weeks, the passive range of motion (ROM) is no more completely recoverable even if normal mobility is restored [133], suggesting the urgency to restore mobility in comatose patients within that time interval.

A multidisciplinary team must undertake management of spasticity, as optimal treatment involves physical therapy in conjunction with pharmacological treatment. A variety of treatment options are available, and clinical experience has shown that a multimodal approach has many benefits in combining physical therapies with surgical and/or pharmacological treatments. The combination of botulinum toxin injections (Botox-A) with physical therapy has shown functional improvements, lending support to the concept that this should be part of a comprehensive plan to treat focal [134] or diffuse spasticity with intrathecal baclofen pump [135]. A comprehensive approach to neurorehabilitation is illustrated

Table 43.1 Comprehensive approaches to neurorehabilitation

1. Adequate nursing of the skin areas more exposed to compression
2. Adequate mobilization from supine to lateral position, at least every 2–3 h
3. Adequate mobilization of limbs and trunk at least 2 h a day
4. Accurate hygiene, mobilization, and stimulation of the mouth, lips, and tongue, also by means of gustatory stimuli
5. Postural changes and drainage of tracheobronchial secretions
6. Positioning splinting of the limbs to prevent muscle contractures and joint ankylosis
7. Gradual recovery of the sitting and standing positions for recovery of trunk control
8. Basal and emotional stimulation during nursing care and by proxy emotional stimuli

Table 43.2 Systematic evaluation of neuromotor and neuropsychological deficits

Disorders of consciousness	Responsiveness evaluation via specific scales and proxy emotional stimulation
Quadriplegia or quadriparesis	Sometimes with pathological postures: decortication or decerebration
Hemiplegia or hemiparesis	Aphasia and/or apraxia (left hemispheric brain damage) hemi-inattention or neglect (right hemispheric brain damage)
Motor coordination deficits and/or balance disorders	Ataxia and postural or intentional tremor
Increased muscle tone	Focal and diffuse spasticity
Parkinsonism	Bradykinesia, rigidity, hypomimia, facial seborrhea, hypersalivation, anti-flexion of the trunk, ocular convergence deficit (as in postencephalitic parkinsonism), resting or postural tremor more rarely
Diffuse myoclonic jerks or intentional myoclonus	Commonly posthypoxic or due to brainstem damage
Cranial nerves or peripheral nervous system deficits	Critical illness polyneuropathy (CIP) and critical illness myoneuropathy, compressive neuropathy (CRIMINE)
Visual disorders and visual field deficits	Amblyopia, strabismus, commonly associated with ocular deviation (diplopia)
Pseudobulbar syndrome with deficit of the most caudal cranial nerves	Anarthria or dysarthria, dysphagia, pneumophonic incoordination, aphonia or dysphonia (as by brainstem damage), sometimes associated with spastic laughing and crying

in Table 43.1 and a systematic evaluation of neuromotor and neuropsychological deficits is suggested in Table 43.2.

Special Considerations in Neurorehabilitation

Hydrotherapy

Hydrotherapy may be useful for balance disorders, gait training, active motor recruitment, and range of motion recovery due to the reduced gravity and massaging action of the water.

Aquatics may enhance health by promoting positive behaviors, physical self-concept, and self-esteem [136].

Occupational Therapy

Occupational therapy involves employing activity-based tasks for recovering functional autonomy. The primary objective is to allow the patient to regain the ability of performing daily hygiene and personal care, as well as dressing. A simulation of the home environment may be beneficial in preparing for home reentry [137].

Urological Rehabilitation

Early removal of the bladder catheter is feasible even in DOC patients as long as there is no evidence of spinal cord injury. Determination of post-micturition of residual urine is useful and can be accomplished utilizing a portable ultrasound scanner [138]. In a few cases, the return of spontaneous micturition recovery may be facilitated by means of intermittent catheterization [139].

Phoniatric Assessment and Rehabilitation

Fiberoptic rhinolaryngoscopy can be used to investigate deglutition, whereas a speech-language pathologist (SLP) can examine the patient's oral motor abilities, any swallowing disorders, and dysphagia. Respiratory therapy aims to improve the drainage of tracheobronchial secretions and the recovery of cough efficacy by employing forced expiration exercises. Tracheal tube removal is generally possible after sufficient improvement of swallowing disorders and resolution of dysphagia with progressive reduction of the tube diameter. Head and trunk dystonia may also cause swallowing disorders and failure of dysphagia training. Achievement of safe oral feeding without risk of aspiration is an important milestone in the recovery of individuals with severe ABI given the symbolic meaning of the nutrition by mouth as a return to life [44, 45].

Swallowing Training

In patients with low responsiveness and unable to assist in their therapy, gentle tactile stimulation of the oropharynx may improve collaboration and motivation, especially when gustatory stimulation is employed. Thermal and proprioceptive stimulation of the mouth, lips, tongue, and palatal region may activate the swallowing reflex. The integration of tube feeding during swallowing training prevents malnourishment, dehydration, and pulmonary infections. Substitution of the nasogastric tube with a percutaneous endoscopic gastrostomy (PEG) facilitates swallowing recovery by reducing the oral dysesthesia created by the feeding tube as well as reducing the risk of tracheobronchial food aspiration due to the abnormal closure of the pharyngoesophageal tract [140]. The success of swallowing training depends on the collaboration of the patient and the severity of cognitive and behavioral disorders [141].

Pharmacotherapy

Pharmacotherapy for individuals with severe ABI consists of symptomatic and syndromic interventions. Unfortunately, although pharmacotherapy is commonly applied during early rehabilitation, few controlled studies have been performed on this topic.

A Cochrane review supports the efficacy of propranolol in controlling agitation [142] and paroxysmal sympathetic hyperactivity, whereas other evidence-based approaches did not confirm any efficacy in modifying the final outcome of severe ABI patients. Several sedative agents have been extensively investigated in the past: barbiturates [143], corticosteroids [144], calcium channel blockers [145], antiepileptic drugs [146], and monoaminergic agonists as amphetamines [147]. Phenobarbital, diazepam, and clonidine have demonstrated deleterious effects on neuronal and neural plasticity and should be avoided [148]. Acute and subacute myoclonic jerks may be successfully treated with piracetam [149–151], clonazepam in increasing dosages, or levetiracetam [152–155]. Oxcarbazepine may substitute carbamazepine for treatment of epilepsy or agitation, because it is less hepatotoxic and bone marrow suppressant, although it can be associated with hyponatremia.

Piracetam has been demonstrated to improve the consciousness level after severe TBI [156, 157] and protect neurons from hypoxia in experimental studies [158, 159]. Positive emission tomography studies also showed that its neuroprotective effects are potentially useful for improved recovery of language disturbances, memory, and learning abilities [160–162], as well as communication between the two hemispheres through the corpus callosum [161, 163]. More recently, acetylcholinesterase inhibitors (AchE-I) have been reported in the treatment of cognitive and behavioral disorders after TBI [164–169]. Memantine, an excitatory amino acid inhibitor, might be of some interest for its efficacy in Alzheimer's disease, although the risk of epileptic seizures has to be carefully considered [170].

Some nonsteroidal anti-inflammatory agents, such as indomethacin, may improve the collaboration and tolerance of the patient by reducing pain during passive range of motion. In fact, gradual assisted verticalization may be facilitated by wearing elastic stockings on the lower limbs and indomethacin therapy, which may counteract orthostatic hypotension [171]. Indomethacin is also able to prevent PAO and its postsurgery reoccurrence [172].

Central and peripheral pain should be monitored by means of the Visual Analogue Scale (VAS) or by the Nociception Coma Scale in noncooperative and nonresponsive patients [173]. Finally, L-Dopa and dopaminergic drugs, especially amantadine, may be considered for enhancing consciousness and verbal communication recovery, as well as for improving cognitive functions in posttraumatic parkinsonism and patients with DOC [174, 175]. Amantadine should be used with caution in epileptic patients with TBI, to improve posttraumatic parkinsonism, based on the dopaminergic nature of the drug.

Stroke Rehabilitation

Stroke presents a major global public health challenge, with 5.5 million people dying from stroke each year [176] and many more living with chronic disability [177]. Specialized treatment in a stroke unit, compared to treatment in a general medical ward, reduces the odds of death or disability at 12 months post-stroke [178]. Early rehabilitation is described as an important goal of stroke unit care; however, there is only limited information about what early rehabilitation entails and who provides it. Exactly how early (even within 24–48 h) rehabilitation should start is controversial [179], and protocols are affected by local practices [180–182].

A systematic review of the literature from 1980 to 2005 was conducted focusing on rehabilitation interventions after neuroinjury [183]. The efficacy of a given intervention was classified as strong (supported by at least two randomized controlled trials [RCTs], moderate [supported by a single RCT], or limited [supported by other types of studies in the absence of RCTs]). The majority of interventions were only supported by limited evidence. However, at least one study showed that neurorehabilitation increases the chance of successful reintegration in a productive society [184].

Neuropsychological Approach to the Brain-Injured Patient

Caregiver

Traumatic brain injury (TBI) occurs within the relational context of family, friendships, and workplaces with such rapid and dramatic changes that relatives can barely perceive the patient's shift from a critical to chronic illness condition [185–187]. Generally, caregivers demonstrate a great willingness to adjust their lives to accommodate the needs of the injured person [188, 189]; they may experience role changes and have to take on more responsibility than before the TBI [190–195] at the expense of considerable physical and social burden [196–200]. Emotional support and practical advice, as well as a clear disclosure of the patent's potential for rehabilitation and improved outcome, are highly valued by family members once the patient reaches the rehabilitative phase [201–203].

An informed assessment of the rehabilitation potential of the patient should be provided to the family in a multidisciplinary meeting and should include details of individualized rehabilitative projects with a variety of media, such as pamphlets illustrating diagnostics and therapeutic schedules, medical literature references, video, and a list of the patient's focused multidisciplinary meetings [204, 205]. The educational material provided to the family and caregiver should be (a) *appropriate*, relevant and pertinent for each patient and caregiver and based on actual needs; (b) *accessible*, use simple language that can be understood by a lay person; and (c) *acceptable*, provided gradually and pertinent to the different rehabilitative phases of the patient. Preformatted TBI rehabilitation programs are now available, such as the Brain Integration Program [206, 207], which provides support to patients recovering from TBI and their caregivers and has shown significant psychological benefit for both.

While the degree of family support and their role as caregivers differs among cultures and financial capabilities [195], the patient's quality of life seems to be multifactorial [196] but, above all, is reliably affected by the efficacy of the neurorehabilitation team [208]. The perceived quality of life should be assessed by utilizing specific tools, such as Qolibri, a recently validated scale for individuals with TBI [209–211].

Patient Assessment

The levels of the cognitive functioning scale (LCF [3] and LCF-revised [LCF-R] [212]) consist of a systematic observation, outlining the patient's neuropsychological features from ICU discharge, through the rehabilitation process, and, when feasible, to reentry into the home. During coma recovery, in addition to qualitative measurement methods, such as LCF-R, which classifies the patient into a defined cognitive-behavioral level, further measures are needed. Standardized behavioral quantitative assessment scales are, in general, employed in the early coma recovery phase (LCF 2–3). The most commonly used are:

- Coma Recovery Scale (CRS) [213] and CRS-R [214]
- Coma/Near Coma Scale (CNC) [215]
- Sensory Stimulation Assessment Measure (SSAM) [216]
- Western Neuro Sensory Stimulation Profile (WNSSP) [217]
- Wessex Head Injury Matrix (WHIM) [218]

Among the serial assessments described above, the Coma Recovery Scale (CRS) [213] and its revised version (CRS-R)

[214, 219] are the most sensitive scales used when the patient is still in a VS or MCS or is recovering from DOC; these scales are an attempt to unify the nomenclature and specific diagnostic criteria for a differential diagnosis for DOC patients [220, 221].

While the above longitudinal assessments of patient behavior and consciousness have been successfully used in a variety of post-comatose patients, they appear to be inconsistent in following the fluctuations seen in these patients; the latency of the performances are typical of the MCS, in which a much wider range of emotional stimulations by proxy may facilitate the patient's responsiveness [205]. The initial rehabilitative phase of all patients with DOC is affected by the persistence of significant comorbidities. Evaluations should be short and frequent, possibly in a quiet environment to verify the *intentionality*, *frequency*, and *consistency* of interactive behaviors. The patient's performance may be impaired by underlying neurological deficits, such as sensorimotor deficits, aphasia, apraxia, and lack of initiation or initiative (inertia); therefore, the evaluation should be limited to commands the patient is actually *able to obey*.

Agitation and restlessness, frequently seen in the early recovery phases of the DOC stage, are specific characteristics of PTA and coincide with level 4–5 of the LCF-R scale (*confused-agitated* or *not agitated*). In this phase, lasting two to four times longer than coma duration [222], the patient is unable to memorize everyday events of the last 24 h [51]. PTA may be a significant tool to predict a patient's cognitive recovery [223] post-TBI [224–227]. Specific tools, such as the Galveston Orientation Amnesia test GOAT [228] or the Westmead Post-Traumatic Amnesia Scale (WPTAS) [229], have been specifically created to measure PTA deficits. Posttraumatic amnesia may also include an excess of behaviors, including psychomotor agitation, which can be observed as a combination of aggression, akathisia, disinhibition, and emotional lability [50]. The reported incidence of psychomotor agitation in the acute coma-emerging stage differs among various studies, from 33 to 50 % [50], due to variation of the criteria used to define agitation and its severity. Early resolution of this phase is associated with improved outcome [26], although the persistence of aggressive behavior can be responsible for poor social integration. The clinical scales that have been validated to assess agitation/aggression following severe TBI include the Agitated Behavior Scale (ABS) [230], the Overt Aggression Scale (OAS) [231], the Neurobehavioral Rating Scale (NBRS) [232], and the Neuropsychiatric Inventory (NPI) [233].

Neuropsychological Treatment

During the ICU stay, when severe ABI patients suffer a lack of consciousness or can give only generalized responses (LCF-R = 1 - 2) several clinical intervention schedules have

been proposed [234]. Pharmacological interventions, sensory stimulation, and physical therapy have been all utilized for rehabilitative purposes [235].

Contradictory data have been reported on the effectiveness of multisensorial stimulation [236–238] versus specific stimulation, such as active music therapy. The latter type of therapy has been useful in improving the patient's collaboration, reducing behavioral disorders, improving initiative in cases of inertia, and calming acutely agitated patients [238, 239].

In the early phase of the ICU stay, rhythmic and balanced stimulation is needed, together with organizing the patient's environment to make it reassuring and familiar and avoiding, as much as possible, intrusive and uncomfortable stimuli to the patient. In the ICU or post-acute rehabilitation setting, restraining noises and confusion, creating an adequate rhythm between brightness and darkness, and alternating between therapeutic measures and periods of relaxation require a very integrated teamwork and specific training for the caregiver. As a general principle, during the early coma recovery stage (LCF-R 4), cognitive-behavioral techniques are rarely applicable in the ICU. Simple stimulation provided from the professional staff and relatives is still applicable and should be pleasant and reassuring.

As far as behavioral nonpharmacological therapy, when self-awareness of cognitive deficits improves [240], a more intensive rehabilitation plan is indicated and should be encouraged. However, lack of self-awareness and motivation to participate in rehabilitation programs [241–243] can severely compromise the patient's quality of life (QoL) [244–246].

In summary, a neuropsychological approach to the severe TBI and ABI patient consists of a gradual but comprehensive holistic treatment plan involving the patient together with his/her caregiver that should be started as soon as feasible in the ICU or immediately after discharge from the acute phase. An intensive rehabilitation plan improves the patient's prognosis and significantly contributes to their social reintegration.

References

1. Teasdale G, Jennett B. Assessment of coma and impaired consciousness. A practical scale. Lancet. 1974;2(7872):81–4.
2. Rappaport M, Hall KM, Hopkins K, Belleza T, Cope DN. Disability Rating Scale for severe head trauma: coma to community. Arch Phys Med Rehabil. 1982;63:118–23.
3. Hagen C, Malkmus D, Durham P. Levels of cognitive functioning. In: Rehabilitation of the head injured adult; comprehensive physical management. Downey: Professional Staff Association of Rancho Los Amigos Hospital, Inc; 1979.
4. Jennett B, Bond M. Assessment of outcome after severe brain damage. Lancet. 1975;1(7905):480–4.
5. Jennett B, MacMillan R. Epidemiology of head injury. Br Med J (Clin Res Ed). 1981;282:101–4.
6. Jennett B. Clinical assessment of consciousness. Introduction of modern concepts in neurotraumatology. Acta Neurochir Suppl. 1986;36:90.

7. Plum F, Posner JB. The diagnosis of stupor and coma. 3rd ed. Philadelphia: FA Davis; 1982.

8. Perkes I, Baguley IJ, Nott MT, Menon DK. A review of paroxysmal sympathetic hyperactivity after acquired brain injury. Ann Neurol. 2010;68:126–35.

9. Andrews K. International Working Party on the management of the vegetative state. Brain Inj. 1996;10(11):797–806.

10. Andrews K, Murphy L, Munday R, Littlewood C. Misdiagnosis of the vegetative state: retrospective study in a rehabilitation unit. BMJ. 1996;313:13–6.

11. Childs N, Mercer WN, Childs HW. Accuracy of diagnosis of the persistent vegetative state. Neurology. 1993;43:1465–7.

12. Estraneo A, Moretta P, Loreto V, Lanzillo B, Santoro L, Trojano L. Late recovery after traumatic, anoxic, or hemorrhagic long-lasting vegetative state. Neurology. 2010;75:239–45.

13. Clauss R, Nel W. Drug induced arousal from the permanent vegetative state. NeuroRehabilitation. 2006;21:23–8.

14. Vespa PM, Nuwer MR, Nenov V, et al. Increased incidence and impact of nonconvulsive and convulsive seizures after traumatic brain injury as detected by continuous electroencephalographic monitoring. J Neurosurg. 1999;91(5):750–60.

15. Gerstenbrand F. Das Traumatische Apallische Syndrom. Vienna/New York: Springer; 1967.

16. von Wild K, Gerstenbrand F, Dolce G, et al. Guidelines on quality management of patients in apallic syndrome (vegetative state). Eur J Trauma Emerg Surg. 2007;33:268–92.

17. Tomaiuolo F, Carlesimo GA, Di Paola M, et al. Gross morphology and morphometric sequelae in the hippocampus, fornix, and corpus callosum of patients with severe non-missile traumatic brain injury without macroscopic detectable lesions: a T1 weighted MRI study. J Neurol Neurosurg Neuropsychol. 2004;75:1314–22.

18. Graham DI, Mclellan D, Adams JH, Doyle D, Kerr A, Murray LS. The neuropathology of the vegetative state and severe disability after non-missile head injury. Acta Neurochir. 1983;32:65–7.

19. Mclellan DR, Adams JH, Graham DI, et al. The structural basis of the vegetative state and prolonged coma after non-missile head injury. In: Papo P, Cohadon F, Massarotti M, editors. Le Coma Traumatique. Padova: Liviana Editrice; 1986. p. 165.

20. Adams JH. Brain damage in fatal non-missile head injury in man. In: Braakman R, editor. Handbook of clinical neurology. Vol. 13(57). Head injury. Amsterdam/New York: Elsevier Science Publishers B; 1990. p. 43.

21. Multi-Society Task Force on PVS. Medical aspects of the persistent vegetative state (1). N Engl J Med. 1994;330:1499–508.

22. Royal College of Physicians. The permanent vegetative state. Review by a working group convened by the Royal College of Physicians and endorsed by the Conference of Medical Royal Colleges and their faculties of the United Kingdom. J R Coll Physicians Lond. 1996;30(2):119–21.

23. Laureys S, Celesia GG, Cohadon F, et al; European Task Force on Disorders of Consciousness. Unresponsive wakefulness syndrome: a new name for the vegetative state or apallic syndrome. BMC Med. 2010;8:68.

24. Formisano R, Pistoia F, Sarà M. Disorders of consciousness: a taxonomy to be changed? Brain Inj. 2011;25:638–9.

25. Beaumont JG, Kenealy PM. Incidence and prevalence of the vegetative and minimally conscious states. Neuropsychol Rehabil. 2005;15(3–4):184–9.

26. Formisano R, Bivona U, Penta F, et al. Early clinical predictive factors during coma recovery. Acta Neurochir Suppl. 2005;93:201–5.

27. Missori P, Miscusi M, Formisano R, et al. Magnetic resonance imaging flow void changes after cerebrospinal fluid shunt in post-traumatic hydrocephalus: clinical correlations and outcome. Neurosurg Rev. 2006;29:224–8.

28. Jennett B, Plum F. Persistent vegetative state after brain damage. Lancet. 1972;1(7753):734–7.

29. Danze F. Coma and the vegetative states. Soins. 1993;(569):4–10.

30. Kelly DF, Gonzalo IT, Cohan P, Berman N, Swerdloff R, Wang C. Hypopituitarism following traumatic brain injury and aneurysmal subarachnoid hemorrhage: a preliminary report. J Neurosurg. 2000;93:743–52.

31. Benvenga S, Campenni A, Ruggeri RM, Trimarchi F. Clinical review 113: hypopituitarism secondary to head trauma. J Clin Endocrinol Metab. 2000;85:1353–61.

32. Masel BE. Rehabilitation and hypopituitarism after traumatic brain injury. Growth Horm IGF Res. 2004;14 Suppl A:S108–13.

33. Agha A, Rogers B, Sherlock M, et al. Anterior pituitary dysfunction in survivors of traumatic brain injury. J Clin Endocrinol Metab. 2004;89:4929–36.

34. Agha A, Phillips J, O'Kelly P, Tormey W, Thompson CJ. The natural history of post-traumatic hypopituitarism: implications for assessment and treatment. Am J Med. 2005;118:1416.

35. Agha A, Thompson CJ. Anterior pituitary dysfunction following traumatic brain injury (TBI). Clin Endocrinol (Oxf). 2006;64:481–8.

36. Aimaretti G, Ghigo E. Traumatic brain injury and hypopituitarism. ScientificWorldJournal. 2005;5:777–81.

37. Aimaretti G, Ambrosio MR, Di Somma C, et al. Hypopituitarism induced by traumatic brain injury in the transition phase. J Endocrinol Invest. 2005;28:984–9.

38. Bondanelli M, Ambrosio MR, Zatelli MC, De Marinis L, degli Uberti EC. Hypopituitarism after traumatic brain injury. Eur J Endocrinol. 2005;152:679–91.

39. Leal-Cerro A, Flores JM, Rincon M, et al. Prevalence of hypopituitarism and growth hormone deficiency in adults long-term after severe traumatic brain injury. Clin Endocrinol (Oxf). 2005;62:525–32.

40. Popovic V. GH deficiency as the most common pituitary defect after TBI: clinical implications. Pituitary. 2005;8:239–43.

41. Popovic V, Aimaretti G, Casanueva FF, Ghigo E. Hypopituitarism following traumatic brain injury (TBI): call for attention. J Endocrinol Invest. 2005;28(5 Suppl):61–4.

42. Schneider HJ, Schneider M, Saller B, et al. Prevalence of anterior pituitary insufficiency 3 and 12 months after traumatic brain injury. Eur J Endocrinol. 2006;154:259–65.

43. Medical Disability Society. Report of a working party on the management of traumatic brain injury. London: The Development Trust for the Young Disabled; 1988.

44. Formisano R, Voogt RD, Buzzi MG, et al. Time interval of oral feeding recovery as a prognostic factor in severe traumatic brain injury. Brain Inj. 2004;18:103–9.

45. Formisano R, Carlesimo GA, Sabbatini M, et al. Clinical predictors and neuropsychological outcome in severe traumatic brain injury patients. Acta Neurochir (Wien). 2004;146:457–62.

46. Mahoney FI, Barthel DW. Functional evaluation: the Barthel Index. Md State Med J. 1965;14:61–5.

47. Reyes RL, Bhattacharya AK, Heller D. Traumatic head injury: restlessness and agitation as prognosticators of physical and psychological improvement in patients. Arch Phys Med Rehabil. 1981;62:20–3.

48. Corrigan JD, Mysiw WJ. Agitation following traumatic head injury: equivocal evidence for a discrete stage of cognitive recovery. Arch Phys Med Rehabil. 1988;69:487–92.

49. Corrigan JD, Bogner JA. Factor structure of the Agitated Behavior Scale. J Clin Exp Neuropsychol. 1994;16:386–92.

50. Sandel ME, Mysiw WJ. The agitated brain injured patient. Part 1: definitions, differential diagnosis, and assessment. Arch Phys Med Rehabil. 1996;77:617–23.

51. Russel WR, Smith A. Post-traumatic amnesia in closed head injury. Arch Neurol. 1961;5:4–17.

52. Gerstenbrand F, Poewe W, Aichner F, Saltuari L. Klüver-Bucy syndrome in man: experiences with posttraumatic cases. Neurosci Behav Rev. 1983;7:413–7.

53. Goscinski I, Kwiatkowski S, Polak J, Orlowiejska M, Partyk A. The Klüver-Bucy syndrome. J Neurosurg Sci. 1997;41:269–72.

54. Formisano R, Saltuari L, Gerstenbrand F. Presence of Klüver-Bucy syndrome as a positive prognostic feature for the remission of traumatic prolonged distirbances of consciousness. Acta Neurol Scand. 1995;91:54–7.

55. Dolce G, Sazbon L. The post-traumatic vegetative state. Stuttgart: Thieme; 2002.

56. Baguley IJ, Nicholls JL, Felmingham KL, Crooks J, Gurka JA, Wade JD. Dysautonomia after traumatic brain injury: a forgotten syndrome? J Neurol Neurosurg Psychiatry. 1999;67:39–43.

57. Intiso D, Formisano R, Grasso MG, et al. Neurovegetative disorders after severe head injury. J Auton Nerv Syst. 1993;43(Suppl):86–7.

58. Sazbon L, Najenson T, Tartakovsky M, Becker E, Grosswasser Z. Widespread periarticular new-bone formation in long-term comatose patients. J Bone Joint Surg Br. 1981;63-B(1):120–5.

59. Ippolito E, Formisano R, Caterini R, Farsetti P, Penta F. Resection of elbow ossification and continuous passive motion in postcomatose patients. J Hand Surg. 1999;24:546–53.

60. Ippolito E, Formisano R, Farsetti P, Caterini R, Penta F. Excision for the treatment of periarticular ossification of the knee in patients who have a traumatic brain injury. J Bone Joint Surg. 1999;81:783–9.

61. Ippolito E, Formisano R, Caterini R, Farsetti P, Penta F. Operative treatment of heterotopic hip ossification in patients with coma after brain injury. Clin Orthop Relat Res. 1999;365:130–8.

62. Kline BL, Morawetz RB, Swaid SN. Indirect injury of the optic nerve. Neurosurgery. 1984;14:756–64.

63. Latronico N, Peli E, Botteri M. Critical illness myopathy and neuropathy. Curr Opin Crit Care. 2005;11:126–32.

64. Jellinger KA. Parkinsonism and persistent vegetative state after head injury. J Neurol Neurosurg Psychiatry. 2004;75:1082–3.

65. Formisano R, Saltuari L, Sailer U, Birbarmer G, Gerstenbrand G. Post-traumatic cerebellar syndrome. New Trends Clin Neuropharmacol. 1987;(1–2):115–8.

66. Levin HS, Madison CF, Bailey CB, Meyers CA, Eisenberg HM, Guinto FC. Mutism after closed head injury. Arch Neurol. 1983;40:601–6.

67. Vogel M, von Cramon D. Articulatory recovery after traumatic mutism. Folia Phonia (Basel). 1983;35:294–309.

68. Bricolo A, Turazzi S, Facciolo F. Combined clinical and EEG examinations for assessment of severity of acute head injuries. Acta Neurochir Suppl (Wien). 1979;28:35–9.

69. Synek VM. EEG abnormality grades and subdivision of prognostic importance in traumatic and anoxic coma in adults. Clin Electroencephalogr. 1998;19:160–6.

70. Facco E. The role of the EEG in brain injury. Intensive Care Med. 1999;25:872–7.

71. Rae-Grant AD, Eckert N, Barbour PI, et al. Outcome of severe brain injury: a multimodality neurophysiologic study. J Trauma. 1996;40:401–7.

72. Gutling E, Gonser A, Imof HG, Landis T. EEG reactivity in the prognosis of severe head injury. Neurology. 1995;45:915–8.

73. Kane NM, Moss TH, Curry SH, Butler SR. Quantitative electroencephalographic evaluation of non-fatal and fatal traumatic coma. Electroencephalogr Clin Neurophysiol. 1998;106:244–50.

74. Klein HJ, Rath SA, Goppel F. The use of EEG spectral analysis after thiopental bolus in the prognostic evaluation of comatose patients with brain injuries. Acta Neurochir Suppl (Wien). 1988;42:31–4.

75. Fischgold H, Matis P, Fischgold H. Obnubilations. Comas et stupeurs. Etudes Electroencephalografiques. Paris : Masson et Cie ; (Niort : impr. Soulisse et Cassegrain). Electroenceph Clin Neurophisiol 1959;(Suppl 11):125.

76. Harada M, Minami R, Hattori E, Nakamura K, Kabashima K. Sleep in brain-damaged patients. An all night study of 105 cases. Kumamoto Med J. 1976;29:110–27.

77. Ron S, Algom D, Hary D, Cohen M. Time-related changes in the distribution of sleep stages in brain injured patients. Electroencephalogr Clin Neurophysiol. 1980;48:432–41.

78. Giubilei F, Formisano R, Fiorini M, et al. Sleep abnormalities in traumatic apallic syndrome. J Neurol Neurosurg Psychiatry. 1995;58:484–6.

79. Valente M, Placidi F, Oliveira AJ, et al. Sleep organization pattern as a prognostic marker at the subacute stage of post-traumatic coma. Clin Neurophysiol. 2002;113:1798–805.

80. Chatrian GE, Bergamasco B, Bricolo A, Frost Jr JD, Prior PF. IFCN recommended standards for electrophysiologic monitoring in comatose and other unresponsive states. Report of an IFCN committee. Electroencephalogr Clin Neurophysiol. 1996;99:103–22.

81. Facco E, Munari M, Baratto F, Dona B, Giron GP. Somatosensory evocated potentials in severe head trauma. Electroencephalogr Clin Neurophysiol. 1990;41:330–41.

82. Greenberg RP, Becher DP, Miller DJ, Mayer DJ. Evaluation of brain function in severe human head trauma with multimodality evoked potentials. Part 2: localization of brain dysfunction and correlation with posttraumatic neurological conditions. J Neurosurg. 1977;47:163–77.

83. Inghilleri M, Formisano R, Berardelli A, Saltuari L, Gerstenbrand F, Manfredi M. Transcranial electrical stimulation in patients with apallic syndrome. Acta Neurol Scand. 1994;89:15–7.

84. Riganello F, Sannita WG. Residual brain processing in the vegetative state. J Psychophysiol. 2009;23:18–26.

85. Daltrozzo J, Wioland N, Mutschler V, Kotchoubey B. Predicting coma and other low responsive patients outcome using event-related brain potentials: a meta-analysis. Clin Neurophysiol. 2007;118:606–14.

86. Fischer C, Luauté J, Némoz C, Morlet D, Kirkorian G, Mauguière F. Editorial response: evoked potentials can be used as a prognosis factor for awakening. Crit Care Med. 2006;34:2025.

87. Fischer C, Morlet D, Bouchet P, Luaute J, Jourdan C, Salord F. Mismatch negativity and late auditory evoked potentials in comatose patients. Clin Neurophysiol. 1999;110:1601–10.

88. Duncan CC, Barry RJ, Connolly JF, et al. Event-related potentials in clinical research: guidelines for eliciting, recording, and quantifying mismatch negativity, P300, and N400. Clin Neurophysiol. 2009;120:1883–908.

89. Marshall LF, Marshall SB, Klauber MR, et al. The diagnosis of head injury requires a classification based on computed axial tomography. J Neurotrauma. 1992;9 Suppl 1:S287–92.

90. Lee B, Newberg A. Neuroimaging in traumatic brain imaging. NeuroRx. 2005;2:372–83.

91. Kampfl A, Schmutzhard E, Pfausler B, et al. Prediction of recovery from post-traumatic vegetative state with cerebral magnetic resonance imaging. Lancet. 1998;351:1763–7.

92. Wilson JT, Wiedmann KD, Hadley DM, Condon B, Teasdale G, Brooks DN. Early and late magnetic resonance imaging and neuropsychological outcome after head injury. J Neurol Neurosurg Psychiatry. 1988;51:391–6.

93. Barzo P, Marmarou A, Fatouros P, Corwin F, Dunbar J. Magnetic resonance imaging-monitored acute blood-brain barrier changes in experimental traumatic brain injury. J Neurosurg. 1996;85:1113–21.

94. Arfanakis K, Hermann BP, Rogers BP, Carew JD, Seidenberg M, Meyerand ME. Diffusion tensor MRI in temporal lobe epilepsy. Magn Reson Imaging. 2002;20:511–9.

95. Goetz P, Blamire A, Rajagopalan B, Cadoux-Hudson T, Young D, Styles P. Increase in apparent diffusion coefficient in normal appearing white matter following human traumatic brain injury correlates with injury severity. J Neurotrauma. 2004;21:645.

96. Shanmuganathan K, Gullapalli RP, Mirvis SE, Roys S, Murthy P. Whole-brain apparent diffusion coefficient in traumatic brain injury: correlation with Glasgow Coma Scale score. AJNR Am J Neuroradiol. 2004;25:539–44.

97. Naganawa S, Sato C, Ishihra S, et al. Serial evaluation of diffusion tensor brain fiber tracking in a patient with severe diffuse axonal injury. AJNR Am J Neuroradiol. 2004;25:1553–6.

98. Huisman TA, Schwamm LH, Schaefer PW, et al. Diffusion tensor imaging as potential biomarker of white matter injury in diffuse axonal injury. AJNR Am J Neuroradiol. 2004;25:370–6.

99. Van Putten HP, Bouwhuis MG, Muizelaar JP, Lyeth BG, Berman RF. Diffusion-weighted imaging of edema following traumatic brain injury in rats: effects of secondary hypoxia. J Neurotrauma. 2005;22:857–72.

100. Cherubini A, Luccichenti G, Peran P, et al. Multimodal fMRI tractography in normal subjects and in clinically recovered traumatic brain injury patients. Neuroimage. 2007;34:1331–41.

101. Garnett MR, Blamire AM, Corkill RG, et al. Abnormal cerebral blood volume in regions of contused and normal appearing brain following traumatic brain injury using perfusion magnetic resonance imaging. J Neurotrauma. 2001;18:585–93.

102. Giugni E, Sabatini U, Hagberg GE, Formisano R, Castriota-Scanderbeg A. Fast detection of diffuse axonal damage in severe traumatic brain injury: comparison between gradientrecalled echo and turbo proton echo-planar spectroscopic imaging MRI sequences. AJNR Am J Neuroradiol. 2005;26:1140–8.

103. Tomaiuolo F, Bivona U, Lerch JP, et al. Memory and anatomical change in severe non missile traumatic brain injury: 1 vs 8 years follow-up. Brain Res Bull. 2012;87:373–82.

104. Owen AM, Coleman MR, Boly M, Davis MH, Laureys S, Pickard JD. Detecting awareness in the vegetative state. Science. 2006;313:1402.

105. Schiff ND. Central thalamic deep-brain stimulation in the severely injured brain: rationale and proposed mechanisms of action. Ann N Y Acad Sci. 2009;1157:101–16.

106. Laureys S. Functional neuroimaging in the vegetative state. NeuroRehabilitation. 2004;19:335–41.

107. Schnakers C, Perrin F, Schabus M, et al. Voluntary brain processing in disorder of consciousness. Neurology. 2008;71:1614–20.

108. Cruse D, Chennu S, Chatelle C, et al. Relationship between etiology and covert cognition in the minimally conscious state. Neurology. 2012;78:816.

109. Monti MM, Vanhaudenhuyse A, Coleman MR, et al. Willful modulation of brain activity in disorders of consciousness. N Engl J Med. 2010;362:579–89.

110. Bruno MA, Vanhaudenhuyse A, Thibaut A, Moonen G, Laureys S. From unresponsive wakefulness to minimally conscious PLUS and functional locked-in syndromes: recent advances in our understanding of disorders of consciousness. J Neurol. 2011; 258(7):1373–84.

111. Formisano R, D'Ippolito M, Catani C. Functional locked-in syndrome as recovery phase of vegetative state. Brain Injury (in press).

112. Jacobs A, Put E, Ingels M, Put T, Bossuyt A. One-year follow-up of technetium-99 m-HMPAO SPECT in mild head injury. J Nucl Med. 1996;37:1605–9.

113. Baulieu F, Rournier P, Baulieu JL, et al. Technetium-99m ECD single photon emission computed tomography in brain trauma : comparison of early scintigraphic findings with long-term neuropsychological outcome. J Neuroimaging. 2001;11:112–20.

114. Oder W, Goldenberg G, Spatt J, Podreka I, Binder H, Deecke L. Behavioural and psychosocial sequelae of severe closed head injury and regional several blood flow: a SPECT study. J Neurol Neurosurg Psychiatry. 1992;55:475–80.

115. Boly M, Faymonville ME, Peigneux P, et al. Auditory processing in severely brain injured patients : differences between the

116. minimally conscious state and the persistent vegetative state. Arch Neurol. 2004;61:233–8.

116. Alavi A. Functional and anatomic studies of head injury. J Neuropsychiatry Clin Neurosci. 1989;1:S45–50.

117. Rao N, Tursky PA, Polcyn RE, Nickels J, Matthews CG, Flynn MM. 18F positron emission computed tomography in closed head injury. Arch Phys Med Rehabil. 1984;65:780–5.

118. Bouma GJ, Muizelaar JP. Cerebral blood flow, cerebral blood volume, and cerebrovascular reactivity after severe head injury. J Neurotrauma. 1992;9 Suppl 1:333–48.

119. Martin NA, Doberstein C, Zane C, Caron MJ, Thomas K, Becker DP. Post-traumatic cerebral arterial spasm: transcranial Doppler ultrasound, cerebral blood flow and angiographic findings. J Neurosurg. 1992;77:575–83.

120. Aaslid R, Huber P, Nornes H. Evaluation of cerebrovascular spasm with trancranial Doppler ultrasound. J Neurosurg. 1984;60: 37–41.

121. International Classification of Functioning, Disability and Health (ICF). World Health Organization. Available at: http://www3.who.int/icf/icftemplate.cfm. Accessed 6 July 2012.

122. Gutenbrunner C, Ward AB, Chamberlain MA. White book on physical and rehabilitation medicine in Europe. J Rehabil Med. 2007;45 Suppl:6–47.

123. Turner-Stokes L, Nair A, Sedki I, Disler PB, Wade DT. Multidisciplinary rehabilitation for acquired brain injury in adults of working age. Cochrane Database Sys Rev. 2005;(3):CD004170.

124. Messerole E, Peine P, Wittkopp S, Marini JJ, Albert RK. The pragmatics of prone positioning. Am J Respir Crit Care Med. 2002;165:1359–63.

125. Kopterides P, Siempos II, Armaganidis A. Prone positioning in hypoxemic respiratory failure: meta-analysis of randomized controlled trials. J Crit Care. 2009;24:89–100.

126. Chang AT, Boots RJ, Hodges PW, Thomas PJ, Paratz JD. Standing with the assistance of a tilt table improves minute ventilation in chronic critically ill patients. Arch Phys Med Rehabil. 2004;85: 1972–6.

127. Winkelman C, Higgins PA, Chen YJ, Levine AD. Cytokines in chronically critically ill patients after activity and rest. Biol Res Nurs. 2007;8:261–71.

128. LeBlanc A, Gogia P, Schneider V, Krebs J, Schonfeld E, Evans H. Calf muscle area and strength changes after five weeks of horizontal bed rest. Am J Sports Med. 1988;16:624–9.

129. Trappe S, Creer A, Minchev K, et al. Human soleus single muscle fiber function with exercise or nutrition countermeasures during 60 days of bed rest. Am J Physiol Regul Integr Comp Physiol. 2008;294:R939–47.

130. Ferrando AA, Paddon-Jones D, Wolfe RR. Bed rest and myopathies. Curr Opin Clin Nutr Metab Care. 2006;9:410–5.

131. Gracies JM. Pathophysiology of spastic paresis. I: paresis and soft tissue changes. Muscle Nerve. 2005;31:535–51.

132. Gracies JM. Pathophysiology of spastic paresis. II: emergence of muscle overactivity. Muscle Nerve. 2005;31:552–71.

133. Bryden J. How many head injured? The epidemiology of post head injury disability. In: Wood RL, Eames P, editors. Models of brain injury rehabilitation. London: Chapman & Hall; 1990.

134. Clemenzi A, Formisano R, Matteis M, et al. Care management of spasticity with botulinum toxin-A in patients with severe acquired brain injury: a 1-year follow-up prospective study. Brain Inj. 2012;26:979–83.

135. Stokic DS, Yablon SA, Hayes A. Comparison of clinical and neurophysiologic responses to intrathecal baclofen bolus administration in moderate to severe spasticity after acquired brain injury. Arch Phy Med Rehabil. 2005;86(9):1801.

136. Driver S, Rees K, O'Connor J, Lox C. Aquatics, health-promoting self-care behaviours and adults with brain injuries. Brain Inj. 2006;20:133–41.

137. Golisz K. Occupational therapy practice guidelines for adults with traumatic brain injury. Bethesda: American Occupational Therapy Association (AOTA) Press; 2009.

138. Formisano R, Penta F, Bivona U, Mastrilli F, Giustini M, Taggi F. Diagnostic-therapeutic protocol of the patient with severe traumatic brain injury and prolonged coma. Rapporti ISTISAN. 2001;9 Suppl(3):1–63.

139. Giannantoni A, Silvestro D, Siracusano S, et al. Urological dysfunction and neurological outcome in coma survivors after traumatic brain injury in the postacute and chronic phase. Arch Phys Med Rehabil. 2011;92:1134–8.

140. Terré R, Mearin F. Prospective evaluation of oro-pharyngeal dysphagia after severe traumatic brain injury. Brain Inj. 2007;21: 1411–7.

141. Winstein CJ. Neurogenic dysphagia. Frequency, progression, and outcome in adults following head injury. Phys Ther. 1983;63: 1992–7.

142. Fleminger S, Greenwood RJ, Olivier DL. Pharmacological management for agitation and aggression in people with acquired brain injury. Cochrane Database Syst Rev. 2006;(4):CD003299.

143. Roberts I. Barbiturates for acute traumatic brain injury. Cochrane Database Syst Rev. 2000;2, CD000033.

144. Alderson P, Roberts I. Corticosteroids for acute traumatic brain injury. Cochrane Database Syst Rev. 2000;2, CD000196.

145. Langham J, Goldfrad C, Teasdale G, et al. Calcium channel blockers for acute traumatic brain injury. Cochrane Database Syst Rev. 2000;2, CD000565.

146. Schierhout G, Roberts I. Anti-epileptic drugs for preventing seizures following acute traumatic brain injury. Cochrane Database Syst Rev. 2000;(2):CD000173.

147. Forsyth RJ, Jayamoni B, Paine TC. Monoaminergic agonists for acute traumatic brain injury. Cochrane Database Syst Rev. 2006;(4):CD003984.

148. Feeney DM, Sutton RL. Pharmacotherapy for recovery of function after brain injury. Crit Rev Neurobiol. 1987;3:135–97.

149. Van Vleymen B, Van Zandijcke M. Piracetam in the treatment of myoclonus: an overview. Acta Neurol Belg. 1996;96:270–80.

150. Ikeda A, Shibasaki H, Tashiro K, Mizuno Y, Kimura J. Clinical trial of piracetam in patients with myoclonus: nationwide multiinstitution study in Japan. The Myoclonus/Piracetam Study Group. Mov Disord. 1996;11:691–700.

151. Guerrini R, De Lorey TM, Bonanni P, et al. Cortical myoclonus in Angelman syndrome. Ann Neurol. 1996;40:39–48.

152. Ben-Menachem E, Falter U. Efficacy and tolerability of levetiracetam 3000 mg/d in patients with refractory partial seizures: a multicenter, double-blind, responder-selected study evaluating monotherapy. European Levetiracetam Study Group. Epilepsia. 2000;41:1276–83.

153. Cereghino JJ, Biton V, Abou-Khalil B, Dreifuss F, Gauer LJ, Leppik I. Levetiracetam for partial seizures: results of a double-blind, randomized clinical trial. Neurology. 2000;55:236–42.

154. Shorvon SD, Lowenthal A, Janz D, Bielen E, Loiseau P. Multicenter, double-blind, randomized, placebo controlled trial of levetiracetam as add-on therapy in patients with refractory partial seizures. European Levetiracetam Study Group. Epilepsia. 2000;41:1179–86.

155. Genton P, Sadzot B, Fejerman N, et al. Levetiracetam in a broad population of patients with refractory epilepsy: interim results of the international SKATE trial. Acta Neurol Scand. 2006;113: 387–94.

156. Schulte EJ, Pfeiffer J. Preliminary experience with Piracetam during intensive care of severe head injuries (author's transl). Med Klin. 1974;69:1235–8.

157. Calliauw L, Marchau M. Clinical trial of piracetam in disorders of consciousness due to head injury. Acta Anaesthesiol Belg. 1975;26:51–60.

158. Gobert JG. Genesis of a drug: Piracetam. Metabolism and biochemical research. J Pharm Belg. 1972;27:281–304.

159. Giurgea C, Mouravieff-Lesuisse F. Central hypoxia models and correlations with aging brain. Neuropsychoparmacology. 1978;2:1623.

160. Heiss WD, Kessler J, Karbe H, Fink GR, Pawlik G. Cerebral glucose metabolism as a predictor of recovery from aphasia in ischemic stroke. Arch Neurol. 1993;50:958–64.

161. Giurgea C, Moyersoons F. The pharmacology of callosal transmission: a general survey. In: Russel I, Van Hof M, Berlucchi G, editors. Structure and function of cerebral commissures. London: Macmillan; 1979. p. 283.

162. Huber W, Willmes K, Poeck K, Van Vleymen B, Deberdt W. Piracetam as an adjuvant to language therapy for aphasia: a randomized double-blind placebo-controlled pilot study. Arch Phys Med Rehabil. 1997;78:245–50.

163. Dimond S. Drugs to improve learning in man: implications and neuropsychological analysis. In: Knight R, Bakker O, editors. The neuropsychology of learning disorders. London: University Park Press; 1979. p. 367.

164. Dixon CE, Ma X, Marion DW. Reduced evoked release of acetylcholine in the rodent neocortex following traumatic brain injury. Brain Res. 1997;749:127–30.

165. Wengel SP, Roccaforte WH, Burke WJ, et al. Behavioral complications associated with donepezil. Am J Psychiatry. 1998;155: 1632–3.

166. Taverni JP, Seliger G, Lichtman SW. Donepezil medicated memory improvement in traumatic brain injury during post acute rehabilitation. Brain Inj. 1998;12:77–80.

167. Whitlock JA. Brain injury, cognitive impairment, and donepezil. J Head Trauma Rehabil. 1999;14:424–7.

168. Whelan FJ, Walker MS, Schultz SK. Donepezil in the treatment of cognitive disfunction associated wuth traumatic brain injury. Ann Clin Psychiatry. 2000;12:131–5.

169. Tenovuo O. Central acetylcholinesterase inhibitors in the treatment of chronic traumatic brain injury clinical experience in 111 patients. Prog Neuropsychopharmacol Biol Psychiatry. 2005;29:61–7.

170. Schneider LS. Discontinuing donepezil or starting memantine for Alzheimer's disease. N Engl J Med. 2012;366:957–9.

171. Kochar MS, Itskovitz HD. Treatment of idiopathic orthostatic hypotension (Shy–Dràger syndrome) with indomethacin. Lancet. 1978;1:1011–4.

172. Singer BJ, Jegasothy GM, Singer KP, Allison GT, Dunne JW. Incidence of ankle contracture after moderate to severe acquired brain injury. Arch Phys Med Rehabil. 2004;85:1465–9.

173. Schnakers C, Chatelle C, Vanhaudenhuyse A, et al. The Nociception Coma Scale: a new tool to assess nociception in disorders of consciousness. Pain. 2010;148:215–9.

174. Haig AJ, Ruess JM. Recovery from vegetative state of six months' duration associated with Sinemet (levodopa/carbidopa). Arch Phys Med Rehabil. 1990;71:1081–3.

175. Giacino JT, Whyte J, Bagiella E, et al. Placebo-controlled trial of amantadine for severe traumatic brain injury. N Engl J Med. 2012;366:819–26.

176. The World Health Report 2003. Shaping the Future. World Health Organization. 2003. Available at: http://www.who.int/whr/2003/en/whr03_en.pdf. Accessed 9 July 2012.

177. Wolfe CD. The impact of stroke. Br Med Bull. 2000;56: 275–86.

178. Organised inpatient (stroke unit) care forv stroke. Stroke Unit Trialists' Collaboration. Cochrane Database Syst Rev. 2000;(2): CD000197.

179. Bernhardt J, Thuy MN, Collier JM, Legg LA. Very early versus delayed mobilization after stroke. Stroke. 2009;40:e489–e490.

180. Langhorne P, Dennis M. Stroke units: an evidence based approach. London: BMJ Books; 1998.

181. Diserens K, Michel P, Bogousslavsky J. Early mobilization after stroke: review of the literature. Cerebrovasc Dis. 2006;22:183–90.

182. Bernhardt J, Indredavik B, Dewey H, et al. Mobilisation 'in bed' is not mobilisation. Cerebrovasc Dis. 2007;24:157–8.

183. Marshall S, Teasell R, Bayona N, et al. Motor impairment rehabilitation post acquired brain injury. Brain Inj. 2007;21:133–60.

184. Cullen N, Chundamala J, Bayley M, Jutai J, Erabi Group. The efficacy of acquired brain injury rehabilitation. Brain Inj. 2007;21:113–32.

185. Jumisko E, Lexell J, Söderberg S. Living with moderate or severe traumatic brain injury: the meaning of family members' experiences. J Fam Nurs. 2007;13:353–69.

186. Duff D. Codman Award paper. Family concerns and responses following a severe traumatic brain injury. Axone. 2002;24:14–22.

187. Engström A, Söderberg S. The experiences of partners of critically ill persons in an intensive care unit. Intensive Crit Care Nurs. 2004;20:299–308.

188. Carson P. Investing in the comeback: parents' experience following traumatic brain injury. J Neurosci Nurs. 1993;25:165–73.

189. Simpson G, Mohr R, Redman A. Cultural variations in the understanding of traumatic brain injury and brain injury rehabilitation. Brain Inj. 2000;14:125–40.

190. Gill DJ, Wells DL. Forever different: experiences of living with a sibling who has a traumatic brain injury. Rehabil Nurs. 2000;25:48–53.

191. Kneafsey R, Gawthorpe D. Head injury: long-term consequences for patients and families and implications for nurses. J Clin Nurs. 2004;13:601–8.

192. Perlesz A, Kinsella G, Crowe S. Impact of traumatic brain injury on the family: a critical review. Rehabil Psychol. 1999;44:6–35.

193. Grant JS, Davis LL. Living with loss: the stroke family caregiver. J Fam Nurs. 1997;1:36–52.

194. Öhman M, Söderberg S. The experiences of close relatives living with a person with serious chronic illness. Qual Health Res. 2004;14:396–410.

195. Smith JE, Smith DL. No map, no guide. Family caregivers' perspectives on their journeys through the system. Care Manag J. 2000;2:27–33.

196. Wells R, Dywan J, Dumas J. Life satisfaction and distress in family caregivers as related to specific behavioural changes after traumatic brain injury. Brain Inj. 2005;19:1105–15.

197. Riley GA. Stress and depression in family cares following traumatic brain injury: the influence of beliefs about difficult behaviours. Clin Rehabil. 2007;21:82–8.

198. Visser-Meily JMA, van Heugten CM, Post MWM, Schepers VM, Lindeman E. Intervention studies for caregivers of stroke survivors, a critical review. Patient Educ Couns. 2005;56:257–67.

199. Geurtsen GJ, Van Heugten CM, Meijer R, Martina JD, Geurts ACH. Prospective study of a community reintegration programme for patients with acquired chronic brain injury: effects on caregivers' emotional burden and family functioning. Brain Inj. 2011;25:691–7.

200. Kreutzer JS, Stejskal TM, Ketchum JM, Marwitz JH, Taylor LA, Menzel JC. A preliminary investigation of brain injury family intervention: impact on the family members. Brain Inj. 2009;23:535–47.

201. Serio CD, Kreutzer JS, Witol AD. Family needs after traumatic brain injury: a factor analytic study of the Family Needs Questionnaire. Brain Inj. 1997;11:1–9.

202. Wood RL, Yurdakul LK. Change in relationship status following traumatic brain injury. Brain Inj. 1997;11:491–501.

203. Morris KC. Psychological distress in carers of head injured individuals: the provision of written information. Brain Inj. 2001;15:239–54.

204. Judd T. Neuropsychotherapy and community integration: brain illness, emotions and behavior. New York: Kluwer Academic/Plenum Publisher; 1999.

205. Formisano R, D'Ippolito M, Risetti M, et al. Vegetative state, minimally conscious state, akinetic mutism and Parkinsonism as a continuum of recovery from disorders of consciousness: an exploratory and preliminary study. Funct Neurol. 2011;26:15–24.

206. Geurtsen GJ, Martina JD, van Heugten CM, Geurts ACH. A prospective study to evaluate a new residential community integration programme for severe chronic brain injury: The Brain Integration Programme. Brain Inj. 2008;22:545–54.

207. Geurtsen GJ, van Heugten CM, Martina JD, Rietveld ACM, Meijer R, Geurts ACH. A prospective study to evaluate a residential community reintegration program for patients with chronic acquired brain injury. Arch Phys Med Rehabil. 2011;92:696–704.

208. Jumisko E, Lexell J, Söderberg S. The experiences of treatment from other people as narrated by people with moderate or severe traumatic brain injury and their close relatives. Disabil Rehabil. 2007;29:1535–43.

209. von Steinbüchel N, Wilson L, Gibbons H, et al. Quality of Life after Brain Injury (QOLIBRI): scale development and metric properties. J Neurotrauma. 2010;27:1167–85.

210. von Steinbüchel N, Wilson L, Gibbons H, et al. Quality of Life after Brain Injury (QOLIBRI): scale validity and correlates of quality of life. J Neurotrauma. 2010;27:1157–65.

211. Truelle JL, Koskinen S, Hawthorne G, et al. Quality of life after traumatic brain injury: the clinical use of the QOLIBRI, a novel disease-specific instrument. Brain Inj. 2010;24:1272–91.

212. Hagen C. LCF-Revised. Downey: Professional Staff Association of Rancho Los Amigos Hospital; 2000.

213. Giacino JT, Kezmarsky MA, De Luca J, et al. Monitoring rate of recovery to predict outcome in minimally responsive patients. Arch Phys Med Rehabil. 1991;72:897–901.

214. Giacino JT, Kalmar K, Whyte J. The JFK Coma Recovery Scale-Revised: measurement characteristics and diagnostic utility. Arch Phys Med Rehabil. 2004;85:2020–9.

215. Rappaport M, Dougherty AM, Kelting DL. Evaluation of coma and vegetative states. Arch Phys Med Rehabil. 1992;73:628–34.

216. Rader MA, Alston JB, Ellis DW. Sensory stimulation of severely brain injured patients. Brain Inj. 1989;3:141–7.

217. Ansell BJ, Keeman JE. The Western Neurosensory Stimulation Profile: a tool for assessing slow-to-recover head-injured patients. Arch Phys Med Rehabil. 1989;70:104–8.

218. Shiel A, Horn SA, Wilson BA, Watson MJ, Campbell MJ, McLellan DL. The Wessex Head Injury Matrix (WHIM) main scale: a preliminary report on a scale to assess and monitor patient recovery after severe head injury. Clin Rehabil. 2000;14:408–16.

219. Lombardi F, Gatta G, Sacco S, Muratori A, Carolei A. The Italian version of the Coma Recovery Scale-Revised (CRS-R). Funct Neurol. 2007;22:47–61.

220. Giacino JT. Disorders of consciousness: differential diagnosis and neuropathologic features. Semin Neurol. 1997;17:105–11.

221. Giacino JT, Ashwal S, Childs N, et al. The minimally conscious state: definition and diagnostic criteria. Neurology. 2002;58:349–53.

222. Jennett B, Frankowski RF. The epidemiology of head injury. In: Vinken PJ, Bruyn GW, Klawans HL, editors. Handbook of clinical neurolgy, vol. 57. Amsterdam: Elsevier Science Publishers; 1990. p. 1.

223. Brooks DN, Aughton ME, Bond MR, Jones P, Rizvi S. Cognitive sequelae in relationship to early indices of severity of brain damage after severe blunt head injury. J Neurol Neurosurg Psychiatry. 1980;43:529–34.

224. Jennett B, Teasdale G, Braakman R, Minderhoud J, Heiden J, Kurze T. Prognosis of patients with severe head injury. Neurosurgery. 1979;4:283–9.

225. Levin HS, Hamilton WJ, Grossman RG. Outcome after head injury. In: Vinken PJ, Bruyn GW, Klawans HL, editors. Handbook of clinical neurolgy, vol. 57. Amsterdam: Elsevier Science Publishers; 1990. p. 367.

226. Bishara SN, Partridge FM, Godfrey HP, Knight RG. Post-traumatic amnesia and Glasgow Coma Scale related to outcome in survivors in a consecutive series of patients with severe closed-head injury. Brain Inj. 1992;6:373–80.

227. Zafonte RD, Mann NR, Millis SR, Black KL, Wood DL, Hammond F. Posttraumatic amnesia: its relation to functional outcome. Arch Phys Med Rehabil. 1997;78:1103–6.

228. Levin HS, O'Donnell VM, Grossmann R. The Galveston Orientation and Amnesia Test: a practical scale to asses cognition after head injury. J Nerv Ment Dis. 1979;167:675–84.

229. Shores EA, Marosszeky JE, Sandanam J, Batchelor J. Preliminary validation of a clinical scale for measuring the duration of post-traumatic amnesia. Med J Aust. 1986;144:569–72.

230. Corrigan JD. Development of a scale for assessment of agitation following traumatic brain injury. J Clin Exp Neuropsychol. 1989;11:261–77.

231. Yudofsky SC, Silver JM, Jackson W, Endicott J, Williams D. The Overt Aggression Scale for the objective rating of verbal and physical aggression. Am J Psychiatry. 1986;143:35–9.

232. Levin HS, High WM, Goethe KE, et al. The neurobehavioural rating scale: assessment of the behavioural sequelae of head injury by the clinician. J Neurol Neurosurg Psychiatry. 1987;50:183–93.

233. Cummings JL, Mega M, Gray K, Rosenberg-Thompson S, Carusi DA, Gornben J. The Neuropsychiatric Inventory: comprehensive assessment of psychopathology in dementia. Neurology. 1994;44:2308–14.

234. Andrews K. Should PVS, patients be treated? Neuropsychol Rehabil. 1993;3:109–19.

235. Giacino JT, Trott CT. Rehabilitative management of patients with disorders of consciousness. J Head Trauma Rehabil. 2004;19:254–65.

236. Wood RL. Critical analysis of the concept of sensory stimulation for patients in vegetative states. Brain Inj. 1991;5:401–9.

237. Doman G, Wilkinson R, Dimancescu MD, Pelligra R. The effect of intense multisensory stimulation on coma arousal and recovery. Special issue: Coma and the persistent vegetative state. Neuropsychol Rehabil. 1993;3:203–12.

238. Lombardi F, De Tanti A, Boldrini P, Perino C, Taricco M. The effectiveness of sensory stimulation programs in patients with severe brain injury (Protocol). The Cochrane Library. 2000;(4).

239. Formisano R, Vinicola V, Penta F, Matteis M, Brunelli S, Weckel JW. Active music therapy in the rehabilitation of severe brain injured patients during coma recovery. Ann Ist Super Sanita. 2001;37:627–30.

240. Prigatano GP. Challenging dogma in neuropsychology and related disciplines. Arch Clin Neuropsychol. 2003;18:811–25.

241. Prigatano GP. Learning from our successes and failures: reflections and comments on "Cognitive Rehabilitation: how it is and how it might be". J Int Neuropsychol Soc. 1997;3:497–9.

242. Bivona U, Ciurli P, Barba C, et al. Executive function and metacognitive self-awareness after severe traumatic brain injury. J Int Neuropsychol Soc. 2008;14:862–8.

243. Ciurli P, Bivona U, Barba C, et al. Metacognitive unawareness correlates with executive function impairment after severe traumatic brain injury. J Int Neuropsychol Soc. 2010;16:360–8.

244. Sherer M, Bergloff P, Levin E, High Jr WM, Oden KE, Nick TG. Impaired awareness and employment outcome after traumatic brain injury. J Head Trauma Rehabil. 1998;13:52–61.

245. Bergquist TF, Jacket MP. Awareness and goal setting with the traumatically brain injured. Brain Inj. 1993;7:275–82.

246. Bogod NM, Mateer CA, Macdonald SWS. Self-awareness after traumatic brain injury: a comparison of measures and their relationships to executive functions. J Int Neuropsychol Soc. 2003;9:450–8.

Brain Death and Management of the Potential Organ Donor

44

Kenneth E. Wood and A. Joseph Layon

Contents

K.E. Wood, DO (✉)
Department of Critical Care Medicine,
The Geisinger Medical Center, 100 North Academy Avenue,
Danville, PA 17822, USA
e-mail: kewood@geisinger.edu

A.J. Layon, MD, FACP
Critical Care Medicine,
Pulmonary and Critical Care Medicine,
The Geisinger Health System, 100 Academy Avenue,
Danville, PA 17822, USA

Temple University School of Medicine,
Philadelphia, PA, USA
e-mail: ajlayon@geisinger.edu

Abstract

A structured and standardized approach to the diagnosis of brain death is essential to ensure that patients are appropriately classified. This involves a physical exam to establish coma and exclude reversible causes of coma, a comprehensive evaluation of the cranial nerves, and an apnea test. The inability to perform any of the physical exam elements necessitates the use of confirmatory studies. Management of the potential organ donor commences after the diagnosis of brain death is established. Donation after cardiac death should be considered in patients whose prognosis is futile and in whom care is to be withdrawn. Specific donor management goals have been established and have been associated with greater organ procurement. Hemodynamic management forms the cornerstone of brain-dead donor management. Echocardiography should be performed in all potential donors to evaluate cardiac function. Fluid resuscitation is frequently necessary as potential donors tend to be intravascularly volume depleted. Vasopressors should be used to support acceptable blood pressure and hemodynamic profiles. Donor lung management should utilize a lung protective strategy with ventilatory manipulations undertaken to ensure adequate systemic oxygenation and lung expansion. A coordinated donor management approach utilizing intensivists and OPO coordinators has been shown to more effectively manage the donation process, resulting in more organs procured and transplanted.

Keywords

Brain death history • Brain death declaration • Brain death physiology • Cardiac donor management • Pulmonary donor management • Consent for organ donation • Infections • Malignant contraindications to organ donation

A.J. Layon et al. (eds.), *Textbook of Neurointensive Care*,
DOI 10.1007/978-1-4471-5226-2_44, © Springer-Verlag London 2013

Introduction

The management of the potential organ donor in critical care units throughout the country represents the most immediate and practical solution to the current crisis in organ donation. Ensuring that there is maximal utilization and optimal management of the existing donor pool can significantly increase the number of donors available for procurement and enable transplantation to save the lives of those with end-stage disease and enhance the quality of life for those individuals maintained on dialysis. Similar to other areas of medicine, the standardization and the elimination of unwarranted variation in the management of the potential organ donor have led to higher rates of procurement, improved quality of organs procured, and improved outcomes in the transplant recipient. A standardized approach to the management of the potential organ donor begins with surveillance to identify patients with severe neurologic injury that will likely progress to brain death and identification of patients that may be potential candidates for donation after cardiac death. The Organ Procurement Organization (OPO) notification process should be standardized and utilize accepted clinical triggers such as the recognition of a non-survivable neurologic injury, initiation of end-of-life discussions with a family, or the consideration of a formal brain death examination. The methodology to determine the diagnosis of brain death should be standardized and followed by a uniform request for consent in all cases of brain death.

In the interval between the suspicion of brain death and the declaration of brain death, it is imperative that the patient be supported such that the brain death examination can be undertaken. Similarly, the brain-dead potential organ donor should be fully supported in the interval between the declaration of brain death and attempting to secure consent from the donor family. The Centers for Medicare and Medicaid Services (CMS) Conditions of Participation require that all potential organ donors be supported during this interval and that a formal request is made in all cases of brain death. Although the patient should be fully supported during this interval, formal donor management commences after consent is obtained. Donor management necessitates an ongoing intensity of support that should be indistinguishable from the management of any other critically ill patient. However, there is a distinct focus shift away from the previously undertaken cerebral protective strategies to that, resulting in the optimization of the donor organs for transplantation. This is a crucial management period for multiple reasons: it facilitates donor somatic survivorship such that procurement may be undertaken, maintains the donor organs in the best possible condition, and mitigates ongoing ischemia–reperfusion injury. The latter has been linked to an inflammatory response which creates an immunologic continuum between the donor and recipient which has been shown to jeopardize organ function in the

recipient. Management of the potential organ donor is effectively the simultaneous medical management of the seven recipients of the donor organs. The cornerstone of donor management is hemodynamic and cardiovascular maintenance which will be the primary focus of this chapter.

Brain Death Physiology

In a landmark manuscript published in 1902, Harvey Cushing described the "Experimental and Clinical Observations Concerning States of Increased Intracranial Tension" [1]. Utilizing an animal model and differentiating local compression from a general compression of the brain, Cushing examined the physiology of intracranial hypertension and its effect upon systemic hemodynamics, which have become known as Cushing's triad (irregular respirations, decreased heart rate, and increased blood pressure). However, in contrast to animal models used by Cushing and others where the experimentation is undertaken in a controlled setting, the physiology of human brain death remains challenging for multiple reasons: the time of actual brain death may be significantly different from the certification time with significant physiologic changes occurring in the interval, treatment of the patient in the period antecedent to brain death and in the immediate post-brain death period may result in abnormalities independent of brain death, and, lastly, there will never be a human model of brain death [2]. As a consequence, an understanding of brain death physiology is derived from animal models and data inferred from human case series.

Similarly, management of the potential organ donor requires not only an implicit understanding of the pathophysiology of brain death but an appreciation of the traumatic or physiologic events that contributed to or precipitated brain death and which may act synergistically with brain death physiology to impair organ function during the management period. This is best exemplified in the cardiovascular system where it is recognized that hemodynamic instability in the potential organ donor is likely reflective of a series of events conspiring to produce coincident cardiac dysfunction and vasodilatation. It has long been recognized that brain injury may lead to cardiac dysfunction which is reflected in EKG abnormalities and cardiac enzymatic elevations [3]. However, recent studies of survivors with severe brain injury have revealed significant cardiovascular dysfunction consequent to brain injury, best exemplified in the subarachnoid (SAH) patient population. Recognizing that the degree of injury in the brain-dead potential organ donor is far greater than in the survivors of severe neurologic injury, it is plausible to assume that the events predating brain death will precipitate cardiac dysfunction to which the brain death event is additive.

In the SAH patient population, the severity of the initial event has been shown to predict the magnitude of cardiac dysfunction [4–6]. A high-grade Hunt–Hess SAH is associated with a greater troponin release as 80 % of Hunt–Hess grade 5 SAH patients will exhibit a troponin release compared to less than 10 % of patients with a Hunt–Hess grade 1 SAH. Temporally, this release occurs early in the days after the initial event. In this population, left ventricular systolic dysfunction is reported to occur in 10–28 % of patients and diastolic dysfunction in 70 % of patients. Diastolic impairment and the associated distortion in the pressure volume relationship of the left ventricle will assume an important role in the volume resuscitation of organ donors and potentially contribute to increased extravascular lung water. The pattern of wall motion abnormalities reported differs appreciably from those related to coronary artery disease, with a pattern of unique apical sparing and frequent involvement of the basal and mid-ventricular portions of the anteroseptal and anterior walls and the mid-ventricular portions for the infero-septal and antero-lateral walls. Importantly, it appears that this myocardial dysfunction is reversible over time which may have implications for the echocardiographic assessment of potential organ donors. In a study comparing sympathetic innervation evaluated with MIBG scanning (meta{123} iodobenzylguanidine) to myocardial vascular perfusion assessed with MIBI scanning (technetium sestamibi) in SAH patients with cardiac dysfunction, an association between regions of contractile dysfunction and abnormalities in sympathetic innervation with normal perfusion was reported. Patients with evidence of global cardiac denervation manifested the lowest cardiac ejection fraction and worst regional wall motion scores compared to patients without evidence of cardiac denervation, whose ejection fraction and wall motion scores were preserved [7]. The preceding is at least partially explained by a catecholamine release hypothesis related to severe brain injury with the resultant effect upon cardiac function. Although not well studied, it would seem likely that similar neurocardiac associations occur in other forms of severe brain injury such as traumatic brain injury. Insofar as severely brain-injured patients that eventuate in brain death undoubtedly have a more severe form of brain injury than those surviving, it would be reasonable to conclude that the antecedent brain injury, in conjunction with the brain death process described later in this chapter, will significantly impact upon cardiac function.

Similar to the earlier recognition of a neurocardiac axis in patients with severe brain injury, there is evidence of endocrine dysfunction in patients with severe brain injury. Given the controversial use of hormone resuscitation therapy (HRT) in the management of potential organ donors, it is important to appreciate that antecedent endocrine dysfunction may be present in advance of brain death and contribute to the instability of potential organ donors. Pre-brain death endocrine dysfunction may be precipitated by direct injury to the hypothalamic–pituitary axis, neuroendocrine effects from catecholamines and cytokines, disruption of the vascular supply,

or from systemic infection or inflammation. In a review of endocrine failure after traumatic brain injury in adults, the estimated incidence of hormonal reduction was adrenal 15 %, thyroid 5–15 %, growth hormone 18 %, vasopressin 3–37 %, and gonadal 25–80 %. Hyperprolactinemia was present in more than 50 % of patients. The authors concluded that severe traumatic brain injury when accompanied by basilar skull fracture, hypothalamic edema, prolonged unresponsiveness, hyponatremia, and/or hypotension was associated with a high incidence of endocrinopathy [8, 9]. As with antecedent cardiac dysfunction, it would seem reasonable that pre-brain death endocrine dysfunction, in conjunction with the brain death process, may contribute to instability during the donor management period.

In concert with the previously described pre-brain death physiology associated with severe brain injury, the brain death process precipitates significant pathophysiologic changes in all organ systems with the most pronounced effect upon the cardiovascular system. The rostral–caudal progression of ischemia contemporarily known as coning is illustrated in Fig. 44.1. Ischemia at the cerebral level produces vagal activation associated with a decreased heart rate, decreased cardiac output, and decreased blood pressure. Although underappreciated, the first signs of incipient herniation may simply be bradycardia in a severely brain-injured patient. Ischemia at the pons level produces the mixed vagal and sympathetic stimulation known as the Cushing's response characterized by bradycardia and hypertension associated with irregular breathing. Further progression of the coning process to involve ischemia of the medulla oblongata is associated with a sympathetic stimulation termed the autonomic storm. During this period, dramatic increases in catecholamines are reported with significant tachycardia and elevations in blood pressure. This represents the severely brain-injured patient's attempt to maintain cerebral perfusion pressure gradients in the face of elevated increased intracranial pressure (ICP) and evolving herniation. During this period, there is ischemic destruction of the hypothalamic–pituitary axis resulting in thermoregulatory impairment and purported endocrine dysfunction. Further progression of ischemia results in spinal cord destruction with herniation and sympathetic deactivation characterized by bradycardia, vasodilatation, and a low cardiac output state. Somatic death after clinical brain death will inevitably occur in the absence of aggressive support. In an era when brain death was not accepted, prolonged survivorship, with a mean duration of 23 days, was noted in a study that aggressively maintained brain-dead patients [10]. Autopsy studies of patients that were declared brain dead revealed histopathologic evidence of necrosis and liquefaction [11].

The catecholamine surge or autonomic storm produces multiple EKG and hemodynamic abnormalities along with biochemical and histologic changes in the cardiac system.

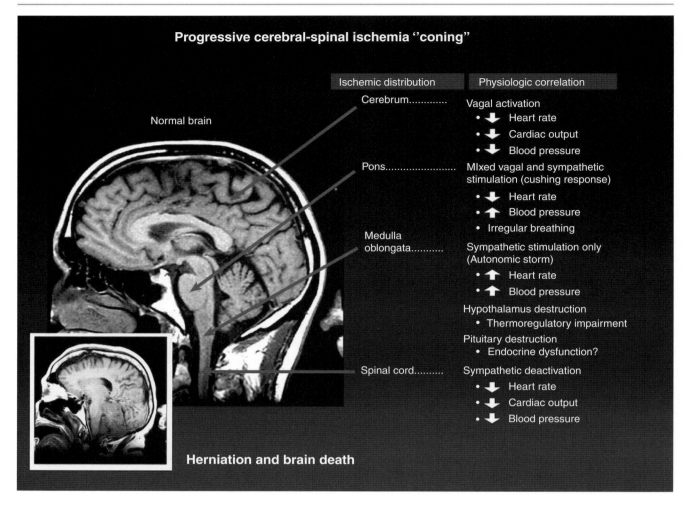

Fig. 44.1 The rostral–caudal progression of ischemia contemporarily known as coning

In a series of sentinel observations and experiments, Novitzky initially defined the cardiovascular pathophysiology associated with brain death [12–17]. Catecholamines induce a sudden increase in cytosolic calcium which jeopardizes ATP production and activates lipases, proteases, and endonucleases. Xanthine oxidase activation reportedly produces free radicals which further impair organ function. Histopathologic changes reported in experimental animals reveal various degrees of focal myocyte necrosis located predominantly in the subendocardial area consisting of contraction bands and myocytolysis with mononuclear cell infiltrates precipitating edema proximate to the necrotic areas. Contraction bands were observed in the smooth muscle of coronary arteries and electron microscopy revealed a hypercontractile state of the sarcomere visualizing mitochondrial deposition of electron dense material and secondary lysosome containing injured mitochondria. The loss of ATP production jeopardizes myocardial energy stores and mediates the transition from the aerobic to anaerobic metabolism compromising myocardial function.

Animal data and observations from human series have defined multiple abnormalities related to the catecholamine surge and brain death including impaired coronary endothelial dysfunction [18], selective expression of inflammatory molecules [19], downregulation of myocardial contractility [20], abnormalities in loading conditions and impaired coronary perfusion [21], abnormalities of left ventricular myocardial gene expression [22], and changes in myocardial beta-adrenergic receptor function and high-energy phosphates along with beta-adrenergic receptor deregulation [23, 24]. From animal models, it appears that a sudden rise in ICP is more provocative of the hyperdynamic–hemodynamic response with significantly higher catecholamine levels and is associated with greater histopathologic damage. A more gradual intracranial pressure increase resulting in brain death is associated with a milder hyperdynamic response, less catecholamine release, and milder ischemic changes in the myocardium [25]. Clinically, this has been correlated with the development of cardiac allograft vasculopathy in the recipient. The coronary artery vasoconstriction, subendocardial ischemia, and focal myocardial necrosis associated with the autonomic storm have been reported to be associated with a high incidence of intimal thickening of the transplanted heart coronary arteries, myocardial infarction, and the need for subsequent revascularization surgery [26].

The hemodynamic abnormalities and their impact are illustrated in a recent study that compared post-brain death cardiac function in a group of potential organ donors whose autonomic storm was attenuated compared to donors whose autonomic system storm was untreated. Using a definition of autonomic storm characterized by a systolic blood pressure greater than or equal to 200 mmHg and tachycardia with heart rates exceeding 140 beats per minute, the authors treated this hemodynamic response, which was observed in 63 % of donors for a mean duration of 1.2 h, with beta-blockers. Treatment resulted in a significantly higher post-brain death left ventricular ejection fraction (63.9 % versus 49.0 %), a higher rate of cardiac transplantation (91.7 % versus 41.2 %), and better heart recipient survival at 2 months (100 % versus 43 %). The authors concluded that treatment of the autonomic storm enabled better cardiac function post-brain death, higher rates of cardiac transplantation, and better recipient outcomes [27]. The study illustrates the significant impact of brain death upon cardiac function. However, recommendations regarding the treatment of the autonomic surge should be viewed with caution as this physiologic compensatory mechanism represents the patient's attempt to maintain cerebral perfusion in the face of herniation. Abolition of this response constitutes active intervention and donor management in patients who have not been declared brain dead which raises significant ethical concerns.

Globally, the intense systemic vasoconstriction of the autonomic storm compromises blood flow in various organs during this period. Subsequently, with herniation/brain death and associated denervation with vasodilatation, there is reperfusion which forms the basis of the global ischemia–reperfusion (IR) injury which is thought to contribute significantly to organ dysfunction in the donor and facilitates the development of an immunologic continuum between the donor and recipient. In addition to the IR injury that occurs with the brain death process, IR may occur antecedent to the brain death event during resuscitation from the initial trauma or may follow brain death during the periods of cold storage and transplantation. Ischemia precipitates the loss of aerobic oxidative metabolism which is associated with cellular energy loss along with changed ion gradients promoting calcium influx. With reperfusion of oxygen-rich blood, there is generation of oxygen radicals, lipid peroxidation, and further membrane permeability to calcium. IR activates the vascular endothelium and donor leukocytes with resultant cytokine expression. This precipitates local inflammation, which is thought to contribute to graft immunogenicity by producing major histocompatibility antigens and adhesion molecules.

In concert with this, there are substantial animal and some human data to support that hypothalamic–pituitary destruction produces an endocrinopathy of brain death which is additive to the issues noted previously. Dominated by the thyroid and adrenal deficiencies, it is proposed that the absence of these key hormones contributes to cellular dysfunction, metabolic abnormalities, and hemodynamic deterioration. Deficiency of thyroid hormone is proposed to impair mitochondrial function and consequently diminish energy substrate with the resultant transition from aerobic to anaerobic metabolism. Proponents of HRT propose that diminished cardiac contractility consequent to low thyroid hormone levels can be reversed with exogenous hormone supplementation. However, significant disparities exist related to hypothalamic–pituitary axis dysfunction when comparing animal and human studies. An abundance of animal data suggest that low circulating thyroid hormone levels are responsible for abnormal energy sources, impaired cardiac function, and hemodynamic instability [14, 15, 28]. Animal studies and some human reports suggest that there is a dramatic reversal of the anaerobic metabolism, improvement in cardiovascular stability, and normalization of lab parameters and EKG changes as well as improved organ suitability for transplantation when the exogenous hormonal therapy is employed [14, 15].

However, it is important to recognize that several studies have failed to define the presence of endocrine dysfunction [29–31], show improvement with the addition of exogenous hormones [32, 33], or correlate hemodynamic instability with hormone levels [30, 31]. Consequently, the use of hormone replacement therapy remains controversial and will be further discussed under cardiovascular management.

The impact of brain death upon graft function and transplanted organs was first recognized in the early 1980s by Cooper and coworkers in a landmark series of experiments and observations related to the pathophysiologic effects of brain death on transplanted organs. During this period, the authors observed that hearts procured from healthy anesthetized baboons that were stored for 48 h, and when subsequently transplanted, functioned immediately with no evidence of cardiac dysfunction. However, hearts procured from brain-dead donors and stored in a similar fashion required several hours to achieve adequate function. The authors recognized that the only difference between the two groups was brain death and determined that the brain death process was a risk factor for poor outcomes after transplantation [28]. These observations began to establish that the brain death process is not static and that the graft is not biologically inert. Tilney and colleagues have proposed the existence of an immunologic continuum between donors and the recipients as a mechanism to understand the influence of brain death on recipient organ function [34, 35]. Utilizing this model, they hypothesize that IR events associated with brain death and pre-/post-brain death events precipitate immunologic and non-immunologic injuries that impact upon short- and long-term graft function. A major component of the immunologic continuum is the IR injury that is proposed to initiate a significant inflammatory response, which triggers and amplifies the acute post-immunologic activity impacting upon multiple organs and contributing to their dysfunction in the short and long term.

Recently, it has been reported that increased plasma interleukin-6 levels in donors have been associated with lower recipient hospital-free survival after cadaveric organ transplantation [36]. Similarly, elevated plasma interleukin-6 levels in donors were associated with greater degrees of preload responsiveness that correlated with fewer organs transplanted [37]. In a study of cardiac donors, serum and myocardial levels of tumor necrosis factor alpha and interleukin-6 were elevated in all donors but were more markedly elevated in the dysfunctional unused donor hearts [38]. An intense inflammatory environment defined by elevated levels of interleukin-1, interleukin-6, tumor necrosis factor alpha, C-reactive protein, and procalcitonin has been reported in potential heart and lung donors. In this study, elevated procalcitonin levels were related to worse cardiac function and potentially thought to attenuate any improvement in cardiac function gained by donor management [39]. Similar elevations of inflammatory markers have been reported in liver transplantation. In a comparison study of hepatic tissue from brain-dead donors and living donors, the authors reported significant elevations in inflammatory cytokines in brain-dead donors compared to living donors. Cellular infiltrates were appreciably increased in parallel to the cytokine levels. This correlated with elevated liver enzymes and bilirubin levels and increased rates of rejection and primary graft nonfunction [40]. Attenuation of the increased inflammatory response with methylprednisolone was shown to significantly decrease soluble interleukins and the inflammatory response which significantly ameliorated IR injury in the posttransplant course, which was accompanied by a decreased incidence of acute rejection [41]. In summary, there is appreciable evidence that brain death and the associated inflammatory response has a substantial impact upon the transplanted organs. Future strategies will likely seek to not simply preserve organs but attenuate the inflammatory response in the donor.

Brain Death Declaration

After the description of "Le coma Depasse" by Mollart and Goulan in 1959, the description and understanding of coma and death had been changed forever [42]. These authors presented 23 cases from their Paris hospital in which they described irreversible or "irretrievable coma." This was coma that was associated with a lack of cognitive and vegetative functions and went beyond any description of coma that had been previously discussed. This description initiated the discussion and formed the basis of what is contemporarily recognized as brain death. The authors defined the necessity of considering the circumstances of the injury, the role of the neurologic examination, the results of electroencephalography (EEG), and the consequence of brain death on other organs. They found that the majority of injuries to the brain were confined to trauma, subarachnoid hemorrhage, meningitis, cerebral venous thrombosis, massive stroke, and brain death after craniotomy for posterior fossa tumor. In this series, they detailed problems including deterioration of pulmonary function, polyuria, hyperglycemia, and tachycardia. It is intriguing that this paper, even though published in a relatively well-known European journal, took more than 15 years before it became known in the United States and Great Britain.

It is significant to note that the paper by Mollart and Goulan was not the first description of brain death [42]. Lofstedt and von Reis described six mechanically ventilated patients with absent reflexes, apnea, hypotension, hypothermia, and polyuria associated with absent angiographic cerebral blood flow [43]. Death was declared when cardiac arrest occurred, between 2 and 26 days after the clinical examination. In 1963, Schwab and associates reported EEG as an adjunct for determining death when cardiac activity was present [44]. These authors proposed the following criteria to determine that the patient was dead: (1) absence of spontaneous respiration for 30 min, (2) no tendon reflexes of any type, (3) no pupillary reflexes, (4) absence of oculocardiac reflex, and (5) 30 min of an isoelectric EEG.

These papers and the recommendations contained therein generated substantial controversy in the organ transplant community, as some were uncomfortable procuring organs for transplantation from donors that were pronounced dead using brain death criteria.

In 1968, Harvard Anesthesiologist Henry Beecher chaired a committee at Harvard Medical School which attempted to define irreversible coma as new criteria for death. The committee defined death as the irreversible loss of all brain function and proposed the criteria necessary to make that determination [45].

The Harvard criteria included non-receptivity and unresponsiveness, no movements or breathing, no reflexes, and a flat EEG. The committee suggested that the tests would be repeated at 24 h and in the absence of hypothermia and central nervous system depressants and with no change in examination, the patient would fulfill criteria for the diagnosis of brain death.

Subsequently, concern regarding the relevance of EEG unfolded, and the Conference of the Royal Colleges and Faculties of the United Kingdom published the *Diagnosis of*

Brain Death first in 1976 and again in 1995, altering the definition from brain death to brain stem death [46]. They determined that if the brain stem was dead, the brain was dead, and if the brain was dead, the patient was dead. The conference required that the etiology of the condition that led to coma be established and a search for reversible factors be undertaken. Examples of "reversible factors" included central nervous system depressant drugs, neuromuscular-blocking agents, respiratory depressants, and metabolic or endocrine disturbances. A period of observation was recommended and the technique for apnea testing was described [46, 47].

The Quality Standards Subcommittee of the American Academy of Neurology formally redefined brain death in 1993, utilizing an evidence-based approach from the literature. They defined criteria for evaluating brain death as the presence of coma and evidence for the cause of the coma, including the absence of confounding factors, such as hypothermia, drugs, and electrolyte or endocrine disturbances. Fulfilling the preceding criteria, brain stem and motor reflexes needed to be absent. An apnea test was finally established as a criteria and part of the exam to define brain death. The Subcommittee recommended a repeat evaluation 6 h after the initial evaluation but recognized that the time was arbitrary and suggested that confirmatory studies should only be required when specific components of clinical testing could not be reliably evaluated [48].

The 1977 NIH-sponsored study [49] is the only prospective attempt to develop guidelines for determination of brain death based on neurologic criteria. Enrollment in this study required demonstration of cerebral unresponsiveness and apnea and at least one isoelectric EEG. This group recommended examinations at least 6 h after the onset of coma and apnea. The examination required demonstration of cerebral unresponsiveness, dilated pupils, absent brain stem reflexes, apnea, and an isoelectric EEG. The apnea examination, as defined in this study, only required that the patient not make any effort to breath over the ventilator. In the United States today, most institutional policies are modeled after the Quality Standards Subcommittee of the American Academy of Neurology [50].

Examination to Determine Brain Death

When the diagnosis of brain death is considered in the appropriate clinical context, a very careful physical exam must be performed. The assessment utilizes a standardized approach ensuring that (1) the major confounding factors must be excluded, (2) the cause of the coma should be established, (3) irreversibility must be ascertained, and (4) brain stem reflexes need to be tested and an apnea test must be performed unless contraindicated.

Brain death testing requires that certain prerequisites are met. These include the following: first, definitive evidence of an acute catastrophic event that involves both cerebral hemispheres or the brain stem in the appropriate clinical context so that irreversibility is assured, and second, complicating medical conditions that potentially could compromise the appropriate clinical assessment must be ruled out. These include electrolyte, acid–base, and endocrine disturbances. There should be no evidence of drug intoxication, neuromuscular-blocking agents, poisoning, or any other agent that might compromise the clinical examination. Additionally, hypothermia needs to be corrected and ideally the patient should have a core temperature between 35 and 38 °C. Frequently, the computerized tomographic (CT) scan of the head will provide evidence for the magnitude of the brain injury. These injuries may include massive intraparenchymal or subarachnoid hemorrhage and/or epidural or subdural hemorrhages with mass effect. The CT scan may also appear slightly less dramatic after a cardiac arrest. Findings may be limited to the loss of sulci and the gray matter–white mater differentiation and effacement of the basilar cisterns, all of which reflect cerebral edema.

The patient must exhibit lack of consciousness. Unresponsiveness usually implies the administration of some painful stimuli. While there are multiple approaches (sternal rubbing, rubbing knuckles on ribs, twisting nipples, and pinprick), these can be construed as somewhat abusive. Perhaps more appropriate, although not accepted as the standard, is to utilize an instrument such as a pen, pencil, or the tip of a Kelly clamp to apply pressure at the lunula (junction of the cuticle and skin of the digit intersect). This pressure will consistently elicit a response in patients with an intact nervous system and it is not construed as potentially "violent" as pinprick or nipple twisting. Furthermore, it does not leave bruising that nipple twisting does and will not cause skin abrasions in the fragile skin of the elderly.

When painful stimulation is applied, there should be no responses such as eye opening or withdrawal and grimacing, although there may be an occasional "spinal" reflex with this stimulus. This spinal reflex is neither reproducible nor purposeful. Spinal movements have been described by Wijdicks [51] as brief, slow movements in upper limbs, flexion of the finger, and arm lifting that is not a decerebrate or decorticate response; these movements are not persistent and usually not reproducible. The precise reflex pathway[s] is not understood; however, these are recognized as spinal reflexes.

Brain Stem Reflexes

Pupillary Response

The pupillary response to light should be absent in both eyes. The pupils in brain-dead patients are most often dilated midposition and usually 4–6 mm. It is important to ensure that there is no preexisting ocular abnormalities and that topical ocular agents have not been instilled. Wijdicks suggests that neuromuscular-blocking agents may cause a nonreactive light reflex [51]. The cranial nerves (CrN) evaluated in the pupil light response are CrN II and III.

Ocular Testing

In the presence of brain death, there should be no ocular movements either to brisk movement of the head from side to side (absence of doll's eyes) or to instillation of cold water into the auditory canals. The nerves stimulated by these maneuvers include CrN VIII (efferent) with CrN III and VI (afferents). Prior to stimulating the oculocephalic reflex, one must ensure that the cervical spine is intact and the test should not be performed when there is known or suspected cervical spine injury. With the head in neutral position, the head is briskly moved, first to the left, and held there for approximately 30 s. If the cranial nerves are intact, the eyes will move from the direct frontal gaze to the left and then back towards the previous midline focus. The same is true when head is moved to the right; if the nerves are intact, the eyes will move from the direct frontal gaze to the right and then back to the previous midline frontal gaze. In the presence of brain death, the eyes will remain in the direction the head is moved.

When there is concern that the cervical spine may not be intact, cold-water calorics should be utilized. The same nerves are tested; however, the risk to the cervical spine is eliminated. Prior to the instillation of iced saline in the auditory canal, one must ensure that the tympanic membranes are intact and that there is no occlusion of the auditory canal. Approximately 50 ml of iced saline is instilled into the auditory canal. The cold stimulus results in sedimentation of the endolymph and stimulation of hair cells in the vestibular apparatus. The response in a comatose patient with an intact neurologic system is a slow deviation of the eyes towards the cold stimulus. In the presence of brain death, the eyes stay fixed in midline position. Wijdicks [51] reports that drugs such as aminoglycosides, tricyclic antidepressants, anticholinergic agents, any antiepileptic drug, and some chemotherapeutic agents may ablate or abolish this caloric response in the presence of an intact brain stem. Basilar fracture may abrogate the response unilaterally on the side of the fracture.

Corneal Reflexes

Corneal reflexes should be evaluated by carefully using a sterile cotton-tipped swab. Blinking requires an intact brain stem. Care must be taken so that the eyelashes are not stimulated. The CrNs involved are V (afferent) and VII (efferent). Blinking that occurs with stimulation of the cornea is not compatible with brain death. Severe facial and ocular trauma can compromise the interpretation of these findings.

Pharyngeal and Tracheal Reflexes

In the intact brain stem, pharyngeal and tracheal reflexes (cough, gag) may be stimulated by passing a catheter through the endotracheal tube into the trachea and suctioning for several seconds. The CrNs involved are CrN IX and CrN X; CrN IX is the afferent to the trachea and CrN X is the efferent from the brain stem back to the trachea. The presence of a cough reflex is not compatible with brain death. Wijdicks comments that the gag response may be difficult to interpret and is unreliable in an intubated patient [51].

Apnea Study

The apnea study is usually the final portion of the clinical examination to determine brain death. There are several techniques that may be used to perform the study. In principle, the arterial CO_2 partial pressure ($PaCO_2$) must rise to at least 60 or 20 mmHg greater than the patient's baseline. This relatively rapid rise in $PaCO_2$ results in a decrease in the cerebral spinal fluid pH, which is sensed by the medullary respiratory center. When the respiratory center is functional, respiratory efforts will result. In the presence of brain death, there will be no respiratory effort.

Initially, one must ensure that the patient's core temperature is ideally above 35 °C and preferably normothermic. The patient must be preoxygenated and stabilized, ensuring correction of any hemodynamic or electrolyte abnormalities. This is especially true when the technique used for the apnea study is removal of the patient from the ventilator with no continuous positive airway pressure (CPAP). Preoxygenation usually requires 10 min of breathing and an FiO_2 of 1.0. Prior to initiation of the procedure, an arterial blood gas analysis must be obtained both to ensure adequate oxygenation and to define a baseline arterial CO_2 value. With the baseline arterial CO_2 value, one can calculate the apnea time required for the $PaCO_2$ to rise to 60 mmHg.

The technique is as follows: the measured $PaCO_2$ value is subtracted from 60 mmHg (delta-CO_2). It is recognized that $PaCO_2$ will climb approximately 3 mmHg, in the first minute of apnea, and thereafter, it will climb by approximately 2 mmHg/min. Therefore, dividing the delta-CO_2 by the lower value of 2 mmHg increase per minute will ensure an adequate apnea time, allowing the $PaCO_2$ to achieve the minimal value of 60 mmHg in the presence of brain death-associated apnea.

Once the time required to achieve the delta value is determined, there are three techniques that may be used for the apnea study. These include:

1. Simply removing the patient from mechanical ventilation and placing a catheter through the ETT while insufflating O_2 at approximately 6 l/min; this will most often ensure adequate apneic oxygenation.

2. Set the mechanical ventilator to spontaneous mode with no backup apneic mode; with this approach, the patient can be maintained on a low level of CPAP to preserve oxygenation. The monitoring modalities of the mechanical ventilator can be used to visualize respiratory efforts if these were to occur.

3. The patient may be taken off mechanical ventilation and connected to a Mapleson D circuit. In addition to the Mapleson D circuit, a Wright's spirometer may be placed in line. With fresh oxygen flow of 6–10 l/min, one can partially close the Mapleson D circuit pop-off valve, ensure that there is some CPAP, and then watch both the bag of the Mapleson D circuit and the Wright's spirometer for respiratory efforts.

Whichever technique is used, the patient is kept off mechanical ventilation for the calculated time to achieve the delta-CO_2 value. Pulse oximetric saturation is followed to ensure that desaturation does not occur. Desaturations, hemodynamic instability, or significant rhythm disturbances necessitate immediate replacement of full mechanical ventilation. Ideally, a blood gas should be drawn at the onset of instability and used for assessment. A $PaCO_2$ greater than or equal to 60 mmHg would be consistent with a failed apnea test. Failure to achieve a $PaCO_2 \geq 60$ mmHg in the absence of any respiratory efforts suggests inadequate time for CO_2 production to achieve threshold. In this case, the test may be re-performed after correcting metabolic/physiologic abnormalities or moving directly to a confirmatory study. At the end of the newly calculated time period, an arterial blood gas analysis is obtained. If the $PaCO_2$ value is greater or equal to 60 mmHg, or has increased more than 20 mmHg above the patients known baseline value, and there have been no respiratory efforts, the result is compatible with brain death.

After the second blood gas is drawn, the patient is reconnected to the mechanical ventilator, and if the $PaCO_2$ from the previous sample is greater than 60 mmHg, the family is notified that the exam is consistent with brain death. After the patient has failed the apnea study, the patient is pronounced clinically brain dead.

Common complications of the apnea study are hypotension and cardiac dysrhythmias. If one is unable to adequately perform the apnea study because of these complications or because of hypoxia, confirmatory tests, such as a radionuclear cerebral blood flow study or a 4-vessel angiogram, will be required.

Finally, there is some question as to the need for two brain death examinations and the interval between exams in adult patients. The latest data suggest that no observation period is required and a single exam will suffice [42].

When a repeat examination is performed, a repeat apnea study is not an absolute requirement, although it is imperative to ensure that institution and state regulations are followed.

Exclusions and Contraindications

Given the dramatic shortage of organs available for donation, exclusions and contraindications should be viewed as absolutely relative or relatively absolute [52]. Consequently, all cases should be reviewed in conjunction with the OPO coordinator to determine suitability. Successful procurement has been undertaken in a broad array of cases that were previously deemed unsuitable including patients with sepsis and bacterial meningitis, provided appropriate anti-infective treatment is undertaken. However, organs should not be procured from potential donors when the etiology of the purported infection has not been determined. An evolving literature suggests that organ procurement from patients with known meningitis that have been appropriately treated has not resulted in significant transmission of the infectious agent nor organ compromise in the recipient [53]. In a retrospective study over 10 years of 39 patients undergoing heart and lung transplantation undertaken with organs from cadaveric donors with bacterial meningitis defined by either positive blood or cerebral spinal fluid cultures and associated clinical signs and symptoms, no contraindications could be defined because none of the recipients died of infection-related causes. Common organisms in the donor were reported to be *Neisseria meningitidis* 53.8 %, *Streptococcus pneumoniae* 41 %, and *Haemophilus influenzae* 5.2 %. Importantly, adequate antibiotic therapy was initiated before organ retrieval and continued after transplantation [54]. Similarly, Satoi reported that liver transplantation from donors with bacterial meningitis was safe and appropriate provided the donor and recipient received adequate antimicrobial therapy. In this study of 34 recipients, there were no infectious complications caused by the meningeal pathogens [55]. Although recommendations are difficult to establish, treatment of the donor for 24–48 h and a minimum 7–10 days for the recipient appears to be adequate.

Frequently, potential organ donors in the intensive care unit are bacteremic from multiple causes that may originate from many sources. Similar to this literature for donors with meningitis, procurement of organs from bacteremic patients has been successfully undertaken and the presence of bacteremia should not preclude donor evaluation. In a study that reviewed heart transplantation from donors that expired from community-acquired infections with severe septic shock, meningitis, and/or pneumonia, no evidence of donor-associated infection and sepsis or rejection was observed in the recipient [56].

In a report of transplantation from bacteremic donors with gram-negative septic shock, all recipients were alive with good graft function at 60 days following transplantation with no infectious complications. The authors recommended that appropriate antibiotics be given for at least 48 h prior to organ retrieval and that recipients receive 7 days of culture-specific antibiotics posttransplantation [57].

Patients with human immunodeficiency virus (HIV) represent an absolute contraindication to donation. However, there are occasionally patients with high-risk social behavior who are HIV seronegative that are considered for possible organ donation. In this circumstance, there should be an extensive review of the medical record, interviews with the family, and active communication with OPO. High-risk patients for HIV are not precluded from donation; however, it is recommended that this information be conveyed to the transplant center who should inform the potential recipient of the risks and benefits of this potential organ use.

Donor malignancy represents another area of concern that warrants careful evaluation when a donor is considered for procurement. Any active non-central nervous system malignancy is viewed as an absolute contraindication to donation. A previous history of choriocarcinoma, lung cancer, melanoma, and patients with previous colon, breast, or kidney cancer similarly are precluded. Donors with a previous history of nonmelanoma skin cancers and a select group of patients with cancer defined in situ or with very low-grade levels of malignancy may be considered as can be patients with a history of previous curative therapy. These cases should be discussed on an individual basis with the OPO and the transplant center. Central nervous system malignancies are not uncommon in the potential organ donor population. Given their rare metastasis and low incidence of development in the recipient, procurement is frequently undertaken. Potential donors with a low-grade tumor, absent craniotomy, and no ventricular shunts are better candidates than those donors with previously defined high-grade malignancy, craniotomy, and shunt placement. It is important to recognize that hemorrhage may occur into primary or metastatic tumors and autopsy should be undertaken when this is a consideration.

Consent

Approaching and obtaining consent from the potential donor's family is an absolute requirement for organ donation. In the case of previously defined first person consent, where an individual firmly establishes their desire to donate via a driver's license or donor card, it is imperative that the first person consent be honored and recognized as the basis for consent. In 1998, the Center for Medicare and Medicaid Services established several parameters governing the organ donation process through the Federal Conditions of Participation. A change in the Conditions of Participation required timely notification of the OPO when death was imminent to ensure that families were provided the opportunity to discuss the option of organ and tissue donation. Similarly, the Conditions of Participation mandated that individuals specially trained in requesting, termed "designated requestors," be responsible for making the request and required that all individuals discussing organ donation with families receive the appropriate training (COP) (42CFR Part 482 {HCFA-3005-F} RIN:0938-A195). The intent of this mandate was to ensure that individuals approaching families and discussing organ donation were trained and sensitive to the family situation. Initially, this is interpreted by some to imply that physicians would be excluded from the request process and only OPO designated requestors could approach the family. Subsequent discussion and policy recommendations which were adopted by the American Medical Association suggested that the designated requestor contact the attending physician before organ donation requests and include the attending physician in the discussion with the family. It is important to appreciate that OPO coordinators, physicians, and nurses may be defined as designated requestors, provided they undertake the appropriate training [58].

Family characteristics and the approach to the consent process have been shown to significantly impact upon the decision to donate. It has been reported that non-donor families are less satisfied with the quality of care, had a lesser degree of understanding of brain death, and remained under the impression that brain-dead patients could survive. These families felt that there was insufficient time and privacy during the request process and that the requestor was not sensitive to their needs. Alternatively, families that consented for donation had a much clearer understanding of brain death and were more satisfied with the overall consent process and their decision making [59]. Siminoff evaluated the roles of pre-request factors and decision process variables in the consent process. This large study of 11,555 deaths with 741 potential donors had a family request rate of 80 % and a final consent rate of 48 %. Family decisions were made early, with 55 % of families making their decision during the initial request. Of those families with an initial favorable view of consent (58 %), 81 % went on to complete the consent with consent not obtained in 19 %. In families who initially had an unfavorable view of the donation process (25 %), consent was eventually obtained in 9 % and no consent was sustained in the remaining 91 %. In the 17 % of families that were undecided during the initial donation request, 47 % went on to consent and consent was not obtained in 53 %. The initial response predicted a final donation decision in 70 % of families. Pre-request factors that were associated with successful consent included patient characteristics of young, white males dying from trauma and family beliefs in donation, prior knowledge of organ donation, the presence of a donor card, explicit discussions, and a belief that the patient would have wished to donate and that the information provided was adequate and the health-care provider was comfortable with questions. There was no association noted between family education and income levels, hospital environmental factors, health-care practitioner-associated demographics, or the health-care practitioner's attitude towards donation. Decision process variables that correlated with donation were the correct initial assessment by the health-care provider, instances when the family raised the donation issue, conversations and time spent with the OPO coordinator, and clear, unambiguous discussions related to cost, funeral homes, and choices. Decision process variables that had a negative correlation with donation included perceptions that the health-care provider was not caring, surprise by the family when the request was made, or feeling harassed and pressured to make a decision. No correlation was found with the overall satisfaction of care, the timing of the request, or the belief that the patient was alive after the declaration of brain death. Hazard ratios for factors that directly related to donation included pre-request characteristics (7.68), optimal request pattern with the health-care provider being a nonphysician and the OPO coordinator (2.96), OPO related factors (3.08), and the topics discussed (5.22) [60].

The request for organ donation has undergone an evolutionary process from random or inconsistent requesting to the use of designated requestors to the use of an effective requestor to the currently recommended process of effective requesting. Key elements of the requesting process recommended by the Institute of Medicine (IOM) include a focus on the family and the continuation of compassionate care with an acknowledgement of the uniqueness of each family and avoiding scripted statements. A determination of the most appropriate requestor and the timing of the request should be individualized and done on a case-by-case basis. Families of patients with protracted intensive care unit stays frequently develop close associations with specific physicians or nurses and may be willing to accept discussions related to impending death and donation at times earlier in the course than families with an acute crisis. The IOM panel recommended that donation be discussed as an opportunity utilizing language that emphasizes the benefit to the transplant recipient and the potential of healing for the donor family. Importantly, the panel recommended that excellent end-of-life care be continued for the family, independent of the donation decision [61].

Although there is some variability, it has generally been accepted that decoupling or separating the request for donation from the declaration of brain death notification be used as the model for requests [62, 63]. In this model, the notification of brain death is both temporally and geographically segregated from the organ donation request. This provides the opportunity for the family to process the notification of brain death before the request is made for consent. Although decoupling traditionally has referred to the temporal and geographic segregation of the two events, others have suggested that the consent may occur after the family has accepted the patient's futility [64]. In conjunction with the decoupling process, factors that have been associated with a successful consent rate include making the request in a private setting and ensuring the engagement of the OPO transplant coordinator. When all three elements are present, the consent rate was reported to be 2.5 times greater than when none of the elements were present [62]. The Council on Scientific Affairs for the American Medical Association recommended that the process focus upon supporting the family of all potential donors be consistent with quality end-of-life principles, decouple discussions of brain death from the organ donation requests, ensure that the opportunity to donate is presented to all families, and do so in a private setting. Ensuring that the OPO transplant coordinator is involved and assists with coordinating the efforts in the intensive care unit was strongly recommended. For those wishing to participate in the request process, special training should be undertaken and certification as a designated requestor obtained.

Medical Management

Hemodynamic and cardiovascular management form the cornerstone of potential organ donor management. A standardized and structured approach to hemodynamic management ensures that the donor somatically survives for procurement and maintains the remainder of potential organs in the best possible condition. Similar to the care of any critical patient, a collaborative approach utilizing the skills of physicians, nurses, respiratory therapists, and the OPO coordinator is pivotal for optimum management. Standardization of donor management from the referral process through consent, followed by management and recovery, has been shown to significantly increase the number of organs recovered and organs transplanted. A 10.3 % increase in organs recovered per 100 donors and a 3.3 % increase in total organs transplanted per 100 donors were reported by Rosendale in a study that emphasized standardization of general medical management, eliminating variability in laboratory and diagnostic studies, along with standardization of respiratory therapy, and IV fluids and medications [65]. The Surgical Trauma Group at the University of Southern California has been instrumental in pioneering the standardized approach to organ donor management. The development of an aggressive organ donor management program was reported to significantly increase the number of organs available for transplantation. Employing a critical care team that accepted potential organ donors for management utilizing pulmonary artery catheters (PAC), fluid resuscitation and use of vasopressors, prevention and treatment of complications associated with brain death, and liberal use of thyroid hormone in unstable donors resulted in a 57 % increase in total referrals, a 19 % increase in potential donors, an 82 % increase in the number of actual donors, and an 87 % decrease in the number of donors lost to hemodynamic instability. Overall, the implementation of this aggressive donor management team resulted in a 71 % increase in the number of organs recovered [66]. In a follow-up study by the same group utilizing an aggressive approach to organ donor management, the authors evaluated the impact of the complications of brain death upon organ retrieval. They hypothesized that brain death-related complications would have no significant impact on the number of organs donated provided there was an aggressive organ donor management protocol in place. With complications defined as the requirement for vasoactive support which occurred in 97.1 %, coagulopathy in 55.1 %, thrombocytopenia in 53.6 %, diabetes insipidus in 46.4 %, cardiac ischemia in 30.4 %, lactic acidosis in 24 %, renal failure in 20.3 %, and adult respiratory distress syndrome noted in 13 %, there was no appreciable impact of the complications on the average number of organs procured. Additional benefits included a dramatic diminution in the number of donors lost to cardiovascular collapse and improvement in conversion rates [67]. In a comparison with other level I trauma centers that did not utilize an aggressive donor management protocol, dramatic benefits were similarly reported which included a significant decrease in the incidence of cardiovascular collapse and the number of organs procured per potential donor [67].

Although the traditional management of the potential organ donor has been taken by the OPO transplant coordinator, there has been an evolution towards a collaborative approach between the intensivist/critical care community and the OPO, as reflected in the previously mentioned studies. Intensivist-led management of potential organ donors has been reported to increase the organs recovered for transplantation. In a study that evaluated the implementation of an intensivist-led donor management program, the overall number of organs recovered for transplantation increased significantly (44 % versus 31 %), which was largely reflective of an increase in the number of lungs procured and transplanted (24 % versus 11 %). No appreciable change occurred in the number of hearts and livers recovered for transplantation. This study is reflective of the enormous impact that a collaborative and partnered approach between intensivists and OPO coordinators can have upon donor management.

Although no clear current consensus exists, the traditional approach to organ donor management was to minimize the time between brain death and procurement because of the perception that prolonged management was detrimental to the donor organs and bed utilization in busy intensive care units necessitated admission for salvageable patients.

However, this concept has recently been challenged as evolving literature reports that a longer period of donor management may be beneficial. In a retrospective study with a mean time from brain death to procurement of 35 h, it was reported that there was no decrease in the procurement to consented ratio with increasing time after brain death. When individual organs were analyzed separately, heart and pancreas procurement improved with an increased management period after brain death and some organs were successfully procured greater than 60 h after brain death [68]. Similarly, in a study of 100 consecutive organ donors whose mean donor management time was 23 h, it was reported that donors managed in excess of 20 h resulted in significantly more heart and lung procurements, more organs procured per donor (4.2 versus 3.2) and more organs transplanted per donor (3.7 versus 2.6). Interestingly, there was no significant difference noted in the obtainment of donor management goals [69].

Specific donor management goals during the donor management period have evolved as a standard. Attainment of these management goals has resulted in a significant increase in the number of organs procured and transplanted per donor. In an initial report by Hagan, consensus was developed for six specific donor management goals amongst six OPO organizations. The following management goals were derived: mean arterial pressure greater than 60 mmHg, central venous pressure less than 10 mmHg (or serum osmolarity 285–295 mMol/kg), sodium less than 155 mMol/l, pH 7.25–7.5, pressors (1 or none – 1 pressor plus vasopressin for diabetes insipidus was deemed appropriate), and PaO_2 greater than 300 mmHg while on 100 % oxygen. These donor management goals were considered a bundle with compliance defined as achieving a minimum of five goals. The number of organs transplanted per donor was 4.87 in those meeting goals and 3.19 in those donors failing to meet the bundle goals for standard criteria donors. No significant change was noted for extended criteria donors [70]. Subsequent studies have sought to refine which of the management goals should receive a higher priority. In a similar consensus-driven study, eight common goals were defined: mean airway pressure, central venous pressure, pH, PaO_2, sodium, glucose, vasopressor use, and urine output. Throughout the study period, there was a dramatic increase in the compliance with donor management goals, which was associated with a significant improvement in organs transplanted per donor. The authors reported that the success of transplantation was predominantly associated with limitations in vasopressor use and achieving adequate PaO_2. Thoracic organs were most sensitive to the donor management goals as there was a dramatic increase in lung transplantation with higher levels of PaO_2. Interestingly, mean arterial pressure, central venous pressure, pH, sodium, and urine output had little effect on the transplantation rate. The authors concluded that goals and standardization of endpoints of donor management are associated with increased rates of transplantation. However, it was evident that not all standard goals are necessary with the most significant parameters being the low use of vasopressors and ensuring adequate oxygenation, which should form the focus of donor management [71]. Similarly, in a study that evaluated ten donor management goals and defined success as the achievement of eight goals, the authors used binary logistic regression to determine the independent predictors of more than four organs transplanted per donor. The authors reported that donors meeting donor management goals had more organs transplanted per donor (4.4 versus 3.3). Independent predictors of transplanting more than four organs were age, serum creatinine, thyroid hormone, and meeting donor management goals. Amongst the individual donor management goals, odds ratios were higher for central venous pressure 4–10 mmHg (OR=1.9), ejection fraction greater than 50 % (OR=4.0), $PaO_2:FiO_2$ greater than 300 (OR=4.6), and a serum sodium 135–168 mEq/l (odds ratio=3.4) [71, 72]. The impact of a structured and standardized approach to organ donor management has similarly been reported to dramatically increase the retrieval rate of lungs and hearts for transplantation. In a study where potential lung donors were aggressively managed through protocol-guided optimization of ventilatory and hemodynamic strategies that consisted of measurements of extravascular lung water, bronchoscopy, and invasive monitoring, a dramatic increase in the rate of lung procurement was reported (40 % versus 27 %) [73]. Similarly, an aggressive and structured approach to the management of potential heart donors reported a significant increase in the numbers of hearts procured with a standardized approach using invasive monitoring and critical care management techniques [74].

Figure 44.2 represents an algorithmic approach to the cardiovascular and hemodynamic management of the potential organ donor. Initial assessments of stability should be undertaken in all potential donors and include echocardiography, mean arterial blood pressure, vasoactive requirements, urine output, and measurement of the left ventricular ejection fraction. Potential organ donors achieving the thresholds identified in Fig. 44.2 should be continuously monitored and formally evaluated for cardiac donation. As depicted in the figure, age plays a major role in the initial cardiac evaluation. Traditionally, cardiac catheterization has been required for potential organ donors over 40 years of age. Given the significant myocardial stress associated with brain death, echocardiography should not be performed immediately after brain death declaration as this may provide misleading information related to cardiac function. Initial attempts at stabilization should include normalizing blood pressure, metabolic abnormalities, and electrolyte disturbances. Transthoracic echocardiography (TTE) should be performed in all patients to evaluate structural abnormalities that may preclude cardiac donation and evaluate the left ventricular ejection fraction. Since

first reported in the evaluation of potential organ donors in 1988, TTE has proven invaluable for evaluation of cardiac function, particularly in circumstances where clinical events might have precluded cardiac utilization. In the original study, 29 % of donor hearts that would have been previously excluded on clinical criteria were procured and successfully transplanted [75]. Echocardiographic abnormalities are reported to be responsible for 26 % of non-used hearts with an odds ratio of 1.48 per 5 % decrease in ejection fraction [76]. Although instrumental in the evaluation of cardiac function in the potential organ donor, several issues warrant consideration regarding echocardiographic evaluation. These include the difficulty in securing the test, technical challenges with imaging in critically ill patients, and the accuracy and impact of the echocardiographic interpretation. As previously described, neurologic events and brain death predispose potential donors to cardiac dysfunction with regional wall motion abnormalities that may be reversible. Similarly, it is important to appreciate that left ventricular ejection fraction is a load-dependent measure of contractility with variance noted when there are changes in preload and afterload [77]. It is also important to recognize that temporal changes occur in left ventricular systolic function. In a study that evaluated sequential echocardiograms in potential organ donors, with ejection fractions less than 50 % or regional wall motion abnormalities on the initial cardiogram, 12 of 13 patients improved after donor management. Utilizing a strategy that employed high-dose corticosteroids and dopamine without the use of thyroid hormone, these 12 donor hearts were transplanted with a survival rate of 92 % with an average follow-up of 16 months [78]. In a series that evaluated clinical characteristics and echocardiographic and pathologic findings of myocardial dysfunction in potential donors, echocardiographic evidence of systolic dysfunction was appreciated in 42 % of potential organ donors. This was not predicted by clinical findings, the EKG findings, or the type of neurologic injury. Histopathologically, there was a very limited correlation to the area of echocardiographic dysfunction in the histopathology of hearts that were not procured. This suggests that brain death is associated with significant myocardial dysfunction and the potential for reversibility needs to be appreciated. Consequently, no heart should be rejected on the basis of a first initial abnormal echocardiogram. In instances where TTE evaluation is difficult, consideration should be given to the use of transesophageal echocardiography (TEE). Limited literature comparing TTE with TEE suggests that the TTE assessment may be inadequate in almost one-third of the patients. A substantial increase in the number of abnormalities was detected with TEE, although no outcome difference was established [79]. Recent literature suggests that more than 50 % of the hearts with initial abnormal function may attain hemodynamic transplantation criteria with aggressive donor management. In this prospective study of 66 potential

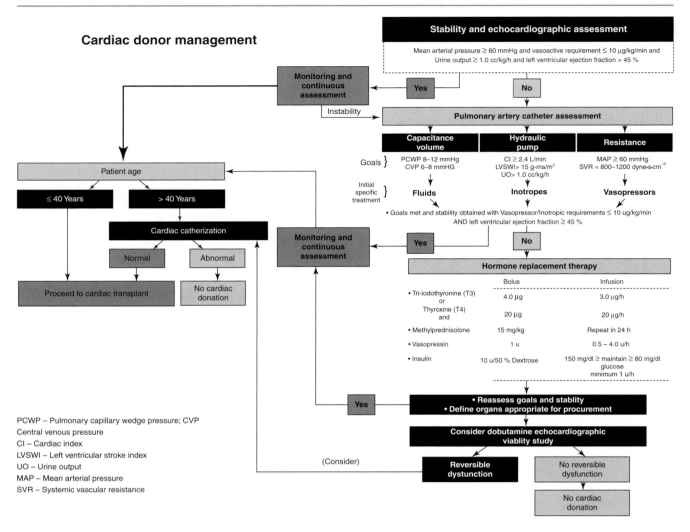

Cardiac donor management

Fig. 44.2 Algorithmic approach to the cardiovascular and hemodynamic management of the potential organ donor (Adapted with permission of the Massachusetts Medical Society from Wood et al. [113])

organ donors, an initial normal left ventricular ejection fraction independently predicted end-assessment hemodynamic suitability for transplantation. An initial abnormal left ventricular systolic function was identified in almost half of donor hearts, of which 58 % achieved hemodynamic stability criteria for procurement [80]. Although there are limited data from small case series, low-dose dobutamine stress tests may be able to detect myocardium that appears dysfunctional in the donor and may be capable of recrudescing function in the recipient [81].

In potential organ donors failing to achieve the stability thresholds identified in Fig. 44.2, direct measurements of intravascular pressures and cardiac function should be undertaken. Traditionally, a PAC has been used to assess cardiac pressures and cardiac output, calculate systemic vascular resistance, and use measured and derived data to manipulate fluid resuscitation and vasoactive support. This approach was pioneered by the donor management program at the

Papworth Hospital in Cambridge, United Kingdom. In a landmark study by Wheeldon, 35 % of potential organ donors were initially deemed unacceptable based upon the following criteria: mean arterial pressure less than 55 mmHg, central venous pressure (CVP) exceeding 15 mmHg, inotropic support requirement exceeding 20 mg/kg/min, pulmonary capillary wedge pressure greater than 15 mmHg, and a left ventricular stroke work index less than 15 g. Utilizing invasive monitoring with a PAC and HRT, 44 of the 52 initially unacceptable donors were successfully procured and transplanted. The authors concluded that 92 % of organs that initially fell outside of transplant acceptance criteria were capable of functional resuscitation and the optimization of cardiovascular performance had significant benefits for the viability of all organs [82]. Given the current speculation regarding the use of PACs, it may be that the dramatic success seen in this and other studies reflect the time, effort, and vigilant commitment to the donor management process as much as the placement of a PAC. Recently, the commonly accepted practice of inferring volume status from pressure measurements has been questioned. In a systematic review of the literature assessing the accuracy of central venous pressure (CVP) to predict fluid responsiveness found an exceedingly poor correlation between CVP and blood volume. The inability of the CVP/change in CVP with fluid challenge to predict a hemodynamic response leads to the conclusion that CVP should not be used to make decisions regarding fluid management [83]. Consequently, other measurements have been proposed to evaluate intravascular volume and fluid responsiveness in critically ill patients which are equally applicable to the management of the potential organ donor. Dynamic changes in the arterial waveform-derived variables have been shown to be accurate predictors of fluid responsiveness in mechanically ventilated patients [84] and have been applied to the management of potential organ donors [37]. In a study that utilized a pulse pressure variation greater than 13 % to define preload responsiveness, 48 % of potential organ donors were characterized as preload responsive. Interleukin-6 and tumor necrosis factor concentrations were greater in preload-responsive donors suggesting that there was inadequate volume resuscitation in the early phase donor management. When comparing preload-responsive donors to those potential organ donors that were not preload responsive (pulse pressure variation less than 13 %), fewer organs were transplanted from the preload-responsive donors as the number of organs transplanted per donor from the preload responsive versus unresponsive donors was 1.8 versus 3.7. As illustrated in Fig. 44.2, it is important to define hemodynamic profiles for optimum management utilizing tools that are both available and familiar.

Hemodynamic instability is reported to occur in a vast majority of potential organ donors and can be sustained in 20 % of donors, despite ongoing vasoactive support [85]. Table 44.1 provides an overview of the broad differential diagnosis of hemodynamic instability in the potential organ donor. Recognizing that the brain death event jeopardizes cardiac function and produces vasodilatation, these are usually coincident events. As previously discussed, a significant number of potential organ donors are hypovolemic after brain death. This may reflect inadequacy of the initial resuscitation, third spacing of fluids secondary to the inflammatory response, or misinterpretation of pressure-derived variables. The previous focus upon minimizing increased intracranial

Table 44.1 Differential diagnosis of hemodynamic instability in the brain-dead patient

Brain stem vasomotor center infarction
Volume depletion from diabetes insipidus
Myocardial injury from catecholamine storm
Reduction in circulating thyroid hormone

pressure with fluid restriction, diuretics, or mannitol will significantly contribute to decreased intravascular volume. Volume depletion may also be precipitated by hyperglycemia-induced osmotic diuresis, diabetes insipidus, or a cold diuresis in the hypothermic patient. Cardiac dysfunction may be consequent to the brain death event, reflective of initial injury to the myocardium, or result from metabolic depression secondary to acidosis, hypophosphatemia, or hypocalcemia. Vasodilatation is a consistent feature in the potential organ donor predominantly related to herniation-mediated denervation and the loss of vasomotor control and autoregulation. However, other contributing factors may include the relative adrenal insufficiency associated with trauma/critical illness, the endocrinopathy of brain death, or a superimposed/acquired sepsis. Ongoing hypotension further compounds the initial ischemia–reperfusion injury, which may result in cardiac arrest and loss of the potential organ donor. Consequently, an aggressive approach to defining the adequacy of intravascular volume, cardiac function, and the degree of vasodilatation is of paramount importance in managing the potential organ donor. Whenever possible, fluid resuscitation in the potential organ donor should be guided by objective measurements and defined endpoints. Traditionally, normal saline has been used as the initial fluid for volume resuscitation to achieve either the previously described central venous pressure endpoints or abolition of preload responsiveness determined by pulse pressure variation. Inadequacy of initial volume resuscitation has been shown to precipitate a significant increase in inflammatory mediators with fewer organs procured and transplanted [37]. Diabetes insipidus is common in potential organ donors and predisposes towards hypernatremia. After achieving intravascular volume repletion, a transition to more hypotonic solutions such as dextrose and water may be undertaken to ensure correction of the serum sodium. Serum sodium levels greater than 155 mMol/l have been shown to adversely affect liver transplantation with a higher incidence of graft loss and metabolic abnormalities. Totsuka reported that serum sodiums greater than 155 mMol/l were associated with a higher incidence of graft loss, compared to donors whose serum sodium was less than 155 mMol/l. In patients who initially had a serum sodium exceeding 155 mMol/l and were effectively treated to achieve a pre-procurement sodium less than 155 mMol/l, graft dysfunction was minimized. Therefore, cautious attention to correcting the serum sodium and appropriately transitioning from normal saline to a hypotonic solution is appropriate once intravascular volume has been repleted and there is evidence of adequate perfusion [86]. Similarly, it is important to recognize that the infusion of significant amounts of hypotonic solutions containing dextrose, which are frequently used to treat diabetes insipidus, may precipitate hyperglycemia, osmotic diuresis, and hyperglycemia-mediated immune dysfunction. Similar to other critical care scenarios, the use of colloid for resuscitation remains controversial. Initial reports suggested that the use of colloid may facilitate minimizing extravascular lung water and result in an increased rate of lung procurement [87].

Frequently, there are antagonistic and competing strategies related to fluid resuscitation in the potential organ donor. Excessive fluid resuscitation with the resultant increase in extravascular lung water has been reported to be the single largest reason for lung procurement failure. In a study of potential organ donors with a lung procurement rate of 17.1 %, progressive pulmonary dysfunction occurred in 31 % of donors who had a significant positive fluid balance of approximately 7,000 ml [88]. Traditionally, there has been an emphasis upon overhydration to maximize renal function. The emphasis upon overhydration stems from a large body of literature originating during the renal transplantation surgery in the recipient, which has emphasized significant positive fluid balance, as evidenced in the following study that evaluated the impact of the timing of maximal crystalloid hydration on early graft function during renal transplantation. Early graft dysfunction was minimized when intraoperative CVP was maintained at 15 mmHg and 3 l of fluid was given with an average infusion rate of 48.3 ml/min during the 48 min of renal ischemia. Older donor management literature suggested that urine output greater than 100 ml/h during the hour prior to explanation and a decrease in the creatinine, reflective of increased hydration, were associated with improved renal function in the recipient [89]. Consequent to these and multiple other studies, there has been an emphasis upon maximal hydration for the organs below the diaphragm, which contrasts with the more minimalist volume resuscitation approach believed to enhance lung procurement. Recently, several studies have sought to clarify the approach to an appropriate fluid balance which will ensure the optimum procurement of both lungs and kidneys. In a study that compared the relationship between HRT and CVP on increasing organs for transplantation, the authors reported that when HRT was infused for greater than 15 h and a CVP was maintained at less than 10 mmHg, there was a dramatic increase in the number of hearts and lungs procured. When a final CVP was less than 10 mmHg, 44 % more hearts, 95 % more lungs, and 13 % more kidneys were transplanted [90]. A similar retrospective study sought to evaluate the impact of a restrictive fluid balance that focused upon increasing lung procurement and evaluating renal function after kidney transplantation. The authors reported that a negative or equal fluid balance with a CVP less than or equal to 6 mmHg had no effect on kidney recipient graft function or the development of delayed graft function. A positive fluid balance between the brain death event and organ procurement did not reduce the risk of graft survivorship of delayed graft function. The authors concluded that a restrictive fluid management approach, focused upon enhancing lung procurement

with a CVP less than 6 mmHg, avoided volume overload, minimized the effects of neurogenic pulmonary edema, and increased the rate of lung procurement without an adverse effect on either kidney graft survivorship or delayed graft function [91]. In summary, fluid resuscitation should be guided by objective measurements and defined endpoints similar to that used in the management of other critically ill patients. Previous strategies that focused upon aggressive overhydration to enhance renal perfusion have been shown to jeopardize pulmonary function and preclude procurement. A moderate or restrictive fluid resuscitative strategy is appropriate for both lung procurement and maintenance of renal function similar to the management approach for other critically ill patients.

In patients failing to achieve stability and defined endpoints in Fig. 44.2, vasopressors are frequently necessary to maintain perfusion pressures and are used in a majority of potential organ donors. Clear recommendations regarding the choice of vasopressors remain handicapped by an absence of controlled trials and perceived negative effects of catecholamines from studies that did not reliably measure the adequacy of intravascular volume. When employed, vasopressor and the endpoints of therapy should be clearly defined and vasopressor use titrated to specific physiologic abnormalities. Once intravascular volume resuscitation has been adequately undertaken, the choice of vasoactive support depends upon the predominant physiologic abnormalities in organ donors. In those with predominant myocardial dysfunction and inadequate flow, despite adequate volume resuscitation, dobutamine should be used for inotropic support. In potential organ donors whose hemodynamic instability is dominated by vasodilatation, vasopressors should be used to maintain mean arterial pressure and ensure adequacy of perfusion pressure gradients. Traditionally, alpha agents such as phenylephrine or norepinephrine were used to maintain vascular tone in the face of brain death-induced vasodilatation. However, recent recommendations have supported the use of vasopressin as a first-line agent to maintain vascular tone [92]. In one of the few large randomized prospective controlled trials of HRT in potential organ donors, the transition from norepinephrine to vasopressin was associated with a significant increase in cardiac output (3.18–3.72 l/min/m²) and a fall in systemic vascular resistance (1,190–964 Dyne CM SEC). Consequently, vasopressin has begun to supplant the use of phenylephrine and norepinephrine for patients whose hemodynamic profile is dominated by vasodilatation. Although not well appreciated, catecholamines have immunomodulatory properties. A large retrospective study conducted by Schnuelle reported that the donor use of dopamine and/or norepinephrine was associated with beneficial results related to acute rejection that were attributed to the immunomodulatory ability of catecholamines. This benefit was dominantly confined to renal graft survivorship, although a potential negative impact of norepinephrine was noted on heart transplantation [93, 94]. Recent literature suggests that the use of low-dose dopamine (4 mcg/kg/min) independent of hemodynamic instability was associated with a decrease in the need for dialysis after kidney transplantation [95]. Similarly, a recent review of donor pretreatment with dopamine on survivorship after heart transplant was reported. In this study, donor dopamine was associated with an improved survival after 3 years (87 % versus 67.8 %). The authors concluded that fewer recipients of a pretreated graft required hemofiltration after transplantation (21.7 % versus 40.4 %) and that treatment of potential brain-dead donors with dopamine of 4 mcg/kg/min did not harm cardiac allographs and improved the clinical course of the recipient [96].

The use of HRT is predicated upon the assumption that the ischemic damage to the hypothalamic–pituitary axis occurring with brain death creates an endocrinopathy dominated by the absence of thyroid and adrenal hormones that contribute to donor instability. Albeit it is beyond the scope of this chapter to review in great detail, it is important to recognize that the anterior pituitary and posterior pituitary have distinct differences in blood supply, innervation, and hormonal production. There is no specific direct arterial blood supply to the anterior pituitary which receives its blood supply via drainage from the hypothalamus. Blood emerging from the hypothalamus empties into a portal system that bathes the anterior pituitary. Blood supply for the posterior pituitary is via the inferior hypophyseal artery and the connection to the hypothalamus is predominantly neuronal. HRT proposes that there is significant damage to the blood supply to the hypothalamic and pituitary areas that precipitate an endocrinopathy with the attendant physiologic sequelae of a low thyroid hormone state and adrenal insufficiency. As previously discussed, there are substantial animal data and some human data to support a state of profound thyroid/adrenal depletion with exogenous supplementation reported to dramatically improve hemodynamic instability and suitability for transplantation [14]. In the original work utilizing HRT, which consisted of thyroid hormone, corticosteroids, and insulin, dramatic improvements in organ donor stability were achieved resulting in significant improvements in transplant suitability, diminutions in the requirements for vasoactive support, and dramatic improvements in cardiac function [15]. Large retrospective reviews of brain-dead donors reported significant benefit through the use of steroids and vasopressin and utilization of either triiodothyronine or thyroxine. In the group of potential organ donors that received HRT, the number of organs procured was significantly higher than the donors that did not receive HRT. This resulted in a 23 % increase in the number of organs procured with dramatic improvements in the likelihood of an organ being transplanted [97]. However, a review of thyroid hormone administration during adult donor care concluded that no publications support the routine administration of thyroid hormone for all donors. Rescue replacement for cardiac inotropic support was supported by some studies, although the methodologic designs were not detailed enough to support a recommendation for routine use [98]. In one of the few prospective randomized double-blind trials, 80 potential cardiac donors were allocated to receive triiodothyronine (0.8 mg/kg/bolus followed by a 0.113 mg/kg/h infusion), methylprednisolone 1,000 mg bolus, both drugs, or placebo following an initial hemodynamic assessment. Independent of the use of HRT, an explicit donor management algorithm with optimization variables was initiated that used vasopressin as the primary vasoactive agent. During the 6-h management period, cardiac index was noted to significantly increase in virtually all donors. However, the administration of thyroid hormone and methylprednisolone, either alone or in combination, did not affect the hemodynamics nor has any impact upon heart retrieval. Importantly, 35 % of the hearts initially deemed marginal or dysfunctional were suitable for transplantation at the end of the assessment. The authors concluded that donor circulatory status can be improved by active management with the potential to increase transplantable hearts when organ acceptance is deferred until a period of resuscitation and assessment is completed. Hemodynamic management utilizing a PAC was felt to be the cornerstone of donor management and the introduction of hormonal therapy was not a substitute for a detailed hemodynamic assessment and management optimization approaches [74]. Consequently, the use of HRT in potential organ donor management remains controversial and of uncertain benefit. Pragmatically, it would appear that this therapy should be utilized in hemodynamically unstable donors with ongoing instability, despite aggressive optimization management.

Management of the potential organ donor with a focus upon optimizing the respiratory status has assumed a greater degree of importance as the overall lung procurement ratings are usually below 20 %. The overall poor procurement rate may be explained by many factors such as an unknown past history; multiple associations with the causative brain death event, including aspiration, pulmonary contusion, shock, and resuscitation; or the complications of mechanical ventilation to include atelectasis, barotrauma, and oxygen toxicity. However, it is important to recognize that several recent studies have shown dramatic increases in the rate of lung procurement when an aggressive strategy focused upon ventilator management and respiratory care was employed.

Pathophysiologically, multiple factors conspire to jeopardize pulmonary function. These include the aforementioned events that transpire before brain death, and similar to the cardiovascular consequences of brain death, pulmonary consequences have been increasingly recognized. Traditionally, this has been dominated by neurogenic pulmonary edema consisting of the initial blast injury associated with brain death. Consequent to the catecholamine surge, there are significant elevations in systemic vascular resistance which result in elevations in left arterial pressure. This represents a transient massive hydrostatic pressure gradient generating fluid flux into the lung that is coupled with structural damage to the capillary endothelium. Against this background of capillary permeability, ongoing fluid resuscitation is purported to increase extravascular lung water, which is associated with changes in the chest x-ray appearance and diminution in lung function which have precluded procurement. Initial work in animal models revealed a dramatic distribution of blood to the right atrium and right ventricle consequent to venoconstriction and augmentation of venous return. Dramatic increases in pulmonary artery pressure were reported that resulted in 72 % of the effective circulating volume contained in the lungs for several minutes during the brain death event [16]. Subsequent to this hydrostatic and capillary burst injury pattern associated with brain death, Fisher recognized the presence of an inflammatory response associated with brain death. In a study that compared inflammatory signals in brain-dead patients compared to controls, dramatic increases in neutrophil concentration and lavage concentrations of interleukin-8 were reported [99]. In a subsequent study by Fisher and colleagues, the magnitude of the inflammatory response in the donor was evaluated in the recipient. The interleukin-8 signal in the donor was found to be correlative with the degree of impairment in graft oxygenation, the development of severe early graft dysfunction, and the early recipient mortality [100]. Avlonitis has proposed that a combination of hydrostatic forces and inflammatory responses conspires to jeopardize pulmonary function during the donor management period. The inflammatory response is derived from events that are antecedent to brain death in conjunction with ischemia–reperfusion injury of brain death. Allowing time for the lung to recover in the immediate brain death period could potentially mitigate the reperfusion injury [101, 102]. Hemodynamic mechanisms of lung injury and systemic response following brain death to the transplant donor.

The criteria for ideal lungs suitable for procurement were defined during the early phase of transplantation and included a PaO_2/FiO_2 ratio greater than 300 mmHg, a clear chest x-ray, PEEP requirements less than or equal to 5 cm of H_2O, age less than 55 years, minimal tobacco abuse, and the absence of significant chest trauma, pulmonary secretions, and aspiration. However, there has been a liberalization of these criteria which were felt to be excessively stringent and capricious. In a large autopsy series of potential donors, 47 % of those potential donors deemed suitable for lung procurement but not procured and had significant pulmonary disease and 25 % had bronchopneumonia. In those potential donors that were deemed not suitable, only 15 % had minor pulmonary abnormalities [103]. Similarly, autopsy assessment of lungs rejected for transplantation reveals that 41 % of rejected lungs

were potentially suitable for transplantation. In this case-matched study of lungs rejected for donation, 83 % were found to have absent or mild pulmonary edema, 74 % had an intact alveolar fluid clearance, and 62 % had normal or only mildly abnormal cytopathology [104]. Similarly, Fisher reported that the traditional criteria were poor discriminators of pulmonary injury and infection, which led to the exclusion of potentially usable lungs. Utilizing bronchial alveolar lavage samplings of inflammatory mediators, there was no difference between those lungs that were accepted and those excluded by clinical criteria [105].

Traditionally, donor lung ventilator management was not aggressively pursued and frequently suboptimal for preservation of lung function. This is illustrated in a study of 34 brain-dead patients, of whom 11 were considered eligible lung donors, yet only two donated lungs. In this potential lung donor population, no ventilator changes were made after brain-dead confirmation, no recruitment maneuvers were undertaken to preserve gas exchange, saline infusions were increased from 187 to 275 ml/h, and CVP was permitted to increase. Forty-five percent of the potential lung donors experienced decrements in the PaO_2/FiO_2 ratio, making them ineligible for donation. In contrast, several studies that focused upon optimization of donor lungs have reported dramatic improvement in the rate of lung procurement. In one of the original studies of lung donor management that included antibiotic therapy, strict fluid management, physiotherapy, bronchoscopy, and pulmonary toilet, along with alterations in ventilator status including the initiation of pressure ventilation, dramatic improvements in lung procurement were reported. In a study population with an initial PaO_2/FiO_2 ratio less than 300 mmHg, 31 % of lungs were clearly unsuitable and were not subjected to aggressive donor management. However, the remaining 69 % were aggressively managed to include manipulations in mechanical ventilation, adjustments in PEEP, and bronchoscopy. Forty-nine percent of those subjected to aggressive donor management were able to achieve a PaO_2/FiO_2 ratio greater than 300 mmHg and were successfully transplanted with outcomes indistinguishable from those with an initially acceptable ratio. Similar outcomes between the ideal and donor management lungs were achieved related to postop gas exchange, ICU length of stay, and short- or medium-term mortality [106]. A subsequent study similarly reported the results of an aggressive donor management program to improve the rate of lung procurement. The San Antonio Lung Transplant (SALT) Donor Management Protocol hypothesized that the implementation of a donor lung management program would increase the rate of lung procurement without adversely impacting the overall survival rate of lung transplant recipients. Elements of the protocol included educational activity to enhance the interaction between transplant pulmonologists and OPO staff related to donor selection and management, emphasis upon every donor as a lung donor, ensuring requests for donation, and educating organ procurement coordinators about donor management strategies. These included the use of recruitment maneuvers which were defined as maintenance of a pressure-controlled ventilation of 25 cm of H_2O and a PEEP of 15 cm of H_2O for 2 h with subsequent transition to conventional volume control ventilation with a tidal volume of 10 ml/kg and a PEEP of 5 cm of H_2O. Fluid balance focused upon minimizing the use of crystalloid solutions and diuretics to maintain a neutral or negative fluid balance. Aspiration risk was minimized by elevating the head of the bed to 30° and inflating the endotracheal balloon to 25 cm of H_2O. Additionally, bronchoscopy with bronchial alveolar lavage was performed on all patients to evaluate the chest x-ray area of infiltrate. Despite poor donors accounting for 76 % of the total donors during the trial period, the pretrial period compared to posttrial period resulted in a dramatic increase in actual lung donors (98 versus 38) and a significant increase in lung transplantations (121 versus 53). The authors concluded that an aggressive protocol focused on lung donor management significantly increased the number of lung donors and transplant procedures without compromising lung function, length of stay, or survival of the recipients [107]. In a recent comparison trial of lung donor management, a significant increase in the rate of lung procurement was reported, with an aggressive lung donor management strategy (40 % versus 27 %). In the control group, donor management commenced within 2 h of consent for donation and continued for approximately 7 h. Management strategies included early bronchoscopy, tidal volumes of 10 ml/kg with a PEEP of 5 cm of H_2O, frequent suctioning, and volume recruitment enabled by turning the potential donor every 2 h. A specific hemodynamic algorithm titrating vasoactive support and fluid resuscitation to a cardiac index of greater than 2.5 l/min/m^2, focusing on a low CVP and pulmonary capillary wedge pressures, was employed. Fluid resuscitation was minimized and colloid solution was preferentially utilized. Donor lungs subjected to this aggressive management approach resulted in a procurement rate of 40 % [73].

Although a lung protective strategy has been adopted by the intensive care community for patients with acute lung injury, traditional donor management has utilized relatively high tidal volumes in an effort to minimize de-recruitment and improve gas exchange. In all likelihood, hyperinflation has cosmetically improved the chest x-ray which is one of the traditional criteria for procurement. However, these traditional concepts were recently challenged in a randomized controlled trial comparing the outcomes of conventional ventilator strategies with tidal volumes of 10–12 ml/kg, PEEP maintenance with 3–5 cm of H_2O, and the performance of apnea tests by disconnecting the ventilator with an open suction to a protective ventilator strategy with tidal volumes of 6–8 ml/kg, PEEP of 8–10 cm of H_2O with apnea tests performed by using continuous positive airway pressure, and closed circuit for suction. In the conventional strategy group, only 54 % of potential donors met lung donor eligibility after a 6-h observation period compared to 95 % in the protective strategy group. Only 27 % of lungs were procured from donors in the conventional strategy group compared to a procurement rate of 54 % in the protective strategy group. Six months survivorship did not differ between those recipients receiving lungs from either category. Similar to data from patients with acute lung injury, a significantly higher level of inflammatory mediators were reported in the conventional ventilator strategy compared to the protective ventilator strategy. This study strongly suggests that hyperinflation has an adverse effect on lung function, compromises eligibility of lung donors, and should be replaced by a protective ventilator strategy similar to patients with acute lung injury. Similar to the evidence supporting aggressive donor cardiac management, an aggressive approach to lung donor management will result in a higher level of lung donor procurement and no donor lung should be rejected upon the initial evaluation. Ongoing assessments for suitability are required in conjunction with aggressive donor management [108].

Supportive Care

Hemodynamic management forms the cornerstone of potential organ donor management. Ensuring adequate perfusion to all organs is the best approach to support liver, kidney, pancreas and small bowel function, anticipating possible procurement. This requires ongoing hemodynamic measurements using the previously described donor management endpoints. Although there are extremely limited data, there is speculation that hepatic glycogen stores may be depleted in the brain death period and that support with enteral nutrition may play an important role in modulating organ function after transplantation [109]. In the absence of contraindications, it is appropriate to continue enteral nutrition carefully following for any evidence of hyperglycemia. As previously mentioned, the liver is explicitly sensitive to hypernatremia in some studies and serum sodium level should be corrected to less than 155 mEq/l. Diabetes insipidus is a frequent complication of brain death secondary to a deficiency of vasopressin after pituitary destruction. Vasopressin absence can contribute to multiple donor management issues, including hyperosmolarity, electrolyte disturbances, and intravascular volume depletion. It is important to differentiate diabetes insipidus from mannitol-induced osmotic diuresis. Diabetes insipidus is generally associated with a serum sodium greater than 150 mEq/l, an elevated serum osmolarity, a urine output exceeding 300 ml/h, and a low urine osmolarity usually less than 200 mOsm/l with an associated normal serum osmolar gap. The preceding serves to differentiate diabetes insipidus from mannitol-induced polyuria. Diabetes insipidus should be treated with hypotonic solutions, and frequently, 5 % dextrose in water is used to match urine output ml for ml. In instances of excessive urine output greater than 200–300 ml/h, desmopressin acetate (DVAVP) or arginine vasopressin may be utilized. Vasopressin exerts its effect on three receptors: V1 receptors on the smooth muscle and is responsible for vasopressor effects, V2 receptors located in the kidney which promote the antidiuretic effect, and V3 receptors in the pituitary which regulate corticotropin-releasing hormone. Arginine vasopressin has antidiuretic and vasopressor effects, whereas DVAVP has greater affinity for the V2 receptor and consequently a predominant antidiuretic effect. Clinically, 1–4 μg of DVAVP is given intravenously following urine osmolarity, urine output, and serum sodium closely. Subsequent dosing is dependent upon the response. In the setting of hypotension, arginine vasopressin is preferred at a dose between 0.01 and 0.04 IU/min. Hyperglycemia is frequent in potential organ donors and frequently necessitates the use of insulin for control. Although the effects of hyperglycemia are not well established, hyperglycemia is believed to impair organ function. Consequently, hyperglycemia should be treated similarly to critically ill patients using an empiric level of 150 mg/dl to initiate therapy. Coagulation abnormalities are frequently common in potential organ donors, and ongoing assessment of coagulopathy and hemoglobin is necessary during the course of donor management. Although there are no outcome data for potential organ donors, the approach advocated is similar to that of other critically ill patients utilizing a transfusion threshold for hemoglobin of 8 mg/dl and normalization of coagulation parameters. Pituitary injury predisposes to thermoregulatory impairment and it is imperative that the donor receive warmed fluids and body temperature be monitored routinely, as hypothermia can further impair coagulation and predispose to cardiac rhythm disturbances.

Donation After Cardiac Death

Donation after cardiac death refers to the recovery of organs from patients that are not brain dead but die secondary to cardiopulmonary causes. This was previously known as a non-heartbeating donor. Donation may occur in several circumstances that are either controlled or uncontrolled. The vast majority of donation after cardiac death occurs during controlled situations when care is withdrawn and the patient is pronounced dead from cardiopulmonary arrest. Uncontrolled donation after cardiac death is far less common and occurs in emergent circumstances such as death from an acute trauma. Prior to 1968, there was no legal definition for

brain death and donation after cardiac death was the primary method for obtaining organs for transplantation. After the acceptance of brain death, donation from brain-dead donors has significantly exceeded those from donation after cardiac death. The Institute of Medicine (IOM) formally evaluated the donation after cardiac death practice into separate reports [110, 111]. Specifically, the IOM stipulated that the decision to withdraw or withhold care be undertaken based upon the patient's wishes and not influenced by any potential for organ donation. It was further recommended that a separate team provide end-of-life care that was distinct from the transplant team. Donation after cardiac death must adhere to the dead donor rule, which stipulates that donor organs may only be procured from dead patients. When undertaking donation after cardiac death, the withdrawal of care should be indistinguishable from the withdrawal of care in any other critically ill patient. Death is declared when there is cessation of cardiopulmonary function and after a period of time to ensure that there is no spontaneous recrudescence of respiratory function. Although the initial 1997 recommendation from the IOM was a 5-min period between the diagnosis of death and the initiation of organ recovery, it is currently recommended that this period be at least 2 min and no more than 5 min [112].

References

1. Cushing H. Some experimental and clinical observations concerning states of increased intracranial tension. Am J Med Sci. 1901; 124:375.
2. Power BM, Van Heerden PV. The physiological changes associated with brain death – current concepts and implications for treatment of the brain dead organ donor. Anaesth Intensive Care. 1995;23:26–36.
3. Kopelnik A, Zaroff JG. Neurocardiogenic injury in neurovascular disorders. Crit Care Clin. 2006;22:733–52.
4. Banki NM, Zaroff JG. Neurogenic cardiac injury. Curr Treat Options Cardiovasc Med. 2003;5:451–8.
5. Banki NM, Kopelnik A, Dae MW, et al. Acute neurocardiogenic injury after subarachnoid hemorrhage. Circulation. 2005;112:3314–9.
6. Tung P, Kopelnik A, Banki N, et al. Predictors of neurocardiogenic injury after subarachnoid hemorrhage. Stroke. 2004;35:548–51.
7. Banki NM, Parmley WW, Foster E, Gress D, Lawton MT. Reversibility of left ventricular systolic dysfunction in humans with subarachnoid hemorrhage. Circulation. 2001;104:11 (Abstracted).
8. Powner DJ, Boccalandro C, Alp MS, Vollmer DG. Endocrine failure after traumatic brain injury in adults. Neurocrit Care. 2006;5: 61–70.
9. Schneider HJ, Kreitschmann-Andermahr I, Ghigo E, Stalla GK, Agha A. Hypothalamopituitary dysfunction following traumatic brain injury and aneurysmal subarachnoid hemorrhage: a systematic review. JAMA. 2007;298:1429–38.
10. Yoshioka T, Sugimoto H, Uenishi M, et al. Prolonged hemodynamic maintenance by the combined administration of vasopressin and epinephrine in brain death: a clinical study. Neurosurgery. 1986;18:565–7.
11. Black PM. Brain death (first of two parts). N Engl J Med. 1978;299:338–44.

12. Novitzky D. Donor management: state of the art. Transplant Proc. 1997;29:3773–5.

13. Novitzky D, Cooper DK, Chaffin JS, Greer AE, DeBault LE, Zuhdi N. Improved cardiac allograft function following triiodothyronine therapy to both donor and recipient. Transplantation. 1990;49:311–6.

14. Novitzky D, Cooper DK, Morrell D, Isaacs S. Change from aerobic to anaerobic metabolism after brain death, and reversal following triiodothyronine therapy. Transplantation. 1988;45:32–6.

15. Novitzky D, Cooper DK, Reichart B. Hemodynamic and metabolic responses to hormonal therapy in brain-dead potential organ donors. Transplantation. 1987;43:852–4.

16. Novitzky D, Wicomb WN, Rose AG, Cooper DK, Reichart B. Pathophysiology of pulmonary edema following experimental brain death in the chacma baboon. Ann Thorac Surg. 1987;43: 288–94.

17. Novitzky D, Wicomb W, Cooper D, Rose AG. Electrocardiographic, hemodynamic and endocrine changes occurring during experimental brain death in the chacma baboon. J Heart Transplant. 1984;IV:63–9.

18. Szabo G, Buhmann V, Bahrle S, Vahl CF, Hagl S. Brain death impairs coronary endothelial function. Transplantation. 2002;73:1846–8.

19. Segel LD, VonHaag DW, Zhang J, Follette DM. Selective overexpression of inflammatory molecules in hearts from brain-dead rats. J Heart Lung Transplant. 2002;21:804–11.

20. Szabo G, Hackert T, Buhmann V, et al. Downregulation of myocardial contractility via intact ventriculo – arterial coupling in the brain dead organ donor. Eur J Cardiothorac Surg. 2001;20:170–6.

21. Szabo G, Hackert T, Buhmann V, Sebening C, Vahl CF, Hagl S. Myocardial performance after brain death: studies in isolated hearts. Ann Transplant. 2000;5:45–50.

22. Yeh Jr T, Wechsler AS, Graham LJ, et al. Acute brain death alters left ventricular myocardial gene expression. J Thorac Cardiovasc Surg. 1999;117:365–74.

23. Bittner HB, Chen EP, Milano CA, et al. Myocardial beta-adrenergic receptor function and high-energy phosphates in brain death – related cardiac dysfunction. Circulation. 1995;92:472–8.

24. D'Amico TA, Meyers CH, Koutlas TC, et al. Desensitization of myocardial beta-adrenergic receptors and deterioration of left ventricular function after brain death. J Thorac Cardiovasc Surg. 1995;110:746–51.

25. Shivalkar B, Van Loon J, Wieland W, et al. Variable effects of explosive or gradual increase of intracranial pressure on myocardial structure and function. Circulation. 1993;87:230–9.

26. Mehra MR, Uber PA, Ventura HO, Scott RL, Park MH. The impact of mode of donor brain death on cardiac allograft vasculopathy: an intravascular ultrasound study. J Am Coll Cardiol. 2004;43:806–10.

27. Audibert G, Charpentier C, Seguin-Devaux C, et al. Improvement of donor myocardial function after treatment of autonomic storm during brain death. Transplantation. 2006;82:1031–6.

28. Cooper DK, Novitzky D, Wicomb WN. The pathophysiological effects of brain death on potential donor organs, with particular reference to the heart. Ann R Coll Surg Engl. 1989;71:261–6.

29. Gramm HJ, Meinhold H, Bickel U, et al. Acute endocrine failure after brain death? Transplantation. 1992;54:851–7.

30. Howlett TA, Keogh AM, Perry L, Touzel R, Rees LH. Anterior and posterior pituitary function in brain-stem-dead donors. A possible role for hormonal replacement therapy. Transplantation. 1989;47:828–34.

31. Powner DJ, Hendrich A, Lagler RG, Ng RH, Madden RL. Hormonal changes in brain dead patients. Crit Care Med. 1990;18:702–8.

32. Goarin JP, Cohen S, Riou B, et al. The effects of triiodothyronine on hemodynamic status and cardiac function in potential heart donors. Anesth Analg. 1996;83:41–7.

33. Randell TT, Hockerstedt KA. Triiodothyronine treatment in brain-dead multiorgan donors – a controlled study. Transplantation. 1992;54:736–8.

34. Gasser M. Organ transplantation from brain dead donors: its impact on short and long term outcome revisited. Transplant Rev. 2001;15:1–10.

35. Pratschke J, Wilhelm MJ, Kusaka M, et al. Brain death and its influence on donor organ quality and outcome after transplantation. Transplantation. 1999;67:343–8.

36. Murugan R, Venkataraman R, Wahed AS, et al. Increased plasma interleukin-6 in donors is associated with lower recipient hospital-free survival after cadaveric organ transplantation. Crit Care Med. 2008;36:1810–6.

37. Murugan R, Venkataraman R, Wahed AS, et al. Preload responsiveness is associated with increased interleukin-6 and lower organ yield from brain-dead donors. Crit Care Med. 2009;37: 2387–93.

38. Birks EJ, Burton PB, Owen V, et al. Elevated tumor necrosis factor-alpha and interleukin-6 in myocardium and serum of malfunctioning donor hearts. Circulation. 2000;102:352–8.

39. Venkateswaran RV, Dronavalli V, Lambert PA, et al. The proinflammatory environment in potential heart and lung donors: prevalence and impact of donor management and hormonal therapy. Transplantation. 2009;88:582–8.

40. Weiss S, Kotsch K, Francuski M, et al. Brain death activates donor organs and is associated with a worse I/R injury after liver transplantation. Am J Transplant. 2007;7:1584–93.

41. Kotsch K, Ulrich F, Reutzel-Selke A, et al. Methylprednisolone therapy in deceased donors reduces inflammation in the donor liver and improves outcome after liver transplantation: a prospective randomized controlled trial. Ann Surg. 2008;248:1042–50.

42. Mollaret P, Goulon M. The depassed coma (preliminary memoir). Rev Neurol (Paris). 1959;101:3–15.

43. Lofstedt S. Intracranial lesions with abolished passage of x-ray contrast throughout the internal carotid arteries. Pacing Clin Electrophysiol. 1956;8:99.

44. Schwab R. EEG as an aid in determining death in the presence of cardiac acuity. Electroencephalogr Clin Neurophysiol. 1963;15: 147.

45. A definition of irreversible coma. Report of the Ad Hoc Committee of the Harvard Medical School to examine the definition of brain death. JAMA. 1968;205:337–40.

46. Diagnosis of brain death. Statement issued by the honorary secretary of the Conference of Medical Royal Colleges and their Faculties in the United Kingdom on 11 October 1976. Br Med J. 1976;2:1187–8.

47. Criteria for the diagnosis of brain stem death. Review by a working group convened by the Royal College of Physicians and endorsed by the Conference of Medical Royal Colleges and their Faculties in the United Kingdom. J R Coll Physicians Lond. 1995;29:381–2.

48. Practice parameters for determining brain death in adults (summary statement). The Quality Standards Subcommittee of the American Academy of Neurology. Neurology. 1995;45:1012–4.

49. An appraisal of the criteria of cerebral death. A summary statement. A collaborative study. JAMA. 1977;237:982–6.

50. Wijdicks EF, Varelas PN, Gronseth GS, Greer DM. American Academy of N. Evidence-based guideline update: determining brain death in adults: report of the Quality Standards Subcommittee of the American Academy of Neurology. Neurology. 2010;74: 1911–8.

51. Wijdicks EF. Clinical diagnosis and confirmatory testing of brain death in adults. In: Brain death. Philadelphia: Lippincott Williams & Wilkins; 2001. p. 61–90.

52. Lutz-Dettinger N, de Jaeger A, Kerremans I. Care of the potential pediatric organ donor. Pediatr Clin North Am. 2001;48:715–49.

53. Lopez-Navidad A, Domingo P, Caballero F, Gonzalez C, Santiago C. Successful transplantation of organs retrieved from donors with bacterial meningitis. Transplantation. 1997;64:365–8.

54. Bahrami T, Vohra HA, Shaikhrezai K, et al. Intrathoracic organ transplantation from donors with meningitis: a single-center 20-year experience. Ann Thorac Surg. 2008;86:1554–6.

55. Satoi S, Bramhall SR, Solomon M, et al. The use of liver grafts from donors with bacterial meningitis. Transplantation. 2001;72:1108–13.

56. Kubak BM, Gregson AL, Pegues DA, et al. Use of hearts transplanted from donors with severe sepsis and infectious deaths. J Heart Lung Transplant. 2009;28:260–5.

57. Cohen J, Michowiz R, Ashkenazi T, Pitlik S, Singer P. Successful organ transplantation from donors with Acinetobacter baumannii septic shock. Transplantation. 2006;81:853–5.

58. Williams MA, Lipsett PA, Rushton CH, Grochowski EC, Berkowitz ID, Mann SL, Shatzer JH, Short MP, Genel M, Council on Scientific Affairs, American Medical Association. The physician's role in discussing organ donation with families. Crit Care Med. 2003;31:1568–73.

59. DeJong W, Franz HG, Wolfe SM, et al. Requesting organ donation: an interview study of donor and nondonor families. Am J Crit Care. 1998;7:13–23.

60. Siminoff LA, Gordon N, Hewlett J, Arnold RM. Factors influencing families' consent for donation of solid organs for transplantation. JAMA. 2001;286:71–7.

61. Childress JF, Liverman CT. Organ donation. Washington DC: The National Academies Press; 2006.

62. Gortmaker SL, Beasley CL, Sheehy E, et al. Improving the request process to increase family consent for organ donation. J Transpl Coord. 1998;8:210–7.

63. Garrison RN, Bentley FR, Raque GH, et al. There is an answer to the shortage of organ donors. Surg Gynecol Obstet. 1991;173:391–6.

64. Siminoff LA, Lawrence RH, Zhang A. Decoupling: what is it and does it really help increase consent to organ donation? Prog Transplant. 2002;12:52–60.

65. Rosendale JD, Chabalewski FL, McBride MA, et al. Increased transplanted organs from the use of a standardized donor management protocol. Am J Transplant. 2002;2:761–8.

66. Salim A, Velmahos GC, Brown C, Belzberg H, Demetriades D. Aggressive organ donor management significantly increases the number of organs available for transplantation. J Trauma. 2005;58:991–4.

67. Salim A, Martin M, Brown C, Rhee P, Demetriades D, Belzberg H. The effect of a protocol of aggressive donor management: implications for the national organ donor shortage. J Trauma. 2006;61:429–33.

68. Inaba K, Branco BC, Lam L, et al. Organ donation and time to procurement: late is not too late. J Trauma. 2010;68:1362–6.

69. Christmas AB, Bogart TA, Etson KE, et al. The reward is worth the wait: a prospective analysis of 100 consecutive organ donors. Am Surg. 2012;78:296–9.

70. Hagan ME, McClean D, Falcone CA, Arrington J, Matthews D, Summe C. Attaining specific donor management goals increases number of organs transplanted per donor: a quality improvement project. Prog Transplant. 2009;19:227–31.

71. Franklin GA, Santos AP, Smith JW, Galbraith S, Harbrecht BG, Garrison RN. Optimization of donor management goals yields increased organ use. Am Surg. 2010;76:587–94.

72. Malinoski DJ, Daly MC, Patel MS, Oley-Graybill C, Foster 3rd CE, Salim A. Achieving donor management goals before deceased donor procurement is associated with more organs transplanted per donor. J Trauma. 2011;71:990–5.

73. Venkateswaran RV, Patchell VB, Wilson IC, et al. Early donor management increases the retrieval rate of lungs for transplantation. Ann Thorac Surg. 2008;85:278–86.

74. Venkateswaran RV, Steeds RP, Quinn DW, et al. The haemodynamic effects of adjunctive hormone therapy in potential heart donors: a prospective randomized double-blind factorially designed controlled trial. Eur Heart J. 2009;30:1771–80.

75. Gilbert EM, Krueger SK, Murray JL, et al. Echocardiographic evaluation of potential cardiac transplant donors. J Thorac Cardiovasc Surg. 1988;95:1003–7.

76. Zaroff JG, Babcock WD, Shiboski SC. The impact of left ventricular dysfunction on cardiac donor transplant rates. J Heart Lung Transplant. 2003;22:334–7.

77. Zaroff J. Echocardiographic evaluation of the potential cardiac donor. J Heart Lung Transplant. 2004;23:S250–2.

78. Zaroff JG, Babcock WD, Shiboski SC, Solinger LL, Rosengard BR. Temporal changes in left ventricular systolic function in heart donors: results of serial echocardiography. J Heart Lung Transplant. 2003;22:383–8.

79. Stoddard MF, Longaker RA. The role of transesophageal echocardiography in cardiac donor screening. Am Heart J. 1993;125:1676–81.

80. Venkateswaran RV, Townend JN, Wilson IC, Mascaro JG, Bonser RS, Steeds RP. Echocardiography in the potential heart donor. Transplantation. 2010;89:894–901.

81. Kouo T, Nishina T, Morita H, et al. Usefulness of low dose dobutamine stress echocardiography for evaluating reversibility of brain death-induced myocardial dysfunction. Am J Cardiol. 1999;84:558–82.

82. Wheeldon DR, Potter CD, Oduro A, Wallwork J, Large SR. Transforming the "unacceptable" donor: outcomes from the adoption of a standardized donor management technique. J Heart Lung Transplant. 1995;14:734–42.

83. Marik PE, Baram M, Vahid B. Does central venous pressure predict fluid responsiveness? A systematic review of the literature and the tale of seven mares. Chest. 2008;134:172–8.

84. Marik PE, Cavallazzi R, Vasu T, Hirani A. Dynamic changes in arterial waveform derived variables and fluid responsiveness in mechanically ventilated patients: a systematic review of the literature. Crit Care Med. 2009;37:2642–7.

85. Whelchel J, Diethelm A, Phillips M. The effect of high dose dopamine in cadaveric donor management in delayed graft function and graft survival following renal transplant. Transplant Proc. 1986;18:523–7.

86. Totsuka E, Dodson F, Urakami A, et al. Influence of high donor serum sodium levels on early postoperative graft function in human liver transplantation: effect of correction of donor hypernatremia. Liver Transpl Surg. 1999;5:421–8.

87. Follette D, Rudich S, Bonacci C, Allen R, Hoso A, Albertson T. Importance of an aggressive multidisciplinary management approach to optimize lung donor procurement. Transplant Proc. 1999;31:169–70.

88. Reilly P, Morgan L, Grossman MD, et al. Lung procurement from solid organ donors – role of fluid resuscitation in procurement failures. Internet J Emerg Intensive Care Med [serial online]. 1999;3(2): http://www.ispub.com/journals/IJEICM/VOl3N2/organ.htm.

89. Lucas BA, Vaughn WK, Spees EK, Sanfilippo F. Identification of donor factors predisposing to high discard rates of cadaver kidneys and increased graft loss within one year posttransplantation – SEOPF 1977–1982. South-Eastern Organ Procurement Foundation. Transplantation. 1987;43:253–8.

90. Abdelnour T, Rieke S. Relationship of hormonal resuscitation therapy and central venous pressure on increasing organs for transplant. J Heart Lung Transplant. 2009;28:480–5.

91. Minambres E, Rodrigo E, Ballesteros MA, et al. Impact of restrictive fluid balance focused to increase lung procurement on renal function after kidney transplantation. Nephrol Dial Transplant. 2010;25:2352–6.

92. Shemie SD, Ross H, Pagliarello J, et al. Organ donor management in Canada: recommendations of the forum on Medical Management to Optimize Donor Organ Potential. CMAJ. 2006;174:S13–32.

93. Schnuelle P, Lorenz D, Mueller A, Trede M, Van Der Woude FJ. Donor catecholamine use reduces acute allograft rejection and improves graft survival after cadaveric renal transplantation. Kidney Int. 1999;56:738–46.

94. Schnuelle P, Berger S, de Boer J, Persijn G, van der Woude FJ. Effects of catecholamine application to brain-dead donors on graft survival in solid organ transplantation. Transplantation. 2001;72: 455–63.

95. Schnuelle P, Gottmann U, Hoeger S, et al. Effects of donor pre-treatment with dopamine on graft function after kidney transplantation: a randomized controlled trial. JAMA. 2009;302:1067–75.

96. Benck U, Hoeger S, Brinkkoetter PT, et al. Effects of donor pre-treatment with dopamine on survival after heart transplantation: a cohort study of heart transplant recipients nested in a randomized controlled multicenter trial. J Am Coll Cardiol. 2011;58: 1768–77.

97. Rosendale JD, Kauffman HM, McBride MA, et al. Aggressive pharmacologic donor management results in more transplanted organs. Transplantation. 2003;75:482–7.

98. Powner DJ, Hernandez M. A review of thyroid hormone administration during adult donor care. Prog Transplant. 2005;15: 2002–7.

99. Fisher AJ, Donnelly SC, Hirani N, et al. Enhanced pulmonary inflammation in organ donors following fatal non-traumatic brain injury. Lancet. 1999;353:1412–3.

100. Fisher A, Donnelly SC, Mirani N, et al. Elevated levels of interleukin-8 in donor lungs is associated with early graft failure after lung transplantation. Am J Respir Crit Care Med. 2001;163: 259–65.

101. Avlonitis VS, Wigfield CH, Golledge HD, Kirby JA, Dark JH. Early hemodynamic injury during donor brain death determines the severity of primary graft dysfunction after lung transplantation. Am J Transplant. 2007;7:83–90.

102. Avlonitis VS, Wigfield CH, Kirby JA, Dark JH. The hemodynamic mechanisms of lung injury and systemic inflammatory response following brain death in the transplant donor. Am J Transplant. 2005;5:684–93.

103. Finfer S, Bohn D, Colpitts D, Cox P, Fleming F, Barker G. Intensive care management of paediatric organ donors and its effect on post-transplant organ function. Intensive Care Med. 1996;22:1424–32.

104. Ware LB, Wang Y, Fang X, et al. Assessment of lungs rejected for transplantation and implications for donor selection. Lancet. 2002;360:619–20.

105. Fisher AJ, Donnelly SC, Pritchard G, Dark JH, Corris PA. Objective assessment of criteria for selection of donor lungs suitable for transplantation. Thorax. 2004;59:434–7.

106. Gabbay E, Williams TJ, Griffiths AP, et al. Maximizing the utilization of donor organs offered for lung transplantation. Am J Respir Crit Care Med. 1999;160:265–71.

107. Angel LF, Levine DJ, Restrepo MI, et al. Impact of a lung transplantation donor-management protocol on lung donation and recipient outcomes. Am J Respir Crit Care Med. 2006;174:710–6.

108. Mascia L, Pasero D, Slutsky AS, et al. Effect of a lung protective strategy for organ donors on eligibility and availability of lungs for transplantation: a randomized controlled trial. JAMA. 2010; 304:2620–7.

109. Singer P, Cohen J, Cynober L. Effect of nutritional state of brain-dead organ donor on transplantation. Nutrition. 2001;17:948–52.

110. Herdman R, Potts J. Non-heart beating organ transplantation: Medical and ethical issues in procurement. Institute of Medicine, National Academy of Sciences. Washington, DC: National Academy Press; 1997.

111. Institute of Medicine. Non-heart beating organ transplantation: Practice and Protocols. Institute of Medicine, National Academy of Sciences. Washington, DC: National Academy Press; 2000.

112. Ethics Committee, American College of Critical Care Medicine, Society of Critical Care Medicine. Recommendations for non-heartbeating organ donation – a position paper by the Ethics Committee, American College of Critical Care Medicine, Society of Critical Care Medicine. Crit Care Med. 2001;29: 1826–31.

113. Wood KE, Becker B, McCarney J, et al. Care of the potential organ donor. N Engl J Med. 2004;351:2730–9.

Ethical Issues in the Neurointensive Care Unit

45

William Allen

Contents

Abstract

Patients present daily in neurosurgical intensive care units with illnesses that require physicians to consider not only diagnostic and therapeutic questions but ethical issues as well. While these ethical concerns are often asked and answered only at an intuitive level, physicians in the intensive care unit face an increasingly complex set of ethical and legal concerns, such as allocation of resources, medical futility, withholding and withdrawal of life-sustaining treatment (LST), and palliative sedation, among others. Adequate answers to such complex issues require critical analysis of issues rather than a merely intuitive approach.

Intensive care services should be allocated by medical need, rather than personal characteristics, behavioral traits, political clout of the referring hospital service, employment status, or degree of medical benefit. An appropriate approach to assessment of patient decisional capacity recognizes that such capacity manifests over a range of functional abilities that are context dependent and therefore requires specific analysis of a patient's ability to make particular decisions about specific options that vary in complexity and comprehensiveness. When harvesting organs from patients declared dead by appropriate criteria, each institution must adopt clear policies that avoid real or apparent conflicts of interests. Those who harvest organs must not be the physician who pronounces death. Decisionally capacitated adult patients have ethical and legal rights to refuse any life-sustaining treatment. There is no ethical or legal difference between withholding life-sustaining treatment and withdrawing life-sustaining treatment. Advance directives should be seen as an occasion to initiate conversation about patient end-of-life wishes rather than as a substitute for such conversations. Attempts to substantively define medical futility have not brought consensus, but procedural approaches to medical futility show some promise. Although physician aid in dying remains illegal in most states, other last-resort options are legally available, although controversial, including voluntary refusal of nutrition and hydration and palliative sedation.

W. Allen, JD, MD
Program for Bioethics, Law, and Medical Professionalism,
University of Florida College of Medicine, 1600 SW Archer Rd,
Suite N1-07, Gainesville, FL 32610, USA
e-mail: wmallen@ufl.edu

A.J. Layon et al. (eds.), *Textbook of Neurointensive Care*,
DOI 10.1007/978-1-4471-5226-2_45, © Springer-Verlag London 2013

Keywords

Ethics • End of life • Futility • Allocation • Decisional capacity • Palliative sedation

Introduction

Patients present daily in neurointensive care units (Neuro ICU) with illnesses that require physicians to consider not only diagnostic and therapeutic questions but ethical issues as well. While these ethical concerns are often asked and answered only at an intuitive level, ICU physicians face an increasingly complex set of ethical and legal concerns, such as allocation of resources, medical futility, withholding and withdrawal of life-sustaining treatment (LST), and palliative sedation, among others. Adequate answers to such complex issues require critical analysis of issues rather than a merely intuitive approach.

Principles of Biomedical Ethics

The most widely utilized approach to modern biomedical ethics in the English-speaking world, principlism, analyzes cases in terms of an attempt to balance four major principles: autonomy, nonmaleficence, beneficence, and (distributive) justice [1]. Autonomy, meaning self-determination, refers to the rights of patients to choose among reasonable medical alternatives or to refuse recommended medical interventions. Nonmaleficence entails the obligation not to inflict harm on the patient, whereas beneficence refers to the physician's positive obligation to promote the good of the patient. Distributive justice expresses the obligation of the physician to distribute fairly and equitably either the benefits of medical interventions or the burdens that may accompany medical care.

No one of these four principles has automatic or absolute priority over the others. In fact, these principles alone are too abstract to be very useful in resolving particular moral problems in actual cases, without appropriate qualification and specification of more concrete norms in the form of rules, recognized exceptions, and a process of balancing conflicting principles and rules. Nonmaleficence, for example, cannot be taken so literally that a physician does not utilize medical treatments that have a risk of harm or even a certainty of harmful "side effects." The obligation to do no harm must be balanced by beneficence in a specific manner so that the balance of medical benefit of an intervention is greater than the risk of harm or the harmful side effects. As a social institution, medicine historically placed most emphasis on nonmaleficence (do no harm) and beneficence (promote the best medical interests of your patient), as well as on the physician's professional autonomy (nonphysicians should not tell physicians how to

practice medicine). In the latter half of the twentieth century, however, patient autonomy has become more widely advocated and incorporated into biomedical ethics as well as in healthcare law. Simultaneously, the dramatic increases in the costs of high-tech medical care and the scarcity of resources such as organs for persons who need transplants have moved distributive justice issues to the forefront of challenging ethical problems in biomedical ethics and society. The issues that arise when treating members of the Jehovah's Witness faith provide a good opportunity for illustrating how to balance the principles of nonmaleficence, beneficence, and autonomy in a concrete context. Following the section on Jehovah's Witnesses, the principle of distributive justice will be addressed as it arises in intensive care medicine.

Jehovah's Witnesses

A distinctive article of Jehovah's Witnesses' faith poses a challenge for physicians providing Witnesses with medical care when blood transfusions are medically indicated. The physician's commitment to the principles of nonmaleficence and beneficence makes the use of blood transfusions seem to be medically necessary when serious morbidity or mortality is at stake. The religious convictions of Jehovah's Witnesses, however, create a conflict between the individual Witness's autonomy-based refusal of blood transfusions and the physician's conception of the patient's best interests as supported by the principle of beneficence. Witnesses interpret the Biblical proscription against eating any animal that has not been drained of blood literally, refusing to accept blood transfusions, since they regard transfusions as "consuming blood." This prohibition extends even to lifesaving transfusions. Although Witnesses are not eager to die, they believe that remaining true to Jehovah's command against consumption of blood, even if it means death, is preferable to the consequences of disobedience to Jehovah's [2]. The refusal of blood transfusion by an adult Jehovah's Witness, even when the risk of death is real, should be respected on the basis of patient autonomy and the common law recognition that "Every human being of adult years and sound mind has a right to determine what shall be done with his own body…" [3].

Although Witnesses do not believe in hell, they still believe that disobedience to God's command could prevent them from eternal life with God. Moreover, the temporal consequences are not trivial. Witnesses who voluntarily accept blood transfusions are shunned by the congregation and even by family members [2]. In order to encourage Witnesses facing the need for transfusion to remain steadfast in the refusal of blood, family and other members of the congregation gather to encourage the Witness to refuse. Thus, when attempting to distinguish whether a Jehovah's Witness's decision to refuse a blood transfusion is an authentic expression of autonomy rather than a product of undue influence from well-meaning family members and elders in their congregation, the physician should at some point speak with the Witness patient alone. In some cases, a Witness will reluctantly accept a transfusion if reassured that the decision and the transfusion will be maintained in strict confidence. If the Witness does accept a transfusion under these conditions, the physician is not obligated to lie about the patient's decision when responding to the family's questions. The physician should simply respond to inquiries from family that all patient information is confidential.

The clearest Jehovah's Witness prohibition is on receiving a blood transfusion from another person or even the patient's own blood that has been separated from continuous circulation. When their own blood remains in continuous circulation through tubing that remains connected to their bodies, such as in cardiopulmonary bypass surgery or in erythrocyte retrieval and salvage, many Jehovah's Witnesses will not consider this as prohibited consumption of blood, and this issue is generally left up to the individual's choice by Jehovah's Witness official doctrine [2]. Acceptance of albumin or plasma is also left up to the individual Witness [2].

Courts have consistently upheld the right to refuse blood transfusions of adult, decisionally capacitated Jehovah's Witnesses. A strategy of waiting until the refusing Witness is unconscious or otherwise incapacitated in order to override the patient's earlier refusal, even if a non-Witness family member authorizes the transfusion, is ethically and legally invalid [4]. When the patient is a minor, however, courts will routinely override the refusals of adult Jehovah's Witness parents and authorize medically necessary transfusions. In some cases, when the minor is close to the age of majority, some courts have determined a Jehovah's Witness 17-year-old who evinces a refusal based on the minor's own independent beliefs rather than parental coercion to be a "mature minor," allowing the minor to refuse blood transfusions. Such decisions are made on a case-by-case basis and depend on the court's examination of the particular minor's maturity [5].

Distributive Justice: Allocation of Intensive Care Resources

Discussion of the principle of justice will begin with a conceptual framework that elucidates the distinction between the formal principle of justice and various material (or substantive) principles. The formal principle of justice may be expressed as follows: treat like cases alike and different cases differently in proportion to their differences. When determining how to distribute benefits (or burdens) fairly, one should make distributions consistently among persons who are in similar situations, and conversely, when persons are in different situations, one should make differing distributions

in proportion to ethically relevant differences. The material principles of justice, by contrast, are those substantive criteria by which persons are determined to be in morally relevant similar or different situations.

Healthcare is allocated at the societal level in the United States according to a variety of material criteria, including need; ability to pay; first come, first served; medical utility; and proximity to services [1]. *In many cases, there is no coherent overarching rationale for the overall pattern of allocation.* Emergency services are de facto allocated by need, since emergency departments are legally required to treat everyone who has an emergent need, although they will collect payment, if they can. Chronic treatment for at least one disease, dialysis for end-stage renal disease (ESRD), is allocated by need, although treatments for other diseases just as fatal are not so consistently allocated according to need. This is a clear violation of the formal principal of justice, since persons similarly situated with medical conditions just as fatal do not necessarily receive the same type of financial coverage that allows them access to care. Oregon has allocated some Medicaid coverage by lottery [6], while Vermont has chosen universal coverage by means of a single-payer system [7]. Massachusetts has approached universal coverage [8], and national legislation has been passed with a similar goal and similar measures to implement access for all US citizens, but some states are resisting expansion of Medicaid coverage, which may leave some US citizens uninsured [9].

A complete discussion of macroallocation at the level of state and national policies is beyond the scope of this chapter. Microallocation of medical resources at the clinical level, however, is impacted by macroallocation at all levels above it. Therefore, allocation decisions by individual clinicians cannot ignore the implications of allocation policies from national and state levels or more regional and local social or political decisions that set allocation policies. Before moving to a discussion of more purely microallocation issues, several points about macroallocation issues at the institutional level are in order. The Task Force on Values, Ethics, and Rationing in Critical Care (VERICC) recognizes that allocation of intensive care resources "necessarily means that beneficial interventions are withheld from some individuals" [10]. Withholding of such beneficial resources should only be considered as a last resort. According to the American Thoracic Society's position on Fair Allocation of Intensive Care Unit Resources, prior to limiting marginally beneficial care on the basis that the benefit does not justify the cost, healthcare institutions must first (1) eliminate waste, (2) eliminate measures that cost more but provide no greater benefit than less expensive interventions of equal effectiveness, (3) implement a closed financial system that insures savings from ICU care will be directed to other healthcare services that are basic to health benefits that should be provided to all members of society, and (4) provide full public disclosure about the limitation of such services, an appeal process, and any available alternative services [11].

The ATS position also states that institutions should match the available supply of intensive care services to medical need by anticipating the demands for intensive care when new services are added to the institution. For example, institutions should not initiate new surgical units whose patients will require intensive care services without planning sufficient new intensive care unit beds to take care of the additional patients requiring intensive care services. There is substantial potential for abuse when expansions of services, based on either expectations of better reimbursement or expectations of greater potential to benefit control such decisions. The ATS position illustrates this potential problem with the example of a proposed expansion of a cardiac surgery program targeting well-insured patients that gives preferential access to limited ICU beds to cardiac surgery patients on the basis that they have greater potential for medical benefit when compared with critically ill uninsured patients from the hospital's emergency department [11].

One of the most basic allocation decisions made by intensive care physicians is admission and discharge to intensive care units. One of the ATS principles states that "Patients should have equal access to ICU care regardless of their personal or behavioral characteristics" [11]. When a patient meets the appropriate threshold of medical need, neither admission to nor discharge from the ICU should be made on the basis of "age, race, ethnic origin, religious belief, sexual or political orientation, perceptions of social worth, how poorly the patient has complied with social norms or with prior medical advice, other self-injurious behavior, or similar personal characteristics or behaviors of the patient's family or friends" ([11], p. 1287).

In addition to the inappropriateness of such criteria as race in allocation decisions, when clinicians' allocation decisions are influenced by social utility criteria such as employment, the disparate impact on racial and ethnic minorities is amplified. One study found that do-not-resuscitate (DNR) orders were negatively correlated with the patient's employment status prior to hospitalization, for example [12]. Another study found that surgical ICU bed admission was influenced by political power of the surgical service rather than patient-centered criteria [13]. Explicit specification of both appropriate and inappropriate allocation criteria in hospital policies and transparent articulation of the reasons for clinical allocation decisions can help to reduce such factors by ensuring that decisions are not made implicitly on unexamined, unspoken, and unjustifiable criteria.

Another criterion that has been suggested, but also heavily critiqued in allocation decisions, is the age of the patient. Typically, if age is used without a critically examined rationale, it is used as a marker of poor prognostic outcome, resulting in medical intervention being withheld. While it is a truism to note that an older person will not, on average, live as long as a younger person, age is not a sufficiently precise

marker for the prognosis of a poor outcome. Chafin and Carlon, for example, found that older critically ill cancer patients in the ICU had a lower mortality rate than that of younger patients [14]. These authors reviewed the records of all cancer patients admitted to the ICU over a 1-year period; patients younger than 65 years of age had a higher proportion of hematologic malignancies, whereas those 65 and older had primarily solid tumors. The length of stay was the same for the two groups, but the average severity of illness was less for the 65 and older group, and mortality was lower. Some studies at the University of Florida have also suggested that chronological age is an inadequate indicator for ethically acceptable rationing of ICU resources [15, 16].

The best case for using age as an ethically appropriate material criterion for allocation decisions is not based on age as a marker for poor prognosis, but rather on other ethical considerations. A different rationale for a limited use of age as an acceptable allocation criterion has been called the "fair innings" argument. It holds that when all other allocation criteria are equal, preference may be given to a younger patient over an older patient because the older patient has already had more time to achieve her life plans or enjoyment. From this perspective it is considered fair to give the young person more time to realize her life goals [17].

The ATS position statement allows for refusal of admission to an ICU on the basis of the patient's inability to benefit from intensive care services; this is really a futility rationale. Specific examples of inability to benefit from intensive care include patients reliably diagnosed as permanently unconscious or those whose irreversible lack of cognitive function has reached such a severe level that the patient would be incapable of appreciating the intervention as a benefit. If patients already admitted to an ICU are reliably diagnosed to have such a condition while in the ICU, discharge from ICU care to another setting, such as a palliative care unit, may be appropriate, unless a brief period of palliative care in the ICU unit is warranted.

Medical need should be the primary material criterion for allocation of intensive care. The ATS position holds that ICU care, like emergency care, should be provided regardless of a patient's ability to pay [11]. Once medical need is established, however, some advocate making allocation decisions by triage that recognizes varying degrees of potential to benefit from intensive care. Sinuff and colleagues studied triage patterns and found that hospital mortality rates are increased for patients denied ICU admission when compared to patients admitted. They concluded that physicians refuse ICU admission on the basis of perceived minimal potential to benefit from critical care. Factors associated with ICU refusal were "age, poor performance status, underlying malignancy (associated with multiple-system organ failure or terminal metastatic disease), and chronic respiratory or cardiac failure" ([18], p. 1594). Such triage is not recommended by the ATS guidelines, which uphold "first come, first served" as the appropriate criterion for allocating ICU care, even when there are differences in the potential for various patients to benefit from care [11].

All of the suggested bases for making relevant distinctions on the basis of greater potential to benefit, such as prognostic scoring systems, are inappropriate because they were based on patients who experienced ICU care, and thus, their use to deny ICU care for someone with a low predicted risk of dying in the hospital makes a category mistake. They do not reliably predict a person's ability to recover without ICU care, since they were based on patients who did receive ICU care [11].

Although the ATS position recommends first come, first served as the most egalitarian material criterion for allocation, they recognize that some exceptions may need to be made when one patient's need consumes so much of a resource that it threatens the availability of that resource for other patients who need it, too. For example, when a patient requires continuous transfusions with no prospect of recovery and those transfusions will exhaust the supply for actual current patients for whom that blood would enable recovery, institutions may ethically allocate the blood to those patients for whom it would be effective. Institutions should specify such policies in advance of the occasion and have clear processes for informing patients prior to the incident about such limits, as well as any available options for transfer to another institution.

All policies of rationing ICU care should be transparent and publicly disclosed, including any financial incentives that may affect such decisions. The fiduciary duty of individual physicians to their patients is crucial, and both financial incentives and policies for allocation of resources have the potential to undermine patient trust in individual physicians as well as institutions. Policies must be prospectively designed and implemented so that the patient's physician is not required to make ad hoc or individual judgments about limiting care. Such policies must include fair procedures for minimizing bias, inaccurate clinical judgments, or conflicts of interest that could undermine patient trust in the fairness of allocation decisions.

In summary, decisions related to limitation of care and end-of-life care are fraught with emotion and difficulty, on the part of both the family and the care providers. The issue of our ultimate terminality cannot be ignored, and the limitation of personal and national resources we are able to utilize for care may well impact these decisions. The problem is not that we recognize these issues exist. Rather, it would be to ignore that they exist; we must have open, transparent, and honest communication about these issues if we are to come to grips with them.

Assessment of Decisional Capacity

One of the prerequisites necessary for ethically and legally valid informed consent is the mental and emotional capacity of a patient to make medical decisions. Competence (or its antonym, incompetence) is frequently used to refer to a patient's decision-making ability. Although the terms competence and capacity are often used interchangeably in clinical contexts, it is helpful to distinguish them for purposes of clarity and precision. An adult person is presumed legally to have the *competence* to make decisions, medical or otherwise, unless a court has declared that person to be incompetent and appointed a guardian of the person to manage the incompetent's affairs and make decisions, including medical decisions. Typically, because of the procedural complexity, expense, and traumatic impact of such a declaration, judicial declarations of incompetence do not occur until a person's mental faculties have so deteriorated that their incompetence is generally seen to be global. Correspondingly, the scope of the appointed guardian's authority to make decisions is usually broad, including management of financial and medical decision-making, as well as other issues such as living arrangements and custodial supervision.

This mechanism of recognizing decisional inability and providing a substitute decision-maker is not necessary for the much wider array of circumstances in which persons who become patients are temporarily or partially unable to make decisions on their own behalf. Therefore, less formal means for recognizing and addressing patients' ability or inability to make medical decisions have evolved that do not require judicial determinations or judicial appointments of authorized decision-makers when patients cannot provide informed consent for themselves. Since many persons lose some or all aspects of decision-making capacity either temporarily (e.g., during general anesthesia) or partially and progressively (e.g., in the early stages of dementia), physicians providing care for such patients must be able to make determinations about patient decisional *capacity* and have readily available authorized decision-makers to provide informed consent or informed refusal on the incapacitated patient's behalf.

Many physicians erroneously believe that if a patient's decisional capacity is in question, a psychiatric consult must be obtained in order to resolve it; this is not necessarily true. There is no reason that psychiatrists alone should be able to make determinations of capacity, for reasons that will become clear in the following discussion. In the average hospital, most patients without capacity are not encountered on a psychiatric ward. Most patients who have impaired decisional capacity frequently have lost capacity due to organic illnesses or injuries or sequelae of etiologies other than mental illness [19].

Two common tendencies in assessment of patient decisional capacity have been widely criticized in the literature as inadequate and inappropriate: the outcomes approach and the category or status approach [20]. Both should be avoided, although each approach may provide some indication that a more appropriate approach to capacity assessment should be considered. The outcomes approach bases the assessment of patient decisional capacity on whether the patient accepts and authorizes the physician's recommendation for or against medical intervention. The most obvious problem with this approach is its over-inclusiveness: it deems patients who are decisionally capacitated as incapacitated simply because their choices do not agree with the physician's conception of the patient's best interest. Although less obvious, this approach is under-inclusive as well. It deems as capacitated patients who are compliant and cooperative even if they do not have decisional capacity as long as they accept the physician's recommendation [20].

The category or status approach to capacity assessment tends to shift the analysis from the presumption that the patient is capacitated unless demonstrated otherwise to a presumption that the patient is incapacitated because the patient has a history of a mental illness or disability or because the patient falls into a category such as adolescent, elderly, or seriously ill. None of these categories, including a history of mental illness or disability, is by itself tantamount to a valid determination or presumption of decisional incapacity [20]. A patient with a history of mental illness may be able to make decisions either because the illness was never sufficiently disabling, or it has subsided, or because treatments, including current medications, sufficiently mitigate the effects of the condition to maintain decisional capacity. Mature minors may have decisional capacity, just as the elderly may retain mental functions in spite of old age. Finally, persons who are seriously ill do not lose mental functioning simply by having serious physiological impairments [19].

An appropriate approach to assessment of patient decisional capacity recognizes that such capacity manifests over a range of functional abilities that are context dependent and therefore require specific analysis of a patient's ability to make particular decisions about specific options that vary in complexity and comprehensiveness. This method is known as the functional approach because it assesses the current functional ability of the patient to make decisions as needed. Decisional capacity may not always be an all or nothing determination. A patient with some compromised mental functioning may be able to make some decisions for herself, yet unable to grasp more complex factors that are necessary to make other decisions [19].

Several factors have been adduced as important to a thorough assessment of patient decisional capacity for particular decision-making. Overall, the best way to approach the issue of a patient's decisional capacity is to determine what information the particular patient would need to be able to comprehend and appreciate in order to provide informed consent or refusal for the particular diagnostic or therapeutic intervention in question. Substantively, this would mean that the patient must be able to comprehend the risks and benefits of physician recommendations and the risks and benefits of medically reasonable alternatives (including the possibility of no treatment) and have the ability to make reasoned choices among those options within the framework of the patient's particular values and worldview [19]. This focus on the patient's ability to comprehend and reason, however, must be augmented by consideration of the patient's emotional state. A patient who is acutely depressed, for example, may be able to comprehend the necessary information to make decisions yet lack the emotional wherewithal to care sufficiently about her own well-being to avoid making harmful decisions resulting from her emotional condition rather than her authentic values.

End-of-Life Issues

Until the latter part of the twentieth century, the traditional definition of death prevailed, namely, the cessation of heartbeat and respiration. The Ad Hoc Committee of the Harvard Medical School to Examine the Definition of Brain Death (1968) marked the beginning of a fairly rapid change, not only in the medical community but also in law, to the definition of death as cessation of function of the entire brain, including the brain stem and autonomic reflexes. Two reasons were cited by the Harvard Committee for this change: (1) the burdens of continued intensive care for those who were not expected to regain meaningful awareness and (2) the growing need for a source of transplantable organs [21]. Issues relating to these two distinct rationales for the change from traditional heart-lung definition of death to brain death will be discussed separately.

Issues of Withholding and Withdrawal of Treatment in Expectation of Organ Donation

One of the major reasons for the Harvard Committee's recommendation of whole-brain death was to allow for persons who would meet criteria for the definition of brain death, but not the heart-lung definition, to be organ donors. The major criterion for a person to be an organ donor has been the "dead-donor rule," which ensures that potential organ donors would not have their organs taken prior to death or have their deaths hastened in order to acquire their organs sooner. By redefining death according to whole-brain criteria rather than cessation of circulation, the Harvard Committee increased the number of available donors and organs for the rapidly increasing numbers of potential transplants for patients in need of them. Nevertheless, the number of persons who will die without organ transplantation has continued to outstrip the available supply of donors.

In spite of the widespread acceptance into the law of the whole-brain death standard, it has continued to receive criticism, for both conceptual and practical reasons. One line of criticism has been from those who argued, from the beginning, that the definition of brain death should include the loss of higher cortical functioning applying to any person who has irretrievably lost consciousness [22]. If the definition of brain death were altered to include such persons, the supply of potential organ donors and organs would be increased.

Controversy over the definition of death has also continued as a result of the introduction of "donation after cardiac death," which has become another way of increasing availability and quality of transplantable organs. The problem has been amplified by the need to keep organs oxygenated as long as possible, which requires an arguably arbitrary way of determining at what point after withdrawal of life support that cardiopulmonary death is deemed to be irreversible. The greater the number of minutes that elapse between withdrawal of life support and the harvesting of the organs, the less viable the organs are. Therefore, the protocols for declaring death of the donor have varied from 2 to 5 min. Of course, when the heart is transplanted, the fact that it can be "restored" in another body makes it difficult to speak coherently about irreversible cessation of cardiac function for the purpose of "donation after cardiac death" [23].

Commentators who recognize these conceptual problems with the definition of death have argued that instead of changing the definition of death again, the organ donation implications could be addressed without regard to a definition of death. They hold that the dead-donor rule is unnecessary if potential donors provide informed consent to be organ donors with the understanding that permanent coma or permanent vegetative state will suffice to qualify them for donation.

Public understanding and acceptance of the ethical rationale for organ donation requires more clarity than is currently the case. One of the problems manifest in the controversial case of Ms. Terri Schiavo was that many in the public did not understand the phenomenon of a permanent vegetative state, especially when they saw brief video clips of a person whose eyes were open and whose reflexive movements were visible, even though sustained expert clinical observation indicated no consciousness or no ability to respond to stimuli. Such factors contribute to confusion, suspicion, and mistrust that decisions to withdraw life-sustaining treatment may be premature because they are based more on the demand for transplant organs than on the prognosis for potential donors. Whichever approach is taken on increasing the pool of organ donors, the public will need clarification about criteria for transplantation, procedures that assure that conflicts of interest are mitigated, and reliable methods of determining the absence of consciousness and irreversibility of lack of consciousness. Each institution must adopt clear policies that avoid real or apparent conflicts of interest. For example, the physician who pronounces death must not be involved in the harvesting of organs [24].

Issues of Withholding and Withdrawal of Life-Sustaining Treatment (LST) Without Organ Donation

Some have continued to argue that the definition of brain death should be expanded to include cessation of function of the higher cortical functions. Legal definitions reflect the "whole-brain death" definition of death, however, as determined by clinical examination and testing. When patients are found by clinical criteria to be brain dead, treatment is generally neither ethically appropriate nor legally required. Physicians generally do not need the consent of family or loved ones to discontinue life-sustaining treatment on patients who meet criteria for whole-brain death, though they should explain carefully the basis for the conclusion of death by whole-brain criteria and its legal authority. It is not uncommon, however, for hospitals to have informal policies of continuing LST for 24–48 h on compassionate grounds for such purposes as allowing family to gather before LST is withdrawn.

Although most states' laws defining brain death do not provide for exceptions based on alternative definitions, a few states do specify exceptions for religions or cultural groups whose views reject brain-based definitions of death in favor of the traditional heart-lung definition. Widespread acceptance of the whole-brain definition of death into almost all state statutes has implications beyond transplantation. Patients determined to meet criteria for brain death are legally dead, and treatment may be discontinued without consent of the patient's authorized decision-maker or family. Statutes in three states require some accommodation for patients whose religious or cultural beliefs hold to the traditional heart-lung circulatory definition of death. New Jersey statutes require that for such patients brain death definitions may not be used, and the physician may not declare death until cardiorespiratory criteria are met [25]. New York statutes also require "reasonable accommodations" for those with religious or moral objections, which must be spelled out in institutional policies that may include continuing life support as well as spelling out limits to such accommodation [26]. California statutes also specify that when a patient meets criteria for brain death, any patient's family should be given a brief period of continuing cardiac support sufficient to gather the family before withdrawal of LST. The California statutes state that accommodation should be made for religious or cultural beliefs within vaguely expressed limits acknowledging the effects on other patients in need of care [27].

Since the whole-brain death definition prevails in state statutes, patients diagnosed in a permanent vegetative state (the so-called cortical or higher brain death) are not included in the definition of brain death. Thus, physicians may not withhold or withdraw life-sustaining treatment (LST) unilaterally on the basis of a definition of the so-called higher brain death, although (as will be discussed subsequently) some argue for unilateral withholding and withdrawal of LST under a futility rationale when they consider permanent vegetative state to be beyond any benefit that treatment can confer. Most state statutes specify that a vegetative state must be permanent in order to qualify for withholding or withdrawal of life-sustaining treatment when the patient's advance directive or authorized decision-maker indicates that the patient would not want treatment under the circumstances, but leave the determination of permanence to clinical criteria. The determination of permanence varies by etiology of injury and length of time since manifestation of the vegetative state. When the source of the brain injury is an anoxic event, the period regarded as reliable for a determination of permanence is 3 months in the vegetative state. For traumatic brain injuries, however, the period before reliable prognosis that the vegetative state will be permanent is 1 year [28, 29].

Some studies have projected misdiagnosis of permanent vegetative states as high as 30–40 % because the criteria for distinguishing permanent vegetative state from the minimally conscious state, such as episodic behavioral responses, can be inconsistent and difficult to reproduce, especially in less intensive medical environments, like chronic care facilities [30].

The Right of Capacitated Adults to Refuse Life-Sustaining Treatment

The many legal rulings that established the right of Jehovah's Witnesses to refuse blood transfusions have helped to pave the way legally for a more general right of all patients to refuse life-sustaining treatments. The Bouvia case helped to articulate the reasons for the application of the more general right as well as other end-of-life concerns.

Elizabeth Bouvia was a 28-year-old woman with quadriplegia and extremely painful arthritis who had spent much of her adult life in hospitals and nursing care facilities. She reached a point that her quality of life had so deteriorated that she refused to eat or drink and refused in advance any artificial nutrition or hydration. The hospital decided that, when she became incapacitated, they would implement tube feedings and hydration to prevent her death from dehydration or malnutrition, arguing that with continued treatment she could live for 15–20 more years. She went to court to assert her right to refuse life-sustaining treatment against her will. Ultimately, the California appellate court ruled that she had the right to refuse LST [31]. Although the court's ruling was not binding outside its jurisdiction, the ethical and legal rationale for it has been influential in characterizing the right of capacitated patients to refuse LST:

> Who shall say what the minimum amount of available life must be? Does it matter if it be 15 to 20 years, 15 to 20 months, or 15 to 20 days, if such life has been physically destroyed and its quality, dignity and purpose gone? As in all matters lines must be drawn at some point, somewhere, but that decision must ultimately belong to the one whose life is in issue.
>
> Here Elizabeth Bouvia's decision to forego medical treatment or life-support through a mechanical means belongs to her. It is not a medical decision for her physicians to make. Neither is it a legal question whose soundness is to be resolved by lawyers or judges. It is not a conditional right subject to approval by ethics committees or courts of law. It is a moral and philosophical decision that, being a competent adult, is hers alone [32].

One thing that we are able to say with some certainty is that the recent "debate" related to health insurance reform and so-called death panels serves no one. The ability of physicians to discuss end-of-life care with patients and families is critical to the care of our patients, the functioning of our profession, and the management of our health system.

Withholding and Withdrawal of Life-Sustaining Treatment

Another important advance in the ethical approach to end-of-life issues has been the recognition that there is no valid ethical distinction between withholding treatment and withdrawal of treatment. Prior to this recognition, the prevailing ethical reasoning was that passive withholding of life support was ethically acceptable but that actively withdrawing life support was unethical. Careful analysis of this issue has resulted in this important change both for conceptual and for practical reasons.

The use of DNR orders provides a good example to illustrate this reasoning. If one tries to classify a DNR order either as passive or as active, it is not entirely clear that it fits neatly into either classification without a plausible argument that it also fits into the other. On first blush it would seem to be passive, because it withholds CPR, a life-sustaining treatment. Yet if you consider it as an order to avoid an intervention that is by default presumed without such an order, the order itself seems to be an active order. In the case of a cardiac arrest for which CPR would be an appropriate intervention, without which an otherwise healthy patient would die, it would be just as wrong to withhold it as it would be to withdraw ventilation from that same patient who needed and wanted temporary respiratory support in order to recover. This recognition helps to illustrate an important bioethics principle. Whether one merely withholds or acts to withdraw LST, one must take responsibility for the result of a deliberate omission as well as an affirmative action when both lead to the same intended outcome. Therefore, at least in the context of withholding or withdrawal of LST, there is no ethical difference between the two.

There are also practical reasons for not distinguishing between withholding and withdrawal of life-sustaining treatment. If withholding life support were acceptable but withdrawing it were not, physicians considering a trial of an intervention that might or might not be effective might hesitate to try it for fear that once life support were begun, it could not ethically be withdrawn. Since withdrawal of LST is ethically acceptable, however, a prospective intervention of plausible but uncertain benefit may be provided for a trial period to ascertain its effectiveness. If it does not prove to be effective, it can be withdrawn, thereby avoiding a prolonged dying process.

The types of treatment typically associated with end-of-life interventions are mechanical ventilation, artificial nutrition and hydration, and dialysis. Another class of interventions not so typically thought of as life-sustaining treatment is Cardiac Implanted Electronic Devices (CIED), such as pacemakers and defibrillators. Although these devices are not typically begun as a part of care in an ICU, increasingly patients in an ICU for other reasons have some form of CIED that needs to be considered in anticipating end-of-life decisions. Both the medical literature and the popular press have carried accounts of the difficulties patients have encountered at the end of life [33].

Twenty percent of implantable cardio-defibrillator device (ICD) patients endure painful shocks in the final weeks of life, causing not only physical pain but emotional stress for both the patient and family members. Many physicians fail to address this problem with patients at the time of implantation. Even patients with DNR orders frequently have not had device deactivation discussed with them as a part of the conversation about their resuscitation choices. Some physicians are uncomfortable initiating conversation about device deactivation. Others simply do not think of it. Still others are unwilling to deactivate such devices because they think it is tantamount to assisted suicide [33].

Careful reflection and analysis, however, demonstrates that activation of CIEDs is a form of invasive life-sustaining treatment that may become more burdensome than beneficial for some patients, just as dialysis or mechanical ventilation might. There is no reason to treat deactivation of such devices any differently than withdrawal of other LST measures. A number of professional and patient advocacy organizations have published a consensus statement in support of the ethical acceptability of withdrawal of such devices, including the Heart Rhythm Society, the American Heart Association, American College of Cardiology, the American Geriatrics Society, the American Academy of Hospice and Palliative Medicine, the American Heart Association, the European Heart Rhythm Association, and the Hospice and Palliative Nurses Association. Among other aspects of consensus, it states:

- Ethically and legally, there are no differences between refusing CIED therapy and requesting withdrawal of CIED therapy.
- Ethically and legally, carrying out a request to withdraw life-sustaining treatment is neither physician-assisted suicide nor euthanasia.
- Clinicians who have conscience-based objections to deactivating a CIED should not be forced to do so, but neither should such clinicians abandon patients who desire deactivation. Clinicians who have conscience-based objections should find a colleague willing to perform device deactivation for the patient [34].

Recognition of the moral equivalence of withholding and withdrawal of LST has been followed by courts in case law as well as statutes. Thus, there is no legal difference between withholding and withdrawing LST [35].

This ethical and legal consensus in medicine and law, however, does not mean that family members of a patient have assimilated the best ethical and legal reasoning that has become the basis for public policy. For many patient family members or friends, the intuitively powerful difference between withholding and withdrawal is very emotionally compelling. Often, even when such family members are able to contemplate withholding life-sustaining treatment, they are more reluctant to withdraw life-sustaining treatment because the act of withdrawal seems to be the most proximate action that leads to the patient's death. Thus, in some cases, it will be easier for a family member to agree to withhold CPR than it will be for the family to agree to withdraw a ventilator, even if the rationale concerning life-sustaining treatment would be the same for both a DNR and withdrawal of other life support measures. When this occurs, sometimes the best that can be achieved is a DNR and an agreement not to escalate care, without an agreement to withdraw other measures of life support. In some cases, this differential in emotional valence will be strong enough to influence decision-making without being absolute. A useful way to negotiate this dynamic is to propose a conditional, time-limited trial of LST long enough to demonstrate any possible benefits, after which treatment will be withdrawn if it has not been effective.

Advance Directives

The term advance directive is a generic way of referring to several distinct types of patient instructions enabling persons to make choices about their medical care prior to losing decisional capacity. The two most basic types focus either on a set of directions about what types of interventions the patient wants to ensure or wants to refuse as the end-of-life approaches or on the capacitated patient's formal appointment of a person to make medical decision on her behalf in the event she loses decisional capacity. These two primary types of advance directive often are combined in a single document, but either type may be utilized alone. The type that provides instructions concerning end-of-life care, whether to accept or to limit life-sustaining treatment (LST), is called a living will. The type in which a patient, while capacitated, designates a person to make medical decisions on her behalf, if she becomes incapacitated, may be referred to by one of several terms: a durable power of attorney for healthcare, a healthcare surrogate, or a healthcare proxy.

State statutes are not consistent in their use of the terms surrogate and proxy, so it is important to know the difference in whichever state one practices. In most states either "surrogate" or "proxy" is used to mean the patient-designated decision-maker, and the other term is used to mean the person with priority order on the statutory next of kin list who becomes a decision-maker when an incapacitated patient has

Fig. 45.1 End of life decision chart

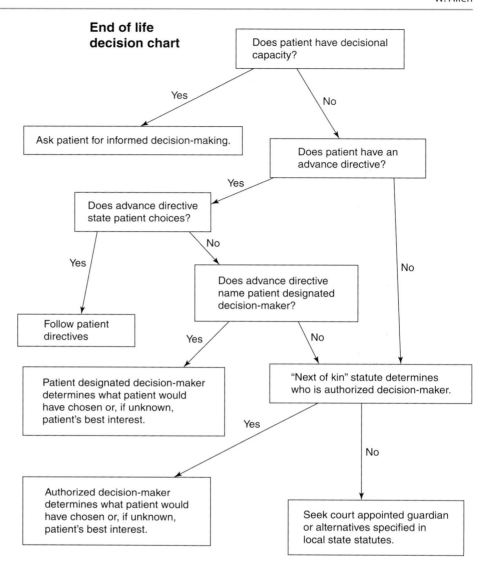

End of life decision chart

not designed a decision-maker. For example, in New York State, the patient designates a healthcare proxy to make decisions on her behalf, but if she has not designated anyone, the New York statute refers to the decision-maker authorized by statute as the healthcare surrogate. In Florida, by contrast, these terms are reversed. Since these terms are used interchangeably in general discussion, it is important to clarify whether someone using one of these terms is referring to a patient-designated decision-maker or a statutorily authorized decision-maker. Although the two types of decision-maker may have the same roles and responsibilities, in some states the patient-designated decision-maker enjoys the presumption of accuracy in representing what the patient would have chosen, while the statutorily authorized "next of kin" decision-maker bears the burden of proof that their decision is what the patient would have chosen (Fig. 45.1).

The term durable power of attorney (DPA), however, always refers to a patient-designated decision-maker.

Physicians must also recognize a crucial distinction as to which type of "power of attorney" is legally effective for enabling an authorized healthcare decision-maker. An ordinary power of attorney ceases to be effective when the person who delegated it loses capacity. Thus, in order to be effective when a person loses capacity, a power of attorney must be a *durable* power of attorney [36]. This means that it does not lose its legal effectiveness when the patient loses capacity. Moreover, in order to be effective for the authorized decision-maker to make healthcare decisions, it must also include healthcare decisions in the scope of its authority. Typically, ordinary powers of attorney do not specify healthcare decisions within their scope of authority. Both laypersons and clinicians are often unaware of this crucial distinction when discussing whether an incapacitated patient has a validly authorized healthcare decision-maker. Some persons may believe they do have such authority because they have been given a general, ordinary power of attorney, when in fact they do not have the authority to make health-care decisions for an incapacitated patient. In order to be legally effective for healthcare decision-making, the power of attorney should state that it is durable and that it pertains to healthcare decisions as well as any other types of authority conveyed (such as financial authority).

The major limitation of living wills is that they may be written before the patient knows what their medical circumstances will be during a time of incapacity, when end-of-life decisions need to be made under specific health conditions. Even so, a person's general indications in their living will as to

what quality of life they value may well provide useful and applicable guidance for end-of-life decision-making. Some people have completed living wills that are more specific as to what types of interventions they want to be withheld or withdrawn when they approach the end of life (Fig. 45.2). These types of living wills may provide more specific guidance about particular circumstances in which they choose to accept or refuse particular interventions. Such specificity about types of treatment to be accepted or rejected may be useful in implementing the patient's choices when the living will was completed with help from a knowledgeable clinician in view of

---

I, _____ , have a right to life-prolonging procedures including food and water [nutrition and hydration]. I also have a right to have life-prolonging procedures stopped or no new ones started. I can choose someone to do this for me if I am unconscious, in a coma, incompetent, or otherwise mentally or physically incapable of making my wishes known.

I understand that treatments or medications which take away pain, suffering, anxiety, or other forms of distress will not be withheld or withdrawn even if they hasten my death.

By signing below, I hereby choose   _____, my   _____ , whose telephone numbers are: and whose address is:

as my designee.

I would like my designee, my health care or residential facility, physician or other health care provider, to read my answers to the following questions and use my answers to help them carry out my wishes if I am unable to do that myself.

1.   If I have a terminal condition, from which I will probably not recover or survive and my death will likely occur within weeks:

a.   I want life-prolonging procedures to be:

_____ Withdrawn   _____ Continued;

b.   I would want artificially administered food and water such as tube or

intravenous feedings to be:

_____ Withheld/Withdrawn   _____ Continued;

c.   If my heart or breathing stopped, I would want my physician to try to restart it through

CPR [cardiopulmonary resuscitation] or other means:

_____ Yes   _____ No.

2.   If I have a medical condition that is steadily getting worse and my physician has told me [or my designee] that there is no reasonable chance of recovery, but I could survive this condition for weeks or even months:

a.   I want life-prolonging procedures to be:

_____ Withdrawn   _____ Continued;

b.   I would want artificially administered food and water such as tube or intravenous feedings to be:

_____ Withheld/Withdrawn   _____ Continued;

c.   If my heart or breathing stopped, I would want my physician to try to restart it

through CPR [cardiopulmonary resuscitation] or other means:

_____ Yes   _____ No.

Fig. 45.2 Sample of "Advance Directive to My Physician" form

3.   If I am in a irreversible coma, persistent vegetative state, or other condition where my physician

has determined that there is no reasonable medical likelihood I will ever be awake or able to

make medical decisions for myself again:

a.   I want life-prolonging procedures to be:

_____ Withdrawn   _____Continued;

b.   I would want artificially administered food and water such as tube or intravenous feedings to be:

_____Withheld/Withdrawn   _____Continued;

c.   If my heart or breathing stopped, I would want my physician to try to restart it through

CPR [cardiopulmonary resuscitation] or other means:

_____Yes   _____No.

4.   If I must live in a hospital or nursing home for the rest of my life because I am unable to feed or groom

myself or take care of my other bodily functions such as responding to my toilet needs:

a.   I want life-prolonging procedures to be:

_____ Withdrawn   _____Continued;

b.   I would want artificially administered food and water such as tube or intravenous feedings to be:

_____Withheld/Withdrawn   _____Continued;

c.   If my heart or breathing stopped, I would want my physician to try to restart it through

CPR [cardiopulmonary resuscitation] or other means:

_____Yes   _____No.

5.   If I have progressive or permanent memory loss such that I am no longer able to recognize my family

and friends or communicate my thoughts to others:

a.   I want life-prolonging procedures to be:

_____ Withdrawn   _____Continued;

b.   I would want artificially administered food and water such as tube or intravenous feedings to be:

_____Withheld/Withdrawn   _____Continued;

c.   If my heart or breathing stopped, I would want my physician to try to restart it through

CPR [cardiopulmonary resuscitation] or other means:

_____Yes   _____No.

6.   If I am in the hospital with a serious condition, and my physician and I have decided to continue

treatment because we believe it may be effective and treatment seems to be going well,

if my heart or breathing unexpectedly stopped, I would want my physician to try to restart it

through CPR or other means:

_____Yes   _____No.

7.   In my current state of health, if my heart or breathing unexpectedly stopped, I would want my

physician to try to restart it through CPR or other means:

_____Yes   _____No.

Fig. 45.2 (continued)

I understand that I can make quality of life choices. I am not asking anyone else to make quality of life choices for me. This document merely directs others to carry out the quality of life choices I have made. If, in the course of making decisions for me, my designee is dissatisfied with any determination of my attending physician, my designee may substitute another attending physician.

If I can not make medical decisions for myself, I want the directions in this Declaration to be accepted and fulfilled as the final expression of my legal right to accept or refuse medical or surgical treatment and to accept the consequences of my decisions.

I understand the full import of this directive and I am emotionally and mentally competent to make this Declaration.

By executing this Declaration, I am revoking all prior Declarations.

Signed _____ Date

Of the City of _____ and State of _____

In signing this Declaration on the date noted above, I state that the Declarant is known to me and I believe the Declarant to be of sound mind. I certify that I am not the Declarant's designee named in this document.

Witness: _____

Current residence of First Witness: _____

_____

In signing this Declaration on the date noted above, I state that the Declarant is known to me and I believe the Declarant to be of sound mind. I certify that I am not the Declarant's spouse, blood relative, or designee named in this document.

Witness: _____

Current residence of Second Witness: _____

_____

Fig. 45.2 (continued)

likely and foreseeable clinical scenarios. Most patients, however, will not have had such expert help when completing a living will, and therefore, they will not be able to specify with precision which specific interventions should be withheld or withdrawn. Even the most well-informed and thoughtful living will may not clearly address questions and issues that were not anticipated at the time it was completed. It may, therefore, be more effective for patients to specify in their living will the quality of life they find acceptable and to authorize their physicians to discontinue LSTs when there is no longer a reasonable possibility of achieving that quality of life.

In addition, a person who completes a living will should be encouraged to designate a decision-maker whom they believe will be able to interpret accurately their living will and to provide additional direction about what the now incapacitated patient would have chosen, based on their knowledge of the patients values and goals. A statutorily authorized next of kin decision-maker may well be able to provide the same function, but someone the patient has specifically chosen for this reasonably increases the probability that the decisions will represent the patient's values. Although a living will alone is legally sufficient to provide consent or refusal for an incapacitated patient on matters that the document addresses, a designated decision-maker named by the patient prior to incapacity can provide a complementary source of authoritative decision-making for issues that the living will may not address. A legally authorized decision-maker can also make end-of-life decisions if there is no living will.

The goal of advance directives is to base decision-making as closely as possible on what the patient would have chosen if decisionally capacitated. This is referred to as the "substituted judgment" standard, which is distinguishable from a "best interest" decision-making standard. For example, while most persons would decide to accept a blood transfusion to save their lives, a particular Jehovah's Witness might refuse a blood transfusion because of her religious convictions. The preferred standard in end-of-life care decisions is the substituted judgment standard rather than the best interest standard. If a particular patient's end-of-life choices or values can be determined, those preferences should be the basis for decision-making, even if they are not what most patients would choose. If a patient's preferences are not known, however, it is acceptable to use a best interest analysis, or what most reasonable patients would choose, as the basis for end-of-life decisions.

Empirical studies of how well advance directives accomplish this goal show that the utility of these measures is still evolving [37]. They have not been a panacea for the challenges of end-of-life decision-making, but as more is learned about how best to approach end-of-life care, advance directives have proven to be a useful tool for facilitating the types of communication and decision-making that help patients, clinicians, and family members. A large study of patients over 60 years of age found that, among those who required decision-making at the end of life, 29.8 % lacked decision-making capacity; of those, two thirds had advance directives. More than 90 % of those who had living wills requested limited care or comfort care. The study found that "83.2 % of subjects who requested limited care and 97.1 % of subjects who requested comfort care received care consistent with their preferences" ([38], p. 1211). Those who had living wills were less likely to receive all care possible than those who did not, and those who had chosen a durable power of attorney for healthcare were less likely to die in a hospital or to receive all care possible than those who did not name a durable power of attorney for healthcare [38].

In spite of the overall usefulness of advance directives, they should not be seen as eliminating the need for conversation between the patient, the authorized decision-maker, and the primary physicians providing medical management of the patient's care. There is a tendency to see a living will as averting the need for conversation with the capacitated patient or her authorized decision-maker, since that has all been settled by the advance directive. Advance directives should be seen instead as an occasion for conversation with a capacitated patient and the patient's authorized decision-maker in order to clarify the patient's choices as expressed in writing or in prior conversations with the decision-maker in case the patient loses capacity. There are frequent aspects of care not clearly anticipated or addressed in advance directives that should be clarified before the patient loses capacity, if possible. Discussing an advance directive also provides the opportunity to ensure that the patient and the patient's authorized decision-maker have actually discussed the patient's values, goals, and choices sufficiently for the decision-maker to reflect the patient's own particular perspectives if the patient becomes incapacitated.

One problem in discussing end-of-life care with patients and their families, particularly on the issue of resuscitation status, has been the public overestimation of the success of CPR. Many have attributed this misperception of the effectiveness of CPR to the unrealistic portrayal of CPR in television and film, which in turn is thought to lead patients and their authorized decision-makers to reject the option of a DNR order when discussing code status. An American study of three popular TV dramas in the middle 1990s showed 75 % of patients surviving the immediate arrest with 67 % surviving to hospital discharge [39]. Another study confirmed that 96 % of respondents had unrealistic expectations of CPR with mean expectations of survival ranging from 65 to 74 %. Those who cited television as their primary source of information about CPR expectations predicted survival in 70 % of cases. Moreover, even those who had some type of medical training predicted a 74 % rate of success [40].

In contrast to the publically perceived rate of CPR success, a study of US Medicare patients over 65 from 1992 to 2005 showed that only 18.3 % survived to hospital discharge. Interestingly, the proportion of deaths in the hospital increased during this period, and the proportion of persons discharged home decreased, with a corresponding increase in persons discharged to locations other than their homes. These data suggest that, in spite of increased availability of DNR orders and other advance care planning measures, CPR continues to be used without long-term benefit in this population [41].

In view of general public misperceptions of the success rate of CPR, evidence-based data about such expectations should be part of conversation about end-of-life care. In discussing DNR status (as well as other LSTs) with patients and families, some phrases and approaches consistently cause problems and should therefore be avoided. The common question "Do you want us to do everything?" implies that whatever "everything" means must have a reasonable likelihood of success or the physician would not be asking the question. Of course, most of the time when that question is asked, it is precisely because the point has been reached at which the physician does not expect the intervention(s) in question to change the outcome of the course of care. Moreover, when the question is put that way, patients or especially patient's decision-makers are predisposed to answer "yes" because to answer otherwise seems to imply that they have not done everything they could for their loved one. Phrasing such as "there is nothing more to do" and "we're going to stop the machines" has also been discouraged by experienced clinicians, since these ways of speaking tend to be heard by patients or decision-makers as abandonment [42]. Even when there is little to no chance for a cure and continued aggressive care is no longer appropriate, palliative care should be offered and provided.

Some physicians are reluctant to initiate conversation with patients about end-of-life issues out of concern that addressing the topic will be too stressful for the patient to think about or discuss. A study of this issue found that 89.7 % of terminally ill patients had little or no stress from a structured interview discussing end-of-life issues. Only 7.1 % reported some stress, and only 1.9 % reported a great deal of stress. Their caregivers reported almost the same rates, showing that there is no need to avoid discussion of end-of-life issues with the patient or his/her caregivers [43].

Another study found that 68 % of the patients who participated received end-of-life care that was consistent with their previously stated choices. Patients whose care reflected their choices were more likely to understand that they had a terminal illness and more likely to have discussed their choices about end-of-life care with a physician. Moreover, patients whose quality of life was highest and whose distress was lowest in the last week of life were those who chose symptom-directed care rather than life-extending measures [44].

In delineating the respective arenas of decision-making entailed in end-of-life care, a distinction should be made between the relative spheres of expertise between the patient and the physician providing care. One author summarized this distinction as follows: "The patient is the expert on his or her values, goals, and preferences, while the physician is the expert on the medical means for honoring the patient's perspective" ([45], p. 849). Therefore, in order to facilitate care plans that implement the patient's goals, the physician needs to elicit those values and goals from the patient, the patient's living will, and the patient's authorized decision-maker.

A key way of determining this is to understand the minimum quality of life the patient is willing to accept in light of the burdens of whatever interventions are needed to attempt to restore or to maintain that quality of life. Both of these items, the patient's minimum acceptable quality of life and the patient's willingness to bear the burdens necessary to achieve it may vary considerably from one person to another. Not only do they vary from one patient to another, but those factors may vary over time even for a single patient. Therefore, it is important to attempt to reassess how the patient perceives those factors as the patient's condition and circumstances change, if the patient retains decisional capacity. Some patients may be willing to tolerate substantial burdens for a defined period of time in order to survive to see a loved one's graduation, marriage, birth, or some other milestone, even if the patient would not want to tolerate those burdens indefinitely [45].

In another study, a majority (55 %) of authorized decision-makers want to make the value-laden decision about whether life-sustaining treatment should be continued or discontinued, although a substantial plurality (40 %) wanted to share that responsibility with the physician, whereas only 5 % wanted to defer that decision to the physician. Regardless of whether they wanted to make the final decision, however, 90 % of authorized decision-makers wanted to hear the physician's opinion about whether or not to discontinue intensive medical interventions. Eliciting authorized decision-makers' expectations about their preferences for the physician's role in making such decisions will help ICU physicians ascertain how much initiative should be taken in helping decision-makers reach a comfortable equilibrium [46].

Perioperative DNR Status

The issue of perioperative DNR status has presented substantial consternation and controversy in recent decades. Procedures entailed in anesthesia or surgery can precipitate arrhythmias, respiratory instability, or both. Anesthesiologists and surgeons are understandably reluctant to withhold interventions that can easily reverse cardiac and respiratory instability precipitated by anesthesia or surgery. Nevertheless, patients who have chosen to decline resuscitation in the event of a cardiac arrest, based on their own assessment of their quality of life and the burdens of LST, may decide to accept surgery to improve some aspect of their condition, even if cure is no longer possible.

Withholding resuscitative measures during surgery may or may not make sense in terms of the patient's goals in accepting surgery and more generally in avoiding what the patient regards as an unacceptable quality of life. If the patient believes that a successful surgery may provide net benefit but also believes that her condition after an arrest and resuscitation would be unacceptable, it is not incoherent to consent to surgery but not consent to resuscitation just because the setting of the arrest has changed to the surgical or recovery suite. This rationale is analogous in many respects to the Jehovah's Witness's refusal of blood products. Just as the Jehovah's Witness consents to surgery with full knowledge of the additional risks of death as a result of declining a standard life-sustaining intervention, the patient who does not want a DNR rescinded accepts the potential benefits of surgery with the additional risk of dying that results from declining resuscitation measures.

Ambiguity about what specific interventions are entailed in resuscitation has led some institutions to develop forms that list specific interventions in order to clarify what should be withheld when an arrest occurs. Truog and coworkers suggest a framework for when such procedure-specific forms should be utilized, and they suggest a different format for a DNR to be used during surgery. They note that clarity is the main virtue of procedure-specific DNRs, which is an important factor on a ward when patients are provided care by a large number of different clinicians who change relatively frequently. For DNRs during surgery, however, they recommend that instead of a procedure-specific DNR, it is better simply to focus on the patient's values and goals, allowing the anesthesiologist to decide during surgery and recovery whether particular interventions will promote the patient's goals in term of outcomes, such as quality of life. In order to arrive at an understanding of the patient's goals and concept of factors relevant to the patient's conception of quality of life, the anesthesiologist and surgeon need to take the time to have a sustained dialogue with the patient, and the patient must gain confidence that the surgeon and anesthesiologist understand their goals well enough to implement their values in the course of care [23]. Layon and Dirk emphasize the importance of this dialogue in the following way: "Quality of life issues demand more of the physician-patient relationship – that physicians communicate more than their knowledge of pathophysiology and pharmacology and that patients communicate more than their symptoms" ([47], p.136).

The American Association of Anesthesiologists (ASA) policy statement recognizes that a policy of automatic suspension of DNR orders during surgery and recovery does not sufficiently respect patient autonomy. Therefore, deliberation with the patient or patient-authorized decision-maker about how to achieve the patient's preferences is a prerequisite to whatever option is mutually agreed about the patient's DNR status during surgery. The ASA also recommends that when anesthesiologists or surgeons have a conscience-based objection to the patient's choice to refuse resuscitation procedures, they should refer the patient to another physician who is willing to perform the procedure in a manner that respects the patient's autonomy [48].

Medical Futility

The debate over medical futility has continued for more than two decades without sufficient consensus to consider it settled, although some progress has been made. A full account of the debate is beyond the scope of this chapter, but a summary of the progress that has been made and some practical recommendations are in order.

In a very general sense, the concept of medical futility is widely accepted: physicians are not required to offer or to provide treatments that provide no medical effect (definition provided next) for the patient, even if the patient demands them. For example, patients who request laetrile as a cancer treatment or antibiotics for a viral infection should be declined because they are known to provide no medical effect on the condition the patient has. Reasons for declining to provide such measures should be explained to a patient who requests them, but the physician is not obligated to provide them even if the patient does not accept that the measures would be ineffective for her condition. This is a legitimate limitation of patient autonomy by the physician's professional autonomy and integrity.

The concept of futility has been more controversial in end-of-life decisions, however, primarily because it has been expanded beyond the question of whether a treatment will have an intended effect. Futility in the context of end-of-life care has been extended to the distinguishable question of whether even a treatment that might achieve the intended medical *effect* should be considered as a legitimate *benefit* for the patient. This second question ventures beyond purely medical expertise about treatment effectiveness into whether the quality of life achieved by an effective treatment produces a quality of life that justifies using the treatment. Critics of this second aspect of the concept of medical futility hold that decisions about whether a patient's quality of life is sufficient to be considered beneficial is not a decision physicians should make unilaterally and that patients are in a better position to decide whether their quality of life is worth the burdens of the treatment in question.

Attempts to define both quantitative and qualitative futility consistently and to operationalize futility in practice have been fraught with difficulty. Schneiderman and colleagues attempted to define clinical futility quantitatively as follows: "…when physicians conclude (either through personal experience, experiences shared with colleagues, or consideration of published empiric data) that in the last 100 cases a medical treatment has been useless, they should regard that treatment as futile" ([49], p. 949). There is more than the numbers to unpack, here, but let's begin with the quantitative aspect. First, the basis for justifying unilateral physician determinations of futility is grounded in the physician's unilateral expertise about the clinical scientific basis for judging what effect a treatment will have. Conceived in this way, a futility determination should be objective, scientific, and quantifiably predictable.

In the decades since this definition was formulated, the claim that clinical medicine should be evidence-based calls into question the breadth of the epistemic sources embraced by Schneiderman's original definition. The last hundred cases "either through personal experience or experiences shared with colleagues" do not sufficiently meet the rigor of the third part of the definition, "consideration of published empiric data" ([50], p. 126). If life or death outcomes or even timing of death outcomes are to be based on the physician's unilateral knowledge of scientific evidence, such unilateral decisions should at least have a more scientific justification than merely personal experience or shared collegial observations without a rigorous evidence base. In an article published 20 years after the original definition, Schneiderman acknowledged that "Physicians should not be free to invoke medical futility unless they can justify it before their peers with good evidence-based data and before society with professional standards of practice" ([50], p.126).

In a major study to assess the accuracy and validity of Acute Physiology and Chronic Health Evaluation (APACHE) III hospital mortality predictions, Zimmerman and coworkers found the APACHE III criteria to be accurate for predictions of group outcomes but cautioned that ICU day 1 mortality estimates, while useful for prediction on a population basis, do not support individual patient predictions for purposes of withholding or withdrawal of LST [51]. After additional data are obtained on individual patients during the course of their subsequent care, such as how they are responding to interventions, such group-predicted outcomes may be a useful basis for attempting to portray to patient's decision-makers potential scenarios for weighing likely outcomes for purposes of decisions about continuing aggressive care or transitioning to palliative care. However, they are not an adequate basis for predictions of individual outcomes sufficient to support unilateral decisions to withhold or to withdraw LST.

The qualitative aspect of futility, according to Schneiderman and coworkers, requires physicians to "distinguish between an effect, which is limited to some part of the patient's body, and a benefit, which appreciably improves the person as a whole" ([49], p. 949). By this definition, a physician unilaterally could withhold or withdraw a treatment that might be effective in producing a physiological effect, such as restoration of cardiac rhythm, but if it "merely preserves permanent unconsciousness or cannot end dependence on intensive medical care, the treatment should be considered futile" ([49], p. 949).

Several physician specialty groups attempted to promulgate definitions of futility that could be applied along these lines, such as "lethal condition futility" or "imminent demise futility" [52]. Halevy and Brody note that lethal condition futility is far too broad, since many persons have meaningful quality of life for a substantial period of time even after they have been diagnosed with a lethal condition [52]. Imminent demise futility is narrower but often is interpreted as "will not leave the hospital."

Once again, a number of persons survive in the hospital for a period of time with what they deem to be an acceptable quality of life. Even when imminent demise is interpreted more narrowly than "will not leave the hospital," some patients or their decision-makers value as a benefit the life-sustaining treatment that allows the patient to survive long enough for visiting family to arrive or some other matter of personal significance. These instances demonstrate that when it comes to goals of care, futility is in the mind of the beholder. It is thus not entirely a matter of an objective, quantifiable fact that should be made unilaterally on the basis of physician expertise alone.

A narrower definition of futility, called physiological futility, defines futility by whether the medical treatment in question will achieve its intended physiological effect. For example, CPR would be futile if there was a hole in the heart wall. Although physiological futility is defensible for unilateral physician decision-making, it is not broad enough to include the types of qualitative futility judgments that Schneiderman and others believe should be made by physicians. Halevy and Brody find that all of the substantive attempts to define futility fail to meet standards of precision, prospectiveness, social acceptability, and sufficient numbers. Finding substantive definitions wanting, they move on to address futility cases procedurally [52].

Houston area hospitals collaboratively agreed to a city-wide process for handling futility cases in common, which later became the basis for the section of the Texas Advance Directives Act (TADA) that allows hospitals and other healthcare facilities unilaterally to withhold or withdraw life-sustaining treatment from patients if they have followed specified procedures designed to provide due process and any other available care options to patients and their authorized decision-makers. Although the Texas statute does not use the term futility, this process-based approach requires a physician who has determined that an intervention is medically inappropriate to submit that determination to an ethics committee for review. The patient's authorized decision-maker must receive 48-h notice of the ethics committee meeting, may attend the meeting, and is entitled to a written explanation of the committee's decision. If the ethics committee agrees with the physician's decision, the provider must continue LST for at least 10 days in order to allow for the patient's decision-maker to find another facility willing to take the patient in transfer and provide continued care. If no other facility agrees to take the patient and the patient's decision-maker cannot obtain a court order to extend the period in view of a possible transfer, the provider facility is allowed legally to discontinue LSTs in spite of the objections of the patient's decision-maker. If the physician and hospital comply with these procedures, they are protected from liability claims [53].

A majority of states have enacted statutory provisions that codify the notion that a physician is not required to provide medically inappropriate treatment. Most of these provisions are sufficiently vague, however, that physicians, hospitals, and other healthcare facilities generally have not relied on them for immunity from liability in order to invoke unilaterally withholding or withdrawal of LST against the wishes of patients' authorized decision-makers. Pope concludes that what distinguishes the Texas statute is its purely procedural character. By arriving at futility procedurally, Texas has avoided uncertainty about substantive definitions or criteria that have otherwise plagued the futility debate [53]. In effect, the fact that no other provider emerges to take the patient in transfer is tantamount to a justification that the hospital invoking futility has met the prevailing standard of care.

Artificial Nutrition and Hydration

For purposes of withholding and withdrawal of treatment in end-of-life decision-making, some have advocated that artificially provided nutrition and hydration (ANH) should not be considered in the same category of interventions as respirators, dialysis, cardiopulmonary resuscitation, or other LSTs. Various reasons for this position have been advanced including the following: (1) ANH is always an essential means of comfort care and must be maintained for palliative purposes even if not for the purpose of prolonging life when other LST measures have been withheld or withdrawn; (2) ANH is an inherent aspect of the symbolism of the most basic humane obligation of caring, providing food and drink, and cannot be humanely withheld; and (3) withholding or withdrawal of ANH creates a slippery slope toward not only withholding ANH from dying patients but also withholding or withdrawal of ordinary nutrition and hydration from non-dying patients whose continued care is perceived to be too costly for society [1].

Well-validated palliative care measures have shown that withholding or withdrawal of ANH need not result in discomfort or distress for the patient, which means that provision of ANH is not always necessary as a comfort measure. The option of withholding or withdrawal of ANH without imposing discomfort on the patient is especially crucial when the provision of ANH would prolong the dying process of a person whose quality of life has deteriorated and other LSTs have been withdrawn in order to mitigate a prolonged dying process. Thus, ANH, which is as invasive, intrusive, and potentially burdensome as other forms of LST, is no different than other forms of LST that may be withheld or withdrawn when patients or their authorized decision-makers believe that the burdens outweigh the benefits of its use. The symbolism of food and water as a basic gesture of humane caring more clearly applies to normal contexts in which persons can swallow ordinary means of nutrition and hydration rather than the provision of ANH for symbolic reasons to a dying patient who does not value the actual burdensome impact of ANH.

Rabenek and colleagues devised an algorithm to capture clinical guidelines combining both medical and ethical rationales for addressing the use of percutaneous endoscopic gastrostomy (PEG) tubes [35]. When a patient has an anorexia-cachexia syndrome refractory to nutritional therapy – such as in advanced cancer or AIDS – they recommend that PEG placement is not indicated and should not be offered unless it is the only way to provide necessary medications. This recommendation would not apply to cases in which nutrition could reverse cachexia, such as a benign esophageal stricture [35]. Moreover, they recommend that in cases of permanent vegetative state the physician should explain why, in spite of the potential for PEG placement to provide their intended physiological function, the PEG will not be able to restore the patient to a condition in which the patient can experience any quality of life and, therefore, recommend against PEG placement. They recommend both offering and recommending a PEG placement in uncomplicated dysphagia cases in which there is no other deficit in quality of life. In cases of complicated dysphasia, in which additional deficits and symptoms are present that compromise the patient's physical or mental quality of life or prolong progressive underlying disease, they recommend that the physician should thoroughly discuss the various benefits and burdens associated with PEG placement in the patient's condition and engage in nondirective counseling to elicit the patient's values rather than making a recommendation. For patients with permanent vegetative states, physicians should offer the procedure and recommend against it. For patients who have dysphagia without other deficits in quality of life, physicians should offer and recommend the procedure. For the remaining patients who have dysphagia with other deficits in quality of life, the physician's role is to provide nondirective counseling regarding the short- and long-term consequences of a trial of PEG tube feeding (Fig. 45.3) [35].

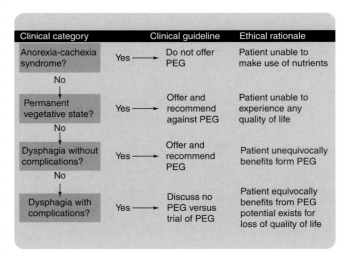

Fig. 45.3 Decision-making algorithm for PEG tube placement (Reprinted with permission of Elsevier from Rabeneck and McCullough [35], p. 9050)

Legally, judicial decisions and statutes have followed the general ethical consensus that ANH is not significantly different from other forms of LST that can be withheld or withdrawn when patients or their authorized decision-makers regard it as more burdensome than beneficial [54]. Following the Schiavo case, however, two states made it substantially more difficult to accomplish withholding or withdrawal of ANH. Patients in North Dakota and Arizona who want to refuse ANH in advance of their incapacity must explicitly state their refusal of ANH in a written advance directive to be sure that their wishes can be carried out [54].

Palliative Sedation, Voluntary Dehydration, and Physician Aid in Dying

Arguments against physician aid in dying have traditionally centered on claims that narrowly circumscribed parameters invoked to justify the practice initially would (1) inevitably expand to include involuntary euthanasia, (2) undermine support for high-quality palliative care, (3) manipulate or coerce patients who did not really want it to acquiesce into accepting aid in dying, (4) result in incapacitated patients receiving it, and (5) result in especially vulnerable groups (racial or ethnic minorities, disabled persons, the elderly,

those without healthcare access) being disproportionately pressured into accepting aid in dying because their costs of their care to society would make them feel that others thought they should choose assisted suicide in order to minimize those costs.

In Oregon a limited form of physician aid in dying designed to address those concerns has been legally available for well over a decade. The Oregon experience provides empirical reassurance that the concerns of critics can be avoided while allowing terminally ill patients to know that, if their quality of life becomes unacceptable, the process of dying need not be protracted. Through the first 12 years of its implementation, a total of 525 patients have died from self-administered prescriptions allowed by the Oregon Death with Dignity Act (DWDA) [55]. During 2010, 96 such prescriptions were written, and 20 of the patients who received them did not take the prescription, ultimately dying of their underlying illnesses [55]. The rate of death from ingesting prescriptions allowed by DWDA in 2010 was 20.8 deaths per 10,000 deaths in Oregon [55]. Similar data from prior years confirm that over a sustained period, the rate of physician-assisted suicides in Oregon is low and stable, mitigating concerns that legalization would lead to a slippery slope (Fig. 45.4) [55]. The substantial number of prescription recipients in each year that have chosen not to ingest their

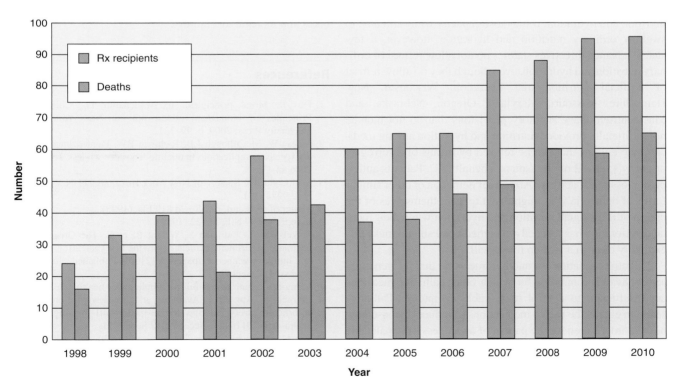

Fig. 45.4 Number of DWDA prescription recipients and deaths as of January 7, 2011, by year, Oregon, 1998–2010 (From Oregon Department of Human Services [55])

medications shows that some patients request them for peace of mind in case their quality of life becomes unacceptable, yet ultimately do not decide to use them.

As in earlier years, more than 90 % in 2010 died at home under hospice care, refuting the concern that physician-assisted suicide undermines availability of good palliative care [55]. Moreover, more than 95 % of 2010 patients who died from DWDA prescriptions had some form of health insurance, which addresses the fear that persons would be coerced to accept it for lack of access to healthcare coverage [55]. One hundred percent of persons who died as a result of DWDA in 2010 were white, tempering the apprehension that racial minorities will be disproportionately affected [55].

Physician aid in dying is not legally available to US patients dying in states other than Washington, Oregon, Montana, and Vermont. Quill suggests voluntary dehydration as a legally available option of last resort for cases in which palliative measures cannot adequately mitigate pain or other debilitating symptoms or cannot address a patient's loss of dignity [56]. Since refusal of artificial nutrition and hydration is legal in all states, a capacitated patient who cannot choose physician aid in dying could nevertheless choose voluntary dehydration if good palliative support is available to mitigate the symptoms entailed in dehydration. The legality of this option is most clear when the patient begins the voluntary refusal of ordinary nutrition and hydration while capacitated and specifies that upon their loss of decisional capacity they refuse both ordinary nutrition and hydration, as well as refusing artificial nutrition and hydration. If they lose capacity while still able to swallow ordinary nutrition and hydration, however, a few states' advance directives statutes do not allow refusal of ordinary nutrition and hydration, even though they do allow refusal of artificial nutrition and hydration. Wisconsin, New Hampshire, Missouri, Maryland, Oregon, Nebraska, and Massachusetts have statutory provisions that do not include non-artificially provided nutrition and hydration among medical interventions that can be refused by means of a surrogate or proxy's refusal on the patient's behalf [54]. Patients anticipating loss of capacity by Alzheimer dementia or other similar forms of dementia who might want to avail themselves of the option of refusing all nutrition and hydration when their mental deterioration has reached a specified point should make this explicitly clear in a written living will.

Palliative sedation is another measure that is generally legally available in cases for which other palliative measures are insufficient to control undesirable symptoms. Palliative sedation entails the use of medications to induce unconsciousness in order to relieve the patient of awareness of unpalatable symptoms such as pain, agitation, myoclonic jerks, seizures, or other stressful symptoms [57]. Although legally available, palliative sedation is ethically controversial. Physicians ethically opposed to physician aid in dying emphasize that only those cases in which the criteria for double effect can be met are ethically appropriate uses of palliative sedation. The double effect doctrine specifies that when two distinct consequences result from a single action, one good consequence and one bad consequence, the action is morally acceptable if it meets four criteria: (1) the action is not inherently bad, (2) the bad consequence is not a means to the good consequence, (3) the actor does not intend the bad consequence, and (4) the bad consequence is not disproportional to the good consequence [58].

In the context of palliative sedation, meeting these criteria would require that sedation for palliative goals is not inherently bad; that hastening the patient's death is not the means of relieving the patient's symptoms (such as pain); that the physician does not intend to hasten the patient's death, even if some suppression of respiratory drive is a foreseeable risk; and that any unintentional hastening of the patient's death as a side effect of suppression of respiration is not disproportional to the goal of relieving the patient's intractable symptoms. Proponents of this rule believe that it can be coherent to speak of consequences that are foreseen but not intended [58].

Critics of the double effect rule maintain that it is not coherent to say that one both foresees a bad consequence as a result of one's actions and yet does not intend that consequence [56]. They hold that it is more coherent to speak of being responsible for foreseeable consequences, good and bad, and some hastening of death as a possible consequence of palliative sedation that does not make it unethical. Generally, such critics support physician aid in dying and see no real ethical difference between physician aid in dying and palliative sedation, other than the longer time it typically takes and its legal availability.

References

1. Part II. Moral principles. In: Beauchamp TL, Childress JF. Principles of biomedical ethics. 6th ed. New York: Oxford University Press; 2009. p. 99–331.
2. Jones JW, McCullough LB, Richman BW. Painted into a corner: unexpected complications in treating Jehovah's witness. J Vasc Surg. 2006;44:435–8.
3. Schloendorff v Society of New York Hospital, 211 N.Y. 125, 105 N.E. 92 (1914).
4. Matter of Dubreuil, 629 So.2d 819 Fla. (1993).
5. In re E.G., 549 N.E.2d 322 (1989).
6. Finkelstein A, Taubman S, Wright B, et al. The Oregon health insurance experiment: evidence from the first year. 2011. Available at: http://www.nber.org/papers/w17190. Published July 2011. Accessed 12 Sept 2011.
7. Vermont's senate passes bill for single-payer health care. National Journal. 27 Apr 2011. Available at: http://www.nationaljournal.com/healthcare/vermont-s-senate-passes-bill-for-single-payer-health-care-20110427. Accessed 12 Sept 2011.
8. Lee C. Massachusetts begins universal health care. Washington Post. Available at: http://www.washingtonpost.com/wp-dyn/content/article/2007/06/30/AR2007063000248.html. Published 1 July 2007. Accessed 12 Sept 2011.
9. Pear R. States' policies on health care exclude poorest. The New York Times. 25 May 2013, p. A1.
10. Truog RD, Brock DW, Cook DJ, et al. Rationing in the intensive care unit. Crit Care Med. 2006;34(4):959.

11. American Thoracic Society. Fair allocation of intensive care unit resources. AM J Respir Crit Care Med. 1997;4:1282–301.
12. Guyatt G, Cook D, Weaver B, et al. The Level of Care Investigators and the Canadian Critical Care Trials Group. Influence of perceived functional and employment status on cardiopulmonary resuscitation directives. J Crit Care. 2003;18:133–41.
13. Marshall MF, Schwenzer KJ, Orsina M, et al. Influence of political power, medical provincialism, and economic incentives on the rationing of surgical intensive care unit beds. Crit Care Med. 1992;20:387–94.
14. Chalfin DB, Carlon GC. Age and utilization of ICU resources of critically ill cancer patients. Crit Care Med. 1990;18:694.
15. Layon AJ, George BE, Hamby B, Gallagher TJ. Do elderly patients over utilize health care resources and benefit less from them than younger patients ? A study of patients who underwent craniotomy for treatment of neoplasm. Crit Care Med. 1995;23:829–34.
16. Stachniak JB, Layon AJ, Day AL, Gallagher TJ. Craniotomy for intracranial aneurysm and subarachnoid hemorrhage – is course, cost, or outcome affected by age? Stroke. 1996;27:276–81.
17. Lockwood M. Quality of life and resource allocation. In: Kuhse H, Singer P, editors. Bioethics: an anthology. 2nd ed. Malden: Blackwell Publishing Ltd.; 2006. p. 451–64.
18. Sinuff T, Kahnamoui K, Cook DJ, Luce JM, Levy MM. Rationing critical care beds: a systematic review. Crit Care Med. 2004;32(7): 1588–97.
19. Applebaum PS. Assessment of patients' competence to consent to treatment. N Engl J Med. 2007;357:1834–40.
20. Boyle RJ. Determining patients' capacity to share in decision making. In: Fletcher J, Lombardo PA, Marshall MF, Miller FG, editors. Introduction to clinical ethics. 2nd ed. Hagerstown: University Publishing Group, Inc; 1997. p. 71–88.
21. Singer P. Is the sanctity of life ethic terminally Ill? In: Kuhse H, Singer P, editors. Bioethics: an anthology. 2nd ed. Malden: Blackwell Publishing Ltd; 2006. p. 344–53.
22. Veatch RM. The impending collapse of the whole-brain definition of death. Hastings Cent Rep. 1993;23(4):18–24.
23. Truog RD, Miller FG. The dead donor rule and organ transplantation. N Engl J Med. 2008;359:674–5.
24. Bernat JL. The boundaries of organ donation after circulatory death. N Engl J Med. 2008;359:669–71.
25. N.J. Stat § 26:6A-5
26. New York State Department of Health. Guidelines for determining brain death. New York State Department of Health; Dec 2005.
27. CAL. HSC. CODE § 1254.4.
28. The Multi-Society Task Force on PVS. Medical aspects of the persistent vegetative state (1). N Engl J Med. 1994;330(21):1499–508.
29. The Multi-Society Task Force on PVS. Medical aspects of the persistent vegetative state (2). N Engl J Med. 1994;330(22):1572–9.
30. Fins JJ, Master MG, Gerber LM, Giacino JT. The minimally conscious state: a diagnosis in search of an epidemiology. Arch Neurol. 2007;64:1400–5.
31. Liang BA, Lin L. Bouvia v. Superior court: quality of life matters. Virtual Mentor. 2005;7(2). Available at: http://virtualmentor.ama-assn.org/2005/02/hlaw1-0502.html. Accessed 21 Sept 2011.
32. Bouvia v Superior Court, 179 Cal. App. 3d 1127, 1135–36, 225 Cal. Rptr. 297. (Ct. App. 1986), review denied (Cal. June 5, 1986).
33. Butler K. What broke my father's heart. The New York Times. 20 June 2010, p. MM38.
34. Lampert R, Hayes DL, Annas GJ, et al. HRS expert consensus statement on the management of cardiovascular implantable electronic devices (CIEDs) in patients nearing end of life or requesting withdrawal of therapy. Heart Rhythm. 2010;7(7):1008–26.
35. Rabaneck L, McCullough LB. Ethically justified, clinically comprehensive guidelines for percutaneous endoscopic gastrostomy tube replacement. Lancet. 1997;349:497.
36. American Bar Association. The rights of older Americans: ABA family legal guide. 3rd ed. Chicago: Random House Reference; 2004.
37. Prendergast TJ. Advance care planning: pitfalls, progress, promise. Crit Care Med. 2001;29:N34–9.
38. Silverira MJ, Kim SYH, Langa KM. Advance directives and outcomes of surrogate decision making before death. N Eng J Med. 2010;362:1211–8.
39. Diem SJ, Lantos JD, Tulsky JA. Cardiopulmonary resuscitation on television – miracles and misinformation. N Eng J Med. 1996;334: 1578–82.
40. Jones GK, Brewer KL, Garrison HG. Public expectations of survival following cardiopulmonary resuscitation. Acad Emerg Med. 2000;7:48–53.
41. Ehlenbach WJ, Barnato AE, Curtis JR, et al. Epidemiologic study of in-hospital cardiopulmonary resuscitation in the elderly. N Engl J Med. 2009;361:122–31.
42. Pantilat SZ. Communicating with seriously ill patients: better words to say. JAMA. 2009;301(12):1279–81.
43. Emanuel EJ, Fairclough DL, Wolfe P, Emanuel LL. Talking with terminally ill patients and their caregivers about death, dying, and bereavement. Arch Intern Med. 2004;164:1999–2004.
44. Mack JW, Weeks JC, Wright AA, Block SD, Prigerson HG. End-of-life discussions, goal attainment, and distress at the end of life: predictors and outcomes of receipt of care consistent with preferences. J Clin Oncol. 2010;28:1203–8.
45. Billings A, Krakauer EL. On patient autonomy and physician responsibility in end-of-life care. Arch Intern Med. 2011;171(9):849–53.
46. Johnson SK, Bautista CA, Hong SY, Weissfeld L, White DB. An empirical study of surrogates' preferred level of control over value-laden life support decisions in intensive care units. AM J Respir Crit Care Med. 2011;183:915–21.
47. Layon AJ, Layon DL. Resuscitation and DNR: ethical aspects for anaesthetists. Can J Anaesth. 1995;42(2):134–40.
48. The American Association of Anesthesiologists. Ethical guidelines for the anesthesia care of patients with no-not-resuscitate orders or other directives that limit treatment. ASA House of Delegates. Available at: http://www.asahq.org/For-Members/Clinical-Information/~/media/For%2520Members/documents/Standards%2520Guidelines%2520S tmts/Ethical%2520Guidelines%2520for%2520the%2520Anesthesia %2520Care%2520of%2520Patients.ashx. Published on 17 Oct 2001. Accessed on 22 Sept 2011.
49. Schneiderman LJ, Jecker NS, Jonsen AR. Medical futility: its meaning and ethical implications. Ann Intern Med. 1990;112(12): 949–54.
50. Schneiderman LJ. Defining medical futility and improving medical care. J Bioeth Inq. 2011;8(2):123–31.
51. Zimmerman JE, Wagner DP, Draper EA, Wright L, Alzola C, Knaus WA. Evaluation of acute physiology and chronic health evaluation III predictions of hospital mortality in an independent database. Crit Care Med. 1998;26(8):1317–26.
52. Brody BA, Halevy A. The role of futility in health care reform. In: Misbin RI, Jennings B, Orentlicher D, Dewar M, editors. Health care crisis? The search for answers. Frederick: University Publishing Group; 1995.
53. Pope TM. Medical futility statutes: no safe harbor to unilaterally refuse life-sustaining treatment. Tenn Law Rev. 2007;75:1.
54. Meisel A, Cerminara K. The right to die. 3rd ed. New York: Aspen Law and Business; 2004.
55. Oregon Department of Human Services. Thirteenth annual report on the Oregon Death with Dignity Act. 13th ed. Salem: Oregon Public Health Division; 2011. Available at: http://public.health.oregon.gov/ProviderPartnerResources/EvaluationResearch/DeathWithDignityAct/Documents/year13.pdf. Accessed on 25 May 2011.
56. Quill TE, Lo B, Brock DW, Meisel A. Last-resort options for palliative sedation. Ann Intern Med. 2009;151:421–4.
57. Lo B, Rubenfeld G. Palliative sedation in dying patients: We turn to it when everything else hasn't worked. JAMA. 2005;294(14):1810–6.
58. Sulmasy DP, Pellegrino ED. The rule of double effect: clearing up the double talk. Arch Intern Med. 1999;159:545–50.

Pharmacotherapy in the Neurosurgical Intensive Care Unit

46

Aimée C. LeClaire, Jennifer R. Bushwitz, and Steven A. Robicsek

Contents

A.C. LeClaire, PharmD, BCPS (✉)
Clinical Pharmacy Services,
Critical Care Clinical Pharmacy Services,
Department of Pharmacy Services,
Shands at the University of Florida,
1432 NW 98th Terrace, Gainesville, FL 32610, USA
e-mail: leclaa@shands.ufl.edu

J.R. Bushwitz, PharmD
Department of Pharmacy Services,
Shands at the University of Florida, 1600 SW Archer Rd,
100316, Gainesville, FL 32610, USA
e-mail: bushj@shands.ufl.edu

S.A. Robicsek, MD, PhD
Department of Anesthesiology,
University of Florida College of Medicine,
1600 SW Archer Road,
100254, Gainesville, FL 32610, USA
e-mail: robicsek@ufl.edu

Abstract

An understanding of the basic pharmacodynamic and pharmacokinetic characteristics of medications is paramount in the management of the critically ill neuroscience patient. Furthermore, the influence or alterations a neurologic disease process or injury may exert on these basic and specific drug principles must be considered when designing pharmacotherapy regimens and monitoring plans. Known potential adverse medication reactions, such as the potential for elevation in intracranial pressure with hydralazine, may be of little clinical concern in the average medical or surgical intensive care unit patient but of more severe consequence in the neurologically injured patient. The critical care pharmacist is a key member of the interdisciplinary team and a valuable resource in navigating the many medication issues or needs of the neuroscience patient.

Keywords

Pharmacokinetics • Pharmacotherapy • Sedatives • Analgesics • Corticosteroids • Vasoactive agents • Antiepileptics • Pharmacist

Introduction

Optimal management of the neurologically injured patient depends on rapid recognition of neurologic issues and knowledge of pharmacodynamic and pharmacokinetic properties of neuroactive drugs. Pharmacologic management is aimed at matching the metabolic needs of the brain and spinal cord with perfusion and oxygenation. Major advances in neurosurgical intensive care have come from a better understanding of the pathophysiologic mechanisms of neuronal injury and the application of medications influencing the central nervous system.

A.J. Layon et al. (eds.), *Textbook of Neurointensive Care*,
DOI 10.1007/978-1-4471-5226-2_46, © Springer-Verlag London 2013

Pharmacokinetic Principles

Pharmacokinetics encompasses drug absorption, distribution, and elimination. Each of these phases of drug movement through the body involves passage across cell membranes. Therefore drug properties, including molecular size and shape, degree of ionization, lipid solubility, and protein binding, all influence drug movement [1]. Drugs may be administered by a variety of routes: enteral (oral, sublingual, rectal), parenteral (subcutaneous, intramuscular, intravenous, intra-arterial, intrathecal), topical, transdermal, and inhalational. Absorption from each of these routes has specific advantages and disadvantages in the intensive care unit. Enteral administration is the safest and most economic means of administering a drug; however, a variety of factors, including extensive hepatic and intestinal metabolism, can influence absorption and introduce variability.

Drug distribution is a dynamic process and is dependent on the degree of protein binding. Within the circulation, the principal proteins that bind drugs are albumin and α_1-acid glycoprotein. High degrees of protein binding of a drug can outweigh solubility for lipophilic drugs, which results in decreased volume of distribution (Vd) since the drug does not easily leave the circulation. The degree of protein binding can influence drug availability and toxicity.

Redistribution is the movement of drug from bound sites to unbound sites. This is usually considered to be a dynamic process by which drug diffuses from receptors into the extracellular space and other tissues, usually *via* the blood. Equilibrium is eventually reached between bound and unbound drug (in both the tissues and blood). Movement from blood to tissues takes time, during which, if blood samples are analyzed, a higher concentration of the drug is found than would be predicted based simply on its Vd and the dose administered; this movement is referred to as the distribution phase.

Figure 46.1 depicts two drugs given intravenously. Drug A is highly distributed, as evidenced by the long, sloping, initial part of the curve. Because drug concentration is measured in the blood compartment, we would expect that as the drug moves from the blood into other tissues, its concentration in the blood would decrease rapidly at first and then more slowly as tissue equilibrium is approached. Drug B has little or no distribution, as might occur with a water-soluble agent. Once blood and tissue equilibrium occurs, drug elimination by either metabolism or excretion accounts for the remainder of the curve.

Drug metabolism may be increased by enzyme induction or be modulated, resulting in increased activity with enhanced clearance of some agents. For example, when given concomitantly with phenytoin or phenobarbital, the clearance of certain nondepolarizing neuromuscular antagonists is accelerated. Phenytoin and phenobarbital both induce

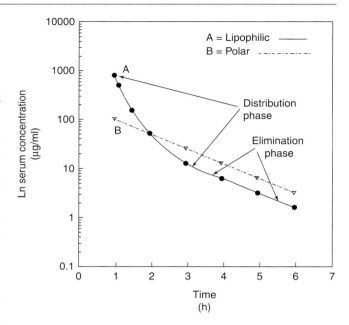

Fig. 46.1 Lipophilic versus polar drug level profiles. *A* hypothetical lipophilic drug profile, with distribution phase and elimination phase, *B* polar drug profile with only elimination phase (Reproduced with permission of Elsevier from Kirby et al. [160, p. 630])

cytochrome P450, specifically P450 2B6 (CYP2B6) enzyme in the liver, which metabolizes vecuronium and rocuronium, and thus shorten the duration of action for any given dose. Enzyme induction generally takes days to weeks to occur and is not usually a concern after the acute administration of barbiturates.

The elimination phase is the linear part of the log concentration versus time curve in Fig. 46.1. The common log or natural log value usually is plotted versus time. Because the decay is so rapid, the decrease in concentration is an exponential function given by the equation

$$C_t = C_0 e^{-kt}$$

where C_t represents the concentration of a drug at a given time, C_0 is the initial concentration, $-k$ is a rate constant, and t is the half-life. By plotting the common log or natural log values of these concentrations, we convert a curve to nearly a straight line. The slope of the latter part of this line then represents the elimination constant for the drug, which is inversely proportional to the half-life ($t_{\frac{1}{2}}$).

Clearance is dependent on the Vd and the elimination constant. As mentioned earlier, the Vd of a drug is dependent on its relative lipid solubility, the degree of protein binding, and its ionization. Ionization has an important role as drugs are generally more soluble in the ionized state. However, they are often not cleared from the body as well, because of difficulty crossing cell membranes. Ionized drugs also tend to be more protein bound and are thus less available to their target tissues.

Weak acids like sodium thiopental (STP) are more ionized and more protein bound in a basic medium. Since a smaller amount of the drug is able to cross cell membranes, the drug effect will be diminished. Therefore, patients maintained in an alkalotic state during hyperventilation therapy for a closed head injury would be expected to have less of an effect from similar levels of sodium thiopental than do non-alkalotic subjects. Increased ionization results in decreased drug availability to cross into the brain. Conversely, on termination of hyperventilation therapy, as the blood becomes less alkalotic, more drug is available for both therapeutic effect and clearance.

With the emergence of more intravenous agents with very short half-lives, the concepts of *context-sensitive* halftime and offset of action become more important. Context-sensitive halftime is the time required for the central compartment drug concentration to decrease by 50 % at the end of infusion as predicted by agent-specific, multicompartment pharmacokinetic models, where "context" refers to the duration of the infusion. Context-sensitive halftime is more useful in predicting the time course of recovery of many agents than is the elimination half-life [2, 3]. For example, barbiturates have a short duration which is dependent on redistribution. This is limited by lean mass and easily overwhelmed by larger cumulative doses. The marked prolongation of recovery time, with increasing duration of pentobarbital infusion, is reflected in an increase in its context-sensitive halftime. At this point the duration of action is no longer related to redistribution but to a high volume of distribution and low clearance. In comparison, the context-sensitive halftime of remifentanil remains virtually constant following prolonged infusions.

Offset of action is defined as the time for resolution of pharmacologic effect once drug administration is discontinued. If the drug concentration is maintained just above the minimum effective concentration, discontinuing the infusion quickly allows the concentration to fall below the minimum effective concentration. If an intermittent bolus technique were used, a comparatively prolonged distribution and elimination would be required for a recently administered bolus dose before offset of action. Continuous infusion administration of propofol provides a good example. Maintenance of the drug level just high enough to provide sedation allows rapid emergence once the infusion is discontinued. However, much more delayed arousal would follow administration of a large bolus (Fig. 46.2).

With redistribution and elimination occurring in accordance with the physiochemical properties of the drug, intravenously administered agents require frequent dosing to maintain the minimum drug effect and concentration at the site of action. To eliminate the "peak and valley" effect of frequent intermittent administration, a continuous infusion technique is preferable [4]. Figure 46.2 shows the

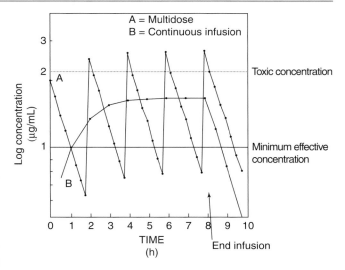

Fig. 46.2 Multidose versus continuous infusions. *A* drug levels from multiple doses of a hypothetical drug, *B* continuous infusions of same hypothetical drug. Note repetitive decay below minimum effective concentration with intermittent dosing (Reproduced with permission of Elsevier from Kirby et al. [160, p. 642])

relationship of multiple injections compared to a continuous infusion of a drug with rapid clearance. It should be noted how continuous infusion dampens the oscillations in serum drug levels that may cause toxicity at the peak or inadequate effect at the trough. Continuous infusions are best suited to drugs with short half-lives and rapid clearance [5]. Since these drugs are eliminated from the blood rapidly, they would require numerous intermittent boluses. Clearly, remifentanil, with a half-life of 5–12 min, is much better administered by continuous infusion rather than intermittent boluses. Alternatively, morphine, with a half-life of 3–7 h, can be delivered by intermittent bolus very effectively.

If the desired effect sought with a particular drug is saturable with a single dose, then no advantage will be obtained with continuous infusion. An example of this behavior would be the histamine$_2$ receptor antagonists (e.g., ranitidine). At the maximal effective drug concentration, no further blockade of acid production occurs regardless of additional drug administration. However, if the process is not saturable – as is the case for most intravenous sedative agents – providing the minimum effective concentration with a continuous infusion will maintain the desired pharmacologic effect.

Maintenance of a particular steady-state drug level is required to sustain the desired pharmacologic effect [4]. To achieve this, the amount of drug entering the body must equal the amount of drug being removed from the body. We know that the concentration at steady state (C_{ss}) is determined by the following relationship:

$$C_{ss} = \frac{X_o}{Cl}$$

where X_o is the amount of drug given per unit time and Cl is the volume of blood cleared of the drug per unit time. Thus, for example, fentanyl (clearance of 12.7 mL/kg/min), administered by continuous infusion at a rate of 2 mcg/kg/h or 0.033 mcg/kg/min, yields a steady-state concentration of 0.0026 mcg/mL (2.6 ng/mL). This value is within the minimum effective concentration range (1–5 ng/mL for analgesia and minimal respiratory depression). Knowledge of the clearance of a drug and the approximate minimum effective concentration in the blood allows prediction of the infusion rate necessary to achieve a particular level.

A steady-state drug concentration can be achieved with a constant infusion, but this is a slow process (curve B in Fig. 46.2). This can be overcome by administering a loading dose (LD) as bolus or as a rapid priming infusion. The loading dose (LD) equals the target plasma concentration (Cp) multiplied by the volume of distribution (Vd):

$$LD = Cp \cdot Vds$$

Thus, from the previous example, the loading dose of fentanyl (in a 70 kg patient using a Vd of 3.2 L/kg) would be

$$LD = (0.0026 \text{ mcg} / \text{mL}) \cdot (70 \text{ kg}) \cdot (3.2 \text{ L} / \text{kg})$$
$$\cdot (1,000 \text{ mL} / \text{L}) = 582 \text{ mcg}$$

The therapeutic index is the ratio of the median lethal dose (LD_{50}) to the median effective dose (ED_{50}) of a drug. Agents with a high therapeutic index can be safely administered in large intermittent doses, since concern about overshooting the target concentration is less significant. If, however, the therapeutic index of an agent is small, continuous infusions minimize the overshoot that occurs with periodic boluses (Fig. 46.2).

Brain and Central Nervous System as Drug Therapy Targets

Drug penetration into the CNS is limited by the blood-brain barrier (BBB) and blood-cerebrospinal-fluid barrier (BCSFB). These barriers are important structures in maintaining brain homeostasis, allowing selective uptake of nutrients, and limiting passage of potentially noxious substances. Disruption of these barriers occurs to a certain extent under pathologic conditions; additionally, the BBB lacks uniformity. Even taking into consideration these elements of enhanced permeability, the overall ability of available medications to reach targets in the CNS is limited [6]. Additionally the need to deliver local drug therapy presents a unique challenge. In order to adequately address the drug therapy needs of patients admitted to the neurosurgical intensive care unit (NICU), utilization of systemic medications and dosing strategies that gain access to the CNS must

sometimes be combined with direct, local administration. Medication considerations for these approaches will be discussed here.

The Effect of Drug Properties on CNS Penetration

The BBB limits systemic medications from freely entering the brain parenchyma. The BBB is predominantly formed by brain capillary endothelial cells (BCEC) joined by tight junctions [6]. Passage across this cell layer is limited, and activity of molecules that are able to cross the BBB is complicated by rapid metabolism and active efflux pumps. One mechanism by which some medications gain access to the CNS is via passive diffusion. The extent to which drug molecules can enter the brain through passive diffusion is dependent upon the medication's physiochemical properties. Ionization, lipophilicity, and molecular weight are the principal determinants of a medication's ability to passively cross the BBB. Highly lipophilic molecules with low molecular weights – for example, less than 500 Da – lack ionization and are able to more readily cross the BBB. It is thought that passage of these molecules is accomplished through small, transiently available pores. Alteration of any of these properties significantly diminishes drug permeability [7].

A number of medications rely partially on passive diffusion to reach their targets in the CNS. BCEC, however, contain a number of active transport systems classified as absorptive-, carrier-, and receptor-mediated transport systems which are the subject of extensive research, with a few being currently utilized in clinical practice. Absorptive-mediated transcytosis occurs as a result of an electrostatic interaction between cationic molecules and the negatively charged BCEC plasma membrane surface. Once initiated, endosome formation and transport occurs. This process is downregulated in the BBB but is the method by which a number of medications including albumin, heparin, and aspirin gain access to the brain parenchyma [6, 7]. Carrier-mediated transport is the principal mechanism by which essential amino acids, vitamins, and some neuropeptides enter the brain. These molecules utilize transporters present on each luminal surface which are carrier specific [8]. Drug molecules with structural similarities to endogenous substances which utilize these transporters to cross the BBB include levodopa, gabapentin, and melphalan [7]. Receptor-mediated endocytosis is the method for a number of large molecules, notably insulin and transferrin, which enter the brain parenchyma [6].

Only a small proportion of commercially available medications are able to take advantage of these entry mechanisms to penetrate the BBB. For all large molecules and over 98 % of small molecules, the BBB remains a significant obstacle [9], and for some, local administration has proved a useful intervention.

Alternative Routes of Administration: Intrathecal and Intracerebroventricular Drug Administration

Medications can be administered directly into the lumbar cistern or the lateral ventricle *via* temporary or implantable devices, or by direct injection in the case of the lumbar cistern. These methods of drug delivery have been utilized for administration of antibiotics, chemotherapy, medications for chronic pain and spasticity, and fibrinolytics [10]. While an effective means of local drug delivery, the ability of locally administered medications to distribute throughout the brain parenchyma is often limited and incompletely understood [9]. Many hydrophilic medications, which lack the physiochemical characteristics which would allow them to freely diffuse into the brain, become trapped within the CNS at high concentrations immediately following administration. For these medications, because the rate of cerebrospinal fluid (CSF) elimination exceeds the rate of medication dissolution, drug elimination is mostly dependent on CSF flow [9, 10]. Patients requiring CSF diversion or those with other pathologies which interfere with the normal outflow of CSF may be at risk for experiencing subtherapeutic drug concentrations across a dosing interval. Theoretical concerns have also been raised that intraventricular administration as a sole method of drug delivery may create a concentration gradient favoring drug flow out of the CNS. This concern has led some to suggest the combination of local and systemic therapy as a more effective means of ensuring therapeutic CNS drug concentrations are maintained [11]. The extent to which this concentration gradient exists and its clinical consequences are unclear.

Pharmaceutical preparation of medications intended for intracerebroventricular or intrathecal use is crucial to ensuring safe and effective drug therapy. Drug volume, sterility, and diluent properties must be considered in conjunction with a medication's pH, osmolarity, and preservatives. Osmolarity and pH may significantly impact drug tolerability as well. CSF does not have the buffering capacity of the blood and is thus more susceptible to alteration in pH resulting from drug administration. Alterations in CSF pH, especially acidification of CSF, may result in adverse CNS effects. Administration of hyper- or hypotonic solutions may cause or worsen neurotoxic effects [10]. Although not all preservatives carry the same risk of neurotoxicity [12, 13], the presence of preservatives and their risk for adverse effects should be investigated prior to drug administration. Ideally, both parent medication and any drug diluents should be preservative-free, as a number of commonly utilized medication preservatives, including benzyl alcohol and chlorobutanol, have demonstrated varying degrees of neurotoxicity in both animal models and human case reports [10, 12].

Direct administration of medications into the CNS remains a complex, incompletely understood intervention. Critical care pharmacists are in a unique position to assist with drug product selection and assessment of the appropriateness of intracerebroventricular or intrathecal drug administration based on a medication's physiochemical properties. Further research is necessary to better understand how best to deliver medication therapy to drug targets in the CNS.

Commonly Used Agents in the Neurointensive Care Unit

Sedatives

The ability to adequately assess neurologic function is paramount in neuro-critical care patients. Thus, deep sedation is reserved for specific indications such as spine instability or severe traumatic brain injury. In the majority of neurologically injured patients, an artificial airway and mechanical ventilation are necessary. The ideal sedative provides sufficient anxiolysis and sedation while still facilitating patient cooperation with care. Whenever possible in these cases, sedation should be titrated to tolerance of the endotracheal tube or tracheostomy tube to maintain the ability to rapidly perform a reliable neurologic examination.

Barbiturates

Barbiturates, namely, pentobarbital (Table 46.1), are not used for routine sedation in the NeuroICU, but rather deep sedation in patients with treatment-refractory status epilepticus or elevated intracranial pressure. In the 1970s, John Michenfelder demonstrated that barbiturates convey cerebral protection in primates during focal ischemia [14, 15]. Barbiturates decrease cerebral metabolic rate for oxygen (CMRO2) up to 50 %, in a dose-dependent fashion, coincident with an isoelectric electroencephalogram (EEG). Additional dosing beyond EEG suppression produces no further reduction in $CMRO_2$, suggesting that the reduction in $CMRO_2$ is secondary to the reduction in neuronal activity. Vasoconstriction occurs primarily in normal areas of the brain, as injured areas remain dilated, resulting in a reverse-steal redistribution of blood flow. Coupled with reduced cerebral blood flow (CBF) and cerebral vasoconstriction, decreased intracranial pressure occurs [16].

Although barbiturates may be neuroprotective in focal ischemia, this has not been demonstrated in global ischemia [17]. Many drug properties have been proposed to explain this phenomenon including decreased cerebral metabolic requirements, improvement of CBF redistribution,

Table 46.1 Sedative characteristics and dosing in the neuroscience intensive care unit

Sedative agent	Onset (min)	Half-life (h)	Dosing (IV bolus)	Dosing (infusion)	Active metabolites
Pentobarbital	1	15–50	5–20 mg/kg	0.5–3 mg/kg/h	N
Diazepam	1–5	20–50	0.03–0.1 mg/kg	–	Y
Lorazepam	5–20	10–16	0.02–0.06 mg/kg	0.01–0.1 mg/kg/h	N
Midazolam	2–5	1–3	0.02–0.08 mg/kg	0.04–0.2 mg/kg/h	Y
Propofol	0.5–1	4–7	–	5–80 mcg/kg/min	N
Dexmedetomidine	20–30	2	1 mcg/kg	0.2–0.7 mcg/kg/h	N
Ketamine	0.5	2–3	0.5–1 mg/kg	15–80 mcg/kg/min	Y

suppression of catecholamine-induced hyperreactivity, loss of thermoregulation, decreased intracerebral edema, decreased intracerebral pressure, decreased CSF secretion, scavenging of free radicals, membrane stabilization, calcium channel antagonism, and alteration of fatty acid metabolism [16].

Barbiturates cause a dose-dependent decrease in blood pressure, attributable to decreased vascular tone, decreased preload, and direct myocardial depression. Barbiturates decrease the mean arterial pressure (MAP) and cardiac output (CO), primarily due to depression of the medullary vasomotor center with a reflex increase in heart rate. The effect on central venous pressure is variable, but most agree that peripheral venous dilation causes reduced filling pressures, which in turn reduces CO and MAP. For this reason, a pulmonary artery catheter – or other invasive monitor – may be beneficial to monitor cardiac output and intravascular volume in patients receiving prolonged barbiturate infusions. Hypotension [18], tachycardia, and lactic acidosis may be severe in hypovolemic patients. Anion gap metabolic acidosis often occurs and is secondary to a low cardiac output state and cerebral ischemia and may be predicted by tachycardia following barbiturate loading [19]. Barbiturates are contraindicated in patients with latent or manifest porphyria (e.g., acute intermittent porphyria, variegate porphyria, and hereditary coproporphyria).

Benzodiazepines

Benzodiazepines potentiate the inhibitory effects of gamma-aminobutyric acid (GABA) by directly binding to one of the GABA receptor subunits, $GABA_A$. Benzodiazepines do not directly activate the GABA receptor but rather *enhance the receptor-binding affinity* of GABA itself. The end result is modulation of GABA-activated influx of chloride ions into the target neuron, resulting in hyperpolarization. The nerve cell is thus made more refractory to any excitatory impulse. In the spinal cord, benzodiazepines also cause increased availability of glycine, which acts as an inhibitory neurotransmitter.

Benzodiazepines are excellent sedatives and also possess anticonvulsant, amnestic, hypnotic, and muscle-relaxant properties. The choice of which benzodiazepine to use is based primarily on pharmacokinetic parameters (Table 46.1).

The elimination half-life of benzodiazepines increases with age and is decreased by agents that induce cytochrome P450. Benzodiazepines alone have very little effect on the respiratory response to carbon dioxide or hypoxia, but the agents do have marked synergistic interactions with opioids. All benzodiazepines are metabolized primarily in the liver and excreted by the kidney. Since the metabolism of lorazepam is not entirely dependent on the hepatic microsomal enzymes, its elimination is less likely, as compared to diazepam, to be prolonged by alterations in hepatic function, age, or drugs such as cimetidine.

Benzodiazepines decrease the $CMRO_2$, CBF, and intracranial pressure (ICP) in the absence of hypoventilation. A decrease in MAP may occur as a result of a decrease in systemic vascular resistance (SVR) with a modest increase in heart rate. Modest respiratory depression will occur with all of the benzodiazepines; patients with chronic obstructive pulmonary disease (COPD) may be more sensitive to the respiratory depressant effects. More dramatic changes are seen with midazolam, possibly due to its high potency and rapid onset. To minimize adverse events, benzodiazepine doses should be reduced in elderly or hypovolemic patients as well as those with concomitant use of other sedatives or narcotics.

Propofol

Benzodiazepines were the mainstay of sedation in the surgical ICU until the introduction of propofol, which gained popularity given its rapid onset and recovery times (Table 46.1). Guidelines recommend propofol as the preferred sedative in mechanically ventilated patients where rapid, frequent neurologic evaluations are desired [20].

Like benzodiazepines, propofol enhances synaptic inhibition mediated by GABA through $GABA_A$ receptors. Propofol decreases the $CMRO_2$, CBF, and ICP but may significantly decrease cerebral perfusion pressure (CPP) due to its effect on MAP. Propofol directly depresses myocardial contractility and decreases SVR, resulting in hypotension. The mean arterial pressure may be decreased by as much as a third regardless of history of cardiovascular disease, as a result of the decrement in CO and SVR [21].

As with other sedative agents, the dose of propofol should be reduced in the elderly, in hypovolemia, or with concomitant use of narcotics or other respiratory depressants. Administration of propofol at high doses and/or for an extended duration has been associated with a clinical presentation aptly called "propofol-related infusion syndrome" (PRIS). The syndrome has most commonly been reported in both critically ill children and adults with acute neurologic illness. PRIS manifests as metabolic acidosis, hypotension, and dyslipidemia and may progress to rhabdomyolysis with acute renal failure and cardiovascular collapse. The exact pathophysiology of PRIS is unknown but is theorized to be associated with mitochondrial toxicity [22, 23]. When PRIS is suspected, propofol should be promptly discontinued and supportive care measures implemented as necessary.

Dexmedetomidine

Alpha-2 receptors are found throughout the peripheral and central nervous systems, predominately on presynaptic sympathetic neurons. Although the exact mechanism through which alpha-2 agonists cause hypotension is not known, it is thought that stimulation of the receptors in the brain and spinal cord decreases sympathetic outflow, resulting in hypotension, bradycardia, sedation, and analgesia [24]. Of the available alpha-2 agonists, dexmedetomidine (Table 46.1) is a much more effective sedative and analgesic agent for reasons including a higher selectivity to alpha$_2$-adrenoceptors ($\alpha_2:\alpha_1 = 1,600:1$) compared to clonidine ($\alpha_2:\alpha_1 = 200:1$,) and a shorter half-life (2 h *versus* clonidine's 6–10 h) [25]. At lower doses, both clonidine and dexmedetomidine produce arousable, effective sedation, and decrease requirements for analgesics with minimal respiratory depression. At doses exceeding 2 mcg/kg, dexmedetomidine can cause deep sedation with respiratory depression. Patients who received dexmedetomidine in the ICU were arousable and alert when stimulated from sedation and quickly returned to their sleep-like state when left alone [26]. Compared to the longer-acting benzodiazepine lorazepam in the sedation of mechanically ventilated patients, dexmedetomidine use resulted in more delirium or coma-free days [27].

Although dexmedetomidine does not appear to have any direct effects on the heart, a biphasic cardiovascular response may occur following intravenous administration [28, 29]. A 2 mcg/kg intravenous administration of dexmedetomidine produces a transient mild hypertension (about a 20 % increase in mean arterial blood pressure) followed by a 30 % decrease in mean arterial blood pressure resulting in values 10 % below baseline [30]. Stimulation of alpha$_2$-adrenoceptor in vascular smooth muscle seems to be responsible for the initial rise in the blood pressure. Even at lower infusion rates, however, the increase in mean arterial pressure over the first 10 min was shown to be in the range of 7 %, with a decrease in heart rate between 16 and 18 % [29]. This initial response is followed by a slight decrease in blood pressure due to the inhibition of the central sympathetic outflow and decreased

norepinephrine release, which is more pronounced in hypovolemic patients [31].

Dexmedetomidine undergoes almost complete hydroxylation through direct glucuronidation and cytochrome P450 metabolism in liver. Metabolites are predominately excreted in the urine; the intrinsic activity of metabolites is unknown. The elimination half-life is approximately 2 h. It may be necessary to decrease the dose in patients with hepatic failure, since they will have lower rates of metabolism of the active drug. In cases of renal failure, accumulation of metabolites may have effects that are presently unknown.

Dexmedetomidine dosing is generally initiated with a loading infusion of 1 mcg/kg over 10 min, followed by a maintenance infusion of between 0.2 and 0.7 mcg/kg/h. Product labeling limits dexmedetomidine infusion to 24 h; however, literature exists that demonstrates dexmedetomidine may be used safely beyond 24 h [27, 32].

Dexmedetomidine should be used cautiously in patients with preexisting severe bradycardia and cardiac conduction system problems, in patients with reduced ventricular function (ejection fraction <30 %), and in patients who are hypovolemic or hypotensive. The drug's effects on CBF and carbon dioxide response are not completely understood.

Ketamine

Ketamine (Table 46.1) is a dissociative anesthetic used to induce anesthesia, sedation, analgesia, and amnesia. Ketamine produces an anesthetic state described as "a dissociation of the limbic from the thalamoneocortical systems" and is characterized by profound analgesia, normal pharyngeal-laryngeal reflexes, normal or slightly enhanced skeletal muscle tone, cardiovascular and respiratory stimulation, and occasionally transient, minimal respiratory depression [33]. In the dissociative state produced by ketamine, it is believed that the brain fails to correctly transduce afferent impulses because of disruption in normal communication between the sensory cortex and the association areas. The result resembles catalepsy in which the eyes may remain open with slow nystagmus and intact corneal reflexes. Patients are generally noncommunicative though they may appear to be awake. Assessing a clear sedation endpoint is often difficult with ketamine administration and poses a unique problem in determining the level of sedation.

Ketamine likely interacts with multiple pharmacologic receptors to produce its effects. Ketamine is a potent, noncompetitive, N-methyl-D-aspartate (NMDA) receptor antagonist; NMDA inhibition produces catalepsy. Ketamine has been shown to interact with sigma receptors, which may mediate the dysphoria that can be induced by ketamine. Analgesia appears to be at least partially mediated by opioid receptors at the brain, spinal cord, and peripheral sites. Ketamine binds preferentially to mu, rather than the delta opioid receptor.

Table 46.2 Opioid characteristics and dosing in the neuroscience intensive care unit

Opioid	Equianalgesic dose	Onset (min)	Half-life (h)	Dosing (IV bolus)	Dosing (infusion)	Active metabolites
Fentanyl	200 mcg	1–2	2–4	25–100 mcg	50–700 mcg/h	N
Hydromorphone	1.5 mg	15	2–3	0.5–2 mg	0.25–1 mg/h	N
Morphine	10 mg	5–10	3–7	1–10 mg	5–35 mg/h	Y

Ketamine is a poor choice for sedation in patients with neurologic injury due to its propensity for delirium as well as a significant increase in CBF (and thus ICP) [34, 35]. This has traditionally precluded use in patients with head injury, hydrocephalus, or intracranial mass. Recent evidence, however, suggests that the elevation in ICP is minimal in the setting of normal ventilation [36–38] and that the corresponding cerebral vasodilation may actually improve cerebral perfusion [37, 39]. As a result, guidelines for ketamine sedation in the emergency department no longer include head injury as a contraindication, but continue to warn against use where structural or other abnormality interferes with normal cerebrospinal fluid movement [40].

Ketamine differs from most anesthetic agents in that it appears to stimulate the cardiovascular system, producing increases in MAP, pulmonary artery pressure, central venous pressure, heart rate, and CO. The central sympathetic stimulation, neuronal release of catecholamines, and inhibition of neuronal uptake of catecholamines usually override the direct myocardial depressant effects of ketamine. These sympathomimetic effects of ketamine administration tend to increase myocardial oxygen demand, and, thus, ketamine should be used cautiously in patients with ischemic heart disease or congestive heart failure. Alpha-receptor antagonists, beta-antagonists, and calcium channel antagonists may unmask the direct myocardial depressant effect of ketamine.

Ketamine is unique in its ability to maintain functional residual capacity (FRC) on induction of anesthesia. In the spontaneously breathing patient, minute ventilation may be maintained at the same level as in the conscious state. Because skeletal muscular tone is maintained during ketamine anesthesia, atelectasis or changes in ventilation-perfusion and FRC do not occur. Ketamine has other beneficial respiratory effects including increased lung compliance, decreased airway resistance, and maintenance of laryngeal tone and reflexes with lower doses. Ketamine is a potent stimulator of salivary and tracheobronchial secretions, and diligent suction of the oral cavity is required in the nonintubated patient to decrease the possibility of coughing and aspiration and to prevent laryngospasm, especially in children. The antisialagogue effects of glycopyrrolate and atropine are effective in reducing these secretions.

Emergence hallucinatory reactions are more common in adults, particularly those between 15 and 65 years of age, who have received rapid administration of high doses of ketamine. The incidence of these reactions can be reduced by premedication with benzodiazepines.

Analgesics

Opioids

Opioids (Table 46.2) are stereospecific agonists acting at receptors in both the central and peripheral nervous system. The different receptors activated by the opioid agents account for the spectrum of responses seen clinically. Mu (μ)-receptor activation by opioids within the brain is not only responsible for the analgesia but also for the ventilatory depression, euphoria, and physical dependence seen with this class of drugs. Kappa (κ)-receptor occupation in the spinal cord results in analgesia as well as ventilatory depression, sedation, and miosis when supraspinal κ receptors are activated. The activation of sigma (σ) receptors results in dysphoria, hallucinations, and vasomotor and ventilatory stimulation. The delta (δ) receptor modulates the effect of the μ receptor, which may account for some of the tolerance seen when narcotics are administered over a prolonged period. Opioids decrease neurotransmission primarily by presynaptic inhibition of neurotransmitter release of acetylcholine, dopamine, norepinephrine, and substance P, as well as by postsynaptic inhibition of neuronal activity [41].

Opioid BBB penetration is affected by lipid solubility and molecular weight. Fentanyl is 800 times more lipid soluble than morphine. For highly lipid-soluble opioids, including fentanyl, the onset of action reflects their circulation time to the central nervous system (CNS) given rapid penetration of cell membranes. Drugs that are much less lipid soluble, like morphine, have a slower onset.

Opioids in blood are bound to proteins such as albumin and α_1-acid glycoprotein. Chronic changes in plasma proteins, such as those seen in debilitated, malnourished, or congestive heart failure patients, can result in higher concentrations of free opioid for a given dose, and the dose required for a given intensity of effect will be less. Protein binding varies considerably between the different narcotic agents.

At lower doses, redistribution plays a significant role in the short duration of effect for several opioids. As higher doses are given, particularly for longer periods of time, the peripheral tissues accumulate the opioid, with a lower concentration gradient between blood and the peripheral tissues. Hence, a lesser amount of drug moves into the tissues, and the decline in plasma (blood) concentrations due to redistribution is of progressively less importance. At that point, most of the decline depends on the elimination processes.

Most opioids are metabolized in the liver. Morphine is conjugated with glucuronic acid, resulting in active (morphine-6-glucuronide) and relatively inactive (morphine-3-glucuronide) metabolites. Fentanyl is also metabolized in the liver (N-dealkylation, hydroxylation, and conjugation), and pharmacokinetics are altered by changes in hepatic blood flow. Fentanyl metabolites are excreted by the kidneys, but since they are pharmacologically inactive, changes in renal function do not prolong the duration of action. Hydromorphone also undergoes hepatic glucuronidation to inactive metabolites.

All opioids produce dose-dependent depression of brainstem ventilatory centers, primarily via the mu receptor [42]. Pontine and medullary centers that regulate the rhythm of ventilation are also affected, possibly via acetylcholine. As with all narcotic agents, doses should be reduced in the elderly or hypovolemic patient, as well as when used concomitantly with sedatives.

In the absence of hypoventilation, opioids decrease CBF and possibly ICP [43]. In humans as well as in animal models, and in the absence of other anesthetics, $CMRO_2$ is either unchanged or decreased in the presence of fentanyl or morphine [44]. Opioids should be used with caution in patients with acute head injury because the alteration in mental status, interference with the pupil neurologic examination (miosis), and ventilatory depression (increasing $PaCO_2$ and thereby increase ICP via vasodilation) that may be noted in head injury can be worsened pharmacologically by opioids. Lack of BBB integrity following head trauma and intracranial surgery may increase sensitivity to opioids [41]. Fentanyl is associated with increases in ICP of 6–9 mmHg despite a constant $PaCO_2$ [45, 46]. These increases in ICP are accompanied by a decrease in MAP and CPP and may be linked, since prevention of hypotension curbs the increase in ICP [47]. When used clinically, there is no evidence that opioids induce major changes in cerebral hemodynamics. Since opioids do not alter cerebrovascular CO_2 reactivity, their use in combination with hypocapnia accounts for a favorable effect on brain volume and ICP [44].

With high doses of μ-receptor agonists, an increase in skeletal muscle activity may be pronounced. This has a variety of manifestations, including glottic closure, truncal rigidity, flexion and, occasionally, flapping of the extremities in a seizure-like movement with no electroencephalographic manifestations of seizures. This rigidity typically occurs at doses that induce apnea and may interfere with positive pressure ventilation due to glottic closure and/or decreased thoracic compliance.

Opioids may cause bradycardia, mediated by the vagal nerve and hypotension likely related to inhibition of certain reflexes modulating sympathetic nervous system activity, thereby reducing sympathetic outflow to vascular smooth muscle in veins and arterioles. Outside the CNS, μ-type opioid receptors mediate the constriction of smooth muscle (e.g., the sphincter of Oddi causing biliary colic, the gastrointestinal tract causing constipation, and the ureter causing renal colic). Opioid-induced biliary tract spasm may be reversed with naloxone (IV/IM 0.2–0.4 mg) or glucagon (IV/IM 0.25–2 mg). Urinary retention, which does not respond to naloxone, may require bladder catheterization. Narcotics may also produce vomiting by activation of the chemoreceptor trigger zone.

Morphine induces the release of histamine from mast cells which may result in hypotension, cutaneous erythema, and pruritus. Direct binding of morphine (and other opioids) to opioid receptors in the medulla oblongata alters sensory modulation and may be the mechanism for pruritus after epidural/intrathecal administration. Antihistamines (e.g., diphenhydramine 12.5–25 mg IV/IM every 6 h as needed) are usually effective in alleviating the symptoms.

Nonsteroidal Anti-inflammatory Drugs

Nonsteroidal anti-inflammatory drugs (NSAIDs) act by inhibiting the enzyme, cyclooxygenase, responsible for prostaglandin synthesis. This inhibition is responsible for decreasing the swelling and pain associated with prostaglandin production. Best results are obtained when these agents are administered before the surgical/painful insult.

NSAIDs do not possess respiratory depressant activity. However, this drug class does inhibit prostaglandin-mediated renal blood flow, particularly in patients with intrinsic renal disease or congestive heart failure, and thus must be used with caution. They also inhibit prostaglandin-mediated platelet aggregation, but, unlike aspirin, the effect is reversible when the drug concentration diminishes. Gastrointestinal adverse events with NSAIDs are common. Due to their acidic nature, NSAIDs are direct irritants to the gastric mucosa. In addition, inhibition of prostaglandin synthesis in the gastrointestinal tract results in increased gastric acid secretion and diminished bicarbonate and mucous production contributing to the risk of ulceration.

Ketorolac, ibuprofen, and diclofenac are all NSAIDs with analgesic, anti-inflammatory, and antipyretic activity. The analgesic potency of 30 mg of intravenous ketorolac is equivalent to 12 mg of morphine with less drowsiness, less nausea and vomiting, and no significant respiratory depression [48]. An initial dose of ketorolac 30–60 mg intravenously may be followed by 15–30 mg every 6 h as needed, not to exceed 5 days of use given the risk for serious gastrointestinal adverse events. Ibuprofen may be alternated with acetaminophen to maintain normothermia in patients with

Table 46.3 Relevant corticosteroid characteristics

Corticosteroid	Equivalent dose	Mineralocorticoid potency	Anti-inflammatory potency	Elimination half-life (h)	Biological half-life (h)
Dexamethasone	0.75	0	25–30	2–4	36–54
Hydrocortisone	20	2	1	1–2	8–12
Methylprednisolone	4	0	5	1–3	18–36

traumatic brain injury. Ibuprofen is typically dosed around 400 mg orally or enterally every 6 h not to exceed 3,200 mg/day. Intravenous diclofenac is available in Europe and has been studied in a small, randomized controlled trial in fever in patients with traumatic brain injury or subarachnoid hemorrhage. Following a 0.2 mg/kg bolus, a continuous infusion of diclofenac ranging between 0.004 and 0.08 mg/kg/h (average 0.03 ± 0.02 mg/kg/h) maintained an afebrile state for a greater percentage of time as compared to treatment with bolus dosed antipyretics [49]. No gastrointestinal or intracranial bleeding was documented during the study.

Corticosteroids

Several synthetic corticosteroids (Table 46.3) are available for use and vary in their relative mineralocorticoid and glucocorticoid potencies. In the NeuroICU, corticosteroids are utilized as anti-inflammatory agents, antiemetics, and as replacement therapy for adrenal and pituitary insufficiency.

Glucocorticoids prevent or suppress inflammation and elements of the immune response when administered at pharmacologic doses. At the molecular level, unbound glucocorticoids readily cross cell membranes and bind with high affinity to cytoplasmic receptors. These receptors interact with transcription factors to modify transcription and, ultimately, protein synthesis. Actions include inhibition of leukocyte infiltration at the site of inflammation, interference with the function of mediators of inflammatory response, and suppression of humoral immune responses.

Dexamethasone is widely used in neurologically injured patients to reduce swelling of the brain when vasogenic edema surrounding brain tumors is present. Response depends on severity and duration of symptoms; however, a decrease in intracranial pressure has been reported as early as 12 h after administration followed by symptom resolution within 24 h [50]. The typical dosing scheme for dexamethasone in cerebral edema is 4 mg given intravenously every 6 h [50, 51]. The management of nausea and vomiting in patients with intracranial pathology may be paramount in patients to avoid additional increases in ICP. There is evidence that dexamethasone (4–10 mg IV) is a useful adjunct in combination with 5-HT3 and dopamine antagonists [52].

Methylprednisolone has been studied in the management of acute spinal cord injury and subsequent neurologic outcomes with widely criticized findings [53–56]. Treatment within 8 h of injury with high-dose methylprednisolone,

30 mg/kg bolus followed by 5.4 mg/kg/h for 23 h, continues to be used by some. However, consensus guidelines for the management of acute spinal cord injury do not recommend the use of methylprednisolone regardless of timing from injury or duration of infusion [57, 58]. Due to increased mortality, methylprednisolone use in patients with traumatic brain injury is similarly not recommended [59].

Hydrocortisone has been shown to hasten septic shock reversal [60, 61]. Guidelines for the management of adrenal insufficiency and sepsis recommend the administration of hydrocortisone at a dose of 50 mg intravenously every 6 h or a continuous infusion of 10 mg/h in patients with septic shock refractory to fluids and vasopressors [62, 63]. Hydrocortisone should be discontinued once vasopressors are no longer necessary to maintain hemodynamics.

The administration of corticosteroids to a critically ill patient is not benign and should be done with caution. Corticosteroids may impair wound healing and contribute to hyperglycemia.

Neuromuscular Antagonists

Depolarizing Neuromuscular Antagonists

Succinylcholine is a short-acting depolarizing neuromuscular blocking agent typically used for endotracheal intubation or short surgical procedures rather than sustained paralysis in the ICU. Intermittent intravenous doses to maintain paralysis range between 0.25 and 1.5 mg/kg; the ED_{95} of this drug is, however, 0.25 mg/kg. Succinylcholine is relatively contraindicated in patients with intracranial lesions. Mild increases in ICP have been demonstrated, persisting as long as 30 min [64]; this can be attenuated by pretreatment with a nondepolarizing neuromuscular blocking agent (NMBA) [65]. The rise in ICP that occurs is not usually clinically significant or dangerous and should be balanced with rapid control of the airway and ventilation. Alternatively, non-histamine-releasing nondepolarizing NMBAs may be used. The rise in ICP associated with the rise in $PaCO_2$ from ineffective mask ventilation may be more detrimental than the small rise in ICP associated with succinylcholine.

Hyperkalemia has been demonstrated following the administration of succinylcholine to patients with muscular dystrophy, following denervation leading to atrophy and upper motor neuron lesions [66]. Excessive potassium release has been detected after a time period ranging from 96 h to up to 6 months of denervation [67]. By way of

Table 46.4 Comparative characteristics of selected nondepolarizing neuromuscular antagonists

Paralytic	Bolus dose (mg/kg)	Duration (min)	Infusion (mcg/kg/min)	Active metabolite	Histamine release	Renal failure effect	Hepatic failure effect
Atracurium	0.4–0.5	25–35	4–12	N[a]	Minimal	–	–
Cisatracurium	0.1–0.2	45–60	2.5–3	N	None	–	–
Pancuronium	0.06–0.1	90–100	1–2	Y	None	++	+
Rocuronium	0.6–1	30	10–12	N	None	–	++
Vecuronium	0.08–0.1	35–45	0.8–1.2	Y	None	++	+

Adapted from American College of Critical Care Medicine of the Society of Critical Care Medicine, American Society of Health-System Pharmacists, American College of Chest Physicians [161]

[a]Laudanosine metabolite can accumulate with prolonged use and may be associated with central nervous system excitation and seizures

contrast, in burn patients, hyperkalemia may be seen 6–7 days after injury. The mechanism of hyperkalemia is thought to occur by increased sensitivity and upregulation of extrajunctional nicotinic cholinergic receptors. This exaggerated response may persist 6–8 months following injury. Pretreatment with nondepolarizing neuromuscular antagonists does not attenuate the magnitude of hyperkalemia.

The metabolism of succinylcholine is accomplished by rapid hydrolysis by plasma cholinesterase to succinylmonocholine. Severe liver dysfunction or the genetic presence of atypical plasma cholinesterase may cause prolongation of neuromuscular blockade.

Nondepolarizing Neuromuscular Antagonists

Numerous nondepolarizing NMBAs (Table 46.4) block acetylcholine from binding to receptors on the motor end plate, thus inhibiting depolarization. In patients without hepatic or renal failure, most of these compounds can be used in intermittent doses or continuous infusion so as to allow for immediate reversal of paralysis for neurologic assessment. Those with long half-lives, such as pancuronium, are usually avoided. Any patient who is pharmacologically paralyzed should be sedated adequately with benzodiazepines or propofol as a precaution to avoid awareness. Prolonged infusion of nondepolarizing NMBAs has been associated with myopathies.

Nondepolarizing NMBAs may be reversed, if necessary, by administering an anticholinesterase agent such as neostigmine or physostigmine. The administration of a muscarinic cholinergic antagonist such as atropine or glycopyrrolate must be given prior to the anticholinesterase agent to avoid profound bradycardia.

Inotropes and Vasoactive Agents

Inotropes

β-Adrenergic receptor agonists are the most potent and widely used inotropes. They work by binding to and stimulating β-adrenergic receptors that are coupled to the formation of the intracellular messenger, adenosine 3′: 5′monophosphate (cyclic AMP). A number of different β-adrenergic agonists are available including the natural catecholamines epinephrine, norepinephrine, and dopamine and the synthetic catecholamines, dobutamine and isoproterenol, as well as the phosphodiesterase inhibitor milrinone. These drugs have varying actions at β_1-, β_2-, and α-receptors and are initially selected based on their relative actions at each receptor type.

Severe ventricular failure usually requires the maximal potency of epinephrine or norepinephrine, frequently in combination with vasodilator therapy. Epinephrine and norepinephrine are also useful when ventricular dysfunction is accompanied by peripheral vasodilation, since they are also potent α-receptor agonists. The vasopressor effect of norepinephrine is greater than that of epinephrine because of the greater potency of epinephrine at β_2-receptors, which produce considerable vasodilation in skeletal muscle. Dobutamine and dopamine are useful when moderate inotropic support is desired. Dobutamine is a β_1-receptor agonist with a minimal α-receptor activity and is therefore useful when further vasoconstriction is undesirable. The use of dopamine as an inotrope at higher doses (>10 mcg/kg/min) is complicated by its activity at α-adrenergic receptors, which may produce undesirable increases in systemic vascular resistance, and by its tendency to increase ventricular filling pressures and to induce tachycardia and atrial arrhythmias. The partial dependence of the inotropic effects of dopamine on endogenous catecholamines may also limit its efficacy in patients with chronic ventricular dysfunction. The use of dopamine or epinephrine as an inotrope in severe left ventricular dysfunction is limited by dose-dependent increases in afterload and preload. These undesirable side effects are the basis for the frequent clinical use of combined inotropic stimulation and afterload reduction with direct-acting vasodilators such as nitroprusside or nitroglycerin or an "inodilators" like milrinone.

Isoproterenol is a nonselective β-receptor agonist that is a potent inotrope (β_1-effect) and peripheral vasodilator (β_2-effect). The potent chronotropic effect of isoproterenol (β_1 and β_2) is not compensated for by the baroreceptor-mediated reflex bradycardia that occurs with β-receptor agonists that also possess intrinsic α-receptor activity such as epinephrine and norepinephrine. Isoproterenol or dobutamine may be useful in patients with severe pulmonary hypertension and right ventricular failure because α-receptor stimulation – minimal to nonexistent in these agents – is a potent mechanism in producing pulmonary vasoconstriction. Isoproterenol is also useful for the treatment of slow ventricular rates or atrioventricular conduction disturbances when other methods have failed because of the positive chronotropic and dromotropic effects of β-adrenergic stimulation.

Milrinone is a selective inhibitor of fraction III of cyclic nucleotide phosphodiesterase (PDE III). The inotropic activity of milrinone appears to be synergistic with that of β-adrenergic agents and may not be associated with increased myocardial oxygen consumption, making this agent particularly useful in patients with severe left ventricular dysfunction. Advantage can be taken of the inotropic activity of milrinone without its vasodilatory activity by combining it with an α-adrenergic vasoconstrictor, usually norepinephrine. Another important application of milrinone in combination with adrenergic agonists is its use in patients with antecedent congestive heart failure. The desensitization of β-adrenergic receptors that occurs in congestive heart failure significantly limits the efficacy of β-adrenergic agonists. Combined therapy with phosphodiesterase inhibitors enhances the inotropic effect of β-adrenergic receptor agonists by potentiating the rise in intracellular cyclic AMP and may permit use of a lower dose of β-adrenergic agonist. Inhibitors of phosphodiesterase also have a positive lusitropic, or myocardial relaxation, effect. This positive lusitropic effect enhances diastolic myocardial relaxation, improves ventricular compliance, facilitates ventricular filling, and decreases ventricular filling pressure and perhaps end-diastolic wall tension at any given filling volume. Thus, myocardial oxygen consumption may be decreased while stroke volume is increased.

Vasopressors

Vasopressors work by increasing afterload and preload by increasing SVR and decreasing venous capacitance, respectively, due to their action at α-adrenergic receptors. While norepinephrine is a mixed agonist, phenylephrine is a pure α_1-agonist useful in the treatment of hypotension secondary to vasodilation. In general, the use of pure α-agonists to increase arterial blood pressure in patients with poor ventricular function or pulmonary hypertension is best avoided because increased afterload without a compensatory increase in contractility results in a decreased stroke volume. If significant arterial vasodilation is combined with poor left ventricular function, norepinephrine, which possesses less β_2-adrenergic activity than epinephrine, may be appropriate. Pure α-receptor agonists are useful in the treatment of

hypotension in patients with good ventricular function; the beneficial increase in coronary and cerebral perfusion pressure usually outweighs the negative effects of decreased CO and increased filling pressures in the patient with coronary artery disease or ventricular hypertrophy.

Vasopressin is an endogenous hormone, also known as antidiuretic hormone, synthesized in the hypothalamus and released from the posterior pituitary to regulate volume status. Increases in plasma osmolality or decreases in blood volume or arterial blood pressure are the triggers for release. The vasopressin 1 (V1) and vasopressin 2 (V2) receptors are the primary sites where vasopressin acts. Binding at the V1 receptor in the vascular smooth muscle causes peripheral vasoconstriction via intracellular calcium release and extracellular calcium influx. The V2 receptors in the renal collecting duct facilitate the retention of water by altering the permeability. Vasopressin has been shown to reduce catecholamine requirements when added to existing therapy but may also be used as initial therapy for septic shock [68–70].

Acute Antihypertensive Agents

Blood pressure regulation is a complex, controversial intervention of importance in the management of critically ill NeuroICU patients [71, 72]. The goal of acute blood pressure control in these patients is most often to prevent secondary injury, such as the prevention of rebleeding in patients with aneurysmal subarachnoid hemorrhage (aSAH) or hematoma expansion in patients with intracerebral hemorrhage. As our understanding of the changes in autoregulation of CBF that occur after injury grows, however, so does our understanding of the relationship between blood pressure and neurologic outcome. At this time, the relationship between these remains controversial. As with other critically ill patient populations, the choice of blood pressure-lowering agent should be patient specific and take into account factors such as comorbid conditions and be modified based on patient response. The ideal agent would have a fast onset and offset and be easily titratable with few adverse effects. A unique adverse effect to consider in patients with neurologic injury is the impact of antihypertensives on ICP. The remainder of this section will discuss the commonly used antihypertensives in the NeuroICU, specifically nicardipine, nitroprusside, labetalol, and hydralazine (Table 46.5), as well as considerations of their impact on ICP.

The Effect of Antihypertensives on ICP

Sodium nitroprusside (SNP), hydralazine, nitroglycerin, and adenosine all cause dilation of the cerebral vasculature, which increases cerebral blood volume and thus increase ICP. Whether these agents result in vasodilation to the same extent in injured and uninjured brain is unclear. The impact of this vasodilation on regional CBF is likewise unclear.

Table 46.5 Characteristics of commonly used agents for blood pressure control in the neuroscience intensive care unit

Antihypertensive	Onset (min)	Duration	Half-life	Dosing (IV bolus)	Dosing (infusion)	Increases ICP	Dose adjust for hepatic dysfunction	Dose adjust for renal dysfunction
Nicardipine	10	0.5–2 h	2 h	–	0.5–15 mg/h	No	Yes	No
Sodium nitroprusside	<2	1–10 min	2 min	–	0.25–3 mcg/kg/min	Yes	No	Yes
Labetalol	2–5	2–4 h	4–8 h	20–80 mg every 10 min up to 300 mg	1–2 mg/min	No	Yes	No
Hydralazine	5–20	2–12 h	2–8 h	10–20 mg every 4–6 h	–	Yes	No	Yes

Thus, the clinical relevance of observed changes in ICP is not fully understood.

Nitroprusside-induced changes in ICP have been well described in animal models. Increases in ICP produced by SNP are maximal during modest decreases (<30 %) in mean arterial pressure. However, with reductions in mean arterial pressure greater than 30 %, ICP is reduced [73, 74]. Slow infusions, hypocarbia, and hyperoxia appear to attenuate SNP-associated changes in ICP. Nitroprusside administered to normocarbic subjects can produce significant increases in intracranial pressure and cause neurologic dysfunction with only slight decreases in blood pressure [75]. Large differences in regional CBF occur experimentally during SNP-induced hypotension which may be the result of impaired autoregulation [76, 77].

Hydralazine's hemodynamic effects on the cerebral vasculature are complex. Its effect on ICP is profound, resulting in an increase in one report of 110 [78]. This change in ICP occurs before detectable changes in systemic blood pressure. Cerebral blood flow, however, does not appear to be impacted to the same extent. This may be the result of vasoconstriction induced by hydralazine-stimulated hyperventilation or a delayed activity on cerebral resistance vessels [78].

Nicardipine

Nicardipine is a dihydropyridine calcium channel antagonist which inhibits calcium influx through voltage-dependent L-type calcium channels [79]. Nicardipine shows selective preference for vascular smooth muscle over cardiac muscle and thus reduces blood pressure via a decrease in SVR with little to no negative inotropic effect. It likewise has no influence on cardiac conduction and minimal effect on left ventricular end-diastolic pressure [80]. Nicardipine has gained popularity in many NeuroICUs due to its quick onset, ease of titration, lack of impact on ICP, and supportive, although scant, body of literature. Because nicardipine is eliminated hepatically via the CYP P450 enzymes 2C8, 2D6, and 3A4, it is susceptible to a number of drug interactions, and dosage adjustments may be necessary in patients with hepatic dysfunction. It is safe to be used in patients with varying degrees of renal dysfunction. It has few unique adverse effects [79].

Sodium Nitroprusside (SNP)

Sodium nitroprusside is a potent vasodilator, with rapid onset and a short duration of action. It is used primarily to manage hypertensive emergencies. SNP undergoes enzymatic degradation in the blood stream to nitric oxide and cyanide. Nitric oxide stimulates the downstream production of cyclic guanosine monophosphate, resulting in peripheral vasodilation in both arterial and venous smooth muscle, although arterial vasodilation predominates. The hypotensive effects of SNP are enhanced by other hypotensive agents. Sympathomimetics that exert a direct stimulatory effect (e.g., epinephrine) are the only class of drugs that effectively increase blood pressure during nitroprusside therapy.

Sodium nitroprusside has a unique side effect: cyanide toxicity. A single molecule of SNP releases five cyanide ions. Cyanide is enzymatically converted to thiocyanate by renal and hepatic rhodanese or reacts with methemoglobin to form cyanomethemoglobin. The enzymatic conversion of cyanide to thiocyanate may be delayed by hypothermia [81]. Both cyanide and thiocyanate are toxic compounds interfering with aerobic metabolism by binding cytochrome c. Both are renally eliminated and may accumulate in patients with renal impairment. Thiocyanate toxicity occurs at plasma levels of between 50 and 100 mcg/mL. Following prolonged infusions, cyanide and thiocyanate may accumulate, causing nausea, tinnitus, and mental status changes. Recognition of subtoxic concentrations can be identified by drug resistance, progressive metabolic acidosis, and increased mixed venous O_2 saturation. Treatment of cyanide toxicity includes cessation of SNP administration, hemodialysis, and/or administration of thiosulfate (150 mg/kg IV). In severe situations, sodium nitrite (5 mg/kg IV) may be considered as well as an infusion of hydroxocobalamin (25 mg/h) [82].

Labetalol

Labetalol is a mixed β_1-, β_2-, and α_1-adrenergic antagonist. When given intravenously it has a sevenfold more potent effect on beta-receptors than on α_1-receptors. Blood pressure reduction primarily results from decreases in SVR and vasodilation. Like nicardipine and SNP, labetalol may be administered as a continuous IV infusion for blood pressure control. Compared to other agents available for IV infusion,

Table 46.6 Drug dosing and monitoring recommendations for selected AEDs

AED	Loading dose	Maintenance dose	Target drug levels	Drug level timing	IV available	Hepatic metabolism	Renal elimination
Phenytoin/fosphenytoin	15–20 mg/kg	5–6 mg/kg/day divided every 8–12 h	Total: 10–20 mcg/mL Free: 1–2 mcg/mL	IV: ≥2 h after a dose PO: ≥4–6 h after a dose	Yes[a]	Yes	No
Levetiracetam	20–30 mg/kg[b]	1,000–3,000 mg/day divided every 8–12 h	Not established	Not established	Yes	No	Yes
Valproic acid/divalproex	30–60 mg/kg	15 mg/kg/day (divided if dose is greater than 250 mg)	Total: 50–100 mcg/mL Unbound: 5–25 mcg/mL	Trough	Yes	Yes	No
Phenobarbital	15–20 mg/kg (given as 5–10 mg/kg every 2–3 h)	2 mg/kg/day	15–40 mcg/mL	Trough	Yes[c]	Yes	Yes
Pentobarbital	5–15 mg/kg	1–10 mg/kg/h continuous infusion	20–50 mcg/mL to achieve EEG suppression	–	Yes	Yes	No
Lacosamide	[b]	200–400 mg/day	Not established	–	Yes	Yes	Yes

[a]Fosphenytoin preferred over IV phenytoin due to risk of arrhythmias and hypotension with propylene glycol carrier in phenytoin
[b]Not routinely recommended
[c]Administered in propylene glycol carrier

labetalol has a much prolonged half-life. Labetalol may also be given in intermittent IV boluses. It is extensively metabolized in the liver and may require dosage adjustments in patients with severe hepatic impairment [83]. Labetalol does not appear to have any effect on ICP [84].

Hydralazine

Hydralazine is a phthalazine derivative that decreases systemic blood pressure by a direct action on arteriolar smooth muscle. Although the precise mechanism of action is not known, it is endothelium dependent, suggesting a role for nitric oxide. Hydralazine also interferes with calcium mobilization. The use of hydralazine is associated with a baroreceptor-mediated increase in sympathetic activity, resulting in increased chronotropic and inotropic activity, an increase in plasma renin activity, and fluid retention. Unlike previously discussed agents, hydralazine is not available to be administered via continuous IV infusion and instead is predominantly administered as intermittent IV boluses for as-needed blood pressure control.

Antiepileptics

Antiepileptic drugs (AEDs) are used in neurointensive care for both the prevention and treatment of seizures and seizure disorders, most notably status epilepticus. The choice of AED will depend largely on the type of seizure being treated and the side effect profiles of available agents. The most efficacious first-line agent for the treatment or prophylaxis of many seizure types remains controversial. Additionally, the

role of combination therapy remains a subject of debate. A discussion of the role of available agents in the management of the major seizure types is beyond the scope of this chapter.

Commonly encountered AEDs in the NeuroICU include phenytoin/fosphenytoin, levetiracetam, valproic acid, the barbiturates phenobarbital and pentobarbital, and occasionally lacosamide (Table 46.6). Many of these agents have complex pharmacokinetics that require drug therapy monitoring. It is important to note that target drug levels for many AEDs have been derived from studies investigating chronic use of these agents. Thus, alternative drug levels may be more appropriate in critically ill patients, specifically those with status epilepticus. Drug levels of AEDs must always be interpreted in the context of a patient's clinical response. This section will focus on the earlier-mentioned AEDs, their side effect profiles, and pharmacokinetic considerations for use.

Phenytoin and Fosphenytoin

Phenytoin (PHT), with its water-soluble prodrug formulation fosphenytoin, remains a frequently used medication. PHT exerts its anticonvulsant effect by limiting the spread of seizure activity. At therapeutic concentrations, PHT selectively prolongs the inactive phase of voltage-activated sodium channels. This reduces repetitive neuronal firing without causing general CNS depression [85].

PHT exhibits complex pharmacokinetics. The most clinically relevant pharmacokinetic principles are its half-life, protein binding, saturable metabolism, and interplay with various CYP enzymes. PHT's long but variable half-life ranges from 7 to 42 h [86]. Loading doses are required to achieve therapeutic concentrations prior to completing 5–7 days of therapy. It is highly protein bound, and dosage adjustments may need to be made in patients with low serum albumin or other alterations in protein binding. Certainly for these patients free, rather than total, serum PHT levels should be followed. PHT undergoes hepatic metabolism. This metabolism is saturable at therapeutic concentrations, giving the drug nonlinear kinetics. The result is that very small changes in drug dose may result in disproportionately large changes in available serum drug concentrations. PHT undergoes metabolism via the CYP enzyme system predominantly via 2C9 and 2C19, making it susceptible to a number of clinically significant drug interactions including those observed with amiodarone [87] and fluconazole [88].

PHT's most important features remain its many side effects. PHT is known to cause cardiac dysrhythmias and cardiac collapse, although many are attributed to IV PHT's propylene glycol carrier; these side effects have been observed with oral formulations and fosphenytoin to a much lesser extent. PHT's adverse effects on the CNS – such as nystagmus, lethargy, and ataxia – are thought to be dose-related phenomena with worsening severity as concentrations rise. Numerous hypersensitivity reactions have been noted with PHT use including Stevens-Johnson syndrome and toxic epidermal necrolysis [89]. PHT may also cause drug fever, an especially important adverse effect in patients with neurologic injury.

Levetiracetam

The precise mechanism by which levetiracetam (LEV) controls seizures has not been fully elucidated. LEV appears to affect a number of different sites including synaptic vesicle protein 2A (SV2A) which may play a role in neuronal cell vesicle exocytosis [90]. Animal models have demonstrated an association between SV2A and epilepsy; however, the extent to which a casual relationship exists is unclear [91]. LEV also appears to decrease levels of interneuronal calcium via a variety of mechanisms, stabilizes the GABAA receptor, inhibits neuronal hypersynchronicity [90], and inhibits delayed rectifier potassium currents [92].

LEV has gained popularity largely because of its relatively benign safety profile. Its most common side effects include headache, fatigue, and drowsiness, with few additional adverse effects noted with escalating doses. While it may cause leukopenia, neutropenia, and thrombocytopenia, such reactions are rare [93]. The paucity of adverse effects has led to the utilization of much higher than the recommended maximum 3,000 mg/day being utilized in clinical practice. In fact, up to 9,000 mg/day have been reported in the treatment of status epilepticus [94]. LEV is eliminated renally and undergoes hydrolysis; it is thus subject to few drug interactions. As more is understood regarding LEV's mechanism of action, its role in therapy is likely to continue to expand.

Valproic Acid/Divalproex

Similar to PHT, valproic acid (VPA) prolongs inactivation of voltage-activated sodium channels at therapeutic concentrations. VPA also slows depolarization by reducing T-type calcium currents and has been associated with increased GABA levels in animal models [95]. This duel mechanism may account for its efficacy in managing multiple types of seizure disorders.

VPA exhibits linear pharmacokinetics within the therapeutic dose range, is highly protein bound and, like PHT, has complex interplay with the CYP enzyme system. Drug level monitoring may be useful in patients receiving VPA, particularly those with low serum albumin or those taking medications which interact with VPA. Because of VPA's complex drug distribution, all drug levels should be drawn as troughs; total and unbound VPA levels are available. VPA is hepatically metabolized but the CYP enzyme system, specifically 2C9 and 2C19, is a minor contributor. VPA does, however, inhibit CYP2C9 and UGT which may have an impact on coadministration of other AEDs including PHT and phenobarbital [85].

VPA has few side effects. Of greatest relevance in intensive care is its ability to cause thrombocytopenia and inhibit platelet aggregation; this appears to be a dose-dependent phenomenon. Elevations in hepatic enzymes are also frequently observed with VPA therapy. Hepatic failure resulting in death has occurred, although it is uncommon and this risk is greatest within the first 6 months of therapy [95].

Barbiturates: Phenobarbital and Pentobarbital

Barbiturates work at the GABAA receptor to prolong the duration of chloride channel opening. This class contains some of the first antiseizure medications available and remains one of the most reliable drug classes. The key features of the barbiturates are their toxicities and side effect profile.

Both phenobarbital and pentobarbital have very long half-lives: 5 and 4 days, respectively, on average. Pentobarbital, in spite of its long half-life, has been observed to often have a short offset of activity which has been attributed to drug reuptake in the tissues. This effect may be lost with prolonged administration. The influence of barbiturates on hemodynamics is described earlier in the chapter.

Lacosamide

Similar to PHT, lacosamide prolongs inactivation of voltage-gated sodium channels [85]. Similar to LEV, lacosamide has generated interest based on its efficacy, limited side effect profile, comparatively simple pharmacokinetics, and the availability of an intravenous formulation. It has been used off label for the treatment of status epilepticus with some success. Few unique adverse effects have been noted with lacosamide. Lacosamide is eliminated by a combination of renal and hepatic impairment that involves CYP2C19.

Treatment and Prophylaxis Against Thrombosis

The treatment and prevention of thromboses in patients with neurologic injury can be a dangerous task, as many patients are at risk for serious complications if bleeding occurs. An understanding of how fibrinolytics, anticoagulants, and antiplatelet agents affect coagulation and bleeding is an important tool in minimizing these risks.

Alteplase

Alteplase, or recombinant tissue plasminogen activator (rtPA), is best known for its role in the treatment of acute ischemic stroke and remains the only Food and Drug Administration (FDA)-approved agent for this indication [96]. While a number of other fibrinolytics have been investigated for use in ischemic stroke, because of the comparative lack of evidence, their use is not recommended outside of clinical trials [97]. The use of alteplase in this capacity will be the focus of this section. In the NeuroICU, it has also been administered intrathecally as a part of the management of intraventricular hemorrhage [98], intravenously and intraarterially for massive and submassive pulmonary embolism [99], and is frequently used for treatment and prophylaxis against occluded catheters [100].

Like endogenous tissue plasminogen activator, rtPA enhances the conversion plasminogen to plasmin which degrades fibrin clots into soluble products. The activity of rtPA is significantly enhanced in the presence of fibrin such that limited systemic proteolysis has been noted. Thus, the majority of plasminogen to plasmin conversion occurs at the site of the thrombus. rtPA has a half-life of less than 5 min and undergoes hepatic metabolism and renal excretion. The principal side effect of alteplase is bleeding, most notably intracerebral hemorrhage. Post-marketing experience has also revealed orolingual angioedema causing partial airway obstruction to be an important adverse effect. While uncommon, angioedema has occurred up to 2 h after alteplase infusions have been completed and mostly in patients concomitantly receiving angiotensin-converting enzyme inhibitors [96]. In addition to bleeding, orolingual angioedema is an important side effect that should be considered when initiating intravenous rtPA [97].

rtPA gained approval for use in ischemic stroke in 1996 largely in response to the results of the NINDS trial which demonstrated improved neurologic outcomes at 3 months compared to placebo [101]. Intravenous rtPA is recommended for selected patients who present within 3 h of onset of ischemic stroke [97] but may still be beneficial in patients who present up to 4.5 h after onset [102, 103]. For ischemic stroke, intravenous rtPA should be administered as a 0.09 mg bolus followed by a 0.81 mg/kg, 1-hour infusion, up to a maximum total dose of 90 mg [96].

Heparin

Heparin, or unfractionated heparin (UFH), is a parenteral anticoagulant frequently used in critical care. Heparin consists of a heterogenous combination of mucopolysaccharides of varying molecular sizes and anticoagulant activity [104]. It exerts its antithrombotic effects by enhancing the ability of antithrombin III (ATIII) to inactivate the active forms of circulating factors IIa (thrombin), IXa, Xa, XIa, and XIIa [104, 105]. Of these factors, it is factors IIa and Xa which are the most affected by heparin administration. Not all heparin molecules are of sufficient length to bind to ATIII and catalyze its activity [106]. The varying molecular sizes and anticoagulant activity of heparin molecules lead to the development of the low-molecular-weight heparins and fondaparinux, which differ principally in their activity against factors IIa and Xa.

Heparin may be administered intravenously or subcutaneously. Heparin is metabolized via the reticuloendothelial system and thus does not require dosage adjustments for either hepatic or renal dysfunction. It is rapidly eliminated from the blood stream with a half-life of 60–90 min when administered as a continuous infusion, although clearance is dose dependent. In addition to its short half-life, one unique advantage of UFH when used in the intensive care unit is its reversibility. Protamine sulfate 1 mg will bind 100 units of heparin to form a stable salt that may be eliminated. The half-life of circulating protamine is 7 min. Subcutaneous doses of heparin may require a protamine continuous infusion due to the prolonged release of heparin from its subcutaneous site. Heparin may be monitored using activated partial thromboplastin time (aPTT) or anti-Xa levels [104].

While the most common side effect of heparin administration is bleeding, its most *important* side effect is heparin-induced thrombocytopenia (HIT). HIT occurs in 1–3 % of patients exposed to heparin for more than 5 days. In HIT, heparin induces an antibody-mediated response which causes platelet activation and thrombosis. Its diagnosis is complex and requires a combination of clinical and laboratory findings [107]. Once a diagnosis has been made – or if strongly suspected – all forms of heparin, including heparin line flushes and heparin-coated catheters [108], must be discontinued. Anticoagulation with a non-heparin anticoagulant should then be initiated, even in the absence of thrombosis [109].

Table 46.7 Available dosage forms of desmopressin (DDAVP) for the treatment of central diabetes insipidus

Dosage form	Starting dose (mg)	Dosing interval	Usual dose range	Approximate dose equivalents (mg)	Onset (min)	Peak (h)	Half-life (h)
Intravenous	0.001	BID	0.002–0.004 mg divided BID	0.001	30	1.5–2	3
Intranasal	0.01	Daily	0.01–0.04 mg divided daily-TID	0.01	15–60	1–5	1.26
Oral	0.05	BID	0.1–1.2 mg/day divided BID-TID	0.2	60	4–7	1.5–2.5

Low-Molecular-Weight Heparins and Fondaparinux

The low-molecular-weight heparins (LMWHs), enoxaparin, dalteparin, and tinzaparin, have a lower molecular weight and contain fewer saccharide chains long enough to adequately bind ATIII and factor IIa compared to UFH. They also have a greater affinity for factor Xa compared to UFH. Fondaparinux is a synthetic compound which specifically binds ATIII and factor Xa. Fondaparinux is derived from a pentasaccharide found in UFH and LMWH. Both LMWHs and fondaparinux demonstrate more predictable anticoagulant effects than UFH. As a result, routine monitoring of aPTT or anti-Xa levels is not recommended [104] but may be warranted in certain clinical scenarios such as pregnancy, renal impairment, or critical illness.

While the LMWHs do display some pharmacodynamic differences, clinically they exhibit similar efficacy and safety profiles and are, for the most part, considered therapeutically interchangeable [110]. All LMWHs are renally eliminated and require dose adjustments for renal impairment. Fondaparinux is also renally eliminated and use is contraindicated in patients with a creatinine clearance less than 30 mL/min. Unlike UFH, the LMWHs and fondaparinux are not easily reversible. No commercially available reversal agents exist, although protamine has been investigated with limited success. LMWHs and fondaparinux are administered subcutaneously in fixed or weight-based dosing regimens [104].

Aspirin and Aspirin/Dipyridamole

Aspirin in the NeuroICU is used primarily for its antithrombotic effects. Aspirin is an inhibitor of cyclooxygenase (COX)-1 and COX-2. Aspirin inhibits platelet aggregation through downstream inhibition of thromboxane A2 (TXA2) and prostacyclin (PGI2). Due to the limited amount of mRNA present in platelets, this inhibition is irreversible and its effects persist for 36 h after drug discontinuation [111]. Aspirin at a dose less than 325 mg/day is recommended as secondary prophylaxis for ischemic stroke from multiple etiologies [112].

Aspirin has also been combined with dipyridamole at a fixed dose under the brand name Aggrenox® (Boehringer Ingelheim Pharmaceuticals, Inc., Ridgefield, CT) for the secondary prevention of ischemic stroke. The mechanism by which dipyridamole inhibits platelet aggregation has not been fully elucidated but may be related to its ability to increase cyclic adenosine monophosphate [113]. Combination aspirin/dipyridamole as Aggrenox® has been shown to be equivalent to aspirin alone as secondary prophylaxis against ischemic stroke. While the combination product does not appear to carry an increased risk of bleeding, a higher incidence of headache and gastrointestinal side effects have been reported compared to aspirin alone [112].

Miscellaneous Agents

Desmopressin

Desmopressin, 1-deamino-8-D-arginine vasopressin, or DDAVP® (Sanofi-Aventis, Paris, France) is a synthetic analogue of vasopressin. Unlike vasopressin, which is a nonselective vasopressin receptor agonist, desmopressin has selective activity at V_2 receptors [114]. Stimulation of V2 receptors causes insertion of water channels in the collecting duct of the kidney, resulting in increased free water absorption and increased circulating levels of factor VIII and von Willebrand factors [115]. The antidiuretic effects of 1 mcg of desmopressin are equivalent to 4 units of vasopressin [116]. In the NeuroICU, desmopressin is used mostly in the treatment of central diabetes insipidus although also occasionally used for its hemostatic effects particularly in hemophiliacs or those with variceal bleeding. Desmopressin has a short half-life usually requiring multiple doses per day. Desmopressin is available in intravenous, subcutaneous, intranasal, and oral dosage forms (Table 46.7). Regarding desmopressin dosing, it is important to note that there is a large degree of interpatient response variability which can make dosage form changes challenging. Desmopressin is renally eliminated and use is contraindicated in patients with a creatinine clearance less than 50 mL/min, although use has been described [116, 117].

Vasopressin Receptor Antagonists: Conivaptan and Tolvaptan

Vasopressin receptor antagonists conivaptan and tolvaptan have been used for the treatment of hyponatremia. Tolvaptan selectively blocks the V_2 receptor and demonstrates 1.8-fold greater affinity for V_2 compared to vasopressin. Conivaptan selectively antagonizes V_{1A} and V_2 receptors. Conivaptan's therapeutic effects are attributed to its activity at the V_2 receptor. Blocking the V_2 receptor prevents passive reabsorption of free water in the collecting duct of the kidney. This results in profound aquaresis, excretion of free water without loss of electrolytes [118]. The degree of aquaresis achieved by V_2 receptor antagonists has resulted in rapid overcorrection of sodium, and caution is warranted when initiating or making modifications to a patient's drug regimen [119]. Because it is available in an intravenous dosage form, conivaptan is more commonly used in the NeuroICU. Conivaptan was approved as a bolus dose followed by a continuous infusion administered for a maximum of 4 days [119]. Clinical experience utilizing conivaptan in intermittent bolus doses has been published [120]. Conivaptan has demonstrated a high degree of inter-patient pharmacokinetic variability. In healthy subjects, the average half-life was 5 h [119]. Tolvaptan is available orally and is more commonly used as long-term maintenance therapy. Like conivaptan, tolvaptan displays wide inter-patient pharmacokinetic variability. Its half-life is approximately 12 h which allows for once-daily administration [121]. Neither drug requires dosage adjustment for renal or hepatic impairment.

Intravenous Immunoglobulin

Intravenous immunoglobulin (IVIG) has been used off-label in the neurosciences for the treatment of a variety of autoimmune neuromuscular disorders, most notably Guillain-Barré syndrome [122]. The mechanism by which IVIG exerts its beneficial effects has not been fully elucidated but is likely multifactorial. Proposed mechanisms of efficacy include suppression of inflammatory cytokine production, neutralization of autoantibodies, inhibition of idiotypic antibody production, and blockade of macrophage Fc receptors [123]. Use of IVIG for many of its off-label indications remains controversial.

IVIG contains purified immunoglobulins from pooled human donors. While IgG is the principal immunoglobulin contained, trace amounts of IgA and IgM are present in most formulations. For this reason, IVIG use should generally be avoided in patients with selective IgA deficiency due to an increased risk of anaphylaxis in these patients who often produce anti-IgA antibodies. A number of different IVIG products are available: BayGam® (Bayer Pharmaceuticals, Wayne, NJ), Carimune® NF (CSL Behring, King of Prussia, PA), Flebogamma® (Grifols Inc., Clayton, NC), Gammagard S/D® (Baxter Healthcare, Deerfield, IL), Gammar-P IV® (Sanofi-Aventis, Paris, France), Gammaked® (Kedrion BioPharma, Fort Lee, NJ), Gammaplex® (Bio Products Laboratory Ltd., Hertfordshire, UK), Gamunex® (Grifols, Inc., Clayton, NC), Iveegam EN®

(Baxter Healthcare, Deerfield, IL), Octagam® (Octapharma, Lachen, Switzerland), Polygam S/D® (Baxter Healthcare, Deerfield, IL), and Vivaglobin® (CSL Behring, King of Prussia, PA) [124, 125]. Differences in the manufacturing process of IVIG have resulted in product variability with unclear clinical significance outside adverse events. Differences in available IVIG products do appear to impact the side effect profile of IVIG [124]. Infusion reactions such as flushing, hyper-/hypotension, and chills are the most common side effects of IVIG and occur to differing degrees with each of the available products. Premedication and slowing the IVIG infusion rate effectively address most of these reactions. The recommended infusion rate for IVIG is product specific. Manufacturing variability also appears to impact the incidence of the development of renal failure after IVIG infusion. IVIG products which utilize sucrose as a stabilizer, such as Carimune® and Gammar-P IV®, have been associated with a higher incidence of renal failure [124]. Aseptic meningitis has also been reported after administration of IVIG but appears to be manufacturer independent. Aseptic meningitis after administration appears to be self-limiting and resolves within 3–5 days of drug discontinuation [125].

Nimodipine

Nimodipine, a calcium channel antagonist, is the only FDA-approved medication for preventing delayed cerebral ischemia and improving neurologic outcomes after aneurysmal subarachnoid hemorrhage (aSAH). Being highly lipophilic, nimodipine readily crosses the BBB and is a potent cerebral vasodilator. In an early study, good-grade aneurysm patients treated with nimodipine had less severe neurologic deficits from vasospasm alone at the end of 21 days of treatment as compared to placebo [126]. Following subarachnoid hemorrhage from an aneurysm, poor-grade evaluations (Hunt and Hess classification ≥3), nimodipine demonstrated improved neurologic outcomes, as defined by Glasgow Outcome Score, at 3 months and has subsequently been considered standard of care in the management of aSAH [127]. Nimodipine is typically administered as 60 mg orally or enterally every 4 h for 21 days. A shorter course of nimodipine given over 15 days in good-grade aneurysms did not lead to any untoward outcomes [128].

Hypotension may occur with nimodipine and is often dose related. Dosing strategies including smaller doses at more frequent intervals, like nimodipine 30 mg every 2 h or 15 mg every hour, may ameliorate the hypotension. In the United States, nimodipine is commercially available as a gelatin capsule, and the contents of the capsule must be aspirated for enteral administration. Serious adverse events, including death, have been reported following inadvertent administration of the oral solution by an intravenous route [129]. When possible, enteral liquid nimodipine doses should be prepared by pharmacy and dispensed in ready-to-use enteral syringes. Outside the capsule in an amber enteral syringe and light-resistant bag, nimodipine is stable for 31 days [130].

Magnesium

Like nimodipine, magnesium has found application in aSAH and the associated cerebral vasospasm primarily for its vasodilatory actions. The mechanism of benefit is proposed to be the antagonism of intracellular calcium influx by magnesium. Cerebral vasospasm incidence has been reduced with the prophylactic administration of magnesium with some outcome benefits also reported [131–137]. Several studies describe a 20–25 mMol intravenous magnesium bolus followed by 24–144 mMol/day continuous intravenous infusion for 7–18 days [131–136, 138–140]. A single study used weight-based dosing, 0.4 mMol/kg intravenous bolus then 1.2 mMol/kg continuous intravenous infusion [137]. Infusion rate may be adapted to target a specific magnesium level, range of 1–2.5 mMol/L (2.4–6 mg/dL) in studies, or remain constant [131–140]. When administered without any titration, 64 mMol/day continuous intravenous infusion is most frequently described in the published literature [131, 133, 139, 140]. For reference, 2 g of magnesium sulfate equates to 8 mMol of magnesium cation.

In numerous patient populations, the administration of high doses of magnesium has been associated with serious adverse events including areflexia, respiratory paralysis, and cardiac arrest and typically correlates with serum magnesium levels above 5 mMol/L (11.3 mg/dL) [141]. Muscle weakness progressing to loss of deep tendon reflexes may be an early clinical sign of magnesium toxicity and should be monitored routinely along with magnesium serum concentrations.

Statins

Hydroxymethylglutaryl-coenzyme A reductase (HMG-CoA) inhibitors, otherwise known as statins, are conventionally used to manage hyperlipidemia; however, the anti-inflammatory and immunomodulating properties of statins have been investigated in numerous conditions, including aSAH, where endothelial dysfunction may cause an imbalance between vasoconstriction and vasodilation resulting in cerebral vasospasm. The proposed mechanism of benefit in cerebral vasospasm is direct upregulation of endothelial nitric oxide synthase [142]. Pravastatin 40 mg orally daily for up to 14 days reduced vasospasm, severe vasospasm, rescue therapy, in-hospital mortality, disability at discharge, and disability at 6 months [143, 144]. Similarly, simvastatin 80 mg orally daily for 14–21 days reduced the incidences of cerebral vasospasm and delayed ischemic neurologic deficits [145, 146], although other studies with simvastatin demonstrated no benefit [147, 148]. Transient elevations in transaminases and creatinine phosphokinase

(CPK) have been reported [145, 146]. At a minimum, liver function tests and CPK should be evaluated prior to beginning treatment with a statin.

Role of the Critical Care Pharmacist

The pharmacist is an essential member of the interdisciplinary critical care team. Guidelines for critical care services and personnel recommend pharmacist evaluation of drugs with regard to dosing and administration, adverse events, drug-drug interactions, and cost-effectiveness in addition to further specialized activities such as nutritional support assessment, emergency event participation, and collaborative clinical research [149].

The position paper on critical care pharmacy services by the Society of Critical Care Medicine and American College of Clinical Pharmacy further outlines fundamental pharmacist activities to include prospective medication review, pharmacokinetic monitoring, policy and procedure development, and quality assurance participation [150].

Critical care clinical pharmacist involvement has demonstrated cost savings across a multitude of intensive care unit populations, including the neurosurgical intensive care unit [151–154]. The influence of the critical care pharmacist is not limited to economics but further extends to patient outcomes. Specifically, critical care pharmacist participation in interdisciplinary patient care has contributed to reduced mortality, hospital length of stay, ventilator-associated pneumonia rates, bleeding complications, and other adverse drug events as well as improved fluid balance in the setting of parenteral nutrition administration [155–159].

While activities may vary with institutional models and critical care populations, the critical care pharmacist clearly impacts healthcare costs and clinical outcomes. Critical care pharmacists contribute to not only the collaborative practice model but also critical care clinical research and the education of other members of the healthcare team at all levels of training and education. The critical care pharmacist is vital to the successful dynamics of interdisciplinary care in the intensive care unit, and pharmacy participation in clinical activities should be routine.

Conclusion

With the elevated severity of injury of patients, including multisystem disorders that may predate the neurologic injury, the pharmacologic agents used for therapy are complex. Recognition that the pharmacokinetic and pharmacodynamic properties of drugs, when the blood-brain barrier is violated, are somewhat unpredictable is necessary. There is an obvious need for a broad knowledge base, understanding of drug-drug interactions, as well as the special considerations necessary in ensuring adequate medication delivery to the central nervous system, when applicable. It is for these reasons that we recommend a critical care pharmacist as an integral member of the ICU team.

Acknowledgment The authors acknowledge the original work and contributions of Dr. Richard J. Rogers and Dr. Hugh C. Hemmings in the first edition of this chapter, which inspired this new second edition chapter.

References

1. Wilkinson GR. Pharmacokinetics. In: Hardman JG, Limbird LL, editors. Goodman & Gilman's the pharmacological basis of therapeutics. 10th ed. New York: McGraw-Hill; 2001. p. 3–30.
2. Bailey JM. Context-sensitive half-times: what are they and how valuable are they in anaesthesiology? Clin Pharmacokinet. 2002;41:793–9.
3. Hughes MA, Glass PS, Jacobs J. Context-sensitive half-time in multicompartment pharmacokinetic models for intravenous anesthetic drugs. Anesthesiology. 1992;76:334–41.
4. White PF. Clinical uses of intravenous anesthetic and analgesic infusions. Anesth Analg. 1989;68:161–71.
5. Rafferty S, Sherry E. Total intravenous anaesthesia with propofol and alfentanil protects against postoperative nausea and vomiting. Can J Anaesth. 1992;39:37–40.
6. De Boer AG, Gaillard PJ. Strategies to improve drug deliver across the blood-brain barrier. Clin Pharmacokinet. 2007;46(7):553–76.
7. Patel MM, Goyal BG, Bhadada SV, et al. Getting into the brain: approaches to enhance brain drug delivery. CNS Drugs. 2009;23(1):35–58.
8. De Boer AG, Gaillard PJ. Drug targeting to the brain. Annu Rev Pharmacol Toxicol. 2007;47:323–55.
9. Pardridge WM. Blood-brain barrier delivery. Drug Discov Today. 2007;12:54–61.
10. Cook AM, Mieure KD, Owen RD, et al. Intracerebroventricular administration of drugs. Pharmacotherapy. 2009;29:832–45.
11. Hirsch BE, Amodio M, Einzig AI, et al. Installation of vancomycin into a cerebrospinal fluid reservoir to clear infection: pharmacokinetic considerations. J Infect Dis. 1991;163:197–200.
12. Jackson GD, Themelis NJ, Messerl SO, et al. Doxapram and potential benzyl alcohol toxicity: a moratorium on clinical investigation? Pediatrics. 1986;78:540–1.
13. Hodgson PS, Neal JM, Pollock JE, et al. The neurotoxicity of drugs given intrathecally (spinal). Anesth Analg. 1999;88(4):797–809.
14. Michenfelder JD, Theye R. Cerebral protection by thiopental during hypoxia. Anesthesiology. 1973;39:510–7.
15. Michenfelder JD, Milde JH, Sundt TM. Cerebral protection by barbiturate anesthesia. Use of middle cerebral artery occlusion in Java monkeys. Arch Neurol. 1976;33:345–50.
16. Baughman VL. Brain protection during neurosurgery. Anaesthesiol Clin North Am. 2002;20:315–27.
17. Brain Resuscitation Clinical Trial 1 Study Group. Randomized clinical study of thiopental loading in comatose survivors of cardiac arrest. N Engl J Med. 1986;314:397–403.
18. Sonntag H, Helberg K, Schenk H, et al. Effects of thiopental (Trapanal®) on coronary blood flow and myocardial metabolism in man. Acta Anaesthesiol Scand. 1975;19:69–78.
19. Robicsek SA, Black S. Acidosis following barbiturate administration for focal ischemia during EC-IC bypass. J Neurosurg Anesthesiol. 2000;12:A-34.
20. Jacobi J, Fraser GL, Coursin DB, et al. Clinical practice guidelines for the sustained use of sedative and analgesics in the critically ill adult. Crit Care Med. 2002;30:119–41.
21. Hug CC, McLeskey CH, Nahrwald ML, et al. Hemodynamic effects of propofol: data from over 25,000 patients. Anesth Analg. 1993;77(Suppl):521.
22. Diedrich DA, Brown DR. Analytic reviews: propofol infusion syndrome in the ICU. J Intensive Care Med. 2011;26:59–72.
23. Fodale V, La Monaca E. Propofol infusion syndrome: an overview of a perplexing disease. Drug Saf. 2008;31:293–303.
24. Hoffman BB, Lefkowitz RJ. Catecholamines, sympathomimetic drugs, and adrenergic receptor antagonists. In: Hardman JG, Limbird LL, editors. Goodman and Gilman's the pharmacological basis of therapeutics. 9th ed. New York: McGraw-Hill; 1996. p. 217–8.
25. Kamibayashi T, Maze M. Clinical uses of alpha2-adrenergic agonists. Anesthesiology. 2000;93:345–9.
26. Venn RM, Bradshaw CJ, Spencer R, Brealey D, Caudwell E, Naughton C, Vedio A, Singer M, Feneck R, Treacher D, Willatts SM, Grounds RM. Preliminary UK experience of dexmedetomidine, a novel agent for postoperative sedation in the intensive care unit. Anaesthesia. 1999;54:1136–42.
27. Riker RR, Shehabi Y, Bokesch PM, et al. Effect of sedation with dexmedetomidine vs lorazepam on acute brain dysfunction in mechanically ventilated patients. JAMA. 2007;298:2644–53.
28. Bloor BC, Ward DS, Belleville JP, Maze M. Effects of intravenous dexmedetomidine in humans. II. Hemodynamic changes. Anesthesiology. 1992;77:1134–42.
29. Hall JE, Uhrich TD, Barney JA, Arain SR, Ebert TJ. Sedative, amnestic, and analgesic properties of small-dose dexmedetomidine infusions. Anesth Analg. 2000;90:699–705.
30. Veselis RA. Anesthetic adjuvants and other CNS drugs. In: Hemmings HC, Hopkins PM, editors. Foundations of anesthesia. London: Mosby; 2000. p. 261–74.
31. Aantaa R, Kanto J, Scheinin M, Kallio A, Scheinin H. Dexmedetomidine, an alpha 2-adrenoceptor agonist, reduces anesthetic requirements for patients undergoing minor gynecologic surgery. Anesthesiology. 1990;73:230–5.
32. Riker RR, Shehabi Y, Bokesch PM, et al. Dexmedetomidine vs midazolam for sedation of critically ill patients. JAMA. 2009;301:489–99.
33. Corssen G, Domino EF. Dissociative anesthesia: further pharmacologic studies and first clinical experience with the phencyclidine derivative CI-581. Anesth Analg Curr Res. 1966;45:29.
34. Sari A, Okuda Y, Takeshita H. Effect of ketamine on cerebral circulation and metabolism. Masui. 1971;20:68–73.
35. Wyte SR, Shapiro HM, Turner P, et al. Ketamine-induced intracranial hypertension. Anesthesiology. 1972;36:174–6.
36. Mayberg TS, Lam AM, Matta BF, et al. Ketamine does not increase cerebral blood flow velocity or intracranial pressure during isoflurane/nitrous oxide anesthesia in patients undergoing craniotomy. Anesth Analg. 1995;81:84–9.
37. Bar-Joseph G, Guilburd Y, Tamir A, et al. Effectiveness of ketamine in decreasing intracranial pressure in children with intracranial hypertension. J Neurosurg Pediatr. 2009;4:40–6.
38. Bourgoin A, Albanese J, Wereszczynski N, et al. Safety of sedation with ketamine in severe head injury patients: comparison with sufentanil. Crit Care Med. 2003;31:711–7.
39. Himmelseher S, Durieux ME. Revising a dogma: ketamine for patients with neurological injury? Anesth Analg. 2005;101:524–34.
40. Green SM, Roback MG, Kennedy RM, Krauss B. Clinical practice guidelines for emergency department ketamine dissociative sedation: 2011 update. Ann Emerg Med. 2011;57:449–61.
41. Stoelting RK. Opioid agonists and antagonists. In: Stoelting RK, editor. Pharmacology and physiology in anesthetic practice. 3rd ed. Philadelphia: Lippincott-Raven Publishers; 1999. p. 77–112.
42. Atcheson R, Lambert DG. Update on opioid receptors. Br J Anaesth. 1994;73:132.

43. Larsen CP, Maxxe RI, Cooperman LH, et al. Effects of anesthetics on cerebral, renal and splanchnic circulation: recent developments. Anesthesiology. 1974;41:161.

44. Black S, Michenfelder J. Cerebral blood flow and metabolism. In: Cucchiara RF, Black S, Michenfelder JD, editors. Clinical neuroanesthesia. 2nd ed. New York: Churchill Livingstone, Inc.; 1998. p. 23–4.

45. Albanese J, Durbec O, Viviand X, et al. Sufentanil increases intracranial pressure in patients with head trauma. Anesthesiology. 1993;79:493.

46. Sperry RJ, Bailey PL, Reichman MV, et al. Fentanyl and sufentanil increase intracranial pressure in head trauma patients. Anesthesiology. 1992;77:416.

47. Werner C, Kochs E, Bause H, et al. Effects of sufentanil on cerebral hemodynamics and intracranial pressure in patients with brain injury. Anesthesiology. 1995;83:721.

48. Buckley MM, Brogen RN. Ketorolac: a review of its pharmacodynamic and pharmacokinetic properties, and therapeutic potential. Drugs. 1990;39:86–109.

49. Cormio M, Citerio G. Continuous low dose diclofenac sodium infusion to control fever in neurosurgical critical care. Neurocrit Care. 2007;6:82–9.

50. Wissinger JP, French LA, Gillingham FJ. The use of dexamethasone in the control of cerebral edema. J Neurol Neurosurg Psychiatry. 1967;30:588.

51. Kotsarini C, Griffiths PD, Wilkinson ID, et al. A systematic review of the literature of the effects of dexamethasone on the brain from in vivo human-based studies: Implications for physiological brain imaging of patients with intracranial tumors. Neurosurgery. 2010;67:1799–815.

52. Eberhart LH, Morin AM, Georgieff M. Dexamethasone for prophylaxis of postoperative nausea and vomiting. A meta-analysis of randomized controlled studies. Anaesthesist. 2000;49:713–20.

53. Bracken MB, Collins WF, Freeman DF, et al. Efficacy of methylprednisolone in acute spinal cord injury. JAMA. 1984;251:45–52.

54. Bracken MB, Shepard MJ, Hellenbrand KG, et al. Methylprednisolone and neurological function 1 year after spinal cord injury: results of the National Acute Spinal Cord Injury Study. J Neurosurg. 1985;63:704–13.

55. Bracken MB, Shepard MJ, Collins WF, et al. A randomized, controlled trial of methylprednisolone or naloxone in the treatment of acute spinal cord injury: results of the Second National Acute Spinal Cord Injury Study (NASCIS-2). N Engl J Med. 1990;322:1405–11.

56. Bracken MB, Shepard MJ, Holford TR, et al. Administration of methylprednisolone for 24 or 48 hours or tirilazad mesylate for 48 hours in the treatment of acute spinal cord injury: results of the Third National Acute Spinal Cord Injury Randomized Controlled Trial – National Acute Spinal Cord Injury Study. JAMA. 1997;277:1597–604.

57. Consortium for Spinal Cord Medicine Clinical Practice Guidelines. Early acute management in adults with spinal cord injury: a clinical practice guideline for health-care professionals. J Spinal Cord Med. 2008;31(4):21–3.

58. The section on disorders of the spine and peripheral nerves of the American Association of Neurological Surgeons and the Congress of Neurological Surgeons. Guidelines for the management of acute cervical spine and spinal cord injuries. 2001;185–202.

59. Bratton SL, Chestnut RM, Ghajar J, et al. for the Brain Trauma Foundation; American Association of Neurological Surgeons; Congress of Neurological Surgeons; Joint Section on Neurotrauma and Critical Care, AANS/CNS. Guidelines for the management of severe traumatic brain injury. XV. Steroids. J Neurotrauma. 2007;24 Suppl 1:S91–5.

60. Annane D, Sebille V, Charpentier C, et al. Effect of treatment with low doses of hydrocortisone and fludrocortisone on morality in patients with septic shock. JAMA. 2002;288:862–71.

61. Sprung CL, Annane D, Keh D, et al. Hydrocortisone therapy for patients with septic shock. N Engl J Med. 2008;358:111–24.

62. Dellinger RP, Levy MM, Carlet JM, et al. Surviving sepsis campaign: international guidelines for the management of severe sepsis and septic shock: 2008. Crit Care Med. 2008;36:296–327.

63. Marik PE, Pastores SM, Annane D, et al. Recommendations for the diagnosis and management of corticosteroid insufficiency in critically ill adult patients: consensus statements from an international task force by the American College of Critical Care Medicine. Crit Care Med. 2008;36:1937–49.

64. Lanier WL, Milde JH, Michenfelder JD. Cerebral stimulation following succinylcholine in dogs. Anesthesiology. 1986;64:551–9.

65. Minton MD, Grosslight K, Stirt JA, Bedford RF. Increases in intracranial pressure from succinylcholine: prevention by prior nondepolarizing blockade. Anesthesiology. 1986;65:165–9.

66. Stoelting RK. Neuromuscular-blocking drugs. In: Stoelting RK, editor. Pharmacology and physiology in anesthetic practice. 3rd ed. Philadelphia: Lippincott-Raven Publishers; 1999. p. 192–3.

67. John DA, Tobey RE, Homer LD, Rice CL. Onset of succinylcholine-induced hyperkalemia following denervation. Anesthesiology. 1976;45:294–9.

68. Szumita PM, Enfanto CM, Greenwood B, et al. Vasopressin for vasopressor-dependent septic shock. Am J Health Syst Pharm. 2005;62:1931–6.

69. Hodges BM, Fraser G. Vasopressin for vasodilatory shock. Hosp Pharm. 2002;37:1149–57.

70. Hall LG, Oyen LJ, Taner CB, et al. Fixed-dose vasopressin compared with titrated dopamine and norepinephrine as initial vasopressor therapy for septic shock. Pharmacotherapy. 2004;24:1002–12.

71. Rose JC, Mayer SA. Optimizing blood pressure in neurologic emergencies. Neurocrit Care. 2004;1:287–99.

72. Talbert RL. The challenge of blood pressure management in neurologic emergencies. Pharmacotherapy. 2006;26:123S–30.

73. Cottrell JE, Patel K, Turndorf H, et al. Intracranial pressure changes induced by sodium nitroprusside in patients with intracranial mass lesions. J Neurosurg. 1978;48:329–31.

74. Turner JM, Powell D, Gibson RM. Intracranial pressure change. Br J Anaesth. 1977;49:419–24.

75. Marsh ML, Shapiro HM, Smith RL, et al. Changes in neurologic status and intracranial pressure associated with sodium nitroprusside administration. Anesthesiology. 1979;51:336.

76. Miletich DJ, Gil KS, Albrecht RF, et al. Intracerebral blood flow distribution during hypotensive anesthesia in the goat. Anesthesiology. 1980;53:210.

77. Hartmann A, Buttinger C, Rommel T, et al. Alteration of intracranial pressure, cerebral blood flow, autoregulation and carbon dioxide-reactivity by hypotensive agents in baboons with intracranial hypertension. Neurochirurgia (Stuttg). 1989;32(2):37–43.

78. Overgaard JRN, Skinh EJ. A paradoxical cerebral hemodynamic effect of hydralazine. Stroke. 1975;6:402–4.

79. Cardene® [package insert]. Deerfield: Baxter Healthcare Corporation; rev 2010.

80. Curran MP, Robinson DM, Keating GM. Intravenous nicardipine: its use in the short-term treatment of hypertension and various other indications. Drugs. 2006;66:1755–82.

81. Moore RA, Geller EA, Gallagher JD, et al. Effect of hypothermic cardiopulmonary bypass on nitroprusside sodium. Clin Pharmacol Ther. 1985;37:680–3.

82. Anagnostou JM, Stoelting RK. Complications of drugs used in anesthesia. In: Benumof JL, Saidman LJ, editors. Anesthesia and perioperative complications. 2nd ed. St. Louis: Mosby, Inc; 1999. p. 161–91.

83. Orlowski JP, Shiesley D, Vidt DG, Barnett GH, Little JR. Labetalol to control blood pressure after cerebrovascular surgery. Crit Care Med. 1988;16:765.

84. Van Aken H, Puchstein C, Schweppe ML, et al. Effect on labetalol on intracranial pressure in dogs with and without intracranial hypertension. Acta Anaesthesiol Scand. 1982;26:615.

85. McNamara JO. Pharmacotherapy of the epilepsies. In: Burton LL, editor. Goodman & Gilman's the pharmacologic basis of therapeutics. 12th ed. New York: McGraw-Hill Companies, Inc; 2011. Web. Accessed July 17, 2011.

86. Dilantin® [package insert]. New York: Pfizer, Inc; rev 2011.

87. McGovern B, Geer VR, LaRaia PJ, et al. Possible interaction between amiodarone and phenytoin. Ann Intern Med. 1984;101:650–1.

88. Diflucan® [package insert]. Deerfield: Baxter Healthcare Corporation; rev 2011.

89. Haruda F. Phenytoin hypersensitivity: 38 cases. Neurology. 1979;29:1480–5.

90. Lyseng-Williams KA. Levetiracetam: a review of its use in epilepsy. Drugs. 2011;71(4):489–514.

91. Rogawski MA, Bazil CW. New molecular targets for antiepileptic drugs: 2, SV2A, and Kv7/KCNQ/M potassium channels. Curr Neurol Neurosci Rep. 2008;8:345–52.

92. Perucca E. Clinical pharmacology and therapeutic use of the new antiepileptic drugs. Fundam Clin Pharmacol. 2011;15:405–17.

93. Gold Standard, Inc. Levetiracetam. Clinical pharmacology [database online]. Available at: http://www.clinicalpharmacology.com. Accessed 17 Jul 2011.

94. Rossetti AO, Bromfield EB. Determinants of success in the use of oral levetiracetam in status epilepticus. Epilepsy Behav. 2006;8:651–4.

95. Depakote® [package insert]. North Chicago: Abbott Laboratories; rev 2010.

96. Activase® [package insert]. San Francisco: Genetech Inc.; 2011.

97. Adams HP, Zoppo G, Alberts ML, et al. Guidelines for the early management of adults with ischemic stroke. Stroke. 2007;38:1655–711.

98. Staykov D, Wagner I, Volbers B, et al. Dose effect of intraventricular fibrinolysis in ventricular hemorrhage. Stroke. 2011;42:2061–4.

99. Konstantinides S, Geibel A, Heusel G, et al. Heparin plus alteplase compared with heparin alone in patients with submassive pulmonary embolism. N Engl J Med. 2002;347:1143–50.

100. CathFlo Activase [package insert]. San Francisco: Genetech Inc.; 2001.

101. Tissue plasminogen activator for acute ischemic stroke. The National Institute of Neurological Disorders and Stroke rt-PA Stroke Study Group. N Engl J Med. 1995;333 24:1581–7.

102. Keyser JD, Gdovinova Z, Uyttenboogaart M, et al. Intravenous alteplase for stroke: beyond the guidelines and in particular clinical situations. Stroke. 2007;38:2612–8.

103. Hacke W, Kaste M, Bluhmki E, et al. Thrombolysis with alteplase 3 to 4.5 hours after acute ischemic stroke. N Engl J Med. 2008;359:1317–29.

104. Hirsh J, Bauer KA, Donati MB, et al. Parenteral anticoagulants: American College of Chest Physicians Evidence-Based Clinical Practice Guidelines (8th Edition). Chest. 2008;133(6 Suppl):141S–59.

105. Rosenberg R, Bauer K. The heparin-antithrombin system: a natural anticoagulant mechanism. 3rd ed. Philadelphia: Lippincott; 1994.

106. Weitz JI. Blood coagulation and anticoagulant, fibrinolytic, and antiplatelet drugs. In: Burton LL, editor. Goodman & Gilman's the pharmacologic basis of therapeutics. 12th ed. New York: McGraw-Hill Companies, Inc; 2011. Web. Accessed August 20, 2011.

107. Shantsila E, Lip GY, Chong BG. Heparin-induced thrombocytopenia: a contemporary clinical approach to diagnosis and management. Chest. 2009;135(6):1651–64.

108. Laster JL, Nichols WK, Silver D. Thrombocytopenia associated with heparin-coated catheters in patients with heparin-associated antiplatelet antibodies. Arch Intern Med. 1989;149:2285–7.

109. Warkentin TE, Greinacher A, Koster A, et al. Treatment and prevention of heparin-induced thrombocytopenia: American College of Chest Physicians Evidence-Based Clinical Practice Guidelines (8th Edition). Chest. 2008;133(6 Suppl):340S–80.

110. Lopez L. Low-molecular-weight heparins are essentially the same for treatment and prevention of venous thromboembolism. Pharmacotherapy. 2001;21(6 Pt 2):56S–61.

111. Gold Standard, Inc. Aspirin. Clinical pharmacology [database online]. Available at: http://www.clinicalpharmacology.com. Accessed 23 Aug 2011.

112. Furie KL, Kasner SE, Adams RJ, et al. Guidelines for the prevention of stroke in patients with stroke or transient ischemic attack. Stroke. 2011;42:227–76.

113. Gold Standard, Inc. Dipyridamole. Clinical pharmacology [database online]. Available at: http://www.clinicalpharmacology.com. Accessed 23 Aug 2011.

114. Robinson AG. The posterior pituitary (neurohypophysis). In: Gardner DG, Shoback D, editors. Greenspan's basic & clinical endocrinology. 9th ed. New York: McGraw-Hill Companies, Inc; 2011. Web. Accessed August 23, 2011.

115. Lethagen S. Desmopressin (DDAVP) and hemostasis. Ann Hematol. 1994;69:173–80.

116. DDAVP® [package insert]. Bridgewater: Sanofi-Aventis; rev 2007.

117. Ruzicka H, Bjorkman S, Lethagen S, et al. Pharmacokinetic and antidiuretic effect of high-dose desmopressin in patients with chronic renal failure. Pharmacol Toxicol. 2003;92:137–42.

118. Polsker GL. Tolvaptan. Drugs. 2010;70(4):443–54.

119. Vaprisol® [package insert]. Deerfield: Astellas Pharma US, Inc; rev 2011.

120. Murphy T, Dhar R, Diringer M. Conivaptan bolus dosing for the correction of hyponatremia in the neurointensive care unit. Neurocrit Care. 2009;11:14–9.

121. Samsca® [package insert]. Tokyo: Otsuka Pharmaceutical Co, Ltd; rev 2009.

122. McDoneld LM, Fields JD, Bourdette DN, et al. Immunomodulatory therapies in neurologic critical care. Neurocrit Care. 2010;12:132–43.

123. Dalakas MC. Mechanisms of action of IVIG and therapeutic considerations in the treatment of acute and chronic demyelinating neuropathies. Neurology. 2002;59(12):S13–21.

124. Siegel J. The product: all intravenous immunoglobulins are not created equivalent. Pharmacotherapy. 2005;25(11 Part 2):78S–84.

125. Gold Standard, Inc. Immune Globulin IV, IVIG, IGIV. Clinical pharmacology [database online]. Available at: http://www.clinicalpharmacology.com. Accessed 23 Aug 2011.

126. Allen GS, Ahn HS, Preziosi TJ, et al. Cerebral arterial spasm – a controlled trial of nimodipine in patients with subarachnoid hemorrhage. N Engl J Med. 1983;308:619–24.

127. Petruck KC, West M, Mohr G, et al. Nimodipine treatment in poor-grade aneurysm patients. Results of a multicenter double-blind placebo-controlled trial. J Neurosurg. 1988;68:505–17.

128. Toyota BD. The efficacy of an abbreviated course of nimodipine in patients with good-grade aneurysmal subarachnoid hemorrhage. J Neurosurg. 1999;90:203–6.

129. Nimodipine [package insert]. Wayne: Bayer HealthCare Pharmaceuticals Inc.; 2008.

130. Green AE, Banks S, Jay M, et al. Stability of nimodipine solution in oral syringes. Am J Health Syst Pharm. 2004;61:493–6.

131. Muroi C, Terzic A, Fortunati M, et al. Magnesium sulfate in the management of patients with aneurysmal subarachnoid hemorrhage: a randomized, placebo-controlled, dose-adapted trial. Surg Neurol. 2008;69:33–9.

132. Chia RY, Hughes RS, Morgan MK. Magnesium: a useful adjunct in the prevention of cerebral vasospasm following aneurysmal subarachnoid haemorrhage. J Clin Neurosci. 2002;9:279–81.

133. van den Bergh WM. Magnesium sulfate in aneurysmal subarachnoid hemorrhage. A randomized controlled trial. Stroke. 2005; 36:1011–5.

134. Wong GKC, Chan MTV, Boet R, et al. Intravenous magnesium sulfate after aneurysmal subarachnoid hemorrhage: a prospective randomized pilot study. J Neurosurg Anesthesiol. 2006;18:142–8.

135. Prevedello DM, Cordeiro JG, de Morais AL, et al. Magnesium sulfate: role as possible attenuating factor in vasospasm morbidity. Surg Neurol. 2006;65 Suppl 1:S1. 14-1:21.

136. Stippler M, Crago E, Levy EI, et al. Magnesium infusion for vasospasm prophylaxis after subarachnoid hemorrhage. J Neurosurg. 2006;105:723–9.

137. Schmid-Elsaesser R, Kunz M, Zausinger S, et al. Intravenous magnesium versus nimodipine in the treatment of patients with aneurysmal subarachnoid hemorrhage: a randomized study. Neurosurgery. 2006;58:1054–65.

138. Boet R, Mee E. Magnesium sulfate in the management of patients with Fisher grade 3 subarachnoid hemorrhage: a pilot study. Neurosurgery. 2000;47:602–7.

139. van den Bergh WM, Albrecht KW, van der Sprenkel Berkelbach JW, et al. Magnesium therapy after aneurysmal subarachnoid haemorrhage a dose-finding study for long term treatment. Acta Neurochir. 2003;145:195–9.

140. van Norden AGW, van den Bergh WM, Rinkel GJE. Dose evaluation for long-term magnesium treatment in aneurysmal subarachnoid hemorrhage. J Clin Pharm Ther. 2005;30:439–42.

141. Noronha JL, Matuschak GM. Magnesium in critical illness: metabolism, assessment, and treatment. Intensive Care Med. 2002;28:667–79.

142. McGirt MJ, Lynch JR, Parra A, et al. Simvastatin increases endothelia nitric oxide synthase and ameliorates cerebral vasospasm resulting from subarachnoid hemorrhage. Stroke. 2002;33:2950–6.

143. Tseng MY, Czosnyka M, Richards H, et al. Effects of acute treatment with pravastatin on cerebral vasospasm, autoregulation and delayed ischemic deficits after aneurysmal subarachnoid hemorrhage: a phase II randomized placebo-controlled trial. Stroke. 2005;36:1627–32.

144. Tseng MY, Hutchinson PJ, Czosnyka M, et al. Effects of acute pravastatin on intensity of rescue therapy, length of inpatient stay, and 6-month outcome in patients after aneurysmal subarachnoid hemorrhage. Stroke. 2007;38:1545–50.

145. Lynch JR, Wang H, McGirt MJ, et al. Simvastatin reduces vasospasm after aneurysmal subarachnoid hemorrhage: results of a pilot randomized controlled trial. Stroke. 2005;36:2024–6.

146. Chou SHY, Smith EE, Badjatia N, et al. A randomized, double-blind, placebo-controlled pilot study of simvastatin in aneurysmal subarachnoid hemorrhage. Stroke. 2008;39:2891–3.

147. Kramer AH, Gurka MJ, Nathan B, et al. Statin use was not associated with less vasospasm or improved outcome after subarachnoid hemorrhage. Neurosurgery. 2008;62:422–30.

148. McGirt MJ, Garces Ambrossi GL, Huang J, et al. Simvastatin for the prevention of symptomatic cerebral vasospasm following aneurysmal subarachnoid hemorrhage: a single-institution prospective cohort study. J Neurosurg. 2009;110:968–74.

149. Haupt MT, Bekes CE, Brilli RJ, et al. Guidelines on critical care services and personnel: recommendations based on a system of categorization of three levels of care. Crit Care Med. 2003;31: 267–83.

150. Rudis MI, Brandl KM. For the Society of Critical Care Medicine and American College of Clinical Pharmacy Task Force on Critical Care Pharmacy Services. Position paper on critical care pharmacy services. Crit Care Med. 2000;28:3746–50.

151. Baldinger SL, Chow MS, Gannon RH, Kelly ET. Cost savings from having a clinical pharmacist work part-time in a medical intensive care unit. Am J Health Syst Pharm. 1997;54:2811–4.

152. Gandhi PJ, Smith BS, Tataronis GR, Maas B. Impact of a pharmacist on drug costs in a coronary care unit. Am J Health Syst Pharm. 2001;58:497–503.

153. Krupicka MI, Bratton SL, Sonnenthal K, Goldstein B. Impact of a pediatric clinical pharmacist in the pediatric intensive care unit. Crit Care Med. 2002;30:919–21.

154. Weant KA, Armitstead JA, Ladha AM, et al. Cost effectiveness of a clinical pharmacist on a neurosurgical team. Neurosurgery. 2009;65:946–51.

155. Leape LL, Cullen DJ, Dempsey Clapp M, et al. Pharmacist participation on physician rounds and adverse drug events in the intensive care unit. JAMA. 1999;282:267–70.

156. Devlin JW, Holbrook AM, Fuller HD. The effect of ICU sedation guidelines and pharmacist interventions on clinical outcomes and drug cost. Ann Pharmacother. 1997;31:689–95.

157. Kaye J, Ashline V, Erickson D, et al. Critical care bug team: a multidisciplinary team approach to reducing ventilator-associated pneumonia. Am J Infect Control. 2000;28:197–201.

158. Broyles JE, Brown RO, Vehe KL, et al. Pharmacist interventions improve fluid balance in fluid-restricted patients requiring parenteral nutrition. DICP. 1991;25:119–22.

159. MacLaren R, Bond CA. Effects of pharmacist participation in intensive care units on clinical and economic outcomes of critically ill patients with thromboembolic or infarction-related events. Pharmacotherapy. 2009;29:761–8.

160. Kirby RR, Gravenstein N, Lobato EB, Gravenstein JS. Clinical anesthesia practice. 2nd ed. Philadelphia: WB Saunders; 2001.

161. American College of Critical Care Medicine of the Society of Critical Care Medicine, American Society of Health-System Pharmacists, American College of Chest Physicians. Clinical practice guidelines for sustained neuromuscular blockade in the adult critically ill patient. Am J Health Syst Pharm. 2002;59: 179–95.

Index

A.J. Layon et al. (eds.), *Textbook of Neurointensive Care*,
DOI 10.1007/978-1-4471-5226-2, © Springer-Verlag London 2013